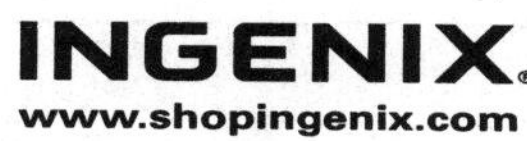

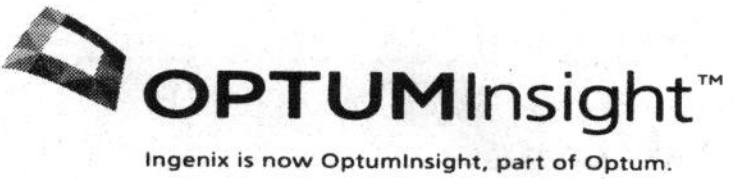

Current Procedural Coding Expert

2012

Notice

American Medical Association Notice

Our Commitment to Accuracy

OptumInsight is committed to producing accurate and reliable materials.

To report corrections, please visit www.ingenixonline.com/accuracy or email accuracy@ingenix.com. You can also reach customer service by calling 1.800.464.3649, option 1.

For Answers to Coding Questions

Try our Ingenix Coding Answers—

Validate your coding accuracy and reduce denials. Find answers to those difficult coding procedures in 48 to 72 hours.

Increase your productivity. Access the tool, and submit your questions online 24 hours a day, seven days a week.

Save time and money associated with researching those hard-to-code procedures.

Use existing site content as a research tool. Quickly access previously submitted questions and answers by other users.

Always know where your questions stand during the Q&A process. Access real-time status of pending questions. Email notifications are delivered when a question is answered.

No subscription necessary. Take advantage of the flexible pricing options based on the number of questions you purchase.

For information, please visit www.shopingenix.com or call customer service at 1.800.464.3649, option 1.

Copyright

Made in the USA

ISBN 978-1-60151-568-1

Acknowledgments

Julie Van, CPC, CPC-P, CEMC, COBGC, CGENSC, *Product Manager*
Karen Schmidt, BSN, *Technical Director*
Stacy Perry, *Manager, Desktop Publishing*
Lisa Singley, *Project Manager*
Wendy Gabbert, CPC, CPC-H, *Clinical/Technical Editor*
Karen H. Kachur, RN, CPC, *Clinical/Technical Editor*
Trudy Whitehead, CPC-H, CMAS, *Clinical/Technical Editor*
Anita Schmidt, RHIT, *Clinical/Technical Editor*
Tracy Betzler, *Desktop Publishing Specialist*
Hope M. Dunn, *Desktop Publishing Specialist*
Kathleen Flynn, *Desktop Publishing Specialist*
Kate Holden, *Editor*

About the Contributors

Wendy Gabbert, CPC, CPC-H, PCS, FCS

Ms. Gabbert has more than 25 years of experience in the health care field. She has extensive background in CPT/HCPCS and ICD-9-CM coding. She served several years as a coding consultant. Her areas of expertise include physician and hospital CPT coding assessments, chargemaster reviews, and the outpatient prospective payment system (OPPS). She is a member of the American Academy of Professional Coders.

Karen H. Kachur, RN, CPC

Ms. Kachur is a clinical/technical editor for Ingenix with expertise in CPT/HCPCS and ICD-9-CM coding, in addition to physician billing, compliance, and fraud and abuse. Prior to joining Ingenix, she worked for many years as a staff RN in a variety of clinical settings, including medicine, surgery, intensive care, and psychiatry. In addition to her clinical background, Ms. Kachur served as assistant director of a hospital utilization management and quality assurance department and has extensive experience as a nurse reviewer for Blue Cross/Blue Shield. She is an active member of the American Academy of Professional Coders.

Trudy Whitehead, CPC-H, CMAS

Ms. Whitehead has more than 20 years of experience in hospital and physician coding and reimbursement. Recently she developed an APC review system for the postpayment review of Medicare FFS APC claims, including workflow, training, and development of an instruction manual as director of ambulatory review systems. She has conducted hospital and insurance bill auditing, managed facility claims processing and claims negotiations, developed outpatient repricer and rules engines, performed hospital chargemaster reviews, and worked on software development. Ms. Whitehead is a member of the American Academy of Professional Coders (AAPC) and the American Association of Medical Audit Specialists.

Contents

Introduction

Welcome to OptumInsight's *Current Procedural Coding Expert* (formerly *CPT® Expert*), an exciting Medicare coding and reimbursement tool and definitive procedure coding source that combines the work of the Centers for Medicare and Medicaid Services, American Medical Association, and OptumInsight experts with the technical components you need for proper reimbursement and coding accuracy.

This new approach to CPT Medicare coding utilizes new, more intuitive ways of communicating the information you need to code claims accurately and efficiently. *Includes* and *Excludes* notes similar to those found in your ICD-9-CM manuals, help determine what services are related to the codes you are reporting. Icons help you crosswalk the code you are reporting to laboratory and radiology procedures necessary for proper reimbursement. CMS-mandated icons and relative value units (RVUs) help you determine which codes are most appropriate for the service you are reporting. In addition, icons denoting codes that apply to Physician Quality Reporting System (PQRS) quality indicators are included along with their denominators. Add to that additional information identifying age and sex edits, ambulatory surgery center (ASC) and ambulatory payment classification (APC) indicators, and Medicare coverage and payment rule citations and *Current Procedural Coding Expert* provides the best in Medicare procedure reporting.

Current Procedural Coding Expert includes the information needed to submit claims to federal contractors and most commercial payers, and is correct at the time of printing. However, CMS, federal contractors, and commercial payers may change payment rules at any time throughout the year. *Current Procedural Coding Expert* includes effective codes that will not be published in the AMA's Physicians' Current Procedural Terminology (CPT) book until the following year. Commercial payers will announce changes through monthly news or information posted on their websites. CMS will post changes in policy on its website at http://www.cms.gov/transmittals. National and local coverage determinations (NCDs and LCDs) provide universal and individual contractor guidelines for specific services. The existence of a procedure code does not imply coverage under any given insurance plan.

Current Procedural Coding Expert is based on the AMA's Physicians' Current Procedural Terminology coding system, which is copyrighted and owned by the physician organization. CPT is the nation's official, Health Information Portability and Accountability Act (HIPAA) compliant code set for procedures and services provided by physicians, ASCs, and hospital outpatient services, as well as laboratories, imaging centers, physical therapy clinics, urgent care centers, and others.

GETTING STARTED WITH *CURRENT PROCEDURAL CODING EXPERT*

Current Procedural Coding Expert is an exciting tool combining the most current material at publication time from the AMA's *CPT 2012*, CMS's online manual system, the Correct Coding Initiative (CCI), CMS fee schedules, official Medicare guidelines for reimbursement and coverage, and OptumInsight's own coding expertise.

Note: The AMA releases code changes quarterly. *Current Procedural Coding Expert* contains the most current information from the AMA, including new, changed, and deleted codes that are released on its website for future inclusion in the CPT book. Some of these changes will not appear in the AMA's CPT book until the following year.

Another feature of *Current Procedural Coding Expert* that differs from the official CPT book is the addition of appendix H, "Glossary." The glossary includes the definition of terms used throughout the manual.

Material is presented in a logical fashion for those billing Medicare, Medicaid, and private payers. The format, based on customer comments, better addresses what customers tell us they need in a comprehensive Medicare procedure coding guide.

Designed to be easy to use and full of information, this product is an excellent companion to your AMA CPT manual and to Medicare, OptumInsight, or other resources.

General Conventions

Sources of information in this book can be determined by color:

- OptumInsight information derived by our experts is in blue ink.
- Medicare-derived information is in red ink.
- Codes, descriptions, and evaluation and management (E/M) guidelines from the American Medical Association are in black ink.

Icons derived from AMA guidelines or coding conventions are presented as circles. Icons derived from federal guidelines, data, or rules are square.

GUIDELINES

Coding guidelines have been incorporated into more specific section notes, code notes, icons, and the glossary. Section notes are listed under a range of codes and apply to all the codes in that range. Code notes are found under individual codes and apply to the single code. Definitions of coding terms are listed in the glossary and can be found in appendix H.

RESEQUENCING OF CPT CODES

The American Medical Association (AMA) introduced a new numbering methodology beginning in 2010. Resequencing is the practice of displaying codes outside of their numerical order according to the description relationship. According to the AMA, there are instances in which a new code is needed within an existing grouping of codes but an unused code number is not available. In these situations, the AMA will resequence the codes. In other words, it will assign a code that is not in numeric sequence with the related codes. However, the code and description will appear in the CPT manual with the other related codes.

An example of resequencing from *Current Procedural Coding Expert* follows:

21555 Excision, tumor, soft tissue of neck or anterior thorax, subcutaneous; less than 3 cm

\# **21552 3 cm or greater**

21556 Excision, tumor, soft tissue of neck or anterior thorax, subfascial (eg, intramuscular); less than 5 cm

\# **21554 5 cm or greater**

Note that codes 21552 and 21554 are out of numeric sequence. However, as they are indented codes, they are in the correct place.

In *Current Procedural Coding Expert* the resequenced codes are listed twice. They appear in their resequenced position as shown above as well as in their original numeric position with a note indicating that the code is out of numerical sequence and where it can be found. (See example below.)

51797 Resequenced code. See code following 51729.

This differs from the AMA CPT book, in which the coder is directed to a code range that contains the resequenced code and description, rather than to a specific location.

Resequenced codes will appear in brackets in the notes and code ranges. For example:

82286-82308 [82652] Chemistry: Bradykinin-Calcitonin
Code [82652] is included in section 82286-82308 Chemistry: Bradykinin-Calcitonin in its resequenced position.

Injection facet joint (64620-64645, [64633, 64634, 64635, 64636])

Codes 64633, 64634, 64635, 64636 are included in code range 64620-64645 in their resequenced position.

Appendix D identifies all CPT codes that are resequenced.

OptumInsight will display the resequenced coding as assigned by the AMA in its CPT products so that the user may understand the code description relationships.

Each particular group of CPT codes in *Current Procedural Coding Expert* is organized in a more intuitive fashion for Medicare billing, being grouped by the Medicare rules and regulations that govern payment of these particular procedures and services, as in this example:

99241–99255 Consultations

CMS 100-1,5,70 Definition of Physician

CMS 100-2,15,30 Physician Services

CMS 100-3,70.1 Consultations with a Beneficiary's Family and Associates

CMS 100-4,12,30.6.10 Consultation Services

ICONS

● **New Codes**
Codes that have been added since the last edition of the book was printed.

▲ **Revised Codes**
Codes that have been revised since the last edition of the book was printed.

Resequenced Codes
Codes that are out of numeric order but apply to the appropriate category.

○ **Reinstated Code**
Codes that have been reinstated since the last edition of the book was printed.

Red Color Bar—Not Covered by Medicare
Services and procedures identified by this color bar are never covered benefits under Medicare. Services and procedures that are not covered may be billed directly to the patient at the time of the service.

Yellow Color Bar—Unlisted Procedure
Unlisted CPT codes report procedures that have not been assigned a specific code number. An unlisted code delays payment due to the extra time necessary for review.

Blue Color Bar—Resequenced Codes
Resequenced codes are codes that are out of numeric sequence—they are indicated with a blue color bar. They are listed twice, in their resequenced position as well as in their original numeric position with a note that the code is out of numerical sequence and where the resequenced code and description can be found.

INCLUDES **Includes notes**
Includes notes identify procedures and services that would be bundled in the procedure code. These are derived from AMA, CMS, CCI, and OptumInsight coding guidelines. This is not meant to be an all-inclusive list.

EXCLUDES **Excludes notes**
Excludes notes may lead the user to other codes. They may identify services that are not bundled and may be separately reported, OR may lead the user to another more appropriate code. These are derived from AMA, CMS CCI, and OptumInsight coding guidelines.

Laboratory/Pathology Crosswalk
This icon denotes CPT codes in the laboratory and pathology section of CPT that may be reported separately with the primary CPT code.

Radiology Crosswalk
This icon denotes codes in the radiology section that may be used with the primary CPT code being reported.

TC **Technical Component Only**
Codes with this icon represent only the technical component (staff and equipment costs) of a procedure or service. Do not use either modifier 26 (physician component) or TC (technical component) with these codes.

26 **Professional Component**
Only codes with this icon represent the physician's work or professional component of a procedure or service. Do not use either modifier 26 (physician component) or TC (technical component) with these codes.

50 **Bilateral Procedure**
This icon identifies codes that can be reported bilaterally when the same surgeon provides the service for the same patient on the same date. Medicare allows payment for both procedures at 150 percent of the usual amount for one procedure. The modifier does not apply to bilateral procedures inclusive to one code.

80 **Assist-at-Surgery Allowed**
Services noted by this icon are allowed an assist at surgery with a Medicare payment equal to 16 percent of the allowed amount for the global surgery for that procedure. No documentation is required.

80 **Assist-at-Surgery Allowed with Documentation**
Services noted by this icon are allowed an assistant at surgery with a Medicare payment equal to 16 percent of the allowed amount for the global surgery for that procedure. Documentation is required.

\+ **Add-on Codes**
This icon identifies procedures reported in addition to the primary procedure. The icon "+" denotes add-on codes. An add-on code is neither a stand-alone code nor subject to multiple procedure rules since it describes work in addition to the primary procedure.

⊘ **Modifier 51 Exempt**
Codes identified by this icon indicate that the procedure should not be reported with modifier 51 (Multiple procedures).

Correct Coding Initiative (CCI)
Current Procedural Coding Expert identifies those codes with corresponding CCI edits. The CCI edits define correct coding practices that serve as the basis of the national Medicare policy for paying claims. The code noted is the major service/procedure. The code may represent a column 1 code within the column 1/column 2 correct coding edits table or a code pair that is mutually exclusive of each other.

CLIA Waived Test
This symbol is used to distinguish those laboratory tests that can be performed using test systems that are waived from regulatory oversight established by the Clinical Laboratory Improvement Amendments of 1988 (CLIA). The applicable CPT code for a CLIA waived test may be reported by providers who perform the testing but do not hold a CLIA license.

(63) **Modifier 63 Exempt**
This icon identifies procedures performed on infants that weigh less than 4 kg. Due to the complexity of performing procedures on infants less than 4 kg, modifier 63 may be added to the surgery codes to inform the payers of the special circumstances involved.

A2–Z3 **ASC Payment Indicators**
This icon identifies ASC status payment indicators. They indicate how the ASC payment rate was derived and/or how the procedure, item, or service is treated under the revised ASC payment system. For more information about these indicators and how they affect billing, consult OptumInsight's *Outpatient Billing Editor.*

- A2 Surgical procedure on ASC list in calendar year (CY) 2007; payment based on OPPS relative payment weight.
- C5 Inpatient procedures.
- F4 Corneal tissue acquisition; hepatitis B vaccine; paid at reasonable cost.
- G2 Non-office-based surgical procedure added in CY 2008 or later; payment based on outpatient prospective payment system (OPPS) relative payment weight.
- H2 Brachytherapy source paid separately when provided integral to a surgical procedure on ASC list; payment contractor-priced.
- J7 OPPS pass-through device paid separately when provided integral to a surgical procedure on ASC list; payment contractor-priced.
- J8 Device-intensive procedure; paid at adjusted rate.
- K2 Drugs and biologicals paid separately when provided integral to a surgical procedure on ASC list; payment based on OPPS rate.
- K7 Unclassified drugs and biologicals; payment contractor-priced.

L1 Influenza vaccine; pneumococcal vaccine. Packaged item/service; no separate payment made.

L6 New technology intraocular lens (NTIOL); special payment.

M5 Quality measurement code used for reporting purposes only; no payment made.

N1 Packaged service/item; no separate payment made.

P2 Office-based surgical procedure added to ASC list in CY 2008 or later with Medicare physician fee schedule (MPFS) nonfacility practice expense (PE) RVUs; payment based on OPPS relative payment weight.

P3 Office-based surgical procedure added to ASC list in CY 2008 or later with MPFS nonfacility PE RVUs; payment based on MPFS nonfacility PE RVUs.

R2 Office-based surgical procedure added to ASC list in CY 2008 or later without MPFS nonfacility PE RVUs; payment based on OPPS relative payment weight.

Z2 Radiology service paid separately when provided integral to a surgical procedure on ASC list; payment based on OPPS relative payment weight.

Z3 Radiology service paid separately when provided integral to a surgical procedure on ASC list; payment based on MPFS nonfacility PE RVUs

⊙ **Moderate Sedation**
This icon identifies procedures that include moderate sedation. Moderate sedation codes should not be reported separately with these procedures.

A **Age Edit**
This icon denotes codes intended for use with a specific age group, such as neonate, newborn, pediatric, and adult. Carefully review the code description to ensure the code you report most appropriately reflects the patient's age.

M **Maternity**
This icon identifies procedures that by definition should be used only for maternity patients generally between 12 and 55 years of age.

♀ **Female Only**
This icon identifies procedures that some payers may consider for females only.

♂ **Male Only**
This icon identifies procedures that some payers may consider for males only.

Facility RVU
This icon precedes the facility RVU from CMS's 2011 physician fee schedule (PFS). It can be found under the code description.

Nonfacility RVU
This icon precedes the nonfacility RVU from CMS's 2012 PFS. It can be found under the code description.

Global Days The global period is the time following surgery during which routine care by the physician is considered postoperative and included in the surgical fee. Office visits or other routine care related to the original surgery cannot be separately reported if provided during the global period. Global days are sometimes referred to as "follow-up days," or FUDs. The statuses are:

000 No follow-up care included in this procedure

010 Normal postoperative care is included in this procedure for ten days

090 Normal postoperative care is included in the procedure for 90 days

MMM Maternity codes; usual global period does not apply

XXX The global concept does not apply to the code

YYY The carrier is to determine whether the global concept applies and establishes postoperative period, if appropriate, at time of pricing

ZZZ The code is related to another service and is always included in the global period of the other service

CMS: This notation indicates that there is a specific CMS guideline pertaining to this code in the CMS Online Manual System which includes the internet-only manual (IOM) *National Coverage Determinations Manual* (NCD). These CMS sources present the rules for submitting these services to the federal government or its contractors and are included in the appendix G of this book.

AMA: This indicates discussion of the code in the American Medical Association's *CPT Assistant* newsletter. Use the citation to find the correct issue.

Drug Not Approved by FDA
The AMA CPT Editorial Panel is publishing new vaccine product codes prior to Food and Drug Administration approval. This symbol indicates which of these codes are pending FDA approval at press time.

PQ **Physician Quality Reporting System (PQRS)**
This icon denotes CPT codes that specifically address one or more of the CMS-determined quality measures. See appendix K for a list of denominators that apply to those codes.

A–Y **OPPS Status Indicators (OPSI)**
Status indicators identify how individual CPT codes are paid or not paid under the latest available hospital outpatient prospective payment system (OPPS). The same status indicator is assigned to all the codes within an ambulatory payment classification (APC). Consult your payer or other resource to learn which CPT codes fall within various APCs.

A Services furnished to a hospital outpatient that are paid under a fee schedule or payment system other than OPPS

B Codes that are not recognized by OPPS when submitted on an outpatient hospital Part B bill type (12x and 13x).

C Inpatient procedures

E Non-allowed item or service

F Corneal tissue acquisition; certain CRNA services and hepatitis B vaccines

G Pass-through drugs and biologicals

H Pass-through device categories

K Nonpass-through drugs and nonimplantable biologics, including therapeutic radiopharmaceuticals

L Influenza vaccine; pneumococcal pneumonia vaccine

M Items and services not billable to the FI/MAC

N Items and services packaged into APC rates

P Partial hospitalization

Q1 STVX-packaged codes

Q2 T-packaged codes

Q3 Codes that may be paid through a composite APC

R Blood and blood products

S Significant procedure, not discounted when multiple

T Significant procedure, multiple reduction applies

U Brachytherapy sources

V Clinic or emergency department visit

X Ancillary service

Y Nonimplantable durable medical equipment

APPENDIXES

Appendix A: Modifiers—This appendix identifies the modifiers. A modifier is a two-position alphabetic or numeric code that is appended to a CPT or HCPCS code to clarify the services being billed. Modifiers provide a means by which a service can be altered without changing the procedure code. They add more information, such as anatomical site, to the code. In addition, they help eliminate the appearance of duplicate billing and unbundling. Modifiers are used to increase the accuracy in reimbursement and coding consistency, ease editing, and capture payment data.

Appendix B: New, Changed, and Deleted Codes—This is a list of new, changed, and deleted CPT codes for the current year.

Appendix C: Crosswalk of Deleted Codes—This appendix is a cross-reference from a deleted CPT code to an active code when one is available. The deleted code cross-reference will also appear under the deleted code description in the tabular section of the book.

Appendix D: Resequenced Codes—This appendix contains a list of codes that are not in numeric order in the book. AMA resequenced some of the code numbers to relocate codes in the same category but not in numeric sequence.

Appendix E: Add-on, Modifier 51 Exempt, Modifier 63 Exempt, and Moderate Sedation Codes—This list includes add-on codes that cannot be reported alone, codes that are exempt from modifier 51, codes that should not be reported with modifier 63, and codes that include moderate sedation.

Appendix F: Place of Service and Type of Service—This appendix contains lists of place-of-service codes that should be used on professional claims and type-of-service codes used by the Medicare Common Working File.

Appendix G: Pub. 100 References—This appendix contains a verbatim printout of the Medicare Internet Only Manual references that pertain to specific codes. The reference, when available, is listed after the header in the CPT section. For example:

60600–60605 CAROTID BODY PROCEDURES

CMS 100-3, 20.18, Carotid Body Resection/Carotid Body Denervation

Since appendix G contains this reference from the *Medicare Claims Processing Manual*, Pub. 100-3 chapter 20, section 20.18, there is no need to search the Medicare website for the applicable reference.

Appendix H: Glossary—This appendix contains general terms and definitions as well as those that would apply to or be helpful for billing and reimbursement.

Appendix I: Listing of Sensory, Motor, and Mixed Nerves—This appendix lists a summary of each sensory, motor, and mixed nerve with its appropriate nerve conduction study code.

Appendix J: Vascular Families—Appendix J contains a table of vascular families starting with the aorta. Additional information can be found in the interventional radiology illustrations located behind the index.

Appendix K: Physician Quality Reporting System (PQRS)—Lists the numerators and denominators applicable to Medicare PQRS.

Appendix L: Medically Unlikely Edits—This appendix contains the published medically unlikely edits (MUEs). These edits establish maximum daily allowable units of service. The edits will be applied to the services provided to the same patient, for the same CPT code, on the same date of service when billed by the same provider. Included are the physician and facility edits.

Appendix M: Inpatient-Only Procedures—This appendix identifies services with the status indicator C. Medicare will not pay an OPPS hospital or ASC when these procedures are performed on a Medicare patient as an outpatient. Physicians should refer to this list when scheduling Medicare patients for surgical procedures. CMS will update this list quarterly.

For more information about ongoing development of the CPT coding system, consult the AMA website at URL http://www.ama-assn.org/.

Note: All data current as of November 7, 2011

Anatomical Illustrations

BODY PLANES AND MOVEMENTS

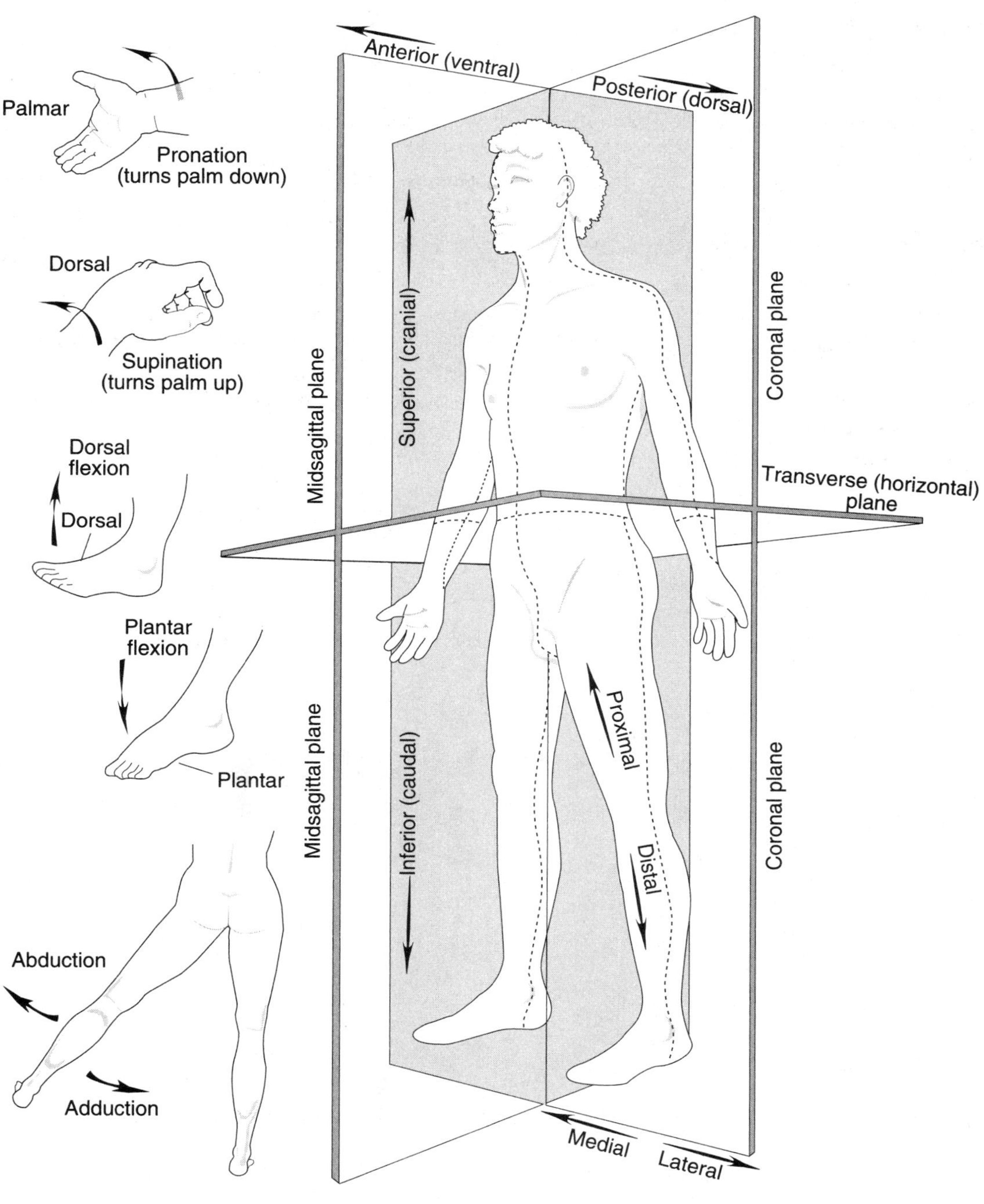

MUSCULOSKELETAL SYSTEM

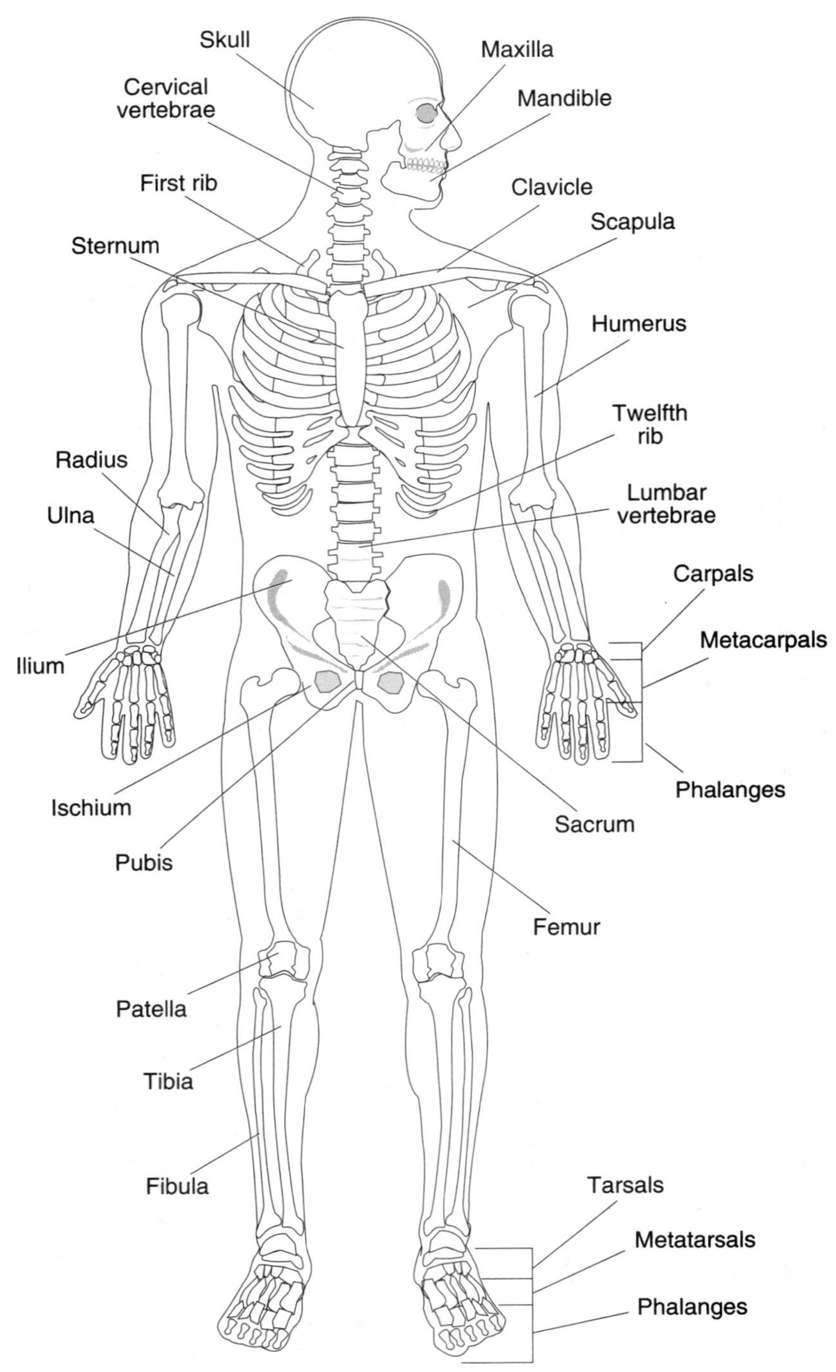

MUSCULOSKELETAL SYSTEM

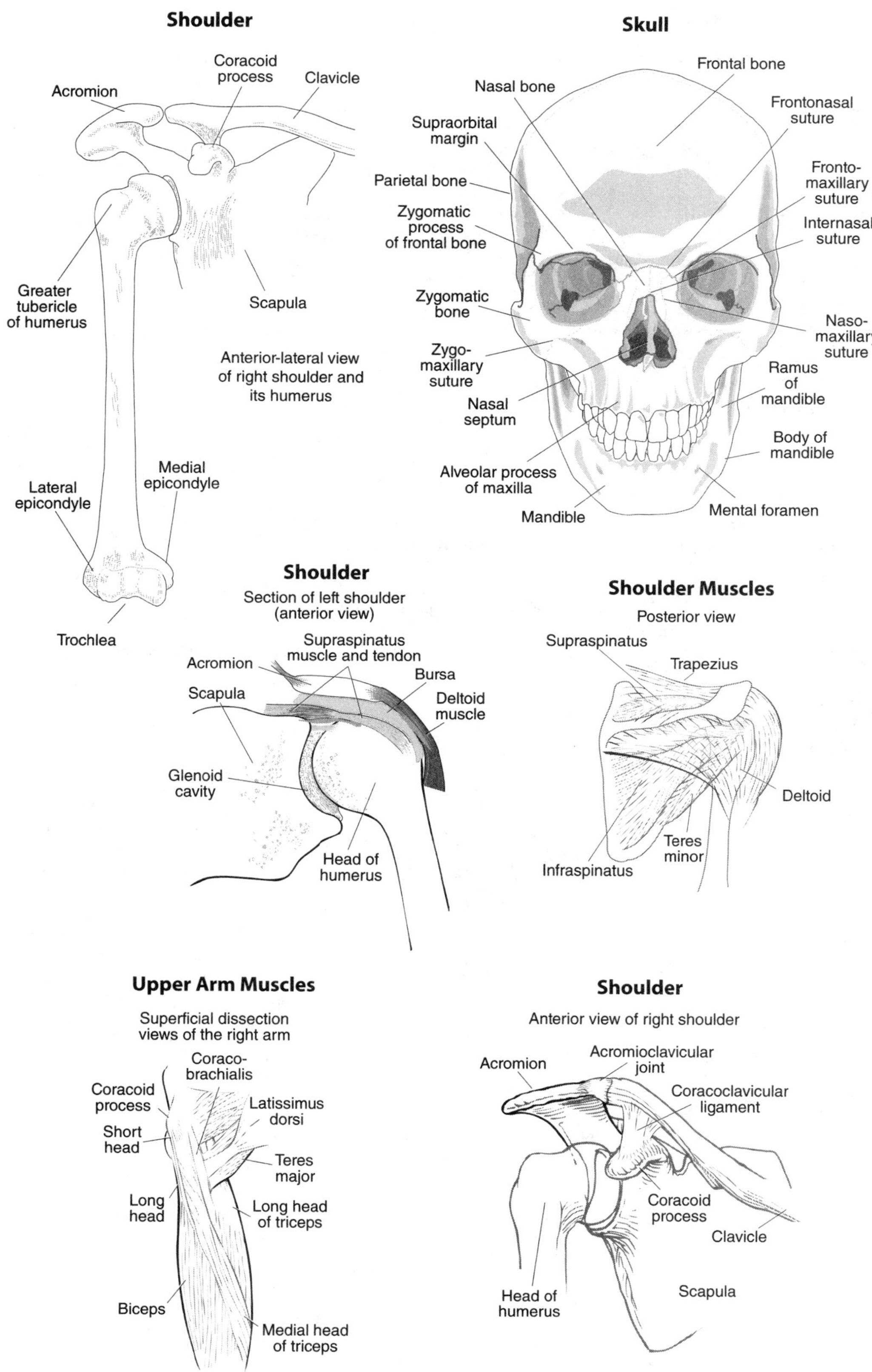

Anatomical Illustrations

MUSCULOSKELETAL SYSTEM

Elbow

Anterior view of right arm and elbow

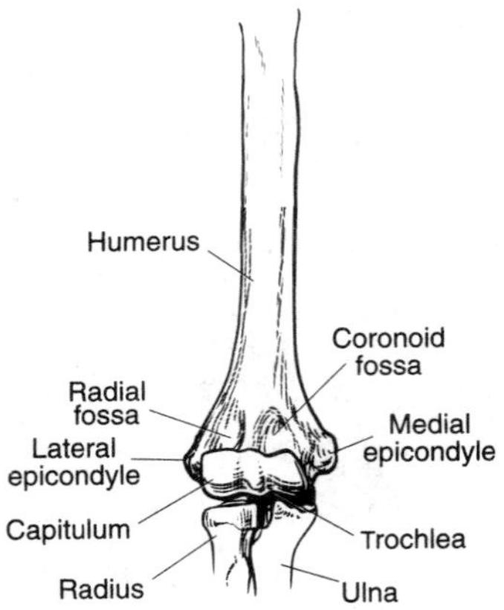

Humerus
Coronoid fossa
Radial fossa
Medial epicondyle
Lateral epicondyle
Capitulum
Trochlea
Radius
Ulna

Elbow

Anterior view of right elbow

Humerus
Joint capsule
Lateral epicondyle
Medial epicondyle
Radial collateral ligament
Ulnar collateral ligament
Radius
Ulna

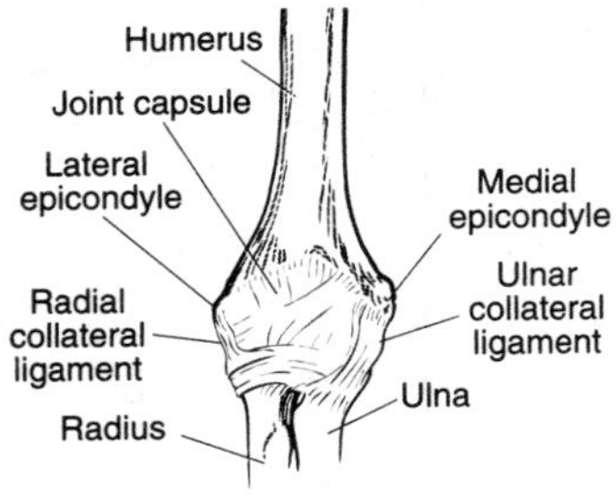

Lateral view of right elbow joint

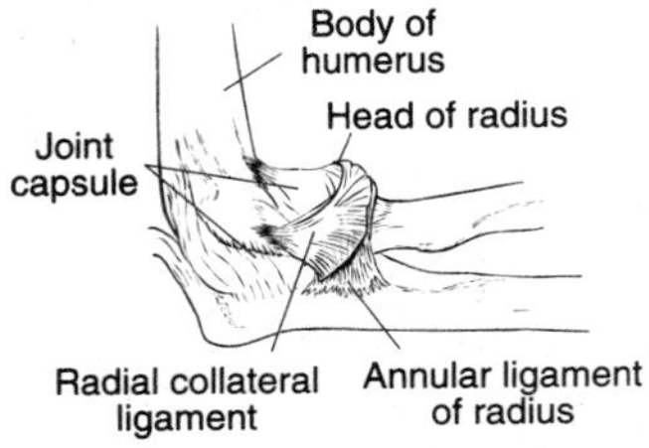

Body of humerus
Head of radius
Joint capsule
Radial collateral ligament
Annular ligament of radius

Elbow

Posterior view of right elbow

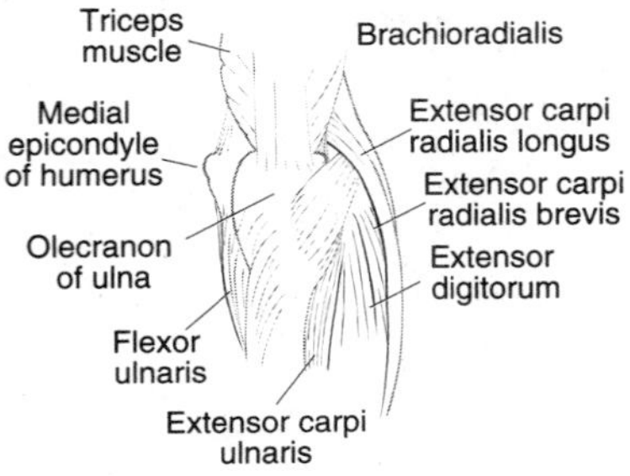

Triceps muscle
Brachioradialis
Medial epicondyle of humerus
Extensor carpi radialis longus
Extensor carpi radialis brevis
Olecranon of ulna
Extensor digitorum
Flexor ulnaris
Extensor carpi ulnaris

Lower Arm

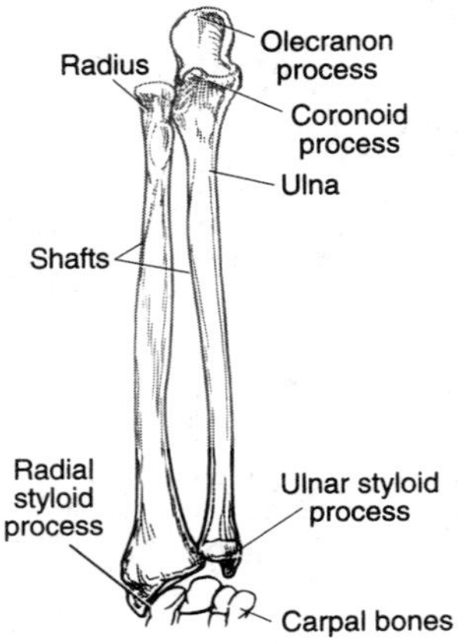

Radius
Olecranon process
Coronoid process
Ulna
Shafts
Radial styloid process
Ulnar styloid process
Carpal bones

Finger

Medial schematic of finger joints

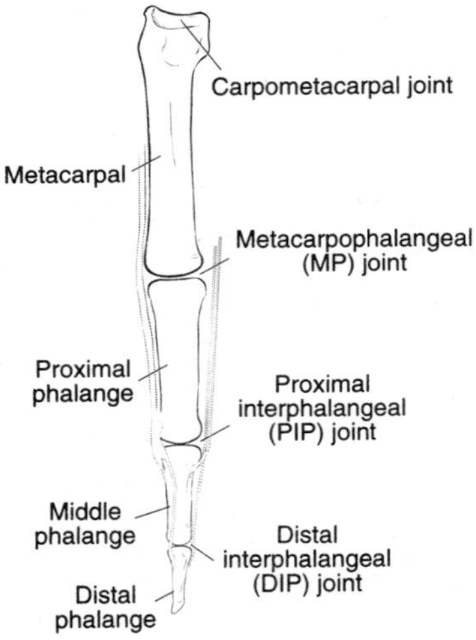

Carpometacarpal joint
Metacarpal
Metacarpophalangeal (MP) joint
Proximal phalange
Proximal interphalangeal (PIP) joint
Middle phalange
Distal interphalangeal (DIP) joint
Distal phalange

Hand

Palmar view

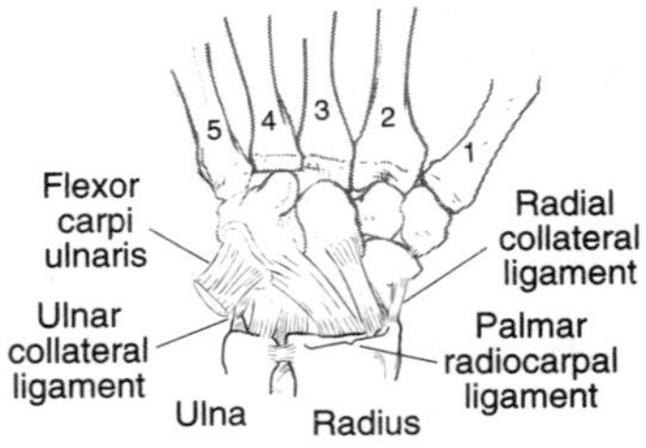

5 4 3 2 1
Flexor carpi ulnaris
Radial collateral ligament
Ulnar collateral ligament
Palmar radiocarpal ligament
Ulna
Radius

Dorsal view

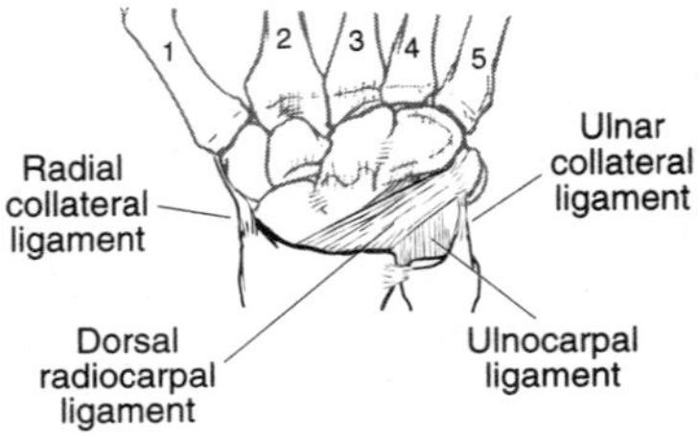

1 2 3 4 5
Radial collateral ligament
Ulnar collateral ligament
Dorsal radiocarpal ligament
Ulnocarpal ligament

Hand

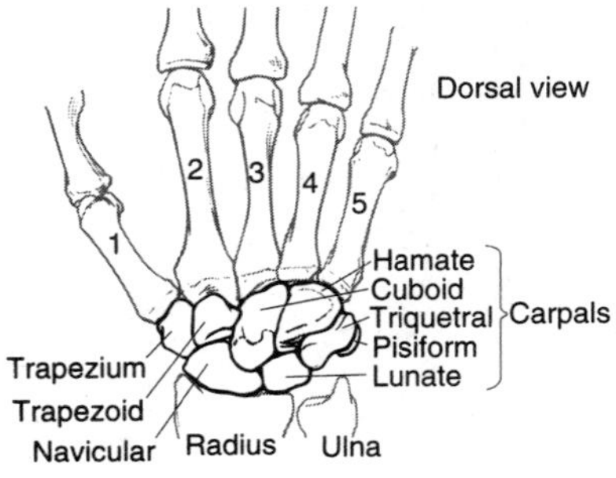

Dorsal view

1 2 3 4 5
Hamate
Cuboid
Triquetral
Pisiform
Lunate
Carpals
Trapezium
Trapezoid
Navicular
Radius
Ulna

MUSCULOSKELETAL SYSTEM

Ankle

Lateral and posterior views of right ankle

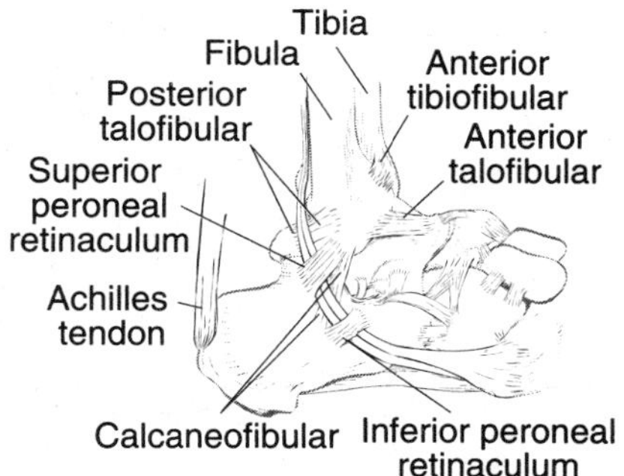

Achilles tendon not shown

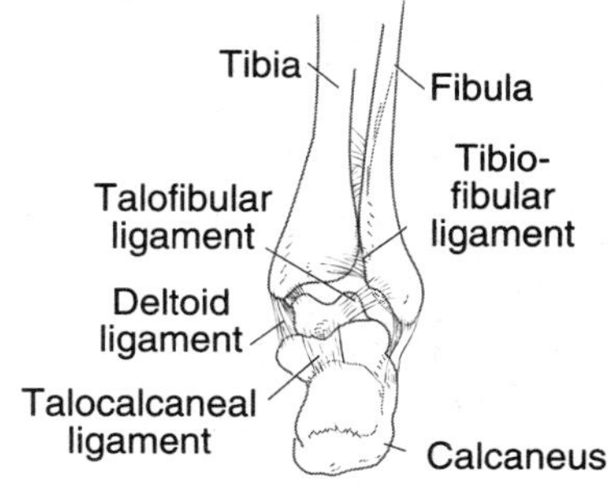

Foot

Select extensors of the foot

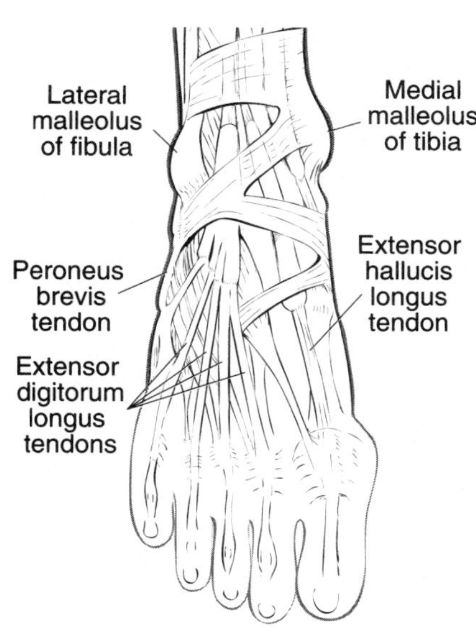

Foot

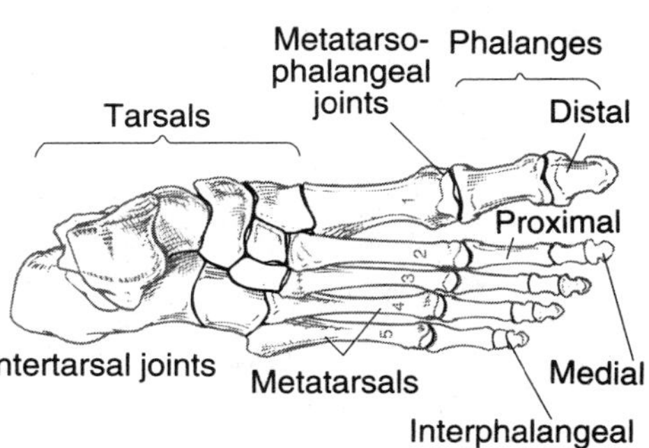

Foot

Tarsals, excluding talus and calcaneus (dark), superior view

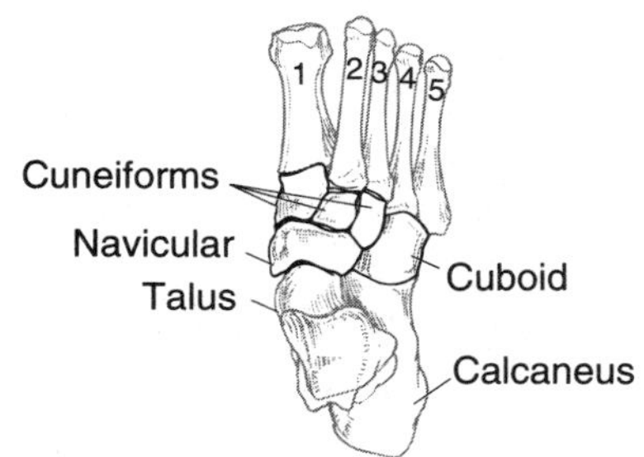

MUSCULOSKELETAL SYSTEM

Leg

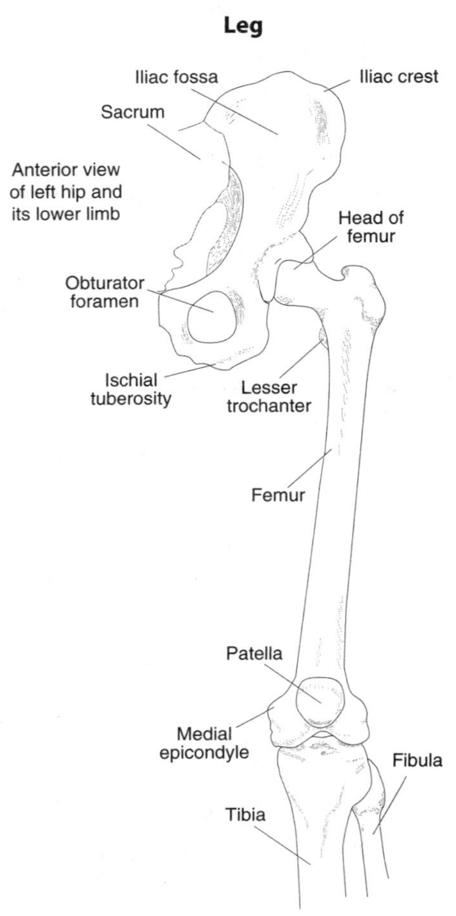

Hip

Iliac crest

Wing of ilium

Greater sciatic notch

Acetabulum

Pubis

Ischial tuberosity

Obturator foramen

Lateral view of right hip socket

Knee

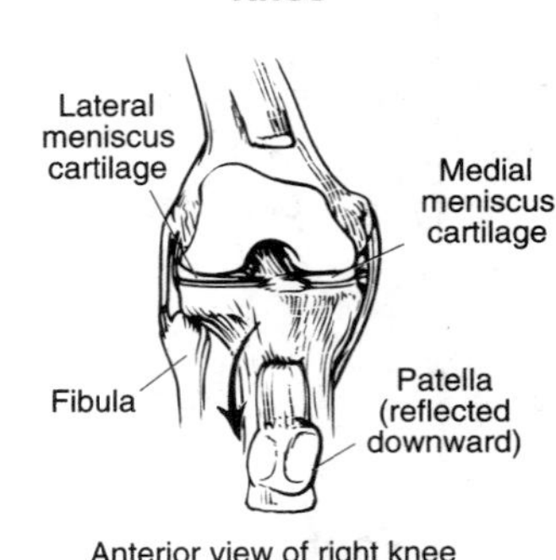

Anterior view of right knee

Lower Leg

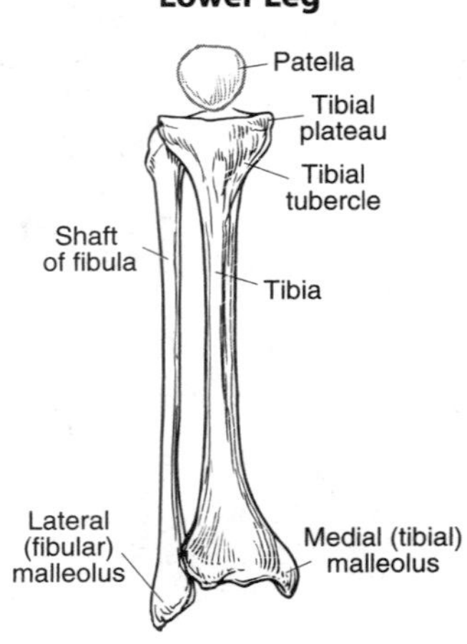

Knee

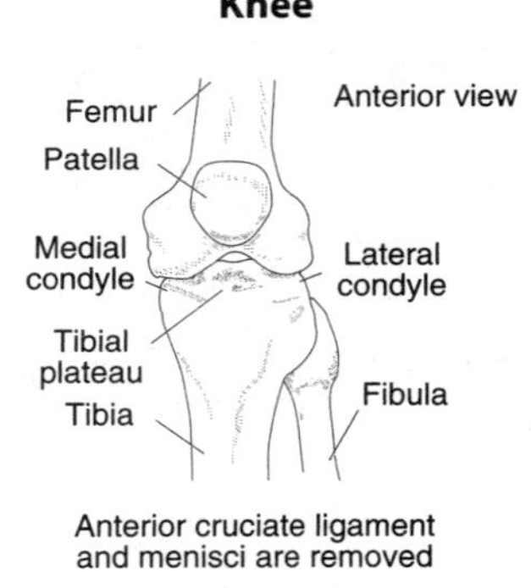

Anterior cruciate ligament and menisci are removed

RULE OF NINES FOR BURNS

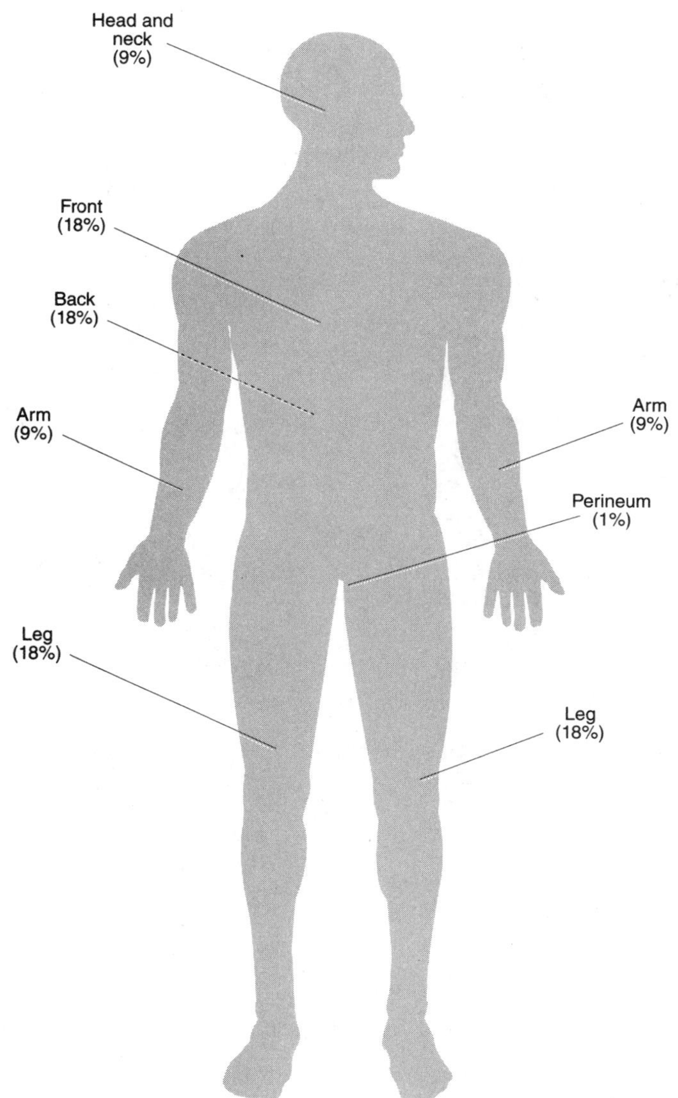

First-degree burns involve surface layers only and tissue destruction is minimal.

Second-degree burns damage deeper epidermal layers and upper layers of the dermis; damage to sweat glands, hair follicles, and sebaceous glands may occur.

Third-degree burns include destruction of both epidermis and dermis and tissue death extends below the hair follicles and sweat glands.

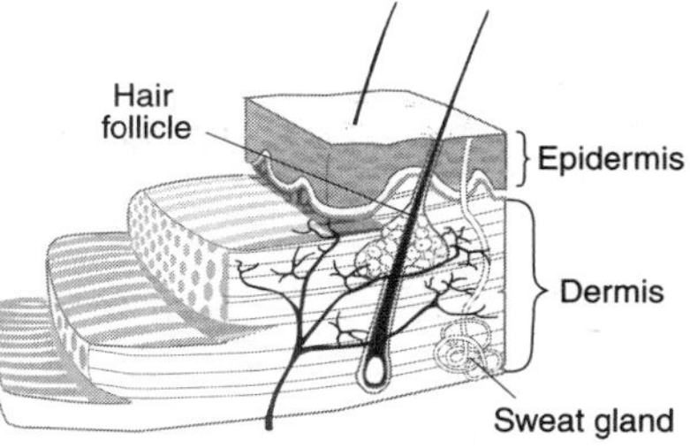

DIGESTIVE SYSTEM

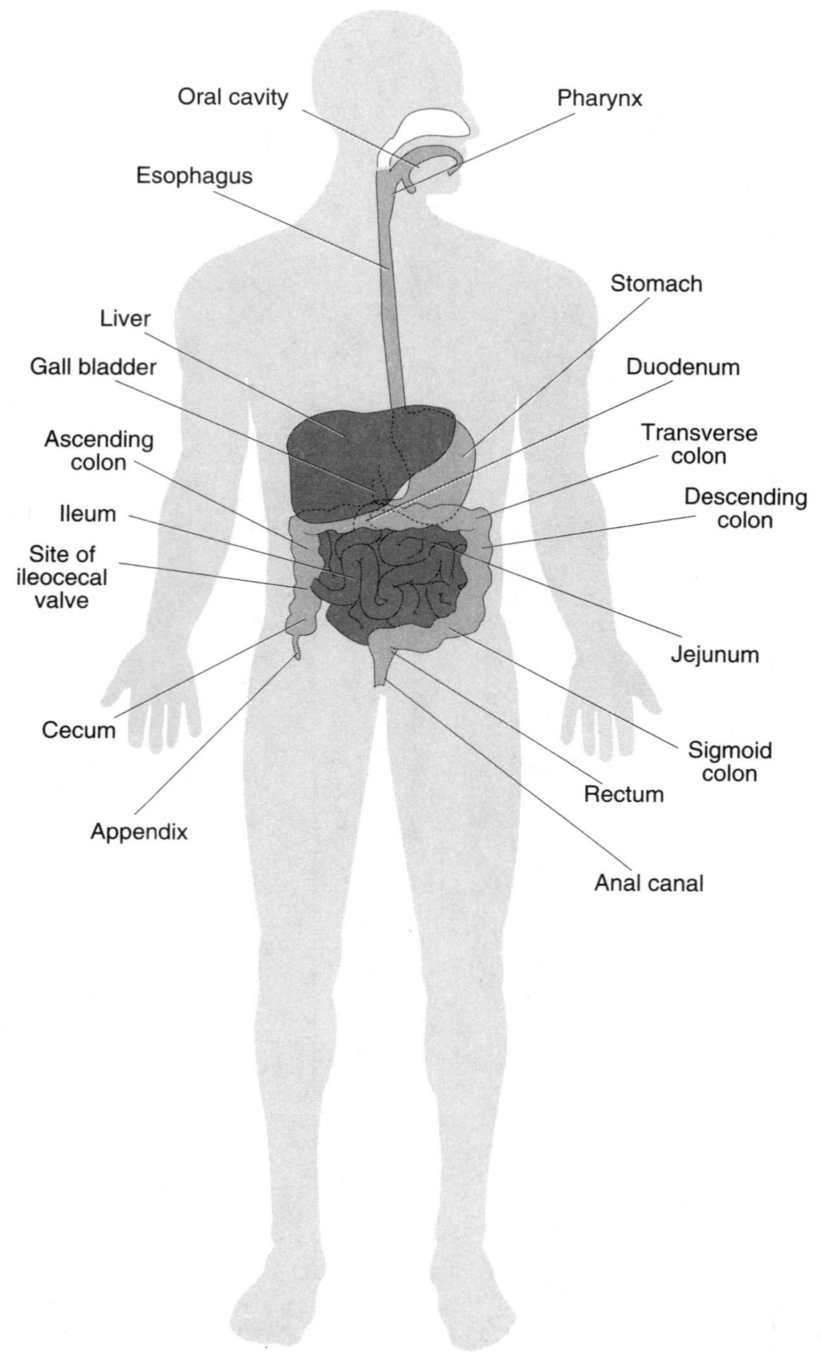

DIGESTIVE SYSTEM

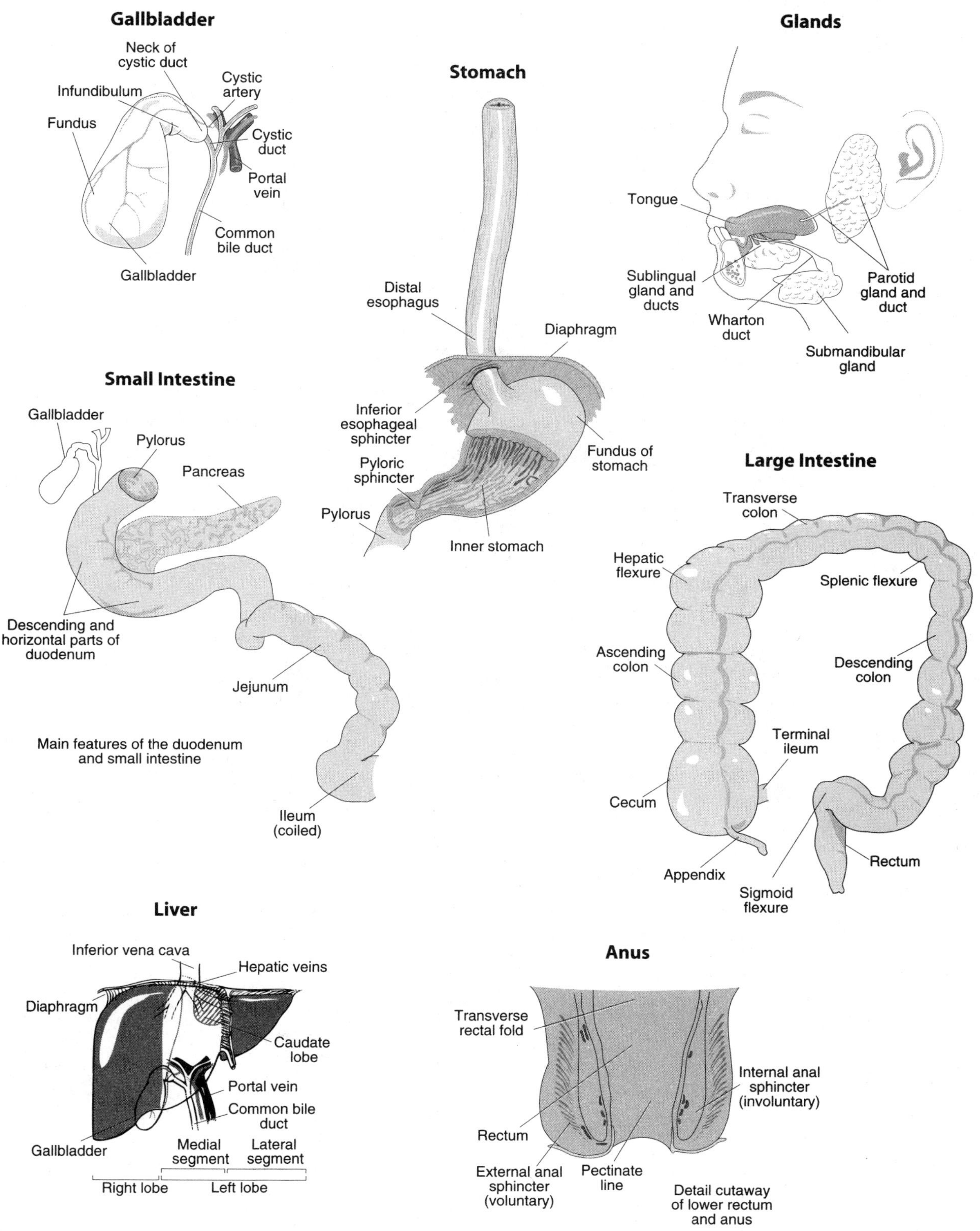

ARTERIAL SYSTEM

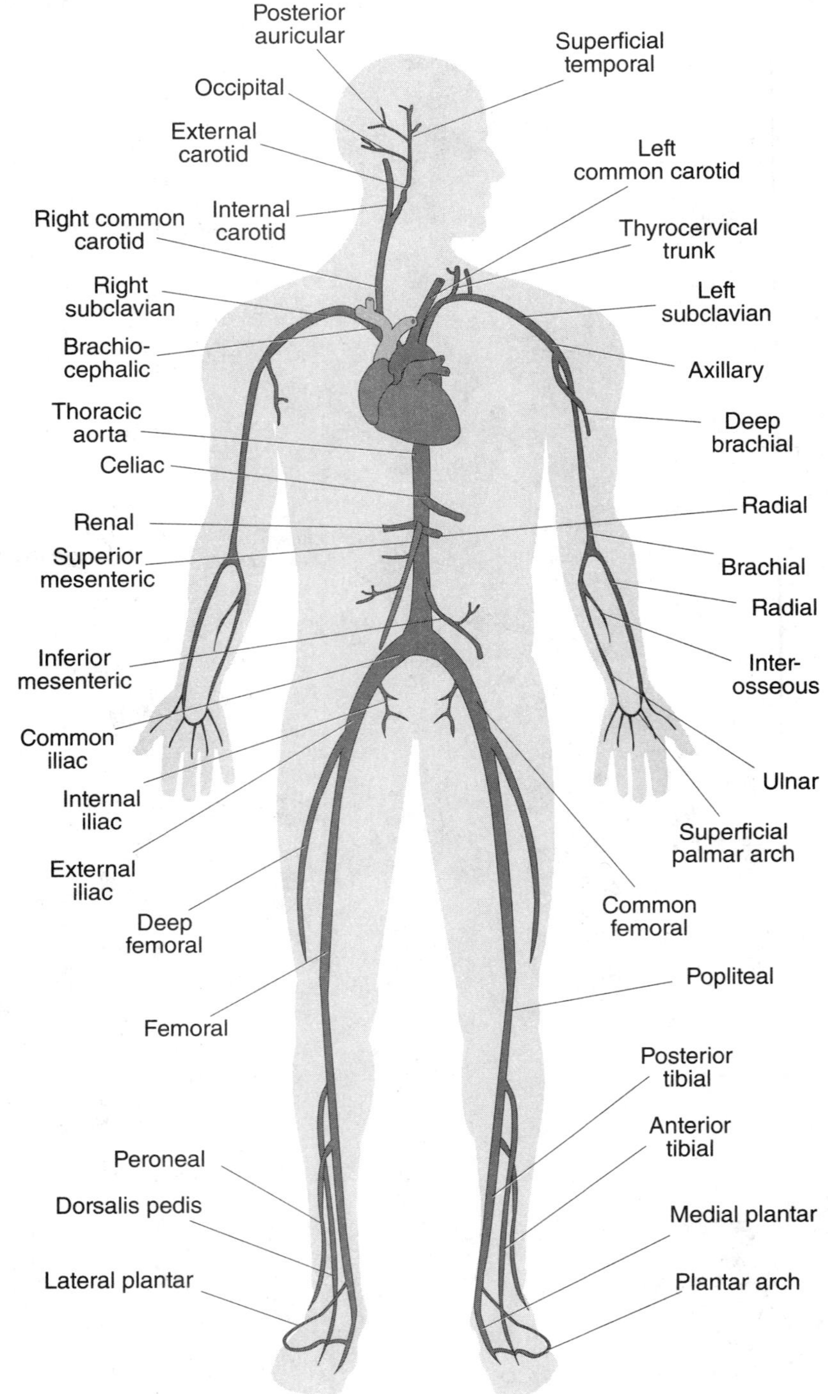

ARTERIAL SYSTEM

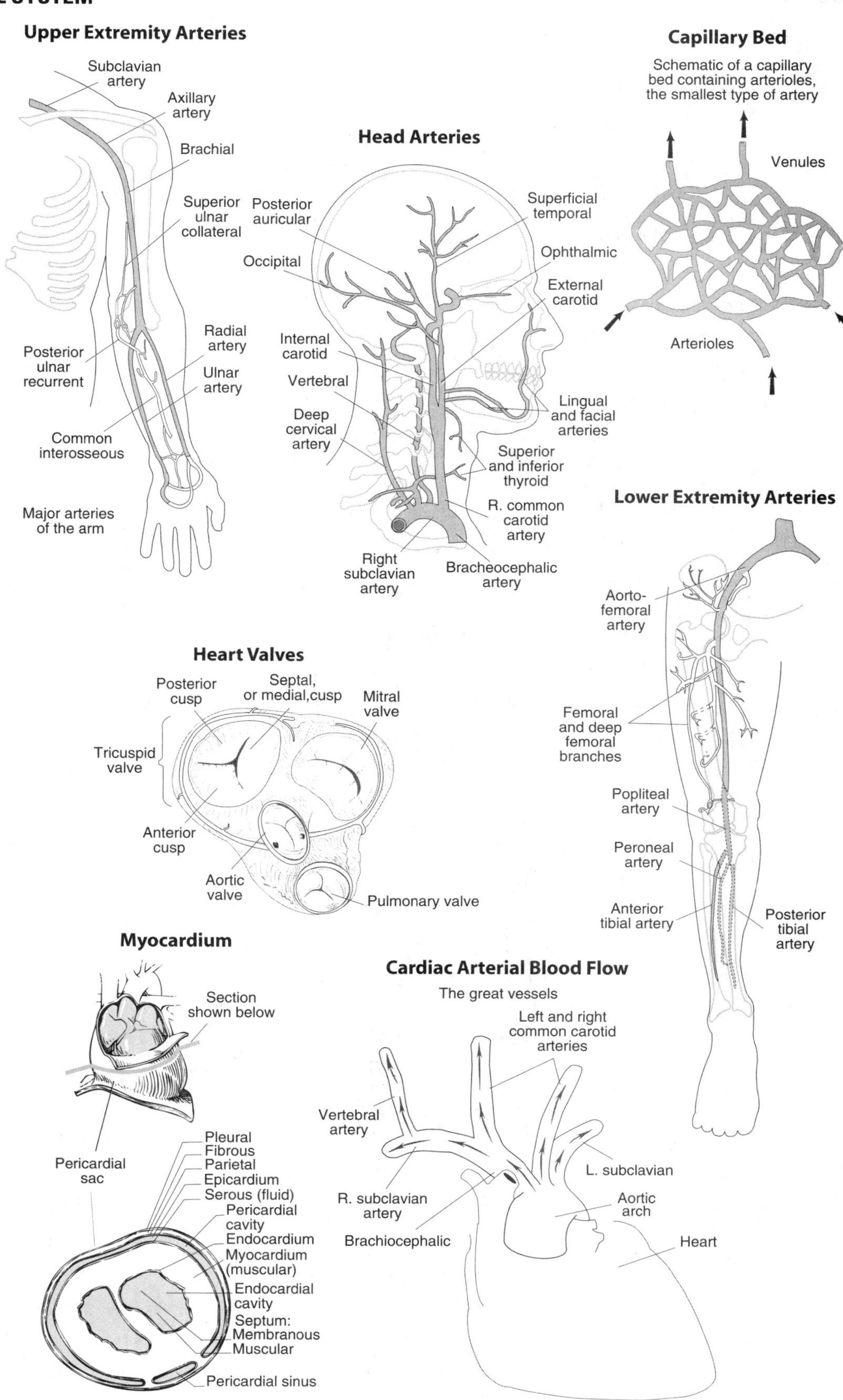

VENOUS SYSTEM

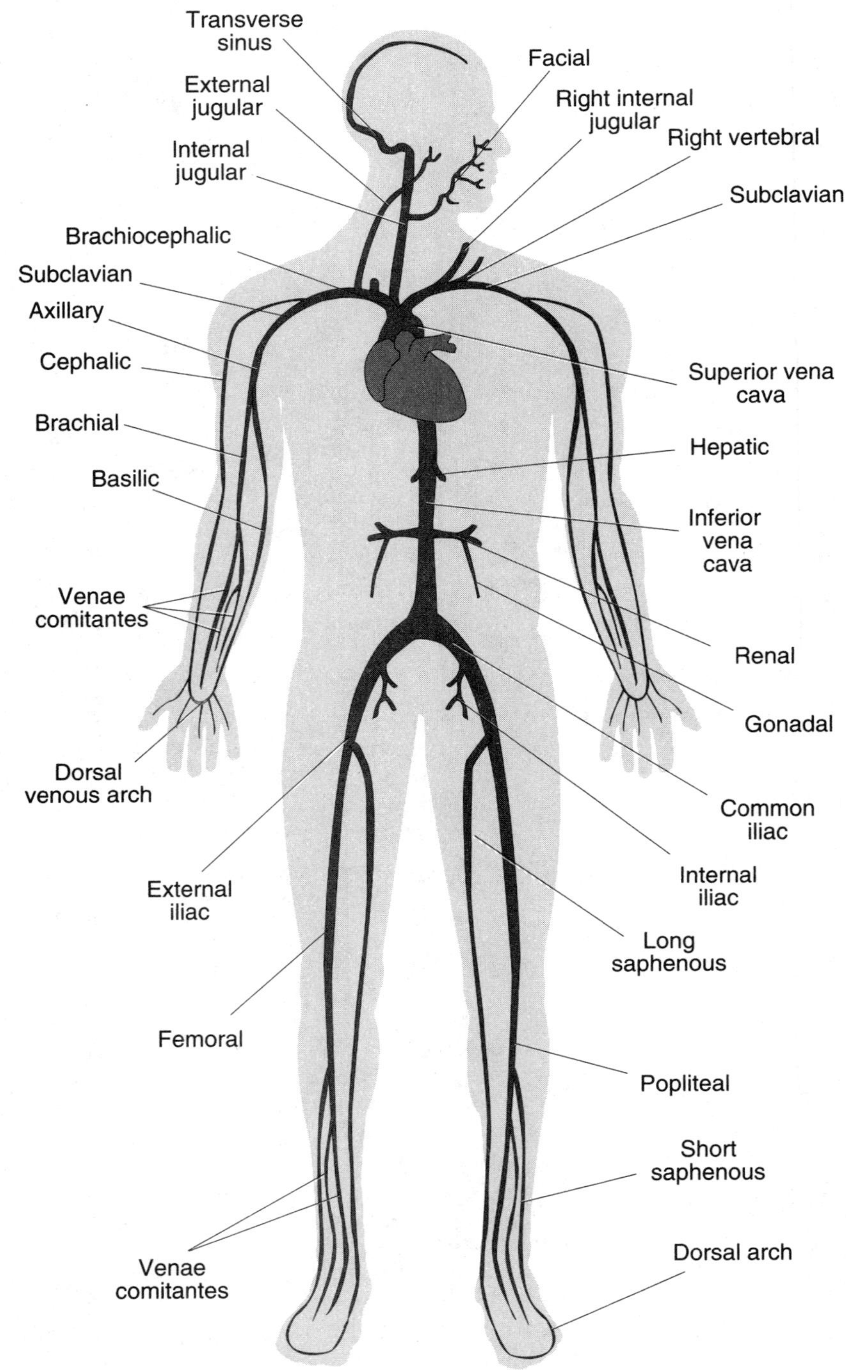

VENOUS SYSTEM

Upper Extremity Veins

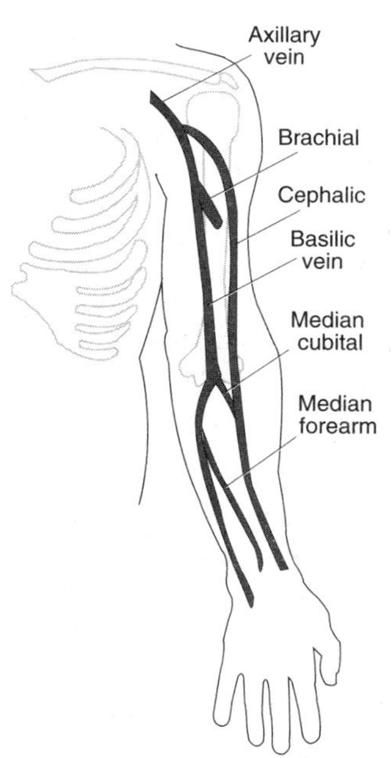

Venae Comitantes

Heart Veins

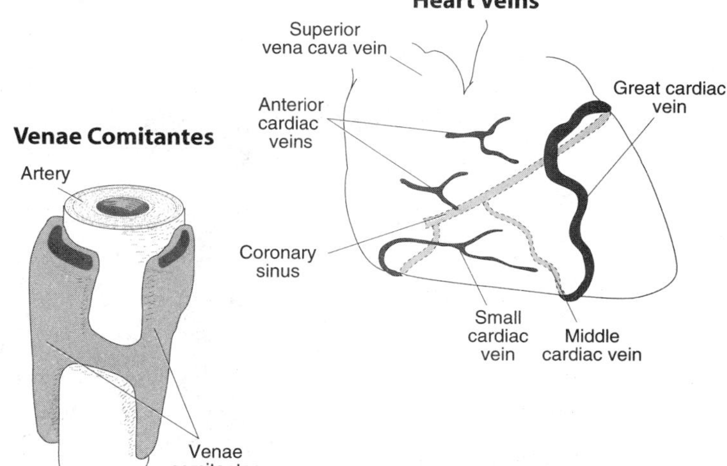

Venous Blood Flow

Venous blood flow is assisted by valves in the lumen of the vessels

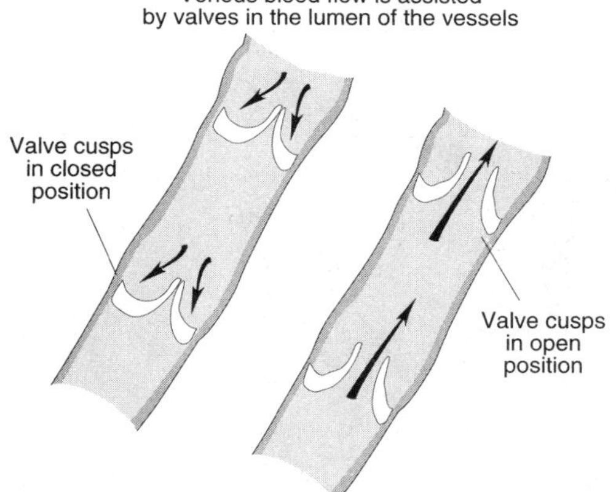

Head Veins

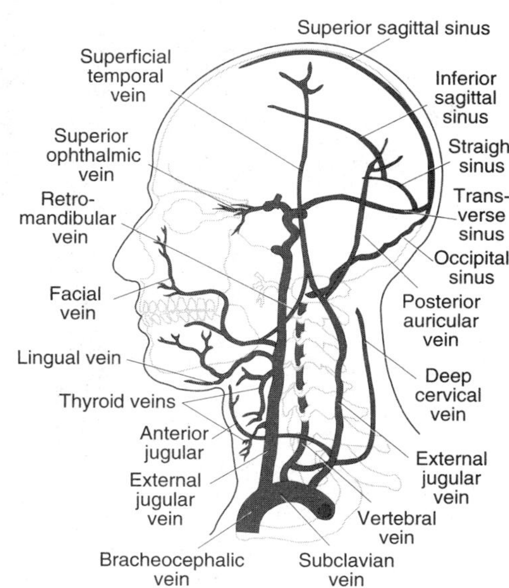

Cardiac Venous Blood Flow

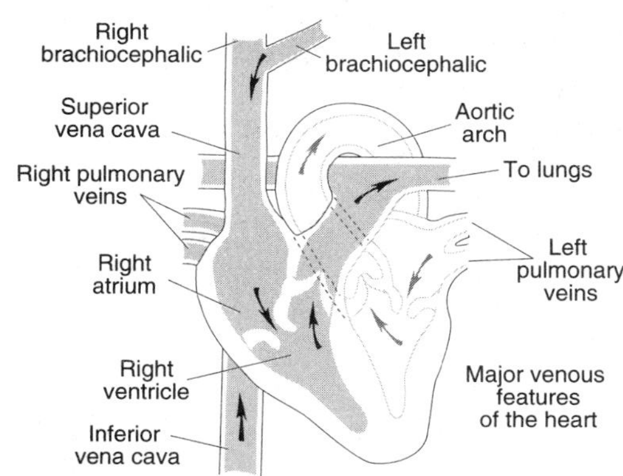

Abdominal Veins

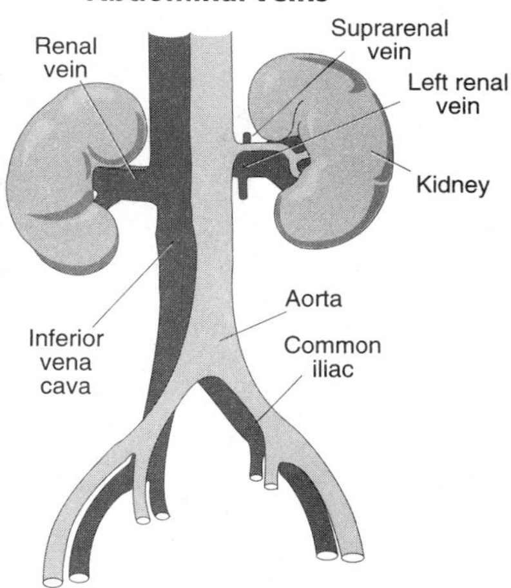

NERVOUS SYSTEM

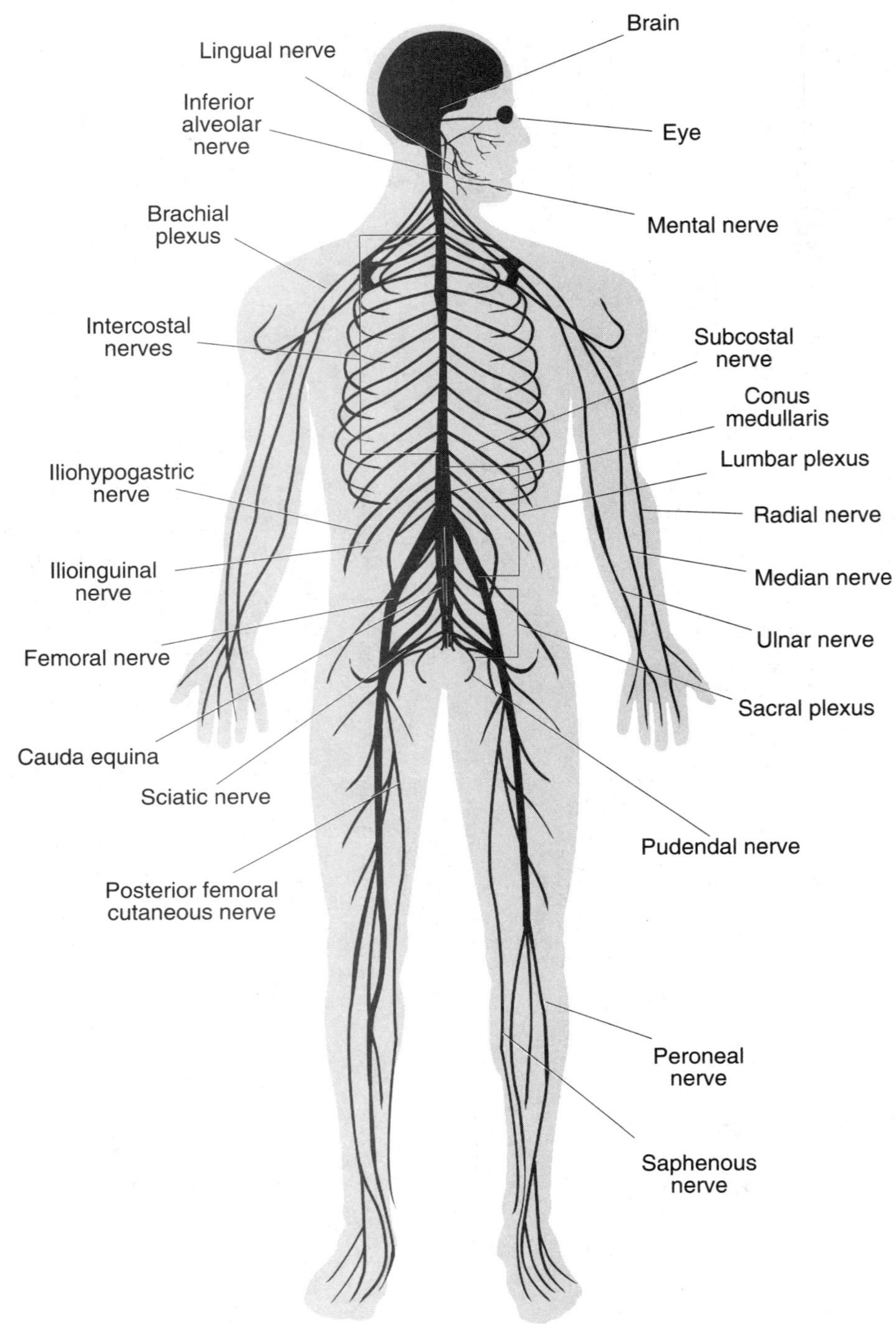

NERVOUS SYSTEM

Brain

Corpus callosum
Cerebrum
Hypothalamus
Optic chiasm
Hypophysis
Mamillary body
Peduncle
Medulla oblangata
Pons
Interventricular foramen
Fornix
Third ventricle
Pineal body
Corpora quadrigemina
Cerebral aqueduct
Vermis
Fourth ventricle
Median aperture
Spinal cord

Cranial Nerves

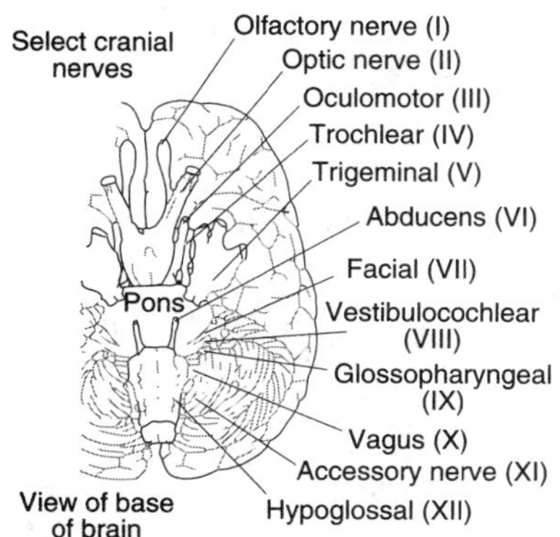

Spinal Cord

Schematic of spinal cord layers

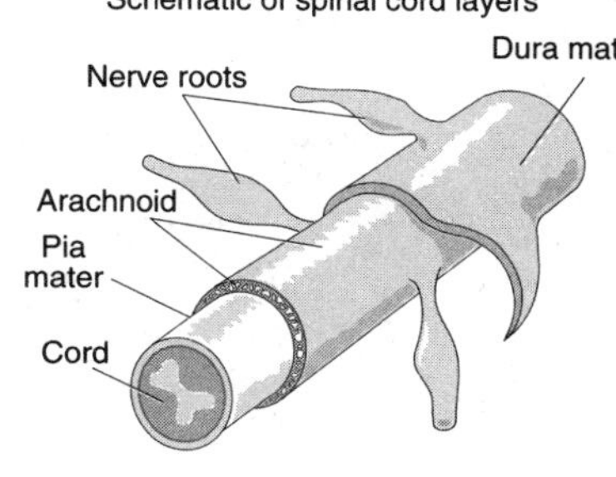

Spinal Column

Cranial Layers

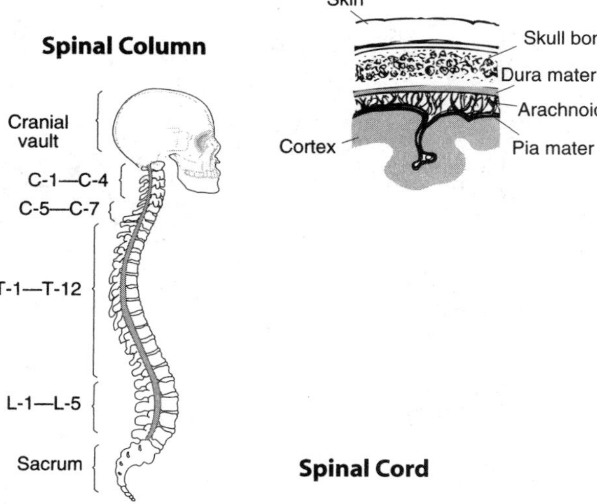

Spinal Cord

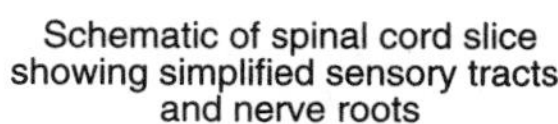
Schematic of spinal cord slice showing simplified sensory tracts and nerve roots

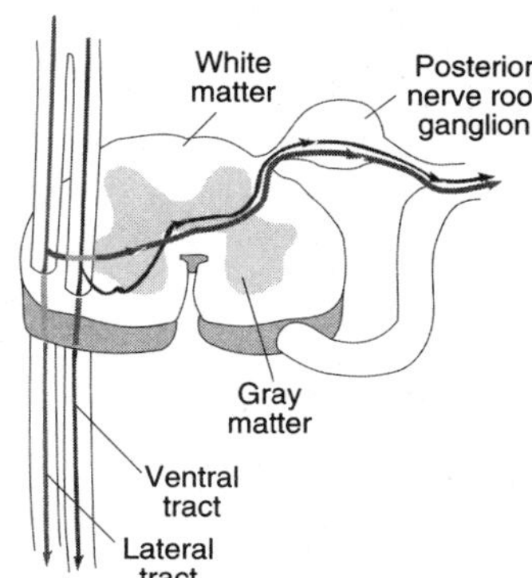

Spinal Cord

Schematic of spinal cord showing nerve roots

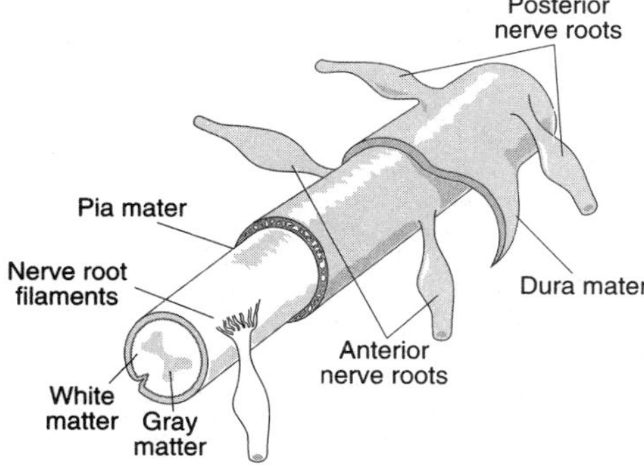

LYMPHATIC SYSTEM

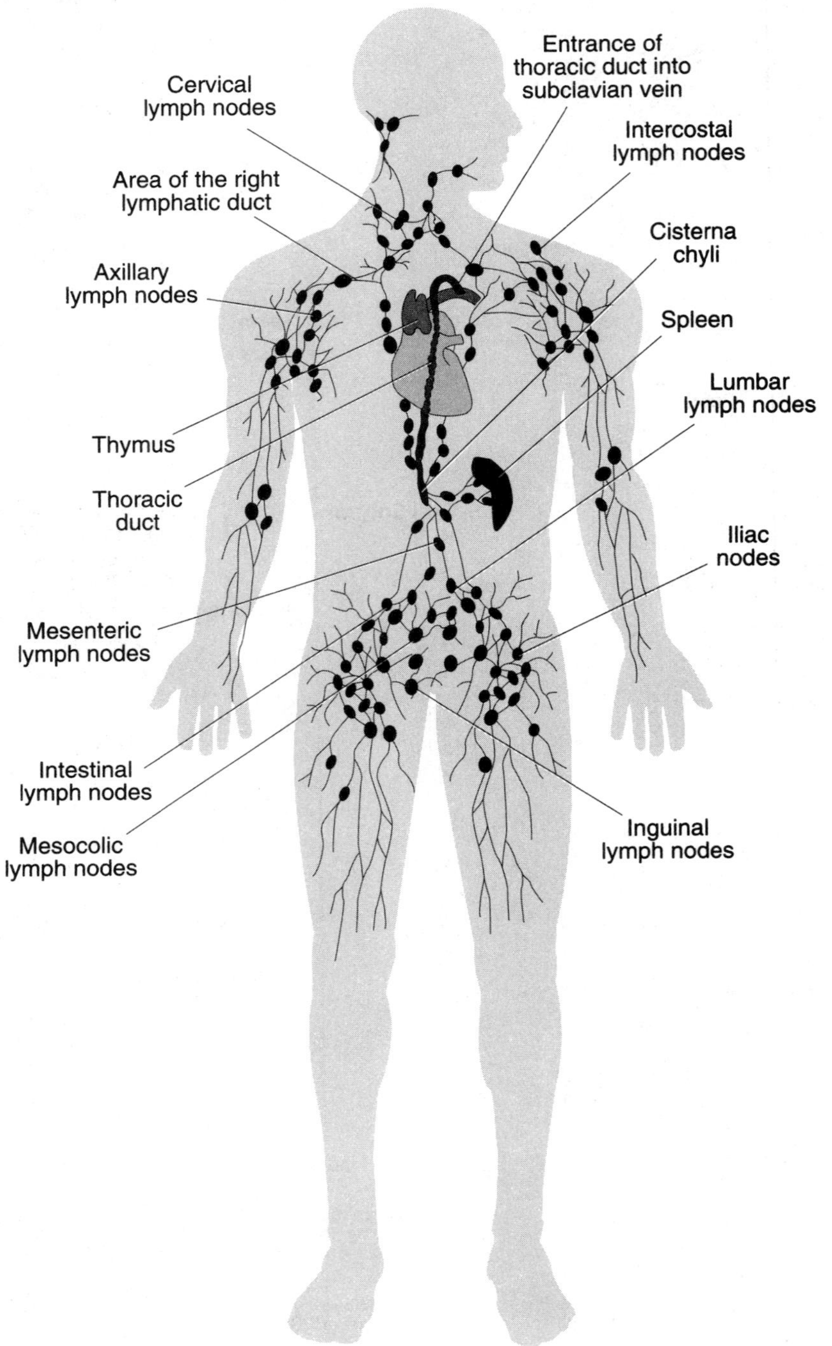

LYMPHATIC SYSTEM

Axillary Lymph Nodes

Sternum
Clavicle
Deltoid
Brachialis
Parasternal nodes
Lateral nodes
Subscapular nodes
Pectoral nodes
Central lymph nodes
Latissimus dorsi muscle
Axillary lymph nodes
Rectus abdominis

Lymphatic Capillaries

Schematic of lymphatic capillaries

Tissue cells
Valves
Endothelial cells

Fluids and particles can enter the capillary through overlapping valves

Lymphatic Drainage

Lymphatic drainage of the colon follows blood supply

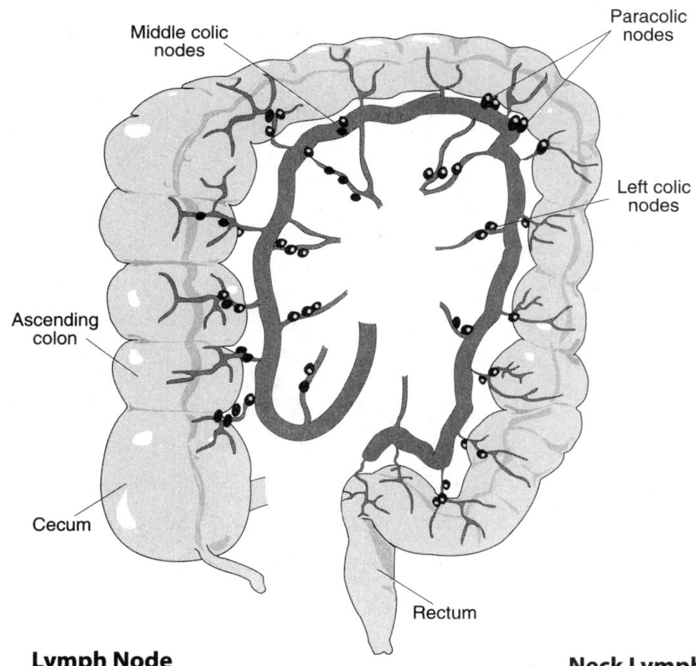

Lymph Node

Schematic of lymph node

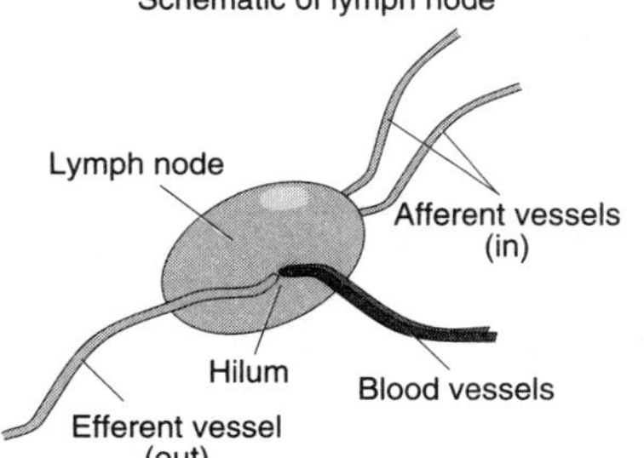

Neck Lymph Nodes

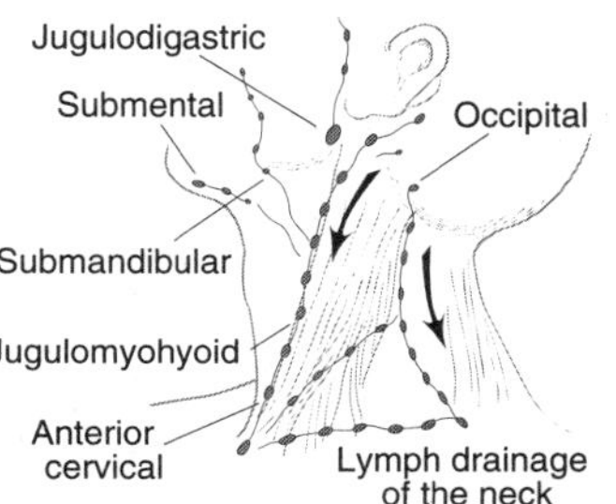

ENDOCRINE SYSTEM

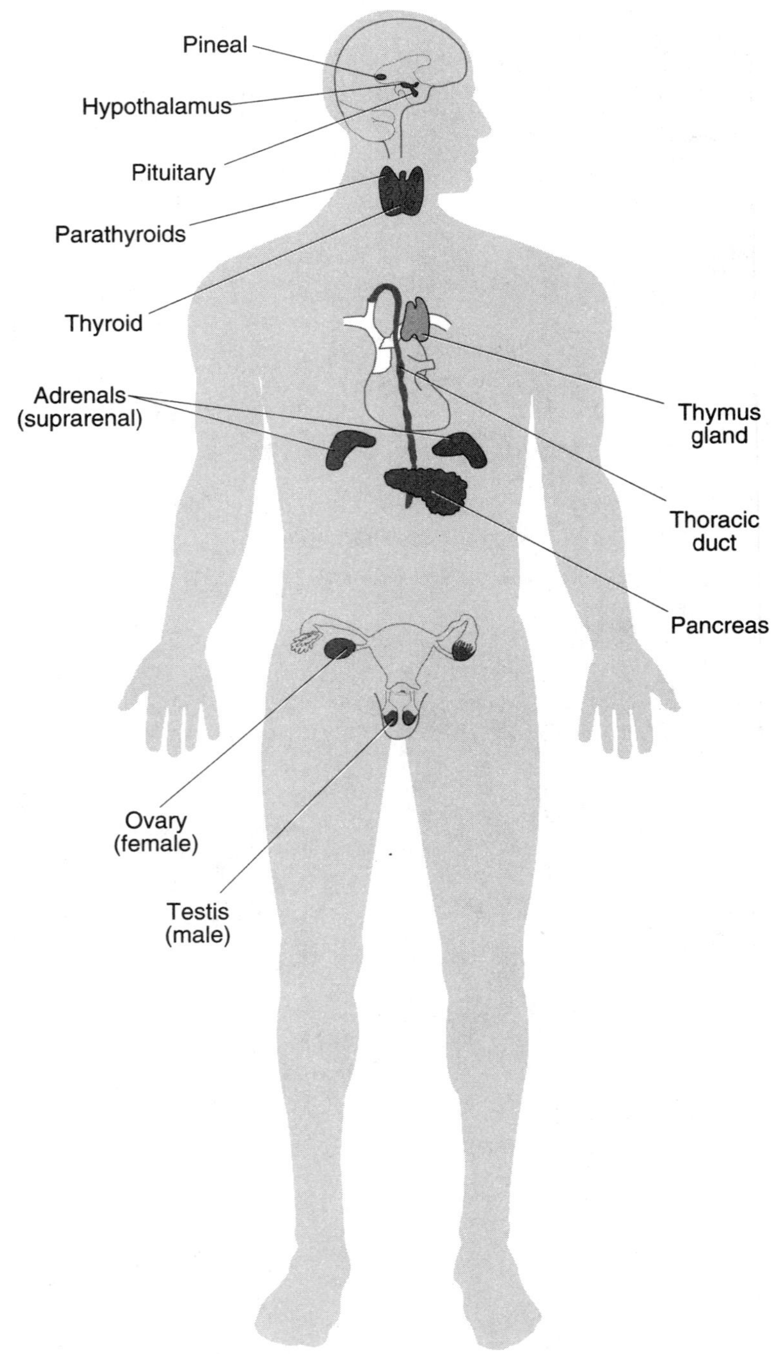

ENDOCRINE SYSTEM

Thyroid Glands

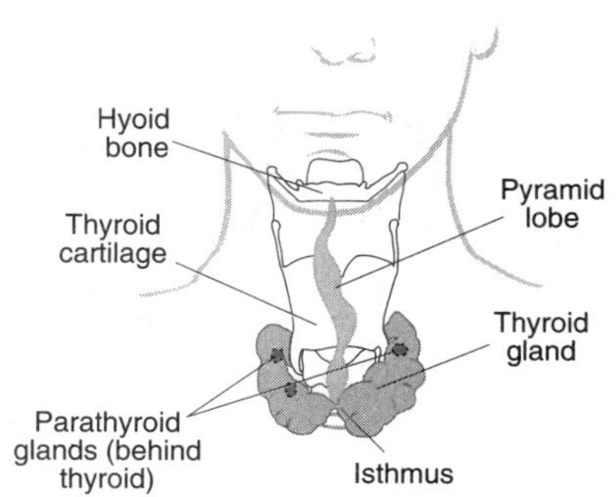

Pituitary Glands

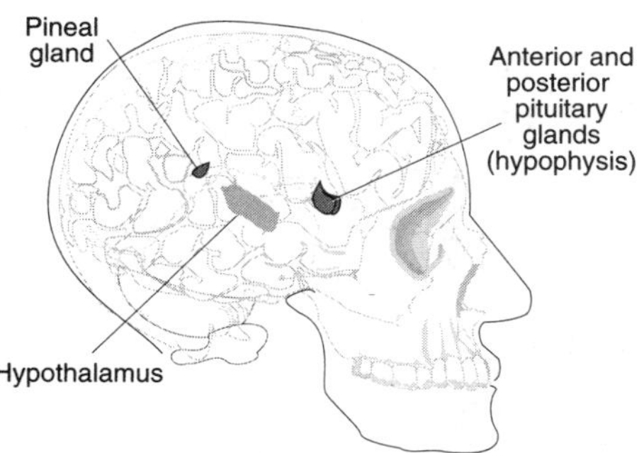

The pituitary gland and its controller, the hypothalamus, control body growth and stimulate and regulate other glands

Thyroid

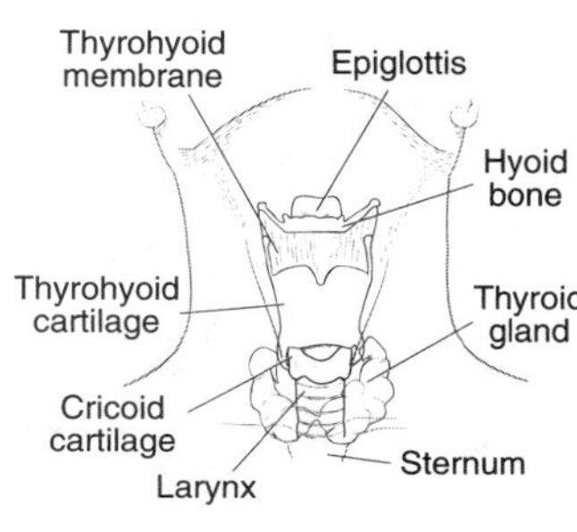

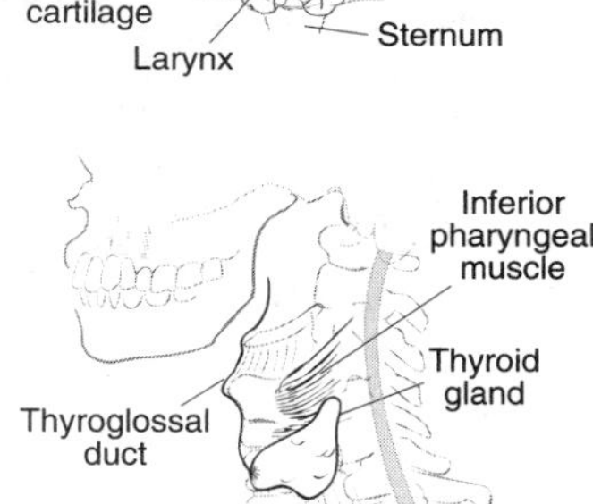

Thyroid

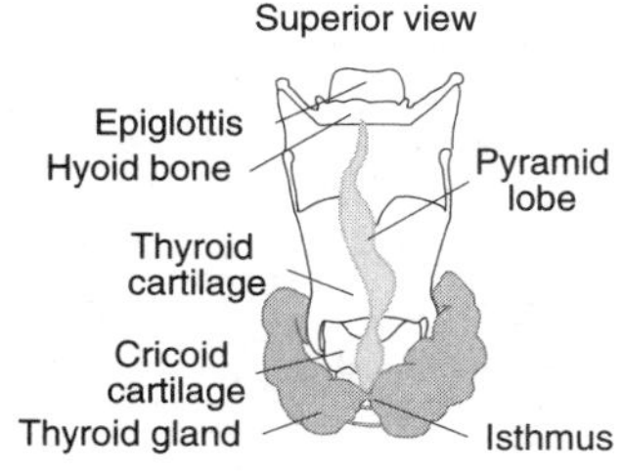

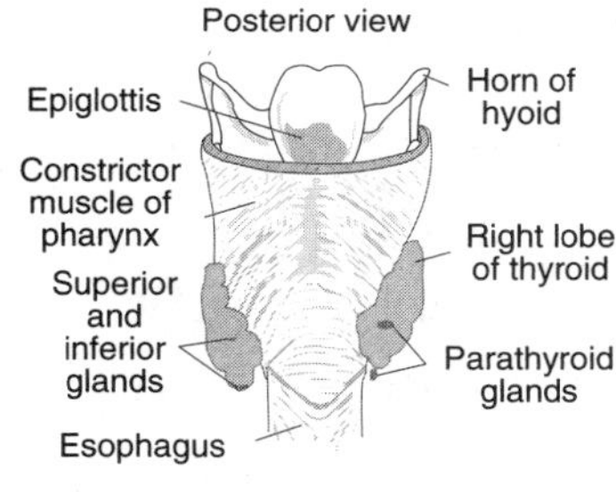

Placenta

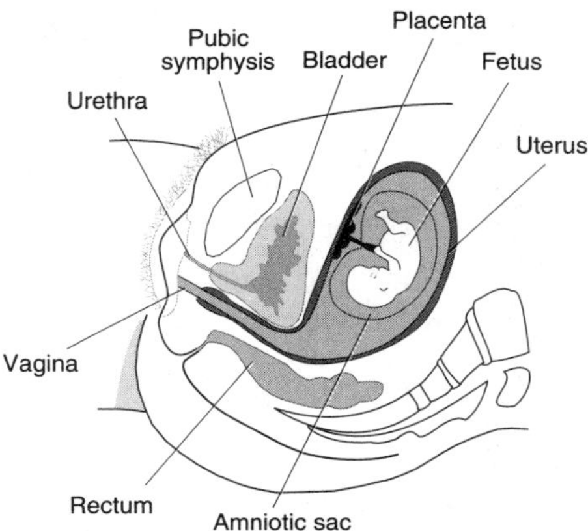

The placenta is considered part of the endocrine system, secreting chorionic gonadotropin, estrogen, progesterone, and somatomammotropin

GENITOURINARY SYSTEM

Kidney

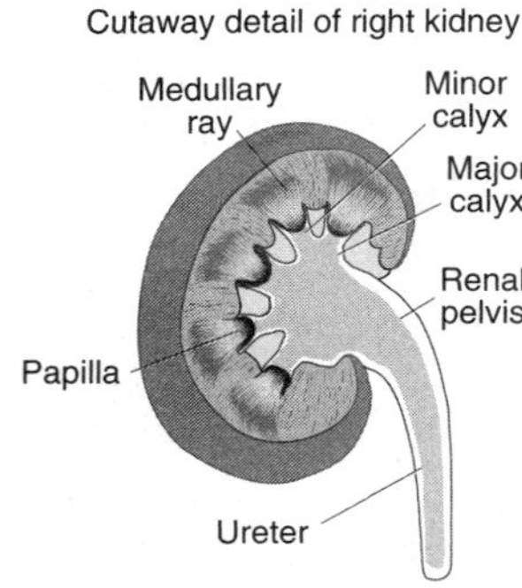

Male Urinary

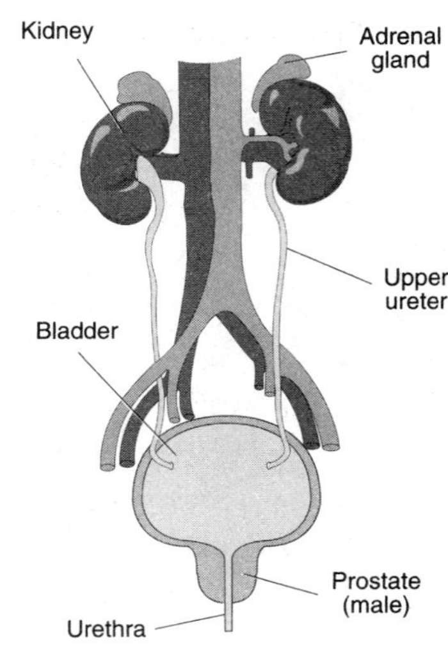

Nephron

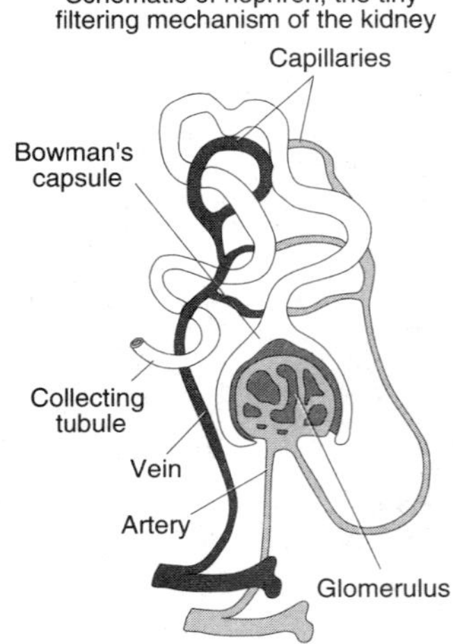

Male Genitourinary

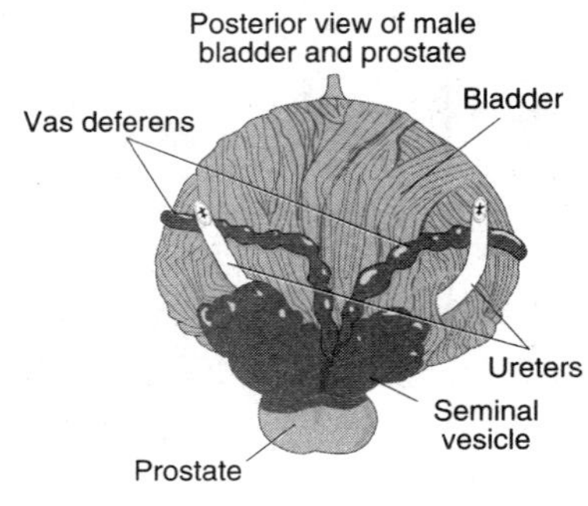

Urinary

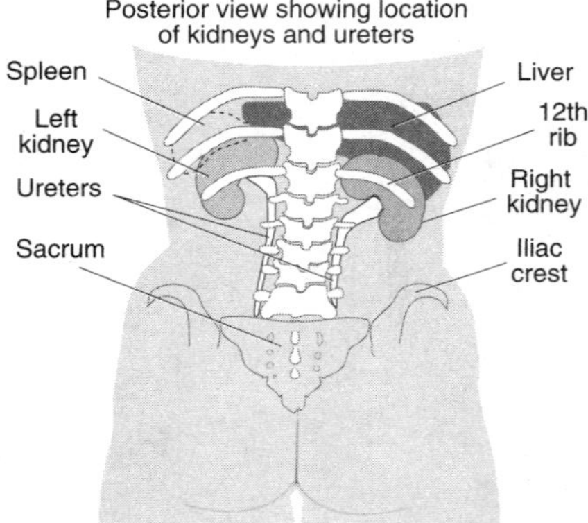

Male Reproductive

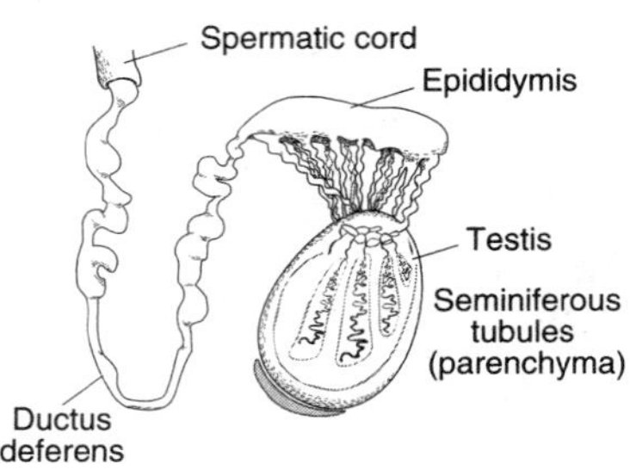

GENITOURINARY SYSTEM

Female Genitourinary

Sideview schematic of female urogenital system

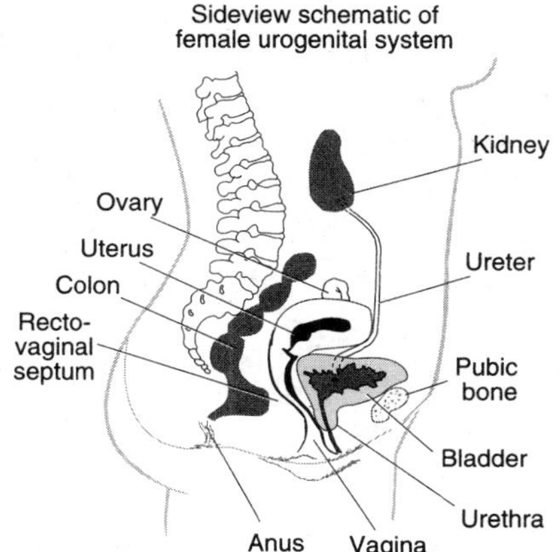

Female Rectoperineal

Lateral schematic showing the female rectoperineal area

Uterus
Rectouterine pouch
Bladder
Cervix
Pubic bone
Rectum
Clitoris
Urethral orifice
Anus
Labia majora
Labia minora
Vaginal canal

Female Bladder

Female Reproductive

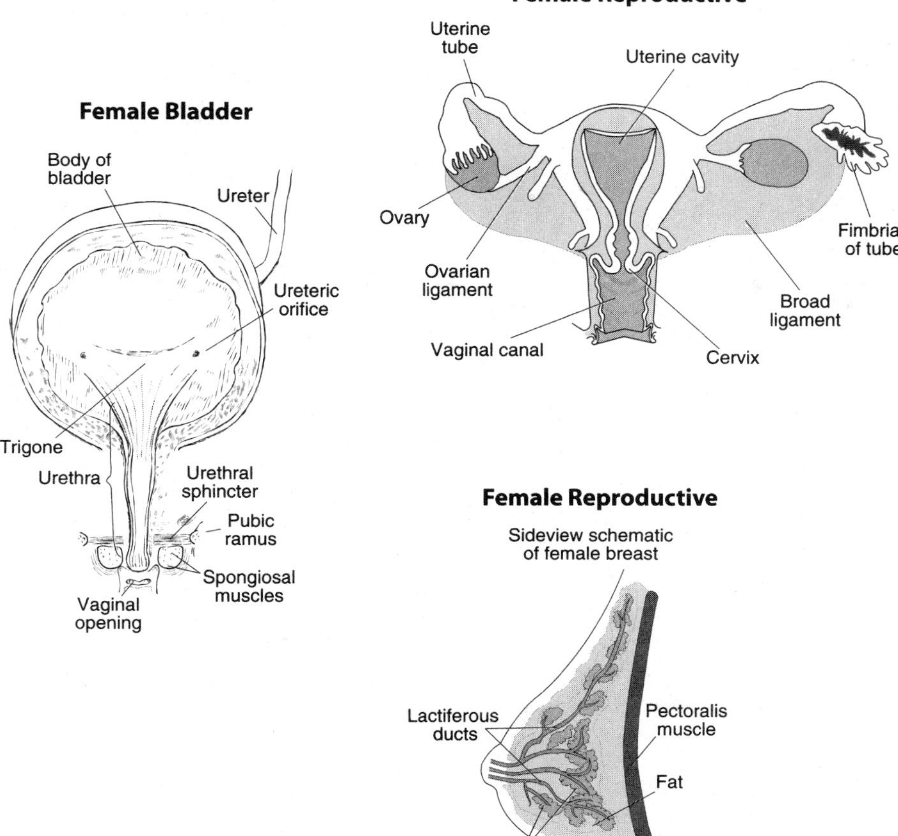

Female Reproductive

Sideview schematic of female breast

Lactiferous ducts
Pectoralis muscle
Fat
Gland lobules

RESPIRATORY SYSTEM

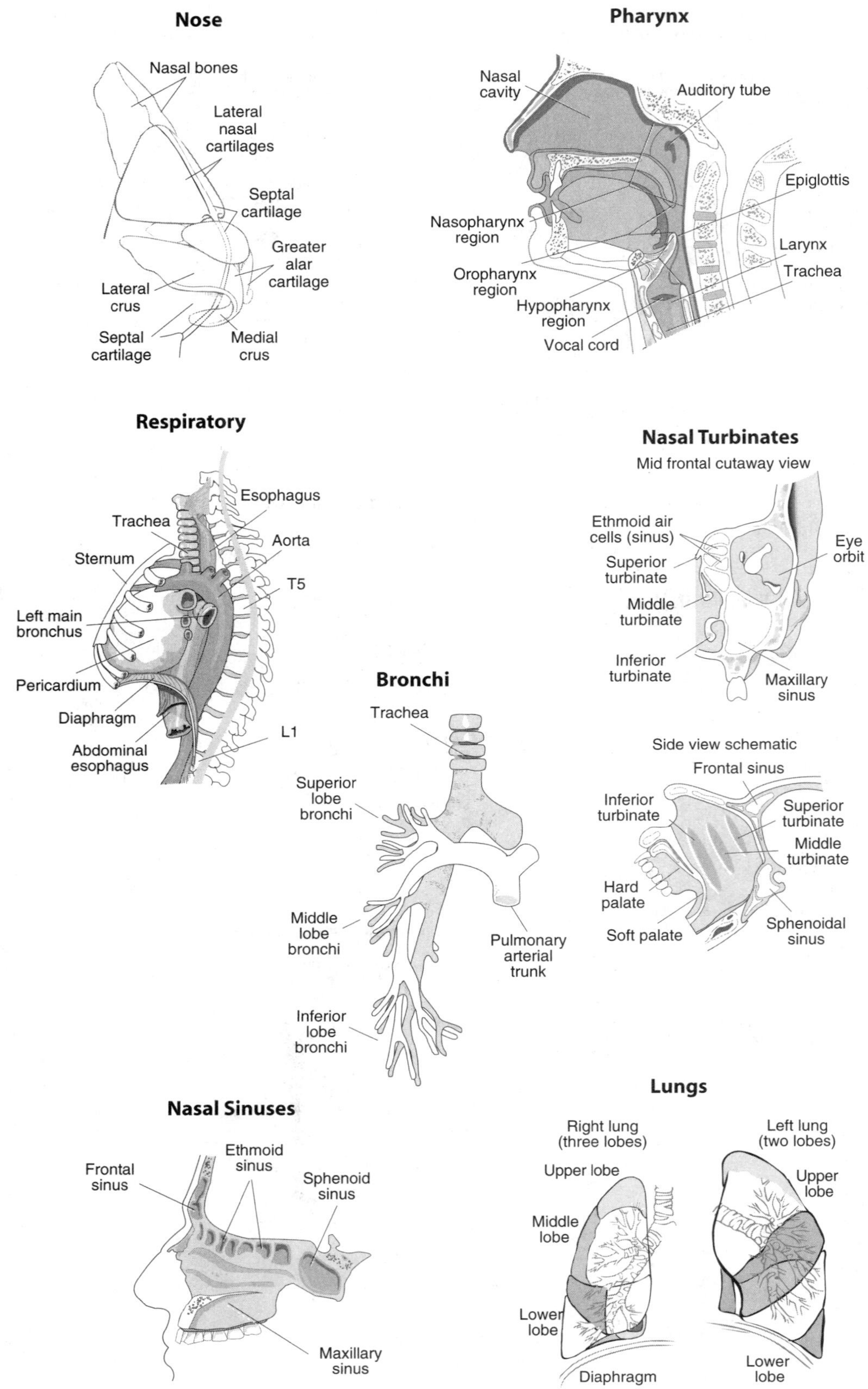

EYE

Eye

Muscles of the right eye

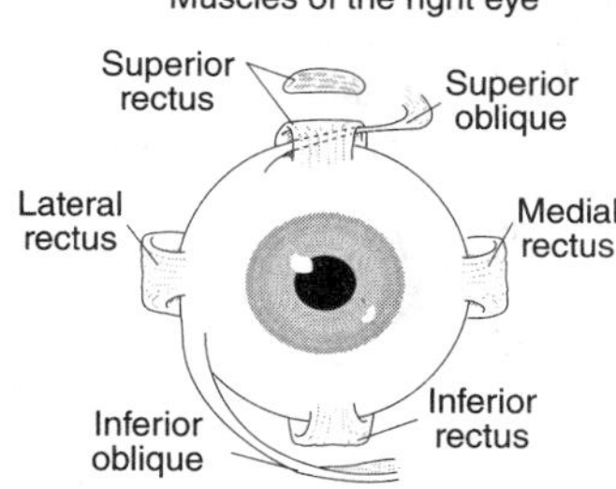

Lacrimal System

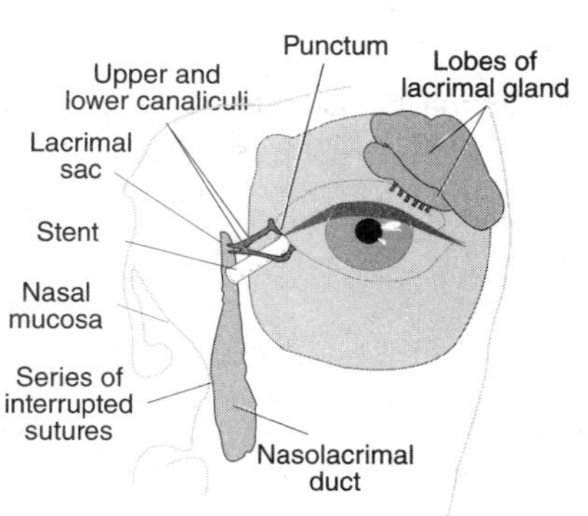

Eye

Anterior and posterior chambers of the eye

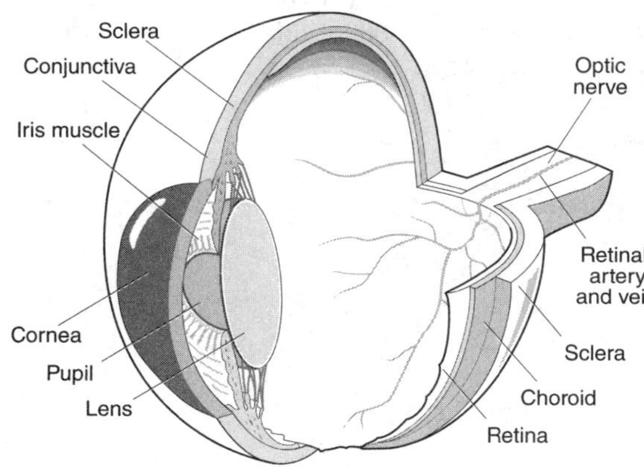

EAR

Ear

Middle ear
Auditory ossicles: Stapes
Semicircular canals
Malleus
Incus
Tympanic membrane (ear drum)
External auditory meatus
Cochlea (in bone)
Pharynx
Auricle (pinna)
Cochlear (round) window
Auditory (eustachian) tube

Middle Ear

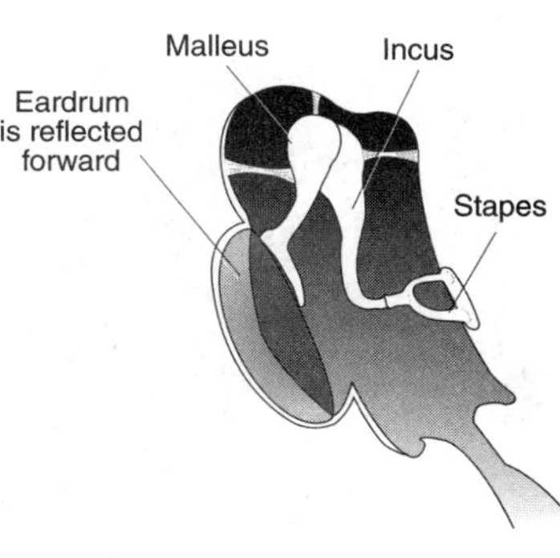

Normal Aortic Arch and Branch Anatomy – Transfemoral Approach

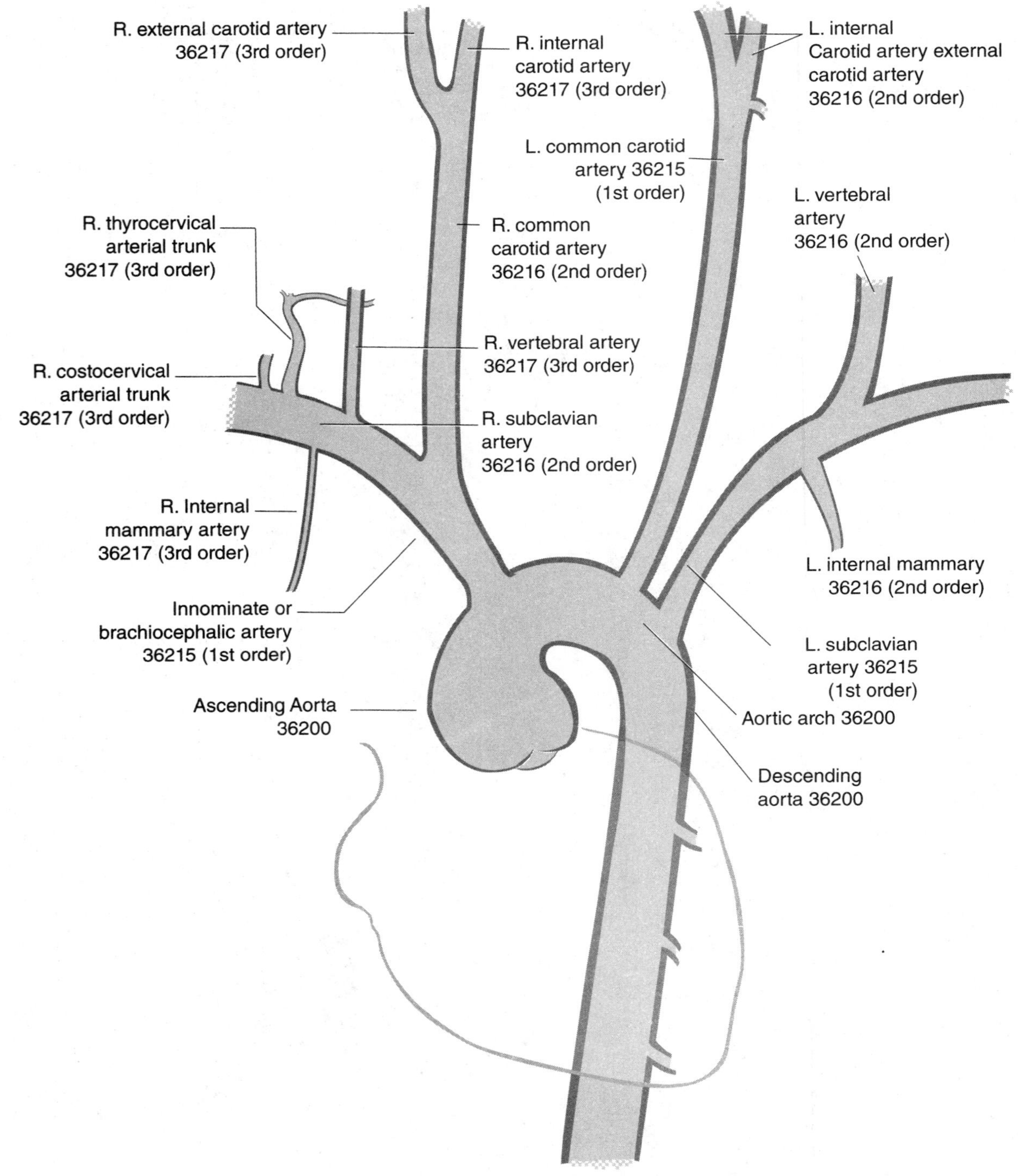

Superior and Inferior Mesenteric Arteries and Branches

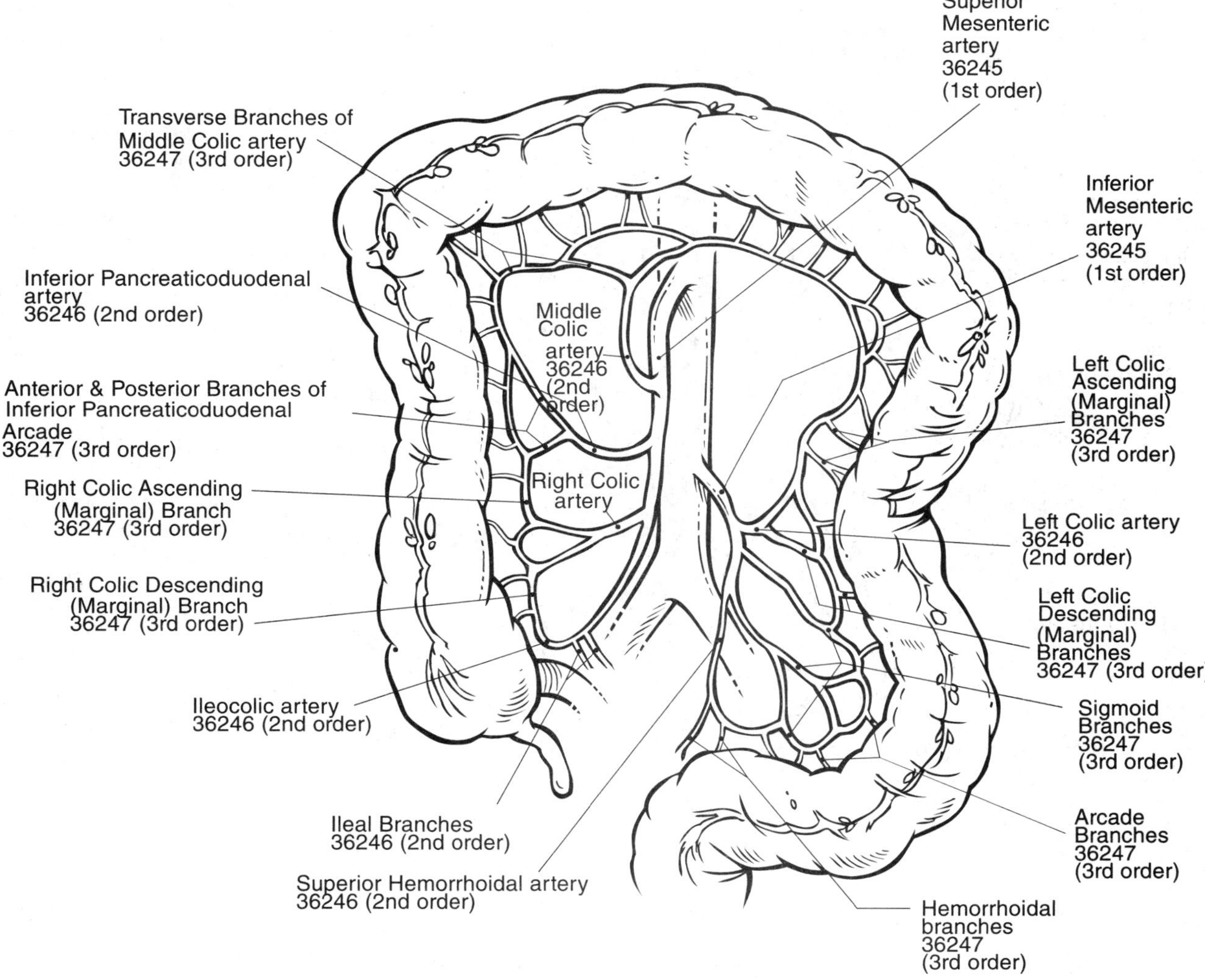

Portal System

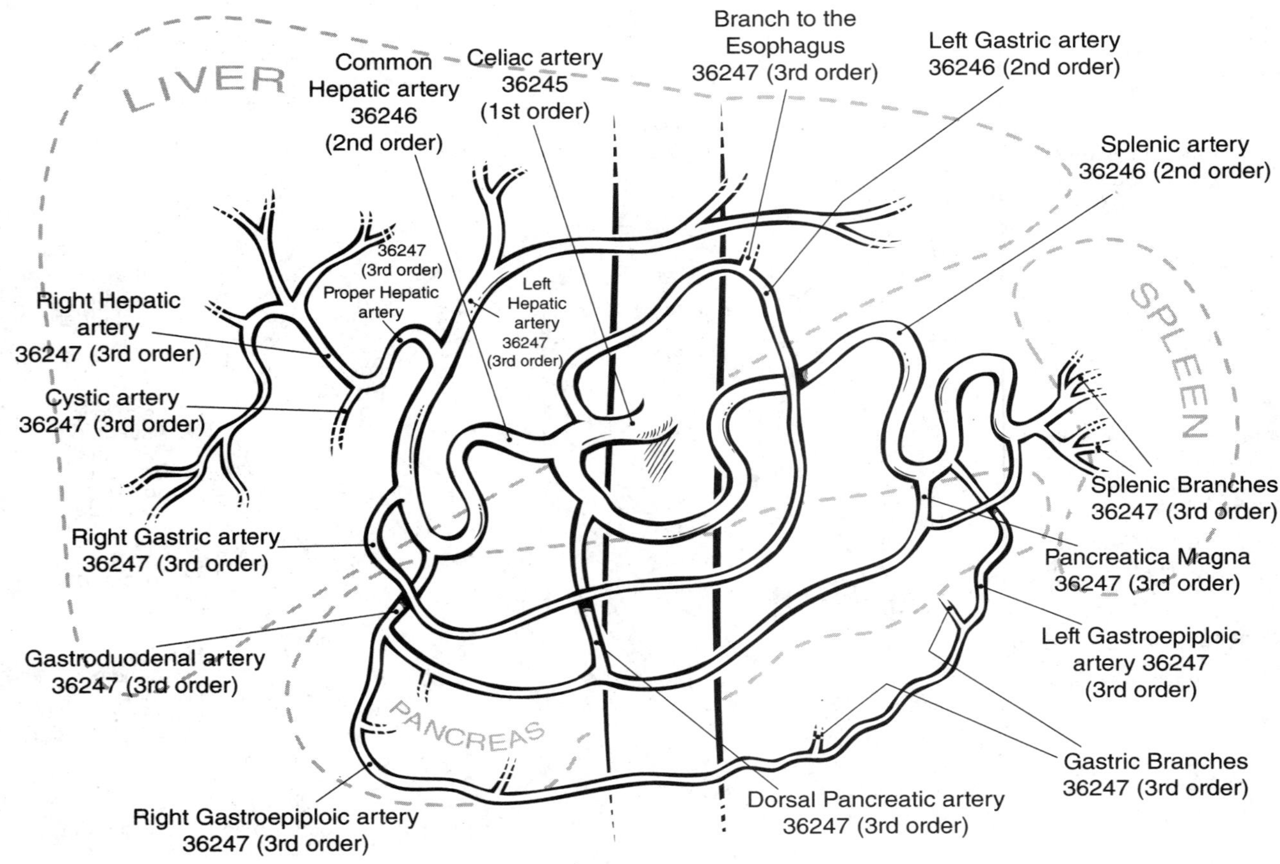

Renal Artery Anatomy–Femoral Approach

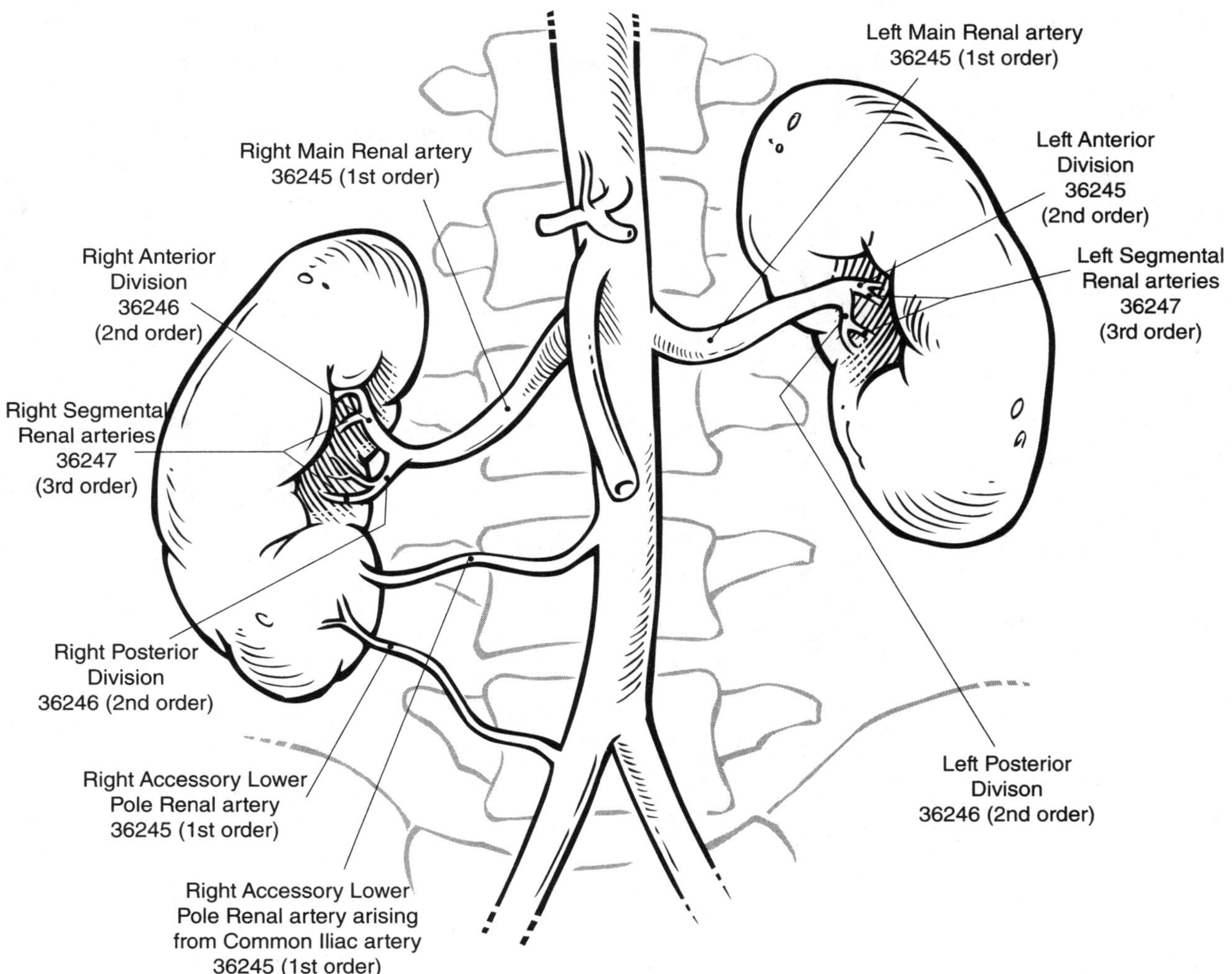

Upper Extremity Arterial Anatomy–Transfemoral or Contralateral Approach

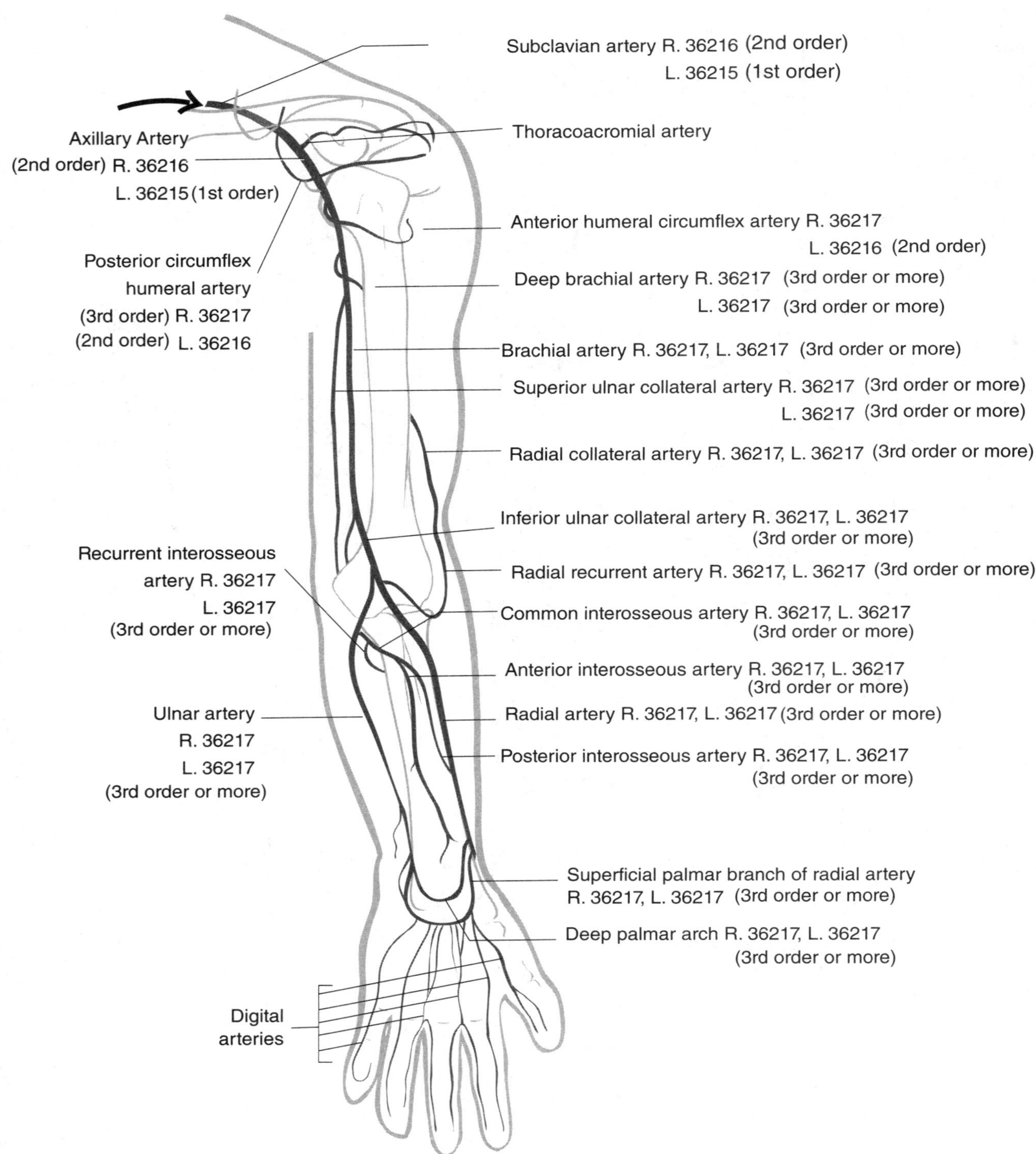

Lower Extremity Arterial Anatomy–Contralateral, Axillary or Brachial Approach

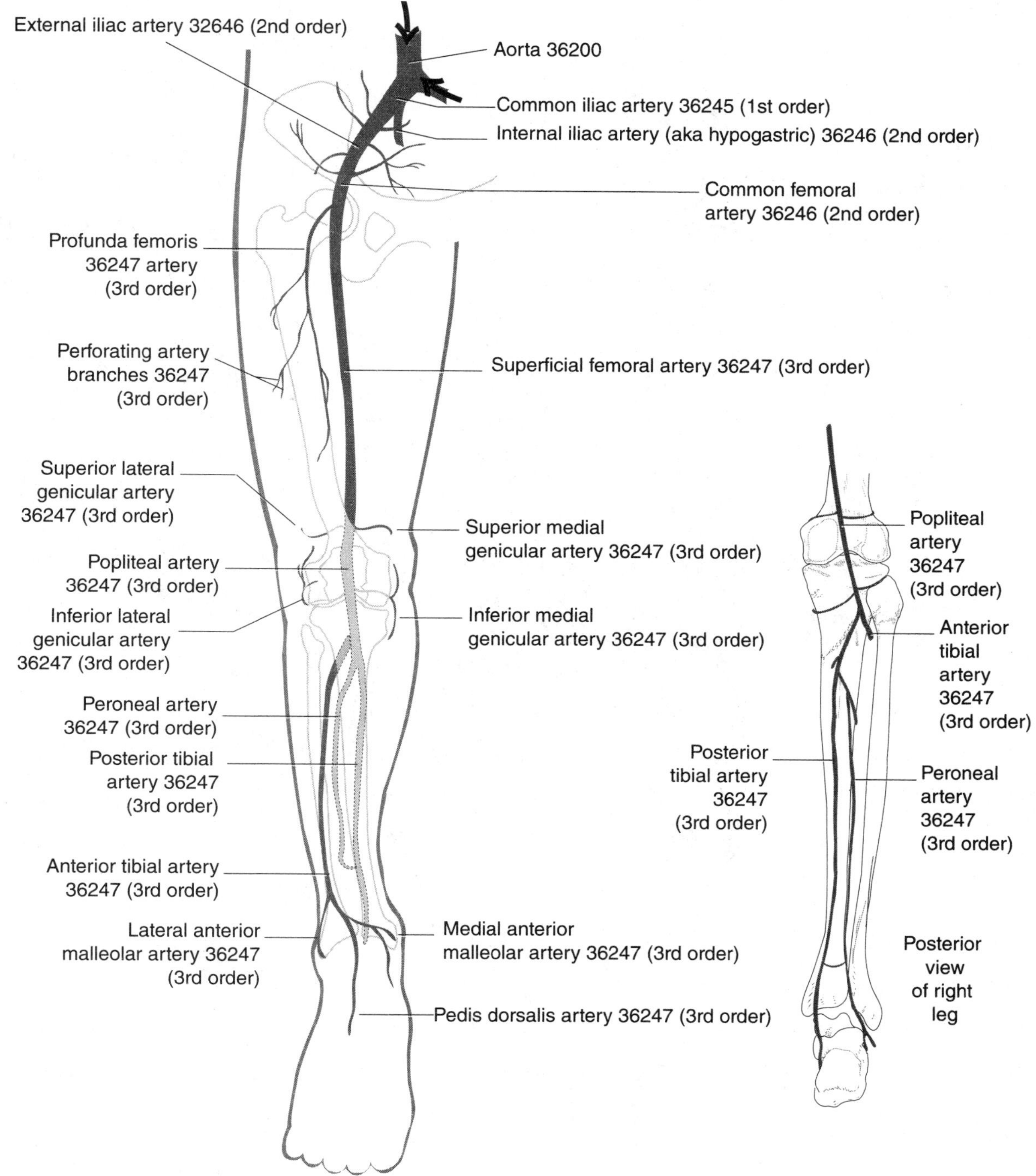

Portal System

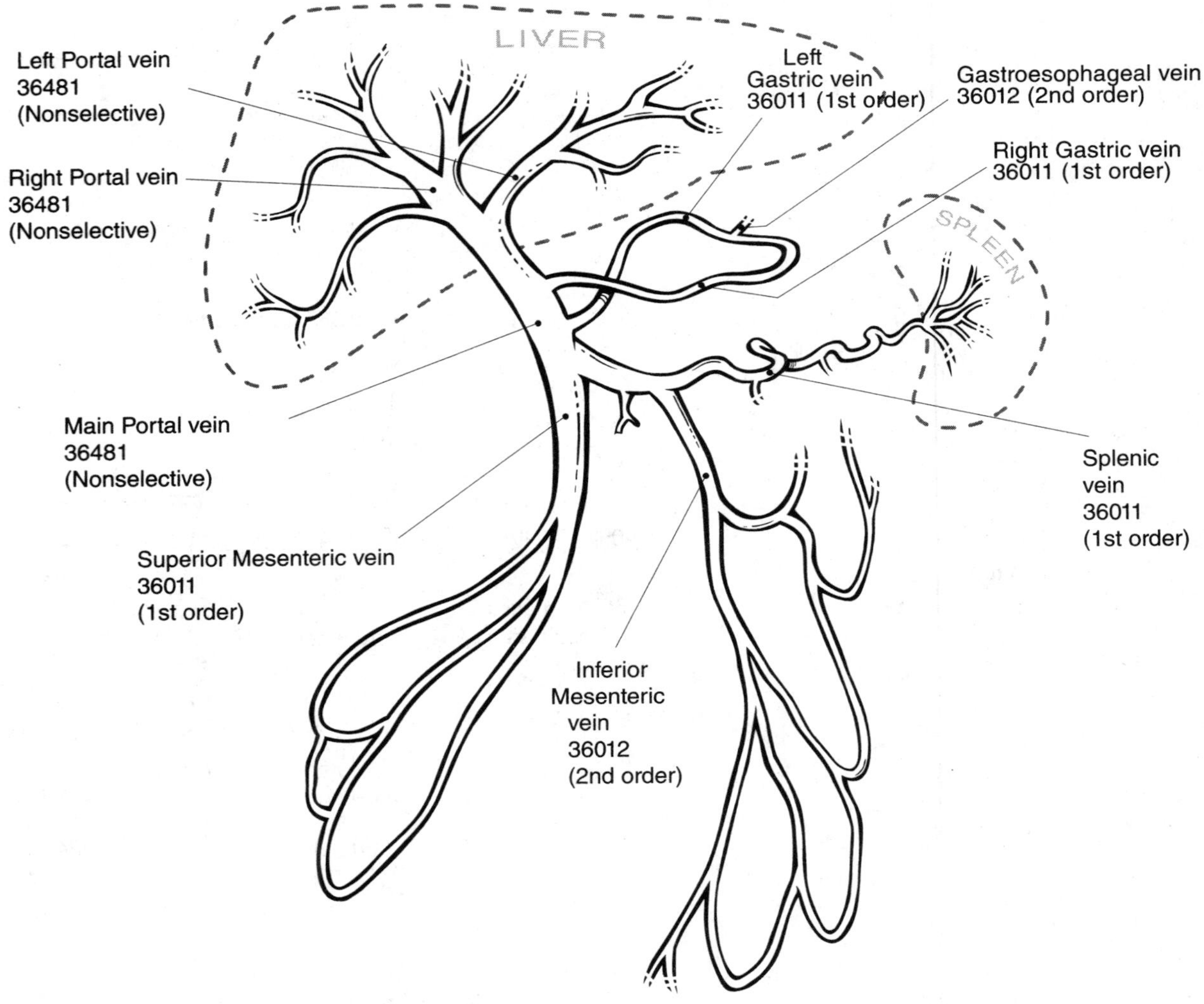

Coronary Arteries Anterior View

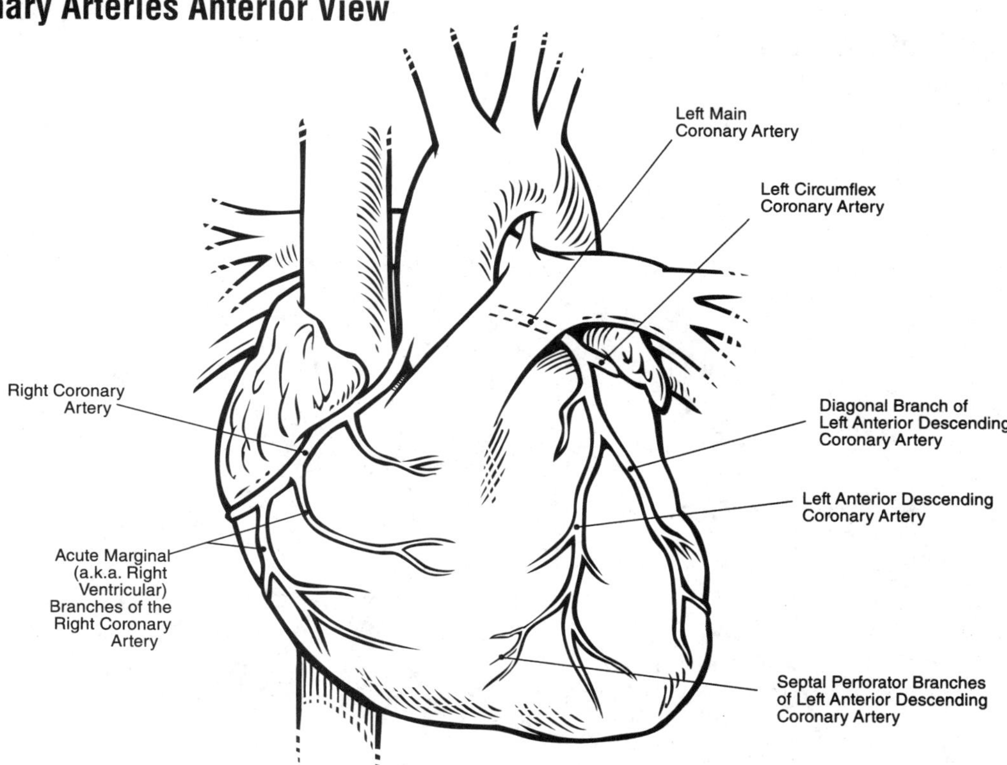

Left Heart Catheterization

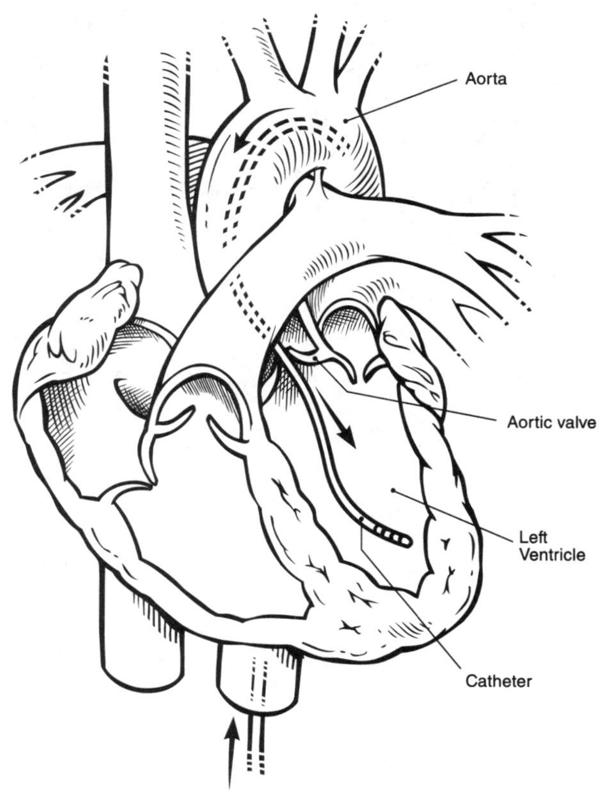

Heart Conduction System

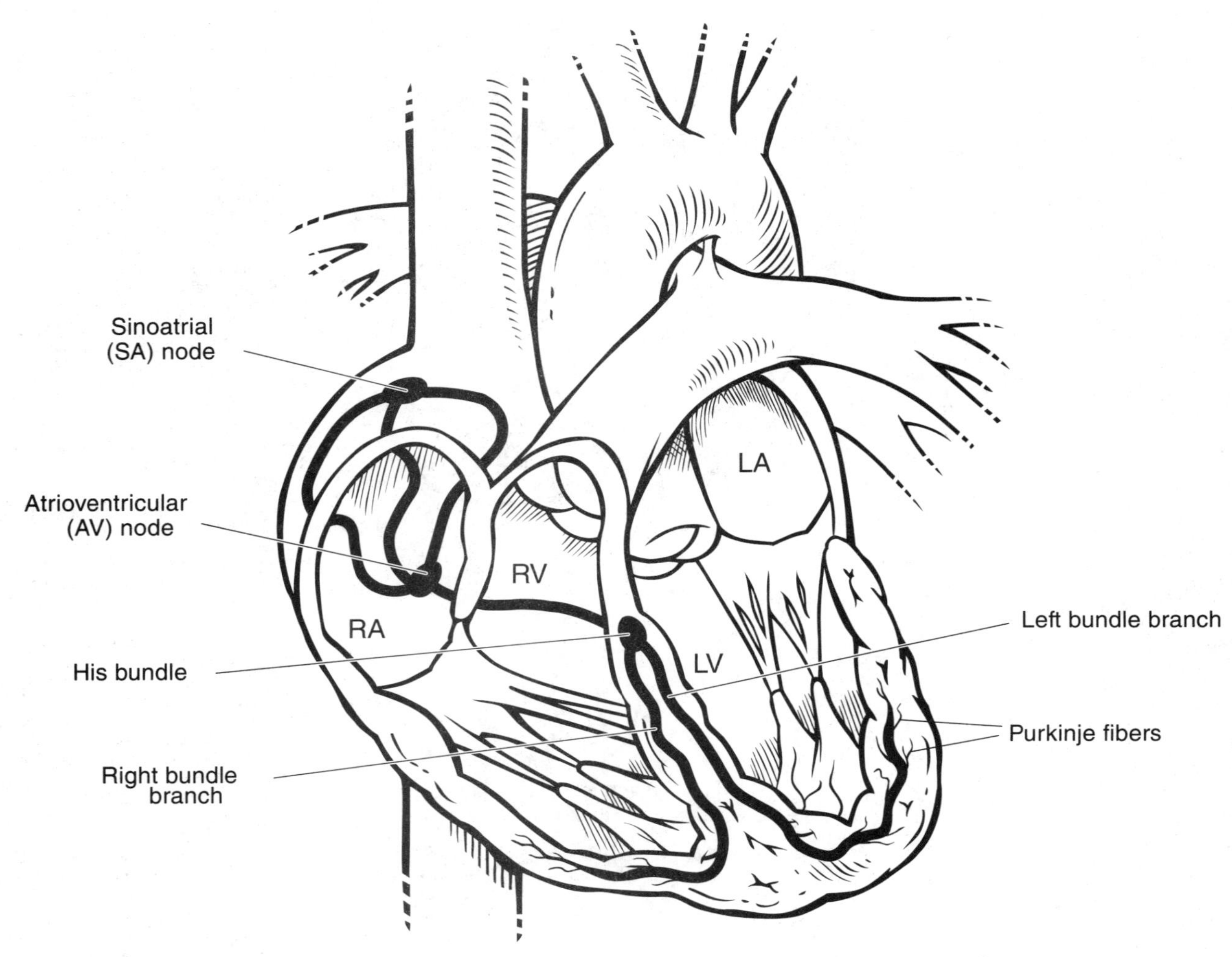

0-Numeric

A

C

 [Resequenced]

D

F

G

I

J

M

P

U

W

Y

Z

00100-00126 Anesthesia for Gland, Cleft Lip, Eyelid, ECT, and Ear Procedures

CMS 100-4,4,10.4 Packaging Rules Under OPPS
CMS 100-4,4,20.6 Modifier Use Under OPPS
CMS 100-4,4,20.6.4 Modifiers for Discontinued Services
CMS 100-4,12,50 Anesthesia Services
CMS 100-4,12,140 Certified Registered Nurse Anesthetist Services
CMS 100-4,12,140.2 Payment for CRNA Services
CMS 100-4,12,140.3.2 Calculation of Anesthesia Time

00100 **Anesthesia for procedures on salivary glands, including biopsy** N PQ
0.00 0.00 Global Days XXX
AMA: 2009, Jan, 11-31; 2008, Jan, 10-25; 2008, Apr, 3-4; 2007, January, 13-27

00102 **Anesthesia for procedures involving plastic repair of cleft lip** N PQ
0.00 0.00 Global Days XXX
AMA: 2009, Jan, 11-31; 2008, Apr, 3-4

00103 **Anesthesia for reconstructive procedures of eyelid (eg, blepharoplasty, ptosis surgery)** N PQ
0.00 0.00 Global Days XXX
AMA: 2009, Jan, 11-31; 2008, Apr, 3-4

00104 **Anesthesia for electroconvulsive therapy** N PQ
0.00 0.00 Global Days XXX
AMA: 2009, Jan, 11-31; 2008, Apr, 3-4

00120 **Anesthesia for procedures on external, middle, and inner ear including biopsy; not otherwise specified** N PQ
0.00 0.00 Global Days XXX
AMA: 2009, Jan, 11-31; 2008, Apr, 3-4

00124 **otoscopy** N PQ
0.00 0.00 Global Days XXX
AMA: 2009, Jan, 11-31; 2008, Apr, 3-4

00126 **tympanotomy** N PQ
0.00 0.00 Global Days XXX
AMA: 2009, Jan, 11-31; 2008, Apr, 3-4

00140-00148 Anesthesia for Eye Procedures

CMS 100-3,230.1 NCD for Treatment of Kidney Stones
CMS 100-4,4,10.4 Packaging Rules Under OPPS
CMS 100-4,4,20.6 Modifier Use Under OPPS
CMS 100-4,4,20.6.4 Modifiers for Discontinued Services
CMS 100-4,12,50 Anesthesia Services
CMS 100-4,12,140 Certified Registered Nurse Anesthetist Services
CMS 100-4,12,140.3.2 Calculation of Anesthesia Time

00140 **Anesthesia for procedures on eye; not otherwise specified** N PQ
0.00 0.00 Global Days XXX
AMA: 2009, Jan, 11-31; 2008, Apr, 3-4

00142 **lens surgery** N PQ
0.00 0.00 Global Days XXX
AMA: 2009, Jan, 11-31; 2008, Apr, 3-4

00144 **corneal transplant** N PQ
0.00 0.00 Global Days XXX
AMA: 2009, Jan, 11-31; 2008, Apr, 3-4

00145 **vitreoretinal surgery** N PQ
0.00 0.00 Global Days XXX
AMA: 2009, Jan, 11-31; 2008, Apr, 3-4

00147 **iridectomy** N PQ
0.00 0.00 Global Days XXX
AMA: 2009, Jan, 11-31; 2008, Apr, 3-4

00148 **ophthalmoscopy** N PQ
0.00 0.00 Global Days XXX
AMA: 2009, Jan, 11-31; 2008, Apr, 3-4

00160-00326 Anesthesia for Face and Head Procedures

CMS 100-4,4,10.4 Packaging Rules Under OPPS
CMS 100-4,4,20.6 Modifier Use Under OPPS
CMS 100-4,12,50 Anesthesia Services
CMS 100-4,12,140 Certified Registered Nurse Anesthetist Services
CMS 100-4,12,140.2 Payment for CRNA Services
CMS 100-4,12,140.3.2 Calculation of Anesthesia Time

00160 **Anesthesia for procedures on nose and accessory sinuses; not otherwise specified** N PQ
0.00 0.00 Global Days XXX
AMA: 2009, Jan, 11-31; 2008, Apr, 3-4

00162 **radical surgery** N PQ
0.00 0.00 Global Days XXX
AMA: 2009, Jan, 11-31; 2008, Apr, 3-4

00164 **biopsy, soft tissue** N PQ
0.00 0.00 Global Days XXX
AMA: 2009, Jan, 11-31; 2008, Apr, 3-4

00170 **Anesthesia for intraoral procedures, including biopsy; not otherwise specified** N PQ
0.00 0.00 Global Days XXX
AMA: 2009, Jan, 11-31; 2008, Apr, 3-4

00172 **repair of cleft palate** N PQ
0.00 0.00 Global Days XXX
AMA: 2009, Jan, 11-31; 2008, Apr, 3-4

00174 **excision of retropharyngeal tumor** N PQ
0.00 0.00 Global Days XXX
AMA: 2009, Jan, 11-31; 2008, Apr, 3-4

00176 **radical surgery** C5 C PQ
0.00 0.00 Global Days XXX
AMA: 2009, Jan, 11-31; 2008, Apr, 3-4

00190 **Anesthesia for procedures on facial bones or skull; not otherwise specified** N PQ
0.00 0.00 Global Days XXX
AMA: 2009, Jan, 11-31; 2008, Apr, 3-4

00192 **radical surgery (including prognathism)** C5 C PQ
0.00 0.00 Global Days XXX
AMA: 2009, Jan, 11-31; 2008, Apr, 3-4

00210 **Anesthesia for intracranial procedures; not otherwise specified** N PQ
0.00 0.00 Global Days XXX
AMA: 2009, Jan, 11-31; 2008, Apr, 3-4

00211 **craniotomy or craniectomy for evacuation of hematoma** C5 C PQ
0.00 0.00 Global Days XXX
AMA: 2009, Jan, 11-31

00212 **subdural taps** N PQ
0.00 0.00 Global Days XXX
AMA: 2009, Jan, 11-31; 2008, Apr, 3-4

00214 **burr holes, including ventriculography** C5 C PQ
0.00 0.00 Global Days XXX
AMA: 2009, Jan, 11-31; 2008, Apr, 3-4

00215 **cranioplasty or elevation of depressed skull fracture, extradural (simple or compound)** C5 C PQ
0.00 0.00 Global Days XXX
AMA: 2009, Jan, 11-31; 2008, Apr, 3-4

00216 **vascular procedures** N PQ
0.00 0.00 Global Days XXX
AMA: 2009, Jan, 11-31; 2008, Apr, 3-4

00218 **procedures in sitting position** N PQ
0.00 0.00 Global Days XXX
AMA: 2009, Jan, 11-31; 2008, Apr, 3-4

00220 cerebrospinal fluid shunting procedures N
0.00 0.00 Global Days XXX
AMA: 2009, Jan, 11-31; 2008, Apr, 3-4

00222 electrocoagulation of intracranial nerve N
0.00 0.00 Global Days XXX
AMA: 2009, Jan, 11-31; 2008, Apr, 3-4

00300 Anesthesia for all procedures on the integumentary system, muscles and nerves of head, neck, and posterior trunk, not otherwise specified N
0.00 0.00 Global Days XXX
AMA: 2009, Jan, 11-31; 2008, Apr, 3-4

00320 Anesthesia for all procedures on esophagus, thyroid, larynx, trachea and lymphatic system of neck; not otherwise specified, age 1 year or older N
0.00 0.00 Global Days XXX
AMA: 2009, Jan, 11-31; 2008, Apr, 3-4

00322 needle biopsy of thyroid N
EXCLUDES *Cervical spine and spinal cord procedures (00600, 00604, 00670)*
0.00 0.00 Global Days XXX
AMA: 2009, Jan, 11-31; 2008, Apr, 3-4

00326 Anesthesia for all procedures on the larynx and trachea in children younger than 1 year of age A N
Do not report with (99100)
0.00 0.00 Global Days XXX
AMA: 2009, Jan, 11-31; 2008, Apr, 3-4

00350-00352 Anesthesia for Neck Vessel Procedures

CMS 100-4,4,10.4	Packaging Rules Under OPPS
CMS 100-4,4,20.6	Modifier Use Under OPPS
CMS 100-4,4,20.6.4	Modifiers for Discontinued Services
CMS 100-4,12,50	Anesthesia Services
CMS 100-4,12,140	Certified Registered Nurse Anesthetist Services
CMS 100-4,12,140.2	Payment for CRNA Services
CMS 100-4,12,140.3.2	Calculation of Anesthesia Time

EXCLUDES *Arteriography (01916)*

00350 Anesthesia for procedures on major vessels of neck; not otherwise specified N
0.00 0.00 Global Days XXX
AMA: 2009, Jan, 11-31; 2008, Apr, 3-4

00352 simple ligation N
0.00 0.00 Global Days XXX
AMA: 2009, Jan, 11-31; 2008, Apr, 3-4

00400-00529 Anesthesia for Chest/Pectoral Girdle Procedures

CMS 100-4,4,10.4	Packaging Rules Under OPPS
CMS 100-4,4,20.6	Modifier Use Under OPPS
CMS 100-4,4,20.6.4	Modifiers for Discontinued Services
CMS 100-4,12,50	Anesthesia Services
CMS 100-4,12,140	Certified Registered Nurse Anesthetist Services
CMS 100-4,12,140.2	Payment for CRNA Services
CMS 100-4,12,140.3.2	Calculation of Anesthesia Time

00400 Anesthesia for procedures on the integumentary system on the extremities, anterior trunk and perineum; not otherwise specified N
0.00 0.00 Global Days XXX
AMA: 2009, Jan, 11-31; 2008, Apr, 3-4

00402 reconstructive procedures on breast (eg, reduction or augmentation mammoplasty, muscle flaps) N
0.00 0.00 Global Days XXX
AMA: 2009, Jan, 11-31; 2008, Apr, 3-4

00404 radical or modified radical procedures on breast N
0.00 0.00 Global Days XXX
AMA: 2009, Jan, 11-31; 2008, Apr, 3-4

00406 radical or modified radical procedures on breast with internal mammary node dissection N
0.00 0.00 Global Days XXX
AMA: 2009, Jan, 11-31; 2008, Apr, 3-4

00410 electrical conversion of arrhythmias N
0.00 0.00 Global Days XXX
AMA: 2009, Jan, 11-31; 2008, Apr, 3-4

00450 Anesthesia for procedures on clavicle and scapula; not otherwise specified N
0.00 0.00 Global Days XXX
AMA: 2009, Jan, 11-31; 2008, Apr, 3-4

00452 radical surgery C5 C
0.00 0.00 Global Days XXX
AMA: 2009, Jan, 11-31; 2008, Apr, 3-4

00454 biopsy of clavicle N
0.00 0.00 Global Days XXX
AMA: 2009, Jan, 11-31; 2008, Apr, 3-4

00470 Anesthesia for partial rib resection; not otherwise specified N
0.00 0.00 Global Days XXX
AMA: 2009, Jan, 11-31; 2008, Apr, 3-4

00472 thoracoplasty (any type) N
0.00 0.00 Global Days XXX
AMA: 2009, Jan, 11-31; 2008, Apr, 3-4

00474 radical procedures (eg, pectus excavatum) C5 C
0.00 0.00 Global Days XXX
AMA: 2009, Jan, 11-31; 2008, Apr, 3-4

00500 Anesthesia for all procedures on esophagus N
0.00 0.00 Global Days XXX
AMA: 2009, Jan, 11-31; 2008, Apr, 3-4

00520 Anesthesia for closed chest procedures; (including bronchoscopy) not otherwise specified N
0.00 0.00 Global Days XXX
AMA: 2009, Jan, 11-31; 2008, Apr, 3-4

00522 needle biopsy of pleura N
0.00 0.00 Global Days XXX
AMA: 2009, Jan, 11-31; 2008, Apr, 3-4

00524 pneumocentesis C5 C
0.00 0.00 Global Days XXX
AMA: 2009, Jan, 11-31; 2008, Apr, 3-4

00528 mediastinoscopy and diagnostic thoracoscopy not utilizing 1 lung ventilation N
EXCLUDES *Tracheobronchial reconstruction (00539)*
0.00 0.00 Global Days XXX
AMA: 2009, Jan, 11-31; 2008, Apr, 3-4

00529 mediastinoscopy and diagnostic thoracoscopy utilizing 1 lung ventilation N
0.00 0.00 Global Days XXX
AMA: 2009, Jan, 11-31; 2008, Apr, 3-4

00530 Anesthesia for Cardiac Pacemaker Procedure

CMS 100-4,4,10.4 Packaging Rules Under OPPS
CMS 100-4,4,20.6 Modifier Use Under OPPS
CMS 100-4,4,20.6.4 Modifiers for Discontinued Services
CMS 100-4,12,50 Anesthesia Services
CMS 100-4,12,140 Certified Registered Nurse Anesthetist Services
CMS 100-4,12,140.2 Payment for CRNA Services
CMS 100-4,12,140.3.2 Calculation of Anesthesia Time

00530 **Anesthesia for permanent transvenous pacemaker insertion** N PQ
0.00 0.00 **Global Days XXX**
AMA: 2009, Jan, 11-31; 2008, Apr, 3-4

00532-00550 Anesthesia for Heart and Lung Procedures

CMS 100-4,4,10.4 Packaging Rules Under OPPS
CMS 100-4,4,20.6 Modifier Use Under OPPS
CMS 100-4,12,50 Anesthesia Services
CMS 100-4,12,140 Certified Registered Nurse Anesthetist Services
CMS 100-4,12,140.2 Payment for CRNA Services
CMS 100-4,12,140.3.2 Calculation of Anesthesia Time

00532 **Anesthesia for access to central venous circulation** N PQ
0.00 0.00 **Global Days XXX**
AMA: 2009, Jan, 11-31; 2008, Apr, 3-4

00534 **Anesthesia for transvenous insertion or replacement of pacing cardioverter-defibrillator** N PQ
EXCLUDES *Transthoracic approach (00560)*
0.00 0.00 **Global Days XXX**
AMA: 2009, Jan, 11-31; 2008, Apr, 3-4

00537 **Anesthesia for cardiac electrophysiologic procedures including radiofrequency ablation** N PQ
0.00 0.00 **Global Days XXX**
AMA: 2009, Jan, 11-31; 2008, Apr, 3-4

00539 **Anesthesia for tracheobronchial reconstruction** N PQ
0.00 0.00 **Global Days XXX**
AMA: 2009, Jan, 11-31; 2008, Apr, 3-4

00540 **Anesthesia for thoracotomy procedures involving lungs, pleura, diaphragm, and mediastinum (including surgical thoracoscopy); not otherwise specified** C5 C PQ
EXCLUDES *Thoracic spine and spinal cord procedures via anterior transthoracic approach (00625-00626)*
0.00 0.00 **Global Days XXX**
AMA: 2009, Jan, 11-31; 2008, Apr, 3-4

00541 **utilizing 1 lung ventilation** N PQ
EXCLUDES *Thoracic spine and spinal cord procedures via anterior transthoracic approach (00625-00626)*
0.00 0.00 **Global Days XXX**
AMA: 2009, Jan, 11-31; 2008, Apr, 3-4

00542 **decortication** C5 C PQ
0.00 0.00 **Global Days XXX**
AMA: 2009, Jan, 11-31; 2008, Apr, 3-4

00546 **pulmonary resection with thoracoplasty** C5 C PQ
0.00 0.00 **Global Days XXX**
AMA: 2009, Jan, 11-31; 2008, Apr, 3-4

00548 **intrathoracic procedures on the trachea and bronchi** N PQ
0.00 0.00 **Global Days XXX**
AMA: 2009, Jan, 11-31; 2008, Apr, 3-4

00550 **Anesthesia for sternal debridement** N PQ
0.00 0.00 **Global Days XXX**
AMA: 2009, Jan, 11-31; 2008, Apr, 3-4

00560-00580 Anesthesia for Open Heart Procedures

CMS 100-3,160.9 Electroencephalographic (EEG) Monitoring During Open-Heart Surgery
CMS 100-4,12,50 Anesthesia Services
CMS 100-4,12,140 Certified Registered Nurse Anesthetist Services
CMS 100-4,12,140.2 Payment for CRNA Services
CMS 100-4,12,140.3.2 Calculation of Anesthesia Time

00560 **Anesthesia for procedures on heart, pericardial sac, and great vessels of chest; without pump oxygenator** C5 C PQ
0.00 0.00 **Global Days XXX**
AMA: 2009, Jan, 11-31; 2008, Apr, 3-4

00561 **with pump oxygenator, younger than 1 year of age** A C5 C PQ
Do not report with (99100, 99116, 99135)
0.00 0.00 **Global Days XXX**
AMA: 2009, Jan, 11-31; 2008, Apr, 3-4

00562 **with pump oxygenator, age 1 year or older, for all non-coronary bypass procedures (eg, valve procedures) or for re-operation for coronary bypass more than 1 month after original operation** A C5 C PQ
0.00 0.00 **Global Days XXX**
AMA: 2009, Jan, 11-31; 2008, Apr, 3-4

00563 **with pump oxygenator with hypothermic circulatory arrest** N PQ
0.00 0.00 **Global Days XXX**
AMA: 2009, Jan, 11-31; 2008, Apr, 3-4

00566 **Anesthesia for direct coronary artery bypass grafting; without pump oxygenator** N PQ
0.00 0.00 **Global Days XXX**
AMA: 2009, Jan, 11-31; 2008, Apr, 3-4

00567 **with pump oxygenator** C5 C PQ
0.00 0.00 **Global Days XXX**
AMA: 2009, Jan, 11-31

00580 **Anesthesia for heart transplant or heart/lung transplant** C5 C PQ
0.00 0.00 **Global Days XXX**
AMA: 2009, Jan, 11-31; 2008, Apr, 3-4

00600-00670 Anesthesia for Spinal Procedures

CMS 100-4,4,10.4 Packaging Rules Under OPPS
CMS 100-4,4,20.6 Modifier Use Under OPPS
CMS 100-4,4,20.6.4 Modifiers for Discontinued Services
CMS 100-4,12,50 Anesthesia Services
CMS 100-4,12,140 Certified Registered Nurse Anesthetist Services
CMS 100-4,12,140.2 Payment for CRNA Services
CMS 100-4,12,140.3.2 Calculation of Anesthesia Time

00600 **Anesthesia for procedures on cervical spine and cord; not otherwise specified** N PQ
EXCLUDES *Percutaneous image-guided spine and spinal cord anesthesia services (01935-01936)*
0.00 0.00 **Global Days XXX**
AMA: 2009, Jan, 11-31; 2008, Jan, 10-25; 2008, Apr, 3-4

00604 **procedures with patient in the sitting position** C5 C PQ
0.00 0.00 **Global Days XXX**
AMA: 2009, Jan, 11-31; 2008, Apr, 3-4

00620 **Anesthesia for procedures on thoracic spine and cord; not otherwise specified** N PQ
0.00 0.00 **Global Days XXX**
AMA: 2009, Jan, 11-31; 2008, Jan, 10-25; 2008, Apr, 3-4; 2007, March, 9-11

00622 thoracolumbar sympathectomy
0.00 0.00 Global Days XXX
AMA: 2009, Jan, 11-31; 2008, Jan, 10-25; 2008, Apr, 3-4; 2007, March, 9-11

00625 **Anesthesia for procedures on the thoracic spine and cord, via an anterior transthoracic approach; not utilizing 1 lung ventilation**
EXCLUDES *Anesthesia services for thoracotomy procedures other than spine (00540-00541)*
0.00 0.00 Global Days XXX
AMA: 2009, Jan, 11-31; 2008, Jan, 10-25; 2008, Apr, 3-4; 2007, March, 9-11

00626 **utilizing 1 lung ventilation**
EXCLUDES *Anesthesia services for thoracotomy procedures other than spine (00540-00541)*
0.00 0.00 Global Days XXX
AMA: 2009, Jan, 11-31; 2008, Jan, 10-25; 2008, Apr, 3-4; 2007, March, 9-11

00630 **Anesthesia for procedures in lumbar region; not otherwise specified**
0.00 0.00 Global Days XXX
AMA: 2009, Jan, 11-31; 2008, Apr, 3-4

00632 **lumbar sympathectomy**
0.00 0.00 Global Days XXX
AMA: 2009, Jan, 11-31; 2008, Apr, 3-4

00634 **chemonucleolysis**
0.00 0.00 Global Days XXX
AMA: 2009, Jan, 11-31; 2008, Apr, 3-4

00635 **diagnostic or therapeutic lumbar puncture**
0.00 0.00 Global Days XXX
AMA: 2009, Jan, 11-31; 2008, Apr, 3-4

00640 **Anesthesia for manipulation of the spine or for closed procedures on the cervical, thoracic or lumbar spine**
0.00 0.00 Global Days XXX
AMA: 2009, Jan, 11-31; 2008, Apr, 3-4

00670 **Anesthesia for extensive spine and spinal cord procedures (eg, spinal instrumentation or vascular procedures)**
0.00 0.00 Global Days XXX
AMA: 2009, Jan, 11-31; 2008, Apr, 3-4

00700-00882 Anesthesia for Abdominal Procedures

CMS 100-4,4,10.4 Packaging Rules Under OPPS
CMS 100-4,4,20.6 Modifier Use Under OPPS
CMS 100-4,4,20.6.4 Modifiers for Discontinued Services
CMS 100-4,12,50 Anesthesia Services
CMS 100-4,12,140 Certified Registered Nurse Anesthetist Services
CMS 100-4,12,140.2 Payment for CRNA Services
CMS 100-4,12,140.3.2 Calculation of Anesthesia Time

00700 **Anesthesia for procedures on upper anterior abdominal wall; not otherwise specified**
0.00 0.00 Global Days XXX
AMA: 2009, Jan, 11-31; 2008, Apr, 3-4

00702 **percutaneous liver biopsy**
0.00 0.00 Global Days XXX
AMA: 2009, Jan, 11-31; 2008, Apr, 3-4

00730 **Anesthesia for procedures on upper posterior abdominal wall**
0.00 0.00 Global Days XXX
AMA: 2009, Jan, 11-31; 2008, Apr, 3-4

00740 **Anesthesia for upper gastrointestinal endoscopic procedures, endoscope introduced proximal to duodenum**
0.00 0.00 Global Days XXX
AMA: 2009, Jan, 11-31; 2008, Apr, 3-4

00750 **Anesthesia for hernia repairs in upper abdomen; not otherwise specified**
0.00 0.00 Global Days XXX
AMA: 2009, Jan, 11-31; 2008, Apr, 3-4

00752 **lumbar and ventral (incisional) hernias and/or wound dehiscence**
0.00 0.00 Global Days XXX
AMA: 2009, Jan, 11-31; 2008, Apr, 3-4

00754 **omphalocele**
0.00 0.00 Global Days XXX
AMA: 2009, Jan, 11-31; 2008, Apr, 3-4

00756 **transabdominal repair of diaphragmatic hernia**
0.00 0.00 Global Days XXX
AMA: 2009, Jan, 11-31; 2008, Apr, 3-4

00770 **Anesthesia for all procedures on major abdominal blood vessels**
0.00 0.00 Global Days XXX
AMA: 2009, Jan, 11-31; 2008, Apr, 3-4

00790 **Anesthesia for intraperitoneal procedures in upper abdomen including laparoscopy; not otherwise specified**
0.00 0.00 Global Days XXX
AMA: 2009, Jan, 11-31; 2008, Apr, 3-4

00792 **partial hepatectomy or management of liver hemorrhage (excluding liver biopsy)**
0.00 0.00 Global Days XXX
AMA: 2009, Jan, 11-31; 2008, Apr, 3-4

00794 **pancreatectomy, partial or total (eg, Whipple procedure)**
0.00 0.00 Global Days XXX
AMA: 2009, Jan, 11-31; 2008, Apr, 3-4

00796 **liver transplant (recipient)**
EXCLUDES *Physiological support during liver harvest (01990)*
0.00 0.00 Global Days XXX
AMA: 2009, Jan, 11-31; 2008, Apr, 3-4

00797 **gastric restrictive procedure for morbid obesity**
0.00 0.00 Global Days XXX
AMA: 2009, Jan, 11-31; 2008, Apr, 3-4

00800 **Anesthesia for procedures on lower anterior abdominal wall; not otherwise specified**
0.00 0.00 Global Days XXX
AMA: 2009, Jan, 11-31; 2008, Apr, 3-4

00802 **panniculectomy**
0.00 0.00 Global Days XXX
AMA: 2009, Jan, 11-31; 2008, Apr, 3-4

00810 **Anesthesia for lower intestinal endoscopic procedures, endoscope introduced distal to duodenum**
0.00 0.00 Global Days XXX
AMA: 2009, Jan, 11-31; 2008, Apr, 3-4

00820 **Anesthesia for procedures on lower posterior abdominal wall**
0.00 0.00 Global Days XXX
AMA: 2009, Jan, 11-31; 2008, Apr, 3-4

00830 **Anesthesia for hernia repairs in lower abdomen; not otherwise specified** N PQ

EXCLUDES *Anesthesia for hernia repairs on infants one year old or younger (00834, 00836)*

0.00 0.00 Global Days XXX

AMA: 2009, Jan, 11-31; 2008, Apr, 3-4

00832 **ventral and incisional hernias** N PQ

EXCLUDES *Anesthesia for hernia repairs on infants one year old or younger (00834, 00836)*

0.00 0.00 Global Days XXX

AMA: 2009, Jan, 11-31; 2008, Apr, 3-4

00834 **Anesthesia for hernia repairs in the lower abdomen not otherwise specified, younger than 1 year of age** A N PQ

Do not report with (99100)

0.00 0.00 Global Days XXX

AMA: 2009, Jan, 11-31; 2008, Apr, 3-4

00836 **Anesthesia for hernia repairs in the lower abdomen not otherwise specified, infants younger than 37 weeks gestational age at birth and younger than 50 weeks gestational age at time of surgery** A N PQ

Do not report with (99100)

0.00 0.00 Global Days XXX

AMA: 2009, Jan, 11-31; 2008, Apr, 3-4

00840 **Anesthesia for intraperitoneal procedures in lower abdomen including laparoscopy; not otherwise specified** N PQ

0.00 0.00 Global Days XXX

AMA: 2009, Jan, 11-31; 2008, Apr, 3-4

00842 **amniocentesis** M ♀ N PQ

0.00 0.00 Global Days XXX

AMA: 2009, Jan, 11-31; 2008, Apr, 3-4

00844 **abdominoperineal resection** C5 C PQ

0.00 0.00 Global Days XXX

AMA: 2009, Jan, 11-31; 2008, Apr, 3-4

00846 **radical hysterectomy** ♀ C5 C PQ

0.00 0.00 Global Days XXX

AMA: 2009, Jan, 11-31; 2008, Apr, 3-4

00848 **pelvic exenteration** C5 C PQ

0.00 0.00 Global Days XXX

AMA: 2009, Jan, 11-31; 2008, Apr, 3-4

00851 **tubal ligation/transection** ♀ N PQ

0.00 0.00 Global Days XXX

AMA: 2009, Jan, 11-31; 2008, Apr, 3-4

00860 **Anesthesia for extraperitoneal procedures in lower abdomen, including urinary tract; not otherwise specified** N PQ

0.00 0.00 Global Days XXX

AMA: 2009, Jan, 11-31; 2008, Apr, 3-4

00862 **renal procedures, including upper one-third of ureter, or donor nephrectomy** N PQ

0.00 0.00 Global Days XXX

AMA: 2009, Jan, 11-31; 2008, Apr, 3-4

00864 **total cystectomy** C5 C PQ

0.00 0.00 Global Days XXX

AMA: 2009, Jan, 11-31; 2008, Apr, 3-4

00865 **radical prostatectomy (suprapubic, retropubic)** ♂ C5 C PQ

0.00 0.00 Global Days XXX

AMA: 2009, Jan, 11-31; 2008, Apr, 3-4

00866 **adrenalectomy** C5 C PQ

0.00 0.00 Global Days XXX

AMA: 2009, Jan, 11-31; 2008, Apr, 3-4

00868 **renal transplant (recipient)** C5 C PQ

EXCLUDES *Anesthesia for donor nephrectomy (00862)*
Harvesting kidney from brain dead patient (01990)

0.00 0.00 Global Days XXX

AMA: 2009, Jan, 11-31; 2008, Apr, 3-4

00870 **cystolithotomy** N PQ

0.00 0.00 Global Days XXX

AMA: 2009, Jan, 11-31; 2008, Apr, 3-4

00872 **Anesthesia for lithotripsy, extracorporeal shock wave; with water bath** N PQ

0.00 0.00 Global Days XXX

AMA: 2009, Jan, 11-31; 2008, Apr, 3-4

00873 **without water bath** N PQ

0.00 0.00 Global Days XXX

AMA: 2009, Jan, 11-31; 2008, Apr, 3-4

00880 **Anesthesia for procedures on major lower abdominal vessels; not otherwise specified** N PQ

0.00 0.00 Global Days XXX

AMA: 2009, Jan, 11-31; 2008, Apr, 3-4

00882 **inferior vena cava ligation** C5 C PQ

0.00 0.00 Global Days XXX

AMA: 2009, Jan, 11-31; 2008, Apr, 3-4

00902-00952 Anesthesia for Genitourinary Procedures

CMS 100-4,4,10.4 Packaging Rules Under OPPS
CMS 100-4,4,20.6 Modifier Use Under OPPS
CMS 100-4,4,20.6.4 Modifiers for Discontinued Services
CMS 100-4,12,50 Anesthesia Services
CMS 100-4,12,140 Certified Registered Nurse Anesthetist Services
CMS 100-4,12,140.2 Payment for CRNA Services
CMS 100-4,12,140.3.2 Calculation of Anesthesia Time

EXCLUDES *Perineal procedures on skin, muscles, and nerves (00300, 00400)*

00902 **Anesthesia for; anorectal procedure** N PQ

0.00 0.00 Global Days XXX

AMA: 2009, Jan, 11-31; 2008, Apr, 3-4

00904 **radical perineal procedure** C5 C PQ

0.00 0.00 Global Days XXX

AMA: 2009, Jan, 11-31; 2008, Apr, 3-4

00906 **vulvectomy** ♀ N PQ

0.00 0.00 Global Days XXX

AMA: 2009, Jan, 11-31; 2008, Apr, 3-4

00908 **perineal prostatectomy** ♂ C5 C PQ

0.00 0.00 Global Days XXX

AMA: 2009, Jan, 11-31; 2008, Apr, 3-4

00910 **Anesthesia for transurethral procedures (including urethrocystoscopy); not otherwise specified** N PQ

0.00 0.00 Global Days XXX

AMA: 2009, Jan, 11-31; 2008, Apr, 3-4

00912 **transurethral resection of bladder tumor(s)** N PQ

0.00 0.00 Global Days XXX

AMA: 2009, Jan, 11-31; 2008, Apr, 3-4

00914 **transurethral resection of prostate** ♂ N PQ

0.00 0.00 Global Days XXX

AMA: 2009, Jan, 11-31; 2008, Apr, 3-4

00916 **post-transurethral resection bleeding** N PQ

0.00 0.00 Global Days XXX

AMA: 2009, Jan, 11-31; 2008, Apr, 3-4

00918 **with fragmentation, manipulation and/or removal of ureteral calculus** N PQ

0.00 0.00 Global Days XXX

AMA: 2009, Jan, 11-31; 2008, Apr, 3-4

00920 **Anesthesia for procedures on male genitalia (including open urethral procedures); not otherwise specified**
0.00 0.00 Global Days XXX
AMA: 2009, Jan, 11-31; 2008, Apr, 3-4

00921 **vasectomy, unilateral or bilateral**
0.00 0.00 Global Days XXX
AMA: 2009, Jan, 11-31; 2008, Apr, 3-4

00922 **seminal vesicles**
0.00 0.00 Global Days XXX
AMA: 2009, Jan, 11-31; 2008, Apr, 3-4

00924 **undescended testis, unilateral or bilateral**
0.00 0.00 Global Days XXX
AMA: 2009, Jan, 11-31; 2008, Apr, 3-4

00926 **radical orchiectomy, inguinal**
0.00 0.00 Global Days XXX
AMA: 2009, Jan, 11-31; 2008, Apr, 3-4

00928 **radical orchiectomy, abdominal**
0.00 0.00 Global Days XXX
AMA: 2009, Jan, 11-31; 2008, Apr, 3-4

00930 **orchiopexy, unilateral or bilateral**
0.00 0.00 Global Days XXX
AMA: 2009, Jan, 11-31; 2008, Apr, 3-4

00932 **complete amputation of penis**
0.00 0.00 Global Days XXX
AMA: 2009, Jan, 11-31; 2008, Apr, 3-4

00934 **radical amputation of penis with bilateral inguinal lymphadenectomy**
0.00 0.00 Global Days XXX
AMA: 2009, Jan, 11-31; 2008, Apr, 3-4

00936 **radical amputation of penis with bilateral inguinal and iliac lymphadenectomy**
0.00 0.00 Global Days XXX
AMA: 2009, Jan, 11-31; 2008, Apr, 3-4

00938 **insertion of penile prosthesis (perineal approach)**
0.00 0.00 Global Days XXX
AMA: 2009, Jan, 11-31; 2008, Apr, 3-4

00940 **Anesthesia for vaginal procedures (including biopsy of labia, vagina, cervix or endometrium); not otherwise specified**
0.00 0.00 Global Days XXX
AMA: 2009, Jan, 11-31; 2008, Apr, 3-4

00942 **colpotomy, vaginectomy, colporrhaphy, and open urethral procedures**
0.00 0.00 Global Days XXX
AMA: 2009, Jan, 11-31; 2008, Apr, 3-4

00944 **vaginal hysterectomy**
0.00 0.00 Global Days XXX
AMA: 2009, Jan, 11-31; 2008, Apr, 3-4

00948 **cervical cerclage**
0.00 0.00 Global Days XXX
AMA: 2009, Jan, 11-31; 2008, Apr, 3-4

00950 **culdoscopy**
0.00 0.00 Global Days XXX
AMA: 2009, Jan, 11-31; 2008, Apr, 3-4

00952 **hysteroscopy and/or hysterosalpingography**
0.00 0.00 Global Days XXX
AMA: 2009, Jan, 11-31; 2008, Apr, 3-4

01112-01522 Anesthesia for Lower Extremity Procedures

CMS 100-4,4,10.4	Packaging Rules Under OPPS
CMS 100-4,4,20.6	Modifier Use Under OPPS
CMS 100-4,4,20.6.4	Modifiers for Discontinued Services
CMS 100-4,12,50	Anesthesia Services
CMS 100-4,12,140	Certified Registered Nurse Anesthetist Services
CMS 100-4,12,140.2	Payment for CRNA Services
CMS 100-4,12,140.3.2	Calculation of Anesthesia Time

01112 **Anesthesia for bone marrow aspiration and/or biopsy, anterior or posterior iliac crest**
0.00 0.00 Global Days XXX
AMA: 2009, Jan, 11-31; 2008, Apr, 3-4

01120 **Anesthesia for procedures on bony pelvis**
0.00 0.00 Global Days XXX
AMA: 2009, Jan, 11-31; 2008, Apr, 3-4

01130 **Anesthesia for body cast application or revision**
0.00 0.00 Global Days XXX
AMA: 2009, Jan, 11-31; 2008, Apr, 3-4

01140 **Anesthesia for interpelviabdominal (hindquarter) amputation**
0.00 0.00 Global Days XXX
AMA: 2009, Jan, 11-31; 2008, Apr, 3-4

01150 **Anesthesia for radical procedures for tumor of pelvis, except hindquarter amputation**
0.00 0.00 Global Days XXX
AMA: 2009, Jan, 11-31; 2008, Apr, 3-4

01160 **Anesthesia for closed procedures involving symphysis pubis or sacroiliac joint**
0.00 0.00 Global Days XXX
AMA: 2009, Jan, 11-31; 2008, Apr, 3-4

01170 **Anesthesia for open procedures involving symphysis pubis or sacroiliac joint**
0.00 0.00 Global Days XXX
AMA: 2009, Jan, 11-31; 2008, Apr, 3-4

01173 **Anesthesia for open repair of fracture disruption of pelvis or column fracture involving acetabulum**
0.00 0.00 Global Days XXX
AMA: 2009, Jan, 11-31; 2008, Apr, 3-4

01180 **Anesthesia for obturator neurectomy; extrapelvic**
0.00 0.00 Global Days XXX
AMA: 2009, Jan, 11-31; 2008, Apr, 3-4

01190 **intrapelvic**
0.00 0.00 Global Days XXX
AMA: 2009, Jan, 11-31; 2008, Apr, 3-4

01200 **Anesthesia for all closed procedures involving hip joint**
0.00 0.00 Global Days XXX
AMA: 2009, Jan, 11-31; 2008, Apr, 3-4

01202 **Anesthesia for arthroscopic procedures of hip joint**
0.00 0.00 Global Days XXX
AMA: 2009, Jan, 11-31; 2008, Apr, 3-4

01210 **Anesthesia for open procedures involving hip joint; not otherwise specified**
0.00 0.00 Global Days XXX
AMA: 2009, Jan, 11-31; 2008, Apr, 3-4

01212 **hip disarticulation**
0.00 0.00 Global Days XXX
AMA: 2009, Jan, 11-31; 2008, Apr, 3-4

01214 **total hip arthroplasty**
0.00 0.00 Global Days XXX
AMA: 2009, Jan, 11-31; 2008, Apr, 3-4

PC/TC Comp Only | ASC Pmt | Bilateral | ♂ Male Only | ♀ Female Only | Facility RVU | Non-Facility RVU
AMA: CPT Asst | MED: Pub 100 | OPPSI | Surg Assist Allowed / w/Doc | Lab Crosswalk | Radiology Crosswalk

01215 revision of total hip arthroplasty
0.00 0.00 Global Days XXX
AMA: 2009, Jan, 11-31; 2008, Apr, 3-4

01220 Anesthesia for all closed procedures involving upper 2/3 of femur
0.00 0.00 Global Days XXX
AMA: 2009, Jan, 11-31; 2008, Apr, 3-4

01230 Anesthesia for open procedures involving upper 2/3 of femur; not otherwise specified
0.00 0.00 Global Days XXX
AMA: 2009, Jan, 11-31; 2008, Apr, 3-4

01232 amputation
0.00 0.00 Global Days XXX
AMA: 2009, Jan, 11-31; 2008, Apr, 3-4

01234 radical resection
0.00 0.00 Global Days XXX
AMA: 2009, Jan, 11-31; 2008, Apr, 3-4

01250 Anesthesia for all procedures on nerves, muscles, tendons, fascia, and bursae of upper leg
0.00 0.00 Global Days XXX
AMA: 2009, Jan, 11-31; 2008, Apr, 3-4

01260 Anesthesia for all procedures involving veins of upper leg, including exploration
0.00 0.00 Global Days XXX
AMA: 2009, Jan, 11-31; 2008, Apr, 3-4

01270 Anesthesia for procedures involving arteries of upper leg, including bypass graft; not otherwise specified
0.00 0.00 Global Days XXX
AMA: 2009, Jan, 11-31; 2008, Apr, 3-4

01272 femoral artery ligation
0.00 0.00 Global Days XXX
AMA: 2009, Jan, 11-31; 2008, Apr, 3-4

01274 femoral artery embolectomy
0.00 0.00 Global Days XXX
AMA: 2009, Jan, 11-31; 2008, Apr, 3-4

01320 Anesthesia for all procedures on nerves, muscles, tendons, fascia, and bursae of knee and/or popliteal area
0.00 0.00 Global Days XXX
AMA: 2009, Jan, 11-31; 2008, Apr, 3-4

01340 Anesthesia for all closed procedures on lower 1/3 of femur
0.00 0.00 Global Days XXX
AMA: 2009, Jan, 11-31; 2008, Apr, 3-4

01360 Anesthesia for all open procedures on lower 1/3 of femur
0.00 0.00 Global Days XXX
AMA: 2009, Jan, 11-31; 2008, Apr, 3-4

01380 Anesthesia for all closed procedures on knee joint
0.00 0.00 Global Days XXX
AMA: 2009, Jan, 11-31; 2008, Apr, 3-4

01382 Anesthesia for diagnostic arthroscopic procedures of knee joint
0.00 0.00 Global Days XXX
AMA: 2009, Jan, 11-31; 2008, Apr, 3-4

01390 Anesthesia for all closed procedures on upper ends of tibia, fibula, and/or patella
0.00 0.00 Global Days XXX
AMA: 2009, Jan, 11-31; 2008, Apr, 3-4

01392 Anesthesia for all open procedures on upper ends of tibia, fibula, and/or patella
0.00 0.00 Global Days XXX
AMA: 2009, Jan, 11-31; 2008, Apr, 3-4

01400 Anesthesia for open or surgical arthroscopic procedures on knee joint; not otherwise specified
0.00 0.00 Global Days XXX
AMA: 2009, Jan, 11-31; 2008, Apr, 3-4

01402 total knee arthroplasty
0.00 0.00 Global Days XXX
AMA: 2009, Jan, 11-31; 2008, Apr, 3-4

01404 disarticulation at knee
0.00 0.00 Global Days XXX
AMA: 2009, Jan, 11-31; 2008, Apr, 3-4

01420 Anesthesia for all cast applications, removal, or repair involving knee joint
0.00 0.00 Global Days XXX
AMA: 2009, Jan, 11-31; 2008, Apr, 3-4

01430 Anesthesia for procedures on veins of knee and popliteal area; not otherwise specified
0.00 0.00 Global Days XXX
AMA: 2009, Jan, 11-31; 2008, Apr, 3-4

01432 arteriovenous fistula
0.00 0.00 Global Days XXX
AMA: 2009, Jan, 11-31; 2008, Apr, 3-4

01440 Anesthesia for procedures on arteries of knee and popliteal area; not otherwise specified
0.00 0.00 Global Days XXX
AMA: 2009, Jan, 11-31; 2008, Apr, 3-4

01442 popliteal thromboendarterectomy, with or without patch graft
0.00 0.00 Global Days XXX
AMA: 2009, Jan, 11-31; 2008, Apr, 3-4

01444 popliteal excision and graft or repair for occlusion or aneurysm
0.00 0.00 Global Days XXX
AMA: 2009, Jan, 11-31; 2008, Apr, 3-4

01462 Anesthesia for all closed procedures on lower leg, ankle, and foot
0.00 0.00 Global Days XXX
AMA: 2009, Jan, 11-31; 2008, Apr, 3-4

01464 Anesthesia for arthroscopic procedures of ankle and/or foot
0.00 0.00 Global Days XXX
AMA: 2009, Jan, 11-31; 2008, Apr, 3-4

01470 Anesthesia for procedures on nerves, muscles, tendons, and fascia of lower leg, ankle, and foot; not otherwise specified
0.00 0.00 Global Days XXX
AMA: 2009, Jan, 11-31; 2008, Apr, 3-4

01472 repair of ruptured Achilles tendon, with or without graft
0.00 0.00 Global Days XXX
AMA: 2009, Jan, 11-31; 2008, Apr, 3-4

01474 gastrocnemius recession (eg, Strayer procedure)
0.00 0.00 Global Days XXX
AMA: 2009, Jan, 11-31; 2008, Apr, 3-4

01480 Anesthesia for open procedures on bones of lower leg, ankle, and foot; not otherwise specified
0.00 0.00 Global Days XXX
AMA: 2009, Jan, 11-31; 2008, Apr, 3-4

01482 radical resection (including below knee amputation)
0.00 0.00 Global Days XXX
AMA: 2009, Jan, 11-31; 2008, Apr, 3-4

01484 osteotomy or osteoplasty of tibia and/or fibula
0.00 0.00 Global Days XXX
AMA: 2009, Jan, 11-31; 2008, Apr, 3-4

01486 total ankle replacement
0.00 0.00 Global Days XXX
AMA: 2009, Jan, 11-31; 2008, Apr, 3-4

01490 Anesthesia for lower leg cast application, removal, or repair
0.00 0.00 Global Days XXX
AMA: 2009, Jan, 11-31; 2008, Apr, 3-4

01500 Anesthesia for procedures on arteries of lower leg, including bypass graft; not otherwise specified
0.00 0.00 Global Days XXX
AMA: 2009, Jan, 11-31; 2008, Apr, 3-4

01502 embolectomy, direct or with catheter
0.00 0.00 Global Days XXX
AMA: 2009, Jan, 11-31; 2008, Apr, 3-4

01520 Anesthesia for procedures on veins of lower leg; not otherwise specified
0.00 0.00 Global Days XXX
AMA: 2009, Jan, 11-31; 2008, Apr, 3-4

01522 venous thrombectomy, direct or with catheter
0.00 0.00 Global Days XXX
AMA: 2009, Jan, 11-31; 2008, Apr, 3-4

01610-01682 Anesthesia for Shoulder Procedures

CMS 100-4,12,50 Anesthesia Services
CMS 100-4,12,140 Certified Registered Nurse Anesthetist Services
CMS 100-4,12,140.2 Payment for CRNA Services
CMS 100-4,12,140.3.2 Calculation of Anesthesia Time

INCLUDES Acromioclavicular joint
Humeral head and neck
Shoulder joint
Sternoclavicular joint

01610 Anesthesia for all procedures on nerves, muscles, tendons, fascia, and bursae of shoulder and axilla
0.00 0.00 Global Days XXX
AMA: 2009, Jan, 11-31; 2008, Apr, 3-4

01620 Anesthesia for all closed procedures on humeral head and neck, sternoclavicular joint, acromioclavicular joint, and shoulder joint
0.00 0.00 Global Days XXX
AMA: 2009, Jan, 11-31; 2008, Apr, 3-4

01622 Anesthesia for diagnostic arthroscopic procedures of shoulder joint
0.00 0.00 Global Days XXX
AMA: 2009, Jan, 11-31; 2008, Apr, 3-4

01630 Anesthesia for open or surgical arthroscopic procedures on humeral head and neck, sternoclavicular joint, acromioclavicular joint, and shoulder joint; not otherwise specified
0.00 0.00 Global Days XXX
AMA: 2009, Jan, 11-31; 2008, Apr, 3-4

01634 shoulder disarticulation
0.00 0.00 Global Days XXX
AMA: 2009, Jan, 11-31; 2008, Apr, 3-4

01636 interthoracoscapular (forequarter) amputation
0.00 0.00 Global Days XXX
AMA: 2009, Jan, 11-31; 2008, Apr, 3-4

01638 total shoulder replacement
0.00 0.00 Global Days XXX
AMA: 2009, Jan, 11-31; 2008, Apr, 3-4

01650 Anesthesia for procedures on arteries of shoulder and axilla; not otherwise specified
0.00 0.00 Global Days XXX
AMA: 2009, Jan, 11-31; 2008, Apr, 3-4

01652 axillary-brachial aneurysm
0.00 0.00 Global Days XXX
AMA: 2009, Jan, 11-31; 2008, Apr, 3-4

01654 bypass graft
0.00 0.00 Global Days XXX
AMA: 2009, Jan, 11-31; 2008, Apr, 3-4

01656 axillary-femoral bypass graft
0.00 0.00 Global Days XXX
AMA: 2009, Jan, 11-31; 2008, Apr, 3-4

01670 Anesthesia for all procedures on veins of shoulder and axilla
0.00 0.00 Global Days XXX
AMA: 2009, Jan, 11-31; 2008, Apr, 3-4

01680 Anesthesia for shoulder cast application, removal or repair; not otherwise specified
0.00 0.00 Global Days XXX
AMA: 2009, Jan, 11-31; 2008, Apr, 3-4

01682 shoulder spica
0.00 0.00 Global Days XXX
AMA: 2009, Jan, 11-31; 2008, Apr, 3-4

01710-01860 Anesthesia for Upper Extremity Procedures

CMS 100-4,12,50 Anesthesia Services
CMS 100-4,12,140 Certified Registered Nurse Anesthetist Services
CMS 100-4,12,140.2 Payment for CRNA Services
CMS 100-4,12,140.3.2 Calculation of Anesthesia Time

01710 Anesthesia for procedures on nerves, muscles, tendons, fascia, and bursae of upper arm and elbow; not otherwise specified
0.00 0.00 Global Days XXX
AMA: 2009, Jan, 11-31; 2008, Apr, 3-4

01712 tenotomy, elbow to shoulder, open
0.00 0.00 Global Days XXX
AMA: 2009, Jan, 11-31; 2008, Apr, 3-4

01714 tenoplasty, elbow to shoulder
0.00 0.00 Global Days XXX
AMA: 2009, Jan, 11-31; 2008, Apr, 3-4

01716 tenodesis, rupture of long tendon of biceps
0.00 0.00 Global Days XXX
AMA: 2009, Jan, 11-31; 2008, Apr, 3-4

01730 Anesthesia for all closed procedures on humerus and elbow
0.00 0.00 Global Days XXX
AMA: 2009, Jan, 11-31; 2008, Apr, 3-4

01732 Anesthesia for diagnostic arthroscopic procedures of elbow joint
0.00 0.00 Global Days XXX
AMA: 2009, Jan, 11-31; 2008, Apr, 3-4

01740 Anesthesia for open or surgical arthroscopic procedures of the elbow; not otherwise specified
0.00 0.00 Global Days XXX
AMA: 2009, Jan, 11-31; 2008, Apr, 3-4

01742 osteotomy of humerus
0.00 0.00 Global Days XXX
AMA: 2009, Jan, 11-31; 2008, Apr, 3-4

01744 repair of nonunion or malunion of humerus
0.00 0.00 Global Days XXX
AMA: 2009, Jan, 11-31; 2008, Apr, 3-4

01756 radical procedures
0.00 0.00 Global Days XXX
AMA: 2009, Jan, 11-31; 2008, Apr, 3-4

01758 excision of cyst or tumor of humerus
0.00 0.00 Global Days XXX
AMA: 2009, Jan, 11-31; 2008, Apr, 3-4

01760 total elbow replacement N PQ
0.00 0.00 Global Days XXX
AMA: 2009, Jan, 11-31; 2008, Apr, 3-4

01770 Anesthesia for procedures on arteries of upper arm and elbow; not otherwise specified N PQ
0.00 0.00 Global Days XXX
AMA: 2009, Jan, 11-31; 2008, Apr, 3-4

01772 embolectomy N PQ
0.00 0.00 Global Days XXX
AMA: 2009, Jan, 11-31; 2008, Apr, 3-4

01780 Anesthesia for procedures on veins of upper arm and elbow; not otherwise specified N PQ
0.00 0.00 Global Days XXX
AMA: 2009, Jan, 11-31; 2008, Apr, 3-4

01782 phleborrhaphy N PQ
0.00 0.00 Global Days XXX
AMA: 2009, Jan, 11-31; 2008, Apr, 3-4

01810 Anesthesia for all procedures on nerves, muscles, tendons, fascia, and bursae of forearm, wrist, and hand N PQ
0.00 0.00 Global Days XXX
AMA: 2009, Jan, 11-31; 2008, Apr, 3-4

01820 Anesthesia for all closed procedures on radius, ulna, wrist, or hand bones N PQ
0.00 0.00 Global Days XXX
AMA: 2009, Jan, 11-31; 2008, Apr, 3-4

01829 Anesthesia for diagnostic arthroscopic procedures on the wrist N PQ
0.00 0.00 Global Days XXX
AMA: 2009, Jan, 11-31; 2008, Apr, 3-4

01830 Anesthesia for open or surgical arthroscopic/endoscopic procedures on distal radius, distal ulna, wrist, or hand joints; not otherwise specified N PQ
0.00 0.00 Global Days XXX
AMA: 2009, Jan, 11-31; 2008, Apr, 3-4

01832 total wrist replacement N PQ
0.00 0.00 Global Days XXX
AMA: 2009, Jan, 11-31; 2008, Apr, 3-4

01840 Anesthesia for procedures on arteries of forearm, wrist, and hand; not otherwise specified N PQ
0.00 0.00 Global Days XXX
AMA: 2009, Jan, 11-31; 2008, Apr, 3-4

01842 embolectomy N PQ
0.00 0.00 Global Days XXX
AMA: 2009, Jan, 11-31; 2008, Apr, 3-4

01844 Anesthesia for vascular shunt, or shunt revision, any type (eg, dialysis) N PQ
0.00 0.00 Global Days XXX
AMA: 2009, Jan, 11-31; 2008, Apr, 3-4

01850 Anesthesia for procedures on veins of forearm, wrist, and hand; not otherwise specified N PQ
0.00 0.00 Global Days XXX
AMA: 2009, Jan, 11-31; 2008, Apr, 3-4

01852 phleborrhaphy N PQ
0.00 0.00 Global Days XXX
AMA: 2009, Jan, 11-31; 2008, Apr, 3-4

01860 Anesthesia for forearm, wrist, or hand cast application, removal, or repair N PQ
0.00 0.00 Global Days XXX
AMA: 2009, Jan, 11-31; 2008, Apr, 3-4

01916-01936 Anesthesia for Interventional Radiology Procedures

CMS 100-4,12,50 Anesthesia Services
CMS 100-4,12,140 Certified Registered Nurse Anesthetist Services
CMS 100-4,12,140.2 Payment for CRNA Services
CMS 100-4,12,140.3.2 Calculation of Anesthesia Time

01916 Anesthesia for diagnostic arteriography/venography N
Do not report with (01924-01926, 01930-01933)
0.00 0.00 Global Days XXX
AMA: 2009, Jan, 11-31; 2008, Apr, 3-4

01920 Anesthesia for cardiac catheterization including coronary angiography and ventriculography (not to include Swan-Ganz catheter) N
0.00 0.00 Global Days XXX
AMA: 2009, Jan, 11-31; 2008, Apr, 3-4

01922 Anesthesia for non-invasive imaging or radiation therapy N
0.00 0.00 Global Days XXX
AMA: 2009, Jan, 11-31; 2008, Apr, 3-4

01924 Anesthesia for therapeutic interventional radiological procedures involving the arterial system; not otherwise specified N PQ
0.00 0.00 Global Days XXX
AMA: 2009, Jan, 11-31; 2008, Apr, 3-4

01925 carotid or coronary N PQ
0.00 0.00 Global Days XXX
AMA: 2009, Jan, 11-31; 2008, Apr, 3-4

01926 intracranial, intracardiac, or aortic N PQ
0.00 0.00 Global Days XXX
AMA: 2009, Jan, 11-31; 2008, Apr, 3-4

01930 Anesthesia for therapeutic interventional radiological procedures involving the venous/lymphatic system (not to include access to the central circulation); not otherwise specified N PQ
0.00 0.00 Global Days XXX
AMA: 2009, Jan, 11-31; 2008, Apr, 3-4

01931 intrahepatic or portal circulation (eg, transvenous intrahepatic portosystemic shunt[s] [TIPS]) N PQ
0.00 0.00 Global Days XXX
AMA: 2009, Jan, 11-31; 2008, Apr, 3-4

01932 intrathoracic or jugular N PQ
0.00 0.00 Global Days XXX
AMA: 2009, Jan, 11-31; 2008, Apr, 3-4

01933 intracranial N PQ
0.00 0.00 Global Days XXX
AMA: 2009, Jan, 11-31; 2008, Apr, 3-4

01935 Anesthesia for percutaneous image guided procedures on the spine and spinal cord; diagnostic N PQ
0.00 0.00 Global Days XXX
AMA: 2009, Jan, 11-31; 2008, Apr, 3-4

01936 therapeutic N PQ
0.00 0.00 Global Days XXX
AMA: 2009, Jan, 11-31; 2008, Apr, 3-4

01951-01953 Anesthesia for Burn Procedures

CMS 100-4,3,20.1.2.8 Special Payments for Burn Cases
CMS 100-4,12,50 Anesthesia Services
CMS 100-4,12,140 Certified Registered Nurse Anesthetist Services
CMS 100-4,12,140.2 Payment for CRNA Services
CMS 100-4,12,140.3.2 Calculation of Anesthesia Time

01951 Anesthesia for second- and third-degree burn excision or debridement with or without skin grafting, any site, for total body surface area (TBSA) treated during anesthesia and surgery; less than 4% total body surface area
0.00 0.00 Global Days XXX
AMA: 2009, Jan, 11-31; 2008, Apr, 3-4

01952 between 4% and 9% of total body surface area
0.00 0.00 Global Days XXX
AMA: 2009, Jan, 11-31; 2008, Apr, 3-4

+ **01953 each additional 9% total body surface area or part thereof (List separately in addition to code for primary procedure)**
Code first (01952)
0.00 0.00 Global Days XXX
AMA: 2009, Jan, 11-31; 2008, Apr, 3-4

01958-01969 Anesthesia for Obstetric Procedures

CMS 100-4,12,50 Anesthesia Services
CMS 100-4,12,140 Certified Registered Nurse Anesthetist Services
CMS 100-4,12,140.2 Payment for CRNA Services
CMS 100-4,12,140.3.2 Calculation of Anesthesia Time

01958 Anesthesia for external cephalic version procedure ♀
0.00 0.00 Global Days XXX
AMA: 2009, Jan, 11-31; 2008, Apr, 3-4

01960 Anesthesia for vaginal delivery only ♀
0.00 0.00 Global Days XXX
AMA: 2009, Jan, 11-31; 2008, Apr, 3-4

01961 Anesthesia for cesarean delivery only ♀
0.00 0.00 Global Days XXX
AMA: 2009, Jan, 11-31; 2008, Apr, 3-4

01962 Anesthesia for urgent hysterectomy following delivery ♀
0.00 0.00 Global Days XXX
AMA: 2009, Jan, 11-31; 2008, Apr, 3-4

01963 Anesthesia for cesarean hysterectomy without any labor analgesia/anesthesia care ♀
0.00 0.00 Global Days XXX
AMA: 2009, Jan, 11-31; 2008, Apr, 3-4

01965 Anesthesia for incomplete or missed abortion procedures ♀
0.00 0.00 Global Days XXX
AMA: 2009, Jan, 11-31; 2008, Apr, 3-4

01966 Anesthesia for induced abortion procedures ♀
0.00 0.00 Global Days XXX
AMA: 2009, Jan, 11-31; 2008, Apr, 3-4

01967 Neuraxial labor analgesia/anesthesia for planned vaginal delivery (this includes any repeat subarachnoid needle placement and drug injection and/or any necessary replacement of an epidural catheter during labor) ♀
0.00 0.00 Global Days XXX
AMA: 2009, Jan, 11-31; 2008, Apr, 3-4

+ **01968 Anesthesia for cesarean delivery following neuraxial labor analgesia/anesthesia (List separately in addition to code for primary procedure performed)** ♀
Code first (01967)
0.00 0.00 Global Days XXX
AMA: 2009, Jan, 11-31; 2008, Apr, 3-4

+ **01969 Anesthesia for cesarean hysterectomy following neuraxial labor analgesia/anesthesia (List separately in addition to code for primary procedure performed)** ♀
Code first (01967)
0.00 0.00 Global Days XXX
AMA: 2009, Jan, 11-31; 2008, Apr, 3-4

01990-01999 Anesthesia Miscellaneous

CMS 100-4,12,50 Anesthesia Services
CMS 100-4,12,140 Certified Registered Nurse Anesthetist Services
CMS 100-4,12,140.2 Payment for CRNA Services
CMS 100-4,12,140.3.2 Calculation of Anesthesia Time

01990 Physiological support for harvesting of organ(s) from brain-dead patient
0.00 0.00 Global Days XXX
AMA: 2009, Jan, 11-31; 2008, Apr, 3-4

01991 Anesthesia for diagnostic or therapeutic nerve blocks and injections (when block or injection is performed by a different provider); other than the prone position
Do not report with (99143-99150)
EXCLUDES *Bier block for pain management (64999)*
IV or intra-arterial injections (96373-96374)
Regional or local anesthesia of arms or legs for surgical procedure
0.00 0.00 Global Days XXX
AMA: 2009, Jan, 11-31; 2008, Apr, 3-4

01992 prone position
Do not report with (99143-99150)
EXCLUDES *Bier block for pain management (64999)*
Pain management via intra-arterial or intravenous therapy (96373-96374)
Regional or local anesthesia of arms or legs for surgical procedure
0.00 0.00 Global Days XXX
AMA: 2009, Jan, 11-31; 2008, Apr, 3-4

01996 Daily hospital management of epidural or subarachnoid continuous drug administration
INCLUDES Continuous epidural or subarachnoid drug services performed after insertion of an epidural or subarachnoid catheter
0.00 0.00 Global Days XXX
AMA: 2009, Jan, 11-31; 2008, Apr, 3-4

01999 Unlisted anesthesia procedure(s)
0.00 0.00 Global Days XXX
AMA: 2009, Jan, 11-31; 2008, Jan, 10-25; 2008, Apr, 3-4; 2007, January, 13-27

26/TC PC/TC Comp Only · A2-Z3 ASC Pmt · 50 Bilateral · ♂ Male Only · ♀ Female Only · Facility RVU · Non-Facility RVU
AMA: CPT Asst · **MED:** Pub 100 · A-Y OPPSI · 80/80 Surg Assist Allowed / w/Doc · Lab Crosswalk · Radiology Crosswalk

10021-10022 Fine Needle Aspiration

CMS 100-4,13,80.1 Supervision and Interpretation Codes
CMS 100-4,13,80.2 S&I Multiple Procedure Reduction

EXCLUDES *Percutaneous localization clip placement during breast biopsy (19295)*
Percutaneous needle biopsy of:
Abdominal or retroperitoneal mass (49180)
Bone (20220, 20225)
Bone marrow (38220-38221)
Breast (19100)
Epididymis (54800)
Kidney (50200)
Liver (47000)
Lung or mediastinum (32405)
Lymph node (38505)
Muscle (20206)
Nucleus pulposus, paravertebral tissue, intervertebral disc (62267)
Pancreas (48102)
Pleura (32400)
Prostate (55700)
Salivary gland (42400)
Spinal cord (62269)
Testis (54500)
Thyroid (60100)

10021 Fine needle aspiration; without imaging guidance P2 T 80
88172-88173
2.07 4.30 Global Days XXX
AMA: 2009, Jan, 11-31; 2008, Jan, 10-25; 2007, January, 13-27

10022 with imaging guidance G2 T 80
88172-88173
76942, 77002, 77012, 77021
1.90 4.02 Global Days XXX
AMA: 2009, Jan, 11-31; 2008, Jan, 10-25; 2007, June, 10-11

10040-10180 Treatment of Fluid-filled Lesions: Skin and Subcutaneous Tissues

CMS 100-4,12,30 Correct Coding Policy
CMS 100-4,13,80.1 Physician Presence
CMS 100-4,13,80.2 S&I Multiple Procedure Reduction

EXCLUDES *Excision benign lesion (11400-11471)*

10040 Acne surgery (eg, marsupialization, opening or removal of multiple milia, comedones, cysts, pustules) P2 T
2.61 3.00 Global Days 010
AMA: 2009, Jan, 11-31

10060 Incision and drainage of abscess (eg, carbuncle, suppurative hidradenitis, cutaneous or subcutaneous abscess, cyst, furuncle, or paronychia); simple or single P3 T
2.77 3.32 Global Days 010
AMA: 2009, Jan, 11-31; 2008, Jan, 10-25; 2007, January, 13-27

10061 complicated or multiple P2 T
5.09 5.81 Global Days 010

10080 Incision and drainage of pilonidal cyst; simple P2 T
2.97 5.12 Global Days 010
AMA: 2007, May, 5-8

10081 complicated P3 T
EXCLUDES *Excision of pilonidal cyst (11770-11772)*
5.02 7.87 Global Days 010
AMA: 2007, May, 5-8

10120 Incision and removal of foreign body, subcutaneous tissues; simple P3 T
2.72 4.10 Global Days 010

10121 complicated A2 T
EXCLUDES *Debridement associated with a fracture or dislocation (11010-11012)*
Exploration penetrating wound (20100-20103)
5.44 7.95 Global Days 010

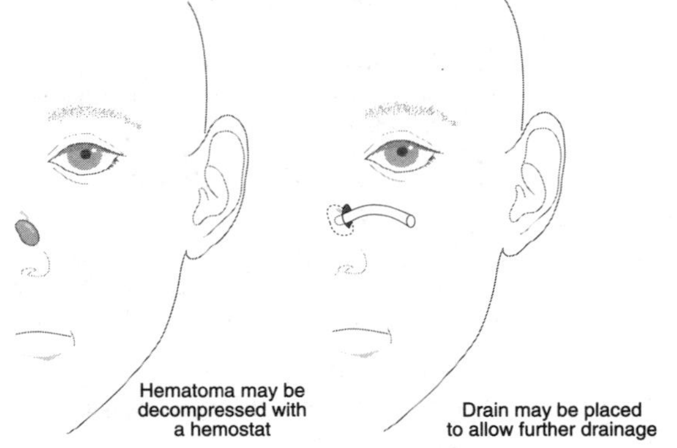

10140 Incision and drainage of hematoma, seroma or fluid collection P3 T
76942, 77012, 77021
3.45 4.68 Global Days 010
AMA: 2009, Jan, 11-31; 2008, Jan, 10-25; 2007, January, 13-27

10160 Puncture aspiration of abscess, hematoma, bulla, or cyst P2 T
76942, 77012, 77021
2.80 3.76 Global Days 010

10180 Incision and drainage, complex, postoperative wound infection A2 T
EXCLUDES *Wound dehiscence (12020-12021, 13160)*
5.24 7.15 Global Days 010
AMA: 2009, Jan, 11-31; 2008, Jan, 10-25

11000-11012 Removal of Foreign Substances and Infected/Devitalized Tissue

CMS 100-4,12,40.1 Global Surgery Package
CMS 100-4,12,40.2 Billing Requirements for Global Surgeries

EXCLUDES *Debridement of:*
Burn (16000-16030)
Deeper tissue (11042-11047 [11045, 11046])
Nails (11720-11721)
Wounds (11042-11047 [11045, 11046])
Dermabrasions (15780-15783)
Pressure ulcer excision (15920-15999)

11000 Debridement of extensive eczematous or infected skin; up to 10% of body surface P3 T
EXCLUDES *Necrotizing soft tissue infection of:*
Abdominal wall (11005-11006)
External genitalia and perineum (11004, 11006)
0.85 1.56 Global Days 000

\+ **11001 each additional 10% of the body surface, or part thereof (List separately in addition to code for primary procedure)** P3 T
EXCLUDES *Necrotizing soft tissue infection of:*
Abdominal wall (11005-11006)
External genitalia and perineum (11004, 11006)
Code first (11000)
0.42 0.62 Global Days ZZZ

11004 **Debridement of skin, subcutaneous tissue, muscle and fascia for necrotizing soft tissue infection; external genitalia and perineum**

EXCLUDES *Skin grafts or flaps (14000-14350, 15040-15770)*

17.09 17.09 Global Days 000

11005 **abdominal wall, with or without fascial closure**

23.02 23.02 Global Days 000

11006 **external genitalia, perineum and abdominal wall, with or without fascial closure**

EXCLUDES *Orchiectomy (54520)*
Testicular transplant (54680)

20.82 20.82 Global Days 000

\+ **11008** **Removal of prosthetic material or mesh, abdominal wall for infection (eg, for chronic or recurrent mesh infection or necrotizing soft tissue infection) (List separately in addition to code for primary procedure)**

INCLUDES Debridement:
- Associated with an open fracture
- Bone
- Extensive eczematous or infected skin
- Muscle
- Skin
- Subcutaneous tissue

EXCLUDES *Insertion of mesh (49568)*
Skin grafts or flaps (14000-14350, 15040-15770)

Code first (10180, 11004-11006)

Do not report with (11000-11001, 11010-11044 [11045, 11046])

8.08 8.08 Global Days ZZZ

11010 **Debridement including removal of foreign material at the site of an open fracture and/or an open dislocation (eg, excisional debridement); skin and subcutaneous tissues**

8.29 14.45 Global Days 010

AMA: 2009, Jan, 11-31; 2008, Jan, 10-25; 2007, January, 13-27

11011 **skin, subcutaneous tissue, muscle fascia, and muscle**

8.86 15.78 Global Days 000

11012 **skin, subcutaneous tissue, muscle fascia, muscle, and bone**

12.57 20.89 Global Days 000

AMA: 2009, Jan, 11-31; 2008, Jan, 10-25; 2007, January, 13-27

11042-11047 [11045, 11046] Removal of Infected/Devitalized Tissue

CMS 100-2,15,260 Covered ASC Procedures
CMS 100-4,12,40.1 Global Surgery Definition
CMS 100-4,12,40.2 Billing Requirements for Global Surgeries
CMS 100-4,14,10 ASC Procedures

INCLUDES Debridement reported by the size and depth
Debridement reported for multiple wounds by adding the total surface area of wounds that are of the same depth
Injuries, wounds, chronic ulcers, infections

EXCLUDES *Active wound care and management (97597-97598)*
Debridement of:
- *Burn (16020-16035)*
- *Dermis/epidermis only (97597-97598)*
- *Eczematous or infected skin (11000-11001)*
- *Nails (11720-11721)*
- *Necrotizing soft tissue of external genitalia or abdominal wall (11004-11006)*

Dermabrasions (15780-15783)
Excision of pressure ulcers (15920-15999)

Code also each additional single wound of different depths

Code also modifier 59 for additional wound debridement

Code also multiple wound groups of different depths.

11042 **Debridement, subcutaneous tissue (includes epidermis and dermis, if performed); first 20 sq cm or less**

1.75 3.18 Global Days 000

\+ # **11045** **each additional 20 sq cm, or part thereof (List separately in addition to code for primary procedure)**

Code first (11042)

0.79 1.20 Global Days ZZZ

11043 **Debridement, muscle and/or fascia (includes epidermis, dermis, and subcutaneous tissue, if performed); first 20 sq cm or less**

4.65 6.80 Global Days 000

AMA: 2009, Jan, 11-31; 2008, Jan, 10-25; 2007, January, 13-27

\+ # **11046** **each additional 20 sq cm, or part thereof (List separately in addition to code for primary procedure)**

Code first (11043)

1.62 2.11 Global Days ZZZ

11044 **Debridement, bone (includes epidermis, dermis, subcutaneous tissue, muscle and/or fascia, if performed); first 20 sq cm or less**

6.95 9.41 Global Days 000

AMA: 2009, Jan, 11-31; 2008, Jan, 10-25; 2007, January, 13-27

11045 Resequenced code, See code following 11042.

11046 Resequenced code, See code following 11043.

\+ **11047** **each additional 20 sq cm, or part thereof (List separately in addition to code for primary procedure)**

Code first (11044)

2.87 3.56 Global Days ZZZ

11055-11057 Excision Benign Hypertrophic Skin Lesions

CMS 100-2,15,290 Routine Foot Care

EXCLUDES *Destruction (17000-17004)*

11055 **Paring or cutting of benign hyperkeratotic lesion (eg, corn or callus); single lesion**

0.59 1.46 Global Days 000

AMA: 2009, Jan, 11-31; 2008, Jan, 10-25; 2007, January, 13-27

11056 2 to 4 lesions P3 T CCI PQ
0.68 1.64 Global Days 000

11057 more than 4 lesions P3 T CCI PQ
1.07 2.05 Global Days 000

11100-11101 Surgical Biopsy Skin and Mucous Membranes

CMS 100-4,12,30 Correct Coding Policy

INCLUDES Attaining tissue for pathologic exam

EXCLUDES *Biopsy of:*
Conjunctiva (68100)
Eyelid (67810)
Unrelated and separately distinct biopsies

11100 **Biopsy of skin, subcutaneous tissue and/or mucous membrane (including simple closure), unless otherwise listed; single lesion** P3 T CCI
1.45 3.05 Global Days 000
AMA: 2008, Feb, 1

\+ 11101 **each separate/additional lesion (List separately in addition to code for primary procedure)** P3 T
Code first (11100)
0.73 0.96 Global Days ZZZ
AMA: 2008, Feb, 1

11200-11201 Skin Tag Removal - All Techniques

CMS 100-4,12,30 Correct Coding Policy
CMS 100-4,12,40.1 Global Surgery Package Definition
CMS 100-4,12,40.2 Billing Requirements for Global Surgeries

INCLUDES Chemical destruction
Electrocauterization
Electrosurgical destruction
Ligature strangulation
Removal with or without local anesthesia
Sharp excision or scissoring

EXCLUDES *Extensive or complicated secondary wound closure (13160)*

11200 **Removal of skin tags, multiple fibrocutaneous tags, any area; up to and including 15 lesions** P2 T CCI
2.12 2.53 Global Days 010
AMA: 2009, Jan, 11-31; 2008, Jan, 10-25; 2007, January, 13-27

\+ 11201 **each additional 10 lesions, or part thereof (List separately in addition to code for primary procedure)** P3 T
Code first (11200)
0.49 0.55 Global Days ZZZ

11300-11313 Skin Lesion Removal: Shaving

CMS 100-4,12,40.1 Global Surgery Package Definition
CMS 100-4,12,40.2 Global Surgery Billing Requirements
CMS 100-4,12,50 Local anesthesia

INCLUDES Local anesthesia
Partial thickness excision by horizontal slicing
Wound cauterization

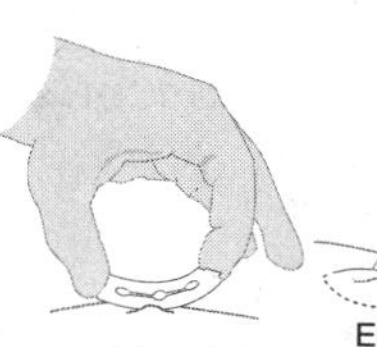
Shave excision of an elevated lesion; technique also used to biopsy

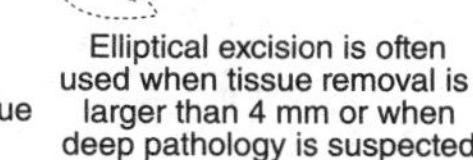
Elliptical excision is often used when tissue removal is larger than 4 mm or when deep pathology is suspected

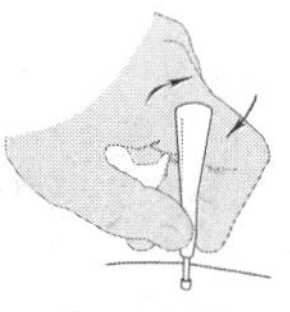
A punch biopsy cuts a core of tissue as the tool is twisted downward

The skin is the largest organ of the human body and accounts for about 20 percent of total body weight. It serves mainly as a protective barrier, a temperature regulator, and as a sensory device. The epidermis is outermost and is the thinnest of the skin layers; the major part of the dermis is high in collagen and is notable for its great elasticity and strength; the major blood and nerve network is found in the middermis. Adnexal structures are the hair follicles, sebaceous glands, sweat glands, and the follicles that produce fingernails and toenails. Lesions are small areas of skin disease and may be solitary or multiple

11300 **Shaving of epidermal or dermal lesion, single lesion, trunk, arms or legs; lesion diameter 0.5 cm or less** P2 T 80 CCI
0.88 2.05 Global Days 000
AMA: 2009, Jan, 11-31; 2008, Jan, 10-25; 2008, Feb, 1; 2007, January, 13-27

11301 **lesion diameter 0.6 to 1.0 cm** P2 T 80 CCI
1.49 2.74 Global Days 000
AMA: 2009, Jan, 11-31; 2008, Jan, 10-25; 2008, Feb, 1; 2007, January, 13-27

11302 **lesion diameter 1.1 to 2.0 cm** P2 T 80 CCI
1.85 3.27 Global Days 000
AMA: 2009, Jan, 11-31; 2008, Jan, 10-25; 2008, Feb, 1; 2007, January, 13-27

11303 **lesion diameter over 2.0 cm** P3 T 80 CCI
2.19 3.86 Global Days 000
AMA: 2009, Jan, 11-31; 2008, Jan, 10-25; 2008, Feb, 1; 2007, January, 13-27

11305 **Shaving of epidermal or dermal lesion, single lesion, scalp, neck, hands, feet, genitalia; lesion diameter 0.5 cm or less** P3 T 80 CCI
0.97 2.04 Global Days 000
AMA: 2009, Jan, 11-31; 2008, Jan, 10-25; 2008, Feb, 1; 2007, January, 13-27

11306 **lesion diameter 0.6 to 1.0 cm** P2 T 80 CCI
1.57 2.80 Global Days 000
AMA: 2009, Jan, 11-31; 2008, Jan, 10-25; 2008, Feb, 1; 2007, January, 13-27

11307 **lesion diameter 1.1 to 2.0 cm** P2 T 80 CCI
1.88 3.29 Global Days 000
AMA: 2009, Jan, 11-31; 2008, Jan, 10-25; 2008, Feb, 1; 2007, January, 13-27

11308 **lesion diameter over 2.0 cm** P3 T 80 CCI
2.16 3.64 Global Days 000
AMA: 2009, Jan, 11-31; 2008, Jan, 10-25; 2008, Feb, 1; 2007, January, 13-27

11310 **Shaving of epidermal or dermal lesion, single lesion, face, ears, eyelids, nose, lips, mucous membrane; lesion diameter 0.5 cm or less** P2 T 80
1.27 2.51 Global Days 000
AMA: 2009, Jan, 11-31; 2008, Jan, 10-25; 2008, Feb, 1; 2007, January, 13-27

11311 **lesion diameter 0.6 to 1.0 cm** P2 T 80
1.86 3.14 Global Days 000
AMA: 2009, Jan, 11-31; 2008, Jan, 10-25; 2008, Feb, 1; 2007, January, 13-27

11312 **lesion diameter 1.1 to 2.0 cm** P3 T 80
2.15 3.64 Global Days 000
AMA: 2009, Jan, 11-31; 2008, Jan, 10-25; 2008, Feb, 1; 2007, January, 13-27

11313 **lesion diameter over 2.0 cm** P2 T 80
2.87 4.52 Global Days 000
AMA: 2009, Jan, 11-31; 2008, Jan, 10-25; 2008, Feb, 1; 2007, January, 13-27

11400-11446 Skin Lesion Removal: Benign

CMS 100-2,16,120 Cosmetic Procedures
CMS 100-4,12,40.1 Global Surgery Package Definition
CMS 100-4,12,40.2 Billing Requirements for Global Surgeries
CMS 100-4,12,50 Local anesthesia

INCLUDES Biopsy on same lesion
Full thickness removal including margins
Lesion measurement before excision at largest diameter plus margin
Local anesthesia
Simple, nonlayered closure

EXCLUDES *Biopsy of eyelid (67810)*
Destruction of eyelid lesion (67850)
Excision and reconstruction of eyelid (67961-67975)
Excision of chalazion (67800-67808)
Eyelid procedures involving more than skin (67800 and subsequent codes)
Shave removal (11300-11313)

Code also complex closure (13100-13153)
Code also each separate lesion
Code also intermediate closure (12031-12057)
Code also modifier 22 if excision is complicated or unusual
Code also reconstruction (15002-15261, 15570-15770)
Do not report with adjacent tissue transfer. Report only adjacent tissue transfer code. (14000-14302)

11400 **Excision, benign lesion including margins, except skin tag (unless listed elsewhere), trunk, arms or legs; excised diameter 0.5 cm or less** P3 T
2.32 3.57 Global Days 010
AMA: 2009, Jan, 11-31; 2008, Jan, 10-25; 2008, Jul, 5-6&15; 2007, January, 13-27

11401 **excised diameter 0.6 to 1.0 cm** P3 T
3.04 4.33 Global Days 010
AMA: 2008, Jul, 5-6&15

11402 **excised diameter 1.1 to 2.0 cm** P3 T
3.34 4.82 Global Days 010
AMA: 2008, Jul, 5-6&15

11403 **excised diameter 2.1 to 3.0 cm** P3 T
4.29 5.56 Global Days 010
AMA: 2008, Jul, 5-6&15

11404 **excised diameter 3.1 to 4.0 cm** A2 T
4.73 6.31 Global Days 010
AMA: 2008, Jul, 5-6&15

11406 **excised diameter over 4.0 cm** A2 T
7.13 9.01 Global Days 010
AMA: 2008, Jul, 5-6&15

11420 **Excision, benign lesion including margins, except skin tag (unless listed elsewhere), scalp, neck, hands, feet, genitalia; excised diameter 0.5 cm or less** P3 T
2.39 3.55 Global Days 010
AMA: 2008, Jul, 5-6&15

11421 **excised diameter 0.6 to 1.0 cm** P3 T
3.25 4.58 Global Days 010
AMA: 2008, Jul, 5-6&15

11422 **excised diameter 1.1 to 2.0 cm** P3 T
3.96 5.10 Global Days 010
AMA: 2008, Jul, 5-6&15

11423 **excised diameter 2.1 to 3.0 cm** P3 T
4.61 5.90 Global Days 010
AMA: 2008, Jul, 5-6&15

11424 **excised diameter 3.1 to 4.0 cm** A2 T
5.25 6.78 Global Days 010
AMA: 2008, Jul, 5-6&15

11426 **excised diameter over 4.0 cm** A2 T
8.00 9.66 Global Days 010
AMA: 2008, Jul, 5-6&15

11440 **Excision, other benign lesion including margins, except skin tag (unless listed elsewhere), face, ears, eyelids, nose, lips, mucous membrane; excised diameter 0.5 cm or less** P3 T
3.01 3.91 Global Days 010
AMA: 2008, Jul, 5-6&15

11441 **excised diameter 0.6 to 1.0 cm** P3 T
3.86 4.90 Global Days 010
AMA: 2008, Jul, 5-6&15

11442 **excised diameter 1.1 to 2.0 cm** P3 T
4.29 5.51 Global Days 010
AMA: 2009, Jan, 11-31; 2008, Jun, 14-15; 2008, Jul, 5-6&15

11443 **excised diameter 2.1 to 3.0 cm** P3 T
5.25 6.56 Global Days 010
AMA: 2008, Jul, 5-6&15

11444 **excised diameter 3.1 to 4.0 cm** A2 T
6.68 8.22 Global Days 010
AMA: 2008, Jul, 5-6&15

11446 **excised diameter over 4.0 cm** A2 T
9.50 11.31 Global Days 010
AMA: 2009, Jan, 11-31; 2008, Jan, 10-25; 2008, Jul, 5-6&15; 2007, January, 13-27

11450-11471 Treatment of Hidradenitis: Excision and Repair

CMS 100-2,15,260 Covered ASC Procedures
CMS 100-4,4,20.5 HCPCS Under OPPS
CMS 100-4,12,90.3 MD Services in ASCs
CMS 100-4,14,10 General ASC Services

Code also closure by skin graft or flap (14000-14350, 15040-15770)

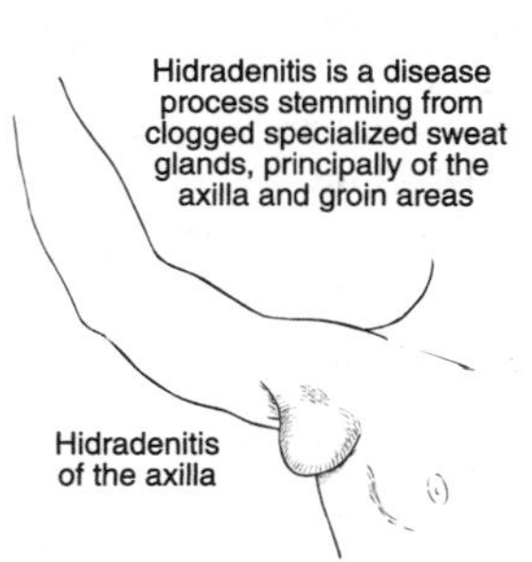

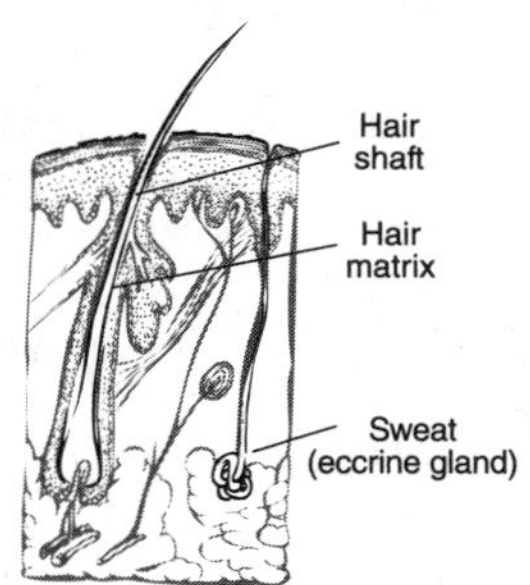

11450 **Excision of skin and subcutaneous tissue for hidradenitis, axillary; with simple or intermediate repair** A2 T CCI
7.27 10.93 Global Days 090

11451 **with complex repair** A2 T 80 CCI
9.40 13.99 Global Days 090

11462 **Excision of skin and subcutaneous tissue for hidradenitis, inguinal; with simple or intermediate repair** A2 T 80 CCI
7.03 10.82 Global Days 090

11463 **with complex repair** A2 T 80 CCI
9.48 14.19 Global Days 090

11470 **Excision of skin and subcutaneous tissue for hidradenitis, perianal, perineal, or umbilical; with simple or intermediate repair** A2 T CCI
8.16 11.90 Global Days 090

11471 **with complex repair** A2 T 80 CCI
10.15 14.81 Global Days 090

11600-11646 Skin Lesion Removal: Malignant

CMS 100-2,15,260 Covered ASC Procedures
CMS 100-4,4,20.5 HCPCS Under OPPS
CMS 100-4,12,90.3 MD Services in ASCs
CMS 100-4,14,10 General ASC Services

INCLUDES Biopsy on same lesion
Excision of additional margin at same operative session
Full thickness removal including margins
Lesion measurement before excision at largest diameter plus margin
Local anesthesia
Simple, nonlayered closure

EXCLUDES *Destruction (17260-17286)*
Excision of additional margin at subsequent operative session (11600-11646)

Code also complex closure (13100-13153)
Code also each separate lesion
Code also intermediate closure (12031-12057)
Code also modifier 58 if re-excision is performed during postoperative period
Code also reconstruction (15002-15261, 15570-15770)
Do not report with adjacent tissue transfer. Report only adjacent tissue transfer code. (14000-14302)

11600 **Excision, malignant lesion including margins, trunk, arms, or legs; excised diameter 0.5 cm or less** P3 T CCI PQ
3.48 5.55 Global Days 010
AMA: 2009, Jan, 11-31; 2008, Jan, 10-25; 2008, Feb, 8-9; 2008, Jul, 5-6&15; 2007, January, 13-27

11601 **excised diameter 0.6 to 1.0 cm** P3 T CCI PQ
4.38 6.67 Global Days 010
AMA: 2008, Feb, 8-9; 2008, Jul, 5-6&15

11602 **excised diameter 1.1 to 2.0 cm** P3 T CCI PQ
4.82 7.27 Global Days 010
AMA: 2008, Feb, 8-9; 2008, Jul, 5-6&15

11603 **excised diameter 2.1 to 3.0 cm** P3 T CCI PQ
5.73 8.26 Global Days 010
AMA: 2008, Feb, 8-9; 2008, Jul, 5-6&15

11604 **excised diameter 3.1 to 4.0 cm** A2 T CCI PQ
6.31 9.18 Global Days 010
AMA: 2008, Feb, 8-9; 2008, Jul, 5-6&15

11606 **excised diameter over 4.0 cm** A2 T CCI PQ
9.33 13.05 Global Days 010
AMA: 2008, Feb, 8-9; 2008, Jul, 5-6&15

11620 **Excision, malignant lesion including margins, scalp, neck, hands, feet, genitalia; excised diameter 0.5 cm or less** P3 T CCI PQ
3.53 5.64 Global Days 010
AMA: 2008, Feb, 8-9; 2008, Jul, 5-6&15

11621 **excised diameter 0.6 to 1.0 cm** P3 T CCI PQ
4.42 6.72 Global Days 010
AMA: 2008, Feb, 8-9; 2008, Jul, 5-6&15

11622 **excised diameter 1.1 to 2.0 cm** P3 T CCI PQ
5.07 7.52 Global Days 010
AMA: 2008, Feb, 8-9; 2008, Jul, 5-6&15

11623 **excised diameter 2.1 to 3.0 cm** P3 T CCI PQ
6.25 8.80 Global Days 010
AMA: 2008, Feb, 8-9; 2008, Jul, 5-6&15

11624 **excised diameter 3.1 to 4.0 cm** A2 T CCI PQ
7.08 9.91 Global Days 010
AMA: 2008, Feb, 8-9; 2008, Jul, 5-6&15

11626 **excised diameter over 4.0 cm** A2 T CCI PQ
8.70 11.97 Global Days 010
AMA: 2008, Feb, 8-9; 2008, Jul, 5-6&15

11640 **Excision, malignant lesion including margins, face, ears, eyelids, nose, lips; excised diameter 0.5 cm or less** P3 T CCI PQ
EXCLUDES *Eyelid excision involving more than skin (67800 and subsequent codes)*
3.68 5.84 Global Days 010
AMA: 2008, Feb, 8-9; 2008, Jul, 5-6&15

11641 **excised diameter 0.6 to 1.0 cm** P3 T CCI PQ
EXCLUDES *Eyelid excision involving more than skin (67800 and subsequent codes)*
4.64 6.99 Global Days 010
AMA: 2008, Feb, 8-9; 2008, Jul, 5-6&15

11642 **excised diameter 1.1 to 2.0 cm** P3 T CCI PQ
EXCLUDES *Eyelid excision involving more than skin (67800 and subsequent codes)*
5.46 7.98 Global Days 010
AMA: 2008, Feb, 8-9; 2008, Jul, 5-6&15

11643 **excised diameter 2.1 to 3.0 cm** P3 T CCI PQ
EXCLUDES *Eyelid excision involving more than skin (67800 and subsequent codes)*
6.83 9.41 Global Days 010
AMA: 2008, Feb, 8-9; 2008, Jul, 5-6&15

11644 **excised diameter 3.1 to 4.0 cm** A2 T CCI PQ
EXCLUDES *Eyelid excision involving more than skin (67800 and subsequent codes)*
8.47 11.61 Global Days 010
AMA: 2008, Feb, 8-9; 2008, Jul, 5-6&15

11646 **excised diameter over 4.0 cm** A2 T PO
EXCLUDES *Eyelid excision involving more than skin (67800 and subsequent codes)*
11.75 15.15 Global Days 010
AMA: 2009, Jan, 11-31; 2008, Jan, 10-25; 2008, Feb, 8-9; 2008, Jul, 5-6&15; 2007, January, 13-27

11719-11765 Nails and Supporting Structures

CMS 100-2,15,290 Foot Care
CMS 100-4,4,20.5 HCPCS Under OPPS
EXCLUDES *Drainage of paronychia or onychia (10060-10061)*

11719 **Trimming of nondystrophic nails, any number** P3 T PO
0.23 0.65 Global Days 000

11720 **Debridement of nail(s) by any method(s); 1 to 5** P3 T PO
0.44 0.92 Global Days 000

11721 **6 or more** P3 T PO
0.74 1.28 Global Days 000

11730 **Avulsion of nail plate, partial or complete, simple; single** P2 T PO
1.50 2.82 Global Days 000
AMA: 2009, Jan, 11-31; 2008, Jan, 10-25; 2007, January, 13-27

+ 11732 **each additional nail plate (List separately in addition to code for primary procedure)** P3 T
Code first (11730)
0.61 1.05 Global Days ZZZ

11740 **Evacuation of subungual hematoma** P2 T PO
0.94 1.39 Global Days 000

11750 **Excision of nail and nail matrix, partial or complete (eg, ingrown or deformed nail), for permanent removal;** P3 T
EXCLUDES *Skin graft (15050)*
5.06 6.40 Global Days 010

11752 **with amputation of tuft of distal phalanx** P3 T
EXCLUDES *Skin graft (15050)*
7.64 9.24 Global Days 010

11755 **Biopsy of nail unit (eg, plate, bed, matrix, hyponychium, proximal and lateral nail folds) (separate procedure)** P3 T 80
2.33 3.90 Global Days 000
AMA: 2009, Jan, 11-31; 2008, Jan, 10-25; 2007, January, 13-27

11760 **Repair of nail bed** G2 T
3.94 6.67 Global Days 010

11762 **Reconstruction of nail bed with graft** P3 T
5.47 8.07 Global Days 010

11765 **Wedge excision of skin of nail fold (eg, for ingrown toenail)** P2 T
INCLUDES Cotting's operation
2.65 4.68 Global Days 010

11770-11772 Treatment Pilonidal Cyst: Excision

CMS 100-2,15,260 Covered ASC Procedures
CMS 100-4,4,20.5 HCPCS Under OPPS
CMS 100-4,12,90.3 MD Services in ASCs
EXCLUDES *Incision of pilonidal cyst (10080-10081)*

11770 **Excision of pilonidal cyst or sinus; simple** A2 T
5.34 7.97 Global Days 010

11771 **extensive** A2 T
12.58 16.50 Global Days 090

11772 **complicated** A2 T
16.67 20.01 Global Days 090

11900-11901 Treatment of Lesions: Injection

CMS 100-4,17,20.5.7 Injection Services
EXCLUDES *Injection of veins (36470-36471)*
Intralesional chemotherapy (96405-96406)

Do not report for local anesthetic injection performed preoperatively

11900 **Injection, intralesional; up to and including 7 lesions** P3 T
0.93 1.64 Global Days 000
AMA: 2009, Jan, 11-31; 2008, Jan, 10-25; 2007, January, 13-27

11901 **more than 7 lesions** P3 T
1.44 2.06 Global Days 000
AMA: 2009, Jan, 11-31; 2008, Jan, 10-25; 2007, January, 13-27

11920-11971 Tattoos, Tissue Expanders, and Dermal Fillers

CMS 100-2,16,10 Exclusions from Coverage
CMS 100-2,16,120 Cosmetic Procedures
CMS 100-2,16,180 Services Related to Noncovered Procedures
CMS 100-4,4,20.5 HCPCS Under OPPS

11920 **Tattooing, intradermal introduction of insoluble opaque pigments to correct color defects of skin, including micropigmentation; 6.0 sq cm or less** P3 T 80
3.45 5.20 Global Days 000

11921 **6.1 to 20.0 sq cm** P3 T 80
4.04 5.98 Global Days 000

+ 11922 **each additional 20.0 sq cm, or part thereof (List separately in addition to code for primary procedure)** P3 T 80
Code first (11921)
0.88 1.82 Global Days ZZZ

11950 **Subcutaneous injection of filling material (eg, collagen); 1 cc or less** P3 T 80
1.43 2.09 Global Days 000

11951 **1.1 to 5.0 cc** P3 T 80
2.23 3.13 Global Days 000

11952 **5.1 to 10.0 cc** P3 T 80
3.06 4.19 Global Days 000

11954 **over 10.0 cc** P2 T 80
3.45 4.74 Global Days 000

11960 **Insertion of tissue expander(s) for other than breast, including subsequent expansion** A2 T
EXCLUDES *Breast reconstruction with tissue expander(s) (19357)*
26.62 26.62 Global Days 090

11970 **Replacement of tissue expander with permanent prosthesis** A2 T 50
18.20 18.20 Global Days 090

11971 **Removal of tissue expander(s) without insertion of prosthesis** A2 T 80 50
9.42 13.95 Global Days 090
AMA: 2009, Jan, 11-31; 2008, Jan, 10-25; 2007, January, 13-27

11975-11983 Drug Implantation

CMS 100-2,15,50 Drugs and Biologicals
CMS 100-2,16,20 General Exclusions

~~11975 Insertion, implantable contraceptive capsules~~
To report, see 11981

11976 **Removal, implantable contraceptive capsules** ♀ P3 T 80
2.84 4.28 Global Days 000

~~11977 Removal with reinsertion, implantable contraceptive capsules~~
To report, see 11976, 11981

11980 Subcutaneous hormone pellet implantation (implantation of estradiol and/or testosterone pellets beneath the skin) P2 X
2.38 3.05 Global Days 000

11981 Insertion, non-biodegradable drug delivery implant P2 X 80
2.41 3.98 Global Days XXX
AMA: 2009, Jan, 11-31; 2007, Dec, 10-179

11982 Removal, non-biodegradable drug delivery implant P2 X 80
2.87 4.47 Global Days XXX

11983 Removal with reinsertion, non-biodegradable drug delivery implant P2 X 80
5.04 6.35 Global Days XXX

12001-12021 Suturing of Superficial Wounds

CMS 100-2,15,260 Covered ASC Procedures
CMS 100-4,4,20.5 HCPCS Under OPPS
CMS 100-4,14,10 ASC Procedures

INCLUDES Administration of local anesthesia
Cauterization without closure
Simple:
Exploration nerves, blood vessels, tendons
Vessel ligation, in wound
Simple repair that involves:
Routine debridement and decontamination
Simple one layer closure
Superficial tissues
Sutures, staples, tissue adhesives
Total length of several repairs in same code category

EXCLUDES *Adhesive strips only (99201-99499 [99224, 99225, 99226])*
Complex repair nerves, blood vessels, tendons (see appropriate anatomical section)
Debridement:
Performed separately, no closure (11042-11047 [11045, 11046])
That requires:
Comprehensive cleaning
Removal of significant tissue
Removal soft tissue and/or bone, no fracture/dislocation (11042-11047 [11045, 11046])
Removal soft tissue and/or bone with open fracture/dislocation (11010-11012)
Deep tissue repair (12031-13153)
Major exploration (20100-20103)
Repair of nerves, blood vessels, tendons (see appropriate anatomical section). Repair of these wounds includes simple and intermediate closure. Report complex closure with modifier 59.
Secondary closure/dehiscense (13160)

Code also modifier 59 added to the less complicated procedure code if reporting more than one classification of wound repair

12001 Simple repair of superficial wounds of scalp, neck, axillae, external genitalia, trunk and/or extremities (including hands and feet); 2.5 cm or less P3 T
1.46 2.75 Global Days 000
AMA: 2009, Jan, 11-31; 2008, Jan, 10-25; 2008, Feb, 8-9; 2007, January, 13-27; 2007, February, 10-11

12002 2.6 cm to 7.5 cm P2 T
1.90 3.28 Global Days 000
AMA: 2009, Jan, 11-31; 2008, Jan, 10-25; 2008, Feb, 8-9; 2007, January, 13-27; 2007, February, 10-11

12004 7.6 cm to 12.5 cm P2 T
2.34 3.87 Global Days 000
AMA: 2009, Jan, 11-31; 2008, Jan, 10-25; 2008, Feb, 8-9; 2007, January, 13-27; 2007, February, 10-11

12005 12.6 cm to 20.0 cm A2 T
3.12 5.00 Global Days 000
AMA: 2009, Jan, 11-31; 2008, Jan, 10-25; 2008, Feb, 8-9; 2007, February, 10-11; 2007, January, 13-27

12006 20.1 cm to 30.0 cm A2 T
3.81 6.03 Global Days 000
AMA: 2009, Jan, 11-31; 2008, Jan, 10-25; 2008, Feb, 8-9; 2007, February, 10-11; 2007, January, 13-27

12007 over 30.0 cm A2 T
4.65 7.00 Global Days 000
AMA: 2009, Jan, 11-31; 2008, Jan, 10-25; 2008, Feb, 8-9; 2007, February, 10-11; 2007, January, 13-27

12011 Simple repair of superficial wounds of face, ears, eyelids, nose, lips and/or mucous membranes; 2.5 cm or less P2 T
1.79 3.30 Global Days 000
AMA: 2009, Jan, 11-31; 2008, Jan, 10-25; 2008, Feb, 8-9; 2007, February, 10-11; 2007, January, 13-27

12013 2.6 cm to 5.0 cm P2 T
2.01 3.61 Global Days 000
AMA: 2009, Jan, 11-31; 2008, Jan, 10-25; 2008, Feb, 8-9; 2007, February, 10-11; 2007, January, 13-27

12014 5.1 cm to 7.5 cm P2 T
2.52 4.24 Global Days 000
AMA: 2009, Jan, 11-31; 2008, Feb, 8-9; 2008, Jan, 10-25; 2007, January, 13-27; 2007, February, 10-11

12015 7.6 cm to 12.5 cm G2 T
3.11 5.22 Global Days 000
AMA: 2009, Jan, 11-31; 2008, Feb, 8-9; 2008, Jan, 10-25; 2007, February, 10-11; 2007, January, 13-27

12016 12.6 cm to 20.0 cm A2 T
4.18 6.47 Global Days 000
AMA: 2009, Jan, 11-31; 2008, Jan, 10-25; 2008, Feb, 8-9; 2007, February, 10-11; 2007, January, 13-27

12017 20.1 cm to 30.0 cm A2 T 80
4.79 4.79 Global Days 000
AMA: 2009, Jan, 11-31; 2008, Jan, 10-25; 2008, Feb, 8-9; 2007, January, 13-27; 2007, February, 10-11

12018 over 30.0 cm A2 T 80
5.56 5.56 Global Days 000
AMA: 2009, Jan, 11-31; 2008, Jan, 10-25; 2008, Feb, 8-9; 2007, February, 10-11; 2007, January, 13-27

12020 Treatment of superficial wound dehiscence; simple closure A2 T
EXCLUDES *Secondary closure major/complex wound (13160)*
5.49 8.05 Global Days 010
AMA: 2009, Jan, 11-31; 2008, Jan, 10-25; 2008, Feb, 8-9; 2007, January, 13-27

12021 with packing A2 T
EXCLUDES *Secondary closure major/complex wound (13160)*
4.13 4.86 Global Days 010
AMA: 2009, Jan, 11-31; 2008, Jan, 10-25; 2008, Feb, 8-9; 2007, January, 13-27

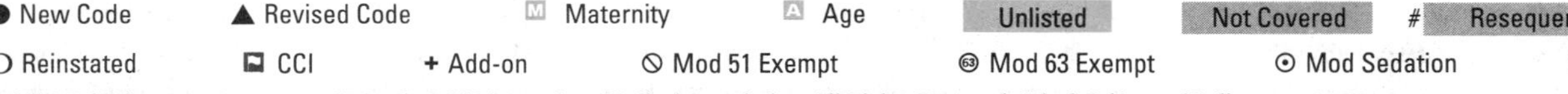

12031-12057 Suturing of Intermediate Wounds

CMS 100-4,4,20.5 HCPCS Under OPPS
CMS 100-4,12,90.3 MD Services in ASCs
CMS 100-4,14,10 General ASC Services

INCLUDES Administration of local anesthesia
Intermediate repair that involves:
Closure of contaminated single layer wound
Layer closure (e.g., subcutaneous tissue, superficial fascia)
Removal foreign material (e.g. gravel, glass)
Routine debridement and decontamination
Simple:
Exploration nerves, blood vessels, tendons in wound
Vessel ligation, in wound
Total length of several repairs in same code category

EXCLUDES *Complex repair nerves, blood vessels, tendons (see appropriate anatomical section)*
Debridement:
Performed separately, no closure (11042-11047 [11045, 11046])
That requires:
Removal soft tissue and/or bone, no fracture/dislocation (11042-11047 [11045, 11046])
Removal soft tissue/bone due to open fracture/dislocation (11010-11012)
Major exploration (20100-20103)
Repair of nerves, blood vessels, tendons (see appropriate anatomical section). Repair of these wounds includes simple and intermediate closure. Report complex closure with modifier 59.
Secondary closure major/complex wound or dehiscense (13160)
Wound repair involving more than layer closure

Code also modifier 59 added to the less complicated procedure code if reporting more than one classification of wound repair

12031 **Repair, intermediate, wounds of scalp, axillae, trunk and/or extremities (excluding hands and feet); 2.5 cm or less** P3 T
4.50 6.91 **Global Days 010**
AMA: 2009, Jan, 11-31; 2008, Jan, 10-25; 2007, February, 10-11; 2007, January, 13-27

12032 **2.6 cm to 7.5 cm** P2 T
5.77 8.95 **Global Days 010**
AMA: 2009, Jan, 11-31; 2008, Jan, 10-25; 2007, January, 13-27; 2007, February, 10-11

12034 **7.6 cm to 12.5 cm** A2 T
6.06 9.08 **Global Days 010**
AMA: 2009, Jan, 11-31; 2008, Jan, 10-25; 2007, January, 13-27; 2007, February, 10-11

12035 **12.6 cm to 20.0 cm** A2 T
7.05 11.11 **Global Days 010**
AMA: 2009, Jan, 11-31; 2008, Jan, 10-25; 2007, February, 10-11; 2007, January, 13-27

12036 **20.1 cm to 30.0 cm** A2 T
8.26 12.34 **Global Days 010**
AMA: 2009, Jan, 11-31; 2008, Jan, 10-25; 2007, February, 10-11; 2007, January, 13-27

12037 **over 30.0 cm** A2 T 80
9.64 13.85 **Global Days 010**
AMA: 2009, Jan, 11-31; 2008, Jan, 10-25; 2007, February, 10-11; 2007, January, 13-27

12041 **Repair, intermediate, wounds of neck, hands, feet and/or external genitalia; 2.5 cm or less** P2 T
4.61 7.05 **Global Days 010**
AMA: 2009, Jan, 11-31; 2008, Jan, 10-25; 2007, January, 13-27; 2007, February, 10-11

12042 **2.6 cm to 7.5 cm** P3 T
5.90 8.49 **Global Days 010**
AMA: 2009, Jan, 11-31; 2008, Jan, 10-25; 2007, February, 10-11; 2007, January, 13-27

12044 **7.6 cm to 12.5 cm** A2 T
6.30 10.36 **Global Days 010**
AMA: 2009, Jan, 11-31; 2008, Jan, 10-25; 2007, February, 10-11; 2007, January, 13-27

12045 **12.6 cm to 20.0 cm** A2 T
7.77 11.51 **Global Days 010**
AMA: 2009, Jan, 11-31; 2008, Jan, 10-25; 2007, February, 10-11; 2007, January, 13-27

12046 **20.1 cm to 30.0 cm** A2 T 80
8.88 13.17 **Global Days 010**
AMA: 2009, Jan, 11-31; 2008, Jan, 10-25; 2007, January, 13-27; 2007, February, 10-11

12047 **over 30.0 cm** A2 T 80
9.98 15.14 **Global Days 010**
AMA: 2009, Jan, 11-31; 2008, Jan, 10-25; 2007, February, 10-11; 2007, January, 13-27

12051 **Repair, intermediate, wounds of face, ears, eyelids, nose, lips and/or mucous membranes; 2.5 cm or less** P3 T
5.09 7.62 **Global Days 010**
AMA: 2009, Jan, 11-31; 2008, Jan, 10-25; 2007, January, 13-27; 2007, February, 10-11

12052 **2.6 cm to 5.0 cm** P2 T
6.10 8.72 **Global Days 010**
AMA: 2009, Jan, 11-31; 2008, Jan, 10-25; 2008, Jul, 5-6&15; 2007, February, 10-11; 2007, January, 13-27

12053 **5.1 cm to 7.5 cm** P2 T
6.41 10.08 **Global Days 010**
AMA: 2009, Jan, 11-31; 2008, Jan, 10-25; 2007, February, 10-11; 2007, January, 13-27

12054 **7.6 cm to 12.5 cm** A2 T
6.74 10.72 **Global Days 010**
AMA: 2009, Jan, 11-31; 2008, Jan, 10-25; 2007, February, 10-11; 2007, January, 13-27

12055 **12.6 cm to 20.0 cm** A2 T
8.72 13.61 **Global Days 010**
AMA: 2009, Jan, 11-31; 2008, Jan, 10-25; 2007, February, 10-11; 2007, January, 13-27

12056 **20.1 cm to 30.0 cm** A2 T 80
10.89 15.86 **Global Days 010**
AMA: 2009, Jan, 11-31; 2008, Jan, 10-25; 2007, January, 13-27; 2007, February, 10-11

12057 **over 30.0 cm** A2 T 80
11.82 18.16 **Global Days 010**
AMA: 2009, Jan, 11-31; 2008, Jan, 10-25; 2007, February, 10-11; 2007, January, 13-27

13100-13160 Suturing of Complicated Wounds

CMS 100-4,4,20.5 HCPCS Under OPPS
CMS 100-4,12,90.3 MD Services in ASCs
CMS 100-4,14,10 General ASC Services

INCLUDES Creation of a limited defect for repair
Debridement complicated wounds/avulsions
More complicated than layered closure
Simple:
Exploration nerves, vessels, tendons in wound
Vessel ligation in wound
Total length of several repairs in same code category
Undermining, stents, retention sutures

EXCLUDES *Complex/secondary wound closure or dehiscence*
Debridement of open fracture/dislocation (15002-15005)
Excision:
Benign lesions (11400-11446)
Malignant lesions (11600-11646)
Extensive exploration (20100-20103)
Repair of nerves, blood vessels, tendons (see appropriate anatomical section). Repair of these wounds includes simple and intermediate closure. Report complex closure with modifier 59.
Surgical preparation of a wound bed (15002-15005)

Code also modifier 59 added to the less complicated procedure code if reporting more than one classification of wound repair

13100 Repair, complex, trunk; 1.1 cm to 2.5 cm A2 T
EXCLUDES *Complex repair 1.0 cm or less (12001, 12031)*
6.91 9.20 **Global Days 010**
AMA: 2009, Jan, 11-31; 2008, Jan, 10-25; 2007, January, 13-27

13101 2.6 cm to 7.5 cm A2 T
8.39 11.68 **Global Days 010**
AMA: 2009, Jan, 11-31; 2008, Jan, 10-25; 2007, January, 13-27

+ **13102 each additional 5 cm or less (List separately in addition to code for primary procedure)** A2 T
Code first (13101)
2.22 3.20 **Global Days ZZZ**
AMA: 2009, Jan, 11-31; 2008, Jan, 10-25; 2007, January, 13-27

13120 Repair, complex, scalp, arms, and/or legs; 1.1 cm to 2.5 cm A2 T
EXCLUDES *Complex repair 1.0 cm or less (12001, 12031)*
7.24 9.56 **Global Days 010**
AMA: 2009, Jan, 11-31; 2008, Jan, 10-25; 2007, January, 13-27

13121 2.6 cm to 7.5 cm A2 T
9.67 13.04 **Global Days 010**
AMA: 2009, Jan, 11-31; 2008, Jan, 10-25; 2007, January, 13-27

+ **13122 each additional 5 cm or less (List separately in addition to code for primary procedure)** A2 T
Code first (13121)
2.54 3.51 **Global Days ZZZ**
AMA: 2009, Jan, 11-31; 2008, Jan, 10-25; 2007, January, 13-27

13131 Repair, complex, forehead, cheeks, chin, mouth, neck, axillae, genitalia, hands and/or feet; 1.1 cm to 2.5 cm A2 T
EXCLUDES *Complex repair 1.0 cm or less (12001, 12011, 12031, 12041, 12051)*
8.13 10.54 **Global Days 010**
AMA: 2009, Jan, 11-31; 2008, Jan, 10-25; 2007, January, 13-27

13132 2.6 cm to 7.5 cm A2 T
13.87 17.05 **Global Days 010**
AMA: 2009, Jan, 11-31; 2008, Jan, 10-25; 2007, January, 13-27

+ **13133 each additional 5 cm or less (List separately in addition to code for primary procedure)** A2 T
Code first (13132)
3.91 4.93 **Global Days ZZZ**
AMA: 2009, Jan, 11-31; 2008, Jan, 10-25; 2007, January, 13-27

13150 Repair, complex, eyelids, nose, ears and/or lips; 1.0 cm or less A2 T
8.12 10.52 **Global Days 010**
AMA: 2009, Jan, 11-31; 2008, Jan, 10-25; 2007, January, 13-27

13151 1.1 cm to 2.5 cm A2 T
9.36 11.92 **Global Days 010**
AMA: 2009, Jan, 11-31; 2008, Jan, 10-25; 2007, January, 13-27

13152 2.6 cm to 7.5 cm A2 T
12.51 16.48 **Global Days 010**
AMA: 2009, Jan, 11-31; 2008, Jan, 10-25; 2007, January, 13-27

+ **13153 each additional 5 cm or less (List separately in addition to code for primary procedure)** A2 T
Code first (13152)
4.23 5.46 **Global Days ZZZ**
AMA: 2009, Jan, 11-31; 2008, Jan, 10-25; 2007, January, 13-27

13160 Secondary closure of surgical wound or dehiscence, extensive or complicated A2 T
EXCLUDES *Packing or simple secondary wound closure (12020-12021)*
23.82 23.82 **Global Days 090**
AMA: 2009, Jan, 11-31; 2008, Jan, 10-25; 2007, January, 13-27

14000-14350 Reposition ContiguousTissue

CMS 100-2,16,120 Cosmetic Procedures
CMS 100-4,4,20.5 HCPCS Under OPPS
CMS 100-4,12,90.3 MD Services in ASCs
CMS 100-4,14,10 Part B ASC Payment

INCLUDES Excision of lesion with repair by adjacent tissue transfer or tissue rearrangement
Z-plasty, W-plasty, VY-plasty, rotation flap, advancement flap, double pedicle flap

EXCLUDES *Closure of wounds using adjacent tissue without additional incisions (13100-13160)*
Full thickness closure of:
Eyelid (67930-67935, 67961-67975)
Lip (40650-40654)

Code also skin graft necessary to repair secondary defect (15040-15731)

Do not report with (11400-11446, 11600-11646)

Example of common Z-plasty. Lesion is removed with oval-shaped incision

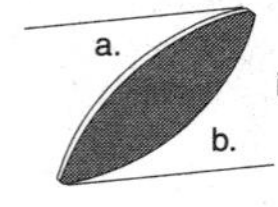

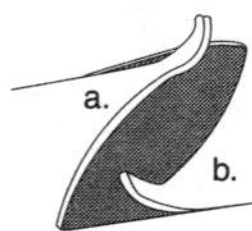

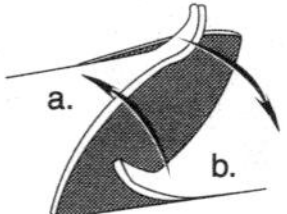

The flaps are then transposed and the repair is closed

An adjacent flap, or other rearrangement flap, is performed to repair a defect of 10 sq cm or less (14000); a larger defect (up to 30 sq cm) is coded 14001

14000 Adjacent tissue transfer or rearrangement, trunk; defect 10 sq cm or less A2 T PQ
INCLUDES Burrow's operation
14.99 18.43 Global Days 090
AMA: 2009, Jan, 11-31; 2008, Jan, 10-25; 2008, Jul, 5-6&15; 2007, January, 13-27

14001 defect 10.1 sq cm to 30.0 sq cm A2 T PQ
19.55 23.67 Global Days 090
AMA: 2009, Jan, 11-31; 2008, Jan, 10-25; 2008, Jul, 5-6&15; 2007, January, 13-27

14020 Adjacent tissue transfer or rearrangement, scalp, arms and/or legs; defect 10 sq cm or less A2 T PQ
17.02 20.67 Global Days 090
AMA: 2009, Jan, 11-31; 2008, Jan, 10-25; 2008, Jul, 5-6&15; 2007, January, 13-27

14021 defect 10.1 sq cm to 30.0 sq cm A2 T PQ
21.57 25.82 Global Days 090
AMA: 2009, Jan, 11-31; 2008, Jan, 10-25; 2008, Jul, 5-6&15; 2007, January, 13-27

14040 Adjacent tissue transfer or rearrangement, forehead, cheeks, chin, mouth, neck, axillae, genitalia, hands and/or feet; defect 10 sq cm or less A2 T PQ
INCLUDES Krimer's palatoplasty
19.02 22.65 Global Days 090
AMA: 2009, Jan, 11-31; 2008, Jan, 10-25; 2008, Jul, 5-6&15; 2007, January, 13-27

14041 defect 10.1 sq cm to 30.0 sq cm A2 T PQ
23.34 27.97 Global Days 090
AMA: 2009, Jan, 11-31; 2008, Jan, 10-25; 2008, Jul, 5-6&15; 2007, January, 13-27

14060 Adjacent tissue transfer or rearrangement, eyelids, nose, ears and/or lips; defect 10 sq cm or less A2 T PQ
INCLUDES Denonvillier's operation
EXCLUDES *Eyelid, full thickness (67961 and subsequent codes)*
20.15 22.99 Global Days 090
AMA: 2009, Jan, 11-31; 2008, Jan, 10-25; 2008, Jul, 5-6&15; 2007, January, 13-27

14061 defect 10.1 sq cm to 30.0 sq cm A2 T PQ
EXCLUDES *Eyelid, full thickness (67961 and subsequent codes)*
24.93 30.02 Global Days 090
AMA: 2009, Jan, 11-31; 2008, Jan, 10-25; 2008, Jul, 5-6&15; 2007, January, 13-27

14301 Adjacent tissue transfer or rearrangement, any area; defect 30.1 sq cm to 60.0 sq cm G2 T 80 PQ
26.63 32.23 Global Days 090

\+ **14302 Adjacent tissue transfer or rearrangement, any area; each additional 30.0 sq cm, or part thereof (List separately in addition to code for primary procedure)** G2 T 80 PQ
Code first 14301
6.65 6.65 Global Days ZZZ

14350 Filleted finger or toe flap, including preparation of recipient site A2 T 80
21.24 21.24 Global Days 090
AMA: 2009, Jan, 11-31; 2008, Jan, 10-25; 2008, Jul, 5-6&15; 2007, January, 13-27

15002-15005 Development of Base for Tissue Grafting

CMS 100-4,3,20.1.2.8 Special Payments for Burn Cases
CMS 100-4,12,90.3 MD Services in ASCs
CMS 100-4,14,10 Part B ASC Payment

INCLUDES Add together the surface area of multiple wounds in the same anatomical locations as indicated in the code description groups, such as face and scalp. Do not add together multiple wounds at different anatomical sites groups such as trunk and face.
Ankle or wrist if code description describes leg or arm
Cleaning and preparing viable tissue for graft or negative pressure wound therapy used to heal the wound primarily
Code selection based on the defect size and location
Percentage applies to children age 9 or younger
Preparation of nonviable, nonchronic wounds for healing primarily
Square centimeters applies to age 10 or older

EXCLUDES *Chronic wound management on wounds left to heal by secondary intention (11042-11047 [11045, 11046], 97597-97598)*
Necrotizing soft tissue infections for specific anatomical locations (11004-11008)

15002 **Surgical preparation or creation of recipient site by excision of open wounds, burn eschar, or scar (including subcutaneous tissues), or incisional release of scar contracture, trunk, arms, legs; first 100 sq cm or 1% of body area of infants and children** A2 T 80
EXCLUDES *Linear scar revision (13100-13153)*
6.70 10.09 Global Days 000
AMA: 2009, Jan, 11-31; 2008, Mar, 14-15; 2008, Jan, 10-25; 2007, January, 13-27

\+ **15003** **each additional 100 sq cm, or part thereof, or each additional 1% of body area of infants and children (List separately in addition to code for primary procedure)** A2 T 80
Code first (15002)
1.35 2.21 Global Days ZZZ
AMA: 2009, Jan, 11-31; 2008, Jan, 10-25; 2007, January, 13-27

15004 **Surgical preparation or creation of recipient site by excision of open wounds, burn eschar, or scar (including subcutaneous tissues), or incisional release of scar contracture, face, scalp, eyelids, mouth, neck, ears, orbits, genitalia, hands, feet and/or multiple digits; first 100 sq cm or 1% of body area of infants and children** A2 T 80
7.99 11.66 Global Days 000
AMA: 2009, Jan, 11-31; 2008, Jan, 10-25; 2007, January, 13-27

\+ **15005** **each additional 100 sq cm, or part thereof, or each additional 1% of body area of infants and children (List separately in addition to code for primary procedure)** A2 T 80
Code first (15004)
2.70 3.65 Global Days ZZZ
AMA: 2009, Jan, 11-31; 2008, Jan, 10-25; 2007, January, 13-27

15040 Obtain Autograft

CMS 100-4,3,20.1.2.8 Special Payments for Burn Cases
CMS 100-4,12,90.3 MD Services in ASCs

INCLUDES Ankle or wrist if code description describes leg or arm
Percentage applies to children age 9 or younger
Square centimeters applies to age 10 or older

15040 **Harvest of skin for tissue cultured skin autograft, 100 sq cm or less** A2 T
3.75 7.54 Global Days 000
AMA: 2009, Jan, 11-31; 2008, Feb, 3-4; 2008, Jan, 10-25; 2007, January, 13-27

15050 Pinch Graft

INCLUDES Autologous skin graft harvest and application
Current graft removal
Fixation and anchoring skin graft
Simple cleaning

Code also graft or flap necessary to repair donor site
Do not report with (97602)

15050 **Pinch graft, single or multiple, to cover small ulcer, tip of digit, or other minimal open area (except on face), up to defect size 2 cm diameter** A2 T
13.25 16.77 Global Days 090
AMA: 2009, Jan, 11-31; 2008, Jan, 10-25; 2007, January, 13-27

15100-15261 Skin Grafts and Replacements

CMS 100-4,3,20.1.2.8 Special Payments for Burn Cases
CMS 100-4,12,90.3 MD Services in ASCs
CMS 100-4,14,10 Part B ASC Payment

INCLUDES Add together the surface area of multiple wounds in the same anatomical locations as indicated in the code description groups, such as face and scalp. Do not add together multiple wounds at different anatomical site groups such as trunk and face.
Ankle or wrist if code description describes leg or arm
Autologous skin graft harvest and application
Code selection based on recipient site location and size and type of graft
Current graft removal
Fixation and anchoring skin graft
Percentage applies to children age 9 or younger
Simple cleaning
Simple tissue debridement
Square centimeters applies to age 10 or older

EXCLUDES *Debridement without immediate primary closure (11042-11047 [11045, 11046], 97597-97598)*

Code also graft or flap necessary to repair donor site
Code also primary procedure requiring skin graft for definitive closure
Do not report with (97602)

15100 **Split-thickness autograft, trunk, arms, legs; first 100 sq cm or less, or 1% of body area of infants and children (except 15050)** A2 T
21.32 25.51 Global Days 090
AMA: 2009, Jan, 11-31; 2008, Feb, 3-4; 2008, Jan, 10-25; 2007, January, 13-27

\+ **15101** **each additional 100 sq cm, or each additional 1% of body area of infants and children, or part thereof (List separately in addition to code for primary procedure)** A2 T
Code first (15100)
3.28 5.52 Global Days ZZZ
AMA: 2009, Jan, 11-31; 2008, Jan, 10-25; 2008, Feb, 3-4; 2007, January, 13-27

15110 **Epidermal autograft, trunk, arms, legs; first 100 sq cm or less, or 1% of body area of infants and children** A2 T
22.17 25.43 Global Days 090
AMA: 2009, Jan, 11-31; 2008, Feb, 3-4; 2008, Jan, 10-25; 2007, January, 13-27

\+ **15111** **each additional 100 sq cm, or each additional 1% of body area of infants and children, or part thereof (List separately in addition to code for primary procedure)** A2 T
Code first (15110)
3.01 3.36 Global Days ZZZ
AMA: 2009, Jan, 11-31; 2008, Jan, 10-25; 2008, Feb, 3-4; 2007, January, 13-27

15115 **Epidermal autograft, face, scalp, eyelids, mouth, neck, ears, orbits, genitalia, hands, feet, and/or multiple digits; first 100 sq cm or less, or 1% of body area of infants and children** A2 T
22.46 25.57 Global Days 090
AMA: 2009, Jan, 11-31; 2008, Jan, 10-25; 2008, Feb, 3-4; 2007, January, 13-27

\+ **15116** **each additional 100 sq cm, or each additional 1% of body area of infants and children, or part thereof (List separately in addition to code for primary procedure)** A2 T
Code first (15115)
4.57 5.03 Global Days ZZZ
AMA: 2009, Jan, 11-31; 2008, Feb, 3-4; 2008, Jan, 10-25; 2007, January, 13-27

15120 **Split-thickness autograft, face, scalp, eyelids, mouth, neck, ears, orbits, genitalia, hands, feet, and/or multiple digits; first 100 sq cm or less, or 1% of body area of infants and children (except 15050)** A2 T
EXCLUDES *Other eyelid repair (67961-67975)*
21.08 25.53 Global Days 090
AMA: 2009, Jan, 11-31; 2008, Feb, 3-4; 2008, Jul, 5-6&15; 2008, Jan, 10-25; 2007, January, 13-27

\+ **15121** **each additional 100 sq cm, or each additional 1% of body area of infants and children, or part thereof (List separately in addition to code for primary procedure)** A2 T
EXCLUDES *Other eyelid repair (67961-67975)*
Code first (15120)
4.00 6.37 Global Days ZZZ
AMA: 2009, Jan, 11-31; 2008, Feb, 3-4; 2008, Jan, 10-25; 2007, January, 13-27

15130 **Dermal autograft, trunk, arms, legs; first 100 sq cm or less, or 1% of body area of infants and children** A2 T
16.78 19.96 Global Days 090
AMA: 2009, Jan, 11-31; 2008, Feb, 3-4; 2008, Jan, 10-25; 2007, January, 13-27

\+ **15131** **each additional 100 sq cm, or each additional 1% of body area of infants and children, or part thereof (List separately in addition to code for primary procedure)** A2 T
Code first (15130)
2.74 3.00 Global Days ZZZ
AMA: 2009, Jan, 11-31; 2008, Jan, 10-25; 2008, Feb, 3-4; 2007, January, 13-27

15135 **Dermal autograft, face, scalp, eyelids, mouth, neck, ears, orbits, genitalia, hands, feet, and/or multiple digits; first 100 sq cm or less, or 1% of body area of infants and children** A2 T
22.69 25.74 Global Days 090
AMA: 2009, Jan, 11-31; 2008, Jan, 10-25; 2008, Feb, 3-4; 2007, January, 13-27

\+ **15136** **each additional 100 sq cm, or each additional 1% of body area of infants and children, or part thereof (List separately in addition to code for primary procedure)** A2 T
Code first (15135)
2.36 2.54 Global Days ZZZ
AMA: 2009, Jan, 11-31; 2008, Feb, 3-4; 2008, Jan, 10-25; 2007, January, 13-27

▲ **15150** **Tissue cultured skin autograft, trunk, arms, legs; first 25 sq cm or less** A2 T
18.61 20.37 Global Days 090
AMA: 2009, Jan, 11-31; 2008, Jan, 10-25; 2008, Feb, 3-4; 2007, January, 13-27

\+ ▲ **15151** **additional 1 sq cm to 75 sq cm (List separately in addition to code for primary procedure)** A2 T
EXCLUDES *Grafts over 75 sq cm (15152)*
Code first (15150)
3.26 3.55 Global Days ZZZ
AMA: 2009, Jan, 11-31; 2008, Feb, 3-4; 2008, Jan, 10-25; 2007, January, 13-27

\+ ▲ **15152** **each additional 100 sq cm, or each additional 1% of body area of infants and children, or part thereof (List separately in addition to code for primary procedure)** A2 T
Code first (15151)
4.60 4.90 Global Days ZZZ
AMA: 2009, Jan, 11-31; 2008, Jan, 10-25; 2008, Feb, 3-4; 2007, January, 13-27

▲ **15155** **Tissue cultured skin autograft, face, scalp, eyelids, mouth, neck, ears, orbits, genitalia, hands, feet, and/or multiple digits; first 25 sq cm or less** A2 T
18.49 20.24 Global Days 090
AMA: 2009, Jan, 11-31; 2008, Feb, 3-4; 2008, Jan, 10-25; 2007, January, 13-27

\+ ▲ **15156** **additional 1 sq cm to 75 sq cm (List separately in addition to code for primary procedure)** A2 T
Code first (15155)
EXCLUDES *Grafts over 75 sq cm (15157)*
5.00 5.27 Global Days ZZZ
AMA: 2009, Jan, 11-31; 2008, Feb, 3-4; 2008, Jan, 10-25; 2007, January, 13-27

\+ ▲ **15157** **each additional 100 sq cm, or each additional 1% of body area of infants and children, or part thereof (List separately in addition to code for primary procedure)** A2 T
Code first (15156)
4.94 5.33 Global Days ZZZ
AMA: 2009, Jan, 11-31; 2008, Feb, 3-4; 2008, Jan, 10-25; 2007, January, 13-27

~~15170~~ ~~**Acellular dermal replacement, trunk, arms, legs; first 100 sq cm or less, or 1% of body area of infants and children**~~
To report, see 15271, 15273

~~15171~~ ~~**each additional 100 sq cm, or each additional 1% of body area of infants and children, or part thereof (List separately in addition to code for primary procedure)**~~
To report, see 15272, 15274

~~15175~~ ~~**Acellular dermal replacement, face, scalp, eyelids, mouth, neck, ears, orbits, genitalia, hands, feet, and/or multiple digits; first 100 sq cm or less, or 1% of body area of infants and children**~~
To report, see 15275, 15277

~~15176~~ ~~**each additional 100 sq cm, or each additional 1% of body area of infants and children, or part thereof (List separately in addition to code for primary procedure)**~~
To report, see 15276, 15278

15200 **Full thickness graft, free, including direct closure of donor site, trunk; 20 sq cm or less** A2 T
19.84 24.37 Global Days 090
AMA: 2009, Jan, 11-31; 2008, Jan, 10-25; 2008, Mar, 14-15; 2008, Feb, 3-4; 2007, January, 13-27

+ **15201** **each additional 20 sq cm, or part thereof (List separately in addition to code for primary procedure)** A2 T
Code first (15200)
2.38 4.43 Global Days ZZZ
AMA: 2009, Jan, 11-31; 2008, Jan, 10-25; 2008, Mar, 14-15; 2008, Feb, 3-4; 2007, January, 13-27

15220 **Full thickness graft, free, including direct closure of donor site, scalp, arms, and/or legs; 20 sq cm or less** A2 T
18.38 22.82 Global Days 090
AMA: 2009, Jan, 11-31; 2008, Mar, 14-15; 2008, Feb, 3-4; 2008, Jan, 10-25; 2007, January, 13-27

+ **15221** **each additional 20 sq cm, or part thereof (List separately in addition to code for primary procedure)** A2 T
Code first (15220)
2.15 4.08 Global Days ZZZ
AMA: 2009, Jan, 11-31; 2008, Feb, 3-4; 2008, Mar, 14-15; 2008, Jan, 10-25; 2007, January, 13-27

15240 **Full thickness graft, free, including direct closure of donor site, forehead, cheeks, chin, mouth, neck, axillae, genitalia, hands, and/or feet; 20 sq cm or less** A2 T
EXCLUDES *Finger tip graft (15050)*
Syndactyly repair fingers (26560-26562)
23.86 27.56 Global Days 090
AMA: 2009, Jan, 11-31; 2008, Mar, 14-15; 2008, Jan, 10-25; 2008, Feb, 3-4; 2007, January, 13-27

+ **15241** **each additional 20 sq cm, or part thereof (List separately in addition to code for primary procedure)** A2 T
Code first (15240)
3.34 5.48 Global Days ZZZ
AMA: 2009, Jan, 11-31; 2008, Feb, 3-4; 2008, Mar, 14-15; 2008, Jan, 10-25; 2007, January, 13-27

15260 **Full thickness graft, free, including direct closure of donor site, nose, ears, eyelids, and/or lips; 20 sq cm or less** A2 T
EXCLUDES *Other eyelid repair (67961-67975)*
25.63 29.84 Global Days 090
AMA: 2009, Jan, 11-31; 2008, Mar, 14-15; 2008, Feb, 3-4; 2008, Jan, 10-25; 2007, January, 13-27

+ **15261** **each additional 20 sq cm, or part thereof (List separately in addition to code for primary procedure)** A2 T
Code first (15260)
EXCLUDES *Other eyelid repair (67961-67975)*
4.23 6.41 Global Days ZZZ
AMA: 2009, Jan, 11-31; 2008, Mar, 14-15; 2008, Jan, 10-25; 2008, Feb, 3-4; 2007, January, 13-27

15271-15278 Skin Substitute Graft Application

INCLUDES Add together the surface area of multiple wounds in the same anatomical locations as indicated in the code description groups, such as face and scalp. Do not add together multiple wounds at different anatomical site groups such as trunk and face.
Ankle or wrist if code description describes leg or arm
Code selection based on defect site location and size
Fixation and anchoring skin graft
Nonautologous human skin such as:
- Accelular
- Biological material used for scaffolding for growing skin
- Cellular
- Dermal
- Epidermal
- Nonhuman grafts

Percentage applies to children age 9 or younger
Removing current graft
Simple cleaning
Simple tissue debridement
Square centimeters applies to age 10 or older

Code also primary procedure requiring skin graft for definitive closure
Code also supply of skin substitute product
Do not report for application of nongraft dressing
Do not report for injected skin substitutes
Do not report with (97602)

● **15271** **Application of skin substitute graft to trunk, arms, legs, total wound surface area up to 100 sq cm; first 25 sq cm or less wound surface area** G2 T
EXCLUDES *Total wound area greater than or equal to 100 sq cm (15273-15274)*
Do not report with (15273-15274)
2.58 4.24 Global Days 000

+ ● **15272** **each additional 25 sq cm wound surface area, or part thereof (List separately in addition to code for primary procedure)** G2 T
EXCLUDES *Total wound area greater than or equal to 100 sq cm (15273-15274)*
Code first (15271)
Do not report with (15273-15274)
0.51 0.80 Global Days ZZZ

● **15273** **Application of skin substitute graft to trunk, arms, legs, total wound surface area greater than or equal to 100 sq cm; first 100 sq cm wound surface area, or 1% of body area of infants and children** G2 T
EXCLUDES *Total wound surface area up to 100 cm (15271-15272)*
Do not report with (15271-15272)
6.15 8.71 Global Days 000

+ ● **15274** **each additional 100 sq cm wound surface area, or part thereof, or each additional 1% of body area of infants and children, or part thereof (List separately in addition to code for primary procedure)** G2 T
EXCLUDES *Total wound surface area up to 100 cm (15271-15272)*
Code first (15273)
1.30 2.05 Global Days ZZZ

● **15275** **Application of skin substitute graft to face, scalp, eyelids, mouth, neck, ears, orbits, genitalia, hands, feet, and/or multiple digits, total wound surface area up to 100 sq cm; first 25 sq cm or less wound surface area** G2 T

EXCLUDES *Total wound area greater than or equal to 100 sq cm (15277-15278)*

Do not report with (15277-15278)

2.99 4.55 Global Days 000

\+ ● **15276** **each additional 25 sq cm wound surface area, or part thereof (List separately in addition to code for primary procedure)** G2 T

EXCLUDES *Total wound area greater than or equal to 100 sq cm (15277-15278)*

Code first (15275)

Do not report with (15277-15278)

0.73 0.99 Global Days ZZZ

● **15277** **Application of skin substitute graft to face, scalp, eyelids, mouth, neck, ears, orbits, genitalia, hands, feet, and/or multiple digits, total wound surface area greater than or equal to 100 sq cm; first 100 sq cm wound surface area, or 1% of body area of infants and children** G2 T

EXCLUDES *Mesh insertion or other implant for open incisional or ventral hernia repair (49560-49566, 49568)*
Total surface area up to 100 sq cm (15275-15276)

Do not report with (15275-15276)

6.35 8.76 Global Days 000

\+ ● **15278** **each additional 100 sq cm wound surface area, or part thereof, or each additional 1% of body area of infants and children, or part thereof (List separately in addition to code for primary procedure)** G2 T

EXCLUDES *Total surface area up to 100 sq cm (15275-15276)*

Code first (15277)

Do not report with (15275-15276)

1.61 2.42 Global Days ZZZ

15300-15366 Homografts

CMS 100-4,3,20.1.2.8 Special Payments for Burn Cases
CMS 100-4,4,20.5 HCPCS Under OPPS

~~15300~~ ~~Allograft skin for temporary wound closure, trunk, arms, legs; first 100 sq cm or less, or 1% of body area of infants and children~~
To report, see 15271, 15273

~~15301~~ ~~each additional 100 sq cm, or each additional 1% of body area of infants and children, or part thereof (List separately in addition to code for primary procedure)~~
To report, see 15272, 15274

~~15320~~ ~~Allograft skin for temporary wound closure, face, scalp, eyelids, mouth, neck, ears, orbits, genitalia, hands, feet, and/or multiple digits; first 100 sq cm or less, or 1% of body area of infants and children~~
To report, see 15275, 15277

~~15321~~ ~~each additional 100 sq cm, or each additional 1% of body area of infants and children, or part thereof (List separately in addition to code for primary procedure)~~
To report, see 15276, 15278

~~15330~~ ~~Acellular dermal allograft, trunk, arms, legs; first 100 sq cm or less, or 1% of body area of infants and children~~
To report, see 15271, 15273

~~15331~~ ~~each additional 100 sq cm, or each additional 1% of body area of infants and children, or part thereof (List separately in addition to code for primary procedure)~~
To report, see 15272, 15274

~~15335~~ ~~Acellular dermal allograft, face, scalp, eyelids, mouth, neck, ears, orbits, genitalia, hands, feet, and/or multiple digits; first 100 sq cm or less, or 1% of body area of infants and children~~
To report, see 15275, 15277

~~15336~~ ~~each additional 100 sq cm, or each additional 1% of body area of infants and children, or part thereof (List separately in addition to code for primary procedure)~~
To report, see 15276, 15278

~~15340~~ ~~Tissue cultured allogeneic skin substitute; first 25 sq cm or less~~
To report, see 15271, 15273, 15275, 15277

~~15341~~ ~~each additional 25 sq cm, or part thereof (List separately in addition to code for primary procedure)~~
To report, see 15272, 15274, 15276, 15278

~~15360~~ ~~Tissue cultured allogeneic dermal substitute, trunk, arms, legs; first 100 sq cm or less, or 1% of body area of infants and children~~
To report, see 15271, 15273

~~15361~~ ~~each additional 100 sq cm, or each additional 1% of body area of infants and children, or part thereof (List separately in addition to code for primary procedure)~~
To report, see 15272, 15274

~~15365~~ ~~Tissue cultured allogeneic dermal substitute, face, scalp, eyelids, mouth, neck, ears, orbits, genitalia, hands, feet, and/or multiple digits; first 100 sq cm or less, or 1% of body area of infants and children~~
To report, see 15275, 15277

~~15366~~ ~~each additional 100 sq cm, or each additional 1% of body area of infants and children, or part thereof (List separately in addition to code for primary procedure)~~
To report, see 15276, 15278

15400-15431 Heterografts

CMS 100-4,3,20.1.2.8 Special Payments for Burn Cases

~~15400~~ ~~Xenograft, skin (dermal), for temporary wound closure, trunk, arms, legs; first 100 sq cm or less, or 1% of body area of infants and children~~
To report, see 15271, 15273

~~15401~~ ~~each additional 100 sq cm, or each additional 1% of body area of infants and children, or part thereof (List separately in addition to code for primary procedure)~~
To report, see 15272, 15274

~~15420~~ ~~Xenograft skin (dermal), for temporary wound closure, face, scalp, eyelids, mouth, neck, ears, orbits, genitalia, hands, feet, and/or multiple digits; first 100 sq cm or less, or 1% of body area of infants and children~~
To report, see 15275, 15277

~~15421 each additional 100 sq cm, or each additional 1% of body area of infants and children, or part thereof (List separately in addition to code for primary procedure)~~

To report, see 15276, 15278

~~15430 Acellular xenograft implant; first 100 sq cm or less, or 1% of body area of infants and children~~

To report, see 15271, 15273, 15275, 15277

~~15431 each additional 100 sq cm, or each additional 1% of body area of infants and children, or part thereof (List separately in addition to code for primary procedure)~~

To report, see 15272, 15274, 15276, 15278

15570-15738 Wound Reconstruction: Skin Flaps

CMS 100-4,3,20.1.2.8 Special Payments for Burn Cases
CMS 100-4,4,20.5 HCPCS Under OPPS

INCLUDES Ankle or wrist if code description describes leg or arm
Code based on recipient site
Fixation and anchoring skin graft
Routine dressing
Simple tissue debridement
Tube formation for later transfer

EXCLUDES *Debridement without immediate primary closure (11042-11047 [11045, 11046], 97597-97598)*
Excision of:
Benign lesion (11400-11471)
Burn eschar or scar (15002-15005)
Malignant lesion (11600-11646)
Microvascular repair (15756-15758)
Primary procedure such as radical mastectomy, extensive tumor removal, orbitectomy (see appropriate anatomical site)

Code also application of extensive immobilization apparatus
Code also repair of donor site with skin grafts or flaps

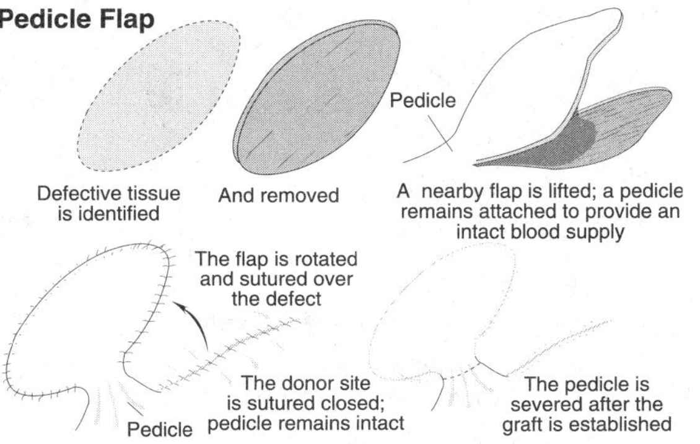

15570 Formation of direct or tubed pedicle, with or without transfer; trunk A2 T CCI
21.75 26.84 Global Days 090

15572 scalp, arms, or legs A2 T CCI
22.00 26.00 Global Days 090

15574 forehead, cheeks, chin, mouth, neck, axillae, genitalia, hands or feet A2 T CCI
22.76 26.94 Global Days 090

15576 eyelids, nose, ears, lips, or intraoral A2 T CCI
20.02 23.87 Global Days 090

15600 Delay of flap or sectioning of flap (division and inset); at trunk A2 T 80 CCI
6.20 9.74 Global Days 090

15610 at scalp, arms, or legs A2 T 80 CCI
7.20 10.42 Global Days 090

15620 at forehead, cheeks, chin, neck, axillae, genitalia, hands, or feet A2 T CCI
9.66 13.03 Global Days 090

15630 at eyelids, nose, ears, or lips A2 T CCI
10.36 13.69 Global Days 090

15650 Transfer, intermediate, of any pedicle flap (eg, abdomen to wrist, Walking tube), any location A2 T 80 CCI
EXCLUDES *Defatting, revision, or rearranging of transferred pedicle flap or skin graft (13100-14302)*
11.50 15.13 Global Days 090

15731 Forehead flap with preservation of vascular pedicle (eg, axial pattern flap, paramedian forehead flap) A2 T 80
EXCLUDES *Muscle, myocutaneous, or fasciocutaneous flap of the head or neck (15732)*
30.40 33.78 Global Days 090

15732 Muscle, myocutaneous, or fasciocutaneous flap; head and neck (eg, temporalis, masseter muscle, sternocleidomastoid, levator scapulae) A2 T CCI
EXCLUDES *Forehead flap with preservation of vascular pedicle (15731)*
34.00 38.75 Global Days 090

15734 trunk A2 T 80 CCI PQ
39.74 44.95 Global Days 090

15736 upper extremity A2 T CCI
34.42 39.61 Global Days 090

15738 lower extremity A2 T 80 CCI PQ
37.23 42.15 Global Days 090
AMA: 2009, Jan, 11-31; 2008, Jan, 10-25; 2007, January, 13-27

15740-15758 Wound Reconstruction: Other

CMS 100-4,3,20.1.2.8 Special Payments for Burn Cases
CMS 104-4,12,30 Correct Coding Policy

INCLUDES Fixation and anchoring skin graft
Routine dressing
Simple tissue debridement

EXCLUDES *Adjacent tissue transfer (14000-14302)*
Skin graft for repair of donor site (15050-15278)
Excision of:
Benign lesion (11400-11471)
Burn eschar or scar (15002-15005)
Malignant lesion (11600-11646)
Flaps without addition of a vascular pedicle (15570-15576)
Primary procedure such as radical mastectomy, extensive tumor removal, orbitectomy (see appropriate anatomical section)

Code also repair of donor site with skin grafts or flaps (14000-14350, 15050-15278)

15740 Flap; island pedicle A2 T CCI
EXCLUDES *V-Y subcutaneous flaps, random island flaps, and other flaps from adjacent areas (14000-14302)*
25.54 30.08 Global Days 090
AMA: 2009, Jan, 11-31; 2008, Jan, 10-25; 2007, January, 13-27

15750 neurovascular pedicle A2 T 80 CCI
EXCLUDES *V-Y subcutaneous flaps, random island flaps, and other flaps from adjacent areas (14000-14302)*
27.17 27.17 Global Days 090

15756 **Free muscle or myocutaneous flap with microvascular anastomosis** C5 C 80

INCLUDES Includes operating microscope (69990)

70.26 70.26 Global Days 090

15757 **Free skin flap with microvascular anastomosis** C5 C 80

INCLUDES Includes operating microscope (69990)

69.00 69.00 Global Days 090

15758 **Free fascial flap with microvascular anastomosis** C5 C 80

INCLUDES Includes operating microscope (69990)

69.14 69.14 Global Days 090

15760-15770 Grafts Comprising Multiple Tissue Types

CMS 100-4,3,20.1.2.8 Special Payments for Burn Cases
CMS 100-4,4,20.5 HCPCS Under OPPS

INCLUDES Fixation and anchoring skin graft
Routine dressing
Simple tissue debridement

EXCLUDES *Adjacent tissue transfer (14000-14302)*
Excision of:
Benign lesion (11400-11471)
Burn eschar or scar (15002-15005)
Malignant lesion (11600-11646)
Flaps without addition of vascular pedicle (15570-15576)
Microvascular repair (15756-15758)
Primary procedure such as extensive tumor removal (see appropriate anatomical site)
Repair of donor site with skin grafts or flaps (14000-14350, 15050-15278)
Skin graft (15050-15278)

15760 **Graft; composite (eg, full thickness of external ear or nasal ala), including primary closure, donor area** A2 T

21.17 25.29 Global Days 090

15770 **derma-fat-fascia** A2 T 80

19.96 19.96 Global Days 090

15775-15839 Plastic, Reconstructive, and Aesthetic Surgery

CMS 100-2,16,10 Exclusions from Coverage
CMS 100-2,16,120 Cosmetic Procedures
CMS 100-2,16,180 Services Related to Noncovered Procedures

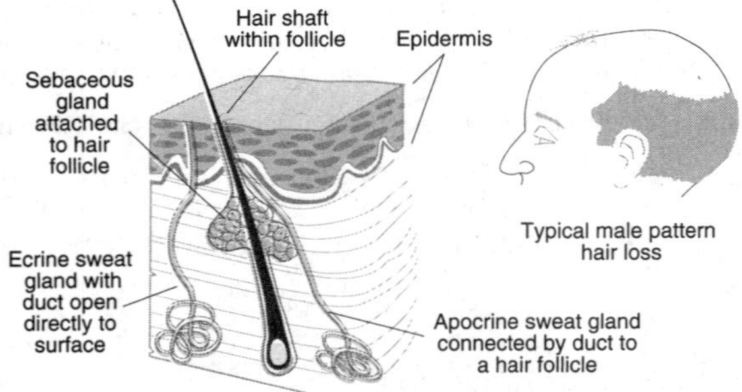

Alopecia means hair loss and the condition is separated into two major categories: that which occurs with associated, visible scalp disease, and that which occurs in the absence of visible disease. Male and female pattern hair loss is of the latter category. Hirsutism is excess hair growth, particularly in women, and is often a sign of a systemic medical syndrome

15775 **Punch graft for hair transplant; 1 to 15 punch grafts** A2 T 80

EXCLUDES *Strip transplant (15220)*

6.26 8.54 Global Days 000

15776 **more than 15 punch grafts** A2 T 80

EXCLUDES *Strip transplant (15220)*

8.66 11.79 Global Days 000

+ ● **15777** **Implantation of biologic implant (eg, acellular dermal matrix) for soft tissue reinforcement (eg, breast, trunk) (List separately in addition to code for primary procedure)** G2 T

EXCLUDES *Application of skin substitute to an external wound (15271-15278)*
Mesh implantation for:
Open repair of ventral or incisional hernia (49568)
Repair of devitalized soft tissue infection (49568)
Repair of pelvic floor (57267)

Code first primary procedure

6.29 6.29 Global Days ZZZ

15780 **Dermabrasion; total face (eg, for acne scarring, fine wrinkling, rhytids, general keratosis)** P3 T 80

18.66 24.50 Global Days 090

AMA: 2009, Jan, 11-31; 2008, Jan, 10-25; 2007, January, 13-27

15781 **segmental, face** P2 T

12.79 16.13 Global Days 090

15782 **regional, other than face** P2 T 80

12.67 17.58 Global Days 090

15783 **superficial, any site (eg, tattoo removal)** P2 T 80

11.09 14.33 Global Days 090

15786 **Abrasion; single lesion (eg, keratosis, scar)** P2 T

4.08 7.21 Global Days 010

+ **15787** **each additional 4 lesions or less (List separately in addition to code for primary procedure)** P3 T

Code first (15786)

0.52 1.44 Global Days ZZZ

15788 **Chemical peel, facial; epidermal** P2 T

7.38 13.50 Global Days 090

15789 **dermal** P2 T

12.51 16.42 Global Days 090

15792 **Chemical peel, nonfacial; epidermal** P2 T 80

7.82 12.86 Global Days 090

15793 **dermal** P2 T 80

10.79 14.40 Global Days 090

15819 **Cervicoplasty** G2 T 80

22.38 22.38 Global Days 090

15820 **Blepharoplasty, lower eyelid;** A2 T 80 50

15.19 16.75 Global Days 090

AMA: 2009, Jan, 11-31; 2008, Jan, 10-25; 2007, January, 13-27

15821 **with extensive herniated fat pad** A2 T 80 50

16.15 17.91 Global Days 090

15822 **Blepharoplasty, upper eyelid;** A2 T 50

11.52 13.05 Global Days 090

15823 **with excessive skin weighting down lid** A2 T 50

16.38 18.13 Global Days 090

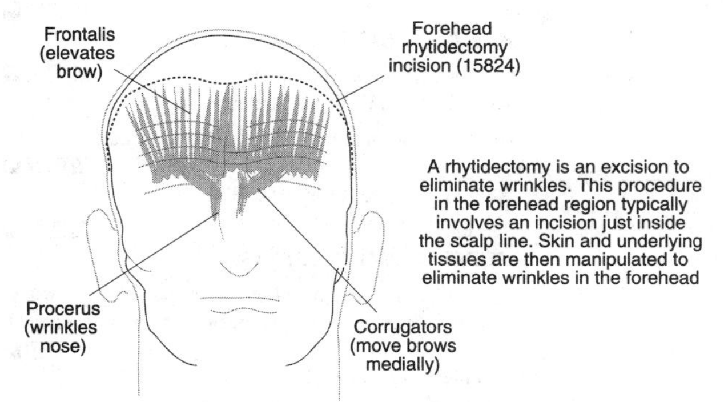

15824 Rhytidectomy; forehead A2 T 80 50

EXCLUDES *Repair of brow ptosis (67900)*

0.00 0.00 Global Days 000

15825 neck with platysmal tightening (platysmal flap, P-flap) A2 T 80 50

0.00 0.00 Global Days 000

15826 glabellar frown lines A2 T 80 50

0.00 0.00 Global Days 000

15828 cheek, chin, and neck A2 T 80 50

0.00 0.00 Global Days 000

15829 superficial musculoaponeurotic system (SMAS) flap A2 T 80 50

0.00 0.00 Global Days 000

15830 Excision, excessive skin and subcutaneous tissue (includes lipectomy); abdomen, infraumbilical panniculectomy A2 T 80

EXCLUDES *Other abdominoplasty (17999)*

Code also (15847)

Do not report with (12031-12032, 12034-12037, 13100-13102, 14000-14001, 14302)

34.64 34.64 Global Days 090

15832 thigh A2 T 80

26.82 26.82 Global Days 090

15833 leg A2 T 80

25.98 25.98 Global Days 090

15834 hip A2 T 80

26.33 26.33 Global Days 090

15835 buttock A2 T 80

25.19 25.19 Global Days 090

15836 arm A2 T 80

22.25 22.25 Global Days 090

15837 forearm or hand G2 T 80

20.96 25.32 Global Days 090

15838 submental fat pad G2 T 80

17.05 17.05 Global Days 090

15839 other area A2 T 80

21.70 25.82 Global Days 090

15840-15845 Reanimation of the Paralyzed Face

CMS 100-2,15,260 Covered ASC Procedures
CMS 100-4,4,20.5 HCPCS Under OPPS
CMS 100-4,12,40.7 Bilateral Procedures
CMS 100-4,12,90.3 MD Services in ASCs

INCLUDES Routine dressing and supplies

EXCLUDES *Intravenous fluorescein evaluation of blood flow in graft or flap (15860)*
Nerve:
Decompression (69720, 69725, 69955)
Pedicle transfer (64905, 64907)
Suture (64831-64876, 69740, 69745)

Code also repair of donor site with skin grafts or flaps

15840 Graft for facial nerve paralysis; free fascia graft (including obtaining fascia) A2 T

30.32 30.32 Global Days 090

15841 free muscle graft (including obtaining graft) A2 T 80

48.08 48.08 Global Days 090

15842 free muscle flap by microsurgical technique G2 T 80

INCLUDES Operating microscope (69990)

73.71 73.71 Global Days 090

15845 regional muscle transfer A2 T 80

29.14 29.14 Global Days 090

15847 Removal of Excess Abdominal Tissue Add-on

+ **15847 Excision, excessive skin and subcutaneous tissue (includes lipectomy), abdomen (eg, abdominoplasty) (includes umbilical transposition and fascial plication) (List separately in addition to code for primary procedure)** A2 T 80

Code first (15830)

EXCLUDES *Abdominal wall hernia repair (49491-49587)*
Other abdominoplasty (17999)

0.00 0.00 Global Days YYY

15850-15852 Suture Removal/Dressing Change: Anesthesia Required

CMS 100-4,12,40.1 Global Surgery Package Definition
CMS 100-4,12,50 Anesthesia Services

15850 Removal of sutures under anesthesia (other than local), same surgeon G2 T

1.15 2.52 Global Days XXX

15851 Removal of sutures under anesthesia (other than local), other surgeon P3 T

1.36 2.86 Global Days 000

15852 Dressing change (for other than burns) under anesthesia (other than local) R2 X

EXCLUDES *Dressing change for burns (16020-16030)*

1.38 1.38 Global Days 000

15860 Injection for Vascular Flow Determination

15860 Intravenous injection of agent (eg, fluorescein) to test vascular flow in flap or graft G2 X 80

3.27 3.27 Global Days 000

15876-15879 Liposuction

CMS 100-2,16,10 Exclusions from Coverage
CMS 100-2,16,120 Cosmetic Procedures
CMS 100-2,16,180 Services Related to Noncovered Procedures
CMS 100-4,12,20.4.3 Payment for Assistant at Surgery

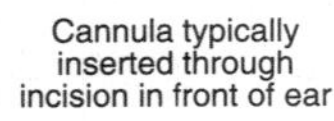

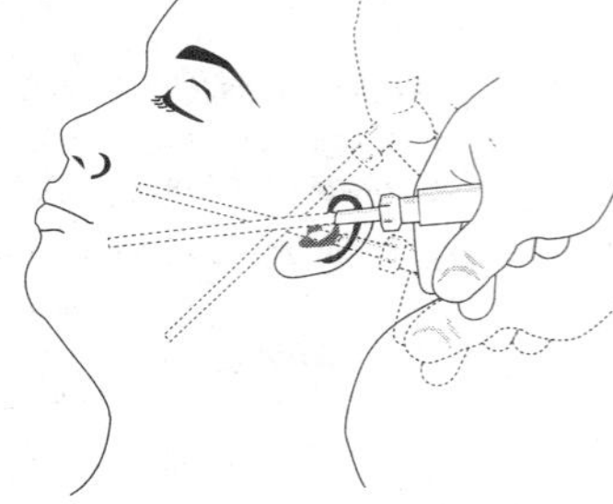

In 15876, a liposuction cannula is inserted through fat deposits creating tunnels and removing excess deposits

15876 **Suction assisted lipectomy; head and neck** A2 T 80
0.00 0.00 Global Days 000

15877 **trunk** A2 T 80
0.00 0.00 Global Days 000
AMA: 2009, Jan, 11-31; 2008, Jan, 10-25; 2007, January, 13-27

15878 **upper extremity** A2 T 80 50
0.00 0.00 Global Days 000

15879 **lower extremity** A2 T 80 50
0.00 0.00 Global Days 000

15920-15999 Treatment of Decubitus Ulcers

CMS 100-3,270.4 Treatment of Decubitus
CMS 100-4,12,20.4.3 Payment for Assistant at Surgery
CMS 100-4,12,40.6 Multiple procedures
CMS 100-4,12,40.8 Co-surgery and team surgery
Code also free skin graft to repair ulcer or donor site

15920 **Excision, coccygeal pressure ulcer, with coccygectomy; with primary suture** A2 T 80
18.00 18.00 Global Days 090

15922 **with flap closure** A2 T 80
23.18 23.18 Global Days 090

15931 **Excision, sacral pressure ulcer, with primary suture;** A2 T
19.96 19.96 Global Days 090

15933 **with ostectomy** A2 T 80
24.76 24.76 Global Days 090

15934 **Excision, sacral pressure ulcer, with skin flap closure;** A2 T
27.22 27.22 Global Days 090

15935 **with ostectomy** A2 T 80
32.74 32.74 Global Days 090

15936 **Excision, sacral pressure ulcer, in preparation for muscle or myocutaneous flap or skin graft closure;** A2 T
Code also any defect repair with:
Muscle or myocutaneous flap (15734, 15738)
Split skin graft (15100-15101)
26.48 26.48 Global Days 090

15937 **with ostectomy** A2 T
Code also any defect repair with:
Muscle or myocutaneous flap (15734, 15738)
Split skin graft (15100-15101)
30.84 30.84 Global Days 090

15940 **Excision, ischial pressure ulcer, with primary suture;** A2 T
20.46 20.46 Global Days 090

15941 **with ostectomy (ischiectomy)** A2 T 80
26.57 26.57 Global Days 090

15944 **Excision, ischial pressure ulcer, with skin flap closure;** A2 T 80
26.59 26.59 Global Days 090

15945 **with ostectomy** A2 T 80
29.43 29.43 Global Days 090

15946 **Excision, ischial pressure ulcer, with ostectomy, in preparation for muscle or myocutaneous flap or skin graft closure** A2 T
Code also any defect repair with:
Muscle or myocutaneous flap (15734, 15738)
Split skin graft (15100-15101)
48.74 48.74 Global Days 090
AMA: 2009, Jan, 11-31; 2008, Jan, 10-25; 2007, January, 13-27

15950 **Excision, trochanteric pressure ulcer, with primary suture;** A2 T
17.16 17.16 Global Days 090

15951 **with ostectomy** A2 T 80
25.89 25.89 Global Days 090

15952 **Excision, trochanteric pressure ulcer, with skin flap closure;** A2 T 80
26.97 26.97 Global Days 090

15953 **with ostectomy** A2 T
29.53 29.53 Global Days 090

15956 **Excision, trochanteric pressure ulcer, in preparation for muscle or myocutaneous flap or skin graft closure;** A2 T
Code also any defect repair with:
Muscle or myocutaneous flap (15734, 15738)
Split skin graft (15100-15101)
34.26 34.26 Global Days 090

15958 **with ostectomy** A2 T
Code also any defect repair with:
Muscle or myocutaneous flap (15734-15738)
Split skin graft (15100-15101)
34.97 34.97 Global Days 090

15999 **Unlisted procedure, excision pressure ulcer** T 80
0.00 0.00 Global Days YYY

16000-16036 Burn Care

CMS 100-4,3,20.1.2.8 Special Payments for Burn Cases

INCLUDES Local care of burn surface only

EXCLUDES *Application of skin grafts including all services described in the following codes (15100-15278)*
Evaluation and management services
Flaps (15570-15650)

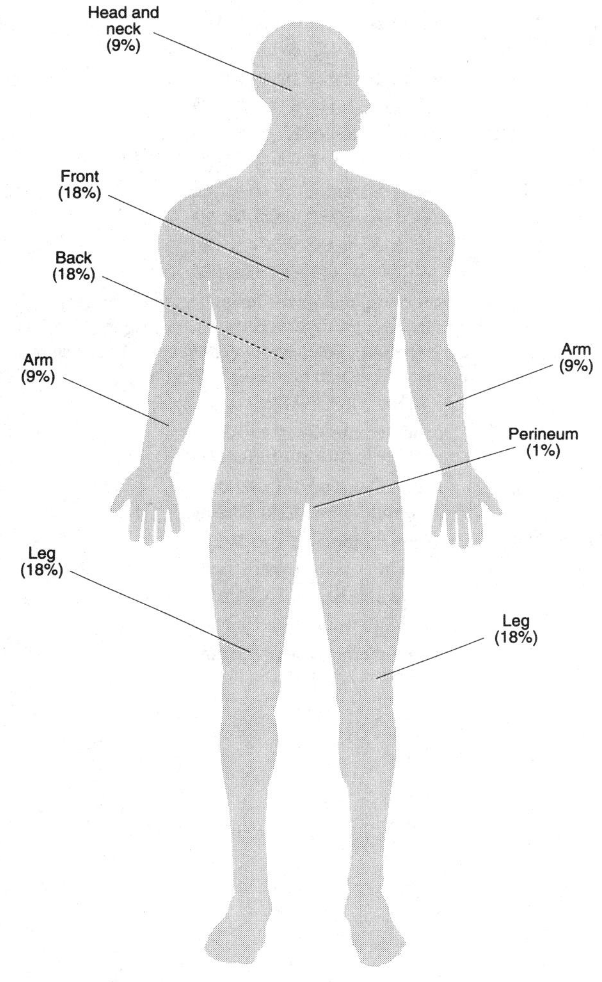

16000 **Initial treatment, first degree burn, when no more than local treatment is required** P3 T
1.35 2.02 Global Days 000

16020 **Dressings and/or debridement of partial-thickness burns, initial or subsequent; small (less than 5% total body surface area)** P3 T
INCLUDES Wound coverage other than skin graft
1.58 2.37 Global Days 000

16025 **medium (eg, whole face or whole extremity, or 5% to 10% total body surface area)** A2 T
INCLUDES Wound coverage other than skin graft
3.29 4.30 Global Days 000
AMA: 2009, Jan, 11-31; 2008, Jun, 14-15

16030 **large (eg, more than 1 extremity, or greater than 10% total body surface area)** A2 T
INCLUDES Wound coverage other than skin graft
3.90 5.31 Global Days 000
AMA: 2009, Jan, 11-31; 2008, Jun, 14-15

16035 **Escharotomy; initial incision** G2 T
EXCLUDES *Debridement or scraping of burn wound (16020-16030)*
5.90 5.90 Global Days 000

+ **16036** **each additional incision (List separately in addition to code for primary procedure)** C5 C
EXCLUDES *Debridement or scraping of burn wound (16020-16030)*
Code first (16035)
2.46 2.46 Global Days ZZZ

17000-17004 Destruction Any Method: Premalignant Lesion

CMS 100-2,16,10 Exclusions from Coverage
CMS 100-2,16,120 Cosmetic Procedures
CMS 100-2,16,180 Services Related to Noncovered Procedures
CMS 100-3,140.5 Laser Procedures
CMS 100-4,4,20.5 HCPCS Under OPPS
CMS 100-4,12,40.6 Multiple procedures

EXCLUDES *Cryotherapy acne (17340)*
Destruction of lesion of:
- *Anus (46900-46917, 46924)*
- *Conjunctiva (68135)*
- *Eyelid (67850)*
- *Penis (54050-54057, 54065)*
- *Vagina (57061, 57065)*
- *Vestibule of mouth (40820)*
- *Vulva (56501, 56515)*

Destruction of plantar warts (17110-17111)
Destruction or excision of skin tags (11200-11201)
Localized chemotherapy treatment (99201-99499 [99224, 99225, 99226])
Paring or excision of benign hyperkeratotic lesion (11055-11057)
Shaving skin lesions (11300-11313)
Treatment of inflammatory skin disease via laser (96920-96922)

17000 **Destruction (eg, laser surgery, electrosurgery, cryosurgery, chemosurgery, surgical curettement), premalignant lesions (eg, actinic keratoses); first lesion** P2 T
1.65 2.38 Global Days 010
AMA: 2009, Jan, 11-31; 2008, Jan, 10-25; 2007, January, 13-27; 2007, February, 10-11

+ **17003** **second through 14 lesions, each (List separately in addition to code for first lesion)** P3 T
Code first (17000)
0.13 0.21 Global Days ZZZ
AMA: 2009, Jan, 11-31; 2008, Jan, 10-25; 2007, January, 13-27; 2007, February, 10-11

⊘ **17004** **Destruction (eg, laser surgery, electrosurgery, cryosurgery, chemosurgery, surgical curettement), premalignant lesions (eg, actinic keratoses), 15 or more lesions** P3 T
Do not report with (17000-17003)
3.90 5.05 Global Days 010
AMA: 2009, Jan, 11-31; 2008, Jan, 10-25; 2007, February, 10-11; 2007, January, 13-27

17106-17250 Destruction Any Method: Vascular Proliferative Lesion

CMS 100-2,16,10 Exclusions from Coverage
CMS 100-2,16,120 Cosmetic Procedures
CMS 100-2,16,180 Services Related to Noncovered Procedures

EXCLUDES *Destruction of lesion of:*
Anus (46900-46917, 46924)
Conjunctiva (68135)
Eyelid (67850)
Penis (54050-54057, 54065)
Vagina (57061, 57065)
Vestibule of mouth (40820)
Vulva (56501, 56515)
Treatment of inflammatory skin disease via laser (96920-96922)

17106 **Destruction of cutaneous vascular proliferative lesions (eg, laser technique); less than 10 sq cm** P2 T
8.12 10.05 Global Days 090
AMA: 2009, Jan, 11-31; 2008, Jun, 14-15; 2008, Jan, 10-25; 2007, April, 11-12

17107 **10.0 to 50.0 sq cm** P2 T
10.41 12.95 Global Days 090
AMA: 2009, Jan, 11-31; 2008, Jun, 14-15; 2008, Jan, 10-25; 2007, April, 11-12

17108 **over 50.0 sq cm** P2 T 80
15.54 18.87 Global Days 090
AMA: 2009, Jan, 11-31; 2008, Jan, 10-25; 2008, Jun, 14-15; 2007, April, 11-12

17110 **Destruction (eg, laser surgery, electrosurgery, cryosurgery, chemosurgery, surgical curettement), of benign lesions other than skin tags or cutaneous vascular proliferative lesions; up to 14 lesions** P2 T
2.05 3.26 Global Days 010
AMA: 2009, Jan, 11-31; 2008, Nov, 10-11; 2008, Jan, 10-25; 2007, February, 10-11; 2007, April, 11-12

17111 **15 or more lesions** P2 T
2.52 3.86 Global Days 010
AMA: 2009, Jan, 11-31; 2008, Jan, 10-25; 2008, Nov, 10-11; 2007, April, 11-12; 2007, February, 10-11

17250 **Chemical cauterization of granulation tissue (proud flesh, sinus or fistula)** P3 T
Do not report with excision/removal codes for the same lesion
1.07 2.29 Global Days 000

17260-17286 Destruction, Any Method: Malignant Lesion

CMS 100-3,140.5 Laser Procedures
CMS 100-4,12,30 Correct Coding Policy

EXCLUDES *Destruction of lesion of:*
Anus (46900-46917, 46924)
Conjunctiva (68135)
Eyelid (67850)
Localized chemotherapy treatment (99201-99499 [99224, 99225, 99226])
Penis (54050-54057, 54065)
Shaving skin lesion (11300-11313)
Vestibule of mouth (40820)
Vulva (56501-56515)
Treatment of inflammatory skin disease via laser (96920-96922)

17260 **Destruction, malignant lesion (eg, laser surgery, electrosurgery, cryosurgery, chemosurgery, surgical curettement), trunk, arms or legs; lesion diameter 0.5 cm or less** P3 T
2.04 2.78 Global Days 010

17261 **lesion diameter 0.6 to 1.0 cm** P2 T
2.72 4.24 Global Days 010

17262 **lesion diameter 1.1 to 2.0 cm** P2 T
3.45 5.15 Global Days 010

17263 **lesion diameter 2.1 to 3.0 cm** P2 T
3.83 5.63 Global Days 010

17264 **lesion diameter 3.1 to 4.0 cm** P2 T
4.09 6.04 Global Days 010

17266 **lesion diameter over 4.0 cm** P3 T
4.76 6.83 Global Days 010

17270 **Destruction, malignant lesion (eg, laser surgery, electrosurgery, cryosurgery, chemosurgery, surgical curettement), scalp, neck, hands, feet, genitalia; lesion diameter 0.5 cm or less** P2 T
2.96 4.42 Global Days 010

17271 **lesion diameter 0.6 to 1.0 cm** P2 T
3.30 4.82 Global Days 010

17272 **lesion diameter 1.1 to 2.0 cm** P2 T
3.80 5.49 Global Days 010

17273 **lesion diameter 2.1 to 3.0 cm** P3 T
4.29 6.12 Global Days 010

17274 **lesion diameter 3.1 to 4.0 cm** P3 T
5.24 7.22 Global Days 010

17276 **lesion diameter over 4.0 cm** P2 T
6.30 8.39 Global Days 010

17280 **Destruction, malignant lesion (eg, laser surgery, electrosurgery, cryosurgery, chemosurgery, surgical curettement), face, ears, eyelids, nose, lips, mucous membrane; lesion diameter 0.5 cm or less** P2 T
2.69 4.15 Global Days 010

17281 **lesion diameter 0.6 to 1.0 cm** P3 T
3.71 5.24 Global Days 010

17282 **lesion diameter 1.1 to 2.0 cm** P3 T
4.28 6.02 Global Days 010

17283 **lesion diameter 2.1 to 3.0 cm** P3 T
5.34 7.22 Global Days 010

17284 **lesion diameter 3.1 to 4.0 cm** P2 T
6.21 8.23 Global Days 010

17286 **lesion diameter over 4.0 cm** P2 T
8.50 10.65 Global Days 010

17311-17315 Mohs Surgery

CMS 100-4,12,40.1 Global Surgery Package Definition

INCLUDES The following surgical/pathological services performed by the same physician:
Evaluation of skin margins by surgeon
Pathology exam on Mohs surgery specimen (88302-88309)
Routine frozen section stain (88314)
Tumor removal, mapping, preparation, and examination of lesion

EXCLUDES *Frozen section if no prior diagnosis determination has been peformed (88331)*

Code also any special histochemical stain on a frozen section, nonroutine (with modifier 59) (88311-88314, 88342)
Code also biopsy if no prior diagnosis determination has been performed (11100-11101)
Code also complex repair (13100-13160)
Code also flaps or grafts (14000-14350, 15050-15770)
Code also intermediate repair (12031-12057)
Code also simple repair (12001-12021)

17311 Mohs micrographic technique, including removal of all gross tumor, surgical excision of tissue specimens, mapping, color coding of specimens, microscopic examination of specimens by the surgeon, and histopathologic preparation including routine stain(s) (eg, hematoxylin and eosin, toluidine blue), head, neck, hands, feet, genitalia, or any location with surgery directly involving muscle, cartilage, bone, tendon, major nerves, or vessels; first stage, up to 5 tissue blocks P2 T PQ
11.24 19.50 Global Days 000

+ **17312 each additional stage after the first stage, up to 5 tissue blocks (List separately in addition to code for primary procedure)** P3 T
Code first 17311
5.97 11.65 Global Days ZZZ

17313 Mohs micrographic technique, including removal of all gross tumor, surgical excision of tissue specimens, mapping, color coding of specimens, microscopic examination of specimens by the surgeon, and histopathologic preparation including routine stain(s) (eg, hematoxylin and eosin, toluidine blue), of the trunk, arms, or legs; first stage, up to 5 tissue blocks P2 T PQ
10.08 17.80 Global Days 000

+ **17314 each additional stage after the first stage, up to 5 tissue blocks (List separately in addition to code for primary procedure)** P3 T
Code first (17313)
5.54 10.80 Global Days ZZZ

+ **17315 Mohs micrographic technique, including removal of all gross tumor, surgical excision of tissue specimens, mapping, color coding of specimens, microscopic examination of specimens by the surgeon, and histopathologic preparation including routine stain(s) (eg, hematoxylin and eosin, toluidine blue), each additional block after the first 5 tissue blocks, any stage (List separately in addition to code for primary procedure)** P3 T
Code first (17311-17314)
1.57 2.33 Global Days ZZZ

17340-17999 Treatment for Active Acne and Permanent Hair Removal

17340 Cryotherapy (CO2 slush, liquid N2) for acne P3 T
1.41 1.48 Global Days 010

17360 Chemical exfoliation for acne (eg, acne paste, acid) P3 T
2.92 3.81 Global Days 010

17380 Electrolysis epilation, each 30 minutes R2 T 80
EXCLUDES *Actinotherapy (96900)*
0.00 0.00 Global Days 000

17999 Unlisted procedure, skin, mucous membrane and subcutaneous tissue T 80
0.00 0.00 Global Days YYY
AMA: 2009, Jan, 11-31; 2008, Jan, 10-25; 2008, Nov, 10-11; 2007, January, 13-27

19000-19030 Treatment of Breast Abscess and Cyst with Injection, Aspiration, Incision

19000 Puncture aspiration of cyst of breast; P3 T
76942, 77021, 77031, 77032
1.28 3.23 Global Days 000
AMA: 2008, Nov, 10-11

+ **19001 each additional cyst (List separately in addition to code for primary procedure)** P3 T
Code first (19000)
76942, 77021, 77031, 77032
0.63 0.77 Global Days ZZZ

19020 Mastotomy with exploration or drainage of abscess, deep A2 T 50
8.85 13.66 Global Days 090

19030 Injection procedure only for mammary ductogram or galactogram N1 N 50
77053-77054
2.25 4.72 Global Days 000

19100-19103 Breast Biopsy

CMS 100-2,15,260 Covered ASC Procedures
CMS 100-3,220.13 Percutaneous Image-guided Breast Biopsy
CMS 100-4,13,80.1 Supervision and Interpretation Codes
CMS 100-4,13,80.2 Physician Presence

INCLUDES Open removal of breast mass without concentration on surgical margins

EXCLUDES *Lesion removal without concentration on surgical margins (19110-19126)*
Partial mastectomy (19301-19302)
Total mastectomy (19303-19307)

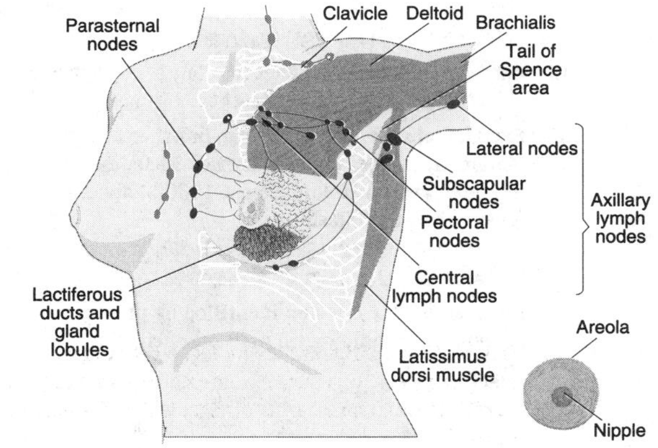

19100 **Biopsy of breast; percutaneous, needle core, not using imaging guidance (separate procedure)** A2 T 50

EXCLUDES *Fine needle aspiration (10021)*
Radiology guided breast biopsy (10022, 19102-19103)

2.03 4.35 Global Days 000
AMA: 2009, Jan, 11-31; 2008, Jan, 10-25; 2008, Nov, 10-11; 2007, January, 13-27

19101 **open, incisional** A2 T 50

6.45 9.92 Global Days 010
AMA: 2009, Jan, 11-31; 2008, Jan, 10-25; 2007, January, 13-27

19102 **percutaneous, needle core, using imaging guidance** A2 T 50

EXCLUDES *Insertion of percutaneous localization clip if appropriate (19295)*

76942, 77002, 77012, 77021, 77031-77032
2.98 6.23 Global Days 000
AMA: 2009, Jan, 11-31; 2008, Jan, 10-25; 2008, Nov, 10-11; 2007, January, 13-27

19103 **percutaneous, automated vacuum assisted or rotating biopsy device, using imaging guidance** A2 T 50

INCLUDES ABBI biopsy

EXCLUDES *Insertion of percutaneous localization clip if appropriate (19295)*

76942, 77012, 77021, 77031-77032
5.57 16.11 Global Days 000
AMA: 2009, Jan, 11-31; 2008, Jan, 10-25; 2008, Nov, 10-11; 2007, January, 13-27

19105 Treatment of Fibroadenoma: Cryoablation

CMS 100-4,13,80.1 Supervision and Interpretation Codes
CMS 100-4,13,80.2 Physician Presence

INCLUDES Adjacent lesions treated with one cryoprobe
Ultrasound guidance

19105 **Ablation, cryosurgical, of fibroadenoma, including ultrasound guidance, each fibroadenoma** P2 T 50

Do not report with (76940, 76942)
5.80 82.53 Global Days 000
AMA: 2007, March, 7-8

19110-19126 Excisional Procedures: Breast

CMS 100-4,12,40.7 Bilateral Procedures

19110 **Nipple exploration, with or without excision of a solitary lactiferous duct or a papilloma lactiferous duct** A2 T 50

9.89 14.06 Global Days 090

19112 **Excision of lactiferous duct fistula** A2 T 80 50

9.03 13.31 Global Days 090

19120 **Excision of cyst, fibroadenoma, or other benign or malignant tumor, aberrant breast tissue, duct lesion, nipple or areolar lesion (except 19300), open, male or female, 1 or more lesions** A2 T 50

11.94 14.21 Global Days 090
AMA: 2009, Jan, 11-31; 2008, Jan, 10-25; 2007, January, 13-27

19125 **Excision of breast lesion identified by preoperative placement of radiological marker, open; single lesion** A2 T 50

13.26 15.76 Global Days 090
AMA: 2009, Jan, 11-31; 2008, Jan, 10-25; 2007, January, 13-27

\+ 19126 **each additional lesion separately identified by a preoperative radiological marker (List separately in addition to code for primary procedure)** A2 T

Code first (19125)
4.70 4.70 Global Days ZZZ
AMA: 2009, Jan, 11-31; 2008, Jan, 10-25; 2007, January, 13-27

19260-19272 Excisional Procedures: Chest Wall

CMS 100-4,12,20.4.3 Payment for Assistant at Surgery

Do not report with (32100, 32422, 32503-32504, 32551)

19260 **Excision of chest wall tumor including ribs** T 80 PQ

35.47 35.47 Global Days 090
AMA: 2007, February, 4-5

19271 **Excision of chest wall tumor involving ribs, with plastic reconstruction; without mediastinal lymphadenectomy** C5 C 80 PQ

48.37 48.37 Global Days 090
AMA: 2007, February, 4-5

19272 **with mediastinal lymphadenectomy** C5 C 80 PQ

53.32 53.32 Global Days 090
AMA: 2007, February, 4-5

19290-19298 Placement of Localization Markers and Brachytherapy Catheters

CMS 100-4,12,40.7 Bilateral Procedures
CMS 100-4,13,80.1 Supervision and Interpretation Codes
CMS 100-4,13,80.2 Physician Presence

19290 **Preoperative placement of needle localization wire, breast;** N1 N 50

76942, 77031-77032
1.87 4.69 Global Days 000

\+ 19291 **each additional lesion (List separately in addition to code for primary procedure)** N1 N

Code first (19290)
76942, 77031-77032
0.92 1.99 Global Days ZZZ

\+ 19295 **Image guided placement, metallic localization clip, percutaneous, during breast biopsy/aspiration (List separately in addition to code for primary procedure)** N1 Q1 80

Code first (10022, 19102-19103)
76942, 77031-77032
2.68 2.68 Global Days ZZZ
AMA: 2009, Jan, 11-31; 2008, Nov, 10-11

19296 **Placement of radiotherapy afterloading expandable catheter (single or multichannel) into the breast for interstitial radioelement application following partial mastectomy, includes imaging guidance; on date separate from partial mastectomy** A2 T 80 50

Code also (C1728)
6.12 120.63 Global Days 000
AMA: 2007, February, 4-5

\+ 19297 **concurrent with partial mastectomy (List separately in addition to code for primary procedure)** A2 T 80

Code also (C1728)
Code first (19301-19302)
2.75 2.75 Global Days ZZZ
AMA: 2007, February, 4-5

⊙ 19298 **Placement of radiotherapy afterloading brachytherapy catheters (multiple tube and button type) into the breast for interstitial radioelement application following (at the time of or subsequent to) partial mastectomy, includes imaging guidance** A2 T 80 50

Code also (C1728)
9.38 34.04 Global Days 000
AMA: 2007, February, 4-5

19300-19307 Mastectomies: Partial, Simple, Radical

CMS 100-4,12,20.4.3 Payment for Assistant at Surgery
CMS 100-4,12,40.7 Bilateral Procedures
EXCLUDES *Instantaneous or postponed insertion of prosthesis (19340, 19342)*

19300 Mastectomy for gynecomastia ♂ A2 T 50
11.87 15.16 Global Days 090
AMA: 2007, February, 4-5

19301 Mastectomy, partial (eg, lumpectomy, tylectomy, quadrantectomy, segmentectomy); A2 T 80 50 PQ
EXCLUDES *Insertion of radiotherapy afterloading balloon or brachytherapy catheters (19296-19298)*
18.81 18.81 Global Days 090
AMA: 2009, Jan, 11-31; 2008, Sep, 5-6; 2007, Dec, 7-8; 2007, February, 4-5

19302 with axillary lymphadenectomy A2 T 80 50 PQ
EXCLUDES *Insertion of radiotherapy afterloading balloon or brachytherapy catheters (19296-19298)*
26.02 26.02 Global Days 090
AMA: 2009, Jan, 11-31; 2008, Jan, 10-25; 2008, Sep, 5-6; 2007, Dec, 7-8; 2007, February, 4-5

19303 Mastectomy, simple, complete A2 T 80 50 PQ
EXCLUDES *Gynecomastia (19300)*
29.14 29.14 Global Days 090
AMA: 2007, February, 4-5

19304 Mastectomy, subcutaneous A2 T 80 50 PQ
16.64 16.64 Global Days 090
AMA: 2009, Jan, 11-31; 2008, Jan, 10-25; 2007, February, 4-5; 2007, Dec, 7-8

19305 Mastectomy, radical, including pectoral muscles, axillary lymph nodes C5 C 80 50 PQ
32.83 32.83 Global Days 090
AMA: 2008, Sep, 5-6; 2007, February, 4-5

19306 Mastectomy, radical, including pectoral muscles, axillary and internal mammary lymph nodes (Urban type operation) C5 C 80 50 PQ
34.74 34.74 Global Days 090
AMA: 2008, Sep, 5-6; 2007, February, 4-5

19307 Mastectomy, modified radical, including axillary lymph nodes, with or without pectoralis minor muscle, but excluding pectoralis major muscle T 80 50 PQ
34.63 34.63 Global Days 090
AMA: 2008, Sep, 5-6; 2007, February, 4-5

19316-19499 Plastic, Reconstructive, and Aesthetic Breast Procedures

CMS 100-2,16,120 Cosmetic Procedures
CMS 100-2,16,180 Services Related to Noncovered Procedures
CMS 100-3,140.2 Breast Reconstruction Following Mastectomy
CMS 100-4,12,40.7 Bilateral Procedures
Code also biologic implant for tissue reinforcement (15777)

19316 Mastopexy A2 T 80 50 PQ
22.99 22.99 Global Days 090

19318 Reduction mammaplasty ♀ A2 T 80 50 PQ
INCLUDES Aries-Pitanguy mammaplasty
Biesenberger mammaplasty
33.23 33.23 Global Days 090
AMA: 2009, Jan, 11-31; 2008, Jan, 10-25; 2007, January, 13-27

19324 Mammaplasty, augmentation; without prosthetic implant A2 T 80 50 PQ
14.31 14.31 Global Days 090

19325 with prosthetic implant A2 T 80 50 PQ
EXCLUDES *Flap or graft (15100-15650)*
Code also (C1789, L8600)
19.32 19.32 Global Days 090

19328 Removal of intact mammary implant A2 T 50 PQ
14.78 14.78 Global Days 090

19330 Removal of mammary implant material A2 T 50 PQ
18.87 18.87 Global Days 090
AMA: 2009, Jan, 11-31; 2008, Jan, 10-25; 2007, January, 13-27

19340 Immediate insertion of breast prosthesis following mastopexy, mastectomy or in reconstruction A2 T 50
EXCLUDES *Supply of prosthetic implant (99070, L8030, L8039, L8600)*
28.10 28.10 Global Days 090
AMA: 2007, February, 4-5

19342 Delayed insertion of breast prosthesis following mastopexy, mastectomy or in reconstruction A2 T 80 50 PQ
EXCLUDES *Preparation of moulage for custom breast implant (19396)*
Code also (C1789, L8600)
27.64 27.64 Global Days 090
AMA: 2007, February, 4-5

19350 Nipple/areola reconstruction A2 T 50 PQ
20.17 24.77 Global Days 090
AMA: 2009, Jan, 11-31; 2008, Jan, 10-25; 2007, January, 13-27

19355 Correction of inverted nipples A2 T 80 50 PQ
16.69 20.67 Global Days 090

19357 Breast reconstruction, immediate or delayed, with tissue expander, including subsequent expansion ♀ A2 T 80 50 PQ
44.79 44.79 Global Days 090

19361 Breast reconstruction with latissimus dorsi flap, without prosthetic implant C5 C 80 50 PQ
EXCLUDES *Implant of prosthesis (19340)*
47.94 47.94 Global Days 090

19364 Breast reconstruction with free flap C5 C 80 50 PQ
INCLUDES Closure of donor site
Harvesting of skin graft
Inset shaping of flap into breast
Microvascular repair
Operating microscope (69990)
82.92 82.92 Global Days 090

19366 Breast reconstruction with other technique A2 T 80 50 PQ
Code also implant of prosthesis if appropriate (19340, 19342)
Code also operating microscope (69990)
40.85 40.85 Global Days 090

19367 Breast reconstruction with transverse rectus abdominis myocutaneous flap (TRAM), single pedicle, including closure of donor site; C5 C 80 50 PQ
53.86 53.86 Global Days 090

19368 with microvascular anastomosis (supercharging) C5 C 80 50 PQ
INCLUDES Operating microscope (69990)
66.42 66.42 Global Days 090

19369 Breast reconstruction with transverse rectus abdominis myocutaneous flap (TRAM), double pedicle, including closure of donor site C5 C 80 50 PQ
61.48 61.48 Global Days 090

19370 **Open periprosthetic capsulotomy, breast** A2 T 50
20.51 20.51 Global Days 090

19371 **Periprosthetic capsulectomy, breast** A2 T 50
23.48 23.48 Global Days 090
AMA: 2009, Jan, 11-31; 2008, Jan, 10-25; 2007, January, 13-27

19380 **Revision of reconstructed breast** A2 T 50
23.13 23.13 Global Days 090

19396 **Preparation of moulage for custom breast implant** G2 T 80 50
4.32 8.26 Global Days 000

19499 **Unlisted procedure, breast** T 80 50
0.00 0.00 Global Days YYY

20005 Incisional Treatment Soft Tissue Abscess

EXCLUDES *Superficial incision and drainage (10040-10160)*

20005 Incision and drainage of soft tissue abscess, subfascial (ie, involves the soft tissue below the deep fascia) A2 T
6.79 8.83 Global Days 010

20100-20103 Exploratory Surgery of Traumatic Wound

INCLUDES Debridement
Extraction of foreign material
Open examination
Tying or coagulation of small vessels

EXCLUDES *Cutaneous/subcutaneous incision and drainage procedures (10060-10061)*
Laparotomy (49000-49010)
Repair of major vessels of:
Abdomen (35221, 35251, 35281)
Chest (35211, 35216, 35241, 35246, 35271, 35276)
Extremity (35206-35207, 35226, 35236, 35256, 35266, 35286)
Neck (35201, 35231, 35261)
Thoracotomy (32100-32160)

20100 Exploration of penetrating wound (separate procedure); neck T 80 50
17.64 17.64 Global Days 010
AMA: 2009, Jan, 11-31; 2008, Jan, 10-25; 2007, January, 13-27

20101 chest T
6.08 12.99 Global Days 010
AMA: 2009, Jan, 11-31; 2008, Jan, 10-25; 2007, January, 13-27

20102 abdomen/flank/back T
7.39 13.97 Global Days 010
AMA: 2009, Jan, 11-31; 2008, Jan, 10-25; 2007, January, 13-27

20103 extremity G2 T 80
10.36 17.16 Global Days 010
AMA: 2009, Jan, 11-31; 2008, Jan, 10-25; 2007, January, 13-27

20150 Epiphyseal Bar Resection

EXCLUDES *Bone marrow aspiration (38220)*

20150 Excision of epiphyseal bar, with or without autogenous soft tissue graft obtained through same fascial incision G2 T 80 50
29.30 29.30 Global Days 090

20200-20206 Muscle Biopsy

EXCLUDES *Removal of muscle tumor (see appropriate anatomic section)*

20200 Biopsy, muscle; superficial A2 T
2.79 6.05 Global Days 000

20205 deep A2 T
4.49 8.21 Global Days 000

20206 Biopsy, muscle, percutaneous needle A2 T
INCLUDES Fluoroscopic guidance (77002)
EXCLUDES *Fine needle aspiration (10021-10022)*
88172-88173
76942, 77012, 77021
1.74 7.25 Global Days 000

20220-20225 Percutaneous Bone Biopsy

CMS 100-3,150.3 Bone (Mineral) Density Studies

EXCLUDES *Bone marrow biopsy (38221)*

20220 Biopsy, bone, trocar, or needle; superficial (eg, ilium, sternum, spinous process, ribs) A2 T
77002, 77012, 77021
2.14 4.89 Global Days 000

20225 deep (eg, vertebral body, femur) A2 T
77002, 77012, 77021
3.27 17.22 Global Days 000

20240-20251 Open Bone Biopsy

CMS 100-3,150.3 Bone (Mineral) Density Studies

EXCLUDES *Sequestrectomy or incision and drainage of bone abscess of:*
Calcaneus (28120)
Carpal bone (25145)
Clavicle (23170)
Humeral head (23174)
Humerus (24134)
Olecranon process (24138)
Radius (24136, 25145)
Scapula (23172)
Skull (61501)
Talus (28120)
Ulna (24138, 24145)

20240 Biopsy, bone, open; superficial (eg, ilium, sternum, spinous process, ribs, trochanter of femur) A2 T
6.52 6.52 Global Days 010
AMA: 2009, Jan, 11-31; 2008, Jan, 10-25; 2007, January, 13-27

20245 deep (eg, humerus, ischium, femur) A2 T
18.47 18.47 Global Days 010

20250 Biopsy, vertebral body, open; thoracic A2 T
11.24 11.24 Global Days 010

20251 lumbar or cervical A2 T 80
12.20 12.20 Global Days 010

20500-20501 Injection Fistula/Sinus Tract

CMS 100-4,13,80.1 Supervision and Interpretation Codes
CMS 100-4,13,80.2 Physician Presence

EXCLUDES *Arthrography injection of:*
Ankle (27648)
Elbow (24220)
Hip (27093, 27095)
Knee (27370)
Sacroiliac joint (27096)
Shoulder (23350)
Temporomandibular joint (TMJ) (21116)
Wrist (25246)

20500 Injection of sinus tract; therapeutic (separate procedure) P3 T
76080
2.57 3.17 Global Days 010

20501 diagnostic (sinogram) N1 N
EXCLUDES *Contrast injection or injections for radiological evaluation of existing gastrostomy, duodenostomy, jejunostomy, gastro-jejunostomy, or cecostomy (or other colonic) tube from percutaneous approach (49465)*
76080
1.12 3.58 Global Days 000

20520-20525 Foreign Body Removal

CMS 100-4,12,30 Correct Coding Policy

20520 **Removal of foreign body in muscle or tendon sheath; simple** P3 T
1.29 5.88 Global Days 010

20525 **deep or complicated** A2 T
7.35 14.19 Global Days 010

20526-20553 Therapeutic Injections: Tendons, Trigger Points

CMS 100-3,150.7 Prolotherapy, Joint Sclerotherapy, and Ligamentous Injections with Sclerosing Agents
CMS 100-4,12,30 Correct Coding Policy
CMS 100-4,13,80.1 Supervision and Interpretation Codes
CMS 100-4,13,80.2 Physician Presence

EXCLUDES *Platelet rich plasma (PRP) injections (0232T)*

20526 **Injection, therapeutic (eg, local anesthetic, corticosteroid), carpal tunnel** P3 T 50
1.66 2.20 Global Days 000
AMA: 2009, Jan, 11-31; 2008, Jan, 10-25; 2007, January, 13-27

● **20527** **Injection, enzyme (eg, collagenase), palmar fascial cord (ie, Dupuytren's contracture)** P3 T 50
EXCLUDES *Post injection palmar fascial cord manipulation (26341)*
1.75 2.23 Global Days 000

20550 **Injection(s); single tendon sheath, or ligament, aponeurosis (eg, plantar "fascia")** P3 T 50
Do not report with (0232T)
76942, 77002, 77021
1.20 1.68 Global Days 000
AMA: 2009, Jan, 11-31; 2009, Jan, 6&9; 2008, Jan, 10-25; 2007, January, 13-27

20551 **single tendon origin/insertion** P3 T
EXCLUDES *Platelet rich plasma injection (0232T)*
76942, 77002, 77021
Do not report with (0232T)
1.24 1.72 Global Days 000
AMA: 2009, Jan, 11-31; 2008, Jan, 10-25; 2007, January, 13-27

20552 **single or multiple trigger point(s), 1 or 2 muscle(s)** P3 T
76942, 77002, 77021
1.09 1.58 Global Days 000
AMA: 2009, Jan, 11-31; 2008, Jan, 10-25; 2007, January, 13-27

20553 **single or multiple trigger point(s), 3 or more muscle(s)** P3 T
76942, 77002, 77021
1.23 1.81 Global Days 000
AMA: 2009, Jan, 11-31; 2008, Jan, 10-25; 2008, Jun, 8-11; 2007, January, 13-27

20555 Placement of Catheters/Needles for Brachytherapy

20555 **Placement of needles or catheters into muscle and/or soft tissue for subsequent interstitial radioelement application (at the time of or subsequent to the procedure)** A2 T 80
EXCLUDES *Interstitial radioelement:*
Devices placed into the breast (19296-19298)
Placement of needle, catheters, or devices into muscle or soft tissue of the head and neck (41019)
Placement of needles or catheters into pelvic organs or genitalia (55920)
Placement of needles or catheters into prostate (55875)
Radioelement application (77776-77778, 77785-77787)
76942, 77002, 77012, 77021
9.69 9.69 Global Days 000
AMA: 2009, Jan, 11-31; 2008, Feb, 8-9; 2008, Jun, 8-11; 2007, Dec, 1-2

20600-20610 Aspiration and/or Injection of Joint

CMS 100-3,150.6 Vitamin B12 Injections to Strenghen Tendons, Ligaments of Foot
CMS 100-3,150.7 Prolotherapy, Joint Sclerotherapy, and Ligamentous Injections with Sclerosing Agents
CMS 100-4,12,30 Correct Coding Policy
CMS 100-4,13,80.1 Supervision and Interpretation Codes
CMS 100-4,13,80.2 Physician Presence

20600 **Arthrocentesis, aspiration and/or injection; small joint or bursa (eg, fingers, toes)** P3 T 50
76942, 77002, 77012, 77021
1.13 1.59 Global Days 000
AMA: 2007, Dec, 10-179

20605 **intermediate joint or bursa (eg, temporomandibular, acromioclavicular, wrist, elbow or ankle, olecranon bursa)** P3 T 50
76942, 77002, 77012, 77021
1.19 1.68 Global Days 000
AMA: 2007, Dec, 10-179

20610 **major joint or bursa (eg, shoulder, hip, knee joint, subacromial bursa)** P3 T 50
76942, 77002, 77012, 77021
1.46 2.05 Global Days 000
AMA: 2009, Jan, 11-31; 2008, Jan, 10-25; 2008, Jun, 8-11; 2008, Jul, 9; 2007, January, 13-27; 2007, Dec, 10-179

20612-20615 Aspiration and/or Injection of Cyst

CMS 100-4,12,30 Correct Coding Policy

20612 **Aspiration and/or injection of ganglion cyst(s) any location** P3 T
1.22 1.73 Global Days 000

20615 **Aspiration and injection for treatment of bone cyst** P3 T
4.68 6.81 Global Days 010

20650-20697 Devices Related to External Fixation

CMS 100-4,12,30 Correct Coding Policy

20650 **Insertion of wire or pin with application of skeletal traction, including removal (separate procedure)** A2 T CCI
4.47 5.84 Global Days 010

20660 **Application of cranial tongs, caliper, or stereotactic frame, including removal (separate procedure)** T CCI
7.16 7.16 Global Days 000
AMA: 2009, Jan, 11-31; 2008, Feb, 8-9; 2008, Jul, 10&13; 2008, Jan, 10-25; 2007, January, 13-27; 2007, Dec, 1-2

20661 **Application of halo, including removal; cranial** C5 C CCI
14.76 14.76 Global Days 090

20662 **pelvic** R2 T 80 CCI
12.78 12.78 Global Days 090

20663 **femoral** R2 T 80 CCI
11.98 11.98 Global Days 090

20664 **Application of halo, including removal, cranial, 6 or more pins placed, for thin skull osteology (eg, pediatric patients, hydrocephalus, osteogenesis imperfecta)** C5 C CCI
25.33 25.33 Global Days 090

20665 **Removal of tongs or halo applied by another physician** G2 X 80 CCI
2.62 3.07 Global Days 010

20670 **Removal of implant; superficial (eg, buried wire, pin or rod) (separate procedure)** A2 T CCI
4.36 11.40 Global Days 010
AMA: 2009, Jan, 11-31; 2009, Jun, 7-8; 2008, Jan, 10-25; 2007, Dec, 7-8

20680 **deep (eg, buried wire, pin, screw, metal band, nail, rod or plate)** A2 T 80 CCI
12.49 18.14 Global Days 090
AMA: 2009, Jun, 7-8

20690 **Application of a uniplane (pins or wires in 1 plane), unilateral, external fixation system** A2 T CCI
17.05 17.05 Global Days 090
AMA: 2009, Jan, 11-31; 2009, Jun, 7-8; 2008, Feb, 8-9; 2008, Jan, 4-5; 2008, Jan, 10-25; 2007, January, 13-27

20692 **Application of a multiplane (pins or wires in more than 1 plane), unilateral, external fixation system (eg, Ilizarov, Monticelli type)** A2 T 80 CCI
32.28 32.28 Global Days 090
AMA: 2009, Jan, 11-31; 2009, Jun, 7-8; 2008, Jan, 10-25; 2008, Jan, 4-5; 2008, Feb, 8-9; 2007, January, 13-27

20693 **Adjustment or revision of external fixation system requiring anesthesia (eg, new pin[s] or wire[s] and/or new ring[s] or bar[s])** A2 T CCI
13.35 13.35 Global Days 090
AMA: 2009, Jun, 7-8; 2009, Jan, 11-31; 2008, Jan, 10-25; 2007, January, 13-27

20694 **Removal, under anesthesia, of external fixation system** A2 T CCI
9.90 12.46 Global Days 090
AMA: 2009, Jan, 11-31; 2009, Jun, 7-8; 2008, Jan, 10-25; 2007, January, 13-27

20696 **Application of multiplane (pins or wires in more than 1 plane), unilateral, external fixation with stereotactic computer-assisted adjustment (eg, spatial frame), including imaging; initial and subsequent alignment(s), assessment(s), and computation(s) of adjustment schedule(s)** G2 T 80
Do not report with (20692, 20697)
32.36 32.36 Global Days 090
AMA: 2009, Jun, 7-8

⊘ **20697** **exchange (ie, removal and replacement) of strut, each** P2 T 80
Do not report with (20692, 20696)
57.20 57.20 Global Days 000
AMA: 2009, Jun, 7-8

20802-20838 Reimplantation Procedures

CMS 100-4,12,30 Correct Coding Policy
CMS 100-4,12,40.1 Global Surgery Package Definition

EXCLUDES *Repair of incomplete amputation (see individual repair codes for bone(s), ligament(s), tendon(s), nerve(s), or blood vessel(s))*

20802 **Replantation, arm (includes surgical neck of humerus through elbow joint), complete amputation** C5 C 80 50 CCI
67.45 67.45 Global Days 090

20805 **Replantation, forearm (includes radius and ulna to radial carpal joint), complete amputation** C5 C 80 50 CCI
84.76 84.76 Global Days 090

20808 **Replantation, hand (includes hand through metacarpophalangeal joints), complete amputation** C5 C 80 50 CCI
117.91 117.91 Global Days 090

20816 **Replantation, digit, excluding thumb (includes metacarpophalangeal joint to insertion of flexor sublimis tendon), complete amputation** C5 C 80 CCI
62.45 62.45 Global Days 090
AMA: 2009, Jan, 11-31; 2008, Jan, 10-25; 2007, January, 13-27

20822 **Replantation, digit, excluding thumb (includes distal tip to sublimis tendon insertion), complete amputation** G2 T 80 CCI
53.25 53.25 Global Days 090

20824 **Replantation, thumb (includes carpometacarpal joint to MP joint), complete amputation** C5 C 80 50 CCI
64.74 64.74 Global Days 090

20827 **Replantation, thumb (includes distal tip to MP joint), complete amputation** C5 C 80 50 CCI
54.99 54.99 Global Days 090

20838 **Replantation, foot, complete amputation** C5 C 80 50 CCI
75.30 75.30 Global Days 090

20900-20926 Bone and Tissue Autografts

CMS 100-4,12,30 Correct Coding Policy

EXCLUDES *Acquisition of autogenous bone graft, cartilage, tendon, fascia lata through distinct incision unless included in the code description*
Bone graft procedures on the spine (20930-20938)
Platelet rich plasma (PRP) injection (0232T)

20900 **Bone graft, any donor area; minor or small (eg, dowel or button)** A2 T 80 CCI
6.50 12.38 Global Days 000
AMA: 2009, Jan, 11-31; 2008, Jan, 10-25; 2007, January, 13-27

20902 **major or large** A2 T 80 CCI
9.30 9.30 Global Days 000
AMA: 2009, Jan, 11-31; 2008, Jan, 10-25; 2007, January, 13-27

20910 **Cartilage graft; costochondral** A2 T 80
EXCLUDES *Graft with ear cartilage (21235)*
13.28 13.28 Global Days 090

20912 **nasal septum** A2 T 80
EXCLUDES *Graft with ear cartilage (21235)*
14.39 14.39 Global Days 090

20920 **Fascia lata graft; by stripper** A2 T
11.84 11.84 Global Days 090

20922 **by incision and area exposure, complex or sheet** A2 T 80
14.59 17.76 Global Days 090

20924 **Tendon graft, from a distance (eg, palmaris, toe extensor, plantaris)** A2 T 80
14.89 14.89 Global Days 090

20926 **Tissue grafts, other (eg, paratenon, fat, dermis)** A2 T
12.88 12.88 Global Days 090
AMA: 2009, Jan, 11-31; 2008, Jan, 10-25; 2007, March, 9-11; 2007, January, 13-27

20930-20938 Bone Allograft and Autograft of Spine

CMS 100-4,12,40.1 Global Surgery Package Definition
EXCLUDES *Bone marrow aspiration for grafting (38220)*

\+ 20930 **Allograft, morselized, or placement of osteopromotive material, for spine surgery only (List separately in addition to code for primary procedure)** N
Code first (22319, 22532-22533, 22548-22558, 22590-22612, 22630, 22800-22812, 0195T-0196T)
0.00 0.00 Global Days XXX
AMA: 2009, Jan, 11-31; 2008, Feb, 8-9; 2008, Jan, 10-25; 2007, January, 13-27; 2007, Dec, 1-2

\+ 20931 **Allograft, structural, for spine surgery only (List separately in addition to code for primary procedure)** N
Code first (22319, 22532-22533, 22548-22558, 22590-22612, 22630, 22800-22812)
3.33 3.33 Global Days ZZZ
AMA: 2009, Jan, 11-31; 2008, Feb, 8-9; 2007, Dec, 1-2

\+ 20936 **Autograft for spine surgery only (includes harvesting the graft); local (eg, ribs, spinous process, or laminar fragments) obtained from same incision (List separately in addition to code for primary procedure)** C5 C
Code first (22319, 22532-22533, 22548-22558, 22590-22612, 22630, 22800-22812, 0195T-0196T)
0.00 0.00 Global Days XXX
AMA: 2009, Jan, 11-31; 2008, Feb, 8-9; 2007, Dec, 1-2

\+ 20937 **morselized (through separate skin or fascial incision) (List separately in addition to code for primary procedure)** C5 C 80
Code first (22319, 22532-22533, 22548-22558, 22590-22612, 22630, 22800-22812, 0195T-0196T)
4.98 4.98 Global Days ZZZ
AMA: 2009, Jan, 11-31; 2008, Feb, 8-9; 2007, Dec, 1-2

\+ 20938 **structural, bicortical or tricortical (through separate skin or fascial incision) (List separately in addition to code for primary procedure)** C5 C 80
Code first (22319, 22532-22533, 22548-22558, 22590-22612, 22630)
5.47 5.47 Global Days ZZZ
AMA: 2009, Jan, 11-31; 2008, Feb, 8-9; 2007, Dec, 1-2

20950 Measurement of Intracompartmental Pressure

CMS 100-4,12,20.4.3 Payment for Assistant at Surgery
CMS 100-4,12,30 Correct Coding Policy

20950 **Monitoring of interstitial fluid pressure (includes insertion of device, eg, wick catheter technique, needle manometer technique) in detection of muscle compartment syndrome** G2 T 80
2.67 7.39 Global Days 000
AMA: 2009, Jan, 11-31; 2008, Jan, 10-25

20955-20973 Bone and Osteocutaneous Grafts

CMS 100-4,12,20.4.3 Payment for Assistant at Surgery
CMS 100-4,12,30 Correct Coding Policy
INCLUDES Operating microscope (69990)

20955 **Bone graft with microvascular anastomosis; fibula** C5 C 80
75.05 75.05 Global Days 090

20956 **iliac crest** C5 C 80
77.83 77.83 Global Days 090

20957 **metatarsal** C5 C 80
79.24 79.24 Global Days 090

20962 **other than fibula, iliac crest, or metatarsal** C5 C 80
66.82 66.82 Global Days 090

20969 **Free osteocutaneous flap with microvascular anastomosis; other than iliac crest, metatarsal, or great toe** C5 C 80
83.13 83.13 Global Days 090

20970 **iliac crest** C5 C 80
82.44 82.44 Global Days 090

20972 **metatarsal** G2 T 80
65.65 65.65 Global Days 090

20973 **great toe with web space** G2 T 80
EXCLUDES *Wrap-around repair (26551)*
80.85 80.85 Global Days 090

20974-20979 Osteogenic Stimulation

CMS 100-3,150.2 Osteogenic Stimulation
CMS 100-4,12,20.4.3 Payment for Assistant at Surgery
CMS 100-4,12,30 Correct Coding Policy

⊘ 20974 **Electrical stimulation to aid bone healing; noninvasive (nonoperative)** A
1.45 2.16 Global Days 000
AMA: 2009, Jan, 11-31; 2008, Jan, 10-25; 2007, January, 13-27

⊘ 20975 **invasive (operative)** N1 N 80
5.21 5.21 Global Days 000

20979 **Low intensity ultrasound stimulation to aid bone healing, noninvasive (nonoperative)** P3 X
0.98 1.56 Global Days 000
AMA: 2009, Jan, 11-31; 2008, Jan, 10-25; 2007, January, 13-27

20982-20999 General Musculoskeletal Procedures

CMS 100-4,12,20.4.3 Payment for Assistant at Surgery
CMS 100-4,12,30 Correct Coding Policy
CMS 100-4,12,40.7 Bilateral Procedures

⊙ 20982 **Ablation, bone tumor(s) (eg, osteoid osteoma, metastasis) radiofrequency, percutaneous, including computed tomographic guidance** G2 T 50
Do not report with (77013)
11.20 111.18 Global Days 000

+ **20985 Computer-assisted surgical navigational procedure for musculoskeletal procedures, image-less (List separately in addition to code for primary procedure)**

EXCLUDES *Image guidance derived from intraoperative and preoperative obtained images (0054T-0055T)*

Code first primary procedure

Do not report with (61781-61783)

4.35 4.35 Global Days ZZZ

AMA: 2007, Dec, 1-2

20999 Unlisted procedure, musculoskeletal system, general

0.00 0.00 Global Days YYY

21010 Temporomandibular Joint Arthrotomy

21010 Arthrotomy, temporomandibular joint

EXCLUDES *Excision of foreign body from dentoalveolar site (41805-41806)*
Soft tissue (subfascial) abscess drainage (20005)
Superficial abscess and hematoma drainage (10060-10061)

21.69 21.69 Global Days 090

21011-21016 Excision Soft Tissue Tumors Face and Scalp

CMS 100-4,4,20.5 HCPCS Under OPPS
CMS 100-4,12,30 Correct Coding Policy
CMS 100-4,12,90.3 MD Services in ASCs
CMS 100-4,14,10 General ASC Services

INCLUDES Any necessary elevation of tissue planes or dissection
Measurement of tumor and necessary margin at greatest diameter prior to excision
Simple and intermediate repairs
Types of excisions:
Fascial or subfascial soft tissue tumors: simple and marginal resection of most often benign and intramuscular tumors found either in or below the deep fascia, not involving bone
Radical resection soft tissue tumor: wide resection of tumor, mostly malignant or aggressive benign, involving large margins of normal tissue and may involve tissue removal from one or more layers
Subcutaneous: simple and marginal resection of most often benign tumors found in the subcutaneous tissue above the deep fascia

EXCLUDES *Complex repair*
Radical resection of cutaneous tumors (e.g., melanoma) (11600-11646)
Significant exploration of vessels or neuroplasty

21011 Excision, tumor, soft tissue of face or scalp, subcutaneous; less than 2 cm

7.72 10.41 Global Days 090

21012 2 cm or greater

10.01 10.01 Global Days 090

21013 Excision, tumor, soft tissue of face and scalp, subfascial (eg, subgaleal, intramuscular); less than 2 cm

12.04 15.60 Global Days 090

21014 2 cm or greater

15.51 15.51 Global Days 090

21015 Radical resection of tumor (eg, malignant neoplasm), soft tissue of face or scalp; less than 2 cm

EXCLUDES *Removal of cranial tumor for osteomyelitis (61501)*

20.32 20.32 Global Days 090

21016 2 cm or greater

30.92 30.92 Global Days 090

21025-21070 Procedures of Cranial and Facial Bones

INCLUDES Any necessary elevation of tissue planes or dissection
Measurement of tumor and necessary margins prior to excision
Radical resection of bone tumor involves resection of the tumor (may include entire bone) and wide margins of normal tissue primarily for malignant or aggressive benign tumors.
Simple and intermediate repairs

EXCLUDES *Radical resection of cutaneous tumors (e.g., melanoma) (11600-11646)*
Significant exploration of vessels, neuroplasty, reconstruction, or complex bone repair

Do not report excision of soft tissue codes when adjacent soft tissue is removed during the bone tumor resection (21011-21016)

21025 Excision of bone (eg, for osteomyelitis or bone abscess); mandible

22.03 26.11 Global Days 090

21026 facial bone(s)

14.65 18.08 Global Days 090

Vestibular incision

Burs, files, and osteotomes used to remove bone

Area of benign bone growth

21029 Removal by contouring of benign tumor of facial bone (eg, fibrous dysplasia)

19.17 22.96 Global Days 090

21030 Excision of benign tumor or cyst of maxilla or zygoma by enucleation and curettage

12.21 15.14 Global Days 090

21031 Excision of torus mandibularis

8.53 11.38 Global Days 090

21032 Excision of maxillary torus palatinus

8.44 11.56 Global Days 090

21034 Excision of malignant tumor of maxilla or zygoma

34.67 39.41 Global Days 090

21040 Excision of benign tumor or cyst of mandible, by enucleation and/or curettage

INCLUDES Removal of benign tumor or cyst without osteotomy

EXCLUDES *Removal of benign tumor or cyst with osteotomy (21046-21047)*

12.21 15.21 Global Days 090

21044 Excision of malignant tumor of mandible;

26.19 26.19 Global Days 090

21045 radical resection

Code also bone graft procedure (21215)

36.54 36.54 Global Days 090

21046 **Excision of benign tumor or cyst of mandible; requiring intra-oral osteotomy (eg, locally aggressive or destructive lesion(s))** A2 T 80
32.35 32.35 Global Days 090

21047 **requiring extra-oral osteotomy and partial mandibulectomy (eg, locally aggressive or destructive lesion(s))** A2 T 80
38.38 38.38 Global Days 090

21048 **Excision of benign tumor or cyst of maxilla; requiring intra-oral osteotomy (eg, locally aggressive or destructive lesion(s))** R2 T 80
33.12 33.12 Global Days 090

21049 **requiring extra-oral osteotomy and partial maxillectomy (eg, locally aggressive or destructive lesion(s))** T 80
36.58 36.58 Global Days 090

21050 **Condylectomy, temporomandibular joint (separate procedure)** A2 T 80 50
25.95 25.95 Global Days 090

21060 **Meniscectomy, partial or complete, temporomandibular joint (separate procedure)** A2 T 80 50
24.49 24.49 Global Days 090

21070 **Coronoidectomy (separate procedure)** A2 T 80 50
18.44 18.44 Global Days 090

21073 Temporomandibular Joint Manipulation with Anesthesia

CMS 100-3,150.1 Manipulation

21073 **Manipulation of temporomandibular joint(s) (TMJ), therapeutic, requiring an anesthesia service (ie, general or monitored anesthesia care)** P3 T 80 50

EXCLUDES *Closed treatment of TMJ dislocation (21480, 21485)*
Manipulation of TMJ without an anesthesia service (97140, 98925-98929, 98943)

7.51 11.40 Global Days 090
AMA: 2009, Jan, 11-31; 2008, Feb, 8-9; 2007, Dec, 1-2

21076-21089 Medical Impressions for Fabrication Maxillofacial Prosthesis

CMS 100-4,12,30 Correct Coding Policy

INCLUDES Design, preparation, and professional services rendered by a physician

EXCLUDES *Application or removal of caliper or tongs (20660, 20665)*
Professional services rendered for outside laboratory designed and prepared prosthesis

21076 **Impression and custom preparation; surgical obturator prosthesis** P3 T 80
24.21 28.76 Global Days 010
AMA: 2009, Jan, 11-31; 2008, Jan, 10-25; 2007, January, 13-27

21077 **orbital prosthesis** P3 T 80 50
61.13 71.74 Global Days 090

21079 **interim obturator prosthesis** P3 T
40.65 48.66 Global Days 090

21080 **definitive obturator prosthesis** P3 T
45.27 54.73 Global Days 090

21081 **mandibular resection prosthesis** P3 T 80
41.44 50.38 Global Days 090

21082 **palatal augmentation prosthesis** P3 T 80
38.83 47.51 Global Days 090

21083 **palatal lift prosthesis** P3 T 80
34.93 44.19 Global Days 090

21084 **speech aid prosthesis** P3 T 80
41.83 51.87 Global Days 090

21085 **oral surgical splint** P3 T 80
18.67 23.81 Global Days 010

21086 **auricular prosthesis** P3 T 80 50
44.94 53.11 Global Days 090

21087 **nasal prosthesis** P3 T 80
44.59 52.92 Global Days 090

21088 **facial prosthesis** R2 T 80
0.00 0.00 Global Days 090

21089 **Unlisted maxillofacial prosthetic procedure** T
0.00 0.00 Global Days YYY
AMA: 2009, Jan, 11-31; 2008, Jan, 10-25; 2007, January, 13-27

21100-21110 Application Fixation Device

CMS 100-4,12,40.1 Global Surgery Package Definition

21100 **Application of halo type appliance for maxillofacial fixation, includes removal (separate procedure)** A2 T 80
11.44 21.23 Global Days 090

21110 **Application of interdental fixation device for conditions other than fracture or dislocation, includes removal** P2 T

EXCLUDES *Removal of interdental fixation by another doctor (20670-20680)*

19.47 23.19 Global Days 090
AMA: 2009, Jan, 11-31; 2008, Jan, 10-25; 2007, January, 13-27

21116 Injection for TMJ Arthrogram

CMS 100-4,13,80.1 Supervision and Interpretation Codes
CMS 100-4,13,80.2 Physician Presence

21116 **Injection procedure for temporomandibular joint arthrography** N1 N
70332
1.23 4.40 Global Days 000

21120-21299 Repair/Reconstruction Craniofacial Bones

CMS 100-2,16,10 Exclusions from Coverage
CMS 100-2,16,120 Cosmetic Procedures
CMS 100-2,16,180 Services Related to Noncovered Procedures
CMS 100-4,12,40.1 Global Surgery Package Definition

EXCLUDES *Cranioplasty (62116, 62120, 62140-62147)*

21120 Genioplasty; augmentation (autograft, allograft, prosthetic material) A2 T
16.10 20.26 Global Days 090

21121 sliding osteotomy, single piece A2 T 80
18.61 22.36 Global Days 090

21122 sliding osteotomies, 2 or more osteotomies (eg, wedge excision or bone wedge reversal for asymmetrical chin) A2 T 80
19.03 19.03 Global Days 090

21123 sliding, augmentation with interpositional bone grafts (includes obtaining autografts) A2 T 80
24.82 24.82 Global Days 090

21125 Augmentation, mandibular body or angle; prosthetic material A2 T 80
23.36 90.17 Global Days 090

21127 with bone graft, onlay or interpositional (includes obtaining autograft) A2 T 80
25.20 120.93 Global Days 090

21137 Reduction forehead; contouring only G2 T 80
22.46 22.46 Global Days 090

21138 contouring and application of prosthetic material or bone graft (includes obtaining autograft) G2 T 80
26.32 26.32 Global Days 090

21139 contouring and setback of anterior frontal sinus wall G2 T 80
31.39 31.39 Global Days 090

21141 Reconstruction midface, LeFort I; single piece, segment movement in any direction (eg, for Long Face Syndrome), without bone graft C5 C 80
41.08 41.08 Global Days 090

21142 2 pieces, segment movement in any direction, without bone graft C5 C 80
41.88 41.88 Global Days 090

21143 3 or more pieces, segment movement in any direction, without bone graft C5 C 80
43.44 43.44 Global Days 090

21145 single piece, segment movement in any direction, requiring bone grafts (includes obtaining autografts) C5 C 80
45.18 45.18 Global Days 090

21146 2 pieces, segment movement in any direction, requiring bone grafts (includes obtaining autografts) (eg, ungrafted unilateral alveolar cleft) C5 C 80
51.65 51.65 Global Days 090

21147 3 or more pieces, segment movement in any direction, requiring bone grafts (includes obtaining autografts) (eg, ungrafted bilateral alveolar cleft or multiple osteotomies) C5 C 80
48.58 48.58 Global Days 090

21150 Reconstruction midface, LeFort II; anterior intrusion (eg, Treacher-Collins Syndrome) G2 T 80
48.69 48.69 Global Days 090

21151 any direction, requiring bone grafts (includes obtaining autografts) C5 C 80
56.69 56.69 Global Days 090

21154 Reconstruction midface, LeFort III (extracranial), any type, requiring bone grafts (includes obtaining autografts); without LeFort I C5 C 80
64.04 64.04 Global Days 090

21155 with LeFort I C5 C 80
63.99 63.99 Global Days 090

21159 Reconstruction midface, LeFort III (extra and intracranial) with forehead advancement (eg, mono bloc), requiring bone grafts (includes obtaining autografts); without LeFort I C5 C 80
73.95 73.95 Global Days 090

21160 with LeFort I C5 C 80
77.26 77.26 Global Days 090

21172 Reconstruction superior-lateral orbital rim and lower forehead, advancement or alteration, with or without grafts (includes obtaining autografts) T 80

EXCLUDES *Frontal or parietal craniotomy for craniosynostosis (61556)*

53.47 53.47 Global Days 090

21175 Reconstruction, bifrontal, superior-lateral orbital rims and lower forehead, advancement or alteration (eg, plagiocephaly, trigonocephaly, brachycephaly), with or without grafts (includes obtaining autografts) T 80

EXCLUDES *Bifrontal craniotomy for craniosynostosis (61557)*

67.67 67.67 Global Days 090

21179 Reconstruction, entire or majority of forehead and/or supraorbital rims; with grafts (allograft or prosthetic material) C5 C 80

EXCLUDES *Extensive craniotomy for numerous suture craniosynostosis (61558-61559)*

42.81 42.81 Global Days 090

21180 with autograft (includes obtaining grafts) C5 C 80

EXCLUDES *Extensive craniotomy for numerous suture craniosynostosis (61558-61559)*

46.37 46.37 Global Days 090

21181 Reconstruction by contouring of benign tumor of cranial bones (eg, fibrous dysplasia), extracranial A2 T 80
20.95 20.95 Global Days 090

21182 Reconstruction of orbital walls, rims, forehead, nasoethmoid complex following intra- and extracranial excision of benign tumor of cranial bone (eg, fibrous dysplasia), with multiple autografts (includes obtaining grafts); total area of bone grafting less than 40 sq cm C5 C 80

EXCLUDES *Removal of benign tumor of the skull (61563-61564)*

57.82 57.82 Global Days 090

21183 total area of bone grafting greater than 40 sq cm but less than 80 sq cm C5 C 80
EXCLUDES *Removal of benign tumor of the skull (61563-61564)*
68.91 68.91 Global Days 090

21184 total area of bone grafting greater than 80 sq cm C5 C 80
EXCLUDES *Removal of benign tumor of the skull (61563-61564)*
70.37 70.37 Global Days 090

21188 Reconstruction midface, osteotomies (other than LeFort type) and bone grafts (includes obtaining autografts) C5 C 80
47.38 47.38 Global Days 090

21193 Reconstruction of mandibular rami, horizontal, vertical, C, or L osteotomy; without bone graft T 80
38.86 38.86 Global Days 090
AMA: 2009, Jan, 11-31; 2008, Jan, 10-25; 2007, January, 13-27

21194 with bone graft (includes obtaining graft) C5 C 80
41.01 41.01 Global Days 090

21195 Reconstruction of mandibular rami and/or body, sagittal split; without internal rigid fixation T 80
39.91 39.91 Global Days 090
AMA: 2009, Jan, 11-31; 2008, Jan, 10-25; 2007, January, 13-27

21196 with internal rigid fixation C5 C 80
43.69 43.69 Global Days 090
AMA: 2009, Jan, 11-31; 2008, Jan, 10-25; 2007, January, 13-27

21198 Osteotomy, mandible, segmental; G2 T 80
EXCLUDES *Total maxillary osteotomy (21141-21160)*
34.38 34.38 Global Days 090

21199 with genioglossus advancement G2 T 80
EXCLUDES *Total maxillary osteotomy (21141-21160)*
30.11 30.11 Global Days 090

21206 Osteotomy, maxilla, segmental (eg, Wassmund or Schuchard) A2 T 80
35.41 35.41 Global Days 090

21208 Osteoplasty, facial bones; augmentation (autograft, allograft, or prosthetic implant) A2 T 80
25.14 56.38 Global Days 090

21209 reduction A2 T 80
19.49 24.74 Global Days 090

21210 Graft, bone; nasal, maxillary or malar areas (includes obtaining graft) A2 T
EXCLUDES *Cleft palate treatment (42200-42225)*
24.95 65.82 Global Days 090

21215 mandible (includes obtaining graft) A2 T
26.73 117.76 Global Days 090

21230 rib cartilage, autogenous, to face, chin, nose or ear (includes obtaining graft) A2 T 80
EXCLUDES *Augmentation graft of the facial bones (21208)*
23.02 23.02 Global Days 090

21235 ear cartilage, autogenous, to nose or ear (includes obtaining graft) A2 T
EXCLUDES *Augmentation graft of the facial bones (21208)*
17.01 21.79 Global Days 090
AMA: 2009, Jan, 11-31; 2008, Jan, 10-25; 2007, March, 9-11

TMJ syndrome is often related to stress and tooth-grinding; in other cases, arthritis, injury, poorly aligned teeth, or ill-fitting dentures may be the cause
Upper joint space
Lower joint space
Articular disc (meniscus)
Cutaway detail
Condyle
Mandible
Cutaway view of temporomandibular joint (TMJ)
Symptoms include facial pain and chewing problems; TMJ syndrome occurs more frequently in women

21240 Arthroplasty, temporomandibular joint, with or without autograft (includes obtaining graft) A2 T 80 50
32.29 32.29 Global Days 090

21242 Arthroplasty, temporomandibular joint, with allograft A2 T 80 50
29.64 29.64 Global Days 090

21243 Arthroplasty, temporomandibular joint, with prosthetic joint replacement A2 T 80 50
49.19 49.19 Global Days 090

21244 Reconstruction of mandible, extraoral, with transosteal bone plate (eg, mandibular staple bone plate) A2 T 80
31.55 31.55 Global Days 090

21245 Reconstruction of mandible or maxilla, subperiosteal implant; partial A2 T 80
26.70 33.51 Global Days 090

21246 complete A2 T 80
24.63 24.63 Global Days 090

21247 Reconstruction of mandibular condyle with bone and cartilage autografts (includes obtaining grafts) (eg, for hemifacial microsomia) C5 C 80
49.67 49.67 Global Days 090

21248 Reconstruction of mandible or maxilla, endosteal implant (eg, blade, cylinder); partial A2 T
EXCLUDES *Midface reconstruction (21141-21160)*
26.15 32.07 Global Days 090

21249 complete A2 T 80
EXCLUDES *Midface reconstruction (21141-21160)*
36.17 43.93 Global Days 090

21255 Reconstruction of zygomatic arch and glenoid fossa with bone and cartilage (includes obtaining autografts) C5 C 80
41.29 41.29 Global Days 090

21256 Reconstruction of orbit with osteotomies (extracranial) and with bone grafts (includes obtaining autografts) (eg, micro-ophthalmia) T 80
35.31 35.31 Global Days 090

21260 Periorbital osteotomies for orbital hypertelorism, with bone grafts; extracranial approach G2 T 80
36.32 36.32 Global Days 090

21261 combined intra- and extracranial approach T 80
64.37 64.37 Global Days 090

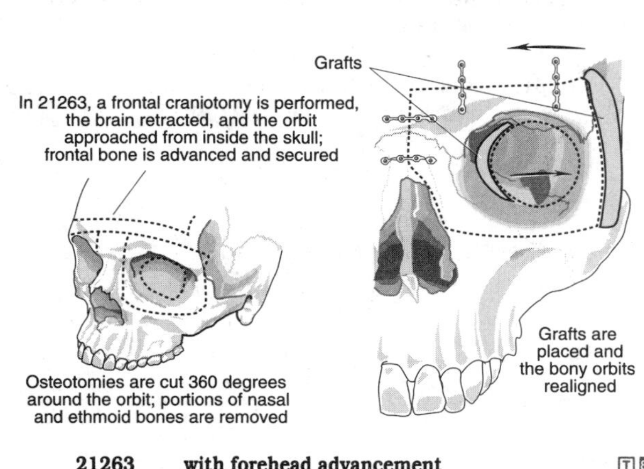

21263 with forehead advancement T 80
55.23 55.23 Global Days 090

21267 Orbital repositioning, periorbital osteotomies, unilateral, with bone grafts; extracranial approach A2 T 80
46.10 46.10 Global Days 090

21268 combined intra- and extracranial approach C5 C 80
53.33 53.33 Global Days 090

21270 Malar augmentation, prosthetic material A2 T 80
EXCLUDES *Bone graft (21210)*
21.69 28.53 Global Days 090

21275 Secondary revision of orbitocraniofacial reconstruction A2 T 80
25.07 25.07 Global Days 090

21280 Medial canthopexy (separate procedure) A2 T 80 50
EXCLUDES *Reconstruction of canthus (67950)*
16.99 16.99 Global Days 090

21282 Lateral canthopexy A2 T 50
11.21 11.21 Global Days 090

21295 Reduction of masseter muscle and bone (eg, for treatment of benign masseteric hypertrophy); extraoral approach A2 T 80
5.45 5.45 Global Days 090

21296 intraoral approach A2 T 80
12.69 12.69 Global Days 090

21299 Unlisted craniofacial and maxillofacial procedure T 80
0.00 0.00 Global Days YYY

21310-21499 Care of Fractures/Dislocations of the Cranial and Facial Bones

CMS 100-4,4,20.5 HCPCS Under OPPS
CMS 100-4,12,40.1 Global Surgery Package Definition
CMS 100-4,12,90.3 MD Services in ASCs
CMS 100-4,14,10 General ASC Services

EXCLUDES *Closed treatment of skull fracture (99201-99499 [99224, 99225, 99226])*
Open treatment of skull fracture (62000-62010)

21310 Closed treatment of nasal bone fracture without manipulation A2 T
0.82 3.68 Global Days 000

21315 Closed treatment of nasal bone fracture; without stabilization A2 T
4.56 8.35 Global Days 010

21320 with stabilization A2 T
4.06 7.70 Global Days 010

21325 Open treatment of nasal fracture; uncomplicated A2 T 80
14.11 14.11 Global Days 090

21330 complicated, with internal and/or external skeletal fixation A2 T 80
17.06 17.06 Global Days 090

21335 with concomitant open treatment of fractured septum A2 T
21.83 21.83 Global Days 090

21336 Open treatment of nasal septal fracture, with or without stabilization A2 T 80
19.40 19.40 Global Days 090

21337 Closed treatment of nasal septal fracture, with or without stabilization A2 T 80
8.81 12.10 Global Days 090

21338 Open treatment of nasoethmoid fracture; without external fixation A2 T 80
22.60 22.60 Global Days 090

21339 with external fixation A2 T 80
23.69 23.69 Global Days 090

21340 Percutaneous treatment of nasoethmoid complex fracture, with splint, wire or headcap fixation, including repair of canthal ligaments and/or the nasolacrimal apparatus A2 T 80
24.27 24.27 Global Days 090

21343 Open treatment of depressed frontal sinus fracture C5 C 80
36.35 36.35 Global Days 090

21344 Open treatment of complicated (eg, comminuted or involving posterior wall) frontal sinus fracture, via coronal or multiple approaches C5 C 80
47.07 47.07 Global Days 090

21345 Closed treatment of nasomaxillary complex fracture (LeFort II type), with interdental wire fixation or fixation of denture or splint A2 T 80
18.97 23.61 Global Days 090

21346 Open treatment of nasomaxillary complex fracture (LeFort II type); with wiring and/or local fixation T PQ
27.50 27.50 Global Days 090

21347 requiring multiple open approaches C5 C 80 PQ
33.16 33.16 Global Days 090

21348 with bone grafting (includes obtaining graft) C5 C 80 PQ
32.67 32.67 Global Days 090

21355 Percutaneous treatment of fracture of malar area, including zygomatic arch and malar tripod, with manipulation A2 T 80
9.64 12.99 Global Days 010

21356 Open treatment of depressed zygomatic arch fracture (eg, Gillies approach) A2 T 80
11.22 14.85 Global Days 010

21360 Open treatment of depressed malar fracture, including zygomatic arch and malar tripod G2 T 80
15.79 15.79 Global Days 090

21365 Open treatment of complicated (eg, comminuted or involving cranial nerve foramina) fracture(s) of malar area, including zygomatic arch and malar tripod; with internal fixation and multiple surgical approaches T 80
33.12 33.12 Global Days 090

21366 with bone grafting (includes obtaining graft) C5 C 80
35.74 35.74 Global Days 090

21385 **Open treatment of orbital floor blowout fracture; transantral approach (Caldwell-Luc type operation)** T 80
20.59 20.59 Global Days 090

21386 **periorbital approach** T 80
19.52 19.52 Global Days 090

21387 **combined approach** T 80
22.13 22.13 Global Days 090

21390 **periorbital approach, with alloplastic or other implant** G2 T 80
23.68 23.68 Global Days 090

21395 **periorbital approach with bone graft (includes obtaining graft)** T 80
29.17 29.17 Global Days 090

21400 **Closed treatment of fracture of orbit, except blowout; without manipulation** A2 T 80
4.58 5.62 Global Days 090

21401 **with manipulation** A2 T 80
9.05 14.45 Global Days 090

21406 **Open treatment of fracture of orbit, except blowout; without implant** G2 T 80
16.58 16.58 Global Days 090

21407 **with implant** G2 T 80
19.31 19.31 Global Days 090

21408 **with bone grafting (includes obtaining graft)** T 80
27.01 27.01 Global Days 090

21421 **Closed treatment of palatal or maxillary fracture (LeFort I type), with interdental wire fixation or fixation of denture or splint** A2 T 80
19.51 23.40 Global Days 090

21422 **Open treatment of palatal or maxillary fracture (LeFort I type);** C5 C 80 PO
19.77 19.77 Global Days 090

21423 **complicated (comminuted or involving cranial nerve foramina), multiple approaches** C5 C 80 PO
23.78 23.78 Global Days 090

21431 **Closed treatment of craniofacial separation (LeFort III type) using interdental wire fixation of denture or splint** C5 C 80
20.16 20.16 Global Days 090

21432 **Open treatment of craniofacial separation (LeFort III type); with wiring and/or internal fixation** C5 C 80 PO
21.27 21.27 Global Days 090

21433 **complicated (eg, comminuted or involving cranial nerve foramina), multiple surgical approaches** C5 C 80 PO
49.21 49.21 Global Days 090

21435 **complicated, utilizing internal and/or external fixation techniques (eg, head cap, halo device, and/or intermaxillary fixation)** C5 C 80 PO
EXCLUDES *Removal of internal or external fixation (20670)*
40.70 40.70 Global Days 090

21436 **complicated, multiple surgical approaches, internal fixation, with bone grafting (includes obtaining graft)** C5 C 80 PO
61.33 61.33 Global Days 090

21440 **Closed treatment of mandibular or maxillary alveolar ridge fracture (separate procedure)** P3 T 80
13.78 16.86 Global Days 090

21445 **Open treatment of mandibular or maxillary alveolar ridge fracture (separate procedure)** A2 T 80
18.27 22.44 Global Days 090

21450 **Closed treatment of mandibular fracture; without manipulation** A2 T 80
14.43 17.79 Global Days 090

21451 **with manipulation** A2 T 80
18.62 22.16 Global Days 090

In 21452, external fixation is necessary
Comminuted fractures
Metal or acrylic bar
Rods and pins placed in drilled holes

21452 **Percutaneous treatment of mandibular fracture, with external fixation** A2 T 80
10.49 18.05 Global Days 090

21453 **Closed treatment of mandibular fracture with interdental fixation** A2 T 80
23.03 26.67 Global Days 090
AMA: 2009, Jan, 11-31; 2008, Jan, 10-25; 2007, Dec, 7-8

21454 **Open treatment of mandibular fracture with external fixation** A2 T 80 PO
17.35 17.35 Global Days 090

21461 **Open treatment of mandibular fracture; without interdental fixation** A2 T PO
27.99 62.71 Global Days 090

21462 **with interdental fixation** A2 T 80 PO
30.54 65.74 Global Days 090

21465 **Open treatment of mandibular condylar fracture** A2 T 80 PO
28.15 28.15 Global Days 090

21470 **Open treatment of complicated mandibular fracture by multiple surgical approaches including internal fixation, interdental fixation, and/or wiring of dentures or splints** T 80 PO
35.74 35.74 Global Days 090
AMA: 2009, Jan, 11-31; 2008, Jan, 10-25; 2007, January, 13-27

21480 **Closed treatment of temporomandibular dislocation; initial or subsequent** A2 T 50
0.95 2.86 Global Days 000

21485 **complicated (eg, recurrent requiring intermaxillary fixation or splinting), initial or subsequent** A2 T 80 50
17.01 20.28 Global Days 090

21490 **Open treatment of temporomandibular dislocation** A2 T 80 50
EXCLUDES *Interdental wiring (21497)*
27.45 27.45 Global Days 090

21495 **Open treatment of hyoid fracture** G2 T 80
EXCLUDES *Closed treatment of larynx fracture (99201-99499 [99224, 99225, 99226])*
Laryngoplasty with open fracture repair (31584)
21.26 21.26 Global Days 090

21497 **Interdental wiring, for condition other than fracture** A2 T 80
17.99 21.53 Global Days 090
AMA: 2009, Jan, 11-31; 2008, Jan, 10-25; 2007, January, 13-27

21499 **Unlisted musculoskeletal procedure, head** T 80
EXCLUDES *Unlisted procedures of craniofacial or maxillofacial areas*
0.00 0.00 Global Days YYY

21501-21510 Surgical Incision for Drainage: Chest and Soft Tissues of Neck

EXCLUDES *Biopsy of the flank or back (21920-21925)*
Simple incision and drainage of abscess or hematoma (10060, 10140)
Tumor removal of flank or back (21930-21935)

21501 **Incision and drainage, deep abscess or hematoma, soft tissues of neck or thorax;** A2 T
EXCLUDES *Deep incision and drainage of posterior spine (22010-22015)*
9.50 13.37 Global Days 090

21502 **with partial rib ostectomy** A2 T 80
15.69 15.69 Global Days 090

21510 **Incision, deep, with opening of bone cortex (eg, for osteomyelitis or bone abscess), thorax** C5 C 80
15.26 15.26 Global Days 090

21550 Soft Tissue Biopsy of Chest or Neck

EXCLUDES *Biopsy of bone (20220-20251)*
Soft tissue needle biopsy (20206)

21550 **Biopsy, soft tissue of neck or thorax** G2 T
4.66 7.69 Global Days 010

21552-21558 [21552, 21554] Excision Soft TissuesTumors Chest and Neck

INCLUDES Any necessary elevation of tissue planes or dissection
Measurement of tumor and necessary margin at greatest diameter prior to excision
Resection without removal of significant normal tissue
Simple and intermediate repairs
Types of Excisions:
Fascial or subfascial soft tissue tumors: simple and marginal resection of most often benign and intramuscular tumors found either in or below the deep fascia, not involving bone
Radical resection soft tissue tumor: wide resection of tumor, mostly malignant or aggressive benign, involving large margins of normal tissue and may involve tissue removal from one or more layers
Subcutaneous: simple and marginal resection of most often benign tumors found in the subcutaneous tissue above the deep fascia

EXCLUDES *Complex repair*
Radical resection of cutaneous tumors (e.g., melanoma) (11600-11646)
Significant exploration of the vessels or neuroplasty

21552 Resequenced code, See code following 21555.

21554 Resequenced code, See code following 21556.

21555 **Excision, tumor, soft tissue of neck or anterior thorax, subcutaneous; less than 3 cm** G2 T
9.12 12.29 Global Days 090
AMA: 2009, Jan, 11-31; 2008, Jan, 10-25; 2007, January, 13-27

\# 21552 **3 cm or greater** G2 T 80
13.19 13.19 Global Days 090

21556 **Excision, tumor, soft tissue of neck or anterior thorax, subfascial (eg, intramuscular); less than 5 cm** G2 T
15.54 15.54 Global Days 090

\# 21554 **5 cm or greater** G2 T 80
21.59 21.59 Global Days 090

21557 **Radical resection of tumor (eg, malignant neoplasm), soft tissue of neck or anterior thorax; less than 5 cm** G2 T 80
27.41 27.41 Global Days 090

21558 **5 cm or greater** G2 T 80
39.92 39.92 Global Days 090

21600-21632 Bony Resection Chest and Neck

21600 **Excision of rib, partial** A2 T 80
EXCLUDES *Extensive debridement (11044, 11047)*
Extensive tumor removal (19260)
16.88 16.88 Global Days 090

21610 **Costotransversectomy (separate procedure)** A2 T 80
34.95 34.95 Global Days 090

21615 **Excision first and/or cervical rib;** C5 C 80 50
19.31 19.31 Global Days 090

21616 **with sympathectomy** C5 C 80 50
25.05 25.05 Global Days 090

21620 **Ostectomy of sternum, partial** C5 C 80
15.36 15.36 Global Days 090

21627 **Sternal debridement** C5 C 80 PQ
EXCLUDES *Debridement with sternotomy closure (21750)*
16.36 16.36 Global Days 090

21630 **Radical resection of sternum;** C5 C 80
37.18 37.18 Global Days 090

21632 **with mediastinal lymphadenectomy** C5 C 80 PQ
36.61 36.61 Global Days 090

21685-21750 Repair/Reconstruction Chest and Soft Tissues Neck

EXCLUDES *Biopsy of flank or back (21920-21925)*
Repair of simple wounds (12001-12007)
Tumor removal of flank or back (21930, 21935)

21685 **Hyoid myotomy and suspension** G2 T 80
29.73 29.73 Global Days 090
AMA: 2009, Jan, 11-31; 2008, Jan, 10-25; 2007, January, 13-27

21700 **Division of scalenus anticus; without resection of cervical rib** A2 T 80
11.57 11.57 Global Days 090

21705 **with resection of cervical rib** C5 C 80
18.50 18.50 Global Days 090

21720 **Division of sternocleidomastoid for torticollis, open operation; without cast application** A2 T 80
EXCLUDES *Transection of spinal accessory and cervical nerves (63191, 64722)*
14.89 14.89 Global Days 090

21725 **with cast application** A2 T 80
EXCLUDES *Transection of spinal accessory and cervical nerves (63191, 64722)*
14.10 14.10 Global Days 090

21740 **Reconstructive repair of pectus excavatum or carinatum; open** C5 C 80 PQ
35.40 35.40 Global Days 090

21742 **minimally invasive approach (Nuss procedure), without thoracoscopy** T 80
0.00 0.00 Global Days 090

21743 **minimally invasive approach (Nuss procedure), with thoracoscopy** T 80
0.00 0.00 Global Days 090

21750 **Closure of median sternotomy separation with or without debridement (separate procedure)** C5 C 80 PQ
20.79 20.79 Global Days 090

21800-21825 Fracture Care: Ribs and Sternum

21800 **Closed treatment of rib fracture, uncomplicated, each** A2 T
3.28 3.19 Global Days 090

21805 **Open treatment of rib fracture without fixation, each** A2 T 80
7.89 7.89 Global Days 090

21810 **Treatment of rib fracture requiring external fixation (flail chest)** C5 C 80
15.21 15.21 Global Days 090

21820 **Closed treatment of sternum fracture** A2 T
4.18 4.09 Global Days 090

21825 **Open treatment of sternum fracture with or without skeletal fixation** C5 C 80
EXCLUDES *Treatment of sternoclavicular dislocation (23520-23532)*
16.46 16.46 Global Days 090

21899 Unlisted Procedures of Chest or Neck

21899 **Unlisted procedure, neck or thorax** T 80
0.00 0.00 Global Days YYY

21920-21925 Biopsy Soft Tissue of Back and Flank

EXCLUDES *Soft tissue needle biopsy (20206)*

21920 **Biopsy, soft tissue of back or flank; superficial** P3 T
EXCLUDES *Needle biopsy (20206)*
4.79 7.67 Global Days 010

21925 **deep** A2 T
EXCLUDES *Needle biopsy (20206)*
10.30 12.96 Global Days 090

21930-21936 Excision Soft Tissue Tumors Back or Flank

INCLUDES Any necessary elevation of tissue planes or dissection
Measurement of tumor and necessary margin at greatest diameter prior to excision
Resection without removal of significant normal tissue
Simple and intermediate repairs
Types of excision:
Fascial or subfascial soft tissue tumors: simple and marginal resection of most often benign and intramuscular tumors found either in or below the deep fascia, not involving bone
Radical resection soft tissue tumor: wide resection of tumor, mostly malignant or aggressive benign, involving large margins of normal tissue and may involve tissue removal from one or more layers
Subcutaneous: simple and marginal resection of most often benign tumors found in the subcutaneous tissue above the deep fascia

EXCLUDES *Complex repair*
Radical resection of cutaneous tumors (e.g., melanoma) (11600-11646)
Significant exploration of the vessels or neuroplasty

21930 **Excision, tumor, soft tissue of back or flank, subcutaneous; less than 3 cm** G2 T
10.77 13.88 Global Days 090
AMA: 2009, Jan, 11-31; 2008, Jan, 10-25; 2007, January, 13-27

21931 **3 cm or greater** G2 T 80
13.89 13.89 Global Days 090

21932 **Excision, tumor, soft tissue of back or flank, subfascial (eg, intramuscular); less than 5 cm** G2 T 80
19.52 19.52 Global Days 090

21933 **5 cm or greater** G2 T 80
21.85 21.85 Global Days 090

21935 **Radical resection of tumor (eg, malignant neoplasm), soft tissue of back or flank; less than 5 cm** G2 T
30.36 30.36 Global Days 090

21936 **5 cm or greater** G2 T 80
41.53 41.53 Global Days 090

22010-22015 Incision for Drainage of Deep Spinal Abscess

EXCLUDES *Incision and drainage of hematoma (10060, 10140)*
Injection:
Chemonucleolysis (62292)
Discography (62290-62291)
Facet joint (64490-64495, [64633, 64634, 64635, 64636])
Myelography (62284)
Needle/trocar biopsy (20220-20225)

22010 **Incision and drainage, open, of deep abscess (subfascial), posterior spine; cervical, thoracic, or cervicothoracic** C5 C 80
27.74 27.74 Global Days 090

22015 **lumbar, sacral, or lumbosacral** C5 C
Do not report with (10180, 22010, 22850, 22852)
27.25 27.25 Global Days 090

22100-22103 Partial Resection Vertebral Component

EXCLUDES *Back or flank biopsy (21920-21925)*
Bone biopsy (20220-20251)
Bone grafting procedures (20930-20938)
Injection
Chemonucleolysis (62292)
Discography (62290-62291)
Facet joint (64490-64495, [64633, 64634, 64635, 64636])
Myelography (62284)
Removal of tumor flank or back (21930)
Soft tissue needle biopsy (20206)

22100 **Partial excision of posterior vertebral component (eg, spinous process, lamina or facet) for intrinsic bony lesion, single vertebral segment; cervical** T 80
26.93 26.93 Global Days 090

22101 **thoracic** T 80
27.06 27.06 Global Days 090

22102 **lumbar** G2 T 80
EXCLUDES *Insertion of posterior spinous process distraction devices (0171T-0172T)*
24.05 24.05 Global Days 090

+ **22103** **each additional segment (List separately in addition to code for primary procedure)** G2 T 80
Code first (22100-22102)
4.22 4.22 Global Days ZZZ

22110-22116 Partial Resection Vertebral Component without Decompression

EXCLUDES *Back or flank biopsy (21920-21925)*
Bone biopsy (20220-20251)
Bone grafting procedures (20930-20938)
Harvest bone graft (20931, 20938)
Injection:
Chemonucleolysis (62292)
Discography (62290-62291)
Facet joint (64490-64495, [64633, 64634, 64635, 64636])
Myelography (62284)
Osteotomy (22210-22226)
Removal of tumor flank or back (21930)
Restoration after vertebral body resection (22585, 63082 or 63086 or 63088 or 63091)
Spinal restoration with graft:
Cervical (20931 or 20938, 22554, 63081)
Lumbar (20931 or 20938, 22558, 63087 or 63090)
Thoracic (20931 or 20938, 22556, 63085 or 63087)
Spinal restoration with prosthesis:
Cervical (20931 or 20938, 22554, 22851, 63081)
Lumbar (20931 or 20938, 22558, 22851, 63087 or 63090)
Thoracic (20931 or 20938, 22556, 22851, 63085 or 63087)
Vertebral corpectomy (63081-63091)

22110 **Partial excision of vertebral body, for intrinsic bony lesion, without decompression of spinal cord or nerve root(s), single vertebral segment; cervical** C5 C 80
31.84 31.84 Global Days 090

22112 **thoracic** C5 C 80
31.27 31.27 Global Days 090

22114 **lumbar** C5 C 80
29.27 29.27 Global Days 090

+ **22116** **each additional vertebral segment (List separately in addition to code for primary procedure)** C5 C 80
Code first (22110-22114)
4.16 4.16 Global Days ZZZ

22206-22216 Spinal Osteotomy: Posterior/Posterolateral Approach

CMS 100-4,12,40.8 Co-surgery and team surgery

EXCLUDES *Decompression of the spinal cord and/or nerve roots (63001-63308)*
Injection:
Chemonucleolysis (62292)
Discography (62290-62292)
Facet joint (64490-64495, [64633, 64634, 64635, 64636])
Myelography (62284)
Repair of vertebral fracture by the anterior approach, see appropriate arthrodesis, bone graft, instrumentation codes, and (63081-63091)

Code also arthrodesis (22590-22632)
Code also bone grafting procedures (20930-20938)
Code also spinal instrumentation (22840-22855)

22206 **Osteotomy of spine, posterior or posterolateral approach, 3 columns, 1 vertebral segment (eg, pedicle/vertebral body subtraction); thoracic** C5 C 80
Do not report with (22207)
Do not report with the following codes if performed at same level (22210-22226, 22830, 63001-63048, 63055-63066, 63075-63091, 63101-63103)
69.30 69.30 Global Days 090
AMA: 2009, Jan, 11-31; 2008, Feb, 8-9; 2007, Dec, 1-2

22207 **lumbar** C5 C 80
Do not report with (22206)
Do not report with the following codes if performed at the same level (22210-22226, 22830, 63001-63048, 63055-63066, 63075-63091, 63101-63103)
70.41 70.41 Global Days 090
AMA: 2009, Jan, 11-31; 2008, Feb, 8-9; 2007, Dec, 1-2

+ **22208** **each additional vertebral segment (List separately in addition to code for primary procedure)** C5 C 80
Code first (22206 or 22207)
Do not report with the following codes if performed at the same level (22210-22226, 22830, 63001-63048, 63055-63066, 63075-63091, 63101-63103)
17.40 17.40 Global Days ZZZ
AMA: 2009, Jan, 11-31; 2008, Feb, 8-9; 2007, Dec, 1-2

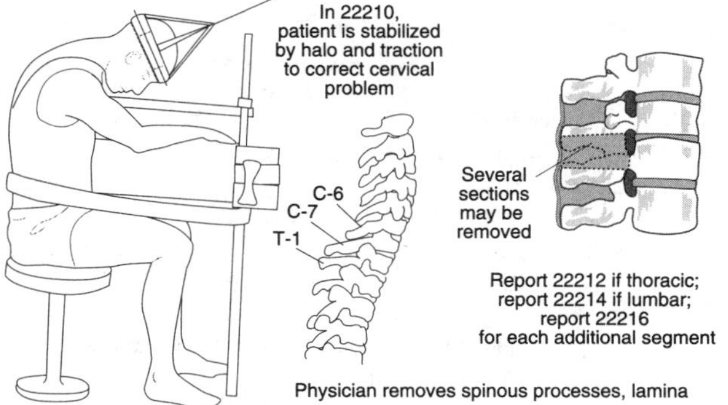

22210 **Osteotomy of spine, posterior or posterolateral approach, 1 vertebral segment; cervical** C5 C 80 PQ
52.13 52.13 Global Days 090
AMA: 2007, Dec, 1-2

22212 **thoracic** C5 C 80
43.25 43.25 Global Days 090
AMA: 2007, Dec, 1-2

22214 **lumbar** C5 C 80 PQ
43.58 43.58 Global Days 090
AMA: 2007, Dec, 1-2

+ **22216** **each additional vertebral segment (List separately in addition to primary procedure)** C5 C 80
Code first (22210-22214)
10.80 10.80 Global Days ZZZ
AMA: 2007, Dec, 1-2

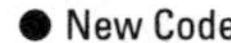

22220-22226 Spinal Osteotomy: Anterior Approach

CMS 100-4,12,40.8 Co-surgery and team surgery

EXCLUDES *Corpectomy (63081-63091)*
Decompression of the spinal cord and/or nerve roots (63001-63308)
Injection:
Chemonucleolysis (62292)
Discography (62290-62291)
Facet joint (64490-64495, [64633], [64634], [64635], [64636])
Myelography (62284)
Needle/trocar biopsy (20220-20225)
Repair of vertebral fracture by the anterior approach, see appropriate arthrodesis, bone graft, instrumentation codes, and (63081-63091)

Code also arthrodesis (22590-22632)
Code also spinal instrumentation (22840-22855)
Code also bone grafting procedures (20930-20938)

22220 **Osteotomy of spine, including discectomy, anterior approach, single vertebral segment; cervical** C5 C 80 PQ
47.66 47.66 Global Days 090

22222 **thoracic** T 80 PQ
44.87 44.87 Global Days 090

22224 **lumbar** C5 C 80 PQ
46.51 46.51 Global Days 090

+ **22226** **each additional vertebral segment (List separately in addition to code for primary procedure)** C5 C 80 PQ
Code first (22220-22224)
10.84 10.84 Global Days ZZZ

22305-22315 Closed Treatment Vertebral Fractures

EXCLUDES *Injection:*
Chemonucleolysis (62292)
Discography (62290-62291)
Facet joint (64490-64495, [64633], [64634], [64635], [64636])
Myelography (62284)

22305 **Closed treatment of vertebral process fracture(s)** A2 T PQ
5.06 5.56 Global Days 090

22310 **Closed treatment of vertebral body fracture(s), without manipulation, requiring and including casting or bracing** A2 T PQ
8.20 8.89 Global Days 090
AMA: 2009, Jan, 11-31; 2008, Jan, 10-25; 2007, January, 13-27

22315 **Closed treatment of vertebral fracture(s) and/or dislocation(s) requiring casting or bracing, with and including casting and/or bracing by manipulation or traction** A2 T PQ
EXCLUDES *Spinal manipulation (97140)*
22.68 25.86 Global Days 090

22318-22319 Open Treatment Odontoid Fracture: Anterior Approach

EXCLUDES *Injection:*
Chemonucleolysis (62292)
Discography (62290-62291)
Facet joint (64490-64495, [64633, 64634, 64635, 64636])
Myelography (62284)
Needle/trocar biopsy (20220-20225)

Code also arthrodesis (22590-22632)
Code also bone grafting procedures (20930-20938)
Code also spinal instrumentation (22840-22855)

22318 **Open treatment and/or reduction of odontoid fracture(s) and or dislocation(s) (including os odontoideum), anterior approach, including placement of internal fixation; without grafting** C5 C 80 PQ
48.18 48.18 Global Days 090

22319 **with grafting** C5 C 80 PQ
53.79 53.79 Global Days 090

22325-22328 Open Treatment Vertebral Fractures: Posterior Approach

EXCLUDES *Corpectomy (63081-63091)*
Injection:
Chemonucleolysis (62292)
Discography (62290-62291)
Facet joint (64490-64495, [64633], [64634], [64635], [64636])
Myelography (62284)
Needle/trocar biopsy (20220-20225)
Spine decompression (63001-63091)
Vertebral fracture care frontal approach (63081-63091)

Code also arthrodesis (22548-22632)
Code also bone grafting procedure (20930-20938)
Code also spinal instrumentation (22840-22855)

22325 **Open treatment and/or reduction of vertebral fracture(s) and/or dislocation(s), posterior approach, 1 fractured vertebra or dislocated segment; lumbar** C5 C 80 PQ
42.33 42.33 Global Days 090

22326 **cervical** C5 C 80 PQ
43.80 43.80 Global Days 090

22327 **thoracic** C5 C 80 PQ
43.59 43.59 Global Days 090

+ **22328** **each additional fractured vertebra or dislocated segment (List separately in addition to code for primary procedure)** C5 C 80
Code first (22325-22327)
8.41 8.41 Global Days ZZZ

22505 Spinal Manipulation with Anesthesia

EXCLUDES *Manipulation not requiring anesthesia (97140)*

22505 **Manipulation of spine requiring anesthesia, any region** A2 T
3.50 3.50 Global Days 010
AMA: 2009, Jan, 11-31; 2008, Jan, 10-25; 2007, January, 13-27

22520-22525 Percutaneous Vertebroplasty/Kyphoplasty

EXCLUDES *Injection:*
Chemonucleolysis (62292)
Discography (62290-62291)
Facet joint (64490-64495, [64633], [64634], [64635], [64636])
Myelography (62284)
Needle/trocar biopsy (20220-20225)

Do not report with the following codes when performed at the same level (20225, 22310-22315, 22325, 22327)

⊙ ▲ **22520** **Percutaneous vertebroplasty (bone biopsy included when performed), 1 vertebral body, unilateral or bilateral injection; thoracic** A2 T CCI PQ
72291-72292
15.06 66.16 Global Days 010

⊙ ▲ **22521** **lumbar** A2 T CCI PQ
72291-72292
14.33 65.86 Global Days 010

+ ▲ **22522** **each additional thoracic or lumbar vertebral body (List separately in addition to code for primary procedure)** A2 T CCI
Code first (22520-22521)
72291-72292
6.66 6.66 Global Days ZZZ

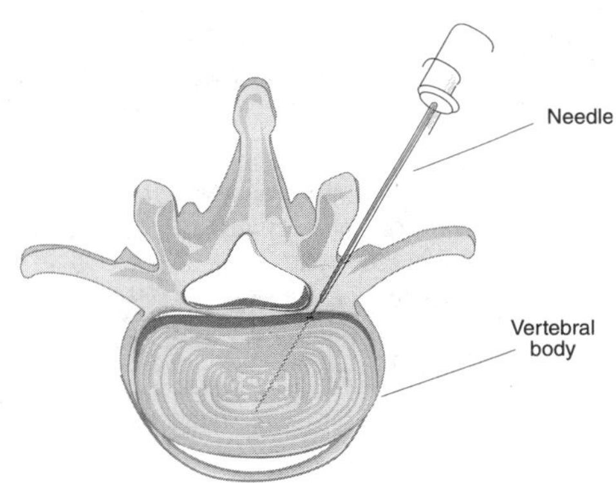

22523 **Percutaneous vertebral augmentation, including cavity creation (fracture reduction and bone biopsy included when performed) using mechanical device, 1 vertebral body, unilateral or bilateral cannulation (eg, kyphoplasty); thoracic** G2 T PQ
72291-72292
16.78 225.00 Global Days 010

22524 **lumbar** G2 T PQ
72291-72292
15.95 223.23 Global Days 010

+ **22525** **each additional thoracic or lumbar vertebral body (List separately in addition to code for primary procedure)** G2 T
Code first (22523-22524)
72291-72292
7.65 139.60 Global Days ZZZ

22526-22527 Percutaneous Annuloplasty

EXCLUDES *Needle/trocar biopsy (20220-20225)*
Injection:
Chemonucleolysis (62292)
Discography (62290-62291)
Facet joint (64490-64495, [64633], [64634], [64635], [64636])
Myelography (62284)
Procedure performed by other methods (22899)

Do not report with (77002, 77003)

⊙ **22526** **Percutaneous intradiscal electrothermal annuloplasty, unilateral or bilateral including fluoroscopic guidance; single level** E
INCLUDES Contrast injection during fluoroscopic guidance/localization (77003)
EXCLUDES *Percutaneous intradiscal annuloplasty other than electrothermal (22899)*
9.74 66.43 Global Days 010
AMA: 2009, Jan, 11-31; 2008, Jan, 10-25; 2007, March, 7-8

+ ⊙ **22527** **1 or more additional levels (List separately in addition to code for primary procedure)** E
INCLUDES Contrast injection during fluoroscopic guidance/localization (77003)
EXCLUDES *Percutaneous intradiscal annuloplasty other than electrothermal (22899)*
Code first (22526, 22527)
4.37 54.25 Global Days ZZZ
AMA: 2007, March, 7-8

22532-22534 Spinal Fusion: Lateral Extracavitary Approach

CMS 100-3,150.2 Osteogenic Stimulation

EXCLUDES *Corpectomy (63101-63103)*
Exploration of spinal fusion (22830)
Fracture care (22305-22328)
Injection:
Chemonucleolysis (62292)
Discography (62290-62291)
Facet joint (64490-64495, [64633], [64634], [64635], [64636])
Myelography (62284)
Laminectomy (63001-63017)
Needle/trocar biopsy (20220-20225)
Osteotomy (22206)

Code also bone grafting procedures (20930-20938)
Code also spinal instrumentation (22840-22855)

22532 **Arthrodesis, lateral extracavitary technique, including minimal discectomy to prepare interspace (other than for decompression); thoracic** C5 C 80 CCI PQ
52.59 52.59 Global Days 090

22533 **lumbar** C5 C 80 CCI PQ
49.54 49.54 Global Days 090

+ **22534** **thoracic or lumbar, each additional vertebral segment (List separately in addition to code for primary procedure)** C5 C 80 CCI PQ
Code first (22532-22533)
10.77 10.77 Global Days ZZZ

22548-22634 Spinal Fusion: Anterior and Posterior Approach

CMS 100-3,150.2 Osteogenic Stimulation

EXCLUDES *Corpectomy (63081-63091)*
Exploration of spinal fusion (22830)
Fracture care (22305-22328)
Facet joint arthrodesis (0219T-0222T)
Injection:
Chemonucleolysis (62292)
Discography (62290-62291)
Facet joint (64490-64495, [64633], [64634], [64635], [64636])
Myelography (62284)
Laminectomy (63001-63017)
Needle/trocar biopsy (20220-20225)
Osteotomy (22206)

Code also bone grafting procedures (20930-20938)

Code also spinal instrumentation (22840-22855)

22548 Arthrodesis, anterior transoral or extraoral technique, clivus-C1-C2 (atlas-axis), with or without excision of odontoid process

EXCLUDES *Laminectomy or laminotomy with disc removal (63020-63042)*

57.75 57.75 Global Days 090

AMA: 2009, Jan, 11-31; 2008, Jan, 10-25; 2007, January, 13-27

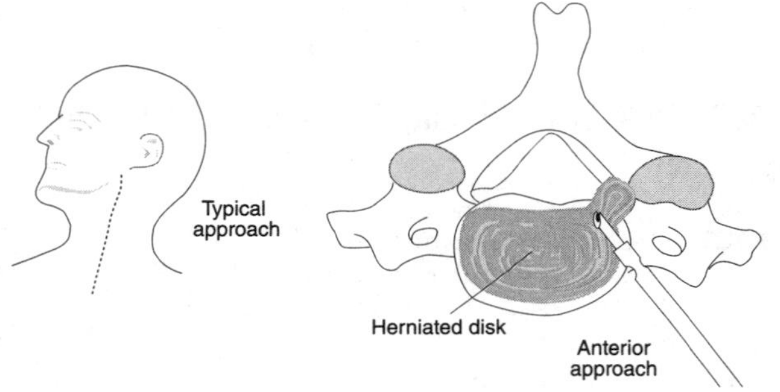

22551 Arthrodesis, anterior interbody, including disc space preparation, discectomy, osteophytectomy and decompression of spinal cord and/or nerve roots; cervical below C2

INCLUDES Operating microscope (69990)

50.98 50.98 Global Days 090

\+ **22552 cervical below C2, each additional interspace (List separately in addition to code for separate procedure)**

INCLUDES Operating microscope (69990)

Code first (22551)

11.68 11.68 Global Days ZZZ

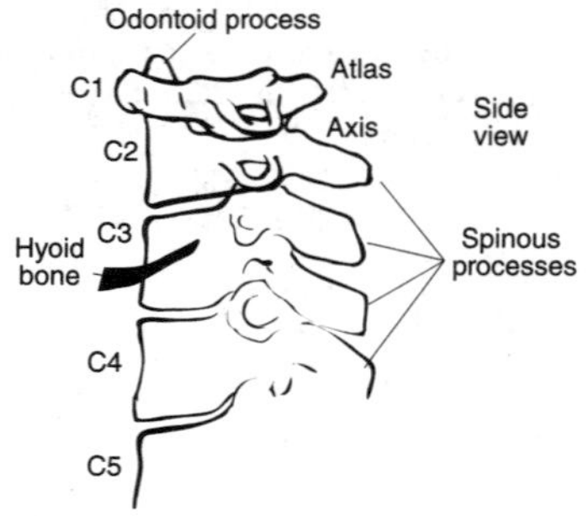

22554 Arthrodesis, anterior interbody technique, including minimal discectomy to prepare interspace (other than for decompression); cervical below C2

EXCLUDES *Anterior discectomy and interbody fusion during the same operative session (regardless if performed by multiple surgeons) (22551)*

Do not report with anterior discectomy (even by another provider) (63075)

37.71 37.71 Global Days 090

AMA: 2009, Jan, 11-31; 2008, Jan, 10-25; 2007, January, 13-27

22556 thoracic

49.13 49.13 Global Days 090

AMA: 2009, Jan, 11-31; 2008, Jan, 10-25; 2007, January, 13-27

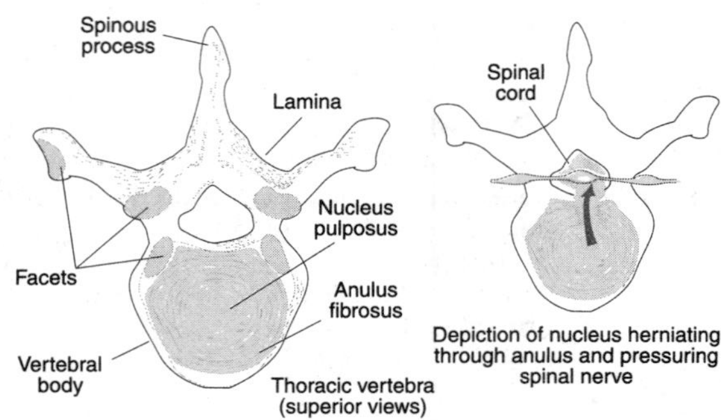

Intervertebral disc displacement and prolapse are major causes of disability among working people. When a disc prolapses, nuclear material bursts through the anulus fibrosus damaging ligaments, nerve roots, and other structures. The herniated matter usually fibroses and shrinks over time

22558 lumbar

45.47 45.47 Global Days 090

AMA: 2009, Jan, 11-31; 2008, Jan, 10-25; 2008, Apr, -11; 2007, January, 13-27; 2007, June, 1-3

\+ **22585 each additional interspace (List separately in addition to code for primary procedure)**

EXCLUDES *Anterior discectomy and interbody fusion during the same operative session (regardless if performed by multiple surgeons) (22552)*

Code first (22554-22558)

Do not report with anterior discectomy (even by another provider) (63075)

10.00 10.00 Global Days ZZZ

AMA: 2009, Jan, 11-31; 2008, Jan, 10-25; 2008, Apr, -11; 2007, June, 1-3; 2007, January, 13-27

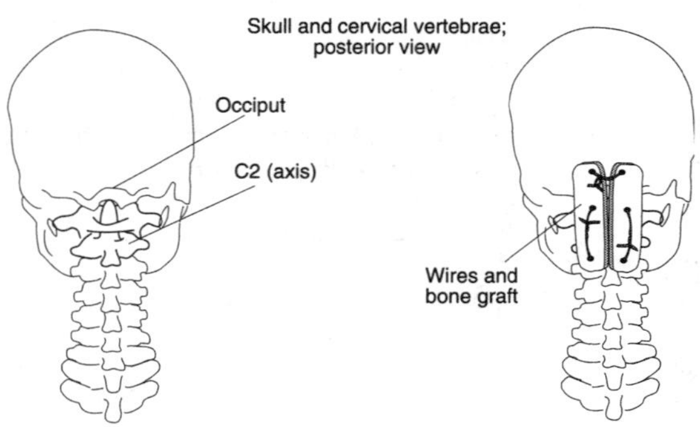

In 22590, the physician fuses skull to C2 (axis) to stabilize cervical vertebrae; anchor holes are drilled in the occiput of the skull

22590 **Arthrodesis, posterior technique, craniocervical (occiput-C2)** C5 C 80 CCI PQ
EXCLUDES *Posterior intrafacet implant insertion (0219T-0222T)*
46.58 46.58 Global Days 090

22595 **Arthrodesis, posterior technique, atlas-axis (C1-C2)** C5 C 80 CCI PQ
EXCLUDES *Posterior intrafacet implant insertion (0219T-0222T)*
44.35 44.35 Global Days 090

22600 **Arthrodesis, posterior or posterolateral technique, single level; cervical below C2 segment** C5 C 80 CCI PQ
EXCLUDES *Posterior intrafacet implant insertion (0219T-0222T)*
37.98 37.98 Global Days 090

▲ 22610 **thoracic (with lateral transverse technique, when performed)** C5 C 80 CCI
EXCLUDES *Posterior intrafacet implant insertion (0219T-0222T)*
37.10 37.10 Global Days 090

▲ 22612 **lumbar (with lateral transverse technique, when performed)** T 80 CCI PQ
EXCLUDES *Fusion of facet joint (0219T-0222T)*
Combined technique at the same interspace and segment (22633)

Do not report with the following code when performed at the same interspace and segment (22630, 22633)
47.12 47.12 Global Days 090
AMA: 2009, Jan, 11-31; 2008, Jan, 10-25; 2008, Apr, -11; 2008, Jul, 7-8&15; 2007, January, 13-27

+ 22614 **each additional vertebral segment (List separately in addition to code for primary procedure)** T 80 CCI PQ
INCLUDES Additional level fusion arthrodesis posterior or posterolateral interbody
EXCLUDES *Additional level interbody arthrodesis combined posterolateral or posterior.with posterior interbody arthrodesis (22634)*
Additional level posterior interbody arthrodesis (22632)

Code first (22600, 22610, 22612, 22630, 22633)
11.64 11.64 Global Days ZZZ

22630 **Arthrodesis, posterior interbody technique, including laminectomy and/or discectomy to prepare interspace (other than for decompression), single interspace; lumbar** C5 C 80 CCI PQ
EXCLUDES *Combined technique at the same interspace and segment (22633)*

Do not report with the following code at the same interspace and segment (22612, 22633)
45.60 45.60 Global Days 090
AMA: 2009, Jan, 11-31; 2008, Jan, 10-25; 2007, January, 13-27

+ 22632 **each additional interspace (List separately in addition to code for primary procedure)** C5 C 80 CCI PQ
INCLUDES Includes posterior interbody fusion arthrodesis, additional level
EXCLUDES *Additional level combined technique (22634)*
Additional level posterior or posteriolateral fusion (22614)

Code first (22612, 22630, 22633)
9.50 9.50 Global Days ZZZ

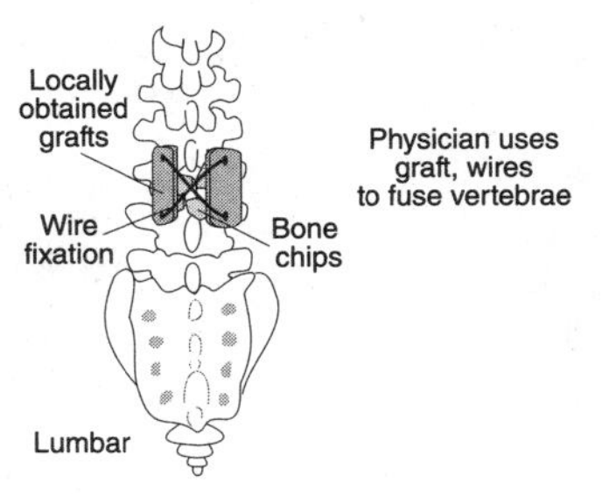

Using a posterior or posterolateral technique the vertebral interbody is fused

● 22633 **Arthrodesis, combined posterior or posterolateral technique with posterior interbody technique including laminectomy and/or discectomy sufficient to prepare interspace (other than for decompression), single interspace and segment; lumbar** C5 C 80
Do not report same level (22612, 22630)
54.76 54.76 Global Days 090

+ ● 22634 **each additional interspace and segment (List separately in addition to code for primary procedure)** C5 C 80
Code first (22633)
14.77 14.77 Global Days ZZZ

22800-22819 Procedures to Correct Anomalous Spinal Vertebrae

EXCLUDES *Facet injection (64490-64495, [64633, 64634, 64635, 64636])*
Code also bone grafting procedures (20930-20938)
Code also spinal instrumentation (22840-22855)

22800 **Arthrodesis, posterior, for spinal deformity, with or without cast; up to 6 vertebral segments** C5 C 80 CCI PQ
39.95 39.95 Global Days 090

22802 **7 to 12 vertebral segments** C5 C 80 CCI PQ
62.06 62.06 Global Days 090
AMA: 2009, Jan, 11-31; 2008, Jan, 10-25; 2007, January, 13-27

22804 **13 or more vertebral segments** C5 C 80 CCI PQ
71.36 71.36 Global Days 090

22808 **Arthrodesis, anterior, for spinal deformity, with or without cast; 2 to 3 vertebral segments** C5 C 80 CCI
INCLUDES Smith-Robinson arthrodesis
53.83 53.83 Global Days 090

22810 **4 to 7 vertebral segments** C5 C 80 CCI
60.02 60.02 Global Days 090
AMA: 2009, Jan, 11-31; 2008, Jan, 10-25; 2007, January, 13-27

22812 **8 or more vertebral segments** C5 C 80 CCI
65.01 65.01 Global Days 090

22818 **Kyphectomy, circumferential exposure of spine and resection of vertebral segment(s) (including body and posterior elements); single or 2 segments** C5 C 80 CCI PQ
EXCLUDES *Arthrodesis (22800-22804)*
63.98 63.98 Global Days 090

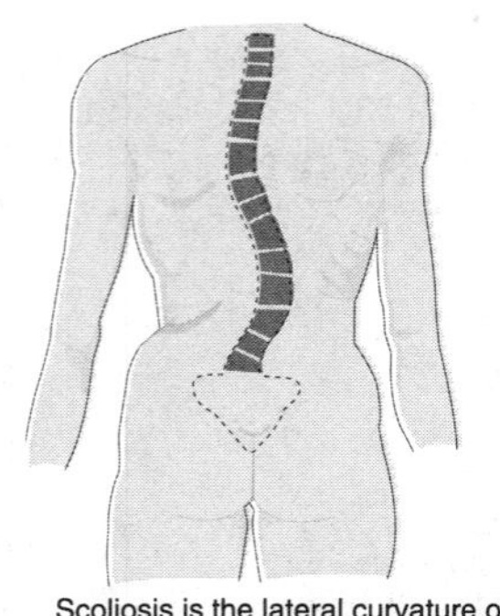

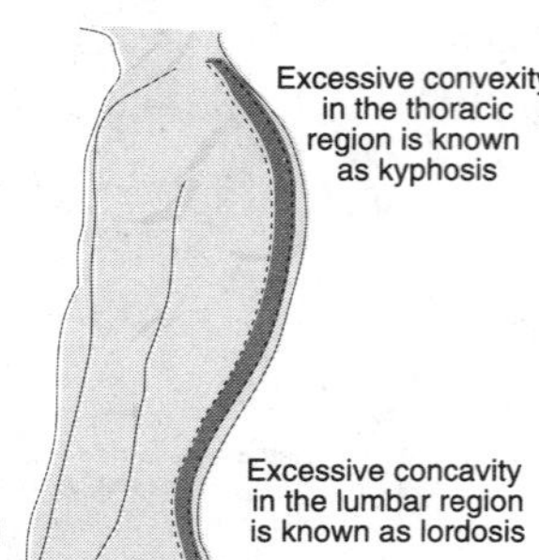

22819 **3 or more segments**

EXCLUDES *Arthrodesis (22800-22804)*

80.91 80.91 Global Days 090

22830 Surgical Exploration Previous Spinal Fusion

CMS 100-3,150.2 Osteogenic Stimulation

EXCLUDES *Arthrodesis (22532-22819)*
Bone grafting procedures (20930-20938)
Facet injection (64490-64495, [64633, 64634, 64635, 64636])
Spinal decompression (63001-63103)

Code also spinal instrumentation (22840-22855)

22830 **Exploration of spinal fusion**

Do not report with (22850, 22852, 22855)

23.91 23.91 Global Days 090

AMA: 2009, Jan, 11-31; 2008, Jan, 10-25; 2007, January, 13-27

22840-22848 Posterior, Anterior, Pelvic Spinal Instrumentation

INCLUDES Removal or revision of previously placed spinal instrumentation during same session as insertion of new instrumentation at levels including all or part of previously instrumented segments (22840-22848)

EXCLUDES *Arthrodesis (22532-22534, 22548-22812)*
Bone grafting procedures (20930-20938)
Exploration of spinal fusion (22830)
Facet injection (64490-64495, [64633], [64634], [64635], [64636])
Fracture treatment (22325-22328)

Do not report removal or reinsertion in addition to insertion of the new instrumentation (22849, 22850, 22852, 22855)

\+ **22840** **Posterior non-segmental instrumentation (eg, Harrington rod technique, pedicle fixation across 1 interspace, atlantoaxial transarticular screw fixation, sublaminar wiring at C1, facet screw fixation) (List separately in addition to code for primary procedure)**

EXCLUDES *Insertion of posterior spinous process distraction devices (0171T-0172T)*

Code first (22100-22102, 22110-22114, 22206-22207, 22210-22214, 22220-22224, 22305-22327, 22532-22533, 22548-22558, 22590-22612, 22630, 22800-22812, 63001-63030, 63040-63042, 63045-63047, 63050-63056, 63064, 63075, 63077, 63081, 63085, 63087, 63090, 63101-63102, 63170-63290, 63300-63307)

22.69 22.69 Global Days ZZZ

AMA: 2009, Jan, 11-31; 2008, Jan, 10-25; 2007, January, 13-27

\+ **22841** **Internal spinal fixation by wiring of spinous processes (List separately in addition to code for primary procedure)**

INCLUDES Hibb's fusion

Code first (22100-22102, 22110-22114, 22206-22207, 22210-22214, 22220-22224, 22305-22327, 22532-22533, 22548-22558, 22590-22612, 22630, 22800-22812, 63001-63030, 63040-63042, 63045-63047, 63050-63056, 63064, 63075, 63077, 63081, 63085, 63087, 63090, 63101-63102, 63170-63290, 63300-63307)

0.00 0.00 Global Days XXX

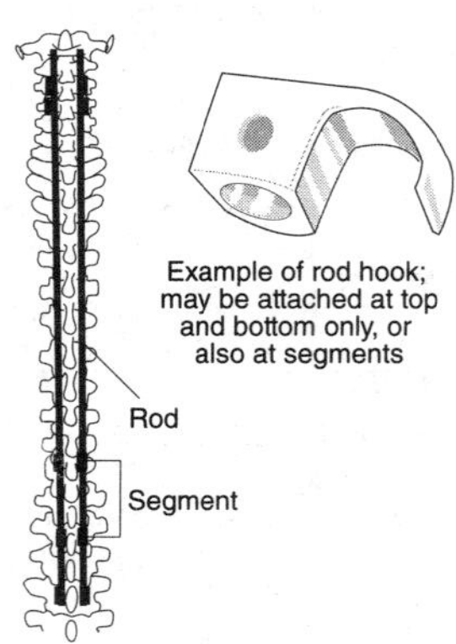

\+ **22842** **Posterior segmental instrumentation (eg, pedicle fixation, dual rods with multiple hooks and sublaminar wires); 3 to 6 vertebral segments (List separately in addition to code for primary procedure)**

Code first (22100-22102, 22110-22114, 22206-22207, 22210-22214, 22220-22224, 22305-22327, 22532-22533, 22548-22558, 22590-22612, 22630, 22800-22812, 63001-63030, 63040-63042, 63045-63047, 63050-63056, 63064, 63075, 63077, 63081, 63085, 63087, 63090, 63101-63102, 63170-63290, 63300-63307)

22.72 22.72 Global Days ZZZ

\+ **22843** **7 to 12 vertebral segments (List separately in addition to code for primary procedure)**

Code first (22100-22102, 22110-22114, 22206-22207, 22210-22214, 22220-22224, 22305-22327, 22532-22533, 22548-22558, 22590-22612, 22630, 22800-22812, 63001-63102, 63170-63290, 63300-63307)

24.14 24.14 Global Days ZZZ

\+ **22844** **13 or more vertebral segments (List separately in addition to code for primary procedure)**

Code first (22100-22102, 22206-22207, 22210-22214, 22210-22214, 22220-22224, 22305-22327, 22532-22533, 22548-22558, 22590-22612, 22630, 22800-22812, 63001-63030, 63040-63042, 63045-63047, 63050-63056, 63064, 63075, 63077, 63081, 63085, 63087, 63090, 63101-63102, 63170-63290, 63300-63307)

29.08 29.08 Global Days ZZZ

\+ **22845** **Anterior instrumentation; 2 to 3 vertebral segments (List separately in addition to code for primary procedure)**

INCLUDES Dwyer instrumentation technique

Code first (22100-22102, 22110-22114, 22206-22207, 22210-22214, 22220-22224, 22305-22327, 22532-22533, 22548-22558, 22590-22612, 22630, 22800-22812, 63001-63030, 63040-63042, 63045-63047, 63050-63056, 63064, 63075, 63077, 63081, 63085, 63087, 63090, 63101-63102, 63170-63290, 63300-63307)

21.92 21.92 Global Days ZZZ

AMA: 2009, Jan, 11-31; 2008, Jan, 10-25; 2007, January, 13-27; 2007, June, 1-3

\+ **22846 4 to 7 vertebral segments (List separately in addition to code for primary procedure)** C5 C 80 PQ

INCLUDES Dwyer instrumentation technique

Code first (22100-22102, 22110-22114, 22206-22207, 22210-22214, 22220-22224, 22305-22327, 22532-22533, 22548-22558, 22590-22612, 22630, 22800-22812, 63001-63030, 63040-63042, 63045-63047, 63050-63056, 63064, 63075, 63077, 63081, 63085, 63087, 63090, 63101-63102, 63170-63290, 63300-63307)

22.74 22.74 Global Days ZZZ

AMA: 2009, Jan, 11-31; 2008, Jan, 10-25

\+ **22847 8 or more vertebral segments (List separately in addition to code for primary procedure)** C5 C 80 PQ

INCLUDES Dwyer instrumentation technique

Code first (22100-22102, 22110-22114, 22206-22207, 22210-22214, 22220-22224, 22305-22327, 22532-22533, 22548-22558, 22590-22612, 22630, 22800-22812, 63001-63030, 63040-63042, 63045-63047, 63050-63056, 63064, 63075, 63077, 63081, 63085, 63087, 63090, 63101-63102, 63170-63290, 63300-63307)

26.24 26.24 Global Days ZZZ

AMA: 2009, Jan, 11-31; 2008, Jan, 10-25

\+ **22848 Pelvic fixation (attachment of caudal end of instrumentation to pelvic bony structures) other than sacrum (List separately in addition to code for primary procedure)** C5 C 80 PQ

Code first (22100-22102, 22110-22114, 22206-22207, 22210-22214, 22220-22224, 22305-22327, 22532-22533, 22548-22558, 22590-22612, 22630, 22800-22812, 63001-63030, 63040-63042, 63045-63047, 63050-63056, 63064, 63075, 63077, 63081, 63085, 63087, 63090, 63101-63102, 63170-63290, 63300-63307)

10.65 10.65 Global Days ZZZ

22849-22855 Miscellaneous Spinal Instrumentation

EXCLUDES *Arthrodesis (22532-22534, 22548-22812)*
Bone grafting procedures (20930-20938)
Exploration of spinal fusion (22830)
Facet injection (64490-64495, [64633], [64634], [64635], [64636])
Fracture treatment (22325-22328)

Do not report Removal or reinsertion in addition to insertion of the new instrumentation (22849, 22850, 22852, 22855)

22849 Reinsertion of spinal fixation device C5 C 80 PQ

Do not report with removal of instrumentation at the same level (22850, 22852, 22855)

38.45 38.45 Global Days 090

22850 Removal of posterior nonsegmental instrumentation (eg, Harrington rod) C5 C 80

21.29 21.29 Global Days 090

\+ **22851 Application of intervertebral biomechanical device(s) (eg, synthetic cage(s), methylmethacrylate) to vertebral defect or interspace (List separately in addition to code for primary procedure)** T 80

EXCLUDES *Application of intervertebral bone device/graft (20930-20938)*
Insertion of posterior spinous process distraction devices (0171T-0172T)

Code first (22100-22102, 22110-22114, 22206-22207, 22210-22214, 22220-22224, 22305-22327, 22532-22533, 22548-22558, 22590-22612, 22630, 22800-22812, 63001-63030, 63040-63042, 63045-63047, 63050-63056, 63064, 63075, 63077, 63081, 63085, 63087, 63090, 63101-63102, 63170-63290, 63300-63307)

12.15 12.15 Global Days ZZZ

AMA: 2009, Jan, 11-31; 2008, Jan, 10-25; 2007, January, 13-27; 2007, June, 1-3

22852 Removal of posterior segmental instrumentation C5 C 80

20.35 20.35 Global Days 090

AMA: 2009, Jan, 11-31; 2008, Jan, 10-25; 2007, January, 13-27

22855 Removal of anterior instrumentation C5 C 80

33.08 33.08 Global Days 090

22856-22899 Artificial Disc Replacement

CMS 100-3,150.10 Lumbar Artificial Disc Replacement (LADR)

INCLUDES Fluoroscopy (76000-76001)

EXCLUDES *Facet injection (64490-64495, [64633], [64634], [64635], [64636])*
Spinal decompression (63001-63048)

22856 Total disc arthroplasty (artificial disc), anterior approach, including discectomy with end plate preparation (includes osteophytectomy for nerve root or spinal cord decompression and microdissection), single interspace, cervical C5 C 80

INCLUDES Operating microscope (69990)
Same level:
Arthrodesis (22554)
Discectomy (63075)
Instrumentation (22845, 22851)

EXCLUDES *Cervical total disc arthroplasty with additional interspace revision (0092T)*

49.17 49.17 Global Days 090

22857 Total disc arthroplasty (artificial disc), anterior approach, including discectomy to prepare interspace (other than for decompression), single interspace, lumbar C5 C 80

INCLUDES Operating microscope (69990)
Same level:
Arthrodesis (22558)
Instrumentation (22845, 22851)
Retroperitoneal exploration (49010)

EXCLUDES *Arthroplasty more than one interspace (0163T)*

48.90 48.90 Global Days 090

AMA: 2007, June, 1-3

22861 Revision including replacement of total disc arthroplasty (artificial disc), anterior approach, single interspace; cervical C5 C 80

INCLUDES Operating microscope (69990)

EXCLUDES *Revision of additional cervical arthroplasty (0098T)*
Same level:
Discectomy (63075)
Instrumentation (22845, 22851)
Removal of artificial disc (22864)

59.03 59.03 Global Days 090

22862 lumbar C5 C 80

INCLUDES Same level:
Arthrodesis (22558)
Instrumentation (22845, 22851)
Removal artificial disc (22865)
Retroperitoneal exploration (49010)

EXCLUDES *Arthroplasty revision more than one interspace (0165T)*

61.82 61.82 Global Days 090

AMA: 2007, June, 1-3

22864 **Removal of total disc arthroplasty (artificial disc), anterior approach, single interspace; cervical** C5 C 80
INCLUDES Operating microscope (69990)
EXCLUDES *Cervical total disc arthroplasty with additional interspace removal (0095T)*
Do not report with (22861)
56.71 56.71 Global Days 090

22865 **lumbar** C5 C 80
EXCLUDES *Arthroplasty more than one level (0164T)*
Do not report with (49010)
60.66 60.66 Global Days 090
AMA: 2007, June, 1-3

22899 **Unlisted procedure, spine** T 80
0.00 0.00 Global Days YYY
AMA: 2009, Jan, 11-31; 2008, Jan, 10-25; 2007, January, 13-27

22900-22999 Musculoskeletal Procedures of Abdomen

INCLUDES Any necessary elevation of tissue planes or dissection
Measurement of tumor and necessary margin at greatest diameter prior to excision
Resection without removal of significant normal tissue
Simple and intermediate repairs
Types of Excision:
Fascial or subfascial soft tissue tumors: simple and marginal resection of most often benign and intramuscular tumors found either in or below the deep fascia, not involving bone
Radical resection soft tissue tumor: wide resection of tumor, mostly malignant or aggressive benign, involving large margins of normal tissue and may involve tissue removal from one or more layers
Subcutaneous: simple and marginal resection of most often benign tumors found in the subcutaneous tissue above the deep fascia

EXCLUDES *Complex repair*
Radical resection of cutaneous tumors (e.g., melanoma) (11600-11646)
Significant exploration of the vessels or neuroplasty

22900 **Excision, tumor, soft tissue of abdominal wall, subfascial (eg, intramuscular); less than 5 cm** G2 T 80
16.10 16.10 Global Days 090

22901 **5 cm or greater** G2 T 80
19.66 19.66 Global Days 090

22902 **Excision, tumor, soft tissue of abdominal wall, subcutaneous; less than 3 cm** G2 T 80
9.60 12.81 Global Days 090

22903 **3 cm or greater** G2 T 80
12.85 12.85 Global Days 090

22904 **Radical resection of tumor (eg, malignant neoplasm), soft tissue of abdominal wall; less than 5 cm** G2 T 80
31.08 31.08 Global Days 090

22905 **5 cm or greater** G2 T 80
39.44 39.44 Global Days 090

22999 **Unlisted procedure, abdomen, musculoskeletal system** T 80
0.00 0.00 Global Days YYY

23000-23044 Surgical Incision Shoulder: Drainage, Foreign Body Removal, Contracture Release

23000 **Removal of subdeltoid calcareous deposits, open** A2 T 80
EXCLUDES *Arthroscopic calcium deposit removal (29999)*
10.74 16.71 Global Days 090

23020 **Capsular contracture release (eg, Sever type procedure)** A2 T 80 50
EXCLUDES *Simple incision and drainage (10040-10160)*
20.24 20.24 Global Days 090

23030 **Incision and drainage, shoulder area; deep abscess or hematoma** A2 T
7.48 12.80 Global Days 010

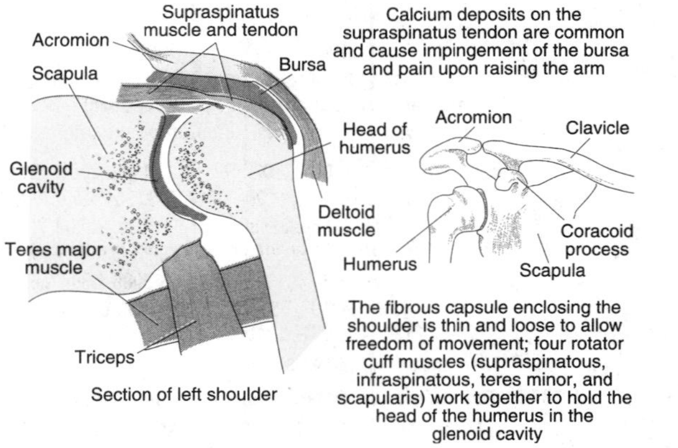

23031 **infected bursa** A2 T 50
6.35 12.16 Global Days 010

23035 **Incision, bone cortex (eg, osteomyelitis or bone abscess), shoulder area** A2 T 80 50
20.00 20.00 Global Days 090

23040 **Arthrotomy, glenohumeral joint, including exploration, drainage, or removal of foreign body** A2 T 80 50
21.09 21.09 Global Days 090

23044 **Arthrotomy, acromioclavicular, sternoclavicular joint, including exploration, drainage, or removal of foreign body** A2 T 50
16.82 16.82 Global Days 090

23065-23066 Shoulder Biopsy

EXCLUDES *Soft tissue needle biopsy (20206)*

23065 **Biopsy, soft tissue of shoulder area; superficial** P3 T 50
5.01 6.45 Global Days 010

23066 **deep** A2 T 50
10.23 15.80 Global Days 090

23071-23078 [23071, 23073] Excision Soft Tissue Tumors of Shoulder

INCLUDES Any necessary elevation of tissue planes or dissection
Measurement of tumor and necessary margin at greatest diameter prior to excision
Resection without removal of significant normal tissue
Simple and intermediate repairs
Types of Excision:
Fascial or subfascial soft tissue tumors: simple and marginal resection of most often benign and intramuscular tumors found either in or below the deep fascia, not involving bone
Radical resection soft tissue tumor: wide resection of tumor, mostly malignant or aggressive benign, involving large margins of normal tissue and may involve tissue removal from one or more layers
Subcutaneous: simple and marginal resection of most often benign tumors found in the subcutaneous tissue above the deep fascia

EXCLUDES *Complex repair*
Significant exploration of the vessels or neuroplasty

23071 *Resequenced code, See code following 23075.*

23073 *Resequenced code, See code following 23076.*

23075 **Excision, tumor, soft tissue of shoulder area, subcutaneous; less than 3 cm** G2 T 50 CCI
9.11 12.91 Global Days 090

\# **23071** **3 cm or greater** G2 T 80 50
12.35 12.35 Global Days 090

23076 **Excision, tumor, soft tissue of shoulder area, subfascial (eg, intramuscular); less than 5 cm** G2 T 50 CCI
15.91 15.91 Global Days 090

\# **23073** **5 cm or greater** G2 T 80 50
20.45 20.45 Global Days 090

23077 **Radical resection of tumor (eg, malignant neoplasm), soft tissue of shoulder area; less than 5 cm** G2 T 80 50 CCI
33.92 33.92 Global Days 090

23078 **5 cm or greater** G2 T 80 50
41.97 41.97 Global Days 090

23100-23195 Bone and Joint Procedures of Shoulder

INCLUDES Acromnioclavicular joint
Clavicle
Head and neck of humerus
Scapula
Shoulder joint
Sternoclavicular joint

23100 **Arthrotomy, glenohumeral joint, including biopsy** A2 T 80 50 CCI
14.56 14.56 Global Days 090

23101 **Arthrotomy, acromioclavicular joint or sternoclavicular joint, including biopsy and/or excision of torn cartilage** A2 T 50 CCI
13.29 13.29 Global Days 090

23105 **Arthrotomy; glenohumeral joint, with synovectomy, with or without biopsy** A2 T 80 50 CCI
18.69 18.69 Global Days 090

23106 **sternoclavicular joint, with synovectomy, with or without biopsy** A2 T 50 CCI
14.39 14.39 Global Days 090

23107 **Arthrotomy, glenohumeral joint, with joint exploration, with or without removal of loose or foreign body** A2 T 80 50 CCI
19.35 19.35 Global Days 090

23120 **Claviculectomy; partial** A2 T 80 CCI
INCLUDES Mumford operation
EXCLUDES *Arthroscopic claviculectomy (29824)*
17.13 17.13 Global Days 090

23125 **total** A2 T 80 50 CCI
20.69 20.69 Global Days 090

23130 **Acromioplasty or acromionectomy, partial, with or without coracoacromial ligament release** A2 T 50 CCI
17.81 17.81 Global Days 090
AMA: 2009, Jan, 11-31; 2008, Jan, 10-25; 2007, January, 13-27

23140 **Excision or curettage of bone cyst or benign tumor of clavicle or scapula;** A2 T 50 CCI
15.50 15.50 Global Days 090

23145 **with autograft (includes obtaining graft)** A2 T 80 50 CCI
20.31 20.31 Global Days 090

23146 **with allograft** A2 T 80 50 CCI
18.02 18.02 Global Days 090

23150 **Excision or curettage of bone cyst or benign tumor of proximal humerus;** A2 T 80 50 CCI
19.30 19.30 Global Days 090

23155 **with autograft (includes obtaining graft)** A2 T 80 50 CCI
23.20 23.20 Global Days 090

23156 **with allograft** A2 T 80 50 CCI
19.81 19.81 Global Days 090

23170 **Sequestrectomy (eg, for osteomyelitis or bone abscess), clavicle** A2 T 50 CCI
16.19 16.19 Global Days 090

23172 **Sequestrectomy (eg, for osteomyelitis or bone abscess), scapula** A2 T 80 50 CCI
16.46 16.46 Global Days 090

23174 **Sequestrectomy (eg, for osteomyelitis or bone abscess), humeral head to surgical neck** A2 T 80 50 CCI
22.16 22.16 Global Days 090

23180 **Partial excision (craterization, saucerization, or diaphysectomy) bone (eg, osteomyelitis), clavicle** A2 T 50 CCI
19.78 19.78 Global Days 090

23182 **Partial excision (craterization, saucerization, or diaphysectomy) bone (eg, osteomyelitis), scapula** A2 T 80 50 CCI
19.30 19.30 Global Days 090

23184 **Partial excision (craterization, saucerization, or diaphysectomy) bone (eg, osteomyelitis), proximal humerus** A2 T 80 50 CCI
21.61 21.61 Global Days 090

23190 **Ostectomy of scapula, partial (eg, superior medial angle)** A2 T 80 50 CCI
16.59 16.59 Global Days 090

23195 **Resection, humeral head** A2 T 80 50 CCI
EXCLUDES *Arthroplasty with replacement with implant (23470)*
22.08 22.08 Global Days 090

23200-23220 Radical Resection of Bone Tumors of Shoulder

INCLUDES Any necessary elevation of tissue planes or dissection
Measurement of tumor and necessary margin at greatest diameter prior to excision
Simple and intermediate repairs

EXCLUDES *Complex repair*
Significant exploration of vessels, neuroplasty, reconstruction, or complex bone repair

Do not report excision of soft tissue codes when adjacent soft tissue is removed during the bone tumor resection (23076-23078 [23071, 23073])

23200 **Radical resection of tumor; clavicle** C5 C 80 50
42.98 42.98 Global Days 090

23210 **scapula** C5 C 80 50
50.38 50.38 Global Days 090

23220 **Radical resection of tumor, proximal humerus** C5 C 80 50
55.24 55.24 Global Days 090

23330-23332 Foreign Body Removal: Shoulder

EXCLUDES *Bursal arthrocentesis or needling (20610)*
K-wire or pin insertion (20650)
K-wire or pin removal (20670, 20680)

23330 **Removal of foreign body, shoulder; subcutaneous** A2 T 80 50
4.46 7.00 Global Days 010

23331 **deep (eg, Neer hemiarthroplasty removal)** A2 T 80 50
17.35 17.35 Global Days 090

23332 **complicated (eg, total shoulder)** C5 C 80 50
25.91 25.91 Global Days 090
AMA: 2009, Jan, 11-31; 2008, Jan, 10-25; 2007, January, 13-27

23350 Injection for Shoulder Arthrogram

23350 **Injection procedure for shoulder arthrography or enhanced CT/MRI shoulder arthrography** N1 N 50
EXCLUDES *Shoulder biopsy (29805-29826)*
73040, 73201-73202, 73222-73223, 77002
1.49 4.32 Global Days 000

23395-23491 Repair/Reconstruction of Shoulder

23395 **Muscle transfer, any type, shoulder or upper arm; single** A2 T 80
37.83 37.83 Global Days 090

23397 **multiple** A2 T 80
33.51 33.51 Global Days 090

23400 **Scapulopexy (eg, Sprengels deformity or for paralysis)** A2 T 80 50
28.49 28.49 Global Days 090

23405 **Tenotomy, shoulder area; single tendon** A2 T 80
18.45 18.45 Global Days 090

23406 **multiple tendons through same incision** A2 T 80
22.84 22.84 Global Days 090

23410 **Repair of ruptured musculotendinous cuff (eg, rotator cuff) open; acute** A2 T 80 50
EXCLUDES *Arthroscopic repair (29827)*
24.16 24.16 Global Days 090
AMA: 2009, Jan, 11-31; 2008, Jan, 10-25; 2007, January, 13-27

23412 **chronic** A2 T 80 50
EXCLUDES *Arthroscopic repair (29827)*
25.11 25.11 Global Days 090
AMA: 2009, Jan, 11-31; 2008, Jan, 10-25; 2007, January, 13-27

23415 **Coracoacromial ligament release, with or without acromioplasty** A2 T 50
EXCLUDES *Arthroscopic repair (29826)*
19.91 19.91 Global Days 090

23420 **Reconstruction of complete shoulder (rotator) cuff avulsion, chronic (includes acromioplasty)** A2 T 80 50
28.50 28.50 Global Days 090
AMA: 2009, Jan, 11-31; 2008, Jan, 10-25; 2007, January, 13-27

23430 **Tenodesis of long tendon of biceps** A2 T 80 50
EXCLUDES *Arthroscopic biceps tenodesis (29828)*
21.92 21.92 Global Days 090

23440 **Resection or transplantation of long tendon of biceps** A2 T 80 50
22.22 22.22 Global Days 090

23450 **Capsulorrhaphy, anterior; Putti-Platt procedure or Magnuson type operation** A2 T 80 50
EXCLUDES *Arthroscopic thermal capsulorrhaphy (29999)*
27.82 27.82 Global Days 090

23455 **with labral repair (eg, Bankart procedure)** A2 T 80 50
EXCLUDES *Arthroscopic repair (29806)*
29.50 29.50 Global Days 090

23460 **Capsulorrhaphy, anterior, any type; with bone block** A2 T 80 50
INCLUDES Bristow procedure
32.02 32.02 Global Days 090

23462 **with coracoid process transfer** A2 T 80 50
EXCLUDES *Open thermal capsulorrhaphy (23929)*
31.50 31.50 Global Days 090

23465 **Capsulorrhaphy, glenohumeral joint, posterior, with or without bone block** A2 T 80 50
EXCLUDES *Sternoclavicular and acromioclavicular joint repair (23530, 23550)*
32.91 32.91 Global Days 090

23466 **Capsulorrhaphy, glenohumeral joint, any type multi-directional instability** A2 T 80 50
32.99 32.99 Global Days 090

23470 **Arthroplasty, glenohumeral joint; hemiarthroplasty** T 80 50
35.56 35.56 Global Days 090

23472 **total shoulder (glenoid and proximal humeral replacement (eg, total shoulder))** C5 C 80 50
EXCLUDES *Proximal humerus osteotomy (24400)*
Removal of total shoulder components (23331-23332)
44.04 44.04 Global Days 090
AMA: 2009, Jan, 11-31; 2008, Jan, 10-25; 2007, January, 13-27

23480 **Osteotomy, clavicle, with or without internal fixation;** A2 T 50
24.04 24.04 Global Days 090

23485 **with bone graft for nonunion or malunion (includes obtaining graft and/or necessary fixation)** A2 T 80 50
28.21 28.21 Global Days 090

23490 **Prophylactic treatment (nailing, pinning, plating or wiring) with or without methylmethacrylate; clavicle** A2 T 80 50
26.05 26.05 Global Days 090

23491 proximal humerus A2 T 80 50
29.76 29.76 Global Days 090

23500-23680 Treatment of Shoulder Fracture/Dislocation

23500 Closed treatment of clavicular fracture; without manipulation A2 T 50
6.42 6.35 Global Days 090

23505 with manipulation A2 T 50
9.57 10.13 Global Days 090

23515 Open treatment of clavicular fracture, includes internal fixation, when performed A2 T 80 50
21.09 21.09 Global Days 090
AMA: 2008, Jan, 4-5

23520 Closed treatment of sternoclavicular dislocation; without manipulation A2 T 80 50
6.73 6.64 Global Days 090

23525 with manipulation A2 T 80 50
10.10 10.90 Global Days 090

23530 Open treatment of sternoclavicular dislocation, acute or chronic; A2 T 80 50
16.51 16.51 Global Days 090

23532 with fascial graft (includes obtaining graft) A2 T 80 50
18.23 18.23 Global Days 090

23540 Closed treatment of acromioclavicular dislocation; without manipulation A2 T 50
6.56 6.50 Global Days 090

23545 with manipulation A2 T 80 50
8.89 9.77 Global Days 090

23550 Open treatment of acromioclavicular dislocation, acute or chronic; A2 T 80 50
16.70 16.70 Global Days 090

23552 with fascial graft (includes obtaining graft) A2 T 80 50
19.29 19.29 Global Days 090

23570 Closed treatment of scapular fracture; without manipulation A2 T 50
6.90 6.72 Global Days 090

23575 with manipulation, with or without skeletal traction (with or without shoulder joint involvement) A2 T 80 50
10.84 11.56 Global Days 090

23585 Open treatment of scapular fracture (body, glenoid or acromion) includes internal fixation, when performed A2 T 80 50
28.78 28.78 Global Days 090
AMA: 2009, Jan, 11-31; 2008, Jan, 10-25; 2007, January, 13-27

23600 Closed treatment of proximal humeral (surgical or anatomical neck) fracture; without manipulation P2 T 50
8.80 9.43 Global Days 090

23605 with manipulation, with or without skeletal traction A2 T 50
12.44 13.56 Global Days 090

23615 Open treatment of proximal humeral (surgical or anatomical neck) fracture, includes internal fixation, when performed, includes repair of tuberosity(s), when performed; A2 T 80 50
25.96 25.96 Global Days 090
AMA: 2008, Jan, 4-5

23616 with proximal humeral prosthetic replacement A2 T 80 50
36.72 36.72 Global Days 090

23620 Closed treatment of greater humeral tuberosity fracture; without manipulation P2 T 50
7.43 7.83 Global Days 090

23625 with manipulation A2 T 50
10.24 10.97 Global Days 090

23630 Open treatment of greater humeral tuberosity fracture, includes internal fixation, when performed A2 T 80 50
22.85 22.85 Global Days 090

23650 Closed treatment of shoulder dislocation, with manipulation; without anesthesia A2 T 50
8.21 8.95 Global Days 090

23655 requiring anesthesia A2 T 50
11.52 11.52 Global Days 090

23660 Open treatment of acute shoulder dislocation A2 T 80 50
EXCLUDES *Chronic dislocation repair (23450-23466)*
17.09 17.09 Global Days 090

23665 Closed treatment of shoulder dislocation, with fracture of greater humeral tuberosity, with manipulation A2 T 50
11.49 12.31 Global Days 090

23670 Open treatment of shoulder dislocation, with fracture of greater humeral tuberosity, includes internal fixation, when performed A2 T 80 50
25.51 25.51 Global Days 090

23675 Closed treatment of shoulder dislocation, with surgical or anatomical neck fracture, with manipulation A2 T 50
14.57 15.94 Global Days 090

23680 Open treatment of shoulder dislocation, with surgical or anatomical neck fracture, includes internal fixation, when performed A2 T 80 50
27.19 27.19 Global Days 090

23700-23929 Other/Unlisted Shoulder Procedures

23700 Manipulation under anesthesia, shoulder joint, including application of fixation apparatus (dislocation excluded) A2 T 50
5.71 5.71 Global Days 010
AMA: 2009, Jan, 11-31; 2009, May, 8-9&11; 2008, Jan, 10-25; 2007, January, 13-27

23800 Arthrodesis, glenohumeral joint; A2 T 80 50
30.10 30.10 Global Days 090

23802 with autogenous graft (includes obtaining graft) A2 T 80
37.44 37.44 Global Days 090

23900 Interthoracoscapular amputation (forequarter) C5 C 80
40.28 40.28 Global Days 090

23920 Disarticulation of shoulder; C5 C 80
32.73 32.73 Global Days 090

23921 secondary closure or scar revision A2 T
12.49 12.49 Global Days 090

23929 Unlisted procedure, shoulder T 80
0.00 0.00 Global Days YYY

23930-24006 Surgical Incision Elbow/Upper Arm

EXCLUDES *Simple incision and drainage procedures (10040-10160)*

23930 Incision and drainage, upper arm or elbow area; deep abscess or hematoma A2 T 50
6.34 10.40 Global Days 010

23931 bursa A2 T 50
4.68 8.38 Global Days 010

23935 Incision, deep, with opening of bone cortex (eg, for osteomyelitis or bone abscess), humerus or elbow
14.78 14.78 Global Days 090

24000 Arthrotomy, elbow, including exploration, drainage, or removal of foreign body
13.96 13.96 Global Days 090

24006 Arthrotomy of the elbow, with capsular excision for capsular release (separate procedure)
20.90 20.90 Global Days 090

24065-24066 Biopsy of Elbow/Upper Arm

24065 Biopsy, soft tissue of upper arm or elbow area; superficial
EXCLUDES *Soft tissue needle biopsy (20206)*
4.97 7.57 Global Days 010

24066 deep (subfascial or intramuscular)
EXCLUDES *Soft tissue needle biopsy (20206)*
12.00 17.97 Global Days 090

24071-24079 [24071, 24073] Excision Soft Tissue Tumors Elbow/Upper Arm

INCLUDES Any necessary elevation of tissue planes or dissection
Measurement of tumor and necessary margin at greatest diameter prior to excision
Resection without removal of significant normal tissue
Types of excision:
Fascial or subfascial soft tissue tumors: simple and marginal resection of most often benign and intramuscular tumors found either in or below the deep fascia, not involving bone
Radical resection of tumor: wide resection of soft tissue tumor, mostly malignant or aggressive benign, involving large margins of normal tissue and may involve tissue removal from one or more layers
Subcutaneous: simple and marginal resection of most often benign tumors found in the subcutaneous tissue above the deep fascia

EXCLUDES *Complex repair*
Radical resection of cutaneous tumors (e.g., melanoma) (11600-11646)
Significant exploration of vessels or neuroplasty

24071 *Resequenced code, See code following 24075*

24073 *Resequenced code, See code following 24076.*

24075 Excision, tumor, soft tissue of upper arm or elbow area, subcutaneous; less than 3 cm
9.65 14.44 Global Days 090

\# **24071** 3 cm or greater
12.01 12.01 Global Days 090

24076 Excision, tumor, soft tissue of upper arm or elbow area, subfascial (eg, intramuscular); less than 5 cm
15.82 15.82 Global Days 090

\# **24073** 5 cm or greater
20.47 20.47 Global Days 090

24077 Radical resection of tumor (eg, malignant neoplasm), soft tissue of upper arm or elbow area; less than 5 cm
30.21 30.21 Global Days 090

24079 5 cm or greater
39.31 39.31 Global Days 090

24100-24149 Bone/Joint Procedures Upper Arm/Elbow

24100 Arthrotomy, elbow; with synovial biopsy only
12.13 12.13 Global Days 090

24101 with joint exploration, with or without biopsy, with or without removal of loose or foreign body
14.61 14.61 Global Days 090

24102 with synovectomy
18.03 18.03 Global Days 090

24105 Excision, olecranon bursa
10.17 10.17 Global Days 090

24110 Excision or curettage of bone cyst or benign tumor, humerus;
17.15 17.15 Global Days 090

24115 with autograft (includes obtaining graft)
21.53 21.53 Global Days 090

24116 with allograft
25.25 25.25 Global Days 090

24120 Excision or curettage of bone cyst or benign tumor of head or neck of radius or olecranon process;
15.45 15.45 Global Days 090

24125 with autograft (includes obtaining graft)
18.06 18.06 Global Days 090

24126 with allograft
18.95 18.95 Global Days 090

24130 Excision, radial head
EXCLUDES *Radial head arthroplasty with implant (24366)*
14.86 14.86 Global Days 090

24134 Sequestrectomy (eg, for osteomyelitis or bone abscess), shaft or distal humerus
21.91 21.91 Global Days 090

24136 Sequestrectomy (eg, for osteomyelitis or bone abscess), radial head or neck
18.19 18.19 Global Days 090

24138 Sequestrectomy (eg, for osteomyelitis or bone abscess), olecranon process
19.67 19.67 Global Days 090

24140 Partial excision (craterization, saucerization, or diaphysectomy) bone (eg, osteomyelitis), humerus
20.72 20.72 Global Days 090

24145 Partial excision (craterization, saucerization, or diaphysectomy) bone (eg, osteomyelitis), radial head or neck
17.41 17.41 Global Days 090

24147 Partial excision (craterization, saucerization, or diaphysectomy) bone (eg, osteomyelitis), olecranon process
18.30 18.30 Global Days 090

24149 Radical resection of capsule, soft tissue, and heterotopic bone, elbow, with contracture release (separate procedure)
EXCLUDES *Capsular and soft tissue release (24006)*
34.39 34.39 Global Days 090

24150-24152 Radical Resection Bone Tumor Upper Arm

INCLUDES Any necessary elevation of tissue planes or dissection
Measurement of tumor and necessary margin at greatest diameter prior to excision
Radical resection of bone tumor: resection of the tumor (may include entire bone) and wide margins of normal tissue primarily for malignant or aggressive benign tumors
Simple and intermediate repairs

EXCLUDES *Complex repair*
Significant exploration of vessels, neuroplasty, reconstruction, or complex bone repair

Do not report excision of soft tissue codes when adjacent soft tissue is removed during the bone tumor resection (24076-24079 [24071, 24073])

24150 Radical resection of tumor, shaft or distal humerus T 80 50
44.41 44.41 Global Days 090

24152 Radical resection of tumor, radial head or neck G2 T 80 50
38.19 38.19 Global Days 090

24155 Elbow Arthrectomy

24155 Resection of elbow joint (arthrectomy) A2 T 80 50
24.96 24.96 Global Days 090

24160-24201 Removal Implant/Foreign Body from Elbow/Upper Arm

EXCLUDES *Bursal or joint arthrocentesis or needling (20605)*
K-wire or pin insertion (20650)
K-wire or pin removal (20670, 20680)

24160 Implant removal; elbow joint A2 T 50
17.73 17.73 Global Days 090

24164 radial head A2 T 50
14.54 14.54 Global Days 090

24200 Removal of foreign body, upper arm or elbow area; subcutaneous P3 T 80 50
4.07 5.98 Global Days 010

24201 deep (subfascial or intramuscular) A2 T 50
10.70 16.25 Global Days 090

24220 Injection for Elbow Arthrogram

24220 Injection procedure for elbow arthrography N1 N 80 50
EXCLUDES *Injection tennis elbow (20550)*
73085
1.98 4.73 Global Days 000

24300-24498 Repair/Reconstruction of Elbow/Upper Arm

24300 Manipulation, elbow, under anesthesia G2 T 50
EXCLUDES *Application of external fixation (20690, 20692)*
11.95 11.95 Global Days 090

24301 Muscle or tendon transfer, any type, upper arm or elbow, single (excluding 24320-24331) A2 T 80
22.09 22.09 Global Days 090

24305 Tendon lengthening, upper arm or elbow, each tendon A2 T 80
16.98 16.98 Global Days 090

24310 Tenotomy, open, elbow to shoulder, each tendon A2 T 80
13.97 13.97 Global Days 090

24320 Tenoplasty, with muscle transfer, with or without free graft, elbow to shoulder, single (Seddon-Brookes type procedure) A2 T 80
22.82 22.82 Global Days 090

24330 Flexor-plasty, elbow (eg, Steindler type advancement); A2 T 80 50
20.99 20.99 Global Days 090

24331 with extensor advancement A2 T 80 50
21.61 21.61 Global Days 090

24332 Tenolysis, triceps G2 T 50
17.87 17.87 Global Days 090

24340 Tenodesis of biceps tendon at elbow (separate procedure) A2 T 80 50
18.01 18.01 Global Days 090

24341 Repair, tendon or muscle, upper arm or elbow, each tendon or muscle, primary or secondary (excludes rotator cuff) A2 T 80 50
21.87 21.87 Global Days 090

24342 Reinsertion of ruptured biceps or triceps tendon, distal, with or without tendon graft A2 T 80 50
22.85 22.85 Global Days 090

24343 Repair lateral collateral ligament, elbow, with local tissue G2 T 80 50
20.66 20.66 Global Days 090

24344 Reconstruction lateral collateral ligament, elbow, with tendon graft (includes harvesting of graft) G2 T 80 50
32.32 32.32 Global Days 090

24345 Repair medial collateral ligament, elbow, with local tissue A2 T 80 50
20.54 20.54 Global Days 090

24346 Reconstruction medial collateral ligament, elbow, with tendon graft (includes harvesting of graft) G2 T 80 50
32.18 32.18 Global Days 090

24357 Tenotomy, elbow, lateral or medial (eg, epicondylitis, tennis elbow, golfer's elbow); percutaneous G2 T 80 50
Do not report with (29837-29838)
12.99 12.99 Global Days 090
AMA: 2008, Jan, 4-5

24358 debridement, soft tissue and/or bone, open G2 T 80 50
Do not report with (29837-29838)
15.33 15.33 Global Days 090
AMA: 2008, Jan, 4-5

24359 debridement, soft tissue and/or bone, open with tendon repair or reattachment G2 T 80 50
Do not report with (29837-29838)
19.30 19.30 Global Days 090
AMA: 2008, Jan, 4-5

24360 Arthroplasty, elbow; with membrane (eg, fascial) A2 T 80 50
26.35 26.35 Global Days 090

24361 with distal humeral prosthetic replacement J8 T 80 50
Code also (C1776)
29.53 29.53 Global Days 090

24362 with implant and fascia lata ligament reconstruction A2 T 80 50
31.10 31.10 Global Days 090

Musculoskeletal System

24150 — 24362

● New Code ▲ Revised Code Maternity Age Unlisted Not Covered # Resequenced
○ Reinstated CCI + Add-on ⊘ Mod 51 Exempt Mod 63 Exempt ⊙ Mod Sedation PQ PQRS

24363 with distal humerus and proximal ulnar prosthetic replacement (eg, total elbow) J8 T 80 50
Code also (C1776)
44.01 44.01 Global Days 090

24365 Arthroplasty, radial head; A2 T 80 50
18.70 18.70 Global Days 090

24366 with implant J8 T 80 50
Code also (C1776)
19.99 19.99 Global Days 090

24400 Osteotomy, humerus, with or without internal fixation A2 T 80 50
24.10 24.10 Global Days 090

24410 Multiple osteotomies with realignment on intramedullary rod, humeral shaft (Sofield type procedure) A2 T 80 50
28.02 28.02 Global Days 090

24420 Osteoplasty, humerus (eg, shortening or lengthening) (excluding 64876) A2 T 80 50
29.04 29.04 Global Days 090

24430 Repair of nonunion or malunion, humerus; without graft (eg, compression technique) A2 T 80 50
31.08 31.08 Global Days 090

24435 with iliac or other autograft (includes obtaining graft) A2 T 80 50
31.64 31.64 Global Days 090

24470 Hemiepiphyseal arrest (eg, cubitus varus or valgus, distal humerus) A2 T 80 50
19.35 19.35 Global Days 090

24495 Decompression fasciotomy, forearm, with brachial artery exploration A2 T 80 50
19.32 19.32 Global Days 090

24498 Prophylactic treatment (nailing, pinning, plating or wiring), with or without methylmethacrylate, humeral shaft A2 T 80 50
25.45 25.45 Global Days 090

24500-24685 Treatment of Fracture/Dislocation of Elbow/Upper Arm

INCLUDES Treatment for either closed or open fractures or dislocations

24500 Closed treatment of humeral shaft fracture; without manipulation A2 T 50
9.40 10.35 Global Days 090

24505 with manipulation, with or without skeletal traction A2 T 50
13.22 14.58 Global Days 090

24515 Open treatment of humeral shaft fracture with plate/screws, with or without cerclage A2 T 80 50
25.72 25.72 Global Days 090

24516 Treatment of humeral shaft fracture, with insertion of intramedullary implant, with or without cerclage and/or locking screws A2 T 80 50 PQ
25.27 25.27 Global Days 090
AMA: 2009, Jun, 7-8

24530 Closed treatment of supracondylar or transcondylar humeral fracture, with or without intercondylar extension; without manipulation A2 T 50
9.98 11.04 Global Days 090

24535 with manipulation, with or without skin or skeletal traction A2 T 50
16.60 17.95 Global Days 090

24538 Percutaneous skeletal fixation of supracondylar or transcondylar humeral fracture, with or without intercondylar extension A2 T 50
21.78 21.78 Global Days 090

24545 Open treatment of humeral supracondylar or transcondylar fracture, includes internal fixation, when performed; without intercondylar extension A2 T 80 50
27.23 27.23 Global Days 090

24546 with intercondylar extension A2 T 80 50
30.62 30.62 Global Days 090

24560 Closed treatment of humeral epicondylar fracture, medial or lateral; without manipulation A2 T 50
8.31 9.32 Global Days 090

24565 with manipulation A2 T 50
14.11 15.36 Global Days 090

24566 Percutaneous skeletal fixation of humeral epicondylar fracture, medial or lateral, with manipulation A2 T 50
20.94 20.94 Global Days 090

24575 Open treatment of humeral epicondylar fracture, medial or lateral, includes internal fixation, when performed A2 T 80 50
21.52 21.52 Global Days 090

24576 Closed treatment of humeral condylar fracture, medial or lateral; without manipulation A2 T 50
8.82 9.82 Global Days 090

24577 with manipulation A2 T 50
14.53 15.86 Global Days 090

24579 Open treatment of humeral condylar fracture, medial or lateral, includes internal fixation, when performed A2 T 80 50
EXCLUDES *Closed treatment without manipulation (24530, 24560, 24576, 24650, 24670)*
Repair with manipulation (24535, 24565, 24577, 24675)
24.50 24.50 Global Days 090

24582 Percutaneous skeletal fixation of humeral condylar fracture, medial or lateral, with manipulation A2 T 50
23.53 23.53 Global Days 090

24586 Open treatment of periarticular fracture and/or dislocation of the elbow (fracture distal humerus and proximal ulna and/or proximal radius); A2 T 80 50
31.95 31.95 Global Days 090

24587 with implant arthroplasty A2 T 80 50
EXCLUDES *Distal humerus arthroplasty (24361)*
31.79 31.79 Global Days 090

24600 Treatment of closed elbow dislocation; without anesthesia A2 T 50
9.67 10.58 Global Days 090

24605 requiring anesthesia A2 T 50
13.66 13.66 Global Days 090

24615 Open treatment of acute or chronic elbow dislocation A2 T 80 50
20.84 20.84 Global Days 090

24620 Closed treatment of Monteggia type of fracture dislocation at elbow (fracture proximal end of ulna with dislocation of radial head), with manipulation A2 T 80 50
16.12 16.12 Global Days 090

24635 Open treatment of Monteggia type of fracture dislocation at elbow (fracture proximal end of ulna with dislocation of radial head), includes internal fixation, when performed A2 T 80 50
20.19 20.19 Global Days 090

24640 Closed treatment of radial head subluxation in child, nursemaid elbow, with manipulation A P2 T 80 50
2.70 3.95 Global Days 010

24650 **Closed treatment of radial head or neck fracture; without manipulation** P2 T 50
6.93 7.58 Global Days 090

24655 **with manipulation** A2 T 50
11.68 12.81 Global Days 090

24665 **Open treatment of radial head or neck fracture, includes internal fixation or radial head excision, when performed;** A2 T 80 50
19.07 19.07 Global Days 090

24666 **with radial head prosthetic replacement** A2 T 80 50
21.48 21.48 Global Days 090

24670 **Closed treatment of ulnar fracture, proximal end (eg, olecranon or coronoid process[es]); without manipulation** A2 T 50
7.60 8.44 Global Days 090

24675 **with manipulation** A2 T 50
12.17 13.32 Global Days 090

24685 **Open treatment of ulnar fracture, proximal end (eg, olecranon or coronoid process[es]), includes internal fixation, when performed** A2 T 80 50

Do not report with (24100-24102)

19.15 19.15 Global Days 090

24800-24999 Other/Unlisted Elbow/Upper Arm Procedures

24800 **Arthrodesis, elbow joint; local** A2 T 80 50
24.07 24.07 Global Days 090

24802 **with autogenous graft (includes obtaining graft)** A2 T 80 50
29.34 29.34 Global Days 090

24900 **Amputation, arm through humerus; with primary closure** C5 C 80 50
21.31 21.31 Global Days 090

24920 **open, circular (guillotine)** C5 C 80 50
19.85 19.85 Global Days 090

24925 **secondary closure or scar revision** A2 T 80 50
16.49 16.49 Global Days 090

24930 **re-amputation** C5 C 80 50
22.54 22.54 Global Days 090

24931 **with implant** C5 C 80 50
22.48 22.48 Global Days 090

24935 **Stump elongation, upper extremity** T 80 50
29.71 29.71 Global Days 090

24940 **Cineplasty, upper extremity, complete procedure** C5 C 80 50
0.00 0.00 Global Days 090

24999 **Unlisted procedure, humerus or elbow** T 80 50
0.00 0.00 Global Days YYY

25000-25001 Incision Tendon Sheath of Wrist

25000 **Incision, extensor tendon sheath, wrist (eg, deQuervains disease)** A2 T 50

EXCLUDES *Carpal tunnel release (64721)*

9.97 9.97 Global Days 090

25001 **Incision, flexor tendon sheath, wrist (eg, flexor carpi radialis)** G2 T 50
10.00 10.00 Global Days 090

25020-25025 Decompression Fasciotomy Forearm/Wrist

25020 **Decompression fasciotomy, forearm and/or wrist, flexor OR extensor compartment; without debridement of nonviable muscle and/or nerve** A2 T 50

EXCLUDES *Brachial artery exploration (24495)*
Superficial incision and drainage (10060-10160)

17.01 17.01 Global Days 090

25023 **with debridement of nonviable muscle and/or nerve** A2 T 80 50

EXCLUDES *Brachial artery exploration (24495)*
Debridement (11000-11044 [11045, 11046])
Superficial incision and drainage (10060-10160)

32.54 32.54 Global Days 090

25024 **Decompression fasciotomy, forearm and/or wrist, flexor AND extensor compartment; without debridement of nonviable muscle and/or nerve** A2 T 50
22.98 22.98 Global Days 090

25025 **with debridement of nonviable muscle and/or nerve** A2 T 80 50
35.74 35.74 Global Days 090

25028-25040 Incision for Drainage/Foreign Body Removal

25028 **Incision and drainage, forearm and/or wrist; deep abscess or hematoma** A2 T 50
15.32 15.32 Global Days 090

25031 **bursa** A2 T 80 50
10.76 10.76 Global Days 090

25035 **Incision, deep, bone cortex, forearm and/or wrist (eg, osteomyelitis or bone abscess)** A2 T 80 50
17.60 17.60 Global Days 090

25040 **Arthrotomy, radiocarpal or midcarpal joint, with exploration, drainage, or removal of foreign body** A2 T 80 50
16.59 16.59 Global Days 090

25065-25066 Biopsy Forearm/Wrist

EXCLUDES *Soft tissue needle biopsy (20206)*

25065 **Biopsy, soft tissue of forearm and/or wrist; superficial** P3 T 50
4.87 7.51 Global Days 010

25066 **deep (subfascial or intramuscular)** A2 T 50
10.67 10.67 Global Days 090

26040-26045 Incision Palmar Fascia

EXCLUDES *Enzyme injection fasciotomy (20527, 26341)*
Fasciectomy (26121, 26123, 26125)

26040 **Fasciotomy, palmar (eg, Dupuytren's contracture); percutaneous** A2 T 50
9.08 9.08 Global Days 090

26045 **open, partial** A2 T 50
13.66 13.66 Global Days 090

25071-25078 [25071, 25073] Excision Soft Tissue Tumors Forearm/Wrist

INCLUDES Any necessary elevation of tissue planes or dissection
Measurement of tumor and necessary margin at greatest diameter prior to excision
Resection without removal of significant normal tissue
Simple and intermediate repairs
Types of excision:
Fascial or subfascial soft tissue tumors: simple and marginal resection of most often benign and intramuscular tumors found either in or below the deep fascia, not involving bone
Radical resection of tumor: wide resection of tumor, mostly malignant or aggressive benign, involving large margins of normal tissue and may involve tissue removal from one or more layers
Subcutaneous: simple and marginal resection of most often benign tumors found in the subcutaneous tissue above the deep fascia

EXCLUDES *Complex repair*
Radical resection of cutaneous tumors (e.g., melanoma) (11600-11646)
Significant exploration of vessels or neuroplasty

25071 Resequenced code, See code following 25075.

25073 Resequenced code, See code following 25076.

25075 **Excision, tumor, soft tissue of forearm and/or wrist area, subcutaneous; less than 3 cm** G2 T 50
9.46 14.28 Global Days 090

\# **25071** **3 cm or greater** G2 T 80 50
12.60 12.60 Global Days 090

25076 **Excision, tumor, soft tissue of forearm and/or wrist area, subfascial (eg, intramuscular); less than 3 cm** G2 T 50
15.22 15.22 Global Days 090

\# **25073** **3 cm or greater** G2 T 80 50
15.75 15.75 Global Days 090

25077 **Radical resection of tumor (eg, malignant neoplasm), soft tissue of forearm and/or wrist area; less than 3 cm** G2 T 50
25.94 25.94 Global Days 090

25078 **3 cm or greater** G2 T 80 50
34.70 34.70 Global Days 090

25085-25240 Procedures of Bones/Joints Lower Arm/Wrist

25085 **Capsulotomy, wrist (eg, contracture)** A2 T 80 50
13.32 13.32 Global Days 090

25100 **Arthrotomy, wrist joint; with biopsy** A2 T 80 50
10.12 10.12 Global Days 090

25101 **with joint exploration, with or without biopsy, with or without removal of loose or foreign body** A2 T 80 50
11.84 11.84 Global Days 090

25105 **with synovectomy** A2 T 80 50
14.21 14.21 Global Days 090

25107 **Arthrotomy, distal radioulnar joint including repair of triangular cartilage, complex** A2 T 80 50
18.11 18.11 Global Days 090

25109 **Excision of tendon, forearm and/or wrist, flexor or extensor, each** G2 T 50
15.67 15.67 Global Days 090

25110 **Excision, lesion of tendon sheath, forearm and/or wrist** A2 T 50
10.14 10.14 Global Days 090

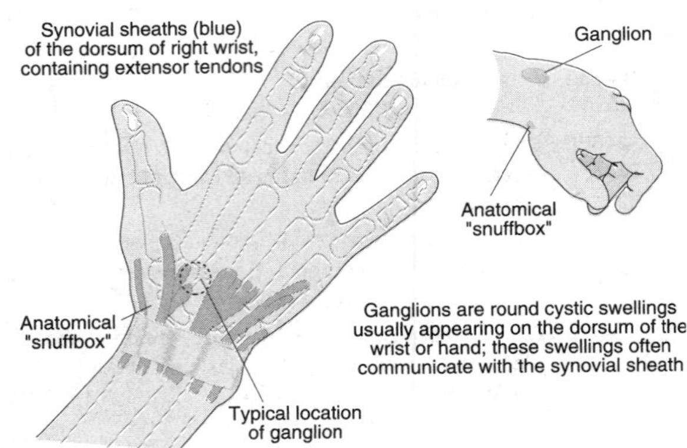

25111 **Excision of ganglion, wrist (dorsal or volar); primary** A2 T 50
EXCLUDES *Excision of ganglion hand or finger (26160)*
9.37 9.37 Global Days 090

25112 **recurrent** A2 T 50
EXCLUDES *Excision of ganglion hand or finger (26160)*
11.35 11.35 Global Days 090

25115 **Radical excision of bursa, synovia of wrist, or forearm tendon sheaths (eg, tenosynovitis, fungus, Tbc, or other granulomas, rheumatoid arthritis); flexors** A2 T 50
EXCLUDES *Finger synovectomy (26145)*
22.71 22.71 Global Days 090

25116 **extensors, with or without transposition of dorsal retinaculum** A2 T 80 50
EXCLUDES *Finger synovectomy (26145)*
18.04 18.04 Global Days 090

25118 **Synovectomy, extensor tendon sheath, wrist, single compartment;** A2 T 50
EXCLUDES *Finger synovectomy (26145)*
11.22 11.22 Global Days 090

25119 **with resection of distal ulna** A2 T 80 50
EXCLUDES *Finger synovectomy (26145)*
14.76 14.76 Global Days 090

25120 **Excision or curettage of bone cyst or benign tumor of radius or ulna (excluding head or neck of radius and olecranon process);** A2 T 80 50
EXCLUDES *Removal of bone cyst or tumor of radial head, neck, or olecranon process (24120-24126)*
15.04 15.04 Global Days 090

25125 **with autograft (includes obtaining graft)** A2 T 80 50
18.16 18.16 Global Days 090

25126 **with allograft** A2 T 80 50
17.88 17.88 Global Days 090

25130 **Excision or curettage of bone cyst or benign tumor of carpal bones;** A2 T 80 50
13.16 13.16 Global Days 090

25135 **with autograft (includes obtaining graft)** A2 T 80 50
16.70 16.70 Global Days 090

25136 **with allograft** A2 T 80 50
14.44 14.44 Global Days 090

25145 **Sequestrectomy (eg, for osteomyelitis or bone abscess), forearm and/or wrist** A2 T 80 50
15.53 15.53 Global Days 090

25150 **Partial excision (craterization, saucerization, or diaphysectomy) of bone (eg, for osteomyelitis); ulna** A2 T 50

16.69 16.69 Global Days 090

25151 **radius** A2 T 80 50

EXCLUDES *Partial removal of radial head, neck, or olecranon process (24145, 24147)*

17.62 17.62 Global Days 090

25170 **Radical resection of tumor, radius or ulna** T 80 50

INCLUDES Any necessary elevation of tissue planes or dissection
Measurement of tumor and necessary margin at greatest diameter prior to excision
Radical resection of tumor: wide resection of soft tissue tumor, mostly malignant or aggressive benign, involving large margins of normal tissue and may involve tissue removal from one or more layers
Resection without removal of significant normal tissue
Simple and intermediate repairs

EXCLUDES *Complex repair*
Significant exploration of vessels, neuroplasty, reconstruction, or complex bone repair

Do not report radical excision of soft tissue codes when adjacent soft tissue is removed during the bone tumor resection (25076-25078 [25071, 25073])

42.43 42.43 Global Days 090

25210 **Carpectomy; 1 bone** A2 T 80

EXCLUDES *Carpectomy with insertion of implant (25441-25445)*

14.39 14.39 Global Days 090

25215 **all bones of proximal row** A2 T 80

18.20 18.20 Global Days 090

25230 **Radial styloidectomy (separate procedure)** A2 T 50

12.67 12.67 Global Days 090

25240 **Excision distal ulna partial or complete (eg, Darrach type or matched resection)** A2 T 80 50

EXCLUDES *Acquisition of fascia for interposition (20920, 20922)*
Implant replacement (25442)

12.66 12.66 Global Days 090

25246 Injection for Wrist Arthrogram

EXCLUDES *Excision of foreign body (20520)*
K-wire, pin, or rod placement or removal (20650, 20670, 20680)

25246 **Injection procedure for wrist arthrography** N1 N 50

73115

2.18 4.84 Global Days 000

25248-25251 Removal Foreign Body of Wrist

EXCLUDES *Excision of superficial foreign body (20520)*
K-wire, pin, or rod placement or removal (20650, 20670, 20680)

25248 **Exploration with removal of deep foreign body, forearm or wrist** A2 T 50

12.45 12.45 Global Days 090

25250 **Removal of wrist prosthesis; (separate procedure)** A2 T 80 50

15.46 15.46 Global Days 090

25251 **complicated, including total wrist** A2 T 80

21.04 21.04 Global Days 090

25259 Manipulation of Wrist with Anesthesia

25259 **Manipulation, wrist, under anesthesia** G2 T 50

EXCLUDES *Application of external fixation (20690, 20692)*

12.03 12.03 Global Days 090

AMA: 2009, Jan, 11-31; 2008, Jan, 10-25; 2007, January, 13-27

25260-25492 Repair/Reconstruction of Forearm/Wrist

25260 **Repair, tendon or muscle, flexor, forearm and/or wrist; primary, single, each tendon or muscle** A2 T

18.95 18.95 Global Days 090

25263 **secondary, single, each tendon or muscle** A2 T 80

18.77 18.77 Global Days 090

25265 **secondary, with free graft (includes obtaining graft), each tendon or muscle** A2 T 80

22.34 22.34 Global Days 090

25270 **Repair, tendon or muscle, extensor, forearm and/or wrist; primary, single, each tendon or muscle** A2 T 80

14.93 14.93 Global Days 090

25272 **secondary, single, each tendon or muscle** A2 T 80

16.76 16.76 Global Days 090

25274 **secondary, with free graft (includes obtaining graft), each tendon or muscle** A2 T 80

20.19 20.19 Global Days 090

25275 **Repair, tendon sheath, extensor, forearm and/or wrist, with free graft (includes obtaining graft) (eg, for extensor carpi ulnaris subluxation)** A2 T 80 50

19.91 19.91 Global Days 090

25280 **Lengthening or shortening of flexor or extensor tendon, forearm and/or wrist, single, each tendon** A2 T 80

16.99 16.99 Global Days 090

25290 **Tenotomy, open, flexor or extensor tendon, forearm and/or wrist, single, each tendon** A2 T

13.51 13.51 Global Days 090

25295 **Tenolysis, flexor or extensor tendon, forearm and/or wrist, single, each tendon** A2 T

15.78 15.78 Global Days 090

AMA: 2009, Jan, 11-31; 2008, Jan, 10-25; 2007, January, 13-27

25300 **Tenodesis at wrist; flexors of fingers** A2 T 80 50

20.52 20.52 Global Days 090

25301 **extensors of fingers** A2 T 80 50

18.94 18.94 Global Days 090

25310 **Tendon transplantation or transfer, flexor or extensor, forearm and/or wrist, single; each tendon** A2 T 80

18.59 18.59 Global Days 090

AMA: 2009, Jan, 11-31; 2008, Jan, 10-25; 2007, January, 13-27

25312 **with tendon graft(s) (includes obtaining graft), each tendon** A2 T 80

21.57 21.57 Global Days 090

25315 **Flexor origin slide (eg, for cerebral palsy, Volkmann contracture), forearm and/or wrist;** A2 T 80 50

23.04 23.04 Global Days 090

25316 **with tendon(s) transfer** A2 T 80 50

26.24 26.24 Global Days 090

25320 **Capsulorrhaphy or reconstruction, wrist, open (eg, capsulodesis, ligament repair, tendon transfer or graft) (includes synovectomy, capsulotomy and open reduction) for carpal instability** A2 T 80 50

29.00 29.00 Global Days 090

25332 Arthroplasty, wrist, with or without interposition, with or without external or internal fixation A2 T 80 50
EXCLUDES *Acquiring fascia for interposition (20920, 20922)*
Arthroplasty with prosthesis (25441-25446)
24.86 24.86 Global Days 090

25335 Centralization of wrist on ulna (eg, radial club hand) A2 T 80 50
26.07 26.07 Global Days 090

25337 Reconstruction for stabilization of unstable distal ulna or distal radioulnar joint, secondary by soft tissue stabilization (eg, tendon transfer, tendon graft or weave, or tenodesis) with or without open reduction of distal radioulnar joint A2 T 50
EXCLUDES *Acquiring fascia lata graft (20920, 20922)*
26.13 26.13 Global Days 090

25350 Osteotomy, radius; distal third A2 T 80 50
20.24 20.24 Global Days 090

25355 middle or proximal third A2 T 80 50
22.89 22.89 Global Days 090

25360 Osteotomy; ulna A2 T 80 50
19.67 19.67 Global Days 090

25365 radius AND ulna A2 T 80 50
27.21 27.21 Global Days 090

25370 Multiple osteotomies, with realignment on intramedullary rod (Sofield type procedure); radius OR ulna A2 T 80 50
27.11 27.11 Global Days 090

25375 radius AND ulna A2 T 80 50
23.33 23.33 Global Days 090

25390 Osteoplasty, radius OR ulna; shortening A2 T 80 50
23.04 23.04 Global Days 090

25391 lengthening with autograft A2 T 80 50
29.65 29.65 Global Days 090

25392 Osteoplasty, radius AND ulna; shortening (excluding 64876) A2 T 80 50
30.20 30.20 Global Days 090

25393 lengthening with autograft A2 T 80 50
33.65 33.65 Global Days 090

25394 Osteoplasty, carpal bone, shortening G2 T 80 50
22.92 22.92 Global Days 090

25400 Repair of nonunion or malunion, radius OR ulna; without graft (eg, compression technique) A2 T 80 50
24.11 24.11 Global Days 090

25405 with autograft (includes obtaining graft) A2 T 80 50
30.90 30.90 Global Days 090

25415 Repair of nonunion or malunion, radius AND ulna; without graft (eg, compression technique) A2 T 80 50
28.90 28.90 Global Days 090

25420 with autograft (includes obtaining graft) A2 T 80 50
34.78 34.78 Global Days 090

25425 Repair of defect with autograft; radius OR ulna A2 T 80 50
29.05 29.05 Global Days 090

25426 radius AND ulna A2 T 80 50
32.90 32.90 Global Days 090

25430 Insertion of vascular pedicle into carpal bone (eg, Hori procedure) G2 T 50
20.61 20.61 Global Days 090

25431 Repair of nonunion of carpal bone (excluding carpal scaphoid (navicular)) (includes obtaining graft and necessary fixation), each bone G2 T 80 50
23.04 23.04 Global Days 090

25440 Repair of nonunion, scaphoid carpal (navicular) bone, with or without radial styloidectomy (includes obtaining graft and necessary fixation) A2 T 80 50
22.64 22.64 Global Days 090

25441 Arthroplasty with prosthetic replacement; distal radius J8 T 80 50
Code also (C1776)
26.50 26.50 Global Days 090

25442 distal ulna J8 T 80 50
Code also (C1776)
23.11 23.11 Global Days 090

25443 scaphoid carpal (navicular) A2 T 80 50
22.88 22.88 Global Days 090

25444 lunate A2 T 80 50
23.35 23.35 Global Days 090

25445 trapezium A2 T 50
21.14 21.14 Global Days 090

25446 distal radius and partial or entire carpus (total wrist) J8 T 80 50
Code also (C1776)
34.40 34.40 Global Days 090

25447 Arthroplasty, interposition, intercarpal or carpometacarpal joints A2 T 80 50
EXCLUDES *Wrist arthroplasty (25332)*
24.23 24.23 Global Days 090

25449 Revision of arthroplasty, including removal of implant, wrist joint A2 T 80 50
30.62 30.62 Global Days 090

25450 Epiphyseal arrest by epiphysiodesis or stapling; distal radius OR ulna A2 T 50
17.94 17.94 Global Days 090

25455 distal radius AND ulna A2 T 50
19.86 19.86 Global Days 090

25490 Prophylactic treatment (nailing, pinning, plating or wiring) with or without methylmethacrylate; radius A2 T 80 50
19.91 19.91 Global Days 090

25491 ulna A2 T 80 50
22.12 22.12 Global Days 090

25492 radius AND ulna A2 T 80 50
26.89 26.89 Global Days 090

25500-25695 Treatment of Fracture/Dislocation of Forearm/Wrist

Code also external fixation application (20690)

25500 Closed treatment of radial shaft fracture; without manipulation P2 T 50
7.18 7.85 Global Days 090

25505 with manipulation A2 T 50
13.44 14.66 Global Days 090

25515 Open treatment of radial shaft fracture, includes internal fixation, when performed A2 T 80 50
19.58 19.58 Global Days 090

25520 Closed treatment of radial shaft fracture and closed treatment of dislocation of distal radioulnar joint (Galeazzi fracture/dislocation) A2 T 50
15.54 16.38 Global Days 090

25525 Open treatment of radial shaft fracture, includes internal fixation, when performed, and closed treatment of distal radioulnar joint dislocation (Galeazzi fracture/dislocation), includes percutaneous skeletal fixation, when performed A2 T 80 50
23.08 23.08 Global Days 090

25526 Open treatment of radial shaft fracture, includes internal fixation, when performed, and open treatment of distal radioulnar joint dislocation (Galeazzi fracture/dislocation), includes internal fixation, when performed, includes repair of triangular fibrocartilage complex [A2] [T] [80] [50] [CCI]
28.21 28.21 Global Days 090

25530 Closed treatment of ulnar shaft fracture; without manipulation [P2] [T] [50] [CCI]
6.83 7.57 Global Days 090

25535 with manipulation [A2] [T] [50] [CCI]
13.23 14.26 Global Days 090

25545 Open treatment of ulnar shaft fracture, includes internal fixation, when performed [A2] [T] [80] [50] [CCI]
18.26 18.26 Global Days 090

25560 Closed treatment of radial and ulnar shaft fractures; without manipulation [P2] [T] [50] [CCI]
7.17 7.95 Global Days 090

25565 with manipulation [A2] [T] [50] [CCI]
13.81 15.21 Global Days 090

25574 Open treatment of radial AND ulnar shaft fractures, with internal fixation, when performed; of radius OR ulna [A2] [T] [80] [50] [CCI]
19.64 19.64 Global Days 090

25575 of radius AND ulna [A2] [T] [80] [50] [CCI]
26.34 26.34 Global Days 090

25600 Closed treatment of distal radial fracture (eg, Colles or Smith type) or epiphyseal separation, includes closed treatment of fracture of ulnar styloid, when performed; without manipulation [P2] [T] [50] [CCI] [PQ]

Do not report with (25650)
8.70 9.29 Global Days 090

25605 with manipulation [A2] [T] [50] [CCI] [PQ]

Do not report with (25650)
15.28 16.23 Global Days 090

25606 Percutaneous skeletal fixation of distal radial fracture or epiphyseal separation [A2] [T] [50] [PQ]

EXCLUDES *Open repair of ulnar styloid fracture (25652)*
Percutaneous repair of ulnar styloid fracture (25651)

Do not report with (25650)
19.43 19.43 Global Days 090

25607 Open treatment of distal radial extra-articular fracture or epiphyseal separation, with internal fixation [A2] [T] [80] [50] [PQ]

EXCLUDES *Open repair of ulnar styloid fracture (25652)*
Percutaneous repair of ulnar styloid fracture (25651)

Do not report with (25650)
21.45 21.45 Global Days 090

25608 Open treatment of distal radial intra-articular fracture or epiphyseal separation; with internal fixation of 2 fragments [A2] [T] [80] [50] [PQ]

EXCLUDES *Open repair of ulnar styloid fracture (25652)*
Percutaneous repair of ulnar styloid fracture (25651)

Do not report with (25609, 25650)
24.06 24.06 Global Days 090

25609 with internal fixation of 3 or more fragments [A2] [T] [80] [50] [PQ]

EXCLUDES *Open repair of ulnar styloid fracture (25652)*
Percutaneous repair of ulnar styloid fracture (25651)

Do not report with (25650)
30.62 30.62 Global Days 090

25622 Closed treatment of carpal scaphoid (navicular) fracture; without manipulation [P2] [T] [50] [CCI]
8.01 8.83 Global Days 090

25624 with manipulation [A2] [T] [80] [50] [CCI]
12.51 13.75 Global Days 090

25628 Open treatment of carpal scaphoid (navicular) fracture, includes internal fixation, when performed [A2] [T] [80] [50] [CCI]
21.10 21.10 Global Days 090

25630 Closed treatment of carpal bone fracture (excluding carpal scaphoid [navicular]); without manipulation, each bone [P2] [T] [50] [CCI]
8.13 8.89 Global Days 090

25635 with manipulation, each bone [A2] [T] [80] [50] [CCI]
11.89 13.11 Global Days 090

25645 Open treatment of carpal bone fracture (other than carpal scaphoid [navicular]), each bone [A2] [T] [80] [50] [CCI]
16.61 16.61 Global Days 090

25650 Closed treatment of ulnar styloid fracture [P2] [T] [50] [CCI]

Do not report with (25600, 25605, 25607-25609)
8.70 9.32 Global Days 090

25651 Percutaneous skeletal fixation of ulnar styloid fracture [G2] [T] [80] [50] [CCI] [PQ]
14.18 14.18 Global Days 090

25652 Open treatment of ulnar styloid fracture [G2] [T] [50] [CCI]
18.20 18.20 Global Days 090

25660 Closed treatment of radiocarpal or intercarpal dislocation, 1 or more bones, with manipulation [A2] [T] [80] [50] [CCI]
11.89 11.89 Global Days 090

25670 Open treatment of radiocarpal or intercarpal dislocation, 1 or more bones [A2] [T] [80] [50] [CCI]
17.70 17.70 Global Days 090

25671 Percutaneous skeletal fixation of distal radioulnar dislocation [A2] [T] [50] [CCI]
15.45 15.45 Global Days 090

25675 Closed treatment of distal radioulnar dislocation with manipulation [A2] [T] [80] [50] [CCI]
11.66 12.75 Global Days 090

25676 Open treatment of distal radioulnar dislocation, acute or chronic [A2] [T] [80] [50] [CCI]
18.43 18.43 Global Days 090

25680 Closed treatment of trans-scaphoperilunar type of fracture dislocation, with manipulation [A2] [T] [80] [50] [CCI]
13.80 13.80 Global Days 090

25685 Open treatment of trans-scaphoperilunar type of fracture dislocation [A2] [T] [80] [50] [CCI]
21.48 21.48 Global Days 090

25690 Closed treatment of lunate dislocation, with manipulation [A2] [T] [80] [50] [CCI]
13.93 13.93 Global Days 090

25695 Open treatment of lunate dislocation [A2] [T] [80] [50] [CCI]
18.50 18.50 Global Days 090

25800-25830 Wrist Fusion

25800 Arthrodesis, wrist; complete, without bone graft (includes radiocarpal and/or intercarpal and/or carpometacarpal joints) A2 T 80 50
21.53 21.53 Global Days 090

25805 with sliding graft A2 T 80 50
24.83 24.83 Global Days 090

25810 with iliac or other autograft (includes obtaining graft) A2 T 80 50
25.52 25.52 Global Days 090

25820 limited, without bone graft (eg, intercarpal or radiocarpal) A2 T 80 50
18.06 18.06 Global Days 090

25825 with autograft (includes obtaining graft) A2 T 80 50
22.23 22.23 Global Days 090

25830 Arthrodesis, distal radioulnar joint with segmental resection of ulna, with or without bone graft (eg, Sauve-Kapandji procedure) A2 T 80 50
27.97 27.97 Global Days 090

25900-25999 Amputation Through Forearm/Wrist

25900 Amputation, forearm, through radius and ulna; C5 C 80 50
21.19 21.19 Global Days 090

25905 open, circular (guillotine) C5 C 80 50
20.84 20.84 Global Days 090

25907 secondary closure or scar revision A2 T 80 50
17.00 17.00 Global Days 090

25909 re-amputation T 80 50
20.37 20.37 Global Days 090

25915 Krukenberg procedure C5 C 80 50
31.12 31.12 Global Days 090

25920 Disarticulation through wrist; C5 C 80 50
20.33 20.33 Global Days 090

25922 secondary closure or scar revision A2 T 80 50
16.71 16.71 Global Days 090

25924 re-amputation C5 C 80 50
18.44 18.44 Global Days 090

25927 Transmetacarpal amputation; C5 C 80 50
23.60 23.60 Global Days 090

25929 secondary closure or scar revision A2 T 80 50
17.59 17.59 Global Days 090

25931 re-amputation G2 T 50
20.19 20.19 Global Days 090

25999 Unlisted procedure, forearm or wrist T 80 50
0.00 0.00 Global Days YYY

26010-26037 Incision Hand/Fingers

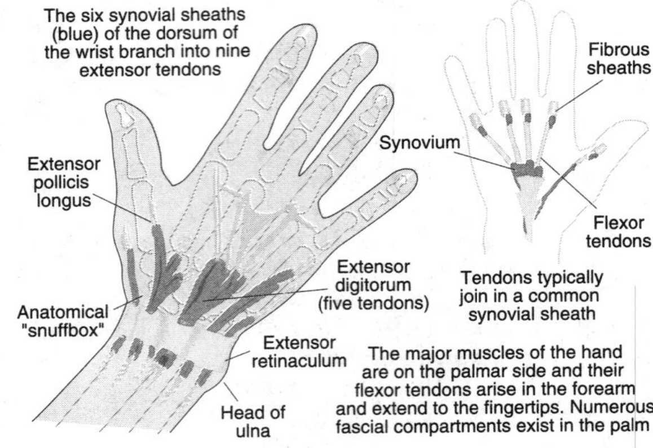

26010 Drainage of finger abscess; simple P2 T
4.01 7.64 Global Days 010

26011 complicated (eg, felon) A2 T
5.42 11.47 Global Days 010

26020 Drainage of tendon sheath, digit and/or palm, each A2 T
12.69 12.69 Global Days 090

26025 Drainage of palmar bursa; single, bursa A2 T 80
12.33 12.33 Global Days 090

26030 multiple bursa A2 T 80
14.48 14.48 Global Days 090

26034 Incision, bone cortex, hand or finger (eg, osteomyelitis or bone abscess) A2 T
15.74 15.74 Global Days 090

26035 Decompression fingers and/or hand, injection injury (eg, grease gun) G2 T 80
24.90 24.90 Global Days 090

26037 Decompressive fasciotomy, hand (excludes 26035) G2 T 80
EXCLUDES *Injection injury (26035)*
16.76 16.76 Global Days 090

26040-26045 Incision Palmar Fascia

EXCLUDES *Enzyme injection fasciotomy (20527, 26341)*
Fasciectomy (26121, 26123, 26125)

26040 Fasciotomy, palmar (eg, Dupuytren's contracture); percutaneous A2 T 50
9.08 9.08 Global Days 090

26045 open, partial A2 T 50
13.66 13.66 Global Days 090

26055-26080 Incision Tendon/Joint of Fingers/Hand

26055 Tendon sheath incision (eg, for trigger finger) A2 T
9.01 16.55 Global Days 090

26060 Tenotomy, percutaneous, single, each digit A2 T 80
EXCLUDES *Arthrocentesis (20610)*
7.80 7.80 Global Days 090

26070 Arthrotomy, with exploration, drainage, or removal of loose or foreign body; carpometacarpal joint A2 T 50
9.10 9.10 Global Days 090

26075 metacarpophalangeal joint, each A2 T 50
9.50 9.50 Global Days 090

26080 interphalangeal joint, each A2 T
11.36 11.36 Global Days 090

26100-26110 Arthrotomy with Biopsy of Joint Hand/Fingers

26100 **Arthrotomy with biopsy; carpometacarpal joint, each** A2 T 80 50
9.68 9.68 Global Days 090

26105 **metacarpophalangeal joint, each** A2 T 80 50
9.81 9.81 Global Days 090

26110 **interphalangeal joint, each** A2 T
9.38 9.38 Global Days 090

26111-26118 [26111, 26113] Excision Soft Tissue Tumors Fingers and Hand

INCLUDES Any necessary elevation of tissue planes or dissection
Measurement of tumor and necessary margin at greatest diameter prior to excision
Resection without removal of significant normal tissue
Simple and intermediate repairs
Type of excisions:
Fascial or subfascial soft tissue tumors: simple and marginal resection of most often benign and intramuscular tumors found either in or below the deep fascia, not involving bone
Radical resection soft tissue tumor: wide resection of tumor, mostly malignant or aggressive benign, involving large margins of normal tissue and may involve tissue removal from one or more layers
Subcutaneous: simple and marginal resection of most often benign tumors found in the subcutaneous tissue above the deep fascia

EXCLUDES *Complex repair*
Radical resection of cutaneous tumors (e.g., melanoma) (11600-11646)
Significant exploration of the vessels or neuroplasty

26111 Resequenced code, See code following 26115.

26113 Resequenced code, See code following 26116.

26115 **Excision, tumor or vascular malformation, soft tissue of hand or finger, subcutaneous; less than 1.5 cm** G2 T
9.92 15.64 Global Days 090

\# 26111 **1.5 cm or greater** G2 T 80
12.40 12.40 Global Days 090

26116 **Excision, tumor, soft tissue, or vascular malformation, of hand or finger, subfascial (eg, intramuscular); less than 1.5 cm** G2 T
15.42 15.42 Global Days 090

\# 26113 **1.5 cm or greater** G2 T 80
16.26 16.26 Global Days 090

26117 **Radical resection of tumor (eg, malignant neoplasm), soft tissue of hand or finger; less than 3 cm** G2 T
21.74 21.74 Global Days 090

26118 **3 cm or greater** G2 T 80
31.51 31.51 Global Days 090

26121-26236 Procedures of Bones, Fascia, Joints and Tendons Hands and Fingers

26121 **Fasciectomy, palm only, with or without Z-plasty, other local tissue rearrangement, or skin grafting (includes obtaining graft)** A2 T 50
EXCLUDES *Enzyme injection fasciotomy (20527, 26341)*
Fasciotomy (26040, 26045)
17.51 17.51 Global Days 090

26123 **Fasciectomy, partial palmar with release of single digit including proximal interphalangeal joint, with or without Z-plasty, other local tissue rearrangement, or skin grafting (includes obtaining graft);** A2 T 50
EXCLUDES *Enzyme injection fasciotomy (20527, 26341)*
Fasciotomy (26040, 26045)
24.38 24.38 Global Days 090

\+ 26125 **each additional digit (List separately in addition to code for primary procedure)** A2 T
EXCLUDES *Enzyme injection fasciotomy (20527, 26341)*
Fasciotomy (26040, 26045)
Code first 26123 (26123)
8.13 8.13 Global Days ZZZ

26130 **Synovectomy, carpometacarpal joint** A2 T 50
13.48 13.48 Global Days 090

26135 **Synovectomy, metacarpophalangeal joint including intrinsic release and extensor hood reconstruction, each digit** A2 T 80
16.14 16.14 Global Days 090

26140 **Synovectomy, proximal interphalangeal joint, including extensor reconstruction, each interphalangeal joint** A2 T
14.79 14.79 Global Days 090

26145 **Synovectomy, tendon sheath, radical (tenosynovectomy), flexor tendon, palm and/or finger, each tendon** A2 T
EXCLUDES *Wrist synovectomy (25115-25116)*
15.01 15.01 Global Days 090

26160 **Excision of lesion of tendon sheath or joint capsule (eg, cyst, mucous cyst, or ganglion), hand or finger** A2 T
EXCLUDES *Trigger finger (26055)*
Wrist ganglion removal (25111-25112)
9.73 16.89 Global Days 090

26170 **Excision of tendon, palm, flexor or extensor, single, each tendon** A2 T 80
Do not report with (26390, 26415)
11.89 11.89 Global Days 090

26180 **Excision of tendon, finger, flexor or extensor, each tendon** A2 T 80
Do not report with (26390, 26415)
12.98 12.98 Global Days 090

26185 **Sesamoidectomy, thumb or finger (separate procedure)** A2 T 80 50
16.25 16.25 Global Days 090

26200 **Excision or curettage of bone cyst or benign tumor of metacarpal;** A2 T 80
13.21 13.21 Global Days 090

26205 **with autograft (includes obtaining graft)** A2 T
17.60 17.60 Global Days 090

26210 **Excision or curettage of bone cyst or benign tumor of proximal, middle, or distal phalanx of finger;** A2 T
12.93 12.93 Global Days 090

26215 **with autograft (includes obtaining graft)** A2 T
16.41 16.41 Global Days 090

26230 **Partial excision (craterization, saucerization, or diaphysectomy) bone (eg, osteomyelitis); metacarpal** A2 T 80
14.62 14.62 Global Days 090

26235 **proximal or middle phalanx of finger** A2 T 80
14.45 14.45 Global Days 090

26236 **distal phalanx of finger** A2 T
12.91 12.91 Global Days 090

26250-26262 Radical Resection Bone Tumor of Hand/Finger

INCLUDES Any necessary elevation of tissue planes or dissection
Measurement of tumor and necessary margin at greatest diameter prior to excision
Radical resection of bone tumor: resection of the tumor (may include entire bone) and wide margins of normal tissue primarily for malignant or aggressive benign tumors
Simple and intermediate repairs

EXCLUDES *Complex repair*
Significant exploration of vessels, neuroplasty, reconstruction, or complex bone repair

Do not report radical excision of soft tissue codes when adjacent soft tissue is removed during the bone tumor resection (26116-26118 [26111, 26113])

26250 **Radical resection of tumor, metacarpal** A2 T 80
30.18 30.18 Global Days 090

26260 **Radical resection of tumor, proximal or middle phalanx of finger** A2 T 80
22.90 22.90 Global Days 090

26262 **Radical resection of tumor, distal phalanx of finger** A2 T 80
18.44 18.44 Global Days 090

26320 Implant Removal Hand/Finger

26320 **Removal of implant from finger or hand** A2 T
EXCLUDES *Excision of foreign body (20520, 20525)*
10.14 10.14 Global Days 090

26340-26548 Repair/Reconstruction of Fingers and Hand

26340 **Manipulation, finger joint, under anesthesia, each joint** G2 T 50
EXCLUDES *Application of external fixation (20690, 20692)*
9.69 9.69 Global Days 090
AMA: 2009, Jan, 11-31; 2008, Jan, 10-25; 2007, January, 13-27

● **26341** **Manipulation, palmar fascial cord (ie, Dupuytren's cord), post enzyme injection (eg, collagenase), single cord** G2 T 50
EXCLUDES *Enzyme injection fasciotomy (20527)*
Code also custom orthotic fabrication and/or fitting
2.19 2.90 Global Days 010

26350 **Repair or advancement, flexor tendon, not in zone 2 digital flexor tendon sheath (eg, no man's land); primary or secondary without free graft, each tendon** A2 T
20.82 20.82 Global Days 090

26352 **secondary with free graft (includes obtaining graft), each tendon** A2 T 80
23.72 23.72 Global Days 090

26356 **Repair or advancement, flexor tendon, in zone 2 digital flexor tendon sheath (eg, no man's land); primary, without free graft, each tendon** A2 T
31.94 31.94 Global Days 090
AMA: 2009, Jan, 11-31; 2008, Jan, 10-25; 2007, January, 13-27

26357 **secondary, without free graft, each tendon** A2 T 80
25.28 25.28 Global Days 090

26358 **secondary, with free graft (includes obtaining graft), each tendon** A2 T 80
26.71 26.71 Global Days 090

26370 **Repair or advancement of profundus tendon, with intact superficialis tendon; primary, each tendon** A2 T 80
22.28 22.28 Global Days 090

26372 **secondary with free graft (includes obtaining graft), each tendon** A2 T 80
25.78 25.78 Global Days 090

26373 **secondary without free graft, each tendon** A2 T 80
24.69 24.69 Global Days 090

26390 **Excision flexor tendon, with implantation of synthetic rod for delayed tendon graft, hand or finger, each rod** A2 T 80
24.26 24.26 Global Days 090

26392 **Removal of synthetic rod and insertion of flexor tendon graft, hand or finger (includes obtaining graft), each rod** A2 T 80
28.65 28.65 Global Days 090

26410 **Repair, extensor tendon, hand, primary or secondary; without free graft, each tendon** A2 T
16.52 16.52 Global Days 090

26412 **with free graft (includes obtaining graft), each tendon** A2 T 80
19.97 19.97 Global Days 090

26415 **Excision of extensor tendon, with implantation of synthetic rod for delayed tendon graft, hand or finger, each rod** A2 T 80
19.93 19.93 Global Days 090

26416 **Removal of synthetic rod and insertion of extensor tendon graft (includes obtaining graft), hand or finger, each rod** A2 T
25.03 25.03 Global Days 090

26418 **Repair, extensor tendon, finger, primary or secondary; without free graft, each tendon** A2 T
16.88 16.88 Global Days 090
AMA: 2009, Jan, 11-31; 2008, Jan, 10-25; 2007, January, 13-27

26420 **with free graft (includes obtaining graft) each tendon** A2 T 80
20.89 20.89 Global Days 090

26426 **Repair of extensor tendon, central slip, secondary (eg, boutonniere deformity); using local tissue(s), including lateral band(s), each finger** A2 T
15.22 15.22 Global Days 090

26428 **with free graft (includes obtaining graft), each finger** A2 T 80
21.98 21.98 Global Days 090

26432 **Closed treatment of distal extensor tendon insertion, with or without percutaneous pinning (eg, mallet finger)** A2 T
14.54 14.54 Global Days 090

26433 **Repair of extensor tendon, distal insertion, primary or secondary; without graft (eg, mallet finger)** A2 T
EXCLUDES *Trigger finger (26055)*
15.54 15.54 Global Days 090

26434 **with free graft (includes obtaining graft)** A2 T 80
EXCLUDES *Trigger finger (26055)*
18.75 18.75 Global Days 090

26437 **Realignment of extensor tendon, hand, each tendon** A2 T
18.12 18.12 Global Days 090

26440 **Tenolysis, flexor tendon; palm OR finger, each tendon** A2 T
18.18 18.18 Global Days 090
AMA: 2009, Jan, 11-31; 2008, Jan, 10-25; 2007, January, 13-27

26442 **palm AND finger, each tendon** A2 T
28.16 28.16 Global Days 090

26445 Tenolysis, extensor tendon, hand OR finger, each tendon
16.91 16.91 Global Days 090
AMA: 2009, Jan, 11-31; 2008, Jan, 10-25; 2007, January, 13-27

26449 Tenolysis, complex, extensor tendon, finger, including forearm, each tendon
20.96 20.96 Global Days 090

26450 Tenotomy, flexor, palm, open, each tendon
11.78 11.78 Global Days 090

26455 Tenotomy, flexor, finger, open, each tendon
11.77 11.77 Global Days 090

26460 Tenotomy, extensor, hand or finger, open, each tendon
11.45 11.45 Global Days 090

26471 Tenodesis; of proximal interphalangeal joint, each joint
17.92 17.92 Global Days 090

26474 of distal joint, each joint
13.95 13.95 Global Days 090

26476 Lengthening of tendon, extensor, hand or finger, each tendon
17.10 17.10 Global Days 090

26477 Shortening of tendon, extensor, hand or finger, each tendon
17.06 17.06 Global Days 090

26478 Lengthening of tendon, flexor, hand or finger, each tendon
18.20 18.20 Global Days 090

26479 Shortening of tendon, flexor, hand or finger, each tendon
18.16 18.16 Global Days 090

26480 Transfer or transplant of tendon, carpometacarpal area or dorsum of hand; without free graft, each tendon
22.01 22.01 Global Days 090

26483 with free tendon graft (includes obtaining graft), each tendon
24.76 24.76 Global Days 090

26485 Transfer or transplant of tendon, palmar; without free tendon graft, each tendon
23.64 23.64 Global Days 090

26489 with free tendon graft (includes obtaining graft), each tendon
26.82 26.82 Global Days 090

26490 Opponensplasty; superficialis tendon transfer type, each tendon
EXCLUDES *Thumb fusion (26820)*
23.07 23.07 Global Days 090

26492 tendon transfer with graft (includes obtaining graft), each tendon
EXCLUDES *Thumb fusion (26820)*
25.59 25.59 Global Days 090

26494 hypothenar muscle transfer
EXCLUDES *Thumb fusion (26820)*
23.19 23.19 Global Days 090

26496 other methods
EXCLUDES *Thumb fusion (26820)*
25.00 25.00 Global Days 090

26497 Transfer of tendon to restore intrinsic function; ring and small finger
25.12 25.12 Global Days 090

26498 all 4 fingers
33.23 33.23 Global Days 090

26499 Correction claw finger, other methods
24.08 24.08 Global Days 090

26500 Reconstruction of tendon pulley, each tendon; with local tissues (separate procedure)
18.34 18.34 Global Days 090

26502 with tendon or fascial graft (includes obtaining graft) (separate procedure)
20.60 20.60 Global Days 090

26508 Release of thenar muscle(s) (eg, thumb contracture)
18.14 18.14 Global Days 090

26510 Cross intrinsic transfer, each tendon
17.41 17.41 Global Days 090

26516 Capsulodesis, metacarpophalangeal joint; single digit
20.49 20.49 Global Days 090

26517 2 digits
24.30 24.30 Global Days 090

26518 3 or 4 digits
24.27 24.27 Global Days 090

26520 Capsulectomy or capsulotomy; metacarpophalangeal joint, each joint
EXCLUDES *Carpometacarpal joint arthroplasty (25447)*
19.05 19.05 Global Days 090

26525 interphalangeal joint, each joint
EXCLUDES *Carpometacarpal joint arthroplasty (25447)*
19.08 19.08 Global Days 090
AMA: 2009, Jan, 11-31; 2008, Jan, 10-25; 2007, January, 13-27

26530 Arthroplasty, metacarpophalangeal joint; each joint
EXCLUDES *Carpometacarpal joint arthroplasty (25447)*
15.71 15.71 Global Days 090

26531 with prosthetic implant, each joint
EXCLUDES *Carpometacarpal joint arthroplasty (25447)*
18.25 18.25 Global Days 090

26535 Arthroplasty, interphalangeal joint; each joint
EXCLUDES *Carpometacarpal joint arthroplasty (25447)*
12.03 12.03 Global Days 090

26536 with prosthetic implant, each joint
EXCLUDES *Carpometacarpal joint arthroplasty (25447)*
20.48 20.48 Global Days 090

26540 Repair of collateral ligament, metacarpophalangeal or interphalangeal joint
19.21 19.21 Global Days 090

26541 Reconstruction, collateral ligament, metacarpophalangeal joint, single; with tendon or fascial graft (includes obtaining graft)
23.34 23.34 Global Days 090

26542 with local tissue (eg, adductor advancement)
19.84 19.84 Global Days 090

26545 Reconstruction, collateral ligament, interphalangeal joint, single, including graft, each joint
20.27 20.27 Global Days 090

26546 Repair non-union, metacarpal or phalanx (includes obtaining bone graft with or without external or internal fixation)
28.91 28.91 Global Days 090

26548 Repair and reconstruction, finger, volar plate, interphalangeal joint
22.28 22.28 Global Days 090

26550-26556 Reconstruction Procedures with Finger and Toe Transplants

26550 Pollicization of a digit A2 T 80
46.83 46.83 Global Days 090

26551 Transfer, toe-to-hand with microvascular anastomosis; great toe wrap-around with bone graft C5 C 80
INCLUDES Operating microscope (69990)
EXCLUDES *Big toe with web space (20973)*
87.08 87.08 Global Days 090

26553 other than great toe, single C5 C 80
INCLUDES Operating microscope (69990)
78.67 78.67 Global Days 090

26554 other than great toe, double C5 C 80
INCLUDES Operating microscope (69990)
93.63 93.63 Global Days 090

26555 Transfer, finger to another position without microvascular anastomosis A2 T 80
39.92 39.92 Global Days 090

26556 Transfer, free toe joint, with microvascular anastomosis C5 C 80
INCLUDES Operating microscope (69990)
EXCLUDES *Big toe to hand transfer (20973)*
84.22 84.22 Global Days 090

26560-26596 Repair of Other Deformities of the Fingers/Hand

26560 Repair of syndactyly (web finger) each web space; with skin flaps A2 T 80
17.02 17.02 Global Days 090

26561 with skin flaps and grafts A2 T 80
27.70 27.70 Global Days 090

26562 complex (eg, involving bone, nails) A2 T 80
37.61 37.61 Global Days 090

26565 metacarpal, each A2 T 80
19.89 19.89 Global Days 090

26567 phalanx of finger, each A2 T 80
19.83 19.83 Global Days 090

26568 Osteoplasty, lengthening, metacarpal or phalanx A2 T 80
26.14 26.14 Global Days 090

26580 Repair cleft hand A2 T 80
INCLUDES Barsky's procedure
44.27 44.27 Global Days 090

26587 Reconstruction of polydactylous digit, soft tissue and bone A2 T 80
EXCLUDES *Soft tissue removal only (11200)*
27.17 27.17 Global Days 090
AMA: 2009, Jan, 11-31; 2008, Jan, 10-25; 2007, January, 13-27

26590 Repair macrodactylia, each digit A2 T 80
37.16 37.16 Global Days 090
AMA: 2009, Jan, 11-31; 2008, Jan, 10-25; 2007, January, 13-27

26591 Repair, intrinsic muscles of hand, each muscle A2 T 80
12.82 12.82 Global Days 090
AMA: 2009, Jan, 11-31; 2008, Jan, 10-25; 2007, January, 13-27

26593 Release, intrinsic muscles of hand, each muscle A2 T
17.48 17.48 Global Days 090

26596 Excision of constricting ring of finger, with multiple Z-plasties A2 T 80
EXCLUDES *Graft repair or scar contracture release (11042, 14040-14041, 15120, 15240)*
21.95 21.95 Global Days 090

26600-26785 Treatment of Fracture/Dislocation of Fingers and Hand

INCLUDES Treatment for open or closed fractures or dislocations

26600 Closed treatment of metacarpal fracture, single; without manipulation, each bone P2 T
7.94 8.48 Global Days 090

26605 with manipulation, each bone A2 T
8.52 9.36 Global Days 090

26607 Closed treatment of metacarpal fracture, with manipulation, with external fixation, each bone A2 T 80
13.30 13.30 Global Days 090

26608 Percutaneous skeletal fixation of metacarpal fracture, each bone A2 T 80 P0
13.97 13.97 Global Days 090

26615 Open treatment of metacarpal fracture, single, includes internal fixation, when performed, each bone A2 T
16.73 16.73 Global Days 090

26641 Closed treatment of carpometacarpal dislocation, thumb, with manipulation P2 T 80
9.65 10.55 Global Days 090

26645 Closed treatment of carpometacarpal fracture dislocation, thumb (Bennett fracture), with manipulation A2 T 80
11.28 12.29 Global Days 090

26650 Percutaneous skeletal fixation of carpometacarpal fracture dislocation, thumb (Bennett fracture), with manipulation A2 T P0
13.99 13.99 Global Days 090

26665 Open treatment of carpometacarpal fracture dislocation, thumb (Bennett fracture), includes internal fixation, when performed A2 T
18.31 18.31 Global Days 090

26670 Closed treatment of carpometacarpal dislocation, other than thumb, with manipulation, each joint; without anesthesia P2 T 80
8.74 9.62 Global Days 090

26675 requiring anesthesia A2 T 80
12.04 13.09 Global Days 090

26676 Percutaneous skeletal fixation of carpometacarpal dislocation, other than thumb, with manipulation, each joint A2 T P0
14.67 14.67 Global Days 090

26685 Open treatment of carpometacarpal dislocation, other than thumb; includes internal fixation, when performed, each joint A2 T
16.84 16.84 Global Days 090

26686 complex, multiple, or delayed reduction A2 T 80
18.20 18.20 Global Days 090

26700 Closed treatment of metacarpophalangeal dislocation, single, with manipulation; without anesthesia P2 T
8.69 9.28 Global Days 090

26705 requiring anesthesia A2 T 80
10.94 11.96 Global Days 090

26706 Percutaneous skeletal fixation of metacarpophalangeal dislocation, single, with manipulation A2 T P0
12.87 12.87 Global Days 090

26715 Open treatment of metacarpophalangeal dislocation, single, includes internal fixation, when performed A2 T 80
16.73 16.73 Global Days 090

26720 Closed treatment of phalangeal shaft fracture, proximal or middle phalanx, finger or thumb; without manipulation, each P2 T
5.32 5.74 Global Days 090

26725 with manipulation, with or without skin or skeletal traction, each P2 T
8.88 9.86 Global Days 090

26727 Percutaneous skeletal fixation of unstable phalangeal shaft fracture, proximal or middle phalanx, finger or thumb, with manipulation, each A2 T PQ
13.74 13.74 Global Days 090

26735 Open treatment of phalangeal shaft fracture, proximal or middle phalanx, finger or thumb, includes internal fixation, when performed, each A2 T
17.39 17.39 Global Days 090

26740 Closed treatment of articular fracture, involving metacarpophalangeal or interphalangeal joint; without manipulation, each P2 T
6.21 6.63 Global Days 090

26742 with manipulation, each A2 T
9.76 10.76 Global Days 090

26746 Open treatment of articular fracture, involving metacarpophalangeal or interphalangeal joint, includes internal fixation, when performed, each A2 T
21.58 21.58 Global Days 090

26750 Closed treatment of distal phalangeal fracture, finger or thumb; without manipulation, each P2 T
5.31 5.34 Global Days 090

26755 with manipulation, each G2 T
7.97 9.17 Global Days 090

26756 Percutaneous skeletal fixation of distal phalangeal fracture, finger or thumb, each A2 T 80
12.24 12.24 Global Days 090

26765 Open treatment of distal phalangeal fracture, finger or thumb, includes internal fixation, when performed, each A2 T
14.53 14.53 Global Days 090

26770 Closed treatment of interphalangeal joint dislocation, single, with manipulation; without anesthesia G2 T
7.32 7.93 Global Days 090

26775 requiring anesthesia P3 T
10.07 11.16 Global Days 090

26776 Percutaneous skeletal fixation of interphalangeal joint dislocation, single, with manipulation A2 T
12.94 12.94 Global Days 090

26785 Open treatment of interphalangeal joint dislocation, includes internal fixation, when performed, single A2 T
15.80 15.80 Global Days 090

26820-26863 Fusion of Joint(s) of Fingers or Hand

26820 Fusion in opposition, thumb, with autogenous graft (includes obtaining graft) A2 T 80
22.86 22.86 Global Days 090

26841 Arthrodesis, carpometacarpal joint, thumb, with or without internal fixation; A2 T 80
21.21 21.21 Global Days 090

26842 with autograft (includes obtaining graft) A2 T 80
22.99 22.99 Global Days 090

26843 Arthrodesis, carpometacarpal joint, digit, other than thumb, each; A2 T 80
21.42 21.42 Global Days 090
AMA: 2009, Jan, 11-31; 2008, Jan, 10-25; 2007, January, 13-27

26844 with autograft (includes obtaining graft) A2 T 80
24.11 24.11 Global Days 090

26850 Arthrodesis, metacarpophalangeal joint, with or without internal fixation; A2 T 80
20.18 20.18 Global Days 090

26852 with autograft (includes obtaining graft) A2 T 80
23.13 23.13 Global Days 090

26860 Arthrodesis, interphalangeal joint, with or without internal fixation; A2 T
16.42 16.42 Global Days 090
AMA: 2009, Jul, 10

\+ **26861** each additional interphalangeal joint (List separately in addition to code for primary procedure) A2 T
Code first (26860)
3.06 3.06 Global Days ZZZ
AMA: 2009, Jul, 10

26862 with autograft (includes obtaining graft) A2 T 80
21.18 21.18 Global Days 090

\+ **26863** with autograft (includes obtaining graft), each additional joint (List separately in addition to code for primary procedure) A2 T 80
Code first (26862)
6.79 6.79 Global Days ZZZ

26910-26989 Amputations and Unlisted Procedures Finger/Hand

26910 Amputation, metacarpal, with finger or thumb (ray amputation), single, with or without interosseous transfer A2 T
EXCLUDES *Repositioning (26550, 26555)*
Transmetacarpal amputation of hand (25927)
20.98 20.98 Global Days 090

26951 Amputation, finger or thumb, primary or secondary, any joint or phalanx, single, including neurectomies; with direct closure A2 T
EXCLUDES *Repair necessitating flaps or grafts (15050-15758)*
Transmetacarpal amputation of hand (25927)
18.89 18.89 Global Days 090

26952 with local advancement flaps (V-Y, hood) A2 T
EXCLUDES *Repair necessitating flaps or grafts (15050-15758)*
Transmetacarpal amputation of hand (25927)
18.90 18.90 Global Days 090

26989 Unlisted procedure, hands or fingers T
0.00 0.00 Global Days YYY

26990-26992 Incision for Drainage of Pelvis or Hip

EXCLUDES *Simple incision and drainage procedures (10040-10160)*

26990 Incision and drainage, pelvis or hip joint area; deep abscess or hematoma A2 T
18.27 18.27 Global Days 090

26991 infected bursa A2 T 80
15.39 20.76 Global Days 090

26992 Incision, bone cortex, pelvis and/or hip joint (eg, osteomyelitis or bone abscess) C5 C 80
28.10 28.10 Global Days 090
AMA: 2009, Jan, 11-31; 2008, Jan, 10-25; 2007, January, 13-27

27000-27006 Tenotomy Procedures of Hip

27000 **Tenotomy, adductor of hip, percutaneous (separate procedure)** A2 T 50
12.80 12.80 Global Days 090

27001 **Tenotomy, adductor of hip, open** A2 T 80 50
15.87 15.87 Global Days 090

27003 **Tenotomy, adductor, subcutaneous, open, with obturator neurectomy** A2 T 80 50
17.36 17.36 Global Days 090

27005 **Tenotomy, hip flexor(s), open (separate procedure)** C5 C 80 50
21.33 21.33 Global Days 090

27006 **Tenotomy, abductors and/or extensor(s) of hip, open (separate procedure)** T 80 50
21.62 21.62 Global Days 090

27025-27036 Surgical Incision of Hip

CMS 100-3,160.1 Induced Lesions of Nerve Tracts

27025 **Fasciotomy, hip or thigh, any type** C5 C 80 50
26.98 26.98 Global Days 090

27027 **Decompression fasciotomy(ies), pelvic (buttock) compartment(s) (eg, gluteus medius-minimus, gluteus maximus, iliopsoas, and/or tensor fascia lata muscle), unilateral** T 80 50
24.61 24.61 Global Days 090

27030 **Arthrotomy, hip, with drainage (eg, infection)** C5 C 80 50
27.45 27.45 Global Days 090

27033 **Arthrotomy, hip, including exploration or removal of loose or foreign body** A2 T 80 50
28.62 28.62 Global Days 090

27035 **Denervation, hip joint, intrapelvic or extrapelvic intra-articular branches of sciatic, femoral, or obturator nerves** A2 T 80 50

EXCLUDES *Transection of obturator nerve (64763, 64766)*

30.23 30.23 Global Days 090

27036 **Capsulectomy or capsulotomy, hip, with or without excision of heterotopic bone, with release of hip flexor muscles (ie, gluteus medius, gluteus minimus, tensor fascia latae, rectus femoris, sartorius, iliopsoas)** C5 C 80 50
29.61 29.61 Global Days 090

27040-27041 Biopsy of Hip/Pelvis

EXCLUDES *Soft tissue needle biopsy (20206)*

27040 **Biopsy, soft tissue of pelvis and hip area; superficial** A2 T 50
5.88 10.02 Global Days 010

27041 **deep, subfascial or intramuscular** A2 T 50
19.91 19.91 Global Days 090

27043-27059 [27043, 27045, 27059] Excision Soft Tissue Tumors Hip/ Pelvis

INCLUDES Any necessary elevation of tissue planes or dissection
Measurement of tumor and necessary margin at greatest diameter prior to excision
Simple and intermediate repairs
Types of Exision:
Fascial or subfascial soft tissue tumors: simple and marginal resection of most often benign and intramuscular tumors found either in or below the deep fascia, not involving bone
Radical resection of tumor: wide resection of tumor, mostly malignant or aggressive benign, involving large margins of normal tissue and may involve tissue removal from one or more layers
Subcutaneous: simple and marginal resection of most often benign tumors found in the subcutaneous tissue above the deep fascia

EXCLUDES *Complex repair*
Radical resection of cutaneous tumors (e.g., melanoma) (11600-11646)
Significant exploration of vessels, neuroplasty, reconstruction, or complex bone repair

27043 ***Resequenced code, See code following 27047.***

27045 ***Resequenced code, See code following 27048.***

27047 **Excision, tumor, soft tissue of pelvis and hip area, subcutaneous; less than 3 cm** G2 T 50
10.99 14.10 Global Days 090

\# **27043** **3 cm or greater** G2 T 50
13.90 13.90 Global Days 090

27048 **Excision, tumor, soft tissue of pelvis and hip area, subfascial (eg, intramuscular); less than 5 cm** G2 T 80 50
17.69 17.69 Global Days 090

\# **27045** **5 cm or greater** G2 T 80 50
22.14 22.14 Global Days 090

27049 **Radical resection of tumor (eg, malignant neoplasm), soft tissue of pelvis and hip area; less than 5 cm** G2 T 80 50
39.46 39.46 Global Days 090

\# **27059** **5 cm or greater** G2 T 80 50
53.12 53.12 Global Days 090

27050-27071 Procedures of Bones and Joints of Hip and Pelvis

27050 **Arthrotomy, with biopsy; sacroiliac joint** A2 T 80 50
11.42 11.42 Global Days 090

27052 **hip joint** A2 T 80 50
16.84 16.84 Global Days 090

27054 **Arthrotomy with synovectomy, hip joint** C5 C 80 50
20.04 20.04 Global Days 090

27057 **Decompression fasciotomy(ies), pelvic (buttock) compartment(s) (eg, gluteus medius-minimus, gluteus maximus, iliopsoas, and/or tensor fascia lata muscle) with debridement of nonviable muscle, unilateral** T 80 50
27.63 27.63 Global Days 090

27059 ***Resequenced code, See code following 27049.***

27060 **Excision; ischial bursa** A2 T 50
13.40 13.40 Global Days 090

27062 **trochanteric bursa or calcification** A2 T 50

EXCLUDES *Arthrocentesis (20610)*

13.33 13.33 Global Days 090

27065 **Excision of bone cyst or benign tumor, wing of ilium, symphysis pubis, or greater trochanter of femur; superficial, includes autograft, when performed** A2 T 80 50
14.92 14.92 Global Days 090

27066 **deep (subfascial), includes autograft, when performed** A2 T 80 50
23.80 23.80 Global Days 090

27067 **with autograft requiring separate incision** A2 T 80 50
30.33 30.33 Global Days 090

27070 **Partial excision, wing of ilium, symphysis pubis, or greater trochanter of femur, (craterization, saucerization) (eg, osteomyelitis or bone abscess); superficial** C5 C 80 50
25.02 25.02 Global Days 090

27071 **deep (subfascial or intramuscular)** C5 C 80 50
26.87 26.87 Global Days 090

27075-27078 Radical Resection Bone Tumor of Hip/Pelvis

INCLUDES Any necessary elevation of tissue planes or dissection
Measurement of tumor and necessary margin at greatest diameter prior to excision
Radical resection of bone tumor: resection of the tumor (may include entire bone) and wide margins of normal tissue primarily for malignant or aggressive benign tumors
Simple and intermediate repairs

EXCLUDES *Complex repair*
Significant exploration of vessels, neuroplasty, reconstruction, or complex bone repair

Do not report radical excision of soft tissue codes when adjacent soft tissue is removed during the bone tumor resection (27048-27049 [27043, 27045, 27059])

27075 **Radical resection of tumor; wing of ilium, 1 pubic or ischial ramus or symphysis pubis** C5 C 80
61.91 61.91 Global Days 090

27076 **ilium, including acetabulum, both pubic rami, or ischium and acetabulum** C5 C 80
72.75 72.75 Global Days 090

27077 **innominate bone, total** C5 C 80
82.98 82.98 Global Days 090

27078 **ischial tuberosity and greater trochanter of femur** C5 C 80
58.60 58.60 Global Days 090

27080 Excision of Coccyx

EXCLUDES *Surgical excision of decubitus ulcers (15920, 15922, 15931-15958)*

27080 **Coccygectomy, primary** A2 T 80
14.83 14.83 Global Days 090

27086-27091 Removal Foreign Body or Hip Prosthesis

27086 **Removal of foreign body, pelvis or hip; subcutaneous tissue** A2 T 80 50
4.37 7.40 Global Days 010

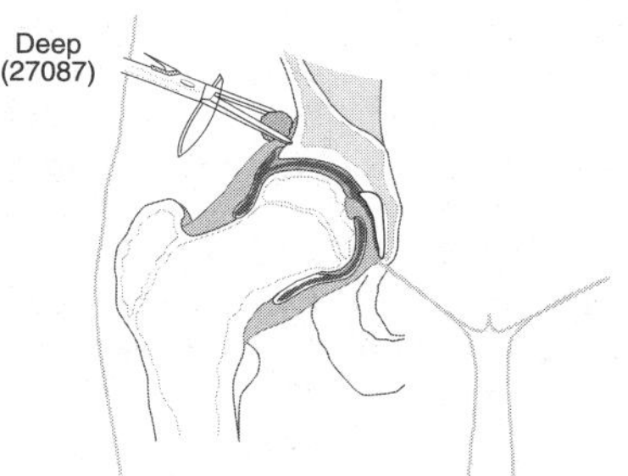

A foreign body is removed from the pelvis or hip

27087 **deep (subfascial or intramuscular)** A2 T 80 50
18.54 18.54 Global Days 090

27090 **Removal of hip prosthesis; (separate procedure)** C5 C 80 50
24.37 24.37 Global Days 090

27091 **complicated, including total hip prosthesis, methylmethacrylate with or without insertion of spacer** C5 C 80 50
47.05 47.05 Global Days 090

27093-27096 Injection for Arthrogram Hip/Sacroiliac Joint

27093 **Injection procedure for hip arthrography; without anesthesia** N1 N 50
73525
2.06 5.73 Global Days 000

27095 **with anesthesia** N1 N 50
73525
2.40 7.09 Global Days 000

▲ 27096 **Injection procedure for sacroiliac joint, anesthetic/steroid, with image guidance (fluoroscopy or CT) including arthrography when performed** B 50
INCLUDES Confirmation of intra-articular needle placement with CT or fluoroscopy
EXCLUDES *Procedure performed without fluoroscopy or CT guidance (20552)*
2.41 5.05 Global Days 000
AMA: 2009, Jan, 11-31; 2008, Jan, 10-25; 2008, Jul, 9; 2007, January, 13-27

27097-27187 Revision/Reconstruction Hip and Pelvis

27097 **Release or recession, hamstring, proximal** A2 T 80 50
19.83 19.83 Global Days 090

27098 **Transfer, adductor to ischium** A2 T 80 50
19.91 19.91 Global Days 090

27100 **Transfer external oblique muscle to greater trochanter including fascial or tendon extension (graft)** A2 T 80 50
INCLUDES Eggers procedure
24.15 24.15 Global Days 090

27105 **Transfer paraspinal muscle to hip (includes fascial or tendon extension graft)** A2 T 80 50
25.36 25.36 Global Days 090

27110 **Transfer iliopsoas; to greater trochanter of femur** A2 T 80 50
28.32 28.32 Global Days 090

27111 to femoral neck A2 T 80 50
24.25 24.25 Global Days 090

27120 Acetabuloplasty; (eg, Whitman, Colonna, Haygroves, or cup type) C5 C 80 50
37.96 37.96 Global Days 090

27122 resection, femoral head (eg, Girdlestone procedure) C5 C 80 50
32.39 32.39 Global Days 090

27125 Hemiarthroplasty, hip, partial (eg, femoral stem prosthesis, bipolar arthroplasty) C5 C 80 50 PQ
EXCLUDES *Total joint following hip fracture (27236)*
33.29 33.29 Global Days 090
AMA: 2009, Jan, 11-31; 2008, Jan, 10-25; 2007, January, 13-27

27130 Arthroplasty, acetabular and proximal femoral prosthetic replacement (total hip arthroplasty), with or without autograft or allograft C5 C 80 50 PQ
42.47 42.47 Global Days 090
AMA: 2007, January, 1-5

27132 Conversion of previous hip surgery to total hip arthroplasty, with or without autograft or allograft C5 C 80 50 PQ
49.47 49.47 Global Days 090

27134 Revision of total hip arthroplasty; both components, with or without autograft or allograft C5 C 80 50 PQ
56.71 56.71 Global Days 090

27137 acetabular component only, with or without autograft or allograft C5 C 80 50 PQ
43.50 43.50 Global Days 090

27138 femoral component only, with or without allograft C5 C 80 50 PQ
45.26 45.26 Global Days 090

27140 Osteotomy and transfer of greater trochanter of femur (separate procedure) C5 C 80 50
26.30 26.30 Global Days 090

27146 Osteotomy, iliac, acetabular or innominate bone; C5 C 80 50
INCLUDES Salter osteotomy
37.61 37.61 Global Days 090
AMA: 2009, Jan, 11-31; 2008, Jan, 10-25; 2007, January, 13-27

27147 with open reduction of hip C5 C 80 50
INCLUDES Pemberton osteotomy
43.18 43.18 Global Days 090

27151 with femoral osteotomy C5 C 80 50
46.29 46.29 Global Days 090

27156 with femoral osteotomy and with open reduction of hip C5 C 80 50
INCLUDES Chiari osteotomy
50.37 50.37 Global Days 090

27158 Osteotomy, pelvis, bilateral (eg, congenital malformation) C5 C 80
41.03 41.03 Global Days 090

27161 Osteotomy, femoral neck (separate procedure) C5 C 80 50
35.75 35.75 Global Days 090

27165 Osteotomy, intertrochanteric or subtrochanteric including internal or external fixation and/or cast C5 C 80 50
40.39 40.39 Global Days 090

27170 Bone graft, femoral head, neck, intertrochanteric or subtrochanteric area (includes obtaining bone graft) C5 C 80 50
34.63 34.63 Global Days 090

27175 Treatment of slipped femoral epiphysis; by traction, without reduction C5 C 80 50
19.52 19.52 Global Days 090

27176 by single or multiple pinning, in situ C5 C 80 50
26.88 26.88 Global Days 090

27177 Open treatment of slipped femoral epiphysis; single or multiple pinning or bone graft (includes obtaining graft) C5 C 80 50
32.67 32.67 Global Days 090

27178 closed manipulation with single or multiple pinning C5 C 80 50
26.84 26.84 Global Days 090

27179 osteoplasty of femoral neck (Heyman type procedure) T 80 50
28.60 28.60 Global Days 090

27181 osteotomy and internal fixation C5 C 80 50
32.90 32.90 Global Days 090

27185 Epiphyseal arrest by epiphysiodesis or stapling, greater trochanter of femur C5 C 50
19.43 19.43 Global Days 090

27187 Prophylactic treatment (nailing, pinning, plating or wiring) with or without methylmethacrylate, femoral neck and proximal femur C5 C 80 50
29.15 29.15 Global Days 090

27193-27269 Treatment of Fracture/Dislocation Hip/Pelvis

27193 Closed treatment of pelvic ring fracture, dislocation, diastasis or subluxation; without manipulation A2 T
13.94 13.77 Global Days 090

27194 with manipulation, requiring more than local anesthesia A2 T 80
20.43 20.43 Global Days 090

27200 Closed treatment of coccygeal fracture P2 T
5.40 5.21 Global Days 090

27202 Open treatment of coccygeal fracture A2 T 80
16.42 16.42 Global Days 090

27215 Open treatment of iliac spine(s), tuberosity avulsion, or iliac wing fracture(s), unilateral, for pelvic bone fracture patterns that do not disrupt the pelvic ring, includes internal fixation, when performed E
18.01 18.01 Global Days 090

27216 Percutaneous skeletal fixation of posterior pelvic bone fracture and/or dislocation, for fracture patterns that disrupt the pelvic ring, unilateral (includes ipsilateral ilium, sacroiliac joint and/or sacrum) E
26.66 26.66 Global Days 090

27217 Open treatment of anterior pelvic bone fracture and/or dislocation for fracture patterns that disrupt the pelvic ring, unilateral, includes internal fixation, when performed (includes pubic symphysis and/or ipsilateral superior/inferior rami) E
25.10 25.10 Global Days 090

27218 Open treatment of posterior pelvic bone fracture and/or dislocation, for fracture patterns that disrupt the pelvic ring, unilateral, includes internal fixation, when performed (includes ipsilateral ilium, sacroiliac joint and/or sacrum) E
34.47 34.47 Global Days 090

27220 Closed treatment of acetabulum (hip socket) fracture(s); without manipulation G2 T 50
15.35 15.49 Global Days 090

27222 with manipulation, with or without skeletal traction C5 C 50
28.72 28.72 Global Days 090

27226 Open treatment of posterior or anterior acetabular wall fracture, with internal fixation C5 C 80 50
30.98 30.98 Global Days 090

27227 Open treatment of acetabular fracture(s) involving anterior or posterior (1) column, or a fracture running transversely across the acetabulum, with internal fixation C5 C 80 50
48.92 48.92 Global Days 090

27228 Open treatment of acetabular fracture(s) involving anterior and posterior (2) columns, includes T-fracture and both column fracture with complete articular detachment, or single column or transverse fracture with associated acetabular wall fracture, with internal fixation C5 C 80 50
55.85 55.85 Global Days 090

27230 Closed treatment of femoral fracture, proximal end, neck; without manipulation A2 T 50 PQ
13.75 13.86 Global Days 090

27232 with manipulation, with or without skeletal traction C5 C 50 PQ
22.46 22.46 Global Days 090

27235 Percutaneous skeletal fixation of femoral fracture, proximal end, neck T 50 PQ
26.72 26.72 Global Days 090

27236 Open treatment of femoral fracture, proximal end, neck, internal fixation or prosthetic replacement C5 C 80 50 PQ
35.18 35.18 Global Days 090
AMA: 2009, Jan, 11-31; 2008, Jan, 10-25; 2007, January, 13-27; 2007, January, 1-5

27238 Closed treatment of intertrochanteric, peritrochanteric, or subtrochanteric femoral fracture; without manipulation A2 T 50 PQ
13.42 13.42 Global Days 090

27240 with manipulation, with or without skin or skeletal traction C5 C 50 PQ
28.16 28.16 Global Days 090

27244 Treatment of intertrochanteric, peritrochanteric, or subtrochanteric femoral fracture; with plate/screw type implant, with or without cerclage C5 C 80 50 PQ
36.17 36.17 Global Days 090

27245 with intramedullary implant, with or without interlocking screws and/or cerclage C5 C 80 50 PQ
36.38 36.38 Global Days 090

27246 Closed treatment of greater trochanteric fracture, without manipulation A2 T 50 PQ
11.28 11.24 Global Days 090

27248 Open treatment of greater trochanteric fracture, includes internal fixation, when performed C5 C 80 50 PQ
21.90 21.90 Global Days 090

27250 Closed treatment of hip dislocation, traumatic; without anesthesia A2 T 50
5.68 5.68 Global Days 000

27252 requiring anesthesia A2 T 50
22.27 22.27 Global Days 090

27253 Open treatment of hip dislocation, traumatic, without internal fixation C5 C 80 50
27.68 27.68 Global Days 090

27254 Open treatment of hip dislocation, traumatic, with acetabular wall and femoral head fracture, with or without internal or external fixation C5 C 80 50
EXCLUDES *Acetabular fracture treatment (27226-27227)*
37.36 37.36 Global Days 090

27256 Treatment of spontaneous hip dislocation (developmental, including congenital or pathological), by abduction, splint or traction; without anesthesia, without manipulation G2 T 80 50
6.94 8.78 Global Days 010

27257 with manipulation, requiring anesthesia A2 T 80 50
9.81 9.81 Global Days 010

27258 Open treatment of spontaneous hip dislocation (developmental, including congenital or pathological), replacement of femoral head in acetabulum (including tenotomy, etc); C5 C 80 50
INCLUDES Lorenz's operation
32.57 32.57 Global Days 090

27259 with femoral shaft shortening C5 C 80 50
45.59 45.59 Global Days 090

27265 Closed treatment of post hip arthroplasty dislocation; without anesthesia A2 T 50
11.68 11.68 Global Days 090

27266 requiring regional or general anesthesia A2 T 50
17.01 17.01 Global Days 090

27267 Closed treatment of femoral fracture, proximal end, head; without manipulation G2 T 80 50
12.66 12.66 Global Days 090
AMA: 2008, Jan, 4-5

27268 with manipulation C5 C 80 50
15.57 15.57 Global Days 090
AMA: 2008, Jan, 4-5

27269 Open treatment of femoral fracture, proximal end, head, includes internal fixation, when performed C5 C 80 50 PQ
Do not report with (27033, 27253)
36.30 36.30 Global Days 090
AMA: 2008, Jan, 4-5

27275 Hip Manipulation with Anesthesia

27275 Manipulation, hip joint, requiring general anesthesia A2 T
5.26 5.26 Global Days 010

27280-27286 Arthrodesis of Hip and Pelvis

27280 Arthrodesis, sacroiliac joint (including obtaining graft) C5 C 80 50
30.35 30.35 Global Days 090

27282 Arthrodesis, symphysis pubis (including obtaining graft) C5 C 80
24.71 24.71 Global Days 090

27284 Arthrodesis, hip joint (including obtaining graft); C5 C 80 50
47.07 47.07 Global Days 090

27286 with subtrochanteric osteotomy C5 C 80 50
48.67 48.67 Global Days 090

27290-27299 Amputations and Unlisted Procedures of Hip and Pelvis

27290 Interpelviabdominal amputation (hindquarter amputation) C5 C 80
INCLUDES Pean's amputation
47.40 47.40 Global Days 090

27295 **Disarticulation of hip** C5 C 80
37.08 37.08 Global Days 090

27299 **Unlisted procedure, pelvis or hip joint** T 80 50
0.00 0.00 Global Days YYY
AMA: 2009, Jan, 11-31; 2008, Jan, 10-25; 2007, January, 13-27

27301-27310 Incisional Procedures Femur or Knee

EXCLUDES *Superficial incision and drainage (10040-10160)*

27301 **Incision and drainage, deep abscess, bursa, or hematoma, thigh or knee region** A2 T 50
14.69 19.66 Global Days 090

27303 **Incision, deep, with opening of bone cortex, femur or knee (eg, osteomyelitis or bone abscess)** C5 C 80 50
18.73 18.73 Global Days 090

27305 **Fasciotomy, iliotibial (tenotomy), open** A2 T 80 50
EXCLUDES *Ober-Yount (gluteal-iliotibial) fasciotomy (27025)*
13.99 13.99 Global Days 090

27306 **Tenotomy, percutaneous, adductor or hamstring; single tendon (separate procedure)** A2 T 80 50
10.45 10.45 Global Days 090

27307 **multiple tendons** A2 T 80 50
13.94 13.94 Global Days 090

27310 **Arthrotomy, knee, with exploration, drainage, or removal of foreign body (eg, infection)** A2 T 80 50
21.43 21.43 Global Days 090

27323-27324 Biopsy Femur or Knee

EXCLUDES *Soft tissue needle biopsy (20206)*

27323 **Biopsy, soft tissue of thigh or knee area; superficial** A2 T 50
5.27 7.98 Global Days 010

27324 **deep (subfascial or intramuscular)** A2 T 50
11.46 11.46 Global Days 090

27325-27326 Neurectomy

27325 **Neurectomy, hamstring muscle** A2 T 80 50
14.98 14.98 Global Days 090

27326 **Neurectomy, popliteal (gastrocnemius)** A2 T 80 50
14.84 14.84 Global Days 090

27327-27329 [27337, 27339] Excision Soft Tissue Tumors Femur/ Knee

INCLUDES Any necessary elevation of tissue planes or dissection
Measurement of tumor and necessary margin at greatest diameter prior to excision
Resection without removal of significant normal tissue
Simple and intermediate repairs
Types of Excision:
Fascial or subfascial soft tissue tumors: simple and marginal resection of most often benign and intramuscular tumors found either in or below the deep fascia, not involving bone
Radical resection of tumor: wide resection of tumor, mostly malignant or aggressive benign, involving large margins of normal tissue and may involve tissue removal from one or more layers
Subcutaneous: simple and marginal resection of most often benign tumors found in the subcutaneous tissue above the deep fascia

EXCLUDES *Complex repair*
Radical resection of cutaneous tumors (e.g., melanoma) (11600-11646)
Significant exploration of vessels or neuroplasty

27327 **Excision, tumor, soft tissue of thigh or knee area, subcutaneous; less than 3 cm** G2 T 50
9.27 13.27 Global Days 090

\# **27337** **3 cm or greater**
12.42 12.42 Global Days 090

27328 **Excision, tumor, soft tissue of thigh or knee area, subfascial (eg, intramuscular); less than 5 cm** G2 T 50
17.85 17.85 Global Days 090

\# **27339** **5 cm or greater**
22.15 22.15 Global Days 090

27329 ***Resequenced code, See code following 27360.***

27330-27360 Resection Procedures Thigh/Knee

27330 **Arthrotomy, knee; with synovial biopsy only** A2 T 50
11.97 11.97 Global Days 090

27331 **including joint exploration, biopsy, or removal of loose or foreign bodies** A2 T 80 50
13.92 13.92 Global Days 090

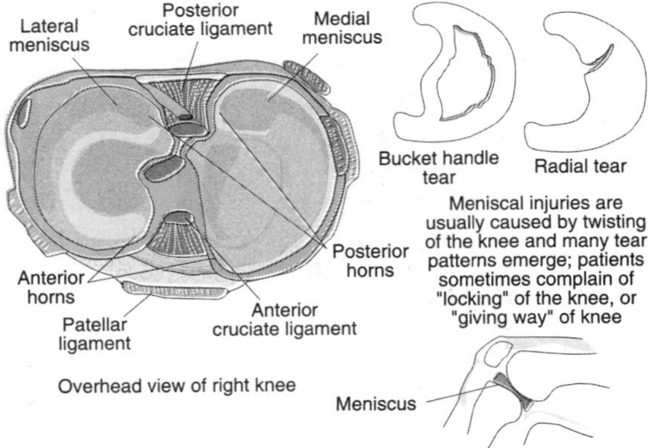

27332 **Arthrotomy, with excision of semilunar cartilage (meniscectomy) knee; medial OR lateral** A2 T 80 50
18.75 18.75 Global Days 090

27333 **medial AND lateral** A2 T 80 50
17.11 17.11 Global Days 090

27334 **Arthrotomy, with synovectomy, knee; anterior OR posterior** A2 T 80 50
20.03 20.03 Global Days 090

27335 **anterior AND posterior including popliteal area** A2 T 80 50
22.43 22.43 Global Days 090

27337 ***Resequenced code, See code following 27327.***

27339 ***Resequenced code, See code following 27328.***

27340 **Excision, prepatellar bursa** A2 T 50
10.83 10.83 Global Days 090

27345 **Excision of synovial cyst of popliteal space (eg, Baker's cyst)** A2 T 80 50
14.11 14.11 Global Days 090

27347 **Excision of lesion of meniscus or capsule (eg, cyst, ganglion), knee** A2 T 80 50
15.44 15.44 Global Days 090

27350 **Patellectomy or hemipatellectomy** A2 T 80 50
19.10 19.10 Global Days 090

27355 **Excision or curettage of bone cyst or benign tumor of femur;** A2 T 80 50
17.67 17.67 Global Days 090

27356 **with allograft** A2 T 80 50
21.61 21.61 Global Days 090

27357 **with autograft (includes obtaining graft)** A2 T 80 50
23.85 23.85 Global Days 090
AMA: 2009, Jan, 11-31; 2008, Jan, 10-25; 2007, January, 13-27

\+ 27358 **with internal fixation (List in addition to code for primary procedure)** A2 T 80
Code first (27355-27357)
8.25 8.25 Global Days ZZZ

27360 **Partial excision (craterization, saucerization, or diaphysectomy) bone, femur, proximal tibia and/or fibula (eg, osteomyelitis or bone abscess)** A2 T 80 50
25.04 25.04 Global Days 090

27329-27365 [27329] Radical Resection Bone Tumor Knee/Thigh

INCLUDES Any necessary elevation of tissue planes or dissection
Measurement of tumor and necessary margin at greatest diameter prior to excision
Radical resection soft tissue tumor: wide resection of tumor, mostly malignant or aggressive benign, involving large margins of normal tissue and may involve tissue removal from one or more layers
Simple and intermediate repairs

EXCLUDES *Complex repair*
Significant exploration of vessels, neuroplasty, reconstruction, or complex bone repair

Do not report radical excision of soft tissue codes when adjacent soft tissue is removed during the bone tumor resection.

\# 27329 **Radical resection of tumor (eg, malignant neoplasm), soft tissue of thigh or knee area; less than 5 cm** G2 T 80 50
30.58 30.58 Global Days 090

27364 **5 cm or greater** G2 T 80 50
46.08 46.08 Global Days 090

27365 **Radical resection of tumor, femur or knee** C5 C 80 50
EXCLUDES *Soft tissue tumor excision thigh or knee area ([27329], 27364)*
59.07 59.07 Global Days 090

27370 Injection for Arthrogram of Knee

27370 **Injection procedure for knee arthrography** N1 N 50
73580
1.54 5.04 Global Days 000

27372 Foreign Body Removal Femur or Knee

27372 **Removal of foreign body, deep, thigh region or knee area** A2 T 80 50
EXCLUDES *Arthroscopic procedures (29870-29887)*
Removal of knee prosthesis (27488)
11.85 17.73 Global Days 090

27380-27499 Repair/Reconstruction of Femur or Knee

27380 **Suture of infrapatellar tendon; primary** A2 T 80 50
17.42 17.42 Global Days 090

27381 **secondary reconstruction, including fascial or tendon graft** A2 T 80 50
23.46 23.46 Global Days 090

27385 **Suture of quadriceps or hamstring muscle rupture; primary** A2 T 80 50
16.94 16.94 Global Days 090

27386 **secondary reconstruction, including fascial or tendon graft** A2 T 80 50
24.39 24.39 Global Days 090

27390 **Tenotomy, open, hamstring, knee to hip; single tendon** A2 T 80
13.06 13.06 Global Days 090

27391 **multiple tendons, 1 leg** A2 T 80
16.84 16.84 Global Days 090

27392 **multiple tendons, bilateral** A2 T 80
20.76 20.76 Global Days 090

27393 **Lengthening of hamstring tendon; single tendon** A2 T 80
14.90 14.90 Global Days 090

27394 **multiple tendons, 1 leg** A2 T 80
19.08 19.08 Global Days 090

27395 **multiple tendons, bilateral** A2 T 80
25.73 25.73 Global Days 090

27396 **Transplant or transfer (with muscle redirection or rerouting), thigh (eg, extensor to flexor); single tendon** A2 T 80
18.01 18.01 Global Days 090

27397 **multiple tendons** A2 T 80
26.78 26.78 Global Days 090

27400 **Transfer, tendon or muscle, hamstrings to femur (eg, Egger's type procedure)** A2 T 80 50
20.29 20.29 Global Days 090

27403 **Arthrotomy with meniscus repair, knee** A2 T 80 50
EXCLUDES *Arthroscopic treatment (29882)*
18.79 18.79 Global Days 090

27405 **Repair, primary, torn ligament and/or capsule, knee; collateral** A2 T 80 50
19.86 19.86 Global Days 090

27407 **cruciate** A2 T 80 50
EXCLUDES *Reconstruction (27427)*
23.05 23.05 Global Days 090

27409 **collateral and cruciate ligaments** A2 T 80 50
EXCLUDES *Reconstruction (27427-27429)*
28.29 28.29 Global Days 090

27412 Autologous chondrocyte implantation, knee T 80 50

Do not report with (20926, 27331, 27570)

EXCLUDES *Obtaining chondrocytes (29870)*

48.57 48.57 Global Days 090

27415 Osteochondral allograft, knee, open T 80 50

EXCLUDES *Arthroscopic procedure (29867)*

Do not report with (27416)

40.28 40.28 Global Days 090

AMA: 2009, Jan, 11-31

27416 Osteochondral autograft(s), knee, open (eg, mosaicplasty) (includes harvesting of autograft[s]) G2 T 80 50

EXCLUDES *Surgical arthroscopy of the knee with osteochondral autograft(s) (29866)*

Do not report with the following procedures in the same compartment (29874, 29877, 29879, 29885-29887)

Do not report with the following procedures performed at the same surgical session (27415, 29870-29871, 29875, 29884)

28.64 28.64 Global Days 090

AMA: 2008, Jan, 4-5

27418 Anterior tibial tubercleplasty (eg, Maquet type procedure) A2 T 80 50

24.46 24.46 Global Days 090

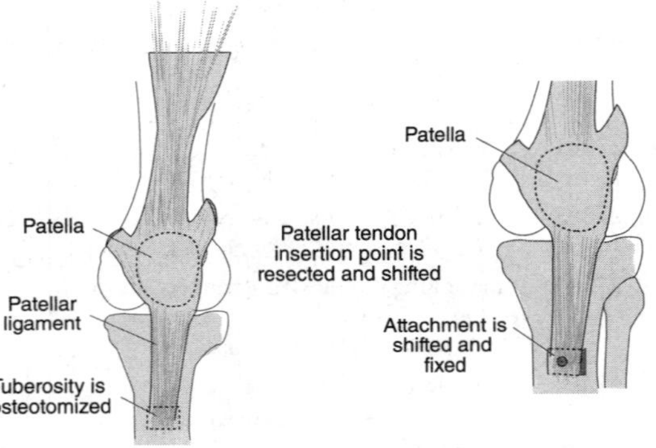

27420 Reconstruction of dislocating patella; (eg, Hauser type procedure) A2 T 80 50

21.80 21.80 Global Days 090

27422 **with extensor realignment and/or muscle advancement or release (eg, Campbell, Goldwaite type procedure)** A2 T 80 50

21.81 21.81 Global Days 090

27424 **with patellectomy** A2 T 80 50

21.88 21.88 Global Days 090

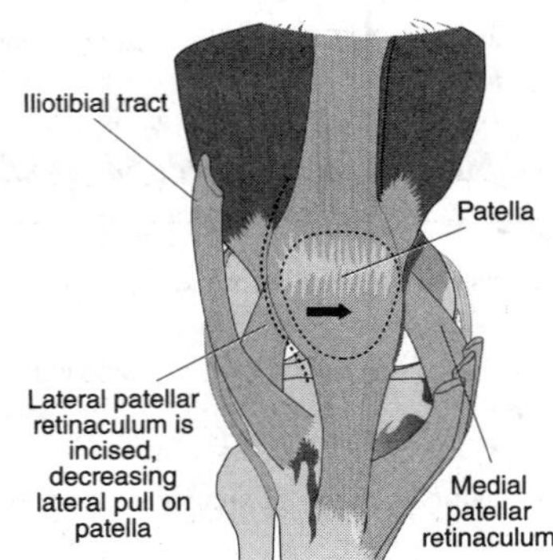

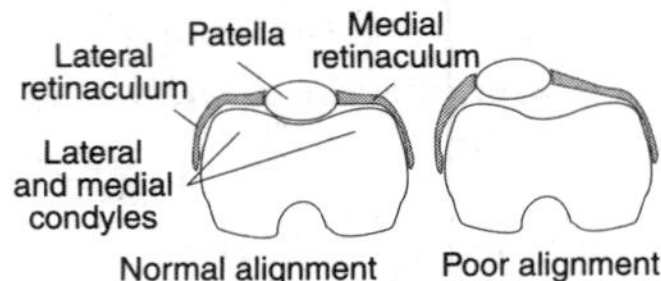

27425 Lateral retinacular release, open A2 T 50

EXCLUDES *Arthroscopic release (29873)*

13.06 13.06 Global Days 090

AMA: 2009, Jan, 11-31; 2008, Jan, 10-25; 2007, January, 13-27

27427 Ligamentous reconstruction (augmentation), knee; extra-articular A2 T 80 50

EXCLUDES *Primary repair of ligament(s) (27405, 27407, 27409)*

21.09 21.09 Global Days 090

27428 **intra-articular (open)** A2 T 80 50

EXCLUDES *Primary repair of ligament(s) (27405, 27407, 27409)*

32.69 32.69 Global Days 090

27429 **intra-articular (open) and extra-articular** A2 T 80 50

EXCLUDES *Primary repair of ligament(s) (27405, 27407, 27409)*

36.69 36.69 Global Days 090

27430 Quadricepsplasty (eg, Bennett or Thompson type) A2 T 80 50

21.72 21.72 Global Days 090

27435 Capsulotomy, posterior capsular release, knee A2 T 80 50

23.69 23.69 Global Days 090

27437 Arthroplasty, patella; without prosthesis A2 T 50

19.35 19.35 Global Days 090

27438 **with prosthesis** A2 T 80 50

24.70 24.70 Global Days 090

27440 Arthroplasty, knee, tibial plateau; G2 T 80 50 PO

23.16 23.16 Global Days 090

27441 **with debridement and partial synovectomy** A2 T 80 50 PO

23.92 23.92 Global Days 090

27442 Arthroplasty, femoral condyles or tibial plateau(s), knee; A2 T 80 50 PO

25.52 25.52 Global Days 090

27443 **with debridement and partial synovectomy** A2 T 80 50 PO

23.93 23.93 Global Days 090

27445 **Arthroplasty, knee, hinge prosthesis (eg, Walldius type)**
EXCLUDES *Removal knee prosthesis (27488)*
Revision knee arthroplasty (27487)
36.86 36.86 Global Days 090

27446 **Arthroplasty, knee, condyle and plateau; medial OR lateral compartment**
EXCLUDES *Removal knee prosthesis (27488)*
Revision knee arthroplasty (27487)
Code also (C1776)
32.59 32.59 Global Days 090

27447 **medial AND lateral compartments with or without patella resurfacing (total knee arthroplasty)**
EXCLUDES *Removal knee prosthesis (27488)*
Revision knee arthroplasty (27487)
45.37 45.37 Global Days 090
AMA: 2007, January, 1-5

27448 **Osteotomy, femur, shaft or supracondylar; without fixation**
24.06 24.06 Global Days 090

27450 **with fixation**
29.89 29.89 Global Days 090

27454 **Osteotomy, multiple, with realignment on intramedullary rod, femoral shaft (eg, Sofield type procedure)**
38.05 38.05 Global Days 090

27455 **Osteotomy, proximal tibia, including fibular excision or osteotomy (includes correction of genu varus [bowleg] or genu valgus [knock-knee]); before epiphyseal closure**
27.63 27.63 Global Days 090

27457 **after epiphyseal closure**
28.27 28.27 Global Days 090

27465 **Osteoplasty, femur; shortening (excluding 64876)**
36.59 36.59 Global Days 090

27466 **lengthening**
34.72 34.72 Global Days 090

27468 **combined, lengthening and shortening with femoral segment transfer**
39.37 39.37 Global Days 090

27470 **Repair, nonunion or malunion, femur, distal to head and neck; without graft (eg, compression technique)**
34.69 34.69 Global Days 090

27472 **with iliac or other autogenous bone graft (includes obtaining graft)**
37.30 37.30 Global Days 090

27475 **Arrest, epiphyseal, any method (eg, epiphysiodesis); distal femur**
19.36 19.36 Global Days 090

27477 **tibia and fibula, proximal**
21.45 21.45 Global Days 090

27479 **combined distal femur, proximal tibia and fibula**
25.34 25.34 Global Days 090

27485 **Arrest, hemiepiphyseal, distal femur or proximal tibia or fibula (eg, genu varus or valgus)**
19.64 19.64 Global Days 090

27486 **Revision of total knee arthroplasty, with or without allograft; 1 component**
41.49 41.49 Global Days 090

27487 **femoral and entire tibial component**
51.95 51.95 Global Days 090

27488 **Removal of prosthesis, including total knee prosthesis, methylmethacrylate with or without insertion of spacer, knee**
35.37 35.37 Global Days 090

27495 **Prophylactic treatment (nailing, pinning, plating, or wiring) with or without methylmethacrylate, femur**
33.20 33.20 Global Days 090

27496 **Decompression fasciotomy, thigh and/or knee, 1 compartment (flexor or extensor or adductor);**
15.65 15.65 Global Days 090

27497 **with debridement of nonviable muscle and/or nerve**
16.79 16.79 Global Days 090

27498 **Decompression fasciotomy, thigh and/or knee, multiple compartments;**
18.74 18.74 Global Days 090

27499 **with debridement of nonviable muscle and/or nerve**
18.82 18.82 Global Days 090

27500-27566 Treatment of Fracture/Dislocation of Femur/Knee

27500 **Closed treatment of femoral shaft fracture, without manipulation**
13.97 15.11 Global Days 090

27501 **Closed treatment of supracondylar or transcondylar femoral fracture with or without intercondylar extension, without manipulation**
14.58 14.73 Global Days 090

27502 **Closed treatment of femoral shaft fracture, with manipulation, with or without skin or skeletal traction**
22.85 22.85 Global Days 090

27503 **Closed treatment of supracondylar or transcondylar femoral fracture with or without intercondylar extension, with manipulation, with or without skin or skeletal traction**
23.50 23.50 Global Days 090

27506 **Open treatment of femoral shaft fracture, with or without external fixation, with insertion of intramedullary implant, with or without cerclage and/or locking screws**
39.37 39.37 Global Days 090
AMA: 2009, Jun, 7-8

27507 **Open treatment of femoral shaft fracture with plate/screws, with or without cerclage**
28.70 28.70 Global Days 090

27508 **Closed treatment of femoral fracture, distal end, medial or lateral condyle, without manipulation**
14.41 15.32 Global Days 090

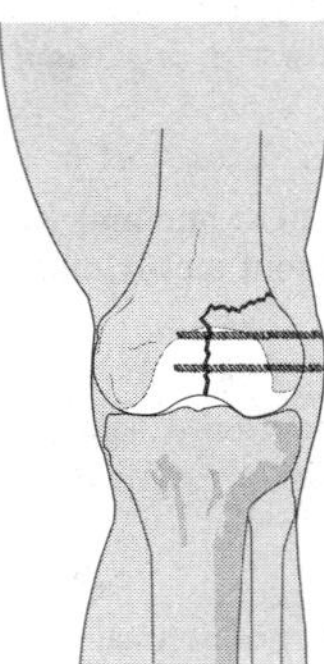

27509 Percutaneous skeletal fixation of femoral fracture, distal end, medial or lateral condyle, or supracondylar or transcondylar, with or without intercondylar extension, or distal femoral epiphyseal separation A2 T 80 50 PQ
18.89 18.89 Global Days 090

27510 Closed treatment of femoral fracture, distal end, medial or lateral condyle, with manipulation A2 T 50
20.37 20.37 Global Days 090

27511 Open treatment of femoral supracondylar or transcondylar fracture without intercondylar extension, includes internal fixation, when performed C5 C 80 50
29.53 29.53 Global Days 090

27513 Open treatment of femoral supracondylar or transcondylar fracture with intercondylar extension, includes internal fixation, when performed C5 C 80 50
36.81 36.81 Global Days 090

27514 Open treatment of femoral fracture, distal end, medial or lateral condyle, includes internal fixation, when performed C5 C 80 50
28.80 28.80 Global Days 090

27516 Closed treatment of distal femoral epiphyseal separation; without manipulation A2 T 50
13.83 14.73 Global Days 090

27517 with manipulation, with or without skin or skeletal traction A2 T 80 50
20.04 20.04 Global Days 090

27519 Open treatment of distal femoral epiphyseal separation, includes internal fixation, when performed C5 C 80 50
26.40 26.40 Global Days 090

27520 Closed treatment of patellar fracture, without manipulation A2 T 50
8.56 9.41 Global Days 090

27524 Open treatment of patellar fracture, with internal fixation and/or partial or complete patellectomy and soft tissue repair T 80 50
22.11 22.11 Global Days 090

27530 Closed treatment of tibial fracture, proximal (plateau); without manipulation A2 T 50
EXCLUDES *Arthroscopic repair (29855-29856)*
8.35 9.03 Global Days 090

27532 with or without manipulation, with skeletal traction A2 T 50
EXCLUDES *Arthroscopic repair (29855-29856)*
16.91 18.01 Global Days 090

27535 Open treatment of tibial fracture, proximal (plateau); unicondylar, includes internal fixation, when performed C5 C 80 50
EXCLUDES *Arthroscopic repair (29855-29856)*
26.52 26.52 Global Days 090

27536 bicondylar, with or without internal fixation C5 C 80 50
EXCLUDES *Arthroscopic repair (29855-29856)*
35.03 35.03 Global Days 090

27538 Closed treatment of intercondylar spine(s) and/or tuberosity fracture(s) of knee, with or without manipulation A2 T 80 50
EXCLUDES *Arthroscopic repair (29850-29851)*
12.92 13.81 Global Days 090

27540 Open treatment of intercondylar spine(s) and/or tuberosity fracture(s) of the knee, includes internal fixation, when performed C5 C 80 50
23.97 23.97 Global Days 090

27550 Closed treatment of knee dislocation; without anesthesia A2 T 80 50
13.42 14.48 Global Days 090

27552 requiring anesthesia A2 T 80 50
18.33 18.33 Global Days 090

27556 Open treatment of knee dislocation, includes internal fixation, when performed; without primary ligamentous repair or augmentation/reconstruction C5 C 80 50
25.98 25.98 Global Days 090

27557 with primary ligamentous repair C5 C 80 50
31.05 31.05 Global Days 090

27558 with primary ligamentous repair, with augmentation/reconstruction C5 C 80 50
35.30 35.30 Global Days 090

27560 Closed treatment of patellar dislocation; without anesthesia A2 T 50
EXCLUDES *Recurrent dislocation (27420-27424)*
10.17 11.01 Global Days 090

27562 requiring anesthesia A2 T 80 50
EXCLUDES *Recurrent dislocation (27420-27424)*
13.99 13.99 Global Days 090

27566 Open treatment of patellar dislocation, with or without partial or total patellectomy A2 T 80 50
EXCLUDES *Recurrent dislocation (27420-27424)*
26.19 26.19 Global Days 090

27570 Knee Manipulation with Anesthesia

27570 Manipulation of knee joint under general anesthesia (includes application of traction or other fixation devices) A2 T
4.39 4.39 Global Days 010

27580 Knee Arthrodesis

27580 Arthrodesis, knee, any technique C5 C 80 50
INCLUDES Albert's operation
42.37 42.37 Global Days 090

27590-27599 Amputations and Unlisted Procedures at Femur or Knee

27590 Amputation, thigh, through femur, any level; C5 C 80 50
24.40 24.40 Global Days 090

27591 immediate fitting technique including first cast C5 C 80 50
25.95 25.95 Global Days 090

27592 open, circular (guillotine) C5 C 80 50
20.68 20.68 Global Days 090

27594 secondary closure or scar revision A2 T 50
15.33 15.33 Global Days 090

27596 re-amputation C5 C 50
21.70 21.70 Global Days 090

27598 Disarticulation at knee C5 C 80 50

INCLUDES Batch-Spittler-McFaddin operation
Callandar knee disarticulation
Gritti amputation

22.06 22.06 Global Days 090

27599 Unlisted procedure, femur or knee T 80 50
0.00 0.00 Global Days YYY
AMA: 2009, Jan, 11-31; 2008, Jan, 4-5; 2008, Mar, 14-15

27600-27602 Decompression Fasciotomy of Leg

EXCLUDES *Fasciotomy with debridement (27892-27894)*
Simple incision and drainage (10140-10160)

27600 Decompression fasciotomy, leg; anterior and/or lateral compartments only A2 T 50
12.43 12.43 Global Days 090

27601 posterior compartment(s) only A2 T 50
12.97 12.97 Global Days 090

27602 anterior and/or lateral, and posterior compartment(s) A2 T 80 50
15.06 15.06 Global Days 090

27603-27612 Incisional Procedures Lower Leg and Ankle

27603 Incision and drainage, leg or ankle; deep abscess or hematoma A2 T 50
11.57 15.80 Global Days 090

27604 infected bursa A2 T 80 50
9.91 13.93 Global Days 090

27605 Tenotomy, percutaneous, Achilles tendon (separate procedure); local anesthesia A2 T 80 50
5.51 10.21 Global Days 010

27606 general anesthesia A2 T 50
8.46 8.46 Global Days 010

27607 Incision (eg, osteomyelitis or bone abscess), leg or ankle A2 T 50
18.06 18.06 Global Days 090

27610 Arthrotomy, ankle, including exploration, drainage, or removal of foreign body A2 T 50
19.19 19.19 Global Days 090

27612 Arthrotomy, posterior capsular release, ankle, with or without Achilles tendon lengthening A2 T 80 50

EXCLUDES *Lengthening or shortening tendon (27685)*

16.42 16.42 Global Days 090

27613-27614 Biopsy Lower Leg and Ankle

EXCLUDES *Needle biopsy (20206)*

27613 Biopsy, soft tissue of leg or ankle area; superficial P3 T 50
4.87 7.49 Global Days 010

27614 deep (subfascial or intramuscular) A2 T 50
12.04 16.99 Global Days 090

27615-27634 [27632, 27634] Excision Soft Tissue Tumors Lower Leg/Ankle

INCLUDES Any necessary elevation of tissue planes or dissection
Measurement of tumor and necessary margin at greatest diameter prior to excision
Resection without removal of significant normal tissue
Simple and intermediate repairs
Types of Excision:
Fascial or subfascial soft tissue tumors: simple and marginal resection of most often benign and intramuscular tumors found either in or below the deep fascia, not involving bone
Radical resection soft tissue tumor: wide resection of tumor, mostly malignant or aggressive benign, involving large margins of normal tissue and may involve tissue removal from one or more layers
Subcutaneous: simple and marginal resection of most often benign tumors found in the subcutaneous tissue above the deep fascia

EXCLUDES *Complex repair*
Radical resection of cutaneous tumors (e.g., melanoma) (11600-11646)
Significant exploration of vessels or neuroplasty

27615 Radical resection of tumor (eg, malignant neoplasm), soft tissue of leg or ankle area; less than 5 cm G2 T 80 50
30.14 30.14 Global Days 090

27616 5 cm or greater G2 T 80 50
37.59 37.59 Global Days 090

27618 Excision, tumor, soft tissue of leg or ankle area, subcutaneous; less than 3 cm G2 T 50
9.14 13.03 Global Days 090

27632 3 cm or greater G2 T 80 50
12.36 12.36 Global Days 090

27619 Excision, tumor, soft tissue of leg or ankle area, subfascial (eg, intramuscular); less than 5 cm G2 T 50
14.34 14.34 Global Days 090

27634 5 cm or greater G2 T 80 50
20.35 20.35 Global Days 090

27620-27641 Bone and Joint Procedures Ankle/Leg

27620 Arthrotomy, ankle, with joint exploration, with or without biopsy, with or without removal of loose or foreign body A2 T 80 50
13.42 13.42 Global Days 090

27625 Arthrotomy, with synovectomy, ankle; A2 T 80 50
16.87 16.87 Global Days 090

27626 including tenosynovectomy A2 T 80 50
18.65 18.65 Global Days 090

27630 Excision of lesion of tendon sheath or capsule (eg, cyst or ganglion), leg and/or ankle A2 T 50
10.85 16.46 Global Days 090

27632 *Resequenced code, See code following 27618.*

27634 *Resequenced code, See code following 27619.*

27635 Excision or curettage of bone cyst or benign tumor, tibia or fibula; A2 T 50
17.41 17.41 Global Days 090

27637 with autograft (includes obtaining graft) A2 T 80 50
22.32 22.32 Global Days 090

27638 with allograft A2 T 80 50
22.75 22.75 Global Days 090

27640 **Partial excision (craterization, saucerization, or diaphysectomy), bone (eg, osteomyelitis); tibia** A2 T 50
EXCLUDES *Excision of exostosis (27635)*
24.76 24.76 Global Days 090

27641 **fibula** A2 T 50
EXCLUDES *Excision of exostosis (27635)*
19.80 19.80 Global Days 090

27645-27647 Radical Resection Bone Tumor Ankle/Leg

INCLUDES Any necessary elevation of tissue planes or dissection
Measurement of tumor and necessary margin at greatest diameter prior to excision
Radical resection of bone tumor: resection of the tumor (may include entire bone) and wide margins of normal tissue primarily for malignant or aggressive benign tumors
Simple and intermediate repairs

EXCLUDES *Complex repair*
Significant exploration of vessels, neuroplasty, reconstruction, or complex bone repair

Do not report radical excision of soft tissue codes when adjacent soft tissue is removed during the bone tumor resection (27615-27619 [27632, 27634])

27645 **Radical resection of tumor; tibia** C5 C 80 50
50.80 50.80 Global Days 090

27646 **fibula** C5 C 80 50
43.97 43.97 Global Days 090

27647 **talus or calcaneus** A2 T 80 50
30.54 30.54 Global Days 090

27648 Injection for Ankle Arthrogram

EXCLUDES *Arthroscopy (29894-29898)*

27648 **Injection procedure for ankle arthrography** N1 N 80 50
73615
1.52 4.82 Global Days 000

27650-27745 Repair/Reconstruction Lower Leg/Ankle

27650 **Repair, primary, open or percutaneous, ruptured Achilles tendon;** A2 T 80 50
19.63 19.63 Global Days 090

27652 **with graft (includes obtaining graft)** A2 T 50
20.54 20.54 Global Days 090

27654 **Repair, secondary, Achilles tendon, with or without graft** A2 T 80 50
20.85 20.85 Global Days 090

27656 **Repair, fascial defect of leg** A2 T 80 50
11.33 18.03 Global Days 090

27658 **Repair, flexor tendon, leg; primary, without graft, each tendon** A2 T 80
11.02 11.02 Global Days 090

27659 **secondary, with or without graft, each tendon** A2 T 80
14.42 14.42 Global Days 090

27664 **Repair, extensor tendon, leg; primary, without graft, each tendon** A2 T 80
10.69 10.69 Global Days 090

27665 **secondary, with or without graft, each tendon** A2 T 80
12.23 12.23 Global Days 090

27675 **Repair, dislocating peroneal tendons; without fibular osteotomy** A2 T 80 50
14.42 14.42 Global Days 090

27676 **with fibular osteotomy** A2 T 80 50
18.20 18.20 Global Days 090

27680 **Tenolysis, flexor or extensor tendon, leg and/or ankle; single, each tendon** A2 T
12.71 12.71 Global Days 090

27681 **multiple tendons (through separate incision(s))** A2 T
15.84 15.84 Global Days 090

27685 **Lengthening or shortening of tendon, leg or ankle; single tendon (separate procedure)** A2 T 80 50
13.67 19.22 Global Days 090

27686 **multiple tendons (through same incision), each** A2 T 50
16.40 16.40 Global Days 090

27687 **Gastrocnemius recession (eg, Strayer procedure)** A2 T 80 50
13.45 13.45 Global Days 090

27690 **Transfer or transplant of single tendon (with muscle redirection or rerouting); superficial (eg, anterior tibial extensors into midfoot)** A2 T 80 50
INCLUDES Toe extensors considered a single tendon with transplant into midfoot
18.60 18.60 Global Days 090

27691 **deep (eg, anterior tibial or posterior tibial through interosseous space, flexor digitorum longus, flexor hallucis longus, or peroneal tendon to midfoot or hindfoot)** A2 T 80 50
INCLUDES Barr procedure
Toe extensors considered a single tendon with transplant into midfoot
22.11 22.11 Global Days 090

\+ 27692 **each additional tendon (List separately in addition to code for primary procedure)** A2 T 80
INCLUDES Toe extensors considered a single tendon with transplant into midfoot

Code first (27690-27691)
3.17 3.17 Global Days ZZZ

Tibia
Fibula
Anterior talofibular
Posterior talofibular
Calcaneus
Calcaneofibular

Lateral view of right ankle showing components of the collateral ligament

The components of the collateral ligament are often affected in sprained ankle type of injuries. Code 27695 reports first time repair of a disrupted collateral ligament. Report 27696 for repair to more than one collateral ligament

27695 **Repair, primary, disrupted ligament, ankle; collateral** A2 T 50
14.23 14.23 Global Days 090
AMA: 2009, Mar, 10-11

27696 **both collateral ligaments** A2 T 50
16.58 16.58 Global Days 090

27698 **Repair, secondary, disrupted ligament, ankle, collateral (eg, Watson-Jones procedure)** A2 T 80 50
18.96 18.96 Global Days 090

27700 **Arthroplasty, ankle;** A2 T 80 50
17.47 17.47 Global Days 090

27702 **with implant (total ankle)** C5 C 80 50
28.71 28.71 Global Days 090

27703 **revision, total ankle** C5 C 80 50 PQ
33.51 33.51 Global Days 090

27704 **Removal of ankle implant** A2 T 50 PQ
16.95 16.95 Global Days 090

27705 **Osteotomy; tibia** A2 T 80 50
EXCLUDES *Genu varus or genu valgus repair (27455-27457)*
22.45 22.45 Global Days 090

27707 **fibula** A2 T 50
EXCLUDES *Genu varus or genu valgus repair (27455-27457)*
11.83 11.83 Global Days 090

27709 **tibia and fibula** A2 T 80 50
EXCLUDES *Genu varus or genu valgus repair (27455-27457)*
34.44 34.44 Global Days 090

27712 **multiple, with realignment on intramedullary rod (eg, Sofield type procedure)** C5 C 80 50
EXCLUDES *Genu varus or genu valgus repair (27455-27457)*
32.42 32.42 Global Days 090

27715 **Osteoplasty, tibia and fibula, lengthening or shortening** C5 C 80 50
INCLUDES Anderson tibial lengthening
31.26 31.26 Global Days 090

27720 **Repair of nonunion or malunion, tibia; without graft, (eg, compression technique)** G2 T 80 50
25.81 25.81 Global Days 090

27722 **with sliding graft** T 80 50
26.03 26.03 Global Days 090

27724 **with iliac or other autograft (includes obtaining graft)** C5 C 80 50
37.44 37.44 Global Days 090

27725 **by synostosis, with fibula, any method** C5 C 80 50
35.75 35.75 Global Days 090

27726 **Repair of fibula nonunion and/or malunion with internal fixation** G2 T 50
Do not report with (27707)
28.30 28.30 Global Days 090
AMA: 2008, Jan, 4-5

27727 **Repair of congenital pseudarthrosis, tibia** C5 C 80 50
29.98 29.98 Global Days 090

27730 **Arrest, epiphyseal (epiphysiodesis), open; distal tibia** A2 T 50
17.12 17.12 Global Days 090

27732 **distal fibula** A2 T 50
11.27 11.27 Global Days 090

27734 **distal tibia and fibula** A2 T 50
17.72 17.72 Global Days 090

27740 **Arrest, epiphyseal (epiphysiodesis), any method, combined, proximal and distal tibia and fibula;** A2 T 80 50
EXCLUDES *Epiphyseal arrest of proximal tibia and fibula (27477)*
18.32 18.32 Global Days 090

27742 **and distal femur** A2 T 80 50
EXCLUDES *Epiphyseal arrest of proximal tibia and fibula (27477)*
22.23 22.23 Global Days 090

27745 **Prophylactic treatment (nailing, pinning, plating or wiring) with or without methylmethacrylate, tibia** A2 T 80 50
22.24 22.24 Global Days 090

27750-27848 Treatment of Fracture/Dislocation Lower Leg/Ankle

INCLUDES Treatment of open or closed fracture or dislocation

27750 **Closed treatment of tibial shaft fracture (with or without fibular fracture); without manipulation** A2 T 50
9.23 10.08 Global Days 090
AMA: 2009, Jan, 11-31; 2008, Jan, 10-25; 2007, January, 13-27

27752 **with manipulation, with or without skeletal traction** A2 T 50
14.57 15.75 Global Days 090

27756 **Percutaneous skeletal fixation of tibial shaft fracture (with or without fibular fracture) (eg, pins or screws)** A2 T 80 50 PQ
16.91 16.91 Global Days 090

27758 **Open treatment of tibial shaft fracture (with or without fibular fracture), with plate/screws, with or without cerclage** A2 T 80 50 PQ
26.18 26.18 Global Days 090
AMA: 2009, Jan, 11-31; 2008, Jan, 10-25; 2007, January, 13-27

27759 **Treatment of tibial shaft fracture (with or without fibular fracture) by intramedullary implant, with or without interlocking screws and/or cerclage** A2 T 80 50 PQ
29.41 29.41 Global Days 090

27760 **Closed treatment of medial malleolus fracture; without manipulation** A2 T 50
8.87 9.75 Global Days 090

27762 **with manipulation, with or without skin or skeletal traction** A2 T 50
12.89 14.08 Global Days 090

27766 **Open treatment of medial malleolus fracture, includes internal fixation, when performed** A2 T 50 PQ
17.91 17.91 Global Days 090

27767 **Closed treatment of posterior malleolus fracture; without manipulation** P2 T 50
Do not report with (27808-27823)
8.20 8.16 Global Days 090

27768 **with manipulation** G2 T 50
Do not report with (27808-27823)
12.66 12.66 Global Days 090

27769 **Open treatment of posterior malleolus fracture, includes internal fixation, when performed** G2 T 50 PQ
Do not report with (27808-27823)
21.33 21.33 Global Days 090

27780 **Closed treatment of proximal fibula or shaft fracture; without manipulation** A2 T 50
8.07 8.89 Global Days 090

27781 **with manipulation** A2 T 50
11.54 12.43 Global Days 090

27784 **Open treatment of proximal fibula or shaft fracture, includes internal fixation, when performed** A2 T 50
21.00 21.00 Global Days 090
AMA: 2009, Jan, 11-31; 2008, Jan, 10-25; 2007, January, 13-27

27786 **Closed treatment of distal fibular fracture (lateral malleolus); without manipulation** A2 T 50
8.32 9.22 Global Days 090

27788 **with manipulation** A2 T 50
11.33 12.38 Global Days 090

27792 Open treatment of distal fibular fracture (lateral malleolus), includes internal fixation, when performed A2 T 50

EXCLUDES *Repair of tibia and fibula shaft fracture (27750-27759)*

19.29 19.29 Global Days 090

AMA: 2009, Mar, 10-11

27808 Closed treatment of bimalleolar ankle fracture (eg, lateral and medial malleoli, or lateral and posterior malleoli or medial and posterior malleoli); without manipulation A2 T 50

8.73 9.73 Global Days 090

27810 with manipulation A2 T 50

12.59 13.82 Global Days 090

27814 Open treatment of bimalleolar ankle fracture (eg, lateral and medial malleoli, or lateral and posterior malleoli, or medial and posterior malleoli), includes internal fixation, when performed A2 T 80 50

22.75 22.75 Global Days 090

27816 Closed treatment of trimalleolar ankle fracture; without manipulation A2 T 50

8.30 9.25 Global Days 090

27818 with manipulation A2 T 50

12.80 14.21 Global Days 090

27822 Open treatment of trimalleolar ankle fracture, includes internal fixation, when performed, medial and/or lateral malleolus; without fixation of posterior lip A2 T 80 50

24.86 24.86 Global Days 090

27823 with fixation of posterior lip A2 T 80 50

28.19 28.19 Global Days 090

27824 Closed treatment of fracture of weight bearing articular portion of distal tibia (eg, pilon or tibial plafond), with or without anesthesia; without manipulation A2 T 50

8.83 9.12 Global Days 090

27825 with skeletal traction and/or requiring manipulation A2 T 80 50

14.55 16.01 Global Days 090

27826 Open treatment of fracture of weight bearing articular surface/portion of distal tibia (eg, pilon or tibial plafond), with internal fixation, when performed; of fibula only A2 T 80 50

24.48 24.48 Global Days 090

27827 of tibia only A2 T 80 50

31.95 31.95 Global Days 090

27828 of both tibia and fibula A2 T 80 50

38.22 38.22 Global Days 090

27829 Open treatment of distal tibiofibular joint (syndesmosis) disruption, includes internal fixation, when performed A2 T 80 50

20.08 20.08 Global Days 090

AMA: 2009, Mar, 10-11

27830 Closed treatment of proximal tibiofibular joint dislocation; without anesthesia A2 T 80 50

10.19 10.94 Global Days 090

27831 requiring anesthesia A2 T 80 50

11.55 11.55 Global Days 090

27832 Open treatment of proximal tibiofibular joint dislocation, includes internal fixation, when performed, or with excision of proximal fibula A2 T 80 50

21.91 21.91 Global Days 090

27840 Closed treatment of ankle dislocation; without anesthesia A2 T 50

10.69 10.69 Global Days 090

27842 requiring anesthesia, with or without percutaneous skeletal fixation A2 T 50

14.46 14.46 Global Days 090

27846 Open treatment of ankle dislocation, with or without percutaneous skeletal fixation; without repair or internal fixation A2 T 80 50

EXCLUDES *Arthroscopy (29894-29898)*

21.63 21.63 Global Days 090

27848 with repair or internal or external fixation A2 T 80 50

EXCLUDES *Arthroscopy (29894-29898)*

24.09 24.09 Global Days 090

27860 Ankle Manipulation with Anesthesia

27860 Manipulation of ankle under general anesthesia (includes application of traction or other fixation apparatus) A2 T 80

5.20 5.20 Global Days 010

27870-27871 Arthrodesis Lower Leg/Ankle

27870 Arthrodesis, ankle, open A2 T 80 50

EXCLUDES *Arthroscopic arthrodesis of ankle (29899)*

30.63 30.63 Global Days 090

27871 Arthrodesis, tibiofibular joint, proximal or distal A2 T 80 50

20.41 20.41 Global Days 090

27880-27889 Amputations of Lower Leg/Ankle

27880 Amputation, leg, through tibia and fibula; C5 C 80 50

INCLUDES Burgess amputation

27.58 27.58 Global Days 090

27881 with immediate fitting technique including application of first cast C5 C 80 50

26.18 26.18 Global Days 090

27882 open, circular (guillotine) C5 C 80 50

18.35 18.35 Global Days 090

27884 secondary closure or scar revision A2 T 50

17.35 17.35 Global Days 090

27886 re-amputation C5 C 50

19.93 19.93 Global Days 090

27888 Amputation, ankle, through malleoli of tibia and fibula (eg, Syme, Pirogoff type procedures), with plastic closure and resection of nerves C5 C 80 50

20.31 20.31 Global Days 090

27889 Ankle disarticulation A2 T 50

19.98 19.98 Global Days 090

27892-27899 Decompression Fasciotomy Lower Leg

EXCLUDES *Decompression fasciotomy without debridement (27600-27602)*

27892 Decompression fasciotomy, leg; anterior and/or lateral compartments only, with debridement of nonviable muscle and/or nerve A2 T 80 50

16.50 16.50 Global Days 090

27893 posterior compartment(s) only, with debridement of nonviable muscle and/or nerve A2 T 80 50

17.63 17.63 Global Days 090

27894 anterior and/or lateral, and posterior compartment(s), with debridement of nonviable muscle and/or nerve A2 T 80 50

25.57 25.57 Global Days 090

27899 **Unlisted procedure, leg or ankle** T 80 50
0.00 0.00 Global Days YYY
AMA: 2009, Jan, 11-31; 2008, Jan, 10-25; 2007, January, 13-27

28001-28008 Surgical Incision Foot/Toe

EXCLUDES *Simple incision and drainage (10060-10160)*

28001 **Incision and drainage, bursa, foot** P3 T
4.98 7.97 Global Days 010

28002 **Incision and drainage below fascia, with or without tendon sheath involvement, foot; single bursal space** A2 T
9.70 13.28 Global Days 010

28003 **multiple areas** A2 T
16.61 20.63 Global Days 090

28005 **Incision, bone cortex (eg, osteomyelitis or bone abscess), foot** A2 T
17.26 17.26 Global Days 090

28008 **Fasciotomy, foot and/or toe** A2 T 50
EXCLUDES *Plantar fascia division (28250)*
Plantar fasciectomy (28060, 28062)
8.66 12.60 Global Days 090

28010-28011 Tenotomy/Toe

EXCLUDES *Open tenotomy (28230-28234)*
Simple incision and drainage (10140-10160)

28010 **Tenotomy, percutaneous, toe; single tendon** P3 T
6.18 6.81 Global Days 090

28011 **multiple tendons** A2 T
8.69 9.66 Global Days 090

28020-28024 Arthrotomy Foot/Toe

EXCLUDES *Simple incision and drainage (10140-10160)*

28020 **Arthrotomy, including exploration, drainage, or removal of loose or foreign body; intertarsal or tarsometatarsal joint** A2 T
10.47 15.39 Global Days 090

28022 **metatarsophalangeal joint** A2 T
9.48 14.02 Global Days 090

28024 **interphalangeal joint** A2 T
8.89 13.22 Global Days 090

28035 Tarsal Tunnel Release

EXCLUDES *Other nerve decompression (64722)*
Other neuroplasty (64704)

28035 **Release, tarsal tunnel (posterior tibial nerve decompression)** A2 T
10.50 15.36 Global Days 090

28039-28047 [28039, 28041] Excision Soft Tissue Tumors Foot/Toe

INCLUDES Any necessary elevation of tissue planes or dissection
Measurement of tumor and necessary margin at greatest diameter prior to excision
Resection without removal of significant normal tissue
Simple and intermediate repairs
Types of Excision:
Fascial or subfascial soft tissue tumors: simple and marginal resection of most often benign and intramuscular tumors found either in or below the deep fascia, not involving bone
Radical resection soft tissue tumor: wide resection of tumor, mostly malignant or aggressive benign, involving large margins of normal tissue and may involve tissue removal from one or more layers
Subcutaneous: simple and marginal resection of most often benign tumors found in the subcutaneous tissue above the deep fascia

EXCLUDES *Complex repair*
Radical resection of cutaneous tumors (e.g., melanoma) (11600-11646)
Significant exploration of vessels, neuroplasty, or reconstruction

28039 ***Resequenced code, See code following 28043.***

28041 ***Resequenced code, See code following 28045.***

28043 **Excision, tumor, soft tissue of foot or toe, subcutaneous; less than 1.5 cm** G2 T 50
7.79 11.41 Global Days 090

\# **28039** **1.5 cm or greater** G2 T 80 50
10.57 15.61 Global Days 090

28045 **Excision, tumor, soft tissue of foot or toe, subfascial (eg, intramuscular); less than 1.5 cm** G2 T 80 50
10.35 14.73 Global Days 090

\# **28041** **1.5 cm or greater** G2 T 80 50
13.91 13.91 Global Days 090

28046 **Radical resection of tumor (eg, malignant neoplasm), soft tissue of foot or toe; less than 3 cm** G2 T 50
21.83 21.83 Global Days 090

28047 **3 cm or greater** G2 T 80 50
30.41 30.41 Global Days 090

28050-28160 Resection Procedures Foot/Toes

28050 **Arthrotomy with biopsy; intertarsal or tarsometatarsal joint** A2 T 50
8.94 13.55 Global Days 090

28052 **metatarsophalangeal joint** A2 T 50
8.24 12.63 Global Days 090

28054 **interphalangeal joint** A2 T 80 50
7.03 11.06 Global Days 090

28055 **Neurectomy, intrinsic musculature of foot** A2 T 80
11.09 11.09 Global Days 090

28060 **Fasciectomy, plantar fascia; partial (separate procedure)** A2 T 50
EXCLUDES *Plantar fasciotomy (28008, 28250)*
10.41 14.93 Global Days 090
AMA: 2009, Jan, 11-31; 2008, Mar, 14-15

28062 **radical (separate procedure)** A2 T
EXCLUDES *Plantar fasciotomy (28008, 28250)*
11.97 17.08 Global Days 090

28070 **Synovectomy; intertarsal or tarsometatarsal joint, each** A2 T
10.40 15.36 Global Days 090

28072 metatarsophalangeal joint, each A2 T
10.01 15.08 Global Days 090

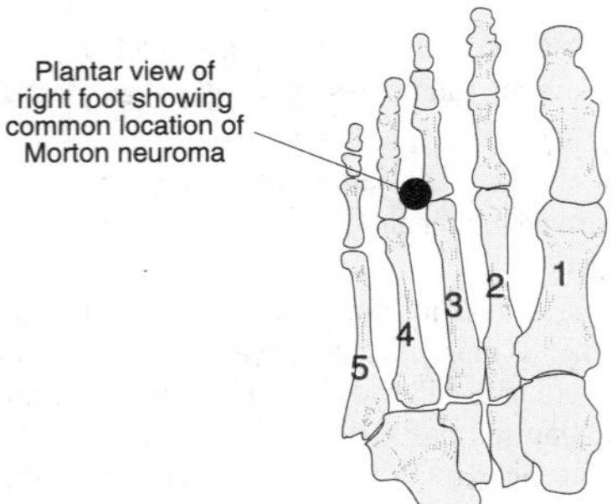

Morton neuroma is a chronic inflammation or irritation of the nerves in the web space between the heads of the metatarsals and phalanges

28080 **Excision, interdigital (Morton) neuroma, single, each** A2 T 80
10.66 15.10 Global Days 090
AMA: 2009, Jan, 6&9

28086 **Synovectomy, tendon sheath, foot; flexor** A2 T 80 50
10.56 15.87 Global Days 090

28088 **extensor** A2 T 80 50
8.77 13.75 Global Days 090

28090 **Excision of lesion, tendon, tendon sheath, or capsule (including synovectomy) (eg, cyst or ganglion); foot** A2 T 50
9.06 13.65 Global Days 090

28092 **toe(s), each** A2 T
7.95 12.35 Global Days 090

28100 **Excision or curettage of bone cyst or benign tumor, talus or calcaneus;** A2 T 80 50
11.94 17.45 Global Days 090

28102 **with iliac or other autograft (includes obtaining graft)** A2 T 80 50
13.91 13.91 Global Days 090

28103 **with allograft** A2 T 80 50
11.76 11.76 Global Days 090

28104 **Excision or curettage of bone cyst or benign tumor, tarsal or metatarsal, except talus or calcaneus;** A2 T 80
10.19 15.00 Global Days 090

28106 **with iliac or other autograft (includes obtaining graft)** A2 T 80
12.76 12.76 Global Days 090

28107 **with allograft** A2 T 80
10.41 15.29 Global Days 090

28108 **Excision or curettage of bone cyst or benign tumor, phalanges of foot** A2 T
EXCLUDES *Hallux valgus (28290)*
8.40 12.64 Global Days 090

28110 **Ostectomy, partial excision, fifth metatarsal head (bunionette) (separate procedure)** A2 T 50
8.50 13.46 Global Days 090
AMA: 2009, Jan, 11-31; 2008, Jan, 10-25; 2007, January, 13-27

28111 **Ostectomy, complete excision; first metatarsal head** A2 T 50
9.81 14.79 Global Days 090

28112 **other metatarsal head (second, third or fourth)** A2 T 50
9.27 14.34 Global Days 090

28113 **fifth metatarsal head** A2 T 80 50
12.54 17.32 Global Days 090

28114 **all metatarsal heads, with partial proximal phalangectomy, excluding first metatarsal (eg, Clayton type procedure)** A2 T 80 50
24.64 31.45 Global Days 090

28116 **Ostectomy, excision of tarsal coalition** A2 T 50
16.84 22.14 Global Days 090

28118 **Ostectomy, calcaneus;** A2 T 80 50
12.12 17.23 Global Days 090

28119 **for spur, with or without plantar fascial release** A2 T 50
10.62 15.31 Global Days 090

28120 **Partial excision (craterization, saucerization, sequestrectomy, or diaphysectomy) bone (eg, osteomyelitis or bossing); talus or calcaneus** A2 T 50
INCLUDES Barker operation
14.41 19.62 Global Days 090

28122 **tarsal or metatarsal bone, except talus or calcaneus** A2 T 80 50
EXCLUDES *Hallux rigidus cheilectomy (28289)*
Partial removal of talus or calcaneus (28120)
13.16 17.74 Global Days 090

28124 **phalanx of toe** P3 T 50
9.70 13.85 Global Days 090

28126 **Resection, partial or complete, phalangeal base, each toe** A2 T
7.34 11.51 Global Days 090

28130 **Talectomy (astragalectomy)** A2 T 80 50
INCLUDES Whitman astragalectomy
EXCLUDES *Calcanectomy (28118)*
19.46 19.46 Global Days 090

28140 **Metatarsectomy** A2 T
13.16 17.81 Global Days 090

28150 **Phalangectomy, toe, each toe** A2 T
8.36 12.59 Global Days 090

28153 **Resection, condyle(s), distal end of phalanx, each toe** A2 T
7.80 12.04 Global Days 090

28160 **Hemiphalangectomy or interphalangeal joint excision, toe, proximal end of phalanx, each** A2 T
8.00 12.31 Global Days 090

28171-28175 Radical Resection Bone Tumor Foot/Toes

INCLUDES Any necessary elevation of tissue planes or dissection
Measurement of tumor and necessary margin at greatest diameter prior to excision
Radical resection of tumor: wide resection of soft tissue tumor, mostly malignant or aggressive benign, involving large margins of normal tissue and may involve tissue removal from one or more layers
Simple and intermediate repairs

EXCLUDES *Complex repair*
Significant exploration of vessels, neuroplasty, reconstruction, or complex bone repair

Do not report radical excision of soft tissue codes when adjacent soft tissue is removed during the bone tumor resection (28045-28047 [28039, 28041])

28171 **Radical resection of tumor; tarsal (except talus or calcaneus)** A2 T 80
EXCLUDES *Talus or calcaneus resection (27647)*
24.72 24.72 Global Days 090

28173 **metatarsal** A2 T
EXCLUDES *Talus or calcaneus resection (27647)*
22.47 22.47 Global Days 090

28175 phalanx of toe A2 T

EXCLUDES *Talus or calcaneus resection (27647)*

14.19 14.19 Global Days 090

28190-28193 Foreign Body Removal: Foot

28190 Removal of foreign body, foot; subcutaneous P3 T 50

3.94 7.43 Global Days 010

28192 deep A2 T 50 PQ

9.31 13.81 Global Days 090

28193 complicated A2 T 50 PQ

10.98 15.66 Global Days 090

28200-28360 Repair/Reconstruction of Foot/Toe

28200 Repair, tendon, flexor, foot; primary or secondary, without free graft, each tendon A2 T

9.30 13.97 Global Days 090

28202 secondary with free graft, each tendon (includes obtaining graft) A2 T 80

12.46 17.30 Global Days 090

28208 Repair, tendon, extensor, foot; primary or secondary, each tendon A2 T

9.04 13.55 Global Days 090

28210 secondary with free graft, each tendon (includes obtaining graft) A2 T 80

11.97 16.64 Global Days 090

28220 Tenolysis, flexor, foot; single tendon P3 T

8.89 13.07 Global Days 090

28222 multiple tendons A2 T

10.36 14.81 Global Days 090

28225 Tenolysis, extensor, foot; single tendon A2 T

7.60 11.85 Global Days 090

28226 multiple tendons A2 T

9.14 13.74 Global Days 090

28230 Tenotomy, open, tendon flexor; foot, single or multiple tendon(s) (separate procedure) P3 T

8.34 12.57 Global Days 090

28232 toe, single tendon (separate procedure) P3 T

7.29 11.44 Global Days 090

28234 Tenotomy, open, extensor, foot or toe, each tendon A2 T

EXCLUDES *Tendon transfer (27690-27691)*

7.84 12.01 Global Days 090

28238 Reconstruction (advancement), posterior tibial tendon with excision of accessory tarsal navicular bone (eg, Kidner type procedure) A2 T 80 50

EXCLUDES *Extensor hallucis longus transfer with big toe fusion (28760)*
Jones procedure (28760)
Subcutaneous tenotomy (28010-28011)
Transfer or transplant of tendon with muscle redirection or rerouting (27690-27692)

14.52 19.87 Global Days 090

28240 Tenotomy, lengthening, or release, abductor hallucis muscle A2 T 50

8.58 12.83 Global Days 090

28250 Division of plantar fascia and muscle (eg, Steindler stripping) (separate procedure) A2 T 80 50

11.76 16.62 Global Days 090

28260 Capsulotomy, midfoot; medial release only (separate procedure) A2 T 80 50

15.30 20.40 Global Days 090

28261 with tendon lengthening A2 T 80 50

22.67 28.40 Global Days 090

28262 extensive, including posterior talotibial capsulotomy and tendon(s) lengthening (eg, resistant clubfoot deformity) A2 T 80 50

34.15 42.18 Global Days 090

28264 Capsulotomy, midtarsal (eg, Heyman type procedure) A2 T 80 50

20.99 27.53 Global Days 090

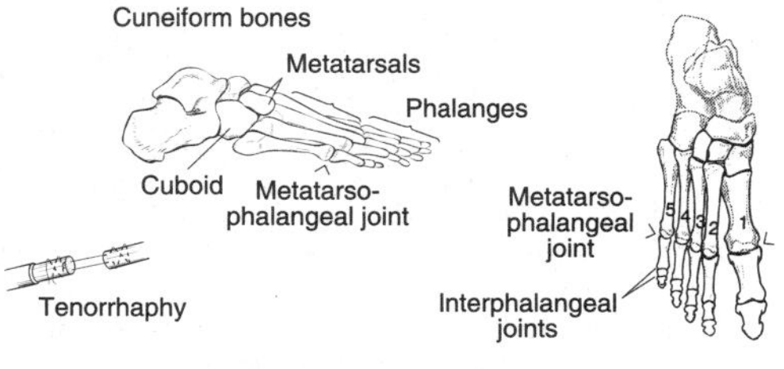

Tarsals, metatarsals, and phalanges

The metatarsophalangeal joint capsule is incised (capsulotomy)

28270 Capsulotomy; metatarsophalangeal joint, with or without tenorrhaphy, each joint (separate procedure) A2 T 50

9.85 14.32 Global Days 090

28272 interphalangeal joint, each joint (separate procedure) P3 T 50

7.48 11.44 Global Days 090

AMA: 2009, Jan, 11-31; 2008, Jan, 10-25; 2007, January, 13-27

28280 Syndactylization, toes (eg, webbing or Kelikian type procedure) A2 T 80 50

10.55 15.44 Global Days 090

28285 Correction, hammertoe (eg, interphalangeal fusion, partial or total phalangectomy) A2 T 50

10.88 15.31 Global Days 090

AMA: 2009, Jan, 11-31; 2008, Jan, 10-25; 2007, January, 13-27

28286 Correction, cock-up fifth toe, with plastic skin closure (eg, Ruiz-Mora type procedure) A2 T

8.86 13.23 Global Days 090

28288 Ostectomy, partial, exostectomy or condylectomy, metatarsal head, each metatarsal head A2 T

12.72 17.69 Global Days 090

28289 Hallux rigidus correction with cheilectomy, debridement and capsular release of the first metatarsophalangeal joint A2 T 80 50

16.19 21.52 Global Days 090

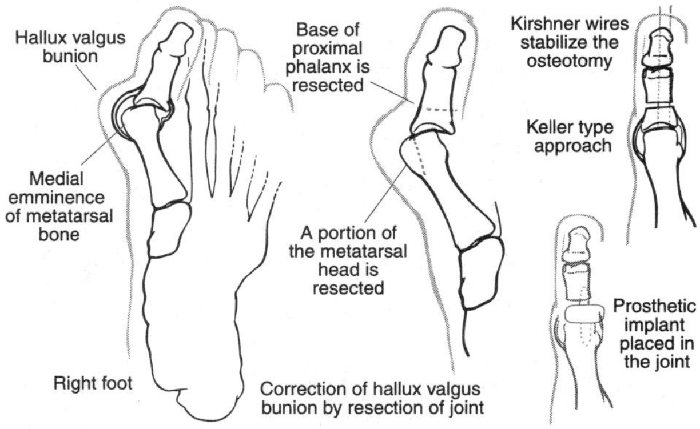

Correction of hallux valgus bunion by resection of joint

28290 Correction, hallux valgus (bunion), with or without sesamoidectomy; simple exostectomy (eg, Silver type procedure) A2 T 50

11.70 17.18 Global Days 090

AMA: 2009, Jan, 11-31; 2008, Jan, 10-25; 2007, January, 28-31

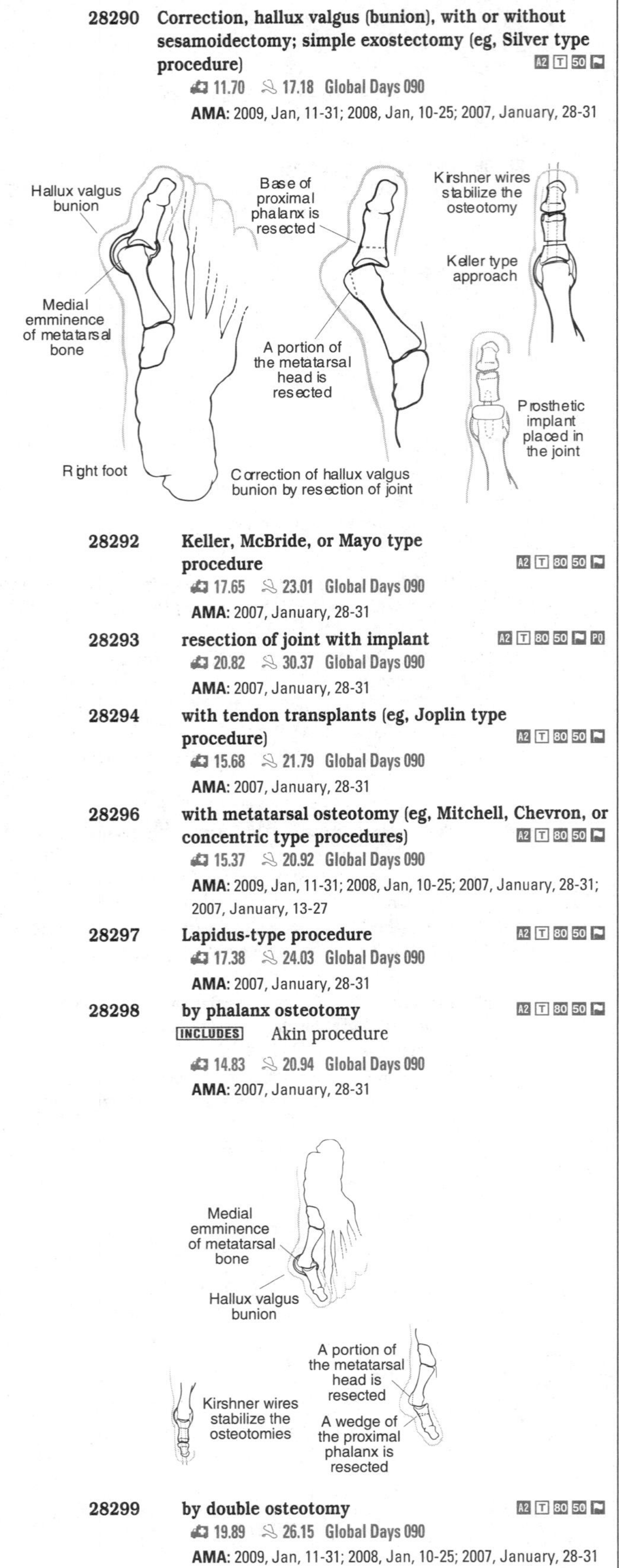

28292 Keller, McBride, or Mayo type procedure A2 T 80 50

17.65 23.01 Global Days 090

AMA: 2007, January, 28-31

28293 resection of joint with implant A2 T 80 50 P0

20.82 30.37 Global Days 090

AMA: 2007, January, 28-31

28294 with tendon transplants (eg, Joplin type procedure) A2 T 80 50

15.68 21.79 Global Days 090

AMA: 2007, January, 28-31

28296 with metatarsal osteotomy (eg, Mitchell, Chevron, or concentric type procedures) A2 T 80 50

15.37 20.92 Global Days 090

AMA: 2009, Jan, 11-31; 2008, Jan, 10-25; 2007, January, 28-31; 2007, January, 13-27

28297 Lapidus-type procedure A2 T 80 50

17.38 24.03 Global Days 090

AMA: 2007, January, 28-31

28298 by phalanx osteotomy A2 T 80 50

INCLUDES Akin procedure

14.83 20.94 Global Days 090

AMA: 2007, January, 28-31

28299 by double osteotomy A2 T 80 50

19.89 26.15 Global Days 090

AMA: 2009, Jan, 11-31; 2008, Jan, 10-25; 2007, January, 28-31

28300 calcaneus (eg, Dwyer or Chambers type procedure), with or without internal fixation A2 T 80 50

19.41 19.41 Global Days 090

28302 talus A2 T 80 50

20.72 20.72 Global Days 090

28304 Osteotomy, tarsal bones, other than calcaneus or talus; A2 T 80 50

17.51 23.60 Global Days 090

28305 with autograft (includes obtaining graft) (eg, Fowler type) A2 T 80 50

18.97 18.97 Global Days 090

28306 Osteotomy, with or without lengthening, shortening or angular correction, metatarsal; first metatarsal A2 T 80 50

11.97 18.02 Global Days 090

28307 first metatarsal with autograft (other than first toe) A2 T 80 50

13.66 20.56 Global Days 090

28308 other than first metatarsal, each A2 T 80 50

11.00 16.35 Global Days 090

28309 multiple (eg, Swanson type cavus foot procedure) A2 T 80 50

26.08 26.08 Global Days 090

28310 Osteotomy, shortening, angular or rotational correction; proximal phalanx, first toe (separate procedure) A2 T

10.39 15.70 Global Days 090

28312 other phalanges, any toe A2 T

9.40 14.80 Global Days 090

28313 Reconstruction, angular deformity of toe, soft tissue procedures only (eg, overlapping second toe, fifth toe, curly toes) A2 T

10.56 15.22 Global Days 090

28315 Sesamoidectomy, first toe (separate procedure) A2 T 50

9.54 13.96 Global Days 090

28320 Repair, nonunion or malunion; tarsal bones A2 T 80

18.16 18.16 Global Days 090

28322 metatarsal, with or without bone graft (includes obtaining graft) A2 T 80

17.02 23.04 Global Days 090

28340 Reconstruction, toe, macrodactyly; soft tissue resection A2 T

12.26 17.04 Global Days 090

28341 requiring bone resection A2 T

14.56 19.71 Global Days 090

28344 Reconstruction, toe(s); polydactyly A2 T

9.24 14.21 Global Days 090

28345 syndactyly, with or without skin graft(s), each web A2 T 80

10.93 15.49 Global Days 090

28360 Reconstruction, cleft foot T 80

31.43 31.43 Global Days 090

28400-28675 Treatment of Fracture/Dislocation of Foot/Toe

28400 Closed treatment of calcaneal fracture; without manipulation A2 T 50

6.64 7.26 Global Days 090

28405 with manipulation A2 T 80 50

INCLUDES Bohler reduction

10.26 11.23 Global Days 090

28406 Percutaneous skeletal fixation of calcaneal fracture, with manipulation A2 T 80 50 PQ
15.58 15.58 Global Days 090

28415 Open treatment of calcaneal fracture, includes internal fixation, when performed; A2 T 80 50 PQ
32.87 32.87 Global Days 090

28420 with primary iliac or other autogenous bone graft (includes obtaining graft) A2 T 80 50 PQ
36.53 36.53 Global Days 090

28430 Closed treatment of talus fracture; without manipulation P2 T 50
6.09 6.86 Global Days 090

28435 with manipulation A2 T 80 50
7.64 8.40 Global Days 090

28436 Percutaneous skeletal fixation of talus fracture, with manipulation A2 T 50 PQ
13.06 13.06 Global Days 090

28445 Open treatment of talus fracture, includes internal fixation, when performed A2 T 80 50 PQ
31.53 31.53 Global Days 090

28446 Open osteochondral autograft, talus (includes obtaining graft[s]) G2 T 80 50

EXCLUDES *Arthroscopically aided osteochondral talus graft (29892)*
Open osteochondral allograft or repairs with industrial grafts (28899)

Do not report with (27705-27707)
35.76 35.76 Global Days 090
AMA: 2008, Jan, 4-5

28450 Treatment of tarsal bone fracture (except talus and calcaneus); without manipulation, each P2 T
5.63 6.33 Global Days 090
AMA: 2009, Jan, 11-31; 2008, Jan, 10-25; 2007, January, 13-27

28455 with manipulation, each P2 T 80
7.66 8.46 Global Days 090

28456 Percutaneous skeletal fixation of tarsal bone fracture (except talus and calcaneus), with manipulation, each A2 T PQ
9.10 9.10 Global Days 090

28465 Open treatment of tarsal bone fracture (except talus and calcaneus), includes internal fixation, when performed, each A2 T PQ
18.19 18.19 Global Days 090

28470 Closed treatment of metatarsal fracture; without manipulation, each P2 T
5.58 6.21 Global Days 090

28475 with manipulation, each P2 T
6.77 7.57 Global Days 090

28476 Percutaneous skeletal fixation of metatarsal fracture, with manipulation, each A2 T 80 PQ
10.21 10.21 Global Days 090

28485 Open treatment of metatarsal fracture, includes internal fixation, when performed, each A2 T PQ
15.51 15.51 Global Days 090

28490 Closed treatment of fracture great toe, phalanx or phalanges; without manipulation P2 T
3.63 4.21 Global Days 090

28495 with manipulation P2 T
4.42 5.20 Global Days 090

28496 Percutaneous skeletal fixation of fracture great toe, phalanx or phalanges, with manipulation A2 T
6.73 12.63 Global Days 090

28505 Open treatment of fracture, great toe, phalanx or phalanges, includes internal fixation, when performed A2 T PQ
14.62 19.58 Global Days 090

28510 Closed treatment of fracture, phalanx or phalanges, other than great toe; without manipulation, each P3 T
3.47 3.56 Global Days 090

28515 with manipulation, each P2 T
4.14 4.65 Global Days 090

28525 Open treatment of fracture, phalanx or phalanges, other than great toe, includes internal fixation, when performed, each A2 T 80 PQ
11.77 16.79 Global Days 090

28530 Closed treatment of sesamoid fracture P3 T 80
2.97 3.33 Global Days 090

28531 Open treatment of sesamoid fracture, with or without internal fixation A2 T PQ
5.66 10.50 Global Days 090

28540 Closed treatment of tarsal bone dislocation, other than talotarsal; without anesthesia P2 T 80
5.38 5.93 Global Days 090

28545 requiring anesthesia A2 T 80
7.44 8.35 Global Days 090

28546 Percutaneous skeletal fixation of tarsal bone dislocation, other than talotarsal, with manipulation A2 T 80
9.74 16.35 Global Days 090

28555 Open treatment of tarsal bone dislocation, includes internal fixation, when performed A2 T 80 PQ
19.80 26.06 Global Days 090

28570 Closed treatment of talotarsal joint dislocation; without anesthesia P2 T 80
4.12 4.77 Global Days 090

28575 requiring anesthesia A2 T 80
9.52 10.47 Global Days 090

28576 Percutaneous skeletal fixation of talotarsal joint dislocation, with manipulation A2 T 80
11.35 11.35 Global Days 090

28585 Open treatment of talotarsal joint dislocation, includes internal fixation, when performed A2 T 80 PQ
20.64 26.05 Global Days 090

28600 Closed treatment of tarsometatarsal joint dislocation; without anesthesia P2 T 80
5.48 6.32 Global Days 090

28605 requiring anesthesia A2 T 80
8.35 9.22 Global Days 090

28606 Percutaneous skeletal fixation of tarsometatarsal joint dislocation, with manipulation A2 T
11.55 11.55 Global Days 090

28615 Open treatment of tarsometatarsal joint dislocation, includes internal fixation, when performed A2 T 80 PQ
23.34 23.34 Global Days 090

28630 Closed treatment of metatarsophalangeal joint dislocation; without anesthesia P2 T 80
3.21 4.51 Global Days 010

28635 requiring anesthesia A2 T 80
3.99 5.27 Global Days 010

28636 Percutaneous skeletal fixation of metatarsophalangeal joint dislocation, with manipulation A2 T
5.79 8.80 Global Days 010

28645 Open treatment of metatarsophalangeal joint dislocation, includes internal fixation, when performed A2 T PQ
14.12 19.00 Global Days 090

28660 **Closed treatment of interphalangeal joint dislocation; without anesthesia** P3 T
2.59 3.35 Global Days 010

28665 **requiring anesthesia** A2 T 80
3.89 4.51 Global Days 010

28666 **Percutaneous skeletal fixation of interphalangeal joint dislocation, with manipulation** A2 T
5.61 5.61 Global Days 010

28675 **Open treatment of interphalangeal joint dislocation, includes internal fixation, when performed** A2 T PQ
12.08 17.18 Global Days 090

28705-28760 Arthrodesis of Foot/Toe

28705 **Arthrodesis; pantalar** A2 T 80 PQ
37.89 37.89 Global Days 090

28715 **triple** A2 T 80 PQ
27.60 27.60 Global Days 090

28725 **subtalar** A2 T 80 PQ
INCLUDES Dunn arthrodesis
Grice arthrosis
21.70 21.70 Global Days 090

28730 **Arthrodesis, midtarsal or tarsometatarsal, multiple or transverse;** A2 T 80 PQ
INCLUDES Lambrinudi arthrodesis
22.17 22.17 Global Days 090

28735 **with osteotomy (eg, flatfoot correction)** A2 T 80 PQ
23.32 23.32 Global Days 090

28737 **Arthrodesis, with tendon lengthening and advancement, midtarsal, tarsal navicular-cuneiform (eg, Miller type procedure)** A2 T 80 PQ
20.09 20.09 Global Days 090

28740 **Arthrodesis, midtarsal or tarsometatarsal, single joint** A2 T 80
18.51 25.09 Global Days 090

28750 **Arthrodesis, great toe; metatarsophalangeal joint** A2 T 80 50
17.67 24.33 Global Days 090

28755 **interphalangeal joint** A2 T 50
9.70 14.79 Global Days 090

28760 **Arthrodesis, with extensor hallucis longus transfer to first metatarsal neck, great toe, interphalangeal joint (eg, Jones type procedure)** A2 T 80 50
EXCLUDES *Hammer toe repair or interphalangeal fusion (28285)*
16.97 23.02 Global Days 090

28800-28825 Amputation Foot/Toe

28800 **Amputation, foot; midtarsal (eg, Chopart type procedure)** C5 C 80 50
16.36 16.36 Global Days 090

28805 **transmetatarsal** T 80 50
22.25 22.25 Global Days 090

28810 **Amputation, metatarsal, with toe, single** A2 T 80
EXCLUDES *Removal of tuft of distal phalanx (11752)*
13.08 13.08 Global Days 090

28820 **Amputation, toe; metatarsophalangeal joint** A2 T
EXCLUDES *Removal of tuft of distal phalanx (11752)*
11.71 16.82 Global Days 090

28825 **interphalangeal joint** A2 T
EXCLUDES *Removal of tuft of distal phalanx (11752)*
11.12 16.18 Global Days 090

28890-28899 Other/Unlisted Procedures Foot/Toe

28890 **Extracorporeal shock wave, high energy, performed by a physician, requiring anesthesia other than local, including ultrasound guidance, involving the plantar fascia** P3 T 50
EXCLUDES *Extracorporeal shock wave therapy of musculoskeletal system not otherwise specified (0019T, 0101T, 0102T)*
6.63 9.90 Global Days 090
AMA: 2009, Jan, 11-31; 2008, Jan, 10-25; 2007, January, 13-27

28899 **Unlisted procedure, foot or toes** T 80
0.00 0.00 Global Days YYY
AMA: 2009, Jan, 6&9; 2008, Jan, 4-5

29000-29086 Casting: Arm/Shoulder/Torso

CMS 100-2,15,100 Surgical Dressings, Splints, Casts, and Devices for Reductions of Fractures/Dislocations
CMS 100-4,4,240 Inpatient Part B Hospital Services Paid Under OPPS
EXCLUDES *Cast or splint material*
Orthotic supervision and training (97760-97762)

29000 **Application of halo type body cast (see 20661-20663 for insertion)** G2 S 80
5.12 9.33 Global Days 000
AMA: 2009, May, 8-9&11

29010 **Application of Risser jacket, localizer, body; only** P3 S 80
4.15 6.38 Global Days 000

29015 **including head** P2 S 80
5.15 8.18 Global Days 000

29020 **Application of turnbuckle jacket, body; only** G2 S 80
4.04 6.42 Global Days 000

29025 **including head** P2 S 80
5.29 8.34 Global Days 000

29035 **Application of body cast, shoulder to hips;** P2 S 80
4.21 7.40 Global Days 000

29040 **including head, Minerva type** G2 S 80
4.40 6.64 Global Days 000

29044 **including 1 thigh** P2 S 80
4.90 8.23 Global Days 000

29046 **including both thighs** G2 S 80
5.30 8.38 Global Days 000

29049 **Application, cast; figure-of-eight** P3 S 80
2.00 2.81 Global Days 000
AMA: 2007, February, 8-9

29055 **shoulder spica** P2 S 80
4.04 6.40 Global Days 000

29058 **plaster Velpeau** P3 S 80
2.32 2.86 Global Days 000

29065 **shoulder to hand (long arm)** P3 S 50
2.01 2.81 Global Days 000

29075 **elbow to finger (short arm)** P3 S 50
1.83 2.63 Global Days 000

29085 **hand and lower forearm (gauntlet)** P3 S 50
1.96 2.77 Global Days 000
AMA: 2009, Jan, 11-31; 2008, Jan, 10-25; 2007, January, 13-27

29086 **finger (eg, contracture)** P3 S 50
1.49 2.25 Global Days 000

29105-29280 Splinting and Strapping: Torso/Upper Extremities

CMS 100-2,15,100 Surgical Dressings, Splints, Casts, and Devices for Reductions of Fractures/Dislocations
CMS 100-4,4,240 Inpatient Part B Hospital Services Paid Under OPPS
EXCLUDES *Orthotic supervision and training (97760-97762)*

29105 **Application of long arm splint (shoulder to hand)** P3 S 50
1.74 2.55 Global Days 000
AMA: 2009, May, 8-9&11

29125 **Application of short arm splint (forearm to hand); static** P3 S 50
1.15 1.88 Global Days 000

29126 **dynamic** P3 S 50
1.43 2.24 Global Days 000

29130 **Application of finger splint; static** P3 S 50
0.83 1.18 Global Days 000

29131 **dynamic** P3 S 50
0.99 1.52 Global Days 000

29200 **Strapping; thorax** P3 S
EXCLUDES *Strapping of low back (29799)*
1.15 1.53 Global Days 000

29240 **shoulder (eg, Velpeau)** P3 S
1.26 1.65 Global Days 000

29260 **elbow or wrist** P3 S 50
1.09 1.51 Global Days 000

29280 **hand or finger** P3 S 50
1.05 1.46 Global Days 000

29305-29450 Casting: Legs

CMS 100-2,15,100 Surgical Dressings, Splints, Casts, and Devices for Reductions of Fractures/Dislocations
CMS 100-4,4,240 Inpatient Part B Hospital Services Paid Under OPPS
EXCLUDES *Cast or splint supplies*
Orthotic supervision and training (97760-97762)

29305 **Application of hip spica cast; 1 leg** P2 S 80
EXCLUDES *Hip spica cast thighs only (29046)*
4.66 7.13 Global Days 000

29325 **1 and 1/2 spica or both legs** P2 S 80
EXCLUDES *Hip spica cast thighs only (29046)*
5.24 7.90 Global Days 000

29345 **Application of long leg cast (thigh to toes);** P3 S 50
2.98 3.98 Global Days 000

29355 **walker or ambulatory type** P3 S 50
3.17 4.14 Global Days 000

29358 **Application of long leg cast brace** P3 S 50
3.05 4.64 Global Days 000

29365 **Application of cylinder cast (thigh to ankle)** P3 S 50
2.59 3.58 Global Days 000

29405 **Application of short leg cast (below knee to toes);** P3 S 50
1.76 2.41 Global Days 000

29425 **walking or ambulatory type** P3 S 50
1.69 2.34 Global Days 000

29435 **Application of patellar tendon bearing (PTB) cast** P3 S 50
2.52 3.50 Global Days 000

29440 **Adding walker to previously applied cast** P3 S 50
1.05 1.66 Global Days 000

29445 **Application of rigid total contact leg cast** P3 S 50
3.13 4.03 Global Days 000

29450 **Application of clubfoot cast with molding or manipulation, long or short leg** P2 S 50
3.37 4.24 Global Days 000

29505-29590 Splinting and Strapping Ankle/Foot/Leg/Toes

CMS 100-2,15,100 Surgical Dressings, Splints, Casts, and Devices for Reductions of Fractures/Dislocations
CMS 100-4,4,240 Inpatient Part B Hospital Services Paid Under OPPS
EXCLUDES *Orthotic supervision and training (97760-97762)*

29505 **Application of long leg splint (thigh to ankle or toes)** P3 S 50
1.43 2.35 Global Days 000
AMA: 2009, May, 8-9&11

29515 **Application of short leg splint (calf to foot)** P3 S 50
1.45 2.07 Global Days 000

29520 **Strapping; hip** P3 S 80
1.05 1.44 Global Days 000

29530 **knee** P3 S
1.10 1.51 Global Days 000

29540 **ankle and/or foot** P3 S
Do not report with (29581, 29582)
0.77 1.07 Global Days 000

29550 **toes** P3 S
0.58 0.90 Global Days 000

29580 **Unna boot** P3 S 50
Do not report with (29581-29582)
1.05 1.53 Global Days 000
AMA: 2009, Jan, 11-31; 2008, Jan, 10-25; 2007, January, 13-27

▲ **29581** **Application of multi-layer compression system; leg (below knee), including ankle and foot** P3 S 80 50
Do not report with (29540, 29580, 29582, 36475, 36478, 97140)
0.37 1.80 Global Days 000

● **29582** **thigh and leg, including ankle and foot, when performed** P3 S 80 50
Do not report with (29540, 29580-29581, 36475, 36478, 97140)
0.45 2.05 Global Days 000

● **29583** **upper arm and forearm** P3 S 80 50
Do not report with (29584, 97140)
0.33 1.27 Global Days 000

● **29584** **upper arm, forearm, hand, and fingers** P3 S 80 50
Do not report with (29583, 97140)
0.45 2.05 Global Days 000

29590 **Denis-Browne splint strapping** P3 S
1.11 1.54 Global Days 000

29700-29799 Casting Services Other Than Application

INCLUDES Casts applied by treating physician

29700 **Removal or bivalving; gauntlet, boot or body cast** P3 S
1.01 1.92 Global Days 000

29705 **full arm or full leg cast** P3 S 50
1.38 1.94 Global Days 000

29710 **shoulder or hip spica, Minerva, or Risser jacket, etc.** P3 S 80 50
2.32 3.19 Global Days 000

Musculoskeletal System 29105 — 29710

29715 turnbuckle jacket P3 S 80
1.61 2.55 Global Days 000

29720 Repair of spica, body cast or jacket P3 S
1.28 2.42 Global Days 000

29730 Windowing of cast P3 S
1.32 1.90 Global Days 000

29740 Wedging of cast (except clubfoot casts) P3 S
1.91 2.67 Global Days 000

29750 Wedging of clubfoot cast P3 S 80 50
2.27 3.02 Global Days 000

29799 Unlisted procedure, casting or strapping S 80
0.00 0.00 Global Days YYY

29800-29999 [29914, 29915, 29916] Arthroscopic Procedures

INCLUDES Diagnostic arthroscopy with surgical arthroscopy

29800 Arthroscopy, temporomandibular joint, diagnostic, with or without synovial biopsy (separate procedure) A2 T 80 50
15.17 15.17 Global Days 090

29804 Arthroscopy, temporomandibular joint, surgical A2 T 80 50
EXCLUDES *Open surgery (21010)*
19.08 19.08 Global Days 090

29805 Arthroscopy, shoulder, diagnostic, with or without synovial biopsy (separate procedure) A2 T 50
EXCLUDES *Open surgery (23065-23066, 23100-23101)*
13.84 13.84 Global Days 090

29806 Arthroscopy, shoulder, surgical; capsulorrhaphy A2 T 50
EXCLUDES *Capsulorrhaphy (29999)*
Open surgery (23450-23466)
31.25 31.25 Global Days 090

29807 repair of SLAP lesion A2 T 50
30.43 30.43 Global Days 090

29819 with removal of loose body or foreign body A2 T 50
EXCLUDES *Open surgery (23040-23044, 23107)*
17.23 17.23 Global Days 090

29820 synovectomy, partial A2 T 80 50
EXCLUDES *Open surgery (23105)*
15.87 15.87 Global Days 090

29821 synovectomy, complete A2 T 80 50
EXCLUDES *Open surgery (23105)*
17.40 17.40 Global Days 090

29822 debridement, limited A2 T 80 50
EXCLUDES *Open surgery (see specific shoulder section)*
16.92 16.92 Global Days 090

29823 debridement, extensive A2 T 80 50
EXCLUDES *Open surgery (see specific shoulder section)*
18.48 18.48 Global Days 090

29824 distal claviculectomy including distal articular surface (Mumford procedure) A2 T 80 50
INCLUDES Mumford procedure
EXCLUDES *Open surgery (23120)*
19.91 19.91 Global Days 090

29825 with lysis and resection of adhesions, with or without manipulation A2 T 80 50
EXCLUDES *Open surgery (see specific shoulder section)*
17.22 17.22 Global Days 090

+ ▲ 29826 decompression of subacromial space with partial acromioplasty, with coracoacromial ligament (ie, arch) release, when performed (List separately in addition to code for primary procedure) A2 T 80 50
Code first (29806-29825, 29827-29828)
EXCLUDES *Open surgery (23130, 23415)*
5.24 5.24 Global Days ZZZ

29827 with rotator cuff repair A2 T 80 50
EXCLUDES *Distal clavicle excision (29824)*
Open surgery or mini open repair (23412)
Subacromial decompression (29826)
31.73 31.73 Global Days 090
AMA: 2009, Jan, 11-31; 2008, Mar, 14-15

29828 biceps tenodesis G2 T 80 50
EXCLUDES *Tenodesis of long tendon of biceps (23430)*
Do not report with (29805, 29820, 29822)
27.13 27.13 Global Days 090
AMA: 2009, Jan, 11-31; 2008, Feb, 8-9

29830 Arthroscopy, elbow, diagnostic, with or without synovial biopsy (separate procedure) A2 T 50
13.33 13.33 Global Days 090

29834 Arthroscopy, elbow, surgical; with removal of loose body or foreign body A2 T 80 50
14.48 14.48 Global Days 090

29835 synovectomy, partial A2 T 80 50
14.86 14.86 Global Days 090

29836 synovectomy, complete A2 T 80 50
17.13 17.13 Global Days 090

29837 debridement, limited A2 T 80 50
15.57 15.57 Global Days 090

29838 debridement, extensive A2 T 80 50
17.38 17.38 Global Days 090

29840 Arthroscopy, wrist, diagnostic, with or without synovial biopsy (separate procedure) A2 T 80 50
13.35 13.35 Global Days 090

29843 Arthroscopy, wrist, surgical; for infection, lavage and drainage A2 T 80 50
14.17 14.17 Global Days 090

29844 synovectomy, partial A2 T 80 50
14.68 14.68 Global Days 090

29845 synovectomy, complete A2 T 80 50
16.92 16.92 Global Days 090
AMA: 2009, Jan, 11-31; 2008, Jan, 10-25; 2007, January, 13-27

29846 excision and/or repair of triangular fibrocartilage and/or joint debridement A2 T 80 50
15.34 15.34 Global Days 090
AMA: 2009, Jan, 11-31; 2008, Jan, 10-25; 2007, January, 13-27

29847 internal fixation for fracture or instability A2 T 80 50
15.93 15.93 Global Days 090

29848 Endoscopy, wrist, surgical, with release of transverse carpal ligament A2 T 50
EXCLUDES *Open surgery (64721)*
14.97 14.97 Global Days 090

29850 Arthroscopically aided treatment of intercondylar spine(s) and/or tuberosity fracture(s) of the knee, with or without manipulation; without internal or external fixation (includes arthroscopy) A2 T 80 50
16.39 16.39 Global Days 090

29851 with internal or external fixation (includes arthroscopy) A2 T 80 50
EXCLUDES *Bone graft (20900, 20902)*
27.37 27.37 Global Days 090

29855 **Arthroscopically aided treatment of tibial fracture, proximal (plateau); unicondylar, includes internal fixation, when performed (includes arthroscopy)** A2 T 80 50
23.11 23.11 Global Days 090

29856 **bicondylar, includes internal fixation, when performed (includes arthroscopy)** A2 T 80 50
EXCLUDES *Bone graft (20900, 20902)*
29.31 29.31 Global Days 090

29860 **Arthroscopy, hip, diagnostic with or without synovial biopsy (separate procedure)** A2 T 80 50
19.49 19.49 Global Days 090

29861 **Arthroscopy, hip, surgical; with removal of loose body or foreign body** A2 T 80 50
21.32 21.32 Global Days 090

29862 **with debridement/shaving of articular cartilage (chondroplasty), abrasion arthroplasty, and/or resection of labrum** A2 T 80 50
24.02 24.02 Global Days 090

29863 **with synovectomy** A2 T 80 50
24.03 24.03 Global Days 090

29914 **with femoroplasty (ie, treatment of cam lesion)** G2 T 80 50
Do not report with (29862-29863)
30.07 30.07 Global Days 090

29915 **with acetabuloplasty (ie, treatment of pincer lesion)** G2 T 80 50
Do not report with (29862-29863)
30.62 30.62 Global Days 090

29916 **with labral repair** G2 T 80 50
EXCLUDES *Labral repair secondary to acetabuloplasty*
Do not report with (29862-29863)
30.62 30.62 Global Days 090

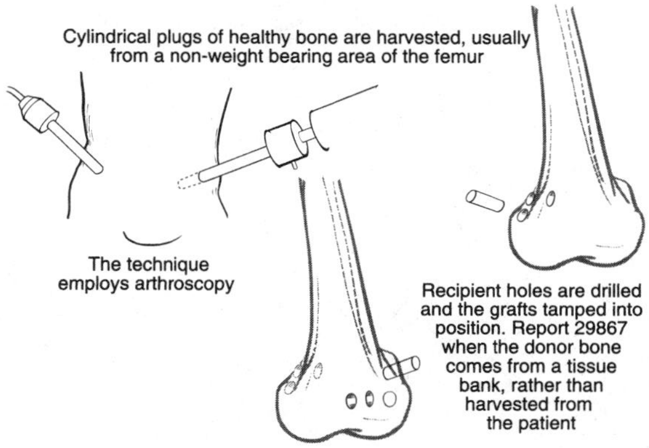

29866 **Arthroscopy, knee, surgical; osteochondral autograft(s) (eg, mosaicplasty) (includes harvesting of the autograft[s])** G2 T 80 50
EXCLUDES *Open osteochondral autograft of the knee (27416)*
Do not report with procedure performed in the same compartment (29874, 29877, 29879, 29885-29887)
Do not report with procedure performed at the same surgical session (29870, 29871, 29875, 29884)
30.81 30.81 Global Days 090

29867 **osteochondral allograft (eg, mosaicplasty)** T 80 50
Do not report with procedures performed in the same compartment (29874, 29877, 29879, 29885-29887)
Do not report with procedures performed at the same surgical session (27415, 27570, 29870-29871, 29875, 29884)
37.49 37.49 Global Days 090

29868 **meniscal transplantation (includes arthrotomy for meniscal insertion), medial or lateral** T 80 50
Do not report with procedure performed in same compartment (29874, 29877, 29881-29882)
Do not report with procedures performed at same surgical session (29870-29871, 29875, 29880, 29883-29884)
49.20 49.20 Global Days 090

29870 **Arthroscopy, knee, diagnostic, with or without synovial biopsy (separate procedure)** A2 T 50
EXCLUDES *Open procedure (27412)*
12.09 17.37 Global Days 090
AMA: 2009, Jan, 11-31; 2007, Dec, 10-179

29871 **Arthroscopy, knee, surgical; for infection, lavage and drainage** A2 T 50
EXCLUDES *Osteochondral graft (27412, 27415, 29866-29867)*
15.08 15.08 Global Days 090
AMA: 2007, Dec, 10-179

29873 **with lateral release** A2 T 50
EXCLUDES *Open procedure (27425)*
15.34 15.34 Global Days 090
AMA: 2007, Dec, 10-179

29874 **for removal of loose body or foreign body (eg, osteochondritis dissecans fragmentation, chondral fragmentation)** A2 T 80 50
15.81 15.81 Global Days 090
AMA: 2007, Dec, 10-179

29875 **synovectomy, limited (eg, plica or shelf resection) (separate procedure)** A2 T 80 50
14.56 14.56 Global Days 090
AMA: 2007, Dec, 10-179

29876 **synovectomy, major, 2 or more compartments (eg, medial or lateral)** A2 T 50
19.27 19.27 Global Days 090
AMA: 2007, Dec, 10-179

29877 **debridement/shaving of articular cartilage (chondroplasty)** A2 T 80 50
18.29 18.29 Global Days 090
AMA: 2009, Jan, 11-31; 2008, Jan, 10-25; 2007, January, 13-27; 2007, Dec, 10-179

29879 **abrasion arthroplasty (includes chondroplasty where necessary) or multiple drilling or microfracture** A2 T 80 50
19.48 19.48 Global Days 090
AMA: 2007, Dec, 10-179

▲ **29880** **with meniscectomy (medial AND lateral, including any meniscal shaving) including debridement/shaving of articular cartilage (chondroplasty), same or separate compartment(s), when performed** A2 T 80 50
16.85 16.85 Global Days 090
AMA: 2007, Dec, 10-179

Musculoskeletal System

29855 — 29880

▲ **29881** **with meniscectomy (medial OR lateral, including any meniscal shaving) including debridement/shaving of articular cartilage (chondroplasty), same or separate compartment(s), when performed** A2 T 80 50
16.16 16.16 Global Days 090
AMA: 2009, Jan, 11-31; 2008, Jan, 10-25; 2007, January, 13-27; 2007, Dec, 10-179

29882 **with meniscus repair (medial OR lateral)** A2 T 50
EXCLUDES *Meniscus transplant (29868)*
20.53 20.53 Global Days 090
AMA: 2009, Jan, 11-31; 2008, Jan, 10-25; 2007, January, 13-27; 2007, Dec, 10-179

29883 **with meniscus repair (medial AND lateral)** A2 T 80 50
EXCLUDES *Meniscus transplant (29868)*
24.75 24.75 Global Days 090
AMA: 2009, Jan, 11-31; 2008, Jan, 10-25; 2007, January, 13-27; 2007, Dec, 10-179

29884 **with lysis of adhesions, with or without manipulation (separate procedure)** A2 T 80 50
18.25 18.25 Global Days 090
AMA: 2007, Dec, 10-179

29885 **drilling for osteochondritis dissecans with bone grafting, with or without internal fixation (including debridement of base of lesion)** A2 T 80 50
22.04 22.04 Global Days 090
AMA: 2007, Dec, 10-179

29886 **drilling for intact osteochondritis dissecans lesion** A2 T 50
18.63 18.63 Global Days 090
AMA: 2007, Dec, 10-179

29887 **drilling for intact osteochondritis dissecans lesion with internal fixation** A2 T 80 50
21.95 21.95 Global Days 090
AMA: 2007, Dec, 10-179

29888 **Arthroscopically aided anterior cruciate ligament repair/augmentation or reconstruction** A2 T 80 50
Do not report with ligamentous reconstruction (27427-27429)
29.13 29.13 Global Days 090
AMA: 2009, Jan, 11-31; 2008, Jan, 10-25; 2007, January, 13-27; 2007, Dec, 10-179

29889 **Arthroscopically aided posterior cruciate ligament repair/augmentation or reconstruction** A2 T 80 50
Do not report with ligamentous reconstruction (27427-27429)
35.63 35.63 Global Days 090
AMA: 2009, Jan, 11-31; 2008, Jan, 10-25; 2007, Dec, 10-179; 2007, January, 13-27

29891 **Arthroscopy, ankle, surgical, excision of osteochondral defect of talus and/or tibia, including drilling of the defect** A2 T 80 50
20.23 20.23 Global Days 090

29892 **Arthroscopically aided repair of large osteochondritis dissecans lesion, talar dome fracture, or tibial plafond fracture, with or without internal fixation (includes arthroscopy)** A2 T 80 50
18.80 18.80 Global Days 090

29893 **Endoscopic plantar fasciotomy** A2 T 50
12.51 17.75 Global Days 090

29894 **Arthroscopy, ankle (tibiotalar and fibulotalar joints), surgical; with removal of loose body or foreign body** A2 T 80 50
15.10 15.10 Global Days 090

29895 **synovectomy, partial** A2 T 80 50
14.36 14.36 Global Days 090

29897 **debridement, limited** A2 T 80 50
15.20 15.20 Global Days 090

29898 **debridement, extensive** A2 T 80 50
16.81 16.81 Global Days 090

29899 **with ankle arthrodesis** A2 T 80 50
EXCLUDES *Open procedure (27870)*
30.67 30.67 Global Days 090

29900 **Arthroscopy, metacarpophalangeal joint, diagnostic, includes synovial biopsy** A2 T 80 50
Do not report with (29901-29902)
13.78 13.78 Global Days 090

29901 **Arthroscopy, metacarpophalangeal joint, surgical; with debridement** A2 T 80 50
15.72 15.72 Global Days 090

29902 **with reduction of displaced ulnar collateral ligament (eg, Stenar lesion)** A2 T 80 50
17.58 17.58 Global Days 090

29904 **Arthroscopy, subtalar joint, surgical; with removal of loose body or foreign body** G2 T 80 50
18.61 18.61 Global Days 090

29905 **with synovectomy** G2 T 80 50
20.14 20.14 Global Days 090

29906 **with debridement** G2 T 80 50
21.20 21.20 Global Days 090

29907 **with subtalar arthrodesis** G2 T 80 50
25.61 25.61 Global Days 090

29914 Resequenced code, See code following 29863.

29915 Resequenced code, See code following 29863.

29916 Resequenced code, See code before 29866.

29999 **Unlisted procedure, arthroscopy** T 80 50
0.00 0.00 Global Days YYY
AMA: 2009, Jan, 11-31; 2009, Mar, 10-11; 2008, Jan, 10-25; 2008, Nov, 10-11; 2007, January, 13-27

30000-30115 I&D, Biopsy, Excision Procedures of the Nose

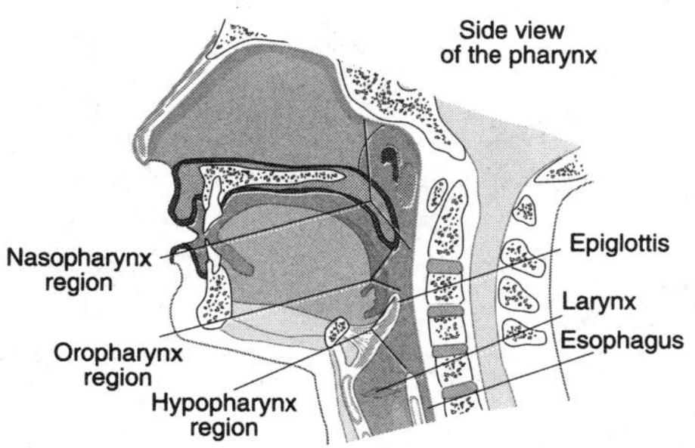

The nasopharynx is the membranous passage above the level of the soft palate; the oropharynx is the region between the soft palate and the upper edge of the epiglottis; the hypopharynx is the region of the epiglottis to the juncture of the larynx and esophagus; the three regions are collectively known as the pharynx

30000 Drainage abscess or hematoma, nasal, internal approach P2 T 80

EXCLUDES *Incision and drainage (10060, 10140)*

3.56 6.97 Global Days 010

30020 Drainage abscess or hematoma, nasal septum P2 T

EXCLUDES *Lateral rhinotomy incision (30118, 30320)*

3.56 6.96 Global Days 010

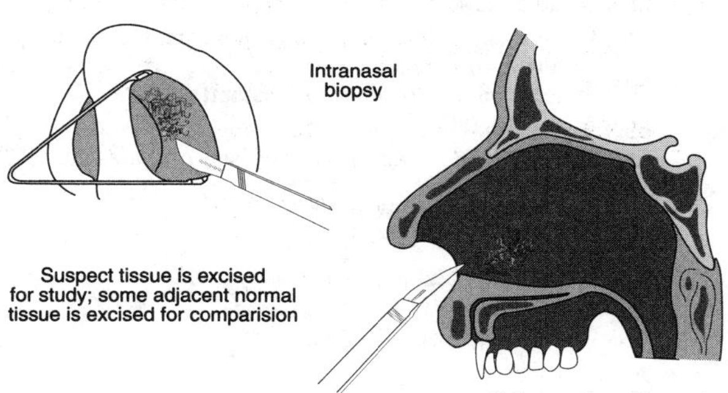

Suspect tissue is excised for study; some adjacent normal tissue is excised for comparision

Only a wedge of tissue is removed for larger lesions

30100 Biopsy, intranasal P3 T

EXCLUDES *Superficial biopsy of nose (11100-11101)*

2.06 4.26 Global Days 000

30110 Excision, nasal polyp(s), simple P3 T 50

3.90 6.91 Global Days 010

30115 Excision, nasal polyp(s), extensive A2 T 50

12.89 12.89 Global Days 090

30117-30118 Destruction Procedures Nose

CMS 100-3,140.5 Laser Procedures

30117 Excision or destruction (eg, laser), intranasal lesion; internal approach A2 T

10.10 26.24 Global Days 090

30118 external approach (lateral rhinotomy) A2 T

22.89 22.89 Global Days 090

30120-30140 Excision Procedures Nose, Turbinate

30120 Excision or surgical planing of skin of nose for rhinophyma A2 T

13.12 15.47 Global Days 090

AMA: 2009, Jan, 11-31; 2008, Jan, 10-25; 2007, May, 9-11

30124 Excision dermoid cyst, nose; simple, skin, subcutaneous P2 T

8.45 8.45 Global Days 090

30125 complex, under bone or cartilage A2 T 80

18.21 18.21 Global Days 090

30130 Excision inferior turbinate, partial or complete, any method A2 T 50

EXCLUDES *Excision middle/superior turbinate(s) (30999)*

Do not report with (30801, 30802, 30930)

11.37 11.37 Global Days 090

AMA: 2009, Jan, 11-31; 2008, Jan, 10-25; 2007, January, 13-27

30140 Submucous resection inferior turbinate, partial or complete, any method A2 T 50

EXCLUDES *Endoscopic resection of concha bullosa of middle turbinate (31240)*
Submucous resection:
Nasal septum (30520)
Superior or middle turbinate (30999)

Do not report with (30801, 30802, 30930)

13.18 13.18 Global Days 090

AMA: 2009, Jan, 11-31; 2008, Mar, 14-15; 2008, Jan, 10-25; 2007, January, 13-27

30150-30160 Surgical Removal: Nose

EXCLUDES *Reconstruction and/or closure (primary or delayed primary intention) (13150-13160, 14060-14302, 15120-15121, 15260-15261, 15760, 20900-20912)*

30150 Rhinectomy; partial A2 T

23.08 23.08 Global Days 090

30160 total A2 T 80

23.19 23.19 Global Days 090

30200-30320 Turbinate Injection, Removal Foreign Substance in the Nose

30200 Injection into turbinate(s), therapeutic P3 T

1.79 3.43 Global Days 000

AMA: 2009, Jan, 11-31; 2008, Jan, 10-25; 2007, January, 13-27

30210 Displacement therapy (Proetz type) P3 T

2.98 4.50 Global Days 010

30220 Insertion, nasal septal prosthesis (button) A2 T

3.76 9.09 Global Days 010

30300 Removal foreign body, intranasal; office type procedure P2 X

3.77 6.95 Global Days 010

30310 requiring general anesthesia A2 T 80

6.18 6.18 Global Days 010

30320 by lateral rhinotomy A2 T 80

13.54 13.54 Global Days 090

30400-30630 Reconstruction or Repair of Nose

EXCLUDES *Bone/tissue grafts (20900-20926, 21210)*

30400 **Rhinoplasty, primary; lateral and alar cartilages and/or elevation of nasal tip** A2 T 80

INCLUDES Carpue's operation

EXCLUDES *Reconstruction of columella (13150-13153)*

30.41 30.41 Global Days 090

30410 **complete, external parts including bony pyramid, lateral and alar cartilages, and/or elevation of nasal tip** A2 T 80

38.34 38.34 Global Days 090

30420 **including major septal repair** A2 T

40.93 40.93 Global Days 090

30430 **Rhinoplasty, secondary; minor revision (small amount of nasal tip work)** A2 T 80

27.92 27.92 Global Days 090

30435 **intermediate revision (bony work with osteotomies)** A2 T 80

33.86 33.86 Global Days 090

30450 **major revision (nasal tip work and osteotomies)** A2 T 80

45.16 45.16 Global Days 090

Cleft lip and cleft palate are described according to length of cleft and whether bilateral or unilateral

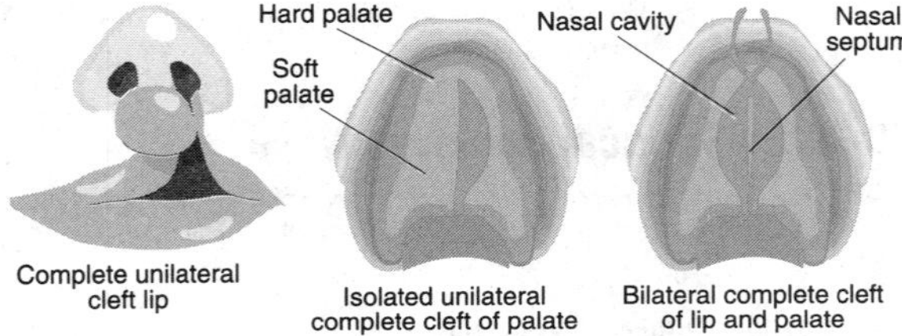

Cleft lip with or without cleft palate is a common birth defect and is seen once or twice per 1000 live births; the condition is twice as common among boys than girls; isolated cleft palate is distinct from cleft lip with or without cleft palate and occurs about once in 2000 births; the condition is more common among girls than boys

30460 **Rhinoplasty for nasal deformity secondary to congenital cleft lip and/or palate, including columellar lengthening; tip only** A2 T 80

22.57 22.57 Global Days 090

30462 **tip, septum, osteotomies** A2 T 80

46.76 46.76 Global Days 090

30465 **Repair of nasal vestibular stenosis (eg, spreader grafting, lateral nasal wall reconstruction)** A2 T 80

29.31 29.31 Global Days 090

30520 **Septoplasty or submucous resection, with or without cartilage scoring, contouring or replacement with graft** A2 T

EXCLUDES *Turbinate resection (30140)*

18.56 18.56 Global Days 090

AMA: 2009, Jan, 11-31; 2008, Jan, 10-25; 2007, January, 13-27

30540 **Repair choanal atresia; intranasal** A2 T 80 63

20.44 20.44 Global Days 090

30545 **transpalatine** A2 T 80 63

27.47 27.47 Global Days 090

30560 **Lysis intranasal synechia** A2 T

4.17 8.19 Global Days 010

30580 **Repair fistula; oromaxillary (combine with 31030 if antrotomy is included)** A2 T

14.74 18.81 Global Days 090

30600 **oronasal** A2 T 80

12.82 17.14 Global Days 090

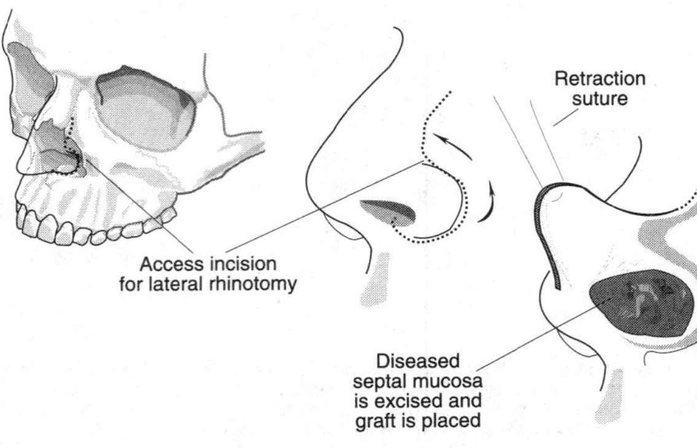

30620 **Septal or other intranasal dermatoplasty (does not include obtaining graft)** A2 T

18.64 18.64 Global Days 090

30630 **Repair nasal septal perforations** A2 T 80

18.67 18.67 Global Days 090

30801-30802 Turbinate Destruction

EXCLUDES *Cautery to stop nasal bleeding (30901-30906)*

Do not report with (30130, 30140)

30801 **Ablation, soft tissue of inferior turbinates, unilateral or bilateral, any method (eg, electrocautery, radiofrequency ablation, or tissue volume reduction); superficial** A2 T

EXCLUDES *Ablation middle/superior turbinates (30999)*

Do not report with (30802)

4.09 6.89 Global Days 010

30802 **intramural (ie, submucosal)** A2 T

5.69 8.75 Global Days 010

AMA: 2009, Jan, 11-31; 2008, Mar, 14-15

30901-30920 Control Nose Bleed

30901 **Control nasal hemorrhage, anterior, simple (limited cautery and/or packing) any method** P3 T 50

1.68 2.86 Global Days 000

30903 **Control nasal hemorrhage, anterior, complex (extensive cautery and/or packing) any method** A2 T 50

2.38 6.06 Global Days 000

30905 **Control nasal hemorrhage, posterior, with posterior nasal packs and/or cautery, any method; initial** A2 T

3.01 7.53 Global Days 000

30906 **subsequent** A2 T

3.93 8.39 Global Days 000

30915 **Ligation arteries; ethmoidal** A2 T

EXCLUDES *External carotid artery (37600)*

17.22 17.22 Global Days 090

30920 **internal maxillary artery, transantral** A2 T

EXCLUDES *External carotid artery (37600)*

24.86 24.86 Global Days 090

30930-30999 Other and Unlisted Procedures of Nose

30930 **Fracture nasal inferior turbinate(s), therapeutic** A2 T 50
EXCLUDES *Fracture of superior or middle turbinate(s) (30999)*

Do not report with (30130, 30140)
3.70 3.70 Global Days 010
AMA: 2009, Jan, 11-31; 2008, Jan, 10-25; 2007, January, 13-27

30999 **Unlisted procedure, nose** T 80
0.00 0.00 Global Days YYY

31000-31230 Opening Sinuses

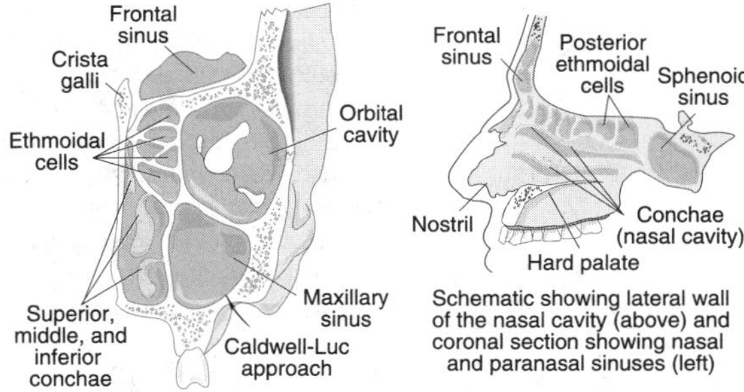

Schematic showing lateral wall of the nasal cavity (above) and coronal section showing nasal and paranasal sinuses (left)

The nasal sinuses are air filled cavities in the cranial bones that bear their names; all are lined with mucous membrane continuous with the nasal cavity and all drain fluids into the nasal cavity. The ethmoid cells vary in size and number and feature very thin septa,or walls. The maxillary sinuses are the largest and are the most frequently infected.

31000 **Lavage by cannulation; maxillary sinus (antrum puncture or natural ostium)** P3 T 50
3.11 5.40 Global Days 010

31002 **sphenoid sinus** R2 T 80 50
5.99 5.99 Global Days 010

31020 **Sinusotomy, maxillary (antrotomy); intranasal** A2 T 50
10.70 14.54 Global Days 090

31030 **radical (Caldwell-Luc) without removal of antrochoanal polyps** A2 T 50
15.51 20.52 Global Days 090

31032 **radical (Caldwell-Luc) with removal of antrochoanal polyps** A2 T 50
17.04 17.04 Global Days 090

31040 **Pterygomaxillary fossa surgery, any approach** R2 T
EXCLUDES *Transantral ligation internal maxillary artery (30920)*

22.62 22.62 Global Days 090

31050 **Sinusotomy, sphenoid, with or without biopsy;** A2 T 50
14.52 14.52 Global Days 090

31051 **with mucosal stripping or removal of polyp(s)** A2 T 50
19.26 19.26 Global Days 090

31070 **Sinusotomy frontal; external, simple (trephine operation)** A2 T 50
INCLUDES Killian operation

EXCLUDES *Intranasal frontal sinusotomy (31276)*

13.13 13.13 Global Days 090

31075 **transorbital, unilateral (for mucocele or osteoma, Lynch type)** A2 T 80 50
23.34 23.34 Global Days 090

31080 **obliterative without osteoplastic flap, brow incision (includes ablation)** A2 T 80 50
INCLUDES Ridell sinusotomy

30.58 30.58 Global Days 090

31081 **obliterative, without osteoplastic flap, coronal incision (includes ablation)** A2 T 80 50
43.06 43.06 Global Days 090

31084 **obliterative, with osteoplastic flap, brow incision** A2 T 80 50
34.58 34.58 Global Days 090

31085 **obliterative, with osteoplastic flap, coronal incision** A2 T 80 50
39.44 39.44 Global Days 090

31086 **nonobliterative, with osteoplastic flap, brow incision** A2 T 80 50
33.41 33.41 Global Days 090

31087 **nonobliterative, with osteoplastic flap, coronal incision** A2 T 80 50
32.31 32.31 Global Days 090

31090 **Sinusotomy, unilateral, 3 or more paranasal sinuses (frontal, maxillary, ethmoid, sphenoid)** A2 T 50
30.42 30.42 Global Days 090

31200 **Ethmoidectomy; intranasal, anterior** A2 T 50
16.54 16.54 Global Days 090

31201 **intranasal, total** A2 T 50
22.02 22.02 Global Days 090

31205 **extranasal, total** A2 T 80 50
26.39 26.39 Global Days 090

31225 **Maxillectomy; without orbital exenteration** C5 C 80 50
55.37 55.37 Global Days 090

31230 **with orbital exenteration (en bloc)** C5 C 80 50
EXCLUDES *Orbital exenteration without maxillectomy (65110-65114)*
Skin grafts (15120-15121)

61.66 61.66 Global Days 090

31231-31235 Nasal Endoscopy, Diagnostic

CMS 100-3,100.2 Endoscopy
CMS 100-4,12,40.6 Multiple procedures
INCLUDES Complete sinus exam (e.g., nasal cavity, turbinates, sphenoethmoidal recess)

31231 **Nasal endoscopy, diagnostic, unilateral or bilateral (separate procedure)** P2 T
2.29 5.79 Global Days 000

31233 **Nasal/sinus endoscopy, diagnostic with maxillary sinusoscopy (via inferior meatus or canine fossa puncture)** A2 T 80 50

Do not report with (31295)
4.11 8.01 Global Days 000

31235 **Nasal/sinus endoscopy, diagnostic with sphenoid sinusoscopy (via puncture of sphenoidal face or cannulation of ostium)** A2 T 80 50

Do not report with (31297)
4.83 9.03 Global Days 000

31237-31240 Nasal Endoscopy, Surgical

CMS 100-3,100.2 Endoscopy

INCLUDES Diagnostic nasal/sinus endoscopy
Unilateral procedure

EXCLUDES *Endoscopic frontal sinus exploration, osteomeatal complex (OMC) resection and/or anterior ethmoidectomy:*
With antrostomy, with/without polyp removal, report all: (31254, 31256, 31276)
With/without polyp removal, report both: (31254, 31276)
Endoscopic frontal sinus exploration, osteomeatal complex (OMC) resection, antrostomy, removal of antral mucosal disease and/or anterior ethmoidectomy, with/without polyp removal, report all: (31254, 31267, 31276)
Endoscopic osteomeatal complex (OMC) resection with antrostomy:
And/or anterior ethmoidectomy, with/without polyp removal, report both: (31254, 31256)
Removal of antral mucosal disease, and/or anterior ethmoidectomy, with/without polyp removal, report both: (31254, 31267)

31237 **Nasal/sinus endoscopy, surgical; with biopsy, polypectomy or debridement (separate procedure)** A2 T 50
5.42 9.78 **Global Days 000**
AMA: 2009, Jan, 11-31; 2008, Jan, 10-25; 2007, January, 13-27

31238 **with control of nasal hemorrhage** A2 T 80 50
5.88 10.04 **Global Days 000**

31239 **with dacryocystorhinostomy** A2 T 80 50
20.20 20.20 **Global Days 010**

31240 **with concha bullosa resection** A2 T 80 50
4.82 4.82 **Global Days 000**

31254-31255 Nasal Endoscopy with Ethmoid Removal

CMS 100-3,100.2 Endoscopy
CMS 100-4,12,40.6 Multiple procedures

INCLUDES Diagnostic nasal/sinus endoscopy
Sinusotomy, when applicable

31254 **Nasal/sinus endoscopy, surgical; with ethmoidectomy, partial (anterior)** A2 T 50

EXCLUDES *Endoscopic exploration frontal sinus, resection osteomeatal complex (OMC), antrostomy:*
And/or anterior ethmoidectomy, with/without polyp removal, report all (31254, 31256, 31276)
Removal of antral mucosal disease and/or anterior ethmoidectomy with/without polyp removal, report all: (31254, 31267, 31276)
Endoscopic frontal sinus exploration, osteomeatal complex (OMC) resection and/or anterior ethmoidectomy, with/without polyp removal, report both: (31254-31276)
Endoscopic resection osteomeatal complex (OMC):
And antrostomy, removal antral mucosal disease, and/or anterior ethmoidectomy, with/without polyp removal, report both: (31254-31276)
Antrostomy, and/or anterior ethmoidectomy, with/without polyp removal, report both (31254, 31256, 31267, 31276)

8.18 8.18 **Global Days 000**
AMA: 2009, Jan, 11-31; 2008, Jan, 10-25; 2007, January, 13-27

31255 **with ethmoidectomy, total (anterior and posterior)** A2 T 50

EXCLUDES *Endoscopic anterior and posterior ethmoidectomy (APE), antrostomy:*
With removal disease of antral mucosa, with/without polyp removal, report both: (31255, 31267)
With/without polyp removal, report both: (31255, 31256)
Endoscopic anterior and posterior ethmoidectomy and sphenoidotomy (APS), antrostomy:
And removal of diseased antral mucosa, with/without polyp removal, report 31255 and 31267 with 31287, or 31288: (31255, 31267, 31287 or 31288)
With/without polyp removal, report 31255 and 31256 with: (31287 or 31288)
Endoscopic anterior and posterior ethmoidectomy and sphenoidotomy (APS), with/without polyp removal (31255, 31287 or 31288)
Endoscopic frontal sinus exploration, anterior and posterior ethmoidectomy and sphenoidotomy (APS):
Antrostomy, removal diseased antral mucosa, with/without polyp removal, report 31255, 31267, and 31276 with: (31287 or 31288)
Antrostomy, with/without polyp removal, report 31255, 31256, and 31276 with: (31287 or 31288)
With/without polyp removal, report 31255 and 31276 with: (31287 or 31288)
Endoscopic frontal sinus exploration, anterior and posterior ethmoidectomy (APE):
Antrostomy, removal diseased antral mucosa, with/without polyp removal, report all: (31255, 31267, 31276)
Antrostomy, with/without polyp removal, report all: (31255, 31256, 31276)
With/without polyp removal, report both: (31255, 31276)

11.98 11.98 **Global Days 000**
AMA: 2009, Jan, 11-31; 2008, Jan, 10-25; 2007, January, 13-27

31256-31267 Nasal Endoscopy with Maxillary Procedures

CMS 100-3,100.2 Endoscopy
CMS 100-4,12,40.6 Multiple procedures

INCLUDES Diagnostic nasal/sinus endoscopy
Sinusotomy, when applicable

Do not report with (31295)

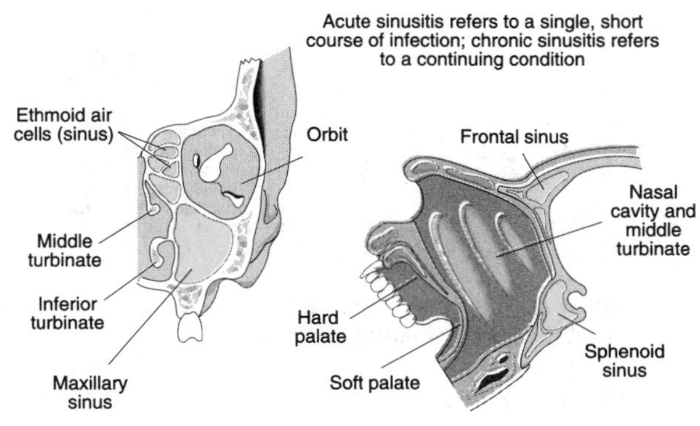

31256 **Nasal/sinus endoscopy, surgical, with maxillary antrostomy;** A2 T 50

EXCLUDES *Endoscopic anterior and posterior ethmoidectomy and sphenoidotomy (APS):*
Antrostomy, with/without polyp removal, report 31255 and 31256 with: (31287 or 31288)
Frontal sinus exploration, and antrostomy, with/without polyp removal, report 31255, 31256, and 31276 with: (31287 or 31288)
Endoscopic anterior and posterior ethmoidectomy (APE):
Antrostomy, with/without polyp removal, report both: (31255, 31256)
Frontal sinus exploration, antrostomy, with/without polyp removal, report all: (31255, 31256, 31276)

5.92 5.92 **Global Days 000**

31267 **with removal of tissue from maxillary sinus** A2 T 50

EXCLUDES *Endoscopic anterior and posterior ethmoidectomy and sphenoidotomy (APS):*
Antrostomy, and removal of diseased antral mucosal, with/without polyp removal, report 31255, 31267 with: (31287 or 31288)
Frontal sinus exploration, antrostomy, and removal of diseased antral mucosa, with/without polyp removal, report 31255, 31267 and 31276 with: (31287 or 31288)
Endoscopic anterior and posterior ethmoidectomy (APE)
Antrostomy, removal of antral mucosal disease, with/without polyp removal, report both: (31255, 31267)
Frontal sinus exploration, antrostomy and removal of antral mucosal disease, with/without polyp removal, report all: (31255, 31267, 31276)

9.50 9.50 **Global Days 000**

AMA: 2009, Jan, 11-31; 2008, Jan, 10-25; 2007, January, 13-27

31276 Nasal Endoscopy with Frontal Sinus Examination

CMS 100-3,100.2 Endoscopy
CMS 100-4,12,40.6 Multiple procedures

INCLUDES Diagnostic nasal/sinus endoscopy
Sinusotomy, when applicable
Unilateral procedure

EXCLUDES *Endoscopic anterior and posterior ethmoidectomy and sphenoidotomy (APS):*
Frontal sinus exploration, with/without polyp removal, report: 31255 and 31276 and (31287 or 31288)
With frontal sinus exploration, antrostomy and removal of antral mucosal disease, with/without polyp removal, report: 31255 and 31267 and 31276 and (31287 or 31288)
With/without polyp removal, with frontal sinus exploration and antrostomy report: 31255 and 31256 and 31276 and (31287 or 31288)
Endoscopic anterior and posterior ethmoidectomy (APE), frontal sinus exploration, with/without polyp removal, report both: (31255, 31276)
Unilateral endoscopy two or more sinuses (31231-31235)

31276 **Nasal/sinus endoscopy, surgical with frontal sinus exploration, with or without removal of tissue from frontal sinus** A2 T 50

Do not report with (31296)

15.12 15.12 **Global Days 000**

31287-31288 Nasal Endoscopy with Sphenoid Procedures

CMS 100-3,100.2 Endoscopy
CMS 100-4,12,40.6 Multiple procedures

Do not report with (31297)

31287 **Nasal/sinus endoscopy, surgical, with sphenoidotomy;** A2 T 80 50

6.96 6.96 **Global Days 000**

31288 **with removal of tissue from the sphenoid sinus** A2 T 80 50

8.07 8.07 **Global Days 000**

31290-31294 Nasal Endoscopy with Repair and Decompression

CMS 100-3,100.2 Endoscopy
CMS 100-4,12,40.6 Multiple procedures

INCLUDES Diagnostic nasal/sinus endoscopy
Sinusotomy, when applicable

31290 **Nasal/sinus endoscopy, surgical, with repair of cerebrospinal fluid leak; ethmoid region** C5 C 80 50
34.60 34.60 Global Days 010

31291 **sphenoid region** C5 C 80 50
36.77 36.77 Global Days 010

31292 **with medial or inferior orbital wall decompression** T 80 50
29.91 29.91 Global Days 010

31293 **with medial orbital wall and inferior orbital wall decompression** T 80 50
32.45 32.45 Global Days 010

31294 **with optic nerve decompression** T 80 50
37.16 37.16 Global Days 010

31295-31297 Nasal Endoscopy with Sinus Ostia Dilation

INCLUDES Any method of tissue displacement
Fluoroscopy, when performed

31295 **Nasal/sinus endoscopy, surgical; with dilation of maxillary sinus ostium (eg, balloon dilation), transnasal or via canine fossa** G2 T 80 50
Do not report with (31233, 31256, 31267)
5.05 63.52 Global Days 000

31296 **with dilation of frontal sinus ostium (eg, balloon dilation)** G2 T 80 50
Do not report with 31276
6.02 64.37 Global Days 000

31297 **with dilation of sphenoid sinus ostium (eg, balloon dilation)** G2 T 80 50
Do not report with (31235, 31287, 31288)
4.95 63.30 Global Days 000

31299 Unlisted Procedures of Accessory Sinuses

31299 **Unlisted procedure, accessory sinuses** T 80
EXCLUDES *Hypophysectomy (61546, 61548)*
0.00 0.00 Global Days YYY

31300-31502 Procedures of the Larynx

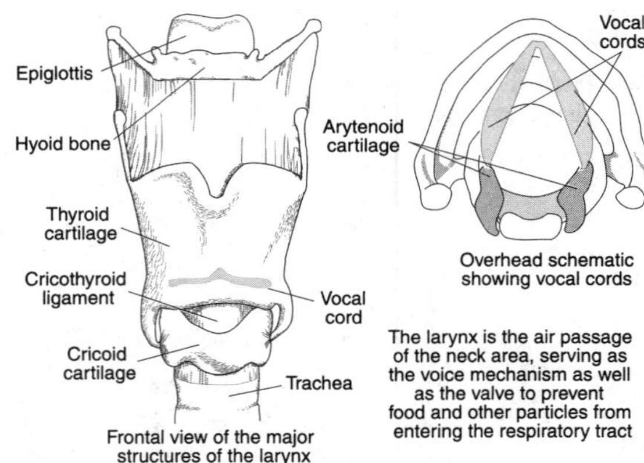

31300 **Laryngotomy (thyrotomy, laryngofissure); with removal of tumor or laryngocele, cordectomy** A2 T 80
37.71 37.71 Global Days 090

31320 **diagnostic** A2 T 80
19.72 19.72 Global Days 090

31360 **Laryngectomy; total, without radical neck dissection** C5 C 80 PQ
61.72 61.72 Global Days 090

31365 **total, with radical neck dissection** C5 C 80 PQ
76.29 76.29 Global Days 090
AMA: 2009, Jan, 11-31; 2008, Jan, 10-25; 2007, January, 13-27

31367 **subtotal supraglottic, without radical neck dissection** C5 C 80 PQ
65.62 65.62 Global Days 090

31368 **subtotal supraglottic, with radical neck dissection** C5 C 80 PQ
72.78 72.78 Global Days 090

31370 **Partial laryngectomy (hemilaryngectomy); horizontal** C5 C 80 PQ
61.72 61.72 Global Days 090

31375 **laterovertical** C5 C 80 PQ
58.56 58.56 Global Days 090

31380 **anterovertical** C5 C 80 PQ
57.72 57.72 Global Days 090

31382 **antero-latero-vertical** C5 C 80 PQ
63.31 63.31 Global Days 090

31390 **Pharyngolaryngectomy, with radical neck dissection; without reconstruction** C5 C 80 PQ
85.08 85.08 Global Days 090

31395 **with reconstruction** C5 C 80 PQ
89.38 89.38 Global Days 090

31400 **Arytenoidectomy or arytenoidopexy, external approach** A2 T 80
EXCLUDES *Endoscopic arytenoidectomy (31560)*
29.96 29.96 Global Days 090

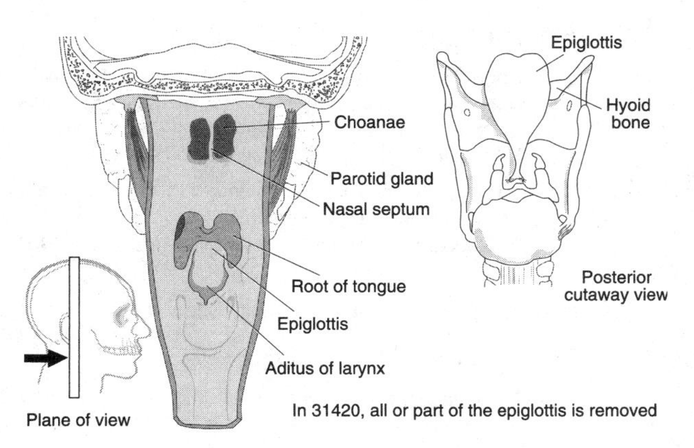

In 31420, all or part of the epiglottis is removed

31420 Epiglottidectomy A2 T 80
24.96 24.96 Global Days 090

⊘ **31500 Intubation, endotracheal, emergency procedure** G2 S
EXCLUDES *Injection of contrast for segmental bronchography (31656)*
3.24 3.24 Global Days 000
AMA: 2007, Jul, 1-4; 2007, April, 3-6

31502 Tracheotomy tube change prior to establishment of fistula tract G2 S
1.03 1.03 Global Days 000

31505-31541 Endoscopy of the Larynx

CMS 100-3,100.2 Endoscopy
CMS 100-4,12,40.6 Multiple procedures

31505 Laryngoscopy, indirect; diagnostic (separate procedure) P2 T
1.47 2.50 Global Days 000

31510 with biopsy A2 T 80
3.63 6.37 Global Days 000

31511 with removal of foreign body A2 T
3.87 6.36 Global Days 000

31512 with removal of lesion A2 T 80
3.92 6.27 Global Days 000

31513 with vocal cord injection A2 T 80
3.97 3.97 Global Days 000

31515 Laryngoscopy direct, with or without tracheoscopy; for aspiration A2 T
3.30 6.28 Global Days 000

31520 diagnostic, newborn A G2 T 80 63
4.70 4.70 Global Days 000

31525 diagnostic, except newborn A2 T
4.79 7.58 Global Days 000

31526 diagnostic, with operating microscope or telescope A2 T
INCLUDES Operating microscope (69990)
4.74 4.74 Global Days 000

31527 with insertion of obturator A2 T 80
5.86 5.86 Global Days 000

31528 with dilation, initial A2 T 80
4.36 4.36 Global Days 000

31529 with dilation, subsequent A2 T 80
4.87 4.87 Global Days 000

31530 Laryngoscopy, direct, operative, with foreign body removal; A2 T
5.96 5.96 Global Days 000

31531 with operating microscope or telescope A2 T 80
INCLUDES Operating microscope (69990)
6.40 6.40 Global Days 000

31535 Laryngoscopy, direct, operative, with biopsy; A2 T
5.71 5.71 Global Days 000

31536 with operating microscope or telescope A2 T
INCLUDES Operating microscope (69990)
6.36 6.36 Global Days 000

31540 Laryngoscopy, direct, operative, with excision of tumor and/or stripping of vocal cords or epiglottis; A2 T
7.30 7.30 Global Days 000

31541 with operating microscope or telescope A2 T
INCLUDES Operating microscope (69990)
7.98 7.98 Global Days 000

31545-31546 Endoscopy of Larynx with Reconstruction

INCLUDES Operating microscope (69990)
EXCLUDES *Vocal cord reconstruction with allograft (31599)*

Do not report with (31540, 31541, 69990)

31545 Laryngoscopy, direct, operative, with operating microscope or telescope, with submucosal removal of non-neoplastic lesion(s) of vocal cord; reconstruction with local tissue flap(s) A2 T 50
10.92 10.92 Global Days 000

31546 reconstruction with graft(s) (includes obtaining autograft) A2 T 50
Do not report with (20926)
16.56 16.56 Global Days 000
AMA: 2009, Jan, 11-31; 2008, Jan, 10-25; 2007, January, 13-27

31560-31571 Endoscopy of Larynx with Arytenoid Removal, Vocal Cord Injection

CMS 100-3,100.2 Endoscopy
CMS 100-4,12,40.6 Multiple procedures

31560 Laryngoscopy, direct, operative, with arytenoidectomy; A2 T 80
9.45 9.45 Global Days 000

31561 with operating microscope or telescope A2 T 80
INCLUDES Operating microscope (69990)
10.32 10.32 Global Days 000

31570 Laryngoscopy, direct, with injection into vocal cord(s), therapeutic; A2 T
6.88 10.25 Global Days 000

31571 with operating microscope or telescope A2 T
INCLUDES Operating microscope (69990)
7.52 7.52 Global Days 000

31575-31579 Endoscopy of Larynx, Flexible Fiberoptic

EXCLUDES *Evaluation by flexible fiberoptic endoscope:*
Sensory assessment (92614-92615)
Swallowing (92612-92613)
Swallowing and sensory assessment (92616-92617)
Flexible fiberoptic endoscopic examination/testing by cine or video recording (92612-92617)

31575 Laryngoscopy, flexible fiberoptic; diagnostic P3 T
2.28 3.44 Global Days 000

31576 with biopsy A2 T
3.70 6.77 Global Days 000

31577 with removal of foreign body A2 T 80
4.45 7.25 Global Days 000

31578 with removal of lesion A2 T 80
5.14 8.45 Global Days 000

31579 Laryngoscopy, flexible or rigid fiberoptic, with stroboscopy P3 T
4.24 6.41 Global Days 000

31580-31599 Larynx Reconstruction

31580 Laryngoplasty; for laryngeal web, 2-stage, with keel insertion and removal A2 T 80
36.52 36.52 Global Days 090

31582 for laryngeal stenosis, with graft or core mold, including tracheotomy A2 T
56.92 56.92 Global Days 090

31584 with open reduction of fracture C5 C 80
45.13 45.13 Global Days 090

31587 Laryngoplasty, cricoid split C5 C 80
29.82 29.82 Global Days 090

31588 Laryngoplasty, not otherwise specified (eg, for burns, reconstruction after partial laryngectomy) A2 T 80
34.16 34.16 Global Days 090
AMA: 2009, Jan, 11-31; 2008, Jan, 10-25; 2007, January, 13-27

31590 Laryngeal reinnervation by neuromuscular pedicle A2 T 80
26.89 26.89 Global Days 090

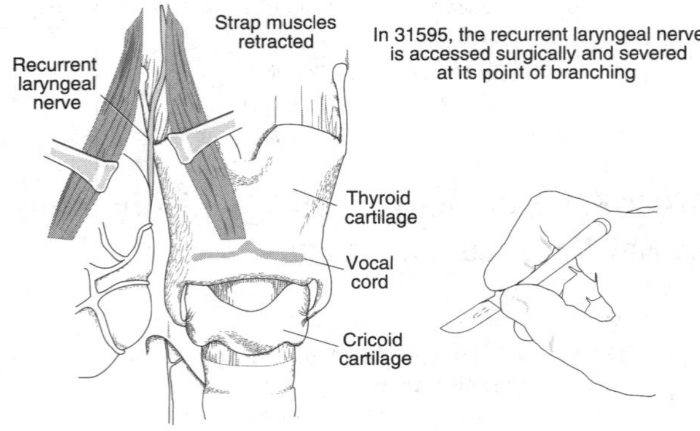

31595 Section recurrent laryngeal nerve, therapeutic (separate procedure), unilateral A2 T 80
22.95 22.95 Global Days 090

31599 Unlisted procedure, larynx T 80
0.00 0.00 Global Days YYY

31600-31610 Stoma Creation: Trachea

EXCLUDES *Aspiration of trachea, direct vision (31515)*
Endotracheal intubation (31500)

31600 Tracheostomy, planned (separate procedure); A T
11.81 11.81 Global Days 000

31601 younger than 2 years A T 80
7.78 7.78 Global Days 000

31603 Tracheostomy, emergency procedure; transtracheal A2 T
6.63 6.63 Global Days 000

31605 cricothyroid membrane G2 T
5.40 5.40 Global Days 000

31610 Tracheostomy, fenestration procedure with skin flaps T
21.32 21.32 Global Days 090

31611-31614 Procedures of the Trachea

31611 Construction of tracheoesophageal fistula and subsequent insertion of an alaryngeal speech prosthesis (eg, voice button, Blom-Singer prosthesis) A2 T 80
16.21 16.21 Global Days 090

31612 Tracheal puncture, percutaneous with transtracheal aspiration and/or injection A2 T 80
EXCLUDES *Tracheal aspiration under direct vision (31515)*
1.41 2.44 Global Days 000

31613 Tracheostoma revision; simple, without flap rotation A2 T
13.57 13.57 Global Days 090

31614 complex, with flap rotation A2 T
22.56 22.56 Global Days 090

31615 Endoscopy Through Tracheostomy

INCLUDES Diagnostic bronchoscopy

⊙ 31615 Tracheobronchoscopy through established tracheostomy incision A2 T
3.83 5.46 Global Days 000

31620 Endobronchial Ultrasound (EBUS)

+ ⊙ 31620 Endobronchial ultrasound (EBUS) during bronchoscopic diagnostic or therapeutic intervention(s) (List separately in addition to code for primary procedure[s]) N1 N
Code first (31622-31646)
2.00 8.32 Global Days ZZZ

31622-31656 Endoscopy of Lung

INCLUDES Diagnostic bronchoscopy with surgical bronchoscopy procedures
Fluoroscopic guidance for codes 31622-31646

⊙ 31622 Bronchoscopy, rigid or flexible, including fluoroscopic guidance, when performed; diagnostic, with cell washing, when performed (separate procedure) A2 T
4.34 9.38 Global Days 000
AMA: 2009, Jan, 11-31; 2008, Jan, 10-25; 2007, January, 13-27

⊙ 31623 with brushing or protected brushings A2 T
4.33 9.94 Global Days 000
AMA: 2009, Jan, 11-31; 2008, May, 9-11; 2008, Jan, 10-25; 2007, January, 13-27

⊙ 31624 with bronchial alveolar lavage A2 T
4.35 9.35 Global Days 000
AMA: 2009, Jan, 11-31; 2008, Jan, 10-25; 2008, May, 9-11; 2007, January, 13-27

⊙ 31625 with bronchial or endobronchial biopsy(s), single or multiple sites A2 T
5.04 10.04 Global Days 000
AMA: 2009, Jan, 11-31; 2008, Jan, 10-25; 2007, January, 13-27

⊙ 31626 with placement of fiducial markers, single or multiple G2 T 80
6.08 13.27 Global Days 000

+ ⊙ 31627 with computer-assisted, image-guided navigation (List separately in addition to code for primary procedure[s]) N1 N 80
INCLUDES 3D reconstruction
Code first (31615, 31622-31631, 31635-31636, 31638-31643)
Do not report with (76376-76377)
2.80 38.66 Global Days ZZZ

⊙ 31628 **with transbronchial lung biopsy(s), single lobe** A2 T

INCLUDES All biopsies taken from lobe

EXCLUDES *Transbronchial biopsies by needle aspiration (31629, 31633)*
Transbronchial biopsies of additional lobe(s) (31632)

5.59 11.52 Global Days 000

AMA: 2009, Jan, 11-31; 2008, May, 9-11; 2008, Jan, 10-25; 2007, January, 13-27

⊙ 31629 **with transbronchial needle aspiration biopsy(s), trachea, main stem and/or lobar bronchus(i)** A2 T

INCLUDES All biopsies from same lobe

EXCLUDES *Transbronchial biopsies of lung (31628, 31632)*
Transbronchial needle biopsies of another lobe(s) (31633)

6.02 18.25 Global Days 000

AMA: 2009, Jan, 11-31; 2008, Jan, 10-25; 2007, January, 13-27

31630 **with tracheal/bronchial dilation or closed reduction of fracture** A2 T

6.02 6.02 Global Days 000

31631 **with placement of tracheal stent(s) (includes tracheal/bronchial dilation as required)** A2 T

EXCLUDES *Bronchial stent placement (31636-31637)*
Revision bronchial or tracheal stent (31638)

6.83 6.83 Global Days 000

+ 31632 **with transbronchial lung biopsy(s), each additional lobe (List separately in addition to code for primary procedure)** G2 T

INCLUDES All biopsies of additional lobe of lung

Code first (31628)

1.45 2.12 Global Days ZZZ

+ 31633 **with transbronchial needle aspiration biopsy(s), each additional lobe (List separately in addition to code for primary procedure)** G2 T

INCLUDES All needle biopsies from another lobe or from trachea

Code first (31629)

1.86 2.59 Global Days ZZZ

AMA: 2009, Jan, 11-31; 2008, Jan, 10-25; 2007, January, 13-27

⊙ 31634 **with balloon occlusion, with assessment of air leak, with administration of occlusive substance (eg, fibrin glue), if performed** G2 T 80

6.33 64.90 Global Days 000

⊙ 31635 **with removal of foreign body** A2 T

EXCLUDES *Removal implanted bronchial valves (0251T, 0252T)*

5.59 10.42 Global Days 000

AMA: 2009, Jan, 11-31; 2008, Jan, 10-25; 2007, January, 13-27

31636 **with placement of bronchial stent(s) (includes tracheal/bronchial dilation as required), initial bronchus** A2 T

6.65 6.65 Global Days 000

+ 31637 **each additional major bronchus stented (List separately in addition to code for primary procedure)** A2 T

Code first (31636)

2.25 2.25 Global Days ZZZ

31638 **with revision of tracheal or bronchial stent inserted at previous session (includes tracheal/bronchial dilation as required)** A2 T

7.65 7.65 Global Days 000

31640 **with excision of tumor** A2 T

7.67 7.67 Global Days 000

31641 **with destruction of tumor or relief of stenosis by any method other than excision (eg, laser therapy, cryotherapy)** A2 T

Code also any photodynamic therapy via bronchoscopy (96570-96571)

7.66 7.66 Global Days 000

31643 **with placement of catheter(s) for intracavitary radioelement application** A2 T

Code also if appropriate (77761-77763, 77785-77787)

5.21 5.21 Global Days 000

⊙ 31645 **with therapeutic aspiration of tracheobronchial tree, initial (eg, drainage of lung abscess)** A2 T

EXCLUDES *Bedside aspiration of trachea, bronchi (31725)*

4.75 9.36 Global Days 000

⊙ 31646 **with therapeutic aspiration of tracheobronchial tree, subsequent** A2 T

EXCLUDES *Bedside aspiration of trachea, bronchi (31725)*

4.13 8.47 Global Days 000

⊙ 31656 **with injection of contrast material for segmental bronchography (fiberscope only)** A2 T 80

71040, 71060

3.23 9.08 Global Days 000

31715-31899 Respiratory Procedures

EXCLUDES *Endotracheal intubation (31500)*
Tracheal aspiration under direct vision (31515)

31715 **Transtracheal injection for bronchography** N1 N 80 50

EXCLUDES *Prolonged services (99354-99360)*

71040, 71060

1.55 1.55 Global Days 000

31717 **Catheterization with bronchial brush biopsy** A2 T

3.23 8.17 Global Days 000

AMA: 2009, Jan, 11-31; 2008, Jan, 10-25; 2007, January, 13-27

31720 **Catheter aspiration (separate procedure); nasotracheal** A2 S

1.51 1.51 Global Days 000

⊙ 31725 **tracheobronchial with fiberscope, bedside** C5 C

2.78 2.78 Global Days 000

31730 **Transtracheal (percutaneous) introduction of needle wire dilator/stent or indwelling tube for oxygen therapy** A2 T

4.35 33.13 Global Days 000

31750 **Tracheoplasty; cervical** A2 T 80

40.83 40.83 Global Days 090

31755 **tracheopharyngeal fistulization, each stage** A2 T 80

51.88 51.88 Global Days 090

31760 **intrathoracic** C5 C 80 PQ

41.37 41.37 Global Days 090

31766 **Carinal reconstruction** C5 C 80 PQ

55.64 55.64 Global Days 090

31770 **Bronchoplasty; graft repair** C5 C 80 PQ

EXCLUDES *Bronchoplasty done with lobectomy (32501)*

40.12 40.12 Global Days 090

31775 **excision stenosis and anastomosis** C5 C 80 PQ

EXCLUDES *Bronchoplasty done with lobectomy (32501)*

41.90 41.90 Global Days 090

31780 **Excision tracheal stenosis and anastomosis; cervical** C5 C 80

35.54 35.54 Global Days 090

31781 **cervicothoracic** C5 C 80
42.05 42.05 Global Days 090

31785 **Excision of tracheal tumor or carcinoma; cervical** T 80
32.10 32.10 Global Days 090

31786 **thoracic** C5 C 80 PQ
43.74 43.74 Global Days 090

31800 **Suture of tracheal wound or injury; cervical** C5 C 80
21.32 21.32 Global Days 090

31805 **intrathoracic** C5 C 80 PQ
24.61 24.61 Global Days 090

31820 **Surgical closure tracheostomy or fistula; without plastic repair** A2 T 80
EXCLUDES *Tracheoesophageal fistula repair (43305, 43312)*
9.86 13.09 Global Days 090

31825 **with plastic repair** A2 T 80
EXCLUDES *Tracheoesophageal fistula repair (43305, 43312)*
14.43 18.11 Global Days 090

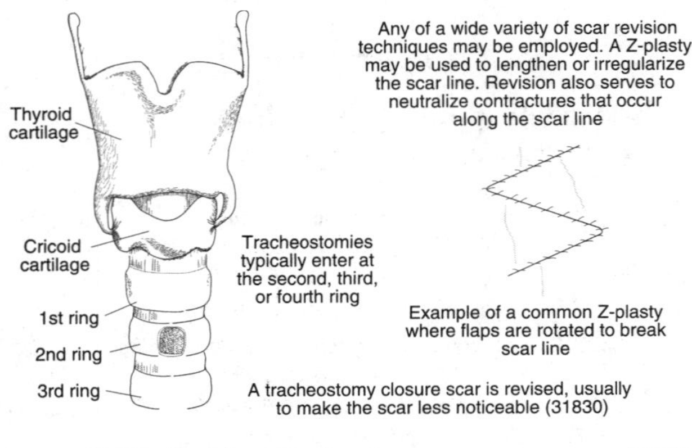

31830 **Revision of tracheostomy scar** A2 T 80
10.24 13.21 Global Days 090

31899 **Unlisted procedure, trachea, bronchi** T 80
0.00 0.00 Global Days YYY

32035-32036 Procedures for Empyema

EXCLUDES *Wound exploration without thoracotomy for penetrating wound of chest (20101)*

32035 **Thoracostomy; with rib resection for empyema** C5 C 80
21.61 21.61 Global Days 090

32036 **with open flap drainage for empyema** C5 C 80
EXCLUDES *Wound exploration due to penetrating trauma without thoracotomy (20101)*
23.40 23.40 Global Days 090

32095-32098 Open Biopsy of Chest and Pleura

INCLUDES Varying amounts of lung tissue excised for analysis
Wedge technique with tissue obtained without precise consideration of margins

EXCLUDES *Percutaneous needle biopsy of pleura, lung, and mediastinum (32400, 32405)*
Thoracoscopy with biopsy (32607-32609)
Thoracoscopy with diagnostic wedge resection resulting in anatomic lung resection (32668)
Thoracotomy with diagnostic wedge resection resulting in anatomic lung resection (32507)

~~32095~~ ~~**Thoracotomy, limited, for biopsy of lung or pleura**~~
To report, see 32096-32098

● **32096** **Thoracotomy, with diagnostic biopsy(ies) of lung infiltrate(s) (eg, wedge, incisional), unilateral** C5 C 80
Code also appropriate add-on code for the more extensive procedure at the same location if diagnostic wedge resection results in the need for further surgery (32507, 32668)
Do not report more than one time per lung
Do not report with (32440-32445, 32488)
24.25 24.25 Global Days 090

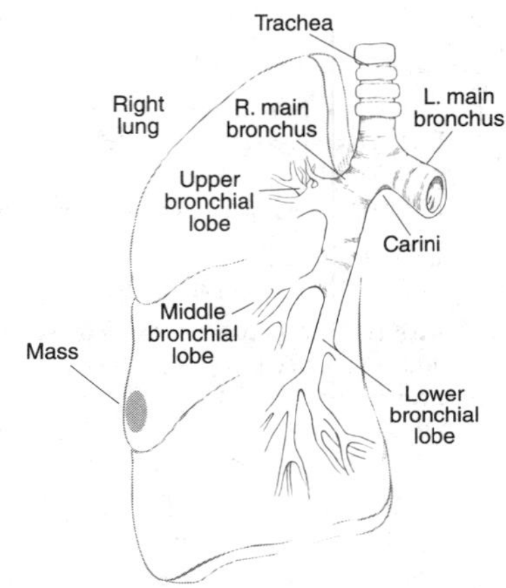

● **32097** **Thoracotomy, with diagnostic biopsy(ies) of lung nodule(s) or mass(es) (eg, wedge, incisional), unilateral** C5 C 80
Code also appropriate add-on code for the more extensive procedure in the same location if diagnostic wedge resection results in the need for further surgery (32507, 32668)
Do not report more than one time per lung
Do not report with (32440-32445, 32488)
24.25 24.25 Global Days 090

● **32098** **Thoracotomy, with biopsy(ies) of pleura** C5 C 80
22.79 22.79 Global Days 090

32100-32160 Open Procedures: Chest

INCLUDES Exploration of penetrating wound of chest

EXCLUDES *Lung resection (32480-32504)*
Wound exploration without thoractomy for penetrating wound of chest (20101)

▲ **32100** **Thoracotomy; with exploration** C5 C 80 PQ
Do not report with (19260, 19271-19272, 32503-32504)
24.96 24.96 Global Days 090
AMA: 2007, March, 1-3

▲ 32110 with control of traumatic hemorrhage and/or repair of lung tear C5 C 80 PQ
43.96 43.96 Global Days 090

▲ 32120 for postoperative complications C5 C 80 PQ
26.34 26.34 Global Days 090

▲ 32124 with open intrapleural pneumonolysis C5 C 80 PQ
28.02 28.02 Global Days 090

▲ 32140 with cyst(s) removal, includes pleural procedure when performed C5 C 80 PQ
29.91 29.91 Global Days 090

▲ 32141 with resection-plication of bullae, includes any pleural procedure when performed C5 C 80 PQ
EXCLUDES *Lung volume reduction (32491)*
45.96 45.96 Global Days 090

▲ 32150 with removal of intrapleural foreign body or fibrin deposit C5 C 80 PQ
30.21 30.21 Global Days 090

▲ 32151 with removal of intrapulmonary foreign body C5 C 80
30.41 30.41 Global Days 090

▲ 32160 with cardiac massage C5 C 80
23.46 23.46 Global Days 090

32200-32320 Open Procedures: Lung

32200 Pneumonostomy; with open drainage of abscess or cyst C5 C 80
75989
34.21 34.21 Global Days 090

⊙ 32201 with percutaneous drainage of abscess or cyst T
75989
5.85 27.30 Global Days 000

32215 Pleural scarification for repeat pneumothorax C5 C 80 PQ
24.06 24.06 Global Days 090

32220 Decortication, pulmonary (separate procedure); total C5 C 80 PQ
47.93 47.93 Global Days 090

32225 partial C5 C 80 PQ
30.03 30.03 Global Days 090

32310 Pleurectomy, parietal (separate procedure) C5 C 80 PQ
27.76 27.76 Global Days 090

32320 Decortication and parietal pleurectomy C5 C 80 PQ
48.13 48.13 Global Days 090

32400-32405 Lung Biopsy

EXCLUDES *Fine needle aspiration biopsy (10022)*
Open lung biopsy (32096-32097)
Open mediastinal biopsy (39000-39010)
Thoracoscopic (VATS) biopsy of lung, pericardium, pleural or mediastinal space (32604-32609)

32400 Biopsy, pleura; percutaneous needle A2 T
76942, 77002, 77012, 77021
2.58 4.38 Global Days 000

~~32402~~ ~~open~~
To report, see 32098

⊙ 32405 Biopsy, lung or mediastinum, percutaneous needle A2 T
76942, 77002, 77012, 77021
3.00 6.82 Global Days 000
AMA: 2009, Jan, 11-31; 2008, Jan, 10-25; 2007, January, 13-27

32420-32422 Needle Insertion: Chest

32420 Pneumocentesis, puncture of lung for aspiration A2 T
3.23 3.23 Global Days 000

32421 Thoracentesis, puncture of pleural cavity for aspiration, initial or subsequent A2 T 50
76942, 77002, 77012
2.24 4.51 Global Days 000

32422 Thoracentesis with insertion of tube, includes water seal (eg, for pneumothorax), when performed (separate procedure) G2 T 50
Do not report with (19260, 19271-19272, 32503-32504)
76942, 77002, 77012
3.61 5.71 Global Days 000

32440-32501 Lung Resection

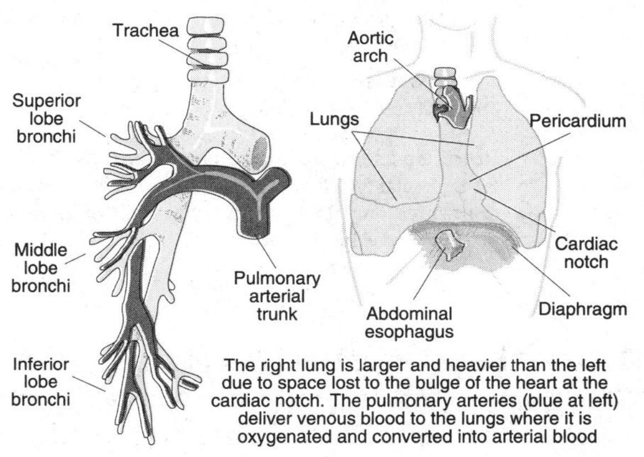

The right lung is larger and heavier than the left due to space lost to the bulge of the heart at the cardiac notch. The pulmonary arteries (blue at left) deliver venous blood to the lungs where it is oxygenated and converted into arterial blood

▲ 32440 Removal of lung, pneumonectomy; C5 C 80 PQ
Code also excision of chest wall tumor (19260-19272)
47.33 47.33 Global Days 090

▲ 32442 with resection of segment of trachea followed by broncho-tracheal anastomosis (sleeve pneumonectomy) C5 C 80 PQ
Code also excision of chest wall tumor (19260-19272)
91.89 91.89 Global Days 090

▲ 32445 extrapleural C5 C 80 PQ
Code also empyemectomy with extrapleural pneumonectomy (32540)
Code also excision of chest wall tumor (19260-19272)
105.81 105.81 Global Days 090

▲ 32480 Removal of lung, other than pneumonectomy; single lobe (lobectomy) C5 C 80 PQ
EXCLUDES *Lung removal with bronchoplasty (32501)*
Code also decortication (32320)
Code also excision of chest wall tumor (19260-19272)
44.75 44.75 Global Days 090

▲ 32482 2 lobes (bilobectomy) C5 C 80 PQ
EXCLUDES *Lung removal with bronchoplasty (32501)*
Code also decortication (32320)
Code also excision of chest wall tumor (19260-19272)
47.88 47.88 Global Days 090
AMA: 2009, Jan, 11-31; 2008, Jan, 10-25; 2007, January, 28-31

▲ 32484 **single segment (segmentectomy)**
EXCLUDES *Lung removal with bronchoplasty (32501)*
Code also decortication (32320)
Code also excision of chest wall tumor (19260-19272)
43.40 43.40 Global Days 090

▲ 32486 **with circumferential resection of segment of bronchus followed by broncho-bronchial anastomosis (sleeve lobectomy)**
Code also decortication (32320)
Code also excision of chest wall tumor (19260-19272)
71.02 71.02 Global Days 090

▲ 32488 **with all remaining lung following previous removal of a portion of lung (completion pneumonectomy)**
Code also decortication (32320)
Code also excision of chest wall tumor (19260-19272)
71.88 71.88 Global Days 090

▲ 32491 **with resection-plication of emphysematous lung(s) (bullous or non-bullous) for lung volume reduction, sternal split or transthoracic approach, includes any pleural procedure, when performed**
44.53 44.53 Global Days 090

~~32500~~ ~~wedge resection, single or multiple~~
To report, see 32505-32507

\+ 32501 **Resection and repair of portion of bronchus (bronchoplasty) when performed at time of lobectomy or segmentectomy (List separately in addition to code for primary procedure)**
Code first (32480-32484)
7.42 7.42 Global Days ZZZ

32503-32504 Excision of Lung Neoplasm

EXCLUDES *Lung resection performed in conjunction with chest wall resection*

Do not report with 19260, 19271-19272, 32100, 32422, 32551 (19260, 19271-19272, 32100, 32422, 32551)

32503 **Resection of apical lung tumor (eg, Pancoast tumor), including chest wall resection, rib(s) resection(s), neurovascular dissection, when performed; without chest wall reconstruction(s)**
54.97 54.97 Global Days 090

32504 **with chest wall reconstruction**
61.96 61.96 Global Days 090

32505-32507 Thoracotomy with Wedge Resection

INCLUDES Wedge technique with tissue obtained with precise consideration of margins and complete resection

Code also resection of chest wall tumor with lung resection when performed (19260-19272)

● 32505 **Thoracotomy; with therapeutic wedge resection (eg, mass, nodule), initial**
Code also a more extensive procedure of the lung when performed on the contralateral lung or different lobe with modifier 59 regardless of intraoperative pathology consultation
Do not report with (32440, 32442, 32445, 32488)
27.98 27.98 Global Days 090

\+ ● 32506 **with therapeutic wedge resection (eg, mass or nodule), each additional resection, ipsilateral (List separately in addition to code for primary procedure)**
Code first (32505)
Code also a more extensive procedure of the lung when performed on the contralateral lung or different lobe with modifier 59
4.72 4.72 Global Days ZZZ

\+ ● 32507 **with diagnostic wedge resection followed by anatomic lung resection (List separately in addition to code for primary procedure)**
INCLUDES Classification as a diagnostic wedge resection if intraoperative pathology consultation dictates more extensive resection in the same anatomical area
EXCLUDES *Diagnostic wedge resection by thoracoscopy (32668)*
Therapeutic wedge resection (32505-32506, 32666-32667)
Code first (32440, 32442, 32445, 32480-32488, 32503-32504)
4.72 4.72 Global Days ZZZ

32540 Removal of Empyema

32540 **Extrapleural enucleation of empyema (empyemectomy)**
EXCLUDES *Lung removal code when empyemectomy is performed with lobectomy (see appropriate lung removal code)*
Code also appropriate removal of lung code when done with lobectomy (32480-32488)
51.81 51.81 Global Days 090

32550-32552 Chest Tube/Catheter

⊙ 32550 **Insertion of indwelling tunneled pleural catheter with cuff**
Code also (C1729)
Do not report with (32421-32422)
75989
6.68 23.63 Global Days 000

⊙ 32551 **Tube thoracostomy, includes water seal (eg, for abscess, hemothorax, empyema), when performed (separate procedure)**
Do not report with (19260, 19271-19272, 32503-32504)
75989
5.06 5.06 Global Days 000

32552 **Removal of indwelling tunneled pleural catheter with cuff**
4.94 5.69 Global Days 010

32553 Intrathoracic Placement Radiation Therapy Devices

⊙ 32553 **Placement of interstitial device(s) for radiation therapy guidance (eg, fiducial markers, dosimeter), percutaneous, intra-thoracic, single or multiple**
EXCLUDES *Percutaneous placement of interstitial device(s) for radiation therapy guidance: intra-abdominal, intrapelvic, and/or retroperitoneal (49411)*
76942, 77002, 77012, 77021
6.14 17.34 Global Days 000

32560-32562 Instillation Drug/Chemical by Chest Tube

EXCLUDES *Insertion of chest tube (32551)*

32560 **Instillation, via chest tube/catheter, agent for pleurodesis (eg, talc for recurrent or persistent pneumothorax)**
2.41 7.55 Global Days 000

32561 **Instillation(s), via chest tube/catheter, agent for fibrinolysis (eg, fibrinolytic agent for break-up of multiloculated effusion); initial day** T 80

Do not report more than one time on the date of initial treatment

2.10 2.78 Global Days 000

32562 **subsequent day** T 80

Do not report more than one time on each day of subsequent treatment

1.88 2.51 Global Days 000

32601-32674 Thoracic Surgery: Video-Assisted (VATS)

CMS 100-3,100.2 Endoscopy
CMS 100-4,12,40.6 Multiple procedures

INCLUDES Diagnostic thoracoscopy in surgical thoracoscopy

▲ **32601** **Thoracoscopy, diagnostic (separate procedure); lungs, pericardial sac, mediastinal or pleural space, without biopsy** T 80

9.35 9.35 Global Days 000

~~32602~~ ~~lungs and pleural space, with biopsy~~

To report, see 32607-32609

~~32603~~ ~~pericardial sac, without biopsy~~

To report, see 32601

32604 **pericardial sac, with biopsy** T 80

EXCLUDES *Open biopsy of pericardium (39010)*

14.57 14.57 Global Days 000

~~32605~~ ~~mediastinal space, without biopsy~~

To report, see 32601

32606 **mediastinal space, with biopsy** T 80

13.96 13.96 Global Days 000

● **32607** **Thoracoscopy; with diagnostic biopsy(ies) of lung infiltrate(s) (eg, wedge, incisional), unilateral** T 80

Do not report more than one time per lung

Do not report with (32440-32445, 32488, 32671)

9.29 9.29 Global Days 000

● **32608** **with diagnostic biopsy(ies) of lung nodule(s) or mass(es) (eg, wedge, incisional), unilateral** T 80

Do not report more than one time per lung

Do not report with (32440-32445, 32488, 32671)

11.41 11.41 Global Days 000

● **32609** **with biopsy(ies) of pleura** T 80

7.89 7.89 Global Days 000

32650 **Thoracoscopy, surgical; with pleurodesis (eg, mechanical or chemical)** C5 C 80

20.13 20.13 Global Days 090

32651 **with partial pulmonary decortication** C5 C 80

32.78 32.78 Global Days 090

32652 **with total pulmonary decortication, including intrapleural pneumonolysis** C5 C 80

49.76 49.76 Global Days 090

32653 **with removal of intrapleural foreign body or fibrin deposit** C5 C 80

31.68 31.68 Global Days 090

32654 **with control of traumatic hemorrhage** C5 C 80

35.32 35.32 Global Days 090

▲ **32655** **with resection-plication of bullae, includes any pleural procedure when performed** C5 C 80

EXCLUDES *Thorascopic lung volume reduction surgery (32672)*

28.77 28.77 Global Days 090

AMA: 2009, Jan, 11-31; 2008, Jan, 10-25; 2007, January, 13-27

32656 **with parietal pleurectomy** C5 C 80

24.07 24.07 Global Days 090

~~32657~~ ~~with wedge resection of lung, single or multiple~~

To report, see 32666-32668

32658 **with removal of clot or foreign body from pericardial sac** C5 C 80

21.61 21.61 Global Days 090

32659 **with creation of pericardial window or partial resection of pericardial sac for drainage** C5 C 80

22.13 22.13 Global Days 090

~~32660~~ ~~with total pericardiectomy~~

32661 **with excision of pericardial cyst, tumor, or mass** C5 C 80

24.15 24.15 Global Days 090

32662 **with excision of mediastinal cyst, tumor, or mass** C5 C 80

27.01 27.01 Global Days 090

AMA: 2009, Jan, 11-31; 2007, Dec, 10-179

▲ **32663** **with lobectomy (single lobe)** C5 C 80 PQ

EXCLUDES *Thoracoscopic segmentectomy (32669)*

42.28 42.28 Global Days 090

32664 **with thoracic sympathectomy** C5 C 80 50

25.61 25.61 Global Days 090

AMA: 2009, Jan, 11-31; 2008, Jan, 10-25; 2007, January, 13-27

32665 **with esophagomyotomy (Heller type)** C5 C 80

EXCLUDES *Exploratory thoracoscopy with and without biopsy (32601-32609)*

36.65 36.65 Global Days 090

● **32666** **with therapeutic wedge resection (eg, mass, nodule), initial unilateral** C5 C 80

Code also a more extensive procedure of the lung when performed on the contralateral lung or different lobe with modifier 59 regardless of pathology consultation

Do not report with (32440-32445, 32488, 32671)

26.17 26.17 Global Days 090

+ ● **32667** **with therapeutic wedge resection (eg, mass or nodule), each additional resection, ipsilateral (List separately in addition to code for primary procedure)** C5 C 80

Code also a more extensive procedure of the lung when performed on the contralateral lung or different lobe with modifier 59 regardless of intraoperative pathology consultation

Code first (32666)

Do not report with (32440-32445, 32488, 32671)

4.72 4.72 Global Days ZZZ

+ ● **32668** **with diagnostic wedge resection followed by anatomic lung resection (List separately in addition to code for primary procedure)** C5 C 80

INCLUDES Classification as a diagnostic wedge resection if intraoperative pathology consultation dictates more extensive resection in the same anatomical area

Code first (32440-32488, 32503-32504, 32663, 32669-32671)

4.75 4.75 Global Days ZZZ

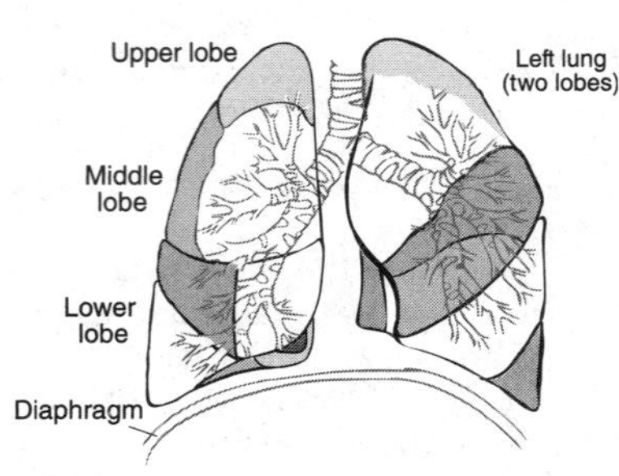

● 32669 with removal of a single lung segment (segmentectomy) C5 C 80
40.30 40.30 Global Days 090

● 32670 with removal of 2 lobes (bilobectomy) C5 C 80
48.09 48.09 Global Days 090

● 32671 with removal of lung (pneumonectomy) C5 C 80
53.40 53.40 Global Days 090

● 32672 with resection-plication for emphysematous lung (bullous or non-bullous) for lung volume reduction (LVRS), unilateral includes any pleural procedure, when performed C5 C 80
45.67 45.67 Global Days 090

● 32673 with resection of thymus, unilateral or bilateral C5 C 80

EXCLUDES *Exploratory thoracoscopy with and without biopsy (32601-32609)*
Open excision mediastinal cyst (39200)
Open excision mediastinal tumor (39220)
Open thymectomy (60520-60522)

35.99 35.99 Global Days 090

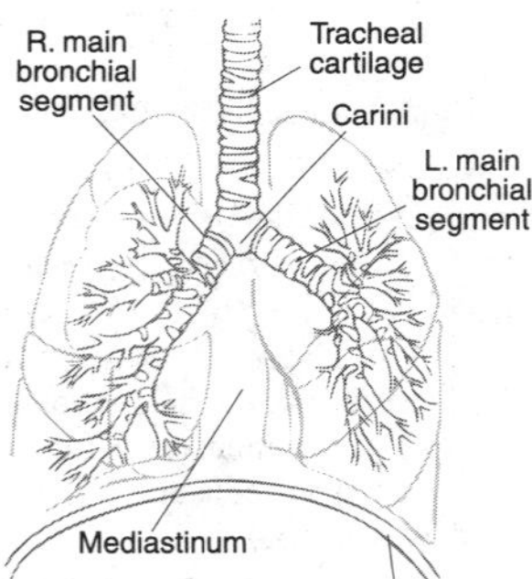

+ ● 32674 with mediastinal and regional lymphadenectomy (List separately in addition to code for primary procedure) C5 C 80

INCLUDES Mediastinal lymph nodes:
Left side:
Aortopulmonary window
Inferior pulmonary ligament
Paraesophageal
Subcarinal
Right side:
Inferior pulmonary ligament
Paraesophageal
Paratracheal
Subcarinal

EXCLUDES *Mediastinal and regional lymphadenectomy by thoracotomy (38746)*

Code first (32440, 32442, 32445, 32480, 32482, 32484, 32486, 32488, 32503-32505, 32663, 32666-32667, 32669-32671)
6.47 6.47 Global Days ZZZ

32800-32820 Chest Repair and Reconstruction Procedures

32800 Repair lung hernia through chest wall C5 C 80 PQ
28.37 28.37 Global Days 090

32810 Closure of chest wall following open flap drainage for empyema (Clagett type procedure) C5 C 80 PQ
27.19 27.19 Global Days 090

32815 Open closure of major bronchial fistula C5 C 80 PQ
83.99 83.99 Global Days 090

32820 Major reconstruction, chest wall (posttraumatic) C5 C 80
40.28 40.28 Global Days 090

32850-32856 Lung Transplant Procedures

INCLUDES Harvesting donor lung(s), cold preservation, preparation of donor lung(s), transplantation into recipient

EXCLUDES *Repairs or resection of donor lung(s) (32491, 32505-32507, 35216, 35276)*

32850 Donor pneumonectomy(s) (including cold preservation), from cadaver donor C5 C
0.00 0.00 Global Days XXX

32851 Lung transplant, single; without cardiopulmonary bypass C5 C 80
99.53 99.53 Global Days 090

32852 with cardiopulmonary bypass C5 C 80
109.09 109.09 Global Days 090

32853 Lung transplant, double (bilateral sequential or en bloc); without cardiopulmonary bypass C5 C 80
137.56 137.56 Global Days 090

32854 with cardiopulmonary bypass C5 C 80
146.52 146.52 Global Days 090

32855 Backbench standard preparation of cadaver donor lung allograft prior to transplantation, including dissection of allograft from surrounding soft tissues to prepare pulmonary venous/atrial cuff, pulmonary artery, and bronchus; unilateral C5 C 80
0.00 0.00 Global Days XXX

32856 bilateral C5 C 80
0.00 0.00 Global Days XXX

32900-32997 Chest and Respiratory Procedures

CMS 100-4,12,40.6 Multiple procedures

32900 Resection of ribs, extrapleural, all stages C5 C 80 PQ
41.80 41.80 Global Days 090

32905 Thoracoplasty, Schede type or extrapleural (all stages); C5 C 80 PQ
40.31 40.31 Global Days 090

32906 with closure of bronchopleural fistula C5 C 80 PQ

EXCLUDES *Open closure of bronchial fistula (32815)*
Resection first rib for thoracic compression (21615, 21616)

49.84 49.84 Global Days 090

32940 Pneumonolysis, extraperiosteal, including filling or packing procedures C5 C 80 PQ
37.17 37.17 Global Days 090

32960 Pneumothorax, therapeutic, intrapleural injection of air G2 T
3.08 4.12 Global Days 000

32997 **Total lung lavage (unilateral)**

EXCLUDES *Broncho-alveolar lavage by bronchoscopy (31624)*

10.49 10.49 Global Days 000

32998-32999 Destruction of Lung Neoplasm

32998 **Ablation therapy for reduction or eradication of 1 or more pulmonary tumor(s) including pleura or chest wall when involved by tumor extension, percutaneous, radiofrequency, unilateral**

76940, 77013, 77022

8.56 86.41 Global Days 000

32999 **Unlisted procedure, lungs and pleura**

0.00 0.00 Global Days YYY

AMA: 2009, Jan, 11-31; 2008, Jan, 10-25; 2008, Jul, 10&13; 2007, January, 13-27

33010-33050 Procedures of the Pericardial Sac

EXCLUDES *Surgical thoracoscopy (video-assisted thoracic surgery [VATS]) procedures of pericardium (32601, 32604, 32658-32659, 32661)*

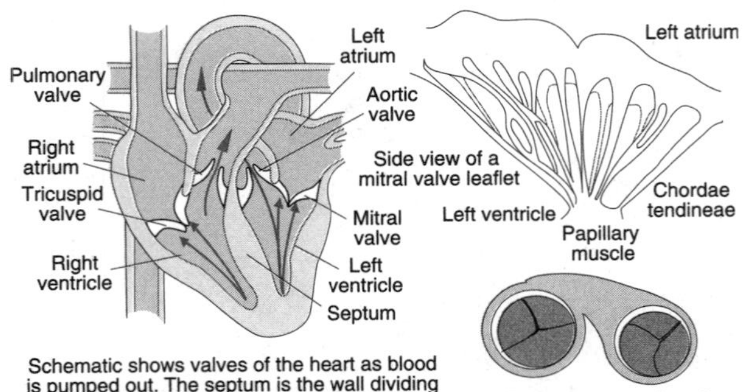

Schematic shows valves of the heart as blood is pumped out. The septum is the wall dividing the left and right ventricles. The papillary muscles and chordae tendineae (above right) function to open and close the atrioventricular valves

Overhead view of aortic (left) and pulmonary valves while closed

⊙ **33010 Pericardiocentesis; initial** A2 T
76930
3.59 3.59 Global Days 000

⊙ **33011 subsequent** A2 T 80
76930
3.62 3.62 Global Days 000

33015 Tube pericardiostomy C5 C
15.35 15.35 Global Days 090

33020 Pericardiotomy for removal of clot or foreign body (primary procedure) C5 C 80 PQ
26.47 26.47 Global Days 090

33025 Creation of pericardial window or partial resection for drainage C5 C 80 PQ
EXCLUDES *Surgical thoracoscopy (video-assisted thoracic surgery [VATS]) creation of pericardial window (32659)*
24.20 24.20 Global Days 090

33030 Pericardiectomy, subtotal or complete; without cardiopulmonary bypass C5 C 80 PQ
INCLUDES Delorme pericardiectomy
59.48 59.48 Global Days 090

33031 with cardiopulmonary bypass C5 C 80 PQ
73.16 73.16 Global Days 090

▲ **33050 Resection of pericardial cyst or tumor** C5 C 80 PQ
EXCLUDES *Open biopsy of pericardium (39010)*
Surgical thoracoscopy (video-assisted thoracic surgery [VATS]) resection of cyst, mass, or tumor of pericardium (32661)
30.34 30.34 Global Days 090

33120-33130 Neoplasms of Heart

33120 Excision of intracardiac tumor, resection with cardiopulmonary bypass C5 C 80 PQ
62.96 62.96 Global Days 090
AMA: 2007, March, 1-3

33130 Resection of external cardiac tumor C5 C 80 PQ
42.10 42.10 Global Days 090
AMA: 2007, March, 1-3

33140-33141 Transmyocardial Revascularization

CMS 100-3,20.6 Transmyocardial Revascularization (TMR) for Severe Angina

33140 Transmyocardial laser revascularization, by thoracotomy; (separate procedure) C5 C 80 PQ
48.08 48.08 Global Days 090
AMA: 2009, Jan, 11-31; 2008, Jan, 10-25; 2007, January, 13-27

\+ **33141 performed at the time of other open cardiac procedure(s) (List separately in addition to code for primary procedure)** C5 C 80 PQ
Code first (33400-33496, 33510-33536, 33542)
4.09 4.09 Global Days ZZZ

33202-33203 Placement Epicardial Leads

Code also insertion of pulse generator when performed by same physician/same surgical session. (33212-33213, [33221], 33240, [33230, 33231])

33202 Insertion of epicardial electrode(s); open incision (eg, thoracotomy, median sternotomy, subxiphoid approach) C5 C PQ
23.50 23.50 Global Days 090

33203 endoscopic approach (eg, thoracoscopy, pericardioscopy) C5 C PQ
24.42 24.42 Global Days 090

33206-33221 [33221] Pacemakers/Implantable Defibrillators

CMS 100-3,20.4 Implantable Automatic Defibrillators
CMS 100-3,20.8 Cardiac Pacemakers
CMS 100-3,20.8.1 Cardiac Pacemaker Evaluation Services
CMS 100-3,20.8.1.1 Transtelephonic Monitoring of Cardiac Pacemakers
CMS 100-3,20.8.2 Self-contained Pacemaker Monitors

INCLUDES Dual lead: device that paces and senses in two heart chambers
Multiple lead: device that paces and senses in three or more heart chambers
Radiological supervision and interpretation for pacemaker or pacing cardioverter defibrillator procedure
Single lead: device that paces and senses in one heart chamber

EXCLUDES *Defibrillator threshold testing (DFT) at the same time as insertion or replacement (93640-93641)*
Upgrade from single to dual pacemaker (33214)

Do not report with codes for device evaluation (93279-93299)

⊙ ▲ **33206 Insertion of new or replacement of permanent pacemaker with transvenous electrode(s); atrial** J8 T PQ
INCLUDES Pulse generator insertion/electrode placement
Code also (C1779, C1785, C1786, C1898, C2619, C2620, C2621)
Code also removal of pacemaker pulse generator when removal and replacement of pulse generator and electrodes is performed (33233, 33234, 33235)
Do not report with ([33227, 33228, 33229])
13.74 13.74 Global Days 090
AMA: 2009, Jan, 11-31; 2008, Jun, 14-15

⊙ ▲ 33207 **ventricular** J8 T CCI PQ

INCLUDES Pulse generator insertion/electrode placement

Code also (C1779, C1785, C1786, C1898, C2619, C2620, C2621)

Code also removal of pacemaker pulse generator when removal and replacement of pulse generator and electrodes is performed (33233 and 33234 or 33235) (33224 or 33225, 33233)

Do not report with ([33227, 33228, 33229])

14.60 14.60 Global Days 090

AMA: 2009, Jan, 11-31; 2008, Jun, 14-15

⊙ ▲ 33208 **atrial and ventricular** J8 T CCI PQ

INCLUDES Pulse generator insertion/electrode placement

Code also (C1779, C1785, C1898, C2619, C2621)

Code also removal of pacemaker pulse generator when removal and replacement of pulse generator and electrodes is performed (33233, 33234, 33235)

Do not report with ([33227, 33228, 33229])

15.76 15.76 Global Days 090

AMA: 2009, Jan, 11-31; 2008, Jan, 10-25; 2008, Jun, 14-15; 2007, January, 13-27

⊙ 33210 **Insertion or replacement of temporary transvenous single chamber cardiac electrode or pacemaker catheter (separate procedure)** G2 T CCI

5.39 5.39 Global Days 000

AMA: 2007, March, 1-3

⊙ 33211 **Insertion or replacement of temporary transvenous dual chamber pacing electrodes (separate procedure)** G2 T CCI

Code also (C1779, C1898)

5.50 5.50 Global Days 000

AMA: 2007, March, 1-3

⊙ ▲ 33212 **Insertion of pacemaker pulse generator only; with existing single lead** J8 T CCI PQ

EXCLUDES *Removal and replacement of pacemaker pulse generator when appropriate ([33227, 33228, 33229])*

Code also (C1786, C2620, C2621)

Code also placement of epicardial leads by same physician/same surgical session (33202-33203)

Do not report with removal and replacement of pacemaker pulse generator (33233)

9.97 9.97 Global Days 090

AMA: 2009, Jan, 11-31; 2008, Jan, 10-25; 2008, Jun, 14-15; 2007, January, 13-27

⊙ ▲ 33213 **with existing dual leads** J8 T CCI PQ

EXCLUDES *Pulse generator replacement ([33227, 33228, 33229])*

Code also (C1785, C2619, C2621)

Code also placement of epicardial leads by same physician/same surgical session (33202-33203)

Do not report with removal and replacement of pacemaker pulse generator (33233)

10.51 10.51 Global Days 090

AMA: 2009, Jan, 11-31; 2008, Jan, 10-25; 2008, Jun, 14-15; 2007, January, 13-27

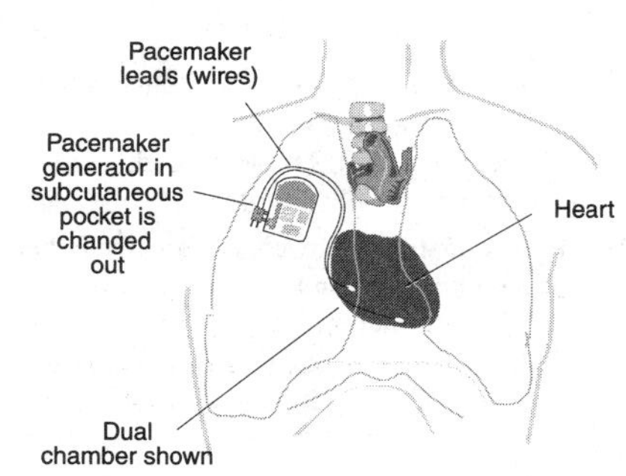

⊙ #● 33221 **with existing multiple leads** J8 T

EXCLUDES *Removal and replacement of pacemaker pulse generator when appropriate ([33227, 33228, 33229])*

Code also placement of epicardial leads by same physician/same surgical session (33202-33203)

Do not report with removal and replacement of the pacemaker pulse generator (33233)

10.52 10.52 Global Days 090

33214-33249 [33227, 33228, 33229, 33230, 33231, 33262, 33263, 33264] Pacemakers/Implantable Defibrillator/Electrode Insertion/Replacement/Revision/Repair

INCLUDES Dual lead: device that paces and senses in two heart chambers

Multiple lead: device that paces and senses in three or more heart chambers

Radiological supervision and interpretation for pacemaker or pacing cardioverter defibrillator procedure

Single lead: device that paces and senses in one heart chamber

Do not report with codes for device evaluation (93279-93299)

⊙ 33214 **Upgrade of implanted pacemaker system, conversion of single chamber system to dual chamber system (includes removal of previously placed pulse generator, testing of existing lead, insertion of new lead, insertion of new pulse generator)** J8 T 80 CCI PQ

Code also (C1779, C1785, C1898, C2619, C2621)

Do not report with ([33227, 33228, 33229])

14.48 14.48 Global Days 090

AMA: 2008, Jun, 14-15

33215 **Repositioning of previously implanted transvenous pacemaker or pacing cardioverter-defibrillator (right atrial or right ventricular) electrode** G2 T CCI PQ

9.15 9.15 Global Days 090

⊙ 33216 **Insertion of a single transvenous electrode, permanent pacemaker or cardioverter-defibrillator** G2 T CCI PQ

EXCLUDES *Insertion or replacement of a lead for a cardiac venous system (33224-33225)*

Code also (C1777, C1779, C1895, C1896, C1898, C1899)

Do not report with (33214)

11.28 11.28 Global Days 090

AMA: 2009, Jan, 11-31; 2008, Jan, 10-25; 2007, January, 13-27

⊙ **33217 Insertion of 2 transvenous electrodes, permanent pacemaker or cardioverter-defibrillator** G2 T PO

EXCLUDES *Insertion or replacement of a lead for a cardiac venous system (33224-33225)*

Code also (C1777, C1779, C1895, C1896, C1898, C1899)

Do not report with (33214)

11.23 11.23 Global Days 090

AMA: 2009, Jan, 11-31; 2008, Jan, 10-25; 2007, January, 13-27

⊙ ▲ **33218 Repair of single transvenous electrode, permanent pacemaker or pacing cardioverter-defibrillator** G2 T PO

Code also for repair one transvenous electrode with replacement pulse generator for permanent pacemaker ([33227, 33228, 33229])

Code also with repair of two transvenous electrodes for replacement of pulse generator for pacing cardioverter-defibrillator ([33262, 33263, 33264])

11.79 11.79 Global Days 090

AMA: 2009, Jan, 11-31; 2008, Jan, 10-25; 2007, January, 13-27

⊙ ▲ **33220 Repair of 2 transvenous electrodes for permanent pacemaker or pacing cardioverter-defibrillator** G2 T PO

Code also for repair two transvenous electrodes with replacement pulse generator for permanent pacemaker ([33228, 33229])

Code also modifier 52 Reduced services, when one electrode of a two-chamber system is repaired

Code also with repair of two transvenous electrodes for replacement of pulse generator for pacing cardioverter-defibrillator ([33263, 33264])

11.89 11.89 Global Days 090

AMA: 2009, Jan, 11-31; 2008, Jun, 14-15

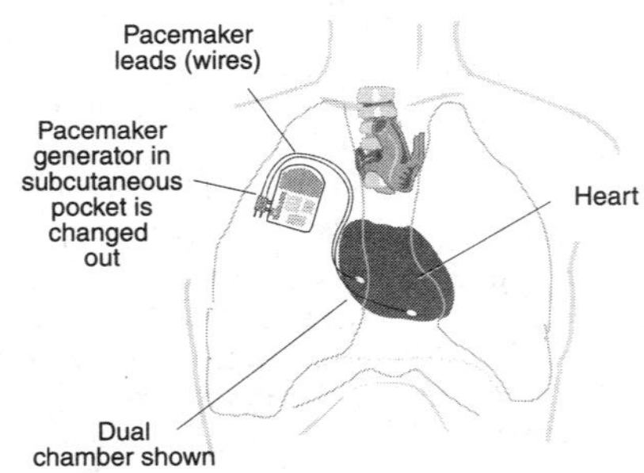

33221 Resequenced Code. See code following 33213.

⊙ **33222 Revision or relocation of skin pocket for pacemaker** A2 T PO

10.40 10.40 Global Days 090

AMA: 2008, Jun, 14-15

⊙ **33223 Revision of skin pocket for cardioverter-defibrillator** A2 T 80 PO

12.44 12.44 Global Days 090

AMA: 2008, Jun, 14-15

▲ **33224 Insertion of pacing electrode, cardiac venous system, for left ventricular pacing, with attachment to previously placed pacemaker or pacing cardioverter-defibrillator pulse generator (including revision of pocket, removal, insertion, and/or replacement of existing generator)** J8 T PO

Code also (C1900)

Code also placement of epicardial electrode when appropriate (33202-33203)

15.23 15.23 Global Days 000

AMA: 2009, Jan, 11-31; 2007, Dec, 10-179

\+ ▲ **33225 Insertion of pacing electrode, cardiac venous system, for left ventricular pacing, at time of insertion of pacing cardioverter-defibrillator or pacemaker pulse generator (including upgrade to dual chamber system and pocket revision) (List separately in addition to code for primary procedure)** J8 03 PO

Code first (33206-33208, 33212-33214 [33221], 33216-33217, 33222, 33233, 33234-33235, 33240, [33230], [33231], 33249)

13.69 13.69 Global Days ZZZ

AMA: 2009, Jan, 11-31; 2007, Dec, 10-179

▲ **33226 Repositioning of previously implanted cardiac venous system (left ventricular) electrode (including removal, insertion and/or replacement of existing generator)** G2 T PO

14.66 14.66 Global Days 000

33227 Resequenced Code. See code following 33233.

33228 Resequenced Code. See code following 33233.

33229 Resequenced Code. See code before 33234.

33230 Resequenced Code. See code following 33240.

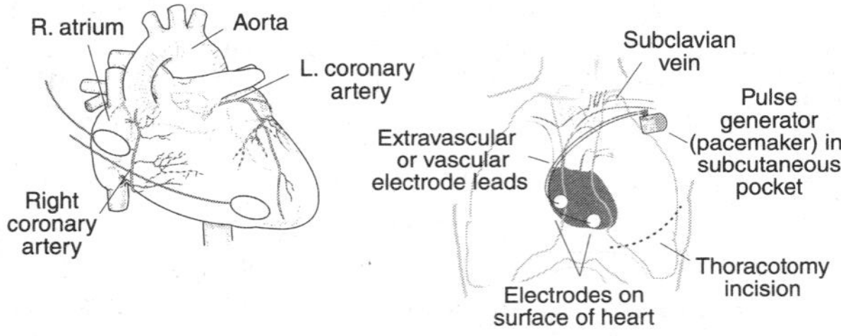

33231 Resequenced Code. See code before 33241.

⊙ ▲ **33233 Removal of permanent pacemaker pulse generator only** A2 T PO

EXCLUDES *Removal and replacement of pacemaker pulse generator and transvenous electrode(s): code 33233 with 33206-33208 and 33234 or 33235 (33206-33208, 33233, 33234 or 33235)*

7.15 7.15 Global Days 090

AMA: 2009, Jan, 11-31; 2008, Jan, 10-25; 2007, January, 13-27

⊙ #● **33227 Removal of permanent pacemaker pulse generator with replacement of pacemaker pulse generator; single lead system** J8 T

Do not report with (33233)

10.04 10.04 Global Days 090

⊙ #● **33228 dual lead system** J8 T

Do not report with (33233)

10.47 10.47 Global Days 090

⊙ #● **33229 multiple lead system** J8 T

Do not report with (33233)

10.90 10.90 Global Days 090

⊙ 33234 **Removal of transvenous pacemaker electrode(s); single lead system, atrial or ventricular** G2 T CCI PQ

Code also pacing electrode insertion in cardiac venous system for pacing of left ventricle during insertion of pulse generator (pacemaker or pacing cardioverter-defibrillator) when performed (33225)

EXCLUDES *Removal and replacement of pacemaker pulse generator and transvenous electrode(s) (33206 or 33207 or 33208, 33233, 33234 or 33235)*

Thoracotomy to remove electrodes (33238)

14.61 14.61 Global Days 090

⊙ 33235 **dual lead system** G2 T CCI PQ

Code also pacing electrode insertion in cardiac venous system for pacing of left ventricle during insertion of pulse generator (pacemaker or pacing cardioverter-defibrillator) when performed

EXCLUDES *Removal and replacement of pacemaker pulse generator and transvenous electrode(s) (33206 or 33207 or 33208, 33233, 33234 or 33235)*

Thoracotomy to remove electrodes (33238, 33243)

19.09 19.09 Global Days 090

33236 **Removal of permanent epicardial pacemaker and electrodes by thoracotomy; single lead system, atrial or ventricular** C5 C 80 CCI PQ

EXCLUDES *Removal of pacing cardioverter-defibrillator electrode(s) by thoracotomy (33243)*

Removal of transvenous pacemaker electrodes, single or dual lead system (33234, 33235)

23.95 23.95 Global Days 090

33237 **dual lead system** C5 C 80 CCI PQ

EXCLUDES *Removal of pacing cardioverter-defibrillator electrode(s) by thoracotomy (33243)*

Removal of transvenous pacemaker electrodes, single or dual lead system (33234, 33235)

25.09 25.09 Global Days 090

33238 **Removal of permanent transvenous electrode(s) by thoracotomy** C5 C 80 CCI PQ

EXCLUDES *Removal of pacing cardioverter-defibrillator electrode(s) by thoracotomy (33243)*

Removal of transvenous pacemaker electrodes, single or dual lead system (33234, 33235)

28.52 28.52 Global Days 090

⊙ ▲ 33240 **Insertion of pacing cardioverter-defibrillator pulse generator only; with existing single lead** J8 T CCI PQ

EXCLUDES *Placement of epicardial leads by same physican/same surgical session (33202-33203)*

Removal and replacement of pacing cardioverter-defibrillator pulse generator ([33262, 33263, 33264])

Code also cardioverter-defibrillator (C1721-C1722, C1882)

11.57 11.57 Global Days 090

AMA: 2009, Jan, 11-31; 2008, Jan, 10-25; 2008, Jun, 14-15; 2007, January, 13-27

⊙ #● 33230 **Insertion of pacing cardioverter-defibrillator pulse generator only; with existing dual leads** J8 T

EXCLUDES *Removal and replacement of pacing cardioverter-defibrillator pulse generator ([33262, 33263, 33264])*

Code also placement of epicardial leads by same physician/same surgical session (33202-33203)

11.32 11.32 Global Days 090

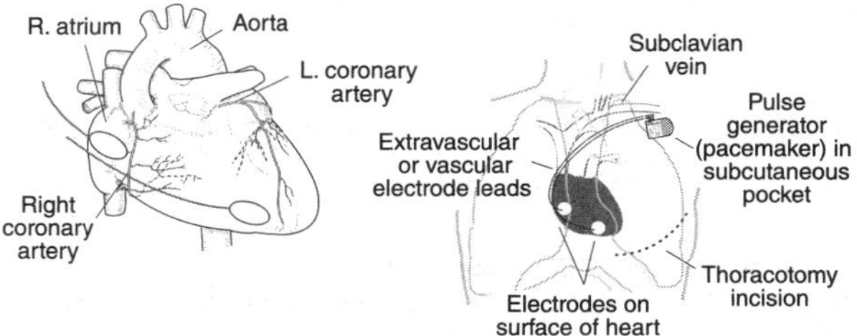

⊙ #● 33231 **with existing multiple leads** J8 T

EXCLUDES *Removal and replacement of pacing cardioverter-defibrillator pulse generator ([33262, 33263, 33264])*

Code also placement of epicardial leads by same physician/same surgical session (33202-33203)

11.75 11.75 Global Days 090

⊙ ▲ 33241 **Removal of pacing cardioverter-defibrillator pulse generator only** G2 T CCI PQ

Code also electrode removal by thoracotomy (33243)

Code also removal with reinsertion of pacing cardioverter-defibrillator with electrodes (33243 or 33244, 33249)

Code also transvenous removal or electrode(s) (33244)

Do not report with ([33262, 33263, 33264])

6.71 6.71 Global Days 090

#● 33262 **Removal of pacing cardioverter-defibrillator pulse generator with replacement of pacing cardioverter-defibrillator pulse generator; single lead system**

EXCLUDES *Repair of cardioverter-defibrillator pulse leads (33218, 33220)*

Code also electrode(s) removal by thoracotomy (33243)

Code also transvenous removal of electrode(s) (33244)

Do not report with (33241)

10.91 10.91 Global Days 090

#● 33263 **dual lead system**

EXCLUDES *Repair of cardioverter-defibrillator pulse generator and/or leads (33218, 33220)*

Code also removal of electrodes by thoracotomy (33243)

Code also transvenous removal of electrodes (33244)

11.34 11.34 Global Days 090

#● 33264 **multiple lead system**

EXCLUDES *Repair of cardioverter-defibrillator pulse generator and/or leads (33218, 33220)*

Code also removal of electrodes by thoracotomy (33243)

Code also transvenous removal of electrodes (33244)

Do not report with (33241)

11.77 11.77 Global Days 090

33243 **Removal of single or dual chamber pacing cardioverter-defibrillator electrode(s); by thoracotomy**

Code also removal and replacement of pacing cardioverter defibrillator system (electrodes and pulse generator) (33241, 33249)

EXCLUDES *Transvenous removal of cardioverter-defibrillator electrode(s) (33244)*

41.42 41.42 Global Days 090

⊙ 33244 **by transvenous extraction**

EXCLUDES *Thoracotomy to remove electrodes (33243)*

Code also transvenous removal and replacement of pacing cardioverter-defibrillator system (electrodes and pulse generator)--report with (33241, 33249)

25.63 25.63 Global Days 090

⊙ ▲ 33249 **Insertion or replacement of permanent pacing cardioverter-defibrillator system with transvenous lead(s), single or dual chamber**

EXCLUDES *Implantable cardioverter defibrillator lead(s) insertion without thoracotomy (33216-33217)*
Upgrade from single-chamber system to dual-chamber system (33214)

Code also cardio-defibrillator (C1721-C1722, C1882)

Code also removal/replacement pacing cardioverter-defibrillator system; report with (33241, 33243 or 33244)

27.19 27.19 Global Days 090

AMA: 2008, May, 9-11; 2008, Jun, 14-15

33250-33251 Surgical Ablation Arrhythmogenic Foci, Supraventricular

INCLUDES Procedures using cryotherapy, laser, microwave, radiofrequency, and ultrasound

33250 **Operative ablation of supraventricular arrhythmogenic focus or pathway (eg, Wolff-Parkinson-White, atrioventricular node re-entry), tract(s) and/or focus (foci); without cardiopulmonary bypass**

EXCLUDES *Pacing and mapping during surgery by other provider (93631)*

44.50 44.50 Global Days 090

33251 **with cardiopulmonary bypass**

49.43 49.43 Global Days 090

33254-33256 Surgical Ablation Arrhythmogenic Foci, Atrial (e.g., Maze)

INCLUDES Excision or isolation of the left atrial appendage
Procedures using cryotherapy, laser, microwave, radiofrequency, and ultrasound

Do not report with (32100, 32551, 33120, 33130, 33210-33211, 33400-33507, 33510-33523, 33533-33548, 33600-33853, 33860-33864, 33910-33920)

33254 **Operative tissue ablation and reconstruction of atria, limited (eg, modified maze procedure)**

41.61 41.61 Global Days 090

AMA: 2007, March, 1-3

33255 **Operative tissue ablation and reconstruction of atria, extensive (eg, maze procedure); without cardiopulmonary bypass**

50.09 50.09 Global Days 090

AMA: 2007, March, 1-3

33256 **with cardiopulmonary bypass**

59.77 59.77 Global Days 090

AMA: 2007, March, 1-3

33257-33259 Surgical Ablation Arrhythmogenic Foci, Atrial, with Other Heart Procedure(s)

Do not report with (32551, 33210-33211, 33254-33256, 33265-33266)

\+ 33257 **Operative tissue ablation and reconstruction of atria, performed at the time of other cardiac procedure(s), limited (eg, modified maze procedure) (List separately in addition to code for primary procedure)**

Code first (33120-33130, 33250-33251, 33261, 33300-33335, 33400-33496, 33500-33507, 33510-33516, 33533-33548, 33600-33619, 33641-33697, 33702-33732, 33735-33767, 33770-33814, 33840-33877, 33910-33922, 33925-33926, 33935, 33945, 33975-33980)

17.76 17.76 Global Days ZZZ

\+ 33258 **Operative tissue ablation and reconstruction of atria, performed at the time of other cardiac procedure(s), extensive (eg, maze procedure), without cardiopulmonary bypass (List separately in addition to code for primary procedure)**

Code first (33130, 33250, 33300, 33310, 33320-33321, 33330, 33332, 33401, 33414-33417, 33420, 33470-33472, 33501-33503, 33510-33516, 33533-33536, 33690, 33735, 33737, 33800-33813, 33840-33852, 33915, 33925)

19.93 19.93 Global Days ZZZ

\+ 33259 **Operative tissue ablation and reconstruction of atria, performed at the time of other cardiac procedure(s), extensive (eg, maze procedure), with cardiopulmonary bypass (List separately in addition to code for primary procedure)**

Code first (33120, 33251, 33261, 33305, 33315, 33322, 33335, 33400, 33403-33413, 33422-33468, 33474-33478, 33496, 33500, 33504-33507, 33510-33516, 33533-33548, 33600-33688, 33692-33722, 33730, 33732, 33736, 33750-33767, 33770-33781, 33786-33788, 33814, 33853, 33860-33877, 33910, 33916-33922, 33926, 33935, 33945, 33975-33980)

25.79 25.79 Global Days ZZZ

33261-33264 Surgical Ablation Arrhythmogenic Foci, Ventricular

33261 **Operative ablation of ventricular arrhythmogenic focus with cardiopulmonary bypass**

49.65 49.65 Global Days 090

33262 Resequenced Code. See code following 33241.

33263 Resequenced Code. See code following 33241.

33264 Resequenced Code. See code before 33243.

33265-33266 Surgical Ablation Arrhythmogenic Foci, Endoscopic

Do not report with (32551, 33210-33211)

33265 **Endoscopy, surgical; operative tissue ablation and reconstruction of atria, limited (eg, modified maze procedure), without cardiopulmonary bypass**

41.16 41.16 Global Days 090

AMA: 2007, March, 1-3

33266 **operative tissue ablation and reconstruction of atria, extensive (eg, maze procedure), without cardiopulmonary bypass**

56.19 56.19 Global Days 090

AMA: 2007, March, 1-3

33282-33284 Implantable Loop Recorder

CMS 100-3,20.15 Electrocardiographic Services

33282 **Implantation of patient-activated cardiac event recorder** J8 S

INCLUDES Initial programming of device

EXCLUDES *Subsequent electronic analysis and/or reprogramming of device (93285, 93291, 93298)*

Code also (C1764)

9.67 9.67 **Global Days 090**

AMA: 2009, Jan, 11-31; 2009, Mar, 5-7; 2009, Feb, 3-12; 2008, Jun, 14-15

33284 **Removal of an implantable, patient-activated cardiac event recorder** G2 T

6.95 6.95 **Global Days 090**

33300-33315 Procedures for Injury of the Heart

33300 **Repair of cardiac wound; without bypass** C5 C 80

73.85 73.85 **Global Days 090**

33305 **with cardiopulmonary bypass** C5 C 80

123.91 123.91 **Global Days 090**

33310 **Cardiotomy, exploratory (includes removal of foreign body, atrial or ventricular thrombus); without bypass** C5 C 80

Do not report with other cardiac procedures unless separate incision into heart is necessary in order to remove thrombus

35.32 35.32 **Global Days 090**

33315 **with cardiopulmonary bypass** C5 C 80

Code also excision of thrombus with cardiopulmonary bypass as appropriate if separate incision is required (33120, 33130, 33420-33430, 33460-33468, 33496, 33542, 33545, 33641-33647, 33670, 33681, 33975-33980)

Do not report with other cardiac procedures unless separate incision into heart is necessary in order to remove thrombus; in this case, append modifier 59

57.71 57.71 **Global Days 090**

33320-33335 Procedures for Injury of the Aorta/Great Vessels

33320 **Suture repair of aorta or great vessels; without shunt or cardiopulmonary bypass** C5 C 80

32.30 32.30 **Global Days 090**

33321 **with shunt bypass** C5 C 80

36.22 36.22 **Global Days 090**

33322 **with cardiopulmonary bypass** C5 C 80

42.24 42.24 **Global Days 090**

33330 **Insertion of graft, aorta or great vessels; without shunt, or cardiopulmonary bypass** C5 C 80

43.33 43.33 **Global Days 090**

33332 **with shunt bypass** C5 C 80

42.62 42.62 **Global Days 090**

33335 **with cardiopulmonary bypass** C5 C 80

57.36 57.36 **Global Days 090**

33400-33415 Aortic Valve Procedures

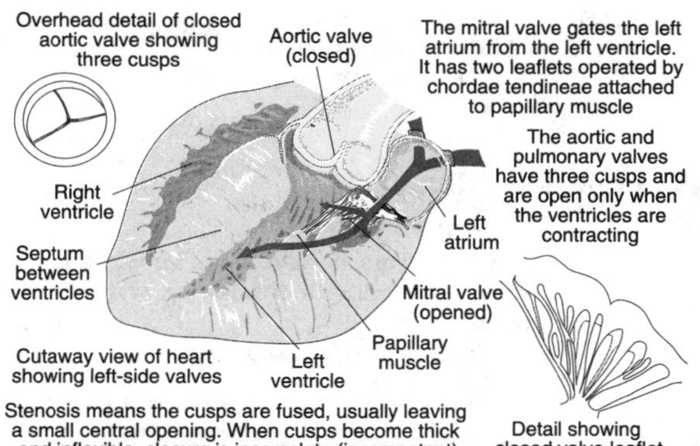

33400 **Valvuloplasty, aortic valve; open, with cardiopulmonary bypass** C5 C 80

69.33 69.33 **Global Days 090**

AMA: 2007, March, 1-3

33401 **open, with inflow occlusion** C5 C 80 63

42.96 42.96 **Global Days 090**

AMA: 2007, March, 1-3

33403 **using transventricular dilation, with cardiopulmonary bypass** C5 C 80 63

45.58 45.58 **Global Days 090**

AMA: 2007, March, 1-3

33404 **Construction of apical-aortic conduit** C5 C 80

53.49 53.49 **Global Days 090**

AMA: 2009, Jan, 11-31; 2008, Jan, 10-25; 2007, January, 13-27; 2007, March, 1-3

33405 **Replacement, aortic valve, with cardiopulmonary bypass; with prosthetic valve other than homograft or stentless valve** C5 C 80

EXCLUDES *Valvotomy of aortic valve:*
With cardiopulmonary bypass (33403)
With inflow occlusion (33401)

69.72 69.72 **Global Days 090**

AMA: 2007, March, 1-3

33406 **with allograft valve (freehand)** C5 C 80

EXCLUDES *Valvotomy of aortic valve:*
With cardiopulmonary bypass (33403)
With inflow occlusion (33401)

87.52 87.52 **Global Days 090**

AMA: 2007, March, 1-3

33410 **with stentless tissue valve** C5 C 80

77.39 77.39 **Global Days 090**

AMA: 2007, March, 1-3

33411 **Replacement, aortic valve; with aortic annulus enlargement, noncoronary sinus** C5 C 80

102.17 102.17 **Global Days 090**

AMA: 2007, March, 1-3

33412 **with transventricular aortic annulus enlargement (Konno procedure)** C5 C 80

96.55 96.55 **Global Days 090**

AMA: 2007, March, 1-3

33413 **by translocation of autologous pulmonary valve with allograft replacement of pulmonary valve (Ross procedure)** C5 C 80

98.49 98.49 **Global Days 090**

AMA: 2007, March, 1-3

33414 **Repair of left ventricular outflow tract obstruction by patch enlargement of the outflow tract**
65.80 65.80 Global Days 090
AMA: 2007, March, 1-3

33415 **Resection or incision of subvalvular tissue for discrete subvalvular aortic stenosis**
62.38 62.38 Global Days 090
AMA: 2007, March, 1-3

33416 Ventriculectomy

CMS 100-3,20.26 Partial Ventriculectomy

33416 **Ventriculomyotomy (-myectomy) for idiopathic hypertrophic subaortic stenosis (eg, asymmetric septal hypertrophy)**
61.83 61.83 Global Days 090
AMA: 2007, March, 1-3

33417 Repair of Supravalvular Stenosis by Aortoplasty

33417 **Aortoplasty (gusset) for supravalvular stenosis**
50.65 50.65 Global Days 090
AMA: 2007, March, 1-3

33420-33468 Mitral and Tricuspid Valve Procedures

INCLUDES Procedures on mitral and tricuspid valves

Code also removal of thrombus through a separate heart incision if applicable (33310, 33315)

33420 **Valvotomy, mitral valve; closed heart**
43.87 43.87 Global Days 090
AMA: 2007, March, 1-3

33422 **open heart, with cardiopulmonary bypass**
51.34 51.34 Global Days 090
AMA: 2007, March, 1-3

33425 **Valvuloplasty, mitral valve, with cardiopulmonary bypass;**
82.80 82.80 Global Days 090
AMA: 2009, Jan, 11-31; 2008, Jan, 10-25; 2007, January, 13-27; 2007, March, 1-3

33426 **with prosthetic ring**
72.72 72.72 Global Days 090
AMA: 2007, March, 1-3

33427 **radical reconstruction, with or without ring**
74.77 74.77 Global Days 090
AMA: 2007, March, 1-3

33430 **Replacement, mitral valve, with cardiopulmonary bypass**
85.46 85.46 Global Days 090
AMA: 2007, March, 1-3

33460 **Valvectomy, tricuspid valve, with cardiopulmonary bypass**
73.80 73.80 Global Days 090
AMA: 2007, March, 1-3

33463 **Valvuloplasty, tricuspid valve; without ring insertion**
93.71 93.71 Global Days 090
AMA: 2007, March, 1-3

33464 **with ring insertion**
74.30 74.30 Global Days 090
AMA: 2007, March, 1-3

33465 **Replacement, tricuspid valve, with cardiopulmonary bypass**
83.75 83.75 Global Days 090
AMA: 2007, March, 1-3

33468 **Tricuspid valve repositioning and plication for Ebstein anomaly**
74.40 74.40 Global Days 090
AMA: 2007, March, 1-3

33470-33474 Pulmonary Valvotomy

INCLUDES Brock's operation

Code also the concurrent ligation/takedown of a systemic-to-pulmonary artery shunt (33924)

33470 **Valvotomy, pulmonary valve, closed heart; transventricular**
37.46 37.46 Global Days 090
AMA: 2007, March, 1-3

33471 **via pulmonary artery**
EXCLUDES *Percutaneous valvuloplasty of pulmonary valve (92990)*
40.40 40.40 Global Days 090
AMA: 2007, March, 1-3

33472 **Valvotomy, pulmonary valve, open heart; with inflow occlusion**
41.01 41.01 Global Days 090
AMA: 2007, March, 1-3

33474 **with cardiopulmonary bypass**
65.24 65.24 Global Days 090
AMA: 2007, March, 1-3

33475-33478 Other Procedures Pulmonary Valve

33475 **Replacement, pulmonary valve**
EXCLUDES *Concurrent ligation/takedown of a systemic-to-pulmonary artery shunt (33924)*
71.23 71.23 Global Days 090
AMA: 2007, March, 1-3

33476 **Right ventricular resection for infundibular stenosis, with or without commissurotomy**
INCLUDES Brock's operation
46.25 46.25 Global Days 090
AMA: 2007, March, 1-3

33478 **Outflow tract augmentation (gusset), with or without commissurotomy or infundibular resection**
Code also 33768 for cavopulmonary anastomosis to a second superior vena cava
48.01 48.01 Global Days 090
AMA: 2007, March, 1-3

33496 Prosthetic Valve Repair

Code also reoperation if performed (33530)

Code also separate incision into heart to remove thrombus if applicable; append modifier 59 to (33315)

33496 **Repair of non-structural prosthetic valve dysfunction with cardiopulmonary bypass (separate procedure)**
50.81 50.81 Global Days 090
AMA: 2007, March, 1-3

33500-33507 Repair Aberrant Coronary Artery Anatomy

INCLUDES Angioplasty and/or endarterectomy

33500 **Repair of coronary arteriovenous or arteriocardiac chamber fistula; with cardiopulmonary bypass** C5 C 80
48.08 48.08 Global Days 090
AMA: 2007, March, 1-3

33501 **without cardiopulmonary bypass** C5 C 80
34.29 34.29 Global Days 090
AMA: 2007, March, 1-3

33502 **Repair of anomalous coronary artery from pulmonary artery origin; by ligation** C5 C 80 63
38.86 38.86 Global Days 090
AMA: 2007, March, 1-3

33503 **by graft, without cardiopulmonary bypass** C5 C 80 63
39.69 39.69 Global Days 090
AMA: 2007, March, 1-3

33504 **by graft, with cardiopulmonary bypass** C5 C 80
44.71 44.71 Global Days 090
AMA: 2007, March, 1-3

33505 **with construction of intrapulmonary artery tunnel (Takeuchi procedure)** C5 C 80 63
62.88 62.88 Global Days 090
AMA: 2007, March, 1-3

33506 **by translocation from pulmonary artery to aorta** C5 C 80 63
62.29 62.29 Global Days 090
AMA: 2007, March, 1-3

33507 **Repair of anomalous (eg, intramural) aortic origin of coronary artery by unroofing or translocation** C5 C 80
52.27 52.27 Global Days 090
AMA: 2007, March, 1-3

33508 Endoscopic Harvesting of Venous Graft

\+ **33508** **Endoscopy, surgical, including video-assisted harvest of vein(s) for coronary artery bypass procedure (List separately in addition to code for primary procedure)** N1 N 80
EXCLUDES *Harvesting of vein of upper extremity (35500)*
Code first (33510-33523)
0.49 0.49 Global Days ZZZ

33510-33516 Coronary Artery Bypass: Venous Grafts

INCLUDES Obtaining saphenous vein grafts
Venous bypass grafting only

EXCLUDES *Arterial bypass (33533-33536)*
Combined arterial-venous bypass (33517-33523, 33533-33535)
Obtaining vein graft:
Femoropopliteal vein (35572)
Upper extremity vein (35500)

33510 **Coronary artery bypass, vein only; single coronary venous graft** C5 C 80 PQ
59.19 59.19 Global Days 090
AMA: 2009, Jan, 11-31; 2008, Jan, 10-25; 2007, January, 13-27; 2007, January, 7-10; 2007, March, 1-3

33511 **2 coronary venous grafts** C5 C 80 PQ
64.98 64.98 Global Days 090
AMA: 2007, March, 1-3; 2007, January, 7-10

33512 **3 coronary venous grafts** C5 C 80 PQ
73.75 73.75 Global Days 090
AMA: 2007, March, 1-3; 2007, January, 7-10

33513 **4 coronary venous grafts** C5 C 80 PQ
75.73 75.73 Global Days 090
AMA: 2007, March, 1-3; 2007, January, 7-10

33514 **5 coronary venous grafts** C5 C 80 PQ
80.06 80.06 Global Days 090
AMA: 2007, January, 7-10; 2007, March, 1-3

33516 **6 or more coronary venous grafts** C5 C 80 PQ
83.46 83.46 Global Days 090
AMA: 2007, January, 7-10; 2007, March, 1-3

33517-33523 Coronary Artery Bypass: Venous AND Arterial Grafts

INCLUDES Obtaining saphenous vein grafts

EXCLUDES *Obtaining artery graft:*
Upper extremity (35600)
Obtaining vein graft:
Femoropopliteal vein graft (35572)
Upper extremity (35500)

Code also (33517-33523)

\+ **33517** **Coronary artery bypass, using venous graft(s) and arterial graft(s); single vein graft (List separately in addition to code for primary procedure)** C5 C 80 PQ
Code first (33533-33536)
5.70 5.70 Global Days ZZZ
AMA: 2007, January, 7-10; 2007, March, 1-3

\+ **33518** **2 venous grafts (List separately in addition to code for primary procedure)** C5 C 80 PQ
Code first (33533-33536)
12.53 12.53 Global Days ZZZ
AMA: 2007, January, 7-10; 2007, March, 1-3

\+ **33519** **3 venous grafts (List separately in addition to code for primary procedure)** C5 C 80 PQ
Code first (33533-33536)
16.59 16.59 Global Days ZZZ
AMA: 2007, March, 1-3; 2007, January, 7-10

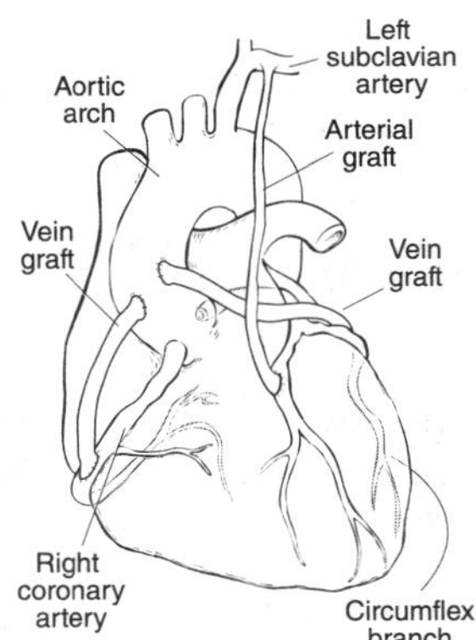

33521: four vein grafts
33522: five vein grafts
33523: six or more

The left internal thoracic (or mammary) artery is the most commonly used arterial graft. Arising from the subclavian artery, each side descends just behind the rib cartilage. The artery is left intact at the subclavian end and anastomosed to the coronary just beyond the occlusion. These codes are not reported alone; code the arterial preparation separately

\+ **33521** **4 venous grafts (List separately in addition to code for primary procedure)** C5 C 80 PQ
Code first (33533-33536)
19.95 19.95 Global Days ZZZ
AMA: 2007, January, 7-10; 2007, March, 1-3

\+ **33522** **5 venous grafts (List separately in addition to code for primary procedure)** C5 C 80 PQ
Code first (33533-33536)
22.44 22.44 Global Days ZZZ
AMA: 2007, January, 7-10; 2007, March, 1-3

+ **33523** **6 or more venous grafts (List separately in addition to code for primary procedure)**

Code first (33533-33536)

25.49 25.49 Global Days ZZZ

AMA: 2007, January, 7-10; 2007, March, 1-3

33530 Reoperative Coronary Artery Bypass Graft or Valve Procedure

+ **33530** **Reoperation, coronary artery bypass procedure or valve procedure, more than 1 month after original operation (List separately in addition to code for primary procedure)**

Code first (33400-33496, 33510-33536, 33863)

15.97 15.97 Global Days ZZZ

AMA: 2009, Jan, 11-31; 2008, Jan, 10-25; 2007, January, 7-10; 2007, January, 13-27

33533-33536 Coronary Artery Bypass: Arterial Grafts

INCLUDES Obtaining arterial graft excluding upper extremity (e.g., epigastric, internal mammary, gastroepiploic and others)

EXCLUDES *Obtaining arterial graft:*
Upper extremity (35600)
Obtaining venous graft:
Femoropopliteal vein (35572)
Upper extremity (35500)
Venous bypass (33510-33516)

Code also (33517-33523)

33533 **Coronary artery bypass, using arterial graft(s); single arterial graft**

57.30 57.30 Global Days 090

AMA: 2007, January, 7-10; 2007, March, 1-3

33534 **2 coronary arterial grafts**

67.25 67.25 Global Days 090

AMA: 2007, January, 7-10; 2007, March, 1-3

33535 **3 coronary arterial grafts**

74.93 74.93 Global Days 090

AMA: 2007, January, 7-10; 2007, March, 1-3

33536 **4 or more coronary arterial grafts**

80.73 80.73 Global Days 090

AMA: 2007, January, 7-10; 2007, March, 1-3

33542-33548 Ventricular Reconstruction

CMS 100-3,20.26 Partial Ventriculectomy

33542 **Myocardial resection (eg, ventricular aneurysmectomy)**

Code also separate incision in heart to remove thrombus

79.83 79.83 Global Days 090

AMA: 2007, March, 1-3

33545 **Repair of postinfarction ventricular septal defect, with or without myocardial resection**

Code also separate incision in heart to remove thrombus

93.94 93.94 Global Days 090

AMA: 2007, March, 1-3

33548 **Surgical ventricular restoration procedure, includes prosthetic patch, when performed (eg, ventricular remodeling, SVR, SAVER, Dor procedures)**

EXCLUDES *Batista procedure or pachopexy (33999)*

Do not report with (33210-33211, 33251, 33310, 33315)

90.70 90.70 Global Days 090

AMA: 2009, Jan, 11-31; 2008, Jan, 10-25; 2007, January, 13-27; 2007, March, 1-3

33572 Endarterectomy with CABG (LAD, RCA, Cx)

+ **33572** **Coronary endarterectomy, open, any method, of left anterior descending, circumflex, or right coronary artery performed in conjunction with coronary artery bypass graft procedure, each vessel (List separately in addition to primary procedure)**

Code first (33510-33516, 33533-33536)

7.06 7.06 Global Days ZZZ

33600-33622 Repair Aberrant Heart Anatomy

Code also the concurrent ligation/takedown of a systemic-to-pulmonary artery shunt (33924)

33600 **Closure of atrioventricular valve (mitral or tricuspid) by suture or patch**

51.96 51.96 Global Days 090

AMA: 2007, March, 1-3

33602 **Closure of semilunar valve (aortic or pulmonary) by suture or patch**

49.68 49.68 Global Days 090

AMA: 2007, March, 1-3

33606 **Anastomosis of pulmonary artery to aorta (Damus-Kaye-Stansel procedure)**

55.28 55.28 Global Days 090

AMA: 2007, March, 1-3

33608 **Repair of complex cardiac anomaly other than pulmonary atresia with ventricular septal defect by construction or replacement of conduit from right or left ventricle to pulmonary artery**

EXCLUDES *Unifocalization of arborization anomalies of pulmonary artery (33925, 33926)*

54.57 54.57 Global Days 090

AMA: 2007, March, 1-3

33610 **Repair of complex cardiac anomalies (eg, single ventricle with subaortic obstruction) by surgical enlargement of ventricular septal defect**

53.78 53.78 Global Days 090

AMA: 2007, March, 1-3

33611 **Repair of double outlet right ventricle with intraventricular tunnel repair;**

61.41 61.41 Global Days 090

AMA: 2007, March, 1-3

33612 **with repair of right ventricular outflow tract obstruction**

60.03 60.03 Global Days 090

AMA: 2007, March, 1-3

33615 **Repair of complex cardiac anomalies (eg, tricuspid atresia) by closure of atrial septal defect and anastomosis of atria or vena cava to pulmonary artery (simple Fontan procedure)**

60.72 60.72 Global Days 090

AMA: 2007, March, 1-3

33617 **Repair of complex cardiac anomalies (eg, single ventricle) by modified Fontan procedure**

Code also 33768 for cavopulmonary anastomosis to a second superior vena cava

65.41 65.41 Global Days 090

AMA: 2007, March, 1-3

33619 **Repair of single ventricle with aortic outflow obstruction and aortic arch hypoplasia (hypoplastic left heart syndrome) (eg, Norwood procedure)**

81.82 81.82 Global Days 090

AMA: 2007, March, 1-3

33620 **Application of right and left pulmonary artery bands (eg, hybrid approach stage 1)**

EXCLUDES *Banding of main pulmonary artery related to septal defect (33690)*

Code also transthoracic insertion of catheter for stent placement with removal of catheter and closure when performed during same session

50.03 50.03 Global Days 090

33621 **Transthoracic insertion of catheter for stent placement with catheter removal and closure (eg, hybrid approach stage 1)**

Code also application of right and left pulmonary artery bands when performed during same session (33620)

Code also stent placement (37207)

26.87 26.87 Global Days 090

33622 **Reconstruction of complex cardiac anomaly (eg, single ventricle or hypoplastic left heart) with palliation of single ventricle with aortic outflow obstruction and aortic arch hypoplasia, creation of cavopulmonary anastomosis, and removal of right and left pulmonary bands (eg, hybrid approach stage 2, Norwood, bidirectional Glenn, pulmonary artery debanding)**

Code also (33768)

Do not report with (33619, 33767, 33822, 33840, 33845, 33851, 33853, 33917)

105.29 105.29 Global Days 090

33641-33645 Closure of Defect: Atrium

33641 **Repair atrial septal defect, secundum, with cardiopulmonary bypass, with or without patch**

49.73 49.73 Global Days 090

AMA: 2007, March, 1-3

33645 **Direct or patch closure, sinus venosus, with or without anomalous pulmonary venous drainage**

Do not report with (33724, 33726)

52.70 52.70 Global Days 090

AMA: 2007, March, 1-3

33647 Closure of Septal Defect: Atrial AND Ventricular

33647 **Repair of atrial septal defect and ventricular septal defect, with direct or patch closure**

EXCLUDES *Tricuspid atresia repair procedures (33615)*

55.71 55.71 Global Days 090

AMA: 2007, March, 1-3

33660-33670 Closure of Defect: Atrioventricular Canal

33660 **Repair of incomplete or partial atrioventricular canal (ostium primum atrial septal defect), with or without atrioventricular valve repair**

53.65 53.65 Global Days 090

AMA: 2007, March, 1-3

33665 **Repair of intermediate or transitional atrioventricular canal, with or without atrioventricular valve repair**

58.54 58.54 Global Days 090

AMA: 2007, March, 1-3

33670 **Repair of complete atrioventricular canal, with or without prosthetic valve**

60.44 60.44 Global Days 090

AMA: 2007, March, 1-3

33675-33677 Closure of Multiple Septal Defects: Ventricle

EXCLUDES *Percutaneous closure (93581)*

Do not report with (32100, 32422, 32551, 33210, 33681, 33684, 33688)

33675 **Closure of multiple ventricular septal defects;**

60.24 60.24 Global Days 090

AMA: 2007, March, 1-3

33676 **with pulmonary valvotomy or infundibular resection (acyanotic)**

63.93 63.93 Global Days 090

AMA: 2007, March, 1-3

33677 **with removal of pulmonary artery band, with or without gusset**

66.43 66.43 Global Days 090

AMA: 2007, March, 1-3

33681-33688 Closure of Septal Defect: Ventricle

EXCLUDES *Repair of pulmonary vein that requires creating an atrial septal defect (33724)*

33681 **Closure of single ventricular septal defect, with or without patch;**

55.81 55.81 Global Days 090

AMA: 2007, March, 1-3

33684 **with pulmonary valvotomy or infundibular resection (acyanotic)**

Code also concurrent ligation/takedown of a systemic-to-pulmonary artery shunt if performed (33924)

57.85 57.85 Global Days 090

AMA: 2007, March, 1-3

33688 **with removal of pulmonary artery band, with or without gusset**

Code also the concurrent ligation/takedown of a systemic-to-pulmonary artery shunt if performed (33924)

57.53 57.53 Global Days 090

AMA: 2007, March, 1-3

33690 Reduce Pulmonary Overcirculation in Septal Defects

33690 **Banding of pulmonary artery**

EXCLUDES *Left and right pulmonary artery banding in a single ventricle (33620)*

36.17 36.17 Global Days 090

AMA: 2007, March, 1-3

33692-33697 Repair of Defects of Tetralogy of Fallot

Code also the concurrent ligation/takedown of a systemic-to-pulmonary artery shunt (33924)

33692 **Complete repair tetralogy of Fallot without pulmonary atresia;**

59.84 59.84 Global Days 090

AMA: 2007, March, 1-3

33694 **with transannular patch**

59.79 59.79 Global Days 090

AMA: 2007, March, 1-3

33697 **Complete repair tetralogy of Fallot with pulmonary atresia including construction of conduit from right ventricle to pulmonary artery and closure of ventricular septal defect**

62.64 62.64 Global Days 090

AMA: 2007, March, 1-3

33702-33722 Repair Anomalies Sinus of Valsalva

33702 Repair sinus of Valsalva fistula, with cardiopulmonary bypass;
47.21 47.21 Global Days 090
AMA: 2007, March, 1-3

33710 with repair of ventricular septal defect
62.76 62.76 Global Days 090
AMA: 2007, March, 1-3

33720 Repair sinus of Valsalva aneurysm, with cardiopulmonary bypass
46.93 46.93 Global Days 090
AMA: 2007, March, 1-3

33722 Closure of aortico-left ventricular tunnel
50.85 50.85 Global Days 090
AMA: 2007, March, 1-3

33724-33732 Repair Aberrant Pulmonary Venous Connection

33724 Repair of isolated partial anomalous pulmonary venous return (eg, Scimitar Syndrome)
Do not report with (32551, 33210-33211)
46.88 46.88 Global Days 090
AMA: 2007, March, 1-3

33726 Repair of pulmonary venous stenosis
Do not report with (32551, 33210-33211)
62.44 62.44 Global Days 090
AMA: 2007, March, 1-3

33730 Complete repair of anomalous pulmonary venous return (supracardiac, intracardiac, or infracardiac types)
EXCLUDES *Partial anomalous pulmonary venous return (33724)*
Repair of pulmonary venous stenosis (33726)
63.29 63.29 Global Days 090
AMA: 2007, March, 1-3

33732 Repair of cor triatriatum or supravalvular mitral ring by resection of left atrial membrane
50.41 50.41 Global Days 090
AMA: 2007, March, 1-3

33735-33737 Creation of Atrial Septal Defect

Code also the concurrent ligation/takedown of a systemic-to-pulmonary artery shunt (33924)

33735 Atrial septectomy or septostomy; closed heart (Blalock-Hanlon type operation)
38.91 38.91 Global Days 090
AMA: 2007, March, 1-3

33736 open heart with cardiopulmonary bypass
42.91 42.91 Global Days 090
AMA: 2007, March, 1-3

33737 open heart, with inflow occlusion
EXCLUDES *Atrial septectomy/septostomy:*
Blade method (92993)
Transvenous balloon method (92992)
40.10 40.10 Global Days 090
AMA: 2007, March, 1-3

33750-33767 Systemic Vessel to Pulmonary Artery Shunts

Code also the concurrent ligation/takedown of a systemic-to-pulmonary artery shunt (33924)

33750 Shunt; subclavian to pulmonary artery (Blalock-Taussig type operation)
41.70 41.70 Global Days 090
AMA: 2007, March, 1-3

33755 ascending aorta to pulmonary artery (Waterston type operation)
40.08 40.08 Global Days 090
AMA: 2007, March, 1-3

33762 descending aorta to pulmonary artery (Potts-Smith type operation)
40.88 40.88 Global Days 090
AMA: 2007, March, 1-3

33764 central, with prosthetic graft
39.14 39.14 Global Days 090
AMA: 2007, March, 1-3

33766 superior vena cava to pulmonary artery for flow to 1 lung (classical Glenn procedure)
41.36 41.36 Global Days 090
AMA: 2007, March, 1-3

33767 superior vena cava to pulmonary artery for flow to both lungs (bidirectional Glenn procedure)
43.38 43.38 Global Days 090
AMA: 2007, March, 1-3

33768 Cavopulmonary Anastomosis to Decrease Volume Load

Do not report with (32551, 33210-33211)

\+ **33768** Anastomosis, cavopulmonary, second superior vena cava (List separately in addition to primary procedure)
Code first (33478, 33617, 33767)
13.26 13.26 Global Days ZZZ
AMA: 2007, March, 1-3

33770-33783 Repair Aberrant Anatomy: Transposition Great Vessels

Code also the concurrent ligation/takedown of a systemic-to-pulmonary artery shunt (33924)

33770 Repair of transposition of the great arteries with ventricular septal defect and subpulmonary stenosis; without surgical enlargement of ventricular septal defect
66.15 66.15 Global Days 090
AMA: 2007, March, 1-3

33771 with surgical enlargement of ventricular septal defect
67.34 67.34 Global Days 090
AMA: 2007, March, 1-3

33774 Repair of transposition of the great arteries, atrial baffle procedure (eg, Mustard or Senning type) with cardiopulmonary bypass;
55.07 55.07 Global Days 090
AMA: 2007, March, 1-3

33775 with removal of pulmonary band
58.23 58.23 Global Days 090
AMA: 2007, March, 1-3

33776 with closure of ventricular septal defect
61.49 61.49 Global Days 090
AMA: 2007, March, 1-3

33777 with repair of subpulmonic obstruction
59.67 59.67 Global Days 090
AMA: 2007, March, 1-3

33778 **Repair of transposition of the great arteries, aortic pulmonary artery reconstruction (eg, Jatene type);**
72.08 72.08 Global Days 090
AMA: 2007, March, 1-3

33779 with removal of pulmonary band
73.71 73.71 Global Days 090
AMA: 2007, March, 1-3

33780 with closure of ventricular septal defect
75.26 75.26 Global Days 090
AMA: 2007, March, 1-3

33781 with repair of subpulmonic obstruction
70.90 70.90 Global Days 090
AMA: 2007, March, 1-3

33782 **Aortic root translocation with ventricular septal defect and pulmonary stenosis repair (ie, Nikaidoh procedure); without coronary ostium reimplantation**

Do not report with (33412-33413, 33608, 33681, 33770-33771, 33778, 33780, 33920)
96.87 96.87 Global Days 090

33783 with reimplantation of 1 or both coronary ostia
104.89 104.89 Global Days 090

33786-33788 Repair Aberrant Anatomy: Truncus Arteriosus

33786 **Total repair, truncus arteriosus (Rastelli type operation)**

Code also the concurrent ligation/takedown of a systemic-to-pulmonary artery shunt (33924)
69.77 69.77 Global Days 090
AMA: 2007, March, 1-3

33788 **Reimplantation of an anomalous pulmonary artery**

EXCLUDES *Pulmonary artery banding (33690)*
46.94 46.94 Global Days 090
AMA: 2007, March, 1-3

33800-33853 Repair Aberrant Anatomy: Aorta

33800 **Aortic suspension (aortopexy) for tracheal decompression (eg, for tracheomalacia) (separate procedure)**
28.39 28.39 Global Days 090
AMA: 2007, March, 1-3

33802 **Division of aberrant vessel (vascular ring);**
32.98 32.98 Global Days 090
AMA: 2007, March, 1-3

33803 with reanastomosis
36.26 36.26 Global Days 090
AMA: 2007, March, 1-3

33813 **Obliteration of aortopulmonary septal defect; without cardiopulmonary bypass**
38.03 38.03 Global Days 090
AMA: 2007, March, 1-3

33814 with cardiopulmonary bypass
48.43 48.43 Global Days 090
AMA: 2007, March, 1-3

33820 **Repair of patent ductus arteriosus; by ligation**
29.67 29.67 Global Days 090
AMA: 2007, March, 1-3

33822 by division, younger than 18 years
31.97 31.97 Global Days 090
AMA: 2007, March, 1-3

33824 by division, 18 years and older
35.66 35.66 Global Days 090
AMA: 2007, March, 1-3

33840 **Excision of coarctation of aorta, with or without associated patent ductus arteriosus; with direct anastomosis**
38.33 38.33 Global Days 090
AMA: 2007, March, 1-3

33845 with graft
41.10 41.10 Global Days 090
AMA: 2007, March, 1-3

33851 repair using either left subclavian artery or prosthetic material as gusset for enlargement
40.32 40.32 Global Days 090
AMA: 2007, March, 1-3

33852 **Repair of hypoplastic or interrupted aortic arch using autogenous or prosthetic material; without cardiopulmonary bypass**

EXCLUDES *Hypoplastic left heart syndrome repair by excision of coarctation of aorta (33619)*
42.29 42.29 Global Days 090
AMA: 2007, March, 1-3

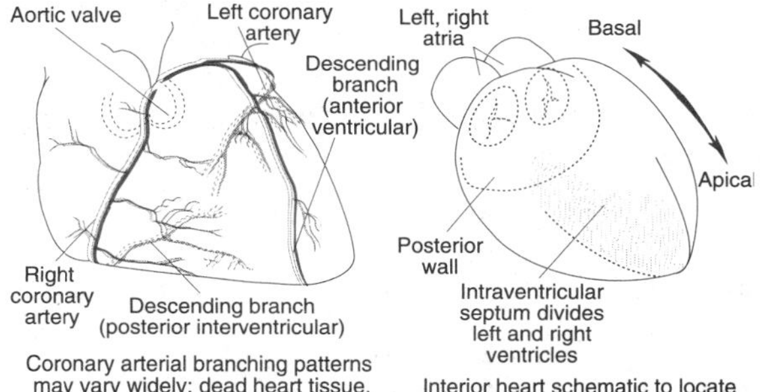

Coronary arterial branching patterns may vary widely; dead heart tissue, usually caused by arterial occlusion, is called a myocardial infarct and about 1.5 million cases are reported annually. Inadequate blood supply can lead to "angina pectoris," or chest pain

Interior heart schematic to locate a myocardial infarction; walls of the left ventrical are much thicker and more than half of MI occurrences will see some degree of transient impairment to the left ventricle

33853 with cardiopulmonary bypass

EXCLUDES *Hypoplastic left heart syndrome repair by excision of coarctation of aorta (33619)*
56.39 56.39 Global Days 090
AMA: 2007, March, 1-3

33860-33877 Aortic Graft Procedures

33860 **Ascending aorta graft, with cardiopulmonary bypass, includes valve suspension, when performed**
97.54 97.54 Global Days 090
AMA: 2007, March, 1-3

33863 **Ascending aorta graft, with cardiopulmonary bypass, with aortic root replacement using valved conduit and coronary reconstruction (eg, Bentall)**

Do not report with (33405, 33406, 33410-33413, 33860)
95.93 95.93 Global Days 090
AMA: 2007, March, 1-3

33864 **Ascending aorta graft, with cardiopulmonary bypass with valve suspension, with coronary reconstruction and valve-sparing aortic root remodeling (eg, David Procedure, Yacoub Procedure)** C5 C 80

Do not report with (33400, 33860-33863)

98.14 98.14 Global Days 090

33870 **Transverse arch graft, with cardiopulmonary bypass** C5 C 80

76.83 76.83 Global Days 090

33875 **Descending thoracic aorta graft, with or without bypass** C5 C 80

83.24 83.24 Global Days 090

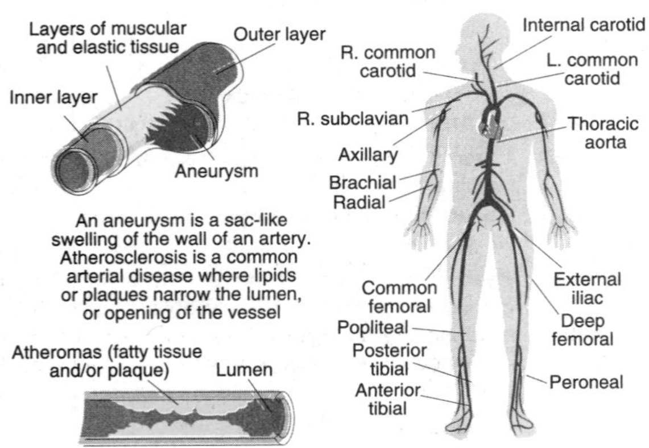

33877 **Repair of thoracoabdominal aortic aneurysm with graft, with or without cardiopulmonary bypass** C5 C 80 P0

110.08 110.08 Global Days 090

33880-33891 Endovascular Repair Aortic Aneurysm: Thoracic

INCLUDES Balloon angioplasty
Introduction, manipulation, placement, and deployment of the device

EXCLUDES *Additional interventional procedures provided during the endovascular repair*
Carotid-carotid bypass (33891)
Guidewire and catheter insertion (36140, 36200-36218)
Open exposure of artery/subsequent closure (34812, 34820, 34833, 34834)
Study, interpretation, and report of implanted wireless pressure sensor in an aneurysmal sac (93982)
Subclavian to carotid artery transposition (33889)
Substantial artery repair/replacement (35226, 35286)
Transcatheter insertion of wireless physiologic sensor in an aneurysmal sac (34806)

33880 **Endovascular repair of descending thoracic aorta (eg, aneurysm, pseudoaneurysm, dissection, penetrating ulcer, intramural hematoma, or traumatic disruption); involving coverage of left subclavian artery origin, initial endoprosthesis plus descending thoracic aortic extension(s), if required, to level of celiac artery origin** C5 C 80 P0

INCLUDES Placement of distal extensions

EXCLUDES *Proximal extensions*

75956

55.45 55.45 Global Days 090

33881 **not involving coverage of left subclavian artery origin, initial endoprosthesis plus descending thoracic aortic extension(s), if required, to level of celiac artery origin** C5 C 80 P0

INCLUDES Placement of distal extensions in distal thoracic aorta

EXCLUDES *Proximal extensions*

75957

47.74 47.74 Global Days 090

33883 **Placement of proximal extension prosthesis for endovascular repair of descending thoracic aorta (eg, aneurysm, pseudoaneurysm, dissection, penetrating ulcer, intramural hematoma, or traumatic disruption); initial extension** C5 C 80 P0

75958

34.60 34.60 Global Days 090

\+ **33884** **each additional proximal extension (List separately in addition to code for primary procedure)** C5 C 80

Code first (33883)

75958

12.61 12.61 Global Days ZZZ

33886 **Placement of distal extension prosthesis(s) delayed after endovascular repair of descending thoracic aorta** C5 C 80 P0

INCLUDES All modules deployed

Do not report with (33880, 33881)

75959

30.04 30.04 Global Days 090

33889 **Open subclavian to carotid artery transposition performed in conjunction with endovascular repair of descending thoracic aorta, by neck incision, unilateral** C5 C 80 50

Do not report with (35694)

24.61 24.61 Global Days 000

33891 **Bypass graft, with other than vein, transcervical retropharyngeal carotid-carotid, performed in conjunction with endovascular repair of descending thoracic aorta, by neck incision** C5 C 80 50 P0

Do not report with (35509, 35601)

30.29 30.29 Global Days 000

33910-33926 Surgical Procedures of Pulmonary Artery

CMS 100-3,240.6 Transvenous (Catheter) Pulmonary Embolectomy

33910 **Pulmonary artery embolectomy; with cardiopulmonary bypass** C5 C 80

78.80 78.80 Global Days 090

AMA: 2007, March, 1-3

33915 **without cardiopulmonary bypass** C5 C 80

41.57 41.57 Global Days 090

AMA: 2007, March, 1-3

33916 **Pulmonary endarterectomy, with or without embolectomy, with cardiopulmonary bypass** C5 C 80

124.01 124.01 Global Days 090

AMA: 2007, March, 1-3

33917 **Repair of pulmonary artery stenosis by reconstruction with patch or graft** C5 C 80

44.47 44.47 Global Days 090

AMA: 2007, March, 1-3

33920 **Repair of pulmonary atresia with ventricular septal defect, by construction or replacement of conduit from right or left ventricle to pulmonary artery**

EXCLUDES *Repair of complicated cardiac anomalies by creating/replacing conduit from ventricle to pulmonary artery (33608)*

Code also the concurrent ligation/takedown of a systemic-to-pulmonary artery shunt (33924)

55.32 55.32 Global Days 090

AMA: 2007, March, 1-3

33922 **Transection of pulmonary artery with cardiopulmonary bypass**

Code also the concurrent ligation/takedown of a systemic-to-pulmonary artery shunt (33924)

44.11 44.11 Global Days 090

\+ **33924** **Ligation and takedown of a systemic-to-pulmonary artery shunt, performed in conjunction with a congenital heart procedure (List separately in addition to code for primary procedure)**

Code first (33470-33475, 33600-33619, 33684-33688, 33692-33697, 33735-33767, 33770-33781, 33786, 33920-33922)

8.65 8.65 Global Days ZZZ

33925 **Repair of pulmonary artery arborization anomalies by unifocalization; without cardiopulmonary bypass**

Do not report with (33697)

52.25 52.25 Global Days 090

33926 **with cardiopulmonary bypass**

Do not report with (33697)

73.64 73.64 Global Days 090

33930-33945 Heart and Heart-Lung Transplants

CMS 100-4,3,90.2 Heart Transplants

CMS 100-4,3,90.2.1 Artificial Hearts and Related Devices

INCLUDES Backbench work to prepare the donor heart and/or lungs for transplantation (33933, 33944)
Harvesting of donor organs with cold preservation (33930, 33940)
Transplantation of heart and/or lungs into recipient (33935, 33945)

EXCLUDES *Implantation/repair/replacement of artificial heart or components (0051T-0053T)*
Procedures performed on donor heart (33300, 33310, 33320, 33400, 33463, 33464, 33510, 33641, 35216, 35276, 35685)

33930 **Donor cardiectomy-pneumonectomy (including cold preservation)**

0.00 0.00 Global Days XXX

33933 **Backbench standard preparation of cadaver donor heart/lung allograft prior to transplantation, including dissection of allograft from surrounding soft tissues to prepare aorta, superior vena cava, inferior vena cava, and trachea for implantation**

0.00 0.00 Global Days XXX

33935 **Heart-lung transplant with recipient cardiectomy-pneumonectomy**

149.54 149.54 Global Days 090

33940 **Donor cardiectomy (including cold preservation)**

0.00 0.00 Global Days XXX

33944 **Backbench standard preparation of cadaver donor heart allograft prior to transplantation, including dissection of allograft from surrounding soft tissues to prepare aorta, superior vena cava, inferior vena cava, pulmonary artery, and left atrium for implantation**

0.00 0.00 Global Days XXX

33945 **Heart transplant, with or without recipient cardiectomy**

146.99 146.99 Global Days 090

33960-33999 Mechanical Circulatory Support

CMS 100-4,3,90.2.1 Artificial Hearts and Related Devices

▲ **33960** **Prolonged extracorporeal circulation for cardiopulmonary insufficiency; initial day**

EXCLUDES *Cannula insertion for prolonged extracorporeal circulation (36822)*

30.02 30.02 Global Days 000

⊘ ▲ **33961** **each subsequent day**

EXCLUDES *Cannula insertion for prolonged extracorporeal circulation (36822)*

Code first (33960)

16.52 16.52 Global Days ZZZ

33967 **Insertion of intra-aortic balloon assist device, percutaneous**

7.94 7.94 Global Days 000

33968 **Removal of intra-aortic balloon assist device, percutaneous**

1.03 1.03 Global Days 000

AMA: 2009, Jan, 11-31; 2008, Jan, 10-25; 2007, January, 13-27

33970 **Insertion of intra-aortic balloon assist device through the femoral artery, open approach**

EXCLUDES *Percutaneous insertion of intra-aortic balloon assist device (33967)*

10.86 10.86 Global Days 000

33971 **Removal of intra-aortic balloon assist device including repair of femoral artery, with or without graft**

21.66 21.66 Global Days 090

33973 **Insertion of intra-aortic balloon assist device through the ascending aorta**

15.76 15.76 Global Days 000

33974 **Removal of intra-aortic balloon assist device from the ascending aorta, including repair of the ascending aorta, with or without graft**

27.06 27.06 Global Days 090

33975 **Insertion of ventricular assist device; extracorporeal, single ventricle**

INCLUDES Replacement of the entire ventricular assist device system, including pump(s) and cannulas
Transthoracic approach

EXCLUDES *Percutaneous approach (0048T)*
Replacement percutaneous transseptal approach (33999)

Code also removal atrial/ventricular thrombi through a separate incision

39.64 39.64 Global Days XXX

AMA: 2009, Jan, 11-31; 2008, Jan, 10-25; 2007, January, 13-27

33976 **extracorporeal, biventricular**

INCLUDES Replacement of the entire ventricular assist device system, including pump(s) and cannulas
Transthoracic approach

EXCLUDES *Percutaneous approach (0048T)*
Replacement percutaneous transseptal approach (33999)

Code also removal atrial/ventricular thrombi through a separate incision

48.52 48.52 Global Days XXX

33977 Removal of ventricular assist device; extracorporeal, single ventricle C5 C 80

INCLUDES Removal of the entire device and the cannulas

EXCLUDES *Replacement percutaneous transseptal approach (33999)*

Code also removal atrial/ventricular thrombi through a separate incision

Do not report removal of the ventricular assist device when performed at the time of of insertion of a new device

35.14 35.14 Global Days XXX

33978 extracorporeal, biventricular C5 C 80

INCLUDES Removal of the entire device and the cannulas

EXCLUDES *Replacement percutaneous transseptal approach (33999)*

Code also removal atrial/ventricular thrombi through a separate incision

Do not report removal of the ventricular assist device when performed at the time of insertion of a new device

41.64 41.64 Global Days XXX

33979 Insertion of ventricular assist device, implantable intracorporeal, single ventricle C5 C 80

INCLUDES Replacement of the entire ventricular assist device system, including pump(s) and cannulas
Transthoracic approach

EXCLUDES *Percutaneous approach (0048T)*
Replacement percutaneous transseptal approach (33999)

Code also removal atrial/ventricular thrombi through a separate incision

60.34 60.34 Global Days XXX

33980 Removal of ventricular assist device, implantable intracorporeal, single ventricle C5 C 80

INCLUDES Removal of the entire device and the cannulas

EXCLUDES *Replacement percutaneous transseptal approach (33999)*

Code also removal atrial/ventricular thrombi through a separate incision

Do not report removal of the ventricular assist device when performed at the time of insertion of a new device

58.65 58.65 Global Days XXX

33981 Replacement of extracorporeal ventricular assist device, single or biventricular, pump(s), single or each pump C5 C 80

INCLUDES Insertion of the new pump with de-airing, connection, and initiation
Removal of the old pump

EXCLUDES *Percutaneous transseptal approach (33999)*

25.39 25.39 Global Days XXX

33982 Replacement of ventricular assist device pump(s); implantable intracorporeal, single ventricle, without cardiopulmonary bypass C5 C 80

INCLUDES New pump insertion with connection, de-airing, and initiation
Removal of the old pump

EXCLUDES *Percutaneous transseptal approach (33999)*

59.41 59.41 Global Days XXX

33983 implantable intracorporeal, single ventricle, with cardiopulmonary bypass C5 C 80

INCLUDES Insertion of the new pump with de-airing, connection, and initiation
Removal of the old pump

EXCLUDES *Percutaneous transseptal approach (33999)*

69.75 69.75 Global Days XXX

33999 Unlisted procedure, cardiac surgery T 80

0.00 0.00 Global Days YYY

AMA: 2009, Jan, 11-31; 2008, Jan, 10-25; 2007, January, 13-27; 2007, March, 1-3

34001-34530 Surgical Revascularization: Veins and Arteries

INCLUDES Repair of blood vessel
Surgeon's component of operative arteriogram

34001 Embolectomy or thrombectomy, with or without catheter; carotid, subclavian or innominate artery, by neck incision C5 C 80 50

30.01 30.01 Global Days 090

34051 innominate, subclavian artery, by thoracic incision C5 C 80 50 PQ

28.48 28.48 Global Days 090

34101 axillary, brachial, innominate, subclavian artery, by arm incision T 80 50

18.79 18.79 Global Days 090

34111 radial or ulnar artery, by arm incision T 80 50

18.81 18.81 Global Days 090

34151 renal, celiac, mesentery, aortoiliac artery, by abdominal incision C5 C 80 50

43.38 43.38 Global Days 090

34201 femoropopliteal, aortoiliac artery, by leg incision T 80 50

31.99 31.99 Global Days 090

34203 popliteal-tibio-peroneal artery, by leg incision T 80 50

29.89 29.89 Global Days 090

34401 Thrombectomy, direct or with catheter; vena cava, iliac vein, by abdominal incision C5 C 80 50

44.42 44.42 Global Days 090

34421 vena cava, iliac, femoropopliteal vein, by leg incision T 80 50

22.76 22.76 Global Days 090

34451 vena cava, iliac, femoropopliteal vein, by abdominal and leg incision C5 C 80 50

45.33 45.33 Global Days 090

34471 subclavian vein, by neck incision
36.65 36.65 Global Days 090

34490 axillary and subclavian vein, by arm incision
19.14 19.14 Global Days 090

34501 **Valvuloplasty, femoral vein**
28.25 28.25 Global Days 090

34502 **Reconstruction of vena cava, any method**
46.80 46.80 Global Days 090

34510 **Venous valve transposition, any vein donor**
35.06 35.06 Global Days 090

34520 **Cross-over vein graft to venous system**
31.20 31.20 Global Days 090

34530 **Saphenopopliteal vein anastomosis**
29.21 29.21 Global Days 090

34800-34834 Endovascular Stent Grafting for Abdominal Aneurysms

CMS 100-3,20.23 Fabric Wrapping of Abdominal Aneurysms

INCLUDES Balloon angioplasty
Introduction, manipulation, placement, and deployment
Open exposure of artery/subsequent closure
Thromboendarterectomy at site of aneurysm

EXCLUDES *Additional interventional procedures*
Guidewire and catheter insertion (36140, 36200, 36245-36248)
Substantial artery repair/replacement (35226, 35286)

75952, 75953

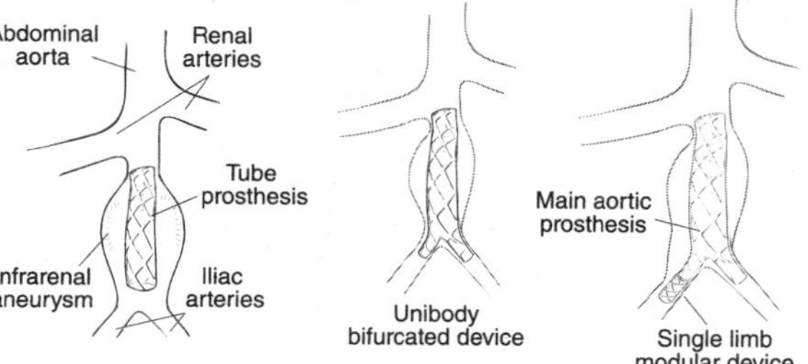

34800 **Endovascular repair of infrarenal abdominal aortic aneurysm or dissection; using aorto-aortic tube prosthesis**
Code also open arterial exposure as appropriate (34812, 34820, 34833, 34834)
75952
34.90 34.90 Global Days 090
AMA: 2009, Jan, 11-31; 2008, Jan, 10-25; 2007, January, 13-27

34802 using modular bifurcated prosthesis (1 docking limb)
Code also open arterial exposure as appropriate (34812, 34820, 34833, 34834)
75952
38.58 38.58 Global Days 090
AMA: 2009, Jan, 11-31; 2008, Jan, 10-25; 2007, January, 13-27

34803 using modular bifurcated prosthesis (2 docking limbs)
EXCLUDES *Use of prosthesis for associated visceral vessels (0078T, 0079T)*
Code also open arterial exposure as appropriate (34812, 34820, 34833, 34834)
75952
39.77 39.77 Global Days 090

34804 using unibody bifurcated prosthesis
Code also open arterial exposure as appropriate (34812, 34820, 34833, 34834)
75952
38.59 38.59 Global Days 090

34805 using aorto-uniiliac or aorto-unifemoral prosthesis
Code also open arterial exposure as appropriate (34812, 34820, 34833, 34834)
75952
36.88 36.88 Global Days 090
AMA: 2009, Jan, 11-31; 2008, Jan, 10-25; 2007, January, 13-27

\+ 34806 **Transcatheter placement of wireless physiologic sensor in aneurysmal sac during endovascular repair, including radiological supervision and interpretation, instrument calibration, and collection of pressure data (List separately in addition to code for primary procedure)**
Code first (33880-33881, 33886, 34800-34805, 34825, 34900)
Code also open arterial exposure as appropriate (34812, 34820, 34833-34834)
Do not report with (93982)
3.17 3.17 Global Days ZZZ

\+ 34808 **Endovascular placement of iliac artery occlusion device (List separately in addition to code for primary procedure)**
Code first (34800, 34805, 34813, 34825, 34826)
Code also open arterial exposure as appropriate (34812, 34820, 34833-34834)
6.34 6.34 Global Days ZZZ

34812 **Open femoral artery exposure for delivery of endovascular prosthesis, by groin incision, unilateral**
Code also as appropriate (34800-34808)
10.42 10.42 Global Days 000
AMA: 2009, Jan, 11-31; 2008, Jan, 10-25; 2007, January, 13-27

\+ 34813 **Placement of femoral-femoral prosthetic graft during endovascular aortic aneurysm repair (List separately in addition to code for primary procedure)**
EXCLUDES *Grafting of femoral artery (35521, 35533, 35539, 35540, 35556, 35558, 35566, 35621, 35646, 35654-35661, 35666, 35700)*
Code first (34812)
7.33 7.33 Global Days ZZZ

34820 **Open iliac artery exposure for delivery of endovascular prosthesis or iliac occlusion during endovascular therapy, by abdominal or retroperitoneal incision, unilateral**
Code also endovascular repair of abdominal aorta aneurysm as appropriate (34800-34808)
15.00 15.00 Global Days 000
AMA: 2009, Jan, 11-31; 2008, Jan, 10-25; 2007, January, 13-27

34825 **Placement of proximal or distal extension prosthesis for endovascular repair of infrarenal abdominal aortic or iliac aneurysm, false aneurysm, or dissection; initial vessel**
Code also endovascular repair of abdominal aorta or iliac aneurysm as appropriate (34800-34805, 34900)
75953
21.63 21.63 Global Days 090

\+ 34826 each additional vessel (List separately in addition to code for primary procedure)
Code also endovascular repair of abdominal aorta or iliac aneurysm as appropriate (34800-34805, 34900)
Code first (34825)
75953
6.34 6.34 Global Days ZZZ

34830 **Open repair of infrarenal aortic aneurysm or dissection, plus repair of associated arterial trauma, following unsuccessful endovascular repair; tube prosthesis** C5 C 80
55.50 55.50 Global Days 090
AMA: 2009, Jan, 11-31; 2008, Oct, 10-11

34831 **aorto-bi-iliac prosthesis** C5 C 80
59.44 59.44 Global Days 090
AMA: 2009, Jan, 11-31; 2008, Oct, 10-11

34832 **aorto-bifemoral prosthesis** C5 C 80
59.67 59.67 Global Days 090
AMA: 2009, Jan, 11-31; 2008, Oct, 10-11

34833 **Open iliac artery exposure with creation of conduit for delivery of aortic or iliac endovascular prosthesis, by abdominal or retroperitoneal incision, unilateral** C5 C 80 50

Do not report with (34820)
18.85 18.85 Global Days 000
AMA: 2009, Jan, 11-31; 2008, Jan, 10-25; 2007, January, 13-27

34834 **Open brachial artery exposure to assist in the deployment of aortic or iliac endovascular prosthesis by arm incision, unilateral** C5 C 80 50
8.50 8.50 Global Days 000

34900 Endovascular Stent Grafting Iliac Artery

INCLUDES Balloon angioplasty
Introduction, manipulation, placement, and deployment

EXCLUDES *Endovascular repair of iliac artery bifurcation (e.g., aneurysm, arteriovenous malformation, pseudoaneurysm, trauma) using bifurcated endoprosthesis (0254T)*
Insertion guidewires, catheters (36200, 36245-36248)
Open exposure femoral or iliac artery (34812, 34820)
Other concurrent interventional procedures
Placement extension prosthesis (34825)
Substantial artery repair/replacement (35206-35286)

34900 **Endovascular repair of iliac artery (eg, aneurysm, pseudoaneurysm, arteriovenous malformation, trauma) using ilio-iliac tube endoprosthesis** C5 C 80 50
75954
27.63 27.63 Global Days 090

35001-35152 Repair Aneurysm, False Aneurysm, Related Arterial Disease

INCLUDES Endarterectomy procedures

EXCLUDES *Endovascular repairs of:*
Abdominal aortic aneurysm (34800-34826)
Aneurysm of iliac artery (34900)
Thoracic aortic aneurysm (33880)
Intracranial aneurysms (61697-61710)
Open repairs thoracic aortic aneurysm (33860-33875)
Repairs related to occlusive disease only (35201-35286)

35001 **Direct repair of aneurysm, pseudoaneurysm, or excision (partial or total) and graft insertion, with or without patch graft; for aneurysm and associated occlusive disease, carotid, subclavian artery, by neck incision** C5 C 80 50
35.22 35.22 Global Days 090

35002 **for ruptured aneurysm, carotid, subclavian artery, by neck incision** C5 C 80 50
38.95 38.95 Global Days 090

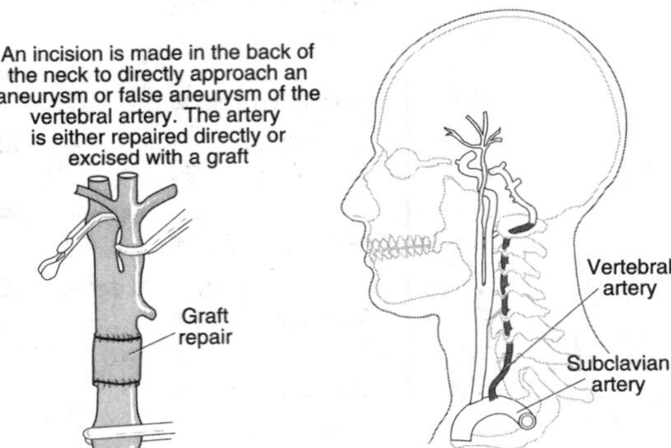

35005 **for aneurysm, pseudoaneurysm, and associated occlusive disease, vertebral artery** C5 C 80 50
33.08 33.08 Global Days 090

35011 **for aneurysm and associated occlusive disease, axillary-brachial artery, by arm incision** T 80 50
31.03 31.03 Global Days 090

35013 **for ruptured aneurysm, axillary-brachial artery, by arm incision** C5 C 80 50
38.45 38.45 Global Days 090

35021 **for aneurysm, pseudoaneurysm, and associated occlusive disease, innominate, subclavian artery, by thoracic incision** C5 C 80 50
37.76 37.76 Global Days 090

35022 **for ruptured aneurysm, innominate, subclavian artery, by thoracic incision** C5 C 80 50
43.66 43.66 Global Days 090

35045 **for aneurysm, pseudoaneurysm, and associated occlusive disease, radial or ulnar artery** T 80 50
30.33 30.33 Global Days 090

35081 **for aneurysm, pseudoaneurysm, and associated occlusive disease, abdominal aorta** C5 C 80
54.50 54.50 Global Days 090
AMA: 2009, Jan, 11-31; 2008, Jan, 10-25; 2007, January, 13-27

35082 **for ruptured aneurysm, abdominal aorta** C5 C 80
68.00 68.00 Global Days 090

35091 **for aneurysm, pseudoaneurysm, and associated occlusive disease, abdominal aorta involving visceral vessels (mesenteric, celiac, renal)** C5 C 80 50
55.92 55.92 Global Days 090

35092 **for ruptured aneurysm, abdominal aorta involving visceral vessels (mesenteric, celiac, renal)** C5 C 80 50
80.96 80.96 Global Days 090

35102 **for aneurysm, pseudoaneurysm, and associated occlusive disease, abdominal aorta involving iliac vessels (common, hypogastric, external)** C5 C 80 50
58.81 58.81 Global Days 090

35103 **for ruptured aneurysm, abdominal aorta involving iliac vessels (common, hypogastric, external)** C5 C 80 50
69.69 69.69 Global Days 090

35111 **for aneurysm, pseudoaneurysm, and associated occlusive disease, splenic artery** C5 C 80 50
41.26 41.26 Global Days 090

35112 **for ruptured aneurysm, splenic artery** C5 C 80 50
55.47 55.47 Global Days 090

35121 for aneurysm, pseudoaneurysm, and associated occlusive disease, hepatic, celiac, renal, or mesenteric artery C5 C 80 50
50.81 50.81 Global Days 090

35122 for ruptured aneurysm, hepatic, celiac, renal, or mesenteric artery C5 C 80 50
64.06 64.06 Global Days 090

35131 for aneurysm, pseudoaneurysm, and associated occlusive disease, iliac artery (common, hypogastric, external) C5 C 80 50 PQ
43.40 43.40 Global Days 090

35132 for ruptured aneurysm, iliac artery (common, hypogastric, external) C5 C 80 50
53.03 53.03 Global Days 090

35141 for aneurysm, pseudoaneurysm, and associated occlusive disease, common femoral artery (profunda femoris, superficial femoral) C5 C 80 50 PQ
34.52 34.52 Global Days 090

35142 for ruptured aneurysm, common femoral artery (profunda femoris, superficial femoral) C5 C 80 50
41.39 41.39 Global Days 090

35151 for aneurysm, pseudoaneurysm, and associated occlusive disease, popliteal artery C5 C 80 50 PQ
38.94 38.94 Global Days 090

35152 for ruptured aneurysm, popliteal artery C5 C 80 50
44.09 44.09 Global Days 090

35180-35190 Repair Arteriovenous Malformations

35180 Repair, congenital arteriovenous fistula; head and neck T 80
27.72 27.72 Global Days 090

35182 thorax and abdomen C5 C 80
53.24 53.24 Global Days 090

35184 extremities T 80
31.77 31.77 Global Days 090

35188 Repair, acquired or traumatic arteriovenous fistula; head and neck A2 T 80
32.95 32.95 Global Days 090

35189 thorax and abdomen C5 C 80
48.03 48.03 Global Days 090

35190 extremities T 80
23.38 23.38 Global Days 090

35201-35286 Surgical Repair Artery or Vein

EXCLUDES *Arteriovenous fistula repair (35180-35190)*

Do not report with a primary open vascular procedure.

35201 Repair blood vessel, direct; neck T 80 50
28.92 28.92 Global Days 090

35206 upper extremity T 80 50
23.85 23.85 Global Days 090

35207 hand, finger A2 T 50
22.23 22.23 Global Days 090

35211 intrathoracic, with bypass C5 C 80 50 PQ
42.24 42.24 Global Days 090

35216 intrathoracic, without bypass C5 C 80 50 PQ
61.62 61.62 Global Days 090

35221 intra-abdominal C5 C 80 50
43.90 43.90 Global Days 090

35226 lower extremity T 80 50
25.92 25.92 Global Days 090

35231 Repair blood vessel with vein graft; neck T 80 50
37.34 37.34 Global Days 090

35236 upper extremity T 80 50
30.34 30.34 Global Days 090

35241 intrathoracic, with bypass C5 C 80 50 PQ
44.19 44.19 Global Days 090

35246 intrathoracic, without bypass C5 C 80 50 PQ
45.35 45.35 Global Days 090

35251 intra-abdominal C5 C 80 50
51.82 51.82 Global Days 090

35256 lower extremity T 80 50
31.59 31.59 Global Days 090

35261 Repair blood vessel with graft other than vein; neck T 80 50
Code also (C1768, L8670)
32.62 32.62 Global Days 090

35266 upper extremity T 80 50
Code also (C1768, L8670)
26.79 26.79 Global Days 090

35271 intrathoracic, with bypass C5 C 80 50 PQ
42.39 42.39 Global Days 090

35276 intrathoracic, without bypass C5 C 80 50 PQ
44.25 44.25 Global Days 090

35281 intra-abdominal C5 C 80 50
49.61 49.61 Global Days 090

35286 lower extremity T 80 50
Code also (C1768, L8670)
29.08 29.08 Global Days 090

35301-35390 Surgical Thromboendarterectomy Peripheral and Visceral Arteries

CMS 100-3,20.1 Vertebral Artery Surgery
CMS 100-3,160.8 Electroencephalographic Monitoring During Cerebral Vasculature Surgery

INCLUDES Obtaining saphenous or arm vein for graft
Thrombectomy/embolectomy

EXCLUDES *Coronary artery bypass procedures (33510-33536, 33572)*
Thromboendarterectomy for vascular occlusion on a different vessel during the same session

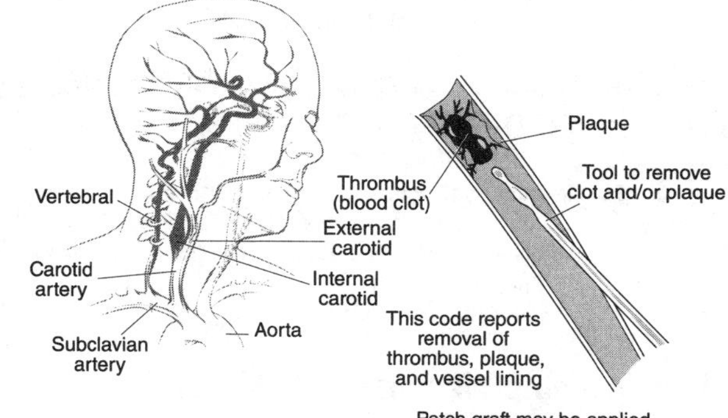

35301 Thromboendarterectomy, including patch graft, if performed; carotid, vertebral, subclavian, by neck incision C5 C 80 50 PQ
32.68 32.68 Global Days 090
AMA: 2007, January, 7-10

35302 superficial femoral artery C5 C 80 50
Do not report with (35500, 37225, 37227)
35.04 35.04 Global Days 090
AMA: 2007, May, 9-11; 2007, January, 7-10

35303 **popliteal artery** C5 C 80 50

Do not report with (35500, 37225, 37227)

38.55 38.55 Global Days 090

AMA: 2007, May, 9-11; 2007, January, 7-10

35304 **tibioperoneal trunk artery** C5 C 80 50

Do not report with (35500, 37229, 37231, 37233, 37235)

39.73 39.73 Global Days 090

AMA: 2007, January, 7-10; 2007, May, 9-11

35305 **tibial or peroneal artery, initial vessel** C5 C 80 50

Do not report with (35500, 37229, 37231, 37233, 37235)

38.33 38.33 Global Days 090

AMA: 2009, Jan, 11-31; 2008, Jan, 10-25; 2007, January, 7-10; 2007, May, 9-11

\+ **35306** **each additional tibial or peroneal artery (List separately in addition to code for primary procedure)** C5 C 80

Code first (35305)

Do not report with (35500, 37229, 37231, 37233, 37235)

13.96 13.96 Global Days ZZZ

AMA: 2007, January, 7-10; 2007, May, 9-11

35311 **subclavian, innominate, by thoracic incision** C5 C 80 50 P0

47.45 47.45 Global Days 090

35321 **axillary-brachial** T 80 50

27.80 27.80 Global Days 090

35331 **abdominal aorta** C5 C 80 50

45.41 45.41 Global Days 090

35341 **mesenteric, celiac, or renal** C5 C 80 50

42.82 42.82 Global Days 090

35351 **iliac** C5 C 80 50

39.94 39.94 Global Days 090

35355 **iliofemoral** C5 C 80 50

32.45 32.45 Global Days 090

35361 **combined aortoiliac** C5 C 80 50

47.97 47.97 Global Days 090

35363 **combined aortoiliofemoral** C5 C 80 50

54.00 54.00 Global Days 090

35371 **common femoral** C5 C 80 50

25.60 25.60 Global Days 090

AMA: 2007, January, 7-10

35372 **deep (profunda) femoral** C5 C 80 50

30.59 30.59 Global Days 090

AMA: 2007, January, 7-10

\+ **35390** **Reoperation, carotid, thromboendarterectomy, more than 1 month after original operation (List separately in addition to code for primary procedure)** C5 C 80

Code first (35301)

4.94 4.94 Global Days ZZZ

35400 Endoscopic Visualization of Vessels

\+ **35400** **Angioscopy (non-coronary vessels or grafts) during therapeutic intervention (List separately in addition to code for primary procedure)** C5 C 80

Code first the therapeutic intervention

4.63 4.63 Global Days ZZZ

35450-35460 Transluminal Angioplasty: Open

35450 **Transluminal balloon angioplasty, open; renal or other visceral artery** C5 C 80 50

75962-75968, 75978

15.89 15.89 Global Days 000

35452 **aortic** C5 C 80 50

75962-75968, 75978

11.01 11.01 Global Days 000

35458 **brachiocephalic trunk or branches, each vessel** T 80 50

Code also (C1725, C1874, C1876, C1885, C2625)

75962-75968, 75978

15.16 15.16 Global Days 000

AMA: 2009, Jan, 11-31; 2008, Jan, 10-25; 2007, January, 13-27

35460 **venous** G2 T 50

Code also (C1725, C1874, C1876, C1885, C2625)

75962-75968, 75978

9.68 9.68 Global Days 000

35471-35476 Transluminal Angioplasty: Percutaneous

CMS 100-3,20.7 Percutaneous Transluminal Angioplasty (PTA)

EXCLUDES *Catheter placement*

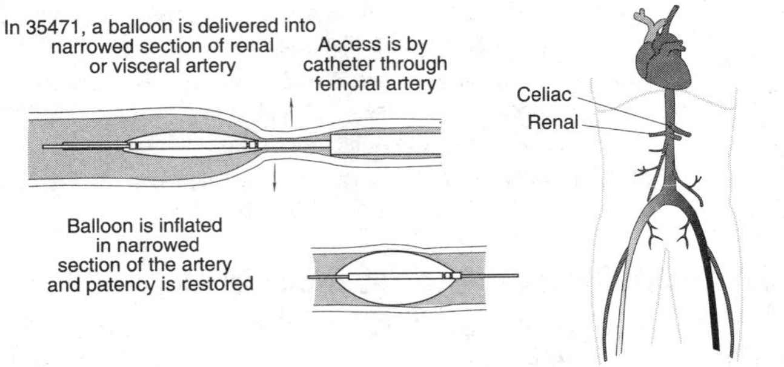

A balloon angioplasty is performed on the renal or visceral artery in a percutaneous procedure

⊙ **35471** **Transluminal balloon angioplasty, percutaneous; renal or visceral artery** T 50

Code also (C1725, C1874, C1876, C1885, C2625)

75966, 75968

16.21 82.31 Global Days 000

⊙ **35472** **aortic** T 80 50

Code also (C1725, C1874, C1876, C1885, C2625)

75966, 75968

11.13 61.20 Global Days 000

⊙ **35475** **brachiocephalic trunk or branches, each vessel** P3 T 50

INCLUDES All work performed for AV shunt to treat lesion(s) from the peri-arterial anastomosis through the axillary vein

EXCLUDES *Removal of arterial plug (36870)*

Code also (C1725, C1874, C1876, C1885, C2625)

75966, 75968

14.74 68.92 Global Days 000

AMA: 2009, Jan, 11-31; 2008, Sep, 10-11

⊙ **35476** **venous** P3 T 50

INCLUDES All services in an AV shunt segment including treatment of multiple distinct lesions

EXCLUDES *Removal of arterial plug (36870)*

Code also (C1725, C1874, C1876, C1885, C2625)

Do not report venous interventional codes for stenosis at the arterial anastomosis (peri-anastomotic or juxta-anastomotic region) (35475)

75978

9.35 52.16 Global Days 000

35500 Obtain Arm Vein for Graft

EXCLUDES *Endoscopic harvest (33508)*
Harvesting of multiple vein segments (35682, 35683)

\+ 35500 **Harvest of upper extremity vein, 1 segment, for lower extremity or coronary artery bypass procedure (List separately in addition to code for primary procedure)** T 80
Code first (33510-33536, 35556, 35566, 35570-35571, 35583-35587)
9.94 9.94 Global Days ZZZ
AMA: 2007, January, 7-10

35501-35571 Arterial Bypass Using Vein Grafts

CMS 100-3,20.1 Vertebral Artery Surgery
CMS 100-3,20.2 Extracranial-intracranial (EC-IC) Arterial Bypass Surgery
CMS 100-3,160.8 Electroencephalographic Monitoring During Cerebral Vasculature Surgery
INCLUDES Obtaining of saphenous vein grafts
EXCLUDES *Obtaining of multiple vein segments (35682, 35683)*
Obtaining vein graft, upper extremity or femoropopliteal (35500, 35572)
Treatment of different sites with different bypass procedures during the same operative session

35501 **Bypass graft, with vein; common carotid-ipsilateral internal carotid** C5 C 80 50
47.42 47.42 Global Days 090
AMA: 2007, January, 7-10

35506 **carotid-subclavian or subclavian-carotid** C5 C 80 50
41.67 41.67 Global Days 090
AMA: 2007, January, 7-10

35508 **carotid-vertebral** C5 C 80 50
INCLUDES Endoscopic procedure
42.30 42.30 Global Days 090

35509 **carotid-contralateral carotid** C5 C 80 50
44.80 44.80 Global Days 090
AMA: 2009, Jan, 11-31; 2008, Jan, 10-25; 2007, May, 9-11; 2007, January, 7-10

35510 **carotid-brachial** C5 C 80 50
38.84 38.84 Global Days 090
AMA: 2009, Jan, 11-31; 2008, Jan, 10-25

35511 **subclavian-subclavian** C5 C 80 50
38.86 38.86 Global Days 090

35512 **subclavian-brachial** C5 C 80 50
38.04 38.04 Global Days 090

35515 **subclavian-vertebral** C5 C 80 50
41.57 41.57 Global Days 090

35516 **subclavian-axillary** C5 C 80 50
38.19 38.19 Global Days 090

35518 **axillary-axillary** C5 C 80 50
36.16 36.16 Global Days 090

35521 **axillary-femoral** C5 C 80 50
EXCLUDES *Synthetic graft (35621)*
38.66 38.66 Global Days 090

35522 **axillary-brachial** C5 C 80 50
36.94 36.94 Global Days 090

35523 **brachial-ulnar or -radial** C5 C 80 50
EXCLUDES *Bypass graft performed with synthetic conduit (37799)*
Do not report with (35206, 35500, 35525, 36838)
39.90 39.90 Global Days 090

35525 **brachial-brachial** C5 C 80 50
35.59 35.59 Global Days 090

35526 **aortosubclavian, aortoinnominate, or aortocarotid** C5 C 80 50 PQ
EXCLUDES *Synthetic graft (35626)*
53.10 53.10 Global Days 090

35531 **aortoceliac or aortomesenteric** C5 C 80 50
62.64 62.64 Global Days 090

35533 **axillary-femoral-femoral** C5 C 80 50
EXCLUDES *Synthetic graft (35654)*
47.52 47.52 Global Days 090

35535 **hepatorenal** C5 C 80 50
Do not report with (35221, 35251, 35281, 35500, 35536, 35560, 35631, 35636)
53.86 53.86 Global Days 090

35536 **splenorenal** C5 C 80 50
53.15 53.15 Global Days 090
AMA: 2009, Jan, 11-31; 2008, Jan, 10-25; 2007, January, 13-27

35537 **aortoiliac** C5 C 80
EXCLUDES *Synthetic graft (35637)*
Do not report with (35538)
65.65 65.65 Global Days 090
AMA: 2007, January, 7-10

35538 **aortobi-iliac** C5 C 80
EXCLUDES *Synthetic graft (35638)*
Do not report with (35537)
73.57 73.57 Global Days 090
AMA: 2007, January, 7-10

35539 **aortofemoral** C5 C 80 50
EXCLUDES *Synthetic graft (35647)*
Do not report with (35540)
68.85 68.85 Global Days 090
AMA: 2007, January, 7-10

35540 **aortobifemoral** C5 C 50
EXCLUDES *Synthetic graft (35646)*
Do not report with (35539)
79.41 79.41 Global Days 090
AMA: 2007, January, 7-10

~~35548~~ ~~**aortoiliofemoral, unilateral**~~
To report, see 35537, 35539, 35565

~~35549~~ ~~**aortoiliofemoral, bilateral**~~
To report, see 35540, 35565

~~35551~~ ~~**aortofemoral-popliteal**~~
To report, see 35539-35540, 35556, 35583

35556 **femoral-popliteal** C5 C 80 50
43.70 43.70 Global Days 090
AMA: 2007, January, 7-10

35558 **femoral-femoral** C5 C 80 50
38.59 38.59 Global Days 090

35560 **aortorenal** C5 C 80 50
53.76 53.76 Global Days 090
AMA: 2009, Jan, 11-31; 2008, Jan, 10-25; 2007, January, 13-27

35563 **ilioiliac** C5 C 80 50
45.64 45.64 Global Days 090

35565 **iliofemoral** C5 C 80 50
41.27 41.27 Global Days 090

35566 **femoral-anterior tibial, posterior tibial, peroneal artery or other distal vessels** C5 C 80 50
52.21 52.21 Global Days 090
AMA: 2007, January, 7-10

35570 **tibial-tibial, peroneal-tibial, or tibial/peroneal trunk-tibial**

Do not report with (35256, 35286)

43.12 43.12 Global Days 090

35571 **popliteal-tibial, -peroneal artery or other distal vessels**

41.66 41.66 Global Days 090

AMA: 2007, January, 7-10

35572 Obtain Femoropopliteal Vein for Graft

\+ **35572** **Harvest of femoropopliteal vein, 1 segment, for vascular reconstruction procedure (eg, aortic, vena caval, coronary, peripheral artery) (List separately in addition to code for primary procedure)**

Code first (33510-33523, 33533-33536, 34502, 34520, 35001, 35002, 35011-35022, 35102-35103, 35121-35152, 35231-35256, 35501-35587, 35879-35907)

10.72 10.72 Global Days ZZZ

AMA: 2009, Jan, 11-31; 2008, Jan, 10-25; 2007, January, 28-31

35583-35587 Lower Extremity Revascularization: In-situ Vein Bypass

INCLUDES Obtaining saphenous vein grafts

EXCLUDES *Obtaining multiple vein segments (35682, 35683)*
Obtaining vein graft, upper extremity or femoropopliteal (35500, 35572)

35583 **In-situ vein bypass; femoral-popliteal**

Code also concurrent aortobifemoral bypass (synthetic) (35646)

Code also concurrent aortofemoral bypass (synthetic) (35647)

Code also concurrent aortobifemoral bypass (vein) (35539)

44.97 44.97 Global Days 090

AMA: 2007, January, 7-10

35585 **femoral-anterior tibial, posterior tibial, or peroneal artery**

52.42 52.42 Global Days 090

AMA: 2007, January, 7-10

35587 **popliteal-tibial, peroneal**

42.96 42.96 Global Days 090

AMA: 2007, January, 7-10

35600 Obtain Arm Artery for Coronary Bypass

EXCLUDES *Arterial reimplantation (35691-35695)*
Transposition of arteries (35691-35695)

\+ **35600** **Harvest of upper extremity artery, 1 segment, for coronary artery bypass procedure (List separately in addition to code for primary procedure)**

Code first (33533-33536)

7.87 7.87 Global Days ZZZ

AMA: 2009, Jan, 11-31; 2008, Jan, 10-25

35601-35671 Arterial Bypass with Synthetic Grafts

CMS 100-3,20.1 Vertebral Artery Surgery

CMS 100-3,20.2 Extracranial-intracranial (EC-IC) Arterial Bypass Surgery

CMS 100-3,160.8 Electroencephalographic Monitoring During Cerebral Vasculature Surgery

EXCLUDES *Transposition and/or reimplantation of arteries (35691-35695)*

35601 **Bypass graft, with other than vein; common carotid-ipsilateral internal carotid**

EXCLUDES *Open transcervical common carotid-common carotid bypass with endovascular repair of descending thoracic aorta (33891)*

44.16 44.16 Global Days 090

AMA: 2007, January, 7-10

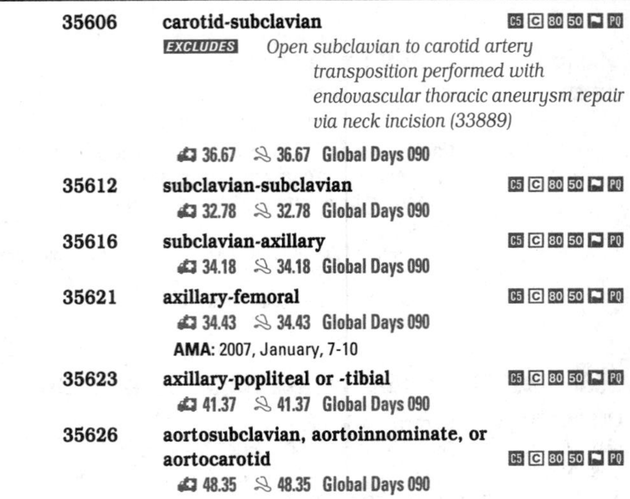

35606 **carotid-subclavian**

EXCLUDES *Open subclavian to carotid artery transposition performed with endovascular thoracic aneurysm repair via neck incision (33889)*

36.67 36.67 Global Days 090

35612 **subclavian-subclavian**

32.78 32.78 Global Days 090

35616 **subclavian-axillary**

34.18 34.18 Global Days 090

35621 **axillary-femoral**

34.43 34.43 Global Days 090

AMA: 2007, January, 7-10

35623 **axillary-popliteal or -tibial**

41.37 41.37 Global Days 090

35626 **aortosubclavian, aortoinnominate, or aortocarotid**

48.35 48.35 Global Days 090

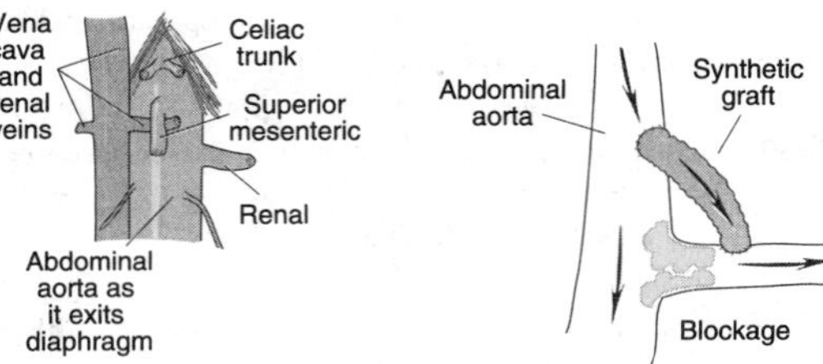

In 35631, a bypass graft of material other than vein is surgically installed from the aorta to the celiac, mesenteric, or renal arteries. The graft is typically placed in an end-to-side fashion on both the aorta and the recipient vessel downstream from the blockage

35631 **aortoceliac, aortomesenteric, aortorenal**

57.55 57.55 Global Days 090

35632 **ilio-celiac**

Do not report with (35221, 35251, 35281, 35531, 35631)

51.15 51.15 Global Days 090

35633 **ilio-mesenteric**

Do not report with (35221, 35251, 35281, 35531, 35631)

56.24 56.24 Global Days 090

35634 **iliorenal**

Do not report with (35221, 35251, 35281, 35536, 35560, 35631)

51.23 51.23 Global Days 090

35636 **splenorenal (splenic to renal arterial anastomosis)**

50.25 50.25 Global Days 090

35637 **aortoiliac**

Do not report with (35638, 35646)

53.87 53.87 Global Days 090

AMA: 2009, Jan, 11-31; 2008, Jan, 10-25; 2007, January, 7-10

35638 **aortobi-iliac**

EXCLUDES *Open placement of aorto-bi-iliac prosthesis after a failed endovascular repair (34831)*

Do not report with (35637, 35646)

54.95 54.95 Global Days 090

AMA: 2009, Jan, 11-31; 2008, Jan, 10-25; 2007, January, 7-10

35642 **carotid-vertebral**

34.65 34.65 Global Days 090

35645 **subclavian-vertebral** C5 C 80 50 CCI PQ
30.06 30.06 Global Days 090

35646 **aortobifemoral** C5 C 80 CCI PQ
EXCLUDES *Bypass graft using vein graft (35540)*
Open placement of aortobifemoral prostheses after a failed endovascular repair (34832)
53.66 53.66 Global Days 090
AMA: 2007, January, 7-10

35647 **aortofemoral** C5 C 80 50 CCI PQ
EXCLUDES *Bypass graft using vein graft (35539)*
48.36 48.36 Global Days 090
AMA: 2007, January, 7-10

35650 **axillary-axillary** C5 C 80 50 CCI PQ
33.36 33.36 Global Days 090

~~35651~~ ~~**aortofemoral-popliteal**~~
To report, see 35646-35647, 35656

35654 **axillary-femoral-femoral** C5 C 80 CCI PQ
42.79 42.79 Global Days 090
AMA: 2007, January, 7-10

35656 **femoral-popliteal** C5 C 80 50 CCI PQ
33.82 33.82 Global Days 090

35661 **femoral-femoral** C5 C 80 50 CCI PQ
33.98 33.98 Global Days 090
AMA: 2007, January, 7-10

35663 **ilioiliac** C5 C 80 50 CCI PQ
39.37 39.37 Global Days 090

35665 **iliofemoral** C5 C 80 50 CCI PQ
36.72 36.72 Global Days 090
AMA: 2007, January, 7-10

35666 **femoral-anterior tibial, posterior tibial, or peroneal artery** C5 C 80 50 CCI PQ
39.77 39.77 Global Days 090

35671 **popliteal-tibial or -peroneal artery** C5 C 80 50 CCI PQ
35.07 35.07 Global Days 090

35681-35683 Arterial Bypass Using Combination Synthetic and Donor Graft

\+ 35681 **Bypass graft; composite, prosthetic and vein (List separately in addition to code for primary procedure)** C5 C 80 CCI
Code first primary procedure
Do not report with (35682, 35683)
2.48 2.48 Global Days ZZZ
AMA: 2009, Jan, 11-31; 2008, Jan, 10-25; 2007, January, 13-27

\+ 35682 **autogenous composite, 2 segments of veins from 2 locations (List separately in addition to code for primary procedure)** C5 C 80 CCI
INCLUDES Harvest and anastomosis of multiple segments of vein from sites other than the limb undergoing bypass for arterial bypass graft conduits
Code first (35556, 35566, 35570, 35571, 35583-35587)
Do not report with (35681, 35683)
11.05 11.05 Global Days ZZZ
AMA: 2009, Jan, 11-31; 2008, Jan, 10-25; 2007, January, 13-27

\+ 35683 **autogenous composite, 3 or more segments of vein from 2 or more locations (List separately in addition to code for primary procedure)** C5 C 80 CCI
INCLUDES Harvest and anastomosis of multiple segments of vein from sites other than the limb undergoing bypass for arterial bypass graft conduits
Code first (35556, 35566, 35570, 35571, 35583-35587)
Do not report with (35681, 35682)
12.84 12.84 Global Days ZZZ
AMA: 2009, Jan, 11-31; 2008, Jan, 10-25; 2007, January, 13-27

35685-35686 Supplemental Procedures

INCLUDES Additional procedures that may be needed with a bypass graft to increase the patency of the graft

EXCLUDES *Composite grafts (35681-35683)*

\+ 35685 **Placement of vein patch or cuff at distal anastomosis of bypass graft, synthetic conduit (List separately in addition to code for primary procedure)** T 80 CCI
Code first (35656, 35666 or 35671)
6.20 6.20 Global Days ZZZ

\+ 35686 **Creation of distal arteriovenous fistula during lower extremity bypass surgery (non-hemodialysis) (List separately in addition to code for primary procedure)** T 80 CCI
Code first (35556, 35566, 35570-35571, 35583-35587, 35623, 35656, 35666, 35671)
5.15 5.15 Global Days ZZZ

35691-35697 Arterial Translocation

CMS 100-3,20.1 Vertebral Artery Surgery
CMS 100-3,20.2 Extracranial-intracranial (EC-IC) Arterial Bypass Surgery
CMS 100-3,160.8 Electroencephalographic Monitoring During Cerebral Vasculature Surgery

35691 **Transposition and/or reimplantation; vertebral to carotid artery** C5 C 80 50 CCI
29.85 29.85 Global Days 090

35693 **vertebral to subclavian artery** C5 C 80 50 CCI
29.49 29.49 Global Days 090

35694 **subclavian to carotid artery** C5 C 80 50 CCI
EXCLUDES *Subclavian to carotid artery transposition procedure (open) with concurrent repair of descending thoracic aorta (endovascular) (33889)*
31.08 31.08 Global Days 090

35695 **carotid to subclavian artery** C5 C 80 50 CCI
32.31 32.31 Global Days 090

\+ 35697 **Reimplantation, visceral artery to infrarenal aortic prosthesis, each artery (List separately in addition to code for primary procedure)** C5 C 80 CCI
Code first primary procedure
Do not report with (33877)
4.61 4.61 Global Days ZZZ

35700 Reoperative Bypass Lower Extremities

\+ 35700 **Reoperation, femoral-popliteal or femoral (popliteal)-anterior tibial, posterior tibial, peroneal artery, or other distal vessels, more than 1 month after original operation (List separately in addition to code for primary procedure)** C5 C 80 CCI
Code first (35556, 35566, 35570-35571, 35583, 35585, 35587, 35656, 35666, 35671)
4.76 4.76 Global Days ZZZ

35701-35761 Arterial Exploration without Repair

35701 **Exploration (not followed by surgical repair), with or without lysis of artery; carotid artery** C5 C 80 50
17.29 17.29 Global Days 090

35721 **femoral artery** C5 C 80 50
14.07 14.07 Global Days 090

35741 **popliteal artery** C5 C 80 50
15.84 15.84 Global Days 090

35761 **other vessels** G2 T 80 50
11.88 11.88 Global Days 090

35800-35860 Arterial Exploration for Postoperative Complication

INCLUDES Return to the operating room for postoperative hemorrhage

35800 **Exploration for postoperative hemorrhage, thrombosis or infection; neck** C5 C 80
21.19 21.19 Global Days 090

35820 **chest** C5 C 80
60.77 60.77 Global Days 090

35840 **abdomen** C5 C 80
34.54 34.54 Global Days 090

35860 **extremity** T 80
25.29 25.29 Global Days 090

35870 Repair Secondary Aortoenteric Fistula

35870 **Repair of graft-enteric fistula** C5 C 80
39.19 39.19 Global Days 090

35875-35876 Removal of Thrombus from Graft

EXCLUDES *Thrombectomy dialysis fistula or graft (36831, 36833)*
Thrombectomy with blood vessel repair, lower extremity, vein graft (35256)
Thrombectomy with blood vessel repair, lower extremity, with/without patch angioplasty (35226)

35875 **Thrombectomy of arterial or venous graft (other than hemodialysis graft or fistula);** A2 T
18.59 18.59 Global Days 090
AMA: 2009, Jan, 11-31; 2008, Jan, 10-25; 2007, January, 13-27

35876 **with revision of arterial or venous graft** A2 T 80
29.58 29.58 Global Days 090

35879-35884 Revision Lower Extremity Bypass Graft

EXCLUDES *Removal of infected graft (35901-35907)*
Revascularization following removal of infected graft(s)

35879 **Revision, lower extremity arterial bypass, without thrombectomy, open; with vein patch angioplasty** T 80 50
28.97 28.97 Global Days 090
AMA: 2007, January, 7-10

35881 **with segmental vein interposition** T 80 50
EXCLUDES *Revision of femoral anastomosis of synthetic arterial bypass graft (35883-35884)*
32.01 32.01 Global Days 090
AMA: 2007, January, 7-10

35883 **Revision, femoral anastomosis of synthetic arterial bypass graft in groin, open; with nonautogenous patch graft (eg, Dacron, ePTFE, bovine pericardium)** T 80 50
Do not report with (35700, 35875-35876, 35884)
37.60 37.60 Global Days 090
AMA: 2009, Jan, 11-31; 2008, Jan, 10-25; 2007, January, 7-10

35884 **with autogenous vein patch graft** T 80 50
Do not report with (35700, 35875-35876, 35883)
38.88 38.88 Global Days 090
AMA: 2009, Jan, 11-31; 2008, Jan, 10-25; 2007, January, 7-10

35901-35907 Removal of Infected Graft

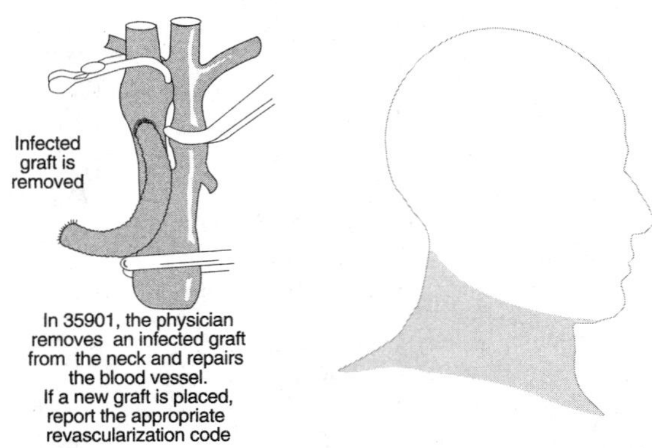

35901 **Excision of infected graft; neck** C5 C 80
15.55 15.55 Global Days 090

35903 **extremity** T 80
17.63 17.63 Global Days 090

35905 **thorax** C5 C 80
52.92 52.92 Global Days 090

35907 **abdomen** C5 C 80
59.61 59.61 Global Days 090

36000 Intravenous Access Established

INCLUDES Venous access for phlebotomy, prophylactic intravenous access, infusion therapy, chemotherapy, hydration, transfusion, drug administration, etc. which is included in the work value of the primary procedure

36000 **Introduction of needle or intracatheter, vein** N1 N
0.29 0.76 Global Days XXX
AMA: 2009, Jan, 11-31; 2008, Jan, 10-25; 2007, Jul, 1-4; 2007, January, 13-27; 2007, February, 10-11

36002 Injection Treatment of Pseudoaneurysm

INCLUDES Insertion of needle or catheter, local anesthesia, injection of contrast, power injections

EXCLUDES *Compression repair pseudoaneurysm, ultrasound guided (76936)*
Medications, contrast material, catheters

Do not report for arteriotomy site sealant

36002 **Injection procedures (eg, thrombin) for percutaneous treatment of extremity pseudoaneurysm** G2 S 50
76942, 77002, 77012, 77021
3.22 4.86 Global Days 000

36005-36015 Insertion Needle or Intracatheter: Venous

INCLUDES Insertion of needle/catheter, local anesthesia, injection of contrast, power injections

EXCLUDES *Medications, contrast materials, catheters*

Code also catheterization of second order vessels (or higher) supplied by the same first order branch, same vascular family

Code also each vascular family (e.g., bilateral procedures are separate vascular families)

36005 Injection procedure for extremity venography (including introduction of needle or intracatheter)
75820, 75822
1.45 10.32 Global Days 000

36010 Introduction of catheter, superior or inferior vena cava
3.65 16.13 Global Days XXX
AMA: 2009, Jan, 7-8; 2009, Jan, 11-31; 2008, Jan, 10-25; 2008, Oct, 10-11; 2007, January, 13-27

36011 Selective catheter placement, venous system; first order branch (eg, renal vein, jugular vein)
4.73 27.05 Global Days XXX

36012 second order, or more selective, branch (eg, left adrenal vein, petrosal sinus)
5.33 26.84 Global Days XXX

36013 Introduction of catheter, right heart or main pulmonary artery
3.91 24.91 Global Days XXX
AMA: 2009, Jan, 7-8; 2009, Jan, 11-31; 2008, Oct, 10-11

36014 Selective catheter placement, left or right pulmonary artery
4.49 25.39 Global Days XXX

36015 Selective catheter placement, segmental or subsegmental pulmonary artery
EXCLUDES *Placement of Swan Ganz/other flow directed catheter for monitoring (93503)*
Selective blood sampling, specific organs (36500)
5.19 27.52 Global Days XXX

36100-36254 Insertion Needle or Intracatheter: Arterial

INCLUDES Introduction of the catheter and catheterization of all lesser order vessels used for the approach
Local anesthesia, placement of catheter/needle, injection of contrast, power injections

EXCLUDES *Angiography (36147, 75600-75774, 75791)*
Angioplasty (35471, 35472, 35475, 37228-37235)
Chemotherapy injections (96401-96549)
Injection procedures for cardiac catheterizations (93452-93568)
Internal mammary artery angiography without left heart catheterization (36216, 36217)
Medications, contrast, catheters
Transcatheter procedures (37200-37208, 61624, 61626)

Code also additional first order or higher catheterization for vascular families if the vascular family is supplied by a first order vessel that is different from one already coded

Code also catheterization of second and third order vessels supplied by the same first order branch, same vascular family (36218, 36248)

75600-75791

36100 Introduction of needle or intracatheter, carotid or vertebral artery
4.87 15.91 Global Days XXX

36120 Introduction of needle or intracatheter; retrograde brachial artery
3.03 13.50 Global Days XXX
AMA: 2009, Jun, 10-11

36140 extremity artery
3.12 14.03 Global Days XXX
AMA: 2009, Jan, 11-31; 2009, Jun, 10-11; 2007, Jul, 1-4; 2007, Dec, 10-179

⊙ **36147 Introduction of needle and/or catheter, arteriovenous shunt created for dialysis (graft/fistula); initial access with complete radiological evaluation of dialysis access, including fluoroscopy, image documentation and report (includes access of shunt, injection[s] of contrast, and all necessary imaging from the arterial anastomosis and adjacent artery through entire venous outflow including the inferior or superior vena cava)**

INCLUDES Access and imaging of the AV shunt
Antegrade and/or retrograde punctures for contrast injection through a needle or catheter for imaging
Catheter manipulation for:
Advancement of the tip of the catheter to the vena cava
Diagnostic imaging of the AV shunt
Visualization of the arterial anastomosis or central veins
Catheterization of all veins in arteriovenous shunt
Diagnostic procedures of all upper and lower arteriovenous fistulae and grafts from the arterial anastomosis to the right atrium
Evaluation of peri-anastomotic portion of the inflow which includes:
Portion of the artery bordering the anastomosis
Portion of the graft or vessel just distal to the anastomosis
Site of the anastomosis

EXCLUDES *Additional catheter work/imaging to evaluate proximal arterial inflow to AV access*
Selective catheter advancement from the AV shunt puncture to the inflow artery (most often AV shunt of upper extremity) (36215)
Ultrasound guidance (76937)

Code also the second shunt catheterization if a need is identified for a therapeutic interventional procedure (36148)

Do not report selective catheterization of inferior/superior vena cava or central veins when performed by direct puncture of the fistula or graft

Do not report with (75791)
5.55 25.77 Global Days XXX

+ ⊙ **36148** **additional access for therapeutic intervention (List separately in addition to code for primary procedure)** N1 N 80

INCLUDES Catheterization of all veins in ateriovenous shunt
Interventional procedures in arteriovenous shunts (arteriovenous fistulae and grafts) considered to be primarily venous
Two vessel segments:
First segment (peripheral) extends from peri-arterial anastomosis through the axillary vein or the complete cephalic vein for cephalic venous outflow
Second segment: veins central to the axillary and cephalic veins (eg, subclavian and innominate veins through the vena cava)

EXCLUDES *Arterial intervention with radiological supervision and interpretation in the peri-anastomotic region (35475, 75962)*
Catheterization for intervention in an accessory vein (36011-36012)
Embolization of an accessory vein (37204, 75894)
Fistula thrombectomy (36870)
Other venous interventional procedures, as appropriate
Radiological supervision and interpretation for venous angioplasty (75978)
Stent placement for central venous stenosis (37206, 75960)
Stent placement from the peri-arterial anastomosis through the axillary and cephalic veins (37205, 75960)
Venous angioplasty, once per vessel only (35476)

Do not report selective catheterization of inferior/superior vena cava or central veins when performed by direct puncture of the fistula or graft

Do not report venous interventional codes for stenosis at the arterial anastomosis (peri-anastomotic or juxta-anastomotic region)

Code first (36147)

1.46 7.93 **Global Days ZZZ**

36160 **Introduction of needle or intracatheter, aortic, translumbar** N1 N

3.87 15.84 **Global Days XXX**

AMA: 2007, Dec, 10-179

⊙ **36200** **Introduction of catheter, aorta** N1 N 50

4.67 19.95 **Global Days 000**

AMA: 2009, Jan, 11-31; 2008, Apr, -11; 2007, Dec, 10-179

36215 **Selective catheter placement, arterial system; each first order thoracic or brachiocephalic branch, within a vascular family** N1 N

INCLUDES Introduction of catheter into the aorta (36200)

EXCLUDES *Placement of catheter for coronary angiography (93454-93461)*

7.33 34.52 **Global Days XXX**

AMA: 2009, Jan, 11-31; 2008, Jan, 10-25; 2007, Dec, 10-179; 2007, January, 13-27

36216 **initial second order thoracic or brachiocephalic branch, within a vascular family** N1 N

8.32 38.35 **Global Days XXX**

AMA: 2007, Dec, 10-179

36217 **initial third order or more selective thoracic or brachiocephalic branch, within a vascular family** N1 N

9.90 63.41 **Global Days XXX**

AMA: 2007, Dec, 10-179

+ **36218** **additional second order, third order, and beyond, thoracic or brachiocephalic branch, within a vascular family (List in addition to code for initial second or third order vessel as appropriate)** N1 N

Code first (36216, 36217)

1.58 5.83 **Global Days ZZZ**

AMA: 2007, Dec, 10-179

⊙ **36245** **Selective catheter placement, arterial system; each first order abdominal, pelvic, or lower extremity artery branch, within a vascular family** N1 N 50

7.41 33.19 **Global Days XXX**

AMA: 2009, Jan, 11-31; 2008, Jan, 10-25; 2007, January, 13-27; 2007, Dec, 10-179; 2007, January, 7-10

⊙ **36246** **initial second order abdominal, pelvic, or lower extremity artery branch, within a vascular family** N1 N 50

8.20 30.53 **Global Days 000**

AMA: 2009, Jan, 11-31; 2008, Jan, 10-25; 2007, January, 13-27; 2007, Dec, 10-179; 2007, January, 7-10

⊙ **36247** **initial third order or more selective abdominal, pelvic, or lower extremity artery branch, within a vascular family** N1 N 50

9.77 51.54 **Global Days 000**

AMA: 2009, Jan, 11-31; 2008, Jan, 10-25; 2007, January, 13-27; 2007, January, 7-10; 2007, Dec, 10-179

+ ⊙ **36248** **additional second order, third order, and beyond, abdominal, pelvic, or lower extremity artery branch, within a vascular family (List in addition to code for initial second or third order vessel as appropriate)** N1 N

Code first (36246, 36247)

1.54 4.70 **Global Days ZZZ**

AMA: 2009, Jan, 11-31; 2008, Jan, 10-25; 2007, January, 13-27; 2007, January, 7-10

⊙ ● **36251** **Selective catheter placement (first-order), main renal artery and any accessory renal artery(s) for renal angiography, including arterial puncture and catheter placement(s), fluoroscopy, contrast injection(s), image postprocessing, permanent recording of images, and radiological supervision and interpretation, including pressure gradient measurements when performed, and flush aortogram when performed; unilateral** N1 02

INCLUDES Closure device placement at vascular access site

8.30 43.20 **Global Days 000**

⊙ ● **36252** **bilateral** N1 02

INCLUDES Closure device placement at vascular access site

10.81 47.42 **Global Days 000**

⊙ ● 36253 **Superselective catheter placement (one or more second order or higher renal artery branches) renal artery and any accessory renal artery(s) for renal angiography, including arterial puncture, catheterization, fluoroscopy, contrast injection(s), image postprocessing, permanent recording of images, and radiological supervision and interpretation, including pressure gradient measurements when performed, and flush aortogram when performed; unilateral** N1 02

INCLUDES Closure device placement at vascular access site

Do not report for same kidney with (36251)

11.55 66.09 Global Days 000

⊙ ● 36254 **bilateral** N1 02

INCLUDES Closure device placement at vascular access site

Do not report with (36252)

12.46 68.76 Global Days 000

36260-36299 Implanted Infusion Pumps: Intra-arterial

CMS 100-3,280.14 Infusion Pumps

36260 **Insertion of implantable intra-arterial infusion pump (eg, for chemotherapy of liver)** A2 T

Code also (C1772, C1891, C2626)

18.85 18.85 Global Days 090

36261 **Revision of implanted intra-arterial infusion pump** A2 T 80

11.80 11.80 Global Days 090

36262 **Removal of implanted intra-arterial infusion pump** A2 T

8.98 8.98 Global Days 090

36299 **Unlisted procedure, vascular injection** N 80

0.00 0.00 Global Days YYY

36400-36425 Specimen Collection: Phlebotomy

EXCLUDES *Collection of specimen from:*
A completely implantable device (36591)
An established catheter (36592)

36400 **Venipuncture, younger than age 3 years, necessitating physician's skill, not to be used for routine venipuncture; femoral or jugular vein** A N1 N

0.57 0.83 Global Days XXX

AMA: 2007, Jul, 1-4

36405 **scalp vein** A N1 N

0.49 0.77 Global Days XXX

AMA: 2007, Jul, 1-4

36406 **other vein** A N1 N

0.26 0.51 Global Days XXX

AMA: 2007, Jul, 1-4

36410 **Venipuncture, age 3 years or older, necessitating physician's skill (separate procedure), for diagnostic or therapeutic purposes (not to be used for routine venipuncture)** A N1 N

0.28 0.52 Global Days XXX

AMA: 2009, Jan, 11-31; 2008, Jan, 10-25; 2007, Jul, 1-4; 2007, January, 13-27; 2007, February, 10-11

36415 **Collection of venous blood by venipuncture** A 63

0.00 0.00 Global Days XXX

AMA: 2009, Jan, 11-31; 2008, Jan, 10-25; 2008, Apr, -9; 2007, Jul, 1-4; 2007, January, 13-27; 2007, February, 10-11

36416 **Collection of capillary blood specimen (eg, finger, heel, ear stick)** N1 N

0.00 0.00 Global Days XXX

AMA: 2008, Apr, -9

36420 **Venipuncture, cutdown; younger than age 1 year** A R2 X 80 63

1.52 1.52 Global Days XXX

AMA: 2007, Jul, 1-4

36425 **age 1 or over** A R2 X

1.18 1.18 Global Days XXX

36430-36460 Transfusions

CMS 100-1,3,20.5 Blood Deductibles
CMS 100-1,3,20.5.2 Part B Blood Deductible
CMS 100-2,1,10 Inpatient Hospital Services Covered Under Part A
CMS 100-3,110.5 Granulocyte Transfulsions
CMS 100-3,110.7 Blood Transfusions
CMS 100-3,110.8 Blood Platelet Transfusions
CMS 100-3,110.16 Nonselective (Random) Transfusions and Living-Related Donor Specific Transfusions (DST) in Kidney Transplantation
CMS 100-4,3,40.2.2 Beneficiary Charges for Part A Services

36430 **Transfusion, blood or blood components** P3 S

1.01 1.01 Global Days XXX

AMA: 2009, Jan, 11-31; 2008, Jan, 10-25; 2007, Jul, 1-4; 2007, January, 13-27

36440 **Push transfusion, blood, 2 years or younger** A R2 S 80

1.67 1.67 Global Days XXX

AMA: 2007, Jul, 1-4

36450 **Exchange transfusion, blood; newborn** A R2 S 80 63

3.20 3.20 Global Days XXX

36455 **other than newborn** A G2 S

3.45 3.45 Global Days XXX

36460 **Transfusion, intrauterine, fetal** A ♀ S 80 63

76941

10.57 10.57 Global Days XXX

36468-36479 Destruction of Veins

CMS 100-2,16,10 Exclusions from Coverage
CMS 100-2,16,120 Cosmetic Procedures
CMS 100-2,16,180 Services Related to Noncovered Procedures

36468 **Single or multiple injections of sclerosing solutions, spider veins (telangiectasia); limb or trunk** R2 T 80

0.00 0.00 Global Days 000

36469 **face** R2 T 80

0.00 0.00 Global Days 000

36470 **Injection of sclerosing solution; single vein** P2 T 50

2.45 4.47 Global Days 010

36471 **multiple veins, same leg** P2 T 50

3.03 5.25 Global Days 010

36475 **Endovenous ablation therapy of incompetent vein, extremity, inclusive of all imaging guidance and monitoring, percutaneous, radiofrequency; first vein treated** A2 T 50

Do not report with (29581-29582, 36000-36005, 36410, 36425, 36478-36479, 37204, 75894, 76000-76001, 76937, 76942, 76998, 77022, 93970-93971)

10.69 53.79 Global Days 000

\+ 36476 **second and subsequent veins treated in a single extremity, each through separate access sites (List separately in addition to code for primary procedure)** A2 T 50

Code first (36475)

Do not report with (29581-29582, 36000-36005, 36410, 36425, 36478-36479, 37204, 75894, 76000-76001, 76937, 76942, 76998, 77022, 93970-93971)

5.25 11.94 Global Days ZZZ

36478 **Endovenous ablation therapy of incompetent vein, extremity, inclusive of all imaging guidance and monitoring, percutaneous, laser; first vein treated** A2 T 50

Do not report with (29581-29582, 36000-36005, 36410, 36425, 36475-36476, 37204, 75894, 76000-76001, 76937, 76942, 76998, 77022, 93970-93971)

10.65 42.57 Global Days 000

+ **36479** **second and subsequent veins treated in a single extremity, each through separate access sites (List separately in addition to code for primary procedure)** A2 T 50

Code first (36478)

Do not report with (29581-29582, 36000-36005, 36410, 36425, 36475-36476, 37204, 75894, 76000-76001, 76937, 76942, 76998, 77022, 93970-93971)

5.25 12.42 Global Days ZZZ

36481-36510 Other Venous Catheterization Procedures

EXCLUDES *Collection of a specimen from:*
A completely implantable device (36591)
An established catheter (36592)

⊙ **36481** **Percutaneous portal vein catheterization by any method** N1 N

75885, 75887

10.66 50.81 Global Days 000

AMA: 2009, Jan, 11-31; 2008, Jan, 10-25; 2007, January, 13-27

36500 **Venous catheterization for selective organ blood sampling** N1 N

EXCLUDES *Inferior or superior vena cava catheterization (36010)*

75893

5.39 5.39 Global Days 000

36510 **Catheterization of umbilical vein for diagnosis or therapy, newborn** A N1 N 80 63

EXCLUDES *Collection of a specimen from:*
Capillary blood (36416)
Venipuncture (36415)

1.81 2.99 Global Days 000

AMA: 2007, Jul, 1-4

36511-36516 Apheresis

CMS 100-1,3,20.5.2 Part B Blood Deductible
CMS 100-3,110.14 Apheresis (Therapeutic Pheresis)

EXCLUDES *Collection of a specimen from:*
A completely implantable device (36591)
An established catheter (36592)

36511 **Therapeutic apheresis; for white blood cells** G2 S

2.81 2.81 Global Days 000

AMA: 2009, Jun, 3-6&11

36512 **for red blood cells** G2 S

2.71 2.71 Global Days 000

AMA: 2009, Jun, 3-6&11

36513 **for platelets** G2 S

2.96 2.96 Global Days 000

AMA: 2009, Mar, 10-11; 2009, Jun, 3-6&11

36514 **for plasma pheresis** G2 S

2.75 15.41 Global Days 000

AMA: 2009, Jun, 3-6&11

36515 **with extracorporeal immunoadsorption and plasma reinfusion** P2 S

2.76 64.38 Global Days 000

AMA: 2009, Jun, 3-6&11

36516 **with extracorporeal selective adsorption or selective filtration and plasma reinfusion** P2 S

2.08 61.94 Global Days 000

AMA: 2009, Jun, 3-6&11

36522 Extracorporeal Photopheresis

CMS 100-3,110.4 Extracorporeal Photopheresis

36522 **Photopheresis, extracorporeal** G2 S

3.00 40.88 Global Days 000

AMA: 2009, Jun, 3-6&11

36555-36571 Placement of Implantable Venous Access Device

INCLUDES Devices that are inserted via cutdown or percutaneous access, either centrally (e.g., femoral, jugular, subclavian veins, or vena cava) or peripherally (e.g., basilic or cephalic)
Devices that terminate in the brachiocephalic (innominate), iliac, or subclavian veins, vena cava, or right atrium

EXCLUDES *Maintenance/refilling of implantable pump/reservoir (96522)*

76937, 77001

⊙ **36555** **Insertion of non-tunneled centrally inserted central venous catheter; younger than 5 years of age** A A2 T P0

EXCLUDES *That by peripheral insertion (36568)*

3.60 8.09 Global Days 000

AMA: 2008, Jun, 8-11; 2007, Jul, 1-4

36556 **age 5 years or older** A A2 T P0

EXCLUDES *That by peripheral insertion (36569)*

3.60 7.00 Global Days 000

AMA: 2008, Jun, 8-11

A tunneled centrally inserted CVC is inserted. Report 36557 for a patient under age 5 and 36558 for patients older than age 5

⊙ **36557** **Insertion of tunneled centrally inserted central venous catheter, without subcutaneous port or pump; younger than 5 years of age** A A2 T 80 50 P0

Code also (C1750-C1752)

9.68 29.62 Global Days 010

AMA: 2008, Jun, 8-11

⊙ **36558** **age 5 years or older** A A2 T 80 50 P0

EXCLUDES *That by peripheral insertion (36571)*

Code also (C1750, C1751, C1752)

8.35 23.64 Global Days 010

AMA: 2008, Jun, 8-11

⊙ **36560** **Insertion of tunneled centrally inserted central venous access device, with subcutaneous port; younger than 5 years of age** A A2 T 80 50 P0

EXCLUDES *That by peripheral insertion (36570)*

Code also (C1751, C1788)

10.77 39.51 Global Days 010

AMA: 2008, Jun, 8-11

⊙ **36561** **age 5 years or older** A A2 T 80 50 CCI PQ

EXCLUDES *That by peripheral insertion (36571)*

Code also (C1751, C1788)

10.61 35.60 **Global Days 010**

AMA: 2008, Jun, 8-11

⊙ **36563** **Insertion of tunneled centrally inserted central venous access device with subcutaneous pump** A2 T 80 CCI PQ

Code also (C1772, C1891, C2626)

11.28 39.54 **Global Days 010**

AMA: 2008, Jun, 8-11

⊙ **36565** **Insertion of tunneled centrally inserted central venous access device, requiring 2 catheters via 2 separate venous access sites; without subcutaneous port or pump (eg, Tesio type catheter)** A2 T 80 50 CCI PQ

Code also (C1750, C1751, C1752)

10.58 30.22 **Global Days 010**

AMA: 2008, Jun, 8-11

⊙ **36566** **with subcutaneous port(s)** A2 T 80 50 CCI PQ

Code also (C1881)

11.39 149.99 **Global Days 010**

AMA: 2008, Jun, 8-11

⊙ **36568** **Insertion of peripherally inserted central venous catheter (PICC), without subcutaneous port or pump; younger than 5 years of age** A A2 T CCI PQ

EXCLUDES *Centrally inserted placement (36555)*

Do not report removal of PICC lines with codes for removal of tunneled central venous catheters; report appropriate E/M code

2.83 8.65 **Global Days 000**

AMA: 2009, Jan, 11-31; 2008, Jan, 10-25; 2008, Jun, 8-11; 2007, January, 13-27

36569 **age 5 years or older** A A2 T CCI PQ

EXCLUDES *Centrally inserted placement (36556)*

Do not report removal of PICC lines with codes for removal of tunneled central venous catheters; report appropriate E/M code

2.71 7.38 **Global Days 000**

AMA: 2009, Jan, 11-31; 2008, Jan, 10-25; 2008, Jun, 8-11; 2007, January, 13-27

⊙ **36570** **Insertion of peripherally inserted central venous access device, with subcutaneous port; younger than 5 years of age** A A2 T 80 50 CCI PQ

EXCLUDES *Centrally inserted placement (36560)*

Code also (C1751, C1788)

9.17 35.20 **Global Days 010**

AMA: 2008, Jun, 8-11

⊙ **36571** **age 5 years or older** A A2 T 80 50 CCI PQ

EXCLUDES *Centrally inserted placement (36561)*

Code also (C1751, C1788)

9.60 38.77 **Global Days 010**

AMA: 2008, Jun, 8-11

36575-36590 Repair, Removal, and Replacement Implantable Venous Access Device

EXCLUDES *Mechanical removal obstructive material, pericatheter/intraluminal (36595, 36596)*

36575 **Repair of tunneled or non-tunneled central venous access catheter, without subcutaneous port or pump, central or peripheral insertion site** A2 T 80 CCI

INCLUDES Repair of the device without replacing any parts

1.06 4.91 **Global Days 000**

AMA: 2008, Jun, 8-11

⊙ **36576** **Repair of central venous access device, with subcutaneous port or pump, central or peripheral insertion site** A2 T 80 CCI

INCLUDES Repair of the device without replacing any parts

5.82 11.27 **Global Days 010**

AMA: 2008, Jun, 8-11

⊙ **36578** **Replacement, catheter only, of central venous access device, with subcutaneous port or pump, central or peripheral insertion site** A2 T 80 CCI PQ

INCLUDES Partial replacement (catheter only)

Code also (C1750, C1751, C1752)

6.48 15.43 **Global Days 010**

AMA: 2008, Jun, 8-11

36580 **Replacement, complete, of a non-tunneled centrally inserted central venous catheter, without subcutaneous port or pump, through same venous access** A2 T CCI PQ

INCLUDES Complete replacement (replace all components/same access site)

1.98 6.45 **Global Days 000**

AMA: 2008, Jun, 8-11

⊙ **36581** **Replacement, complete, of a tunneled centrally inserted central venous catheter, without subcutaneous port or pump, through same venous access** A2 T 80 CCI PQ

INCLUDES Complete replacement (replace all components/same access site)

Code also (C1750, C1751, C1752)

5.91 22.75 **Global Days 010**

AMA: 2008, Jun, 8-11

⊙ **36582** **Replacement, complete, of a tunneled centrally inserted central venous access device, with subcutaneous port, through same venous access** A2 T 80 CCI PQ

INCLUDES Complete replacement (replace all components/same access site)

Code also (C1751, C1788, C1881)

9.19 33.21 **Global Days 010**

AMA: 2008, Jun, 8-11

⊙ **36583** **Replacement, complete, of a tunneled centrally inserted central venous access device, with subcutaneous pump, through same venous access** A2 T 80 CCI PQ

INCLUDES Complete replacement (replace all components/same access site)

Code also (C1772, C1891, C2626)

9.64 35.28 **Global Days 010**

AMA: 2008, Jun, 8-11

36584 **Replacement, complete, of a peripherally inserted central venous catheter (PICC), without subcutaneous port or pump, through same venous access** A2 T CCI PQ

INCLUDES Complete replacement (replace all components/same access site)

1.96 6.11 **Global Days 000**

AMA: 2008, Jun, 8-11

⊙ **36585** **Replacement, complete, of a peripherally inserted central venous access device, with subcutaneous port, through same venous access** A2 T 80 CCI PQ

INCLUDES Complete replacement (replace all components/same access site)

Code also (C1751, C1788)

8.38 33.57 **Global Days 010**

AMA: 2008, Jun, 8-11

36589 **Removal of tunneled central venous catheter, without subcutaneous port or pump**

INCLUDES Complete removal/all components

EXCLUDES *Non-tunneled central venous catheter removal; report appropriate E/M code*

4.18 4.96 Global Days 010

AMA: 2008, Jun, 8-11

⊙ **36590** **Removal of tunneled central venous access device, with subcutaneous port or pump, central or peripheral insertion**

INCLUDES Complete removal/all components

Do not report with non-tunneled central venous catheter removal; report appropriate E/M code

6.12 8.67 Global Days 010

AMA: 2008, Jun, 8-11

36591-36592 Obtain Blood Specimen from Implanted Device or Catheter

36591 **Collection of blood specimen from a completely implantable venous access device**

EXCLUDES *Collection of:*

Capillary blood specimen (36416)

Venous blood specimen by venipuncture (36415)

Do not report with any other service except for a laboratory service

0.68 0.68 Global Days XXX

AMA: 2008, Apr, -9

36592 **Collection of blood specimen using established central or peripheral catheter, venous, not otherwise specified**

EXCLUDES *Collection of blood from an established arterial catheter (37799)*

Do not report with any other service except for a laboratory service

0.77 0.77 Global Days XXX

AMA: 2008, Apr, -9

36593-36596 Restore Patency of Occluded Catheter or Device

EXCLUDES *Venous catheterization (36010-36012)*

36593 **Declotting by thrombolytic agent of implanted vascular access device or catheter**

0.88 0.88 Global Days XXX

AMA: 2008, Apr, -9

36595 **Mechanical removal of pericatheter obstructive material (eg, fibrin sheath) from central venous device via separate venous access**

EXCLUDES *Venous catheterization (36010-36012)*

Do not report with (36593)

75901

5.53 17.04 Global Days 000

36596 **Mechanical removal of intraluminal (intracatheter) obstructive material from central venous device through device lumen**

EXCLUDES *Venous catheterization (36010-36012)*

Do not report with (36593)

75902

1.35 4.00 Global Days 000

36597-36598 Repositioning or Assessment of In Situ Venous Access Device

36597 **Repositioning of previously placed central venous catheter under fluoroscopic guidance**

76000

1.81 3.68 Global Days 000

36598 **Contrast injection(s) for radiologic evaluation of existing central venous access device, including fluoroscopy, image documentation and report**

EXCLUDES *Complete venography studies (75820, 75825, 75827)*

Do not report with (36595-36596, 76000)

1.26 3.32 Global Days 000

36600-36660 Insertion Needle or Catheter: Artery

36600 **Arterial puncture, withdrawal of blood for diagnosis**

Do not report with critical care services

0.45 0.91 Global Days XXX

AMA: 2007, Jul, 1-4; 2007, February, 10-11

⊘ **36620** **Arterial catheterization or cannulation for sampling, monitoring or transfusion (separate procedure); percutaneous**

1.51 1.51 Global Days 000

AMA: 2007, Jul, 1-4

36625 **cutdown**

3.20 3.20 Global Days 000

36640 **Arterial catheterization for prolonged infusion therapy (chemotherapy), cutdown**

EXCLUDES *Intraarterial chemotherapy (96420-96425)*
Transcatheter embolization (75894)

Code also (C1751)

3.85 3.85 Global Days 000

36660 **Catheterization, umbilical artery, newborn, for diagnosis or therapy**

2.26 2.26 Global Days 000

AMA: 2007, Jul, 1-4

36680 Percutaneous Placement of Catheter/Needle into Bone Marrow Cavity

36680 **Placement of needle for intraosseous infusion**

1.77 1.77 Global Days 000

36800-36821 Vascular Access for Hemodialysis

36800 **Insertion of cannula for hemodialysis, other purpose (separate procedure); vein to vein**

Code also (C1750, C1752)

4.87 4.87 Global Days 000

36810 **arteriovenous, external (Scribner type)**

Code also (C1750, C1752)

6.41 6.41 Global Days 000

36815 **arteriovenous, external revision, or closure**

4.55 4.55 Global Days 000

36818 **Arteriovenous anastomosis, open; by upper arm cephalic vein transposition**

INCLUDES Two incisions in the upperarm-a medial incision over the brachial artery and a lateral incision for exposure of part of the vein

20.57 20.57 Global Days 090

36819 by upper arm basilic vein transposition A2 T 80 CCI PQ
22.74 22.74 Global Days 090

36820 by forearm vein transposition A2 T 80 50 CCI PQ
24.69 24.69 Global Days 090

36821 direct, any site (eg, Cimino type) (separate procedure) A2 T 80 CCI PQ
21.19 21.19 Global Days 090

36822-36823 Vascular Access for Extracorporeal Circulation

EXCLUDES *Maintenance for prolonged extracorporeal circulation (33960, 33961)*

36822 **Insertion of cannula(s) for prolonged extracorporeal circulation for cardiopulmonary insufficiency (ECMO) (separate procedure)** C5 C CCI
EXCLUDES *Maintenance for prolonged circulation (33960, 33961)*
11.68 11.68 Global Days 090
AMA: 2009, Jan, 11-31; 2008, Jan, 10-25; 2007, January, 13-27

36823 **Insertion of arterial and venous cannula(s) for isolated extracorporeal circulation including regional chemotherapy perfusion to an extremity, with or without hyperthermia, with removal of cannula(s) and repair of arteriotomy and venotomy sites** C5 C CCI
INCLUDES Chemotherapy perfusion
Do not report with (96409-96425)
39.81 39.81 Global Days 090

36825-36835 Permanent Vascular Access Procedures

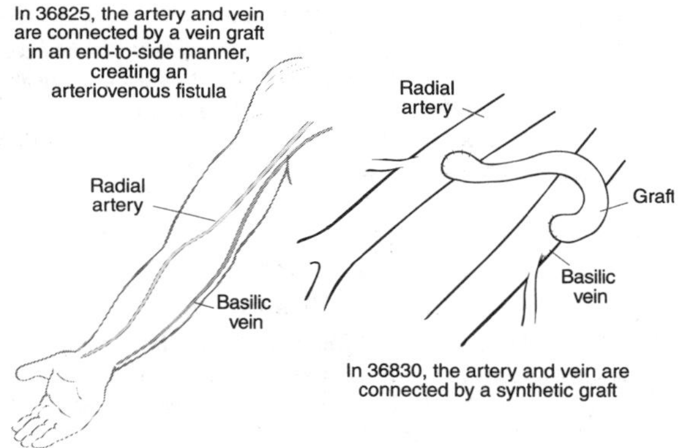

36825 **Creation of arteriovenous fistula by other than direct arteriovenous anastomosis (separate procedure); autogenous graft** A2 T 80 CCI PQ
EXCLUDES *Direct arteriovenous (AV) anastomosis (36821)*
24.02 24.02 Global Days 090

36830 **nonautogenous graft (eg, biological collagen, thermoplastic graft)** A2 T 80 CCI PQ
EXCLUDES *Direct arteriovenous (AV) anastomosis (36821)*
20.19 20.19 Global Days 090

36831 **Thrombectomy, open, arteriovenous fistula without revision, autogenous or nonautogenous dialysis graft (separate procedure)** A2 T 80 CCI
14.04 14.04 Global Days 090
AMA: 2009, Jan, 11-31; 2008, Jan, 10-25; 2007, January, 13-27

36832 **Revision, open, arteriovenous fistula; without thrombectomy, autogenous or nonautogenous dialysis graft (separate procedure)** A2 T 80 CCI
INCLUDES Revision of an arteriovenous access fistula or graft
17.81 17.81 Global Days 090
AMA: 2009, Jan, 11-31; 2008, Jan, 10-25; 2007, January, 13-27

36833 **with thrombectomy, autogenous or nonautogenous dialysis graft (separate procedure)** A2 T 80 CCI
20.13 20.13 Global Days 090
AMA: 2009, Jan, 11-31; 2008, Jan, 10-25; 2007, January, 13-27

36835 **Insertion of Thomas shunt (separate procedure)** A2 T CCI
Code also (C1750, C1752)
15.01 15.01 Global Days 090

36838 DRIL Procedure for Ischemic Steal Syndrome

INCLUDES Banding/ligation angioacess arteriovenous (AV) fistula
Ligation artery of extremity
Open revision arteriovenous (AV) fistula
Subclavian-brachial or axilary-brachial bypass grafts

Do not report with (35512, 35522-35523, 36832, 37607, 37618)

36838 **Distal revascularization and interval ligation (DRIL), upper extremity hemodialysis access (steal syndrome)** T 80 50 CCI
35.53 35.53 Global Days 090

36860-36870 Restore Patency of Occluded Cannula or Arteriovenous Fistula

36860 **External cannula declotting (separate procedure); without balloon catheter** A2 T CCI
76000
3.24 6.13 Global Days 000

36861 **with balloon catheter** A2 T CCI
Code also (C1757)
76000
4.64 4.64 Global Days 000

⊙ 36870 **Thrombectomy, percutaneous, arteriovenous fistula, autogenous or nonautogenous graft (includes mechanical thrombus extraction and intra-graft thrombolysis)** A2 T 50 CCI
INCLUDES Declotting using thrombolytics
Moving thrombus using a mechanical methodolgy including using a balloon catheter
Removal of arterial plug (36870)
EXCLUDES *Catheterization for arteriovenous (AV) shunt (36147-36148)*
Do not report with (36593)
75791
9.07 57.04 Global Days 090

37140-37181 Open Decompression of Portal Circulation

EXCLUDES *Peritoneal-venous shunt (49425)*

37140 **Venous anastomosis, open; portocaval** C5 C CCI
66.38 66.38 Global Days 090

37145 **renoportal** C5 C 80 CCI
62.22 62.22 Global Days 090

37160 **caval-mesenteric** C5 C 80 CCI
63.14 63.14 Global Days 090

37180 **splenorenal, proximal** C5 C 80 CCI
61.02 61.02 Global Days 090

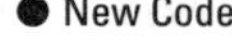

37181 **splenorenal, distal (selective decompression of esophagogastric varices, any technique)**

EXCLUDES *Percutaneous procedure (37182)*

66.62 66.62 Global Days 090

37182-37183 Transvenous Decompression of Portal Circulation

Do not report with (75885, 75887)

37182 **Insertion of transvenous intrahepatic portosystemic shunt(s) (TIPS) (includes venous access, hepatic and portal vein catheterization, portography with hemodynamic evaluation, intrahepatic tract formation/dilatation, stent placement and all associated imaging guidance and documentation)**

EXCLUDES *Open procedure (37140)*

25.09 25.09 Global Days 000

AMA: 2009, Jan, 11-31; 2008, Jan, 10-25; 2007, January, 13-27

⊙ 37183 **Revision of transvenous intrahepatic portosystemic shunt(s) (TIPS) (includes venous access, hepatic and portal vein catheterization, portography with hemodynamic evaluation, intrahepatic tract recanulization/dilatation, stent placement and all associated imaging guidance and documentation)**

EXCLUDES *Arteriovenous (AV) aneurysm repair (36832)*

11.85 168.80 Global Days 000

AMA: 2009, Jan, 11-31; 2008, Jan, 10-25; 2007, January, 13-27

37184-37188 Removal of Thrombus from Vessel: Percutaneous

INCLUDES Fluoroscopic guidance
Injection(s) of thrombolytics during the procedure
Postprocedure evaluation
Pretreatment planning

EXCLUDES *Continuous infusion of thrombolytics prior to and after the procedure (37201, 75896, 75898)*
Diagnostic studies
Mechanical thrombectomy, coronary (92973)
Other interventions performed percutaneously (e.g., balloon angioplasty)
Percutaneous thrombectomy of an arteriovenous fistula (36870)
Placement of catheters
Radiological supervision/interpretation

⊙ 37184 **Primary percutaneous transluminal mechanical thrombectomy, noncoronary, arterial or arterial bypass graft, including fluoroscopic guidance and intraprocedural pharmacological thrombolytic injection(s); initial vessel**

EXCLUDES *Mechanical thrombectomy of another vascular family, separate access site, append modifier 51 to code, as appropriate*
Seconday mechanical thrombectomy for treating of embolus/thrombus complicating another percutaneous intervention (37186)

Code also (C1757)

Do not report with (76000-76001, 96374, 99143-99150)

13.71 70.14 Global Days 000

+ ⊙ 37185 **second and all subsequent vessel(s) within the same vascular family (List separately in addition to code for primary mechanical thrombectomy procedure)**

INCLUDES Treatment of second and all succeeding vessel(s) in same vascular family

EXCLUDES *Intravenous drug injections administered subsequent to an initial service*
Mechanical thrombectomy for embolus/thrombus complicating another percutaneous interventional procedure (37186)
Mechanical thrombectomy of another vascular family/separate access site, append modifier 51 to code as appropriate

Code first (37184)

Do not report with (76000-76001, 96375)

5.07 22.91 Global Days ZZZ

+ ⊙ 37186 **Secondary percutaneous transluminal thrombectomy (eg, nonprimary mechanical, snare basket, suction technique), noncoronary, arterial or arterial bypass graft, including fluoroscopic guidance and intraprocedural pharmacological thrombolytic injections, provided in conjunction with another percutaneous intervention other than primary mechanical thrombectomy (List separately in addition to code for primary procedure)**

INCLUDES Removal of small emboli/thrombi prior to or after another percutaneous procedure

Code first primary procedure

Do not report with (76000-76001, 96375)

7.72 45.06 Global Days ZZZ

AMA: 2009, Jan, 11-31; 2008, May, 9-11

⊙ 37187 **Percutaneous transluminal mechanical thrombectomy, vein(s), including intraprocedural pharmacological thrombolytic injections and fluoroscopic guidance**

INCLUDES Secondary or subsequent intravenous injection after another initial service

Code also (C1757)

Do not report with (76000-76001, 96375)

12.35 66.56 Global Days 000

⊙ 37188 **Percutaneous transluminal mechanical thrombectomy, vein(s), including intraprocedural pharmacological thrombolytic injections and fluoroscopic guidance, repeat treatment on subsequent day during course of thrombolytic therapy**

Code also (C1757)

Do not report with (76000-76001, 96375)

8.79 56.08 Global Days 000

37191-37193 Vena Cava Filters

⊙ ● 37191 **Insertion of intravascular vena cava filter, endovascular approach including vascular access, vessel selection, and radiological supervision and interpretation, intraprocedural roadmapping, and imaging guidance (ultrasound and fluoroscopy), when performed**

EXCLUDES *Open ligation of inferior vena cava via laparotomy or retroperitoneal approach (37619)*

7.07 78.51 Global Days 000

⊙ ● 37192 **Repositioning of intravascular vena cava filter, endovascular approach including vascular access, vessel selection, and radiological supervision and interpretation, intraprocedural roadmapping, and imaging guidance (ultrasound and fluoroscopy), when performed** T

Do not report with (37191)

10.96 52.67 Global Days 000

⊙ ● 37193 **Retrieval (removal) of intravascular vena cava filter, endovascular approach including vascular access, vessel selection, and radiological supervision and interpretation, intraprocedural roadmapping, and imaging guidance (ultrasound and fluoroscopy), when performed** T

Do not report with (37203, 75961)

10.95 50.26 Global Days 000

37195 Intravenous Cerebral Thrombolysis

37195 **Thrombolysis, cerebral, by intravenous infusion** T 80

0.00 0.00 Global Days XXX

37200-37203 Transcatheter Procedures: Infusions, Biopsy, Foreign Body Removal

37200 **Transcatheter biopsy** 62 T

75970

6.65 6.65 Global Days 000

37201 **Transcatheter therapy, infusion for thrombolysis other than coronary** 62 T

EXCLUDES *Thrombolysis of coronary vessels (92975-92977)*

75896

8.28 8.28 Global Days 000

AMA: 2009, Jan, 11-31; 2008, Jan, 10-25; 2007, January, 13-27

37202 **Transcatheter therapy, infusion other than for thrombolysis, any type (eg, spasmolytic, vasoconstrictive)** 62 T

EXCLUDES *Thrombolysis of coronary vessels (92975-92977)*

Code also for nitroglycerin infusion done with a cardiac catheterization

75896

9.98 9.98 Global Days 000

AMA: 2009, Jan, 11-31; 2008, Jan, 10-25; 2007, January, 13-27

⊙ 37203 **Transcatheter retrieval, percutaneous, of intravascular foreign body (eg, fractured venous or arterial catheter)** 62 T

EXCLUDES *Vena cava filter removal (37193)*

75961

7.82 39.74 Global Days 000

AMA: 2009, Jan, 11-31; 2009, Jan, 7-8; 2008, Oct, 10-11

37204 Therapeutic Embolization (Except UFE)

CMS 100-3,20.28 Therapeutic Embolization

INCLUDES Ob/Gyn procedures except uterine fibroid embolization

EXCLUDES *Embolization/uterine fibroids (37210)*
Transcatheter occlusion or embolization for treatment of a tumor, vascular malformation, or hemorrhage (61624, 61626)

37204 **Transcatheter occlusion or embolization (eg, for tumor destruction, to achieve hemostasis, to occlude a vascular malformation), percutaneous, any method, non-central nervous system, non-head or neck** 62 T

75894

26.86 26.86 Global Days 000

AMA: 2009, Jan, 11-31; 2008, Feb, 5-6; 2008, Jan, 10-25; 2007, January, 13-27; 2007, January, 7-10

37205-37208 Insertion Intravascular Stent

EXCLUDES *Placement stent(s):*
Extracranial vertebral or intrathoracic carotid artery (0075T, 0076T)
Femoral, iliac, popliteal, tibial/peroneal arteries (37221, 37223, 37226, 37227, 37230, 37231, 37234, 37235)
Intracoronary (92980, 92981)
Intracranial (61635)
Intravascular cervical carotid artery (37215-37216)
Selective catheter placement (36215-36248)

37205 **Transcatheter placement of an intravascular stent(s) (except coronary, carotid, vertebral, iliac, and lower extremity arteries), percutaneous; initial vessel** T 80

INCLUDES All AV stent placement services from the peri-arterial anastomosis through the axillary and cephalic veins even if multiple stents are placed or there are multiple lesions

Code also (C1874, C1875, C1876, C1877, C2617, C2625)

Code also additional stent placement for central venous stenosis (37206, 75960)

75960

12.99 127.67 Global Days 000

\+ 37206 **each additional vessel (List separately in addition to code for primary procedure)** T 80

Code also (C1874, C1875, C1876, C1877, C2617, C2625)

75960

Code first (37205)

6.43 76.33 Global Days ZZZ

37207 **Transcatheter placement of an intravascular stent(s) (except coronary, carotid, vertebral, iliac and lower extremity arteries), open; initial vessel** 62 T 80 50

Code also (C1874, C1875, C1876, C1877, C2617, C2625)

75960

13.11 13.11 Global Days 000

\+ 37208 **each additional vessel (List separately in addition to code for primary procedure)** 62 T 80

Code also (C1874, C1875, C1876, C1877, C2617, C2625)

Code first (37207)

75960

6.33 6.33 Global Days ZZZ

37209 Replace Intravascular Catheter

37209 **Exchange of a previously placed intravascular catheter during thrombolytic therapy** T

Code also (C1750, C1751, C1752)

75900

3.38 3.38 Global Days 000

● New Code ▲ Revised Code Maternity Age Unlisted Not Covered # Resequenced
○ Reinstated CCI + Add-on ⊘ Mod 51 Exempt Mod 63 Exempt ⊙ Mod Sedation PQRS

37210 Therapeutic Embolization, Uterine Fibroid

CMS 100-3,20.28 Therapeutic Embolization

INCLUDES Access and imaging
Angiography follow-up evaluation
Transcatheter therapy, radiological supervision and interpretation
Vascular access procedures

EXCLUDES *Ob/Gyn procedures other than UFE*
Transcatheter embolization for conditions other than CNS/head or neck (37204)

Do not report with (36200, 36245-36248, 37204, 75894, 75898)

⊙ 37210 **Uterine fibroid embolization (UFE, embolization of the uterine arteries to treat uterine fibroids, leiomyomata), percutaneous approach inclusive of vascular access, vessel selection, embolization, and all radiological supervision and interpretation, intraprocedural roadmapping, and imaging guidance necessary to complete the procedure** ♀ G2 T P0

15.74 107.58 **Global Days 000**

AMA: 2009, Jan, 11-31; 2008, Jan, 10-25; 2008, Feb, 5-6; 2007, January, 7-10

37215-37216 Stenting of Carotid Artery with/without Insertion Distal Embolic Protection Device

INCLUDES Carotid stenting, if required
Ipsilateral diagnostic imaging/supervision and interpretation
Ipsilateral selective carotid catheterization

EXCLUDES *Carotid catheterization and imaging, if carotid stenting not required*
Percutaneous placement intravascular stents besides coronary, carotid, vertebral (37205, 37206)
Transcatheter placement extracranial vertebral or intrathoracic carotid artery stents (0075T, 0076T)

Do not report with (75671, 75680)

⊙ 37215 **Transcatheter placement of intravascular stent(s), cervical carotid artery, percutaneous; with distal embolic protection** C5 C 80

33.19 33.19 **Global Days 090**

⊙ 37216 **without distal embolic protection** E

29.97 29.97 **Global Days 090**

37220-37235 Endovascular Revascularization

INCLUDES Percutaneous and open interventional and associated procedures for lower extremity occlusive disease; unilateral
Accessing the vessel
Arteriotomy closure by suturing of puncture or by pressure and application of arterial closure device
Atherectomy (e.g., directional, laser, rotational)
Balloon angioplasty (e.g., cryoplasty, cutting balloon, low-profile)
Catheterization of the vessel (selective)
Embolic protection
Imaging once procedure is complete
Radiological supervision and interpretation of intervention(s)
Stenting (e.g., bare metal, balloon-expandable, covered, drug-eluting, self-expanding)
Transversing of the lesion
Reporting the most comprehensive treatment in a given vessel according to the following hierarchy:
1. Stent and atherectomy
2. Atherectomy
3. Stent
4. PTA
Revascularization procedures for three arterial vascular territories:
Femoral/popliteal vascular territory including the common, deep, and superficial femoral arteries, and the popliteal artery (one extremity = a single vessel) (37224-37227)
Iliac vascular territory: common iliac, external iliac, internal iliac (37220-37223)
Tibial/peroneal territory: includes anterior tibial, peroneal artery, posterior tibial (37228-37235)

EXCLUDES *Mechanical thrombectomy and/thrombolysis*

Code also add-on codes for different vessels, but not different lesions in the same vessel; and for multiple territories in the same leg

Code also extensive repair or replacement of artery (35226, 35286)

Code also modifer 59 for a bilateral procedure

Code first one primary code for the intial service in each leg

Do not report more than one code for: vessels in the femoral/popliteal territory (report the most complex service for more than one lesion in the territory); when a contigious lesion that spans from one territory to another an be opened with a single procedure; or when more than one stent is deployed in the same vessel

Do not report more than one code from this family for each lower extremity vessel treated.

⊙ 37220 **Revascularization, endovascular, open or percutaneous, iliac artery, unilateral, initial vessel; with transluminal angioplasty** G2 T 50

Code also (C1725, C1885)

12.57 96.94 **Global Days 000**

⊙ 37221 **with transluminal stent placement(s), includes angioplasty within the same vessel, when performed** G2 T 80 50

Code also (C1874-C1877, C2617-C2625)

15.31 144.77 **Global Days 000**

+ ⊙ 37222 **Revascularization, endovascular, open or percutaneous, iliac artery, each additional ipsilateral iliac vessel; with transluminal angioplasty (List separately in addition to code for primary procedure)** G2 T 80 50

Code also (C1725, C1885)

Code first (37220, 37221)

5.70 27.81 **Global Days ZZZ**

+ ⊙ 37223 **with transluminal stent placement(s), includes angioplasty within the same vessel, when performed (List separately in addition to code for primary procedure)** G2 T 80 50

Code also (C1874-C1877, C2617, C2625)

Code first (37221)

6.47 79.34 **Global Days ZZZ**

⊙ **37224** **Revascularization, endovascular, open or percutaneous, femoral, popliteal artery(s), unilateral; with transluminal angioplasty** T 80 50
Code also (C1725-C1885)
13.84 116.60 Global Days 000

⊙ **37225** **with atherectomy, includes angioplasty within the same vessel, when performed** T 80 50
18.70 331.12 Global Days 000

⊙ **37226** **with transluminal stent placement(s), includes angioplasty within the same vessel, when performed** T 80 50
Code also (C1874-C1877, C2617, C2625)
15.37 279.32 Global Days 000

⊙ **37227** **with transluminal stent placement(s) and atherectomy, includes angioplasty within the same vessel, when performed** T 80 50
Code also (C1874-C1877, C2617, C2625)
22.58 447.86 Global Days 000

⊙ **37228** **Revascularization, endovascular, open or percutaneous, tibial, peroneal artery, unilateral, initial vessel; with transluminal angioplasty** T 80 50
Code also (C1725, C1885)
16.93 166.63 Global Days 000

⊙ **37229** **with atherectomy, includes angioplasty within the same vessel, when performed** T 80 50
21.88 327.47 Global Days 000

⊙ **37230** **with transluminal stent placement(s), includes angioplasty within the same vessel, when performed** T 80 50
Code also (C1874-C1877, C2617, C2625)
21.10 259.40 Global Days 000

⊙ **37231** **with transluminal stent placement(s) and atherectomy, includes angioplasty within the same vessel, when performed** T 80 50
Code also (C1874-C1877, C2617, C2625)
22.93 417.05 Global Days 000

+ ⊙ **37232** **Revascularization, endovascular, open or percutaneous, tibial/peroneal artery, unilateral, each additional vessel; with transluminal angioplasty (List separately in addition to code for primary procedure)** T 80 50
Code also (C1725, C1885)
Code first (37228-37231)
6.12 37.26 Global Days ZZZ

+ ⊙ **37233** **with atherectomy, includes angioplasty within the same vessel, when performed (List separately in addition to code for primary procedure)** T 80 50
Code first (37229, 37231)
10.07 45.23 Global Days ZZZ

+ ⊙ **37234** **with transluminal stent placement(s), includes angioplasty within the same vessel, when performed (List separately in addition to code for primary procedure)** T 80 50
Code also (C1874-C1877, C2617, C2625)
Code first (37229-37231)
8.38 119.34 Global Days ZZZ

+ ⊙ **37235** **with transluminal stent placement(s) and atherectomy, includes angioplasty within the same vessel, when performed (List separately in addition to code for primary procedure)** T 80 50
Code also (C1874-C1877, C2617, C2625)
Code first (37231)
11.89 127.30 Global Days ZZZ

37250-37251 Intravascular Ultrasound: Noncoronary

CMS 100-3,220.5 Ultrasound Diagnostic Procedures

INCLUDES Manipulation and repositioning of the transducer prior to and after therapeutic interventional procedures

EXCLUDES *Selective catheter placement for access (36215-36248)*
Transcatheter procedures (37200-37208, 61624, 61626)

+ **37250** **Intravascular ultrasound (non-coronary vessel) during diagnostic evaluation and/or therapeutic intervention; initial vessel (List separately in addition to code for primary procedure)** N1 N 80
Code first primary procedure
75945-75946
3.29 3.29 Global Days ZZZ

+ **37251** **each additional vessel (List separately in addition to code for primary procedure)** N1 N 80
Code first (37250)
75945-75946
2.47 2.47 Global Days ZZZ

37500-37501 Vascular Endoscopic Procedures

INCLUDES Diagnostic endoscopy

EXCLUDES *Open procedure (37760)*

37500 **Vascular endoscopy, surgical, with ligation of perforator veins, subfascial (SEPS)** A2 T 50
21.21 21.21 Global Days 090

37501 **Unlisted vascular endoscopy procedure** T 50
0.00 0.00 Global Days YYY

37565-37606 Ligation Procedures: Jugular Vein, Carotid Arteries

CMS 100-3,160.8 Electroencephalographic Monitoring During Cerebral Vasculature Surgery

EXCLUDES *Arterial balloon occlusion, endovascular, temporary (61623)*
For treatment intracranial aneurysm (61703)
Suture of arteries and veins (35201-35286)
Transcatheter arterial embolization/occlusion, permanent (61624, 61626)

37565 **Ligation, internal jugular vein** T 80
22.00 22.00 Global Days 090

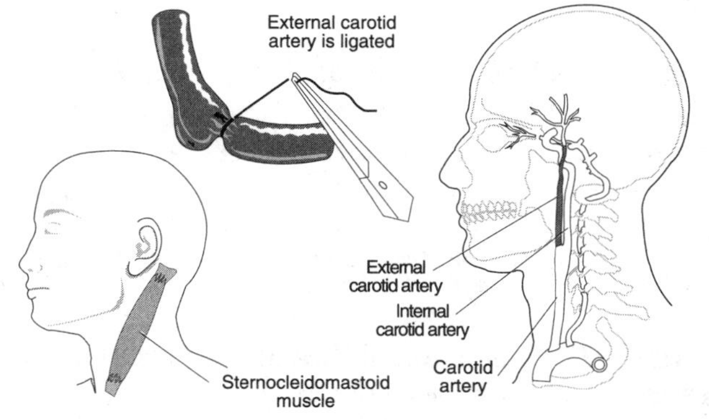

37600 **Ligation; external carotid artery** T 80
21.53 21.53 Global Days 090

37605 **internal or common carotid artery** T 80
24.69 24.69 Global Days 090

37606 **internal or common carotid artery, with gradual occlusion, as with Selverstone or Crutchfield clamp**
16.98 16.98 Global Days 090

37607-37609 Ligation Hemodialysis Angioaccess or Temporal Artery

EXCLUDES *Suture of arteries and veins (35201-35286)*

37607 **Ligation or banding of angioaccess arteriovenous fistula**
11.57 11.57 Global Days 090

37609 **Ligation or biopsy, temporal artery**
6.25 9.34 Global Days 010

37615-37618 Arterial Ligation, Major Vessel, for Injury/Rupture

EXCLUDES *Suture of arteries and veins (35201-35286)*

37615 **Ligation, major artery (eg, post-traumatic, rupture); neck**
INCLUDES Touroff ligation
15.27 15.27 Global Days 090

37616 **chest**
INCLUDES Bardenheurer operation
33.00 33.00 Global Days 090

37617 **abdomen**
39.87 39.87 Global Days 090

37618 **extremity**
11.72 11.72 Global Days 090

37619-37620 Ligation, Any Method, Inferior Vena Cava

EXCLUDES *Suture of arteries and veins (35201-35286)*

● 37619 **Ligation of inferior vena cava**
EXCLUDES *Endovascular delivery of inferior vena cava filter (37191)*
48.78 48.78 Global Days 090

~~37620 **Interruption, partial or complete, of inferior vena cava by suture, ligation, plication, clip, extravascular, intravascular (umbrella device)**~~
To report, see 37191, 37619

37650-37660 Venous Ligation, Femoral and Common Iliac

EXCLUDES *Suture of arteries and veins (35201-35286)*

37650 **Ligation of femoral vein**
16.35 16.35 Global Days 090

37660 **Ligation of common iliac vein**
38.37 38.37 Global Days 090

37700-37785 Treatment of Varicose Veins of Legs

EXCLUDES *Suture of arteries and veins (35201-35286)*

37700 **Ligation and division of long saphenous vein at saphenofemoral junction, or distal interruptions**
INCLUDES Babcock operation

Do not report with (37718, 37722)
7.76 7.76 Global Days 090
AMA: 2009, Jan, 11-31; 2008, Jan, 10-25; 2007, January, 13-27

37718 **Ligation, division, and stripping, short saphenous vein**

Do not report with (37735, 37780)
13.41 13.41 Global Days 090

37722 **Ligation, division, and stripping, long (greater) saphenous veins from saphenofemoral junction to knee or below**
EXCLUDES *Ligation/division/stripping short saphenous vein (37718)*

Do not report with (37700, 37735)
14.85 14.85 Global Days 090

37735 **Ligation and division and complete stripping of long or short saphenous veins with radical excision of ulcer and skin graft and/or interruption of communicating veins of lower leg, with excision of deep fascia**

Do not report with (37700, 37718, 37722, 37780)
19.28 19.28 Global Days 090

37760 **Ligation of perforator veins, subfascial, radical (Linton type), including skin graft, when performed, open, 1 leg**
EXCLUDES *Ligation of subfascial perforator veins, endoscopic (37500)*

Do not report with (76937, 76942, 76998, 93971)
19.18 19.18 Global Days 090

37761 **Ligation of perforator vein(s), subfascial, open, including ultrasound guidance, when performed, 1 leg**
EXCLUDES *Ligation of subfascial perforator veins, endoscopic (37500)*

Do not report with (76937, 76942, 76998, 93971)
16.88 16.88 Global Days 090

37765 **Stab phlebectomy of varicose veins, 1 extremity; 10-20 stab incisions**
EXCLUDES *Fewer than 10 incisions (37799)*
13.88 20.14 Global Days 090

37766 **more than 20 incisions**
EXCLUDES *Fewer than 10 incisions (37799)*
16.95 23.82 Global Days 090

37780 **Ligation and division of short saphenous vein at saphenopopliteal junction (separate procedure)**
7.91 7.91 Global Days 090
AMA: 2009, Jan, 11-31; 2008, Jan, 10-25; 2007, January, 13-27

37785 **Ligation, division, and/or excision of varicose vein cluster(s), 1 leg**
8.02 10.87 Global Days 090

37788-37790 Treatment of Vascular Disease of the Penis

37788 **Penile revascularization, artery, with or without vein graft** ♂
41.15 41.15 Global Days 090

37790 **Penile venous occlusive procedure** ♂
14.28 14.28 Global Days 090

37799 Unlisted Vascular Surgery Procedures

37799 **Unlisted procedure, vascular surgery**
0.00 0.00 Global Days YYY
AMA: 2009, Jan, 11-31; 2008, Jan, 10-25; 2007, January, 13-27

38100-38200 Splenic Procedures

38100 **Splenectomy; total (separate procedure)** C5 C 80 PQ
33.56 33.56 Global Days 090

38101 **partial (separate procedure)** C5 C 80 PQ
33.87 33.87 Global Days 090

+ **38102** **total, en bloc for extensive disease, in conjunction with other procedure (List in addition to code for primary procedure)** C5 C 80
Code first primary procedure
7.67 7.67 Global Days ZZZ

38115 **Repair of ruptured spleen (splenorrhaphy) with or without partial splenectomy** C5 C 80 PQ
37.02 37.02 Global Days 090

38120 **Laparoscopy, surgical, splenectomy** T 80 PQ
INCLUDES Diagnostic laparoscopy
30.75 30.75 Global Days 090

38129 **Unlisted laparoscopy procedure, spleen** T 80
0.00 0.00 Global Days YYY

38200 **Injection procedure for splenoportography** N1 N 80
75810
4.29 4.29 Global Days 000

38204-38215 Hematopoietic Stem Cell Procedures

CMS 100-3,110.8.1 Stem Cell Transplantation

INCLUDES Preservation, preparation, purification before transplant or reinfusion:
Bone marrow
Stem cells
Reporting each code no more than once per day

Do not report with flow cytometry (88182, 88184-88189)

38204 **Management of recipient hematopoietic progenitor cell donor search and cell acquisition** N1 N
2.96 2.96 Global Days XXX
AMA: 2009, Jun, 3-6&11

38205 **Blood-derived hematopoietic progenitor cell harvesting for transplantation, per collection; allogeneic** B 80
2.31 2.31 Global Days 000
AMA: 2009, Jun, 3-6&11

38206 **autologous** G2 S 80
2.36 2.36 Global Days 000
AMA: 2009, Jun, 3-6&11

38207 **Transplant preparation of hematopoietic progenitor cells; cryopreservation and storage** S
88240
1.35 1.35 Global Days XXX
AMA: 2009, Jun, 3-6&11

▲ **38208** **thawing of previously frozen harvest, without washing, per donor** S
88241
0.86 0.86 Global Days XXX
AMA: 2009, Jun, 3-6&11

▲ **38209** **thawing of previously frozen harvest, with washing, per donor** S
0.36 0.36 Global Days XXX
AMA: 2009, Jun, 3-6&11

38210 **specific cell depletion within harvest, T-cell depletion** S
2.39 2.39 Global Days XXX
AMA: 2009, Jun, 3-6&11

38211 **tumor cell depletion** S
2.17 2.17 Global Days XXX
AMA: 2009, Jun, 3-6&11

38212 **red blood cell removal** S
1.42 1.42 Global Days XXX
AMA: 2009, Jun, 3-6&11

38213 **platelet depletion** S
0.36 0.36 Global Days XXX
AMA: 2009, Jun, 3-6&11

38214 **plasma (volume) depletion** S
1.23 1.23 Global Days XXX
AMA: 2009, Jun, 3-6&11

38215 **cell concentration in plasma, mononuclear, or buffy coat layer** S
1.42 1.42 Global Days XXX
AMA: 2009, Jun, 3-6&11

38220-38242 Bone Marrow Procedures

CMS 100-1,5,90.2 Laboratory Defined
CMS 100-2,15,80 Diagnostic Test Requirements
CMS 100-2,15,80.1 Payment for Clinical Laboratory Services
CMS 100-3,110.8.1 Stem Cell Transplantation
CMS 100-4,3,90.3 Stem Cell Transplantation
CMS 100-4,3,90.3.1 Allogeneic Stem Cell Transplantation
CMS 100-4,3,90.3.3 Billing for Stem Cell Transplantation
CMS 100-4,32,90 Billing for Stem Cell Transplantation

EXCLUDES *Expansion and thawing of blood-derived stem cell specimens for transplantation (38208-38209)*
Modification, treatment, processing of bone marrow/blood-derived stem cell specimens for transplantation (38210-38213)
Storage, freezing, and cryopreservation of blood-derived stem cell specimens for transplantation (38207)

38220 **Bone marrow; aspiration only** P3 T 80 50
1.78 4.69 Global Days XXX
AMA: 2009, Jan, 11-31; 2009, Jun, 3-6&11; 2008, Jan, 10-25; 2007, January, 13-27; 2007, June, 10-11

38221 **biopsy, needle or trocar** P3 T 80 50
88305
2.19 4.87 Global Days XXX
AMA: 2009, Jun, 3-6&11

▲ **38230** **Bone marrow harvesting for transplantation; allogeneic** G2 S 80
Autologous blood-derived hematopoietic progenitor cell harvesting for transplant (38206)
86812-86822, 88240-88241
5.45 5.45 Global Days 000
AMA: 2009, Jun, 3-6&11

● **38232** **autologous** G2 S 80
5.45 5.45 Global Days 000

38240 **Bone marrow or blood-derived peripheral stem cell transplantation; allogeneic** S 80
86812-86822, 88240-88241
3.64 3.64 Global Days XXX
AMA: 2009, Jun, 3-6&11

38241 **autologous** G2 S 80
86812-86822, 88240-88241
3.63 3.63 Global Days XXX
AMA: 2009, Jun, 3-6&11

38242 **allogeneic donor lymphocyte infusions** R2 S 80
86812-86822, 88240-88241
2.77 2.77 Global Days 000
AMA: 2009, Jun, 3-6&11

38300-38382 Incision Lymphatic Vessels

38300 **Drainage of lymph node abscess or lymphadenitis; simple** A2 T
5.49 8.28 Global Days 010

38305 **extensive** A2 T
13.54 13.54 Global Days 090

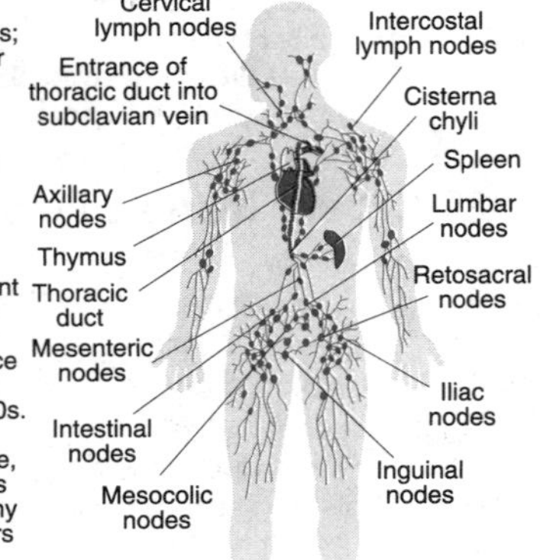

38308 **Lymphangiotomy or other operations on lymphatic channels** A2 T 80
13.18 13.18 Global Days 090

38380 **Suture and/or ligation of thoracic duct; cervical approach** C5 C 80
17.03 17.03 Global Days 090

38381 **thoracic approach** C5 C 80 PQ
24.10 24.10 Global Days 090

38382 **abdominal approach** C5 C 80
20.82 20.82 Global Days 090

38500-38555 Biopsy/Excision Lymphatic Vessels

CMS 100-4,12,30 Correct Coding Policy

EXCLUDES *Injection for sentinel node identification (38792)*
Percutaneous needle biopsy retroperitoneal mass (49180)

38500 **Biopsy or excision of lymph node(s); open, superficial** A2 T 50

Do not report with (38700-38780)
7.42 9.68 Global Days 010
AMA: 2009, Jan, 7-8; 2009, Jan, 11-31; 2008, Jan, 10-25; 2008, Sep, 5-6; 2007, January, 13-27; 2007, Dec, 7-8

38505 **by needle, superficial (eg, cervical, inguinal, axillary)** A2 T 50
EXCLUDES *Fine needle aspiration (10021-10022)*

76942, 77012, 77021
88172, 88173
2.11 3.70 Global Days 000
AMA: 2009, Jan, 7-8

38510 **open, deep cervical node(s)** A2 T 50
12.42 15.36 Global Days 010
AMA: 2009, Jan, 11-31; 2008, Jan, 10-25; 2007, January, 13-27

38520 **open, deep cervical node(s) with excision scalene fat pad** A2 T 50
13.71 13.71 Global Days 090
AMA: 2009, Jan, 11-31; 2008, Jan, 10-25; 2007, January, 13-27

38525 **open, deep axillary node(s)** A2 T 50
12.68 12.68 Global Days 090
AMA: 2009, Jan, 11-31; 2008, Jan, 10-25; 2008, Sep, 5-6; 2007, January, 13-27; 2007, Dec, 7-8

38530 **open, internal mammary node(s)** A2 T 80 50
EXCLUDES *Fine needle aspiration (10022)*

Do not report with (38720-38746)
16.13 16.13 Global Days 090
AMA: 2008, Sep, 5-6

38542 **Dissection, deep jugular node(s)** A2 T 80 50
EXCLUDES *Complete cervical lymphadenectomy (38720)*

15.37 15.37 Global Days 090

38550 **Excision of cystic hygroma, axillary or cervical; without deep neurovascular dissection** A2 T 80
14.76 14.76 Global Days 090

38555 **with deep neurovascular dissection** A2 T 80
29.38 29.38 Global Days 090

38562-38564 Limited Lymphadenectomy: Staging

38562 **Limited lymphadenectomy for staging (separate procedure); pelvic and para-aortic** C5 C 80
EXCLUDES *Prostatectomy (55812, 55842)*
Radioactive substance inserted into prostate (55862)

20.55 20.55 Global Days 090
AMA: 2009, Jan, 11-31; 2008, Jan, 10-25; 2007, January, 13-27

38564 **retroperitoneal (aortic and/or splenic)** C5 C 80
20.58 20.58 Global Days 090

38570-38589 Laparoscopic Lymph Node Procedures

INCLUDES Diagnostic laparoscopy

EXCLUDES *Laparoscopy with draining of lymphocele to peritoneal cavity (49323)*
Limited lymphadenectomy:
Pelvic (38562)
Retroperitoneal (38564)

38570 **Laparoscopy, surgical; with retroperitoneal lymph node sampling (biopsy), single or multiple** A2 T 80
15.70 15.70 Global Days 010

38571 **with bilateral total pelvic lymphadenectomy** A2 T 80 PQ
23.39 23.39 Global Days 010

38572 **with bilateral total pelvic lymphadenectomy and peri-aortic lymph node sampling (biopsy), single or multiple** A2 T 80 PQ
27.88 27.88 Global Days 010

38589 **Unlisted laparoscopy procedure, lymphatic system** T 80 50
0.00 0.00 Global Days YYY

38700-38780 Lymphadenectomy Procedures

INCLUDES Lymph node biopsy/excision

EXCLUDES *Excision of lymphadematous skin and subcutaneous tissue (15004-15005)*
Limited lymphadenectomy
Pelvic (38562)
Retroperitoneal (38564)
Repair of lymphadematous skin and tissue (15570-15650)

Do not report with (38500)

38700 **Suprahyoid lymphadenectomy** G2 T 80 50 PQ
23.95 23.95 Global Days 090

38720 **Cervical lymphadenectomy (complete)** T 80 50 PQ
40.01 40.01 Global Days 090
AMA: 2009, Jan, 11-31; 2008, Jan, 10-25; 2007, January, 13-27

38724 **Cervical lymphadenectomy (modified radical neck dissection)** C5 C 80 50 PQ
43.22 43.22 Global Days 090
AMA: 2009, Jan, 11-31; 2008, Jan, 10-25; 2007, January, 13-27

38740 **Axillary lymphadenectomy; superficial** A2 T 80 50 CCI PQ
20.11 20.11 Global Days 090

38745 **complete** A2 T 80 50 CCI PQ
25.48 25.48 Global Days 090

+ ▲ 38746 **Thoracic lymphadenectomy by thoracotomy, mediastinal and regional lymphadenectomy (List separately in addition to code for primary procedure)** C5 C 80 CCI PQ

INCLUDES Left side
Aortopulmonary window
Inferior pulmonary ligament
Paraesophageal
Subcarinal
Mediastinal lymph nodes
Right side
Inferior pulmonary ligament
Paraesophageal
Paratracheal
Subcarinal

EXCLUDES *Thoracoscopic mediastinal and regional lymphadenectomy (32674)*

Code first primary procedure (32440-32488, 32503-32505)
6.61 6.61 Global Days ZZZ

+ 38747 **Abdominal lymphadenectomy, regional, including celiac, gastric, portal, peripancreatic, with or without para-aortic and vena caval nodes (List separately in addition to code for primary procedure)** C5 C 80 CCI PQ
Code first primary procedure
7.79 7.79 Global Days ZZZ

38760 **Inguinofemoral lymphadenectomy, superficial, including Cloquets node (separate procedure)** A2 T 80 50 CCI PQ
24.65 24.65 Global Days 090
AMA: 2009, Jan, 7-8

38765 **Inguinofemoral lymphadenectomy, superficial, in continuity with pelvic lymphadenectomy, including external iliac, hypogastric, and obturator nodes (separate procedure)** C5 C 80 50 CCI PQ

INCLUDES Lymph node biopsy/excision

EXCLUDES *Limited lymphadenectomy*
Pelvic (38562)
Retroperitoneal (38564)

37.67 37.67 Global Days 090
AMA: 2009, Jan, 7-8

38770 **Pelvic lymphadenectomy, including external iliac, hypogastric, and obturator nodes (separate procedure)** C5 C 80 50 CCI PQ

INCLUDES Lymph node biopsy/excision

EXCLUDES *Limited lymphadenectomy*
Pelvic (38562)
Retroperitoneal (38564)

23.59 23.59 Global Days 090

38780 **Retroperitoneal transabdominal lymphadenectomy, extensive, including pelvic, aortic, and renal nodes (separate procedure)** C5 C 80 CCI PQ

INCLUDES Lymph node biopsy/excision

EXCLUDES *Limited lymphadenectomy*
Pelvic (38562)
Retroperitoneal (38564)

30.27 30.27 Global Days 090

38790-38999 Cannulation/Injection/Other Procedures

38790 **Injection procedure; lymphangiography** N1 N 50 CCI
75801-75807
2.47 2.47 Global Days 000

▲ 38792 **radioactive tracer for identification of sentinel node** N1 01 50 CCI

EXCLUDES *Sentinel node excision (38500-38542)*
Sentinal node(s) identification (mapping) intraoperative with nonradioactive dye injection (38900)

78195
1.20 1.20 Global Days 000
AMA: 2008, Sep, 5-6; 2008, Jan, 10-25; 2007, Dec, 7-8

38794 **Cannulation, thoracic duct** N1 N 80 CCI
8.66 8.66 Global Days 090

+ 38900 **Intraoperative identification (eg, mapping) of sentinel lymph node(s) includes injection of non-radioactive dye, when performed (List separately in addition to code for primary procedure)** N1 N 80 50

EXCLUDES *Injection of tracer for sentinel node identification (38792)*

Code first (19302, 19307, 38500, 38510, 38520, 38525, 38530, 38542, 38740, 38745)
3.97 3.97 Global Days ZZZ

38999 **Unlisted procedure, hemic or lymphatic system** S 80
0.00 0.00 Global Days YYY
AMA: 2009, Jan, 11-31; 2008, Jan, 10-25; 2007, January, 13-27

39000-39499 Surgical Procedures: Mediastinum

39000 **Mediastinotomy with exploration, drainage, removal of foreign body, or biopsy; cervical approach** C5 C 80 CCI PQ
14.99 14.99 Global Days 090

39010 **transthoracic approach, including either transthoracic or median sternotomy** C5 C 80 CCI PQ

EXCLUDES *Video-assisted thoracic surgery (VATS) pericardial biopsy (32604)*

23.97 23.97 Global Days 090

▲ 39200 **Resection of mediastinal cyst** C5 C 80 CCI PQ
26.56 26.56 Global Days 090

▲ 39220 **Resection of mediastinal tumor** C5 C 80 CCI PQ

EXCLUDES *Thymectomy (60520)*
Thyroidectomy, substernal (60270)
Video-assisted thoracic surgery (VATS) resection cyst, mass, or tumor of mediastinum (32662)

34.27 34.27 Global Days 090

▲ 39400 **Mediastinoscopy, includes biopsy(ies), when performed** T CCI
15.29 15.29 Global Days 010

39499 **Unlisted procedure, mediastinum** C5 C 80
0.00 0.00 Global Days YYY

39501-39599 Surgical Procedures: Diaphragm

EXCLUDES *Laparoscopic repair of diaphragmatic (esophageal hiatal) hernias and fundoplication (43280-43282)*
Transabdominal repair of diaphragmatic hernia (43325)

39501 **Repair, laceration of diaphragm, any approach** C5 C 80 CCI PQ
25.07 25.07 Global Days 090

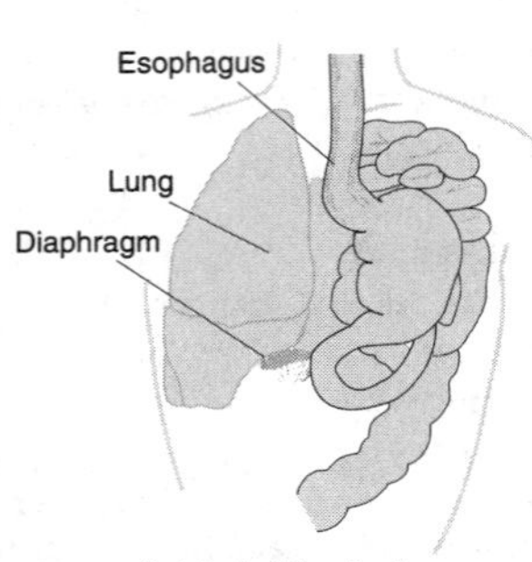

A defect of the diaphragm can allow abdominal contents to herniate into the thoracic cavity

Code 39503 reports the repair of a diaphragmatic hernia in a neonate. The nature of the repair may necessitate the creation of a ventral hernia (an opening in the anterior abdomen to accommodate the viscera). A chest tube may or may not be required

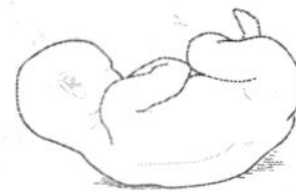

The code is reserved for procedures on neonates

39503 **Repair, neonatal diaphragmatic hernia, with or without chest tube insertion and with or without creation of ventral hernia** A C5 C 80 63 PQ
178.97 178.97 Global Days 090
AMA: 2008, Jun, 3-6

39540 **Repair, diaphragmatic hernia (other than neonatal), traumatic; acute** C5 C 80 PQ
25.59 25.59 Global Days 090
AMA: 2008, Jun, 3-6

39541 **chronic** C5 C 80 PQ
27.81 27.81 Global Days 090
AMA: 2008, Jun, 3-6

39545 **Imbrication of diaphragm for eventration, transthoracic or transabdominal, paralytic or nonparalytic** C5 C 80 PQ
26.96 26.96 Global Days 090

39560 **Resection, diaphragm; with simple repair (eg, primary suture)** C5 C 80 PQ
23.34 23.34 Global Days 090

39561 **with complex repair (eg, prosthetic material, local muscle flap)** C5 C 80 PQ
36.84 36.84 Global Days 090

39599 **Unlisted procedure, diaphragm** C5 C 80
0.00 0.00 Global Days YYY

40490-40799 Resection and Repair Procedures of the Lips

EXCLUDES *Procedures on the skin of lips (10040-17999 [11045, 11046])*

40490 Biopsy of lip P3 T
2.20 3.82 Global Days 000

40500 Vermilionectomy (lip shave), with mucosal advancement A2 T
10.92 15.14 Global Days 090

40510 Excision of lip; transverse wedge excision with primary closure A2 T
EXCLUDES *Excision of mucous lesions (40810-40816)*
10.65 14.46 Global Days 090

40520 V-excision with primary direct linear closure A2 T
EXCLUDES *Excision of mucous lesions (40810-40816)*
10.78 14.74 Global Days 090

40525 full thickness, reconstruction with local flap (eg, Estlander or fan) A2 T
16.72 16.72 Global Days 090

40527 full thickness, reconstruction with cross lip flap (Abbe-Estlander) A2 T 80
EXCLUDES *Cleft lip repair with cross lip pedicle flap (40761)*
18.80 18.80 Global Days 090

40530 Resection of lip, more than 1/4, without reconstruction A2 T
EXCLUDES *Reconstruction (13131-13153)*
12.16 16.27 Global Days 090

40650 Repair lip, full thickness; vermilion only A2 T 80
8.82 12.85 Global Days 090
AMA: 2009, Jan, 11-31; 2008, Jan, 10-25; 2007, January, 13-27

40652 up to half vertical height A2 T 80
10.65 14.70 Global Days 090
AMA: 2009, Jan, 11-31; 2008, Jan, 10-25; 2007, January, 13-27

40654 over 1/2 vertical height, or complex A2 T
12.79 17.12 Global Days 090

40700 Plastic repair of cleft lip/nasal deformity; primary, partial or complete, unilateral A2 T 80
EXCLUDES *Cleft lip repair with cross lip pedicle flap (Abbe-Estlander type) (40761)*
Rhinoplasty for nasal deformity secondary to congenital cleft lip (30460, 30462)
28.39 28.39 Global Days 090

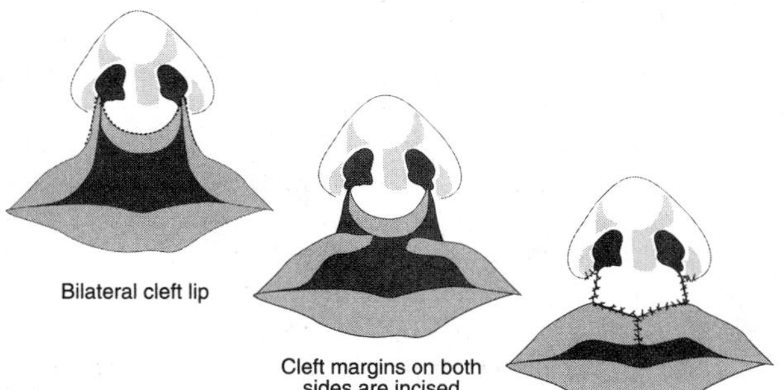

40701 primary bilateral, 1-stage procedure A2 T 80
EXCLUDES *Cleft lip repair with cross lip pedicle flap (Abbe-Estlander type) (40761)*
Rhinoplasty for nasal deformity secondary to congenital cleft lip (30460, 30462)
34.83 34.83 Global Days 090

40702 primary bilateral, 1 of 2 stages A2 T 80
EXCLUDES *Cleft lip repair with cross lip pedicle flap (Abbe-Estlander type) (40761)*
Rhinoplasty for nasal deformity secondary to congenital cleft lip (30460, 30462)
24.24 24.24 Global Days 090

40720 secondary, by recreation of defect and reclosure A2 T 80 50
EXCLUDES *Cleft lip repair with cross lip pedicle flap (Abbe-Estlander type) (40761)*
Rhinoplasty for nasal deformity secondary to congenital cleft lip (30460, 30462)
30.94 30.94 Global Days 090

40761 with cross lip pedicle flap (Abbe-Estlander type), including sectioning and inserting of pedicle A2 T
EXCLUDES *Cleft palate repair (42200-42225)*
Other reconstructive procedures (14060, 14061, 15120-15261, 15574, 15576, 15630)
30.83 30.83 Global Days 090

40799 Unlisted procedure, lips T 80
0.00 0.00 Global Days YYY

40800-40819 Incision and Resection of Buccal Cavity

INCLUDES Mucosal/submucosal tissue of lips/cheeks
Oral cavity outside the dentoalveolar structures

40800 Drainage of abscess, cyst, hematoma, vestibule of mouth; simple P2 T
3.91 6.24 Global Days 010

40801 complicated A2 T
6.58 9.32 Global Days 010

40804 Removal of embedded foreign body, vestibule of mouth; simple P2 X 80
4.00 6.49 Global Days 010

40805 complicated P3 T 80
6.71 10.61 Global Days 010

40806 Incision of labial frenum (frenotomy) P3 T 80
1.13 4.43 Global Days 000

40808 Biopsy, vestibule of mouth P3 T
3.24 5.55 Global Days 010

40810 Excision of lesion of mucosa and submucosa, vestibule of mouth; without repair P3 T
3.84 6.17 Global Days 010

40812 with simple repair P3 T
5.85 8.51 Global Days 010

40814 with complex repair A2 T
9.08 11.39 Global Days 090

40816 complex, with excision of underlying muscle A2 T
9.50 12.02 Global Days 090

40818 Excision of mucosa of vestibule of mouth as donor graft A2 T 80
8.09 10.55 Global Days 090

40819 Excision of frenum, labial or buccal (frenumectomy, frenulectomy, frenectomy) A2 T 80
7.01 9.14 Global Days 090

40820 Destruction of Lesion of Buccal Cavity

CMS 100-3,140.5 Laser Procedures

INCLUDES Mucosal/submucosal tissue of lips/cheeks
Oral cavity outside the dentoalveolar structures

40820 **Destruction of lesion or scar of vestibule of mouth by physical methods (eg, laser, thermal, cryo, chemical)** P3 T
5.21 7.99 Global Days 010

40830-40899 Repair Procedures of the Buccal Cavity

INCLUDES Mucosal/submucosal tissue of lips/cheeks
Oral cavity outside the dentoalveolar structures

EXCLUDES *Skin grafts (15002-15630)*

40830 **Closure of laceration, vestibule of mouth; 2.5 cm or less** G2 T 80
4.95 7.84 Global Days 010

40831 **over 2.5 cm or complex** A2 T 80
6.73 9.95 Global Days 010

40840 **Vestibuloplasty; anterior** A2 T 80
18.25 23.68 Global Days 090

40842 **posterior, unilateral** A2 T 80
18.79 23.71 Global Days 090

40843 **posterior, bilateral** A2 T 80
25.54 32.20 Global Days 090

40844 **entire arch** A2 T 80
33.21 40.64 Global Days 090

40845 **complex (including ridge extension, muscle repositioning)** A2 T 80
36.66 43.66 Global Days 090

40899 **Unlisted procedure, vestibule of mouth** T 80
0.00 0.00 Global Days YYY

41000-41018 Surgical Incision of Floor of Mouth or Tongue

EXCLUDES *Frenoplasty (41520)*

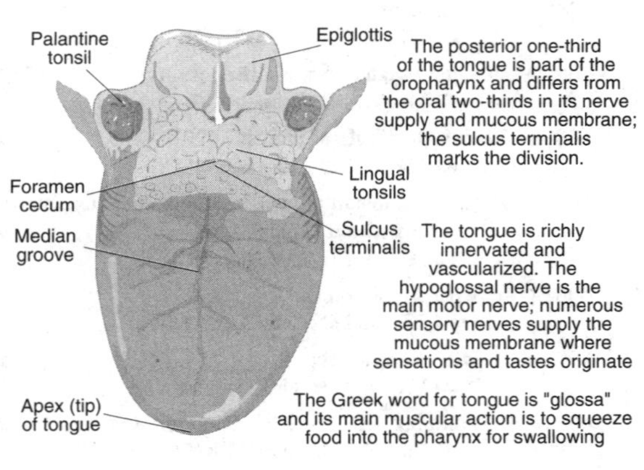

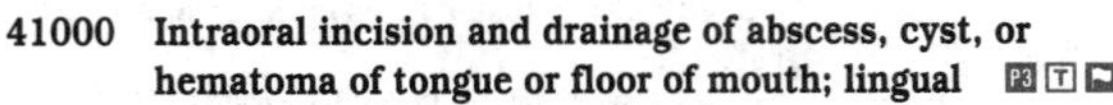

41000 **Intraoral incision and drainage of abscess, cyst, or hematoma of tongue or floor of mouth; lingual** P3 T
3.35 4.83 Global Days 010

41005 **sublingual, superficial** A2 T 80
3.81 6.64 Global Days 010

41006 **sublingual, deep, supramylohyoid** A2 T 80
7.79 10.67 Global Days 090

41007 **submental space** A2 T 80
7.45 10.74 Global Days 090

41008 **submandibular space** A2 T 80
7.97 11.16 Global Days 090

41009 **masticator space** A2 T 80
8.67 11.83 Global Days 090

41010 **Incision of lingual frenum (frenotomy)** A2 T 80
3.33 6.24 Global Days 010

41015 **Extraoral incision and drainage of abscess, cyst, or hematoma of floor of mouth; sublingual** A2 T 80
10.11 12.63 Global Days 090

41016 **submental** A2 T 80
10.39 12.98 Global Days 090

41017 **submandibular** A2 T 80
10.42 13.04 Global Days 090

41018 **masticator space** A2 T 80
12.20 14.70 Global Days 090

41019 Placement of Devices for Brachytherapy

41019 **Placement of needles, catheters, or other device(s) into the head and/or neck region (percutaneous, transoral, or transnasal) for subsequent interstitial radioelement application** G2 T 80

EXCLUDES *Application of interstitial radioelements (77776-77787)*
Intracranial brachytherapy radiation sources with stereotactic insertion (61770)

76942, 77002, 77012, 77021
13.46 13.46 Global Days 000

41100-41599 Resection and Repair of the Tongue

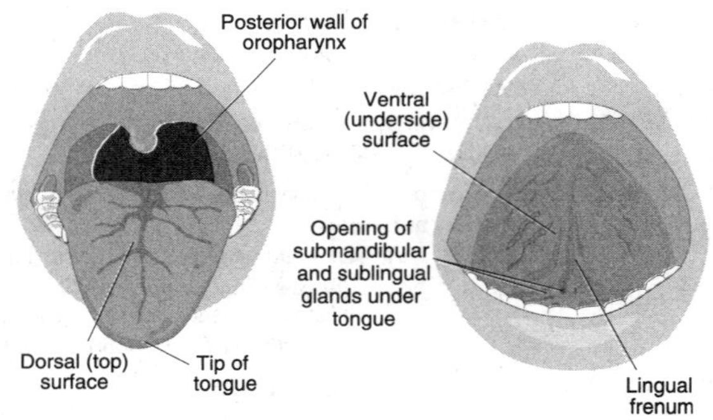

Anterior (front) two-thirds of tongue comprises most of easily visible portions; the base, or root, comprises the remainder of tongue

41100 **Biopsy of tongue; anterior 2/3** P3 T
3.26 5.07 Global Days 010

41105 **posterior 1/3** P3 T
3.35 5.13 Global Days 010

41108 **Biopsy of floor of mouth** P3 T
2.72 4.45 Global Days 010

41110 **Excision of lesion of tongue without closure** P3 T
4.00 6.44 Global Days 010

41112 **Excision of lesion of tongue with closure; anterior 2/3** A2 T
7.58 9.98 Global Days 090

41113 **posterior 1/3** A2 T
8.36 10.87 Global Days 090

41114 with local tongue flap A2 T 80
INCLUDES Excision lesion of tongue with closure anterior/posterior two-thirds (41112-41113)

Do not report with (41112-41113)
19.00 19.00 Global Days 090

41115 Excision of lingual frenum (frenectomy) P3 T 80
4.44 7.54 Global Days 010

41116 Excision, lesion of floor of mouth A2 T
6.63 9.92 Global Days 090

41120 Glossectomy; less than 1/2 tongue A2 T 80
31.78 31.78 Global Days 090

41130 hemiglossectomy C5 C 80 PQ
39.29 39.29 Global Days 090

41135 partial, with unilateral radical neck dissection C5 C 80 PQ
64.44 64.44 Global Days 090

41140 complete or total, with or without tracheostomy, without radical neck dissection C5 C 80 PQ
INCLUDES Regnolli's excision
65.76 65.76 Global Days 090

41145 complete or total, with or without tracheostomy, with unilateral radical neck dissection C5 C 80 PQ
82.90 82.90 Global Days 090

41150 composite procedure with resection floor of mouth and mandibular resection, without radical neck dissection C5 C 80 PQ
65.83 65.83 Global Days 090

41153 composite procedure with resection floor of mouth, with suprahyoid neck dissection C5 C 80 PQ
71.21 71.21 Global Days 090

41155 composite procedure with resection floor of mouth, mandibular resection, and radical neck dissection (Commando type) C5 C 80 PQ
89.28 89.28 Global Days 090
AMA: 2009, Jan, 11-31; 2008, Jan, 10-25; 2007, January, 13-27

41250 Repair of laceration 2.5 cm or less; floor of mouth and/or anterior 2/3 of tongue A2 T 80
4.51 7.64 Global Days 010

41251 posterior 1/3 of tongue A2 T 80
5.24 8.23 Global Days 010

41252 Repair of laceration of tongue, floor of mouth, over 2.6 cm or complex A2 T 80
6.36 9.41 Global Days 010

41500 Fixation of tongue, mechanical, other than suture (eg, K-wire) A2 T 80
13.91 13.91 Global Days 090

41510 Suture of tongue to lip for micrognathia (Douglas type procedure) A2 T 80
12.51 12.51 Global Days 090

41512 Tongue base suspension, permanent suture technique G2 T 80
EXCLUDES *Mechanical fixation of tongue, other than suture (41500)*
Suture tongue to lip for micrognathia (41510)
18.84 18.84 Global Days 090

41520 Frenoplasty (surgical revision of frenum, eg, with Z-plasty) A2 T 80
EXCLUDES *Frenotomy (40806, 41010)*
7.59 10.35 Global Days 090

41530 Submucosal ablation of the tongue base, radiofrequency, 1 or more sites, per session P2 T 80
12.29 99.39 Global Days 010

41599 Unlisted procedure, tongue, floor of mouth T 80
0.00 0.00 Global Days YYY
AMA: 2009, Jan, 11-31; 2008, Jan, 10-25; 2007, January, 13-27

41800-41899 Procedures of the Teeth and Supporting Structures

CMS 100-2,15,150 Dental Services

41800 Drainage of abscess, cyst, hematoma from dentoalveolar structures A2 T
4.30 7.80 Global Days 010

41805 Removal of embedded foreign body from dentoalveolar structures; soft tissues P3 T 80
5.05 7.25 Global Days 010

41806 bone P3 T 80
7.86 10.70 Global Days 010

Gingival recession
Excessive mucosal growth

Gingivitis is an inflammatory response to bacteria on the teeth; it is characterized by tender, red, swollen gums and can lead to gingival recession

41820 Gingivectomy, excision gingiva, each quadrant A2 T 80
0.00 0.00 Global Days 000

41821 Operculectomy, excision pericoronal tissues G2 T 80
0.00 0.00 Global Days 000

41822 Excision of fibrous tuberosities, dentoalveolar structures P3 T 80
5.35 8.54 Global Days 010

41823 Excision of osseous tuberosities, dentoalveolar structures P3 T 80
9.55 12.61 Global Days 090

41825 Excision of lesion or tumor (except listed above), dentoalveolar structures; without repair P3 T
EXCLUDES *Lesion destruction nonexcisional (41850)*
3.69 6.26 Global Days 010

41826 with simple repair P3 T
EXCLUDES *Lesion destruction nonexcisional (41850)*
6.24 9.12 Global Days 010

41827 with complex repair A2 T
EXCLUDES *Lesion destruction nonexcisional (41850)*
9.14 13.00 Global Days 090

41828 Excision of hyperplastic alveolar mucosa, each quadrant (specify) P3 T 80
6.28 8.96 Global Days 010

41830 Alveolectomy, including curettage of osteitis or sequestrectomy P3 T 80
8.35 11.51 Global Days 010

41850 Destruction of lesion (except excision), dentoalveolar structures R2 T 80
0.00 0.00 Global Days 000

41870 Periodontal mucosal grafting G2 T 80
0.00 0.00 Global Days 000

41872 Gingivoplasty, each quadrant (specify) P3 T 80
8.70 12.37 Global Days 090

41874 Alveoloplasty, each quadrant (specify) P3 T 80
EXCLUDES *Fracture reduction (21421-21490)*
Laceration closure (40830, 40831)
Maxilla osteotomy, segmental (21206)
7.51 10.93 Global Days 090

41899 Unlisted procedure, dentoalveolar structures T 80
0.00 0.00 Global Days YYY

42000-42299 Procedures of the Palate and Uvula

42000 Drainage of abscess of palate, uvula A2 T 80
3.13 4.72 Global Days 010

42100 Biopsy of palate, uvula P3 T
3.29 4.50 Global Days 010

42104 Excision, lesion of palate, uvula; without closure P3 T
4.19 6.45 Global Days 010

42106 with simple primary closure P3 T
5.33 8.08 Global Days 010

42107 with local flap closure A2 T
EXCLUDES *Mucosal graft (40818)*
Skin graft (14040-14302)
10.38 13.77 Global Days 090

42120 Resection of palate or extensive resection of lesion A2 T 80
EXCLUDES *Reconstruction of palate with extraoral tissue (14040-14302, 15050, 15120, 15240, 15576)*
29.99 29.99 Global Days 090

42140 Uvulectomy, excision of uvula A2 T
4.74 7.74 Global Days 090

42145 Palatopharyngoplasty (eg, uvulopalatopharyngoplasty, uvulopharyngoplasty) A2 T
EXCLUDES *Removal of exostosis of the bony palate (21031, 21032)*
21.27 21.27 Global Days 090
AMA: 2009, Jan, 11-31; 2008, Jan, 10-25; 2007, January, 13-27

42160 Destruction of lesion, palate or uvula (thermal, cryo or chemical) P3 T 80
4.48 7.08 Global Days 010

42180 Repair, laceration of palate; up to 2 cm A2 T 80
5.56 7.39 Global Days 010

42182 over 2 cm or complex A2 T 80
7.78 9.72 Global Days 010

42200 Palatoplasty for cleft palate, soft and/or hard palate only A2 T 80
25.84 25.84 Global Days 090

42205 Palatoplasty for cleft palate, with closure of alveolar ridge; soft tissue only A2 T 80
26.13 26.13 Global Days 090

42210 with bone graft to alveolar ridge (includes obtaining graft) A2 T 80
33.24 33.24 Global Days 090

42215 Palatoplasty for cleft palate; major revision A2 T 80
20.40 20.40 Global Days 090

42220 secondary lengthening procedure A2 T 80
15.72 15.72 Global Days 090

42225 attachment pharyngeal flap G2 T 80
27.15 27.15 Global Days 090
AMA: 2009, Jan, 11-31; 2008, Jan, 10-25; 2007, January, 13-27

42226 Lengthening of palate, and pharyngeal flap A2 T 80
27.38 27.38 Global Days 090

42227 Lengthening of palate, with island flap G2 T 80
25.90 25.90 Global Days 090

42235 Repair of anterior palate, including vomer flap A2 T 80
EXCLUDES *Oronasal fistula repair (30600)*
22.38 22.38 Global Days 090

42260 Repair of nasolabial fistula A2 T 80
EXCLUDES *Cleft lip repair (40700-40761)*
19.93 24.58 Global Days 090

42280 Maxillary impression for palatal prosthesis P3 T 80
3.31 4.91 Global Days 010

42281 Insertion of pin-retained palatal prosthesis G2 T 80
4.60 6.23 Global Days 010

42299 Unlisted procedure, palate, uvula T 80
0.00 0.00 Global Days YYY
AMA: 2009, Jan, 11-31; 2008, Jan, 10-25; 2007, January, 13-27

42300-42699 Procedures of the Salivary Ducts and Glands

42300 Drainage of abscess; parotid, simple A2 T
4.63 6.35 Global Days 010

42305 parotid, complicated A2 T 80
12.91 12.91 Global Days 090

42310 Drainage of abscess; submaxillary or sublingual, intraoral A2 T 80
3.79 4.92 Global Days 010

42320 submaxillary, external A2 T 80
5.33 7.60 Global Days 010

42330 Sialolithotomy; submandibular (submaxillary), sublingual or parotid, uncomplicated, intraoral P3 T
4.98 7.02 Global Days 010

42335 submandibular (submaxillary), complicated, intraoral P3 T
7.78 11.31 Global Days 090

42340 parotid, extraoral or complicated intraoral A2 T 80
10.19 14.10 Global Days 090

42400 Biopsy of salivary gland; needle P3 T
EXCLUDES *Fine needle aspiration (10021, 10022)*
88172, 88173
76942, 77002, 77012, 77021
1.67 3.23 Global Days 000

42405 incisional A2 T
76942, 77002, 77012, 77021
6.78 8.97 Global Days 010

42408 Excision of sublingual salivary cyst (ranula) A2 T 80
9.87 13.74 Global Days 090

42409 Marsupialization of sublingual salivary cyst (ranula) A2 T 80
6.75 10.14 Global Days 090

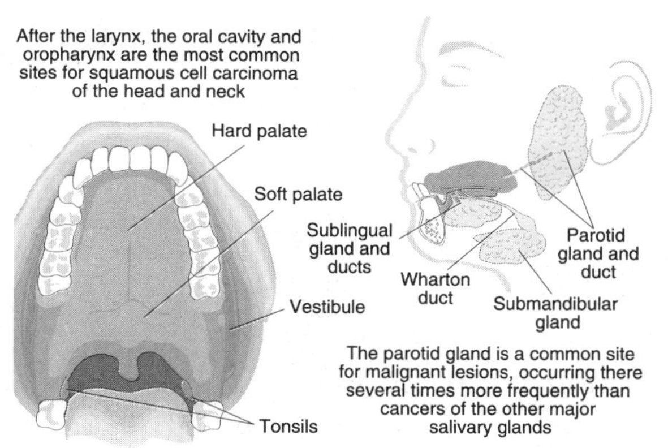

42410 **Excision of parotid tumor or parotid gland; lateral lobe, without nerve dissection** A2 T 80

EXCLUDES *Facial nerve suture or graft (64864, 64865, 69740, 69745)*

18.69 18.69 Global Days 090

42415 **lateral lobe, with dissection and preservation of facial nerve** A2 T 80

EXCLUDES *Facial nerve suture or graft (64864, 64865, 69740, 69745)*

31.88 31.88 Global Days 090

42420 **total, with dissection and preservation of facial nerve** A2 T 80

EXCLUDES *Facial nerve suture or graft (64864, 64865, 69740, 69745)*

35.87 35.87 Global Days 090

42425 **total, en bloc removal with sacrifice of facial nerve** A2 T 80

EXCLUDES *Facial nerve suture or graft (64864, 64865, 69740, 69745)*

25.18 25.18 Global Days 090

42426 **total, with unilateral radical neck dissection** C5 C 80

EXCLUDES *Facial nerve suture or graft (64864, 64865, 69740, 69745)*

40.63 40.63 Global Days 090

42440 **Excision of submandibular (submaxillary) gland** A2 T 80

12.52 12.52 Global Days 090

42450 **Excision of sublingual gland** A2 T 80

10.84 13.67 Global Days 090

42500 **Plastic repair of salivary duct, sialodochoplasty; primary or simple** A2 T 80

10.33 13.07 Global Days 090

42505 **secondary or complicated** A2 T

13.64 16.75 Global Days 090

42507 **Parotid duct diversion, bilateral (Wilke type procedure);** A2 T 80

15.60 15.60 Global Days 090

42508 **with excision of 1 submandibular gland** A2 T 80

21.67 21.67 Global Days 090

42509 **with excision of both submandibular glands** A2 T 80

26.27 26.27 Global Days 090

42510 **with ligation of both submandibular (Wharton's) ducts** A2 T 80

19.06 19.06 Global Days 090

42550 **Injection procedure for sialography** N1 N

70390

1.84 4.05 Global Days 000

42600 **Closure salivary fistula** A2 T 80

10.58 14.60 Global Days 090

42650 **Dilation salivary duct** P3 T

1.77 2.53 Global Days 000

42660 **Dilation and catheterization of salivary duct, with or without injection** P3 T 80

2.32 3.18 Global Days 000

42665 **Ligation salivary duct, intraoral** A2 T 80

6.30 9.55 Global Days 090

42699 **Unlisted procedure, salivary glands or ducts** T 80

0.00 0.00 Global Days YYY

42700-42999 Procedures of the Adenoids/Throat/Tonsils

42700 **Incision and drainage abscess; peritonsillar** A2 T

4.14 5.76 Global Days 010

42720 **retropharyngeal or parapharyngeal, intraoral approach** A2 T 80

11.81 13.68 Global Days 010

42725 **retropharyngeal or parapharyngeal, external approach** A2 T 80

24.34 24.34 Global Days 090

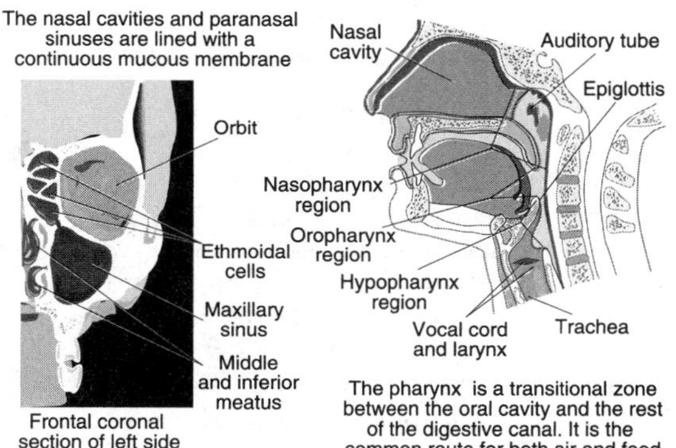

42800 **Biopsy; oropharynx** P3 T

EXCLUDES *Laryngoscopy with biopsy (31510, 31535, 31536)*

3.41 4.84 Global Days 010

42802 **hypopharynx** A2 T

EXCLUDES *Laryngoscopy with biopsy (31510, 31535, 31536)*

4.09 7.18 Global Days 010

42804 **nasopharynx, visible lesion, simple** A2 T

EXCLUDES *Laryngoscopy with biopsy (31510, 31535, 31536)*

3.47 6.07 Global Days 010

42806 **nasopharynx, survey for unknown primary lesion** A2 T

EXCLUDES *Laryngoscopy with biopsy (31510, 31535, 31536)*

4.05 6.82 Global Days 010

42808 **Excision or destruction of lesion of pharynx, any method** A2 T

4.91 6.90 Global Days 010

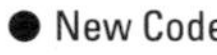

42809 **Removal of foreign body from pharynx** [G2] [X]
3.96 5.18 Global Days 010

42810 **Excision branchial cleft cyst or vestige, confined to skin and subcutaneous tissues** [A2] [T] [80]
8.78 11.83 Global Days 090

42815 **Excision branchial cleft cyst, vestige, or fistula, extending beneath subcutaneous tissues and/or into pharynx** [A2] [T] [80]
16.88 16.88 Global Days 090

42820 **Tonsillectomy and adenoidectomy; younger than age 12** [A] [A2] [T] [80]
8.77 8.77 Global Days 090
AMA: 2009, Jan, 11-31; 2008, Mar, 14-15; 2008, May, 9-11; 2008, Jan, 10-25; 2007, January, 13-27

42821 **age 12 or over** [A] [A2] [T] [80]
9.11 9.11 Global Days 090
AMA: 2009, Jan, 11-31; 2008, May, 9-11; 2008, Mar, 14-15

42825 **Tonsillectomy, primary or secondary; younger than age 12** [A] [A2] [T] [80]
7.33 7.33 Global Days 090
AMA: 2009, Jan, 11-31; 2008, Mar, 14-15

42826 **age 12 or over** [A] [A2] [T]
7.62 7.62 Global Days 090
AMA: 2009, Jan, 11-31; 2008, Mar, 14-15

42830 **Adenoidectomy, primary; younger than age 12** [A] [A2] [T] [80]
6.30 6.30 Global Days 090

42831 **age 12 or over** [A] [A2] [T] [80]
6.78 6.78 Global Days 090

42835 **Adenoidectomy, secondary; younger than age 12** [A] [A2] [T] [80]
5.80 5.80 Global Days 090

42836 **age 12 or over** [A] [A2] [T] [80]
7.30 7.30 Global Days 090

42842 **Radical resection of tonsil, tonsillar pillars, and/or retromolar trigone; without closure** [T] [80]
29.97 29.97 Global Days 090

42844 **closure with local flap (eg, tongue, buccal)** [T] [80]
41.30 41.30 Global Days 090

42845 **closure with other flap** [C5] [C] [80]
Code also closure with other flap(s)
Code also radical neck dissection when combined (38720)
66.77 66.77 Global Days 090

Tonsillar tags or polyps are removed
Snare
Electrocautery tool

In 42860, tags or polyps on the tonsil are removed, usually by simple cauterization or snare

42860 **Excision of tonsil tags** [A2] [T] [80]
5.73 5.73 Global Days 090

42870 **Excision or destruction lingual tonsil, any method (separate procedure)** [A2] [T] [80]
EXCLUDES *Nasopharynx resection (juvenile angiofibroma) by transzygomatic/bicoronal approach (61586, 61600)*
17.63 17.63 Global Days 090

Side view of the pharynx
Nasopharynx region
Oropharynx region
Hypopharynx region
Epiglottis
Larynx
Esophagus

The nasopharynx is the membranous passage above the level of the soft palate; the oropharynx is the region between the soft palate and the upper edge of the epiglottis; the hypopharynx is the region of the epiglottis to the juncture of the larynx and esophagus; the three regions are collectively known as the pharynx

42890 **Limited pharyngectomy** [A2] [T] [80]
Code also radical neck dissection when combined (38720)
42.53 42.53 Global Days 090

42892 **Resection of lateral pharyngeal wall or pyriform sinus, direct closure by advancement of lateral and posterior pharyngeal walls** [A2] [T] [80]
Code also radical neck dissection when combined (38720)
56.43 56.43 Global Days 090

42894 **Resection of pharyngeal wall requiring closure with myocutaneous or fasciocutaneous flap or free muscle, skin, or fascial flap with microvascular anastomosis** [C5] [C] [80]
EXCLUDES *Flap used for reconstruction (15732, 15734, 15756-15758)*
Limited pharyngectomy with radical neck dissection (38720, 42890)
Code also radical neck dissection when combined (38720)
71.08 71.08 Global Days 090
AMA: 2009, Jan, 11-31; 2008, Jan, 10-25

42900 **Suture pharynx for wound or injury** [A2] [T] [80]
10.24 10.24 Global Days 010

42950 **Pharyngoplasty (plastic or reconstructive operation on pharynx)** [A2] [T] [80]
EXCLUDES *Pharyngeal flap (42225)*
24.12 24.12 Global Days 090

42953 **Pharyngoesophageal repair** [C5] [C] [80]
Code also closure using myocutaneous or other flap
29.22 29.22 Global Days 090

42955 **Pharyngostomy (fistulization of pharynx, external for feeding)** [A2] [T] [80]
22.82 22.82 Global Days 090

42960 **Control oropharyngeal hemorrhage, primary or secondary (eg, post-tonsillectomy); simple** [A2] [T] [80]
5.11 5.11 Global Days 010

42961 **complicated, requiring hospitalization** [C5] [C] [80]
12.71 12.71 Global Days 090

42962 **with secondary surgical intervention** [A2] [T]
15.67 15.67 Global Days 090

42970 **Control of nasopharyngeal hemorrhage, primary or secondary (eg, postadenoidectomy); simple, with posterior nasal packs, with or without anterior packs and/or cautery**
12.10 12.10 Global Days 090

42971 **complicated, requiring hospitalization**
13.82 13.82 Global Days 090

42972 **with secondary surgical intervention**
15.46 15.46 Global Days 090

42999 **Unlisted procedure, pharynx, adenoids, or tonsils**
0.00 0.00 Global Days YYY

43020-43135 Incision/Resection of Esophagus

EXCLUDES *Gastrointestinal reconstruction for previous esophagectomy (43360, 43361)*
Gastrotomy with intraluminal tube insertion (43510)

43020 **Esophagotomy, cervical approach, with removal of foreign body**
EXCLUDES *Laparotomy with esophageal intubation (43510)*
16.13 16.13 Global Days 090

43030 **Cricopharyngeal myotomy**
EXCLUDES *Laparotomy with esophageal intubation (43510)*
15.61 15.61 Global Days 090

43045 **Esophagotomy, thoracic approach, with removal of foreign body**
EXCLUDES *Laparotomy with esophageal intubation (43510)*
39.22 39.22 Global Days 090

43100 **Excision of lesion, esophagus, with primary repair; cervical approach**
EXCLUDES *Wide excision of malignant lesion of cervical esophagus, with total laryngectomy:*
With radical neck dissection (31365, 43107, 43116, 43124)
Without radical neck dissection (31360, 43107, 43116, 43124)
18.83 18.83 Global Days 090

43101 **thoracic or abdominal approach**
EXCLUDES *Wide excision of malignant lesion of cervical esophagus with total laryngectomy:*
With radical neck dissection (31365, 43107, 43116, 43124)
Without radical neck dissection (31360, 43107, 43116, 43124)
30.32 30.32 Global Days 090

43107 **Total or near total esophagectomy, without thoracotomy; with pharyngogastrostomy or cervical esophagogastrostomy, with or without pyloroplasty (transhiatal)**
75.68 75.68 Global Days 090

43108 **with colon interposition or small intestine reconstruction, including intestine mobilization, preparation and anastomosis(es)**
131.29 131.29 Global Days 090

43112 **Total or near total esophagectomy, with thoracotomy; with pharyngogastrostomy or cervical esophagogastrostomy, with or without pyloroplasty**
80.50 80.50 Global Days 090

43113 **with colon interposition or small intestine reconstruction, including intestine mobilization, preparation, and anastomosis(es)**
134.16 134.16 Global Days 090

43116 **Partial esophagectomy, cervical, with free intestinal graft, including microvascular anastomosis, obtaining the graft and intestinal reconstruction**
INCLUDES Operating microscope (69990)
EXCLUDES *Free jejunal graft with microvascular anastomosis done by a different physician (43496)*
Code also modifier 52 if intestinal or free jejunal graft with microvascular anastomosis is done by another physician
154.34 154.34 Global Days 090

43117 **Partial esophagectomy, distal 2/3, with thoracotomy and separate abdominal incision, with or without proximal gastrectomy; with thoracic esophagogastrostomy, with or without pyloroplasty (Ivor Lewis)**
EXCLUDES *Esophagogastrectomy (lower third) and vagotomy (43122)*
Total esophagectomy with gastropharyngostomy (43107, 43124)
73.56 73.56 Global Days 090

43118 **with colon interposition or small intestine reconstruction, including intestine mobilization, preparation, and anastomosis(es)**
EXCLUDES *Esophagogastrectomy (lower third) and vagotomy (43122)*
Total esophagectomy with gastropharyngostomy (43107, 43124)
111.46 111.46 Global Days 090

43121 **Partial esophagectomy, distal 2/3, with thoracotomy only, with or without proximal gastrectomy, with thoracic esophagogastrostomy, with or without pyloroplasty**
85.70 85.70 Global Days 090

43122 **Partial esophagectomy, thoracoabdominal or abdominal approach, with or without proximal gastrectomy; with esophagogastrostomy, with or without pyloroplasty**
75.57 75.57 Global Days 090

43123 **with colon interposition or small intestine reconstruction, including intestine mobilization, preparation, and anastomosis(es)**
138.11 138.11 Global Days 090

43124 **Total or partial esophagectomy, without reconstruction (any approach), with cervical esophagostomy**
114.08 114.08 Global Days 090

43130 **Diverticulectomy of hypopharynx or esophagus, with or without myotomy; cervical approach**
23.64 23.64 Global Days 090

43135 **thoracic approach**
44.36 44.36 Global Days 090

43200-43259 Endoscopic Procedures: Upper GI

CMS 100-3,100.2 Endoscopy
INCLUDES Diagnostic endoscopy with surgical endoscopy
Code also appropriate endoscopy of each anatomic site examined

⊙ 43200 **Esophagoscopy, rigid or flexible; diagnostic, with or without collection of specimen(s) by brushing or washing (separate procedure)**
3.14 6.53 Global Days 000
AMA: 2009, Jan, 11-31; 2008, Jan, 10-25; 2008, Oct, 6-7; 2007, January, 13-27

⊙ **43201** **with directed submucosal injection(s), any substance** A2 T
EXCLUDES *Injection sclerosis of esophageal varices (43204)*
3.84 9.27 Global Days 000
AMA: 2008, Oct, 6-7

⊙ **43202** **with biopsy, single or multiple** A2 T
3.46 8.60 Global Days 000
AMA: 2008, Oct, 6-7

⊙ **43204** **with injection sclerosis of esophageal varices** A2 T
6.57 6.57 Global Days 000
AMA: 2008, Oct, 6-7

⊙ **43205** **with band ligation of esophageal varices** A2 T 80
6.71 6.71 Global Days 000
AMA: 2008, Oct, 6-7

⊙ **43215** **with removal of foreign body** A2 T
INCLUDES Removal of esophageal stent
74235
4.63 4.63 Global Days 000
AMA: 2008, Oct, 6-7

⊙ **43216** **with removal of tumor(s), polyp(s), or other lesion(s) by hot biopsy forceps or bipolar cautery** A2 T 80
4.32 6.40 Global Days 000
AMA: 2008, Oct, 6-7

⊙ **43217** **with removal of tumor(s), polyp(s), or other lesion(s) by snare technique** A2 T
5.11 11.47 Global Days 000
AMA: 2008, Oct, 6-7

⊙ **43219** **with insertion of plastic tube or stent** A2 T
5.13 5.13 Global Days 000
AMA: 2008, Oct, 6-7

⊙ **43220** **with balloon dilation (less than 30 mm diameter)** A2 T
EXCLUDES *Dilation of esophagus:*
- *With balloon 30 mm diameter or larger (43458)*
- *Without visualization (43450-43453)*

Fiberoptic esophagogastroscopy:
- *Diagnostic (43200, 43235)*
- *With biopsy or collection of specimen (43200, 43202, 43235, 43239)*
- *With removal of foreign body (43215, 43247)*
- *With removal of polyps(s) (43217, 43251)*

74360
3.80 3.80 Global Days 000
AMA: 2009, Jan, 11-31; 2008, Jan, 10-25; 2008, Oct, 6-7; 2007, January, 13-27

⊙ **43226** **with insertion of guide wire followed by dilation over guide wire** A2 T
74360
4.23 4.23 Global Days 000
AMA: 2008, Oct, 6-7

⊙ **43227** **with control of bleeding (eg, injection, bipolar cautery, unipolar cautery, laser, heater probe, stapler, plasma coagulator)** A2 T
6.31 6.31 Global Days 000
AMA: 2008, Oct, 6-7

⊙ **43228** **with ablation of tumor(s), polyp(s), or other lesion(s), not amenable to removal by hot biopsy forceps, bipolar cautery or snare technique** A2 T
Code also esophagoscopic photodynamic therapy if performed (96570, 96571)
6.67 6.67 Global Days 000
AMA: 2008, Oct, 6-7

⊙ **43231** **with endoscopic ultrasound examination** A2 T 80
Do not report with (76975)
5.70 5.70 Global Days 000
AMA: 2009, Mar, 8-9; 2008, Oct, 6-7

⊙ **43232** **with transendoscopic ultrasound-guided intramural or transmural fine needle aspiration/biopsy(s)** A2 T 80
Do not report with (76942, 76975)
88172-88173
7.79 7.79 Global Days 000
AMA: 2009, Jan, 11-31; 2009, Mar, 8-9; 2008, Jan, 10-25; 2008, Oct, 6-7; 2007, January, 13-27

⊙ **43234** **Upper gastrointestinal endoscopy, simple primary examination (eg, with small diameter flexible endoscope) (separate procedure)** A2 T
3.62 8.51 Global Days 000
AMA: 2009, Jan, 11-31; 2008, Jan, 10-25; 2007, May, 9-11

⊙ **43235** **Upper gastrointestinal endoscopy including esophagus, stomach, and either the duodenum and/or jejunum as appropriate; diagnostic, with or without collection of specimen(s) by brushing or washing (separate procedure)** A2 T
4.35 8.95 Global Days 000
AMA: 2009, May, 8-9&11; 2009, Jan, 11-31; 2008, Jan, 10-25; 2008, Oct, 6-7; 2007, January, 13-27

⊙ **43236** **with directed submucosal injection(s), any substance** A2 T
EXCLUDES *Injection sclerosis of varices, esophageal/gastric (43243)*
5.24 11.38 Global Days 000
AMA: 2008, Oct, 6-7

⊙ **43237** **with endoscopic ultrasound examination limited to the esophagus** A2 T 80
Do not report with (76942, 76975)
7.00 7.00 Global Days 000
AMA: 2009, Mar, 8-9; 2008, Oct, 6-7

⊙ **43238** **with transendoscopic ultrasound-guided intramural or transmural fine needle aspiration/biopsy(s), esophagus (includes endoscopic ultrasound examination limited to the esophagus)** A2 T 80
Do not report with (76942, 76975)
8.74 8.74 Global Days 000
AMA: 2009, Mar, 8-9; 2008, Oct, 6-7

⊙ **43239** **with biopsy, single or multiple** A2 T
5.13 10.34 Global Days 000
AMA: 2009, Jan, 11-31; 2008, Jan, 10-25; 2008, Oct, 6-7; 2007, January, 13-27

⊙ **43240** **with transmural drainage of pseudocyst** A2 T
11.84 11.84 Global Days 000
AMA: 2008, Oct, 6-7

⊙ **43241** **with transendoscopic intraluminal tube or catheter placement** A2 T
4.66 4.66 Global Days 000
AMA: 2008, Oct, 6-7

⊙ **43242** **with transendoscopic ultrasound-guided intramural or transmural fine needle aspiration/biopsy(s) (includes endoscopic ultrasound examination of the esophagus, stomach, and either the duodenum and/or jejunum as appropriate)**

EXCLUDES *Fine needle biopsy/aspiration, transendoscopic, of only the esophagus (43238)*

Do not report with (76942, 76975)

88172-88173

12.63 12.63 Global Days 000

AMA: 2009, Mar, 8-9; 2008, Oct, 6-7

⊙ **43243** **with injection sclerosis of esophageal and/or gastric varices**

7.98 7.98 Global Days 000

AMA: 2008, Oct, 6-7

⊙ **43244** **with band ligation of esophageal and/or gastric varices**

8.81 8.81 Global Days 000

AMA: 2008, Oct, 6-7

⊙ **43245** **with dilation of gastric outlet for obstruction (eg, balloon, guide wire, bougie)**

Do not report with (43256)

5.62 5.62 Global Days 000

AMA: 2009, Jan, 11-31; 2008, Jan, 10-25; 2008, Oct, 6-7; 2007, January, 13-27

⊙ **43246** **with directed placement of percutaneous gastrostomy tube**

EXCLUDES *Percutaneous insertion of gastrostomy tube, nonendoscopic (49440)*

7.52 7.52 Global Days 000

AMA: 2009, Jan, 11-31; 2008, Jan, 10-25; 2008, Oct, 6-7; 2007, January, 13-27

⊙ **43247** **with removal of foreign body**

INCLUDES Removal of esophageal stent

74235

5.99 5.99 Global Days 000

AMA: 2009, Jan, 11-31; 2008, Oct, 6-7; 2008, Jan, 10-25; 2007, Dec, 7-8

⊙ **43248** **with insertion of guide wire followed by dilation of esophagus over guide wire**

5.63 5.63 Global Days 000

AMA: 2009, Jan, 11-31; 2008, Jan, 10-25; 2008, Oct, 6-7; 2007, January, 13-27

⊙ **43249** **with balloon dilation of esophagus (less than 30 mm diameter)**

5.19 5.19 Global Days 000

AMA: 2008, Oct, 6-7

⊙ **43250** **with removal of tumor(s), polyp(s), or other lesion(s) by hot biopsy forceps or bipolar cautery**

5.65 5.65 Global Days 000

AMA: 2009, Jan, 11-31; 2008, Oct, 6-7; 2008, Jan, 10-25; 2007, January, 13-27

⊙ **43251** **with removal of tumor(s), polyp(s), or other lesion(s) by snare technique**

6.52 6.52 Global Days 000

AMA: 2008, Oct, 6-7

⊙ **43255** **with control of bleeding, any method**

8.43 8.43 Global Days 000

AMA: 2008, Oct, 6-7

⊙ **43256** **with transendoscopic stent placement (includes predilation)**

Code also (C1874, C1875, C1876, C1877, C2617, C2625)

7.59 7.59 Global Days 000

AMA: 2008, Oct, 6-7

⊙ **43257** **with delivery of thermal energy to the muscle of lower esophageal sphincter and/or gastric cardia, for treatment of gastroesophageal reflux disease**

9.58 9.58 Global Days 000

AMA: 2008, Oct, 6-7

⊙ **43258** **with ablation of tumor(s), polyp(s), or other lesion(s) not amenable to removal by hot biopsy forceps, bipolar cautery or snare technique**

EXCLUDES *Esophagoscopy with injection sclerosis of esophageal varices (43204)*
Upper gastrointestinal endoscopy with injection sclerosis of esophageal varices (43243)

7.97 7.97 Global Days 000

AMA: 2008, Oct, 6-7

⊙ **43259** **with endoscopic ultrasound examination, including the esophagus, stomach, and either the duodenum and/or jejunum as appropriate**

Do not report with (76975)

9.06 9.06 Global Days 000

AMA: 2009, Mar, 8-9; 2008, Oct, 6-7

43260-43273 Endoscopic Procedures: ERCP

INCLUDES Diagnostic endoscopy with surgical endoscopy

Code also appropriate endoscopy of each anatomic site examined.

⊙ **43260** **Endoscopic retrograde cholangiopancreatography (ERCP); diagnostic, with or without collection of specimen(s) by brushing or washing (separate procedure)**

74328-74330

10.34 10.34 Global Days 000

AMA: 2009, Jan, 11-31; 2008, May, 9-11

⊙ **43261** **with biopsy, single or multiple**

74328-74330

10.86 10.86 Global Days 000

⊙ **43262** **with sphincterotomy/papillotomy**

74328-74330

12.77 12.77 Global Days 000

AMA: 2009, Jul, 10

⊙ **43263** **with pressure measurement of sphincter of Oddi (pancreatic duct or common bile duct)**

74328-74330

12.60 12.60 Global Days 000

⊙ **43264** **with endoscopic retrograde removal of calculus/calculi from biliary and/or pancreatic ducts**

Code also sphincterotomy, when performed (43262)

74328-74330

15.31 15.31 Global Days 000

AMA: 2009, Jan, 11-31; 2007, Dec, 10-179

⊙ **43265** **with endoscopic retrograde destruction, lithotripsy of calculus/calculi, any method**

Code also sphincterotomy, when performed (43262)

74328-74330

17.17 17.17 Global Days 000

⊙ **43267** **with endoscopic retrograde insertion of nasobiliary or nasopancreatic drainage tube**

Code also sphincterotomy, when performed (43262)

74328-74330

12.71 12.71 Global Days 000

⊙ **43268** **with endoscopic retrograde insertion of tube or stent into bile or pancreatic duct**

Code also sphincterotomy, when performed (43262)

74328-74330

12.94 12.94 Global Days 000

AMA: 2009, Jan, 11-31; 2008, Jan, 10-25; 2007, January, 13-27

⊙ **43269** **with endoscopic retrograde removal of foreign body and/or change of tube or stent** A2 T PQ
Code also sphincterotomy, when performed (43262)
74328-74330
14.14 14.14 Global Days 000

⊙ **43271** **with endoscopic retrograde balloon dilation of ampulla, biliary and/or pancreatic duct(s)** A2 T PQ
Code also sphincterotomy, when performed (43262)
74328-74330
12.75 12.75 Global Days 000

⊙ **43272** **with ablation of tumor(s), polyp(s), or other lesion(s) not amenable to removal by hot biopsy forceps, bipolar cautery or snare technique** A2 T 80 PQ
74328-74330
12.76 12.76 Global Days 000

+ ⊙ **43273** **Endoscopic cannulation of papilla with direct visualization of common bile duct(s) and/or pancreatic duct(s) (List separately in addition to code(s) for primary procedure)** G2 T 80
Code first (43260-43265, 43267-43272)
3.79 3.79 Global Days ZZZ
AMA: 2009, Jul, 10

43279-43289 Laparoscopic Procedures of Esophagus

43279 **Laparoscopy, surgical, esophagomyotomy (Heller type), with fundoplasty, when performed** C5 C 80 PQ
EXCLUDES *Esophagomyotomy, open method (43330-43331)*
Do not report with (43280)
37.92 37.92 Global Days 090

43280 **Laparoscopy, surgical, esophagogastric fundoplasty (eg, Nissen, Toupet procedures)** T 80 PQ
EXCLUDES *Esophagogastric fundoplasty, open method (43327-43328)*
Do not report with (43279)
31.68 31.68 Global Days 090

43281 **Laparoscopy, surgical, repair of paraesophageal hernia, includes fundoplasty, when performed; without implantation of mesh** T 80 PQ
EXCLUDES *Transabdominal repair of paraesophageal hiatal hernia (43332-43333)*
Transthoracic repair of diaphragmatic hernia (43334-43335)
Do not report with (43280, 43450, 43453, 43456, 43458, 49568)
45.68 45.68 Global Days 090

43282 **with implantation of mesh** C5 C 80 PQ
EXCLUDES *Transabdominal paraesophageal hernia repair (43332-43333)*
Transthoracic paraesophageal hernia repair (43334-43335)
Do not report with (43280, 43450, 43453, 43456, 43458, 49568)
51.37 51.37 Global Days 090

+ **43283** **Laparoscopy, surgical, esophageal lengthening procedure (eg, Collis gastroplasty or wedge gastroplasty) (List separately in addition to code for primary procedure)** C5 C 80
Code first (43280-43282)
4.74 4.74 Global Days ZZZ

43289 **Unlisted laparoscopy procedure, esophagus** T 80 50
0.00 0.00 Global Days YYY

43300-43425 Open Esophageal Repair Procedures

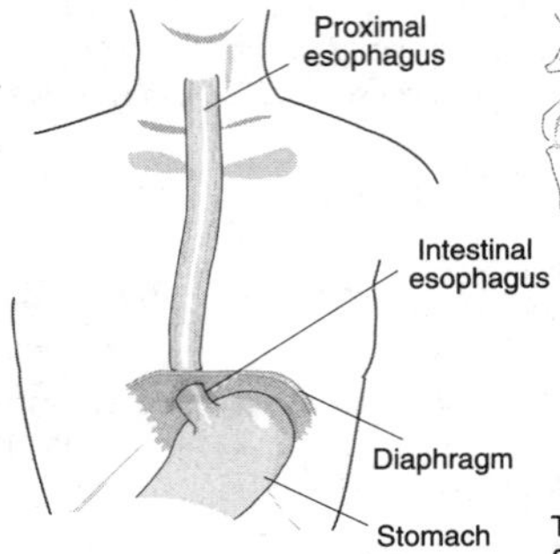

Sections of stomach or bowel are commonly used to repair a resected portion of the esophagus

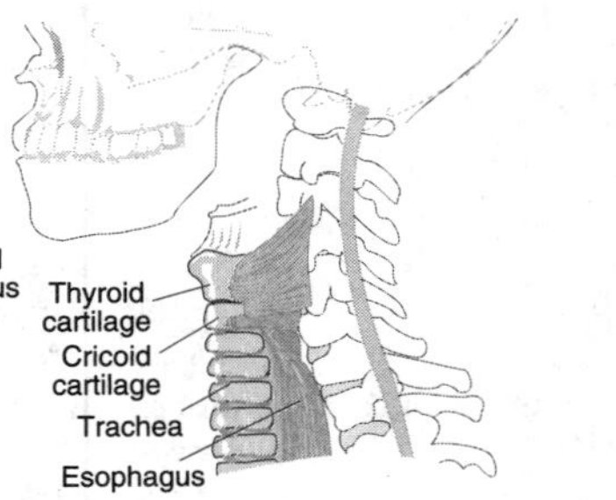

The esophagus is a muscular tube that delivers food from the oral cavity to the stomach. It spans the cervical, thoracic, and abdominal regions and numerous surgical approaches may be used

43300 **Esophagoplasty (plastic repair or reconstruction), cervical approach; without repair of tracheoesophageal fistula** C5 C 80 PQ
18.52 18.52 Global Days 090

43305 **with repair of tracheoesophageal fistula** C5 C 80 PQ
32.84 32.84 Global Days 090

43310 **Esophagoplasty (plastic repair or reconstruction), thoracic approach; without repair of tracheoesophageal fistula** C5 C 80 PQ
44.79 44.79 Global Days 090

43312 **with repair of tracheoesophageal fistula** C5 C 80 PQ
48.50 48.50 Global Days 090

43313 **Esophagoplasty for congenital defect (plastic repair or reconstruction), thoracic approach; without repair of congenital tracheoesophageal fistula** C5 C 80 63 PQ
85.04 85.04 Global Days 090

43314 **with repair of congenital tracheoesophageal fistula** C5 C 80 63 PQ
86.11 86.11 Global Days 090

43320 **Esophagogastrostomy (cardioplasty), with or without vagotomy and pyloroplasty, transabdominal or transthoracic approach** C5 C 80 PQ
EXCLUDES *Laparoscopic approach (43280)*
40.73 40.73 Global Days 090

▲ **43325** **Esophagogastric fundoplasty; with fundic patch (Thal-Nissen procedure)** C5 C 80 PQ
EXCLUDES *Myotomy, cricopharyngeal (43030)*
39.63 39.63 Global Days 090

43327 **Esophagogastric fundoplasty partial or complete; laparotomy** C5 C 80
24.17 24.17 Global Days 090

43328 **thoracotomy** C5 C 80
35.39 35.39 Global Days 090

43330 **Esophagomyotomy (Heller type); abdominal approach** C5 C 80 PQ
EXCLUDES *Esophagomyotomy, laparoscopic method (43279)*
38.42 38.42 Global Days 090

43331 **thoracic approach** C5 C 80 PQ
EXCLUDES *Thoracoscopy with esophagomyotomy (32665)*
40.46 40.46 Global Days 090

43332 **Repair, paraesophageal hiatal hernia (including fundoplication), via laparotomy, except neonatal; without implantation of mesh or other prosthesis** C5 C 80
EXCLUDES *Neonatal diaphragmatic hernia repair (39503)*
34.41 34.41 Global Days 090

43333 **with implantation of mesh or other prosthesis** C5 C 80
EXCLUDES *Neonatal diaphragmatic hernia repair (39503)*
37.34 37.34 Global Days 090

43334 **Repair, paraesophageal hiatal hernia (including fundoplication), via thoracotomy, except neonatal; without implantation of mesh or other prosthesis** C5 C 80
EXCLUDES *Neonatal diaphragmatic hernia repair (39503)*
37.65 37.65 Global Days 090

43335 **with implantation of mesh or other prosthesis** C5 C 80
EXCLUDES *Neonatal diaphragmatic hernia repair (39503)*
40.55 40.55 Global Days 090

43336 **Repair, paraesophageal hiatal hernia, (including fundoplication), via thoracoabdominal incision, except neonatal; without implantation of mesh or other prosthesis** C5 C 80
EXCLUDES *Neonatal diaphragmatic hernia repair (39503)*
44.49 44.49 Global Days 090

43337 **with implantation of mesh or other prosthesis** C5 C 80
EXCLUDES *Neonatal diaphragmatic hernia repair (39503)*
48.70 48.70 Global Days 090

\+ 43338 **Esophageal lengthening procedure (eg, Collis gastroplasty or wedge gastroplasty) (List separately in addition to code for primary procedure)** C5 C 80
Code first (43280, 43327-43337)
3.89 3.89 Global Days ZZZ

43340 **Esophagojejunostomy (without total gastrectomy); abdominal approach** C5 C 80 PQ
40.30 40.30 Global Days 090

43341 **thoracic approach** C5 C 80 PQ
42.43 42.43 Global Days 090

43350 **Esophagostomy, fistulization of esophagus, external; abdominal approach** C5 C 80 PQ
36.95 36.95 Global Days 090

43351 **thoracic approach** C5 C 80 PQ
39.59 39.59 Global Days 090

43352 **cervical approach** C5 C 80 PQ
32.15 32.15 Global Days 090

43360 **Gastrointestinal reconstruction for previous esophagectomy, for obstructing esophageal lesion or fistula, or for previous esophageal exclusion; with stomach, with or without pyloroplasty** C5 C 80 PQ
70.64 70.64 Global Days 090

43361 **with colon interposition or small intestine reconstruction, including intestine mobilization, preparation, and anastomosis(es)** C5 C 80 PQ
78.81 78.81 Global Days 090

43400 **Ligation, direct, esophageal varices** C5 C 80 PQ
44.00 44.00 Global Days 090

43401 **Transection of esophagus with repair, for esophageal varices** C5 C 80 PQ
45.22 45.22 Global Days 090

43405 **Ligation or stapling at gastroesophageal junction for pre-existing esophageal perforation** C5 C 80 PQ
43.23 43.23 Global Days 090

43410 **Suture of esophageal wound or injury; cervical approach** C5 C 80 PQ
32.38 32.38 Global Days 090

43415 **transthoracic or transabdominal approach** C5 C 80 PQ
75.24 75.24 Global Days 090

43420 **Closure of esophagostomy or fistula; cervical approach** T 80 PQ
EXCLUDES *Transabdominal paraesophageal hiatal hernia repair (43332-43333)*
Transabdominal paraesophageal hiatal hernia repair (43334-43335)
30.40 30.40 Global Days 090

43425 **transthoracic or transabdominal approach** C5 C 80 PQ
EXCLUDES *Transabdominal paraesophageal hiatal hernia repair (43332-43333)*
Transthoracic diaphragmatic hernia repair (43334-43335)
43.17 43.17 Global Days 090

43450-43458 Esophageal Dilation

43450 **Dilation of esophagus, by unguided sound or bougie, single or multiple passes** A2 T
74220, 74360
2.67 4.70 Global Days 000
AMA: 2009, Jan, 11-31; 2008, Jan, 10-25; 2007, January, 13-27

⊙ 43453 **Dilation of esophagus, over guide wire** A2 T
EXCLUDES *Dilation performed with direct visualization (43220)*
Esophagus dilation performed by dilator or balloon (43220, 43458)
74220, 74360
2.88 8.89 Global Days 000
AMA: 2009, Jan, 11-31; 2008, Jan, 10-25; 2007, January, 13-27

⊙ 43456 **Dilation of esophagus, by balloon or dilator, retrograde** A2 T
74220, 74360
4.63 18.05 Global Days 000

⊙ 43458 **Dilation of esophagus with balloon (30 mm diameter or larger) for achalasia** A2 T
EXCLUDES *Balloon dilation less than 30 mm diameter (43220)*
74220, 74360
5.41 11.64 Global Days 000
AMA: 2009, Jan, 11-31; 2008, Jan, 10-25; 2008, Oct, 6-7; 2007, January, 13-27

43460-43499 Other/Unlisted Esophageal Procedures

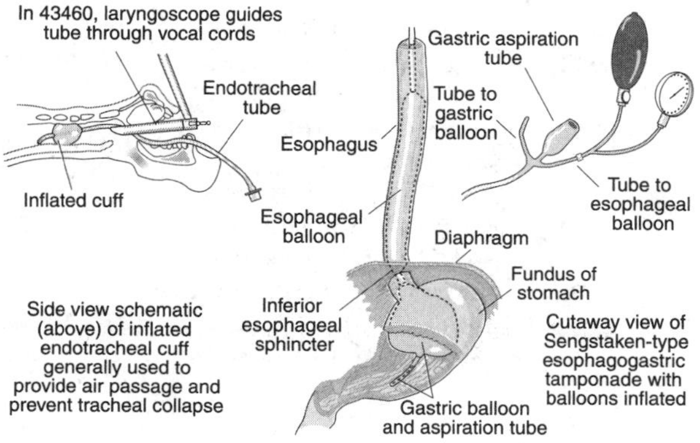

Side view schematic (above) of inflated endotracheal cuff generally used to provide air passage and prevent tracheal collapse

Cutaway view of Sengstaken-type esophagogastric tamponade with balloons inflated

43460 **Esophagogastric tamponade, with balloon (Sengstaken type)**

EXCLUDES *Removal of foreign body of the esophagus with balloon catheter (43215, 43247, 74235)*

6.65 6.65 Global Days 000

43496 **Free jejunum transfer with microvascular anastomosis**

INCLUDES Operating microscope (69990)

0.00 0.00 Global Days 090

43499 **Unlisted procedure, esophagus**

0.00 0.00 Global Days YYY

AMA: 2009, Jan, 11-31; 2008, Jan, 10-25; 2007, May, 9-11

43500-43641 Open Gastric Incisional and Resection Procedures

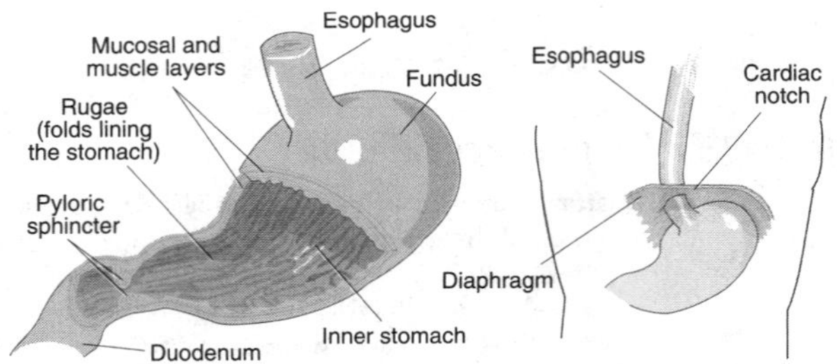

The stomach is a highly distensible organ that serves as a reservoir to mix food and break it down with digestive juices. The esophagus pierces the diaphragm at the cardiac notch, where the stomach begins. The pyloric sphincter marks the inferior border of the stomach. The vagal nerve trunks run down the front and back of the esophagus and serve the stomach by controlling secretion of digestive acids

43500 **Gastrotomy; with exploration or foreign body removal**

22.94 22.94 Global Days 090

43501 **with suture repair of bleeding ulcer**

39.33 39.33 Global Days 090

43502 **with suture repair of pre-existing esophagogastric laceration (eg, Mallory-Weiss)**

44.44 44.44 Global Days 090

43510 **with esophageal dilation and insertion of permanent intraluminal tube (eg, Celestin or Mousseaux-Barbin)**

28.12 28.12 Global Days 090

43520 **Pyloromyotomy, cutting of pyloric muscle (Fredet-Ramstedt type operation)**

20.32 20.32 Global Days 090

43605 **Biopsy of stomach, by laparotomy**

24.40 24.40 Global Days 090

43610 **Excision, local; ulcer or benign tumor of stomach**

28.60 28.60 Global Days 090

43611 **malignant tumor of stomach**

35.50 35.50 Global Days 090

43620 **Gastrectomy, total; with esophagoenterostomy**

57.42 57.42 Global Days 090

43621 **with Roux-en-Y reconstruction**

65.99 65.99 Global Days 090

43622 **with formation of intestinal pouch, any type**

67.04 67.04 Global Days 090

43631 **Gastrectomy, partial, distal; with gastroduodenostomy**

INCLUDES Billroth operation

42.34 42.34 Global Days 090

43632 **with gastrojejunostomy**

INCLUDES Polya anastomosis

59.00 59.00 Global Days 090

43633 **with Roux-en-Y reconstruction**

55.86 55.86 Global Days 090

43634 **with formation of intestinal pouch**

61.86 61.86 Global Days 090

\+ **43635** **Vagotomy when performed with partial distal gastrectomy (List separately in addition to code[s] for primary procedure)**

Code first as appropriate (43631-43634)

3.28 3.28 Global Days ZZZ

43640 **Vagotomy including pyloroplasty, with or without gastrostomy; truncal or selective**

EXCLUDES *Pyloroplasty (43800)*
Vagotomy (64752-64760)

34.35 34.35 Global Days 090

43641 **parietal cell (highly selective)**

EXCLUDES *Upper gastrointestinal endoscopy (43234-43259)*

34.96 34.96 Global Days 090

43644-43645 Laparoscopic Gastric Bypass with Small Bowel Resection

CMS 100-3,40.5 Treatment of Obesity
CMS 100-3,100.1 Bariatric Surgery for Treatment of Morbid Obesity
CMS 100-3,100.8 Intestinal Bypass Surgery

INCLUDES Diagnostic laparoscopy (49320)

EXCLUDES *Endoscopy, upper gastrointestinal, (esophagus / stomach / duodenum / jejunum) (43235-43259)*

43644 **Laparoscopy, surgical, gastric restrictive procedure; with gastric bypass and Roux-en-Y gastroenterostomy (roux limb 150 cm or less)**

EXCLUDES *Open method (43846)*
Roux limb greater than 150 cm (43645)

Do not report with (43846, 49320)

50.60 50.60 Global Days 090

43645 **with gastric bypass and small intestine reconstruction to limit absorption**

Do not report with (43847, 49320)

54.14 54.14 Global Days 090

43647-43659 Other and Unlisted Laparoscopic Gastric Procedures

INCLUDES Diagnostic laparoscopy (49320)

EXCLUDES *Endoscopy, upper gastrointestinal, (esophagus/stomach/duodenum/jejunum) (43235-43259)*

43647 Laparoscopy, surgical; implantation or replacement of gastric neurostimulator electrodes, antrum S 80

EXCLUDES *Electronic analysis/programming gastric neurostimulator pulse generator (95980-95982)*
Insertion/replacement gastric neurostimulator pulse generator (64590)
Laparoscopy with implantation, removal, or revision of gastric neurostimulator electrodes on the lesser curvature of the stomach (43659)
Open method (43881)

Code also (C1778, C1897, L8680)

0.00 0.00 Global Days YYY

AMA: 2009, Jan, 11-31; 2008, Jan, 8-9; 2007, March, 4-5

43648 revision or removal of gastric neurostimulator electrodes, antrum T 80

EXCLUDES *Electronic analysis/programming gastric neurostimulator (95980-95982)*
Laparoscopy with implantation, removal, or revision of gastric neurostimulator electrodes on the lesser curvature of the stomach (43659)
Open method (43882)
Revision/removal gastric neurostimulator pulse generator (64595)

0.00 0.00 Global Days YYY

AMA: 2007, March, 4-5

43651 Laparoscopy, surgical; transection of vagus nerves, truncal T 80 PQ

19.09 19.09 Global Days 090

43652 transection of vagus nerves, selective or highly selective T 80 PQ

22.30 22.30 Global Days 090

43653 gastrostomy, without construction of gastric tube (eg, Stamm procedure) (separate procedure) A2 T 80 PQ

16.68 16.68 Global Days 090

43659 Unlisted laparoscopic procedure, stomach T 80 50

0.00 0.00 Global Days YYY

AMA: 2009, Jan, 11-31; 2008, Jan, 10-25; 2007, Dec, 10-179; 2007, January, 13-27

43752-43761 Nonsurgical Gastric Tube Procedures

CMS 100-4,20,50.3 Payment for Replacement of Parenteral and Enteral Pumps
CMS 100-4,20,100.2.2 Medical Necessity for Parenteral and Enteral Nutrition Therapy

43752 Naso- or oro-gastric tube placement, requiring physician's skill and fluoroscopic guidance (includes fluoroscopy, image documentation and report) G2 03 PQ

EXCLUDES *Percutaneous insertion of gastrostomy tube (43246, 49440)*
Placement of enteric tube (44500, 74340)

Do not report with (99291-99292, 99468-99469, 99471-99472, 99478-99479)

1.19 1.19 Global Days 000

AMA: 2009, Jan, 11-31; 2008, Jan, 10-25; 2007, Jul, 1-4; 2007, January, 13-27; 2007, February, 10-11

43753 Gastric intubation and aspiration(s) therapeutic, necessitating physician's skill (eg, for gastrointestinal hemorrhage), including lavage if performed G2 X 80

0.60 0.60 Global Days 000

43754 Gastric intubation and aspiration, diagnostic; single specimen (eg, acid analysis) G2 X 80

EXCLUDES *Naso- or orogastric tube placement with fluoroscopic guidance (43752)*

82930

0.94 2.49 Global Days 000

43755 collection of multiple fractional specimens with gastric stimulation, single or double lumen tube (gastric secretory study) (eg, histamine, insulin, pentagastrin, calcium, secretin), includes drug administration G2 S 80

EXCLUDES *Naso- or orogastric tube placement under fluoroscopic guidance (43752)*

Code also drugs or substances administered

82930

1.71 3.76 Global Days 000

43756 Duodenal intubation and aspiration, diagnostic, includes image guidance; single specimen (eg, bile study for crystals or afferent loop culture) G2 X 80

89049-89240

1.53 6.92 Global Days 000

43757 collection of multiple fractional specimens with pancreatic or gallbladder stimulation, single or double lumen tube, includes drug administration G2 X 80

Code also drugs or substances administered

89049-89240

2.32 9.77 Global Days 000

43760 Change of gastrostomy tube, percutaneous, without imaging or endoscopic guidance A2 T

EXCLUDES *Fluoroscopically guided gastrostomy replacement (49450)*
Gastrostomy tube, placed endoscopically (43246)

1.45 13.62 Global Days 000

AMA: 2009, Jan, 11-31; 2008, Apr, -11

43761 Repositioning of a naso- or oro-gastric feeding tube, through the duodenum for enteric nutrition A2 T

EXCLUDES *Gastrostomy tube converted endoscopically to jejunostomy tube (44373)*
Introduction of long gastrointestinal tube into the duodenum (44500)

Do not report with (44500, 49446)

76000

3.05 3.48 Global Days 000

AMA: 2008, Jun, 8-11

43770-43775 Laparoscopic Bariatric Procedures

CMS 100-3,100.1 Bariatric Surgery for Treatment of Morbid Obesity

INCLUDES Diagnostic laparoscopy (49320)
Stomach/duodenum/jejunum/ileum
Subsequent band adjustments (change of the gastric band component diameter by injection/aspriation of fluid through the subcutaneous port component) during the postoperative period

43770 Laparoscopy, surgical, gastric restrictive procedure; placement of adjustable gastric restrictive device (eg, gastric band and subcutaneous port components) T 80 PQ

Code also modifier 52 for placement of individual component

32.63 32.63 Global Days 090

AMA: 2009, Jan, 11-31; 2008, Jan, 10-25; 2007, January, 13-27

Digestive

43647 — 43770

43771 **revision of adjustable gastric restrictive device component only** C5 C 80 PQ
37.09 37.09 Global Days 090

43772 **removal of adjustable gastric restrictive device component only** C5 C 80 PQ
27.89 27.89 Global Days 090

43773 **removal and replacement of adjustable gastric restrictive device component only** C5 C 80 PQ
Do not report with (43772)
37.07 37.07 Global Days 090

43774 **removal of adjustable gastric restrictive device and subcutaneous port components** C5 C 80 PQ
EXCLUDES *Removal/replacement of subcutaneous port components and gastric band (43659)*
28.07 28.07 Global Days 090
AMA: 2009, Jan, 11-31; 2008, Jan, 10-25; 2007, January, 13-27

43775 **longitudinal gastrectomy (ie, sleeve gastrectomy)** E PQ
EXCLUDES *Open gastric restrictive procedure for morbid obesity, without gastric bypass, other than vertical-banded gastroplasty (43843)*
37.75 37.75 Global Days XXX

43800-43840 Open Gastric Incisional/Repair/Resection Procedures

43800 **Pyloroplasty** C5 C 80 PQ
EXCLUDES *Vagotomy with pyloroplasty (43640)*
27.14 27.14 Global Days 090

43810 **Gastroduodenostomy** C5 C 80 PQ
29.63 29.63 Global Days 090

43820 **Gastrojejunostomy; without vagotomy** C5 C 80 PQ
38.93 38.93 Global Days 090

43825 **with vagotomy, any type** C5 C 80 PQ
38.02 38.02 Global Days 090

43830 **Gastrostomy, open; without construction of gastric tube (eg, Stamm procedure) (separate procedure)** T 80 PQ
20.39 20.39 Global Days 090

43831 **neonatal, for feeding** A T 80 PQ
EXCLUDES *Change of gastrostomy tube (43760)*
17.35 17.35 Global Days 090

43832 **with construction of gastric tube (eg, Janeway procedure)** C5 C 80 PQ
EXCLUDES *Endoscopic placement of percutaneous gastrostomy tube (43246)*
30.77 30.77 Global Days 090

43840 **Gastrorrhaphy, suture of perforated duodenal or gastric ulcer, wound, or injury** C5 C 80 PQ
39.52 39.52 Global Days 090

43842-43848 Open Bariatric Procedures for Morbid Obesity

CMS 100-3,40.5 Treatment of Obesity
CMS 100-3,100.1 Bariatric Surgery for Treatment of Morbid Obesity
CMS 100-3,100.8 Intestinal Bypass Surgery

43842 **Gastric restrictive procedure, without gastric bypass, for morbid obesity; vertical-banded gastroplasty** E
33.60 33.60 Global Days 090

43843 **other than vertical-banded gastroplasty** C5 C 80 PQ
INCLUDES Laparoscopic longitudinal gastrectomy (ie, sleeve gastrectomy) (43775)
37.27 37.27 Global Days 090

43845 **Gastric restrictive procedure with partial gastrectomy, pylorus-preserving duodenoileostomy and ileoileostomy (50 to 100 cm common channel) to limit absorption (biliopancreatic diversion with duodenal switch)** C5 C 80 PQ
Do not report with (43633, 43847, 44130, 49000)
57.04 57.04 Global Days 090

43846 **Gastric restrictive procedure, with gastric bypass for morbid obesity; with short limb (150 cm or less) Roux-en-Y gastroenterostomy** C5 C 80 PQ
EXCLUDES *Gastric bypass with Roux-en-Y gastroenterostomy performed laparoscopically (43644)*
More than 150 cm (43847)
47.50 47.50 Global Days 090

43847 **with small intestine reconstruction to limit absorption** C5 C 80 PQ
52.44 52.44 Global Days 090

43848 **Revision, open, of gastric restrictive procedure for morbid obesity, other than adjustable gastric restrictive device (separate procedure)** C5 C 80 PQ
EXCLUDES *Gastric restrictive port procedures (43886-43888)*
Procedures for adjustable gastric restrictive devices (43770-43774)
56.28 56.28 Global Days 090

43850-43882 Open Gastric Procedures: Closure/Implantation/Replacement/Revision

43850 **Revision of gastroduodenal anastomosis (gastroduodenostomy) with reconstruction; without vagotomy** C5 C 80 PQ
47.42 47.42 Global Days 090

43855 **with vagotomy** C5 C 80 PQ
49.26 49.26 Global Days 090

43860 **Revision of gastrojejunal anastomosis (gastrojejunostomy) with reconstruction, with or without partial gastrectomy or intestine resection; without vagotomy** C5 C 80 PQ
47.63 47.63 Global Days 090

43865 **with vagotomy** C5 C 80 PQ
49.83 49.83 Global Days 090

43870 **Closure of gastrostomy, surgical** A2 T 80 PQ
20.77 20.77 Global Days 090

43880 **Closure of gastrocolic fistula** C5 C 80 PQ
46.55 46.55 Global Days 090

43881 **Implantation or replacement of gastric neurostimulator electrodes, antrum, open** C5 C 80
EXCLUDES *Electronic analysis and programming (95980-95982)*
Insertion of gastric neurostimulator pulse generator (64590)
Laparotomy with implantation, replacement, revision, or removal of gastric stimulation electrodes, lesser curvature (43999)
Revision/removal gastric neurostimulator pulse generator (64595)
Revision/removal performed laparoscopically (43648)
0.00 0.00 Global Days YYY
AMA: 2007, March, 4-5

26/TC PC/TC Comp Only | A2-Z3 ASC Pmt | 50 Bilateral | ♂ Male Only | ♀ Female Only | Facility RVU | Non-Facility RVU
AMA: CPT Asst | **MED:** Pub 100 | A-Y OPPSI | 80/80 Surg Assist Allowed / w/Doc | Lab Crosswalk | Radiology Crosswalk

43882 **Revision or removal of gastric neurostimulator electrodes, antrum, open** C5 C 80

EXCLUDES *Electronic analysis and programming (95980-95982)*
Insertion of gastric neurostimulator pulse generator (64590)
Laparotomy with implantation, replacement, revision, or removal of gastric stimulation electrodes, lesser curvature (43999)
Revision/removal gastric neurostimulator pulse generator (64595)
Revision/removal performed laparoscopically (43648)

0.00 0.00 Global Days YYY
AMA: 2007, March, 4-5

43886-43999 Bariatric Procedures: Removal/Replacement/Revision Port Components

CMS 100-3,40.5 Treatment of Obesity
CMS 100-3,100.1 Bariatric Surgery for Treatment of Morbid Obesity

43886 **Gastric restrictive procedure, open; revision of subcutaneous port component only** G2 T 80 PQ
10.52 10.52 Global Days 090

43887 **removal of subcutaneous port component only** G2 T 80 PQ

EXCLUDES *Gastric band and subcutaneous port components:*
Removal and replacement (43659)
Removal performed laparoscopically (43774)

9.53 9.53 Global Days 090

43888 **removal and replacement of subcutaneous port component only** G2 T 80 PQ

EXCLUDES *Gastric band and subcutaneous port components:*
Removal and replacement (43659)
Removal performed laparoscopically (43774)

Do not report with (43774, 43887)
13.37 13.37 Global Days 090

43999 **Unlisted procedure, stomach** T 80
0.00 0.00 Global Days YYY

44005-44130 Incisional and Resection Procedures of Bowel

44005 **Enterolysis (freeing of intestinal adhesion) (separate procedure)** C5 C 80 CCI PQ

EXCLUDES *Enterolysis performed laparoscopically (44180)*

Do not report with (45136)
31.93 31.93 Global Days 090
AMA: 2009, Jan, 11-31; 2008, Jan, 10-25; 2007, January, 13-27

44010 **Duodenotomy, for exploration, biopsy(s), or foreign body removal** C5 C 80 CCI PQ
25.28 25.28 Global Days 090

\+ **44015** **Tube or needle catheter jejunostomy for enteral alimentation, intraoperative, any method (List separately in addition to primary procedure)** C5 C 80 CCI
Code first the primary procedure
4.18 4.18 Global Days ZZZ
AMA: 2009, Jan, 11-31; 2008, Jan, 10-25; 2007, January, 13-27

44020 **Enterotomy, small intestine, other than duodenum; for exploration, biopsy(s), or foreign body removal** C5 C 80 CCI PQ
28.42 28.42 Global Days 090

In 44021, a select portion of intestine is surgically approached and incised. A tube is inserted into the bowel lumen and threaded distally, often to a point of obstruction. The tube is used to decompress the bowel segment it passes through, often during or immediately following surgery for bowel obstruction

44021 **for decompression (eg, Baker tube)** C5 C 80 CCI PQ
28.65 28.65 Global Days 090

44025 **Colotomy, for exploration, biopsy(s), or foreign body removal** C5 C 80 CCI PQ

INCLUDES Amussat's operation

EXCLUDES *Intestine exteriorization (Mikulicz resection with crushing of spur) (44602-44605)*

28.86 28.86 Global Days 090

44050 **Reduction of volvulus, intussusception, internal hernia, by laparotomy** C5 C 80 CCI PQ
27.29 27.29 Global Days 090

44055 **Correction of malrotation by lysis of duodenal bands and/or reduction of midgut volvulus (eg, Ladd procedure)** C5 C 80 63 CCI PQ
43.69 43.69 Global Days 090

44100 **Biopsy of intestine by capsule, tube, peroral (1 or more specimens)** A2 T CCI PQ
3.38 3.38 Global Days 000

44110 **Excision of 1 or more lesions of small or large intestine not requiring anastomosis, exteriorization, or fistulization; single enterotomy** C5 C 80 CCI PQ
24.79 24.79 Global Days 090

44111 **multiple enterotomies** C5 C 80 CCI PQ
28.71 28.71 Global Days 090

44120 **Enterectomy, resection of small intestine; single resection and anastomosis** C5 C 80 CCI PQ
Do not report with (45136)
35.67 35.67 Global Days 090

\+ **44121** **each additional resection and anastomosis (List separately in addition to code for primary procedure)** C5 C 80 CCI
Code first single resection of small intestine (44120)
7.08 7.08 Global Days ZZZ

44125 **with enterostomy** C5 C 80 CCI PQ
34.49 34.49 Global Days 090

44126 **Enterectomy, resection of small intestine for congenital atresia, single resection and anastomosis of proximal segment of intestine; without tapering** C5 C 80 63 CCI PQ
71.82 71.82 Global Days 090

44127 **with tapering** C5 C 80 63 CCI PQ
83.08 83.08 Global Days 090

+ **44128** **each additional resection and anastomosis (List separately in addition to code for primary procedure)**

Code first single resection of small intestine (44126, 44127)

7.12 7.12 Global Days ZZZ

44130 **Enteroenterostomy, anastomosis of intestine, with or without cutaneous enterostomy (separate procedure)**

38.16 38.16 Global Days 090

44132-44137 Intestine Transplant Procedures

CMS 100-3,260.5 Intestinal and Multi-Visceral Transplantation

CMS 100-4,3,90.6 Intestinal and Multi-Visceral Transplants

44132 **Donor enterectomy (including cold preservation), open; from cadaver donor**

INCLUDES Graft:
Cold preservation
Harvest

0.00 0.00 Global Days XXX

44133 **partial, from living donor**

INCLUDES Donor care
Graft:
Cold preservation
Harvest

EXCLUDES *Preparation/reconstruction of backbench intestinal graft (44715, 44720, 44721)*

0.00 0.00 Global Days XXX

44135 **Intestinal allotransplantation; from cadaver donor**

INCLUDES Allograft transplantation
Recipient care

0.00 0.00 Global Days XXX

44136 **from living donor**

INCLUDES Allograft transplantation
Recipient care

0.00 0.00 Global Days XXX

44137 **Removal of transplanted intestinal allograft, complete**

EXCLUDES *Partial removal of transplant allograft (44120, 44121, 44140)*

0.00 0.00 Global Days XXX

44139-44160 Colon Resection Procedures

+ **44139** **Mobilization (take-down) of splenic flexure performed in conjunction with partial colectomy (List separately in addition to primary procedure)**

Code first partial colectomy (44140-44147)

3.54 3.54 Global Days ZZZ

44140 **Colectomy, partial; with anastomosis**

EXCLUDES *Partial colectomy with anastomosis performed laparoscopically (44204)*

39.18 39.18 Global Days 090

AMA: 2008, Nov, 7-9

44141 **with skin level cecostomy or colostomy**

53.18 53.18 Global Days 090

AMA: 2008, Nov, 7-9

44143 **with end colostomy and closure of distal segment (Hartmann type procedure)**

EXCLUDES *Laparoscopic method (44206)*

48.65 48.65 Global Days 090

AMA: 2008, Nov, 7-9

44144 **with resection, with colostomy or ileostomy and creation of mucofistula**

51.64 51.64 Global Days 090

AMA: 2008, Nov, 7-9

44145 **with coloproctostomy (low pelvic anastomosis)**

EXCLUDES *Laparoscopic method (44207)*

48.54 48.54 Global Days 090

AMA: 2008, Nov, 7-9

44146 **with coloproctostomy (low pelvic anastomosis), with colostomy**

EXCLUDES *Laparoscopic method (44208)*

61.86 61.86 Global Days 090

AMA: 2008, Nov, 7-9

44147 **abdominal and transanal approach**

56.45 56.45 Global Days 090

AMA: 2008, Nov, 7-9

44150 **Colectomy, total, abdominal, without proctectomy; with ileostomy or ileoproctostomy**

INCLUDES Lane's operation

EXCLUDES *Laparoscopic method (44210)*

54.66 54.66 Global Days 090

AMA: 2008, Nov, 7-9

44151 **with continent ileostomy**

62.48 62.48 Global Days 090

AMA: 2008, Nov, 7-9

44155 **Colectomy, total, abdominal, with proctectomy; with ileostomy**

INCLUDES Miles' colectomy

EXCLUDES *Laparoscopic method (44212)*

60.90 60.90 Global Days 090

AMA: 2008, Nov, 7-9

44156 **with continent ileostomy**

67.43 67.43 Global Days 090

AMA: 2008, Nov, 7-9

44157 **with ileoanal anastomosis, includes loop ileostomy, and rectal mucosectomy, when performed**

63.58 63.58 Global Days 090

AMA: 2008, Nov, 7-9

44158 **with ileoanal anastomosis, creation of ileal reservoir (S or J), includes loop ileostomy, and rectal mucosectomy, when performed**

EXCLUDES *Laparoscopic method (44211)*

65.20 65.20 Global Days 090

AMA: 2008, Nov, 7-9

44160 **Colectomy, partial, with removal of terminal ileum with ileocolostomy**

EXCLUDES *Laparoscopic method (44205)*

36.27 36.27 Global Days 090

AMA: 2008, Nov, 7-9

44180 Laparoscopic Enterolysis

INCLUDES Diagnostic laparoscopy (49320)

44180 **Laparoscopy, surgical, enterolysis (freeing of intestinal adhesion) (separate procedure)**

EXCLUDES *Laparoscopic salpingolysis/ovariolysis (58660)*

26.89 26.89 Global Days 090

44186-44238 Laparoscopic Enterostomy Procedures

INCLUDES Diagnostic laparoscopy when performed with a surgical laparoscopy

44186 **Laparoscopy, surgical; jejunostomy (eg, for decompression or feeding)** T 80 PQ
19.09 19.09 Global Days 090

44187 **ileostomy or jejunostomy, non-tube** C5 C 80 PQ
EXCLUDES *Open method (44310)*
32.39 32.39 Global Days 090

44188 **Laparoscopy, surgical, colostomy or skin level cecostomy** C5 C 80 PQ
EXCLUDES *Open method (44320)*
Do not report with (44970)
35.86 35.86 Global Days 090
AMA: 2009, Jan, 11-31; 2008, Jan, 10-25; 2007, January, 13-27

44202 **Laparoscopy, surgical; enterectomy, resection of small intestine, single resection and anastomosis** C5 C 80 PQ
EXCLUDES *Open method (44120)*
40.54 40.54 Global Days 090

\+ **44203** **each additional small intestine resection and anastomosis (List separately in addition to code for primary procedure)** C5 C 80
EXCLUDES *Open method (44121)*
Code first single resection of small intestine (44202)
7.10 7.10 Global Days ZZZ

44204 **colectomy, partial, with anastomosis** C5 C 80 PQ
EXCLUDES *Open method (44140)*
45.06 45.06 Global Days 090
AMA: 2009, Jan, 11-31; 2008, Jan, 10-25; 2007, January, 13-27

44205 **colectomy, partial, with removal of terminal ileum with ileocolostomy** C5 C 80 PQ
EXCLUDES *Open method (44160)*
39.20 39.20 Global Days 090

44206 **colectomy, partial, with end colostomy and closure of distal segment (Hartmann type procedure)** T 80 PQ
EXCLUDES *Open method (44143)*
51.41 51.41 Global Days 090

44207 **colectomy, partial, with anastomosis, with coloproctostomy (low pelvic anastomosis)** T 80 PQ
EXCLUDES *Open method (44145)*
53.54 53.54 Global Days 090

44208 **colectomy, partial, with anastomosis, with coloproctostomy (low pelvic anastomosis) with colostomy** T 80 PQ
EXCLUDES *Open method (44146)*
58.25 58.25 Global Days 090

44210 **colectomy, total, abdominal, without proctectomy, with ileostomy or ileoproctostomy** C5 C 80 PQ
EXCLUDES *Open method (44150)*
52.59 52.59 Global Days 090

44211 **colectomy, total, abdominal, with proctectomy, with ileoanal anastomosis, creation of ileal reservoir (S or J), with loop ileostomy, includes rectal mucosectomy, when performed** C5 C 80 PQ
EXCLUDES *Open method (44157, 44158)*
65.75 65.75 Global Days 090

44212 **colectomy, total, abdominal, with proctectomy, with ileostomy** C5 C 80 PQ
EXCLUDES *Open method (44155)*
60.47 60.47 Global Days 090

\+ **44213** **Laparoscopy, surgical, mobilization (take-down) of splenic flexure performed in conjunction with partial colectomy (List separately in addition to primary procedure)** T 80
EXCLUDES *Open method (44139)*
Code first partial colectomy (44204-44208)
5.54 5.54 Global Days ZZZ
AMA: 2009, Jan, 11-31; 2008, Jan, 10-25; 2007, January, 13-27

44227 **Laparoscopy, surgical, closure of enterostomy, large or small intestine, with resection and anastomosis** C5 C 80 PQ
EXCLUDES *Open method (44625, 44626)*
48.87 48.87 Global Days 090

44238 **Unlisted laparoscopy procedure, intestine (except rectum)** T 80 50
0.00 0.00 Global Days YYY

44300-44346 Open Enterostomy Procedures

44300 **Placement, enterostomy or cecostomy, tube open (eg, for feeding or decompression) (separate procedure)** C5 C 80 PQ
EXCLUDES *Other colonic tube(s) placed percutaneously with fluoroscopic imaging guidance (49441-49442)*
24.62 24.62 Global Days 090
AMA: 2009, Jan, 11-31; 2008, Jan, 10-25; 2007, January, 13-27

44310 **Ileostomy or jejunostomy, non-tube** C5 C 80 PQ
EXCLUDES *Laparoscopic method (44187)*
Do not report with (44144, 44150-44151, 44155-44156, 45113, 45119, 45136)
30.52 30.52 Global Days 090
AMA: 2009, Jan, 11-31; 2008, Jan, 10-25; 2007, January, 13-27

44312 **Revision of ileostomy; simple (release of superficial scar) (separate procedure)** A2 T 80 PQ
17.33 17.33 Global Days 090

44314 **complicated (reconstruction in-depth) (separate procedure)** C5 C 80 PQ
29.50 29.50 Global Days 090

44316 **Continent ileostomy (Kock procedure) (separate procedure)** C5 C 80 PQ
EXCLUDES *Fiberoptic evaluation (44385)*
41.20 41.20 Global Days 090

44320 **Colostomy or skin level cecostomy;** C5 C 80 PQ
EXCLUDES *Laparoscopic method (44188)*
Do not report with (44141, 44144, 44146, 44605, 45110, 45119, 45126, 45563, 45805, 45825, 50810, 51597, 57307, 58240)
35.13 35.13 Global Days 090

44322 **with multiple biopsies (eg, for congenital megacolon) (separate procedure)** C5 C 80 PQ
29.18 29.18 Global Days 090

44340 **Revision of colostomy; simple (release of superficial scar) (separate procedure)** A2 T PQ
18.17 18.17 Global Days 090

44345 **complicated (reconstruction in-depth) (separate procedure)** C5 C 80 PQ
30.77 30.77 Global Days 090

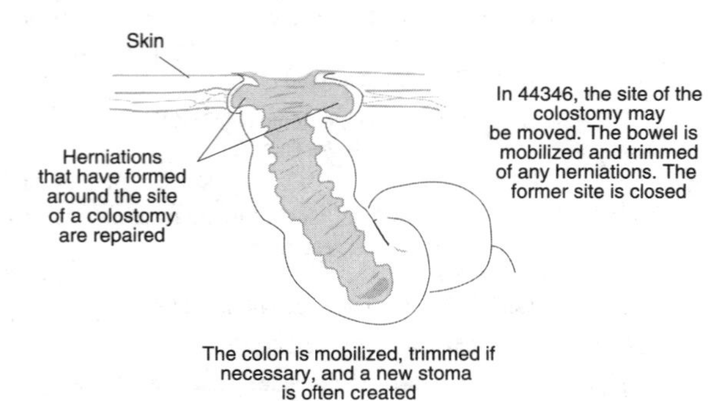

44346 with repair of paracolostomy hernia (separate procedure)
34.55 34.55 Global Days 090

44360-44386 Endoscopy of Small Intestine

CMS 100-3,100.2 Endoscopy

INCLUDES Diagnostic endoscopy performed with a surgical endoscopy

EXCLUDES *Endoscopy, upper gastrointestinal (43234-43258)*

⊙ **44360** Small intestinal endoscopy, enteroscopy beyond second portion of duodenum, not including ileum; diagnostic, with or without collection of specimen(s) by brushing or washing (separate procedure)
4.70 4.70 Global Days 000

⊙ **44361** with biopsy, single or multiple
5.17 5.17 Global Days 000

⊙ **44363** with removal of foreign body
6.18 6.18 Global Days 000

⊙ **44364** with removal of tumor(s), polyp(s), or other lesion(s) by snare technique
6.60 6.60 Global Days 000

⊙ **44365** with removal of tumor(s), polyp(s), or other lesion(s) by hot biopsy forceps or bipolar cautery
5.91 5.91 Global Days 000

⊙ **44366** with control of bleeding (eg, injection, bipolar cautery, unipolar cautery, laser, heater probe, stapler, plasma coagulator)
7.75 7.75 Global Days 000

⊙ **44369** with ablation of tumor(s), polyp(s), or other lesion(s) not amenable to removal by hot biopsy forceps, bipolar cautery or snare technique
7.93 7.93 Global Days 000

⊙ **44370** with transendoscopic stent placement (includes predilation)
Code also (C1874, C1875, C1876, C1877, C2617, C2625)
8.55 8.55 Global Days 000

⊙ **44372** with placement of percutaneous jejunostomy tube
7.64 7.64 Global Days 000

⊙ **44373** with conversion of percutaneous gastrostomy tube to percutaneous jejunostomy tube
EXCLUDES *Jejunostomy, fiberoptic, through stoma (43235)*
6.15 6.15 Global Days 000

⊙ **44376** Small intestinal endoscopy, enteroscopy beyond second portion of duodenum, including ileum; diagnostic, with or without collection of specimen(s) by brushing or washing (separate procedure)
9.07 9.07 Global Days 000

⊙ **44377** with biopsy, single or multiple
9.59 9.59 Global Days 000

⊙ **44378** with control of bleeding (eg, injection, bipolar cautery, unipolar cautery, laser, heater probe, stapler, plasma coagulator)
12.30 12.30 Global Days 000

⊙ **44379** with transendoscopic stent placement (includes predilation)
Code also (C1874, C1875, C1876, C1877, C2617, C2625)
13.08 13.08 Global Days 000

⊙ **44380** Ileoscopy, through stoma; diagnostic, with or without collection of specimen(s) by brushing or washing (separate procedure)
2.04 2.04 Global Days 000

⊙ **44382** with biopsy, single or multiple
2.46 2.46 Global Days 000

⊙ **44383** with transendoscopic stent placement (includes predilation)
Code also (C1874, C1875, C1876, C1877, C2617, C2625)
4.91 4.91 Global Days 000

⊙ **44385** Endoscopic evaluation of small intestinal (abdominal or pelvic) pouch; diagnostic, with or without collection of specimen(s) by brushing or washing (separate procedure)
3.16 7.74 Global Days 000

⊙ **44386** with biopsy, single or multiple
3.78 10.61 Global Days 000

44388-44397 Colonoscopy Via Stoma

CMS 100-3,100.2 Endoscopy

INCLUDES Diagnostic endoscopy when performed with a surgical endoscopy

EXCLUDES *Colonoscopy via rectum (45330-45392)*

⊙ **44388** Colonoscopy through stoma; diagnostic, with or without collection of specimen(s) by brushing or washing (separate procedure)
4.96 10.60 Global Days 000
AMA: 2009, Jan, 11-31; 2008, Jan, 10-25

⊙ **44389** with biopsy, single or multiple
5.53 12.05 Global Days 000

⊙ **44390** with removal of foreign body
6.51 13.55 Global Days 000

⊙ **44391** with control of bleeding (eg, injection, bipolar cautery, unipolar cautery, laser, heater probe, stapler, plasma coagulator)
7.49 15.21 Global Days 000

⊙ **44392** with removal of tumor(s), polyp(s), or other lesion(s) by hot biopsy forceps or bipolar cautery
6.55 13.29 Global Days 000

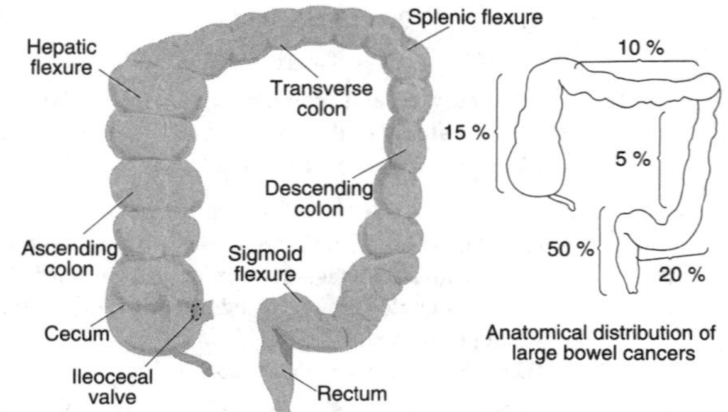

Cancer of the colon and rectum is a major cause of mortality in the U.S. with about 140,000 new cases identified annually; peak incidence is about 70 years of age; rectal cancer is more common among men, colon cancer among women

⊙ 44393 with ablation of tumor(s), polyp(s), or other lesion(s) not amenable to removal by hot biopsy forceps, bipolar cautery or snare technique
8.29 15.26 Global Days 000

⊙ 44394 with removal of tumor(s), polyp(s), or other lesion(s) by snare technique
7.64 15.11 Global Days 000

⊙ 44397 with transendoscopic stent placement (includes predilation)
Code also (C1874, C1875, C1876, C1877, C2617, C2625)
8.22 8.22 Global Days 000

44500 Gastrointestinal Intubation

⊘ ⊙ 44500 Introduction of long gastrointestinal tube (eg, Miller-Abbott) (separate procedure)
EXCLUDES *Placement of oro- or naso-gastric tube (43752)*
74340
0.72 0.72 Global Days 000

44602-44680 Open Repair Procedures of Intestines

44602 Suture of small intestine (enterorrhaphy) for perforated ulcer, diverticulum, wound, injury or rupture; single perforation
41.01 41.01 Global Days 090

44603 multiple perforations
47.11 47.11 Global Days 090

44604 Suture of large intestine (colorrhaphy) for perforated ulcer, diverticulum, wound, injury or rupture (single or multiple perforations); without colostomy
30.87 30.87 Global Days 090

44605 with colostomy
38.29 38.29 Global Days 090

44615 Intestinal stricturoplasty (enterotomy and enterorrhaphy) with or without dilation, for intestinal obstruction
31.45 31.45 Global Days 090

44620 Closure of enterostomy, large or small intestine;
25.34 25.34 Global Days 090

44625 with resection and anastomosis other than colorectal
EXCLUDES *Laparoscopic method (44227)*
29.84 29.84 Global Days 090

44626 with resection and colorectal anastomosis (eg, closure of Hartmann type procedure)
EXCLUDES *Laparoscopic method (44227)*
46.95 46.95 Global Days 090

44640 Closure of intestinal cutaneous fistula
41.03 41.03 Global Days 090

44650 Closure of enteroenteric or enterocolic fistula
42.44 42.44 Global Days 090

44660 Closure of enterovesical fistula; without intestinal or bladder resection
EXCLUDES *Closure of fistula:*
Gastrocolic (43880)
Rectovesical (45800, 45805)
Renocolic (50525, 50526)
39.24 39.24 Global Days 090

44661 with intestine and/or bladder resection
EXCLUDES *Closure of fistula:*
Gastrocolic (43880)
Rectovesical (45800, 45805)
Renocolic (50525, 50526)
45.49 45.49 Global Days 090

44680 Intestinal plication (separate procedure)
INCLUDES Noble intestinal plication
31.43 31.43 Global Days 090

44700-44701 Other Intestinal Procedures

44700 Exclusion of small intestine from pelvis by mesh or other prosthesis, or native tissue (eg, bladder or omentum)
EXCLUDES *Therapeutic radiation clinical treatment (77261-77799 [77424, 77425])*
29.80 29.80 Global Days 090

\+ 44701 Intraoperative colonic lavage (List separately in addition to code for primary procedure)
Code first as appropriate (44140, 44145, 44150, 44604)
Do not report with (44300, 44950-44960)
4.91 4.91 Global Days ZZZ

44715-44799 Backbench Transplant Procedures

CMS 100-3,260.5 Intestinal and Multi-Visceral Transplantation
CMS 100-4,3,90.6 Intestinal and Multi-Visceral Transplants

44715 Backbench standard preparation of cadaver or living donor intestine allograft prior to transplantation, including mobilization and fashioning of the superior mesenteric artery and vein
INCLUDES Mobilization/fashioning of superior mesenteric vein/artery
0.00 0.00 Global Days XXX

44720 Backbench reconstruction of cadaver or living donor intestine allograft prior to transplantation; venous anastomosis, each
7.23 7.23 Global Days XXX

44721 arterial anastomosis, each
11.28 11.28 Global Days XXX

44799 Unlisted procedure, intestine
EXCLUDES *Unlisted intestinal procedure performed laparoscopically (44238)*
Unlisted rectal procedure (45499, 45999)
0.00 0.00 Global Days YYY
AMA: 2009, Jan, 11-31; 2008, Jan, 10-25; 2008, Nov, 10-11; 2008, May, 9-11; 2007, January, 13-27

44800-44899 Meckel's Diverticulum and Mesentery Procedures

44800 Excision of Meckel's diverticulum (diverticulectomy) or omphalomesenteric duct
22.31 22.31 Global Days 090

44820 Excision of lesion of mesentery (separate procedure)
EXCLUDES *Resection of intestine (44120-44128, 44140-44160)*
24.53 24.53 Global Days 090

44850 Suture of mesentery (separate procedure)
EXCLUDES *Internal hernia repair/reduction (44050)*
21.89 21.89 Global Days 090

44899 **Unlisted procedure, Meckel's diverticulum and the mesentery** C5 C 80
0.00 0.00 Global Days YYY

44900-44979 Open and Endoscopic Appendix Procedures

44900 **Incision and drainage of appendiceal abscess; open** C5 C 80
22.55 22.55 Global Days 090

⊙ **44901** **percutaneous** T
75989
4.99 27.60 Global Days 000

44950 **Appendectomy;** T 80
INCLUDES Battle's operation
18.75 18.75 Global Days 090
AMA: 2008, Nov, 7-9

\+ **44955** **when done for indicated purpose at time of other major procedure (not as separate procedure) (List separately in addition to code for primary procedure)** T 80
Code first primary procedure
2.46 2.46 Global Days ZZZ
AMA: 2008, Nov, 7-9

44960 **for ruptured appendix with abscess or generalized peritonitis** C5 C 80
INCLUDES Battle's operation
25.50 25.50 Global Days 090
AMA: 2008, Nov, 7-9

44970 **Laparoscopy, surgical, appendectomy** T 80
INCLUDES Diagnostic laparoscopy (49320)
17.48 17.48 Global Days 090
AMA: 2009, Jan, 11-31; 2008, Jan, 10-25; 2007, January, 13-27

44979 **Unlisted laparoscopy procedure, appendix** T 80 50
0.00 0.00 Global Days YYY

45000-45190 Open and Transrectal Procedures of Rectum

45000 **Transrectal drainage of pelvic abscess** A2 T
12.34 12.34 Global Days 090

45005 **Incision and drainage of submucosal abscess, rectum** A2 T
4.64 7.88 Global Days 010

45020 **Incision and drainage of deep supralevator, pelvirectal, or retrorectal abscess** A2 T
EXCLUDES *Incision and drainage of perianal, ischiorectal, intramural abscess (46050, 46060)*
16.58 16.58 Global Days 090

45100 **Biopsy of anorectal wall, anal approach (eg, congenital megacolon)** A2 T
EXCLUDES *Biopsy performed endoscopically (45305)*
8.72 8.72 Global Days 090

45108 **Anorectal myomectomy** A2 T
10.72 10.72 Global Days 090

45110 **Proctectomy; complete, combined abdominoperineal, with colostomy** C5 C 80
EXCLUDES *Laparoscopic method (45395)*
54.20 54.20 Global Days 090

45111 **partial resection of rectum, transabdominal approach** C5 C 80
INCLUDES Luschka proctectomy
31.87 31.87 Global Days 090

45112 **Proctectomy, combined abdominoperineal, pull-through procedure (eg, colo-anal anastomosis)** C5 C 80
EXCLUDES *Proctectomy for colo-anal anastomosis with creation of colonic pouch or reservoir (45119)*
55.17 55.17 Global Days 090

45113 **Proctectomy, partial, with rectal mucosectomy, ileoanal anastomosis, creation of ileal reservoir (S or J), with or without loop ileostomy** C5 C 80
57.99 57.99 Global Days 090

45114 **Proctectomy, partial, with anastomosis; abdominal and transsacral approach** C5 C 80
52.90 52.90 Global Days 090

45116 **transsacral approach only (Kraske type)** C5 C 80
45.95 45.95 Global Days 090

45119 **Proctectomy, combined abdominoperineal pull-through procedure (eg, colo-anal anastomosis), with creation of colonic reservoir (eg, J-pouch), with diverting enterostomy when performed** C5 C 80
EXCLUDES *Laparoscopic method (45397)*
57.09 57.09 Global Days 090

45120 **Proctectomy, complete (for congenital megacolon), abdominal and perineal approach; with pull-through procedure and anastomosis (eg, Swenson, Duhamel, or Soave type operation)** C5 C 80
46.14 46.14 Global Days 090

45121 **with subtotal or total colectomy, with multiple biopsies** C5 C 80
50.61 50.61 Global Days 090

45123 **Proctectomy, partial, without anastomosis, perineal approach** C5 C 80
32.62 32.62 Global Days 090

45126 **Pelvic exenteration for colorectal malignancy, with proctectomy (with or without colostomy), with removal of bladder and ureteral transplantations, and/or hysterectomy, or cervicectomy, with or without removal of tube(s), with or without removal of ovary(s), or any combination thereof** C5 C 80
84.05 84.05 Global Days 090

45130 **Excision of rectal procidentia, with anastomosis; perineal approach** C5 C 80
INCLUDES Altemeier procedure
31.89 31.89 Global Days 090

45135 **abdominal and perineal approach** C5 C 80 PQ
INCLUDES Altemeier procedure
39.78 39.78 Global Days 090

45136 **Excision of ileoanal reservoir with ileostomy** C5 C 80 PQ
Do not report with (44005, 44120, 44310)
53.13 53.13 Global Days 090

45150 **Division of stricture of rectum** A2 T 80 PQ
11.50 11.50 Global Days 090

45160 **Excision of rectal tumor by proctotomy, transsacral or transcoccygeal approach** A2 T 80 PQ
29.60 29.60 Global Days 090
AMA: 2008, Jan, 6-7

45171 **Excision of rectal tumor, transanal approach; not including muscularis propria (ie, partial thickness)** G2 T 80 PQ
EXCLUDES *Transanal destruction of rectal tumor (45190)*
Transanal endoscopic microsurgical tumer excision (TEMS) (0184T)
17.85 17.85 Global Days 090

45172 **including muscularis propria (ie, full thickness)** G2 T 80 PQ
EXCLUDES *Transanal destruction of rectal tumor (45190)*
Transanal endoscopic microsurgical tumor excision (TEMS) (0184T)
24.13 24.13 Global Days 090

45190 **Destruction of rectal tumor (eg, electrodesiccation, electrosurgery, laser ablation, laser resection, cryosurgery) transanal approach** A2 T PQ
EXCLUDES *Transanal endoscopic microsurgical tumor excision (TEMS) (0184T)*
Transanal excision of rectal tumor (45171-45172)
20.13 20.13 Global Days 090

45300-45327 Rigid Proctosigmoidoscopy Procedures

CMS 100-3,100.2 Endoscopy
INCLUDES Exam of:
Rectum
Sigmoid colon
EXCLUDES *Computed tomographic colonography (74261-74263)*

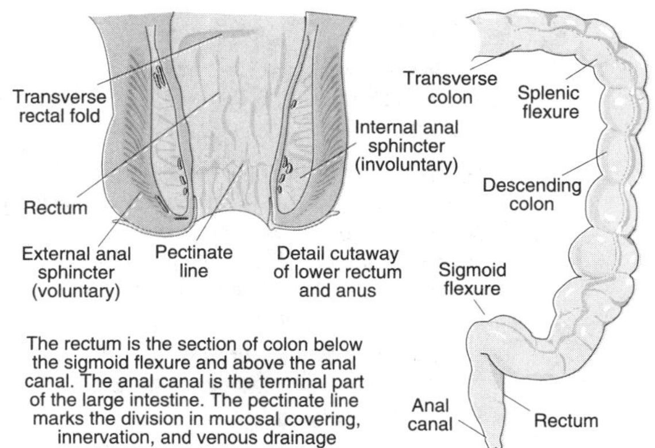

The rectum is the section of colon below the sigmoid flexure and above the anal canal. The anal canal is the terminal part of the large intestine. The pectinate line marks the division in mucosal covering, innervation, and venous drainage

45300 **Proctosigmoidoscopy, rigid; diagnostic, with or without collection of specimen(s) by brushing or washing (separate procedure)** P3 T
1.57 3.56 Global Days 000
AMA: 2008, Jan, 6-7

⊙ 45303 **with dilation (eg, balloon, guide wire, bougie)** P2 T
74360
2.68 27.69 Global Days 000
AMA: 2008, Jan, 6-7

⊙ 45305 **with biopsy, single or multiple** A2 T
2.33 5.74 Global Days 000
AMA: 2008, Jan, 6-7

⊙ 45307 **with removal of foreign body** A2 T 80
3.04 6.68 Global Days 000
AMA: 2008, Jan, 6-7

⊙ 45308 **with removal of single tumor, polyp, or other lesion by hot biopsy forceps or bipolar cautery** A2 T
2.56 6.08 Global Days 000
AMA: 2008, Jan, 6-7

⊙ 45309 **with removal of single tumor, polyp, or other lesion by snare technique** A2 T
2.74 6.55 Global Days 000
AMA: 2008, Jan, 6-7

⊙ 45315 **with removal of multiple tumors, polyps, or other lesions by hot biopsy forceps, bipolar cautery or snare technique** A2 T
3.24 6.78 Global Days 000
AMA: 2008, Jan, 6-7

⊙ 45317 **with control of bleeding (eg, injection, bipolar cautery, unipolar cautery, laser, heater probe, stapler, plasma coagulator)** A2 T
3.47 7.04 Global Days 000
AMA: 2008, Jan, 6-7

⊙ 45320 **with ablation of tumor(s), polyp(s), or other lesion(s) not amenable to removal by hot biopsy forceps, bipolar cautery or snare technique (eg, laser)** A2 T
3.18 7.03 Global Days 000
AMA: 2008, Jan, 6-7

⊙ 45321 **with decompression of volvulus** A2 T
3.18 3.18 Global Days 000
AMA: 2008, Jan, 6-7

⊙ 45327 **with transendoscopic stent placement (includes predilation)** A2 T
Code also (C1874, C1875, C1876, C1877, C2617, C2625)
3.61 3.61 Global Days 000
AMA: 2008, Jan, 6-7

45330-45345 Flexible Sigmoidoscopy Procedures

CMS 100-3,100.2 Endoscopy
INCLUDES Exam of:
Entire rectum
Entire sigmoid colon
Portion of descending colon (may include)
EXCLUDES *Computed tomographic colonography (74261-74263)*

45330 **Sigmoidoscopy, flexible; diagnostic, with or without collection of specimen(s) by brushing or washing (separate procedure)** P3 T
1.89 4.20 Global Days 000
AMA: 2009, Jan, 11-31; 2008, Jan, 10-25; 2007, May, 9-11

45331 **with biopsy, single or multiple** A2 T
2.27 5.03 Global Days 000
AMA: 2009, Jan, 11-31; 2008, Jan, 10-25; 2007, January, 28-31

⊙ 45332 **with removal of foreign body** A2 T
3.32 8.81 Global Days 000

⊙ 45333 **with removal of tumor(s), polyp(s), or other lesion(s) by hot biopsy forceps or bipolar cautery** A2 T
3.29 8.93 Global Days 000

⊙ **45334** **with control of bleeding (eg, injection, bipolar cautery, unipolar cautery, laser, heater probe, stapler, plasma coagulator)** A2 T
Facility RVU 4.89 Non-Facility RVU 4.89 Global Days 000
AMA: 2009, Jan, 11-31; 2008, Jan, 10-25; 2007, January, 28-31

⊙ **45335** **with directed submucosal injection(s), any substance** A2 T
Facility RVU 2.76 Non-Facility RVU 8.14 Global Days 000
AMA: 2009, Jan, 11-31; 2008, Jan, 10-25; 2007, January, 13-27

⊙ **45337** **with decompression of volvulus, any method** A2 T
Facility RVU 4.24 Non-Facility RVU 4.24 Global Days 000

⊙ **45338** **with removal of tumor(s), polyp(s), or other lesion(s) by snare technique** A2 T
Facility RVU 4.22 Non-Facility RVU 9.65 Global Days 000

⊙ **45339** **with ablation of tumor(s), polyp(s), or other lesion(s) not amenable to removal by hot biopsy forceps, bipolar cautery or snare technique** A2 T
Facility RVU 5.56 Non-Facility RVU 10.22 Global Days 000

⊙ **45340** **with dilation by balloon, 1 or more strictures** A2 T
Do not report with (45345)
Facility RVU 3.47 Non-Facility RVU 14.49 Global Days 000

⊙ **45341** **with endoscopic ultrasound examination** A2 T
Do not report with (76942, 76975)
Facility RVU 4.68 Non-Facility RVU 4.68 Global Days 000
AMA: 2009, Mar, 8-9

⊙ **45342** **with transendoscopic ultrasound guided intramural or transmural fine needle aspiration/biopsy(s)** A2 T
EXCLUDES *Transrectal ultrasound with rigid probe device (76872)*
Do not report with (76942, 76975)
Lab Crosswalk *88172-88173*
Facility RVU 7.15 Non-Facility RVU 7.15 Global Days 000
AMA: 2009, Mar, 8-9

⊙ **45345** **with transendoscopic stent placement (includes predilation)** A2 T
Code also (C1874, C1875, C1876, C1877, C2617, C2625)
Facility RVU 5.19 Non-Facility RVU 5.19 Global Days 000

45355-45392 Flexible and Rigid Colonoscopy Procedures

CMS 100-3,100.2 Endoscopy
INCLUDES Exam of:
Entire colon (rectum to cecum)
Terminal ileum (may include)
EXCLUDES *Computed tomographic colonography (74261-74263)*
Code also modifer 53 (physician), or 73, 74 (facility) for an incomplete colonoscopy

⊙ **45355** **Colonoscopy, rigid or flexible, transabdominal via colotomy, single or multiple** A2 T P0
EXCLUDES *Colonoscopy, fiberoptic, past 25 cm to splenic flexure (45330-45345)*
Facility RVU 6.09 Non-Facility RVU 6.09 Global Days 000

⊙ **45378** **Colonoscopy, flexible, proximal to splenic flexure; diagnostic, with or without collection of specimen(s) by brushing or washing, with or without colon decompression (separate procedure)** A2 T P0
Facility RVU 6.48 Non-Facility RVU 11.84 Global Days 000

⊙ **45379** **with removal of foreign body** A2 T
Facility RVU 8.10 Non-Facility RVU 15.12 Global Days 000

⊙ **45380** **with biopsy, single or multiple** A2 T P0
Facility RVU 7.75 Non-Facility RVU 14.12 Global Days 000
AMA: 2009, Jan, 11-31; 2008, Jan, 10-25; 2007, January, 13-27

⊙ **45381** **with directed submucosal injection(s), any substance** A2 T P0
Facility RVU 7.35 Non-Facility RVU 14.08 Global Days 000
AMA: 2009, Jan, 11-31; 2008, Jan, 10-25; 2007, January, 13-27

⊙ **45382** **with control of bleeding (eg, injection, bipolar cautery, unipolar cautery, laser, heater probe, stapler, plasma coagulator)** A2 T
Facility RVU 9.87 Non-Facility RVU 18.44 Global Days 000

⊙ **45383** **with ablation of tumor(s), polyp(s), or other lesion(s) not amenable to removal by hot biopsy forceps, bipolar cautery or snare technique** A2 T P0
Facility RVU 10.02 Non-Facility RVU 17.01 Global Days 000

⊙ **45384** **with removal of tumor(s), polyp(s), or other lesion(s) by hot biopsy forceps or bipolar cautery** A2 T P0
Facility RVU 8.08 Non-Facility RVU 14.01 Global Days 000
AMA: 2009, Jan, 11-31; 2008, Jan, 10-25; 2007, January, 13-27

⊙ **45385** **with removal of tumor(s), polyp(s), or other lesion(s) by snare technique** A2 T P0
EXCLUDES *Endoscopy, small intestine/stomal (44360-44393)*
Facility RVU 9.19 Non-Facility RVU 15.89 Global Days 000
AMA: 2009, Jan, 11-31; 2008, Jan, 10-25; 2007, January, 13-27

⊙ **45386** **with dilation by balloon, 1 or more strictures** A2 T
Do not report with (45387)
Facility RVU 7.94 Non-Facility RVU 20.23 Global Days 000

⊙ **45387** **with transendoscopic stent placement (includes predilation)** A2 T
Code also (C1874, C1875, C1876, C1877, C2617, C2625)
Facility RVU 10.30 Non-Facility RVU 10.30 Global Days 000

⊙ **45391** **with endoscopic ultrasound examination** A2 T
Do not report with (45330, 45341-45342, 45378, 76872)
Facility RVU 8.81 Non-Facility RVU 8.81 Global Days 000

⊙ **45392** **with transendoscopic ultrasound guided intramural or transmural fine needle aspiration/biopsy(s)** A2 T
Do not report with (45330, 45341-45342, 45378, 76872)
Facility RVU 11.34 Non-Facility RVU 11.34 Global Days 000

45395-45499 Laparoscopic Procedures of Rectum

INCLUDES Diagnostic laparoscopy (49320)

45395 **Laparoscopy, surgical; proctectomy, complete, combined abdominoperineal, with colostomy** C5 C 80 P0
EXCLUDES *Open method (45110)*
Facility RVU 58.25 Non-Facility RVU 58.25 Global Days 090

45397 **proctectomy, combined abdominoperineal pull-through procedure (eg, colo-anal anastomosis), with creation of colonic reservoir (eg, J-pouch), with diverting enterostomy, when performed** C5 C 80 P0
EXCLUDES *Open method (45119)*
Facility RVU 62.86 Non-Facility RVU 62.86 Global Days 090
AMA: 2009, Jan, 11-31; 2008, Jan, 10-25; 2007, January, 13-27

45400 **proctopexy (for prolapse)** C5 C 80 P0
EXCLUDES *Open method (45540, 45541)*
Facility RVU 33.77 Non-Facility RVU 33.77 Global Days 090

45402 **proctopexy (for prolapse), with sigmoid resection** C5 C 80 P0
EXCLUDES *Open method (45550)*
Facility RVU 44.79 Non-Facility RVU 44.79 Global Days 090

45499 **Unlisted laparoscopy procedure, rectum** T 80

EXCLUDES *Unlisted rectal procedure performed via open technique (45999)*

0.00 0.00 Global Days YYY

45500-45825 Open Repairs of Rectum

45500 **Proctoplasty; for stenosis** A2 T 80 PQ

15.30 15.30 Global Days 090

45505 **for prolapse of mucous membrane** A2 T PQ

17.16 17.16 Global Days 090

45520 **Perirectal injection of sclerosing solution for prolapse** P2 T PQ

1.17 4.44 Global Days 000

AMA: 2009, Jan, 11-31; 2008, Jan, 10-25; 2007, January, 13-27

45540 **Proctopexy (eg, for prolapse); abdominal approach** C5 C 80 PQ

EXCLUDES *Laparoscopic method (45400)*

30.97 30.97 Global Days 090

45541 **perineal approach** G2 T 80 PQ

27.08 27.08 Global Days 090

45550 **with sigmoid resection, abdominal approach** C5 C 80 PQ

INCLUDES Frickman proctopexy

EXCLUDES *Laparoscopic method (45402)*

42.83 42.83 Global Days 090

45560 **Repair of rectocele (separate procedure)** A2 T 80 PQ

EXCLUDES *Posterior colporrhaphy with rectocele repair (57250)*

20.56 20.56 Global Days 090

45562 **Exploration, repair, and presacral drainage for rectal injury;** C5 C 80 PQ

32.46 32.46 Global Days 090

45563 **with colostomy** C5 C 80 PQ

INCLUDES Maydl colostomy

47.91 47.91 Global Days 090

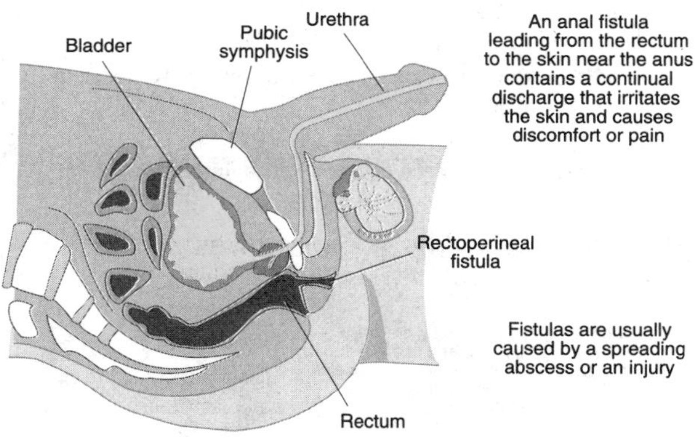

45800 **Closure of rectovesical fistula;** C5 C 80 PQ

35.13 35.13 Global Days 090

45805 **with colostomy** C5 C 80 PQ

42.52 42.52 Global Days 090

45820 **Closure of rectourethral fistula;** C5 C 80 PQ

EXCLUDES *Closure of fistula, rectovaginal (57300-57308)*

34.29 34.29 Global Days 090

45825 **with colostomy** C5 C 80 PQ

EXCLUDES *Closure of fistula, rectovaginal (57300-57308)*

42.82 42.82 Global Days 090

45900-45999 Closed Procedures of Rectum With Anesthesia

45900 **Reduction of procidentia (separate procedure) under anesthesia** A2 T 80

5.90 5.90 Global Days 010

45905 **Dilation of anal sphincter (separate procedure) under anesthesia other than local** A2 T

4.94 4.94 Global Days 010

45910 **Dilation of rectal stricture (separate procedure) under anesthesia other than local** A2 T

5.74 5.74 Global Days 010

45915 **Removal of fecal impaction or foreign body (separate procedure) under anesthesia** A2 T

6.58 9.52 Global Days 010

AMA: 2009, Jan, 11-31; 2008, Jan, 10-25; 2007, January, 13-27

45990 **Anorectal exam, surgical, requiring anesthesia (general, spinal, or epidural), diagnostic** A2 T 80

INCLUDES Diagnostic:
- Anoscopy
- Proctoscopy, rigid

Exam:
- Pelvic (when performed)
- Perineal, external
- Rectal, digital

Do not report with (45300-45327, 46600, 57410, 99170)

3.14 3.14 Global Days 000

AMA: 2009, Jan, 11-31; 2008, Jan, 10-25; 2007, January, 13-27

45999 **Unlisted procedure, rectum** T 80

EXCLUDES *Unlisted rectal procedure performed laparscopically (45499)*

0.00 0.00 Global Days YYY

46020-46083 Surgical Incision of Anus

EXCLUDES *Cryosurgical destruction of hemorrhoid(s) (46999)*
Fistulotomy, subcutaneous (46270)
Hemorrhoidopexy ([46947])
Injection of hemorrhoid(s) (46500)
Thermal energy destruction of internal hemorrhoid(s) (46930)

46020 **Placement of seton** A2 T

Do not report with (46060, 46280, 46600, 0249T)

6.81 7.97 Global Days 010

46030 **Removal of anal seton, other marker** A2 T 80

2.64 4.03 Global Days 010

46040 **Incision and drainage of ischiorectal and/or perirectal abscess (separate procedure)** A2 T

12.01 15.39 Global Days 090

46045 **Incision and drainage of intramural, intramuscular, or submucosal abscess, transanal, under anesthesia** A2 T

12.51 12.51 Global Days 090

46050 **Incision and drainage, perianal abscess, superficial** A2 T

EXCLUDES *Incision and drainage abscess*
Ischiorectal/intramural (46060)
Supralevator/pelvirectal/retrorectal (45020)

2.85 5.82 Global Days 010

46060 **Incision and drainage of ischiorectal or intramural abscess, with fistulectomy or fistulotomy, submuscular, with or without placement of seton**
EXCLUDES *Incision and drainage abscess: Supralevator/pelvirectal/retrorectal (45020)*
Do not report with (46020)
13.78 13.78 Global Days 090

46070 **Incision, anal septum (infant)**
EXCLUDES *Anoplasty (46700-46705)*
6.95 6.95 Global Days 090

46080 **Sphincterotomy, anal, division of sphincter (separate procedure)**
4.66 7.21 Global Days 010

46083 **Incision of thrombosed hemorrhoid, external**
3.13 5.19 Global Days 010
AMA: 2009, Jan, 11-31; 2008, Jan, 10-25; 2007, January, 13-27

46200-46262 [46220, 46320, 46945, 46946] Anal Resection and Hemorrhoidectomies

EXCLUDES *Cryosurgical destruction of hemorrhoid(s) (46999)*
Hemorrhoidopexy ([46947])
Injection of hemorrhoid(s) (46500)
Thermal energy destruction of internal hemorrhoid(s) (46930)

46200 **Fissurectomy, including sphincterotomy, when performed**
9.39 12.69 Global Days 090

46220 ***Resequenced code, See code before 46230.***

46221 **Hemorrhoidectomy, internal, by rubber band ligation(s)**
EXCLUDES *Ligation of hemorrhoidal vascular bundles including ultrasound guidance (0249T)*
Do not report with (0249T)
5.57 7.78 Global Days 010

\# **46945** **Hemorrhoidectomy, internal, by ligation other than rubber band; single hemorrhoid column/group**
EXCLUDES *Other hemorrhoid procedures:*
Destruction (46930)
Excision (46250-46262)
Injection sclerosing solution (46500)
Do not report with (0249T)
6.57 8.88 Global Days 090

\# **46946** **2 or more hemorrhoid columns/groups**
Do not report with (0249T)
6.58 9.07 Global Days 090

\# **46220** **Excision of single external papilla or tag, anus**
3.47 5.97 Global Days 010

46230 **Excision of multiple external papillae or tags, anus**
5.05 7.93 Global Days 010

\# **46320** **Excision of thrombosed hemorrhoid, external**
3.24 5.32 Global Days 010

46250 **Hemorrhoidectomy, external, 2 or more columns/groups**
EXCLUDES *Hemorrhoidectomy, external, single column/group (46999)*
Do not report with (0249T)
9.12 13.31 Global Days 090

46255 **Hemorrhoidectomy, internal and external, single column/group;**
Do not report with (0249T)
10.28 14.66 Global Days 090

46257 **with fissurectomy**
Do not report with (0249T)
12.22 12.22 Global Days 090

46258 **with fistulectomy, including fissurectomy, when performed**
Do not report with (0249T)
13.51 13.51 Global Days 090

46260 **Hemorrhoidectomy, internal and external, 2 or more columns/groups;**
INCLUDES Whitehead hemorrhoidectomy
Do not report with (0249T)
13.76 13.76 Global Days 090

46261 **with fissurectomy**
Do not report with (0249T)
15.25 15.25 Global Days 090

46262 **with fistulectomy, including fissurectomy, when performed**
Do not report with (0249T)
16.07 16.07 Global Days 090

46270-46320 Resection of Anal Fistula

46270 **Surgical treatment of anal fistula (fistulectomy/fistulotomy); subcutaneous**
11.32 14.59 Global Days 090

46275 **intersphincteric**
11.98 15.44 Global Days 090

46280 **transsphincteric, suprasphincteric, extrasphincteric or multiple, including placement of seton, when performed**
Do not report with (46020)
13.59 13.59 Global Days 090

46285 **second stage**
11.91 15.23 Global Days 090

46288 **Closure of anal fistula with rectal advancement flap**
15.87 15.87 Global Days 090

46320 ***Resequenced code, See code following 46230.***

46500 Other Hemorrhoid Procedures

Varicose veins commonly develop in the lower legs, particularly in the elderly, when impaired valves cause the vessels to swell and become inflamed; the risk of clot formation increases with inflamed veins; thrombophlebitis is the inflammation which may result in blood clots in veins

Rectum

Anal sphincter

Internal hemorrhoid

External hemorrhoid

Valve cusps become incompetent in the varicose vein causing blood to pool

Thrombus (blood clot)

Varicose veins and hemorrhoids (varicose rectal veins) are often associated; internal hemorrhoids (also called piles) are varicosities of the tributaries of the superior rectal veins and are covered by mucous membranes; external hemorrhoids are of the inferior rectal veins and are covered by skin

46500 **Injection of sclerosing solution, hemorrhoids**
3.77 6.81 Global Days 010

46505 Chemodenervation Anal Sphincter

46505 **Chemodenervation of internal anal sphincter**
EXCLUDES *Chemodenervation of:*
Extremity/trunk muscles (64614)
Muscles/facial nerve (64612)
Neck muscles (64613)
Other peripheral nerve/branch (64640)
Pudendal nerve (64630)
Code also drug(s)/substance(s) given
7.00 8.34 Global Days 010

46600-46615 Anoscopic Procedures

CMS 100-3,100.2 Endoscopy
EXCLUDES *Delivery of thermal energy via anoscope to the muscle of the anal canal (0288T)*

46600 **Anoscopy; diagnostic, with or without collection of specimen(s) by brushing or washing (separate procedure)**
EXCLUDES *High-resolution anoscopy (HRA), diagnostic (0226T)*
Do not report with (46020, 0249T)
1.18 2.56 Global Days 000

46604 **with dilation (eg, balloon, guide wire, bougie)**
INCLUDES Diagnostic anosocpy (46600)
1.94 17.72 Global Days 000

46606 **with biopsy, single or multiple**
INCLUDES Diagnostic anoscopy (46600)
EXCLUDES *High resolution anoscopy (HRA) with biopsy (0227T)*
2.25 6.60 Global Days 000

46608 **with removal of foreign body**
INCLUDES Diagnostic anoscopy (46600)
2.36 6.83 Global Days 000

46610 **with removal of single tumor, polyp, or other lesion by hot biopsy forceps or bipolar cautery**
INCLUDES Diagnostic anoscopy (46600)
2.38 6.64 Global Days 000

46611 **with removal of single tumor, polyp, or other lesion by snare technique**
INCLUDES Diagnostic anoscopy (46600)
2.42 5.16 Global Days 000

46612 **with removal of multiple tumors, polyps, or other lesions by hot biopsy forceps, bipolar cautery or snare technique**
INCLUDES Diagnostic anoscopy (46600)
2.78 7.79 Global Days 000

46614 **with control of bleeding (eg, injection, bipolar cautery, unipolar cautery, laser, heater probe, stapler, plasma coagulator)**
INCLUDES Diagnostic anoscopy (46600)
1.91 3.75 Global Days 000

46615 **with ablation of tumor(s), polyp(s), or other lesion(s) not amenable to removal by hot biopsy forceps, bipolar cautery or snare technique**
INCLUDES Diagnostic anoscopy (46600)
2.77 4.29 Global Days 000

46700-46947 [46947] Anal Repairs and Stapled Hemorrhoidpexy

46700 **Anoplasty, plastic operation for stricture; adult**
18.97 18.97 Global Days 090

46705 **infant**
EXCLUDES *Anal septum incision (46070)*
14.87 14.87 Global Days 090

46706 **Repair of anal fistula with fibrin glue**
4.86 4.86 Global Days 010

46707 **Repair of anorectal fistula with plug (eg, porcine small intestine submucosa [SIS])**
13.70 13.70 Global Days 090

46710 **Repair of ileoanal pouch fistula/sinus (eg, perineal or vaginal), pouch advancement; transperineal approach**
31.96 31.96 Global Days 090

46712 **combined transperineal and transabdominal approach**
59.34 59.34 Global Days 090

46715 **Repair of low imperforate anus; with anoperineal fistula (cut-back procedure)**
14.33 14.33 Global Days 090

46716 **with transposition of anoperineal or anovestibular fistula**
33.40 33.40 Global Days 090

46730 **Repair of high imperforate anus without fistula; perineal or sacroperineal approach**
52.41 52.41 Global Days 090

46735 **combined transabdominal and sacroperineal approaches**
59.34 59.34 Global Days 090

46740 **Repair of high imperforate anus with rectourethral or rectovaginal fistula; perineal or sacroperineal approach**
62.26 62.26 Global Days 090

46742 **combined transabdominal and sacroperineal approaches**
70.75 70.75 Global Days 090

46744 **Repair of cloacal anomaly by anorectovaginoplasty and urethroplasty, sacroperineal approach**
97.67 97.67 Global Days 090

46746 **Repair of cloacal anomaly by anorectovaginoplasty and urethroplasty, combined abdominal and sacroperineal approach;**
102.94 102.94 Global Days 090

46748 **with vaginal lengthening by intestinal graft or pedicle flaps**
111.54 111.54 Global Days 090

46750 **Sphincteroplasty, anal, for incontinence or prolapse; adult**
22.31 22.31 Global Days 090

46751 **child**
17.73 17.73 Global Days 090

46753 **Graft (Thiersch operation) for rectal incontinence and/or prolapse**
17.06 17.06 Global Days 090

46754 **Removal of Thiersch wire or suture, anal canal**
6.73 8.70 Global Days 010

46760 **Sphincteroplasty, anal, for incontinence, adult; muscle transplant**
31.78 31.78 Global Days 090

46761 levator muscle imbrication (Park posterior anal repair) A2 T 80 PQ
27.24 27.24 Global Days 090

46762 implantation artificial sphincter A2 T 80 PQ
26.90 26.90 Global Days 090

\# 46947 Hemorrhoidopexy (eg, for prolapsing internal hemorrhoids) by stapling A2 T
11.13 11.13 Global Days 090
AMA: 2009, Jan, 11-31; 2008, Jan, 10-25; 2007, January, 13-27

46900-46999 Destruction Procedures: Anus

46900 Destruction of lesion(s), anus (eg, condyloma, papilloma, molluscum contagiosum, herpetic vesicle), simple; chemical P2 T
4.05 6.99 Global Days 010

46910 electrodesiccation P3 T
3.95 7.39 Global Days 010

46916 cryosurgery P2 T
4.27 6.84 Global Days 010

46917 laser surgery A2 T
3.92 13.65 Global Days 010

46922 surgical excision A2 T
3.95 7.73 Global Days 010

46924 Destruction of lesion(s), anus (eg, condyloma, papilloma, molluscum contagiosum, herpetic vesicle), extensive (eg, laser surgery, electrosurgery, cryosurgery, chemosurgery) A2 T
5.41 15.75 Global Days 010

46930 Destruction of internal hemorrhoid(s) by thermal energy (eg, infrared coagulation, cautery, radiofrequency) P3 T 80
EXCLUDES *Other hemorrhoid procedures:*
Cryosurgery destruction (46999)
Destruction with heat (46930)
Excision ([46320], 46250-46262)
Hemorrhoidopexy ([46947])
Incision (46083)
Injection sclerosing solution (46500)
Ligation (46221, [46945, 46946])
4.40 6.10 Global Days 090

46940 Curettage or cautery of anal fissure, including dilation of anal sphincter (separate procedure); initial P3 T
4.29 6.63 Global Days 010

46942 subsequent P3 T 80
3.84 6.20 Global Days 010

46945 *Resequenced code, See code following 46221.*

46946 *Resequenced code, See code following 46221.*

46947 *Resequenced code, See code following 46762.*

46999 Unlisted procedure, anus T 80
0.00 0.00 Global Days YYY

47000-47001 Needle Biopsy of Liver

EXCLUDES *Fine needle aspiration (10021, 10022)*

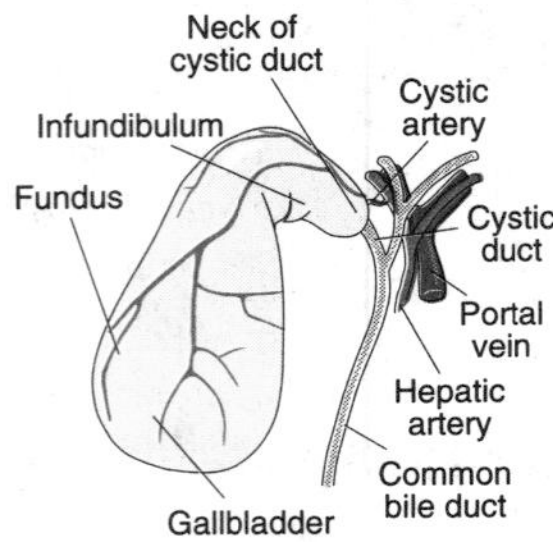

The liver is divided into four lobes for descriptive purposes, although the left and right halves are functionally separate, each receiving its own arterial supply and venous drainage. The liver is the largest gland in the body and serves many metabolic purposes including secretion of bile. The gallbladder is located on the visceral side of the quadrate lobe and stores bile between active phases of digestion; positions of the sac and its structures vary

⊙ 47000 Biopsy of liver, needle; percutaneous A2 T
88172-88173
76942, 77002, 77012, 77021
3.01 7.85 Global Days 000
AMA: 2009, Jan, 11-31; 2008, Jan, 10-25; 2007, June, 10-11

\+ 47001 when done for indicated purpose at time of other major procedure (List separately in addition to code for primary procedure) N1 N
Code first primary procedure
88172-88173
76942, 77002
3.02 3.02 Global Days ZZZ
AMA: 2009, Jan, 11-31; 2008, Jan, 10-25; 2007, June, 10-11

47010-47130 Open Incisional and Resection Procedures of Liver

47010 Hepatotomy; for open drainage of abscess or cyst, 1 or 2 stages C5 C 80 PQ
34.94 34.94 Global Days 090

⊙ 47011 for percutaneous drainage of abscess or cyst, 1 or 2 stages T
75989
5.41 5.41 Global Days 000

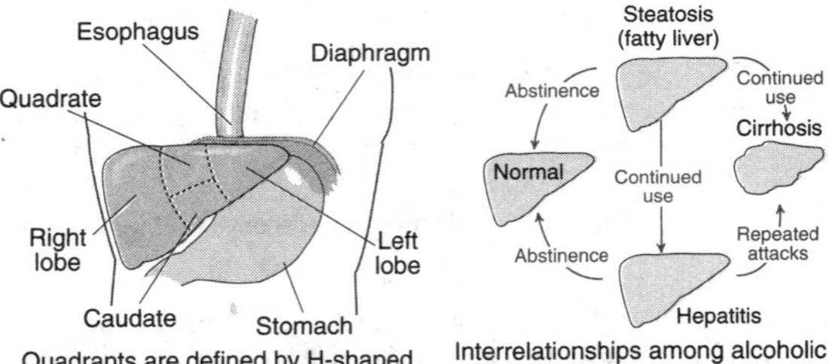

Quadrants are defined by H-shaped grooves on the visceral side

Interrelationships among alcoholic steatosis, hepatitis, and cirrhosis

The liver is the largest gland in the body and serves many metabolic purposes including secretion of bile. Chronic alcohol use leads to three similar forms of alcoholic liver disease: steatosis (fatty liver), hepatitis, and cirrhosis. The conditions have many overlapping features and each may occur without involvement of alcohol. Alcoholic cirrhosis accounts for about 60 percent of all cirrhosis cases and the risk appears to rise with the amount of alcohol consumed daily. The liver tends to shrink and become fibrotic

47015 Laparotomy, with aspiration and/or injection of hepatic parasitic (eg, amoebic or echinococcal) cyst(s) or abscess(es) C5 C 80
33.83 33.83 Global Days 090

47100 **Biopsy of liver, wedge** C5 C 80 PQ
24.57 24.57 Global Days 090

47120 **Hepatectomy, resection of liver; partial lobectomy** C5 C 80 PQ
67.67 67.67 Global Days 090
AMA: 2009, Jan, 11-31; 2008, Jan, 10-25; 2007, January, 13-27

47122 **trisegmentectomy** C5 C 80 PQ
99.73 99.73 Global Days 090

47125 **total left lobectomy** C5 C 80 PQ
89.28 89.28 Global Days 090

47130 **total right lobectomy** C5 C 80 PQ
95.97 95.97 Global Days 090

47133-47147 Liver Transplant Procedures

CMS 100-3,260.1 Adult Liver Transplantation
CMS 100-3,260.2 Pediatric Liver Transplantation
CMS 100-4,3,90.4 Liver Transplants
CMS 100-4,3,90.4.1 Standard Liver Acquisition Charge
CMS 100-4,3,90.4.2 Billing for Liver Transplant and Acquisition Services
CMS 100-4,3,90.6 Intestinal and Multi-Visceral Transplants

47133 **Donor hepatectomy (including cold preservation), from cadaver donor** C5 C
INCLUDES Graft:
Cold preservation
Harvest
0.00 0.00 Global Days XXX

47135 **Liver allotransplantation; orthotopic, partial or whole, from cadaver or living donor, any age** C5 C 80 PQ
INCLUDES Partial/whole recipient hepatectomy
Partial/whole transplant of allograft
Recipient care
142.83 142.83 Global Days 090

47136 **heterotopic, partial or whole, from cadaver or living donor, any age** C5 C 80 PQ
INCLUDES Partial/whole recipient hepatectomy
Partial/whole transplant of allograft
Recipient care
120.64 120.64 Global Days 090

47140 **Donor hepatectomy (including cold preservation), from living donor; left lateral segment only (segments II and III)** C5 C 80 PQ
INCLUDES Donor care
Graft:
Cold preservation
Harvest
102.25 102.25 Global Days 090

47141 **total left lobectomy (segments II, III and IV)** C5 C 80 PQ
INCLUDES Donor care
Graft:
Cold preservation
Harvest
114.16 114.16 Global Days 090

47142 **total right lobectomy (segments V, VI, VII and VIII)** C5 C 80 PQ
INCLUDES Donor care
Graft:
Cold preservation
Harvest
137.06 137.06 Global Days 090

47143 **Backbench standard preparation of cadaver donor whole liver graft prior to allotransplantation, including cholecystectomy, if necessary, and dissection and removal of surrounding soft tissues to prepare the vena cava, portal vein, hepatic artery, and common bile duct for implantation; without trisegment or lobe split** C5 C 80
Do not report with (47120-47125, 47600, 47610)
0.00 0.00 Global Days XXX

47144 **with trisegment split of whole liver graft into 2 partial liver grafts (ie, left lateral segment [segments II and III] and right trisegment [segments I and IV through VIII])** C5 C 80
Do not report with (47120-47125, 47600, 47610)
0.00 0.00 Global Days 090

47145 **with lobe split of whole liver graft into 2 partial liver grafts (ie, left lobe [segments II, III, and IV] and right lobe [segments I and V through VIII])** C5 C 80
Do not report with (47120-47125, 47600, 47610)
0.00 0.00 Global Days XXX

47146 **Backbench reconstruction of cadaver or living donor liver graft prior to allotransplantation; venous anastomosis, each** C5 C 80
Do not report with (47120-47125, 47600, 47610)
9.64 9.64 Global Days XXX

47147 **arterial anastomosis, each** C5 C 80
Do not report with (47120-47125, 47600, 47610)
11.24 11.24 Global Days XXX

47300-47362 Open Repair of Liver

47300 **Marsupialization of cyst or abscess of liver** C5 C 80 PQ
33.01 33.01 Global Days 090

47350 **Management of liver hemorrhage; simple suture of liver wound or injury** C5 C 80 PQ
40.02 40.02 Global Days 090

47360 **complex suture of liver wound or injury, with or without hepatic artery ligation** C5 C 80 PQ
54.28 54.28 Global Days 090

47361 **exploration of hepatic wound, extensive debridement, coagulation and/or suture, with or without packing of liver** C5 C 80 PQ
87.87 87.87 Global Days 090

47362 **re-exploration of hepatic wound for removal of packing** C5 C 80 PQ
42.10 42.10 Global Days 090

47370-47379 Laparoscopic Ablation Liver Tumors

47370 **Laparoscopy, surgical, ablation of 1 or more liver tumor(s); radiofrequency** T 80 PQ
INCLUDES Diagnostic laparoscopy
76940
35.96 35.96 Global Days 090

47371 **cryosurgical** T 80 PQ
INCLUDES Diagnostic laparoscopy
76940
36.77 36.77 Global Days 090

47379 **Unlisted laparoscopic procedure, liver** T 80
0.00 0.00 Global Days YYY
AMA: 2009, Jan, 11-31; 2008, Jan, 10-25; 2007, January, 13-27; 2007, Dec, 10-179

● New Code ▲ Revised Code Maternity Age Unlisted Not Covered # Resequenced
○ Reinstated CCI + Add-on Mod 51 Exempt Mod 63 Exempt Mod Sedation PQ PQRS

47380-47399 Open and Percutaneous Ablation of Liver Tumors

47380 **Ablation, open, of 1 or more liver tumor(s); radiofrequency**
76940
41.72 41.72 Global Days 090

47381 **cryosurgical**
76940
43.28 43.28 Global Days 090

⊙ 47382 **Ablation, 1 or more liver tumor(s), percutaneous, radiofrequency**
76940, 77013, 77022
23.10 144.30 Global Days 010

47399 **Unlisted procedure, liver**
0.00 0.00 Global Days YYY

47400-47490 Surgical Incision Biliary Tract

47400 **Hepaticotomy or hepaticostomy with exploration, drainage, or removal of calculus**
62.82 62.82 Global Days 090

47420 **Choledochotomy or choledochostomy with exploration, drainage, or removal of calculus, with or without cholecystotomy; without transduodenal sphincterotomy or sphincteroplasty**
39.12 39.12 Global Days 090

47425 **with transduodenal sphincterotomy or sphincteroplasty**
39.81 39.81 Global Days 090

47460 **Transduodenal sphincterotomy or sphincteroplasty, with or without transduodenal extraction of calculus (separate procedure)**
37.15 37.15 Global Days 090

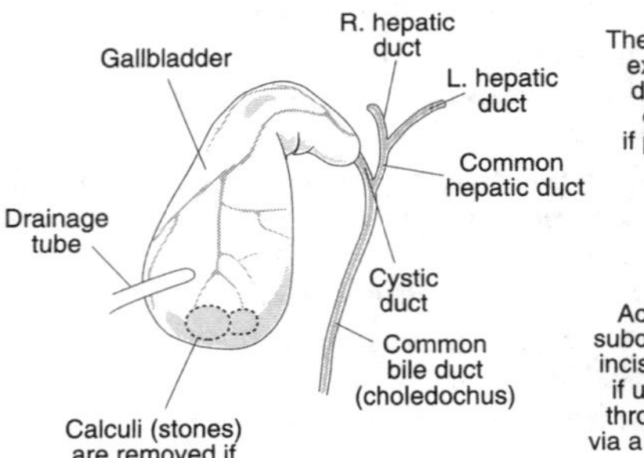

47480 **Cholecystotomy or cholecystostomy, open, with exploration, drainage, or removal of calculus (separate procedure)**
EXCLUDES *Percutaneous cholecystostomy (47490)*
25.42 25.42 Global Days 090

47490 **Cholecystostomy, percutaneous, complete procedure, including imaging guidance, catheter placement, cholecystogram when performed, and radiological supervision and interpretation**
Do not report with (47505, 74305, 75989, 76942, 77002, 77012, 77021)
10.17 10.17 Global Days 010

47500-47530 Injection/Insertion Procedures of Biliary Tract

47500 **Injection procedure for percutaneous transhepatic cholangiography**
74320
2.88 2.88 Global Days 000

47505 **Injection procedure for cholangiography through an existing catheter (eg, percutaneous transhepatic or T-tube)**
Do not report with (47490)
74305
1.11 1.11 Global Days 000

47510 **Introduction of percutaneous transhepatic catheter for biliary drainage**
75980
13.93 13.93 Global Days 090

47511 **Introduction of percutaneous transhepatic stent for internal and external biliary drainage**
75982
17.15 17.15 Global Days 090

⊙ 47525 **Change of percutaneous biliary drainage catheter**
Code also (C1729)
75984
2.67 15.09 Global Days 000

47530 **Revision and/or reinsertion of transhepatic tube**
75984
10.45 42.41 Global Days 090

47550-47556 Endoscopic Procedures of the Biliary Tract

CMS 100-3,100.2 Endoscopy

+ 47550 **Biliary endoscopy, intraoperative (choledochoscopy) (List separately in addition to code for primary procedure)**
Code first primary procedure
4.84 4.84 Global Days ZZZ

47552 **Biliary endoscopy, percutaneous via T-tube or other tract; diagnostic, with or without collection of specimen(s) by brushing and/or washing (separate procedure)**
9.33 9.33 Global Days 000
AMA: 2009, Jan, 11-31

47553 **with biopsy, single or multiple**
INCLUDES Diagnostic endoscopy
9.33 9.33 Global Days 000
AMA: 2009, Jan, 11-31

47554 **with removal of calculus/calculi**
INCLUDES Diagnostic endoscopy
14.46 14.46 Global Days 000
AMA: 2009, Jan, 11-31

47555 **with dilation of biliary duct stricture(s) without stent**
INCLUDES Diagnostic endoscopy
11.05 11.05 Global Days 000
AMA: 2009, Jan, 11-31

47556 **with dilation of biliary duct stricture(s) with stent** A2 T CCI

INCLUDES Diagnostic endoscopy

EXCLUDES *Endoscopic retrograde cholangiopancreatography (ERCP) (43260-43272, 74363)*

74363, 75982

12.52 12.52 Global Days 000

AMA: 2009, Jan, 11-31

47560-47579 Laparoscopic Gallbladder Procedures

CMS 100-3,100.13 Laparoscopic Cholecystectomy

INCLUDES Diagnostic laparoscopy

47560 **Laparoscopy, surgical; with guided transhepatic cholangiography, without biopsy** A2 T 80 CCI PQ

7.86 7.86 Global Days 000

47561 **with guided transhepatic cholangiography with biopsy** A2 T 80 CCI PQ

8.61 8.61 Global Days 000

47562 **cholecystectomy** G2 T 80 CCI PQ

21.85 21.85 Global Days 090

AMA: 2009, Jan, 11-31; 2007, Dec, 10-179

47563 **cholecystectomy with cholangiography** G2 T 80 CCI PQ

20.93 20.93 Global Days 090

AMA: 2009, Jan, 11-31; 2008, Jan, 10-25; 2007, Dec, 10-179; 2007, January, 13-27

47564 **cholecystectomy with exploration of common duct** G2 T 80 CCI PQ

31.90 31.90 Global Days 090

AMA: 2009, Jan, 11-31; 2007, Dec, 10-179

47570 **cholecystoenterostomy** C5 C 80 CCI PQ

22.60 22.60 Global Days 090

47579 **Unlisted laparoscopy procedure, biliary tract** T 80 50

0.00 0.00 Global Days YYY

47600-47620 Open Gallbladder Procedures

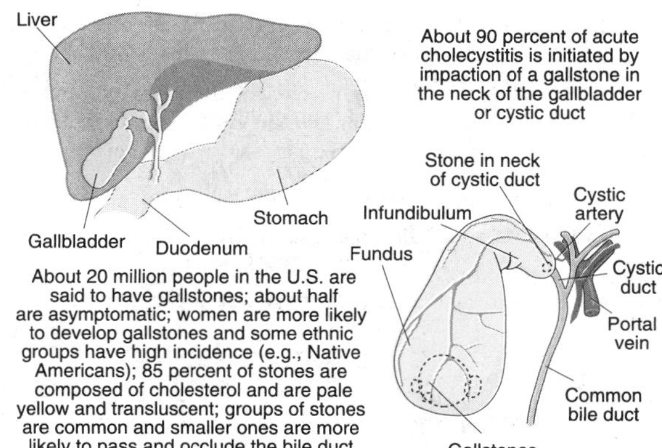

47600 **Cholecystectomy;** C5 C 80 CCI PQ

EXCLUDES *Laparoscopic method (47562-47564)*

31.54 31.54 Global Days 090

47605 **with cholangiography** C5 C 80 CCI PQ

EXCLUDES *Laparoscopic method (47563-47564)*

28.64 28.64 Global Days 090

AMA: 2009, Jan, 11-31; 2008, Jan, 10-25; 2007, January, 13-27

47610 **Cholecystectomy with exploration of common duct;** C5 C 80 CCI PQ

EXCLUDES *Laparoscopic method (47564)*

Code also biliary endoscopy when performed in conjunction with cholecystectomy with exploration of common duct (47550)

36.58 36.58 Global Days 090

AMA: 2009, Jan, 11-31; 2008, Jan, 10-25; 2007, January, 13-27

47612 **with choledochoenterostomy** C5 C 80 CCI PQ

36.96 36.96 Global Days 090

47620 **with transduodenal sphincterotomy or sphincteroplasty, with or without cholangiography** C5 C 80 CCI PQ

39.97 39.97 Global Days 090

47630-47999 Open Resection and Repair of Biliary Tract

47630 **Biliary duct stone extraction, percutaneous via T-tube tract, basket, or snare (eg, Burhenne technique)** A2 T CCI PQ

74327

16.16 16.16 Global Days 090

AMA: 2009, Jan, 11-31; 2008, Jan, 10-25; 2007, January, 13-27

47700 **Exploration for congenital atresia of bile ducts, without repair, with or without liver biopsy, with or without cholangiography** C5 C 80 63 CCI PQ

30.70 30.70 Global Days 090

47701 **Portoenterostomy (eg, Kasai procedure)** C5 C 80 63 CCI PQ

51.00 51.00 Global Days 090

47711 **Excision of bile duct tumor, with or without primary repair of bile duct; extrahepatic** C5 C 80 CCI PQ

EXCLUDES *Anastamosis (47760-47800)*

45.37 45.37 Global Days 090

47712 **intrahepatic** C5 C 80 CCI PQ

EXCLUDES *Anastomosis (47760-47800)*

58.28 58.28 Global Days 090

47715 **Excision of choledochal cyst** C5 C 80 CCI PQ

38.72 38.72 Global Days 090

47720 **Cholecystoenterostomy; direct** C5 C 80 CCI PQ

EXCLUDES *Laparoscopic method (47570)*

33.55 33.55 Global Days 090

47721 **with gastroenterostomy** C5 C 80 CCI PQ

39.44 39.44 Global Days 090

47740 **Roux-en-Y** C5 C 80 CCI PQ

38.19 38.19 Global Days 090

47741 **Roux-en-Y with gastroenterostomy** C5 C 80 CCI PQ

43.00 43.00 Global Days 090

47760 **Anastomosis, of extrahepatic biliary ducts and gastrointestinal tract** C5 C 80 CCI PQ

65.37 65.37 Global Days 090

47765 **Anastomosis, of intrahepatic ducts and gastrointestinal tract** C5 C 80 CCI PQ

INCLUDES Longmire anastomosis

88.13 88.13 Global Days 090

47780 **Anastomosis, Roux-en-Y, of extrahepatic biliary ducts and gastrointestinal tract** C5 C 80 CCI PQ

71.68 71.68 Global Days 090

47785 **Anastomosis, Roux-en-Y, of intrahepatic biliary ducts and gastrointestinal tract** C5 C 80 CCI PQ

94.10 94.10 Global Days 090

47800 **Reconstruction, plastic, of extrahepatic biliary ducts with end-to-end anastomosis** C5 C 80
46.06 46.06 Global Days 090

47801 **Placement of choledochal stent** C5 C 80
30.03 30.03 Global Days 090

47802 **U-tube hepaticoenterostomy** C5 C 80
44.47 44.47 Global Days 090

47900 **Suture of extrahepatic biliary duct for pre-existing injury (separate procedure)** C5 C 80
39.70 39.70 Global Days 090

47999 **Unlisted procedure, biliary tract** T
0.00 0.00 Global Days YYY

48000-48548 Open Procedures of the Pancreas

EXCLUDES *Peroral pancreatic procedures performed endoscopically (43260-43272)*

48000 **Placement of drains, peripancreatic, for acute pancreatitis;** C5 C 80
53.92 53.92 Global Days 090

48001 **with cholecystostomy, gastrostomy, and jejunostomy** C5 C 80
67.37 67.37 Global Days 090

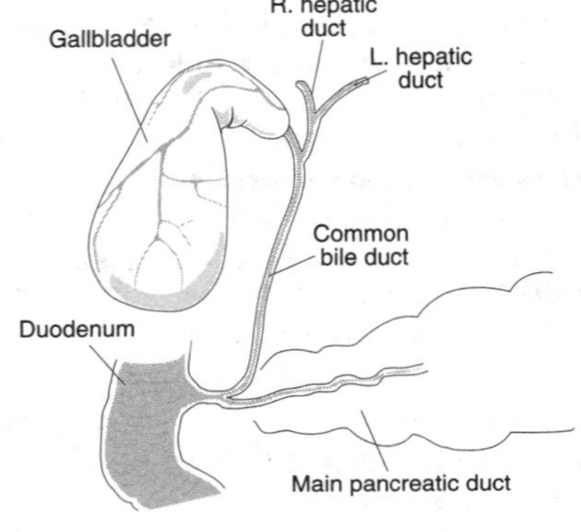

In 48020, a calculus (stone) is surgically removed from the pancreas. This is ordinarily from the main pancreatic duct with access from the duodenum

48020 **Removal of pancreatic calculus** C5 C 80
34.33 34.33 Global Days 090

48100 **Biopsy of pancreas, open (eg, fine needle aspiration, needle core biopsy, wedge biopsy)** C5 C 80
25.84 25.84 Global Days 090

48102 **Biopsy of pancreas, percutaneous needle** A2 T
EXCLUDES *Aspiration, fine needle (10022)*
88172, 88173
76942, 77002, 77012, 77021
7.17 15.97 Global Days 010

48105 **Resection or debridement of pancreas and peripancreatic tissue for acute necrotizing pancreatitis** C5 C 80
83.20 83.20 Global Days 090

48120 **Excision of lesion of pancreas (eg, cyst, adenoma)** C5 C 80
32.13 32.13 Global Days 090

48140 **Pancreatectomy, distal subtotal, with or without splenectomy; without pancreaticojejunostomy** C5 C 80
45.41 45.41 Global Days 090

48145 **with pancreaticojejunostomy** C5 C 80
47.56 47.56 Global Days 090

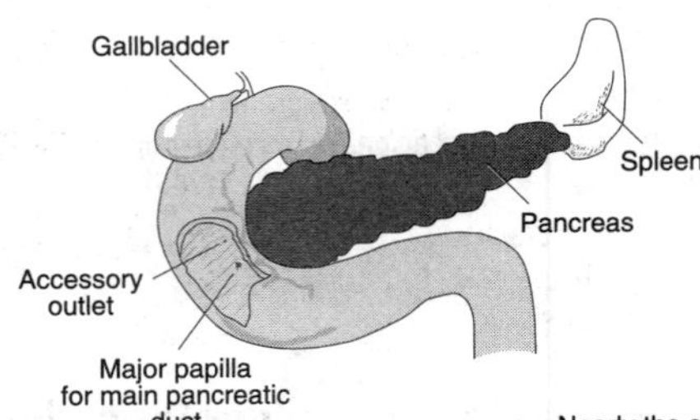

Nearly the entire pancreas is resected. The complex where the pancreatic ducts enter the duodenum is preserved (48146)

48146 **Pancreatectomy, distal, near-total with preservation of duodenum (Child-type procedure)** C5 C 80
54.71 54.71 Global Days 090

48148 **Excision of ampulla of Vater** C5 C 80
36.34 36.34 Global Days 090

48150 **Pancreatectomy, proximal subtotal with total duodenectomy, partial gastrectomy, choledochoenterostomy and gastrojejunostomy (Whipple-type procedure); with pancreatojejunostomy** C5 C 80
90.23 90.23 Global Days 090

48152 **without pancreatojejunostomy** C5 C 80
84.19 84.19 Global Days 090

48153 **Pancreatectomy, proximal subtotal with near-total duodenectomy, choledochoenterostomy and duodenojejunostomy (pylorus-sparing, Whipple-type procedure); with pancreatojejunostomy** C5 C 80
90.10 90.10 Global Days 090

48154 **without pancreatojejunostomy** C5 C 80
84.52 84.52 Global Days 090

48155 **Pancreatectomy, total** C5 C 80
52.85 52.85 Global Days 090

48160 **Pancreatectomy, total or subtotal, with autologous transplantation of pancreas or pancreatic islet cells** E
0.00 0.00 Global Days XXX

+ 48400 **Injection procedure for intraoperative pancreatography (List separately in addition to code for primary procedure)** C5 C 80
Code first primary procedure
74300-74305
3.24 3.24 Global Days ZZZ
AMA: 2009, Jan, 11-31; 2007, Dec, 10-179

48500 **Marsupialization of pancreatic cyst** C5 C 80
33.50 33.50 Global Days 090

48510 **External drainage, pseudocyst of pancreas; open** C5 C 80
31.52 31.52 Global Days 090

⊙ 48511 **percutaneous** T
75989
5.86 27.75 Global Days 000

48520 **Internal anastomosis of pancreatic cyst to gastrointestinal tract; direct** C5 C 80
31.94 31.94 Global Days 090

48540 **Roux-en-Y** C5 C 80
38.16 38.16 Global Days 090

48545 **Pancreatorrhaphy for injury** C5 C 80
39.15 39.15 Global Days 090

48547 **Duodenal exclusion with gastrojejunostomy for pancreatic injury** C5 C 80
52.20 52.20 Global Days 090

48548 **Pancreaticojejunostomy, side-to-side anastomosis (Puestow-type operation)** C5 C 80 PQ
48.52 48.52 Global Days 090

48550-48999 Pancreas Transplant Procedures

CMS 100-3,260.3 Pancreas Transplants
CMS 100-4,3,90.5 Pancreas Transplants with Kidney Transplants

48550 **Donor pancreatectomy (including cold preservation), with or without duodenal segment for transplantation** E
INCLUDES Graft:
Cold preservation
Harvest (with or without duodenal segment)
0.00 0.00 Global Days XXX

48551 **Backbench standard preparation of cadaver donor pancreas allograft prior to transplantation, including dissection of allograft from surrounding soft tissues, splenectomy, duodenotomy, ligation of bile duct, ligation of mesenteric vessels, and Y-graft arterial anastomoses from iliac artery to superior mesenteric artery and to splenic artery** C5 C 80
Do not report with (35531, 35563, 35685, 38100-38102, 44010, 44820, 44850, 47460, 47505-47525, 47550-47556, 48100-48120, 48545)
0.00 0.00 Global Days XXX

48552 **Backbench reconstruction of cadaver donor pancreas allograft prior to transplantation, venous anastomosis, each** C5 C 80
Do not report with (35531, 35563, 35685, 38100-38102, 44010, 44820, 44850, 47460, 47505-47525, 47550-47556, 48100-48120, 48545)
6.90 6.90 Global Days XXX

48554 **Transplantation of pancreatic allograft** C5 C 80 PQ
INCLUDES Allograft transplant
Recipient care
74.59 74.59 Global Days 090

48556 **Removal of transplanted pancreatic allograft** C5 C 80 PQ
37.10 37.10 Global Days 090

48999 **Unlisted procedure, pancreas** T 80
0.00 0.00 Global Days YYY
AMA: 2009, Jan, 11-31; 2007, Dec, 10-179

49000-49084 Exploratory and Drainage Procedures: Abdomen/Peritoneum

49000 **Exploratory laparotomy, exploratory celiotomy with or without biopsy(s) (separate procedure)** C5 C 80 PQ
EXCLUDES *Exploration of penetrating wound without laparotomy (20102)*
22.51 22.51 Global Days 090
AMA: 2009, Jan, 11-31; 2008, Jan, 10-25; 2008, Nov, 7-9; 2007, January, 13-27

49002 **Reopening of recent laparotomy** C5 C 80 PQ
EXCLUDES *Hepatic wound re-exploration for packing removal (47362)*
30.43 30.43 Global Days 090
AMA: 2008, Nov, 7-9

49010 **Exploration, retroperitoneal area with or without biopsy(s) (separate procedure)** C5 C 80 PQ
EXCLUDES *Exploration of penetrating wound without laparotomy (20102)*
27.59 27.59 Global Days 090
AMA: 2007, June, 1-3

49020 **Drainage of peritoneal abscess or localized peritonitis, exclusive of appendiceal abscess; open** C5 C 80 PQ
EXCLUDES *Appendiceal abscess (44900)*
46.39 46.39 Global Days 090

⊙ 49021 **percutaneous** T
75989
4.94 26.47 Global Days 000

49040 **Drainage of subdiaphragmatic or subphrenic abscess; open** C5 C 80 PQ
29.27 29.27 Global Days 090

⊙ 49041 **percutaneous** T
75989
5.85 27.41 Global Days 000

49060 **Drainage of retroperitoneal abscess; open** C5 C PQ
EXCLUDES *Drainage performed laparoscopically (49323)*
32.23 32.23 Global Days 090
AMA: 2009, Jan, 11-31; 2008, Jan, 10-25; 2007, January, 13-27

⊙ 49061 **percutaneous** T
EXCLUDES *Drainage performed laparoscopically (49323)*
75989
5.40 26.81 Global Days 000
AMA: 2009, Jan, 11-31; 2008, Jan, 10-25; 2007, January, 13-27

49062 **Drainage of extraperitoneal lymphocele to peritoneal cavity, open** C5 C 80
21.77 21.77 Global Days 090
AMA: 2009, Jan, 11-31; 2008, Jan, 10-25; 2007, January, 13-27

~~49080~~ ~~**Peritoneocentesis, abdominal paracentesis, or peritoneal lavage (diagnostic or therapeutic); initial**~~
To report, see 49082-49084

~~49081~~ ~~**subsequent**~~
To report, see 49082-49084

● 49082 **Abdominal paracentesis (diagnostic or therapeutic); without imaging guidance** G2 T
2.05 4.81 Global Days 000

● 49083 **with imaging guidance** G2 T
Do not report with (76942, 77002, 77012, 77021)
3.16 9.09 Global Days 000

● 49084 **Peritoneal lavage, including imaging guidance, when performed** G2 T
Do not report with (76942, 77002, 77012, 77021)
2.89 2.89 Global Days 000

49180 Biopsy of Mass: Abdomen/Retroperitoneum

49180 **Biopsy, abdominal or retroperitoneal mass, percutaneous needle** A2 T
EXCLUDES *Aspiration, fine needle (10021, 10022)*
Lysis of intestinal adhesions (44005)
76942, 77002, 77012, 77021
88172, 88173
2.54 4.74 Global Days 000

49203-49205 Open Destruction or Excision: Abdominal Tumors

EXCLUDES *Cryoablation of renal tumor (50250, 50593)*
Lysis of intestinal adhesions (44005)
Primary, recurrent ovarian, uterine, or tubal resection (58957-58958)

Code also colectomy (44140)
Code also small bowel resection (44120)
Code also total nephrectomy (50220 or 50240)
Code also vena caval resection with reconstruction (37799)
Do not report with (38770, 38780, 49000, 49010, 49215, 50010, 50205, 50225, 50236, 50250, 50290, 58900-58960)

49203 **Excision or destruction, open, intra-abdominal tumors, cysts or endometriomas, 1 or more peritoneal, mesenteric, or retroperitoneal primary or secondary tumors; largest tumor 5 cm diameter or less** C5 C 80 PQ
34.91 34.91 Global Days 090

49204 **largest tumor 5.1-10.0 cm diameter** C5 C 80 PQ
44.46 44.46 Global Days 090

49205 **largest tumor greater than 10.0 cm diameter** C5 C 80 PQ
51.01 51.01 Global Days 090

49215 Resection Presacral/Sacrococcygeal Tumor

49215 **Excision of presacral or sacrococcygeal tumor** C5 C 80 63 PQ
64.30 64.30 Global Days 090

49220-49255 Other Open Abdominal Procedures

EXCLUDES *Lysis of intestinal adhesions (44005)*

49220 **Staging laparotomy for Hodgkins disease or lymphoma (includes splenectomy, needle or open biopsies of both liver lobes, possibly also removal of abdominal nodes, abdominal node and/or bone marrow biopsies, ovarian repositioning)** C5 C 80 PQ
28.36 28.36 Global Days 090

49250 **Umbilectomy, omphalectomy, excision of umbilicus (separate procedure)** A2 T PQ
17.04 17.04 Global Days 090

49255 **Omentectomy, epiploectomy, resection of omentum (separate procedure)** C5 C 80 PQ
23.11 23.11 Global Days 090

49320-49329 Laparoscopic Procedures of the Abdomen/Peritoneum/Omentum

INCLUDES Diagnostic laparoscopy

EXCLUDES *Fulguration/excision of lesions of ovary/pelvic viscera/peritoneal surface, performed laparoscopically (58662)*

49320 **Laparoscopy, abdomen, peritoneum, and omentum, diagnostic, with or without collection of specimen(s) by brushing or washing (separate procedure)** A2 T 80 PQ
9.59 9.59 Global Days 010
AMA: 2009, Jan, 11-31; 2008, Jan, 10-25; 2007, March, 4-5; 2007, January, 13-27

49321 **Laparoscopy, surgical; with biopsy (single or multiple)** A2 T 80 PQ
10.15 10.15 Global Days 010

49322 **with aspiration of cavity or cyst (eg, ovarian cyst) (single or multiple)** A2 T 80 PQ
10.89 10.89 Global Days 010

49323 **with drainage of lymphocele to peritoneal cavity** T 80 PQ
EXCLUDES *Retroperitoneal abscess drainage:*
Open (49060)
Percutaneous (49061)
18.91 18.91 Global Days 090
AMA: 2009, Jan, 11-31; 2008, Jan, 10-25; 2007, January, 13-27

49324 **with insertion of tunneled intraperitoneal catheter** G2 T 80
EXCLUDES *Open approach (49421)*
Code also insertion of subcutaneous extension to intraperitoneal cannula with remote chest exit site, when appropriate (49435)
11.55 11.55 Global Days 010

49325 **with revision of previously placed intraperitoneal cannula or catheter, with removal of intraluminal obstructive material if performed** G2 T 80
12.33 12.33 Global Days 010

\+ **49326** **with omentopexy (omental tacking procedure) (List separately in addition to code for primary procedure)** G2 T 80
Code first laparoscopy with permanent intraperitoneal cannula or catheter insertion or revision of previously placed catheter/cannula (49324, 49325)
5.53 5.53 Global Days ZZZ

\+ **49327** **with placement of interstitial device(s) for radiation therapy guidance (eg, fiducial markers, dosimeter), intra-abdominal, intrapelvic, and/or retroperitoneum, including imaging guidance, if performed, single or multiple (List separately in addition to code for primary procedure)** G2 T 80
EXCLUDES *Open approach (49412)*
Percutaneous approach (49411)
Code first laparoscopic abdominal, pelvic or retroperitoneal procedures
3.83 3.83 Global Days ZZZ

49329 **Unlisted laparoscopy procedure, abdomen, peritoneum and omentum** T 80 50
0.00 0.00 Global Days YYY
AMA: 2009, Jan, 11-31; 2008, Jan, 10-25; 2007, January, 13-27

49400-49436 Peritoneal Procedures: Insertion/Modifications/Removal

49400 **Injection of air or contrast into peritoneal cavity (separate procedure)** N1 N
Code also (49446)
2.82 4.30 Global Days 000

49402 **Removal of peritoneal foreign body from peritoneal cavity** A2 T
EXCLUDES *Enterolysis (44005)*
24.93 24.93 Global Days 090

⊙ **49411** **Placement of interstitial device(s) for radiation therapy guidance (eg, fiducial markers, dosimeter), percutaneous, intra-abdominal, intra-pelvic (except prostate), and/or retroperitoneum, single or multiple** P3 X 80
EXCLUDES *Placement (percutaneous) of interstitial device(s) for intrathoracic radiation therapy guidance (32553)*
Code also supply of device
76942, 77002, 77012, 77021
5.70 16.30 Global Days 000

+ **49412** **Placement of interstitial device(s) for radiation therapy guidance (eg, fiducial markers, dosimeter), open, intra-abdominal, intrapelvic, and/or retroperitoneum, including image guidance, if performed, single or multiple (List separately in addition to code for primary procedure)** C5 C 80

EXCLUDES *Laparoscopic approach (49327)*
Percutaneous approach (49411)

Code first open abdominal, pelvic or retroperitoneal procedure(s)

2.38 2.38 Global Days ZZZ

⊙ **49418** **Insertion of tunneled intraperitoneal catheter (eg, dialysis, intraperitoneal chemotherapy instillation, management of ascites), complete procedure, including imaging guidance, catheter placement, contrast injection when performed, and radiological supervision and interpretation, percutaneous** G2 T 80

6.77 46.82 Global Days 000

49419 **Insertion of tunneled intraperitoneal catheter, with subcutaneous port (ie, totally implantable)** A2 T

EXCLUDES *Removal of catheter/cannula (49422)*

Code also (C1788)

12.96 12.96 Global Days 090

49421 **Insertion of tunneled intraperitoneal catheter for dialysis, open** A2 T

EXCLUDES *Laparoscopic approach (49324)*

Code also insertion of subcutaneous extension to intraperitoneal cannula with remote chest exit site, when appropriate (49435)

7.34 7.34 Global Days 000

AMA: 2009, Jan, 11-31; 2008, Jan, 10-25; 2007, January, 13-27

49422 **Removal of tunneled intraperitoneal catheter** A2 T

EXCLUDES *Removal temporary catheter or cannula (Use appropriate E/M code)*

11.23 11.23 Global Days 010

49423 **Exchange of previously placed abscess or cyst drainage catheter under radiological guidance (separate procedure)** G2 T 80

Code also drainage catheter (C1729)

75984

2.16 16.86 Global Days 000

49424 **Contrast injection for assessment of abscess or cyst via previously placed drainage catheter or tube (separate procedure)** N1 N 80

76080

1.15 4.44 Global Days 000

AMA: 2009, Jan, 11-31; 2008, Jan, 10-25; 2007, January, 13-27

49425 **Insertion of peritoneal-venous shunt** C5 C 80

22.12 22.12 Global Days 090

49426 **Revision of peritoneal-venous shunt** A2 T

EXCLUDES *Shunt patency test (78291)*

18.59 18.59 Global Days 090

49427 **Injection procedure (eg, contrast media) for evaluation of previously placed peritoneal-venous shunt** N1 N 80

75809, 78291

1.33 1.33 Global Days 000

49428 **Ligation of peritoneal-venous shunt** C5 C

14.09 14.09 Global Days 010

49429 **Removal of peritoneal-venous shunt** G2 T

13.07 13.07 Global Days 010

+ **49435** **Insertion of subcutaneous extension to intraperitoneal cannula or catheter with remote chest exit site (List separately in addition to code for primary procedure)** G2 T 80

Code first permanent insertion of intraperitoneal catheter/cannula (49324, 49421)

3.53 3.53 Global Days ZZZ

49436 **Delayed creation of exit site from embedded subcutaneous segment of intraperitoneal cannula or catheter** G2 T 80

5.45 5.45 Global Days 010

49440-49442 Insertion of Percutaneous Gastrointestinal Tube

Do not report with (43752)

⊙ **49440** **Insertion of gastrostomy tube, percutaneous, under fluoroscopic guidance including contrast injection(s), image documentation and report** G2 T 80 PQ

EXCLUDES *Gastrostomy tube to gastrojejunostomy tube when gastrostomy first placed, report 49440 and (49446)*

6.67 31.99 Global Days 010

AMA: 2009, Jan, 11-31; 2008, Jan, 8-9; 2008, Jun, 8-11; 2007, Dec, 10-179

⊙ **49441** **Insertion of duodenostomy or jejunostomy tube, percutaneous, under fluoroscopic guidance including contrast injection(s), image documentation and report** G2 T 80 PQ

EXCLUDES *Gastrostrostomy tube to gastrojejunostomy tube conversion (49446)*

7.59 35.46 Global Days 010

AMA: 2009, Jan, 11-31; 2008, Jan, 8-9; 2008, Jun, 8-11; 2007, Dec, 10-179

⊙ **49442** **Insertion of cecostomy or other colonic tube, percutaneous, under fluoroscopic guidance including contrast injection(s), image documentation and report** G2 T 80 PQ

6.36 29.01 Global Days 010

AMA: 2009, Jan, 11-31; 2008, Jan, 8-9; 2008, Jun, 8-11; 2007, Dec, 10-179

49446 Percutaneous Conversion: Gastrostomy to Gastro-jejunostomy Tube

⊙ **49446** **Conversion of gastrostomy tube to gastro-jejunostomy tube, percutaneous, under fluoroscopic guidance including contrast injection(s), image documentation and report** G2 T 80 PQ

EXCLUDES *Gastrostomy tube to gastrojejunostomy tube conversion when gastrostomy tube first placed, report 49446 and (49440)*

4.86 29.96 Global Days 000

AMA: 2009, Jan, 11-31; 2008, Jun, 8-11; 2007, Dec, 10-179

49450-49452 Replacement Gastrointestinal Tube

EXCLUDES *Placement of new tube whether gastrostomy, jejunostomy, duodenostomy, gastro-jejunostomy, or cecostomy at different percutaneous site (49440-49442)*

49450 **Replacement of gastrostomy or cecostomy (or other colonic) tube, percutaneous, under fluoroscopic guidance including contrast injection(s), image documentation and report** G2 T 80 PQ

EXCLUDES *Change of gastrostomy tube, percutaneous, without imaging or endoscopic guidance (43760)*

1.98 20.53 Global Days 000

AMA: 2008, Jun, 8-11

49451 **Replacement of duodenostomy or jejunostomy tube, percutaneous, under fluoroscopic guidance including contrast injection(s), image documentation and report** G2 T 80 PQ

2.73 21.61 Global Days 000

AMA: 2009, Jan, 11-31; 2008, Jan, 8-9; 2008, Jun, 8-11; 2007, Dec, 10-179

49452 **Replacement of gastro-jejunostomy tube, percutaneous, under fluoroscopic guidance including contrast injection(s), image documentation and report** G2 T 80 PQ

4.20 26.68 Global Days 000

AMA: 2008, Jun, 8-11

49460-49465 Removal of Obstruction/Injection for Contrast Through Gastrointestinal Tube

49460 **Mechanical removal of obstructive material from gastrostomy, duodenostomy, jejunostomy, gastro-jejunostomy, or cecostomy (or other colonic) tube, any method, under fluoroscopic guidance including contrast injection(s), if performed, image documentation and report** G2 T 80 PQ

Do not report with (49450-49452, 49465)

1.43 22.99 Global Days 000

AMA: 2008, Jun, 8-11

49465 **Contrast injection(s) for radiological evaluation of existing gastrostomy, duodenostomy, jejunostomy, gastro-jejunostomy, or cecostomy (or other colonic) tube, from a percutaneous approach including image documentation and report** N1 Q1 80 PQ

Do not report with (49450-49460)

0.90 5.13 Global Days 000

AMA: 2008, Jun, 8-11

49491-49492 Inguinal Hernia Repair on Premature Infant

INCLUDES Hernia repairs done on preterm infants younger than or equal to 50 weeks postconception age but younger than 6 months of age since birth
Initial repair: no previous repair required
Mesh or other prosthesis

EXCLUDES *Abdominal wall debridement (11042, 11043)*
Intra-abdominal hernia repair/reduction (44050)

Code also repair or excision of testicle(s), intestine, ovaries if performed (44120, 54520, 58940)

49491 **Repair, initial inguinal hernia, preterm infant (younger than 37 weeks gestation at birth), performed from birth up to 50 weeks postconception age, with or without hydrocelectomy; reducible** A T 80 50

22.46 22.46 Global Days 090

AMA: 2009, Jan, 11-31; 2008, Jun, 3-6; 2008, Jan, 10-25

49492 **incarcerated or strangulated** A T 80 50

27.85 27.85 Global Days 090

AMA: 2008, Jun, 3-6

49495-49557 Hernia Repair: Femoral/Inguinal/Lumbar

INCLUDES Initial repair: no previous repair required
Mesh or other prosthesis
Recurrent repair: required previous repair(s)

EXCLUDES *Abdominal wall debridement (11042, 11043)*
Intra-abdominal hernia repair/reduction (44050)

Code also repair or excision of testicle(s), intestine, ovaries if performed (44120, 54520, 58940)

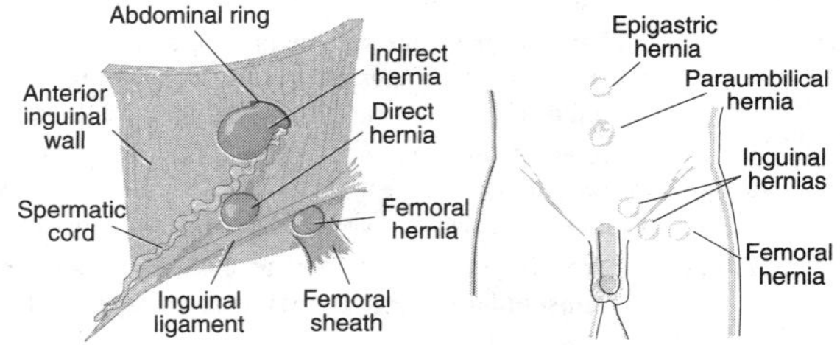

A hernia is a protrusion, usually through an abdominal wall containment. Often, hernias are congenital. Groin hernias are common among both sexes and all age groups. In males, indirect hernias are often associated with incomplete closure of the path the testicle takes as it descends just prior to birth (the processus vaginalis). Direct hernias simply protrude through the wall. Femoral hernias occur below the inguinal ligament. Strangulation and necrosis of the protruding bowel section can occur. Umbilical hernias are often linked to incomplete closure of the umbilicus.

49495 **Repair, initial inguinal hernia, full term infant younger than age 6 months, or preterm infant older than 50 weeks postconception age and younger than age 6 months at the time of surgery, with or without hydrocelectomy; reducible** A A2 T 80 50

INCLUDES Hernia repairs done on preterm infants older than 50 weeks postconception age and younger than 6 months

11.88 11.88 Global Days 090

AMA: 2009, Jan, 11-31; 2008, Jan, 10-25; 2008, Jun, 3-6; 2007, January, 13-27

49496 incarcerated or strangulated

INCLUDES Hernia repairs done on preterm infants older than 50 weeks postconception age and younger than 6 months

17.49 17.49 Global Days 090

AMA: 2009, Jan, 11-31; 2008, Jan, 10-25; 2008, Jun, 3-6; 2007, January, 13-27

49500 **Repair initial inguinal hernia, age 6 months to younger than 5 years, with or without hydrocelectomy; reducible**

INCLUDES Repairs performed on patients 6 months to younger than 5 years old

11.93 11.93 Global Days 090

AMA: 2009, Jan, 11-31; 2008, Jan, 10-25; 2008, Jun, 3-6; 2007, January, 13-27

49501 incarcerated or strangulated

INCLUDES Repairs performed on patients 6 months to younger than 5 years old

17.61 17.61 Global Days 090

AMA: 2009, Jan, 11-31; 2008, Jan, 10-25; 2008, Jun, 3-6; 2007, January, 13-27

49505 **Repair initial inguinal hernia, age 5 years or older; reducible**

INCLUDES MacEwen hernia repair

Code also when performed:
- Excision of hydrocele (55040)
- Excision of spermatocele (54840)
- Simple orchiectomy (54520)

15.15 15.15 Global Days 090

AMA: 2009, Jan, 11-31; 2008, Jan, 10-25; 2008, Jun, 3-6; 2007, January, 13-27

49507 incarcerated or strangulated

Code also when performed:
- Excision of hydrocele (55040)
- Excision of spermatocele (54840)
- Simple orchiectomy (54520)

17.14 17.14 Global Days 090

AMA: 2009, Jan, 11-31; 2008, Jan, 10-25; 2008, Jun, 3-6; 2007, January, 13-27

49520 **Repair recurrent inguinal hernia, any age; reducible**

18.41 18.41 Global Days 090

AMA: 2009, Jan, 11-31; 2008, Jan, 10-25; 2008, Jun, 3-6; 2007, January, 13-27

49521 incarcerated or strangulated

20.92 20.92 Global Days 090

AMA: 2009, Jan, 11-31; 2008, Jan, 10-25; 2008, Jun, 3-6; 2007, January, 13-27

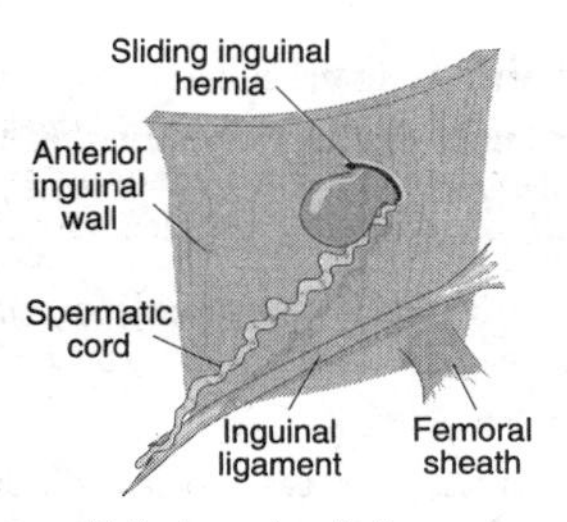

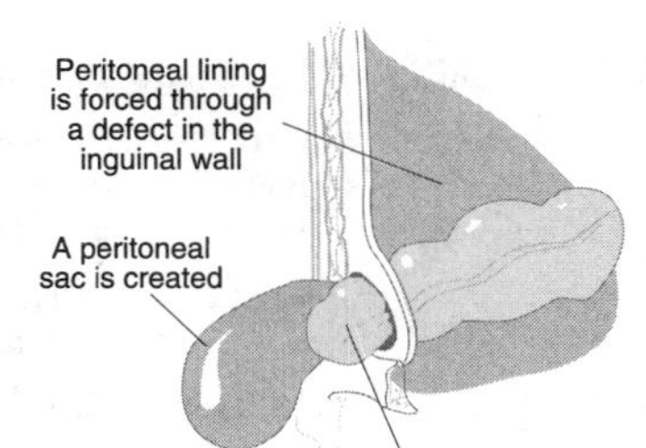

In 49525, a sliding inguinal hernia (depicted above, right) is repaired in a patient of any age

49525 **Repair inguinal hernia, sliding, any age**

EXCLUDES *Inguinal hernia repair, incarcerated/strangulated (49496, 49501, 49507, 49521)*

16.70 16.70 Global Days 090

AMA: 2009, Jan, 11-31; 2008, Jan, 10-25; 2008, Jun, 3-6; 2007, January, 13-27

49540 **Repair lumbar hernia**

19.59 19.59 Global Days 090

AMA: 2008, Jun, 3-6

49550 **Repair initial femoral hernia, any age; reducible**

16.78 16.78 Global Days 090

AMA: 2008, Jun, 3-6

49553 incarcerated or strangulated

18.41 18.41 Global Days 090

AMA: 2008, Jun, 3-6

49555 **Repair recurrent femoral hernia; reducible**

17.46 17.46 Global Days 090

AMA: 2008, Jun, 3-6

49557 incarcerated or strangulated

21.08 21.08 Global Days 090

AMA: 2008, Jun, 3-6

49560-49568 Hernia Repair: Incisional/Ventral

INCLUDES Initial repair: no previous repair required
Recurrent repair: required previous repair(s)

EXCLUDES *Abdominal wall debridement (11042, 11043)*
Intra-abdominal hernia repair/reduction (44050)

Code also repair or excision of testicle(s), intestine, ovaries if performed (44120, 54520, 58940)

49560 **Repair initial incisional or ventral hernia; reducible**

Code also implantation of mesh or other prosthesis if performed (49568)

21.49 21.49 Global Days 090

AMA: 2008, Jun, 3-6

49561 incarcerated or strangulated

Code also implantation of mesh or other prosthesis if performed (49568)

27.11 27.11 Global Days 090

AMA: 2008, Jun, 3-6

49565 **Repair recurrent incisional or ventral hernia; reducible**

Code also implantation of mesh or other prosthesis if performed (49568)

22.40 22.40 Global Days 090

AMA: 2008, Jun, 3-6

49566 incarcerated or strangulated

Code also implantation of mesh or other prosthesis if performed (49568)

27.42 27.42 Global Days 090

AMA: 2008, Jun, 3-6

\+ **49568** **Implantation of mesh or other prosthesis for open incisional or ventral hernia repair or mesh for closure of debridement for necrotizing soft tissue infection (List separately in addition to code for the incisional or ventral hernia repair)**

Code first (11004-11006, 49560-49566)

7.83 7.83 Global Days ZZZ

AMA: 2009, Jan, 11-31; 2008, Jan, 10-25; 2008, Jun, 3-6; 2007, January, 13-27

49570-49590 Hernia Repair: Epigastric/Lateral Ventral/Umbilical

INCLUDES Mesh or other prosthesis

EXCLUDES *Abdominal wall debridement (11042, 11043)*
Intra-abdominal hernia repair/reduction (44050)

Code also repair or excision of testicle(s), intestine, ovaries if performed (44120, 54520, 58940)

49570 Repair epigastric hernia (eg, preperitoneal fat); reducible (separate procedure) A2 T 80 50 PQ
12.13 12.13 Global Days 090
AMA: 2008, Jun, 3-6

49572 incarcerated or strangulated A2 T 80 50
14.99 14.99 Global Days 090
AMA: 2008, Jun, 3-6

49580 Repair umbilical hernia, younger than age 5 years; reducible A A2 T 80
9.66 9.66 Global Days 090
AMA: 2008, Jun, 3-6

49582 incarcerated or strangulated A A2 T 80
14.03 14.03 Global Days 090
AMA: 2008, Jun, 3-6

49585 Repair umbilical hernia, age 5 years or older; reducible A A2 T 80
INCLUDES Mayo hernia repair
12.94 12.94 Global Days 090
AMA: 2008, Jun, 3-6

49587 incarcerated or strangulated A A2 T 80
13.90 13.90 Global Days 090
AMA: 2008, Jun, 3-6

49590 Repair spigelian hernia A2 T 80 50
16.66 16.66 Global Days 090
AMA: 2008, Jun, 3-6

49600-49611 Repair Birth Defect Abdominal Wall: Omphalocele/Gastroschisis

INCLUDES Mesh or other prosthesis

EXCLUDES *Abdominal wall debridement (11042, 11043)*
Intra-abdominal hernia repair/reduction (44050)
Repair hiatal or diaphragmatic hernia (39503, 43332)
Repair of:
Diaphragmatic or hiatal hernia (43332-43337)
Omentum (49999)

49600 Repair of small omphalocele, with primary closure A2 T 80 63
21.34 21.34 Global Days 090
AMA: 2008, Jun, 3-6

49605 Repair of large omphalocele or gastroschisis; with or without prosthesis C5 C 80 63
144.58 144.58 Global Days 090
AMA: 2008, Jun, 3-6

49606 with removal of prosthesis, final reduction and closure, in operating room C5 C 80 63
33.04 33.04 Global Days 090
AMA: 2008, Jun, 3-6

49610 Repair of omphalocele (Gross type operation); first stage C5 C 80 63
20.05 20.05 Global Days 090
AMA: 2008, Jun, 3-6

49611 second stage C5 C 80 63
15.95 15.95 Global Days 090
AMA: 2009, Jan, 11-31; 2008, Jan, 10-25; 2008, Jun, 3-6

49650-49659 Laparoscopic Hernia Repair

INCLUDES Diagnostic laparoscopy

49650 Laparoscopy, surgical; repair initial inguinal hernia A2 T 80 50
12.46 12.46 Global Days 090
AMA: 2008, Jun, 3-6

49651 repair recurrent inguinal hernia A2 T 80 50
16.22 16.22 Global Days 090
AMA: 2008, Jun, 3-6

49652 Laparoscopy, surgical, repair, ventral, umbilical, spigelian or epigastric hernia (includes mesh insertion, when performed); reducible G2 T 80 50
Do not report with (44180, 49568)
20.09 20.09 Global Days 090

49653 incarcerated or strangulated G2 T 80 50
Do not report with (44180, 49568)
25.09 25.09 Global Days 090

49654 Laparoscopy, surgical, repair, incisional hernia (includes mesh insertion, when performed); reducible G2 T 80 50
Do not report with (44180, 49568)
22.82 22.82 Global Days 090

49655 incarcerated or strangulated G2 T 80 50
Do not report with (44180, 49568)
27.86 27.86 Global Days 090

49656 Laparoscopy, surgical, repair, recurrent incisional hernia (includes mesh insertion, when performed); reducible G2 T 80 50
Do not report with (44180, 49568)
24.67 24.67 Global Days 090

49657 incarcerated or strangulated G2 T 80 50
Do not report with (44180, 49568)
35.44 35.44 Global Days 090

49659 Unlisted laparoscopy procedure, hernioplasty, herniorrhaphy, herniotomy T 80 50
0.00 0.00 Global Days YYY
AMA: 2009, Jan, 7-8; 2009, Jan, 11-31; 2008, Jan, 10-25; 2008, Jun, 3-6; 2007, January, 13-27

49900 Surgical Repair Abdominal Wall

EXCLUDES *Abdominal wall debridement (11042, 11043)*
Suture of ruptured diaphragm (39540, 39541)

49900 Suture, secondary, of abdominal wall for evisceration or dehiscence C5 C 80
23.79 23.79 Global Days 090

49904-49999 Harvesting of Omental Flap

49904 Omental flap, extra-abdominal (eg, for reconstruction of sternal and chest wall defects) C5 C
INCLUDES Harvest and transfer
EXCLUDES *Omental flap harvest by second surgeon: both surgeons code 49904 with modifier 62*
42.98 42.98 Global Days 090

\+ **49905 Omental flap, intra-abdominal (List separately in addition to code for primary procedure)** C5 C 80
Code first primary procedure
Do not report with (44700)
10.33 10.33 Global Days ZZZ
AMA: 2009, Jan, 11-31; 2008, Jan, 10-25; 2007, January, 13-27

49906 **Free omental flap with microvascular anastomosis**

INCLUDES Operating microscope (69990)

0.00 0.00 Global Days 090

49999 **Unlisted procedure, abdomen, peritoneum and omentum**

0.00 0.00 Global Days YYY

AMA: 2008, Jun, 3-6

50010-50045 Kidney Procedures for Exploration or Drainage

EXCLUDES Retroperitoneal
Abscess drainage (49060)
Exploration (49010)
Tumor/cyst excision (49203-49205)

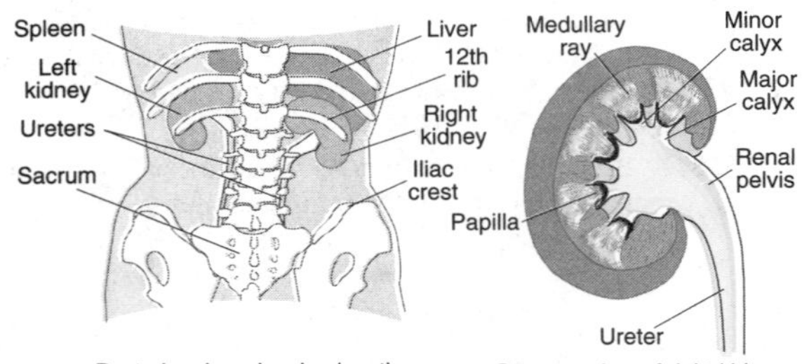

Posterior view showing location of kidneys and ureters

Cutaway view of right kidney showing internal structures

The kidneys remove waste products of protein metabolism and other excess materials and fluids from the blood. Variations in kidney anatomy are fairly common, though abnormalities can complicate procedures. "Pyelo" refers to the renal pelvis, an important access site to the inner kidney. Each kidney is imbedded in a mass of peritoneal fat that helps to enclose and position it

50010 **Renal exploration, not necessitating other specific procedures**
EXCLUDES Laparoscopic ablation of mass lesions of kidney (50542)
21.67 21.67 Global Days 090

50020 **Drainage of perirenal or renal abscess; open**
30.95 30.95 Global Days 090

⊙ **50021** **percutaneous**
75989
4.93 28.11 Global Days 000

50040 **Nephrostomy, nephrotomy with drainage**
27.41 27.41 Global Days 090

50045 **Nephrotomy, with exploration**
EXCLUDES Renal endoscopy through nephrotomy (50570-50580)
27.52 27.52 Global Days 090

50060-50081 Treatment of Kidney Stones

CMS 100-3,230.1 Treatment of Kidney Stones

EXCLUDES Retroperitoneal:
Abscess drainage (49060)
Exploration (49010)
Tumor/cyst excision (49203-49205)

50060 **Nephrolithotomy; removal of calculus**
33.73 33.73 Global Days 090

50065 **secondary surgical operation for calculus**
35.66 35.66 Global Days 090

50070 **complicated by congenital kidney abnormality**
36.04 36.04 Global Days 090

50075 **removal of large staghorn calculus filling renal pelvis and calyces (including anatrophic pyelolithotomy)**
43.18 43.18 Global Days 090

50080 **Percutaneous nephrostolithotomy or pyelostolithotomy, with or without dilation, endoscopy, lithotripsy, stenting, or basket extraction; up to 2 cm**
EXCLUDES Nephrostomy without nephrostolithotomy (50040, 50395, 52334)
25.78 25.78 Global Days 090
AMA: 2009, Jun, 10-11

50081 **over 2 cm**
EXCLUDES Nephrostomy without nephrostolithotomy (50040, 50395, 52334)
76000, 76001
37.84 37.84 Global Days 090
AMA: 2009, Jun, 10-11

50100 Repair of Anomalous Vessels of the Kidney

EXCLUDES Retroperitoneal:
Abscess drainage (49060)
Exploration (49010)
Tumor/cyst excision (49203-49205)

50100 **Transection or repositioning of aberrant renal vessels (separate procedure)**
26.49 26.49 Global Days 090

50120-50135 Procedures of Renal Pelvis

EXCLUDES Retroperitoneal:
Abscess drainage (49060)
Exploration (49010)
Tumor/cyst excision (49203-49205)

50120 **Pyelotomy; with exploration**
INCLUDES Gol-Vernet pyelotomy
EXCLUDES Renal endoscopy through pyelotomy (50570-50580)
28.04 28.04 Global Days 090

50125 **with drainage, pyelostomy**
30.42 30.42 Global Days 090

50130 **with removal of calculus (pyelolithotomy, pelviolithotomy, including coagulum pyelolithotomy)**
30.58 30.58 Global Days 090

50135 **complicated (eg, secondary operation, congenital kidney abnormality)**
33.18 33.18 Global Days 090

50200-50205 Biopsy of Kidney

CMS 100-3,190.4 Electron Microscope

EXCLUDES Laparoscopic renal mass lesion ablation (50542)
Retroperitoneal tumor/cyst excision (49203-49205)

⊙ **50200** **Renal biopsy; percutaneous, by trocar or needle**
EXCLUDES Evaluation of fine needle aspirate (88172, 88173)
Fine needle aspiration (10022)
76942, 77002, 77012, 77021
4.26 17.81 Global Days 000

50205 **by surgical exposure of kidney**
22.03 22.03 Global Days 090

50220-50240 Nephrectomy Procedures

EXCLUDES Retroperitoneal tumor/cyst excision (49203-49205)

50220 **Nephrectomy, including partial ureterectomy, any open approach including rib resection;**
30.89 30.89 Global Days 090

50225 **complicated because of previous surgery on same kidney** C5 C 80 50 PQ
35.39 35.39 Global Days 090

50230 **radical, with regional lymphadenectomy and/or vena caval thrombectomy** C5 C 80 50 PQ
EXCLUDES *Vena caval resection with reconstruction (37799)*
37.93 37.93 Global Days 090

50234 **Nephrectomy with total ureterectomy and bladder cuff; through same incision** C5 C 80 PQ
38.51 38.51 Global Days 090

50236 **through separate incision** C5 C 80 PQ
43.41 43.41 Global Days 090

50240 **Nephrectomy, partial** C5 C 80 PQ
EXCLUDES *Laparoscopic partial nephrectomy (50543)*
39.19 39.19 Global Days 090

50250-50290 Open Removal Kidney Lesions

50250 **Ablation, open, 1 or more renal mass lesion(s), cryosurgical, including intraoperative ultrasound guidance and monitoring, if performed** C5 C 80
EXCLUDES *Laparoscopic renal mass lesion ablation (50542)*
Percutaneous renal tumor ablation (50592-50593)
Open destruction or excision intra-abdominal tumors (49203-49205)
36.17 36.17 Global Days 090
AMA: 2009, Jan, 11-31; 2008, Jan, 10-25; 2007, January, 13-27

50280 **Excision or unroofing of cyst(s) of kidney** C5 C 80
EXCLUDES *Renal cyst laparoscopic ablation (50541)*
28.27 28.27 Global Days 090

50290 **Excision of perinephric cyst** C5 C 80
EXCLUDES *Open destruction or excision intra-abdominal tumors (49203-49205)*
26.28 26.28 Global Days 090

50300-50380 Kidney Transplant Procedures

CMS 100-3,20.3 Thoracic Duct Drainage (TDD) in Renal Transplants
CMS 100-3,110.16 Nonselective (Random) Transfusions and Living-Related Donor Specific Transfusions (DST) in Kidney Transplantation
CMS 100-3,190.1 Histocompatibility Testing
CMS 100-3,260.7 Lymphocyte Immune Globulin, Anti-Thymocyte Globulin (Equine)
CMS 100-4,3,90.1 Kidney Transplant - General
CMS 100-4,3,90.1.1 Standard Kidney Acquisition Charge
CMS 100-4,3,90.1.2 Billing for Kidney Transplant and Acquisition Services

EXCLUDES *Lymphocele drainage to peritoneal cavity performed laparoscopically (49323)*

50300 **Donor nephrectomy (including cold preservation); from cadaver donor, unilateral or bilateral** C5 C
INCLUDES Graft:
Cold preservation
Harvesting
0.00 0.00 Global Days XXX

50320 **open, from living donor** C5 C 80 50 PQ
INCLUDES Donor care
Graft:
Cold preservation
Harvesting
EXCLUDES *Donor nephrectomy performed laparoscopically (50547)*
42.03 42.03 Global Days 090

50323 **Backbench standard preparation of cadaver donor renal allograft prior to transplantation, including dissection and removal of perinephric fat, diaphragmatic and retroperitoneal attachments, excision of adrenal gland, and preparation of ureter(s), renal vein(s), and renal artery(s), ligating branches, as necessary** C5 C 80
Do not report with (60540, 60545)
0.00 0.00 Global Days XXX

50325 **Backbench standard preparation of living donor renal allograft (open or laparoscopic) prior to transplantation, including dissection and removal of perinephric fat and preparation of ureter(s), renal vein(s), and renal artery(s), ligating branches, as necessary** C5 C 80
0.00 0.00 Global Days XXX

50327 **Backbench reconstruction of cadaver or living donor renal allograft prior to transplantation; venous anastomosis, each** C5 C 80
6.34 6.34 Global Days XXX

50328 **arterial anastomosis, each** C5 C 80
5.55 5.55 Global Days XXX

50329 **ureteral anastomosis, each** C5 C 80
5.15 5.15 Global Days XXX

50340 **Recipient nephrectomy (separate procedure)** C5 C 80 50 PQ
27.61 27.61 Global Days 090

50360 **Renal allotransplantation, implantation of graft; without recipient nephrectomy** C5 C 80 PQ
INCLUDES Allograft transplantation
Recipient care
74.88 74.88 Global Days 090

50365 **with recipient nephrectomy** C5 C 80 50 PQ
INCLUDES Allograft transplantation
Recipient care
84.01 84.01 Global Days 090

50370 **Removal of transplanted renal allograft** C5 C 80 PQ
34.91 34.91 Global Days 090

50380 **Renal autotransplantation, reimplantation of kidney** C5 C 80 PQ
INCLUDES Reimplantation of autograft
Code also nephrolithotomy (50060-50075)
Code also partial nephrectomy (50240, 50543)
58.85 58.85 Global Days 090

50382-50386 Removal With/Without Replacement Internal Ureteral Stent

INCLUDES Radiological supervision and interpretation

⊙ 50382 **Removal (via snare/capture) and replacement of internally dwelling ureteral stent via percutaneous approach, including radiological supervision and interpretation** G2 T 50 PQ
EXCLUDES *Removal and replacement of an internally dwelling ureteral stent using a transurethral approach (50385)*
Do not report with (50395)
8.11 36.97 Global Days 000
AMA: 2008, Oct, 8-9

⊙ 50384 **Removal (via snare/capture) of internally dwelling ureteral stent via percutaneous approach, including radiological supervision and interpretation** G2 T 50 PQ

EXCLUDES *Removal of an internally dwelling ureteral stent using a transurethral approach (50386)*

Do not report with (50395)

7.37 30.32 Global Days 000

AMA: 2008, Oct, 8-9

⊙ 50385 **Removal (via snare/capture) and replacement of internally dwelling ureteral stent via transurethral approach, without use of cystoscopy, including radiological supervision and interpretation** G2 T 80 50 PQ

6.92 35.89 Global Days 000

AMA: 2008, Oct, 8-9

⊙ 50386 **Removal (via snare/capture) of internally dwelling ureteral stent via transurethral approach, without use of cystoscopy, including radiological supervision and interpretation** P2 T 80 50 PQ

5.23 23.32 Global Days 000

AMA: 2008, Oct, 8-9

50387 Remove/Replace Accessible Ureteral Stent

CMS 100-4,4,61.2 Requirements for Specific Procedures to be Reported With Device Codes

EXCLUDES *Removal and replacement of ureterostomy tube or externally accessible ureteral stent via ileal conduit (50688)*

Removal without replacement of externally accessible ureteral stent without fluoroscopic guidance (99201-99499 [99224, 99225, 99226])

⊙ 50387 **Removal and replacement of externally accessible transnephric ureteral stent (eg, external/internal stent) requiring fluoroscopic guidance, including radiological supervision and interpretation** G2 T 80 50 PQ

Code also (C1875, C1877, C2617, C2625)

2.94 17.17 Global Days 000

50389-50398 Percutaneous and Injection Procedures With/Without Indwelling Tube/Catheter Access

50389 **Removal of nephrostomy tube, requiring fluoroscopic guidance (eg, with concurrent indwelling ureteral stent)** G2 T 50 PQ

EXCLUDES *Nephrostomy tube removal without fluoroscopic guidance (99201-99499 [99224, 99225, 99226])*

1.61 9.32 Global Days 000

50390 **Aspiration and/or injection of renal cyst or pelvis by needle, percutaneous** A2 T 50

88172-88173

74425, 74470, 76942, 77002, 77012, 77021

2.87 2.87 Global Days 000

AMA: 2008, Oct, 8-9

50391 **Instillation(s) of therapeutic agent into renal pelvis and/or ureter through established nephrostomy, pyelostomy or ureterostomy tube (eg, anticarcinogenic or antifungal agent)** P3 T

2.93 3.66 Global Days 000

50392 **Introduction of intracatheter or catheter into renal pelvis for drainage and/or injection, percutaneous** A2 T 50

74475, 76942, 77012

5.29 5.29 Global Days 000

AMA: 2008, Oct, 8-9

50393 **Introduction of ureteral catheter or stent into ureter through renal pelvis for drainage and/or injection, percutaneous** A2 T 50

74480, 76942, 77002, 77012

6.43 6.43 Global Days 000

50394 **Injection procedure for pyelography (as nephrostogram, pyelostogram, antegrade pyeloureterograms) through nephrostomy or pyelostomy tube, or indwelling ureteral catheter** N1 N 50

74425

1.47 3.02 Global Days 000

50395 **Introduction of guide into renal pelvis and/or ureter with dilation to establish nephrostomy tract, percutaneous** A2 T 50

EXCLUDES *Percutaneous nephrostolithotomy (50080, 50081)*

Renal endoscopy (50551-50561)

Retrograde percutaneous nephrostomy (52334)

74475, 74480, 74485

5.34 5.34 Global Days 000

AMA: 2009, Jan, 7-8

50396 **Manometric studies through nephrostomy or pyelostomy tube, or indwelling ureteral catheter** A2 T 80 50

74425, 74475, 74480

3.45 3.45 Global Days 000

50398 **Change of nephrostomy or pyelostomy tube** A2 T 50

Code also (C1729)

75984

2.16 15.56 Global Days 000

50400-50540 Open Surgical Procedures of Kidney

50400 **Pyeloplasty (Foley Y-pyeloplasty), plastic operation on renal pelvis, with or without plastic operation on ureter, nephropexy, nephrostomy, pyelostomy, or ureteral splinting; simple** C5 C 80

EXCLUDES *Laparoscopic pyeloplasty (50544)*

34.26 34.26 Global Days 090

50405 **complicated (congenital kidney abnormality, secondary pyeloplasty, solitary kidney, calycoplasty)** C5 C 80

EXCLUDES *Laparoscopic pyeloplasty (50544)*

41.34 41.34 Global Days 090

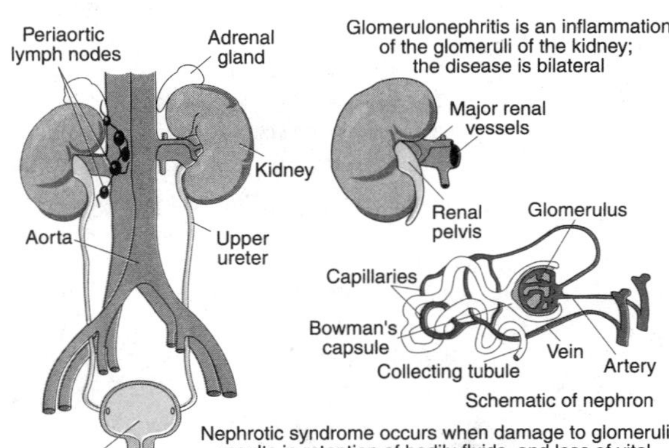

50500 **Nephrorrhaphy, suture of kidney wound or injury** C5 C 80

37.47 37.47 Global Days 090

50520 Closure of nephrocutaneous or pyelocutaneous fistula C5 C 80
30.60 30.60 Global Days 090

50525 Closure of nephrovisceral fistula (eg, renocolic), including visceral repair; abdominal approach C5 C 80
41.58 41.58 Global Days 090

50526 thoracic approach C5 C 80
41.66 41.66 Global Days 090

50540 Symphysiotomy for horseshoe kidney with or without pyeloplasty and/or other plastic procedure, unilateral or bilateral (1 operation) C5 C 80
33.79 33.79 Global Days 090

50541-50549 Laparoscopic Surgical Procedures of the Kidney

INCLUDES Diagnostic laparoscopy

EXCLUDES *Laparoscopic drainage of lymphocele to peritoneal cavity (49323)*

50541 Laparoscopy, surgical; ablation of renal cysts T 80
27.24 27.24 Global Days 090

50542 ablation of renal mass lesion(s), including intraoperative ultrasound guidance and monitoring, when performed T 80

EXCLUDES *Open ablation of renal mass lesions (50250)*
Percutaneous ablation of renal tumors (50592-50593)

34.56 34.56 Global Days 090
AMA: 2009, Jan, 11-31; 2008, Jan, 10-25; 2007, January, 13-27

50543 partial nephrectomy T 80 50 PQ

EXCLUDES *Partial nephrectomy, open approach (50240)*

44.12 44.12 Global Days 090

50544 pyeloplasty T 80
36.96 36.96 Global Days 090

50545 radical nephrectomy (includes removal of Gerota's fascia and surrounding fatty tissue, removal of regional lymph nodes, and adrenalectomy) C5 C 80 50 PQ

EXCLUDES *Radical nephrectomy, open approach (50230)*

39.77 39.77 Global Days 090

50546 nephrectomy, including partial ureterectomy C5 C 80 50 PQ
35.58 35.58 Global Days 090

50547 donor nephrectomy (including cold preservation), from living donor C5 C 80 50 PQ

INCLUDES Donor care
Graft:
Cold preservation
Harvesting

EXCLUDES *Backbench reconstruction renal allograft prior to transplantation (50327-50329)*
Backbench standard preparation of living donor renal allograft prior to transplantation (50325)
Donor nephrectomy, open approach (50320)

47.09 47.09 Global Days 090

50548 nephrectomy with total ureterectomy C5 C 80 50 PQ

EXCLUDES *Nephrectomy, open approach (50234, 50236)*

39.92 39.92 Global Days 090

50549 Unlisted laparoscopy procedure, renal T 80 50
0.00 0.00 Global Days YYY
AMA: 2009, Jan, 11-31; 2008, Jan, 10-25; 2007, January, 13-27

50551-50562 Endoscopic Procedures of Kidney via Established Nephrostomy/Pyelostomy Access

EXCLUDES *Materials and supplies (99070)*

50551 Renal endoscopy through established nephrostomy or pyelostomy, with or without irrigation, instillation, or ureteropyelography, exclusive of radiologic service; A2 T 80 50
8.74 10.69 Global Days 000

50553 with ureteral catheterization, with or without dilation of ureter A2 T 50
9.36 11.43 Global Days 000

50555 with biopsy A2 T 80 50
10.13 12.23 Global Days 000

50557 with fulguration and/or incision, with or without biopsy A2 T 80 50
10.27 12.45 Global Days 000

50561 with removal of foreign body or calculus A2 T 80 50
11.72 14.14 Global Days 000

50562 with resection of tumor G2 T 80
17.27 17.27 Global Days 090

50570-50580 Endoscopic Procedures of Kidney via Nephrotomy/Pyelotomy Access

EXCLUDES *Materials and supplies (99070)*
Nephrotomy (50045)
Pyelotomy (50120)

50570 Renal endoscopy through nephrotomy or pyelotomy, with or without irrigation, instillation, or ureteropyelography, exclusive of radiologic service; G2 T 80 50
14.58 14.58 Global Days 000

50572 with ureteral catheterization, with or without dilation of ureter G2 T 80 50
15.80 15.80 Global Days 000

50574 with biopsy G2 T 80 50
16.80 16.80 Global Days 000

50575 with endopyelotomy (includes cystoscopy, ureteroscopy, dilation of ureter and ureteral pelvic junction, incision of ureteral pelvic junction and insertion of endopyelotomy stent) G2 T 50
21.22 21.22 Global Days 000
AMA: 2009, Jan, 11-31; 2008, Jan, 10-25; 2007, January, 13-27

50576 with fulguration and/or incision, with or without biopsy G2 T 80 50
16.75 16.75 Global Days 000

50580 with removal of foreign body or calculus G2 T 80 50
18.03 18.03 Global Days 000

50590-50593 Noninvasive and Minimally Invasive Procedures of the Kidney

CMS 100-3,230.1 Treatment of Kidney Stones

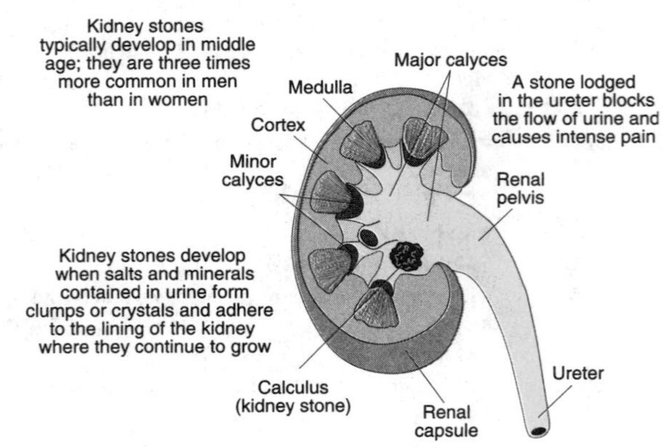

50590 **Lithotripsy, extracorporeal shock wave**
16.74 24.14 Global Days 090
AMA: 2009, Jan, 11-31; 2008, Jan, 10-25; 2007, January, 13-27

⊙ **50592** **Ablation, 1 or more renal tumor(s), percutaneous, unilateral, radiofrequency**
76940, 77013, 77022
10.70 96.49 Global Days 010

⊙ **50593** **Ablation, renal tumor(s), unilateral, percutaneous, cryotherapy**
76940, 77013, 77022
14.09 137.79 Global Days 010

50600-50940 Open and Injection Procedures of Ureter

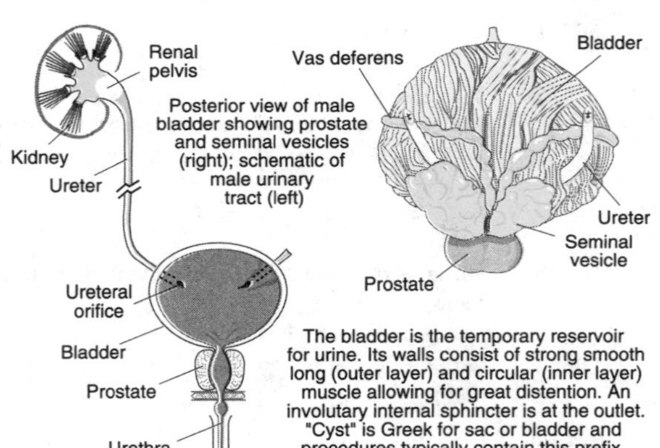

50600 **Ureterotomy with exploration or drainage (separate procedure)**
EXCLUDES *Ureteral endoscopy through ureterotomy (50970-50980)*
27.74 27.74 Global Days 090

50605 **Ureterotomy for insertion of indwelling stent, all types**
28.73 28.73 Global Days 090

50610 **Ureterolithotomy; upper 1/3 of ureter**
EXCLUDES *Cystotomy with calculus basket extraction of ureteral calculus (51065)*
Transvesical ureterolithotomy (51060)
Ureteral calculus manipulation/extraction performed endoscopically (50080, 50081, 50561, 50961, 50980, 52320-52330, 52352, 52353)
Ureterolithotomy performed laparoscopically (50945)
27.98 27.98 Global Days 090

50620 **middle 1/3 of ureter**
EXCLUDES *Cystotomy with calculus basket extraction of ureteral calculus (51065)*
Transvesical ureterolithotomy (51060)
Ureteral calculus manipulation/extraction performed endoscopically (50080, 50081, 50561, 50961, 50980, 52320-52330, 52352, 52353)
Ureterolithotomy performed laparoscopically (50945)
26.76 26.76 Global Days 090

50630 **lower 1/3 of ureter**
EXCLUDES *Cystotomy with calculus basket extraction of ureteral calculus (51065)*
Transvesical ureterolithotomy (51060)
Ureteral calculus manipulation/extraction performed endoscopically (50080, 50081, 50561, 50961, 50980, 52320-52330, 52352, 52353)
Ureterolithotomy performed laparoscopically (50945)
26.33 26.33 Global Days 090

50650 **Ureterectomy, with bladder cuff (separate procedure)**
EXCLUDES *Ureterocele (51535, 52300)*
30.66 30.66 Global Days 090

50660 **Ureterectomy, total, ectopic ureter, combination abdominal, vaginal and/or perineal approach**
EXCLUDES *Ureterocele (51535, 52300)*
33.80 33.80 Global Days 090

50684 **Injection procedure for ureterography or ureteropyelography through ureterostomy or indwelling ureteral catheter**
74425
1.48 3.77 Global Days 000

50686 **Manometric studies through ureterostomy or indwelling ureteral catheter**
2.71 4.20 Global Days 000

50688 **Change of ureterostomy tube or externally accessible ureteral stent via ileal conduit**
Code also (C1729, C1758, C2617, C2625)
75984
2.36 2.36 Global Days 010

50690 **Injection procedure for visualization of ileal conduit and/or ureteropyelography, exclusive of radiologic service**
74425
2.06 2.88 Global Days 000

50700 **Ureteroplasty, plastic operation on ureter (eg, stricture)**
27.37 27.37 Global Days 090

50715 **Ureterolysis, with or without repositioning of ureter for retroperitoneal fibrosis**
34.95 34.95 Global Days 090

50722 **Ureterolysis for ovarian vein syndrome**
31.11 31.11 Global Days 090

50725 **Ureterolysis for retrocaval ureter, with reanastomosis of upper urinary tract or vena cava**
32.43 32.43 Global Days 090

50727 **Revision of urinary-cutaneous anastomosis (any type urostomy);**
15.01 15.01 Global Days 090

50728 **with repair of fascial defect and hernia**
20.57 20.57 Global Days 090

50740 **Ureteropyelostomy, anastomosis of ureter and renal pelvis**
35.93 35.93 Global Days 090

50750 **Ureterocalycostomy, anastomosis of ureter to renal calyx**
34.17 34.17 Global Days 090

50760 **Ureteroureterostomy**
33.34 33.34 Global Days 090

50770 **Transureteroureterostomy, anastomosis of ureter to contralateral ureter**
33.84 33.84 Global Days 090

50780 **Ureteroneocystostomy; anastomosis of single ureter to bladder**
INCLUDES Minor procedures to prevent vesicoureteral reflux
EXCLUDES *Cystourethroplasty with ureteroneocystostomy (51820)*
32.73 32.73 Global Days 090

50782 **anastomosis of duplicated ureter to bladder**
INCLUDES Minor procedures to prevent vesicoureteral reflux
33.95 33.95 Global Days 090

50783 **with extensive ureteral tailoring**
INCLUDES Minor procedures to prevent vesicoureteral reflux
33.04 33.04 Global Days 090

50785 **with vesico-psoas hitch or bladder flap**
INCLUDES Minor procedures to prevent vesicoureteral reflux
35.81 35.81 Global Days 090

50800 **Ureteroenterostomy, direct anastomosis of ureter to intestine**
EXCLUDES *Cystectomy with ureterosigmoidostomy/ureteroileal conduit (51580-51595)*
27.40 27.40 Global Days 090

50810 **Ureterosigmoidostomy, with creation of sigmoid bladder and establishment of abdominal or perineal colostomy, including intestine anastomosis**
EXCLUDES *Cystectomy with ureterosigmoidostomy/ureteroileal conduit (51580-51595)*
40.92 40.92 Global Days 090

50815 **Ureterocolon conduit, including intestine anastomosis**
EXCLUDES *Cystectomy with ureterosigmoidostomy/ureteroileal conduit (51580-51595)*
36.16 36.16 Global Days 090

50820 **Ureteroileal conduit (ileal bladder), including intestine anastomosis (Bricker operation)**
EXCLUDES *Cystectomy with ureterosigmoidostomy/ureteroileal conduit (51580-51595)*
38.95 38.95 Global Days 090

50825 **Continent diversion, including intestine anastomosis using any segment of small and/or large intestine (Kock pouch or Camey enterocystoplasty)**
49.09 49.09 Global Days 090

50830 **Urinary undiversion (eg, taking down of ureteroileal conduit, ureterosigmoidostomy or ureteroenterostomy with ureteroureterostomy or ureteroneocystostomy)**
53.16 53.16 Global Days 090

50840 **Replacement of all or part of ureter by intestine segment, including intestine anastomosis**
36.39 36.39 Global Days 090

50845 **Cutaneous appendico-vesicostomy**
INCLUDES Mitrofanoff operation
36.99 36.99 Global Days 090

50860 **Ureterostomy, transplantation of ureter to skin**
27.93 27.93 Global Days 090

50900 **Ureterorrhaphy, suture of ureter (separate procedure)**
25.02 25.02 Global Days 090

50920 **Closure of ureterocutaneous fistula**
26.08 26.08 Global Days 090

50930 **Closure of ureterovisceral fistula (including visceral repair)**
36.15 36.15 Global Days 090

50940 **Deligation of ureter**
EXCLUDES *Ureteroplasty/ureterolysis (50700-50860)*
26.20 26.20 Global Days 090

50945-50949 Laparoscopic Procedures of Ureter

INCLUDES Diagnostic laparoscopy
EXCLUDES *Ureteroneocystostomy, open approach (50780-50785)*

50945 **Laparoscopy, surgical; ureterolithotomy**
28.81 28.81 Global Days 090
AMA: 2009, Jan, 11-31; 2008, Jan, 10-25; 2007, January, 13-27

50947 **ureteroneocystostomy with cystoscopy and ureteral stent placement**
40.86 40.86 Global Days 090

50948 **ureteroneocystostomy without cystoscopy and ureteral stent placement**
37.79 37.79 Global Days 090

50949 **Unlisted laparoscopy procedure, ureter**
0.00 0.00 Global Days YYY

50951-50961 Endoscopic Procedures of Ureter via Established Ureterostomy Access

50951 **Ureteral endoscopy through established ureterostomy, with or without irrigation, instillation, or ureteropyelography, exclusive of radiologic service;**
9.11 11.17 Global Days 000
AMA: 2009, Jan, 11-31; 2008, Jan, 10-25; 2007, March, 9-11

50953 **with ureteral catheterization, with or without dilation of ureter**
10.08 11.85 Global Days 000
AMA: 2007, March, 9-11

● New Code ▲ Revised Code Maternity Age Unlisted Not Covered # Resequenced
○ Reinstated CCI + Add-on ⊘ Mod 51 Exempt Mod 63 Exempt ⊙ Mod Sedation PQRS

50955 with biopsy A2 T 80 50
10.85 12.76 Global Days 000
AMA: 2007, March, 9-11

50957 with fulguration and/or incision, with or without biopsy A2 T 80 50
10.51 12.73 Global Days 000
AMA: 2007, March, 9-11

50961 with removal of foreign body or calculus A2 T 80 50
9.43 11.49 Global Days 000
AMA: 2009, Jan, 11-31; 2008, Jan, 10-25; 2007, March, 9-11; 2007, April, 11-12

50970-50980 Endoscopic Procedures of Ureter via Ureterotomy

EXCLUDES *Ureterotomy (50600)*

50970 Ureteral endoscopy through ureterotomy, with or without irrigation, instillation, or ureteropyelography, exclusive of radiologic service; A2 T 80 50
11.00 11.00 Global Days 000

50972 with ureteral catheterization, with or without dilation of ureter A2 T 80 50
10.63 10.63 Global Days 000

50974 with biopsy A2 T 80 50
14.04 14.04 Global Days 000

50976 with fulguration and/or incision, with or without biopsy A2 T 80 50
13.83 13.83 Global Days 000

50980 with removal of foreign body or calculus A2 T 80 50
10.57 10.57 Global Days 000

51020-51080 Open Incisional Procedures of Bladder

51020 Cystotomy or cystostomy; with fulguration and/or insertion of radioactive material A2 T 80
13.92 13.92 Global Days 090

51030 with cryosurgical destruction of intravesical lesion A2 T 80
13.75 13.75 Global Days 090

51040 Cystostomy, cystotomy with drainage A2 T 80
8.60 8.60 Global Days 090

51045 Cystotomy, with insertion of ureteral catheter or stent (separate procedure) A2 T 80
14.50 14.50 Global Days 090

51050 Cystolithotomy, cystotomy with removal of calculus, without vesical neck resection A2 T 80
14.00 14.00 Global Days 090

51060 Transvesical ureterolithotomy T 80
17.23 17.23 Global Days 090

51065 Cystotomy, with calculus basket extraction and/or ultrasonic or electrohydraulic fragmentation of ureteral calculus A2 T 80
17.13 17.13 Global Days 090

51080 Drainage of perivesical or prevesical space abscess A2 T 80
12.08 12.08 Global Days 090

51100-51102 Bladder Aspiration Procedures

76942, 77002, 77012

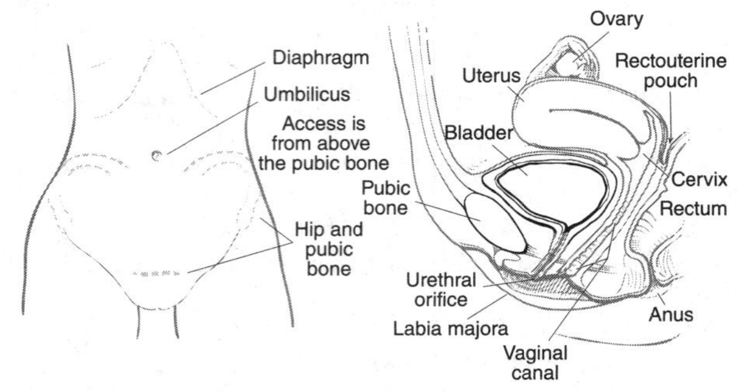

51100 Aspiration of bladder; by needle P3 T
1.15 1.82 Global Days 000
AMA: 2008, Jun, 8-11

51101 by trocar or intracatheter P2 T
1.56 3.76 Global Days 000
AMA: 2008, Jun, 8-11

51102 with insertion of suprapubic catheter A2 T
4.34 6.81 Global Days 000
AMA: 2008, Jun, 8-11; 2007, Dec, 10-179

51500-51597 Open Excisional Procedures of Bladder

51500 Excision of urachal cyst or sinus, with or without umbilical hernia repair A2 T 80
19.84 19.84 Global Days 090

51520 Cystotomy; for simple excision of vesical neck (separate procedure) A2 T 80
17.52 17.52 Global Days 090

51525 for excision of bladder diverticulum, single or multiple (separate procedure) C5 C 80
EXCLUDES *Transurethral resection (52305)*
25.48 25.48 Global Days 090

51530 for excision of bladder tumor C5 C 80
EXCLUDES *Transurethral resection (52234-52240)*
23.25 23.25 Global Days 090

51535 Cystotomy for excision, incision, or repair of ureterocele G2 T 80 50
EXCLUDES *Transurethral excision (52300)*
22.96 22.96 Global Days 090

51550 Cystectomy, partial; simple C5 C 80 PQ
28.62 28.62 Global Days 090

51555 complicated (eg, postradiation, previous surgery, difficult location) C5 C 80 PQ
37.59 37.59 Global Days 090

51565 Cystectomy, partial, with reimplantation of ureter(s) into bladder (ureteroneocystostomy) C5 C 80 PQ
38.32 38.32 Global Days 090

51570 Cystectomy, complete; (separate procedure) C5 C 80 PQ
43.68 43.68 Global Days 090

51575 with bilateral pelvic lymphadenectomy, including external iliac, hypogastric, and obturator nodes C5 C 80 PQ
53.92 53.92 Global Days 090

51580 **Cystectomy, complete, with ureterosigmoidostomy or ureterocutaneous transplantations;** C5 C 80
56.15 56.15 Global Days 090

51585 **with bilateral pelvic lymphadenectomy, including external iliac, hypogastric, and obturator nodes** C5 C 80
62.51 62.51 Global Days 090

51590 **Cystectomy, complete, with ureteroileal conduit or sigmoid bladder, including intestine anastomosis;** C5 C 80
57.22 57.22 Global Days 090

51595 **with bilateral pelvic lymphadenectomy, including external iliac, hypogastric, and obturator nodes** C5 C 80
64.85 64.85 Global Days 090

51596 **Cystectomy, complete, with continent diversion, any open technique, using any segment of small and/or large intestine to construct neobladder** C5 C 80
69.66 69.66 Global Days 090

51597 **Pelvic exenteration, complete, for vesical, prostatic or urethral malignancy, with removal of bladder and ureteral transplantations, with or without hysterectomy and/or abdominoperineal resection of rectum and colon and colostomy, or any combination thereof** C5 C 80
EXCLUDES *Pelvic exenteration for gynecologic malignancy (58240)*
67.91 67.91 Global Days 090

51600-51720 Injection/Insertion/Instillation Procedures of Bladder

51600 **Injection procedure for cystography or voiding urethrocystography** N1 N
74430, 74455
1.30 5.65 Global Days 000

51605 **Injection procedure and placement of chain for contrast and/or chain urethrocystography** N1 N
74430
1.13 1.13 Global Days 000

51610 **Injection procedure for retrograde urethrocystography** N1 N
74450
1.89 3.22 Global Days 000

51700 **Bladder irrigation, simple, lavage and/or instillation** P3 T
1.31 2.49 Global Days 000

51701 **Insertion of non-indwelling bladder catheter (eg, straight catheterization for residual urine)** P2 X
EXCLUDES *Catheterization for specimen collection (P9612)*
Do not report with insertion of catheter as an inclusive component of another procedure
0.81 1.68 Global Days 000
AMA: 2009, Jan, 11-31; 2008, Jan, 10-25; 2007, Jul, 1-4; 2007, January, 28-31

51702 **Insertion of temporary indwelling bladder catheter; simple (eg, Foley)** P2 X
Do not report with insertion of catheter as an inclusive component of another procedure
0.89 2.17 Global Days 000
AMA: 2009, Jan, 11-31; 2008, Jan, 10-25; 2007, Jul, 1-4; 2007, January, 28-31; 2007, January, 13-27

51703 **complicated (eg, altered anatomy, fractured catheter/balloon)** P2 T
2.41 3.93 Global Days 000
AMA: 2007, January, 28-31

51705 **Change of cystostomy tube; simple** P3 T
1.51 2.61 Global Days 000
AMA: 2009, Jan, 11-31; 2008, Jan, 10-25; 2007, January, 28-31; 2007, Dec, 10-179

51710 **complicated** A2 T
Code also (C2627)
75984
2.31 2.71 Global Days 000
AMA: 2007, Dec, 10-179

51715 **Endoscopic injection of implant material into the submucosal tissues of the urethra and/or bladder neck** A2 T 80
Code also (L8603, L8604, L8606)
5.93 8.63 Global Days 000

51720 **Bladder instillation of anticarcinogenic agent (including retention time)** P3 T
2.38 3.27 Global Days 000
AMA: 2009, Jan, 11-31; 2008, Jan, 10-25; 2007, January, 13-27

51725-51798 [51797] Uroflowmetric Evaluations

CMS 100-3,230.2 Uroflowmetric Evaluations

51725 **Simple cystometrogram (CMG) (eg, spinal manometer)** P3 T 80
5.87 5.87 Global Days 000

51726 **Complex cystometrogram (ie, calibrated electronic equipment);** A2 T
8.61 8.61 Global Days 000

51727 **with urethral pressure profile studies (ie, urethral closure pressure profile), any technique** P2 T 80
9.28 9.28 Global Days 000

51728 **with voiding pressure studies (ie, bladder voiding pressure), any technique** P2 T 80
9.24 9.24 Global Days 000

51729 **with voiding pressure studies (ie, bladder voiding pressure) and urethral pressure profile studies (ie, urethral closure pressure profile), any technique** P2 T 80
10.08 10.08 Global Days 000

+ # **51797** **Voiding pressure studies, intra-abdominal (ie, rectal, gastric, intraperitoneal) (List separately in addition to code for primary procedure)** P3 T 80
Code first (51728-51729)
3.63 3.63 Global Days ZZZ
AMA: 2009, Jan, 11-31; 2008, Jan, 10-25; 2007, January, 13-27

51736 **Simple uroflowmetry (UFR) (eg, stop-watch flow rate, mechanical uroflowmeter)** P3 X 80
0.64 0.64 Global Days XXX

51741 **Complex uroflowmetry (eg, calibrated electronic equipment)** P3 T
0.74 0.74 Global Days XXX

51784 **Electromyography studies (EMG) of anal or urethral sphincter, other than needle, any technique** P2 T
5.92 5.92 Global Days 000

51785 **Needle electromyography studies (EMG) of anal or urethral sphincter, any technique** A2 T 80
7.01 7.01 Global Days 000
AMA: 2009, Jan, 11-31; 2008, Jan, 10-25; 2007, January, 13-27

51792 **Stimulus evoked response (eg, measurement of bulbocavernosus reflex latency time)** P2 T 80
6.61 6.61 Global Days 000

51797 Resequenced code, See code following 51729.

51798 **Measurement of post-voiding residual urine and/or bladder capacity by ultrasound, non-imaging** P3 X 80
0.57 0.57 Global Days XXX

51800-51980 Open Repairs Urinary System

51800 **Cystoplasty or cystourethroplasty, plastic operation on bladder and/or vesical neck (anterior Y-plasty, vesical fundus resection), any procedure, with or without wedge resection of posterior vesical neck** C5 C 80 PQ
30.94 30.94 Global Days 090

51820 **Cystourethroplasty with unilateral or bilateral ureteroneocystostomy** C5 C 80 PQ
31.77 31.77 Global Days 090

51840 **Anterior vesicourethropexy, or urethropexy (eg, Marshall-Marchetti-Krantz, Burch); simple** C5 C 80
EXCLUDES *Pereyra type urethropexy (57289)*
19.67 19.67 Global Days 090
AMA: 2009, Jan, 11-31; 2008, Jan, 10-25; 2007, January, 13-27

51841 **complicated (eg, secondary repair)** C5 C 80
EXCLUDES *Pereyra type urethropexy (57289)*
23.37 23.37 Global Days 090

51845 **Abdomino-vaginal vesical neck suspension, with or without endoscopic control (eg, Stamey, Raz, modified Pereyra)** ♀ T 80
17.50 17.50 Global Days 090

51860 **Cystorrhaphy, suture of bladder wound, injury or rupture; simple** T 80
22.16 22.16 Global Days 090

51865 **complicated** C5 C 80
26.56 26.56 Global Days 090

51880 **Closure of cystostomy (separate procedure)** A2 T 80
13.92 13.92 Global Days 090

51900 **Closure of vesicovaginal fistula, abdominal approach** ♀ C5 C 80 PQ
EXCLUDES *Vesicovaginal fistula closure, vaginal approach (57320-57330)*
24.51 24.51 Global Days 090

51920 **Closure of vesicouterine fistula;** ♀ C5 C 80 PQ
EXCLUDES *Enterovesical fistula closure (44660, 44661)*
Rectovesical fistula closure (45800-45805)
22.43 22.43 Global Days 090

51925 **with hysterectomy** ♀ C5 C 80 PQ
EXCLUDES *Enterovesical fistula closure (44660, 44661)*
Rectovesical fistula closure (45800-45805)
30.23 30.23 Global Days 090

51940 **Closure, exstrophy of bladder** C5 C 80
EXCLUDES *Epispadias reconstruction with exstropy of bladder (54390)*
48.16 48.16 Global Days 090

51960 **Enterocystoplasty, including intestinal anastomosis** C5 C 80 PQ
41.20 41.20 Global Days 090

51980 **Cutaneous vesicostomy** C5 C 80
21.08 21.08 Global Days 090

51990-51999 Laparoscopic Procedures of Urinary System

INCLUDES Diagnostic laparoscopy

51990 **Laparoscopy, surgical; urethral suspension for stress incontinence** T 80
22.50 22.50 Global Days 090

51992 **sling operation for stress incontinence (eg, fascia or synthetic)** ♀ A2 T 80
EXCLUDES *Removal/revision of sling for stress incontinence (57287)*
Sling operation for stress incontinence, open approach (57288)
25.39 25.39 Global Days 090

51999 **Unlisted laparoscopy procedure, bladder** T 80
0.00 0.00 Global Days YYY

52000-52318 Endoscopic Procedures via Urethra: Bladder and Urethra

52000 **Cystourethroscopy (separate procedure)** A2 T
3.74 6.09 Global Days 000
AMA: 2009, Jan, 11-31; 2008, Jan, 10-25; 2007, January, 13-27

52001 **Cystourethroscopy with irrigation and evacuation of multiple obstructing clots** A2 T
Do not report with (52000)
8.52 11.06 Global Days 000

52005 **Cystourethroscopy, with ureteral catheterization, with or without irrigation, instillation, or ureteropyelography, exclusive of radiologic service;** A2 T
INCLUDES Howard test
3.95 8.29 Global Days 000
AMA: 2009, Jan, 11-31; 2008, Jan, 10-25; 2007, January, 13-27

52007 **with brush biopsy of ureter and/or renal pelvis** A2 T 50
4.92 14.27 Global Days 000

52010 **Cystourethroscopy, with ejaculatory duct catheterization, with or without irrigation, instillation, or duct radiography, exclusive of radiologic service** ♂ A2 T
74440
4.88 11.45 Global Days 000

52204 **Cystourethroscopy, with biopsy(s)** A2 T
4.20 11.60 Global Days 000
AMA: 2009, Jan, 11-31; 2008, Jan, 10-25; 2007, January, 13-27

52214 **Cystourethroscopy, with fulguration (including cryosurgery or laser surgery) of trigone, bladder neck, prostatic fossa, urethra, or periurethral glands** A2 T
6.02 18.82 Global Days 000

52224 **Cystourethroscopy, with fulguration (including cryosurgery or laser surgery) or treatment of MINOR (less than 0.5 cm) lesion(s) with or without biopsy** A2 T
5.03 19.96 Global Days 000
AMA: 2009, Jan, 11-31; 2009, Jun, 10-11; 2008, Jan, 10-25; 2007, Dec, 7-8

52234 **Cystourethroscopy, with fulguration (including cryosurgery or laser surgery) and/or resection of; SMALL bladder tumor(s) (0.5 up to 2.0 cm)** A2 T
EXCLUDES *Bladder tumor excision through cystotomy (51530)*
7.30 7.30 Global Days 000
AMA: 2009, Jan, 11-31; 2009, Jun, 10-11; 2008, Jan, 10-25; 2007, January, 13-27; 2007, Dec, 7-8

52235 **MEDIUM bladder tumor(s) (2.0 to 5.0 cm)** A2 T
EXCLUDES *Bladder tumor excision through cystotomy (51530)*
8.57 8.57 Global Days 000
AMA: 2009, Jun, 10-11

52240 **LARGE bladder tumor(s)** A2 T
EXCLUDES *Bladder tumor excision through cystotomy (51530)*
14.95 14.95 Global Days 000
AMA: 2009, Jun, 10-11

52250 **Cystourethroscopy with insertion of radioactive substance, with or without biopsy or fulguration** A2 T
7.20 7.20 Global Days 000

52260 **Cystourethroscopy, with dilation of bladder for interstitial cystitis; general or conduction (spinal) anesthesia** A2 T
6.25 6.25 Global Days 000
AMA: 2009, Jan, 11-31; 2008, Jan, 10-25; 2007, January, 13-27

52265 **local anesthesia** P3 T
4.86 11.46 Global Days 000

52270 **Cystourethroscopy, with internal urethrotomy; female** ♀ A2 T
5.40 10.97 Global Days 000

52275 **male** ♂ A2 T
7.38 14.88 Global Days 000

52276 **Cystourethroscopy with direct vision internal urethrotomy** A2 T
7.89 7.89 Global Days 000
AMA: 2009, May, 8-9&11

52277 **Cystourethroscopy, with resection of external sphincter (sphincterotomy)** A2 T 80
9.67 9.67 Global Days 000

52281 **Cystourethroscopy, with calibration and/or dilation of urethral stricture or stenosis, with or without meatotomy, with or without injection procedure for cystography, male or female** A2 T
4.54 8.36 Global Days 000
AMA: 2009, Jan, 11-31; 2008, Jan, 10-25; 2007, June, 10-11

52282 **Cystourethroscopy, with insertion of permanent urethral stent** A2 T
EXCLUDES *Placement of temporary prostatic urethral stent (53855)*
10.03 10.03 Global Days 000

52283 **Cystourethroscopy, with steroid injection into stricture** A2 T
5.97 8.22 Global Days 000

52285 **Cystourethroscopy for treatment of the female urethral syndrome with any or all of the following: urethral meatotomy, urethral dilation, internal urethrotomy, lysis of urethrovaginal septal fibrosis, lateral incisions of the bladder neck, and fulguration of polyp(s) of urethra, bladder neck, and/or trigone** ♀ A2 T
5.82 8.32 Global Days 000

52290 **Cystourethroscopy; with ureteral meatotomy, unilateral or bilateral** A2 T
7.25 7.25 Global Days 000

52300 **with resection or fulguration of orthotopic ureterocele(s), unilateral or bilateral** A2 T 80
8.45 8.45 Global Days 000

52301 **with resection or fulguration of ectopic ureterocele(s), unilateral or bilateral** A2 T 80
8.69 8.69 Global Days 000

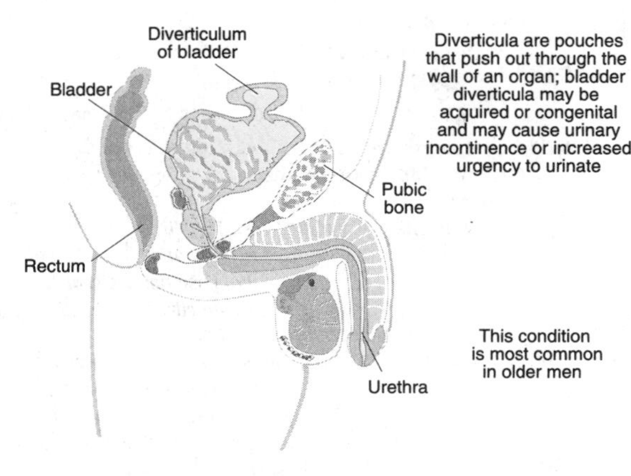

52305 **with incision or resection of orifice of bladder diverticulum, single or multiple** A2 T
8.28 8.28 Global Days 000

52310 **Cystourethroscopy, with removal of foreign body, calculus, or ureteral stent from urethra or bladder (separate procedure); simple** A2 T
4.51 7.28 Global Days 000

52315 **complicated** A2 T
8.14 12.48 Global Days 000

52317 **Litholapaxy: crushing or fragmentation of calculus by any means in bladder and removal of fragments; simple or small (less than 2.5 cm)** A2 T
10.31 25.25 Global Days 000

52318 **complicated or large (over 2.5 cm)** A2 T
14.05 14.05 Global Days 000

52320-52355 Endoscopic Procedures via Urethra: Renal Pelvis and Ureter

INCLUDES Diagnostic cystourethroscopy with therapeutic cystourethroscopy
Insertion/removal of temporary ureteral catheter

EXCLUDES *Diagnostic cystourethroscopy only (52000)*
Self-retaining/indwelling ureteral stent removal by cystourethroscope (52310, 52315)

Code also the insertion of an indwelling stent performed in addition to other procedures within this section (52332)

Do not report with (52005)

52320 **Cystourethroscopy (including ureteral catheterization); with removal of ureteral calculus** A2 T 50
Do not report with (52000)
7.31 7.31 Global Days 000
AMA: 2009, Jan, 11-31; 2008, Jan, 10-25; 2007, January, 13-27

52325 **with fragmentation of ureteral calculus (eg, ultrasonic or electro-hydraulic technique)** A2 T 50
Do not report with (52000)
9.53 9.53 Global Days 000
AMA: 2009, Jan, 11-31; 2007, Dec, 10-179

52327 **with subureteric injection of implant material** A2 T 50
Do not report with (52000)
7.80 7.80 Global Days 000

52330 **with manipulation, without removal of ureteral calculus** A2 T 50
Do not report with (52000)
7.83 17.04 Global Days 000
AMA: 2009, Jan, 11-31; 2008, Jan, 10-25; 2007, January, 13-27

52332 **Cystourethroscopy, with insertion of indwelling ureteral stent (eg, Gibbons or double-J type)** A2 T 50

Do not report with (52000)

4.62 14.93 Global Days 000

AMA: 2009, Jan, 11-31; 2008, Jan, 10-25; 2007, January, 13-27

52334 **Cystourethroscopy with insertion of ureteral guide wire through kidney to establish a percutaneous nephrostomy, retrograde** A2 T 50

EXCLUDES *Cystourethroscopy with incision/fulguration/resection of congenital posterior urethral valves/obstructive hypertrophic mucosal folds (52400)*

Cystourethroscopy with pyeloscopy and/or ureteroscopy (52351-52355)

Nephrostomy tract establishment only (50395)

Percutaneous nephrostolithotomy (50080, 50081)

Do not report with (52000)

7.62 7.62 Global Days 000

52341 **Cystourethroscopy; with treatment of ureteral stricture (eg, balloon dilation, laser, electrocautery, and incision)** A2 T 50

INCLUDES Diagnostic cystourethroscopy with ureteroscopy/pyeloscopy

Do not report with (52000, 52341)

8.59 8.59 Global Days 000

52342 **with treatment of ureteropelvic junction stricture (eg, balloon dilation, laser, electrocautery, and incision)** A2 T 50

INCLUDES Diagnostic cystourethroscopy with ureteroscopy/pyeloscopy

Do not report with (52000, 52351)

9.33 9.33 Global Days 000

AMA: 2009, Jan, 11-31; 2008, Jan, 10-25; 2007, January, 13-27

52343 **with treatment of intra-renal stricture (eg, balloon dilation, laser, electrocautery, and incision)** A2 T 50

INCLUDES Diagnostic cystourethroscopy with ureteroscopy/pyeloscopy

Do not report with (52000, 52351)

10.39 10.39 Global Days 000

52344 **Cystourethroscopy with ureteroscopy; with treatment of ureteral stricture (eg, balloon dilation, laser, electrocautery, and incision)** A2 T 50

INCLUDES Diagnostic cystourethroscopy with ureteroscopy/pyeloscopy

Do not report with (52351)

11.29 11.29 Global Days 000

52345 **with treatment of ureteropelvic junction stricture (eg, balloon dilation, laser, electrocautery, and incision)** A2 T 80

INCLUDES Diagnostic cystourethroscopy with ureteroscopy/pyeloscopy

Do not report with (52351)

12.03 12.03 Global Days 000

52346 **with treatment of intra-renal stricture (eg, balloon dilation, laser, electrocautery, and incision)** A2 T 80

INCLUDES Diagnostic cystourethroscopy with ureteroscopy/pyeloscopy

EXCLUDES *Cystourethroscopy with transurethral resection or incision of ejaculatory ducts (52402)*

Do not report with (52351)

13.61 13.61 Global Days 000

52351 **Cystourethroscopy, with ureteroscopy and/or pyeloscopy; diagnostic** A2 T

Do not report with (52341-52346, 52352-52355)

74485

9.32 9.32 Global Days 000

52352 **with removal or manipulation of calculus (ureteral catheterization is included)** A2 T 50

INCLUDES Diagnostic cystourethroscopy with ureteroscopy/pyeloscopy

Do not report with (52351)

10.95 10.95 Global Days 000

AMA: 2009, Jan, 11-31; 2008, Jan, 10-25; 2007, June, 10-11

52353 **with lithotripsy (ureteral catheterization is included)** A2 T 50

INCLUDES Diagnostic cystourethroscopy with ureteroscopy/pyeloscopy

Do not report with (52351)

12.56 12.56 Global Days 000

AMA: 2009, Jan, 11-31; 2007, Dec, 10-179

52354 **with biopsy and/or fulguration of ureteral or renal pelvic lesion** A2 T 50

INCLUDES Diagnostic cystourethroscopy with ureteroscopy/pyeloscopy

Do not report with (52351)

11.63 11.63 Global Days 000

52355 **with resection of ureteral or renal pelvic tumor** A2 T 50

INCLUDES Diagnostic cystourethroscopy with ureteroscopy/pyeloscopy

Do not report with (52351)

13.85 13.85 Global Days 000

52400-52700 Endoscopic Procedures via Urethra: Prostate and Vesical Neck

52400 **Cystourethroscopy with incision, fulguration, or resection of congenital posterior urethral valves, or congenital obstructive hypertrophic mucosal folds** A2 T

14.20 14.20 Global Days 090

52402 **Cystourethroscopy with transurethral resection or incision of ejaculatory ducts** ♂ A2 T 80

7.91 7.91 Global Days 000

52450 **Transurethral incision of prostate** ♂ A2 T PO

13.92 13.92 Global Days 090

AMA: 2009, Jan, 11-31; 2008, Jan, 10-25; 2007, January, 13-27

52500 **Transurethral resection of bladder neck (separate procedure)** A2 T

14.47 14.47 Global Days 090

AMA: 2009, Jan, 11-31; 2009, May, 8-9&11; 2008, Jan, 10-25; 2007, January, 13-27

52601 **Transurethral electrosurgical resection of prostate, including control of postoperative bleeding, complete (vasectomy, meatotomy, cystourethroscopy, urethral calibration and/or dilation, and internal urethrotomy are included)**

EXCLUDES *Excision of prostate (55801-55845)*

24.90 24.90 Global Days 090

52630 **Transurethral resection; residual or regrowth of obstructive prostate tissue including control of postoperative bleeding, complete (vasectomy, meatotomy, cystourethroscopy, urethral calibration and/or dilation, and internal urethrotomy are included)**

EXCLUDES *Excision of prostate (55801-55845)*

11.87 11.87 Global Days 090

52640 **of postoperative bladder neck contracture**

EXCLUDES *Excision of prostate (55801-55845)*

9.22 9.22 Global Days 090

52647 **Laser coagulation of prostate, including control of postoperative bleeding, complete (vasectomy, meatotomy, cystourethroscopy, urethral calibration and/or dilation, and internal urethrotomy are included if performed)**

19.17 56.56 Global Days 090

AMA: 2009, Jan, 11-31; 2008, Jan, 10-25; 2007, January, 13-27

52648 **Laser vaporization of prostate, including control of postoperative bleeding, complete (vasectomy, meatotomy, cystourethroscopy, urethral calibration and/or dilation, internal urethrotomy and transurethral resection of prostate are included if performed)**

20.45 58.06 Global Days 090

AMA: 2009, Jan, 11-31; 2008, Jan, 10-25; 2007, January, 13-27

52649 **Laser enucleation of the prostate with morcellation, including control of postoperative bleeding, complete (vasectomy, meatotomy, cystourethroscopy, urethral calibration and/or dilation, internal urethrotomy and transurethral resection of prostate are included if performed)**

Do not report with (52000, 52276, 52281, 52601, 52647-52648, 53020, 55250)

24.71 24.71 Global Days 090

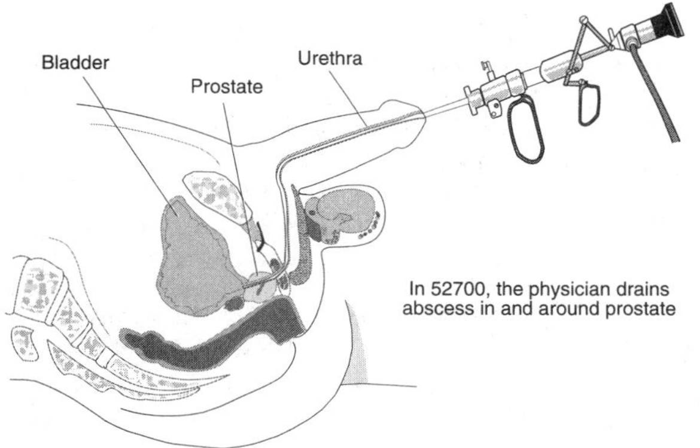

52700 **Transurethral drainage of prostatic abscess**

EXCLUDES *Litholapaxy (52317, 52318)*

13.12 13.12 Global Days 090

53000-53520 Open Surgical Procedures of Urethra

53000 **Urethrotomy or urethrostomy, external (separate procedure); pendulous urethra**

EXCLUDES *Endoscopic procedures; cystoscopy, urethroscopy, cystourethroscopy (52000-52700)*
Urethrocystography injection procedure (51600-51610)

4.41 4.41 Global Days 010

53010 **perineal urethra, external**

EXCLUDES *Endoscopic procedures; cystoscopy, urethroscopy, cystourethroscopy (52000-52700)*
Urethrocystography injection procedure (51600-51610)

8.74 8.74 Global Days 090

53020 **Meatotomy, cutting of meatus (separate procedure); except infant**

2.88 2.88 Global Days 000

53025 **infant**

2.01 2.01 Global Days 000

53040 **Drainage of deep periurethral abscess**

EXCLUDES *Incision and drainage of subcutaneous abscess (10060, 10061)*

11.63 11.63 Global Days 090

53060 **Drainage of Skene's gland abscess or cyst**

4.99 5.56 Global Days 010

53080 **Drainage of perineal urinary extravasation; uncomplicated (separate procedure)**

12.57 12.57 Global Days 090

53085 **complicated**

19.27 19.27 Global Days 090

53200 **Biopsy of urethra**

4.20 4.61 Global Days 000

53210 **Urethrectomy, total, including cystostomy; female**

22.92 22.92 Global Days 090

53215 **male**

27.49 27.49 Global Days 090

53220 **Excision or fulguration of carcinoma of urethra**

13.49 13.49 Global Days 090

53230 **Excision of urethral diverticulum (separate procedure); female**

18.08 18.08 Global Days 090

53235 **male**

18.78 18.78 Global Days 090

53240 **Marsupialization of urethral diverticulum, male or female**

12.61 12.61 Global Days 090

53250 **Excision of bulbourethral gland (Cowper's gland)**

12.53 12.53 Global Days 090

53260 **Excision or fulguration; urethral polyp(s), distal urethra**

EXCLUDES *Endoscopic method (52214, 52224)*

5.36 6.00 Global Days 010

53265 **urethral caruncle**

EXCLUDES *Endoscopic method (52214, 52224)*

5.52 6.50 Global Days 010

53270 **Skene's glands** ♀ A2 T
EXCLUDES *Endoscopic method (52214, 52224)*
5.61 6.26 Global Days 010

53275 **urethral prolapse** ♀ A2 T
EXCLUDES *Endoscopic method (52214, 52224)*
7.80 7.80 Global Days 010

53400 **Urethroplasty; first stage, for fistula, diverticulum, or stricture (eg, Johannsen type)** A2 T 80
EXCLUDES *Hypospadias repair (54300-54352)*
23.81 23.81 Global Days 090

53405 **second stage (formation of urethra), including urinary diversion** A2 T 80
EXCLUDES *Hypospadias repair (54300-54352)*
25.90 25.90 Global Days 090

53410 **Urethroplasty, 1-stage reconstruction of male anterior urethra** ♂ A2 T 80
EXCLUDES *Hypospadias repair (54300-54352)*
28.96 28.96 Global Days 090

53415 **Urethroplasty, transpubic or perineal, 1-stage, for reconstruction or repair of prostatic or membranous urethra** ♂ C5 C 80
33.51 33.51 Global Days 090

53420 **Urethroplasty, 2-stage reconstruction or repair of prostatic or membranous urethra; first stage** ♂ A2 T
24.59 24.59 Global Days 090

53425 **second stage** ♂ A2 T 80
27.78 27.78 Global Days 090

53430 **Urethroplasty, reconstruction of female urethra** ♀ A2 T 80
28.64 28.64 Global Days 090

53431 **Urethroplasty with tubularization of posterior urethra and/or lower bladder for incontinence (eg, Tenago, Leadbetter procedure)** A2 T 80
34.15 34.15 Global Days 090

53440 **Sling operation for correction of male urinary incontinence (eg, fascia or synthetic)** ♂ J8 S 80
Code also (C1762, C1763, C1771, C1781, C2631)
22.70 22.70 Global Days 090

53442 **Removal or revision of sling for male urinary incontinence (eg, fascia or synthetic)** ♂ A2 T 80
23.13 23.13 Global Days 090

53444 **Insertion of tandem cuff (dual cuff)** J8 S 80
Code also (C1815)
23.50 23.50 Global Days 090

53445 **Insertion of inflatable urethral/bladder neck sphincter, including placement of pump, reservoir, and cuff** J8 S 80
Code also (C1815)
22.73 22.73 Global Days 090

53446 **Removal of inflatable urethral/bladder neck sphincter, including pump, reservoir, and cuff** A2 T 80
19.06 19.06 Global Days 090

53447 **Removal and replacement of inflatable urethral/bladder neck sphincter including pump, reservoir, and cuff at the same operative session** J8 S 80
Code also (C1815)
23.99 23.99 Global Days 090

53448 **Removal and replacement of inflatable urethral/bladder neck sphincter including pump, reservoir, and cuff through an infected field at the same operative session including irrigation and debridement of infected tissue** C5 C 80
Do not report with (11042, 11043)
37.91 37.91 Global Days 090

53449 **Repair of inflatable urethral/bladder neck sphincter, including pump, reservoir, and cuff** A2 T 80
18.15 18.15 Global Days 090

53450 **Urethromeatoplasty, with mucosal advancement** A2 T
EXCLUDES *Meatotomy (53020, 53025)*
12.13 12.13 Global Days 090

53460 **Urethromeatoplasty, with partial excision of distal urethral segment (Richardson type procedure)** A2 T 80
13.55 13.55 Global Days 090

53500 **Urethrolysis, transvaginal, secondary, open, including cystourethroscopy (eg, postsurgical obstruction, scarring)** ♀ T 80
EXCLUDES *Retropubic approach (53899)*
Do not report with (52000)
22.30 22.30 Global Days 090

53502 **Urethrorrhaphy, suture of urethral wound or injury, female** ♀ A2 T
14.38 14.38 Global Days 090

53505 **Urethrorrhaphy, suture of urethral wound or injury; penile** ♂ A2 T 80
14.41 14.41 Global Days 090

53510 **perineal** A2 T 80
18.70 18.70 Global Days 090

53515 **prostatomembranous** ♂ A2 T 80
23.52 23.52 Global Days 090

53520 **Closure of urethrostomy or urethrocutaneous fistula, male (separate procedure)** ♂ A2 T
EXCLUDES *Closure of fistula:*
Urethrorectal (45820, 45825)
Urethrovaginal (57310)
16.48 16.48 Global Days 090

53600-53665 Urethral Dilation

EXCLUDES *Endoscopic procedures; cystoscopy, urethroscopy, cystourethroscopy (52000-52700)*
Urethral catheterization (51701-51703)
Urethrocystography injection procedure (51600-51610)

74485

53600 **Dilation of urethral stricture by passage of sound or urethral dilator, male; initial** ♂ P3 T
1.89 2.48 Global Days 000

53601 **subsequent** ♂ P3 T
1.57 2.41 Global Days 000

53605 **Dilation of urethral stricture or vesical neck by passage of sound or urethral dilator, male, general or conduction (spinal) anesthesia** ♂ A2 T
EXCLUDES *Procedure performed under local anesthesia (53600-53601, 53620-53621)*
1.90 1.90 Global Days 000

53620 **Dilation of urethral stricture by passage of filiform and follower, male; initial** ♂ P3 T
2.59 3.50 Global Days 000

53621 **subsequent** ♂ P3 T
2.13 3.29 Global Days 000

53660 **Dilation of female urethra including suppository and/or instillation; initial** ♀ P3 T
1.23 2.12 Global Days 000

53661 **subsequent** ♀ P3 T
1.20 2.09 Global Days 000

53665 **Dilation of female urethra, general or conduction (spinal) anesthesia** ♀ A2 T CCI

EXCLUDES *Procedure performed under local anesthesia (53660-53661)*

74485

1.14 1.14 Global Days 000

53850-53899 Endoscopic Procedures via Urethra: Prostate

EXCLUDES *Endoscopic procedures; cystoscopy, urethroscopy, cystourethroscopy (52000-52700)*

Urethrocystography injection procedure (51600-51610)

53850 **Transurethral destruction of prostate tissue; by microwave thermotherapy** ♂ P3 T CCI

81020

16.84 63.46 Global Days 090

53852 **by radiofrequency thermotherapy** ♂ P3 T CCI

81020

18.43 61.25 Global Days 090

53855 **Insertion of a temporary prostatic urethral stent, including urethral measurement** ♂ P2 T 80

EXCLUDES *Permanent urethral stent insertion (52282)*

2.39 22.23 Global Days 000

53860 **Transurethral radiofrequency micro-remodeling of the female bladder neck and proximal urethra for stress urinary incontinence** ♀ G2 T 80

6.88 44.81 Global Days 090

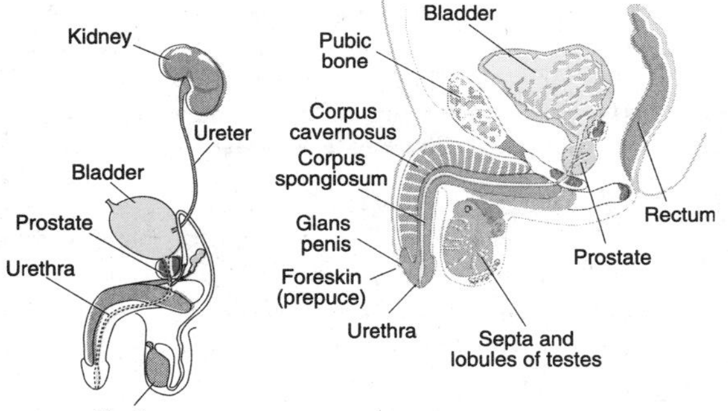

53899 **Unlisted procedure, urinary system** T 80

81020

0.00 0.00 Global Days YYY

AMA: 2009, Jan, 11-31; 2008, Jan, 10-25; 2007, January, 13-27

Urinary System

53665 — 53899

54000-54015 Procedures of Penis: Incisional

EXCLUDES *Debridement of abdominal perineal gangrene (11004-11006)*

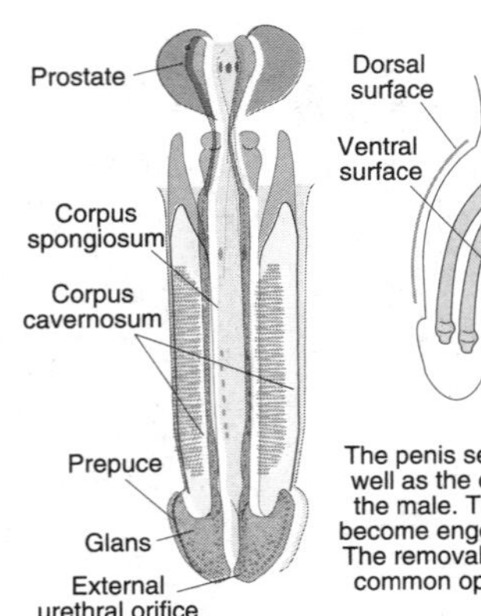

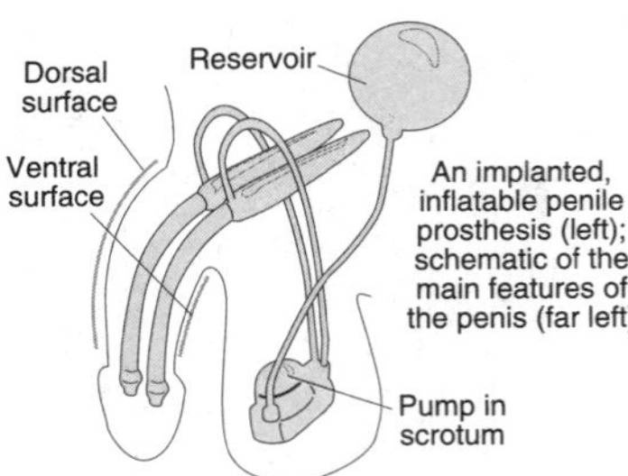

An implanted, inflatable penile prosthesis (left); schematic of the main features of the penis (far left)

The penis serves as the organ of copulation as well as the outlet for seminal fluid and urine in the male. Three cylindrical bodies, or corpora, become engorged with blood to form an erection. The removal of the prepuce by circumcision is a common operation on infant and young males

54000 **Slitting of prepuce, dorsal or lateral (separate procedure); newborn** A ♂ A2 T 80 63
3.19 4.46 Global Days 010

54001 **except newborn** ♂ A2 T
4.12 5.56 Global Days 010

54015 **Incision and drainage of penis, deep** ♂ A2 T 80
EXCLUDES *Abscess, skin/subcutaneous (10060-10160)*
9.12 9.12 Global Days 010

54050-54065 Destruction of Penis Lesions: Multiple Methods

CMS 100-3,140.5 Laser Procedures
EXCLUDES *Excision/destruction other lesions (11420-11426, 11620-11626, 17000-17250, 17270-17276)*

54050 **Destruction of lesion(s), penis (eg, condyloma, papilloma, molluscum contagiosum, herpetic vesicle), simple; chemical** ♂ P3 T
3.08 3.86 Global Days 010

54055 **electrodesiccation** ♂ P3 T
2.72 3.50 Global Days 010

54056 **cryosurgery** ♂ P2 T
3.28 4.17 Global Days 010

54057 **laser surgery** ♂ A2 T
2.78 4.07 Global Days 010

54060 **surgical excision** ♂ A2 T
3.87 5.40 Global Days 010

54065 **Destruction of lesion(s), penis (eg, condyloma, papilloma, molluscum contagiosum, herpetic vesicle), extensive (eg, laser surgery, electrosurgery, cryosurgery, chemosurgery)** ♂ A2 T
5.09 6.51 Global Days 010

54100-54115 Procedures of Penis: Excisional

54100 **Biopsy of penis; (separate procedure)** ♂ A2 T
3.74 5.88 Global Days 000

54105 **deep structures** ♂ A2 T
6.31 7.91 Global Days 010

54110 **Excision of penile plaque (Peyronie disease);** ♂ A2 T 80
18.48 18.48 Global Days 090

54111 **with graft to 5 cm in length** ♂ A2 T 80
23.73 23.73 Global Days 090
AMA: 2009, Jan, 11-31; 2008, Jan, 10-25; 2007, January, 13-27

54112 **with graft greater than 5 cm in length** ♂ A2 T 80
27.79 27.79 Global Days 090

54115 **Removal foreign body from deep penile tissue (eg, plastic implant)** ♂ A2 T 80
12.56 13.39 Global Days 090

54120-54135 Amputation of Penis

EXCLUDES *Lymphadenectomy (separate procedure) (38760-38770)*

54120 **Amputation of penis; partial** ♂ A2 T 80
18.73 18.73 Global Days 090

54125 **complete** ♂ C5 C 80
24.09 24.09 Global Days 090

54130 **Amputation of penis, radical; with bilateral inguinofemoral lymphadenectomy** ♂ C5 C 80
35.35 35.35 Global Days 090

54135 **in continuity with bilateral pelvic lymphadenectomy, including external iliac, hypogastric and obturator nodes** ♂ C5 C 80
45.94 45.94 Global Days 090

54150-54164 Circumcision Procedures

54150 **Circumcision, using clamp or other device with regional dorsal penile or ring block** A ♂ A2 T 80 63
Code also modifier 52 when performed without dorsal penile or ring block
2.92 4.78 Global Days 000
AMA: 2009, Mar, 3,4&7; 2009, Jan, 11-31; 2008, Jan, 10-25; 2007, Jul, 5; 2007, January, 13-27; 2007, May, 9-11

54160 **Circumcision, surgical excision other than clamp, device, or dorsal slit; neonate (28 days of age or less)** A ♂ A2 T 63
4.26 6.62 Global Days 010
AMA: 2009, Jan, 11-31; 2008, Jan, 10-25; 2007, Jul, 5; 2007, May, 9-11; 2007, January, 13-27

54161 **older than 28 days of age** ♂ A2 T
5.85 5.85 Global Days 010
AMA: 2009, Jan, 11-31; 2008, Jan, 10-25; 2007, Jul, 5; 2007, May, 9-11; 2007, January, 13-27

54162 **Lysis or excision of penile post-circumcision adhesions** ♂ A2 T
5.89 7.76 Global Days 010

54163 **Repair incomplete circumcision** ♂ A2 T
6.50 6.50 Global Days 010

54164 **Frenulotomy of penis** ♂ A2 T
Do not report with (54150, 54160-54163)
5.74 5.74 Global Days 010

54200-54250 Evaluation and Treatment of Erectile Abnormalities

54200 **Injection procedure for Peyronie disease;** ♂ P3 T
2.50 3.21 Global Days 010

54205 **with surgical exposure of plaque** ♂ A2 T 80
15.82 15.82 Global Days 090

54220 **Irrigation of corpora cavernosa for priapism** ♂ A2 T
4.00 6.10 Global Days 000

54230 **Injection procedure for corpora cavernosography** ♂ N1 N
74445
2.36 2.86 Global Days 000

54231 **Dynamic cavernosometry, including intracavernosal injection of vasoactive drugs (eg, papaverine, phentolamine)**
3.46 4.16 Global Days 000

54235 **Injection of corpora cavernosa with pharmacologic agent(s) (eg, papaverine, phentolamine)**
2.18 2.67 Global Days 000
AMA: 2009, Jan, 11-31; 2008, Jan, 10-25; 2007, January, 13-27

54240 **Penile plethysmography**
2.94 2.94 Global Days 000

54250 **Nocturnal penile tumescence and/or rigidity test**
3.58 3.58 Global Days 000

54300-54390 Hypospadias Repair and Related Procedures

EXCLUDES *Other urethroplasties (53400-53430)*
Revascularization of penis (37788)

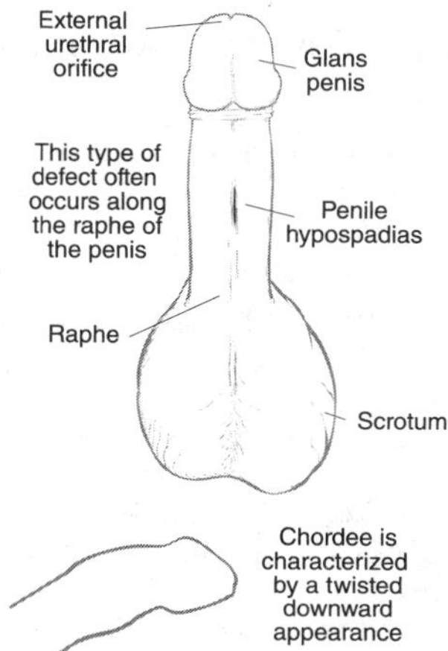

Plastic repair is performed on the penis. Report 54300 to straighten chordee and 54304 to otherwise address chordee and or hypospadias repair

54300 **Plastic operation of penis for straightening of chordee (eg, hypospadias), with or without mobilization of urethra**
19.08 19.08 Global Days 090

54304 **Plastic operation on penis for correction of chordee or for first stage hypospadias repair with or without transplantation of prepuce and/or skin flaps**
22.29 22.29 Global Days 090

54308 **Urethroplasty for second stage hypospadias repair (including urinary diversion); less than 3 cm**
21.83 21.83 Global Days 090

54312 **greater than 3 cm**
24.33 24.33 Global Days 090

54316 **Urethroplasty for second stage hypospadias repair (including urinary diversion) with free skin graft obtained from site other than genitalia**
30.42 30.42 Global Days 090

54318 **Urethroplasty for third stage hypospadias repair to release penis from scrotum (eg, third stage Cecil repair)**
20.78 20.78 Global Days 090

54322 **1-stage distal hypospadias repair (with or without chordee or circumcision); with simple meatal advancement (eg, Magpi, V-flap)**
23.21 23.21 Global Days 090

54324 **with urethroplasty by local skin flaps (eg, flip-flap, prepucial flap)**
INCLUDES Browne's operation
28.79 28.79 Global Days 090

54326 **with urethroplasty by local skin flaps and mobilization of urethra**
27.81 27.81 Global Days 090

54328 **with extensive dissection to correct chordee and urethroplasty with local skin flaps, skin graft patch, and/or island flap**
EXCLUDES *Urethroplasty/straightening of chordee (54308)*
27.81 27.81 Global Days 090
AMA: 2009, Jan, 11-31; 2008, Jan, 10-25; 2007, January, 13-27

54332 **1-stage proximal penile or penoscrotal hypospadias repair requiring extensive dissection to correct chordee and urethroplasty by use of skin graft tube and/or island flap**
30.10 30.10 Global Days 090
AMA: 2009, Jan, 11-31; 2008, Jan, 10-25; 2007, January, 13-27

54336 **1-stage perineal hypospadias repair requiring extensive dissection to correct chordee and urethroplasty by use of skin graft tube and/or island flap**
34.81 34.81 Global Days 090
AMA: 2009, Jan, 11-31; 2008, Jan, 10-25; 2007, January, 13-27

54340 **Repair of hypospadias complications (ie, fistula, stricture, diverticula); by closure, incision, or excision, simple**
16.84 16.84 Global Days 090

54344 **requiring mobilization of skin flaps and urethroplasty with flap or patch graft**
28.17 28.17 Global Days 090

54348 **requiring extensive dissection and urethroplasty with flap, patch or tubed graft (includes urinary diversion)**
29.66 29.66 Global Days 090

54352 **Repair of hypospadias cripple requiring extensive dissection and excision of previously constructed structures including re-release of chordee and reconstruction of urethra and penis by use of local skin as grafts and island flaps and skin brought in as flaps or grafts**
42.11 42.11 Global Days 090

54360 **Plastic operation on penis to correct angulation**
21.43 21.43 Global Days 090

54380 **Plastic operation on penis for epispadias distal to external sphincter;**
INCLUDES Lowsley's operation
26.24 26.24 Global Days 090

54385 **with incontinence**
29.51 29.51 Global Days 090

54390 **with exstrophy of bladder**
37.17 37.17 Global Days 090

54400-54417 Procedures to Treat Impotence

CMS 100-3,230.4 Diagnosis and Treatment of Impotence

EXCLUDES *Other urethroplasties (53400-53430)*
Revascularization of penis (37788)

54400 Insertion of penile prosthesis; non-inflatable (semi-rigid) ♂ J8 S

EXCLUDES *Replacement/removal penile prosthesis (54415, 54416)*

Code also (C2622)

15.72 15.72 Global Days 090

54401 inflatable (self-contained) ♂ J8 S PO

EXCLUDES *Replacement/removal penile prosthesis (54415, 54416)*

Code also (C1813)

19.49 19.49 Global Days 090

54405 Insertion of multi-component, inflatable penile prosthesis, including placement of pump, cylinders, and reservoir ♂ J8 S 80 PO

Code also (C1813)

Code also modifier 52 for reduced services

23.97 23.97 Global Days 090

54406 Removal of all components of a multi-component, inflatable penile prosthesis without replacement of prosthesis ♂ A2 T 80 PO

Code also modifier 52 for reduced services

21.64 21.64 Global Days 090

54408 Repair of component(s) of a multi-component, inflatable penile prosthesis ♂ A2 T 80 PO

23.42 23.42 Global Days 090

54410 Removal and replacement of all component(s) of a multi-component, inflatable penile prosthesis at the same operative session ♂ J8 S 80 PO

Code also (C1813)

25.50 25.50 Global Days 090

54411 Removal and replacement of all components of a multi-component inflatable penile prosthesis through an infected field at the same operative session, including irrigation and debridement of infected tissue ♂ C5 C 80

Code also modifier 52 for reduced services

Do not report with (11042, 11043)

30.36 30.36 Global Days 090

54415 Removal of non-inflatable (semi-rigid) or inflatable (self-contained) penile prosthesis, without replacement of prosthesis ♂ A2 T 80 PO

15.67 15.67 Global Days 090

54416 Removal and replacement of non-inflatable (semi-rigid) or inflatable (self-contained) penile prosthesis at the same operative session ♂ J8 S 80 PO

Code also (C1813, C2622)

21.06 21.06 Global Days 090

54417 Removal and replacement of non-inflatable (semi-rigid) or inflatable (self-contained) penile prosthesis through an infected field at the same operative session, including irrigation and debridement of infected tissue ♂ C5 C 80

Do not report with (11042, 11043)

26.62 26.62 Global Days 090

54420-54450 Other Procedures of the Penis

EXCLUDES *Other urethroplasties (53400-53430)*
Revascularization of penis (37788)

54420 Corpora cavernosa-saphenous vein shunt (priapism operation), unilateral or bilateral ♂ A2 T 80

20.93 20.93 Global Days 090

54430 Corpora cavernosa-corpus spongiosum shunt (priapism operation), unilateral or bilateral ♂ C5 C 80

19.01 19.01 Global Days 090

54435 Corpora cavernosa-glans penis fistulization (eg, biopsy needle, Winter procedure, rongeur, or punch) for priapism ♂ A2 T

12.37 12.37 Global Days 090

54440 Plastic operation of penis for injury ♂ A2 T 80

0.00 0.00 Global Days 090

54450 Foreskin manipulation including lysis of preputial adhesions and stretching ♂ A2 T

1.70 2.08 Global Days 000

54500-54560 Testicular Procedures: Incisional

EXCLUDES *Debridement of abdominal perineal gangrene (11004-11006)*

54500 Biopsy of testis, needle (separate procedure) ♂ A2 T 80 50

EXCLUDES *Fine needle aspiration (10021, 10022)*

88172, 88173

2.21 2.21 Global Days 000

54505 Biopsy of testis, incisional (separate procedure) ♂ A2 T 80 50

Code also vasotomy for vasogram, seminal vesiculogram, epididymogram when combined (55300)

6.24 6.24 Global Days 010

54512 Excision of extraparenchymal lesion of testis ♂ A2 T 50

15.99 15.99 Global Days 090

AMA: 2009, Jan, 11-31; 2008, Jan, 10-25; 2007, January, 13-27

54520 Orchiectomy, simple (including subcapsular), with or without testicular prosthesis, scrotal or inguinal approach ♂ A2 T 50

INCLUDES Huggins' orchiectomy

EXCLUDES *Lymphadenectomy, radical retroperitoneal (38780)*

Code also hernia repair if performed (49505, 49507)

9.71 9.71 Global Days 090

54522 Orchiectomy, partial ♂ A2 T 80 50

EXCLUDES *Lymphadenectomy, radical retroperitoneal (38780)*

17.38 17.38 Global Days 090

54530 Orchiectomy, radical, for tumor; inguinal approach ♂ A2 T 80 50

EXCLUDES *Lymphadenectomy, radical retroperitoneal (38780)*

15.02 15.02 Global Days 090

54535 with abdominal exploration ♂ T 80 50

EXCLUDES *Lymphadenectomy, radical retroperitoneal (38780)*

21.94 21.94 Global Days 090

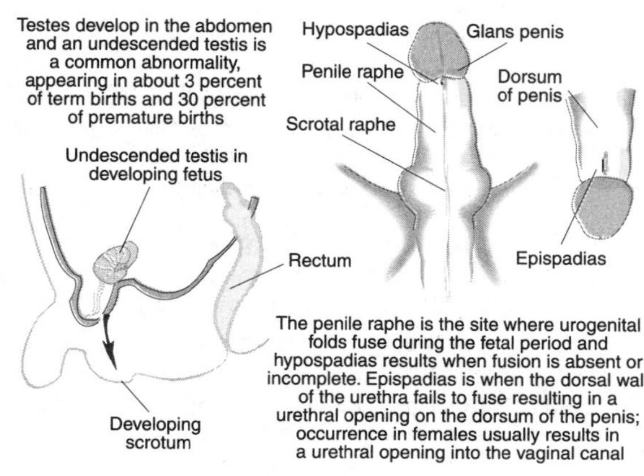

54550 **Exploration for undescended testis (inguinal or scrotal area)** ♂ A2 T 80 50
14.55 14.55 Global Days 090
AMA: 2007, Jul, 5

54560 **Exploration for undescended testis with abdominal exploration** ♂ G2 T 80 50
21.33 21.33 Global Days 090
AMA: 2007, Jul, 5

54600-54699 Open and Laparoscopic Testicular Procedures

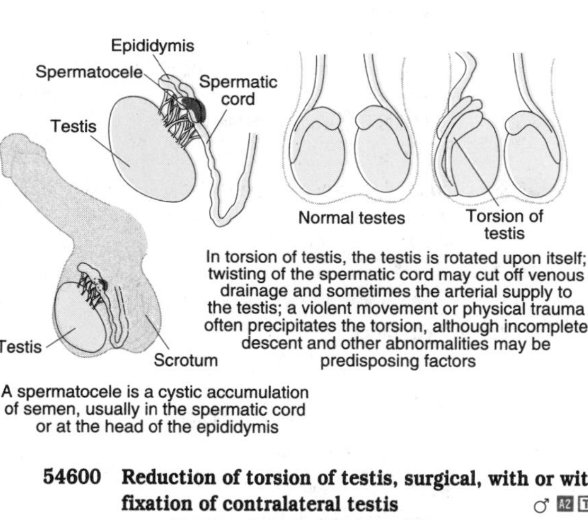

54600 **Reduction of torsion of testis, surgical, with or without fixation of contralateral testis** ♂ A2 T 50
13.41 13.41 Global Days 090
AMA: 2009, Jan, 11-31; 2008, Jan, 10-25; 2007, January, 13-27

54620 **Fixation of contralateral testis (separate procedure)** ♂ A2 T 50
8.90 8.90 Global Days 010

54640 **Orchiopexy, inguinal approach, with or without hernia repair** ♂ A2 T 80 50
INCLUDES Bevan's operation
Koop inguinal orchiopexy
Prentice orchiopexy
EXCLUDES *Repair inguinal hernia with inguinal orchiopexy (49495-49525)*
14.17 14.17 Global Days 090
AMA: 2009, Jan, 11-31; 2008, Jan, 10-25; 2008, Jun, 3-6; 2007, January, 13-27

54650 **Orchiopexy, abdominal approach, for intra-abdominal testis (eg, Fowler-Stephens)** ♂ T 80 50
EXCLUDES *Laparoscopic orchiopexy (54692)*
21.02 21.02 Global Days 090

54660 **Insertion of testicular prosthesis (separate procedure)** ♂ A2 T 80 50
10.56 10.56 Global Days 090

54670 **Suture or repair of testicular injury** ♂ A2 T 80 50
12.00 12.00 Global Days 090

54680 **Transplantation of testis(es) to thigh (because of scrotal destruction)** ♂ A2 T 80 50
23.22 23.22 Global Days 090

54690 **Laparoscopy, surgical; orchiectomy** ♂ A2 T 80 50
INCLUDES Diagnostic laparoscopy
21.63 21.63 Global Days 090

54692 **orchiopexy for intra-abdominal testis** ♂ G2 T 50
INCLUDES Diagnostic laparoscopy
22.50 22.50 Global Days 090

54699 **Unlisted laparoscopy procedure, testis** ♂ T 80 50
0.00 0.00 Global Days YYY

54700-54901 Open Procedures of the Epididymis

54700 **Incision and drainage of epididymis, testis and/or scrotal space (eg, abscess or hematoma)** ♂ A2 T
EXCLUDES *Debridement of genitalia for necrotizing soft tissue infection (11004-11006)*
6.34 6.34 Global Days 010

54800 **Biopsy of epididymis, needle** ♂ A2 T 80
EXCLUDES *Fine needle aspiration (10021, 10022)*
88172, 88173
3.87 3.87 Global Days 000
AMA: 2007, Jul, 5

54830 **Excision of local lesion of epididymis** ♂ A2 T 80
11.06 11.06 Global Days 090

54840 **Excision of spermatocele, with or without epididymectomy** ♂ A2 T
9.54 9.54 Global Days 090

54860 **Epididymectomy; unilateral** ♂ A2 T
12.42 12.42 Global Days 090

54861 **bilateral** ♂ A2 T 80
16.75 16.75 Global Days 090

54865 **Exploration of epididymis, with or without biopsy** ♂ A2 T 80
10.63 10.63 Global Days 090
AMA: 2007, Jul, 5

54900 **Epididymovasostomy, anastomosis of epididymis to vas deferens; unilateral** ♂ A2 T 80
EXCLUDES *Operating microscope (69990)*
22.95 22.95 Global Days 090
AMA: 2009, Jan, 11-31; 2008, Jan, 10-25; 2007, January, 13-27

54901 **bilateral** ♂ A2 T 80
EXCLUDES *Operating microscope (69990)*
30.81 30.81 Global Days 090
AMA: 2009, Jan, 11-31; 2008, Jan, 10-25; 2007, January, 13-27

55000-55180 Procedures of the Tunica Vaginalis and Scrotum

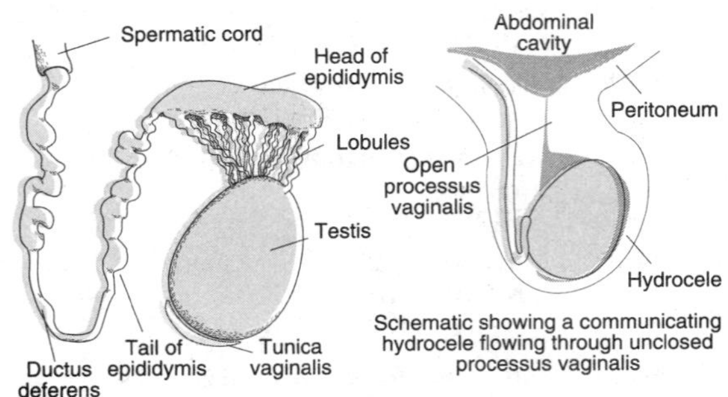

The tunica vaginalis is a closed sac within the scrotum and is the lower remnant of the path taken by the testis as it descends from the abdomen just prior to birth. The presence of fluid in this pathway is called a hydrocele. The testes, or testicles, are the male reproductive organs. Each produces sperm and male sex hormones

55000 Puncture aspiration of hydrocele, tunica vaginalis, with or without injection of medication ♂ P3 T
2.51 3.52 Global Days 000

55040 Excision of hydrocele; unilateral ♂ A2 T
EXCLUDES *Repair of hernia with hydrocelectomy (49495-49501)*
10.07 10.07 Global Days 090
AMA: 2008, Jun, 3-6

55041 bilateral ♂ A2 T
EXCLUDES *Repair of hernia with hydrocelectomy (49495-49501)*
15.13 15.13 Global Days 090

55060 Repair of tunica vaginalis hydrocele (Bottle type) ♂ A2 T 80 50
11.29 11.29 Global Days 090

55100 Drainage of scrotal wall abscess ♂ A2 T
EXCLUDES *Debridement of genitalia for necrotizing soft tissue infection (11004-11006)*
Incision and drainage of scrotal space (54700)
4.94 6.46 Global Days 010

55110 Scrotal exploration ♂ A2 T
11.52 11.52 Global Days 090

55120 Removal of foreign body in scrotum ♂ A2 T 80
10.66 10.66 Global Days 090

55150 Resection of scrotum ♂ A2 T 80
EXCLUDES *Lesion excision of skin of scrotum (11420-11426, 11620-11626)*
14.57 14.57 Global Days 090

55175 Scrotoplasty; simple ♂ A2 T 80
10.78 10.78 Global Days 090

55180 complicated ♂ A2 T 80
20.58 20.58 Global Days 090

55200-55680 Procedures of Other Male Genital Ducts and Glands

55200 Vasotomy, cannulization with or without incision of vas, unilateral or bilateral (separate procedure) ♂ A2 T 80
8.22 13.41 Global Days 090

55250 Vasectomy, unilateral or bilateral (separate procedure), including postoperative semen examination(s) ♂ A2 T
6.74 11.86 Global Days 090
AMA: 2009, Jan, 11-31; 2008, Jan, 10-25; 2007, January, 13-27

55300 Vasotomy for vasograms, seminal vesiculograms, or epididymograms, unilateral or bilateral ♂ N1 N 80
Code also biopsy of testis when combined (54505)
74440
5.48 5.48 Global Days 000

55400 Vasovasostomy, vasovasorrhaphy ♂ A2 T 80 50
EXCLUDES *Operating microscope (69990)*
14.80 14.80 Global Days 090
AMA: 2009, Jan, 11-31; 2008, Jan, 10-25; 2007, January, 13-27

55450 Ligation (percutaneous) of vas deferens, unilateral or bilateral (separate procedure) ♂ P3 T 80
7.59 10.83 Global Days 010

55500 Excision of hydrocele of spermatic cord, unilateral (separate procedure) ♂ A2 T 80
11.73 11.73 Global Days 090

55520 Excision of lesion of spermatic cord (separate procedure) ♂ A2 T 80
13.21 13.21 Global Days 090
AMA: 2009, Jan, 11-31; 2008, Jan, 10-25; 2007, January, 13-27

55530 Excision of varicocele or ligation of spermatic veins for varicocele; (separate procedure) ♂ A2 T 50
10.51 10.51 Global Days 090

55535 abdominal approach ♂ A2 T 80 50
12.72 12.72 Global Days 090

55540 with hernia repair ♂ A2 T 50
15.74 15.74 Global Days 090

55550 Laparoscopy, surgical, with ligation of spermatic veins for varicocele ♂ A2 T 80 50
INCLUDES Diagnostic laparoscopy
12.62 12.62 Global Days 090

55559 Unlisted laparoscopy procedure, spermatic cord ♂ T 80 50
0.00 0.00 Global Days YYY

55600 Vesiculotomy; ♂ A2 T 80 50
12.50 12.50 Global Days 090

55605 complicated ♂ C5 C 80 50
15.27 15.27 Global Days 090

55650 Vesiculectomy, any approach ♂ C5 C 80 50
21.20 21.20 Global Days 090

55680 Excision of Mullerian duct cyst ♂ A2 T 80
EXCLUDES *Injection procedure (52010, 55300)*
10.18 10.18 Global Days 090

55700-55725 Procedures of Prostate: Incisional

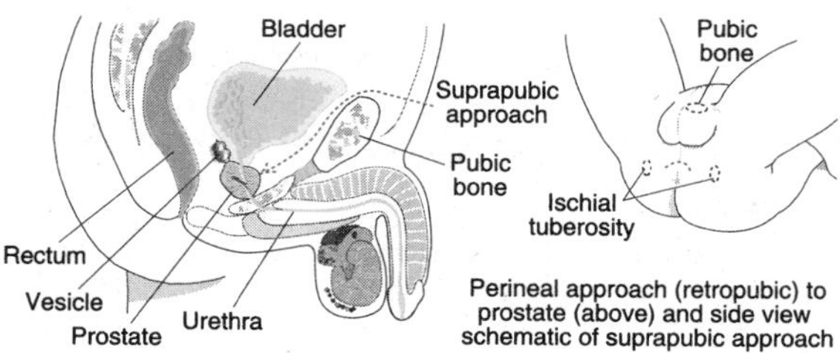

Perineal approach (retropubic) to prostate (above) and side view schematic of suprapubic approach

The walnut-sized prostate gland secretes a thin, milky fluid that mixes with spermatic fluids during ejaculation; its secretion constitutes about one-third of the volume of seminal fluid. The prostate is palpable via the rectum. Some procedures are via the urethra, which can be dilated to accommodate instruments. The seminal vesicles may also be palpated via the rectum. Each is a long, coiled tube which secretes a thick fluid that mixes with sperm as it passes along the ejaculatory ducts. The ejaculatory ducts are the union of the seminal vesicles and the sperm-carrying ductus deferens

55700 Biopsy, prostate; needle or punch, single or multiple, any approach ♂ A2 T

EXCLUDES *Fine needle aspiration (10021, 10022)*
Needle biopsy of prostate, saturation sampling for prostate mapping (55706)

88172, 88173
76942
4.12 6.59 Global Days 000

55705 incisional, any approach ♂ A2 T
7.91 7.91 Global Days 010

55706 Biopsies, prostate, needle, transperineal, stereotactic template guided saturation sampling, including imaging guidance ♂ G2 T 80

Do not report with (55700)
10.98 10.98 Global Days 010

55720 Prostatotomy, external drainage of prostatic abscess, any approach; simple ♂ A2 T 80

EXCLUDES *Drainage of prostatic abscess, transurethral (52700)*

13.37 13.37 Global Days 090

55725 complicated ♂ A2 T 80

EXCLUDES *Drainage of prostatic abscess, transurethral (52700)*

17.54 17.54 Global Days 090

55801-55845 Open Prostatectomy

EXCLUDES *Node dissection, independent (38770-38780)*
Pelvic limited lymphadenectomy for staging (separate procedure) (38562)
Transurethral prostate
Destruction (53850-53852)
Resection (52601-52640)

55801 Prostatectomy, perineal, subtotal (including control of postoperative bleeding, vasectomy, meatotomy, urethral calibration and/or dilation, and internal urethrotomy) ♂ C5 C 80 PQ
32.32 32.32 Global Days 090

55810 Prostatectomy, perineal radical; ♂ C5 C 80 PQ

INCLUDES Walsh modified radical prostatectomy

39.00 39.00 Global Days 090

55812 with lymph node biopsy(s) (limited pelvic lymphadenectomy) ♂ C5 C 80 PQ
47.65 47.65 Global Days 090

55815 with bilateral pelvic lymphadenectomy, including external iliac, hypogastric and obturator nodes ♂ C5 C 80 PQ

EXCLUDES *Perineal radical prostatectomy when performed on a separate day from bilateral pelvic lymphadenectomy (38770, 55810)*

52.22 52.22 Global Days 090

55821 Prostatectomy (including control of postoperative bleeding, vasectomy, meatotomy, urethral calibration and/or dilation, and internal urethrotomy); suprapubic, subtotal, 1 or 2 stages ♂ C5 C 80 PQ
25.90 25.90 Global Days 090

55831 retropubic, subtotal ♂ C5 C 80 PQ
28.00 28.00 Global Days 090

55840 Prostatectomy, retropubic radical, with or without nerve sparing; ♂ C5 C 80 PQ

EXCLUDES *Prostatectomy, radical retropubic, performed laparoscopically (55866)*

39.62 39.62 Global Days 090

55842 with lymph node biopsy(s) (limited pelvic lymphadenectomy) ♂ C5 C 80 PQ
42.45 42.45 Global Days 090

55845 with bilateral pelvic lymphadenectomy, including external iliac, hypogastric, and obturator nodes ♂ C5 C 80 PQ

EXCLUDES *Radical retropubic prostatectomy when performed on a separate day from bilateral pelvic lymphadenectomy (38770, 55840)*

48.45 48.45 Global Days 090

55860-55865 Prostate Exposure for Radiation Source Application

55860 Exposure of prostate, any approach, for insertion of radioactive substance; ♂ G2 T
77776-77778
25.89 25.89 Global Days 090

55862 with lymph node biopsy(s) (limited pelvic lymphadenectomy) ♂ C5 C 80
32.51 32.51 Global Days 090

55865 with bilateral pelvic lymphadenectomy, including external iliac, hypogastric and obturator nodes ♂ C5 C 80
39.55 39.55 Global Days 090

55866 Laparoscopic Prostatectomy

55866 Laparoscopy, surgical prostatectomy, retropubic radical, including nerve sparing, includes robotic assistance, when performed ♂ C5 C 80 PQ

INCLUDES Diagnostic laparoscopy

EXCLUDES *Open method (55840)*

51.37 51.37 Global Days 090

55870-55899 Miscellaneous Prostate Procedures

55870 Electroejaculation ♂ P3 T

EXCLUDES *Artificial insemination (58321-58322)*

4.24 5.21 Global Days 000

55873 Cryosurgical ablation of the prostate (includes ultrasonic guidance and monitoring) ♂ J8 T PQ

Code also (C2618)
23.77 197.23 Global Days 090

55875 **Transperineal placement of needles or catheters into prostate for interstitial radioelement application, with or without cystoscopy** ♂ A2 03 80

EXCLUDES *The placement of needles or catheters into the pelvic organs and/or genitalia (except for the prostate) for interstitial radioelement application (55920)*

76965, 77776-77787

22.56 22.56 Global Days 090

AMA: 2008, Jun, 8-11; 2007, March, 7-8; 2007, May, 1-2

55876 **Placement of interstitial device(s) for radiation therapy guidance (eg, fiducial markers, dosimeter), prostate (via needle, any approach), single or multiple** ♂ P3 X

Code also supply of device

76942, 77002, 77012, 77021

2.98 4.02 Global Days 000

AMA: 2007, May, 1-2

55899 **Unlisted procedure, male genital system** ♂ T 80

0.00 0.00 Global Days YYY

AMA: 2007, May, 1-2

55920 Insertion Brachytherapy Catheters/Needles Pelvis/Genitalia, Male/Female

55920 **Placement of needles or catheters into pelvic organs and/or genitalia (except prostate) for subsequent interstitial radioelement application** G2 T 80

EXCLUDES *Insertion of Heyman capsules for purposes of brachytherapy (58346)*
Insertion of vaginal ovoids and/or uterine tandems for purposes of brachytherapy (57155)
Placement of catheters or needles, prostate (55875)

12.81 12.81 Global Days 000

55970-55980 Transsexual Surgery

CMS 100-2,16,180 Services Related to Noncovered Procedures
CMS 100-3,140.3 Transexual Surgery

55970 **Intersex surgery; male to female** ♂ E

0.00 0.00 Global Days XXX

55980 **female to male** ♀ E

0.00 0.00 Global Days XXX

56405-56420 Incision and Drainage of Abscess

EXCLUDES *Incision and drainage Skene's gland cyst/abscess (53060)*
Incision and drainage subcutaneous abscess/cyst/furuncle (10040, 10060, 10061)

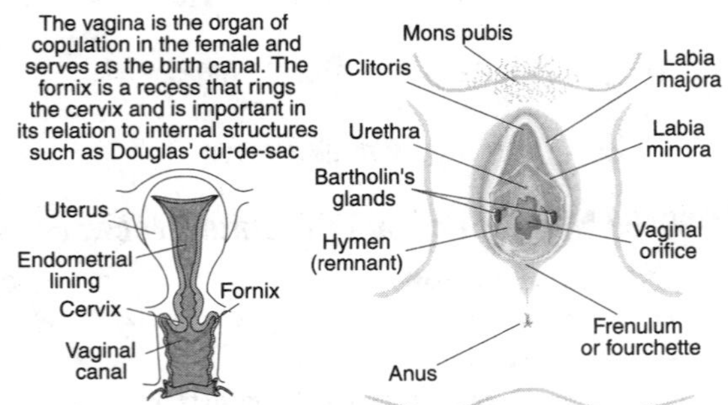

The external female genital region is collectively known as the vulva, or sometimes, the pudendum. A Bartholin's gland is located on either side of the orifice. The perineum is the space between the anus and the vagina, but is often generally defined as the entire pelvic floor and its related structures. Introitus is a general term for the vaginal entrance

56405 **Incision and drainage of vulva or perineal abscess** ♀ P3 T

3.23 3.27 Global Days 010

56420 **Incision and drainage of Bartholin's gland abscess** ♀ P3 T

2.73 3.65 Global Days 010

56440-56442 Other Female Genital Incisional Procedures

EXCLUDES *Incision and drainage subcutaneous abscess/cyst/furuncle (10040, 10060, 10061)*

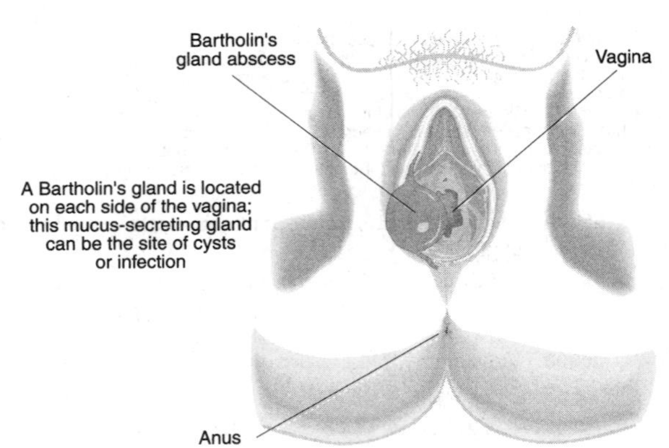

56440 **Marsupialization of Bartholin's gland cyst** ♀ A2 T

5.46 5.46 Global Days 010

56441 **Lysis of labial adhesions** ♀ A2 T 80

4.12 4.30 Global Days 010

56442 **Hymenotomy, simple incision** ♀ A2 T 80

1.44 1.44 Global Days 000

56501-56515 Destruction of Vulvar Lesions, Any Method

CMS 100-3,140.5 Laser Procedures

EXCLUDES *Excision/fulguration/destruction*
Skene's glands (53270)
Urethral caruncle (53265)

56501 **Destruction of lesion(s), vulva; simple (eg, laser surgery, electrosurgery, cryosurgery, chemosurgery)** ♀ P3 T

3.42 3.90 Global Days 010

56515 **extensive (eg, laser surgery, electrosurgery, cryosurgery, chemosurgery)** ♀ A2 T

5.93 6.68 Global Days 010

56605-56606 Vulvar and Perineal Biopsies

EXCLUDES *Excision local lesion (11420-11426, 11620-11626)*

56605 **Biopsy of vulva or perineum (separate procedure); 1 lesion** ♀ P3 T

1.80 2.46 Global Days 000

AMA: 2008, Jun, 3-6

\+ 56606 **each separate additional lesion (List separately in addition to code for primary procedure)** ♀ P3 T

Code first (56605)

0.87 1.11 Global Days ZZZ

56620-56640 Vulvectomy Procedures

INCLUDES Removal of:
Greater than 80% of the vulvar area - complete procedure
Less than 80% of the vulvar area - partial procedure
Skin and deep subcutaneous tissue - radical procedure
Skin and superficial subcutaneous tissues - simple procedure

EXCLUDES *Skin graft (15004-15005, 15120, 15121, 15240, 15241)*

56620 Vulvectomy simple; partial ♀ A2 T 80
15.04 15.04 Global Days 090

56625 complete ♀ A2 T 80
17.99 17.99 Global Days 090

56630 Vulvectomy, radical, partial; ♀ C5 C 80 PQ
26.49 26.49 Global Days 090

56631 with unilateral inguinofemoral lymphadenectomy ♀ C5 C 80 PQ
INCLUDES Bassett's operation
33.59 33.59 Global Days 090

56632 with bilateral inguinofemoral lymphadenectomy ♀ C5 C 80 PQ
INCLUDES Bassett's operation
39.04 39.04 Global Days 090

56633 Vulvectomy, radical, complete; ♀ C5 C 80 PQ
INCLUDES Bassett's operation
34.42 34.42 Global Days 090

56634 with unilateral inguinofemoral lymphadenectomy ♀ C5 C 80 PQ
INCLUDES Bassett's operation
36.51 36.51 Global Days 090

56637 with bilateral inguinofemoral lymphadenectomy ♀ C5 C 80 PQ
INCLUDES Bassett's operation
42.78 42.78 Global Days 090

56640 Vulvectomy, radical, complete, with inguinofemoral, iliac, and pelvic lymphadenectomy ♀ C5 C 80 50 PQ
INCLUDES Bassett's operation
EXCLUDES *Lymphadenectomy (38760-38780)*
42.66 42.66 Global Days 090

56700-56740 Other Excisional Procedures: External Female Genitalia

56700 Partial hymenectomy or revision of hymenal ring ♀ A2 T 80
5.60 5.60 Global Days 010

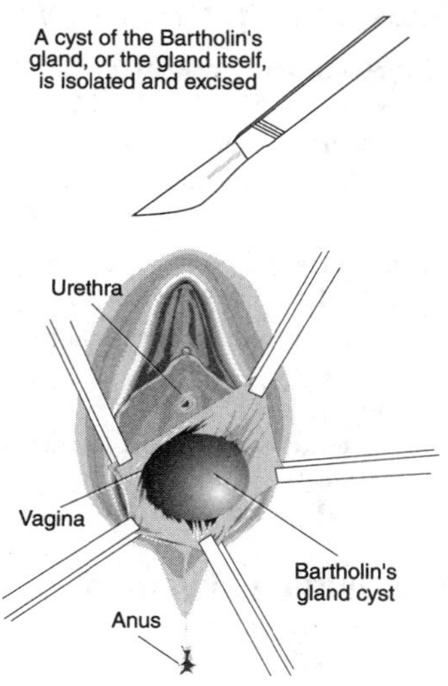

56740 Excision of Bartholin's gland or cyst ♀ A2 T
EXCLUDES *Excision/fulguration/marsupialization:*
Skene's glands (53270)
Urethral carcinoma (53220)
Urethral caruncle (53265)
Urethral diverticulum (53230, 53240)
8.88 8.88 Global Days 010

56800-56810 Repair/Reconstruction External Female Genitalia

EXCLUDES *Repair of urethra for mucosal prolapse (53275)*

56800 Plastic repair of introitus ♀ A2 T 80
INCLUDES Emmet's operation
7.18 7.18 Global Days 010

56805 Clitoroplasty for intersex state ♀ G2 T 80
34.28 34.28 Global Days 090

56810 Perineoplasty, repair of perineum, nonobstetrical (separate procedure) ♀ A2 T 80
INCLUDES Emmet's operation
EXCLUDES *Genitalia wound repair (12001-12007, 12041-12047, 13131-13133)*
Introitus plastic repair (56800)
Sphincteroplasty, anal (46750, 46751)
Vaginal/perineum recent injury repair, nonobstetrical (57210)
Vulva/perineum episiorrhaphy/episioperineorrhaphy for recent injury, nonobstetrical (57210)
7.74 7.74 Global Days 010

56820-56821 Vulvar Colposcopy with/without Biopsy

EXCLUDES *Colposcopic procedures and/or examinations:*
Cervix (57452-57461)
Vagina (57420, 57421)

56820 Colposcopy of the vulva; ♀ P3 T
2.55 3.30 Global Days 000

56821 with biopsy(s) ♀ P3 T
3.42 4.37 Global Days 000

57000-57023 Incisional Procedures: Vagina

57000 **Colpotomy; with exploration** ♀ A2 T 80
5.51 5.51 Global Days 010

57010 **with drainage of pelvic abscess** ♀ A2 T 80
INCLUDES Laroyenne operation
12.97 12.97 Global Days 090

57020 **Colpocentesis (separate procedure)** ♀ A2 T 80
2.44 2.80 Global Days 000

57022 **Incision and drainage of vaginal hematoma; obstetrical/postpartum** ♀ A2 T 80
5.01 5.01 Global Days 010

57023 **non-obstetrical (eg, post-trauma, spontaneous bleeding)** ♀ A2 T 80
9.29 9.29 Global Days 010

57061-57065 Destruction of Vaginal Lesions, Any Method

CMS 100-3,140.5 Laser Procedures

57061 **Destruction of vaginal lesion(s); simple (eg, laser surgery, electrosurgery, cryosurgery, chemosurgery)** ♀ P3 T
2.93 3.40 Global Days 010
AMA: 2009, Jan, 11-31; 2008, Jan, 10-25; 2007, January, 13-27

57065 **extensive (eg, laser surgery, electrosurgery, cryosurgery, chemosurgery)** ♀ A2 T
5.11 5.73 Global Days 010
AMA: 2009, Jan, 11-31; 2008, Jan, 10-25; 2007, January, 13-27

57100-57135 Excisional Procedures: Vagina

57100 **Biopsy of vaginal mucosa; simple (separate procedure)** ♀ P3 T
1.96 2.62 Global Days 000

57105 **extensive, requiring suture (including cysts)** ♀ A2 T
3.73 4.03 Global Days 010

57106 **Vaginectomy, partial removal of vaginal wall;** ♀ T 80
14.37 14.37 Global Days 090

57107 **with removal of paravaginal tissue (radical vaginectomy)** ♀ T 80
41.87 41.87 Global Days 090

57109 **with removal of paravaginal tissue (radical vaginectomy) with bilateral total pelvic lymphadenectomy and para-aortic lymph node sampling (biopsy)** ♀ T 80
47.88 47.88 Global Days 090

57110 **Vaginectomy, complete removal of vaginal wall;** ♀ C5 C 80
26.79 26.79 Global Days 090

57111 **with removal of paravaginal tissue (radical vaginectomy)** ♀ C5 C 80
48.02 48.02 Global Days 090

57112 **with removal of paravaginal tissue (radical vaginectomy) with bilateral total pelvic lymphadenectomy and para-aortic lymph node sampling (biopsy)** ♀ C5 C 80
48.62 48.62 Global Days 090

57120 **Colpocleisis (Le Fort type)** ♀ T 80
15.24 15.24 Global Days 090

57130 **Excision of vaginal septum** ♀ A2 T 80
4.77 5.32 Global Days 010

57135 **Excision of vaginal cyst or tumor** ♀ A2 T
5.14 5.71 Global Days 010

57150-57180 Irrigation/Insertion/Introduction Vaginal Medication or Supply

57150 **Irrigation of vagina and/or application of medicament for treatment of bacterial, parasitic, or fungoid disease** ♀ P3 T
0.87 1.38 Global Days 000

⊙ **57155** **Insertion of uterine tandem and/or vaginal ovoids for clinical brachytherapy** ♀ A2 T
EXCLUDES *The placement of needles or catheters into the pelvic organs and/or genitalia (except for the prostate) for interstitial radioelement application (55920)*
77761-77763, 77785-77787
8.20 12.65 Global Days 000

57156 **Insertion of a vaginal radiation afterloading apparatus for clinical brachytherapy** ♀ G2 T 80
4.16 5.59 Global Days 000

57160 **Fitting and insertion of pessary or other intravaginal support device** ♀ P3 T
1.41 2.28 Global Days 000
AMA: 2009, Jan, 11-31; 2008, Jan, 10-25; 2007, January, 13-27

57170 **Diaphragm or cervical cap fitting with instructions** ♀ P2 T 80
1.44 1.86 Global Days 000

57180 **Introduction of any hemostatic agent or pack for spontaneous or traumatic nonobstetrical vaginal hemorrhage (separate procedure)** ♀ A2 T
3.16 4.21 Global Days 010

57200-57335 Vaginal Repair and Reconstruction

CMS 100-3,230.10 Incontinence Control Devices

EXCLUDES *Marshall-Marchetti-Kranz type urethral suspension, abdominal approach (51840, 51841)*
Urethral suspension performed laparoscopically (51990)

57200 **Colporrhaphy, suture of injury of vagina (nonobstetrical)** ♀ A2 T 80
8.88 8.88 Global Days 090

57210 **Colpoperineorrhaphy, suture of injury of vagina and/or perineum (nonobstetrical)** ♀ A2 T 80
10.91 10.91 Global Days 090

57220 **Plastic operation on urethral sphincter, vaginal approach (eg, Kelly urethral plication)** ♀ A2 T 80
9.54 9.54 Global Days 090

57230 **Plastic repair of urethrocele** ♀ A2 T 80
11.88 11.88 Global Days 090

57240 **Anterior colporrhaphy, repair of cystocele with or without repair of urethrocele** ♀ A2 T 80
19.80 19.80 Global Days 090

57250 **Posterior colporrhaphy, repair of rectocele with or without perineorrhaphy** ♀ A2 T 80
EXCLUDES *Rectocele repair (separate procedure) without posterior colporrhaphy (45560)*
20.05 20.05 Global Days 090

57260 **Combined anteroposterior colporrhaphy;** ♀ A2 T 80
24.72 24.72 Global Days 090

57265 **with enterocele repair** ♀ A2 T 80
27.15 27.15 Global Days 090

+ **57267** **Insertion of mesh or other prosthesis for repair of pelvic floor defect, each site (anterior, posterior compartment), vaginal approach (List separately in addition to code for primary procedure)** ♀ A2 T 80
Code first (45560, 57240-57265, 57285)
7.67 7.67 Global Days ZZZ
AMA: 2009, Jan, 11-31; 2008, Jan, 10-25; 2007, January, 13-27

57268 **Repair of enterocele, vaginal approach (separate procedure)** ♀ A2 T 80
14.38 14.38 Global Days 090

57270 **Repair of enterocele, abdominal approach (separate procedure)** ♀ C5 C 80
23.81 23.81 Global Days 090

57280 **Colpopexy, abdominal approach** ♀ C5 C 80
28.44 28.44 Global Days 090

57282 **Colpopexy, vaginal; extra-peritoneal approach (sacrospinous, iliococcygeus)** ♀ T 80
14.93 14.93 Global Days 090

57283 **intra-peritoneal approach (uterosacral, levator myorrhaphy)** ♀ T 80
Do not report with (57556, 58263, 58270, 58280, 58292, 58294)
20.59 20.59 Global Days 090

57284 **Paravaginal defect repair (including repair of cystocele, if performed); open abdominal approach** ♀ T 80
Do not report with (51840-51841, 51990, 57240, 57260-57265, 58152, 58267)
24.35 24.35 Global Days 090
AMA: 2009, Jan, 11-31; 2008, Jan, 10-25; 2007, January, 13-27

57285 **vaginal approach** ♀ T 80
Do not report with (51990, 57240, 57260-57265, 58267)
20.08 20.08 Global Days 090

57287 **Removal or revision of sling for stress incontinence (eg, fascia or synthetic)** ♀ G2 T 80
20.23 20.23 Global Days 090
AMA: 2009, Jan, 11-31; 2008, Jan, 10-25

57288 **Sling operation for stress incontinence (eg, fascia or synthetic)** ♀ A2 T 80
INCLUDES Millin-Read operation
EXCLUDES *Sling operation for stress incontinence performed laparoscopically (51992)*
Code also (C1762, C1763, C1771, C1781, C2631)
21.16 21.16 Global Days 090
AMA: 2009, Jan, 11-31; 2008, Jan, 10-25; 2007, January, 13-27

57289 **Pereyra procedure, including anterior colporrhaphy** ♀ A2 T 80
21.36 21.36 Global Days 090

57291 **Construction of artificial vagina; without graft** ♀ A2 T 80
INCLUDES McIndoe vaginal construction
18.30 18.30 Global Days 090

57292 **with graft** ♀ T 80
24.50 24.50 Global Days 090

57295 **Revision (including removal) of prosthetic vaginal graft; vaginal approach** ♀ G2 T 80
EXCLUDES *Laparoscopic approach (57426)*
14.29 14.29 Global Days 090

57296 **open abdominal approach** ♀ C5 C 80
EXCLUDES *Laparoscopic approach (57426)*
28.39 28.39 Global Days 090

57300 **Closure of rectovaginal fistula; vaginal or transanal approach** ♀ A2 T 80
16.44 16.44 Global Days 090

57305 **abdominal approach** ♀ C5 C 80
27.32 27.32 Global Days 090

57307 **abdominal approach, with concomitant colostomy** ♀ C5 C 80
31.15 31.15 Global Days 090

57308 **transperineal approach, with perineal body reconstruction, with or without levator plication** ♀ C5 C 80
19.10 19.10 Global Days 090

57310 **Closure of urethrovaginal fistula;** ♀ T 80
13.57 13.57 Global Days 090

57311 **with bulbocavernosus transplant** ♀ C5 C 80
15.44 15.44 Global Days 090

57320 **Closure of vesicovaginal fistula; vaginal approach** ♀ G2 T 80
EXCLUDES *Cystostomy, concomitant (51020-51040, 51101-51102)*
15.78 15.78 Global Days 090

57330 **transvesical and vaginal approach** ♀ T 80
EXCLUDES *Vesicovaginal fistula closure, abdominal approach (51900)*
21.75 21.75 Global Days 090

57335 **Vaginoplasty for intersex state** ♀ T 80
33.58 33.58 Global Days 090

57400-57415 Treatment of Vaginal Disorders Under Anesthesia

57400 **Dilation of vagina under anesthesia (other than local)** ♀ A2 T 80
3.98 3.98 Global Days 000

57410 **Pelvic examination under anesthesia (other than local)** ♀ A2 T
3.19 3.19 Global Days 000

57415 **Removal of impacted vaginal foreign body (separate procedure) under anesthesia (other than local)** ♀ A2 T 80
EXCLUDES *Removal of impacted vaginal foreign body without anesthesia (99201-99499 [99224, 99225, 99226])*
4.75 4.75 Global Days 010

57420-57426 Endoscopic Vaginal Procedures

57420 **Colposcopy of the entire vagina, with cervix if present;** ♀ P3 T
EXCLUDES *Colposcopic procedures and/or examinations:*
Cervix (57452-57461)
Vulva (56820-56821)
Endometrial sampling (biopsy) performed at the same time as colposcopy (58110)
2.68 3.45 Global Days 000

57421 **with biopsy(s) of vagina/cervix** ♀ P3 T
EXCLUDES *Colposcopic procedures and/or examinations:*
Cervix (57452-57461)
Vulva (56820-56821)
Endometrial sampling (biopsy) performed at the same time as colposcopy (58110)
3.66 4.64 Global Days 000
AMA: 2009, Jan, 11-31; 2008, Jan, 10-25; 2007, January, 13-27

57423 Paravaginal defect repair (including repair of cystocele, if performed), laparoscopic approach

Do not report with (49320, 51840-51841, 51990, 57240, 57260, 58152, 58267)

27.46 27.46 Global Days 090

57425 Laparoscopy, surgical, colpopexy (suspension of vaginal apex)

28.91 28.91 Global Days 090

57426 Revision (including removal) of prosthetic vaginal graft, laparoscopic approach

EXCLUDES *Open abdominal approach (57296)*
Vaginal approach (57295)

25.44 25.44 Global Days 090

57452-57461 Endoscopic Cervical Procedures

EXCLUDES *Colposcopic procedures and/or examinations:*
Vagina (57420-57421)
Vulva (56820-56821)

Code also endometrial sampling (biopsy) performed at the same time as colposcopy (58110)

57452 Colposcopy of the cervix including upper/adjacent vagina;

Do not report with (57454-57461)

2.73 3.23 Global Days 000

57454 with biopsy(s) of the cervix and endocervical curettage

4.06 4.57 Global Days 000

57455 with biopsy(s) of the cervix

3.31 4.26 Global Days 000

57456 with endocervical curettage

Do not report with (57461)

3.09 4.03 Global Days 000

AMA: 2009, Jan, 11-31; 2008, Jan, 10-25; 2007, January, 13-27

57460 with loop electrode biopsy(s) of the cervix

4.88 8.58 Global Days 000

AMA: 2009, Jan, 11-31; 2008, Jan, 10-25; 2007, January, 13-27

57461 with loop electrode conization of the cervix

Do not report with (57456)

5.63 9.67 Global Days 000

AMA: 2009, Jan, 11-31; 2008, Jan, 10-25; 2007, January, 13-27

57500-57556 Cervical Procedures: Multiple Techniques

EXCLUDES *Destruction/excision of endometriomas, open method (49203-49205, 58957-58958)*
Radical surgical procedures (58200-58240)

57500 Biopsy of cervix, single or multiple, or local excision of lesion, with or without fulguration (separate procedure)

2.26 3.85 Global Days 000

57505 Endocervical curettage (not done as part of a dilation and curettage)

2.74 3.04 Global Days 010

AMA: 2009, Jan, 11-31; 2008, Jan, 10-25; 2007, January, 13-27

57510 Cautery of cervix; electro or thermal

3.44 3.91 Global Days 010

57511 cryocautery, initial or repeat

3.95 4.34 Global Days 010

57513 laser ablation

3.97 4.29 Global Days 010

57520 Conization of cervix, with or without fulguration, with or without dilation and curettage, with or without repair; cold knife or laser

EXCLUDES *Dilation and curettage, diagnostic/therapeutic, nonobstetrical (58120)*

8.13 9.12 Global Days 090

57522 loop electrode excision

7.27 7.86 Global Days 090

AMA: 2009, Jan, 11-31; 2008, Jan, 10-25; 2007, January, 13-27

57530 Trachelectomy (cervicectomy), amputation of cervix (separate procedure)

10.28 10.28 Global Days 090

57531 Radical trachelectomy, with bilateral total pelvic lymphadenectomy and para-aortic lymph node sampling biopsy, with or without removal of tube(s), with or without removal of ovary(s)

51.57 51.57 Global Days 090

57540 Excision of cervical stump, abdominal approach;

23.26 23.26 Global Days 090

57545 with pelvic floor repair

24.54 24.54 Global Days 090

57550 Excision of cervical stump, vaginal approach;

12.20 12.20 Global Days 090

57555 with anterior and/or posterior repair

17.94 17.94 Global Days 090

57556 with repair of enterocele

EXCLUDES *Insertion of hemostatic agent/pack for spontaneous/traumatic nonobstetrical vaginal hemorrhage (57180)*
Intrauterine device insertion (58300)

16.86 16.86 Global Days 090

57558-57800 Cervical Procedures: Dilation, Suturing, or Instrumentation

EXCLUDES *Destruction/excision of endometriomas, open method (49203-49205, 58957-58958)*

57558 Dilation and curettage of cervical stump

EXCLUDES *Radical surgical procedures (58200-58240)*

3.40 3.73 Global Days 010

57700 Cerclage of uterine cervix, nonobstetrical

INCLUDES McDonald cerclage
Shirodker operation

9.29 9.29 Global Days 090

57720 Trachelorrhaphy, plastic repair of uterine cervix, vaginal approach

INCLUDES Emmet operation

9.18 9.18 Global Days 090

57800 Dilation of cervical canal, instrumental (separate procedure)

1.44 1.79 Global Days 000

58100-58120 Procedures Involving the Endometrium

CMS 100-3,230.6 Vabra Aspirator

58100 Endometrial sampling (biopsy) with or without endocervical sampling (biopsy), without cervical dilation, any method (separate procedure)

EXCLUDES *Endocervical curettage only (57505)*
Endometrial sampling (biopsy) performed in conjunction with colposcopy (58110)

2.62 3.27 Global Days 000

\+ 58110 **Endometrial sampling (biopsy) performed in conjunction with colposcopy (List separately in addition to code for primary procedure)**

Code first colposcopy (57420-57421, 57452-57461)

1.22 1.43 Global Days ZZZ

58120 **Dilation and curettage, diagnostic and/or therapeutic (nonobstetrical)**

EXCLUDES *Postpartum hemorrhage (59160)*

6.50 7.63 Global Days 010

AMA: 2009, Jan, 11-31; 2008, Jan, 10-25; 2007, January, 13-27

58140-58146 Myomectomy Procedures

58140 **Myomectomy, excision of fibroid tumor(s) of uterus, 1 to 4 intramural myoma(s) with total weight of 250 g or less and/or removal of surface myomas; abdominal approach**

27.42 27.42 Global Days 090

AMA: 2009, Jan, 11-31; 2008, Jan, 10-25; 2007, January, 13-27

58145 **vaginal approach**

16.24 16.24 Global Days 090

58146 **Myomectomy, excision of fibroid tumor(s) of uterus, 5 or more intramural myomas and/or intramural myomas with total weight greater than 250 g, abdominal approach**

Do not report with (58140-58145, 58140-58145)

34.51 34.51 Global Days 090

AMA: 2009, Jan, 11-31; 2008, Jan, 10-25; 2007, January, 13-27

58150-58294 Abdominal and Vaginal Hysterectomies

CMS 100-3,230.3 Sterilization

EXCLUDES *Destruction/excision of endometriomas, open method (49203-49205, 58957-58958)*
Paracentesis (49082-49084)
Pelvic laparotomy (49000)
Secondary closure disruption or evisceration of abdominal wall (49900)

58150 **Total abdominal hysterectomy (corpus and cervix), with or without removal of tube(s), with or without removal of ovary(s);**

29.73 29.73 Global Days 090

AMA: 2009, Jan, 11-31; 2008, Jan, 10-25; 2007, January, 13-27

58152 **with colpo-urethrocystopexy (eg, Marshall-Marchetti-Krantz, Burch)**

EXCLUDES *Urethrocystopexy without hysterectomy (51840, 51841)*

37.23 37.23 Global Days 090

58180 **Supracervical abdominal hysterectomy (subtotal hysterectomy), with or without removal of tube(s), with or without removal of ovary(s)**

28.55 28.55 Global Days 090

58200 **Total abdominal hysterectomy, including partial vaginectomy, with para-aortic and pelvic lymph node sampling, with or without removal of tube(s), with or without removal of ovary(s)**

39.23 39.23 Global Days 090

58210 **Radical abdominal hysterectomy, with bilateral total pelvic lymphadenectomy and para-aortic lymph node sampling (biopsy), with or without removal of tube(s), with or without removal of ovary(s)**

INCLUDES Wertheim hysterectomy

EXCLUDES *Chemotherapy (96401-96549)*
Hysterectomy, radical, with transposition of ovary(s) (58825)

52.55 52.55 Global Days 090

58240 **Pelvic exenteration for gynecologic malignancy, with total abdominal hysterectomy or cervicectomy, with or without removal of tube(s), with or without removal of ovary(s), with removal of bladder and ureteral transplantations, and/or abdominoperineal resection of rectum and colon and colostomy, or any combination thereof**

EXCLUDES *Chemotherapy (96401-96549)*
Pelvic exenteration for male genital malignancy or lower urinary tract (51597)

83.38 83.38 Global Days 090

58260 **Vaginal hysterectomy, for uterus 250 g or less;**

24.69 24.69 Global Days 090

58262 **with removal of tube(s), and/or ovary(s)**

27.54 27.54 Global Days 090

58263 **with removal of tube(s), and/or ovary(s), with repair of enterocele**

29.61 29.61 Global Days 090

58267 **with colpo-urethrocystopexy (Marshall-Marchetti-Krantz type, Pereyra type) with or without endoscopic control**

31.55 31.55 Global Days 090

58270 **with repair of enterocele**

EXCLUDES *Vaginal hysterectomy with repair of enterocele and removal of tubes and/or ovaries (58263)*

26.32 26.32 Global Days 090

58275 **Vaginal hysterectomy, with total or partial vaginectomy;**

29.40 29.40 Global Days 090

58280 **with repair of enterocele**

31.45 31.45 Global Days 090

58285 **Vaginal hysterectomy, radical (Schauta type operation)**

39.17 39.17 Global Days 090

58290 **Vaginal hysterectomy, for uterus greater than 250 g;**

34.37 34.37 Global Days 090

58291 **with removal of tube(s) and/or ovary(s)**

37.23 37.23 Global Days 090

58292 **with removal of tube(s) and/or ovary(s), with repair of enterocele**

39.29 39.29 Global Days 090

58293 **with colpo-urethrocystopexy (Marshall-Marchetti-Krantz type, Pereyra type) with or without endoscopic control**

40.86 40.86 Global Days 090

58294 **with repair of enterocele**

36.42 36.42 Global Days 090

58300-58323 Contraception and Reproduction Procedures

58300 **Insertion of intrauterine device (IUD)**

EXCLUDES *Insertion non-biodegradeable contraceptive drug delivery implant (11981)*
Removal of implantable contraceptive capsules (11976, 11981)

1.50 2.08 Global Days XXX

AMA: 2009, Jan, 11-31; 2008, Jan, 10-25; 2007, January, 13-27

58301 **Removal of intrauterine device (IUD)** ♀ P3 T 80

EXCLUDES *Insertion and/or removal of implantable contraceptive capsules (11976, 11981)*

2.03 2.85 Global Days 000

AMA: 2009, Jan, 11-31; 2008, Jan, 10-25; 2007, January, 13-27

58321 **Artificial insemination; intra-cervical** ♀ P3 T 80

1.37 2.20 Global Days 000

58322 **intra-uterine** ♀ P3 T 80

1.75 2.57 Global Days 000

58323 **Sperm washing for artificial insemination** ♀ P3 T 80

0.37 0.49 Global Days 000

58340-58350 Fallopian Tube Patency and Brachytherapy Procedures

58340 **Catheterization and introduction of saline or contrast material for saline infusion sonohysterography (SIS) or hysterosalpingography** ♀ N1 N

74740, 76831

1.72 3.58 Global Days 000

AMA: 2009, Mar, 10-11

58345 **Transcervical introduction of fallopian tube catheter for diagnosis and/or re-establishing patency (any method), with or without hysterosalpingography** ♀ R2 T 80 50

74742

8.35 8.35 Global Days 010

AMA: 2009, Mar, 10-11

58346 **Insertion of Heyman capsules for clinical brachytherapy** ♀ A2 T

EXCLUDES *The placement of needles or catheters into the pelvic organs and/or genitalia (except for the prostate) for interstitial radioelement application (55920)*

77761-77763, 77785-77787

13.21 13.21 Global Days 090

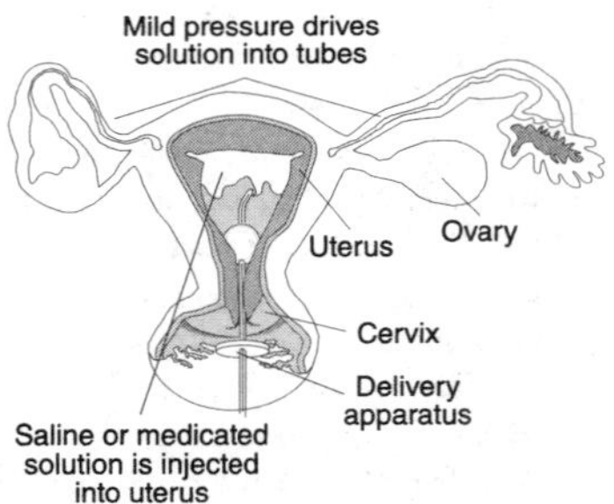

58350 **Chromotubation of oviduct, including materials** ♀ A2 T

EXCLUDES *Materials and supplies provided by the physician (99070)*

2.36 2.89 Global Days 010

AMA: 2009, Jan, 11-31; 2008, Jan, 10-25; 2007, January, 13-27

58353-58356 Ablation of Endometrium

EXCLUDES *Destruction/excision of endometriomas, open method (49203-49205, 58957-58958)*

58353 **Endometrial ablation, thermal, without hysteroscopic guidance** ♀ A2 T

EXCLUDES *Endometrial ablation performed hysteroscopically (58563)*

6.56 31.14 Global Days 010

AMA: 2009, Jan, 11-31; 2008, Jan, 10-25; 2007, January, 13-27

58356 **Endometrial cryoablation with ultrasonic guidance, including endometrial curettage, when performed** ♀ P3 T 80

Code also (C2618)

Do not report with (58100, 58120, 58340, 76700, 76856)

10.36 58.07 Global Days 010

58400-58540 Uterine Repairs: Vaginal and Abdominal

58400 **Uterine suspension, with or without shortening of round ligaments, with or without shortening of sacrouterine ligaments; (separate procedure)** ♀ C5 C 80

INCLUDES Alexander's operation
Baldy-Webster operation
Manchester colporrhaphy

EXCLUDES *Anastomosis of tubes to uterus (58752)*

13.09 13.09 Global Days 090

58410 **with presacral sympathectomy** ♀ C5 C 80

INCLUDES Alexander's operation

EXCLUDES *Anastomosis of tubes to uterus (58752)*

24.00 24.00 Global Days 090

AMA: 2009, Jan, 11-31; 2008, Jan, 10-25; 2007, March, 9-11

58520 **Hysterorrhaphy, repair of ruptured uterus (nonobstetrical)** ♀ C5 C 80

24.11 24.11 Global Days 090

58540 **Hysteroplasty, repair of uterine anomaly (Strassman type)** ♀ C5 C 80

INCLUDES Strassman type

EXCLUDES *Vesicouterine fistula closure (51920)*

27.13 27.13 Global Days 090

58541-58554 Laparoscopic Procedures of the Uterus

INCLUDES Diagnostic laparoscopy

EXCLUDES *Hysteroscopy (58555-58565)*

58541 **Laparoscopy, surgical, supracervical hysterectomy, for uterus 250 g or less;** ♀ T 80

Do not report with (49320, 57000, 57180, 57410, 58140-58146, 58545-58546, 58561, 58661, 58670-58671)

25.74 25.74 Global Days 090

58542 **with removal of tube(s) and/or ovary(s)** ♀ T 80

Do not report with (49320, 57000, 57180, 57410, 58140-58146, 58545-58546, 58561, 58661, 58670-58671)

28.75 28.75 Global Days 090

58543 **Laparoscopy, surgical, supracervical hysterectomy, for uterus greater than 250 g;** ♀ T 80

Do not report with (49320, 57000, 57180, 57410, 58140-58146, 58545-58546, 58561, 58661, 58670-58671)

29.23 29.23 Global Days 090

58544 **with removal of tube(s) and/or ovary(s)** ♀ T 80

Do not report with (49320, 57000, 57180, 57410, 58140-58146, 58545-58546, 58561, 58661, 58670-58671)

31.65 31.65 Global Days 090

58545 **Laparoscopy, surgical, myomectomy, excision; 1 to 4 intramural myomas with total weight of 250 g or less and/or removal of surface myomas** ♀ A2 T 80

26.71 26.71 Global Days 090

58546 **5 or more intramural myomas and/or intramural myomas with total weight greater than 250 g** ♀ A2 T 80

33.67 33.67 Global Days 090

AMA: 2009, Jan, 11-31; 2008, Jan, 10-25; 2007, January, 13-27

58548 **Laparoscopy, surgical, with radical hysterectomy, with bilateral total pelvic lymphadenectomy and para-aortic lymph node sampling (biopsy), with removal of tube(s) and ovary(s), if performed** ♀ C5 C 80

Do not report with (38570-38572, 58210, 58285, 58550-58554)

53.81 53.81 Global Days 090

58550 **Laparoscopy, surgical, with vaginal hysterectomy, for uterus 250 g or less;** ♀ A2 T 80

Do not report with (49320, 57000, 57180, 57410, 58140-58146, 58545-58546, 58561, 58661, 58670-58671)

26.36 26.36 Global Days 090

58552 **with removal of tube(s) and/or ovary(s)** ♀ G2 T 80

Do not report with (49320, 57000, 57180, 57410, 58140-58146, 58545-58546, 58561, 58661, 58670-58671)

29.28 29.28 Global Days 090

58553 **Laparoscopy, surgical, with vaginal hysterectomy, for uterus greater than 250 g;** ♀ T 80

Do not report with (49320, 57000, 57180, 57410, 58140-58146, 58545-58546, 58561, 58661, 58670-58671)

33.90 33.90 Global Days 090

58554 **with removal of tube(s) and/or ovary(s)** ♀ T 80

Do not report with (49320, 57000, 57180, 57410, 58140-58146, 58545-58546, 58561, 58661, 58670-58671)

39.21 39.21 Global Days 090

58555-58565 Hysteroscopy

INCLUDES Diagnostic hysteroscopy

EXCLUDES *Laparoscopy (58541-58554, 58570-58578)*

Some common sites of endometriosis, in descending order of frequency: (1) ovary, (2) cul de sac, (3) uterosacral ligaments, (4) broad ligaments, (5) fallopian tube, (6) uterovesical fold, (7) round ligament, (8) vermiform appendix, (9) vagina, (10) rectovaginal septum

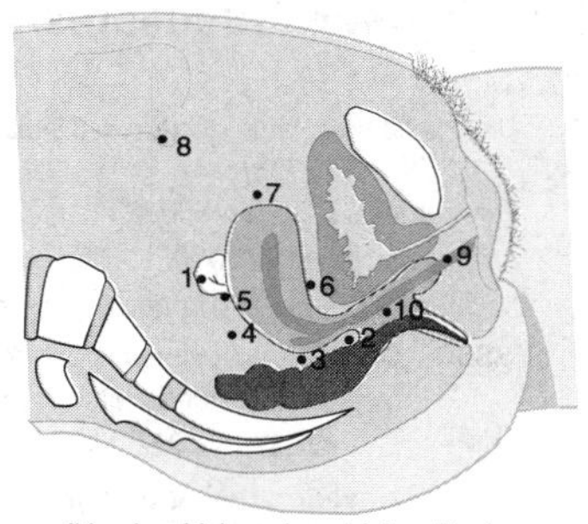

Endometriosis is a benign condition in which endometrial matter is present outside of the endometrial cavity; it is estimated that 15 percent of women have some degree of the disease; occurrence is most common in the ovaries and about 60 percent of patients will have ovarian involvement, many with cyst development

58555 **Hysteroscopy, diagnostic (separate procedure)** ♀ A2 T 80

5.67 8.56 Global Days 000

58558 **Hysteroscopy, surgical; with sampling (biopsy) of endometrium and/or polypectomy, with or without D & C** ♀ A2 T

7.97 11.27 Global Days 000

AMA: 2009, Jan, 11-31; 2008, Jan, 10-25; 2007, January, 13-27

58559 **with lysis of intrauterine adhesions (any method)** ♀ A2 T

10.26 10.26 Global Days 000

58560 **with division or resection of intrauterine septum (any method)** ♀ A2 T 80

11.57 11.57 Global Days 000

58561 **with removal of leiomyomata** ♀ A2 T 80

16.36 16.36 Global Days 000

58562 **with removal of impacted foreign body** ♀ A2 T

8.67 11.72 Global Days 000

AMA: 2009, Jan, 11-31; 2008, Jan, 10-25

58563 **with endometrial ablation (eg, endometrial resection, electrosurgical ablation, thermoablation)** ♀ A2 T 80

10.25 51.18 Global Days 000

AMA: 2009, Jan, 11-31; 2008, Jan, 10-25; 2007, January, 13-27

58565 **with bilateral fallopian tube cannulation to induce occlusion by placement of permanent implants** ♀ A2 T

Do not report with (57800, 58555)

12.96 56.83 Global Days 090

58570-58579 Other Uterine Endoscopy

INCLUDES Diagnostic laparoscopy

EXCLUDES *Hysteroscopy (58555-58565)*

58570 **Laparoscopy, surgical, with total hysterectomy, for uterus 250 g or less;** ♀ T 80

Do not report with (49320, 57000, 57180, 57410, 58140-58146, 58150, 58545, 58546, 58561, 58661, 58670, 58671)

27.68 27.68 Global Days 090

58571 **with removal of tube(s) and/or ovary(s)** ♀ T 80

Do not report with (49320, 57100, 57180, 57410, 58140-58146, 58150, 58545, 58546, 58561, 58661, 58670, 58671)

30.77 30.77 Global Days 090

58572 **Laparoscopy, surgical, with total hysterectomy, for uterus greater than 250 g;** ♀ T 80

Do not report with (49320, 57000, 57180, 57410, 58140-58146, 58150, 58545, 58546, 58561, 58661, 58670, 58671)

34.46 34.46 Global Days 090

58573 **with removal of tube(s) and/or ovary(s)** ♀ T 80

Do not report with (49320, 57000, 57180, 57410, 58140-58146, 58150, 58545, 58546, 58561, 58661, 58670, 58671)

39.40 39.40 Global Days 090

58578 **Unlisted laparoscopy procedure, uterus** ♀ T 80 50

0.00 0.00 Global Days YYY

AMA: 2009, Jan, 11-31; 2008, Jan, 10-25; 2007, March, 9-11

58579 **Unlisted hysteroscopy procedure, uterus** ♀ T 80 50

0.00 0.00 Global Days YYY

58600-58615 Sterilization by Tubal Interruption

CMS 100-3,230.3 Sterilization

EXCLUDES *Destruction/excision of endometriomas, open method (49203-49205, 58957-58958)*

58600 **Ligation or transection of fallopian tube(s), abdominal or vaginal approach, unilateral or bilateral** ♀ G2 T 80

INCLUDES Madlener operation

10.89 10.89 Global Days 090

58605 **Ligation or transection of fallopian tube(s), abdominal or vaginal approach, postpartum, unilateral or bilateral, during same hospitalization (separate procedure)** ♀ C5 C 80

EXCLUDES *Laparoscopic methods (58670, 58671)*

9.83 9.83 Global Days 090

+ **58611** **Ligation or transection of fallopian tube(s) when done at the time of cesarean delivery or intra-abdominal surgery (not a separate procedure) (List separately in addition to code for primary procedure)**

Code first primary procedure

2.31 2.31 Global Days ZZZ

58615 **Occlusion of fallopian tube(s) by device (eg, band, clip, Falope ring) vaginal or suprapubic approach**

EXCLUDES *Laparoscopic method (58671)*
Lysis of adnexal adhesions (58740)

7.33 7.33 Global Days 010

58660-58679 Endoscopic Procedures Fallopian Tubes and/or Ovaries

CMS 100-3,230.3 Sterilization

INCLUDES Diagnostic laparoscopy

EXCLUDES *Laparoscopy with biopsy of fallopian tube or ovary (49321)*
Laparoscopy with ovarian cyst aspiration (49322)

58660 **Laparoscopy, surgical; with lysis of adhesions (salpingolysis, ovariolysis) (separate procedure)**

20.06 20.06 Global Days 090

AMA: 2009, Jan, 11-31; 2008, Jan, 10-25; 2007, January, 13-27

58661 **with removal of adnexal structures (partial or total oophorectomy and/or salpingectomy)**

19.20 19.20 Global Days 010

AMA: 2009, Jan, 11-31; 2008, Jan, 10-25; 2007, January, 13-27

58662 **with fulguration or excision of lesions of the ovary, pelvic viscera, or peritoneal surface by any method**

21.04 21.04 Global Days 090

58670 **with fulguration of oviducts (with or without transection)**

10.92 10.92 Global Days 090

58671 **with occlusion of oviducts by device (eg, band, clip, or Falope ring)**

10.91 10.91 Global Days 090

58672 **with fimbrioplasty**

21.98 21.98 Global Days 090

58673 **with salpingostomy (salpingoneostomy)**

23.89 23.89 Global Days 090

AMA: 2009, Jan, 11-31; 2008, Jan, 10-25; 2007, January, 13-27

58679 **Unlisted laparoscopy procedure, oviduct, ovary**

0.00 0.00 Global Days YYY

58700-58770 Open Procedures Fallopian Tubes, with/without Ovaries

EXCLUDES *Destruction/excision of endometriomas, open method (49203-49205, 58957-58958)*

58700 **Salpingectomy, complete or partial, unilateral or bilateral (separate procedure)**

23.11 23.11 Global Days 090

58720 **Salpingo-oophorectomy, complete or partial, unilateral or bilateral (separate procedure)**

21.53 21.53 Global Days 090

AMA: 2009, Jan, 11-31; 2008, Jan, 10-25; 2007, January, 13-27

58740 **Lysis of adhesions (salpingolysis, ovariolysis)**

EXCLUDES *Excision/fulguration of lesions performed laparoscopically (58662)*
Laparoscopic method (58660)

26.14 26.14 Global Days 090

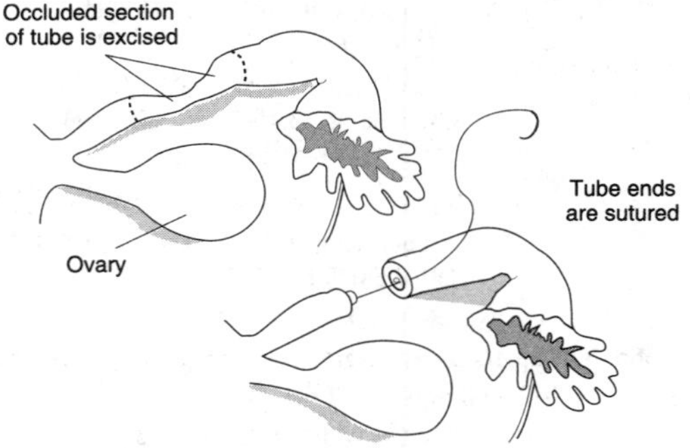

58750 **Tubotubal anastomosis**

26.95 26.95 Global Days 090

58752 **Tubouterine implantation**

25.41 25.41 Global Days 090

58760 **Fimbrioplasty**

EXCLUDES *Laparoscopic method (58672)*

24.22 24.22 Global Days 090

58770 **Salpingostomy (salpingoneostomy)**

EXCLUDES *Laparoscopic method (58673)*

25.35 25.35 Global Days 090

58800-58925 Open Procedures: Ovary

CMS 100-3,230.3 Sterilization

EXCLUDES *Destruction/excision of endometriomas, open method (49203-49205, 58957-58958)*
Paracentesis (49082-49084)
Pelvic laparotomy (49000)
Secondary closure disruption or evisceration (49900)

58800 **Drainage of ovarian cyst(s), unilateral or bilateral (separate procedure); vaginal approach**

8.92 9.52 Global Days 090

58805 **abdominal approach**

12.02 12.02 Global Days 090

58820 **Drainage of ovarian abscess; vaginal approach, open**

9.34 9.34 Global Days 090

58822 **abdominal approach**

22.00 22.00 Global Days 090

⊙ **58823** **Drainage of pelvic abscess, transvaginal or transrectal approach, percutaneous (eg, ovarian, pericolic)**

75989

5.02 27.24 Global Days 000

58825 **Transposition, ovary(s)**

21.13 21.13 Global Days 090

58900 **Biopsy of ovary, unilateral or bilateral (separate procedure)**

EXCLUDES *Laparoscopy with biopsy of fallopian tube or ovary (49321)*

13.20 13.20 Global Days 090

58920 **Wedge resection or bisection of ovary, unilateral or bilateral**

20.88 20.88 Global Days 090

58925 **Ovarian cystectomy, unilateral or bilateral**
22.05 22.05 Global Days 090

58940-58960 Removal Ovary(s) with/without Multiple Procedures for Malignancy

EXCLUDES *Chemotherapy (96401-96549)*
Destruction/excision of tumors, cysts, or endometriomas, open method (49203-49205)
Paracentesis (49082-49084)
Pelvic laparotomy (49000)

58940 **Oophorectomy, partial or total, unilateral or bilateral;**
EXCLUDES *Oophorectomy with concomitant debulking for ovarian malignancy (58952)*
15.42 15.42 Global Days 090

58943 **for ovarian, tubal or primary peritoneal malignancy, with para-aortic and pelvic lymph node biopsies, peritoneal washings, peritoneal biopsies, diaphragmatic assessments, with or without salpingectomy(s), with or without omentectomy**
33.75 33.75 Global Days 090

58950 **Resection (initial) of ovarian, tubal or primary peritoneal malignancy with bilateral salpingo-oophorectomy and omentectomy;**
32.28 32.28 Global Days 090

58951 **with total abdominal hysterectomy, pelvic and limited para-aortic lymphadenectomy**
EXCLUDES *Resection/tumor debulking of recurrent ovarian/tubal/primary peritoneal/uterine malignancy (58957, 58958)*
41.45 41.45 Global Days 090
AMA: 2009, Jan, 11-31; 2008, Jan, 10-25; 2007, January, 13-27

58952 **with radical dissection for debulking (ie, radical excision or destruction, intra-abdominal or retroperitoneal tumors)**
EXCLUDES *Resection/tumor debulking of recurrent ovarian/tubal/primary peritoneal/uterine malignancy (58957, 58958)*
46.84 46.84 Global Days 090
AMA: 2009, Jan, 11-31; 2008, Jan, 10-25; 2007, January, 13-27

58953 **Bilateral salpingo-oophorectomy with omentectomy, total abdominal hysterectomy and radical dissection for debulking;**
57.93 57.93 Global Days 090

58954 **with pelvic lymphadenectomy and limited para-aortic lymphadenectomy**
62.78 62.78 Global Days 090

58956 **Bilateral salpingo-oophorectomy with total omentectomy, total abdominal hysterectomy for malignancy**
Do not report with (49255, 58150, 58180, 58262-58263, 58550, 58661, 58700, 58720, 58900, 58925, 58940, 58957-58958)
39.58 39.58 Global Days 090

58957 **Resection (tumor debulking) of recurrent ovarian, tubal, primary peritoneal, uterine malignancy (intra-abdominal, retroperitoneal tumors), with omentectomy, if performed;**
Do not report with (38770, 38780, 44005, 49000, 49203-49215, 49255, 58900-58960)
45.22 45.22 Global Days 090

58958 **with pelvic lymphadenectomy and limited para-aortic lymphadenectomy**
Do not report with (38770, 38780, 44005, 49000, 49203-49215, 49255, 58900-58960)
49.69 49.69 Global Days 090

58960 **Laparotomy, for staging or restaging of ovarian, tubal, or primary peritoneal malignancy (second look), with or without omentectomy, peritoneal washing, biopsy of abdominal and pelvic peritoneum, diaphragmatic assessment with pelvic and limited para-aortic lymphadenectomy**
Do not report with (58957, 58958)
27.68 27.68 Global Days 090

58970-58999 Procedural Components: In Vitro Fertilization

58970 **Follicle puncture for oocyte retrieval, any method**
76948
5.66 6.32 Global Days 000

58974 **Embryo transfer, intrauterine**
0.00 0.00 Global Days 000

58976 **Gamete, zygote, or embryo intrafallopian transfer, any method**
EXCLUDES *Adnexal procedures performed laparoscopically (58660-58673)*
6.09 7.09 Global Days 000

58999 **Unlisted procedure, female genital system (nonobstetrical)**
0.00 0.00 Global Days YYY

59000-59001 Aspiration of Amniotic Fluid

CMS 100-3,220.5 Ultrasound Diagnostic Procedures
EXCLUDES *Intrauterine fetal transfusion (36460)*
Unlisted fetal invasive procedure (59897)

59000 **Amniocentesis; diagnostic**
76946
2.44 3.80 Global Days 000

59001 **therapeutic amniotic fluid reduction (includes ultrasound guidance)**
5.46 5.46 Global Days 000

59012-59076 Fetal Testing and Treatment

EXCLUDES *Intrauterine fetal transfusion (36460)*
Newborn circumcision (54150, 54160)
Unlisted fetal invasive procedures (59897)

59012 **Cordocentesis (intrauterine), any method**
76941
6.05 6.05 Global Days 000

59015 **Chorionic villus sampling, any method**
76945
3.99 4.68 Global Days 000

59020 **Fetal contraction stress test**
2.10 2.10 Global Days 000

59025 **Fetal non-stress test**
1.42 1.42 Global Days 000
AMA: 2009, Jan, 11-31; 2008, Jan, 10-25; 2007, January, 13-27

59030 **Fetal scalp blood sampling**
Code also modifier 76 or 77, as appropriate, for repeat fetal scalp blood sampling
2.91 2.91 Global Days 000

Maternity Care/Delivery
58925 — 59030

● New Code ▲ Revised Code Maternity Age Unlisted Not Covered # Resequenced
○ Reinstated CCI + Add-on Mod 51 Exempt Mod 63 Exempt Mod Sedation PQRS

59050 **Fetal monitoring during labor by consulting physician (ie, non-attending physician) with written report; supervision and interpretation** M ♀ M 80
1.53 1.53 Global Days XXX

59051 **interpretation only** M ♀ B 80
1.27 1.27 Global Days XXX

59070 **Transabdominal amnioinfusion, including ultrasound guidance** M ♀ G2 T 80
9.42 12.38 Global Days 000
AMA: 2009, Jan, 11-31; 2008, Jan, 10-25; 2007, January, 13-27

59072 **Fetal umbilical cord occlusion, including ultrasound guidance** M ♀ G2 T
15.66 15.66 Global Days 000
AMA: 2009, Jan, 11-31; 2008, Jan, 10-25; 2007, January, 13-27

59074 **Fetal fluid drainage (eg, vesicocentesis, thoracocentesis, paracentesis), including ultrasound guidance** M ♀ G2 T 80
9.59 12.65 Global Days 000
AMA: 2009, Jan, 11-31; 2008, Jan, 10-25; 2007, January, 13-27

59076 **Fetal shunt placement, including ultrasound guidance** M ♀ G2 T 80
15.58 15.58 Global Days 000
AMA: 2009, Jan, 11-31; 2008, Jan, 10-25; 2007, January, 13-27

59100-59151 Tubal Pregnancy/Hysterotomy Procedures

CMS 100-3,230.3 Sterilization

59100 **Hysterotomy, abdominal (eg, for hydatidiform mole, abortion)** M ♀ G2 T 80
Code also ligation of fallopian tubes when performed at the same time as hysterotomy (58611)
25.06 25.06 Global Days 090

59120 **Surgical treatment of ectopic pregnancy; tubal or ovarian, requiring salpingectomy and/or oophorectomy, abdominal or vaginal approach** M ♀ 05 C 80
23.92 23.92 Global Days 090

59121 **tubal or ovarian, without salpingectomy and/or oophorectomy** M ♀ 05 C 80
23.94 23.94 Global Days 090

59130 **abdominal pregnancy** M ♀ 05 C 80
24.46 24.46 Global Days 090

59135 **interstitial, uterine pregnancy requiring total hysterectomy** M ♀ 05 C 80
24.87 24.87 Global Days 090

59136 **interstitial, uterine pregnancy with partial resection of uterus** M ♀ 05 C 80
26.26 26.26 Global Days 090

59140 **cervical, with evacuation** M ♀ 05 C 80
10.72 10.72 Global Days 090

59150 **Laparoscopic treatment of ectopic pregnancy; without salpingectomy and/or oophorectomy** M ♀ G2 T 80
23.15 23.15 Global Days 090

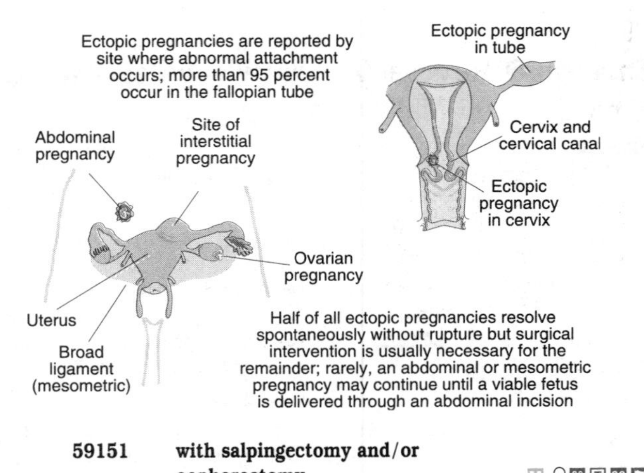

59151 **with salpingectomy and/or oophorectomy** M ♀ G2 T 80
22.53 22.53 Global Days 090

59160-59200 Procedures of Uterus Prior To/After Delivery

59160 **Curettage, postpartum** M ♀ A2 T 80
5.26 6.19 Global Days 010
AMA: 2009, Jan, 11-31; 2008, Jan, 10-25; 2007, January, 13-27

59200 **Insertion of cervical dilator (eg, laminaria, prostaglandin) (separate procedure)** M ♀ P3 T
EXCLUDES *Fetal transfusion, intrauterine (36460)*
Hypertonic solution/prostaglandin introduction for labor initiation (59850-59857)
1.36 2.19 Global Days 000

59300-59350 Postpartum Vaginal/Cervical/Uterine Repairs

EXCLUDES *Nonpregnancy-related cerclage (57700)*

59300 **Episiotomy or vaginal repair, by other than attending physician** M ♀ P3 T 80
4.45 5.78 Global Days 000

59320 **Cerclage of cervix, during pregnancy; vaginal** M ♀ A2 T 80
4.59 4.59 Global Days 000
AMA: 2009, Jan, 11-31; 2008, Jan, 10-25; 2007, January, 13-27; 2007, February, 10-11

59325 **abdominal** M ♀ 05 C 80
6.45 6.45 Global Days 000
AMA: 2009, Jan, 11-31; 2008, Jan, 10-25; 2007, January, 13-27; 2007, February, 10-11

59350 **Hysterorrhaphy of ruptured uterus** M ♀ 05 C 80
8.45 8.45 Global Days 000

59400-59410 Vaginal Delivery: Comprehensive and Component Services

CMS 100-2,15,20.1 Physician Expense for Surgery, Childbirth, and Treatment for Infertility

CMS 100-2,15,180 Nurse-Midwife (CNM) Services

INCLUDES Admission history
Admission to hospital
Artificial rupture of membranes
Management of uncomplicated labor
Physical exam
Vaginal delivery with or without episiotomy or forceps

EXCLUDES *Medical complications of pregnancy:*
Cardiac problems
Diabetes
Hyperemesis
Hypertension
Neurological problems
Premature rupture of membranes
Pre-term labor
Toxemia
Medical problems complicating labor and delivery
Newborn circumcision (54150, 54160)
Surgical complications of pregnancy:
Appendectomy
Bartholin cyst
Hernia
Ovarian cyst

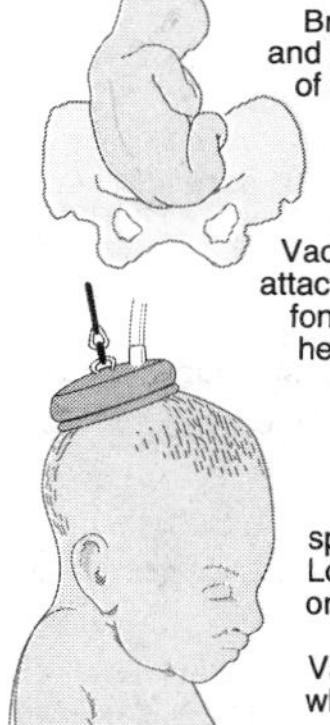

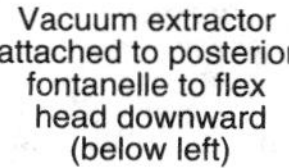

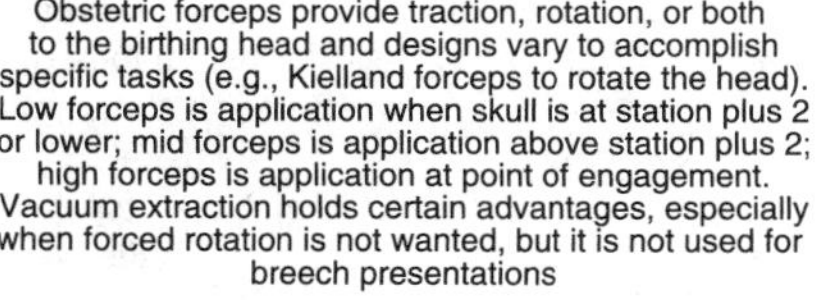

Breech presentation (left) and Simpson forceps delivery of aftercoming head (right)

Vacuum extractor attached to posterior fontanelle to flex head downward (below left)

Obstetric forceps provide traction, rotation, or both to the birthing head and designs vary to accomplish specific tasks (e.g., Kielland forceps to rotate the head). Low forceps is application when skull is at station plus 2 or lower; mid forceps is application above station plus 2; high forceps is application at point of engagement. Vacuum extraction holds certain advantages, especially when forced rotation is not wanted, but it is not used for breech presentations

59400 **Routine obstetric care including antepartum care, vaginal delivery (with or without episiotomy, and/or forceps) and postpartum care** M ♀ B

INCLUDES Biweekly visits to 36 weeks gestation
Fetal heart tones
Hospital/office visits following cesarean section or vaginal delivery
Initial/subsequent history
Monthly visits up to 28 weeks gestation
Physical exams
Recording of weight/blood pressures
Routine chemical urinalysis
Weekly visits until delivery

62.30 62.30 **Global Days MMM**

AMA: 2009, Jan, 11-31; 2008, Jan, 10-25; 2007, January, 13-27

59409 **Vaginal delivery only (with or without episiotomy and/or forceps);** M ♀ T 80

EXCLUDES *Inpatient management after delivery/discharge services (99231-99233, 99238-99239)*

24.51 24.51 **Global Days MMM**

AMA: 2009, Jun, 10-11; 2009, Jan, 11-31; 2008, Jan, 10-25; 2007, January, 13-27; 2007, Dec, 10-179

59410 **including postpartum care** M ♀ B

INCLUDES Hospital/office visits following cesarean section or vaginal delivery

31.14 31.14 **Global Days MMM**

59412-59414 Other Maternity Services

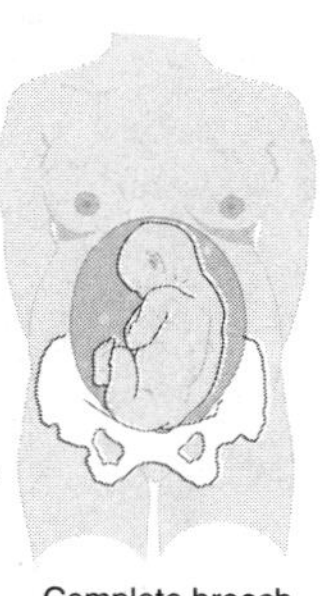

Complete breech presentation at term

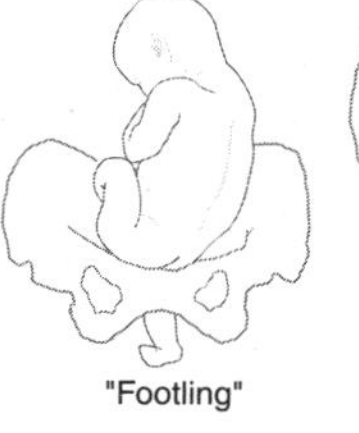

"Footling"

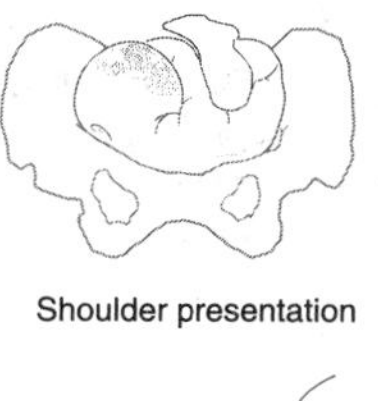

Shoulder presentation

Malposition and malpresentation occur when the fetus is in any presentation other than vertex; breech is most common at about 3 percent of deliveries; prematurity is a major predisposing factor

Brow presentation

59412 **External cephalic version, with or without tocolysis** M ♀ 62 T 80

Code also delivery code(s)

3.12 3.12 **Global Days MMM**

59414 **Delivery of placenta (separate procedure)** M ♀ 62 T 80

2.76 2.76 **Global Days MMM**

AMA: 2009, Jan, 11-31; 2008, Jan, 10-25; 2007, January, 13-27

59425-59430 Prenatal and Postpartum Visits

CMS 100-2,15,20.1 Physician Expense for Surgery, Childbirth, and Treatment for Infertility
CMS 100-2,15,180 Nurse-Midwife (CNM) Services

INCLUDES Physician providing all or a portion of antepartum/postpartum care, but no delivery due to
- Referral to another physician for delivery
- Termination of pregnancy by abortion

EXCLUDES *Antepartum care, 1-3 visits (99201-99499 [99224, 99225, 99226])*
Medical complications of pregnancy:
- *Cardiac problems*
- *Diabetes*
- *Hyperemesis*
- *Hypertension*
- *Neurological problems*
- *Premature rupture of membranes*
- *Pre-term labor*
- *Toxemia*

Newborn circumcision (54150, 54160)
Surgical complications of pregnancy:
- *Appendectomy*
- *Bartholin cyst*
- *Hernia*
- *Ovarian cyst*

59425 Antepartum care only; 4-6 visits M ♀ B 80

INCLUDES Biweekly visits to 36 weeks gestation
Fetal heart tones
Initial/subsequent history
Monthly visits up to 28 weeks gestation
Physical exams
Recording of weight/blood pressures
Routine chemical urinalysis
Weekly visits until delivery

10.71 **13.63** **Global Days MMM**
AMA: 2009, Jan, 11-31; 2008, Jan, 10-25; 2007, January, 13-27

59426 7 or more visits M ♀ B 80

INCLUDES Biweekly visits to 36 weeks gestation
Fetal heart tones
Initial/subsequent history
Monthly visits up to 28 weeks gestation
Physical exams
Recording of weight/blood pressures
Routine chemical urinalysis
Weekly visits until delivery

18.89 **24.38** **Global Days MMM**
AMA: 2009, Jan, 11-31; 2008, Jan, 10-25; 2007, January, 13-27

59430 Postpartum care only (separate procedure) M ♀ B

INCLUDES Office/other outpatient visits following cesarean section or vaginal delivery

4.21 **5.32** **Global Days MMM**
AMA: 2009, Jan, 11-31; 2008, Jan, 10-25; 2007, January, 13-27

59510-59525 Cesarean Section Delivery: Comprehensive and Components of Care

INCLUDES Classic cesarean section
Low cervical cesarean section

EXCLUDES *Infant standby attendance (99360)*
Medical complications of pregnancy:
- *Cardiac problems*
- *Diabetes*
- *Hyperemesis*
- *Hypertension*
- *Neurological problems*
- *Premature rupture of membranes*
- *Pre-term labor*
- *Toxemia*

Newborn circumcision (54150, 54160)
Surgical complications of pregnancy:
- *Appendectomy*
- *Bartholin cyst*
- *Hernia*
- *Ovarian cyst*

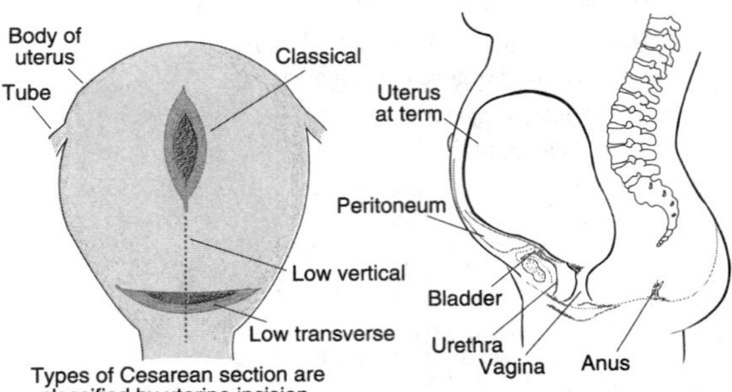

Cesarean section is delivery through incisions in the anterior abdominal and uterine walls and is indicated for numerous conditions in both the fetus and the mother. Although other approaches may be warranted, low transverse is preferred to decrease chance of uterine rupture during future pregnancies

59510 Routine obstetric care including antepartum care, cesarean delivery, and postpartum care M ♀ B

INCLUDES Admission history
Admission to hospital
Biweekly visits to 36 weeks gestation
Cesarean delivery
Fetal heart tones
Hospital/office visits following cesarean section
Initial/subsequent history
Management of uncomplicated labor
Monthly visits up to 28 weeks gestation
Physical exam
Recording of weight/blood pressures
Routine chemical urinalysis
Weekly visits until delivery

EXCLUDES *Medical problems complicating labor and delivery*

69.09 **69.09** **Global Days MMM**
AMA: 2009, Jan, 11-31; 2008, Jan, 10-25; 2007, January, 13-27

59514 Cesarean delivery only;

INCLUDES
Admission history
Admission to hospital
Cesarean delivery
Management of uncomplicated labor
Physical exam

EXCLUDES
Inpatient management after delivery/discharge services (99231-99233, 99238-99239)
Medical problems complicating labor and delivery

27.67 27.67 Global Days MMM

AMA: 2009, Jan, 11-31; 2008, Jan, 10-25; 2007, January, 13-27

59515 including postpartum care

INCLUDES
Admission history
Admission to hospital
Cesarean delivery
Hospital/office visits following cesarean section or vaginal delivery
Management of uncomplicated labor
Physical exam

EXCLUDES
Medical problems complicating labor and delivery

37.72 37.72 Global Days MMM

\+ **59525 Subtotal or total hysterectomy after cesarean delivery (List separately in addition to code for primary procedure)**

Code first cesarean delivery (59510, 59514, 59515, 59618, 59620, 59622)

14.65 14.65 Global Days ZZZ

59610-59614 Vaginal Delivery After Prior Cesarean Section: Comprehensive and Components of Care

CMS 100-2,15,20.1 Physician Expense for Surgery, Childbirth, and Treatment for Infertility
CMS 100-2,15,180 Nurse-Midwife (CNM) Services

INCLUDES
Admission history
Admission to hospital
Management of uncomplicated labor
Patients with previous cesarean delivery who present with the expectation of a vaginal delivery
Physical exam
Successful vaginal delivery after previous cesarean delivery (VBAC)
Vaginal delivery with or without episiotomy or forceps

EXCLUDES
Elective cesarean delivery (59510, 59514, 59515)
Medical complications of pregnancy:
Cardiac problems
Diabetes
Hyperemesis
Hypertension
Neurological problems
Premature rupture of membranes
Pre-term labor
Toxemia
Medical problems complicating labor and delivery
Newborn circumcision (54150, 54160)
Surgical complications of pregnancy:
Appendectomy
Bartholin cyst
Hernia
Ovarian cyst

59610 Routine obstetric care including antepartum care, vaginal delivery (with or without episiotomy, and/or forceps) and postpartum care, after previous cesarean delivery

INCLUDES
Biweekly visits to 36 weeks gestation
Fetal heart tones
Hospital/office visits following cesarean section or vaginal delivery
Initial/subsequent history
Monthly visits up to 28 weeks gestation
Physical exams
Recording of weight/blood pressures
Routine chemical urinalysis
Weekly visits until delivery

65.46 65.46 Global Days MMM

59612 Vaginal delivery only, after previous cesarean delivery (with or without episiotomy and/or forceps);

EXCLUDES
Inpatient management after delivery/discharge services (99231-99233, 99238-99239)

27.57 27.57 Global Days MMM

59614 including postpartum care

INCLUDES
Hospital/office visits following cesarean section or vaginal delivery

34.11 34.11 Global Days MMM

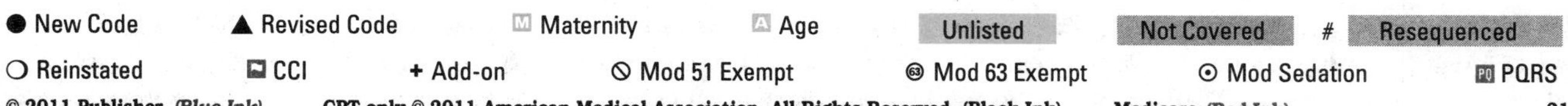

59618-59622 Cesarean Section After Attempted Vaginal Birth/Prior C-Section

INCLUDES Admission history
Admission to hospital
Cesarean delivery
Cesarean delivery following an unsuccessful vaginal delivery attempt after previous cesarean delivery
Management of uncomplicated labor
Patients with previous cesarean delivery who present with the expectation of a vaginal delivery
Physical exam

EXCLUDES *Elective cesarean delivery (59510, 59514, 59515)*
Medical complications of pregnancy:
Cardiac problems
Diabetes
Hyperemesis
Hypertension
Neurological problems
Premature rupture of membranes
Pre-term labor
Toxemia
Medical problems complicating labor and delivery
Newborn circumcision (54150, 54160)
Surgical complications of pregnancy:
Appendectomy
Bartholin cyst
Hernia
Ovarian cyst

59618 **Routine obstetric care including antepartum care, cesarean delivery, and postpartum care, following attempted vaginal delivery after previous cesarean delivery** M ♀ B 80
INCLUDES Biweekly visits to 36 weeks gestation
Fetal heart tones
Hospital/office visits following cesarean section or vaginal delivery
Initial/subsequent history
Monthly visits up to 28 weeks gestation
Physical exams
Recording of weight/blood pressures
Routine chemical urinalysis
Weekly visits until delivery
70.19 70.19 Global Days MMM

59620 **Cesarean delivery only, following attempted vaginal delivery after previous cesarean delivery;** M ♀ C5 C 80
EXCLUDES *Inpatient management after delivery/discharge services (99231-99233, 99238-99239)*
28.72 28.72 Global Days MMM

59622 **including postpartum care** M ♀ B 80
INCLUDES Hospital/office visits following cesarean section or vaginal delivery
38.90 38.90 Global Days MMM

59812-59830 Treatment of Miscarriage

EXCLUDES *Medical treatment of spontaneous complete abortion, any trimester (99201-99233 [99224, 99225, 99226])*

59812 **Treatment of incomplete abortion, any trimester, completed surgically** M ♀ A2 T
INCLUDES Surgical treatment of spontaneous abortion
8.86 9.52 Global Days 090

59820 **Treatment of missed abortion, completed surgically; first trimester** M ♀ A2 T
10.70 11.40 Global Days 090

59821 **second trimester** M ♀ A2 T 80
10.74 11.49 Global Days 090

59830 **Treatment of septic abortion, completed surgically** M ♀ C5 C 80
13.13 13.13 Global Days 090

59840-59866 Elective Abortions

CMS 100-3,140.1 Abortion
CMS 100-4,3,100.1 Billing for Abortion Services

59840 **Induced abortion, by dilation and curettage** M ♀ A2 T 80
6.21 6.46 Global Days 010
AMA: 2009, Jan, 11-31; 2008, Jan, 10-25; 2007, January, 13-27

59841 **Induced abortion, by dilation and evacuation** M ♀ A2 T 80
10.84 11.48 Global Days 010

59850 **Induced abortion, by 1 or more intra-amniotic injections (amniocentesis-injections), including hospital admission and visits, delivery of fetus and secundines;** M ♀ C5 C 80
EXCLUDES *Cervical dilator insertion (59200)*
10.19 10.19 Global Days 090

59851 **with dilation and curettage and/or evacuation** M ♀ C5 C 80
EXCLUDES *Cervical dilator insertion (59200)*
12.01 12.01 Global Days 090

59852 **with hysterotomy (failed intra-amniotic injection)** M ♀ C5 C 80
EXCLUDES *Cervical dilator insertion (59200)*
14.76 14.76 Global Days 090

59855 **Induced abortion, by 1 or more vaginal suppositories (eg, prostaglandin) with or without cervical dilation (eg, laminaria), including hospital admission and visits, delivery of fetus and secundines;** M ♀ C5 C 80
12.50 12.50 Global Days 090

59856 **with dilation and curettage and/or evacuation** M ♀ C5 C 80
14.68 14.68 Global Days 090

59857 **with hysterotomy (failed medical evacuation)** M ♀ C5 C 80
15.16 15.16 Global Days 090

59866 **Multifetal pregnancy reduction(s) (MPR)** M ♀ G2 T 80
6.32 6.32 Global Days 000

59870-59899 Miscellaneous Obstetrical Procedures

59870 **Uterine evacuation and curettage for hydatidiform mole** M ♀ A2 T 80
14.22 14.22 Global Days 090
AMA: 2009, Jan, 11-31; 2008, Jan, 10-25; 2007, January, 13-27

59871 **Removal of cerclage suture under anesthesia (other than local)** M ♀ A2 T 80
4.04 4.04 Global Days 000
AMA: 2007, February, 10-11

59897 **Unlisted fetal invasive procedure, including ultrasound guidance, when performed** ♀ T
0.00 0.00 Global Days YYY

59898 **Unlisted laparoscopy procedure, maternity care and delivery** M ♀ T 80 50
0.00 0.00 Global Days YYY

59899 **Unlisted procedure, maternity care and delivery** M ♀ T 80
0.00 0.00 Global Days YYY
AMA: 2009, Jan, 11-31; 2008, Jan, 10-25; 2007, January, 13-27

60000 I&D of Infected Thyroglossal Cyst

60000 **Incision and drainage of thyroglossal duct cyst, infected** A2 T 80

4.36 4.85 Global Days 010

60100 Core Needle Biopsy: Thyroid

EXCLUDES *Fine needle aspiration (10021-10022)*

60100 **Biopsy thyroid, percutaneous core needle** P3 T

88172-88173

76942, 77002, 77012, 77021

2.32 3.26 Global Days 000

AMA: 2009, Jan, 11-31; 2008, Jun, 8-11; 2008, Jan, 10-25; 2007, June, 10-11

60200 Surgical Removal Thyroid Cyst or Mass; Division of Isthmus

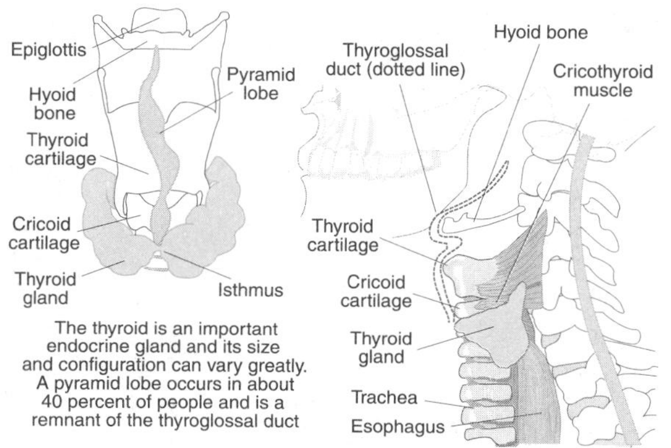

The thyroid is an important endocrine gland and its size and configuration can vary greatly. A pyramid lobe occurs in about 40 percent of people and is a remnant of the thyroglossal duct

60200 **Excision of cyst or adenoma of thyroid, or transection of isthmus** A2 T 80 PQ

19.54 19.54 Global Days 090

60210-60225 Subtotal Thyroidectomy

CMS 100-4,12,40.7 Bilateral Procedures

60210 **Partial thyroid lobectomy, unilateral; with or without isthmusectomy** G2 T 80 PQ

20.91 20.91 Global Days 090

60212 **with contralateral subtotal lobectomy, including isthmusectomy** G2 T 80 PQ

29.88 29.88 Global Days 090

60220 **Total thyroid lobectomy, unilateral; with or without isthmusectomy** G2 T 80 PQ

21.02 21.02 Global Days 090

60225 **with contralateral subtotal lobectomy, including isthmusectomy** G2 T 80 PQ

27.45 27.45 Global Days 090

60240-60271 Complete Thyroidectomy Procedures

60240 **Thyroidectomy, total or complete** T 80 PQ

EXCLUDES *Subtotal or partial thyroidectomy (60271)*

27.19 27.19 Global Days 090

60252 **Thyroidectomy, total or subtotal for malignancy; with limited neck dissection** T 80 PQ

38.87 38.87 Global Days 090

AMA: 2009, Jan, 11-31; 2008, Jan, 10-25; 2007, January, 13-27

60254 **with radical neck dissection** C5 C 80 PQ

49.43 49.43 Global Days 090

AMA: 2009, Jan, 11-31; 2008, Jan, 10-25; 2007, January, 13-27

60260 **Thyroidectomy, removal of all remaining thyroid tissue following previous removal of a portion of thyroid** T 80 50 PQ

32.39 32.39 Global Days 090

60270 **Thyroidectomy, including substernal thyroid; sternal split or transthoracic approach** C5 C 80 PQ

40.46 40.46 Global Days 090

60271 **cervical approach** T 80 PQ

31.24 31.24 Global Days 090

60280-60300 Treatment of Cyst/Sinus of Thyroid

60280 **Excision of thyroglossal duct cyst or sinus;** A2 T 80 PQ

EXCLUDES *Thyroid ultrasound (76536)*

13.23 13.23 Global Days 090

60281 **recurrent** A2 T 80 PQ

EXCLUDES *Thyroid ultrasound (76536)*

17.59 17.59 Global Days 090

60300 **Aspiration and/or injection, thyroid cyst** P3 T

EXCLUDES *Fine needle aspiration (10021-10022)*

76942, 77012

1.45 3.35 Global Days 000

60500-60512 Parathyroid Procedures

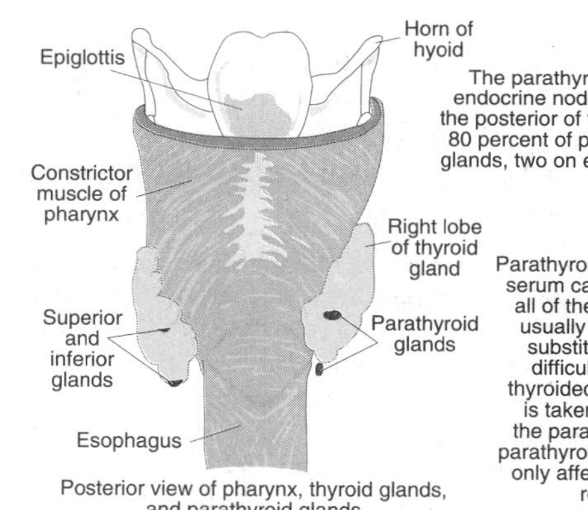

Posterior view of pharynx, thyroid glands, and parathyroid glands

60500 **Parathyroidectomy or exploration of parathyroid(s);** T 80 PQ

28.40 28.40 Global Days 090

60502 **re-exploration** T 80 PQ

37.64 37.64 Global Days 090

60505 **with mediastinal exploration, sternal split or transthoracic approach** C5 C 80 PQ

41.33 41.33 Global Days 090

\+ 60512 **Parathyroid autotransplantation (List separately in addition to code for primary procedure)** T 80

Code first (60212, 60225, 60240, 60252, 60254, 60260, 60270-60271, 60500, 60502, 60505)

7.15 7.15 Global Days ZZZ

60520-60522 Thymus Procedures

60520 **Thymectomy, partial or total; transcervical approach (separate procedure)** T 80 PQ

30.45 30.45 Global Days 090

60521 **sternal split or transthoracic approach, without radical mediastinal dissection (separate procedure)** C5 C 80 PO
33.91 33.91 Global Days 090
AMA: 2009, Jan, 11-31; 2007, Dec, 10-179

60522 **sternal split or transthoracic approach, with radical mediastinal dissection (separate procedure)** C5 C 80 PO
EXCLUDES *Surgical thoracoscopy (video-assisted thoracic surgery (VATS) thymectomy (32673)*
41.23 41.23 Global Days 090

60540-60545 Adrenal Gland Procedures

EXCLUDES *Laparoscopic approach (60650)*
Removal of remote or disseminated pheochromocytoma (49203-49205)

Do not report with (50323)

60540 **Adrenalectomy, partial or complete, or exploration of adrenal gland with or without biopsy, transabdominal, lumbar or dorsal (separate procedure);** C5 C 80 50 PO
31.06 31.06 Global Days 090

60545 **with excision of adjacent retroperitoneal tumor** C5 C 80 PO
35.64 35.64 Global Days 090

60600-60605 Carotid Body Procedures

CMS 100-3,20.18 Carotid Body Resection/Carotid Body Denervation

60600 **Excision of carotid body tumor; without excision of carotid artery** C5 C 80 PO
42.46 42.46 Global Days 090

60605 **with excision of carotid artery** C5 C 80 PO
48.20 48.20 Global Days 090

60650-60699 Laparoscopic and Unlisted Procedures

INCLUDES Diagnostic laparoscopy

60650 **Laparoscopy, surgical, with adrenalectomy, partial or complete, or exploration of adrenal gland with or without biopsy, transabdominal, lumbar or dorsal** C5 C 80 50 PO
34.99 34.99 Global Days 090

60659 **Unlisted laparoscopy procedure, endocrine system** T 80 50
0.00 0.00 Global Days YYY

60699 **Unlisted procedure, endocrine system** T 80
0.00 0.00 Global Days YYY
AMA: 2009, Jan, 11-31; 2008, Jan, 10-25; 2007, January, 13-27; 2007, Dec, 10-179

61000-61253 Transcranial Access via Puncture, Burr Hole, Twist Hole, or Trephine

EXCLUDES *Injection for:*
Cerebral angiography (36100-36218)

61000 Subdural tap through fontanelle, or suture, infant, unilateral or bilateral; initial
EXCLUDES *Injection for:*
Pneumoenephalography (61055)
Ventriculography (61026, 61120)
3.23 3.23 Global Days 000

61001 subsequent taps
3.44 3.44 Global Days 000

61020 Ventricular puncture through previous burr hole, fontanelle, suture, or implanted ventricular catheter/reservoir; without injection
4.07 4.07 Global Days 000

61026 with injection of medication or other substance for diagnosis or treatment
3.81 3.81 Global Days 000

61050 Cisternal or lateral cervical (C1-C2) puncture; without injection (separate procedure)
3.07 3.07 Global Days 000

61055 with injection of medication or other substance for diagnosis or treatment (eg, C1-C2)
INCLUDES Injection for pneumoencephalography
EXCLUDES *Radiology procedures*
4.00 4.00 Global Days 000

61070 Puncture of shunt tubing or reservoir for aspiration or injection procedure
75809
2.52 2.52 Global Days 000
AMA: 2009, Jan, 11-31; 2008, Jul, 10&13; 2008, Sep, 10-11

61105 Twist drill hole for subdural or ventricular puncture
13.62 13.62 Global Days 090

⊘ 61107 Twist drill hole(s) for subdural, intracerebral, or ventricular puncture; for implanting ventricular catheter, pressure recording device, or other intracerebral monitoring device
EXCLUDES *Intracranial neuroendoscopic ventricular catheter insertion or reinsertion (62160)*
9.36 9.36 Global Days 000
AMA: 2007, June, 10-11

61108 for evacuation and/or drainage of subdural hematoma
26.72 26.72 Global Days 090

61120 Burr hole(s) for ventricular puncture (including injection of gas, contrast media, dye, or radioactive material)
21.98 21.98 Global Days 090

61140 Burr hole(s) or trephine; with biopsy of brain or intracranial lesion
37.26 37.26 Global Days 090

61150 with drainage of brain abscess or cyst
40.03 40.03 Global Days 090

61151 with subsequent tapping (aspiration) of intracranial abscess or cyst
29.34 29.34 Global Days 090

61154 Burr hole(s) with evacuation and/or drainage of hematoma, extradural or subdural
37.53 37.53 Global Days 090

61156 Burr hole(s); with aspiration of hematoma or cyst, intracerebral
36.80 36.80 Global Days 090

61210 for implanting ventricular catheter, reservoir, EEG electrode(s), pressure recording device, or other cerebral monitoring device (separate procedure)
EXCLUDES *Intracranial neuroendoscopic ventricular insertion (62160)*
10.94 10.94 Global Days 000
AMA: 2009, Jan, 11-31; 2008, May, 9-11; 2008, Jul, 4; 2007, June, 10-11

61215 Insertion of subcutaneous reservoir, pump or continuous infusion system for connection to ventricular catheter
EXCLUDES *Chemotherapy (96450)*
Refilling and maintenance of implantable infusion pump (95990)
14.95 14.95 Global Days 090

61250 Burr hole(s) or trephine, supratentorial, exploratory, not followed by other surgery
25.55 25.55 Global Days 090

61253 Burr hole(s) or trephine, infratentorial, unilateral or bilateral
EXCLUDES *Burr hole or trephine followed by craniotomy at same operative session (61304-61321)*
24.63 24.63 Global Days 090
AMA: 2009, Jan, 11-31; 2008, Jan, 10-25; 2007, January, 13-27

61304-61323 Craniectomy/Craniotomy: By Indication/Specific Area of Brain

EXCLUDES *Injection for:*
Cerebral angiography (36100-36218)
Pneumoencephalography (61055)
Ventriculography (61026, 61120)

61304 Craniectomy or craniotomy, exploratory; supratentorial
48.53 48.53 Global Days 090

61305 infratentorial (posterior fossa)
59.44 59.44 Global Days 090

61312 Craniectomy or craniotomy for evacuation of hematoma, supratentorial; extradural or subdural
61.52 61.52 Global Days 090

61313 intracerebral
58.70 58.70 Global Days 090

61314 Craniectomy or craniotomy for evacuation of hematoma, infratentorial; extradural or subdural
54.04 54.04 Global Days 090

61315 intracerebellar
61.24 61.24 Global Days 090

+ 61316 Incision and subcutaneous placement of cranial bone graft (List separately in addition to code for primary procedure)
Code first (61304, 61312-61313, 61322-61323, 61340, 61570-61571, 61680-61705)
2.60 2.60 Global Days ZZZ

61320 Craniectomy or craniotomy, drainage of intracranial abscess; supratentorial
56.32 56.32 Global Days 090

61321 infratentorial
62.85 62.85 Global Days 090

61322 Craniectomy or craniotomy, decompressive, with or without duraplasty, for treatment of intracranial hypertension, without evacuation of associated intraparenchymal hematoma; without lobectomy
EXCLUDES *Subtemporal decompression (61340)*
Do not report with (61313)
70.08 70.08 Global Days 090

61323 with lobectomy
EXCLUDES *Subtemporal decompression (61340)*
Do not report with (61313)
70.50 70.50 Global Days 090

61330-61530 Craniectomy/Craniotomy/Decompression Brain By Surgical Approach/Specific Area of Brain

EXCLUDES *Injection for:*
Cerebral angiography (36100-36218)
Pneumoencephalography (61055)
Ventriculography (61026, 61120)

61330 Decompression of orbit only, transcranial approach
INCLUDES Naffziger operation
53.20 53.20 Global Days 090

61332 Exploration of orbit (transcranial approach); with biopsy
59.43 59.43 Global Days 090

61333 with removal of lesion
60.80 60.80 Global Days 090

61334 with removal of foreign body
36.42 36.42 Global Days 090

61340 Subtemporal cranial decompression (pseudotumor cerebri, slit ventricle syndrome)
EXCLUDES *Decompression craniotomy or craniectomy for intracranial hypertension, without hematoma removal (61322-61323)*
42.70 42.70 Global Days 090

61343 Craniectomy, suboccipital with cervical laminectomy for decompression of medulla and spinal cord, with or without dural graft (eg, Arnold-Chiari malformation)
64.92 64.92 Global Days 090

61345 Other cranial decompression, posterior fossa
EXCLUDES *Kroenlein procedure (67445)*
Orbital decompression using a lateral wall approach (67445)
60.36 60.36 Global Days 090

61440 Craniotomy for section of tentorium cerebelli (separate procedure)
59.24 59.24 Global Days 090

61450 Craniectomy, subtemporal, for section, compression, or decompression of sensory root of gasserian ganglion
INCLUDES Frazier-Spiller procedure
Hartley-Krause
Krause decompression
Taarnhoj procedure
56.83 56.83 Global Days 090

61458 Craniectomy, suboccipital; for exploration or decompression of cranial nerves
INCLUDES Jannetta decompression
59.36 59.36 Global Days 090

61460 for section of 1 or more cranial nerves
62.06 62.06 Global Days 090

61470 for medullary tractotomy
52.77 52.77 Global Days 090

61480 for mesencephalic tractotomy or pedunculotomy
48.58 48.58 Global Days 090

61490 Craniotomy for lobotomy, including cingulotomy
56.06 56.06 Global Days 090

61500 Craniectomy; with excision of tumor or other bone lesion of skull
39.55 39.55 Global Days 090

61501 for osteomyelitis
34.22 34.22 Global Days 090

61510 Craniectomy, trephination, bone flap craniotomy; for excision of brain tumor, supratentorial, except meningioma
64.66 64.66 Global Days 090

61512 for excision of meningioma, supratentorial
75.54 75.54 Global Days 090

61514 for excision of brain abscess, supratentorial
56.38 56.38 Global Days 090

61516 for excision or fenestration of cyst, supratentorial
EXCLUDES *Craniopharyngioma (61545)*
Pituitary tumor removal (61546, 61548)
54.90 54.90 Global Days 090

\+ 61517 Implantation of brain intracavitary chemotherapy agent (List separately in addition to code for primary procedure)
EXCLUDES *Intracavity radioelement source or ribbon implantation (77785-77787)*
Code first (61510, 61518)
2.58 2.58 Global Days ZZZ

61518 Craniectomy for excision of brain tumor, infratentorial or posterior fossa; except meningioma, cerebellopontine angle tumor, or midline tumor at base of skull
81.67 81.67 Global Days 090

61519 meningioma
87.27 87.27 Global Days 090

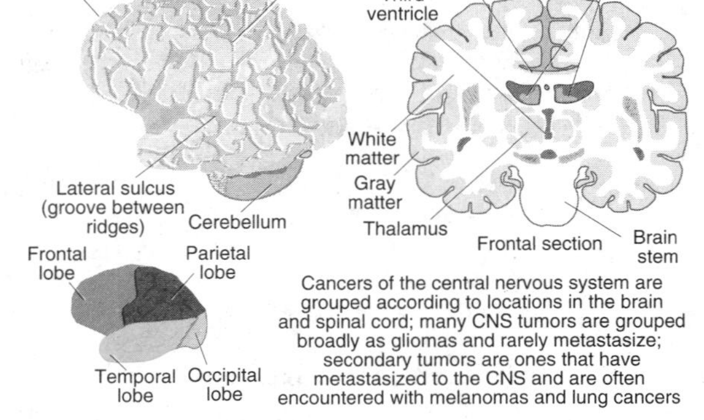

Cancers of the central nervous system are grouped according to locations in the brain and spinal cord; many CNS tumors are grouped broadly as gliomas and rarely metastasize; secondary tumors are ones that have metastasized to the CNS and are often encountered with melanomas and lung cancers

61520 cerebellopontine angle tumor
111.12 111.12 Global Days 090

61521 midline tumor at base of skull
94.18 94.18 Global Days 090

61522 **Craniectomy, infratentorial or posterior fossa; for excision of brain abscess** C5 C 80
64.73 64.73 Global Days 090

61524 **for excision or fenestration of cyst** C5 C 80
61.53 61.53 Global Days 090

61526 **Craniectomy, bone flap craniotomy, transtemporal (mastoid) for excision of cerebellopontine angle tumor;** C5 C PQ
107.61 107.61 Global Days 090

61530 **combined with middle/posterior fossa craniotomy/craniectomy** C5 C PQ
89.19 89.19 Global Days 090

61531-61545 Procedures for Seizures/Implanted Electrodes/Choroid Plexus/Craniopharyngioma

CMS 100-3,160.5 Stereotaxic Depth Electrode Implantation

EXCLUDES *Craniotomy for:*
Multiple subpial transections during procedure (61567)
Selective amygdalohippocampectomy (61566)
Injection for:
Cerebral angiography (36100-36218)
Pneumoencephalography (61055)
Ventriculography (61026, 61120)

61531 **Subdural implantation of strip electrodes through 1 or more burr or trephine hole(s) for long-term seizure monitoring** C5 C 80
EXCLUDES *Craniotomy for intracranial arteriovenous malformation removal (61680-61692)*
Stereotactic insertion of electrodes (61760)
36.13 36.13 Global Days 090

61533 **Craniotomy with elevation of bone flap; for subdural implantation of an electrode array, for long-term seizure monitoring** C5 C 80
EXCLUDES *Continuous EEG observation (95950-95954)*
45.05 45.05 Global Days 090

61534 **for excision of epileptogenic focus without electrocorticography during surgery** C5 C 80
48.65 48.65 Global Days 090

61535 **for removal of epidural or subdural electrode array, without excision of cerebral tissue (separate procedure)** C5 C 80
29.54 29.54 Global Days 090

61536 **for excision of cerebral epileptogenic focus, with electrocorticography during surgery (includes removal of electrode array)** C5 C 80
76.39 76.39 Global Days 090

61537 **for lobectomy, temporal lobe, without electrocorticography during surgery** C5 C 80
72.61 72.61 Global Days 090

61538 **for lobectomy, temporal lobe, with electrocorticography during surgery** C5 C 80
78.69 78.69 Global Days 090

61539 **for lobectomy, other than temporal lobe, partial or total, with electrocorticography during surgery** C5 C 80
69.76 69.76 Global Days 090

61540 **for lobectomy, other than temporal lobe, partial or total, without electrocorticography during surgery** C5 C 80
64.63 64.63 Global Days 090

61541 **for transection of corpus callosum** C5 C 80
63.54 63.54 Global Days 090

61542 **for total hemispherectomy** C5 C 80
65.01 65.01 Global Days 090

61543 **for partial or subtotal (functional) hemispherectomy** C5 C 80
64.08 64.08 Global Days 090

61544 **for excision or coagulation of choroid plexus** C5 C 80
55.46 55.46 Global Days 090

61545 **for excision of craniopharyngioma** C5 C 80
94.15 94.15 Global Days 090

61546-61548 Removal Pituitary Gland/Tumor

EXCLUDES *Injection for:*
Cerebral angiography (36100-36218)
Pneumoencephalography (61055)
Ventriculography (61026, 61120)

61546 **Craniotomy for hypophysectomy or excision of pituitary tumor, intracranial approach** C5 C 80
68.22 68.22 Global Days 090

61548 **Hypophysectomy or excision of pituitary tumor, transnasal or transseptal approach, nonstereotactic** C5 C 80 PQ
INCLUDES Operating microscope (69990)
46.12 46.12 Global Days 090

61550-61559 Craniosynostosis Procedures

EXCLUDES *Injection for:*
Cerebral angiography (36100-36218)
Pneumoencephalography (61055)
Ventriculography (61026, 61120)
Orbital hypertelorism reconstruction (21260-21263)
Reconstruction (21172-21180)

61550 **Craniectomy for craniosynostosis; single cranial suture** C5 C 80
30.05 30.05 Global Days 090

61552 **multiple cranial sutures** C5 C 80
37.75 37.75 Global Days 090

61556 **Craniotomy for craniosynostosis; frontal or parietal bone flap** C5 C 80
50.19 50.19 Global Days 090

61557 **bifrontal bone flap** C5 C 80
49.80 49.80 Global Days 090

61558 **Extensive craniectomy for multiple cranial suture craniosynostosis (eg, cloverleaf skull); not requiring bone grafts** C5 C 80
55.57 55.57 Global Days 090

61559 **recontouring with multiple osteotomies and bone autografts (eg, barrel-stave procedure) (includes obtaining grafts)** C5 C 80
55.09 55.09 Global Days 090

61563-61564 Removal Cranial Bone Tumor With/Without Optic Nerve Decompression

EXCLUDES *Injection for:*
Cerebral angiography (36100-36218)
Pneumoencephalography (61055)
Ventriculography (61026, 61120)
Reconstruction (21181-21183)

61563 **Excision, intra and extracranial, benign tumor of cranial bone (eg, fibrous dysplasia); without optic nerve decompression** C5 C 80
58.60 58.60 Global Days 090

61564 **with optic nerve decompression** C5 C 80
71.23 71.23 Global Days 090

61566-61567 Craniotomy for Seizures

EXCLUDES *Injection for:*
Cerebral angiography (36100-36218)
Pneumoencephalography (61055)
Ventriculography (61026, 61120)

61566 **Craniotomy with elevation of bone flap; for selective amygdalohippocampectomy** C5 C 80
66.60 66.60 Global Days 090

61567 **for multiple subpial transections, with electrocorticography during surgery** C5 C 80
75.99 75.99 Global Days 090

61570-61571 Removal of Foreign Body from Brain

EXCLUDES *Injection for:*
Cerebral angiography (36100-36218)
Pneumoencephalography (61055)
Ventriculography (61026, 61120)
Sequestrectomy for osteomyelitis (61501)

61570 **Craniectomy or craniotomy; with excision of foreign body from brain** C5 C 80
55.11 55.11 Global Days 090

61571 **with treatment of penetrating wound of brain** C5 C 80
58.86 58.86 Global Days 090

61575-61576 Transoral Approach Posterior Cranial Fossa/Upper Cervical Cord

EXCLUDES *Arthrodesis (22548)*
Injection for:
Cerebral angiography (36100-36218)
Pneumoencephalography (61055)
Ventriculography (61026, 61120)

61575 **Transoral approach to skull base, brain stem or upper spinal cord for biopsy, decompression or excision of lesion;** C5 C 80
73.79 73.79 Global Days 090

61576 **requiring splitting of tongue and/or mandible (including tracheostomy)** C5 C 80
110.45 110.45 Global Days 090

61580-61598 Surgical Approach: Cranial Fossae

EXCLUDES *Definitive surgery (61600-61616)*
Injection for:
Cerebral angiography (36100-36218)
Pneumoencephalography (61055)
Ventriculography (61026, 61120)
Primary closure (15732, 15756-15758)
Repair and/or reconstruction (61618-61619)

61580 **Craniofacial approach to anterior cranial fossa; extradural, including lateral rhinotomy, ethmoidectomy, sphenoidectomy, without maxillectomy or orbital exenteration** C5 C 50
73.57 73.57 Global Days 090

61581 **extradural, including lateral rhinotomy, orbital exenteration, ethmoidectomy, sphenoidectomy and/or maxillectomy** C5 C 50
80.33 80.33 Global Days 090

61582 **extradural, including unilateral or bifrontal craniotomy, elevation of frontal lobe(s), osteotomy of base of anterior cranial fossa** C5 C 80
89.96 89.96 Global Days 090

61583 **intradural, including unilateral or bifrontal craniotomy, elevation or resection of frontal lobe, osteotomy of base of anterior cranial fossa** C5 C 80
85.85 85.85 Global Days 090

61584 **Orbitocranial approach to anterior cranial fossa, extradural, including supraorbital ridge osteotomy and elevation of frontal and/or temporal lobe(s); without orbital exenteration** C5 C 80 50
84.56 84.56 Global Days 090

61585 **with orbital exenteration** C5 C 80 50
95.04 95.04 Global Days 090

61586 **Bicoronal, transzygomatic and/or LeFort I osteotomy approach to anterior cranial fossa with or without internal fixation, without bone graft** C5 C 80
71.50 71.50 Global Days 090

61590 **Infratemporal pre-auricular approach to middle cranial fossa (parapharyngeal space, infratemporal and midline skull base, nasopharynx), with or without disarticulation of the mandible, including parotidectomy, craniotomy, decompression and/or mobilization of the facial nerve and/or petrous carotid artery** C5 C 80 50
90.97 90.97 Global Days 090

61591 **Infratemporal post-auricular approach to middle cranial fossa (internal auditory meatus, petrous apex, tentorium, cavernous sinus, parasellar area, infratemporal fossa) including mastoidectomy, resection of sigmoid sinus, with or without decompression and/or mobilization of contents of auditory canal or petrous carotid artery** C5 C 80 50 PQ
92.23 92.23 Global Days 090

61592 **Orbitocranial zygomatic approach to middle cranial fossa (cavernous sinus and carotid artery, clivus, basilar artery or petrous apex) including osteotomy of zygoma, craniotomy, extra- or intradural elevation of temporal lobe** C5 C 80 50
93.86 93.86 Global Days 090

61595 **Transtemporal approach to posterior cranial fossa, jugular foramen or midline skull base, including mastoidectomy, decompression of sigmoid sinus and/or facial nerve, with or without mobilization** C5 C 50 PQ
70.26 70.26 Global Days 090

61596 **Transcochlear approach to posterior cranial fossa, jugular foramen or midline skull base, including labyrinthectomy, decompression, with or without mobilization of facial nerve and/or petrous carotid artery** C5 C 80 50 PQ
73.83 73.83 Global Days 090

61597 **Transcondylar (far lateral) approach to posterior cranial fossa, jugular foramen or midline skull base, including occipital condylectomy, mastoidectomy, resection of C1-C3 vertebral body(s), decompression of vertebral artery, with or without mobilization** C5 C 80 50
86.09 86.09 Global Days 090

61598 **Transpetrosal approach to posterior cranial fossa, clivus or foramen magnum, including ligation of superior petrosal sinus and/or sigmoid sinus** C5 C 80 PQ
82.82 82.82 Global Days 090

61600-61616 Definitive Procedures: Cranial Fossae

EXCLUDES Injection for:
Cerebral angiography (36100-36218)
Pneumoencephalography (61055)
Ventriculography (61026, 61120)
Primary closure (15732, 15756-15758)
Repair and/or reconstruction (61618-61619)
Surgical approach (61580-61598)

61600 **Resection or excision of neoplastic, vascular or infectious lesion of base of anterior cranial fossa; extradural** C5 C 80 CCI
63.53 63.53 Global Days 090

61601 **intradural, including dural repair, with or without graft** C5 C 80 CCI
71.03 71.03 Global Days 090

61605 **Resection or excision of neoplastic, vascular or infectious lesion of infratemporal fossa, parapharyngeal space, petrous apex; extradural** C5 C 80 CCI
65.24 65.24 Global Days 090

61606 **intradural, including dural repair, with or without graft** C5 C 80 CCI PQ
88.84 88.84 Global Days 090

61607 **Resection or excision of neoplastic, vascular or infectious lesion of parasellar area, cavernous sinus, clivus or midline skull base; extradural** C5 C 80 CCI
85.41 85.41 Global Days 090

61608 **intradural, including dural repair, with or without graft** C5 C 80 CCI
96.02 96.02 Global Days 090

\+ **61609** **Transection or ligation, carotid artery in cavernous sinus; without repair (List separately in addition to code for primary procedure)** C5 C 80 CCI
Code first (61605-61608)
17.58 17.58 Global Days ZZZ

\+ **61610** **with repair by anastomosis or graft (List separately in addition to code for primary procedure)** C5 C 80 CCI
Code first (61605-61608)
53.02 53.02 Global Days ZZZ

\+ **61611** **Transection or ligation, carotid artery in petrous canal; without repair (List separately in addition to code for primary procedure)** C5 C 80 CCI
Code first (61605-61608)
11.16 11.16 Global Days ZZZ

\+ **61612** **with repair by anastomosis or graft (List separately in addition to code for primary procedure)** C5 C 80 CCI
Code first (61605-61608)
41.65 41.65 Global Days ZZZ

61613 **Obliteration of carotid aneurysm, arteriovenous malformation, or carotid-cavernous fistula by dissection within cavernous sinus** C5 C 80 50 CCI
96.97 96.97 Global Days 090

61615 **Resection or excision of neoplastic, vascular or infectious lesion of base of posterior cranial fossa, jugular foramen, foramen magnum, or C1-C3 vertebral bodies; extradural** C5 C 80 CCI
68.27 68.27 Global Days 090

61616 **intradural, including dural repair, with or without graft** C5 C 80 CCI PQ
98.38 98.38 Global Days 090

61618-61619 Reconstruction Post-Surgical Cranial Fossae Defects

EXCLUDES Definitive surgery (61600-61616)
Injection for:
Cerebral angiography (36100-36218)
Pneumoencephalography (61055)
Ventriculography (61026, 61120)
Primary closure (15732, 15756-15758)
Surgical approach (61580-61598)

61618 **Secondary repair of dura for cerebrospinal fluid leak, anterior, middle or posterior cranial fossa following surgery of the skull base; by free tissue graft (eg, pericranium, fascia, tensor fascia lata, adipose tissue, homologous or synthetic grafts)** C5 C 80 CCI PQ
38.53 38.53 Global Days 090
AMA: 2009, Jan, 11-31; 2008, Jan, 10-25; 2007, January, 13-27

61619 **by local or regionalized vascularized pedicle flap or myocutaneous flap (including galea, temporalis, frontalis or occipitalis muscle)** C5 C 80 CCI PQ
43.91 43.91 Global Days 090
AMA: 2009, Jan, 11-31; 2008, Jan, 10-25; 2007, January, 13-27

61623-61642 Neurovascular Interventional Procedures

CMS 100-2,16,10 Exclusions from Coverage
CMS 100-2,16,180 Services Related to Noncovered Procedures
CMS 100-3,20.28 Therapeutic Embolization
CMS 100-4,4,61.1 Hospital Requirement for Device Codes on OPPS Claims
CMS 100-4,4,61.2 Requirements for Specific Procedures to be Reported With Device Codes

61623 **Endovascular temporary balloon arterial occlusion, head or neck (extracranial/intracranial) including selective catheterization of vessel to be occluded, positioning and inflation of occlusion balloon, concomitant neurological monitoring, and radiologic supervision and interpretation of all angiography required for balloon occlusion and to exclude vascular injury post occlusion** T CCI PQ
Code also (C2628)
16.40 16.40 Global Days 000

61624 **Transcatheter permanent occlusion or embolization (eg, for tumor destruction, to achieve hemostasis, to occlude a vascular malformation), percutaneous, any method; central nervous system (intracranial, spinal cord)** C5 C CCI
EXCLUDES Transcatheter occlusion or embolization other than head or neck (37204)
75894
32.51 32.51 Global Days 000
AMA: 2009, Jan, 11-31; 2008, Jan, 10-25; 2007, January, 13-27

61626 **non-central nervous system, head or neck (extracranial, brachiocephalic branch)** T CCI
EXCLUDES Transcatheter occlusion or embolization other than head or neck (37204)
Code also (C1769, C1887, C2628)
75894
25.18 25.18 Global Days 000

61630 **Balloon angioplasty, intracranial (eg, atherosclerotic stenosis), percutaneous** C5 C 80

INCLUDES Diagnostic arteriogram if stent or angioplasty is necessary
Radiology services for arteriography of target vascular family
Selective catheterization of the target vascular family

EXCLUDES *Diagnostic arteriogram if stent or angioplasty is not necessary (use applicable code for selective catheterization and radiology services)*

37.03 37.03 Global Days XXX

61635 **Transcatheter placement of intravascular stent(s), intracranial (eg, atherosclerotic stenosis), including balloon angioplasty, if performed** C5 C 80

INCLUDES Diagnostic arteriogram if stent or angioplasty is necessary
Radiology services for arteriography of target vascular family
Selective catheterization of the target vascular family

EXCLUDES *Diagnostic arteriogram if stent or angioplasty is not necessary (use applicable code for selective catheterization and radiology services)*

40.56 40.56 Global Days XXX

61640 **Balloon dilatation of intracranial vasospasm, percutaneous; initial vessel** E

INCLUDES Angiography after dilation of vessel
Fluoroscopic guidance
Injection of contrast material
Roadmapping
Selective catheterization of target vessel
Vessel analysis

18.22 18.22 Global Days 000

\+ 61641 **each additional vessel in same vascular family (List separately in addition to code for primary procedure)** E

INCLUDES Angiography after dilation of vessel
Fluoroscopic guidance
Injection of contrast material
Roadmapping
Selective catheterization of target vessel
Vessel analysis

Code first (61640)

6.41 6.41 Global Days ZZZ

\+ 61642 **each additional vessel in different vascular family (List separately in addition to code for primary procedure)** E

INCLUDES Angiography after dilation of vessel
Fluoroscopic guidance
Injection of contrast material
Roadmapping
Selective catheterization of target vessel
Vessel analysis

Code first (61640)

12.81 12.81 Global Days ZZZ

61680-61692 Surgical Treatment of Arteriovenous Malformation of the Brain

CMS 100-4,12,30 Correct Coding Policy

INCLUDES Craniotomy

61680 **Surgery of intracranial arteriovenous malformation; supratentorial, simple** C5 C 80

66.94 66.94 Global Days 090

61682 **supratentorial, complex** C5 C 80

124.13 124.13 Global Days 090

61684 **infratentorial, simple** C5 C 80

84.01 84.01 Global Days 090

61686 **infratentorial, complex** C5 C 80

133.39 133.39 Global Days 090

61690 **dural, simple** C5 C 80

64.64 64.64 Global Days 090

61692 **dural, complex** C5 C 80

108.35 108.35 Global Days 090

61697-61703 Surgical Treatment Brain Aneurysm

INCLUDES Craniotomy

61697 **Surgery of complex intracranial aneurysm, intracranial approach; carotid circulation** C5 C 80 PQ

INCLUDES Aneurysms bigger than 15 mm
Calcification of the aneurysm neck
Inclusion of normal vessels in aneurysm neck
Surgery needing temporary vessel occlusion, trapping, or cardiopulmonary bypass to treat aneurysm

124.87 124.87 Global Days 090

61698 **vertebrobasilar circulation** C5 C 80

INCLUDES Aneurysm bigger than 15 mm
Calcification of aneurysm neck
Inclusion of normal vessels into aneurysm neck
Surgery needing temporary vessel occlusion, trapping, or cardiopulmonary bypass to treat aneurysm

136.75 136.75 Global Days 090

61700 **Surgery of simple intracranial aneurysm, intracranial approach; carotid circulation** C5 C 80 PQ

101.32 101.32 Global Days 090

AMA: 2009, Jan, 11-31; 2008, Jan, 10-25; 2007, January, 13-27

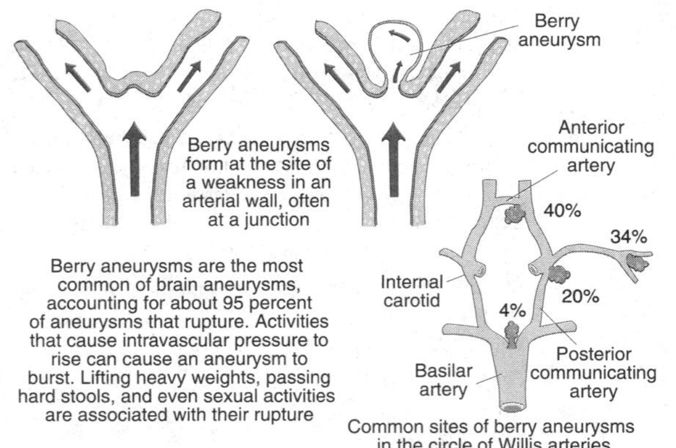

Common sites of berry aneurysms in the circle of Willis arteries

61702 **vertebrobasilar circulation** C5 C 80

118.87 118.87 Global Days 090

61703 **Surgery of intracranial aneurysm, cervical approach by application of occluding clamp to cervical carotid artery (Selverstone-Crutchfield type)**

EXCLUDES *Cervical approach for direct ligation of carotid artery (37600-37606)*

40.21 40.21 Global Days 090

61705-61710 Other Procedures for Aneurysm, Arteriovenous Malformation, and Carotid-Cavernous Fistula

INCLUDES Craniotomy

EXCLUDES *Ligation or gradual occlusion of internal common carotid artery (37605-37606)*

61705 **Surgery of aneurysm, vascular malformation or carotid-cavernous fistula; by intracranial and cervical occlusion of carotid artery**

76.78 76.78 Global Days 090

61708 **by intracranial electrothrombosis**

EXCLUDES *Ligation or gradual occlusion of internal or common carotid artery (37605-37606)*

61.03 61.03 Global Days 090

61710 **by intra-arterial embolization, injection procedure, or balloon catheter**

58.57 58.57 Global Days 090

61711 Extracranial-Intracranial Bypass

INCLUDES Craniotomy

61711 **Anastomosis, arterial, extracranial-intracranial (eg, middle cerebral/cortical) arteries**

EXCLUDES *Carotid or vertebral thromboendarterectomy (35301)*
Operating microscope (69990)

77.18 77.18 Global Days 090

61720-61791 Stereotactic Procedures of the Brain

CMS 100-3,160.4 Stereotactic Cingulotomy as a Means of Psychosurgery--Not Covered
CMS 100-3,160.5 Stereotaxic Depth Electrode Implantation

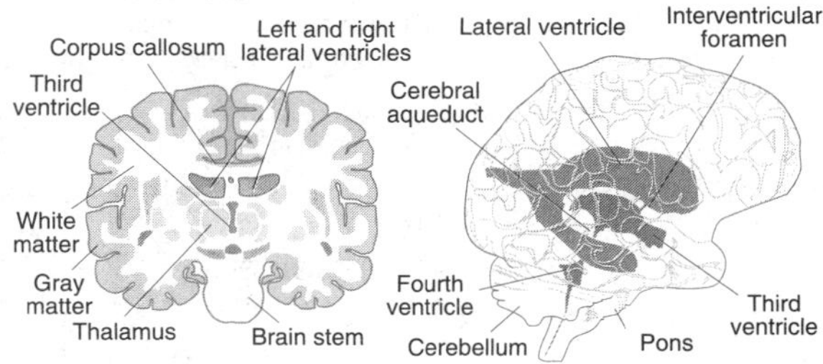

Frontal secion of the brain (left) and lateral view schematic showing the ventricular system in blue (right)

Cerebral spinal fluid (CSF) is secreted in the ventricles and flows generally from the laterals into the third ventricle via the interventricular foramina, and into the fourth ventricle via the cerebral aqueduct. Many brain disorders upset ventricular fluid pressures and shunts are employed to restore balance

61720 **Creation of lesion by stereotactic method, including burr hole(s) and localizing and recording techniques, single or multiple stages; globus pallidus or thalamus**

37.18 37.18 Global Days 090

61735 **subcortical structure(s) other than globus pallidus or thalamus**

46.48 46.48 Global Days 090

61750 **Stereotactic biopsy, aspiration, or excision, including burr hole(s), for intracranial lesion;**

41.55 41.55 Global Days 090

61751 **with computed tomography and/or magnetic resonance guidance**

70450, 70460, 70470, 70551-70553

40.65 40.65 Global Days 090

AMA: 2009, Jan, 11-31; 2008, Jan, 10-25; 2007, January, 13-27

61760 **Stereotactic implantation of depth electrodes into the cerebrum for long-term seizure monitoring**

46.49 46.49 Global Days 090

61770 **Stereotactic localization, including burr hole(s), with insertion of catheter(s) or probe(s) for placement of radiation source**

47.58 47.58 Global Days 090

+ 61781 **Stereotactic computer-assisted (navigational) procedure; cranial, intradural (List separately in addition to code for primary procedure)**

Code first primary procedure

Do not report with (61720-61791, 61796-61799, 61863-61868, 62201, 77371-77373, 77432)

6.98 6.98 Global Days ZZZ

+ 61782 **cranial, extradural (List separately in addition to code for primary procedure)**

Code first primary procedure

Do not report with (61781)

5.73 5.73 Global Days ZZZ

+ 61783 **spinal (List separately in addition to code for primary procedure)**

Code first primary procedure

Do not report with (63620-63621)

6.98 6.98 Global Days ZZZ

61790 **Creation of lesion by stereotactic method, percutaneous, by neurolytic agent (eg, alcohol, thermal, electrical, radiofrequency); gasserian ganglion**

25.69 25.69 Global Days 090

61791 **trigeminal medullary tract**

32.86 32.86 Global Days 090

61796-61800 Stereotactic Radiosurgery (SRS): Brain

INCLUDES Planning, dosimetry, targeting, positioning or blocking performed by the neurosurgen

EXCLUDES *Intensity modulated beam delivery plan and treatment (77301, 77418)*
Stereotactic body radiation therapy (77373, 77435)
Treatment planning, physics and dosimetry, and treatment delivery performed by the oncologist

Do not report more than once per lesion for a course of treatment

Do not report radiation treatment management and radiosurgery by the same physician (77427-77435)

Do not report with (20660)

61796 **Stereotactic radiosurgery (particle beam, gamma ray, or linear accelerator); 1 simple cranial lesion**

INCLUDES Lesions less than 3.5 cm

EXCLUDES *Brainstem lesions or lesions located <= 5 mm from the optic nerve, chasm, or tract (61798-61799)*

Do not report more than once per treatment

Do not report with (61798)

29.22 29.22 Global Days 090

● New Code ▲ Revised Code Maternity Age Unlisted Not Covered # Resequenced
❍ Reinstated CCI + Add-on Mod 51 Exempt Mod 63 Exempt Mod Sedation PQRS

+ **61797** **each additional cranial lesion, simple (List separately in addition to code for primary procedure)** B 80

INCLUDES Lesions < 3.5 cm

EXCLUDES *Brainstem lesions or lesions located <= 5 mm from the optic nerve, chasm, or tract (61798-61799)*

Code first (61796 or 61798)

Do not report 61797 and 61799 more than four times in total per treatment course

6.42 6.42 Global Days ZZZ

61798 **1 complex cranial lesion** B 80

INCLUDES All lesions involved in therapeutic lesion creation procedures
Arteriovenous malformations, cavernous sinus, parasellar, glomus, pineal region, pituary tumors, and Schwannomas
Brainstem lesions or lesions located <= 5 mm from the optic nerve, chasm, or tract
Lesions >= 3.5 cm

Do not report more than once per lesion per treatment course

Do not report with (61796)

39.39 39.39 Global Days 090

+ **61799** **each additional cranial lesion, complex (List separately in addition to code for primary procedure)** B 80

INCLUDES All lesions created in therapeutic lesion creation procedures
Brainstem lesions or lesions located <= 5 mm from the optic nerve, chasm, or tract
Lesions >= 3.5 cm

Code first (61798)

Do not report more than once per lesion per treatment course

Do not report 61797 and 61799 more than four times in total per treatment course

Do not report with (61795)

8.87 8.87 Global Days ZZZ

+ **61800** **Application of stereotactic headframe for stereotactic radiosurgery (List separately in addition to code for primary procedure)** B 80

Code first (61796, 61798)

4.48 4.48 Global Days ZZZ

61850-61888 Intracranial Neurostimulation

CMS 100-3,160.2 Treatment of Motor Function Disorders with Electric Nerve Stimulation
CMS 100-3,160.7 Electrical Nerve Stimulators
CMS 100-4,32,50 Deep Brain Stimulation for Essential Tremor and Parkinson's Disease

INCLUDES Microelectrode recording by same physician, if provided

EXCLUDES *Electronic analysis and reprogramming of neurostimulator pulse generator (95970-95975)*
Neurophysiological mapping by another physician (95961-95962)

61850 **Twist drill or burr hole(s) for implantation of neurostimulator electrodes, cortical** C5 C 80

29.06 29.06 Global Days 090

61860 **Craniectomy or craniotomy for implantation of neurostimulator electrodes, cerebral, cortical** C5 C 80

46.31 46.31 Global Days 090

61863 **Twist drill, burr hole, craniotomy, or craniectomy with stereotactic implantation of neurostimulator electrode array in subcortical site (eg, thalamus, globus pallidus, subthalamic nucleus, periventricular, periaqueductal gray), without use of intraoperative microelectrode recording; first array** C5 C 80 50

44.47 44.47 Global Days 090

+ **61864** **each additional array (List separately in addition to primary procedure)** C5 C 80

Code first (61863)

8.46 8.46 Global Days ZZZ

61867 **Twist drill, burr hole, craniotomy, or craniectomy with stereotactic implantation of neurostimulator electrode array in subcortical site (eg, thalamus, globus pallidus, subthalamic nucleus, periventricular, periaqueductal gray), with use of intraoperative microelectrode recording; first array** C5 C 80 50 P0

67.60 67.60 Global Days 090

+ **61868** **each additional array (List separately in addition to primary procedure)** C5 C 80

Code first (61867)

14.88 14.88 Global Days ZZZ

61870 **Craniectomy for implantation of neurostimulator electrodes, cerebellar; cortical** C5 C 80

35.06 35.06 Global Days 090

61875 **subcortical** C5 C 80

30.46 30.46 Global Days 090

61880 **Revision or removal of intracranial neurostimulator electrodes** G2 T 80 50

16.79 16.79 Global Days 090

61885 **Insertion or replacement of cranial neurostimulator pulse generator or receiver, direct or inductive coupling; with connection to a single electrode array** J8 S 80 50

EXCLUDES *Percutaneous procedure to place cranial nerve neurostimulator electrode(s) (64553)*
Revision or removal of cranial nerve neurostimulator electrode(s) (64569)

Code also (C1767, C1820, L8685, L8686)

15.68 15.68 Global Days 090

61886 **with connection to 2 or more electrode arrays** J8 S 80

EXCLUDES *Percutaneous procedure to place cranial nerve neurostimulator electrode(s) (64553)*
Revision or replacement cranial nerve neurostimulator electrode array (64569)

Code also (C1767, L8687, L8688)

24.97 24.97 Global Days 090

61888 **Revision or removal of cranial neurostimulator pulse generator or receiver** A2 T 50

Do not report with (61885-61886)

11.50 11.50 Global Days 010

62000-62148 Repair of Skull and/or Cerebrospinal Fluid Leaks

62000 **Elevation of depressed skull fracture; simple, extradural** T

26.23 26.23 Global Days 090

62005 **compound or comminuted, extradural** C5 C 80

37.47 37.47 Global Days 090

62010 **with repair of dura and/or debridement of brain** C5 C 80

45.21 45.21 Global Days 090

62100 Craniotomy for repair of dural/cerebrospinal fluid leak, including surgery for rhinorrhea/otorrhea C5 C 80

EXCLUDES *Repair of spinal fluid leak (63707, 63709)*

47.50 47.50 Global Days 090

62115 Reduction of craniomegalic skull (eg, treated hydrocephalus); not requiring bone grafts or cranioplasty C5 C 80

36.42 36.42 Global Days 090

62116 with simple cranioplasty C5 C 80

52.47 52.47 Global Days 090

62117 requiring craniotomy and reconstruction with or without bone graft (includes obtaining grafts) C5 C 80

47.02 47.02 Global Days 090

62120 Repair of encephalocele, skull vault, including cranioplasty C5 C 80

50.43 50.43 Global Days 090

62121 Craniotomy for repair of encephalocele, skull base C5 C 80

49.81 49.81 Global Days 090

62140 Cranioplasty for skull defect; up to 5 cm diameter C5 C 80

30.84 30.84 Global Days 090

62141 larger than 5 cm diameter C5 C 80

33.83 33.83 Global Days 090

62142 Removal of bone flap or prosthetic plate of skull C5 C 80

26.31 26.31 Global Days 090

62143 Replacement of bone flap or prosthetic plate of skull C5 C 80

30.82 30.82 Global Days 090

62145 Cranioplasty for skull defect with reparative brain surgery C5 C 80

41.84 41.84 Global Days 090

62146 Cranioplasty with autograft (includes obtaining bone grafts); up to 5 cm diameter C5 C 80

36.79 36.79 Global Days 090

62147 larger than 5 cm diameter C5 C 80

43.21 43.21 Global Days 090

\+ 62148 Incision and retrieval of subcutaneous cranial bone graft for cranioplasty (List separately in addition to code for primary procedure) C5 C

Code first (62140-62147)

3.75 3.75 Global Days ZZZ

62160-62165 Neuroendoscopic Brain Procedures

INCLUDES Diagnostic endoscopy

\+ 62160 Neuroendoscopy, intracranial, for placement or replacement of ventricular catheter and attachment to shunt system or external drainage (List separately in addition to code for primary procedure) N1 N

Code first (61107, 61210, 62220-62230, 62258)

5.64 5.64 Global Days ZZZ

AMA: 2009, Jan, 11-31; 2008, Jan, 10-25; 2008, May, 9-11; 2007, June, 10-11

62161 Neuroendoscopy, intracranial; with dissection of adhesions, fenestration of septum pellucidum or intraventricular cysts (including placement, replacement, or removal of ventricular catheter) C5 C 80

44.80 44.80 Global Days 090

62162 with fenestration or excision of colloid cyst, including placement of external ventricular catheter for drainage C5 C 80

55.97 55.97 Global Days 090

62163 with retrieval of foreign body C5 C 80

36.24 36.24 Global Days 090

62164 with excision of brain tumor, including placement of external ventricular catheter for drainage C5 C 80

61.59 61.59 Global Days 090

62165 with excision of pituitary tumor, transnasal or trans-sphenoidal approach C5 C 80

45.98 45.98 Global Days 090

62180-62258 Cerebrospinal Fluid Diversion Procedures

62180 Ventriculocisternostomy (Torkildsen type operation) C5 C 80

47.36 47.36 Global Days 090

62190 Creation of shunt; subarachnoid/subdural-atrial, -jugular, -auricular C5 C

27.29 27.29 Global Days 090

62192 subarachnoid/subdural-peritoneal, -pleural, other terminus C5 C 80

28.86 28.86 Global Days 090

62194 Replacement or irrigation, subarachnoid/subdural catheter A2 T 80

12.29 12.29 Global Days 010

62200 Ventriculocisternostomy, third ventricle; C5 C 80

INCLUDES Dandy ventriculocisternostomy

40.71 40.71 Global Days 090

62201 stereotactic, neuroendoscopic method C5 C

EXCLUDES *Intracranial neuroendoscopic surgery (62161-62165)*

35.55 35.55 Global Days 090

AMA: 2009, Jan, 11-31; 2008, Jan, 10-25; 2007, Aug, 15

62220 Creation of shunt; ventriculo-atrial, -jugular, -auricular C5 C 80

EXCLUDES *Intracranial neuroendoscopic ventricular catheter placement (62160)*

30.21 30.21 Global Days 090

AMA: 2007, June, 10-11

62223 ventriculo-peritoneal, -pleural, other terminus C5 C 80 PQ

EXCLUDES *Intracranial neuroendoscopic ventricular catheter placement (62160)*

31.23 31.23 Global Days 090

AMA: 2007, June, 10-11

62225 Replacement or irrigation, ventricular catheter A2 T

EXCLUDES *Intracranial neuroendoscopic ventricular catheter placement (62160)*

15.40 15.40 Global Days 090

AMA: 2007, June, 10-11

62230 Replacement or revision of cerebrospinal fluid shunt, obstructed valve, or distal catheter in shunt system A2 T 80 PQ

EXCLUDES *Intracranial neuroendoscopic ventricular catheter placement (62160)*

24.91 24.91 Global Days 090

AMA: 2007, June, 10-11

62252 Reprogramming of programmable cerebrospinal shunt P3 S 80

EXCLUDES *Intracranial neuroendoscopic ventricular catheter insertion (62160)*
Percutaneous irrigation or aspiraton of shunt reservoir (61070)

2.66 2.66 Global Days XXX

62256 **Removal of complete cerebrospinal fluid shunt system; without replacement** C5 C 80

EXCLUDES *Intracranial neuroendoscopic ventricular catheter insertion (62160)*
Percutaneous irrigation or aspiration of shunt reservoir (61070)
Reprogramming cerebrospinal fluid (SCF) shunt (62252)

17.69 17.69 Global Days 090

62258 **with replacement by similar or other shunt at same operation** C5 C 80

EXCLUDES *Intracranial neuroendoscopic ventricular catheter placement (62160)*
Percutaneous irrigation or aspiration of shunt reservoir (61070)
Reprogramming of a cerebrospinal fluid (CSF) shunt (62252)

33.30 33.30 Global Days 090
AMA: 2007, June, 10-11

62263-62264 Lysis of Epidural Lesions with Injection of Solution/Mechanical Methods

INCLUDES Fluoroscopic guidance and epidurography (72275, 77003)

62263 **Percutaneous lysis of epidural adhesions using solution injection (eg, hypertonic saline, enzyme) or mechanical means (eg, catheter) including radiologic localization (includes contrast when administered), multiple adhesiolysis sessions; 2 or more days** A2 T PQ

INCLUDES All adhesiolysis treatments, injections, and infusions during course of treatment
Contrast injection during fluoroscopic guidance/localization
Fluoroscopic guidance and epidurography (72275, 77003)
Percutaneous epidural catheter insertion and removal for neurolytic agent injections during serialized treatment sessions

Do not report more than once for the complete series spanning two or more treatment days
10.01 20.08 Global Days 010
AMA: 2009, Jan, 11-31; 2008, Jan, 10-25; 2008, Jun, 8-11; 2008, Jul, 9; 2007, January, 13-27

62264 **1 day** A2 T PQ

INCLUDES Contrast injection during fluoroscopic guidance/localization
Multiple treatment sessions performed on the same day

Do not report with (62263)
7.02 12.74 Global Days 010
AMA: 2009, Jan, 11-31; 2008, Jan, 10-25; 2008, Jul, 9; 2008, Jun, 8-11; 2007, January, 13-27

62267-62269 Percutaneous Procedures of Spinal Cord

EXCLUDES *Fluoroscopic guidance and localization unless a formal contrast study is performed (77003)*

62267 **Percutaneous aspiration within the nucleus pulposus, intervertebral disc, or paravertebral tissue for diagnostic purposes** G2 T 80

INCLUDES Contrast injection during fluoroscopic guidance/localization

Do not report with (10022, 20225, 62287, 62290-62291)
77003
4.64 7.27 Global Days 000

62268 **Percutaneous aspiration, spinal cord cyst or syrinx** A2 T
76942, 77002, 77012
7.64 8.72 Global Days 000

62269 **Biopsy of spinal cord, percutaneous needle** A2 T 80

EXCLUDES *Fine needle aspiration (10021-10022)*
76942, 77002, 77012
7.78 9.21 Global Days 000

62270-62272 Spinal Puncture, Subarachnoid Space, Diagnostic/Therapeutic

INCLUDES Contrast injection during fluoroscopic guidance/localization

EXCLUDES *Fluoroscopic guidance and localization unless a formal contrast study is performed (77003)*

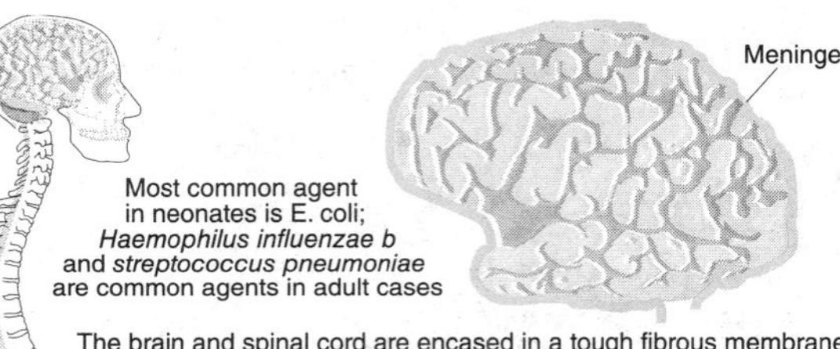

The brain and spinal cord are encased in a tough fibrous membrane known as the meninges and meningitis is an inflammation of that tissue and commonly affects the underlying central nervous system tissues and fluids; causes are numerous and classification is based on type of infection; purulent refers to forms usually caused by bacteria; chronic meningitis is usually caused by mycobacteria and fungi; aseptic or abacterial meningitis is commonly associated with a viral infection and is reported with the underlying disease. Encephalitis is inflammation of the brain and is also usually associated with a viral infection and also is reported with the underlying disease

62270 **Spinal puncture, lumbar, diagnostic** A2 T

INCLUDES Contrast injection during fluoroscopic guidance/localization

2.30 4.61 Global Days 000
AMA: 2007, Jul, 1-4

62272 **Spinal puncture, therapeutic, for drainage of cerebrospinal fluid (by needle or catheter)** A2 T

INCLUDES Contrast injection during fluoroscopic guidance/localization

2.50 5.88 Global Days 000

62273 Epidural Blood Patch

EXCLUDES *Fluoroscopic guidance and localization unless a formal contrast study is performed (77003)*
Injection of diagnostic or therapeutic material (62310-62311, 62318-62319)

62273 Injection, epidural, of blood or clot patch A2 T
INCLUDES Contrast injection during fluoroscopic guidance/localization
3.33 5.08 Global Days 000

62280-62282 Neurolysis

INCLUDES Contrast injection during fluoroscopic guidance/localization

EXCLUDES *Fluoroscopic guidance and localization unless a formal contrast study is performed (77003)*
Injection of diagnostic or therapeutic material only (62310-62311, 62318-62319)

62280 Injection/infusion of neurolytic substance (eg, alcohol, phenol, iced saline solutions), with or without other therapeutic substance; subarachnoid A2 T PQ
4.92 9.86 Global Days 010
AMA: 2008, Jul, 9

62281 epidural, cervical or thoracic A2 T PQ
4.49 7.36 Global Days 010
AMA: 2008, Jul, 9

62282 epidural, lumbar, sacral (caudal) A2 T PQ
EXCLUDES *Fluoroscopic guidance and localization unless a formal contrast study is performed (77003)*
4.18 8.68 Global Days 010
AMA: 2009, Jan, 11-31; 2008, Jan, 10-25; 2008, Jul, 9; 2007, January, 13-27

62284-62294 Injection/Aspiration of Spine, Diagnostic/Therapeutic

62284 Injection procedure for myelography and/or computed tomography, spinal (other than C1-C2 and posterior fossa) N1 N
EXCLUDES *Injection at C1-C2 (61055)*
72126, 72129, 72132, 72240, 72255, 72265, 72270
2.52 5.92 Global Days 000
AMA: 2009, Jan, 11-31; 2008, Jan, 10-25; 2007, January, 13-27

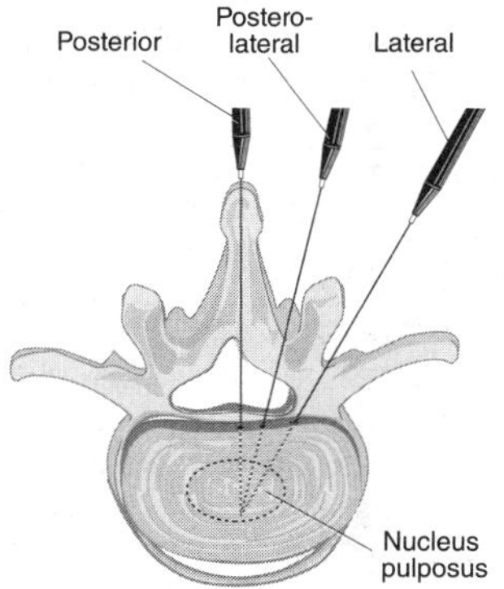

▲ 62287 Decompression procedure, percutaneous, of nucleus pulposus of intervertebral disc, any method utilizing needle based technique to remove disc material under fluoroscopic imaging or other form of indirect visualization, with the use of an endoscope, with discography and/or epidural injection(s) at the treated level(s), when performed, single or multiple levels, lumbar A2 T
INCLUDES Endoscopic approach
EXCLUDES *Percutaneous decompression of nucleus pulposus of an intervetebral disc, non-needle based technique (0274T, 0275T)*
Do not report with (62267, 62290, 62311, 72295, 77003, 77012)
16.46 16.46 Global Days 090
AMA: 2009, Jan, 11-31; 2008, Jun, 8-11; 2008, Jan, 10-25; 2007, January, 13-27

62290 Injection procedure for discography, each level; lumbar N1 N
72295
5.08 10.11 Global Days 000
AMA: 2009, Jan, 11-31; 2008, Jan, 10-25; 2007, January, 13-27

62291 cervical or thoracic N1 N
72285
4.89 9.60 Global Days 000

62292 Injection procedure for chemonucleolysis, including discography, intervertebral disc, single or multiple levels, lumbar R2 T 80
16.82 16.82 Global Days 090
AMA: 2009, Jan, 11-31; 2008, Jan, 10-25; 2007, January, 13-27

62294 Injection procedure, arterial, for occlusion of arteriovenous malformation, spinal A2 T
23.82 23.82 Global Days 090

62310-62319 Injection/Infusion Diagnostic/Therapeutic Material

INCLUDES Contrast injection during fluoroscopic guidance/localization

EXCLUDES *Daily management of continuous epidural or subarachnoid drug administration (01996)*
Epidurography (72275)
Fluoroscopic guidance and localization unless a formal contrast study is performed (77003)
Transforaminal epidural injection (64479-64484)

Do not report more than once, even when catheter tip or substance injected moves into another spinal region

▲ 62310 Injection(s), of diagnostic or therapeutic substance(s) (including anesthetic, antispasmodic, opioid, steroid, other solution), not including neurolytic substances, including needle or catheter placement, includes contrast for localization when performed, epidural or subarachnoid; cervical or thoracic A2 T
Placement and use of a catheter to administer epidural or subarachnoid injection(s), even if more than one injection on a single calendar day
Placement of catheter into the epidural space and then removing the catheter after injecting substance(s) at one or more levels

Do not report with (62318)
3.15 7.25 Global Days 000
AMA: 2009, Jan, 11-31; 2008, Jan, 10-25; 2008, Jul, 9; 2008, Nov, 10-11; 2007, January, 13-27

▲ 62311 **lumbar or sacral (caudal)** A2 T

INCLUDES Placement and use of a catheter to administer epidural or subarachnoid injection(s), even if more than one injection on a single calendar day

Placement of catheter into the epidural space and then removing the catheter after injecting substance(s) at one or more levels

Do not report with (62319)

2.58 6.14 Global Days 000

AMA: 2009, Jan, 11-31; 2008, Jan, 10-25; 2008, Nov, 10-11; 2008, Jul, 9; 2007, January, 13-27

▲ 62318 **Injection(s), including indwelling catheter placement, continuous infusion or intermittent bolus, of diagnostic or therapeutic substance(s) (including anesthetic, antispasmodic, opioid, steroid, other solution), not including neurolytic substances, includes contrast for localization when performed, epidural or subarachnoid; cervical or thoracic** A2 T PQ

Do not report with (62310)

INCLUDES Placement of catheter into the epidural space with delivery of substances for more than one calendar day, either continuously or by intermittent bolus

2.99 7.38 Global Days 000

AMA: 2009, Jan, 11-31; 2008, Jan, 10-25; 2008, Jul, 9; 2008, Nov, 10-11; 2007, January, 13-27

▲ 62319 **lumbar or sacral (caudal)** A2 T PQ

Do not report with (62311)

INCLUDES Placement of catheter into the epidural space with delivery of substances for more than one calendar day, either continuously or by intermittent bolus

2.85 5.44 Global Days 000

AMA: 2009, Jan, 11-31; 2008, Jan, 10-25; 2008, Jul, 9; 2008, Nov, 10-11; 2007, January, 13-27

62350-62370 Procedures Related to Epidural and Intrathecal Catheters

CMS 100-3,280.14 Infusion Pumps

EXCLUDES *Infusion pump refilling and maintenance without reprogramming (95990-95991)*

Percutaneous insertion of intrathecal or epidural catheter (62270-62273, 62280-62284, 62310-62319)

62350 **Implantation, revision or repositioning of tunneled intrathecal or epidural catheter, for long-term medication administration via an external pump or implantable reservoir/infusion pump; without laminectomy** A2 T

11.72 11.72 Global Days 010

62351 **with laminectomy** T 80

25.76 25.76 Global Days 090

62355 **Removal of previously implanted intrathecal or epidural catheter** A2 T 80

7.67 7.67 Global Days 010

62360 **Implantation or replacement of device for intrathecal or epidural drug infusion; subcutaneous reservoir** A2 T 80

9.09 9.09 Global Days 010

62361 **nonprogrammable pump** J8 T 80

Code also (C1891, C2626)

10.29 10.29 Global Days 010

62362 **programmable pump, including preparation of pump, with or without programming** J8 T 80

Code also (C1772)

11.43 11.43 Global Days 010

AMA: 2009, Jan, 11-31; 2008, Jan, 10-25; 2007, January, 13-27

62365 **Removal of subcutaneous reservoir or pump, previously implanted for intrathecal or epidural infusion** A2 T 80

8.65 8.65 Global Days 010

▲ 62367 **Electronic analysis of programmable, implanted pump for intrathecal or epidural drug infusion (includes evaluation of reservoir status, alarm status, drug prescription status); without reprogramming or refill** P3 S

0.73 1.20 Global Days XXX

62368 **with reprogramming** P3 S

1.00 1.62 Global Days XXX

AMA: 2009, Jan, 11-31; 2008, Jan, 10-25; 2007, January, 13-27

● 62369 **with reprogramming and refill** P3 S

1.03 3.66 Global Days XXX

● 62370 **with reprogramming and refill (requiring physician's skill)** P3 S

1.38 3.83 Global Days XXX

63001-63048 Posterior Midline Approach: Laminectomy/Laminotomy/Decompression

INCLUDES Endoscopic assistance through open and direct visualization

Percutaneous laminotomy/hemilaminectomy with imaging guidance and/or endoscope only (0274T, 0275T)

EXCLUDES *Arthrodesis (22590-22614)*

63001 **Laminectomy with exploration and/or decompression of spinal cord and/or cauda equina, without facetectomy, foraminotomy or discectomy (eg, spinal stenosis), 1 or 2 vertebral segments; cervical** T 80 PQ

36.55 36.55 Global Days 090

AMA: 2009, Jan, 11-31; 2008, Jan, 10-25; 2007, January, 13-27; 2007, June, 1-3

63003 **thoracic** T 80 PQ

36.60 36.60 Global Days 090

AMA: 2009, Jan, 11-31; 2008, Jan, 10-25; 2007, January, 13-27; 2007, June, 1-3

63005 **lumbar, except for spondylolisthesis** T 80 PQ

34.81 34.81 Global Days 090

AMA: 2009, Jan, 11-31; 2008, Jan, 10-25; 2007, January, 13-27; 2007, June, 1-3

63011 **sacral** T 80 PQ

32.03 32.03 Global Days 090

AMA: 2009, Jan, 11-31; 2008, Jan, 10-25; 2007, January, 13-27; 2007, June, 1-3

63012 **Laminectomy with removal of abnormal facets and/or pars inter-articularis with decompression of cauda equina and nerve roots for spondylolisthesis, lumbar (Gill type procedure)** T 80 PQ

35.22 35.22 Global Days 090

AMA: 2009, Jan, 11-31; 2008, Jan, 10-25; 2007, January, 13-27; 2007, June, 1-3

63015 **Laminectomy with exploration and/or decompression of spinal cord and/or cauda equina, without facetectomy, foraminotomy or discectomy (eg, spinal stenosis), more than 2 vertebral segments; cervical** T 80 PQ

43.89 43.89 Global Days 090

AMA: 2009, Jan, 11-31; 2008, Jan, 10-25; 2007, January, 13-27; 2007, June, 1-3

63016 **thoracic**
44.79 44.79 Global Days 090
AMA: 2009, Jan, 11-31; 2008, Jan, 10-25; 2007, January, 13-27; 2007, June, 1-3

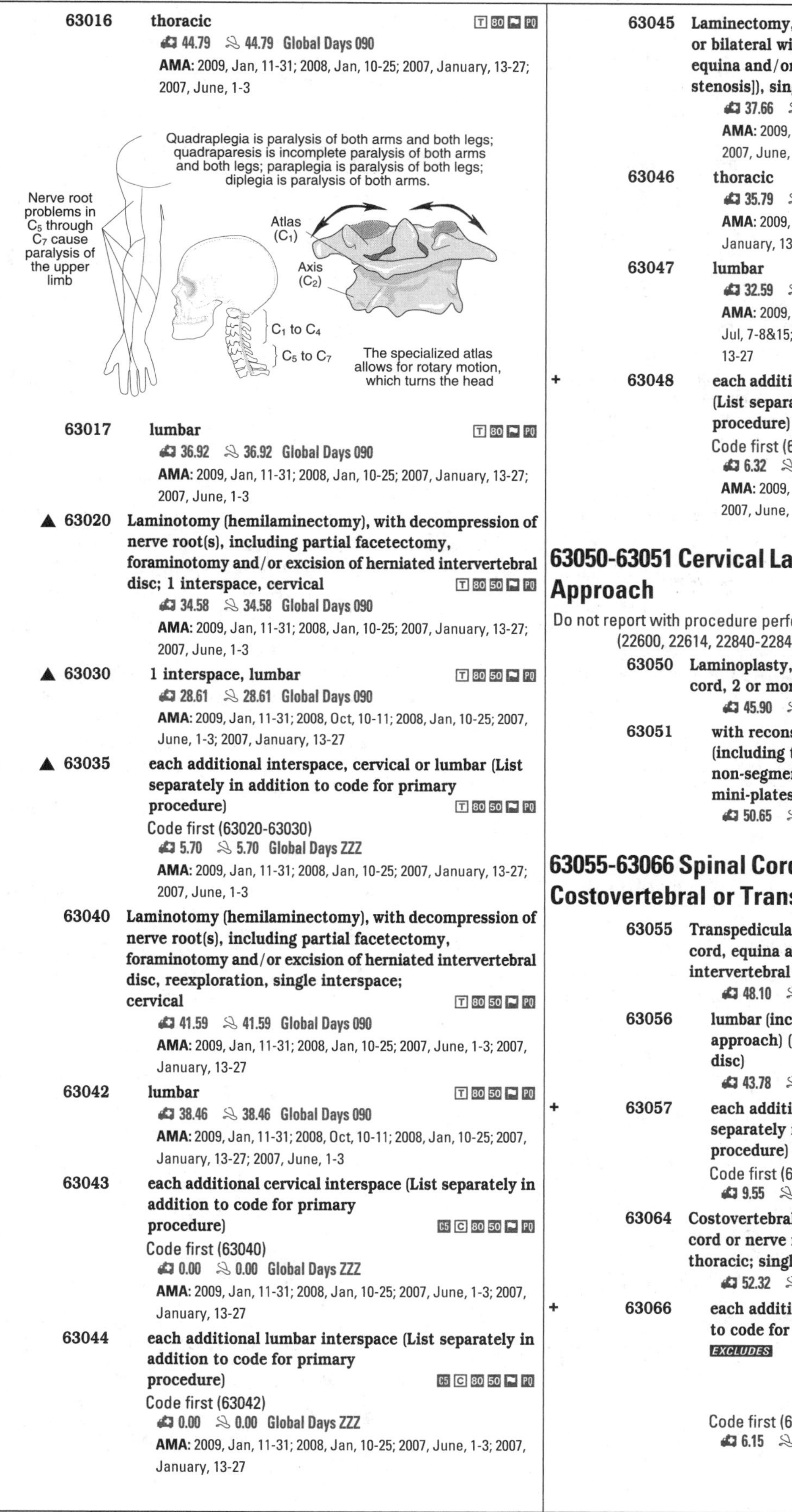

63017 **lumbar**
36.92 36.92 Global Days 090
AMA: 2009, Jan, 11-31; 2008, Jan, 10-25; 2007, January, 13-27; 2007, June, 1-3

▲ **63020** **Laminotomy (hemilaminectomy), with decompression of nerve root(s), including partial facetectomy, foraminotomy and/or excision of herniated intervertebral disc; 1 interspace, cervical**
34.58 34.58 Global Days 090
AMA: 2009, Jan, 11-31; 2008, Jan, 10-25; 2007, January, 13-27; 2007, June, 1-3

▲ **63030** **1 interspace, lumbar**
28.61 28.61 Global Days 090
AMA: 2009, Jan, 11-31; 2008, Oct, 10-11; 2008, Jan, 10-25; 2007, June, 1-3; 2007, January, 13-27

+ ▲ **63035** **each additional interspace, cervical or lumbar (List separately in addition to code for primary procedure)**
Code first (63020-63030)
5.70 5.70 Global Days ZZZ
AMA: 2009, Jan, 11-31; 2008, Jan, 10-25; 2007, January, 13-27; 2007, June, 1-3

63040 **Laminotomy (hemilaminectomy), with decompression of nerve root(s), including partial facetectomy, foraminotomy and/or excision of herniated intervertebral disc, reexploration, single interspace; cervical**
41.59 41.59 Global Days 090
AMA: 2009, Jan, 11-31; 2008, Jan, 10-25; 2007, June, 1-3; 2007, January, 13-27

63042 **lumbar**
38.46 38.46 Global Days 090
AMA: 2009, Jan, 11-31; 2008, Oct, 10-11; 2008, Jan, 10-25; 2007, January, 13-27; 2007, June, 1-3

+ **63043** **each additional cervical interspace (List separately in addition to code for primary procedure)**
Code first (63040)
0.00 0.00 Global Days ZZZ
AMA: 2009, Jan, 11-31; 2008, Jan, 10-25; 2007, June, 1-3; 2007, January, 13-27

+ **63044** **each additional lumbar interspace (List separately in addition to code for primary procedure)**
Code first (63042)
0.00 0.00 Global Days ZZZ
AMA: 2009, Jan, 11-31; 2008, Jan, 10-25; 2007, June, 1-3; 2007, January, 13-27

63045 **Laminectomy, facetectomy and foraminotomy (unilateral or bilateral with decompression of spinal cord, cauda equina and/or nerve root[s], [eg, spinal or lateral recess stenosis]), single vertebral segment; cervical**
37.66 37.66 Global Days 090
AMA: 2009, Jan, 11-31; 2008, Jan, 10-25; 2007, January, 13-27; 2007, June, 1-3

63046 **thoracic**
35.79 35.79 Global Days 090
AMA: 2009, Jan, 11-31; 2008, Jan, 10-25; 2007, June, 1-3; 2007, January, 13-27

63047 **lumbar**
32.59 32.59 Global Days 090
AMA: 2009, Jan, 11-31; 2008, Oct, 10-11; 2008, Apr, -11; 2008, Jul, 7-8&15; 2008, Jan, 10-25; 2007, June, 1-3; 2007, January, 13-27

+ **63048** **each additional segment, cervical, thoracic, or lumbar (List separately in addition to code for primary procedure)**
Code first (63045-63047)
6.32 6.32 Global Days ZZZ
AMA: 2009, Jan, 11-31; 2008, Jan, 10-25; 2007, January, 13-27; 2007, June, 1-3

63050-63051 Cervical Laminoplasty: Posterior Midline Approach

Do not report with procedure performed on the same vertebral segment(s) (22600, 22614, 22840-22842, 63001, 63015, 63045, 63048, 63295)

63050 **Laminoplasty, cervical, with decompression of the spinal cord, 2 or more vertebral segments;**
45.90 45.90 Global Days 090

63051 **with reconstruction of the posterior bony elements (including the application of bridging bone graft and non-segmental fixation devices (eg, wire, suture, mini-plates), when performed)**
50.65 50.65 Global Days 090

63055-63066 Spinal Cord/Nerve Root Decompression: Costovertebral or Transpedicular Approach

63055 **Transpedicular approach with decompression of spinal cord, equina and/or nerve root(s) (eg, herniated intervertebral disc), single segment; thoracic**
48.10 48.10 Global Days 090

63056 **lumbar (including transfacet, or lateral extraforaminal approach) (eg, far lateral herniated intervertebral disc)**
43.78 43.78 Global Days 090

+ **63057** **each additional segment, thoracic or lumbar (List separately in addition to code for primary procedure)**
Code first (63055-63056)
9.55 9.55 Global Days ZZZ

63064 **Costovertebral approach with decompression of spinal cord or nerve root(s) (eg, herniated intervertebral disc), thoracic; single segment**
52.32 52.32 Global Days 090

+ **63066** **each additional segment (List separately in addition to code for primary procedure)**
EXCLUDES *Laminectomy with intraspinal thoracic lesion removal (63266, 63271, 63276, 63281, 63286)*
Code first (63064)
6.15 6.15 Global Days ZZZ

63075-63078 Discectomy: Anterior or Anterolateral Approach

INCLUDES Operating microscope (69990)

63075 **Discectomy, anterior, with decompression of spinal cord and/or nerve root(s), including osteophytectomy; cervical, single interspace**

EXCLUDES *Anterior cervical discectomy and anterior interbody fusion at same level during same operative session (22551)*

Do not report with anterior interbody arthrodesis (even by another provider) (22554)

40.70 40.70 Global Days 090

AMA: 2009, Jan, 11-31; 2008, Jan, 10-25; 2007, January, 13-27

+ 63076 **cervical, each additional interspace (List separately in addition to code for primary procedure)**

EXCLUDES *Anterior cervical discectomy and anterior interbody fusion at same level during same session (22552)*

Code first (63075)

Do not report with anterior interbody arthodesis (even by another provider) (22554)

7.43 7.43 Global Days ZZZ

AMA: 2009, Jan, 11-31; 2008, Jan, 10-25; 2007, January, 13-27

63077 **thoracic, single interspace**

44.21 44.21 Global Days 090

AMA: 2009, Jan, 11-31; 2008, Jan, 10-25; 2007, January, 13-27

+ 63078 **thoracic, each additional interspace (List separately in addition to code for primary procedure)**

Code first (63077)

5.74 5.74 Global Days ZZZ

AMA: 2009, Jan, 11-31; 2008, Jan, 10-25; 2007, January, 13-27

63081-63091 Vertebral Corpectomy, All Levels, Anterior Approach

INCLUDES Disc removal at the level below and/or above vertebral segment

EXCLUDES *Arthrodesis (22548-22812)*

Code also reconstruction (20930-20938, 22548-22812, 22840-22855)

63081 **Vertebral corpectomy (vertebral body resection), partial or complete, anterior approach with decompression of spinal cord and/or nerve root(s); cervical, single segment**

EXCLUDES *Transoral approach (61575-61576)*

52.38 52.38 Global Days 090

+ 63082 **cervical, each additional segment (List separately in addition to code for primary procedure)**

EXCLUDES *Transoral approach (61575-61576)*

Code first (63081)

7.98 7.98 Global Days ZZZ

63085 **Vertebral corpectomy (vertebral body resection), partial or complete, transthoracic approach with decompression of spinal cord and/or nerve root(s); thoracic, single segment**

56.06 56.06 Global Days 090

+ 63086 **thoracic, each additional segment (List separately in addition to code for primary procedure)**

Code first (63085)

5.69 5.69 Global Days ZZZ

63087 **Vertebral corpectomy (vertebral body resection), partial or complete, combined thoracolumbar approach with decompression of spinal cord, cauda equina or nerve root(s), lower thoracic or lumbar; single segment**

70.54 70.54 Global Days 090

+ 63088 **each additional segment (List separately in addition to code for primary procedure)**

Code first (63087)

7.65 7.65 Global Days ZZZ

63090 **Vertebral corpectomy (vertebral body resection), partial or complete, transperitoneal or retroperitoneal approach with decompression of spinal cord, cauda equina or nerve root(s), lower thoracic, lumbar, or sacral; single segment**

58.02 58.02 Global Days 090

+ 63091 **each additional segment (List separately in addition to code for primary procedure)**

Code first (63090)

5.29 5.29 Global Days ZZZ

63101-63103 Corpectomy Lateral Extracavitary Approach

63101 **Vertebral corpectomy (vertebral body resection), partial or complete, lateral extracavitary approach with decompression of spinal cord and/or nerve root(s) (eg, for tumor or retropulsed bone fragments); thoracic, single segment**

68.65 68.65 Global Days 090

63102 **lumbar, single segment**

66.18 66.18 Global Days 090

+ 63103 **thoracic or lumbar, each additional segment (List separately in addition to code for primary procedure)**

Code first (63101-63102)

8.66 8.66 Global Days ZZZ

63170-63295 Laminectomies

63170 **Laminectomy with myelotomy (eg, Bischof or DREZ type), cervical, thoracic, or thoracolumbar**

46.93 46.93 Global Days 090

63172 **Laminectomy with drainage of intramedullary cyst/syrinx; to subarachnoid space**

41.65 41.65 Global Days 090

63173 **to peritoneal or pleural space**

51.08 51.08 Global Days 090

63180 **Laminectomy and section of dentate ligaments, with or without dural graft, cervical; 1 or 2 segments**

43.58 43.58 Global Days 090

63182 **more than 2 segments**

47.37 47.37 Global Days 090

63185 **Laminectomy with rhizotomy; 1 or 2 segments**

INCLUDES Dana rhizotomy
Stoffel rhizotomy

35.10 35.10 Global Days 090

63190 **more than 2 segments**

37.32 37.32 Global Days 090

63191 **Laminectomy with section of spinal accessory nerve**

EXCLUDES *Division of sternocleidomastoid muscle for torticollis (21720)*

36.48 36.48 Global Days 090

63194 **Laminectomy with cordotomy, with section of 1 spinothalamic tract, 1 stage; cervical** C5 C 80 PQ
37.41 37.41 Global Days 090

63195 **thoracic** C5 C 80 PQ
45.34 45.34 Global Days 090

63196 **Laminectomy with cordotomy, with section of both spinothalamic tracts, 1 stage; cervical** C5 C 80 PQ
40.94 40.94 Global Days 090

63197 **thoracic** C5 C 80 PQ
50.60 50.60 Global Days 090

63198 **Laminectomy with cordotomy with section of both spinothalamic tracts, 2 stages within 14 days; cervical** C5 C 80 PQ
INCLUDES Keen laminectomy
46.70 46.70 Global Days 090

63199 **thoracic** C5 C 80 PQ
55.50 55.50 Global Days 090

63200 **Laminectomy, with release of tethered spinal cord, lumbar** C5 C 80 PQ
45.16 45.16 Global Days 090

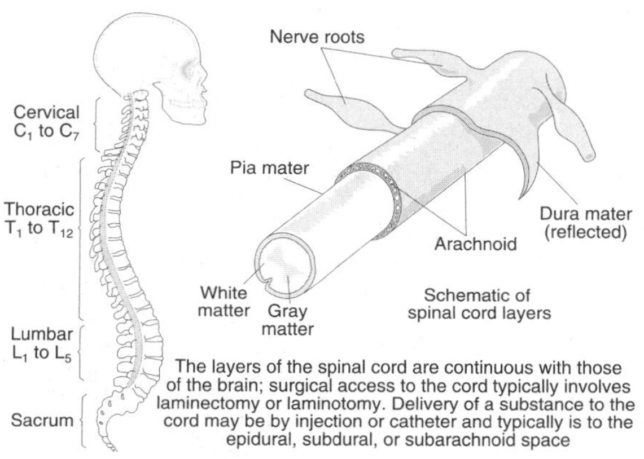

The layers of the spinal cord are continuous with those of the brain; surgical access to the cord typically involves laminectomy or laminotomy. Delivery of a substance to the cord may be by injection or catheter and typically is to the epidural, subdural, or subarachnoid space

63250 **Laminectomy for excision or occlusion of arteriovenous malformation of spinal cord; cervical** C5 C 80
87.75 87.75 Global Days 090

63251 **thoracic** C5 C 80
89.80 89.80 Global Days 090

63252 **thoracolumbar** C5 C 80
89.76 89.76 Global Days 090

63265 **Laminectomy for excision or evacuation of intraspinal lesion other than neoplasm, extradural; cervical** C5 C 80
49.38 49.38 Global Days 090

63266 **thoracic** C5 C 80
50.91 50.91 Global Days 090

63267 **lumbar** C5 C 80 PQ
40.76 40.76 Global Days 090

63268 **sacral** C5 C 80
42.88 42.88 Global Days 090

63270 **Laminectomy for excision of intraspinal lesion other than neoplasm, intradural; cervical** C5 C 80
61.37 61.37 Global Days 090

63271 **thoracic** C5 C 80
61.23 61.23 Global Days 090

63272 **lumbar** C5 C 80
56.35 56.35 Global Days 090

63273 **sacral** C5 C 80
54.85 54.85 Global Days 090

63275 **Laminectomy for biopsy/excision of intraspinal neoplasm; extradural, cervical** C5 C 80
53.18 53.18 Global Days 090

63276 **extradural, thoracic** C5 C 80 PQ
52.80 52.80 Global Days 090

63277 **extradural, lumbar** C5 C 80
45.93 45.93 Global Days 090

63278 **extradural, sacral** C5 C 80
46.85 46.85 Global Days 090

63280 **intradural, extramedullary, cervical** C5 C 80
62.49 62.49 Global Days 090

63281 **intradural, extramedullary, thoracic** C5 C 80
62.02 62.02 Global Days 090

63282 **intradural, extramedullary, lumbar** C5 C 80
58.36 58.36 Global Days 090

63283 **intradural, sacral** C5 C 80
56.11 56.11 Global Days 090

63285 **intradural, intramedullary, cervical** C5 C 80
77.28 77.28 Global Days 090

63286 **intradural, intramedullary, thoracic** C5 C 80
75.88 75.88 Global Days 090

63287 **intradural, intramedullary, thoracolumbar** C5 C 80
81.19 81.19 Global Days 090

63290 **combined extradural-intradural lesion, any level** C5 C 80
EXCLUDES *Drainage intermedullary cyst or syrinx (63172-63173)*
82.57 82.57 Global Days 090

+ 63295 **Osteoplastic reconstruction of dorsal spinal elements, following primary intraspinal procedure (List separately in addition to code for primary procedure)** C5 C 80
Code first (63172-63173, 63185, 63190, 63200-63290)
Do not report with procedure performed at the same vertebral segment(s) (22590-22614, 22840-22844, 63050-63051)
9.84 9.84 Global Days ZZZ

63300-63308 Vertebral Corpectomy for Intraspinal Lesion: Anterior/Anterolateral Approach

EXCLUDES *Arthrodesis (22548-22585)*
Spinal reconstruction (20930-20938)

63300 **Vertebral corpectomy (vertebral body resection), partial or complete, for excision of intraspinal lesion, single segment; extradural, cervical** C5 C 80
54.32 54.32 Global Days 090

63301 **extradural, thoracic by transthoracic approach** C5 C 80
64.75 64.75 Global Days 090

63302 **extradural, thoracic by thoracolumbar approach** C5 C 80
64.00 64.00 Global Days 090

63303 **extradural, lumbar or sacral by transperitoneal or retroperitoneal approach** C5 C 80
65.59 65.59 Global Days 090

63304 **intradural, cervical** C5 C 80
69.41 69.41 Global Days 090

63305 **intradural, thoracic by transthoracic approach** C5 C 80
73.38 73.38 Global Days 090

63306 **intradural, thoracic by thoracolumbar approach** C5 C 80
65.33 65.33 Global Days 090

63307 **intradural, lumbar or sacral by transperitoneal or retroperitoneal approach**
71.00 71.00 Global Days 090

\+ 63308 **each additional segment (List separately in addition to codes for single segment)**
Code first (63300-63307)
9.51 9.51 Global Days ZZZ

63600-63615 Stereotactic Procedures of the Spinal Cord

63600 **Creation of lesion of spinal cord by stereotactic method, percutaneous, any modality (including stimulation and/or recording)**
27.19 27.19 Global Days 090

63610 **Stereotactic stimulation of spinal cord, percutaneous, separate procedure not followed by other surgery**
12.77 19.32 Global Days 000

63615 **Stereotactic biopsy, aspiration, or excision of lesion, spinal cord**
36.30 36.30 Global Days 090

63620-63621 Stereotactic Radiosurgery (SRS): Spine

INCLUDES Computer assisted planning
Planning dosimetry, targeting, positioning, or blocking by neurosurgeon

EXCLUDES *Arteriovenous malformations (see Radiation Oncology Section)*
Intensity modulated beam delivery plan and treatment (77301, 77418)
Stereotactic body radiation therapy (77373, 77435)
Treatment planning, physics, dosimetry, treatment delivery and management provided by the oncologist (77261-77790 [77424, 77425])

Do not report stereotactic radiosurgery services with radiation treatment management by the same physician (77427-77432)
Do not report with (61781-61783)

63620 **Stereotactic radiosurgery (particle beam, gamma ray, or linear accelerator); 1 spinal lesion**
Do not report more than once per treatment course
32.08 32.08 Global Days 090

\+ 63621 **each additional spinal lesion (List separately in addition to code for primary procedure)**
Code first (63620)
Do not report more than twice per entire treatment course
7.38 7.38 Global Days ZZZ

63650-63688 Spinal Neurostimulation

CMS 100-3,160.2 Treatment of Motor Function Disorders with Electric Nerve Stimulation
CMS 100-3,160.7 Electrical Nerve Stimulators
EXCLUDES *Analysis and programming of neurostimulator pulse generator (95970-95975)*

63650 **Percutaneous implantation of neurostimulator electrode array, epidural**
INCLUDES The following are components of a neurostimulator system:
Collection of contacts of which four or more provide the electrical stimulation in the epidural space
Contacts on a catheter-type lead (array)
Extension
External controller
Implanted neurostimulator

Code also (C1778, C1897, L8680)
12.55 12.55 Global Days 010
AMA: 2009, Jan, 11-31; 2008, Jan, 10-25; 2007, January, 13-27

63655 **Laminectomy for implantation of neurostimulator electrodes, plate/paddle, epidural**
INCLUDES The following are components of a neurostimulator system:
Collection of contacts of which four or more provide the electrical stimulation in the epidural space
Contacts on a plate or paddle-shaped surface for systems placed by open exposure
Extension
External controller
Implanted neurostimulator

Code also (C1778, C1897, L8680)
24.47 24.47 Global Days 090

63661 **Removal of spinal neurostimulator electrode percutaneous array(s), including fluoroscopy, when performed**
INCLUDES The following are components of a neurostimulator system:
Collection of contacts of which four or more provide the electrical stimulation in the epidural space
Contacts on a catheter-type lead (array)
Extension
External controller
Implanted neurostimulator

Do not report when removing or replacing a temporary array placed percutaneously for an external generator
9.56 17.67 Global Days 010

63662 **Removal of spinal neurostimulator electrode plate/paddle(s) placed via laminotomy or laminectomy, including fluoroscopy, when performed**
INCLUDES The following are components of a neurostimulator system:
Collection of contacts of which four or more provide the electrical stimulation in the epidural space
Contacts on a catheter-type lead (array)
Extension
External controller
Implanted neurostimulator

23.09 23.09 Global Days 090

63663 **Revision including replacement, when performed, of spinal neurostimulator electrode percutaneous array(s), including fluoroscopy, when performed**
INCLUDES The following are components of a neurostimulator system:
Collection of contacts of which four or more provide the electrical stimulation in the epidural space
Contacts on a catheter-type lead (array)
Extension
External controller
Implanted neurostimulator

Do not report when removing or replacing a temporary array placed percutaneously for an external generator
Do not report with (63661-63662)
13.95 25.13 Global Days 010

63664 **Revision including replacement, when performed, of spinal neurostimulator electrode plate/paddle(s) placed via laminotomy or laminectomy, including fluoroscopy, when performed** J8 S 80

INCLUDES The following are components of a neurostimulator system:
Collection of contacts of which four or more provide the electrical stimulation in the epidural space
Contacts on a catheter-type lead (array)
Extension
External controller
Implanted neurostimulator

Do not report with (63661-63662)

23.65 23.65 Global Days 090

63685 **Insertion or replacement of spinal neurostimulator pulse generator or receiver, direct or inductive coupling** J8 S 80

Code also (C1767, C1820, L8685-L8688)

Do not report with 63688 for the same pulse generator or receiver

10.67 10.67 Global Days 010

63688 **Revision or removal of implanted spinal neurostimulator pulse generator or receiver** A2 T

Do not report with 63685 for the same pulse generator or receiver

10.81 10.81 Global Days 010

63700-63706 Repair Congenital Neural Tube Defects

EXCLUDES *Complex skin repair (see appropriate integumentary closure code)*

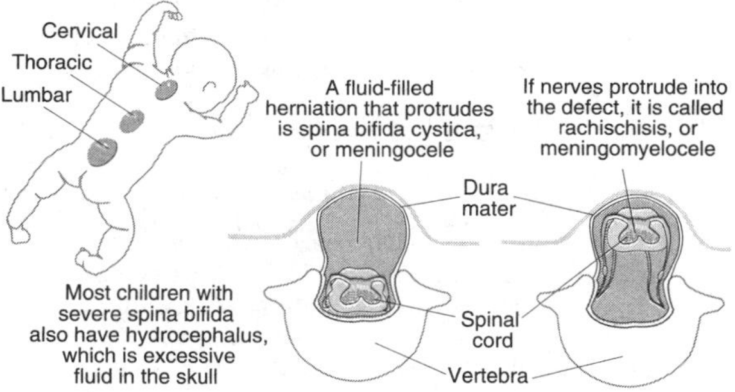

63700 **Repair of meningocele; less than 5 cm diameter** C5 C 80

38.17 38.17 Global Days 090

63702 **larger than 5 cm diameter** C5 C 80

42.01 42.01 Global Days 090

63704 **Repair of myelomeningocele; less than 5 cm diameter** C5 C 80

48.31 48.31 Global Days 090

63706 **larger than 5 cm diameter** C5 C 80

54.12 54.12 Global Days 090

63707-63710 Repair Dural Cerebrospinal Fluid Leak

63707 **Repair of dural/cerebrospinal fluid leak, not requiring laminectomy** C5 C 80

26.94 26.94 Global Days 090

63709 **Repair of dural/cerebrospinal fluid leak or pseudomeningocele, with laminectomy** C5 C 80

32.50 32.50 Global Days 090

63710 **Dural graft, spinal** C5 C 80

EXCLUDES *Laminectomy and section of dentate ligament (63180, 63182)*

32.67 32.67 Global Days 090

63740-63746 Cerebrospinal Fluid (CSF) Shunt: Lumbar

EXCLUDES *Placement of subarachnoid catheter with reservoir and/or pump:*
Not requiring laminectomy (62350, 62360-62362)
With laminectomy (62351, 62360-62362)

63740 **Creation of shunt, lumbar, subarachnoid-peritoneal, -pleural, or other; including laminectomy** C5 C 80

27.96 27.96 Global Days 090

63741 **percutaneous, not requiring laminectomy** T 80

18.62 18.62 Global Days 090

63744 **Replacement, irrigation or revision of lumbosubarachnoid shunt** A2 T 80

19.92 19.92 Global Days 090

63746 **Removal of entire lumbosubarachnoid shunt system without replacement** A2 T 80

17.61 17.61 Global Days 090

64400-64455 Nerve Blocks

EXCLUDES *Epidural or subarachnoid injection (62310-62319)*
Nerve destruction (62280-62282, 64600-64681 [64633, 64634, 64635, 64636])

64400 **Injection, anesthetic agent; trigeminal nerve, any division or branch** P3 T 50

2.00 3.47 Global Days 000

AMA: 2009, Jan, 11-31; 2008, Jan, 10-25; 2008, Jun, 8-11; 2007, January, 13-27

64402 **facial nerve** P3 T 50

2.20 3.48 Global Days 000

AMA: 2009, Jan, 11-31; 2008, Jan, 10-25; 2008, Jun, 8-11; 2007, January, 13-27

64405 **greater occipital nerve** P3 T 50

1.82 2.85 Global Days 000

AMA: 2009, Jan, 11-31; 2008, Jan, 10-25; 2008, Jun, 8-11; 2007, January, 13-27

64408 **vagus nerve** P3 T 80 50

2.31 3.15 Global Days 000

AMA: 2009, Jan, 11-31; 2008, Jan, 10-25; 2008, Jun, 8-11; 2007, January, 13-27

64410 **phrenic nerve** A2 T 80 50

2.57 4.47 Global Days 000

AMA: 2009, Jan, 11-31; 2008, Jun, 8-11; 2008, Jan, 10-25; 2007, January, 13-27

64412 **spinal accessory nerve** P3 T 50

2.18 4.37 Global Days 000

AMA: 2009, Jan, 11-31; 2008, Jan, 10-25; 2008, Jun, 8-11; 2007, January, 13-27; 2007, Aug, 15

64413 **cervical plexus** P3 T 50

2.36 3.63 Global Days 000

AMA: 2009, Jan, 11-31; 2008, Jun, 8-11; 2008, Jan, 10-25; 2007, Aug, 15; 2007, January, 13-27

64415 **brachial plexus, single** A2 T 50

1.96 3.65 Global Days 000

AMA: 2009, Jan, 11-31; 2008, Jan, 10-25; 2008, Jun, 8-11; 2007, January, 13-27

64416 **brachial plexus, continuous infusion by catheter (including catheter placement)**

Do not report with (01996)

2.38 2.38 Global Days 000

AMA: 2009, Jan, 11-31; 2008, Jun, 8-11; 2008, Jan, 10-25; 2007, January, 13-27

64417 **axillary nerve**

2.09 3.91 Global Days 000

AMA: 2009, Jan, 11-31; 2008, Jan, 10-25; 2008, Jun, 8-11; 2007, January, 13-27

64418 **suprascapular nerve**

2.18 4.08 Global Days 000

AMA: 2009, Jan, 11-31; 2008, Jan, 10-25; 2008, Jun, 8-11; 2007, January, 13-27; 2007, Aug, 15

64420 **intercostal nerve, single**

2.00 3.70 Global Days 000

AMA: 2009, Jan, 11-31; 2008, Jan, 10-25; 2008, Jun, 8-11; 2007, January, 13-27

64421 **intercostal nerves, multiple, regional block**

2.77 5.22 Global Days 000

AMA: 2009, Jan, 11-31; 2008, Jan, 10-25; 2008, Jun, 8-11; 2007, January, 13-27

64425 **ilioinguinal, iliohypogastric nerves**

2.80 3.95 Global Days 000

AMA: 2009, Jan, 11-31; 2008, Jan, 10-25; 2008, Jun, 8-11; 2007, January, 13-27

64430 **pudendal nerve**

2.43 4.13 Global Days 000

AMA: 2009, Jan, 11-31; 2008, Jan, 10-25; 2008, Jun, 8-11; 2007, January, 13-27

64435 **paracervical (uterine) nerve** ♀

2.47 4.13 Global Days 000

AMA: 2009, Jan, 11-31; 2008, Jan, 10-25; 2008, Jun, 8-11; 2007, January, 13-27

64445 **sciatic nerve, single**

2.18 4.00 Global Days 000

AMA: 2008, Jun, 8-11

64446 **sciatic nerve, continuous infusion by catheter (including catheter placement)**

Do not report with (01996)

2.40 2.40 Global Days 000

AMA: 2008, Jun, 8-11

64447 **femoral nerve, single**

Do not report with (01996)

1.95 3.65 Global Days 000

AMA: 2008, Jun, 8-11

64448 **femoral nerve, continuous infusion by catheter (including catheter placement)**

Do not report with (01996)

2.14 2.14 Global Days 000

AMA: 2008, Jun, 8-11

64449 **lumbar plexus, posterior approach, continuous infusion by catheter (including catheter placement)**

Do not report with (01996)

2.48 2.48 Global Days 000

AMA: 2008, Jun, 8-11

64450 **other peripheral nerve or branch**

EXCLUDES *Morton's neuroma (64455, 64632)*

2.03 3.10 Global Days 000

AMA: 2009, Jan, 6&9; 2009, Jan, 11-31; 2008, Jan, 10-25; 2008, Jun, 8-11; 2007, January, 13-27

64455 **Injection(s), anesthetic agent and/or steroid, plantar common digital nerve(s) (eg, Morton's neuroma)**

Do not report with (64632)

1.06 1.42 Global Days 000

AMA: 2009, Jan, 6&9

64479-64484 Transforaminal Injection

INCLUDES Imaging guidance (fluoroscopy or CT) and contrast injection

EXCLUDES *Epidural or subarachnoid injection (62310-62319)*
Nerve destruction (62280-62282, 64600-64681 [64633, 64634, 64635, 64636])

The articular facet joints of a single vertebral level are injected with an anesthetic agent or steroid. Report code 64479 for a single level cervical or thoracic injection. Report 64480 for each additional level in the cervical or thoracic regions

64479 **Injection(s), anesthetic agent and/or steroid, transforaminal epidural, with imaging guidance (fluoroscopy or CT); cervical or thoracic, single level**

EXCLUDES *Transforaminal epidural injection under ultrasound guidance (0228T)*

3.94 7.66 Global Days 000

AMA: 2008, Jul, 9; 2008, Jun, 8-11; 2008, Nov, 10-11

+ **64480** **cervical or thoracic, each additional level (List separately in addition to code for primary procedure)**

EXCLUDES *Transforaminal epidural injection at T12-L1 level (64479)*
Transforaminal epidural injection under ultrasound guidance (0229T)

Code first (64479)

1.95 3.67 Global Days ZZZ

AMA: 2009, Jan, 11-31; 2008, Jan, 10-25; 2008, Jul, 9; 2008, Jun, 8-11; 2008, Nov, 10-11; 2007, January, 13-27

64483 **lumbar or sacral, single level**

EXCLUDES *Transforaminal epidural injection under ultrasound guidance (0230T)*

3.29 7.11 Global Days 000

AMA: 2008, Jun, 8-11; 2008, Jul, 9; 2008, Nov, 10-11

+ **64484** **lumbar or sacral, each additional level (List separately in addition to code for primary procedure)**

EXCLUDES *Transforaminal epidural injection under ultrasound guidance (0231T)*

Code first (64483)

1.55 2.94 Global Days ZZZ

AMA: 2009, Jan, 11-31; 2008, Jan, 10-25; 2008, Jun, 8-11; 2008, Nov, 10-11; 2008, Jul, 9; 2007, January, 13-27

64490-64495 Paraspinal Nerve Injections

INCLUDES Image guidance (CT or fluoroscopy) and any contrast injection

EXCLUDES *Injection without imaging (20552-20553)*
Ultrasonic guidance (0213T-0218T)

64490 **Injection(s), diagnostic or therapeutic agent, paravertebral facet (zygapophyseal) joint (or nerves innervating that joint) with image guidance (fluoroscopy or CT), cervical or thoracic; single level** G2 T 80 50
INCLUDES Injection of T12-L1 joint and nerves that innervate that joint
3.26 5.94 Global Days 000

+ 64491 **second level (List separately in addition to code for primary procedure)** G2 T 80 50
Code first (64490)
1.82 2.89 Global Days ZZZ

+ 64492 **third and any additional level(s) (List separately in addition to code for primary procedure)** G2 T 80 50
Code first (64490)
Do not report more than one time per day
1.84 2.91 Global Days ZZZ

64493 **Injection(s), diagnostic or therapeutic agent, paravertebral facet (zygapophyseal) joint (or nerves innervating that joint) with image guidance (fluoroscopy or CT), lumbar or sacral; single level** G2 T 80 50
2.74 5.32 Global Days 000

+ 64494 **second level (List separately in addition to code for primary procedure)** G2 T 80 50
Code first (64493)
1.54 2.64 Global Days ZZZ

+ 64495 **third and any additional level(s) (List separately in addition to code for primary procedure)** G2 T 80 50
Code first (64493)
Do not report more than one time per day
1.57 2.66 Global Days ZZZ

64505-64530 Sympathetic Nerve Blocks

64505 **Injection, anesthetic agent; sphenopalatine ganglion** P3 T
2.46 2.95 Global Days 000
AMA: 2009, Jan, 11-31; 2008, Jun, 8-11; 2008, Jan, 10-25; 2007, January, 13-27

64508 **carotid sinus (separate procedure)** P3 T 80
2.26 2.53 Global Days 000
AMA: 2008, Jun, 8-11

64510 **stellate ganglion (cervical sympathetic)** A2 T
2.13 3.97 Global Days 000
AMA: 2008, Jun, 8-11

64517 **superior hypogastric plexus** A2 T
3.69 5.42 Global Days 000
AMA: 2009, Jan, 11-31; 2008, Jan, 10-25; 2008, Jun, 8-11; 2007, January, 13-27

64520 **lumbar or thoracic (paravertebral sympathetic)** A2 T
2.36 5.81 Global Days 000
AMA: 2008, Jun, 8-11

64530 **celiac plexus, with or without radiologic monitoring** A2 T PQ
2.73 5.92 Global Days 000
AMA: 2009, Jan, 11-31; 2008, Jan, 10-25; 2008, Jun, 8-11; 2007, January, 13-27

64550 Transcutaneous Electrical Nerve Stimulation

CMS 100-3,160.2 Treatment of Motor Function Disorders with Electric Nerve Stimulation
CMS 100-3,160.7.1 Assessing Patients Suitability for Electrical Nerve Stimulation Therapy
CMS 100-3,160.13 Supplies Used for Transcutaneous Electrical Nerve Stimulation and Neuromuscular Electrical Stimulation (NMES)
CMS 100-3,280.13 Transcutaneous Electrical Nerve Stimulators (TENS)
CMS 100-4,4,20.5 HCPCS Under OPPS

EXCLUDES *Analysis and programming neurostimulator pulse generator (95970-95975)*
Implantation of electrode array(s), either trial or permanent, with pulse generator for peripheral subcutaneous field stimulation (0282T-0284T)

64550 **Application of surface (transcutaneous) neurostimulator** A
0.26 0.47 Global Days 000
AMA: 2009, Jan, 11-31; 2008, Jan, 10-25; 2007, January, 13-27

64553-64570 Electrical Nerve Stimulation: Insertion/Replacement/Removal/Revision

CMS 100-3,160.2 Treatment of Motor Function Disorders with Electric Nerve Stimulation
CMS 100-3,160.7 Electrical Nerve Stimulators
CMS 100-3,160.7.1 Assessing Patients Suitability for Electrical Nerve Stimulation Therapy
CMS 100-3,160.12 Neuromuscular Electrical Stimulation (NMES)
CMS 100-3,160.13 Supplies Used for Transcutaneous Electrical Nerve Stimulation and Neuromuscular Electrical Stimulation (NMES)
CMS 100-4,32,40 Sacral Nerve Stimulation

INCLUDES Simple and complex neurostimulators

EXCLUDES *Analysis and programming of neurostimulator pulse generator (95970-95975)*
Implantation of electrode array(s), either trial or permanent, with pulse generator for peripheral subcutaneous field stimulation (0282T-0284T)

▲ 64553 **Percutaneous implantation of neurostimulator electrode array; cranial nerve** J8 S 80
EXCLUDES *Open procedure (61885-61886)*
Code also (C1778, C1897, L8680)
4.90 6.43 Global Days 010

▲ 64555 **peripheral nerve (excludes sacral nerve)** J8 S
Code also (C1778, C1897, L8680)
Do not report with (64566)
4.33 5.81 Global Days 010

~~64560~~ ~~autonomic nerve~~

▲ 64561 **sacral nerve (transforaminal placement)** J8 S 50 PQ
Code also (C1778, C1897, L8680)
11.83 26.18 Global Days 010

▲ 64565 **neuromuscular** J8 S
Code also (C1778, C1897, L8680)
3.72 5.28 Global Days 010
AMA: 2009, Jan, 11-31; 2008, Jan, 10-25; 2007, January, 13-27

64566 **Posterior tibial neurostimulation, percutaneous needle electrode, single treatment, includes programming** G2 T 80
Do not report with (64555, 95970-95972)
0.87 3.93 Global Days 000

64568 **Incision for implantation of cranial nerve (eg, vagus nerve) neurostimulator electrode array and pulse generator** J8 S 80 50
Do not report with (61885-61886, 64570)
Code also (C1767, C1778, C1820, C1897, L8680, L8685-L8688)
18.73 18.73 Global Days 090

64569 **Revision or replacement of cranial nerve (eg, vagus nerve) neurostimulator electrode array, including connection to existing pulse generator** G2 T 80 50

EXCLUDES *Replacement of pulse generator (61885)*

Do not report with (61888, 64570)

20.55 20.55 Global Days 090

64570 **Removal of cranial nerve (eg, vagus nerve) neurostimulator electrode array and pulse generator** G2 T 80 50

Do not report with (61888)

16.59 16.59 Global Days 090

64575-64595 Implantation/Revision/Removal Neurostimulators: Incisional

INCLUDES Simple and complex neurostimulators

EXCLUDES *Implantation of electrode array(s), either trial or permanent, with pulse generator for peripheral subcutaneous field stimulation (0282T-0284T)*

▲ 64575 **Incision for implantation of neurostimulator electrode array; peripheral nerve (excludes sacral nerve)** J8 S

Code also (C1778, C1897, L8680)

8.81 8.81 Global Days 090

~~64577~~ ~~**autonomic nerve**~~

▲ 64580 **neuromuscular** J8 S 80

Code also (C1778, C1897, L8680)

8.97 8.97 Global Days 090

▲ 64581 **sacral nerve (transforaminal placement)** J8 S

Code also (C1778, C1897, L8680)

20.10 20.10 Global Days 090

▲ 64585 **Revision or removal of peripheral neurostimulator electrode array** A2 T

4.37 7.99 Global Days 010

64590 **Insertion or replacement of peripheral or gastric neurostimulator pulse generator or receiver, direct or inductive coupling** J8 S

Code also (C1767, C1820, L8685-L8688)

Do not report with (64595)

4.83 8.11 Global Days 010

AMA: 2007, March, 4-5; 2007, April, 7-10

64595 **Revision or removal of peripheral or gastric neurostimulator pulse generator or receiver** A2 T

Do not report with (64590)

3.83 7.86 Global Days 010

AMA: 2009, Jan, 11-31; 2008, Jan, 8-9; 2007, April, 7-10; 2007, March, 4-5

64600-64610 Neurolysis Trigeminal Nerve

CMS 100-3,160.1 Induced Lesions of Nerve Tracts

INCLUDES Injection of therapeutic medication

EXCLUDES *Treatments that do not destroy the target nerve (64999)*

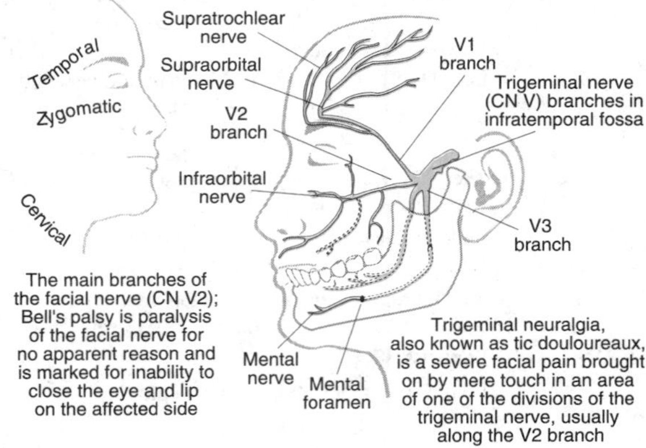

64600 **Destruction by neurolytic agent, trigeminal nerve; supraorbital, infraorbital, mental, or inferior alveolar branch** A2 T

6.46 12.06 Global Days 010

AMA: 2008, Jun, 8-11

64605 **second and third division branches at foramen ovale** A2 T 80 PQ

9.89 17.25 Global Days 010

AMA: 2008, Jun, 8-11

64610 **second and third division branches at foramen ovale under radiologic monitoring** A2 T PQ

14.36 22.19 Global Days 010

AMA: 2008, Jun, 8-11

64611-64614 Chemical Denervation Procedures

CMS 100-3,160.1 Induced Lesions of Nerve Tracts

INCLUDES Injection of therapeutic medication

EXCLUDES *Electromyography or muscle electric stimulation guidance (95873-95874)*
Nerve destruction of:
Anal sphincter (46505)
Extraocular muscles to treat strabismus (67345)
Treatments that do not destroy the target nerve (64999)

64611 **Chemodenervation of parotid and submandibular salivary glands, bilateral** P3 T 80

Code also modifier 52 for injection of fewer than four salivary glands

2.68 2.99 Global Days 010

64612 **Chemodenervation of muscle(s); muscle(s) innervated by facial nerve (eg, for blepharospasm, hemifacial spasm)** P3 T 50

4.71 5.13 Global Days 010

AMA: 2009, Jan, 11-31; 2009, Jan, 7-8; 2008, Jan, 10-25; 2008, Jun, 8-11; 2007, January, 13-27

64613 **neck muscle(s) (eg, for spasmodic torticollis, spasmodic dysphonia)** P3 T 50

4.40 4.88 Global Days 010

AMA: 2009, Jan, 7-8; 2009, Jan, 11-31; 2008, Jan, 10-25; 2008, Jun, 8-11; 2007, January, 13-27

64614 **extremity(s) and/or trunk muscle(s) (eg, for dystonia, cerebral palsy, multiple sclerosis)** P3 T 50
4.59 5.22 Global Days 010
AMA: 2009, Jan, 11-31; 2008, Jan, 10-25; 2008, Jun, 8-11; 2007, January, 13-27

64620-64640 [64633, 64634, 64635, 64636] Neurolysis: Intercostal, Facet Joint, and Pudendal Nerve

CMS 100-3,160.1 Induced Lesions of Nerve Tracts

INCLUDES Injection of therapeutic medication

EXCLUDES *Treatments that do not destroy the target nerve (64999)*

64620 **Destruction by neurolytic agent, intercostal nerve** A2 T PQ
5.09 6.62 Global Days 010
AMA: 2008, Jun, 8-11

64622 ~~Destruction by neurolytic agent, paravertebral facet joint nerve; lumbar or sacral, single level~~
To report, see 64635

64623 ~~lumbar or sacral, each additional level (List separately in addition to code for primary procedure)~~
To report, see 64636

64626 ~~cervical or thoracic, single level~~
To report, see 64633

64627 ~~cervical or thoracic, each additional level (List separately in addition to code for primary procedure)~~
To report, see 64634

#● 64633 **Destruction by neurolytic agent, paravertebral facet joint nerve(s), with imaging guidance (fluoroscopy or CT); cervical or thoracic, single facet joint** G2 T 50
INCLUDES Imaging guidance (fluoroscopy or CT) and contrast injection
Paravertebral facet destruction of T12-L1 joint or nerve(s) that innervate that joint
EXCLUDES *Destruction of paravertebral facet joint nerve(s) without imaging guidance (64999)*
Do not report with (77003, 77012)
6.92 13.29 Global Days 010

\+ #● 64634 **cervical or thoracic, each additional facet joint (List separately in addition to code for primary procedure)** G2 T 50
INCLUDES Imaging guidance (fluoroscopy or CT) and contrast injection
EXCLUDES *Destruction of paravertebral facet joint nerve(s) without imaging guidance (64999)*
Code first ([64633])
Do not report with (77003, 77012)
2.07 6.09 Global Days ZZZ

#● 64635 **lumbar or sacral, single facet joint** G2 T 50
INCLUDES Imaging guidance (fouroscopy or CT) and contrast injection
EXCLUDES *Destruction of paravertebral facet joint nerve(s) without imaging guidance (64999)*
Do not report with (77003, 77012)
6.78 13.06 Global Days 010

\+ #● 64636 **lumbar or sacral, each additional facet joint (List separately in addition to code for primary procedure)** G2 T 50
INCLUDES Imaging guidance (fluoroscopy or CT) with contrast injection
EXCLUDES *Destruction of paravertebral facet joint nerve(s) without imaging guidance (64999)*
Code first ([64635])
Do not report with (77003, 77012)
1.80 5.48 Global Days ZZZ

64630 **Destruction by neurolytic agent; pudendal nerve** A2 T 80
5.60 6.77 Global Days 010
AMA: 2008, Jun, 8-11

64632 **plantar common digital nerve** P3 T 80 50
Do not report with (64455)
2.04 2.50 Global Days 010
AMA: 2009, Jan, 6&9

64633 *Resequenced Code. See code following 64620.*

64634 *Resequenced Code. See code following 64620.*

64635 *Resequenced Code. See code following 64620.*

64636 *Resequenced Code. See code before 64630.*

64640 **other peripheral nerve or branch** P3 T 50
4.99 6.46 Global Days 010
AMA: 2008, Jun, 8-11

64650-64653 Chemical Denervation Eccrine Glands

INCLUDES Injection of therapeutic medication

EXCLUDES *Treatments that do not destroy the target nerve (64999)*

64650 **Chemodenervation of eccrine glands; both axillae** P3 T 80
1.18 3.21 Global Days 000
AMA: 2008, Jun, 8-11

64653 **other area(s) (eg, scalp, face, neck), per day** P3 T 80
EXCLUDES *Hands or feet (64999)*
1.55 3.78 Global Days 000
AMA: 2008, Jun, 8-11

64680-64681 Neurolysis: Celiac Plexus, Superior Hypogastric Plexus

INCLUDES Injection of therapeutic medication
Only for lesions that abut the dura matter or that affect the spinal neural tissue
Planning, dosimetry, targeting, positioning, or blocking performed by the surgeon
Radiation treatment management by the same physician (77427-77432)

EXCLUDES *Treatments that do not destroy the target nerve (64999)*

Do not report more than once per lesion per course of treatment

64680 **Destruction by neurolytic agent, with or without radiologic monitoring; celiac plexus** A2 T PQ
4.89 9.57 Global Days 010
AMA: 2009, Jan, 11-31; 2008, Jan, 10-25; 2008, Jun, 8-11; 2007, January, 13-27

64681 **superior hypogastric plexus** A2 T PQ
5.86 11.17 Global Days 010
AMA: 2009, Jan, 11-31; 2007, Dec, 10-179

64702-64727 Decompression and/or Transposition of Nerve

INCLUDES External neurolysis and/or transposition to repair or restore a nerve
Neuroplasty with nerve wrapping
Surgical decompression/freeing of nerve from scar tissue

EXCLUDES *Facial nerve decompression (69720)*
Neuroplasty with operating microscope (64727)
Percutaneous neurolysis (62263-62264, 62280-62282)

64702 **Neuroplasty; digital, 1 or both, same digit** A2 T
14.61 14.61 Global Days 090
AMA: 2009, Jan, 11-31; 2008, Jan, 10-25; 2007, January, 13-27

64704 **nerve of hand or foot** A2 T 80
9.29 9.29 Global Days 090
AMA: 2009, Jan, 11-31; 2008, Jan, 10-25; 2007, January, 13-27

64708 **Neuroplasty, major peripheral nerve, arm or leg, open; other than specified** A2 T 80
14.54 14.54 Global Days 090
AMA: 2009, Jan, 11-31; 2008, Jan, 10-25; 2007, January, 13-27

64712 **sciatic nerve** A2 T 80
16.39 16.39 Global Days 090
AMA: 2009, Jan, 11-31; 2008, Jan, 10-25; 2007, January, 13-27

64713 **brachial plexus** A2 T 80
22.40 22.40 Global Days 090
AMA: 2009, Jan, 11-31; 2008, Jan, 10-25; 2007, January, 13-27

64714 **lumbar plexus** A2 T 80
19.61 19.61 Global Days 090
AMA: 2009, Jan, 11-31; 2008, Jan, 10-25; 2007, January, 13-27

64716 **Neuroplasty and/or transposition; cranial nerve (specify)** A2 T 80
15.87 15.87 Global Days 090
AMA: 2009, Jan, 11-31; 2008, Jan, 10-25; 2007, January, 13-27

64718 **ulnar nerve at elbow** A2 T 80
17.35 17.35 Global Days 090
AMA: 2009, Jan, 11-31; 2009, Mar, 10-11; 2008, Jan, 10-25; 2007, January, 13-27

64719 **ulnar nerve at wrist** A2 T
11.70 11.70 Global Days 090
AMA: 2009, Jan, 11-31; 2009, Mar, 10-11; 2008, Jan, 10-25; 2007, January, 13-27

64721 **median nerve at carpal tunnel** A2 T 50
EXCLUDES *Arthroscopic procedure (29848)*
12.49 12.57 Global Days 090
AMA: 2009, Jan, 11-31; 2008, Jan, 10-25; 2007, January, 13-27

64722 **Decompression; unspecified nerve(s) (specify)** A2 T 80
10.51 10.51 Global Days 090
AMA: 2009, Jan, 11-31; 2008, Jan, 10-25; 2007, January, 13-27

64726 **plantar digital nerve** A2 T
7.97 7.97 Global Days 090
AMA: 2009, Jan, 11-31; 2008, Jan, 10-25; 2007, January, 13-27

\+ **64727** **Internal neurolysis, requiring use of operating microscope (List separately in addition to code for neuroplasty) (Neuroplasty includes external neurolysis)** A2 T
INCLUDES Operating microscope (69990)
Code first neuroplasty (64702-64721)
5.46 5.46 Global Days ZZZ
AMA: 2009, Jan, 11-31; 2008, Jan, 10-25; 2007, January, 13-27

64732-64772 Surgical Avulsion/Transection of Nerve

CMS 100-3,160.1 Induced Lesions of Nerve Tracts

EXCLUDES *Stereotactic lesion of gasserian ganglion (61790)*

64732 **Transection or avulsion of; supraorbital nerve** A2 T 80
12.82 12.82 Global Days 090

64734 **infraorbital nerve** A2 T 80
13.13 13.13 Global Days 090

64736 **mental nerve** A2 T 80
13.85 13.85 Global Days 090

64738 **inferior alveolar nerve by osteotomy** A2 T 80
14.83 14.83 Global Days 090

64740 **lingual nerve** A2 T 80
13.66 13.66 Global Days 090

64742 **facial nerve, differential or complete** A2 T 80
13.70 13.70 Global Days 090

64744 **greater occipital nerve** A2 T 80 50
14.20 14.20 Global Days 090

64746 **phrenic nerve** A2 T 80 P0
EXCLUDES *Section of recurrent unilateral laryngeal nerve (31595)*
12.96 12.96 Global Days 090

64752 **vagus nerve (vagotomy), transthoracic** C5 C 80
15.35 15.35 Global Days 090

64755 **vagus nerves limited to proximal stomach (selective proximal vagotomy, proximal gastric vagotomy, parietal cell vagotomy, supra- or highly selective vagotomy)** C5 C 80
EXCLUDES *Laparoscopic procedure (43652)*
26.77 26.77 Global Days 090

64760 **vagus nerve (vagotomy), abdominal** C5 C 80
EXCLUDES *Laparoscopic procedure (43651)*
14.87 14.87 Global Days 090

64761 **pudendal nerve** G2 T 80 50
13.50 13.50 Global Days 090

64763 **Transection or avulsion of obturator nerve, extrapelvic, with or without adductor tenotomy** G2 T 80 50
15.25 15.25 Global Days 090

64766 **Transection or avulsion of obturator nerve, intrapelvic, with or without adductor tenotomy** G2 T 80 50
17.36 17.36 Global Days 090

64771 **Transection or avulsion of other cranial nerve, extradural** A2 T 80
17.58 17.58 Global Days 090

64772 **Transection or avulsion of other spinal nerve, extradural** A2 T 80
EXCLUDES *Removal of tender scar and soft tissue including neuroma if necessary (11400-11446, 13100-13153)*
17.10 17.10 Global Days 090

64774-64823 Excisional Nerve Procedures

EXCLUDES *Morton neuroma excision (28080)*

64774 **Excision of neuroma; cutaneous nerve, surgically identifiable** A2 T
12.27 12.27 Global Days 090

64776 **digital nerve, 1 or both, same digit** A2 T 80
11.50 11.50 Global Days 090

+ 64778 digital nerve, each additional digit (List separately in addition to code for primary procedure) A2 T
Code first (64776)
5.40 5.40 Global Days ZZZ

64782 hand or foot, except digital nerve A2 T
13.28 13.28 Global Days 090

+ 64783 hand or foot, each additional nerve, except same digit (List separately in addition to code for primary procedure) A2 T
Code first (64782)
6.43 6.43 Global Days ZZZ

64784 major peripheral nerve, except sciatic A2 T 80
21.61 21.61 Global Days 090

64786 sciatic nerve A2 T 80
31.64 31.64 Global Days 090

+ 64787 Implantation of nerve end into bone or muscle (List separately in addition to neuroma excision) A2 T 80
Code first (64774-64786)
7.22 7.22 Global Days ZZZ

64788 Excision of neurofibroma or neurolemmoma; cutaneous nerve A2 T
11.67 11.67 Global Days 090

64790 major peripheral nerve A2 T 80
24.46 24.46 Global Days 090

64792 extensive (including malignant type) A2 T 80
34.86 34.86 Global Days 090

64795 Biopsy of nerve A2 T
5.71 5.71 Global Days 000

64802 Sympathectomy, cervical A2 T 80 50
15.93 15.93 Global Days 090

64804 Sympathectomy, cervicothoracic T 80 50
23.42 23.42 Global Days 090

64809 Sympathectomy, thoracolumbar C5 C 80 50
INCLUDES Leriche sympathectomy
21.81 21.81 Global Days 090

64818 Sympathectomy, lumbar C5 C 80 50
19.80 19.80 Global Days 090

64820 Sympathectomy; digital arteries, each digit G2 T
INCLUDES Operating microscope (69990)
22.35 22.35 Global Days 090
AMA: 2009, Jan, 11-31; 2008, Jan, 10-25; 2007, January, 13-27

64821 radial artery A2 T 50
INCLUDES Operating microscope (69990)
20.76 20.76 Global Days 090

64822 ulnar artery G2 T 50
INCLUDES Operating microscope (69990)
20.20 20.20 Global Days 090

64823 superficial palmar arch G2 T 50
INCLUDES Operating microscope (69990)
22.94 22.94 Global Days 090

64831-64907 Nerve Repair: Suture and Nerve Grafts

64831 Suture of digital nerve, hand or foot; 1 nerve A2 T
20.15 20.15 Global Days 090

+ 64832 each additional digital nerve (List separately in addition to code for primary procedure) A2 T 80
Code first (64831)
10.10 10.10 Global Days ZZZ

64834 Suture of 1 nerve; hand or foot, common sensory nerve A2 T 80
21.79 21.79 Global Days 090

64835 median motor thenar A2 T 80
23.83 23.83 Global Days 090

64836 ulnar motor A2 T 80
23.84 23.84 Global Days 090

+ 64837 Suture of each additional nerve, hand or foot (List separately in addition to code for primary procedure) A2 T 80
Code first (64834-64836)
10.46 10.46 Global Days ZZZ

64840 Suture of posterior tibial nerve A2 T 80
25.84 25.84 Global Days 090

64856 Suture of major peripheral nerve, arm or leg, except sciatic; including transposition A2 T
29.94 29.94 Global Days 090

64857 without transposition A2 T 80
31.13 31.13 Global Days 090

64858 Suture of sciatic nerve A2 T 80
32.09 32.09 Global Days 090

+ 64859 Suture of each additional major peripheral nerve (List separately in addition to code for primary procedure) A2 T 80
Code first (64856-64857)
7.82 7.82 Global Days ZZZ

64861 Suture of; brachial plexus A2 T 80
39.14 39.14 Global Days 090

64862 lumbar plexus A2 T 80
45.01 45.01 Global Days 090

64864 Suture of facial nerve; extracranial A2 T 80
25.97 25.97 Global Days 090

64865 infratemporal, with or without grafting A2 T 80
33.57 33.57 Global Days 090

64866 Anastomosis; facial-spinal accessory C5 C 80
33.80 33.80 Global Days 090

64868 facial-hypoglossal C5 C 80
INCLUDES Korte-Ballance anastomosis
30.67 30.67 Global Days 090

64870 facial-phrenic A2 T 80
31.10 31.10 Global Days 090

+ 64872 Suture of nerve; requiring secondary or delayed suture (List separately in addition to code for primary neurorrhaphy) A2 T 80
Code first (64831-64865)
3.48 3.48 Global Days ZZZ

+ 64874 requiring extensive mobilization, or transposition of nerve (List separately in addition to code for nerve suture) A2 T 80
Code first (64831-64865)
4.98 4.98 Global Days ZZZ

+ 64876 requiring shortening of bone of extremity (List separately in addition to code for nerve suture) A2 T 80
Code first (64831-64865)
5.44 5.44 Global Days ZZZ

64885 Nerve graft (includes obtaining graft), head or neck; up to 4 cm in length A2 T 80
32.77 32.77 Global Days 090
AMA: 2009, Jan, 11-31; 2008, Jan, 10-25; 2007, January, 13-27

64886 more than 4 cm length A2 T 80
38.29 38.29 Global Days 090
AMA: 2009, Jan, 11-31; 2008, Jan, 10-25; 2007, January, 13-27

64890 Nerve graft (includes obtaining graft), single strand, hand or foot; up to 4 cm length A2 T 80
33.00 33.00 Global Days 090

64891 more than 4 cm length A2 T 80
32.93 32.93 Global Days 090

64892 Nerve graft (includes obtaining graft), single strand, arm or leg; up to 4 cm length A2 T 80
32.06 32.06 Global Days 090

64893 more than 4 cm length A2 T 80
34.12 34.12 Global Days 090

64895 Nerve graft (includes obtaining graft), multiple strands (cable), hand or foot; up to 4 cm length A2 T 80
40.49 40.49 Global Days 090

64896 more than 4 cm length A2 T 80
47.41 47.41 Global Days 090

64897 Nerve graft (includes obtaining graft), multiple strands (cable), arm or leg; up to 4 cm length A2 T 80
38.77 38.77 Global Days 090

64898 more than 4 cm length A2 T 80
42.08 42.08 Global Days 090

+ 64901 Nerve graft, each additional nerve; single strand (List separately in addition to code for primary procedure) A2 T 80
Code first (64885-64893)
18.71 18.71 Global Days ZZZ

+ 64902 multiple strands (cable) (List separately in addition to code for primary procedure) A2 T 80
Code first (64885-64886, 64895-64898)
21.63 21.63 Global Days ZZZ

64905 Nerve pedicle transfer; first stage A2 T 80
30.66 30.66 Global Days 090

64907 second stage A2 T 80
32.78 32.78 Global Days 090

64910-64999 Nerve Repair: Synthetic and Vein Grafts

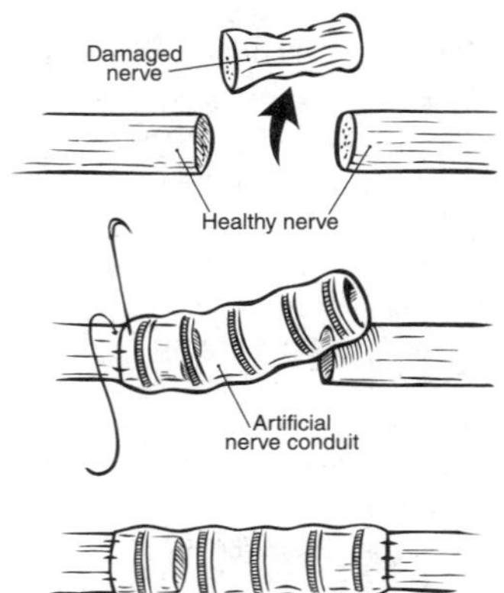

A synthetic "bridge" is affixed to each end of a severed nerve with sutures
This procedure is performed using an operating microscope

64910 Nerve repair; with synthetic conduit or vein allograft (eg, nerve tube), each nerve G2 T 80
24.40 24.40 Global Days 090

64911 with autogenous vein graft (includes harvest of vein graft), each nerve T 80
Do not report with (64910-64911)
30.49 30.49 Global Days 090

64999 Unlisted procedure, nervous system T 80
0.00 0.00 Global Days YYY
AMA: 2009, Jan, 11-31; 2008, Jan, 10-25; 2008, Jul, 9; 2008, Sep, 10-11; 2007, January, 13-27; 2007, Dec, 7-8

65091-65093 Surgical Removal of Eyeball Contents

CMS 100-2,15,120 Prosthetic Devices
CMS 100-4,12,30 Correct Coding Policy
INCLUDES Operating microscope (69990)

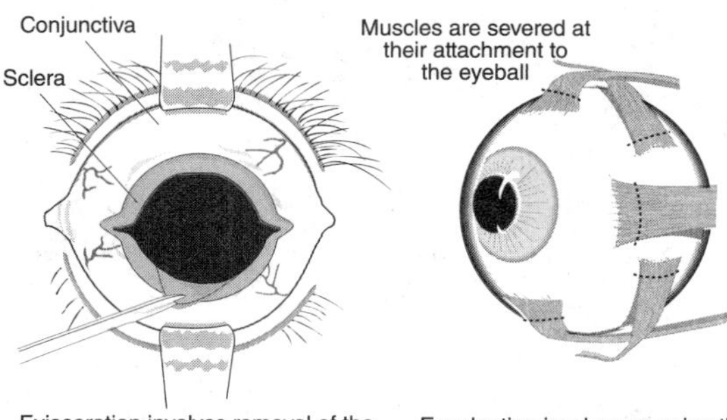

Evisceration involves removal of the contents of the eyeball: the vitreous; retina; choroid; lens; iris; and ciliary muscle. Only the scleral shell remains. A temporary or permanent implant is usually inserted

Enucleation involves severing the extraorbital muscles and optic nerve with removal of the eyeball. An implant is usually inserted and, if permanent, may involve attachment to the severed extraorbital muscles

65091 **Evisceration of ocular contents; without implant** A2 T 80 50
18.77 18.77 Global Days 090

65093 **with implant** A2 T 50
18.64 18.64 Global Days 090

65101-65105 Surgical Removal of Eyeball

CMS 100-2,15,120 Prosthetic Devices
CMS 100-4,12,30 Correct Coding Policy
INCLUDES Operating microscope (69990)
EXCLUDES *Conjunctivoplasty following enucleation (68320-68340)*

65101 **Enucleation of eye; without implant** A2 T 50
21.84 21.84 Global Days 090

65103 **with implant, muscles not attached to implant** A2 T 50
22.80 22.80 Global Days 090

65105 **with implant, muscles attached to implant** A2 T 80 50
25.16 25.16 Global Days 090

65110-65114 Surgical Removal of Orbital Contents

CMS 100-2,15,120 Prosthetic Devices
CMS 100-4,12,30 Correct Coding Policy
INCLUDES Operating microscope (69990)
EXCLUDES *Free full thickness graft (15260-15261)*
Repair more extensive than skin (67930-67975)
Skin graft (15120-15121)

65110 **Exenteration of orbit (does not include skin graft), removal of orbital contents; only** A2 T 80 50
35.20 35.20 Global Days 090

65112 **with therapeutic removal of bone** A2 T 80 50
41.02 41.02 Global Days 090

65114 **with muscle or myocutaneous flap** A2 T 80 50
43.01 43.01 Global Days 090

65125-65175 Implant Procedures: Insertion, Removal, and Revision

CMS 100-2,15,120 Prosthetic Devices
CMS 100-4,12,30 Correct Coding Policy
INCLUDES Operating microscope (69990)
EXCLUDES *Orbit implant insertion outside muscle cone (67550)*
Orbital implant removal or revision outside muscle cone (67560)

65125 **Modification of ocular implant with placement or replacement of pegs (eg, drilling receptacle for prosthesis appendage) (separate procedure)** G2 T 50
8.65 13.37 Global Days 090

65130 **Insertion of ocular implant secondary; after evisceration, in scleral shell** A2 T 50
21.66 21.66 Global Days 090

65135 **after enucleation, muscles not attached to implant** A2 T 50
21.98 21.98 Global Days 090

65140 **after enucleation, muscles attached to implant** A2 T 50
23.31 23.31 Global Days 090

65150 **Reinsertion of ocular implant; with or without conjunctival graft** A2 T 80 50
16.31 16.31 Global Days 090

65155 **with use of foreign material for reinforcement and/or attachment of muscles to implant** A2 T 50
25.11 25.11 Global Days 090

65175 **Removal of ocular implant** A2 T 50
18.95 18.95 Global Days 090

65205-65265 Foreign Body Removal By Area of Eye

CMS 100-4,12,30 Correct Coding Policy
INCLUDES Operating microscope (69990)
EXCLUDES *Removal:*
Anterior segment implant (65920)
Orbital implant outside muscle cone (67560)
Posterior segment implant (67120)
Removal of foreign body:
Eyelid (67938)
Frontal approach (67413)
Lacrimal system (68530)
Lateral approach (67430)
Transcranial approach (61334)

65205 **Removal of foreign body, external eye; conjunctival superficial** P3 S 50
70030, 76529
1.27 1.61 Global Days 000
AMA: 2009, Jan, 11-31; 2008, Jan, 10-25; 2007, January, 13-27

65210 **conjunctival embedded (includes concretions), subconjunctival, or scleral nonperforating** P3 S 50
70030, 76529
1.57 2.01 Global Days 000

65220 **corneal, without slit lamp** G2 S 50
EXCLUDES *Repair of corneal wound with foreign body (65275)*
70030, 76529
1.24 1.68 Global Days 000

65222 **corneal, with slit lamp** P3 S 50
EXCLUDES *Repair of corneal wound with foreign body (65275)*
70030, 76529
1.71 2.21 Global Days 000

65235 **Removal of foreign body, intraocular; from anterior chamber of eye or lens** A2 T 80 50

70030, 76529

20.54 20.54 Global Days 090

65260 **from posterior segment, magnetic extraction, anterior or posterior route** A2 T 80 50

70030, 76529

26.95 26.95 Global Days 090

65265 **from posterior segment, nonmagnetic extraction** A2 T 80 50

70030, 76529

32.43 32.43 Global Days 090

65270-65290 Laceration Repair External Eye

CMS 100-4,12,30 Correct Coding Policy

INCLUDES Conjunctival flap
Operating microscope (69990)
Restoration of anterior chamber with air or saline injection

EXCLUDES *Repair:*
Ciliary body or iris (66680)
Eyelid laceration (12011-12018, 12051-12057, 13150-13160, 67930, 67935)
Lacrimal system injury (68700)
Surgical wound (66250)
Treatment of orbit fracture (21385-21408)

65270 **Repair of laceration; conjunctiva, with or without nonperforating laceration sclera, direct closure** A2 T 80 50

4.10 7.70 Global Days 010

65272 **conjunctiva, by mobilization and rearrangement, without hospitalization** A2 T 50

9.88 14.18 Global Days 090

65273 **conjunctiva, by mobilization and rearrangement, with hospitalization** C5 C 50

10.74 10.74 Global Days 090

65275 **cornea, nonperforating, with or without removal foreign body** A2 T 80 50

13.37 16.60 Global Days 090

65280 **cornea and/or sclera, perforating, not involving uveal tissue** A2 T 80 50

20.00 20.00 Global Days 090

65285 **cornea and/or sclera, perforating, with reposition or resection of uveal tissue** A2 T 50

32.31 32.31 Global Days 090

65286 **application of tissue glue, wounds of cornea and/or sclera** P2 T 50

14.38 20.34 Global Days 090

65290 **Repair of wound, extraocular muscle, tendon and/or Tenon's capsule** A2 T 50

14.64 14.64 Global Days 090

65400-65600 Removal Corneal Lesions

CMS 100-4,12,30 Correct Coding Policy

INCLUDES Operating microscope (69990)

65400 **Excision of lesion, cornea (keratectomy, lamellar, partial), except pterygium** A2 T 50

17.47 19.65 Global Days 090

65410 **Biopsy of cornea** A2 T 80 50

3.14 4.25 Global Days 000

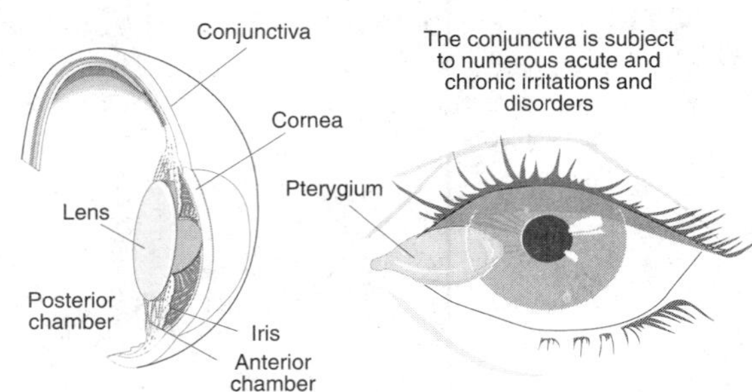

Keratitis is an often painful inflammation of the cornea, the clear membrane covering the anterior segment of the eye

A pterygium is a wedge of excess tissue extending from the medial canthus toward the cornea

65420 **Excision or transposition of pterygium; without graft** A2 T 50

10.87 14.85 Global Days 090

AMA: 2009, Jan, 11-31; 2007, Dec, 10-179

65426 **with graft** A2 T 50

13.88 18.84 Global Days 090

AMA: 2009, Jun, 9&11

65430 **Scraping of cornea, diagnostic, for smear and/or culture** P3 S 50

3.04 3.35 Global Days 000

65435 **Removal of corneal epithelium; with or without chemocauterization (abrasion, curettage)** P3 T 50

2.06 2.35 Global Days 000

65436 **with application of chelating agent (eg, EDTA)** P3 T 50

10.96 11.40 Global Days 090

65450 **Destruction of lesion of cornea by cryotherapy, photocoagulation or thermocauterization** G2 S 50

9.29 9.40 Global Days 090

65600 **Multiple punctures of anterior cornea (eg, for corneal erosion, tattoo)** P3 T 50

9.98 11.42 Global Days 090

65710-65757 Corneal Transplants

CMS 100-3,80.7 Refractive Keratoplasty
CMS 100-4,12,30 Correct Coding Policy

INCLUDES Operating microscope (69990)

EXCLUDES *Processing, preserving, and transporting corneal tissue (V2785)*

Do not report with (92025)

65710 **Keratoplasty (corneal transplant); anterior lamellar** A2 T 80 50

INCLUDES Use and preparation of fresh or preserved graft

EXCLUDES *Refractive keratoplasty surgery (65760, 65765, 65767)*

32.15 32.15 Global Days 090

65730 **penetrating (except in aphakia or pseudophakia)** A2 T 80 50

INCLUDES Use and preparation of fresh or preserved graft

EXCLUDES *Refractive keratoplasty surgery (65760, 65765, 65767)*

35.66 35.66 Global Days 090

65750 **penetrating (in aphakia)** A2 T 80 50 CCI
INCLUDES Use and preparation of fresh or preserved graft
EXCLUDES *Refractive keratoplasty surgery (65760, 65765, 65767)*
35.75 35.75 Global Days 090

65755 **penetrating (in pseudophakia)** A2 T 80 50 CCI
INCLUDES Use and preparation of fresh or preserved graft
EXCLUDES *Refractive keratoplasty surgery (65760, 65765, 65767)*
35.71 35.71 Global Days 090

65756 **endothelial** G2 T 80 50
Code also if appropriate (65757)
33.32 33.32 Global Days 090

\+ 65757 **Backbench preparation of corneal endothelial allograft prior to transplantation (List separately in addition to code for primary procedure)** N1 N 80
Code first (65756)
0.00 0.00 Global Days ZZZ

65760-65775 Corneal Refractive Procedures

CMS 100-3,80.7 Refractive Keratoplasty
INCLUDES Operating microscope (69990)

65760 **Keratomileusis** E
Do not report with (92025)
0.00 0.00 Global Days XXX

65765 **Keratophakia** E
Do not report with (92025)
0.00 0.00 Global Days XXX

65767 **Epikeratoplasty** E
Do not report with (92025)
0.00 0.00 Global Days XXX

65770 **Keratoprosthesis** J8 T 80 50 CCI
Code also (C1818, L8609)
Do not report with (92025)
45.31 45.31 Global Days 090

65771 **Radial keratotomy** E
Do not report with (92025)
0.00 0.00 Global Days XXX

65772 **Corneal relaxing incision for correction of surgically induced astigmatism** A2 T 50 CCI
11.73 13.01 Global Days 090

65775 **Corneal wedge resection for correction of surgically induced astigmatism** A2 T 50 CCI
EXCLUDES *Fitting of contact lens to treat disease (92071-92072)*
15.56 15.56 Global Days 090

65778-65782 Corneal Surface Reconstruction

CMS 100-4,4,200.4 Billing for Amniotic Membrane
CMS 100-4,12,30 Correct Coding Policy
INCLUDES Operating microscope (69990)
EXCLUDES *Obtaining conjunctival allograft from a live donor (68371)*

65778 **Placement of amniotic membrane on the ocular surface for wound healing; self-retaining** N1 Q2 80 50
EXCLUDES *Placement of amniotic membrane with tissue glue (66999)*
Do not report with (65430, 65435, 65780)
2.15 39.74 Global Days 010

65779 **single layer, sutured** G2 T 80 50
EXCLUDES *Placement of amniotic membrane with tissue glue (66999)*
Do not report with (65430, 65435, 65780)
8.48 35.38 Global Days 010

65780 **Ocular surface reconstruction; amniotic membrane transplantation, multiple layers** A2 T 50 CCI
EXCLUDES *Placement of amniotic membrane without ocular surface reconstruction using:*
Self-retaining technique (65778)
Single layer suture technique (65779)
Tissue glue (66999)
25.71 25.71 Global Days 090
AMA: 2009, Jan, 11-31; 2009, Jun, 9&11; 2008, Jan, 10-25; 2007, January, 13-27

65781 **limbal stem cell allograft (eg, cadaveric or living donor)** A2 T 80 50 CCI
37.63 37.63 Global Days 090

65782 **limbal conjunctival autograft (includes obtaining graft)** A2 T 50 CCI
34.44 34.44 Global Days 090
AMA: 2009, Jan, 11-31; 2008, Jan, 10-25; 2007, January, 13-27

65800-66030 Anterior Chamber Procedures

INCLUDES Operating microscope (69990)

65800 **Paracentesis of anterior chamber of eye (separate procedure); with diagnostic aspiration of aqueous** A2 T 50 CCI
3.82 4.34 Global Days 000

65805 **with therapeutic release of aqueous** A2 T 50 CCI
3.89 4.81 Global Days 000

65810 **with removal of vitreous and/or discission of anterior hyaloid membrane, with or without air injection** A2 T 50 CCI
13.54 13.54 Global Days 090

65815 **with removal of blood, with or without irrigation and/or air injection** A2 T 50 CCI
EXCLUDES *Injection only (66020-66030)*
Removal of blood clot only (65930)
14.07 18.67 Global Days 090

65820 **Goniotomy** A2 T 80 50 63 CCI
INCLUDES Barkan's operation
Code also ophthalmic endoscope if used (66990)
21.10 21.10 Global Days 090

65850 **Trabeculotomy ab externo** A2 T 50 CCI
24.85 24.85 Global Days 090

65855 **Trabeculoplasty by laser surgery, 1 or more sessions (defined treatment series)** P3 T 50 CCI
EXCLUDES *Re-treatment after several months for more extensive disease*
Trabeculectomy ab externo (66170)
8.74 9.92 Global Days 010
AMA: 2009, Jan, 11-31; 2008, Jan, 10-25; 2007, January, 13-27

65860 **Severing adhesions of anterior segment, laser technique (separate procedure)** P3 T 80 50 CCI
8.22 9.82 Global Days 090

65865 **Severing adhesions of anterior segment of eye, incisional technique (with or without injection of air or liquid) (separate procedure); goniosynechiae** A2 T 50 CCI
EXCLUDES *Laser trabeculectomy (65855)*
13.33 13.33 Global Days 090

65870 **anterior synechiae, except goniosynechiae** A2 T 50 CCI
17.42 17.42 Global Days 090

65875 posterior synechiae A2 T 50

Code also ophthalmic endoscope if used (66990)

18.27 18.27 Global Days 090

65880 corneovitreal adhesions A2 T 50

18.68 18.68 Global Days 090

65900 Removal of epithelial downgrowth, anterior chamber of eye A2 T 80 50

27.16 27.16 Global Days 090

65920 Removal of implanted material, anterior segment of eye A2 T 50

Code also ophthalmic endoscope if used (66990)

22.77 22.77 Global Days 090

65930 Removal of blood clot, anterior segment of eye A2 T 50

18.86 18.86 Global Days 090

66020 Injection, anterior chamber of eye (separate procedure); air or liquid A2 T 50

3.70 5.27 Global Days 010

66030 medication A2 T 50

3.21 4.79 Global Days 010

66130 Excision Scleral Lesion

CMS 100-4,12,30 Correct Coding Policy

INCLUDES Operating microscope (69990)

EXCLUDES *Intraocular foreign body removal (65235)*
Scleral procedures with retinal procedures (67101-67228)
Surgery on posterior sclera (67250, 67255)

66130 Excision of lesion, sclera A2 T 80 50

17.15 20.79 Global Days 090

66150-66185 Procedures for Glaucoma

INCLUDES Operating microscope (69990)

EXCLUDES *Intraocular foreign body removal (65235)*
Scleral procedures with retinal procedures (67101-67228)
Surgery on posterior sclera (67250, 67255)

66150 Fistulization of sclera for glaucoma; trephination with iridectomy A2 T 50

24.65 24.65 Global Days 090

66155 thermocauterization with iridectomy A2 T 50

24.62 24.62 Global Days 090

66160 sclerectomy with punch or scissors, with iridectomy A2 T 50

INCLUDES Knapp's operation

27.80 27.80 Global Days 090

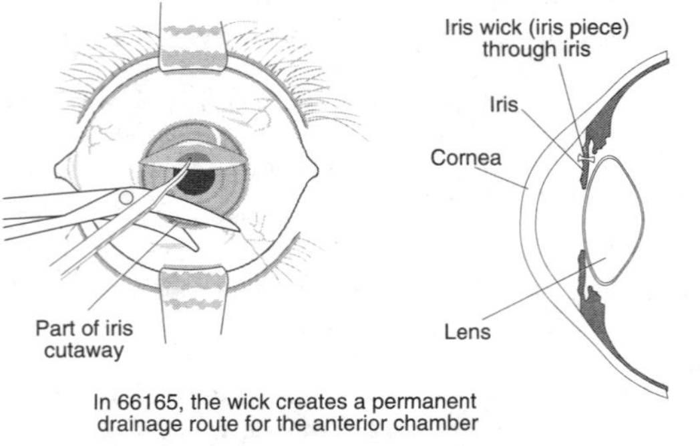

In 66165, the wick creates a permanent drainage route for the anterior chamber

66165 iridencleisis or iridotasis A2 T 80 50

24.16 24.16 Global Days 090

66170 trabeculectomy ab externo in absence of previous surgery A2 T 80 50

EXCLUDES *Repair of surgical wound (66250)*
Trabeculectomy ab externo (65850)

34.63 34.63 Global Days 090

66172 trabeculectomy ab externo with scarring from previous ocular surgery or trauma (includes injection of antifibrotic agents) A2 T 80 50

43.68 43.68 Global Days 090

66174 Transluminal dilation of aqueous outflow canal; without retention of device or stent A2 T 80 50

28.72 28.72 Global Days 090

66175 with retention of device or stent A2 T 80 50

32.56 32.56 Global Days 090

66180 Aqueous shunt to extraocular reservoir (eg, Molteno, Schocket, Denver-Krupin) A2 T 80 50

33.77 33.77 Global Days 090

66185 Revision of aqueous shunt to extraocular reservoir A2 T 80 50

EXCLUDES *Implanted shunt removal (67120)*

22.08 22.08 Global Days 090

66220-66225 Staphyloma Repair

INCLUDES Operating microscope (69990)

EXCLUDES *Scleral procedures with retinal procedures (67101-67228)*
Surgery on posterior sclera (67250, 67255)

66220 Repair of scleral staphyloma; without graft A2 T 80 50

21.48 21.48 Global Days 090

66225 with graft A2 T 50

EXCLUDES *Scleral reinforcement (67250, 67255)*

27.81 27.81 Global Days 090

66250 Anterior Segment Operative Wound Revision or Repair

INCLUDES Operating microscope (69990)

66250 Revision or repair of operative wound of anterior segment, any type, early or late, major or minor procedure A2 T 50

16.57 22.07 Global Days 090

66500-66505 Iridotomy With/Without Transfixion

CMS 100-4,12,30 Correct Coding Policy

INCLUDES Operating microscope (69990)

EXCLUDES *Photocoagulation iridotomy (66761)*

66500 Iridotomy by stab incision (separate procedure); except transfixion A2 T 50

9.97 9.97 Global Days 090

66505 with transfixion as for iris bombe A2 T 50

10.93 10.93 Global Days 090

66600-66635 Iridectomy Procedures

CMS 100-4,12,30 Correct Coding Policy

INCLUDES Operating microscope (69990)

EXCLUDES *Photocoagulation coreoplasty (66762)*

66600 Iridectomy, with corneoscleral or corneal section; for removal of lesion A2 T 50

23.40 23.40 Global Days 090

66605 with cyclectomy A2 T 50

29.73 29.73 Global Days 090

66625 peripheral for glaucoma (separate procedure) A2 T 50
12.44 12.44 Global Days 090

66630 sector for glaucoma (separate procedure) A2 T 50
16.73 16.73 Global Days 090

66635 optical (separate procedure) A2 T 50
16.16 16.16 Global Days 090

66680-66770 Other Procedures of the Uveal Tract

CMS 100-4,12,30 Correct Coding Policy

INCLUDES Operating microscope (69990)

66680 **Repair of iris, ciliary body (as for iridodialysis)** A2 T 50
15.45 15.45 Global Days 090

66682 **Suture of iris, ciliary body (separate procedure) with retrieval of suture through small incision (eg, McCannel suture)** A2 T 50
18.82 18.82 Global Days 090

66700 **Ciliary body destruction; diathermy** A2 T 80 50
INCLUDES Heine's operation
11.20 12.81 Global Days 090

66710 cyclophotocoagulation, transscleral A2 T 50
11.72 13.08 Global Days 090
AMA: 2009, Jan, 11-31; 2008, Jan, 10-25; 2007, January, 13-27

66711 cyclophotocoagulation, endoscopic A2 T 50
INCLUDES Operating microscope (66990)
17.95 17.95 Global Days 090
AMA: 2009, Jan, 11-31; 2008, Jan, 10-25; 2007, January, 13-27

⊙ 66720 cryotherapy A2 T 50
12.20 13.62 Global Days 090

66740 cyclodialysis A2 T 50
11.06 12.31 Global Days 090

66761 **Iridotomy/iridectomy by laser surgery (eg, for glaucoma) (per session)** P3 T 50
7.48 9.07 Global Days 010

66762 **Iridoplasty by photocoagulation (1 or more sessions) (eg, for improvement of vision, for widening of anterior chamber angle)** P3 T 50
12.29 13.70 Global Days 090

66770 **Destruction of cyst or lesion iris or ciliary body (nonexcisional procedure)** P3 T 50
EXCLUDES *Excision:*
Epithelial downgrowth (65900)
Iris, ciliary body lesion (66600-66605)
13.57 14.85 Global Days 090

66820-66825 Post-Cataract Surgery Procedures

INCLUDES Operating microscope (69990)

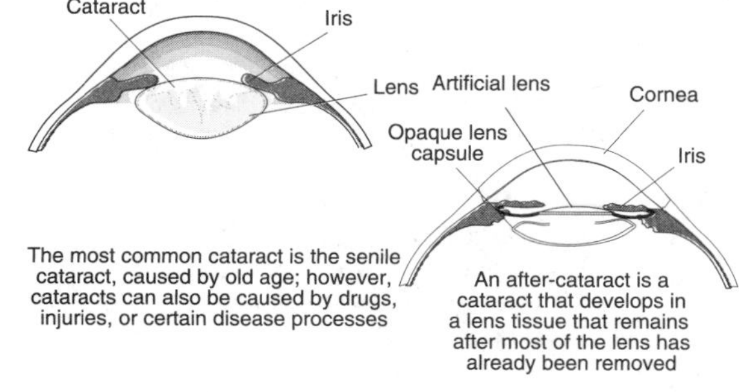

66820 **Discission of secondary membranous cataract (opacified posterior lens capsule and/or anterior hyaloid); stab incision technique (Ziegler or Wheeler knife)** G2 T 50
11.50 11.50 Global Days 090

66821 laser surgery (eg, YAG laser) (1 or more stages) A2 T 50
9.04 9.59 Global Days 090

66825 **Repositioning of intraocular lens prosthesis, requiring an incision (separate procedure)** A2 T 80 50 PQ
21.95 21.95 Global Days 090

66830-66940 Cataract Extraction; Without Insertion Intraocular Lens

CMS 100-3,80.10 Phacoemulsification Procedure--Cataract Extraction

CMS 100-3,80.11 Vitrectomy

CMS 100-4,12,30 Correct Coding Policy

INCLUDES Anterior and/or posterior capsulotomy
Enzymatic zonulysis
Iridectomy/iridotomy
Lateral canthotomy
Medications
Operating microscope (69990)
Subconjunctival injection
Subtenon injection
Use of viscoelastic material

EXCLUDES *Removal of intralenticular foreign body without lens excision (65235)*
Repair of surgical laceration (66250)

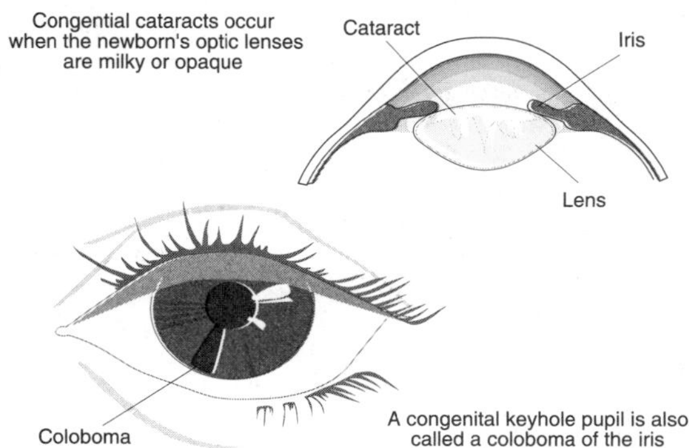

66830 Removal of secondary membranous cataract (opacified posterior lens capsule and/or anterior hyaloid) with corneo-scleral section, with or without iridectomy (iridocapsulotomy, iridocapsulectomy) A2 T 50
INCLUDES Graefe's operation
20.06 20.06 Global Days 090

66840 Removal of lens material; aspiration technique, 1 or more stages A2 T 50 PQ
INCLUDES Fukala's operation
20.75 20.75 Global Days 090
AMA: 2009, Jan, 7-8

66850 phacofragmentation technique (mechanical or ultrasonic) (eg, phacoemulsification), with aspiration A2 T 50 PQ
23.02 23.02 Global Days 090
AMA: 2009, Jan, 7-8

66852 pars plana approach, with or without vitrectomy A2 T 80 50 PQ
24.97 24.97 Global Days 090
AMA: 2009, Jan, 7-8

66920 intracapsular A2 T 80 50 PQ
21.22 21.22 Global Days 090

66930 intracapsular, for dislocated lens A2 T 80 50 PQ
24.12 24.12 Global Days 090

66940 extracapsular (other than 66840, 66850, 66852) A2 T 80 50 PQ
23.01 23.01 Global Days 090
AMA: 2009, Jan, 7-8

66982-66986 Cataract Extraction: With Insertion Intraocular Lens

CMS 100-3,80.10 Phacoemulsification Procedure--Cataract Extraction
CMS 100-3,80.12 Intraocular Lenses (IOLs)
CMS 100-4,12,30 Correct Coding Policy

INCLUDES Anterior or posterior capsulotomy
Enzymatic zonulysis
Iridectomy/iridotomy
Lateral canthotomy
Medications
Operating microscope (69990)
Subconjunctival injection
Subtenon injection
Use of viscoelastic material

EXCLUDES *Intraocular lens supplied by physician*

66982 Extracapsular cataract removal with insertion of intraocular lens prosthesis (1-stage procedure), manual or mechanical technique (eg, irrigation and aspiration or phacoemulsification), complex, requiring devices or techniques not generally used in routine cataract surgery (eg, iris expansion device, suture support for intraocular lens, or primary posterior capsulorrhexis) or performed on patients in the amblyogenic developmental stage A2 T 50 PQ
76519
30.98 30.98 Global Days 090
AMA: 2009, Jan, 11-31; 2008, Jan, 10-25; 2007, January, 13-27

66983 Intracapsular cataract extraction with insertion of intraocular lens prosthesis (1 stage procedure) A2 T 50 PQ
76519
21.06 21.06 Global Days 090

66984 Extracapsular cataract removal with insertion of intraocular lens prosthesis (1 stage procedure), manual or mechanical technique (eg, irrigation and aspiration or phacoemulsification) A2 T 50 PQ
EXCLUDES *Complex extracapsular cataract removal (66982)*
76519
22.35 22.35 Global Days 090

66985 Insertion of intraocular lens prosthesis (secondary implant), not associated with concurrent cataract removal A2 T 50
EXCLUDES *Insertion of lens at the time of cataract procedure (66982-66984)*
Secondary suture (66682)
Code also ophthalmic endoscope if used (66990)
76519
22.27 22.27 Global Days 090

66986 Exchange of intraocular lens A2 T 50
Code also ophthalmic endoscope if used (66990)
76519
26.35 26.35 Global Days 090

66990-66999 Ophthalmic Endoscopy

CMS 100-3,80.10 Phacoemulsification Procedure--Cataract Extraction
CMS 100-3,80.11 Vitrectomy
CMS 100-4,12,30 Correct Coding Policy
INCLUDES Operating microscope (69990)

+ **66990** Use of ophthalmic endoscope (List separately in addition to code for primary procedure) N1 N
Code first (65820, 65875, 65920, 66985-66986, 67036, 67039-67043, 67112-67113)
2.55 2.55 Global Days ZZZ
AMA: 2009, Jan, 11-31; 2008, Jan, 10-25; 2008, Oct, 1-5; 2007, January, 13-27

66999 Unlisted procedure, anterior segment of eye T 80 50
0.00 0.00 Global Days YYY

67005-67015 Vitrectomy: Partial and Subtotal

CMS 100-3,80.11 Vitrectomy
CMS 100-4,12,30 Correct Coding Policy
INCLUDES Operating microscope (69990)

67005 Removal of vitreous, anterior approach (open sky technique or limbal incision); partial removal A2 T 50
EXCLUDES *Anterior chamber vitrectomy by paracentesis (65810)*
Severing of corneovitreal adhesions (65880)
14.12 14.12 Global Days 090

67010 subtotal removal with mechanical vitrectomy A2 T 50
EXCLUDES *Anterior chamber vitrectomy by paracentesis (65810)*
Severing of corneovitreal adhesions (65880)
15.75 15.75 Global Days 090

67015 Aspiration or release of vitreous, subretinal or choroidal fluid, pars plana approach (posterior sclerotomy) A2 T 50
16.83 16.83 Global Days 090

67025-67028 Intravitreal Injection/Implantation

CMS 100-3,80.11 Vitrectomy
CMS 100-4,12,30 Correct Coding Policy
INCLUDES Operating microscope (69990)

67025 **Injection of vitreous substitute, pars plana or limbal approach (fluid-gas exchange), with or without aspiration (separate procedure)** A2 T 50
18.65 21.34 Global Days 090

67027 **Implantation of intravitreal drug delivery system (eg, ganciclovir implant), includes concomitant removal of vitreous** A2 T 80 50
EXCLUDES *Removal of drug delivery system (67121)*
25.18 25.18 Global Days 090
AMA: 2009, Jan, 11-31; 2007, Dec, 10-179

67028 **Intravitreal injection of a pharmacologic agent (separate procedure)** P3 T 50
3.06 3.40 Global Days 000

67030-67031 Incision of Vitreous Strands/Membranes

CMS 100-4,12,30 Correct Coding Policy
INCLUDES Operating microscope (69990)

67030 **Discission of vitreous strands (without removal), pars plana approach** A2 T 50
14.95 14.95 Global Days 090

67031 **Severing of vitreous strands, vitreous face adhesions, sheets, membranes or opacities, laser surgery (1 or more stages)** A2 T 50
10.31 11.22 Global Days 090

67036-67043 Pars Plana Mechanical Vitrectomy

CMS Vitrectomy
CMS 100-4,12,30 Correct Coding Policy
INCLUDES Operating microscope (69990)
EXCLUDES *Foreign body removal (65260, 65265)*
Lens removal (66850)
Vitrectomy in retinal detachment (67108, 67113)

Code also ophthalmic endoscope if used (66990)

67036 **Vitrectomy, mechanical, pars plana approach;** A2 T 80 50
Code also placement of intraocular radiation source applicator (0190T)
27.89 27.89 Global Days 090
AMA: 2008, Jan, 6-7; 2008, Oct, 1-5

67039 **with focal endolaser photocoagulation** A2 T 80 50
36.55 36.55 Global Days 090
AMA: 2009, Jan, 11-31; 2008, Jan, 10-25; 2008, Oct, 1-5; 2007, January, 13-27

67040 **with endolaser panretinal photocoagulation** A2 T 80 50 PQ
41.29 41.29 Global Days 090
AMA: 2009, Jan, 11-31; 2008, Oct, 1-5; 2008, Jan, 10-25; 2007, Jul, 12-13

67041 **with removal of preretinal cellular membrane (eg, macular pucker)** G2 T 80 50
38.51 38.51 Global Days 090
AMA: 2008, Oct, 1-5

67042 **with removal of internal limiting membrane of retina (eg, for repair of macular hole, diabetic macular edema), includes, if performed, intraocular tamponade (ie, air, gas or silicone oil)** G2 T 80 50
44.02 44.02 Global Days 090
AMA: 2008, Oct, 1-5

67043 **with removal of subretinal membrane (eg, choroidal neovascularization), includes, if performed, intraocular tamponade (ie, air, gas or silicone oil) and laser photocoagulation** G2 T 80 50
47.17 47.17 Global Days 090
AMA: 2008, Oct, 1-5

67101-67115 Detached Retina Repair

CMS 100-4,12,30 Correct Coding Policy
INCLUDES Operating microscope (69990)

67101 **Repair of retinal detachment, 1 or more sessions; cryotherapy or diathermy, with or without drainage of subretinal fluid** P3 T 50
19.90 23.02 Global Days 090

67105 **photocoagulation, with or without drainage of subretinal fluid** P2 T 50
18.69 20.88 Global Days 090

67107 **Repair of retinal detachment; scleral buckling (such as lamellar scleral dissection, imbrication or encircling procedure), with or without implant, with or without cryotherapy, photocoagulation, and drainage of subretinal fluid** A2 T 80 50
INCLUDES Gonin's operation
35.97 35.97 Global Days 090

67108 **with vitrectomy, any method, with or without air or gas tamponade, focal endolaser photocoagulation, cryotherapy, drainage of subretinal fluid, scleral buckling, and/or removal of lens by same technique** A2 T 80 50
46.71 46.71 Global Days 090
AMA: 2009, Jan, 11-31; 2008, Oct, 1-5; 2008, Jan, 10-25; 2007, Jul, 12-13

67110 **by injection of air or other gas (eg, pneumatic retinopexy)** P3 T 50
22.38 25.08 Global Days 090

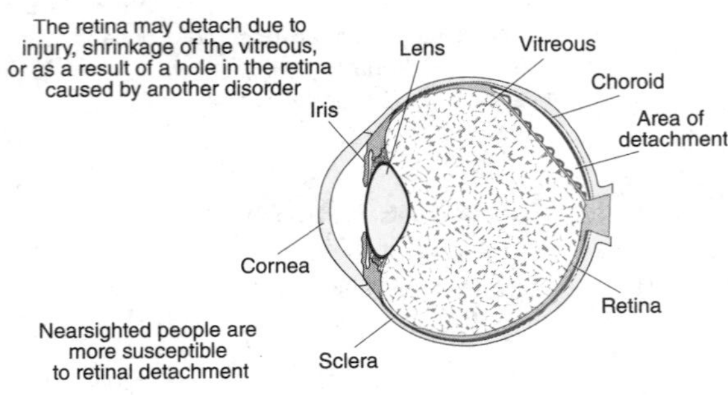

In retinal detachment, the photosensitive retinal layer of the eye separates from the blood-rich choroid layer; this can damage the retina and lead to blindness if not repaired

67112 **by scleral buckling or vitrectomy, on patient having previous ipsilateral retinal detachment repair(s) using scleral buckling or vitrectomy techniques** A2 T 80 50

EXCLUDES *Aspiration or drainage of subretinal or subchoroidal fluid (67015)*

Code also ophthalmic endoscope if used (66990)
38.55 38.55 Global Days 090
AMA: 2009, Jan, 7-8; 2008, Oct, 1-5

67113 **Repair of complex retinal detachment (eg, proliferative vitreoretinopathy, stage C-1 or greater, diabetic traction retinal detachment, retinopathy of prematurity, retinal tear of greater than 90 degrees), with vitrectomy and membrane peeling, may include air, gas, or silicone oil tamponade, cryotherapy, endolaser photocoagulation, drainage of subretinal fluid, scleral buckling, and/or removal of lens** G2 T 80 50

EXCLUDES *Ophthalmic endoscope (66990)*
Vitrectomy for other than retinal detachment, pars plana approach (67036-67043)

50.73 50.73 Global Days 090
AMA: 2008, Oct, 1-5

67115 **Release of encircling material (posterior segment)** A2 T 50
14.39 14.39 Global Days 090

67120-67121 Removal of Previously Implanted Prosthetic Device

CMS 100-4,12,30 Correct Coding Policy
INCLUDES Operating microscope (69990)

EXCLUDES *Foreign body removal (65260, 65265)*
Removal of implanted material anterior segment (65920)

67120 **Removal of implanted material, posterior segment; extraocular** A2 T 50
16.60 19.44 Global Days 090

67121 **intraocular** A2 T 80 50
26.85 26.85 Global Days 090

67141-67145 Retinal Detachment: Preventative Procedures

CMS 100-4,12,30 Correct Coding Policy
INCLUDES Operating microscope (69990)
Treatment at one or more sessions that may occur at different encounters

Do not report more than one time during a defined period of treatment

67141 **Prophylaxis of retinal detachment (eg, retinal break, lattice degeneration) without drainage, 1 or more sessions; cryotherapy, diathermy** A2 T 50
14.37 15.40 Global Days 090
AMA: 2008, Oct, 1-5

67145 **photocoagulation (laser or xenon arc)** P3 T 50
14.41 15.26 Global Days 090
AMA: 2008, Oct, 1-5

67208-67218 Destruction of Retinal Lesions

CMS 100-3,140.5 Laser Procedures
CMS 100-4,12,30 Correct Coding Policy
INCLUDES Operating microscope (69990)
Treatment at one or more sessions that may occur at different encounters

Do not report more than one time during a defined period of treatment

67208 **Destruction of localized lesion of retina (eg, macular edema, tumors), 1 or more sessions; cryotherapy, diathermy** P2 T 50
16.25 16.86 Global Days 090
AMA: 2008, Oct, 1-5

67210 **photocoagulation** P3 T 50
14.81 15.40 Global Days 090
AMA: 2008, Oct, 1-5

67218 **radiation by implantation of source (includes removal of source)** A2 T 50
38.93 38.93 Global Days 090
AMA: 2008, Oct, 1-5

67220-67225 Destruction of Choroidal Lesions

CMS 100-3,80.2 Photodynamic Therapy
CMS 100-3,80.3 Photosensitive Drugs
CMS 100-3,140.5 Laser Procedures
CMS 100-4,12,30 Correct Coding Policy
INCLUDES Operating microscope (69990)

67220 **Destruction of localized lesion of choroid (eg, choroidal neovascularization); photocoagulation (eg, laser), 1 or more sessions** P2 T 50

INCLUDES Treatment at one or more sessions that may occur at different encounters

Do not report more than once during a defined period of treatment
15.89 17.03 Global Days 090
AMA: 2009, Jan, 11-31; 2008, Jan, 10-25; 2008, Oct, 1-5; 2007, January, 13-27

67221 **photodynamic therapy (includes intravenous infusion)** P3 T
6.27 8.41 Global Days 000
AMA: 2009, Jan, 11-31; 2008, Jan, 10-25; 2007, January, 13-27

+ 67225 **photodynamic therapy, second eye, at single session (List separately in addition to code for primary eye treatment)** P3 T

Code first (67221)
0.79 0.84 Global Days ZZZ
AMA: 2009, Jan, 11-31; 2008, Jan, 10-25; 2007, January, 13-27

67227-67229 Destruction Retinopathy

CMS 100-4,12,30 Correct Coding Policy

INCLUDES Operating microscope (69990)

Treatment at one or more sessions that may occur at different encounters

Do not report more than one time during a defined period of treatment

67227 **Destruction of extensive or progressive retinopathy (eg, diabetic retinopathy), 1 or more sessions, cryotherapy, diathermy** A2 T 50

16.05 17.19 Global Days 090

AMA: 2009, Jan, 11-31; 2008, Jan, 10-25; 2008, Oct, 1-5; 2007, January, 13-27

67228 **Treatment of extensive or progressive retinopathy, 1 or more sessions; (eg, diabetic retinopathy), photocoagulation** P2 T 50

28.43 30.62 Global Days 090

AMA: 2008, Oct, 1-5

67229 **preterm infant (less than 37 weeks gestation at birth), performed from birth up to 1 year of age (eg, retinopathy of prematurity), photocoagulation or cryotherapy** R2 T 50

31.53 31.53 Global Days 090

AMA: 2008, Oct, 1-5

67250-67255 Reinforcement of Posterior Sclera

CMS 100-4,12,30 Correct Coding Policy

INCLUDES Operating microscope (69990)

EXCLUDES *Removal of lesion of sclera (66130)*

Repair scleral staphyloma (66220, 66225)

67250 **Scleral reinforcement (separate procedure); without graft** A2 T 50

22.95 22.95 Global Days 090

67255 **with graft** A2 T 80 50

24.99 24.99 Global Days 090

67299 Unlisted Posterior Segment Procedure

67299 **Unlisted procedure, posterior segment** T 80 50

0.00 0.00 Global Days YYY

AMA: 2009, Jan, 11-31; 2007, Dec, 10-179

67311-67334 Strabismus Procedures on Extraocular Muscles

CMS 100-4,12,30 Correct Coding Policy

INCLUDES Operating microscope (69990)

Code also adjustable sutures (67335)

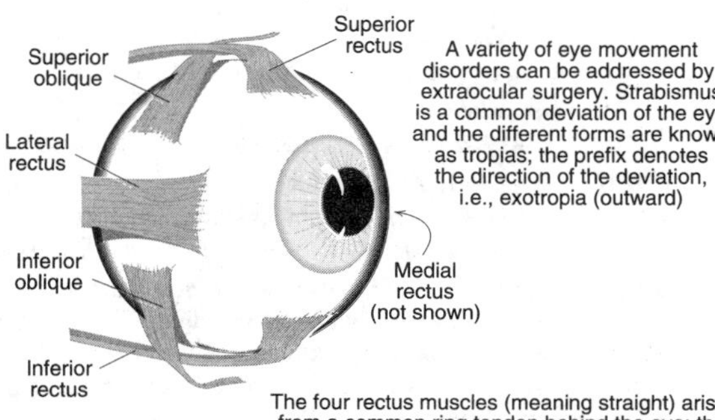

67311 **Strabismus surgery, recession or resection procedure; 1 horizontal muscle** A2 T 50

17.60 17.60 Global Days 090

AMA: 2009, Jan, 11-31; 2008, Jan, 10-25; 2007, January, 13-27

67312 **2 horizontal muscles** A2 T 50

21.28 21.28 Global Days 090

AMA: 2009, Jan, 11-31; 2008, Jan, 10-25; 2007, January, 13-27

67314 **1 vertical muscle (excluding superior oblique)** A2 T 50

19.80 19.80 Global Days 090

67316 **2 or more vertical muscles (excluding superior oblique)** A2 T 80 50

23.93 23.93 Global Days 090

67318 **Strabismus surgery, any procedure, superior oblique muscle** A2 T 50

19.81 19.81 Global Days 090

+ **67320** **Transposition procedure (eg, for paretic extraocular muscle), any extraocular muscle (specify) (List separately in addition to code for primary procedure)** A2 T

Code first (67311-67318)

9.09 9.09 Global Days ZZZ

+ **67331** **Strabismus surgery on patient with previous eye surgery or injury that did not involve the extraocular muscles (List separately in addition to code for primary procedure)** A2 T

Code first (67311-67318)

9.10 9.10 Global Days ZZZ

+ **67332** **Strabismus surgery on patient with scarring of extraocular muscles (eg, prior ocular injury, strabismus or retinal detachment surgery) or restrictive myopathy (eg, dysthyroid ophthalmopathy) (List separately in addition to code for primary procedure)** A2 T

Code first (67311-67318)

9.89 9.89 Global Days ZZZ

+ **67334** **Strabismus surgery by posterior fixation suture technique, with or without muscle recession (List separately in addition to code for primary procedure)** A2 T

Code first (67311-67318)

8.49 8.49 Global Days ZZZ

67335-67399 Other Procedures of Extraocular Muscles

CMS 100-4,12,30 Correct Coding Policy

INCLUDES Operating microscope (69990)

+ **67335** **Placement of adjustable suture(s) during strabismus surgery, including postoperative adjustment(s) of suture(s) (List separately in addition to code for specific strabismus surgery)** A2 T

Code first (67311-67334)

4.44 4.44 Global Days ZZZ

+ **67340** **Strabismus surgery involving exploration and/or repair of detached extraocular muscle(s) (List separately in addition to code for primary procedure)** A2 T 80

INCLUDES Hummelsheim operation

Code first (67311-67334)

10.10 10.10 Global Days ZZZ

67343 **Release of extensive scar tissue without detaching extraocular muscle (separate procedure)** A2 T 50

Code also 67311-67340 if these procedures are performed on other than the affected muscle

19.42 19.42 Global Days 090

67345 **Chemodenervation of extraocular muscle** P3 T 50
EXCLUDES *Nerve destruction for blepharospasm and other neurological disorders (64612-64613)*
6.53 7.21 Global Days 010

67346 **Biopsy of extraocular muscle** A2 T 80 50
EXCLUDES *Repair laceration extraocular muscle, tendon, or Tenon's capsule (65290)*
6.06 6.06 Global Days 000

67399 **Unlisted procedure, ocular muscle** T 80 50
0.00 0.00 Global Days YYY

67400-67415 Frontal Orbitotomy

CMS 100-4,12,30 Correct Coding Policy
INCLUDES Operating microscope (69990)

67400 **Orbitotomy without bone flap (frontal or transconjunctival approach); for exploration, with or without biopsy** A2 T 50
27.53 27.53 Global Days 090

67405 **with drainage only** A2 T 50
22.94 22.94 Global Days 090
AMA: 2009, Jun, 10-11

67412 **with removal of lesion** A2 T 50
25.18 25.18 Global Days 090

67413 **with removal of foreign body** A2 T 80 50
25.44 25.44 Global Days 090

67414 **with removal of bone for decompression** 62 T 80 50
38.25 38.25 Global Days 090
AMA: 2009, Jan, 11-31; 2008, Jan, 10-25; 2007, January, 13-27

67415 **Fine needle aspiration of orbital contents** A2 T 80 50
EXCLUDES *Decompression optic nerve (67570)*
Exenteration, enucleation, and repair (65101-65114)
3.08 3.08 Global Days 000

67420-67450 Lateral Orbitotomy

CMS 100-4,12,30 Correct Coding Policy
INCLUDES Operating microscope (69990)
EXCLUDES *Eyeball removal or repair after removal (65091-65175)*
Orbital implant (67550, 67560)
Transcranial approach orbitotomy (61330-61334)

67420 **Orbitotomy with bone flap or window, lateral approach (eg, Kroenlein); with removal of lesion** A2 T 80 50
48.26 48.26 Global Days 090

67430 **with removal of foreign body** A2 T 80 50
35.17 35.17 Global Days 090

67440 **with drainage** A2 T 80 50
34.86 34.86 Global Days 090

67445 **with removal of bone for decompression** A2 T 80 50
EXCLUDES *Decompression optic nerve sheath (67570)*
41.82 41.82 Global Days 090

67450 **for exploration, with or without biopsy** A2 T 80 50
36.23 36.23 Global Days 090

67500-67515 Eye Injections

CMS 100-4,12,30 Correct Coding Policy
INCLUDES Operating microscope (69990)

67500 **Retrobulbar injection; medication (separate procedure, does not include supply of medication)** 62 S 50
2.18 2.39 Global Days 000

67505 **alcohol** P3 T 50
2.44 2.67 Global Days 000

67515 **Injection of medication or other substance into Tenon's capsule** P3 T 50
EXCLUDES *Subconjunctival injection (68200)*
2.65 2.87 Global Days 000

67550-67560 Orbital Implant

CMS 100-4,12,30 Correct Coding Policy
INCLUDES Operating microscope (69990)
EXCLUDES *Fracture repair malar area, orbit (21355-21408)*
Ocular implant inside muscle cone (65093-65105, 65130-65175)

67550 **Orbital implant (implant outside muscle cone); insertion** A2 T 50
28.73 28.73 Global Days 090

67560 **removal or revision** A2 T 80 50
28.55 28.55 Global Days 090

67570-67599 Other and Unlisted Orbital Procedures

CMS 100-4,12,30 Correct Coding Policy
INCLUDES Operating microscope (69990)

67570 **Optic nerve decompression (eg, incision or fenestration of optic nerve sheath)** A2 T 80 50
36.31 36.31 Global Days 090

67599 **Unlisted procedure, orbit** T 80 50
0.00 0.00 Global Days YYY

67700-67715 Incisional Procedures of Eyelids

CMS 100-4,12,30 Correct Coding Policy
INCLUDES Operating microscope (69990)

67700 **Blepharotomy, drainage of abscess, eyelid** P2 T 50
3.40 7.73 Global Days 010

67710 **Severing of tarsorrhaphy** P3 T 50
2.89 6.52 Global Days 010

67715 **Canthotomy (separate procedure)** A2 T 50
EXCLUDES *Canthoplasty (67950)*
Symblepharon division (68340)
3.25 6.91 Global Days 010

67800-67808 Excision of Chalazion (Meibomian Cyst)

CMS 100-4,12,30 Correct Coding Policy
INCLUDES Lesion removal deeper than skin
Operating microscope (69990)
EXCLUDES *Blepharoplasty, graft, or reconstructive procedures (67930-67975)*
Lesion excision of skin (11310-11313, 11440-11446, 11640-11646, 17000-17004)

67800 **Excision of chalazion; single** P3 T
3.06 3.73 Global Days 010
AMA: 2009, Jan, 11-31; 2008, Jan, 10-25; 2007, January, 13-27

67801 **multiple, same lid** P3 T
4.00 4.81 Global Days 010

67805 **multiple, different lids** P3 T
4.93 5.97 Global Days 010
AMA: 2009, Jan, 11-31; 2008, Jan, 10-25; 2007, January, 13-27

67808 **under general anesthesia and/or requiring hospitalization, single or multiple** A2 T
10.93 10.93 Global Days 090

67810-67875 Other Eyelid Procedures

CMS 100-4,12,30 Correct Coding Policy

INCLUDES Operating microscope (69990)

67810 Biopsy of eyelid P3 T 50
2.67 6.35 Global Days 000
AMA: 2009, Jan, 11-31; 2008, Jan, 10-25; 2007, January, 13-27

67820 Correction of trichiasis; epilation, by forceps only P3 S 50
1.57 1.49 Global Days 000
AMA: 2009, Jan, 11-31; 2008, Jan, 10-25; 2007, January, 13-27

67825 epilation by other than forceps (eg, by electrosurgery, cryotherapy, laser surgery) P3 T 50
3.60 3.80 Global Days 010
AMA: 2009, Jan, 11-31; 2008, Jan, 10-25; 2007, January, 13-27

67830 incision of lid margin A2 T 50
4.11 7.77 Global Days 010

67835 incision of lid margin, with free mucous membrane graft A2 T 80 50
13.10 13.10 Global Days 090

67840 Excision of lesion of eyelid (except chalazion) without closure or with simple direct closure P3 T 50
EXCLUDES *Eyelid removal and reconstruction (67961, 67966)*
4.66 8.02 Global Days 010

67850 Destruction of lesion of lid margin (up to 1 cm) P3 T 50
EXCLUDES *Mohs micro procedures (17311-17315)*
Topical chemotherapy (99201-99215)
4.01 6.31 Global Days 010

67875 Temporary closure of eyelids by suture (eg, Frost suture) G2 T 50
2.89 5.01 Global Days 000

67880-67882 Suturing of the Eyelids

CMS 100-4,12,30 Correct Coding Policy

INCLUDES Operating microscope (69990)

EXCLUDES *Canthoplasty (67950)*
Canthotomy (67715)
Severing of tarsorrhaphy (67710)

67880 Construction of intermarginal adhesions, median tarsorrhaphy, or canthorrhaphy; A2 T 50
10.87 13.43 Global Days 090

67882 with transposition of tarsal plate A2 T 50
14.05 16.66 Global Days 090

67900-67912 Repair of Ptosis/Retraction Eyelids, Eyebrows

CMS 100-2,16,120 Cosmetic Procedures
CMS 100-4,12,30 Correct Coding Policy

INCLUDES Operating microscope (69990)

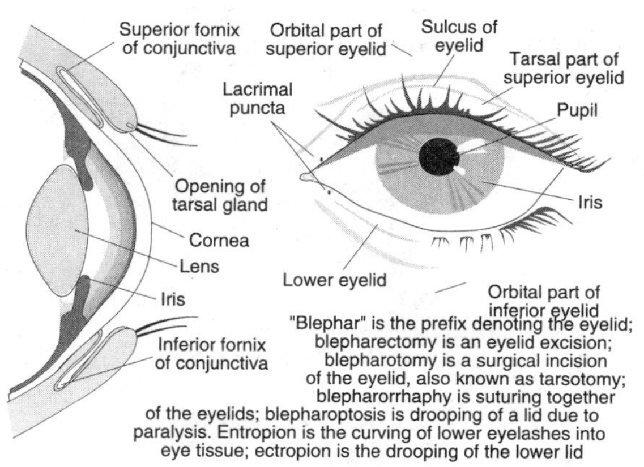

"Blephar" is the prefix denoting the eyelid; blepharectomy is an eyelid excision; blepharotomy is a surgical incision of the eyelid, also known as tarsotomy; blepharorrhaphy is suturing together of the eyelids; blepharoptosis is drooping of a lid due to paralysis. Entropion is the curving of lower eyelashes into eye tissue; ectropion is the drooping of the lower lid

67900 Repair of brow ptosis (supraciliary, mid-forehead or coronal approach) A2 T 50
EXCLUDES *Forehead rhytidectomy (15824)*
15.11 18.86 Global Days 090
AMA: 2009, Jan, 11-31; 2008, Jan, 10-25; 2007, January, 13-27

67901 Repair of blepharoptosis; frontalis muscle technique with suture or other material (eg, banked fascia) A2 T 50
17.18 21.86 Global Days 090

67902 frontalis muscle technique with autologous fascial sling (includes obtaining fascia) A2 T 50
21.53 21.53 Global Days 090

67903 (tarso) levator resection or advancement, internal approach A2 T 50
14.50 17.68 Global Days 090

67904 (tarso) levator resection or advancement, external approach A2 T 50
INCLUDES Everbusch's operation
17.74 21.60 Global Days 090

67906 superior rectus technique with fascial sling (includes obtaining fascia) A2 T 50
14.34 14.34 Global Days 090

67908 conjunctivo-tarso-Muller's muscle-levator resection (eg, Fasanella-Servat type) A2 T 50
12.70 14.60 Global Days 090

67909 Reduction of overcorrection of ptosis A2 T 50
13.09 15.88 Global Days 090

67911 Correction of lid retraction A2 T 50
EXCLUDES *Graft harvest (20920, 20922, 20926)*
Mucous membrane graft repair of trichiasis (67835)
16.66 16.66 Global Days 090

67912 Correction of lagophthalmos, with implantation of upper eyelid lid load (eg, gold weight) A2 T 50
14.40 25.86 Global Days 090
AMA: 2009, Jan, 11-31; 2008, Jan, 10-25; 2007, January, 13-27

67914-67924 Repair Ectropion/Entropion

CMS 100-4,12,30 Correct Coding Policy

INCLUDES Operating microscope (69990)

EXCLUDES *Cicatricial ectropion or entropion with scar excision or graft (67961-67966)*

67914 **Repair of ectropion; suture** A2 T 50
8.55 11.40 Global Days 090

67915 **thermocauterization** P3 T 50
7.43 10.07 Global Days 090

67916 **excision tarsal wedge** A2 T 50
12.76 15.80 Global Days 090
AMA: 2009, Jan, 11-31; 2008, Jan, 10-25; 2007, January, 13-27

67917 **extensive (eg, tarsal strip operations)** A2 T 50
EXCLUDES *Repair of everted punctum (68705)*
14.12 17.29 Global Days 090
AMA: 2009, Jan, 11-31; 2008, Jan, 10-25; 2007, January, 13-27

67921 **Repair of entropion; suture** A2 T 50
8.08 10.92 Global Days 090

67922 **thermocauterization** P3 T 50
7.13 9.72 Global Days 090

67923 **excision tarsal wedge** A2 T 50
13.85 16.75 Global Days 090

67924 **extensive (eg, tarsal strip or capsulopalpebral fascia repairs operation)** A2 T 50
13.36 17.28 Global Days 090

67930-67935 Repair Eyelid Wound

CMS 100-4,12,30 Correct Coding Policy

INCLUDES Operating microscope (69990)

EXCLUDES *Blepharoplasty for entropion or ectropion (67916-67917, 67923-67924)*
Correction of lid retraction and blepharoptosis (67901-67911)
Free graft (15120-15121, 15260-15261)
Graft preparation (15004)
Plastic repair of lacrimal canaliculi (68700)
Procedures more extensive than skin repair (12011-12018, 12051-12057, 13150-13153)
Removal of eyelid lesion (67800-67810, 67840-67850)
Repair involving skin and subcutaneous tissue (12011, 12051-12057, 13150-13153)
Repair of blepharochalasis (15820-15823)
Skin adjacent tissue transfer (14060-14061)
Tarsorrhaphy, canthorrhaphy (67880, 67882)

67930 **Suture of recent wound, eyelid, involving lid margin, tarsus, and/or palpebral conjunctiva direct closure; partial thickness** P3 T 50
7.26 10.81 Global Days 010

67935 **full thickness** A2 T 50
13.30 17.62 Global Days 090

67938-67999 Eyelid Reconstruction/Repair/Removal Deep Foreign Body

CMS 100-4,12,30 Correct Coding Policy

INCLUDES Operating microscope (69990)

EXCLUDES *Blepharoplasty for entropion or ectropion (67916-67917, 67923-67924)*
Correction of lid retraction and blepharoptosis (67901-67911)
Free graft (15120-15121, 15260-15261)
Graft preparation (15004)
Plastic repair of lacrimal canaliculi (68700)
Procedures more extensive than skin repair (12011-12018, 12051-12053, 13150-13153)
Removal of eyelid lesion (67800-67810, 67840-67850)
Repair of blepharochalasis (15820-15823)
Skin adjacent tissue transfer (14060-14061)
Tarsorrhaphy, canthoplasty (67880, 67882)

67938 **Removal of embedded foreign body, eyelid** P2 S 50
3.40 7.04 Global Days 010

67950 **Canthoplasty (reconstruction of canthus)** A2 T 50
13.78 16.90 Global Days 090

67961 **Excision and repair of eyelid, involving lid margin, tarsus, conjunctiva, canthus, or full thickness, may include preparation for skin graft or pedicle flap with adjacent tissue transfer or rearrangement; up to 1/4 of lid margin** A2 T 80 50
EXCLUDES *Canthoplasty (67950)*
Delay flap (15630)
Flap attachment (15650)
Free skin grafts (15120-15121, 15260-15261)
Tubed pedicle flap preparation (15576)
13.54 16.98 Global Days 090

67966 **over 1/4 of lid margin** A2 T 50
EXCLUDES *Canthoplasty (67950)*
Delay flap (15630)
Flap attachment (15650)
Free skin grafts (15120-15121, 15260-15261)
Tubed pedicle flap preparation (15576)
19.54 22.72 Global Days 090

67971 **Reconstruction of eyelid, full thickness by transfer of tarsoconjunctival flap from opposing eyelid; up to 2/3 of eyelid, 1 stage or first stage** A2 T 50
INCLUDES Dupuy-Dutemp reconstruction
Landboldt's operation
21.68 21.68 Global Days 090

67973 **total eyelid, lower, 1 stage or first stage** A2 T 80 50
INCLUDES Landboldt's operation
27.97 27.97 Global Days 090

67974 **total eyelid, upper, 1 stage or first stage** A2 T 80 50
INCLUDES Landboldt's operation
27.90 27.90 Global Days 090

67975 **second stage** A2 T 50
INCLUDES Landboldt's operation
20.51 20.51 Global Days 090

67999 **Unlisted procedure, eyelids** T 80 50
0.00 0.00 Global Days YYY
AMA: 2009, Jan, 11-31; 2008, Jan, 10-25; 2007, January, 13-27

68020-68200 Conjunctival Biopsy/Injection/Treatment of Lesions

CMS 100-4,12,30 Correct Coding Policy

INCLUDES Operating microscope (69990)

68020 **Incision of conjunctiva, drainage of cyst** P3 T 50
3.23 3.48 Global Days 010

68040 **Expression of conjunctival follicles (eg, for trachoma)** P3 S 50
1.59 1.93 Global Days 000

68100 **Biopsy of conjunctiva** P3 T 50
2.87 4.92 Global Days 000

68110 **Excision of lesion, conjunctiva; up to 1 cm** P3 T 50
4.41 6.61 Global Days 010

68115 **over 1 cm** A2 T 50
5.32 8.96 Global Days 010

68130 **with adjacent sclera** A2 T 50
11.61 15.23 Global Days 090

68135 **Destruction of lesion, conjunctiva** P3 T 50
4.39 4.55 Global Days 010

68200 **Subconjunctival injection** P3 S 50
EXCLUDES *Retrobulbar or Tenon's capsule injection (67500-67515)*
1.03 1.24 Global Days 000
AMA: 2009, Jan, 11-31; 2008, Jan, 10-25; 2007, January, 13-27

68320-68340 Conjunctivoplasty Procedures

CMS 100-4,12,30 Correct Coding Policy

INCLUDES Operating microscope (69990)

EXCLUDES *Laceration repair (65270-65273)*

68320 **Conjunctivoplasty; with conjunctival graft or extensive rearrangement** A2 T 50
16.00 21.30 Global Days 090
AMA: 2009, Jan, 11-31; 2008, Jan, 10-25; 2007, Dec, 10-179; 2007, January, 13-27

68325 **with buccal mucous membrane graft (includes obtaining graft)** A2 T 50
19.65 19.65 Global Days 090

68326 **Conjunctivoplasty, reconstruction cul-de-sac; with conjunctival graft or extensive rearrangement** A2 T 50
19.24 19.24 Global Days 090

68328 **with buccal mucous membrane graft (includes obtaining graft)** A2 T 80 50
21.21 21.21 Global Days 090

68330 **Repair of symblepharon; conjunctivoplasty, without graft** A2 T 80 50
13.71 17.82 Global Days 090

68335 **with free graft conjunctiva or buccal mucous membrane (includes obtaining graft)** A2 T 50
19.30 19.30 Global Days 090

68340 **division of symblepharon, with or without insertion of conformer or contact lens** A2 T 80 50
11.87 16.03 Global Days 090

68360-68399 Conjunctival Transplant and Unlisted Procedures

CMS 100-4,12,30 Correct Coding Policy

INCLUDES Operating microscope (69990)

68360 **Conjunctival flap; bridge or partial (separate procedure)** A2 T 50
EXCLUDES *Conjunctival flap for injury (65280, 65285)*
Conjunctival foreign body removal (65205, 65210)
Surgical wound (66250)
12.24 15.66 Global Days 090

68362 **total (such as Gunderson thin flap or purse string flap)** A2 T 50
EXCLUDES *Conjunctival flap for injury (65280, 65285)*
Conjunctival foreign body removal (65205, 65210)
Surgical wound (66250)
19.56 19.56 Global Days 090

68371 **Harvesting conjunctival allograft, living donor** A2 T 50
11.65 11.65 Global Days 010

68399 **Unlisted procedure, conjunctiva** T 80 50
0.00 0.00 Global Days YYY

68400-68899 Nasolacrimal System Procedures

CMS 100-4,12,30 Correct Coding Policy

INCLUDES Operating microscope (69990)

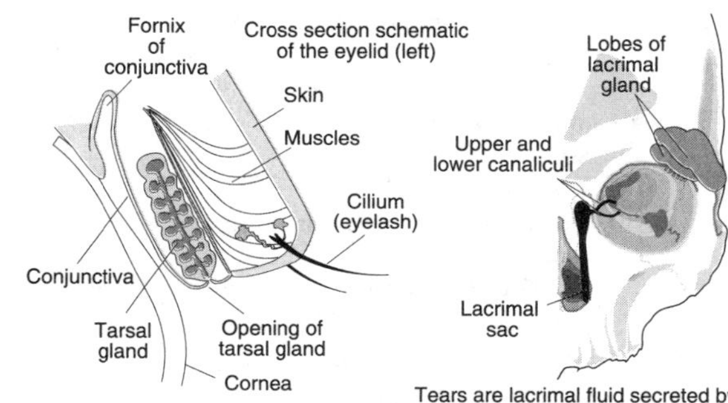

The eyelid is a moveable fold covered by skin externally and highly vascularized conjunctiva internally. The tarsal glands secrete lubricant to the edges of the eyelid

Tears are lacrimal fluid secreted by the almond-sized lacrimal gland through ducts into the fornix of the conjunctiva; fluid is drained through the puncta and into the lacrimal sac and into the nose

68400 **Incision, drainage of lacrimal gland** P2 T 50
3.96 8.24 Global Days 010

68420 **Incision, drainage of lacrimal sac (dacryocystotomy or dacryocystostomy)** P3 T 50
4.92 9.22 Global Days 010

68440 **Snip incision of lacrimal punctum** P3 T 50
2.92 3.06 Global Days 010

68500 **Excision of lacrimal gland (dacryoadenectomy), except for tumor; total** A2 T 50
29.54 29.54 Global Days 090

68505 **partial** A2 T 50
28.98 28.98 Global Days 090

68510 **Biopsy of lacrimal gland** A2 T 80 50
8.82 13.23 Global Days 000

68520 **Excision of lacrimal sac (dacryocystectomy)** A2 T 80 50
19.97 19.97 Global Days 090

68525 Biopsy of lacrimal sac A2 T 50
8.01 8.01 Global Days 000

68530 Removal of foreign body or dacryolith, lacrimal passages P2 T 50
INCLUDES Meller's excision
7.73 12.59 Global Days 010

68540 Excision of lacrimal gland tumor; frontal approach A2 T 50
26.88 26.88 Global Days 090

68550 involving osteotomy A2 T 50
28.16 28.16 Global Days 090

68700 Plastic repair of canaliculi A2 T 50
18.00 18.00 Global Days 090

68705 Correction of everted punctum, cautery P3 T 50
4.94 6.95 Global Days 010

68720 Dacryocystorhinostomy (fistulization of lacrimal sac to nasal cavity) A2 T 80 50
22.28 22.28 Global Days 090
AMA: 2009, Jan, 11-31; 2008, Jan, 10-25; 2007, January, 13-27

68745 Conjunctivorhinostomy (fistulization of conjunctiva to nasal cavity); without tube A2 T 80 50
22.67 22.67 Global Days 090

68750 with insertion of tube or stent A2 T 80 50
23.45 23.45 Global Days 090

68760 Closure of the lacrimal punctum; by thermocauterization, ligation, or laser surgery P3 T 50
4.33 5.91 Global Days 010

68761 by plug, each P3 T 80 50
3.49 4.30 Global Days 010
AMA: 2009, Jan, 11-31; 2008, Jan, 10-25; 2007, January, 13-27; 2007, January, 28-31

68770 Closure of lacrimal fistula (separate procedure) A2 T 80 50
18.52 18.52 Global Days 090

68801 Dilation of lacrimal punctum, with or without irrigation P2 S 50
3.15 3.63 Global Days 010

68810 Probing of nasolacrimal duct, with or without irrigation; A2 T 50
EXCLUDES *Ophthalmological exam under anesthesia (92018)*
5.56 7.08 Global Days 010
AMA: 2008, Oct, 1-5

68811 requiring general anesthesia A2 T 50
EXCLUDES *Ophthalmological exam under anesthesia (92018)*
6.14 6.14 Global Days 010
AMA: 2009, Jan, 11-31; 2008, Jan, 10-25; 2008, Oct, 1-5; 2007, January, 13-27

68815 with insertion of tube or stent A2 T 50
EXCLUDES *Ophthalmological exam under anesthesia (92018)*
7.62 13.06 Global Days 010
AMA: 2009, Jan, 11-31; 2008, Jan, 10-25; 2008, Oct, 1-5; 2007, January, 13-27

68816 with transluminal balloon catheter dilation G2 T 50
7.46 21.16 Global Days 010
AMA: 2008, Oct, 1-5

68840 Probing of lacrimal canaliculi, with or without irrigation P3 S 50
3.42 3.74 Global Days 010

68850 Injection of contrast medium for dacryocystography N1 N 50
70170, 78660
1.58 1.73 Global Days 000
AMA: 2009, Jan, 11-31; 2008, Jan, 10-25; 2007, January, 13-27

68899 Unlisted procedure, lacrimal system T 80 50
0.00 0.00 Global Days YYY

69000-69020 Treatment Abscess/Hematoma External

69000 Drainage external ear, abscess or hematoma; simple P2 T
3.57 5.57 Global Days 010
AMA: 2009, Jan, 11-31; 2008, Jan, 10-25; 2007, January, 13-27

69005 complicated P3 T
4.72 6.44 Global Days 010

69020 Drainage external auditory canal, abscess P2 T
4.32 7.08 Global Days 010
AMA: 2009, Jan, 11-31; 2008, Jan, 10-25; 2007, January, 13-27

69090 Cosmetic Ear Piercing

CMS 100-2,16,10 Exclusions from Coverage
CMS 100-2,16,120 Cosmetic Procedures

69090 Ear piercing E
0.00 0.00 Global Days XXX

69100-69222 Excisional Procedures External Ear/Auditory Canal

CMS 100-4,12,30 Correct Coding Policy
EXCLUDES *Reconstruction of ear (see integumentary section codes)*

69100 Biopsy external ear P3 T
1.46 3.02 Global Days 000

69105 Biopsy external auditory canal P3 T
1.91 4.27 Global Days 000

69110 Excision external ear; partial, simple repair A2 T
9.78 13.76 Global Days 090

69120 complete amputation A2 T
12.11 12.11 Global Days 090

69140 Excision exostosis(es), external auditory canal A2 T 80
26.54 26.54 Global Days 090

69145 Excision soft tissue lesion, external auditory canal A2 T
7.53 11.98 Global Days 090

69150 **Radical excision external auditory canal lesion; without neck dissection**
EXCLUDES *Skin graft (15004-15261)*
Temporal bone resection (69535)
31.48 31.48 Global Days 090

69155 **with neck dissection**
50.21 50.21 Global Days 090

69200 **Removal foreign body from external auditory canal; without general anesthesia**
1.72 3.74 Global Days 000

69205 **with general anesthesia**
3.04 3.04 Global Days 010

69210 **Removal impacted cerumen (separate procedure), 1 or both ears**
0.96 1.51 Global Days 000
AMA: 2009, Jan, 11-31; 2008, Jan, 10-25; 2007, January, 13-27

69220 **Debridement, mastoidectomy cavity, simple (eg, routine cleaning)**
1.86 4.17 Global Days 000

69222 **Debridement, mastoidectomy cavity, complex (eg, with anesthesia or more than routine cleaning)**
4.15 6.70 Global Days 010

69300 Plastic Surgery for Prominent Ears

CMS 100-2,16,120 Cosmetic Procedures
CMS 100-2,16,180 Services Related to Noncovered Procedures
EXCLUDES *Suture of laceration of external ear (12011-14302)*

⊙ 69300 **Otoplasty, protruding ear, with or without size reduction**
14.26 21.48 Global Days YYY

69310-69399 Reconstruction Auditory Canal: Postaural Approach

CMS 100-4,12,30 Correct Coding Policy
EXCLUDES *Suture of laceration of external ear (12011-14302)*

69310 **Reconstruction of external auditory canal (meatoplasty) (eg, for stenosis due to injury, infection) (separate procedure)**
32.83 32.83 Global Days 090

69320 **Reconstruction external auditory canal for congenital atresia, single stage**
EXCLUDES *Other reconstruction surgery with graft (13150-15760, 21230-21235)*
Tympanoplasty (69631, 69641)
46.22 46.22 Global Days 090

69399 **Unlisted procedure, external ear**
0.00 0.00 Global Days YYY

69400-69405 Treatment of Eustachian Tube Obstruction

CMS 100-4,12,30 Correct Coding Policy

69400 **Eustachian tube inflation, transnasal; with catheterization**
1.86 4.46 Global Days 000

69401 **without catheterization**
1.49 2.62 Global Days 000

69405 **Eustachian tube catheterization, transtympanic**
5.79 7.87 Global Days 010

69420-69450 Ear Drum Procedures

CMS 100-4,12,30 Correct Coding Policy

69420 **Myringotomy including aspiration and/or eustachian tube inflation**
3.64 5.82 Global Days 010

69421 **Myringotomy including aspiration and/or eustachian tube inflation requiring general anesthesia**
4.52 4.52 Global Days 010

69424 **Ventilating tube removal requiring general anesthesia**
Do not report with (69205, 69210, 69420-69421, 69433-69676, 69710-69745, 69801-69930)
1.87 3.92 Global Days 000
AMA: 2009, Jan, 11-31; 2008, Jan, 10-25; 2007, January, 13-27

69433 **Tympanostomy (requiring insertion of ventilating tube), local or topical anesthesia**
3.94 6.07 Global Days 010

69436 **Tympanostomy (requiring insertion of ventilating tube), general anesthesia**
4.87 4.87 Global Days 010
AMA: 2009, Mar, 10-11; 2008, Sep, 10-11

69440 **Middle ear exploration through postauricular or ear canal incision**
EXCLUDES *Atticotomy (69601-69605)*
20.80 20.80 Global Days 090
AMA: 2008, Sep, 10-11

69450 **Tympanolysis, transcanal**
16.45 16.45 Global Days 090
AMA: 2008, Sep, 10-11

69501-69535 Transmastoid Excision

CMS 100-4,12,30 Correct Coding Policy
EXCLUDES *Mastoidectomy cavity debridement (69220, 69222)*
Skin graft (15004-15770)

69501 **Transmastoid antrotomy (simple mastoidectomy)**
22.05 22.05 Global Days 090

69502 **Mastoidectomy; complete**
29.25 29.25 Global Days 090

69505 **modified radical**
36.38 36.38 Global Days 090

69511 **radical**
EXCLUDES *Debridement of mastoid cavity (69220, 69222)*
Skin graft (15004-15278)
37.28 37.28 Global Days 090

69530 **Petrous apicectomy including radical mastoidectomy**
49.86 49.86 Global Days 090

69535 **Resection temporal bone, external approach**
EXCLUDES *Middle fossa approach (69950-69970)*
80.21 80.21 Global Days 090

69540-69554 Polyp and Glomus Tumor Removal

CMS 100-4,12,30 Correct Coding Policy

69540 **Excision aural polyp**
3.87 6.38 Global Days 010

69550 **Excision aural glomus tumor; transcanal**
31.49 31.49 Global Days 090

69552 **transmastoid**
47.33 47.33 Global Days 090

Auditory System
69150 — 69552

69554 extended (extratemporal)
75.46 75.46 Global Days 090

69601-69605 Revised Mastoidectomy

CMS 100-4,12,30 Correct Coding Policy

EXCLUDES *Skin graft (15120-15121, 15260-15261)*

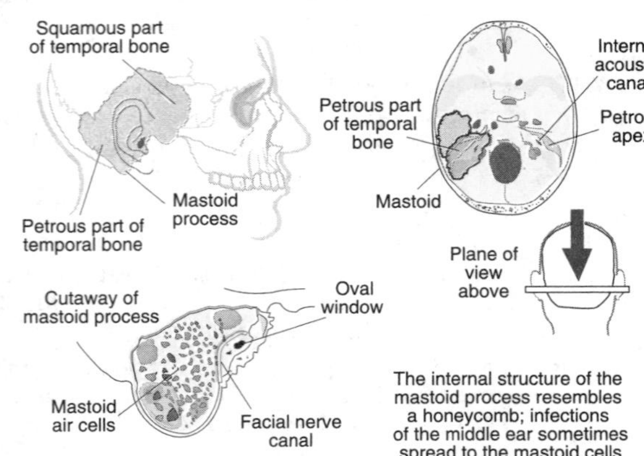

The internal structure of the mastoid process resembles a honeycomb; infections of the middle ear sometimes spread to the mastoid cells

69601 **Revision mastoidectomy; resulting in complete mastoidectomy**
31.53 31.53 Global Days 090

69602 **resulting in modified radical mastoidectomy**
32.83 32.83 Global Days 090

69603 **resulting in radical mastoidectomy**
38.14 38.14 Global Days 090

69604 **resulting in tympanoplasty**
EXCLUDES *Secondary tympanoplasty following mastoidectomy (69631-69632)*
33.62 33.62 Global Days 090

69605 **with apicectomy**
47.09 47.09 Global Days 090

69610-69646 Eardrum Repair with/without Other Procedures

CMS 100-4,12,30 Correct Coding Policy

69610 **Tympanic membrane repair, with or without site preparation of perforation for closure, with or without patch**
8.78 11.66 Global Days 010
AMA: 2009, Jan, 11-31; 2008, Jan, 10-25; 2007, January, 13-27

69620 **Myringoplasty (surgery confined to drumhead and donor area)**
14.71 21.02 Global Days 090
AMA: 2009, Jan, 11-31; 2008, Jan, 10-25; 2007, January, 13-27

69631 **Tympanoplasty without mastoidectomy (including canalplasty, atticotomy and/or middle ear surgery), initial or revision; without ossicular chain reconstruction**
26.69 26.69 Global Days 090
AMA: 2009, Jan, 11-31; 2008, Jan, 10-25; 2007, March, 9-11; 2007, January, 13-27

69632 **with ossicular chain reconstruction (eg, postfenestration)**
32.53 32.53 Global Days 090

69633 **with ossicular chain reconstruction and synthetic prosthesis (eg, partial ossicular replacement prosthesis [PORP], total ossicular replacement prosthesis [TORP])**
31.45 31.45 Global Days 090

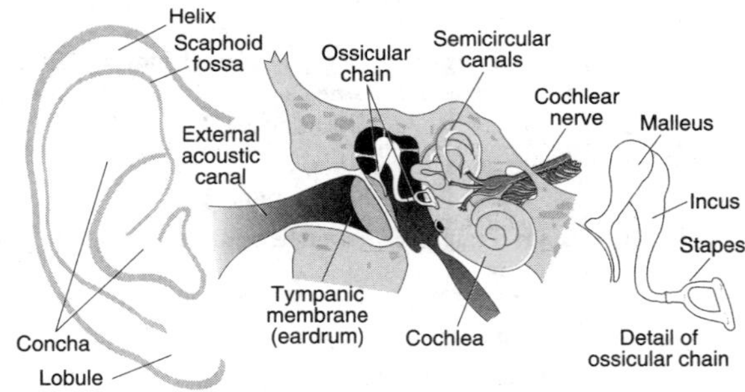

The tympanic membrane is a thin, sensitive tissue and is the gateway to the middle ear; the membrane vibrates in response to sound waves and the movement is transmitted via the ossicular chain to the internal ear. Many surgeries to the middle ear involve repair to the tympanic membrane and reconstruction to the various components of the ossicular chain

69635 **Tympanoplasty with antrotomy or mastoidotomy (including canalplasty, atticotomy, middle ear surgery, and/or tympanic membrane repair); without ossicular chain reconstruction**
36.91 36.91 Global Days 090

69636 **with ossicular chain reconstruction**
41.69 41.69 Global Days 090

69637 **with ossicular chain reconstruction and synthetic prosthesis (eg, partial ossicular replacement prosthesis [PORP], total ossicular replacement prosthesis [TORP])**
41.56 41.56 Global Days 090

69641 **Tympanoplasty with mastoidectomy (including canalplasty, middle ear surgery, tympanic membrane repair); without ossicular chain reconstruction**
31.42 31.42 Global Days 090

69642 **with ossicular chain reconstruction**
40.30 40.30 Global Days 090

69643 **with intact or reconstructed wall, without ossicular chain reconstruction**
36.86 36.86 Global Days 090

69644 **with intact or reconstructed canal wall, with ossicular chain reconstruction**
44.68 44.68 Global Days 090

69645 **radical or complete, without ossicular chain reconstruction**
43.87 43.87 Global Days 090

69646 **radical or complete, with ossicular chain reconstruction**
46.52 46.52 Global Days 090

69650-69662 Stapes Procedures

CMS 100-4,12,30 Correct Coding Policy

69650 **Stapes mobilization**
24.18 24.18 Global Days 090

69660 **Stapedectomy or stapedotomy with reestablishment of ossicular continuity, with or without use of foreign material;**
27.95 27.95 Global Days 090

69661 **with footplate drill out**
36.38 36.38 Global Days 090

69662 Revision of stapedectomy or stapedotomy A2 T 50
34.82 34.82 Global Days 090

69666-69700 Other Inner Ear Procedures

CMS 100-4,12,30 Correct Coding Policy

69666 Repair oval window fistula A2 T 80 50
24.28 24.28 Global Days 090

69667 Repair round window fistula A2 T 80 50
24.34 24.34 Global Days 090

69670 Mastoid obliteration (separate procedure) A2 T 80 50
28.46 28.46 Global Days 090

69676 Tympanic neurectomy A2 T 50
25.13 25.13 Global Days 090

69700 Closure postauricular fistula, mastoid (separate procedure) A2 T 50
20.75 20.75 Global Days 090

69710-69718 Procedures Related to Hearing Aids/Auditory Implants

CMS 100-2,16,100 Hearing Devices
CMS 100-2,16,180 Services Related to Noncovered Procedures

69710 Implantation or replacement of electromagnetic bone conduction hearing device in temporal bone E
INCLUDES Removal of existing device when performing replacement procedure
0.00 0.00 Global Days XXX

69711 Removal or repair of electromagnetic bone conduction hearing device in temporal bone A2 T 80 50
26.06 26.06 Global Days 090

69714 Implantation, osseointegrated implant, temporal bone, with percutaneous attachment to external speech processor/cochlear stimulator; without mastoidectomy J8 T 50
Code also (L8690)
32.36 32.36 Global Days 090

69715 with mastoidectomy J8 T 50
Code also (L8690)
40.00 40.00 Global Days 090

69717 Replacement (including removal of existing device), osseointegrated implant, temporal bone, with percutaneous attachment to external speech processor/cochlear stimulator; without mastoidectomy J8 T 50
Code also (L8690)
34.12 34.12 Global Days 090

69718 with mastoidectomy J8 T 50
Code also (L8690)
40.43 40.43 Global Days 090

69720-69799 Procedures of the Facial Nerve

CMS 100-4,12,30 Correct Coding Policy
EXCLUDES *Extracranial suture of facial nerve (64864)*

69720 Decompression facial nerve, intratemporal; lateral to geniculate ganglion A2 T 80 50 PQ
35.74 35.74 Global Days 090

69725 including medial to geniculate ganglion T 80 50
56.56 56.56 Global Days 090

69740 Suture facial nerve, intratemporal, with or without graft or decompression; lateral to geniculate ganglion A2 T 80 50
35.16 35.16 Global Days 090

69745 including medial to geniculate ganglion A2 T 80 50
EXCLUDES *Extracranial suture of facial nerve (64864)*
37.47 37.47 Global Days 090

69799 Unlisted procedure, middle ear T 80 50
0.00 0.00 Global Days YYY

69801-69915 Procedures of the Labyrinth

CMS 100-4,12,30 Correct Coding Policy

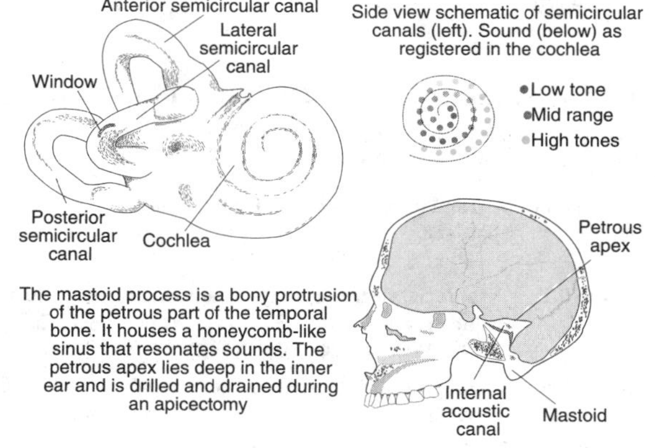

69801 Labyrinthotomy, with perfusion of vestibuloactive drug(s); transcanal P3 T 80 50
Do not report more than once per day
Do not report when performed on the same ear (69420-69421, 69433-69436)
6.33 5.99 Global Days 000
AMA: 2009, Jan, 11-31; 2008, Jan, 10-25; 2007, Dec, 7-8

~~69802~~ ~~with mastoidectomy~~
To report, see 69501-69511, 69601-69605, 69635-69646, 69801, 69905-69910

69805 Endolymphatic sac operation; without shunt A2 T 80 50
31.73 31.73 Global Days 090

69806 with shunt A2 T 50
28.46 28.46 Global Days 090

69820 Fenestration semicircular canal A2 T 80 50
INCLUDES Lempert's fenestration
25.92 25.92 Global Days 090

69840 Revision fenestration operation A2 T 80 50
26.82 26.82 Global Days 090

69905 Labyrinthectomy; transcanal A2 T 50
27.74 27.74 Global Days 090

69910 with mastoidectomy A2 T 80 50
30.68 30.68 Global Days 090

69915 Vestibular nerve section, translabyrinthine approach A2 T 80 50
EXCLUDES *Transcranial approach (69950)*
46.29 46.29 Global Days 090

69930-69949 Cochlear Implantation

CMS 100-2,16,100 Hearing Devices
CMS 100-3,50.3 Cochlear Implantation
CMS 100-4,32,100 Billing Requirements for Cochlear Implantation

69930 Cochlear device implantation, with or without mastoidectomy J8 T 80 50

Code also (L8614)

36.91 36.91 Global Days 090

69949 Unlisted procedure, inner ear T 80 50

0.00 0.00 Global Days YYY

69950-69979 Inner Ear Procedures via Craniotomy

CMS 100-4,12,30 Correct Coding Policy
EXCLUDES *External approach (69535)*

69950 Vestibular nerve section, transcranial approach C5 C 80 50

53.75 53.75 Global Days 090

69955 Total facial nerve decompression and/or repair (may include graft) T 80 50

59.54 59.54 Global Days 090

69960 Decompression internal auditory canal T 80 50

57.86 57.86 Global Days 090

69970 Removal of tumor, temporal bone T 80 50

64.48 64.48 Global Days 090

69979 Unlisted procedure, temporal bone, middle fossa approach T 80 50

0.00 0.00 Global Days YYY

69990 Operating Microscope

CMS 100-4,12,30 Correct Coding Policy
EXCLUDES *Magnifying loupes*

Code first primary procedure

\+ **69990 Microsurgical techniques, requiring use of operating microscope (List separately in addition to code for primary procedure)** N1 N 80

Code first primary procedure

Do not report with (15756-15758, 15842, 19364, 19368, 20955-20962, 20969-20973, 22551, 22552, 22856-22861, 26551-26554, 26556, 31526, 31531, 31536, 31541, 31545-31546, 31561, 31571, 43116, 43496, 49906, 61548, 63075-63078, 64727, 64820-64823, 65091-68850, 0184T, 0226T, 0227T)

6.43 6.43 Global Days ZZZ

AMA: 2009, Mar, 10-11; 2009, Jan, 11-31; 2008, Jan, 6-7; 2008, Jan, 10-25; 2008, Sep, 10-11; 2007, January, 13-27

70010-70015 Radiography: Neurodiagnostic

CMS 100-2,6,10 Medical and Other Services Furnished to Inpatients
CMS 100-2,15,80 Diagnostic Test Requirements
CMS 100-4,3,10.4 Payment of Nonphysician Services for Inpatients
CMS 100-4,13,100 Interpretation of Diagnostic Tests

EXCLUDES *Intrathecal injection procedures (61055, 62284)*

70010 **Myelography, posterior fossa, radiological supervision and interpretation** N1 Q2 80 CCI PQ
2.78 2.78 Global Days XXX

70015 **Cisternography, positive contrast, radiological supervision and interpretation** N1 Q2 80 CCI PQ
4.60 4.60 Global Days XXX

70030-70390 Radiography: Head, Neck, Orofacial Structures

CMS 100-2,6,10 Medical and Other Services Furnished to Inpatients
CMS 100-2,15,80 Diagnostic Test Requirements
CMS 100-4,3,10.4 Payment of Nonphysician Services for Inpatients
CMS 100-4,13,10 ICD-9-CM Coding for Diagnostic Tests
CMS 100-4,13,100 Interpretation of Diagnostic Tests

INCLUDES Minimum number of views or more views when needed to adequately complete the study
Radiographs that have to be repeated during the encounter due to substandard quality; only one unit of service is reported
Obtaining more films after review of initial films, based on the discretion of the radiologist, an order for the test, and a change in the patient's condition

Do not report with a second interpretation by the requesting physician (included in E/M service)

70030 **Radiologic examination, eye, for detection of foreign body** Z3 X 80
0.86 0.86 Global Days XXX

70100 **Radiologic examination, mandible; partial, less than 4 views** Z3 X 80
1.03 1.03 Global Days XXX

70110 **complete, minimum of 4 views** Z3 X 80 CCI
1.19 1.19 Global Days XXX

70120 **Radiologic examination, mastoids; less than 3 views per side** Z3 X 80
1.09 1.09 Global Days XXX

70130 **complete, minimum of 3 views per side** Z2 X 80 CCI
1.71 1.71 Global Days XXX

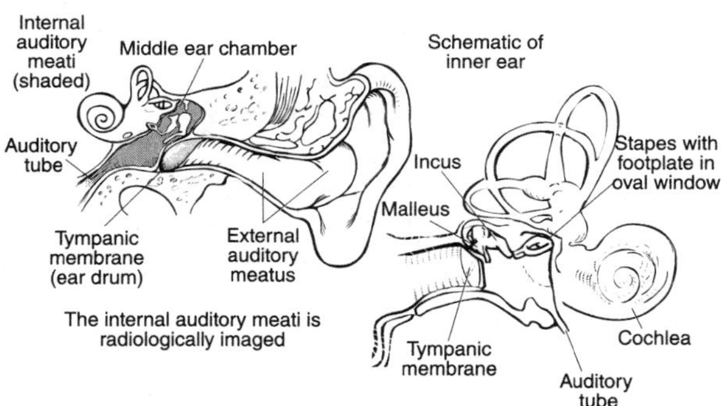

The internal auditory meati is radiologically imaged

70134 **Radiologic examination, internal auditory meati, complete** Z3 X 80
1.68 1.68 Global Days XXX

An x-ray of the facial bones is performed

70140 **Radiologic examination, facial bones; less than 3 views** Z3 X 80
0.91 0.91 Global Days XXX

70150 **complete, minimum of 3 views** Z3 X 80 CCI
1.28 1.28 Global Days XXX

70160 **Radiologic examination, nasal bones, complete, minimum of 3 views** Z3 X 80
1.00 1.00 Global Days XXX

70170 **Dacryocystography, nasolacrimal duct, radiological supervision and interpretation** N1 Q2 80 CCI PQ
EXCLUDES *Procedure (68850)*
0.00 0.00 Global Days XXX

70190 **Radiologic examination; optic foramina** Z3 X 80
1.08 1.08 Global Days XXX

An x-ray of the orbits is performed

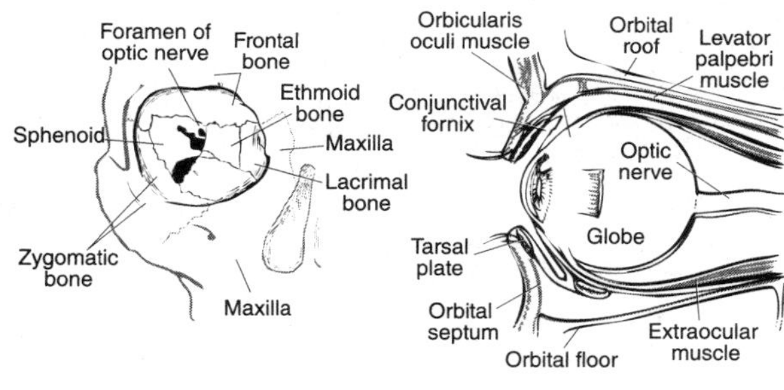

70200 **orbits, complete, minimum of 4 views** Z3 X 80
1.31 1.31 Global Days XXX

70210 **Radiologic examination, sinuses, paranasal, less than 3 views** Z3 X 80
0.93 0.93 Global Days XXX

70220 **Radiologic examination, sinuses, paranasal, complete, minimum of 3 views** Z3 X 80 CCI
1.18 1.18 Global Days XXX

70240 **Radiologic examination, sella turcica** Z3 X 80
0.90 0.90 Global Days XXX

70250 **Radiologic examination, skull; less than 4 views** Z3 X 80
1.11 1.11 Global Days XXX

70260 **complete, minimum of 4 views** Z3 X 80 CCI
1.42 1.42 Global Days XXX

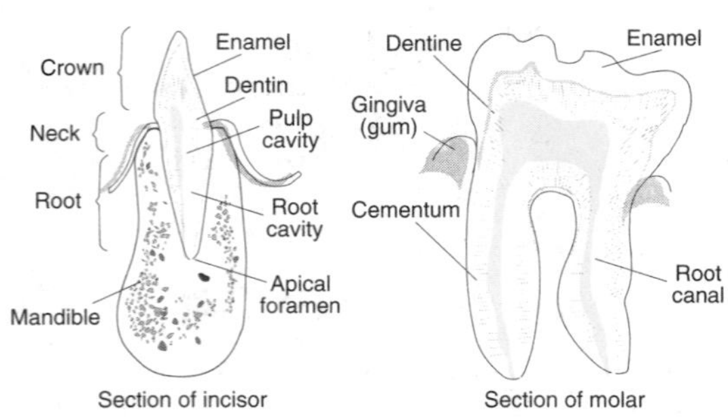

Section of incisor Section of molar

Normal adult dentition numbers 16 teeth in each jaw: four incisors, two canines, four premolars, and six molars. A common tooth eruption problem occurs with the third molars (wisdom teeth) which may be malposed and become impacted. Caries means "rotten" and is a decalcification of tooth enamel and sometimes penetration into the dentin and pulp. Disease processes may cause resorption of the dentin and cementum

70300 **Radiologic examination, teeth; single view**
0.44 0.44 Global Days XXX

70310 **partial examination, less than full mouth**
1.13 1.13 Global Days XXX

70320 **complete, full mouth**
1.54 1.54 Global Days XXX

70328 **Radiologic examination, temporomandibular joint, open and closed mouth; unilateral**
0.93 0.93 Global Days XXX

70330 **bilateral**
1.46 1.46 Global Days XXX

70332 **Temporomandibular joint arthrography, radiological supervision and interpretation**
Do not report with fluoroscopic guidance (77002)
2.25 2.25 Global Days XXX
AMA: 2009, Jan, 11-31; 2008, Jun, 8-11; 2008, Jan, 10-25; 2007, February, 10-11

70336 **Magnetic resonance (eg, proton) imaging, temporomandibular joint(s)**
12.19 12.19 Global Days XXX
AMA: 2009, Jan, 11-31; 2008, Jan, 10-25; 2007, January, 13-27

70350 **Cephalogram, orthodontic**
0.64 0.64 Global Days XXX

▲ **70355** **Orthopantogram (eg, panoramic x-ray)**
0.63 0.63 Global Days XXX

70360 **Radiologic examination; neck, soft tissue**
0.81 0.81 Global Days XXX

70370 **pharynx or larynx, including fluoroscopy and/or magnification technique**
2.58 2.58 Global Days XXX

70371 **Complex dynamic pharyngeal and speech evaluation by cine or video recording**
2.80 2.80 Global Days XXX

70373 **Laryngography, contrast, radiological supervision and interpretation**
2.39 2.39 Global Days XXX

70380 **Radiologic examination, salivary gland for calculus**
1.21 1.21 Global Days XXX

70390 **Sialography, radiological supervision and interpretation**
3.07 3.07 Global Days XXX

70450-70492 Computerized Tomography: Head, Neck, Face

CMS 100-2,6,10 Medical and Other Services Furnished to Inpatients
CMS 100-2,15,80 Diagnostic Test Requirements
CMS 100-3,220.1 Computerized Tomography
CMS 100-4,3,10.4 Payment of Nonphysician Services for Inpatients
CMS 100-4,13,10 ICD-9-CM Coding for Diagnostic Tests
CMS 100-4,13,100 Interpretation of Diagnostic Tests

INCLUDES Imaging using tomographic technique enhanced by computer imaging to create a cross-sectional plane of the body

EXCLUDES *3D rendering (76376, 76377)*

70450 **Computed tomography, head or brain; without contrast material**
5.42 5.42 Global Days XXX
AMA: 2009, Jan, 11-31; 2008, Jan, 10-25; 2007, January, 13-27

70460 **with contrast material(s)**
7.08 7.08 Global Days XXX
AMA: 2009, Jan, 11-31; 2008, Jan, 10-25; 2007, January, 13-27

70470 **without contrast material, followed by contrast material(s) and further sections**
7.57 7.57 Global Days XXX
AMA: 2009, Jan, 11-31; 2008, Jan, 10-25; 2007, January, 13-27

70480 **Computed tomography, orbit, sella, or posterior fossa or outer, middle, or inner ear; without contrast material**
8.90 8.90 Global Days XXX
AMA: 2009, Jan, 11-31

70481 **with contrast material(s)**
10.32 10.32 Global Days XXX
AMA: 2009, Jan, 11-31; 2008, Apr, -11

70482 **without contrast material, followed by contrast material(s) and further sections**
11.54 11.54 Global Days XXX

70486 **Computed tomography, maxillofacial area; without contrast material**
7.37 7.37 Global Days XXX
AMA: 2009, Jan, 11-31; 2008, Jan, 10-25; 2007, January, 13-27

70487 **with contrast material(s)**
8.87 8.87 Global Days XXX

70488 **without contrast material, followed by contrast material(s) and further sections**
10.73 10.73 Global Days XXX

70490 **Computed tomography, soft tissue neck; without contrast material**
EXCLUDES *CT of the cervical spine (72125)*
7.18 7.18 Global Days XXX

70491 **with contrast material(s)**
EXCLUDES *CT of the cervical spine (72126)*
8.66 8.66 Global Days XXX

70492 **without contrast material followed by contrast material(s) and further sections**
EXCLUDES *CT of the cervical spine (72127)*
10.41 10.41 Global Days XXX

70496-70498 Computerized Tomographic Angiography: Head and Neck

CMS 100-2,6,10 Medical and Other Services Furnished to Inpatients
CMS 100-2,15,80 Diagnostic Test Requirements
CMS 100-3,220.1 Computerized Tomography
CMS 100-4,3,10.4 Payment of Nonphysician Services for Inpatients
CMS 100-4,13,10 ICD-9-CM Coding for Diagnostic Tests
CMS 100-4,13,30 Computerized Axial Tomography (CT) Procedures
CMS 100-4,13,100 Interpretation of Diagnostic Tests

INCLUDES Multiple rapid thin section CT scans to create cross-sectional images of bones, organs and tissues

70496 **Computed tomographic angiography, head, with contrast material(s), including noncontrast images, if performed, and image postprocessing** Z2 03 80
16.51 16.51 Global Days XXX
AMA: 2007, January, 28-31

70498 **Computed tomographic angiography, neck, with contrast material(s), including noncontrast images, if performed, and image postprocessing** Z2 03 80 PQ
16.94 16.94 Global Days XXX
AMA: 2007, January, 28-31

70540-70543 Magnetic Resonance Imaging: Face, Neck, Orbits

CMS 100-2,6,10 Medical and Other Services Furnished to Inpatients
CMS 100-2,15,80 Diagnostic Test Requirements
CMS 100-3,220.2 Magnetic Resonance Imaging
CMS 100-4,3,10.4 Payment of Nonphysician Services for Inpatients
CMS 100-4,13,40 Magnetic Resonance Imaging (MRI) Procedures
CMS 100-4,13,100 Interpretation of Diagnostic Tests

INCLUDES Application of an external magnetic field that forces alignment of hydrogen atom nuclei in soft tissues which converts to sets of tomographic images that can be displayed as three-dimensional images
Maximum frequency with which codes may be reported for each imaging session (once)

EXCLUDES *Magnetic resonance angiography head/neck (70544-70549)*

70540 **Magnetic resonance (eg, proton) imaging, orbit, face, and/or neck; without contrast material(s)** Z2 03 80
13.65 13.65 Global Days XXX
AMA: 2007, March, 7-8

70542 **with contrast material(s)** Z2 03 80
15.33 15.33 Global Days XXX

70543 **without contrast material(s), followed by contrast material(s) and further sequences** Z2 03 80
19.40 19.40 Global Days XXX

70544-70549 Magnetic Resonance Angiography: Head and Neck

CMS 100-2,6,10 Medical and Other Services Furnished to Inpatients
CMS 100-2,15,80 Diagnostic Test Requirements
CMS 100-3,220.3 Magnetic Resonance Angiography
CMS 100-4,3,10.4 Payment of Nonphysician Services for Inpatients
CMS 100-4,13,10 ICD-9-CM Coding for Diagnostic Tests
CMS 100-4,13,40.1.1 Magnetic Resonance Angiography
CMS 100-4,13,40.1.1 Magnetic Resonance Angiography Coverage Summary
CMS 100-4,13,100 Interpretation of Diagnostic Tests

INCLUDES Use of magnetic fields and radio waves to produce detailed cross-sectional images of internal body structures

70544 **Magnetic resonance angiography, head; without contrast material(s)** Z2 03 80
15.19 15.19 Global Days XXX
AMA: 2007, January, 28-31

70545 **with contrast material(s)** Z2 03 80
14.94 14.94 Global Days XXX
AMA: 2007, January, 28-31

70546 **without contrast material(s), followed by contrast material(s) and further sequences** Z2 03 80
23.34 23.34 Global Days XXX
AMA: 2007, January, 28-31

70547 **Magnetic resonance angiography, neck; without contrast material(s)** Z2 03 80 PQ
15.17 15.17 Global Days XXX
AMA: 2007, January, 28-31

70548 **with contrast material(s)** Z2 03 80 PQ
16.03 16.03 Global Days XXX
AMA: 2007, January, 28-31

70549 **without contrast material(s), followed by contrast material(s) and further sequences** Z2 03 80 PQ
23.39 23.39 Global Days XXX
AMA: 2007, January, 28-31

70551-70553 Magnetic Resonance Imaging: Brain and Brain Stem

CMS 100-2,6,10 Medical and Other Services Furnished to Inpatients
CMS 100-2,15,80 Diagnostic Test Requirements
CMS 100-3,220.2 Magnetic Resonance Imaging
CMS 100-4,3,10.4 Payment of Nonphysician Services for Inpatients
CMS 100-4,13,10 ICD-9-CM Coding for Diagnostic Tests
CMS 100-4,13,20.1 Professional Component (PC)
CMS 100-4,13,40 Magnetic Resonance Imaging (MRI) Procedures
CMS 100-4,13,100 Interpretation of Diagnostic Tests

INCLUDES Application of an external magnetic field that forces alignment of hydrogen atom nuclei in soft tissues which converts to sets of tomographic images that can be displayed as three-dimensional images

EXCLUDES *Magnetic spectroscopy (76390)*

70551 **Magnetic resonance (eg, proton) imaging, brain (including brain stem); without contrast material** Z2 03 80 PQ
14.25 14.25 Global Days XXX
AMA: 2009, Jan, 11-31; 2008, Jan, 10-25; 2007, January, 13-27; 2007, February, 6-7

70552 **with contrast material(s)** Z2 03 80 PQ
15.92 15.92 Global Days XXX
AMA: 2009, Jan, 11-31; 2008, Jan, 10-25; 2007, January, 13-27; 2007, February, 6-7

70553 **without contrast material, followed by contrast material(s) and further sequences** Z2 03 80 PQ
19.34 19.34 Global Days XXX
AMA: 2009, Jan, 11-31; 2008, Jan, 10-25; 2007, January, 13-27; 2007, February, 6-7

70554-70555 Magnetic Resonance Imaging: Brain Mapping

INCLUDES Neuroimaging technique using MRI to identify and map signals related to brain activity

Do not report with the following codes unless a separate diagnostic MRI is performed (70551-70553)

70554 **Magnetic resonance imaging, brain, functional MRI; including test selection and administration of repetitive body part movement and/or visual stimulation, not requiring physician or psychologist administration** Z2 03 80

EXCLUDES *Testing performed by a physician or psychologist (70555)*

Do not report with functional brain mapping (96020)
15.91 15.91 Global Days XXX
AMA: 2009, Jan, 11-31; 2007, February, 6-7; 2007, March, 7-8

70555 **requiring physician or psychologist administration of entire neurofunctional testing**

EXCLUDES *Testing performed by a technologist, nonphysician, or nonpsychologist (70554)*

Code also (96020)

0.00 0.00 Global Days XXX

AMA: 2007, February, 6-7; 2007, March, 7-8

70557-70559 Magnetic Resonance Imaging: Intraoperative

EXCLUDES *Frequency greater than one for each code per operative session*
Intracranial lesion stereotaxic biopsy with magnetic resonance guidance (61751)

Code also only if a separate report is generated (70557-70559)

Do not report with (61751, 77021, 77022)

70557 **Magnetic resonance (eg, proton) imaging, brain (including brain stem and skull base), during open intracranial procedure (eg, to assess for residual tumor or residual vascular malformation); without contrast material**

0.00 0.00 Global Days XXX

70558 **with contrast material(s)**

0.00 0.00 Global Days XXX

70559 **without contrast material(s), followed by contrast material(s) and further sequences**

0.00 0.00 Global Days XXX

71010-71130 Radiography: Thorax

CMS 100-2,6,10 Medical and Other Services Furnished to Inpatients
CMS 100-2,15,80 Diagnostic Test Requirements
CMS 100-4,3,10.4 Payment of Nonphysician Services for Inpatients
CMS 100-4,13,10 ICD-9-CM Coding for Diagnostic Tests
CMS 100-4,13,100 Interpretation of Diagnostic Tests

EXCLUDES *Needle placement guidance (76942, 77002)*

71010 **Radiologic examination, chest; single view, frontal**

EXCLUDES *Concurrent computer-aided detection (0174T)*

Do not report with (99291-99292)

Do not report with remotely performed CAD (0175T)

0.70 0.70 Global Days XXX

AMA: 2009, Jan, 11-31; 2008, Jan, 10-25; 2007, Jul, 6-10; 2007, February, 10-11; 2007, Jul, 1-4

71015 **stereo, frontal**

Do not report with (99291-99292)

0.91 0.91 Global Days XXX

AMA: 2007, Jul, 1-4; 2007, February, 10-11

71020 **Radiologic examination, chest, 2 views, frontal and lateral;**

EXCLUDES *Concurrent computer-aided detection (0174T)*

Do not report with (99291-99292)

Do not report with remotely performed CAD (0175T)

0.91 0.91 Global Days XXX

AMA: 2007, Jul, 1-4; 2007, Jul, 6-10; 2007, February, 10-11

71021 **with apical lordotic procedure**

Do not report with remotely performed CAD (0175T)

EXCLUDES *Concurrent computer-aided detection (0174T)*

1.13 1.13 Global Days XXX

71022 **with oblique projections**

Do not report with remotely performed CAD (0175T)

EXCLUDES *Concurrent computer-aided detection (0174T)*

1.42 1.42 Global Days XXX

AMA: 2007, Jul, 6-10

71023 **with fluoroscopy**

2.03 2.03 Global Days XXX

AMA: 2009, Jan, 11-31; 2008, Jan, 10-25; 2008, Jun, 8-11; 2007, January, 13-27

71030 **Radiologic examination, chest, complete, minimum of 4 views;**

Do not report with remotely performed CAD (0175T)

EXCLUDES *Concurrent computer-aided detection (0174T)*

1.38 1.38 Global Days XXX

AMA: 2007, Jul, 6-10

71034 **with fluoroscopy**

EXCLUDES *Separate fluoroscopy of chest (76000)*

2.61 2.61 Global Days XXX

AMA: 2009, Jan, 11-31; 2008, Jan, 10-25; 2008, Jun, 8-11; 2007, January, 13-27

71035 **Radiologic examination, chest, special views (eg, lateral decubitus, Bucky studies)**

1.07 1.07 Global Days XXX

71040 **Bronchography, unilateral, radiological supervision and interpretation**

EXCLUDES *Procedure (31656, 31715)*

2.88 2.88 Global Days XXX

71060 **Bronchography, bilateral, radiological supervision and interpretation**

EXCLUDES *Procedure (31656, 31715)*

4.25 4.25 Global Days XXX

~~71090~~ ~~**Insertion pacemaker, fluoroscopy and radiography, radiological supervision and interpretation**~~

To report, see 33206-33249, or 76000

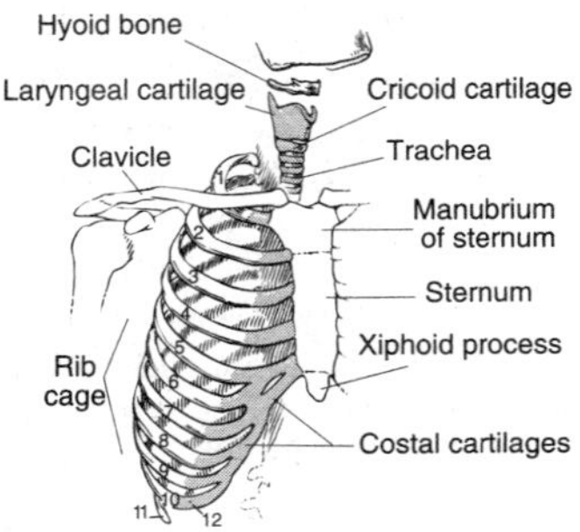

An x-ray of the ribs is performed unilaterally (71100-71101) or bilaterally (71110-71111)

71100 **Radiologic examination, ribs, unilateral; 2 views**

0.98 0.98 Global Days XXX

71101 **including posteroanterior chest, minimum of 3 views**

1.18 1.18 Global Days XXX

71110 **Radiologic examination, ribs, bilateral; 3 views**

1.22 1.22 Global Days XXX

71111 **including posteroanterior chest, minimum of 4 views**

1.59 1.59 Global Days XXX

71120 **Radiologic examination; sternum, minimum of 2 views** Z3 X 80
0.95 0.95 Global Days XXX

71130 **sternoclavicular joint or joints, minimum of 3 views** Z3 X 80
1.12 1.12 Global Days XXX

71250-71270 Computerized Tomography: Thorax

CMS 100-2,6,10 Medical and Other Services Furnished to Inpatients
CMS 100-2,15,80 Diagnostic Test Requirements
CMS 100-3,220.1 Computerized Tomography
CMS 100-4,3,10.4 Payment of Nonphysician Services for Inpatients
CMS 100-4,13,10 ICD-9-CM Coding for Diagnostic Tests
CMS 100-4,13,30 Computerized Axial Tomography (CT) Procedures
CMS 100-4,13,100 Interpretation of Diagnostic Tests

INCLUDES Imaging using tomographic technique enhanced by computer imaging to create a cross-sectional plane of the body

EXCLUDES *3D rendering (76376, 76377)*
Cardiac computed tomography of the heart (75571-75574)

71250 **Computed tomography, thorax; without contrast material** Z2 03 80
6.92 6.92 Global Days XXX
AMA: 2009, Jan, 11-31; 2008, Jan, 10-25; 2007, Jul, 12-13

71260 **with contrast material(s)** Z3 03 80
8.60 8.60 Global Days XXX
AMA: 2009, Jan, 11-31; 2009, Jun, 9&11; 2008, Jan, 10-25; 2007, Jul, 12-13

71270 **without contrast material, followed by contrast material(s) and further sections** Z2 03 80
10.52 10.52 Global Days XXX
AMA: 2009, Jan, 11-31; 2008, Jan, 10-25; 2007, Jul, 12-13; 2007, January, 13-27

71275 Computerized Tomographic Angiography: Thorax

CMS 100-2,6,10 Medical and Other Services Furnished to Inpatients
CMS 100-2,15,80 Diagnostic Test Requirements
CMS 100-3,220.1 Computerized Tomography
CMS 100-4,3,10.4 Payment of Nonphysician Services for Inpatients
CMS 100-4,13,10 ICD-9-CM Coding for Diagnostic Tests
CMS 100-4,13,30 Computerized Axial Tomography (CT) Procedures
CMS 100-4,13,100 Interpretation of Diagnostic Tests

INCLUDES Multiple rapid thin section CT scans to create cross-sectional images of bones, organs and tissues

EXCLUDES *Computed tomographic angiography of coronary arteries that includes calcification score and/or cardiac morphology (75574)*

71275 **Computed tomographic angiography, chest (noncoronary), with contrast material(s), including noncontrast images, if performed, and image postprocessing** Z2 03 80
13.12 13.12 Global Days XXX
AMA: 2009, Jan, 11-31; 2009, Jun, 9&11; 2008, Jan, 10-25; 2007, March, 7-8; 2007, January, 28-31; 2007, January, 13-27

71550-71552 Magnetic Resonance Imaging: Thorax

CMS 100-2,6,10 Medical and Other Services Furnished to Inpatients
CMS 100-2,15,80 Diagnostic Test Requirements
CMS 100-3,220.2 Magnetic Resonance Imaging
CMS 100-4,3,10.4 Payment of Nonphysician Services for Inpatients
CMS 100-4,13,10 ICD-9-CM Coding for Diagnostic Tests
CMS 100-4,13,40 Magnetic Resonance Imaging (MRI) Procedures
CMS 100-4,13,100 Interpretation of Diagnostic Tests

INCLUDES Application of an external magnetic field that forces alignment of hydrogen atom nuclei in soft tissues which converts to sets of tomographic images that can be displayed as three-dimensional images

EXCLUDES *MRI of the breast (77058, 77059)*

71550 **Magnetic resonance (eg, proton) imaging, chest (eg, for evaluation of hilar and mediastinal lymphadenopathy); without contrast material(s)** Z2 03 80
15.68 15.68 Global Days XXX

71551 **with contrast material(s)** Z2 03 80
17.56 17.56 Global Days XXX

71552 **without contrast material(s), followed by contrast material(s) and further sequences** Z2 03 80
22.55 22.55 Global Days XXX

71555 Magnetic Resonance Angiography: Thorax

CMS 100-2,6,10 Medical and Other Services Furnished to Inpatients
CMS 100-2,15,80 Diagnostic Test Requirements
CMS 100-3,220.3 Magnetic Resonance Angiography
CMS 100-4,3,10.4 Payment of Nonphysician Services for Inpatients
CMS 100-4,13,10 ICD-9-CM Coding for Diagnostic Tests
CMS 100-4,13,40.1.1 Magnetic Resonance Angiography
CMS 100-4,13,40.1.1 Magnetic Resonance Angiography Coverage Summary
CMS 100-4,13,100 Interpretation of Diagnostic Tests

71555 **Magnetic resonance angiography, chest (excluding myocardium), with or without contrast material(s)** B 80
15.34 15.34 Global Days XXX
AMA: 2008, Jul, 3&14; 2007, January, 28-31

72010-72120 Radiography: Spine

CMS 100-2,6,10 Medical and Other Services Furnished to Inpatients
CMS 100-2,15,80 Diagnostic Test Requirements
CMS 100-4,3,10.4 Payment of Nonphysician Services for Inpatients
CMS 100-4,13,10 ICD-9-CM Coding for Diagnostic Tests
CMS 100-4,13,100 Interpretation of Diagnostic Tests

INCLUDES Minimum number of views or more views when needed to adequately complete the study
Radiographs that have to be repeated during the encounter due to substandard quality; only one unit of service is reported

EXCLUDES *Obtaining more films after review of initial films, based on the discretion of the radiologist, an order for the test, and a change in the patient's condition*

Do not report with a second interpretation by the requesting physician (included in E/M service)

72010 **Radiologic examination, spine, entire, survey study, anteroposterior and lateral** Z3 X 80
2.32 2.32 Global Days XXX
AMA: 2009, Jan, 11-31; 2008, Jan, 10-25; 2007, January, 13-27; 2007, January, 28-31

72020 **Radiologic examination, spine, single view, specify level** Z3 X 80
0.71 0.71 Global Days XXX

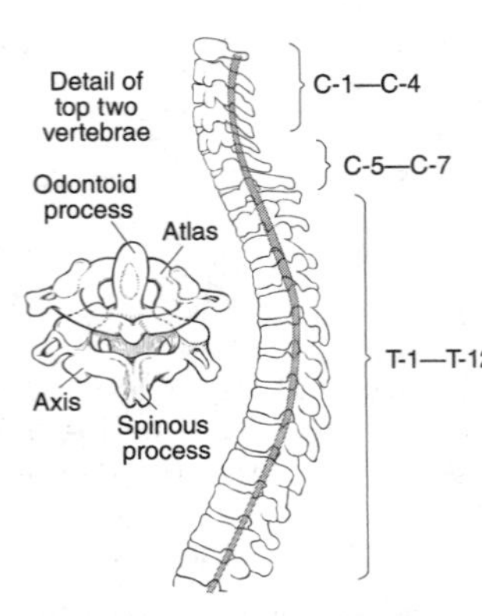

An x-ray of the cervical spine is performed

72040 **Radiologic examination, spine, cervical; 2 or 3 views**
1.19 1.19 Global Days XXX

72050 **minimum of 4 views**
1.60 1.60 Global Days XXX

72052 **complete, including oblique and flexion and/or extension studies**
2.05 2.05 Global Days XXX

72069 **Radiologic examination, spine, thoracolumbar, standing (scoliosis)**
1.14 1.14 Global Days XXX

72070 **Radiologic examination, spine; thoracic, 2 views**
1.01 1.01 Global Days XXX

72072 **thoracic, 3 views**
1.12 1.12 Global Days XXX

72074 **thoracic, minimum of 4 views**
1.33 1.33 Global Days XXX

72080 **thoracolumbar, 2 views**
1.10 1.10 Global Days XXX

72090 **scoliosis study, including supine and erect studies**
1.52 1.52 Global Days XXX

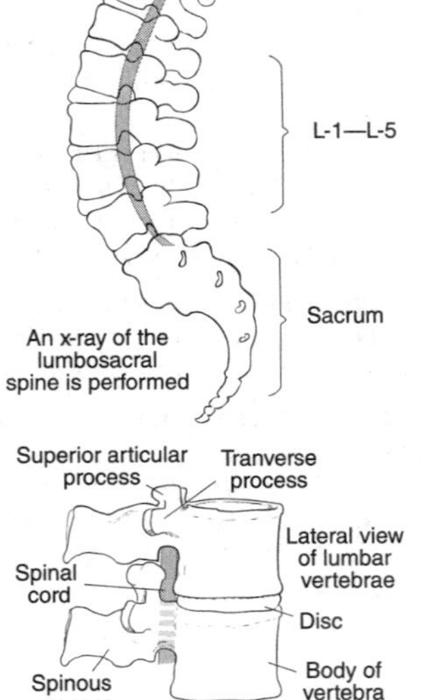

An x-ray of the lumbosacral spine is performed

72100 **Radiologic examination, spine, lumbosacral; 2 or 3 views**
1.11 1.11 Global Days XXX

72110 **minimum of 4 views**
1.51 1.51 Global Days XXX

▲ **72114** **complete, including bending views, minimum of 6 views**
1.97 1.97 Global Days XXX

▲ **72120** **bending views only, 2 or 3 views**
1.32 1.32 Global Days XXX

72125-72133 Computerized Tomography: Spine

CMS 100-2,6,10 Medical and Other Services Furnished to Inpatients
CMS 100-2,15,80 Diagnostic Test Requirements
CMS 100-3,220.1 Computerized Tomography
CMS 100-4,13,10 ICD-9-CM Coding for Diagnostic Tests
CMS 100-4,13,30 Computerized Axial Tomography (CT) Procedures
CMS 100-4,13,100 Interpretation of Diagnostic Tests

INCLUDES Imaging using tomographic technique enhanced by computer imaging to create a cross-sectional plane of the body

EXCLUDES *3D rendering (76376, 76377)*

Code also intrathecal injection procedure when performed (61055, 62284)

72125 **Computed tomography, cervical spine; without contrast material**
7.04 7.04 Global Days XXX

72126 **with contrast material**
8.61 8.61 Global Days XXX

72127 **without contrast material, followed by contrast material(s) and further sections**
10.33 10.33 Global Days XXX

72128 **Computed tomography, thoracic spine; without contrast material**
6.93 6.93 Global Days XXX

72129 **with contrast material**
8.61 8.61 Global Days XXX

72130 **without contrast material, followed by contrast material(s) and further sections**
10.40 10.40 Global Days XXX

72131 **Computed tomography, lumbar spine; without contrast material**
6.91 6.91 Global Days XXX

72132 **with contrast material**
8.59 8.59 Global Days XXX

72133 **without contrast material, followed by contrast material(s) and further sections**
10.39 10.39 Global Days XXX

72141-72158 Magnetic Resonance Imaging: Spine

CMS 100-2,6,10 Medical and Other Services Furnished to Inpatients
CMS 100-2,15,80 Diagnostic Test Requirements
CMS 100-3,220.2 Magnetic Resonance Imaging
CMS 100-4,3,10.4 Payment of Nonphysician Services for Inpatients
CMS 100-4,13,10 ICD-9-CM Coding for Diagnostic Tests
CMS 100-4,13,40 Magnetic Resonance Imaging (MRI) Procedures
CMS 100-4,13,100 Interpretation of Diagnostic Tests

INCLUDES Application of an external magnetic field that forces alignment of hydrogen atom nuclei in soft tissues which converts to sets of tomographic images that can be displayed as three-dimensional images

Code also intrathecal injection procedure when performed (61055, 62284)

72141 **Magnetic resonance (eg, proton) imaging, spinal canal and contents, cervical; without contrast material** Z2 03 80 CCI
12.76 12.76 Global Days XXX

72142 **with contrast material(s)** Z2 03 80 CCI
EXCLUDES *MRI of cervical spinal canal performed without contrast followed by repeating the study with contrast (72156)*
16.17 16.17 Global Days XXX

72146 **Magnetic resonance (eg, proton) imaging, spinal canal and contents, thoracic; without contrast material** Z2 03 80 CCI
12.86 12.86 Global Days XXX

72147 **with contrast material(s)** Z2 03 80 CCI
EXCLUDES *MRI of thoracic spinal canal performed without contrast followed by repeating the study with contrast (72157)*
14.43 14.43 Global Days XXX
AMA: 2009, Jan, 11-31; 2008, Jan, 10-25; 2007, January, 13-27

72148 **Magnetic resonance (eg, proton) imaging, spinal canal and contents, lumbar; without contrast material** Z2 03 80 CCI
12.69 12.69 Global Days XXX
AMA: 2009, Jan, 11-31; 2008, Jan, 10-25; 2007, January, 13-27

72149 **with contrast material(s)** Z2 03 80 CCI
EXCLUDES *MRI of lumbar spinal canal performed without contrast followed by repeating the study with contrast (72158)*
15.78 15.78 Global Days XXX

72156 **Magnetic resonance (eg, proton) imaging, spinal canal and contents, without contrast material, followed by contrast material(s) and further sequences; cervical** Z2 03 80 CCI
19.32 19.32 Global Days XXX

72157 **thoracic** Z2 03 80 CCI
18.10 18.10 Global Days XXX

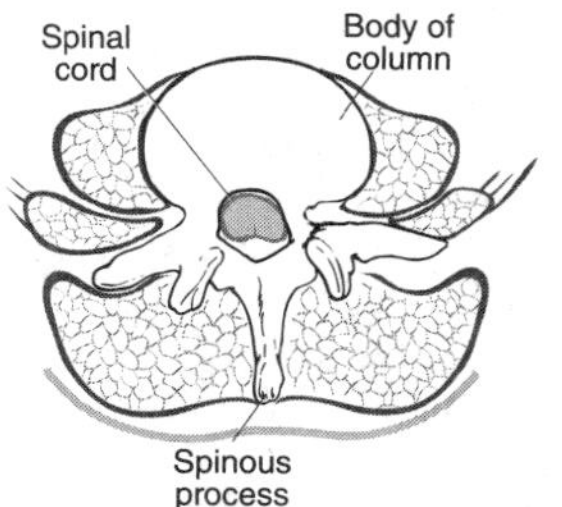

Superior view of thoracic spine and surrounding paraspinal muscles

An MRI of the lumbar spinal canal and its contents is performed without contrast material, and then with contrast. Report 72158 for the lumbar spine

72158 **lumbar** Z2 03 80 CCI
19.00 19.00 Global Days XXX

72159 Magnetic Resonance Angiography: Spine

CMS 100-2,6,10 Medical and Other Services Furnished to Inpatients
CMS 100-2,15,80 Diagnostic Test Requirements
CMS 100-3,220.3 Magnetic Resonance Angiography
CMS 100-4,3,10.4 Payment of Nonphysician Services for Inpatients
CMS 100-4,13,10 ICD-9-CM Coding for Diagnostic Tests
CMS 100-4,13,40 Magnetic Resonance Imaging (MRI) Procedures
CMS 100-4,13,100 Interpretation of Diagnostic Tests

Code also intrathecal injection procedure when performed (61055, 62284)

72159 **Magnetic resonance angiography, spinal canal and contents, with or without contrast material(s)** B 80
15.95 15.95 Global Days XXX
AMA: 2007, January, 28-31

72170-72190 Radiography: Pelvis

CMS 100-2,6,10 Medical and Other Services Furnished to Inpatients
CMS 100-2,15,80 Diagnostic Test Requirements
CMS 100-4,3,10.4 Payment of Nonphysician Services for Inpatients
CMS 100-4,13,10 ICD-9-CM Coding for Diagnostic Tests
CMS 100-4,13,100 Interpretation of Diagnostic Tests

INCLUDES Minimum number of views or more views when needed to adequately complete the study
Radiographs that have to be repeated during the encounter due to substandard quality; only one unit of service is reported

EXCLUDES *Obtaining more films after review of initial films, based on the discretion of the radiologist, an order for the test, and a change in the patient's condition*
Pelvimetry (74710)

Do not report with a second interpretation by the requesting physician (included in E/M service)

72170 **Radiologic examination, pelvis; 1 or 2 views** Z3 X 80
0.80 0.80 Global Days XXX
AMA: 2009, Jan, 11-31; 2008, Jan, 10-25; 2007, January, 13-27

72190 **complete, minimum of 3 views** Z3 X 80 CCI
1.29 1.29 Global Days XXX

72191 Computerized Tomographic Angiography: Pelvis

CMS 100-2,6,10 Medical and Other Services Furnished to Inpatients
CMS 100-2,15,80 Diagnostic Test Requirements
CMS 100-3,220.1 Computerized Tomography
CMS 100-4,3,10.4 Payment of Nonphysician Services for Inpatients
CMS 100-4,13,10 ICD-9-CM Coding for Diagnostic Tests
CMS 100-4,13,30 Computerized Axial Tomography (CT) Procedures
CMS 100-4,13,100 Interpretation of Diagnostic Tests

INCLUDES Multiple rapid thin section CT scans to create cross-sectional images of bones, organs and tissues

EXCLUDES *Combined computed tomographic angiography study of abdomen and pelvis (74174)*
CTA aorto-iliofemoral runoff (75635)

Do not report with (73706, 75635)

72191 **Computed tomographic angiography, pelvis, with contrast material(s), including noncontrast images, if performed, and image postprocessing** Z2 03 80
13.51 13.51 Global Days XXX
AMA: 2007, January, 28-31

72192-72194 Computerized Tomography: Pelvis

CMS 100-2,6,10 Medical and Other Services Furnished to Inpatients
CMS 100-2,15,80 Diagnostic Test Requirements
CMS 100-3,220.1 Computerized Tomography
CMS 100-4,3,10.4 Payment of Nonphysician Services for Inpatients
CMS 100-4,13,10 ICD-9-CM Coding for Diagnostic Tests
CMS 100-4,13,30 Computerized Axial Tomography (CT) Procedures
CMS 100-4,13,100 Interpretation of Diagnostic Tests

EXCLUDES *3D rendering (76376, 76377)*
Combined CT of abdomen and pelvis (74176-74178)
Computed tomographic colonography, diagnostic (74261-74262)
Computed tomographic colonography, screening (74263)

Do not report with (74261-74263)

72192 **Computed tomography, pelvis; without contrast material** Z2 03 80
6.69 6.69 Global Days XXX
AMA: 2009, Jan, 11-31; 2008, Jan, 10-25; 2007, March, 9-11

72193 **with contrast material(s)** Z3 03 80
8.14 8.14 Global Days XXX
AMA: 2007, March, 9-11

72194 **without contrast material, followed by contrast material(s) and further sections** Z2 03 80
10.44 10.44 Global Days XXX
AMA: 2009, Jan, 11-31; 2008, Jan, 10-25; 2007, March, 9-11

72195-72197 Magnetic Resonance Imaging: Pelvis

CMS 100-2,6,10 Medical and Other Services Furnished to Inpatients
CMS 100-2,15,80 Diagnostic Test Requirements
CMS 100-3,220.2 Magnetic Resonance Imaging
CMS 100-4,3,10.4 Payment of Nonphysician Services for Inpatients
CMS 100-4,13,10 ICD-9-CM Coding for Diagnostic Tests
CMS 100-4,13,40 Magnetic Resonance Imaging (MRI) Procedures
CMS 100-4,13,100 Interpretation of Diagnostic Tests

INCLUDES Application of an external magnetic field that forces alignment of hydrogen atom nuclei in soft tissues which converts to sets of tomographic images that can be displayed as three-dimensional images

72195 **Magnetic resonance (eg, proton) imaging, pelvis; without contrast material(s)** Z2 03 80
14.16 14.16 Global Days XXX
AMA: 2009, Jan, 11-31; 2008, Jan, 10-25; 2007, January, 13-27

72196 **with contrast material(s)** Z2 03 80
15.72 15.72 Global Days XXX
AMA: 2009, Jan, 11-31; 2008, Jan, 10-25; 2007, January, 13-27

72197 **without contrast material(s), followed by contrast material(s) and further sequences** Z2 03 80
19.82 19.82 Global Days XXX

72198 Magnetic Resonance Angiography: Pelvis

CMS 100-2,6,10 Medical and Other Services Furnished to Inpatients
CMS 100-2,15,80 Diagnostic Test Requirements
CMS 100-3,220.3 Magnetic Resonance Angiography
CMS 100-4,3,10.4 Payment of Nonphysician Services for Inpatients
CMS 100-4,13,10 ICD-9-CM Coding for Diagnostic Tests
CMS 100-4,13,40.1.1 Magnetic Resonance Angiography
CMS 100-4,13,40.1.1 Magnetic Resonance Angiography Coverage Summary
CMS 100-4,13,100 Interpretation of Diagnostic Tests

INCLUDES Use of magnetic fields and radio waves to produce detailed cross-sectional images of internal body structures

72198 **Magnetic resonance angiography, pelvis, with or without contrast material(s)** B 80
15.35 15.35 Global Days XXX
AMA: 2007, January, 28-31

72200-72220 Radiography: Pelvisacral

CMS 100-2,6,10 Medical and Other Services Furnished to Inpatients
CMS 100-2,15,80 Diagnostic Test Requirements
CMS 100-4,3,10.4 Payment of Nonphysician Services for Inpatients
CMS 100-4,13,10 ICD-9-CM Coding for Diagnostic Tests
CMS 100-4,13,100 Interpretation of Diagnostic Tests

INCLUDES Minimum number of views or more views when needed to adequately complete the study
Radiographs that have to be repeated during the encounter due to substandard quality; only one unit of service is reported

EXCLUDES *Obtaining more films after review of initial films, based on the discretion of the radiologist, an order for the test, and a change in the patient's condition*

Do not report with second interpretation by the requesting physician (included in E/M service)

72200 **Radiologic examination, sacroiliac joints; less than 3 views** Z3 X 80
0.90 0.90 Global Days XXX

72202 **3 or more views** Z3 X 80
1.04 1.04 Global Days XXX

72220 **Radiologic examination, sacrum and coccyx, minimum of 2 views** Z3 X 80
0.87 0.87 Global Days XXX

72240-72270 Myelography with Contrast: Spinal Cord

CMS 100-2,6,10 Medical and Other Services Furnished to Inpatients
CMS 100-2,15,80 Diagnostic Test Requirements
CMS 100-4,3,10.4 Payment of Nonphysician Services for Inpatients
CMS 100-4,13,10 ICD-9-CM Coding for Diagnostic Tests
CMS 100-4,13,100 Interpretation of Diagnostic Tests

INCLUDES Fluoroscopic guidance for subarachnoid puncture for diagnostic radiographic myelography (77003)

Code also injection procedure (61055, 62284)

Do not report with (77003)

72240 **Myelography, cervical, radiological supervision and interpretation** N1 Q2 80 P0
4.10 4.10 Global Days XXX

72255 **Myelography, thoracic, radiological supervision and interpretation** N1 Q2 80 P0
3.90 3.90 Global Days XXX

72265 **Myelography, lumbosacral, radiological supervision and interpretation** N1 02 80 PQ
3.95 3.95 Global Days XXX

72270 **Myelography, 2 or more regions (eg, lumbar/thoracic, cervical/thoracic, lumbar/cervical, lumbar/thoracic/cervical), radiological supervision and interpretation** N1 02 80 PQ
6.18 6.18 Global Days XXX

72275 Radiography: Epidural Space

CMS 100-2,15,80 Diagnostic Test Requirements
CMS 100-4,3,10.4 Payment of Nonphysician Services for Inpatients
CMS 100-4,13,10 ICD-9-CM Coding for Diagnostic Tests
CMS 100-4,13,100 Interpretation of Diagnostic Tests

INCLUDES Epidurogram, documentation of images, formal written report
Fluoroscopic guidance (77003)

Code also injection procedure as appropriate (62280-62282, 62310-62319, 64479-64484)

72275 **Epidurography, radiological supervision and interpretation** N1 N PQ
3.54 3.54 Global Days XXX
AMA: 2008, Jun, 8-11; 2008, Jul, 9

72285 Radiography: Intervertebral Disc (Cervical/Thoracic)

CMS 100-2,6,10 Medical and Other Services Furnished to Inpatients
CMS 100-2,15,80 Diagnostic Test Requirements
CMS 100-4,3,10.4 Payment of Nonphysician Services for Inpatients
CMS 100-4,13,10 ICD-9-CM Coding for Diagnostic Tests
CMS 100-4,13,100 Interpretation of Diagnostic Tests

Code also discography injection procedure

72285 **Discography, cervical or thoracic, radiological supervision and interpretation** N1 02 80 PQ
3.97 3.97 Global Days XXX

72291-72292 Radiography: Percutaneous Vertebral Augmentation

Code also percutaneous vertebroplasty/vertebral augmentation procedure(s) as appropriate (22520-22525, 0200T-0201T)

72291 **Radiological supervision and interpretation, percutaneous vertebroplasty, vertebral augmentation, or sacral augmentation (sacroplasty), including cavity creation, per vertebral body or sacrum; under fluoroscopic guidance** N1 N 80 PQ
0.00 0.00 Global Days XXX
AMA: 2007, March, 7-8

72292 **under CT guidance** N1 N 80
0.00 0.00 Global Days XXX
AMA: 2007, March, 7-8

72295 Radiography: Intervertebral Disc (Lumbar)

CMS 100-2,6,10 Medical and Other Services Furnished to Inpatients
CMS 100-2,15,80 Diagnostic Test Requirements
CMS 100-4,3,10.4 Payment of Nonphysician Services for Inpatients
CMS 100-4,13,10 ICD-9-CM Coding for Diagnostic Tests
CMS 100-4,13,100 Interpretation of Diagnostic Tests

Code also discography injection procedure (62291)

72295 **Discography, lumbar, radiological supervision and interpretation** N1 02 80 PQ
3.51 3.51 Global Days XXX
AMA: 2009, Jan, 11-31; 2008, Jan, 10-25; 2007, January, 13-27

73000-73085 Radiography: Shoulder and Upper Arm

CMS 100-2,15,80 Diagnostic Test Requirements
CMS 100-4,3,10.4 Payment of Nonphysician Services for Inpatients
CMS 100-4,13,10 ICD-9-CM Coding for Diagnostic Tests
CMS 100-4,13,100 Interpretation of Diagnostic Tests

INCLUDES Minimum number of views or more views when needed to adequately complete the study
Radiographs that have to be repeated during the encounter due to substandard quality; only one unit of service is reported

EXCLUDES *Obtaining more films after review of initial films, based on the discretion of the radiologist, an order for the test, and a change in the patient's condition*
Stress views of upper body joint(s), when performed (77071)

Do not report with a second interpretation by the requesting physician (included in E/M service)

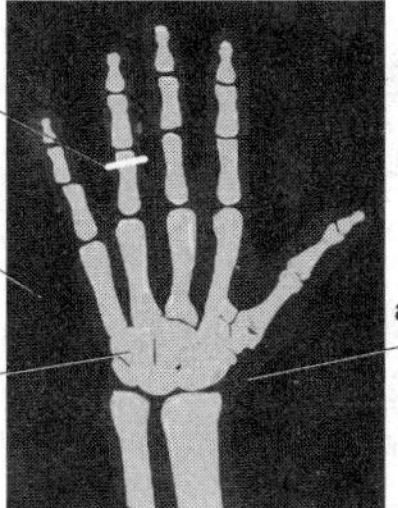

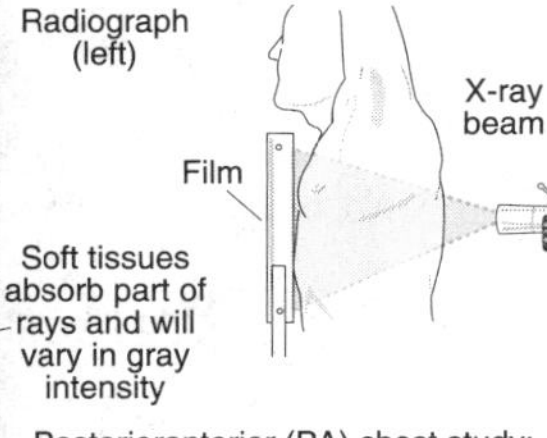

Posterioranterior (PA) chest study; lateral views also common

Traditional diagnostic radiography is defined by the x-ray. Radiographs, or x-rays, are "shadowgrams" of body structures and tissues and show radiopaque matter, such as bone, to be whiter and radiolucent substances, such as air, to be blacker. Each study is oriented by the direction path of the x-ray beam: e.g., PA, the most common, means the beam travels from posterior to anterior. Contrast agents are commonly used to highlight particular areas or structures

73000 **Radiologic examination; clavicle, complete** Z3 X 80
0.87 0.87 Global Days XXX

73010 **scapula, complete** Z3 X 80
0.95 0.95 Global Days XXX

73020 **Radiologic examination, shoulder; 1 view** Z3 X 80
0.72 0.72 Global Days XXX

73030 **complete, minimum of 2 views** Z3 X 80
0.93 0.93 Global Days XXX

73040 **Radiologic examination, shoulder, arthrography, radiological supervision and interpretation** N1 02 80 PQ
Code also arthrography injection procedure (23350)
Do not report with (77002)
3.24 3.24 Global Days XXX
AMA: 2009, Jan, 11-31; 2008, Jan, 10-25; 2008, Jun, 8-11; 2007, February, 10-11

73050 **Radiologic examination; acromioclavicular joints, bilateral, with or without weighted distraction** Z3 X 80
1.21 1.21 Global Days XXX

73060 **humerus, minimum of 2 views** Z3 X 80
0.88 0.88 Global Days XXX

73070 **Radiologic examination, elbow; 2 views** Z3 X 80
0.86 0.86 Global Days XXX

73080 **complete, minimum of 3 views** Z3 X 80
1.02 1.02 Global Days XXX

73085 **Radiologic examination, elbow, arthrography, radiological supervision and interpretation** N1 02 80 PQ
Do not report with (77002)
Code also arthrography injection procedure (24220)
3.03 3.03 Global Days XXX
AMA: 2008, Jun, 8-11; 2007, February, 10-11

73090-73140 Radiography: Forearm and Hand

CMS 100-2,15,80 Diagnostic Test Requirements
CMS 100-4,3,10.4 Payment of Nonphysician Services for Inpatients
CMS 100-4,13,10 ICD-9-CM Coding for Diagnostic Tests
CMS 100-4,13,100 Interpretation of Diagnostic Tests

INCLUDES Minimum number of views or more views when needed to adequately complete the study
Radiographs that have to be repeated during the encounter due to substandard quality; only one unit of service is reported

EXCLUDES *Obtaining more films after review of initial films, based on the discretion of the radiologist, an order for the test, and a change in the patient's condition*

Code also stress views of upper body joint(s), when performed (77071)

Do not report with a second interpretation by the requesting physician (included in E/M service)

73090 Radiologic examination; forearm, 2 views
0.83 0.83 Global Days XXX

73092 upper extremity, infant, minimum of 2 views
0.84 0.84 Global Days XXX

73100 Radiologic examination, wrist; 2 views
0.96 0.96 Global Days XXX

73110 complete, minimum of 3 views
1.12 1.12 Global Days XXX
AMA: 2009, Jan, 11-31; 2008, Jan, 10-25; 2007, January, 13-27

73115 Radiologic examination, wrist, arthrography, radiological supervision and interpretation
Code also arthrography injection procedure (25246)
Do not report with (77002)
3.40 3.40 Global Days XXX
AMA: 2008, Jun, 8-11; 2007, February, 10-11

73120 Radiologic examination, hand; 2 views
0.84 0.84 Global Days XXX

73130 minimum of 3 views
0.97 0.97 Global Days XXX

73140 Radiologic examination, finger(s), minimum of 2 views
0.99 0.99 Global Days XXX
AMA: 2007, January, 28-31

73200-73202 Computerized Tomography: Shoulder, Arm, Hand

CMS 100-2,6,10 Medical and Other Services Furnished to Inpatients
CMS 100-2,15,80 Diagnostic Test Requirements
CMS 100-3,220.1 Computerized Tomography
CMS 100-4,3,10.4 Payment of Nonphysician Services for Inpatients
CMS 100-4,13,10 ICD-9-CM Coding for Diagnostic Tests
CMS 100-4,13,30 Computerized Axial Tomography (CT) Procedures
CMS 100-4,13,100 Interpretation of Diagnostic Tests

INCLUDES Imaging using tomographic technique enhanced by computer imaging to create a cross-sectional plane of the body
Intravascular injection of contrast material
Intravascular, intrathecal, or intra-articular contrast materials when noted in code descriptor

EXCLUDES *3D rendering (76376-76377)*

73200 Computed tomography, upper extremity; without contrast material
6.82 6.82 Global Days XXX

73201 with contrast material(s)
8.36 8.36 Global Days XXX

73202 without contrast material, followed by contrast material(s) and further sections
10.73 10.73 Global Days XXX

73206 Computerized Tomographic Angiography: Shoulder, Arm, and Hand

CMS 100-2,6,10 Medical and Other Services Furnished to Inpatients
CMS 100-2,15,80 Diagnostic Test Requirements
CMS 100-3,220.1 Computerized Tomography
CMS 100-4,3,10.4 Payment of Nonphysician Services for Inpatients
CMS 100-4,13,10 ICD-9-CM Coding for Diagnostic Tests
CMS 100-4,13,30 Computerized Axial Tomography (CT) Procedures
CMS 100-4,13,100 Interpretation of Diagnostic Tests

INCLUDES Intravascular injection of contrast material
Intravascular, intrathecal, or intra-articular contrast materials when noted in code descriptor
Multiple rapid thin section CT scans to create cross-sectional images of bones, organs and tissues

73206 Computed tomographic angiography, upper extremity, with contrast material(s), including noncontrast images, if performed, and image postprocessing
11.95 11.95 Global Days XXX
AMA: 2007, January, 28-31

73218-73223 Magnetic Resonance Imaging: Shoulder, Arm, Hand

CMS 100-2,6,10 Medical and Other Services Furnished to Inpatients
CMS 100-2,15,80 Diagnostic Test Requirements
CMS 100-3,220.2 Magnetic Resonance Imaging
CMS 100-4,3,10.4 Payment of Nonphysician Services for Inpatients
CMS 100-4,13,10 ICD-9-CM Coding for Diagnostic Tests
CMS 100-4,13,30 Computerized Axial Tomography (CT) Procedures
CMS 100-4,13,100 Interpretation of Diagnostic Tests

INCLUDES Application of an external magnetic field that forces alignment of hydrogen atom nuclei in soft tissues which converts to sets of tomographic images that can be displayed as three-dimensional images
Intravascular injection of contrast material
Intravascular, intrathecal, or intra-articular contrast materials when noted in code descriptor

73218 Magnetic resonance (eg, proton) imaging, upper extremity, other than joint; without contrast material(s)
14.04 14.04 Global Days XXX

73219 with contrast material(s)
15.48 15.48 Global Days XXX

73220 without contrast material(s), followed by contrast material(s) and further sequences
19.70 19.70 Global Days XXX

73221 Magnetic resonance (eg, proton) imaging, any joint of upper extremity; without contrast material(s)
13.38 13.38 Global Days XXX

73222 with contrast material(s)
14.51 14.51 Global Days XXX

73223 without contrast material(s), followed by contrast material(s) and further sequences
18.61 18.61 Global Days XXX

73225 Magnetic Resonance Angiography: Shoulder, Arm, Hand

CMS 100-2,6,10 Medical and Other Services Furnished to Inpatients
CMS 100-2,15,80 Diagnostic Test Requirements
CMS 100-3,220.3 Magnetic Resonance Angiography
CMS 100-4,3,10.4 Payment of Nonphysician Services for Inpatients
CMS 100-4,13,10 ICD-9-CM Coding for Diagnostic Tests
CMS 100-4,13,40.1.1 Magnetic Resonance Angiography
CMS 100-4,13,40.1.1 Magnetic Resonance Angiography Coverage Summary
CMS 100-4,13,100 Interpretation of Diagnostic Tests

INCLUDES Intravascular injection of contrast material
Intravascular, intrathecal, or intra-articular contrast materials when noted in code descriptor
Use of magnetic fields and radio waves to produce detailed cross-sectional images of internal body structures

73225 **Magnetic resonance angiography, upper extremity, with or without contrast material(s)** B 80
15.34 15.34 Global Days XXX
AMA: 2007, January, 28-31

73500-73550 Radiography: Pelvic Region and Thigh

CMS 100-2,6,10 Medical and Other Services Furnished to Inpatients
CMS 100-2,15,80 Diagnostic Test Requirements
CMS 100-4,3,10.4 Payment of Nonphysician Services for Inpatients
CMS 100-4,13,10 ICD-9-CM Coding for Diagnostic Tests
CMS 100-4,13,100 Interpretation of Diagnostic Tests

EXCLUDES *Stress views any joint (77071)*

73500 **Radiologic examination, hip, unilateral; 1 view** Z3 X 80
0.82 0.82 Global Days XXX

73510 **complete, minimum of 2 views** Z3 X 80
1.18 1.18 Global Days XXX
AMA: 2009, Jan, 11-31; 2008, Jan, 10-25; 2007, January, 13-27

73520 **Radiologic examination, hips, bilateral, minimum of 2 views of each hip, including anteroposterior view of pelvis** Z3 X 80
1.24 1.24 Global Days XXX
AMA: 2009, Jan, 11-31; 2008, Jan, 10-25; 2007, January, 13-27

73525 **Radiologic examination, hip, arthrography, radiological supervision and interpretation** N1 Q2 80 PQ
Do not report with (77002)
3.13 3.13 Global Days XXX
AMA: 2008, Jun, 8-11; 2007, February, 10-11

73530 **Radiologic examination, hip, during operative procedure** N1 N 80
0.00 0.00 Global Days XXX

73540 **Radiologic examination, pelvis and hips, infant or child, minimum of 2 views** A Z3 X 80
1.33 1.33 Global Days XXX

~~**73542** **Radiological examination, sacroiliac joint arthrography, radiological supervision and interpretation**~~
To report, see 27096

73550 **Radiologic examination, femur, 2 views** Z3 X 80
0.86 0.86 Global Days XXX

73560-73660 Radiography: Lower Leg, Ankle, and Foot

CMS 100-2,15,80 Diagnostic Test Requirements
CMS 100-4,3,10.4 Payment of Nonphysician Services for Inpatients
CMS 100-4,13,10 ICD-9-CM Coding for Diagnostic Tests
CMS 100-4,13,100 Interpretation of Diagnostic Tests

EXCLUDES *Stress views, any joint (77071)*

73560 **Radiologic examination, knee; 1 or 2 views** Z3 X 80
0.94 0.94 Global Days XXX

73562 **3 views** Z3 X 80
1.12 1.12 Global Days XXX

73564 **complete, 4 or more views** Z3 X 80
1.31 1.31 Global Days XXX
AMA: 2009, Jan, 11-31; 2008, Jan, 10-25; 2007, January, 13-27

73565 **both knees, standing, anteroposterior** Z3 X 80
1.07 1.07 Global Days XXX

73580 **Radiologic examination, knee, arthrography, radiological supervision and interpretation** N1 Q2 80 PQ
Do not report with (77002)
4.07 4.07 Global Days XXX
AMA: 2008, Jun, 8-11; 2007, February, 10-11

73590 **Radiologic examination; tibia and fibula, 2 views** Z3 X 80
0.83 0.83 Global Days XXX

73592 **lower extremity, infant, minimum of 2 views** A Z3 X 80
0.97 0.97 Global Days XXX

73600 **Radiologic examination, ankle; 2 views** Z3 X 80
0.87 0.87 Global Days XXX

73610 **complete, minimum of 3 views** Z3 X 80
1.00 1.00 Global Days XXX

73615 **Radiologic examination, ankle, arthrography, radiological supervision and interpretation** N1 Q2 80 PQ
Do not report with (77002)
3.26 3.26 Global Days XXX
AMA: 2008, Jun, 8-11; 2007, February, 10-11

73620 **Radiologic examination, foot; 2 views** Z3 X 80
0.82 0.82 Global Days XXX

73630 **complete, minimum of 3 views** Z3 X 80
0.95 0.95 Global Days XXX

73650 **Radiologic examination; calcaneus, minimum of 2 views** Z3 X 80
0.85 0.85 Global Days XXX

73660 **toe(s), minimum of 2 views** Z3 X 80
0.90 0.90 Global Days XXX

73700-73702 Computerized Tomography: Leg, Ankle, and Foot

CMS 100-2,6,10 Medical and Other Services Furnished to Inpatients
CMS 100-2,15,80 Diagnostic Test Requirements
CMS 100-3,220.1 Computerized Tomography
CMS 100-4,3,10.4 Payment of Nonphysician Services for Inpatients
CMS 100-4,13,10 ICD-9-CM Coding for Diagnostic Tests
CMS 100-4,13,100 Interpretation of Diagnostic Tests

EXCLUDES *Stress views, any joint (77071)*

73700 **Computed tomography, lower extremity; without contrast material** Z2 Q3 80
6.83 6.83 Global Days XXX
AMA: 2007, March, 9-11

73701 **with contrast material(s)** Z3 Q3 80
8.45 8.45 Global Days XXX
AMA: 2007, March, 9-11

73702 **without contrast material, followed by contrast material(s) and further sections** Z2 Q3 80
EXCLUDES *3D rendering (76376, 76377)*
10.72 10.72 Global Days XXX
AMA: 2007, March, 9-11

73706 Computerized Tomographic Angiography: Leg, Ankle, and Foot

CMS 100-2,6,10 Medical and Other Services Furnished to Inpatients
CMS 100-2,15,80 Diagnostic Test Requirements
CMS 100-4,3,10.4 Payment of Nonphysician Services for Inpatients
CMS 100-4,13,10 ICD-9-CM Coding for Diagnostic Tests
CMS 100-4,13,100 Interpretation of Diagnostic Tests
EXCLUDES *Stress views, any joint (77071)*

73706 **Computed tomographic angiography, lower extremity, with contrast material(s), including noncontrast images, if performed, and image postprocessing** Z2 03 80
EXCLUDES *Computed tomographic angiography aorto-iliofemoral runoff (75635)*
13.24 13.24 Global Days XXX
AMA: 2009, Jan, 11-31; 2007, January, 28-31

73718-73723 Magnetic Resonance Imaging: Leg, Ankle, and Foot

CMS 100-2,6,10 Medical and Other Services Furnished to Inpatients
CMS 100-2,15,80 Diagnostic Test Requirements
CMS 100-3,220.2 Magnetic Resonance Imaging
CMS 100-4,3,10.4 Payment of Nonphysician Services for Inpatients
CMS 100-4,13,10 ICD-9-CM Coding for Diagnostic Tests
CMS 100-4,13,40 Magnetic Resonance Imaging (MRI) Procedures
CMS 100-4,13,100 Interpretation of Diagnostic Tests
EXCLUDES *Stress views, any joint (77071)*

73718 **Magnetic resonance (eg, proton) imaging, lower extremity other than joint; without contrast material(s)** Z2 03 80
13.85 13.85 Global Days XXX

73719 **with contrast material(s)** Z2 03 80
15.52 15.52 Global Days XXX

73720 **without contrast material(s), followed by contrast material(s) and further sequences** Z2 03 80
19.80 19.80 Global Days XXX

73721 **Magnetic resonance (eg, proton) imaging, any joint of lower extremity; without contrast material** Z2 03 80
13.67 13.67 Global Days XXX
AMA: 2009, Jan, 11-31; 2008, Jan, 10-25; 2007, January, 13-27

73722 **with contrast material(s)** Z2 03 80
14.84 14.84 Global Days XXX

73723 **without contrast material(s), followed by contrast material(s) and further sequences** Z2 03 80
18.63 18.63 Global Days XXX

73725 Magnetic Resonace Angiography: Leg, Ankle, and Foot

CMS 100-2,6,10 Medical and Other Services Furnished to Inpatients
CMS 100-2,15,80 Diagnostic Test Requirements
CMS 100-3,220.3 Magnetic Resonance Angiography
CMS 100-4,3,10.4 Payment of Nonphysician Services for Inpatients
CMS 100-4,13,10 ICD-9-CM Coding for Diagnostic Tests
CMS 100-4,13,40.1.1 Magnetic Resonance Angiography
CMS 100-4,13,40.1.1 Magnetic Resonance Angiography Coverage Summary
CMS 100-4,13,100 Interpretation of Diagnostic Tests

73725 **Magnetic resonance angiography, lower extremity, with or without contrast material(s)** B 80
15.39 15.39 Global Days XXX
AMA: 2007, January, 28-31

74000-74022 Radiography: Abdomen--General

CMS 100-2,15,80 Diagnostic Test Requirements
CMS 100-4,3,10.4 Payment of Nonphysician Services for Inpatients
CMS 100-4,13,10 ICD-9-CM Coding for Diagnostic Tests
CMS 100-4,13,100 Interpretation of Diagnostic Tests

74000 **Radiologic examination, abdomen; single anteroposterior view** Z3 X 80
0.74 0.74 Global Days XXX

74010 **anteroposterior and additional oblique and cone views** Z3 X 80
1.15 1.15 Global Days XXX
AMA: 2007, January, 28-31

74020 **complete, including decubitus and/or erect views** Z3 X 80
1.20 1.20 Global Days XXX

74022 **complete acute abdomen series, including supine, erect, and/or decubitus views, single view chest** Z3 X 80
1.44 1.44 Global Days XXX

74150-74170 Computerized Tomography: Abdomen–General

CMS 100-2,6,10 Medical and Other Services Furnished to Inpatients
CMS 100-2,15,80 Diagnostic Test Requirements
CMS 100-3,220.1 Computerized Tomography
CMS 100-4,3,10.4 Payment of Nonphysician Services for Inpatients
CMS 100-4,13,10 ICD-9-CM Coding for Diagnostic Tests
CMS 100-4,13,30 Computerized Axial Tomography (CT) Procedures
CMS 100-4,13,100 Interpretation of Diagnostic Tests
EXCLUDES *3D rendering (76376-76377)*
Combined CT of abdomen and pelvis (74176-74178)
Computed tomographic colonography, diagnostic (74261-74262)
Computed tomographic colonography, screening (74263)

Do not report with computed tomographic colonography (74261-74263)

74150 **Computed tomography, abdomen; without contrast material** Z2 03 80
6.82 6.82 Global Days XXX
AMA: 2009, Jan, 11-31; 2008, Jan, 10-25; 2007, January, 13-27

74160 **with contrast material(s)** Z2 03 80
9.30 9.30 Global Days XXX

74170 **without contrast material, followed by contrast material(s) and further sections** Z2 03 80
12.32 12.32 Global Days XXX

74174-74175 Computerized Tomographic Angiography: Abdomen and Pelvis

CMS 100-2,6,10 Medical and Other Services Furnished to Inpatients
CMS 100-2,15,80 Diagnostic Test Requirements
CMS 100-3,220.1 Computerized Tomography
CMS 100-4,3,10.4 Payment of Nonphysician Services for Inpatients
CMS 100-4,13,10 ICD-9-CM Coding for Diagnostic Tests
CMS 100-4,13,30 Computerized Axial Tomography (CT) Procedures
CMS 100-4,13,100 Interpretation of Diagnostic Tests
EXCLUDES *Computed tomographic angiography aorto-iliofemoral runoff (75635)*

● **74174** **Computed tomographic angiography, abdomen and pelvis, with contrast material(s), including noncontrast images, if performed, and image postprocessing** Z3 S 80
Do not report with (72191, 73706, 74175, 75635, 76376-76377)
16.51 16.51 Global Days XXX

74175 **Computed tomographic angiography, abdomen, with contrast material(s), including noncontrast images, if performed, and image postprocessing** Z2 Q3 80

EXCLUDES *Combined computed tomographic angiography study of abdomen and pelvis (74174)*

14.36 14.36 Global Days XXX

AMA: 2007, January, 28-31

74176-74178 Computerized Tomography: Abdomen and Pelvis

Do not report more than once for each combined examination of the abdomen and pelvis

Do not report with (72192-72194, 74150-74170)

74176 **Computed tomography, abdomen and pelvis; without contrast material** Z3 Q3

6.64 6.64 Global Days XXX

74177 **with contrast material(s)** Z2 Q3

10.51 10.51 Global Days XXX

74178 **without contrast material in 1 or both body regions, followed by contrast material(s) and further sections in 1 or both body regions** Z3 Q3

13.35 13.35 Global Days XXX

74181-74183 Magnetic Resonance Imaging: Abdomen–General

CMS 100-2,6,10 Medical and Other Services Furnished to Inpatients
CMS 100-2,15,80 Diagnostic Test Requirements
CMS 100-3,220.2 Magnetic Resonance Imaging
CMS 100-4,3,10.4 Payment of Nonphysician Services for Inpatients
CMS 100-4,13,10 ICD-9-CM Coding for Diagnostic Tests
CMS 100-4,13,40 Magnetic Resonance Imaging (MRI) Procedures
CMS 100-4,13,100 Interpretation of Diagnostic Tests

74181 **Magnetic resonance (eg, proton) imaging, abdomen; without contrast material(s)** Z2 Q3 80

12.60 12.60 Global Days XXX

AMA: 2009, May, 8-9&11; 2009, Jul, 10; 2009, Jan, 11-31; 2008, Jan, 10-25

74182 **with contrast material(s)** Z2 Q3 80

17.17 17.17 Global Days XXX

AMA: 2009, May, 8-9&11; 2009, Jul, 10

74183 **without contrast material(s), followed by with contrast material(s) and further sequences** Z2 Q3 80

19.86 19.86 Global Days XXX

AMA: 2009, May, 8-9&11; 2009, Jul, 10

74185 Magnetic Resonance Angiography: Abdomen–General

CMS 100-2,6,10 Medical and Other Services Furnished to Inpatients
CMS 100-2,15,80 Diagnostic Test Requirements
CMS 100-3,220.3 Magnetic Resonance Angiography
CMS 100-4,3,10.4 Payment of Nonphysician Services for Inpatients
CMS 100-4,13,10 ICD-9-CM Coding for Diagnostic Tests
CMS 100-4,13,40.1.1 Magnetic Resonance Angiography
CMS 100-4,13,100 Interpretation of Diagnostic Tests

74185 **Magnetic resonance angiography, abdomen, with or without contrast material(s)** B 80

15.32 15.32 Global Days XXX

AMA: 2007, January, 28-31

74190 Peritoneography

CMS 100-2,15,80 Diagnostic Test Requirements
CMS 100-4,3,10.4 Payment of Nonphysician Services for Inpatients
CMS 100-4,13,10 ICD-9-CM Coding for Diagnostic Tests
CMS 100-4,13,100 Interpretation of Diagnostic Tests

74190 **Peritoneogram (eg, after injection of air or contrast), radiological supervision and interpretation** N1 Q2 80 PQ

EXCLUDES *Computed tomography, pelvis or abdomen (72192, 74150)*

Code also injection procedure (49400)

0.00 0.00 Global Days XXX

74210-74235 Radiography: Throat and Esophagus

CMS 100-2,15,80 Diagnostic Test Requirements
CMS 100-4,3,10.4 Payment of Nonphysician Services for Inpatients
CMS 100-4,13,10 ICD-9-CM Coding for Diagnostic Tests
CMS 100-4,13,100 Interpretation of Diagnostic Tests

EXCLUDES *Percutaneous placement of gastrostomy tube, endoscopic (43246)*
Percutaneous placement of gastrostomy tube, fluoroscopic guidance (49440)

74210 **Radiologic examination; pharynx and/or cervical esophagus** Z2 S 80 PQ

2.37 2.37 Global Days XXX

74220 **esophagus** Z2 S 80 PQ

2.72 2.72 Global Days XXX

74230 **Swallowing function, with cineradiography/videoradiography** Z3 S 80 PQ

2.76 2.76 Global Days XXX

74235 **Removal of foreign body(s), esophageal, with use of balloon catheter, radiological supervision and interpretation** N1 N 80 PQ

Code also esophagoscopy/upper GI endoscopy (43215, 43247)

0.00 0.00 Global Days XXX

74240-74283 Radiography: Intestines

CMS 100-2,6,10 Medical and Other Services Furnished to Inpatients
CMS 100-2,15,80 Diagnostic Test Requirements
CMS 100-4,3,10.4 Payment of Nonphysician Services for Inpatients
CMS 100-4,13,10 ICD-9-CM Coding for Diagnostic Tests
CMS 100-4,13,100 Interpretation of Diagnostic Tests

EXCLUDES *Percutaneous placement of gastrostomy tube, endoscopic (43246)*
Percutaneous placement of gastrostomy tube, fluoroscopic guidance (49440)

74240 **Radiologic examination, gastrointestinal tract, upper; with or without delayed films, without KUB** Z2 S 80 PQ

3.43 3.43 Global Days XXX

74241 **with or without delayed films, with KUB** Z2 S 80 PQ

3.59 3.59 Global Days XXX

74245 **with small intestine, includes multiple serial films** Z2 S 80 PQ

5.35 5.35 Global Days XXX

74246 **Radiological examination, gastrointestinal tract, upper, air contrast, with specific high density barium, effervescent agent, with or without glucagon; with or without delayed films, without KUB** Z2 S 80 PQ

INCLUDES Moynihan test

3.85 3.85 Global Days XXX

74247 **with or without delayed films, with KUB** Z2 S 80 PQ

4.28 4.28 Global Days XXX

74249 **with small intestine follow-through** Z2 S 80 PQ

5.78 5.78 Global Days XXX

74250 **Radiologic examination, small intestine, includes multiple serial films;**
3.25 3.25 Global Days XXX

74251 **via enteroclysis tube**
11.58 11.58 Global Days XXX

74260 **Duodenography, hypotonic**
9.64 9.64 Global Days XXX

74261 **Computed tomographic (CT) colonography, diagnostic, including image postprocessing; without contrast material**

Do not report with (72192-72194, 74150-74170, 74263, 76376-76377)

15.89 15.89 Global Days XXX

74262 **with contrast material(s) including non-contrast images, if performed**

Do not report with (72192-72194, 74150-74170, 74263, 76376-76377)

18.54 18.54 Global Days XXX

74263 **Computed tomographic (CT) colonography, screening, including image postprocessing**

Do not report with (72192-72194, 74150-74170, 74261-74262, 76376-76377)

23.77 23.77 Global Days XXX

74270 **Radiologic examination, colon; contrast (eg, barium) enema, with or without KUB**
4.68 4.68 Global Days XXX
AMA: 2009, Jan, 11-31; 2008, Jan, 10-25; 2007, January, 13-27

74280 **air contrast with specific high density barium, with or without glucagon**
6.48 6.48 Global Days XXX

74283 **Therapeutic enema, contrast or air, for reduction of intussusception or other intraluminal obstruction (eg, meconium ileus)**
6.08 6.08 Global Days XXX

74290-74330 Radiography: Biliary Tract

CMS 100-2,15,80	Diagnostic Test Requirements
CMS 100-4,3,10.4	Payment of Nonphysician Services for Inpatients
CMS 100-4,13,10	ICD-9-CM Coding for Diagnostic Tests
CMS 100-4,13,100	Interpretation of Diagnostic Tests

EXCLUDES *Percutaneous placement of gastrostomy tube, endoscopic (43246)*
Percutaneous placement of gastrostomy tube, fluoroscopic guidance (49440)

74290 **Cholecystography, oral contrast;**
2.08 2.08 Global Days XXX

74291 **additional or repeat examination or multiple day examination**
2.01 2.01 Global Days XXX

74300 **Cholangiography and/or pancreatography; intraoperative, radiological supervision and interpretation**
0.00 0.00 Global Days XXX
AMA: 2009, Jan, 11-31; 2008, Jan, 10-25; 2007, January, 13-27

\+ **74301** **additional set intraoperative, radiological supervision and interpretation (List separately in addition to code for primary procedure)**
Code first primary procedure (74300)
0.00 0.00 Global Days ZZZ

74305 **through existing catheter, radiological supervision and interpretation**
EXCLUDES *Percutaneous biliary duct stone extraction (47630, 74327)*

Code also (47505, 47560-47561, 47563, 48400)
0.00 0.00 Global Days XXX

74320 **Cholangiography, percutaneous, transhepatic, radiological supervision and interpretation**
INCLUDES Needle placement with fluoroscopic guidance (77002)

3.11 3.11 Global Days XXX
AMA: 2008, Jun, 8-11; 2007, February, 10-11

74327 **Postoperative biliary duct calculus removal, percutaneous via T-tube tract, basket, or snare (eg, Burhenne technique), radiological supervision and interpretation**
Code also percutaneous biliary duct stone extraction (47630)
4.16 4.16 Global Days XXX

74328 **Endoscopic catheterization of the biliary ductal system, radiological supervision and interpretation**
Code also ERCP (43260-43272)
0.00 0.00 Global Days XXX
AMA: 2009, Jan, 11-31; 2008, May, 9-11

74329 **Endoscopic catheterization of the pancreatic ductal system, radiological supervision and interpretation**
Code also ERCP (43260-43272)
0.00 0.00 Global Days XXX

74330 **Combined endoscopic catheterization of the biliary and pancreatic ductal systems, radiological supervision and interpretation**
Code also ERCP (43260-43272)
0.00 0.00 Global Days XXX

74340-74363 Radiography: Bilidigestive Intubation

CMS 100-2,15,80	Diagnostic Test Requirements
CMS 100-4,3,10.4	Payment of Nonphysician Services for Inpatients
CMS 100-4,13,10	ICD-9-CM Coding for Diagnostic Tests
CMS 100-4,13,100	Interpretation of Diagnostic Tests

EXCLUDES *Percutaneous insertion of gastrostomy tube, endoscopic (43246)*
Percutaneous placement of gastrotomy tube, fluoroscopic guidance (49440)

74340 **Introduction of long gastrointestinal tube (eg, Miller-Abbott), including multiple fluoroscopies and films, radiological supervision and interpretation**
Code also placement of tube (44500)
0.00 0.00 Global Days XXX

74355 **Percutaneous placement of enteroclysis tube, radiological supervision and interpretation**
INCLUDES Needle placement with fluoroscopic guidance (77002)

0.00 0.00 Global Days XXX
AMA: 2008, Jun, 8-11; 2007, February, 10-11

74360 **Intraluminal dilation of strictures and/or obstructions (eg, esophagus), radiological supervision and interpretation**
0.00 0.00 Global Days XXX
AMA: 2008, Oct, 6-7

74363 **Percutaneous transhepatic dilation of biliary duct stricture with or without placement of stent, radiological supervision and interpretation**
EXCLUDES *Surgical procedure (47510, 47511, 47555, 47556)*

0.00 0.00 Global Days XXX

74400-74775 Radiography: Urogenital

CMS 100-2,15,80 Diagnostic Test Requirements
CMS 100-4,3,10.4 Payment of Nonphysician Services for Inpatients
CMS 100-4,13,10 ICD-9-CM Coding for Diagnostic Tests
CMS 100-4,13,100 Interpretation of Diagnostic Tests

74400 **Urography (pyelography), intravenous, with or without KUB, with or without tomography** Z2 S 80
3.37 3.37 Global Days XXX

74410 **Urography, infusion, drip technique and/or bolus technique;** Z2 S 80
3.41 3.41 Global Days XXX

74415 **with nephrotomography** Z2 S 80
4.11 4.11 Global Days XXX

74420 **Urography, retrograde, with or without KUB** Z2 S 80
0.00 0.00 Global Days XXX
AMA: 2009, Jan, 11-31; 2008, Jan, 10-25; 2007, January, 13-27

74425 **Urography, antegrade (pyelostogram, nephrostogram, loopogram), radiological supervision and interpretation** N1 Q2 80 PQ
0.00 0.00 Global Days XXX

74430 **Cystography, minimum of 3 views, radiological supervision and interpretation** N1 Q2 80 PQ
1.51 1.51 Global Days XXX

74440 **Vasography, vesiculography, or epididymography, radiological supervision and interpretation** ♂ N1 Q2 80 PQ
2.49 2.49 Global Days XXX

74445 **Corpora cavernosography, radiological supervision and interpretation** ♂ N1 Q2 80 PQ
INCLUDES Needle placement with fluoroscopic guidance (77002)
0.00 0.00 Global Days XXX
AMA: 2008, Jun, 8-11; 2007, February, 10-11

74450 **Urethrocystography, retrograde, radiological supervision and interpretation** N1 Q2 80 PQ
0.00 0.00 Global Days XXX

74455 **Urethrocystography, voiding, radiological supervision and interpretation** N1 Q2 80 PQ
2.65 2.65 Global Days XXX

74470 **Radiologic examination, renal cyst study, translumbar, contrast visualization, radiological supervision and interpretation** N1 Q2 80 PQ
INCLUDES Needle placement with fluoroscopic guidance (77002)
0.00 0.00 Global Days XXX
AMA: 2008, Jun, 8-11; 2007, February, 10-11

74475 **Introduction of intracatheter or catheter into renal pelvis for drainage and/or injection, percutaneous, radiological supervision and interpretation** N1 Q2 80 PQ
INCLUDES Needle placement with fluoroscopic guidance (77002)
3.15 3.15 Global Days XXX
AMA: 2008, Jun, 8-11; 2007, February, 10-11

74480 **Introduction of ureteral catheter or stent into ureter through renal pelvis for drainage and/or injection, percutaneous, radiological supervision and interpretation** N1 Q2 80 PQ
EXCLUDES *Code also ureter/pelvis transurethral surgery (52320-52355)*
3.15 3.15 Global Days XXX

74485 **Dilation of nephrostomy, ureters, or urethra, radiological supervision and interpretation** N1 Q2 80 PQ
EXCLUDES *Change of pyelostomy/nephrostomy tube (50398)*
Ureter dilation without radiologic guidance (52341, 52344)
3.15 3.15 Global Days XXX
AMA: 2009, Jan, 7-8

74710 **Pelvimetry, with or without placental localization** ♀ Z3 X 80
EXCLUDES *Imaging procedures on abdomen and pelvis (72170-72190, 74000-74170)*
1.13 1.13 Global Days XXX

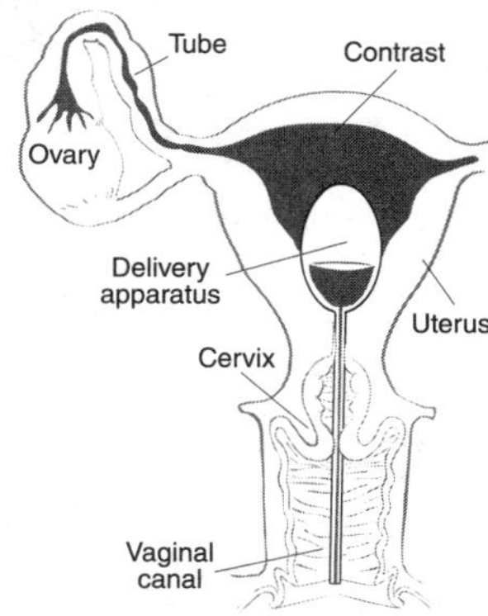

Hysterosalpingography (imaging of the uterus and tubes) is performed. Report for radiological supervision and interpretation

74740 **Hysterosalpingography, radiological supervision and interpretation** ♀ N1 Q2 80 PQ
EXCLUDES *Imaging procedures on abdomen and pelvis (72170-72190, 74000-74170)*
Code also injection of saline/contrast (58340)
2.38 2.38 Global Days XXX
AMA: 2009, Mar, 10-11

74742 **Transcervical catheterization of fallopian tube, radiological supervision and interpretation** ♀ N1 N 80 PQ
EXCLUDES *Imaging procedures on abdomen and pelvis (72170-72190, 74000-74170)*
Code also (58345)
0.00 0.00 Global Days XXX
AMA: 2009, Mar, 10-11

74775 **Perineogram (eg, vaginogram, for sex determination or extent of anomalies)** M ♀ Z2 S 80
EXCLUDES *Imaging procedures on abdomen and pelvis (72170-72190, 74000-74170)*
0.00 0.00 Global Days XXX

75557-75565 Magnetic Resonance Imaging: Heart Structure and Physiology

CMS 100-2,15,80 Diagnostic Test Requirements
CMS 100-3,220.2 Magnetic Resonance Imaging
CMS 100-4,3,10.4 Payment of Nonphysician Services for Inpatients
CMS 100-4,13,10 ICD-9-CM Coding for Diagnostic Tests
CMS 100-4,13,40 Magnetic Resonance Imaging (MRI) Procedures

INCLUDES Physiologic evaluation of cardiac function

EXCLUDES *Cardiac catheterization procedures (93451-93572)*

Code also separate vascular injection (36000-36299)
Do not report with (76376-76377)
Do not report with more than one code in this group per session

75557 **Cardiac magnetic resonance imaging for morphology and function without contrast material;** Z2 03 80
12.19 12.19 Global Days XXX
AMA: 2008, Jul, 3&14

75559 **with stress imaging** Z2 03 80
INCLUDES Pharmacologic wall motion stress evaluation without contrast
Code also for stress testing when performed (93015-93018)
Code also stress test (93015-93018)
17.27 17.27 Global Days XXX
AMA: 2008, Jul, 3&14

75561 **Cardiac magnetic resonance imaging for morphology and function without contrast material(s), followed by contrast material(s) and further sequences;** Z2 03 80
16.42 16.42 Global Days XXX
AMA: 2008, Jul, 3&14

75563 **with stress imaging** Z2 03 80
INCLUDES Pharmacologic perfusion stress evaluation with contrast
Code also stress test (93015-93018)
Code also stress testing codes as appropriate (93015-93018)
19.75 19.75 Global Days XXX
AMA: 2008, Jul, 3&14

\+ **75565** **Cardiac magnetic resonance imaging for velocity flow mapping (List separately in addition to code for primary procedure)** N1 N 80
Code also to report flow with pharmacologic perfusion stress with contrast with (75563)
Code also for flow with pharmacologic wall motion stress evaluation without contrast with (75559)
Code first (75557, 75559, 75561, 75563)
1.94 1.94 Global Days ZZZ

75571-75574 Computed Tomographic Imaging: Heart

75571 **Computed tomography, heart, without contrast material, with quantitative evaluation of coronary calcium** Z2 X 80
3.36 3.36 Global Days XXX

75572 **Computed tomography, heart, with contrast material, for evaluation of cardiac structure and morphology (including 3D image postprocessing, assessment of cardiac function, and evaluation of venous structures, if performed)** Z2 S 80
9.21 9.21 Global Days XXX

75573 **Computed tomography, heart, with contrast material, for evaluation of cardiac structure and morphology in the setting of congenital heart disease (including 3D image postprocessing, assessment of LV cardiac function, RV structure and function and evaluation of venous structures, if performed)** Z2 S 80
12.64 12.64 Global Days XXX

75574 **Computed tomographic angiography, heart, coronary arteries and bypass grafts (when present), with contrast material, including 3D image postprocessing (including evaluation of cardiac structure and morphology, assessment of cardiac function, and evaluation of venous structures, if performed)** Z2 S 80
13.64 13.64 Global Days XXX

75600-75791 Radiography: Arterial

CMS 100-2,15,80 Diagnostic Test Requirements
CMS 100-4,3,10.4 Payment of Nonphysician Services for Inpatients
CMS 100-4,13,10 ICD-9-CM Coding for Diagnostic Tests
CMS 100-4,13,100 Interpretation of Diagnostic Tests

INCLUDES Diagnostic angiography specifically included in the interventional code description
The following diagnostic procedures with interventional supervision and interpretation:
Angiography
Contrast injection
Fluoroscopic guidance for intervention
Post-angioplasty/atherectomy/stent angiography
Roadmapping
Vessel measurement

EXCLUDES *Catheterization codes for diagnostic angiography of lower extremity when an access site other than the site used for the therapy is required*
Diagnostic angiogram during a separate encounter from the interventional procedure
Diagnostic angiography with interventional procedure if:
1. No previous catheter-based angiogram is accessible and a complete diagnostic procedure is performed and the decision to proceed with an interventional procedure is based on the diagnostic service, OR
2. The previous diagnostic angiogram is accessible but the documentation in the medical record specifies that:
A. the patient's condition has changed
B. there is insufficient imaging of the patient's anatomy and/or disease, OR
C. there is a clinical change during the procedure that necessitates a new examination away from the site of the intervention
3. Modifier 59 is appended to the code(s) for the diagnostic radiological supervision and interpretation service to indicate the guidelines were met
Intra-arterial procedures (36100-36248)
Intravenous procedures (36000, 36005-36015)

75600 **Aortography, thoracic, without serialography, radiological supervision and interpretation** N1 Q2 80 PO
EXCLUDES *Injection procedure (93567)*
7.21 7.21 Global Days XXX

75605 **Aortography, thoracic, by serialography, radiological supervision and interpretation** N1 Q2 80 PO
EXCLUDES *Injection procedure (93567)*
5.48 5.48 Global Days XXX
AMA: 2009, Jan, 11-31; 2008, Jan, 10-25; 2007, January, 13-27

75625 **Aortography, abdominal, by serialography, radiological supervision and interpretation** N1 Q2 80 PO
EXCLUDES *Injection procedure (93567)*
5.53 5.53 Global Days XXX
AMA: 2009, Jan, 11-31; 2008, Apr, -11; 2008, Jan, 10-25; 2007, January, 13-27; 2007, Dec, 10-179

75630 **Aortography, abdominal plus bilateral iliofemoral lower extremity, catheter, by serialography, radiological supervision and interpretation**
6.49 6.49 Global Days XXX
AMA: 2009, Jan, 11-31; 2008, Jan, 10-25; 2008, Apr, -11; 2007, January, 13-27

75635 **Computed tomographic angiography, abdominal aorta and bilateral iliofemoral lower extremity runoff, with contrast material(s), including noncontrast images, if performed, and image postprocessing**
Do not report with (72191, 73706, 74174-74175)
14.76 14.76 Global Days XXX
AMA: 2007, January, 28-31

75650 **Angiography, cervicocerebral, catheter, including vessel origin, radiological supervision and interpretation**
6.09 6.09 Global Days XXX

75658 **Angiography, brachial, retrograde, radiological supervision and interpretation**
6.27 6.27 Global Days XXX

75660 **Angiography, external carotid, unilateral, selective, radiological supervision and interpretation**
6.67 6.67 Global Days XXX

75662 **Angiography, external carotid, bilateral, selective, radiological supervision and interpretation**
7.92 7.92 Global Days XXX

75665 **Angiography, carotid, cerebral, unilateral, radiological supervision and interpretation**
6.92 6.92 Global Days XXX

75671 **Angiography, carotid, cerebral, bilateral, radiological supervision and interpretation**
8.15 8.15 Global Days XXX

75676 **Angiography, carotid, cervical, unilateral, radiological supervision and interpretation**
6.53 6.53 Global Days XXX

75680 **Angiography, carotid, cervical, bilateral, radiological supervision and interpretation**
7.45 7.45 Global Days XXX

75685 **Angiography, vertebral, cervical, and/or intracranial, radiological supervision and interpretation**
6.62 6.62 Global Days XXX

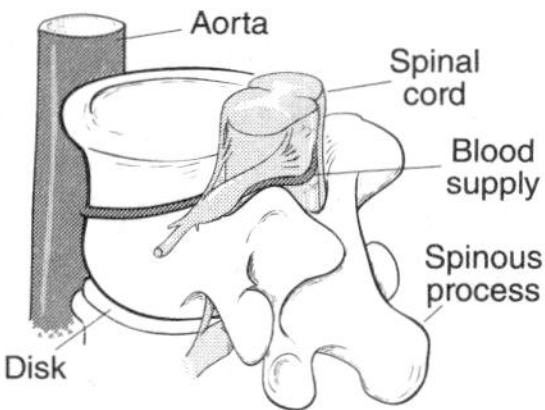

An angiography of a specific area of the spine is performed

75705 **Angiography, spinal, selective, radiological supervision and interpretation**
7.95 7.95 Global Days XXX

75710 **Angiography, extremity, unilateral, radiological supervision and interpretation**
6.13 6.13 Global Days XXX
AMA: 2009, Jan, 11-31; 2008, Jan, 10-25; 2007, January, 13-27

75716 **Angiography, extremity, bilateral, radiological supervision and interpretation**
7.22 7.22 Global Days XXX
AMA: 2009, Jan, 11-31; 2008, Jan, 10-25; 2008, Apr, -11; 2007, January, 13-27; 2007, Dec, 10-179

~~75722~~ ~~**Angiography, renal, unilateral, selective (including flush aortogram), radiological supervision and interpretation**~~
To report, see 36251, 36253

~~75724~~ ~~**Angiography, renal, bilateral, selective (including flush aortogram), radiological supervision and interpretation**~~
To report, see 36252, 36254

75726 **Angiography, visceral, selective or supraselective (with or without flush aortogram), radiological supervision and interpretation**
EXCLUDES *Selective angiography, each additional visceral vessel studied after basic examination (75774)*
6.10 6.10 Global Days XXX

75731 **Angiography, adrenal, unilateral, selective, radiological supervision and interpretation**
5.90 5.90 Global Days XXX

75733 **Angiography, adrenal, bilateral, selective, radiological supervision and interpretation**
7.08 7.08 Global Days XXX

75736 **Angiography, pelvic, selective or supraselective, radiological supervision and interpretation**
6.02 6.02 Global Days XXX

75741 **Angiography, pulmonary, unilateral, selective, radiological supervision and interpretation**
EXCLUDES *Injection procedure (93568)*
5.66 5.66 Global Days XXX

75743 **Angiography, pulmonary, bilateral, selective, radiological supervision and interpretation**
EXCLUDES *Injection procedure (93568)*
6.45 6.45 Global Days XXX

75746 **Angiography, pulmonary, by nonselective catheter or venous injection, radiological supervision and interpretation**
EXCLUDES *Code also injection procedure, catheter introduction (93451, 93453-93461, 93530-93533, 93563-93564, 93568)*
5.89 5.89 Global Days XXX

75756 **Angiography, internal mammary, radiological supervision and interpretation**
EXCLUDES *Injection procedure, catheter introduction (93451-93462, 93530-93533, 93563-93564, 93567-93568)*
6.46 6.46 Global Days XXX

+ 75774 **Angiography, selective, each additional vessel studied after basic examination, radiological supervision and interpretation (List separately in addition to code for primary procedure)**
EXCLUDES *Angiography (36147, 75600-75756, 75791)*
Catheterizations (36215-36248)
Injection procedure, catheter introduction (93451-93462, 93530-93533, 93563-93568)
Code first initial vessel
3.89 3.89 Global Days ZZZ
AMA: 2009, Jan, 11-31; 2007, Dec, 10-179

75791 **Angiography, arteriovenous shunt (eg, dialysis patient fistula/graft), complete evaluation of dialysis access, including fluoroscopy, image documentation and report (includes injections of contrast and all necessary imaging from the arterial anastomosis and adjacent artery through entire venous outflow including the inferior or superior vena cava), radiological supervision and interpretation** N1 Q2 80 PQ

INCLUDES Radiological evaluation performed via existing access into the shunt or from an access that is not a direct puncture of the shunt

EXCLUDES *Catheter introduction, when performed (36140, 36215-36217, 36245-36247)*
Radiological evaluation with introduction of needle/catheter, AV dialysis shunt, complete procedure (36147)

10.00 10.00 Global Days XXX

75801-75893 Radiography: Lymphatic and Venous

CMS 100-2,15,80 Diagnostic Test Requirements
CMS 100-4,3,10.4 Payment of Nonphysician Services for Inpatients
CMS 100-4,13,10 ICD-9-CM Coding for Diagnostic Tests
CMS 100-4,13,100 Interpretation of Diagnostic Tests

INCLUDES Diagnostic venography specifically included in the interventional code description
The following diagnostic procedures with interventional supervision and interpretation:
Contrast injection
Fluoroscopic guidance for intervention
Post-angioplasty/venography
Roadmapping
Venography
Vessel measurement

EXCLUDES *Diagnostic venogram during a separate encounter from the interventional procedure*
Diagnostic venography with interventional procedure if:
1. No previous catheter-based venogram is accessible and a complete diagnostic procedure is performed and the decision to proceed with an interventional procedure is based on the diagnostic service, OR
2. The previous diagnostic venogram is accessible but the documentation in the medical record specifies that:
A. The patient's condition has changed
B. There is insufficient imaging of the patient's anatomy and/or disease, OR
C. There is a clinical change during the procedure that necessitates a new examination away from the site of the intervention
Intravenous procedures (36000-36015, 36400-36510)
Lymphatic injection procedures (38790)

75801 **Lymphangiography, extremity only, unilateral, radiological supervision and interpretation** N1 Q2 80 PQ
0.00 0.00 Global Days XXX

75803 **Lymphangiography, extremity only, bilateral, radiological supervision and interpretation** N1 Q2 80 PQ
0.00 0.00 Global Days XXX

75805 **Lymphangiography, pelvic/abdominal, unilateral, radiological supervision and interpretation** N1 Q2 80 PQ
0.00 0.00 Global Days XXX

75807 **Lymphangiography, pelvic/abdominal, bilateral, radiological supervision and interpretation** N1 Q2 80 PQ
0.00 0.00 Global Days XXX

75809 **Shuntogram for investigation of previously placed indwelling nonvascular shunt (eg, LeVeen shunt, ventriculoperitoneal shunt, indwelling infusion pump), radiological supervision and interpretation** N1 Q2 80 PQ
INCLUDES Needle placement with fluoroscopic guidance (77002)

Code also surgical procedure (49427, 61070)
3.09 3.09 Global Days XXX
AMA: 2009, Jan, 11-31; 2008, Jul, 10&13; 2008, Sep, 10-11; 2008, Jun, 8-11; 2007, February, 10-11

75810 **Splenoportography, radiological supervision and interpretation** N1 Q2 80 PQ
INCLUDES Needle placement with fluoroscopic guidance (77002)
0.00 0.00 Global Days XXX
AMA: 2008, Jun, 8-11; 2007, February, 10-11

75820 **Venography, extremity, unilateral, radiological supervision and interpretation** N1 Q2 80
3.78 3.78 Global Days XXX
AMA: 2009, Jan, 11-31; 2008, May, 9-11; 2008, Jan, 10-25; 2007, January, 13-27

75822 **Venography, extremity, bilateral, radiological supervision and interpretation** N1 Q2 80
4.65 4.65 Global Days XXX

75825 **Venography, caval, inferior, with serialography, radiological supervision and interpretation** N1 Q2 80 PQ
5.31 5.31 Global Days XXX
AMA: 2009, Jan, 11-31; 2009, Jan, 7-8; 2008, Oct, 10-11

75827 **Venography, caval, superior, with serialography, radiological supervision and interpretation** N1 Q2 80 PQ
5.40 5.40 Global Days XXX

75831 **Venography, renal, unilateral, selective, radiological supervision and interpretation** N1 Q2 80 PQ
5.59 5.59 Global Days XXX

75833 **Venography, renal, bilateral, selective, radiological supervision and interpretation** N1 Q2 80 PQ
6.36 6.36 Global Days XXX

75840 **Venography, adrenal, unilateral, selective, radiological supervision and interpretation** N1 Q2 80 PQ
5.55 5.55 Global Days XXX

75842 **Venography, adrenal, bilateral, selective, radiological supervision and interpretation** N1 Q2 80 PQ
6.45 6.45 Global Days XXX

75860 **Venography, venous sinus (eg, petrosal and inferior sagittal) or jugular, catheter, radiological supervision and interpretation** N1 Q2 80 PQ
5.48 5.48 Global Days XXX

75870 **Venography, superior sagittal sinus, radiological supervision and interpretation** N1 Q2 80 PQ
5.42 5.42 Global Days XXX

75872 **Venography, epidural, radiological supervision and interpretation** N1 Q2 80 PQ
8.18 8.18 Global Days XXX

75880 **Venography, orbital, radiological supervision and interpretation** N1 Q2 80 PQ
3.94 3.94 Global Days XXX

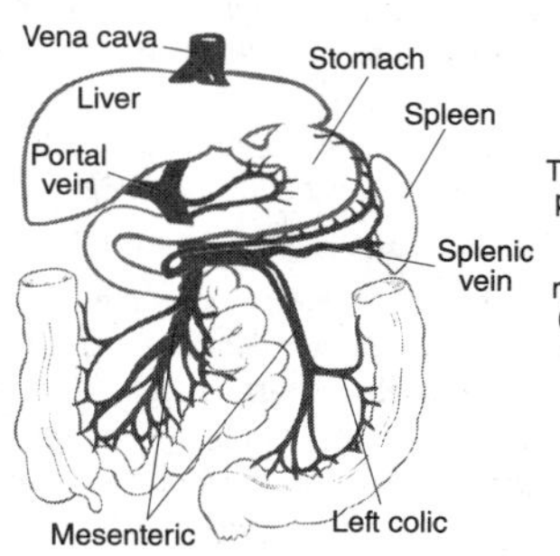

The portal vein is accessed by needle, percutaneously and through the liver, and contrast is delivered into the lumen. Measurement of blood movement through the vein are made (hemodynamic studies). Images are taken. Code 75885 reports the radiological supervision and interpretation of the studies

Schematic showing the portal vein

75885 Percutaneous transhepatic portography with hemodynamic evaluation, radiological supervision and interpretation

INCLUDES Needle placement with fluoroscopic guidance (77002)

5.84 5.84 Global Days XXX

AMA: 2009, Jan, 11-31; 2008, Jan, 10-25; 2008, Jun, 8-11; 2007, February, 10-11; 2007, January, 13-27

75887 Percutaneous transhepatic portography without hemodynamic evaluation, radiological supervision and interpretation

INCLUDES Needle placement with fluoroscopic guidance (77002)

5.84 5.84 Global Days XXX

AMA: 2009, Jan, 11-31; 2008, Jan, 10-25; 2008, Jun, 8-11; 2007, January, 13-27; 2007, February, 10-11

75889 Hepatic venography, wedged or free, with hemodynamic evaluation, radiological supervision and interpretation

5.43 5.43 Global Days XXX

75891 Hepatic venography, wedged or free, without hemodynamic evaluation, radiological supervision and interpretation

5.44 5.44 Global Days XXX

75893 Venous sampling through catheter, with or without angiography (eg, for parathyroid hormone, renin), radiological supervision and interpretation

Code also surgical procedure (36500)

4.53 4.53 Global Days XXX

75894-75946 Transcatheter Procedures

CMS 100-2,15,80 Diagnostic Test Requirements
CMS 100-3,20.28 Therapeutic Embolization
CMS 100-4,3,10.4 Payment of Nonphysician Services for Inpatients
CMS 100-4,13,10 ICD-9-CM Coding for Diagnostic Tests
CMS 100-4,13,100 Interpretation of Diagnostic Tests

INCLUDES The following diagnostic procedures with interventional supervision and interpretation:
- Angiography/venography
- Completion angiography/venography except for those services allowed by 75898
- Contrast injection
- Fluoroscopic guidance for intervention
- Roadmapping
- Vessel measurement

Transurethral approach to the removal or replacement of an internally dwelling ureteral stent (50385-50386)

EXCLUDES *Diagnostic angiography/venography performed at the same session as transcatheter therapy unless it is specifically included in the code descriptor or is excluded in the venography/angiography notes (75600-75893)*

Replacement of gastrostomy, duodenostomy, jejunostomy, gastrojejunostomy, or cecostomy tube, percutaneously, including guidance via fluoroscopy (49450-49452)

75894 Transcatheter therapy, embolization, any method, radiological supervision and interpretation

Code also obstetrical or postpartum hemorrhage embolization (37204)

Code also uterine fibroid embolization (37210)

0.00 0.00 Global Days XXX

AMA: 2008, Feb, 5-6; 2007, January, 7-10

75896 Transcatheter therapy, infusion, any method (eg, thrombolysis other than coronary), radiological supervision and interpretation

EXCLUDES *Coronary disease infusion (92975, 92977)*

0.00 0.00 Global Days XXX

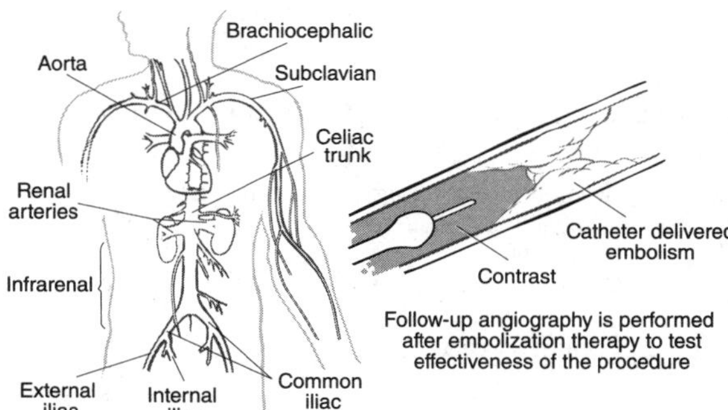

Follow-up angiography is performed after embolization therapy to test effectiveness of the procedure

75898 Angiography through existing catheter for follow-up study for transcatheter therapy, embolization or infusion

0.00 0.00 Global Days XXX

AMA: 2009, Jan, 11-31; 2007, Dec, 10-179; 2007, January, 7-10

75900 Exchange of a previously placed intravascular catheter during thrombolytic therapy with contrast monitoring, radiological supervision and interpretation

Code also surgical procedure (37209)

0.00 0.00 Global Days XXX

Radiology

75885 — 75900

75901 **Mechanical removal of pericatheter obstructive material (eg, fibrin sheath) from central venous device via separate venous access, radiologic supervision and interpretation** N1 N 80 PO

EXCLUDES *Venous catheterization (36010-36012)*

Code also surgical procedure (36595)
5.18 5.18 Global Days XXX

75902 **Mechanical removal of intraluminal (intracatheter) obstructive material from central venous device through device lumen, radiologic supervision and interpretation** N1 N 80 PO

EXCLUDES *Venous catheterization (36010-36012)*

Code also surgical procedure (36596)
2.31 2.31 Global Days XXX

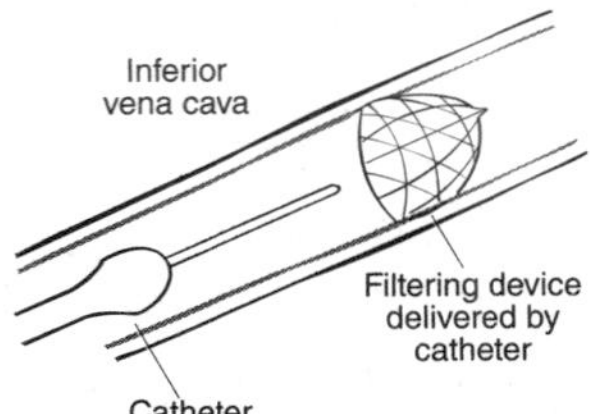

A filtering device is placed by catheter into the inferior vena cava (IVC). Code 75940 reports radiological supervision and interpretation of procedure

~~75940 Percutaneous placement of IVC filter, radiological supervision and interpretation~~
To report, see 37191

75945 **Intravascular ultrasound (non-coronary vessel), radiological supervision and interpretation; initial vessel** N1 Q2 80
0.00 0.00 Global Days XXX

+ **75946** **each additional non-coronary vessel (List separately in addition to code for primary procedure)** N1 N 80
Code first initial vessel (75945)
0.00 0.00 Global Days ZZZ

75952-75959 Endovascular Aneurysm Repair

CMS 100-4,3,10.4 Payment of Nonphysician Services for Inpatients

INCLUDES The following diagnostic procedures with interventional supervision and interpretation:
- Angiography/venography
- Completion angiography/venography except for those services allowed by 75898
- Contrast injection
- Fluoroscopic guidance for intervention
- Roadmapping
- Vessel measurement

EXCLUDES *Diagnostic angiography/venography performed at the same session as transcatheter therapy unless it is specifically included in the code descriptor or is excluded in the venography/angiography notes (75600-75893)*

75952 **Endovascular repair of infrarenal abdominal aortic aneurysm or dissection, radiological supervision and interpretation** C5 C 80 PO

EXCLUDES *Endovascular repair of abdominal aortic aneurysm, radiologic supervision and interpretation (0080T-0081T)*
Implantation endovascular grafts (34800-34805)

0.00 0.00 Global Days XXX

75953 **Placement of proximal or distal extension prosthesis for endovascular repair of infrarenal aortic or iliac artery aneurysm, pseudoaneurysm, or dissection, radiological supervision and interpretation** C5 C 80 PO

EXCLUDES *Placement of endovascular extension prostheses (34825, 34826)*

0.00 0.00 Global Days XXX

75954 **Endovascular repair of iliac artery aneurysm, pseudoaneurysm, arteriovenous malformation, or trauma, using ilio-iliac tube endoprosthesis, radiological supervision and interpretation** C5 C 80 PO

EXCLUDES *Endovascular repair of iliac artery aneurysm, arteriovenous malformation, pseudoaneurysm, or trauma with bifurcated endoprosthesis, radiological supervision and interpretation (0255T)*
Placement of endovascular graft (34900)

0.00 0.00 Global Days XXX

75956 **Endovascular repair of descending thoracic aorta (eg, aneurysm, pseudoaneurysm, dissection, penetrating ulcer, intramural hematoma, or traumatic disruption); involving coverage of left subclavian artery origin, initial endoprosthesis plus descending thoracic aortic extension(s), if required, to level of celiac artery origin, radiological supervision and interpretation** C5 C 80 PO

Code also endovascular graft implantation (33880)
0.00 0.00 Global Days XXX

75957 **not involving coverage of left subclavian artery origin, initial endoprosthesis plus descending thoracic aortic extension(s), if required, to level of celiac artery origin, radiological supervision and interpretation** C5 C 80 PO

Code also endovascular graft implantation (33881)
0.00 0.00 Global Days XXX

75958 **Placement of proximal extension prosthesis for endovascular repair of descending thoracic aorta (eg, aneurysm, pseudoaneurysm, dissection, penetrating ulcer, intramural hematoma, or traumatic disruption), radiological supervision and interpretation** C5 C 80 PO

INCLUDES Corresponding services for placement of each proximal thoracic endovascular extension

Code also placement of proximal endovascular extension (33883, 33884)
0.00 0.00 Global Days XXX

75959 **Placement of distal extension prosthesis(s) (delayed) after endovascular repair of descending thoracic aorta, as needed, to level of celiac origin, radiological supervision and interpretation** C5 C 80 PO

INCLUDES Corresponding services for placement of distal thoracic endovascular extension(s) placed during procedure following the principal procedure

Code also placement of distal endovascular extension (33886)

Do not report with endovascular repair (75956, 75957)
0.00 0.00 Global Days XXX

75960-75961 Transcatheter Insertion and Removal

CMS 100-2,15,80 Diagnostic Test Requirements
CMS 100-4,3,10.4 Payment of Nonphysician Services for Inpatients
CMS 100-4,13,10 ICD-9-CM Coding for Diagnostic Tests
CMS 100-4,13,100 Interpretation of Diagnostic Tests

INCLUDES The following diagnostic procedures with interventional supervision and interpretation:
- Angiography/venography
- Completion angiography/venography except for those services allowed by 75898
- Contrast injection
- Fluoroscopic guidance for intervention
- Roadmapping
- Vessel measurement

EXCLUDES *Diagnostic angiography/venography performed at the same session as transcatheter therapy unless it is specifically included in the code descriptor or is excluded in the venography/angiography notes (75600-75893)*

75960 Transcatheter introduction of intravascular stent(s) (except coronary, carotid, vertebral, iliac, and lower extremity artery), percutaneous and/or open, radiological supervision and interpretation, each vessel N1 N 80 CCI PQ

INCLUDES Placement of stent with radiological supervision and interpretation in:
- *Femoral/popliteal arteries (37224-37227)*
- *Iliac artery (37220-37223)*
- *Tibial/peroneal artery (37228-37235)*

Transcatheter placement of extracranial vertebral/intrathoracic carotid artery stent(s) radiologic supervision and interpretation (0075T, 0076T)

Code also surgical procedure (37205-37208)

4.73 4.73 **Global Days XXX**

75961 Transcatheter retrieval, percutaneous, of intravascular foreign body (eg, fractured venous or arterial catheter), radiological supervision and interpretation N1 N 80 CCI PQ

EXCLUDES *Vena cava filter removal (37193)*

Code also surgical procedure (37203)

10.15 10.15 **Global Days XXX**

AMA: 2009, Jan, 11-31; 2009, Jan, 7-8; 2008, Oct, 10-11

75962-75978 Percutaneous Transluminal Angioplasty

CMS 100-3,20.7 Percutaneous Transluminal Angioplasty (PTA)
CMS 100-4,3,10.4 Payment of Nonphysician Services for Inpatients

INCLUDES The following diagnostic procedures with interventional supervision and interpretation:
- Angiography/venography
- Completion angiography/venography except for those services allowed by 75898
- Contrast injection
- Fluoroscopic guidance for intervention
- Roadmapping
- Vessel measurement

EXCLUDES *Diagnostic angiography/venography performed at the same session as transcatheter therapy unless it is specifically included in the code descriptor or is excluded in the venography/angiography notes (75600-75893)*

Radiological supervision and interpretation for transluminal balloon angioplasty in:
- *Femoral/popliteal arteries (37224-37227)*
- *Iliac artery (37220-37223)*
- *Tibial/peroneal artery (37228-37235)*

▲ **75962 Transluminal balloon angioplasty, peripheral artery other than renal, or other visceral artery, iliac or lower extremity, radiological supervision and interpretation** N1 Q2 80 CCI PQ

EXCLUDES *Angioplasty with radiological supervision and interpretation femoral, iliac, popliteal, tibial/peroneal arteries (37220-37735)*

Code also angioplasty catheter (C1725, C1885)
Code also surgical procedure (35458, 35475)

5.27 5.27 **Global Days XXX**

AMA: 2009, Jan, 11-31; 2007, Dec, 10-179

+ ▲ **75964 Transluminal balloon angioplasty, each additional peripheral artery other than renal, or other visceral artery, iliac or lower extremity, radiological supervision and interpretation (List separately in addition to code for primary procedure)** N1 N 80 CCI

Code first primary procedure (75962)

3.41 3.41 **Global Days ZZZ**

AMA: 2009, Jan, 11-31; 2007, Dec, 10-179

75966 Transluminal balloon angioplasty, renal or other visceral artery, radiological supervision and interpretation N1 Q2 80 CCI PQ

Code also angioplasty catheter (C1725, C1885)

6.43 6.43 **Global Days XXX**

+ **75968 Transluminal balloon angioplasty, each additional visceral artery, radiological supervision and interpretation (List separately in addition to code for primary procedure)** N1 N 80 CCI

EXCLUDES *Percutaneous transluminal coronary angioplasty (92982-92984)*

Code first primary procedure (75966)

3.29 3.29 **Global Days ZZZ**

75970 Transcatheter biopsy, radiological supervision and interpretation N1 N 80 CCI PQ

EXCLUDES *Injection procedure only for transcatheter therapy or biopsy (36100-36299)*
Percutaneous needle biopsy
- *Pancreas (48102)*
- *Retroperitoneal lymph node/mass (49180)*

Transcatheter renal/ureteral biopsy (52007)

0.00 0.00 **Global Days XXX**

75978 **Transluminal balloon angioplasty, venous (eg, subclavian stenosis), radiological supervision and interpretation**

Code also angioplasty catheter (C1725, C1885)

5.39 5.39 Global Days XXX

75980-75989 Percutaneous Drainage

CMS 100-3,220.1 Computerized Tomography
CMS 100-3,220.5 Ultrasound Diagnostic Procedures
CMS 100-4,3,10.4 Payment of Nonphysician Services for Inpatients

INCLUDES The following diagnostic procedures with interventional supervision and interpretation:
- Angiography/venography
- Completion angiography/venography except for those services allowed by 75898
- Contrast injection
- Fluoroscopic guidance for intervention
- Roadmapping
- Vessel measurement

EXCLUDES *Diagnostic angiography/venography performed at the same session as transcatheter therapy unless it is specifically included in the code descriptor or is excluded in the venography/angiography notes (75600-75893)*

75980 **Percutaneous transhepatic biliary drainage with contrast monitoring, radiological supervision and interpretation**

INCLUDES Needle placement with fluoroscopic guidance (77002)

0.00 0.00 Global Days XXX

AMA: 2008, Jun, 8-11; 2007, February, 10-11

75982 **Percutaneous placement of drainage catheter for combined internal and external biliary drainage or of a drainage stent for internal biliary drainage in patients with an inoperable mechanical biliary obstruction, radiological supervision and interpretation**

INCLUDES Needle placement with fluoroscopic guidance (77002)

0.00 0.00 Global Days XXX

AMA: 2008, Jun, 8-11; 2007, February, 10-11

75984 **Change of percutaneous tube or drainage catheter with contrast monitoring (eg, genitourinary system, abscess), radiological supervision and interpretation**

EXCLUDES *Change only of nephrostomy/pyelostomy tube (50398)*
Change only of percutaneous biliary drainage catheter (47525)
Cholecystostomy, percutaneous (47490)
Introduction procedure only for percutaneous biliary drainage (47510, 47511)
Nephrostolithotomy/pyelostolithotomy, percutaneous (50080, 50081)
Percutaneous replacement of gastrointestinal tube using fluoroscopic guidance (49450-49452)

3.40 3.40 Global Days XXX

75989 **Radiological guidance (ie, fluoroscopy, ultrasound, or computed tomography), for percutaneous drainage (eg, abscess, specimen collection), with placement of catheter, radiological supervision and interpretation**

INCLUDES Needle placement with fluoroscopic guidance (77002)

Do not report with (47490)

3.89 3.89 Global Days XXX

AMA: 2008, Jun, 8-11; 2007, February, 10-11

76000-76140 Miscellaneous Techniques

CMS 100-4,3,10.4 Payment of Nonphysician Services for Inpatients

EXCLUDES *Arthrography:*
- *Ankle (73615)*
- *Elbow (73085)*
- *Hip (73525)*
- *Knee (73580)*
- *Shoulder (73040)*
- *Wrist (73115)*

CT cerebral perfusion test (0042T)

76000 **Fluoroscopy (separate procedure), up to 1 hour physician time, other than 71023 or 71034 (eg, cardiac fluoroscopy)**

1.93 1.93 Global Days XXX

AMA: 2009, Jan, 11-31; 2008, Jan, 10-25; 2008, Jul, 9; 2008, Jun, 8-11; 2007, January, 13-27

76001 **Fluoroscopy, physician time more than 1 hour, assisting a nonradiologic physician (eg, nephrostolithotomy, ERCP, bronchoscopy, transbronchial biopsy)**

0.00 0.00 Global Days XXX

AMA: 2009, Jan, 11-31; 2008, Jun, 8-11; 2008, Jul, 9

76010 **Radiologic examination from nose to rectum for foreign body, single view, child**

0.81 0.81 Global Days XXX

76080 **Radiologic examination, abscess, fistula or sinus tract study, radiological supervision and interpretation**

EXCLUDES *Contrast injections, radiology evaluation, and guidance via fluoroscopy of gastrostomy, duodenostomy, jejunostomy, gastro-jejunostomy, or cecostomy tube (49465)*

1.82 1.82 Global Days XXX

AMA: 2009, Jan, 11-31; 2009, Jan, 7-8; 2008, Jan, 10-25; 2007, January, 13-27

76098 **Radiological examination, surgical specimen**

0.55 0.55 Global Days XXX

76100 **Radiologic examination, single plane body section (eg, tomography), other than with urography**

3.35 3.35 Global Days XXX

76101 **Radiologic examination, complex motion (ie, hypercycloidal) body section (eg, mastoid polytomography), other than with urography; unilateral**

EXCLUDES *Panoramic x-ray (70355)*

Do not report more than once per day

EXCLUDES *Nephrotomography (74415)*

4.92 4.92 Global Days XXX

76102 **bilateral**

EXCLUDES *Nephrotomography (74415)*
Panoramic x-ray (70355)

Do not report more than once a day

6.64 6.64 Global Days XXX

76120 **Cineradiography/videoradiography, except where specifically included**

2.29 2.29 Global Days XXX

+ 76125 **Cineradiography/videoradiography to complement routine examination (List separately in addition to code for primary procedure)**

Code first primary procedure

0.00 0.00 Global Days ZZZ

76140 **Consultation on X-ray examination made elsewhere, written report** E
0.00 0.00 Global Days XXX
AMA: 2009, Jan, 11-31; 2008, Jan, 10-25; 2007, Jul, 12-13

76376-76377 Three-dimensional Manipulation

CMS 100-4,3,10.4 Payment of Nonphysician Services for Inpatients

EXCLUDES *Arthrography:*
Ankle (73615)
Elbow (73085)
Hip (73525)
Knee (73580)
Shoulder (73040)
Wrist (73115)
Computer-aided detection of MRI data for lesion, breast MRI (0159T)
CT cerebral perfusion test (0042T)

76376 **3D rendering with interpretation and reporting of computed tomography, magnetic resonance imaging, ultrasound, or other tomographic modality; not requiring image postprocessing on an independent workstation** N1 N 80
INCLUDES Concurrent physician supervision of image postprocessing 3D manipulation of volumetric data set/image rendering
Code also base imaging procedures
Do not report with (31627, 70496, 70498, 70544-70549, 71275, 71555, 72159, 72191, 72198, 73206, 73225, 73706, 73725, 74174-74175, 74185, 74261-74263, 75557-75565, 75571-75574, 75635, 76377, 78000-78999, 0159T)
1.96 1.96 Global Days XXX
AMA: 2009, May, 8-9&11; 2009, Jun, 9&11; 2009, Jan, 11-31; 2009, Jul, 10; 2008, Jan, 10-25; 2008, Jul, 3&14; 2007, January, 28-31; 2007, January, 13-27

76377 **requiring image postprocessing on an independent workstation** N1 N 80
Code also base imaging procedures
Do not report with (70496, 70498, 70544-70549, 71275, 71555, 72159, 72191, 72198, 73206, 73225, 73706, 73725, 74174-74175, 74185, 74261-74263, 75557, 75559, 75561, 75563, 75565, 75571-75574, 75635, 76376, 78000-78999, 0159T)
2.57 2.57 Global Days XXX
AMA: 2009, May, 8-9&11; 2009, Jun, 9&11; 2009, Jan, 11-31; 2009, Jul, 10; 2008, Jan, 10-25; 2008, Jul, 3&14; 2007, January, 13-27; 2007, January, 28-31

76380 Computerized Tomography: Delimited

CMS 100-3,220.1 Computerized Tomography

EXCLUDES *Arthrography:*
Ankle (73615)
Elbow (73085)
Hip (73525)
Knee (73580)
Shoulder (73040)
Wrist (73115)
CT cerebral perfusion test (0042T)

76380 **Computed tomography, limited or localized follow-up study** Z2 S 80
5.32 5.32 Global Days XXX
AMA: 2007, Jul, 12-13

76390-76499 Magnetic Resonance Spectroscopy

CMS 100-3,220.2.1 Magnetic Resonance Spectroscopy

EXCLUDES *Arthrography:*
Ankle (73615)
Elbow (73085)
Hip (73525)
Knee (73580)
Shoulder (73040)
Wrist (73115)
CT cerebral perfusion test (0042T)

76390 **Magnetic resonance spectroscopy** E
EXCLUDES *MRI*
14.25 14.25 Global Days XXX

76496 **Unlisted fluoroscopic procedure (eg, diagnostic, interventional)** Z2 X 80 PQ
0.00 0.00 Global Days XXX

76497 **Unlisted computed tomography procedure (eg, diagnostic, interventional)** Z2 S 80
0.00 0.00 Global Days XXX
AMA: 2009, Jan, 11-31; 2008, Jan, 10-25; 2007, January, 13-27

76498 **Unlisted magnetic resonance procedure (eg, diagnostic, interventional)** Z2 S 80
0.00 0.00 Global Days XXX
AMA: 2009, May, 8-9&11; 2008, Jul, 3&14

76499 **Unlisted diagnostic radiographic procedure** Z2 X 80
0.00 0.00 Global Days XXX
AMA: 2009, Jan, 11-31; 2008, Mar, 14-15; 2008, Jan, 10-25; 2007, January, 13-27

76506 Ultrasound: Brain

CMS 100-3,220.5 Ultrasound Diagnostic Procedures

INCLUDES Required permanent documentation of ultrasound images except when diagnostic purpose is biometric measurement
Written documentation

EXCLUDES *Doppler study of vessels, other than color flow (93880-93990)*
Focused ultrasound ablation of uterine leiomyomata (0071T-0072T)
Noninvasive vascular studies, diagnostic (93880-93990)
Ultrasound exam that does not include thorough assessment of organ or site, recorded image, and written report

76506 **Echoencephalography, real time with image documentation (gray scale) (for determination of ventricular size, delineation of cerebral contents, and detection of fluid masses or other intracranial abnormalities), including A-mode encephalography as secondary component where indicated** Z2 S 80
3.71 3.71 Global Days XXX
AMA: 2007, March, 7-8

76510-76529 Ultrasound: Eyes

CMS 100-3,220.5 Ultrasound Diagnostic Procedures
CMS 100-3,230.1 NCD for Treatment of Kidney Stones

INCLUDES Required permanent documentation of ultrasound images except when diagnostic purpose is biometric measurement
Written documentation

EXCLUDES *Doppler study of vessels, other than color flow (93880-93990)*
Focused ultrasound ablation of uterine leiomyomata (0071T-0072T)
Ultrasound exam that does not include thorough assessment of organ or site, recorded image, and written report

76510 **Ophthalmic ultrasound, diagnostic; B-scan and quantitative A-scan performed during the same patient encounter** Z3 T 80
5.07 5.07 Global Days XXX

76511 **quantitative A-scan only**
2.97 2.97 Global Days XXX

76512 **B-scan (with or without superimposed non-quantitative A-scan)**
2.73 2.73 Global Days XXX

76513 **anterior segment ultrasound, immersion (water bath) B-scan or high resolution biomicroscopy**
EXCLUDES *Computerized ophthalmic testing other than by ultrasound (92132-92134)*
2.70 2.70 Global Days XXX

76514 **corneal pachymetry, unilateral or bilateral (determination of corneal thickness)**
0.43 0.43 Global Days XXX
AMA: 2009, Jan, 11-31; 2008, Jan, 10-25; 2007, January, 13-27

76516 **Ophthalmic biometry by ultrasound echography, A-scan;**
2.22 2.22 Global Days XXX
AMA: 2009, Jan, 11-31; 2008, Jan, 10-25; 2007, January, 13-27

76519 **with intraocular lens power calculation**
EXCLUDES *Partial coherence interferometry (92136)*
2.40 2.40 Global Days XXX
AMA: 2009, Jan, 11-31; 2008, Jan, 10-25; 2007, January, 13-27

76529 **Ophthalmic ultrasonic foreign body localization**
2.27 2.27 Global Days XXX

76536-76800 Ultrasound: Neck, Thorax, Abdomen, and Spine

CMS 100-2,15,80 Diagnostic Test Requirements
CMS 100-3,220.5 Ultrasound Diagnostic Procedures
CMS 100-4,3,10.4 Payment of Nonphysician Services for Inpatients

INCLUDES Required permanent documentation of ultrasound images except when diagnostic purpose is biometric measurement
Written documentation

EXCLUDES *Focused ultrasound ablation of uterine leiomyomata (0071T-0072T)*
Ultrasound exam that does not include thorough assessment of organ or site, recorded image, and written report

76536 **Ultrasound, soft tissues of head and neck (eg, thyroid, parathyroid, parotid), real time with image documentation**
3.62 3.62 Global Days XXX
AMA: 2009, May, 7&10; 2007, March, 7-8

76604 **Ultrasound, chest (includes mediastinum), real time with image documentation**
2.63 2.63 Global Days XXX
AMA: 2009, May, 7&10; 2007, March, 7-8

76645 **Ultrasound, breast(s) (unilateral or bilateral), real time with image documentation**
2.91 2.91 Global Days XXX
AMA: 2007, March, 7-8

76700 **Ultrasound, abdominal, real time with image documentation; complete**
INCLUDES Real time scans of:
- Common bile duct
- Gall bladder
- Inferior vena cava
- Kidneys
- Liver
- Pancreas
- Spleen
- Upper abdominal aorta

4.22 4.22 Global Days XXX
AMA: 2009, May, 7&10; 2007, March, 7-8

76705 **limited (eg, single organ, quadrant, follow-up)**
3.23 3.23 Global Days XXX
AMA: 2009, Jan, 11-31; 2009, May, 7&10; 2009, Feb, 22; 2008, Jan, 10-25; 2007, January, 13-27

76770 **Ultrasound, retroperitoneal (eg, renal, aorta, nodes), real time with image documentation; complete**
INCLUDES Complete assessment of kidneys and bladder if history indicates urinary pathology
Real time scans of:
- Abdominal aorta
- Common iliac artery origins
- Inferior vena cava
- Kidneys

4.00 4.00 Global Days XXX
AMA: 2007, March, 7-8

76775 **limited**
3.30 3.30 Global Days XXX
AMA: 2009, Jan, 11-31; 2009, Feb, 22; 2008, Jan, 10-25; 2007, January, 13-27

76776 **Ultrasound, transplanted kidney, real time and duplex Doppler with image documentation**
EXCLUDES *Transplanted kidney ultrasound without duplex doppler (76775)*

Do not report with abdominal/pelvic/scrotal contents/retroperitoneal duplex scan (93975, 93976)
4.59 4.59 Global Days XXX
AMA: 2007, March, 7-8

76800 **Ultrasound, spinal canal and contents**
3.94 3.94 Global Days XXX
AMA: 2009, Jan, 11-31; 2008, Jan, 10-25; 2007, January, 13-27

76801-76802 Ultrasound: Pregnancy Less Than 14 Weeks

CMS 100-2,15,80 Diagnostic Test Requirements
CMS 100-3,220.5 Ultrasound Diagnostic Procedures
CMS 100-4,3,10.4 Payment of Nonphysician Services for Inpatients

INCLUDES Determination of the number of gestational sacs and fetuses
Gestational sac/fetal measurement appropriate for gestational (younger than 14 weeks 0 days)
Inspection of the maternal uterus and adnexa
Quality analysis of amniotic fluid volume/gestational sac shape
Visualization of fetal and placental anatomic formation
Written documentation of each component of exam

EXCLUDES *Focused ultrasound ablation of uterine leiomyomata (0071T-0072T)*
Ultrasound exam that does not include thorough assessment of organ or site, recorded image, and written report

76801 **Ultrasound, pregnant uterus, real time with image documentation, fetal and maternal evaluation, first trimester (< 14 weeks 0 days), transabdominal approach; single or first gestation** ♀
EXCLUDES *Fetal nuchal translucency measurement, first trimester (76813)*
3.87 3.87 Global Days XXX
AMA: 2009, Jan, 11-31; 2008, Jan, 10-25; 2007, January, 13-27

\+ 76802 **each additional gestation (List separately in addition to code for primary procedure)** ♀
EXCLUDES *Fetal nuchal translucency measurement, first trimester (76814)*

Code first single/first gestation (76801)
2.04 2.04 Global Days ZZZ
AMA: 2009, Jan, 11-31; 2008, Jan, 10-25; 2007, January, 13-27

76805-76810 Ultrasound: Pregnancy of 14 Weeks or More

CMS 100-2,15,80 Diagnostic Test Requirements
CMS 100-3,220.5 Ultrasound Diagnostic Procedures
CMS 100-4,3,10.4 Payment of Nonphysician Services for Inpatients

INCLUDES Determination of the number of gestational/chorionic sacs and fetuses
Evaluation of:
Amniotic fluid
Four chambered heart
Intracranial, spinal, abdominal anatomy
Placenta location
Umbilical cord insertion site
Examination of maternal adnexa if visible
Gestational sac/fetal measurement appropriate for gestational (older than or equal to 14 weeks 0 days)
Written documentation of each component of exam

EXCLUDES *Focused ultrasound ablation of uterine leiomyomata (0071T-0072T)*
Ultrasound exam that does not include thorough assessment of organ or site, recorded image, and written report

76805 Ultrasound, pregnant uterus, real time with image documentation, fetal and maternal evaluation, after first trimester (> or = 14 weeks 0 days), transabdominal approach; single or first gestation M ♀ Z2 S 80 CCI
4.48 4.48 Global Days XXX

+ **76810 each additional gestation (List separately in addition to code for primary procedure)** M ♀ Z3 S 80 CCI
Code first single/first gestation (76805)
2.93 2.93 Global Days ZZZ

76811-76812 Ultrasound: Pregnancy, with Additional Studies of Fetus

CMS 100-3,220.5 Ultrasound Diagnostic Procedures
CMS 100-4,3,10.4 Payment of Nonphysician Services for Inpatients

INCLUDES Determination of the number of gestational/chorionic sacs and fetuses
Evaluation of:
Abdominal organ specific anatomy
Amniotic fluid
Chest anatomy
Face
Fetal brain/ventricles
Four chambered heart
Heart/outflow tracts and chest anatomy
Intracranial, spinal, abdominal anatomy
Limbs including number, length, and architecture
Other fetal anatomy as indicated
Placenta
Umbilical cord insertion site
Examination of maternal adnexa if visible
Gestational sac/fetal measurement appropriate for gestational (older than or equal to 14 weeks 0 days)
Written documentation of each component of exam

EXCLUDES *Focused ultrasound ablation of uterine leiomyomata (0071T-0072T)*
Ultrasound exam that does not include thorough assessment organ or site, recorded image, and written report

76811 Ultrasound, pregnant uterus, real time with image documentation, fetal and maternal evaluation plus detailed fetal anatomic examination, transabdominal approach; single or first gestation M ♀ Z3 S 80 CCI
5.68 5.68 Global Days XXX

+ **76812 each additional gestation (List separately in addition to code for primary procedure)** M ♀ Z2 S 80 CCI
Code first single/first gestation (76811)
6.26 6.26 Global Days ZZZ

76813-76828 Ultrasound: Other Fetal Evaluations

CMS 100-2,15,80 Diagnostic Test Requirements
CMS 100-3,220.5 Ultrasound Diagnostic Procedures
CMS 100-4,3,10.4 Payment of Nonphysician Services for Inpatients

INCLUDES Required permanent documentation of ultrasound images except when diagnostic purpose is biometric measurement
Written documentation

EXCLUDES *Focused ultrasound ablation of uterine leiomyomata (0071T-0072T)*
Ultrasound exam that does not include thorough assessment of organ or site, recorded image, and written report

76813 Ultrasound, pregnant uterus, real time with image documentation, first trimester fetal nuchal translucency measurement, transabdominal or transvaginal approach; single or first gestation ♀ Z2 S 80
3.76 3.76 Global Days XXX
AMA: 2007, March, 7-8

+ **76814 each additional gestation (List separately in addition to code for primary procedure)** ♀ Z3 S 80
Code first single/first gestation (76813)
2.42 2.42 Global Days XXX
AMA: 2007, March, 7-8

76815 Ultrasound, pregnant uterus, real time with image documentation, limited (eg, fetal heart beat, placental location, fetal position and/or qualitative amniotic fluid volume), 1 or more fetuses M ♀ Z2 S 80 CCI
INCLUDES Focused "quick look" exam of one or more elements
Reporting only once per exam, instead of per element
EXCLUDES *Fetal nuchal translucency measurement, first trimester (76813, 76814)*
2.74 2.74 Global Days XXX
AMA: 2009, Jan, 11-31; 2008, Jan, 10-25; 2007, January, 13-27

76816 Ultrasound, pregnant uterus, real time with image documentation, follow-up (eg, re-evaluation of fetal size by measuring standard growth parameters and amniotic fluid volume, re-evaluation of organ system(s) suspected or confirmed to be abnormal on a previous scan), transabdominal approach, per fetus M ♀ Z2 S 80 CCI
Code also modifier 59 for examination of each additional fetus in a multiple pregnancy
3.58 3.58 Global Days XXX

76817 Ultrasound, pregnant uterus, real time with image documentation, transvaginal M ♀ Z2 S 80 CCI
EXCLUDES *Transvaginal ultrasound, non-obstetrical (76830)*
Code also transabdominal obstetrical ultrasound, if performed
3.09 3.09 Global Days XXX

76818 Fetal biophysical profile; with non-stress testing M ♀ Z3 S 80 CCI
Code also modifier 59 for each additional fetus
3.69 3.69 Global Days XXX
AMA: 2009, Jan, 11-31; 2008, Jan, 10-25; 2007, January, 13-27

76819 without non-stress testing M ♀ Z3 S 80 CCI
EXCLUDES *Amniotic fluid index without non-stress test (76815)*
Code also modifier 59 for each additional fetus
2.73 2.73 Global Days XXX
AMA: 2009, Jan, 11-31; 2008, Jan, 10-25; 2007, January, 13-27

76820 Doppler velocimetry, fetal; umbilical artery ♀ Z3 S 80
1.30 1.30 Global Days XXX

76821 middle cerebral artery ♀ Z2 S 80
2.92 2.92 Global Days XXX

76825 **Echocardiography, fetal, cardiovascular system, real time with image documentation (2D), with or without M-mode recording;** M ♀ Z3 S 80
6.58 6.58 Global Days XXX

76826 **follow-up or repeat study** M ♀ Z3 S 80
3.87 3.87 Global Days XXX

76827 **Doppler echocardiography, fetal, pulsed wave and/or continuous wave with spectral display; complete** M ♀ Z3 S 80
1.91 1.91 Global Days XXX

76828 **follow-up or repeat study** M ♀ Z3 S 80
EXCLUDES *Color mapping (93325)*
1.39 1.39 Global Days XXX

76830-76873 Ultrasound: Male and Female Genitalia

CMS 100-2,15,80 Diagnostic Test Requirements
CMS 100-3,220.5 Ultrasound Diagnostic Procedures
CMS 100-4,3,10.4 Payment of Nonphysician Services for Inpatients

INCLUDES Required permanent documentation of ultrasound images except when diagnostic purpose is biometric measurement
Written documentation

EXCLUDES *Focused ultrasound ablation of uterine leiomyomata (0071T-0072T)*
Ultrasound exam that does not include thorough assessment of organ or site, recorded image, and written report

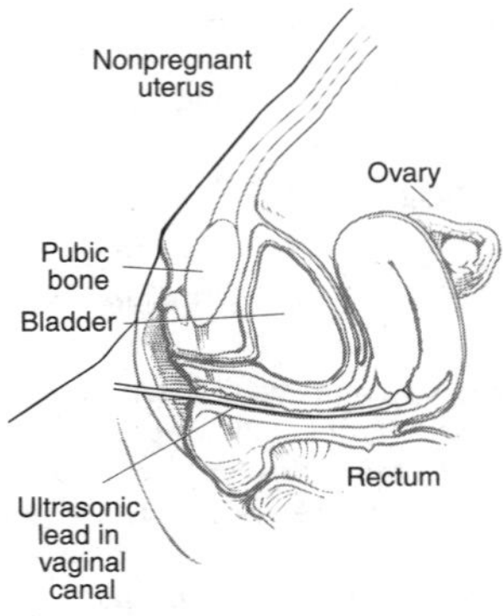

Ultrasound is performed in real time with image documentation by a transvaginal approach

76830 **Ultrasound, transvaginal** ♀ Z2 S 80
EXCLUDES *Transvaginal ultrasound, obstetric (76817)*
Code also transabdominal non-obstetrical ultrasound, if performed
3.79 3.79 Global Days XXX
AMA: 2009, Feb, 22; 2009, Jan, 11-31; 2008, Jan, 10-25; 2007, January, 13-27

76831 **Saline infusion sonohysterography (SIS), including color flow Doppler, when performed** ♀ Z3 Q3 80
Code also saline introduction for saline infusion sonohysterography (58340)
3.83 3.83 Global Days XXX
AMA: 2009, Mar, 10-11

76856 **Ultrasound, pelvic (nonobstetric), real time with image documentation; complete** Z2 Q3 80
INCLUDES Total examination of the female pelvic anatomy which includes:
Bladder measurement
Description and measurement of the uterus and adnexa
Description of any pelvic pathology
Measurement of the endometrium
Total examination of the male pelvis which includes:
Bladder measurement
Description of any pelvic pathology
Evaluation of prostate and seminal vesicles
3.75 3.75 Global Days XXX
AMA: 2009, Jan, 11-31; 2009, Feb, 22; 2008, Jan, 10-25; 2007, March, 7-8; 2007, January, 13-27

76857 **limited or follow-up (eg, for follicles)** Z2 Q3 80
INCLUDES Focused evaluation limited to:
Evaluation of one or more elements listed in 76856 and/or
Reevaluation of one or more pelvic abnormalities previously documented on ultrasound
Urinary bladder alone
EXCLUDES *Bladder volume or post-voided residual measurement without imaging the bladder (51798)*
Urinary bladder and kidneys (76770)
2.98 2.98 Global Days XXX
AMA: 2009, Jan, 11-31; 2009, May, 7&10; 2009, Feb, 22; 2008, Jan, 10-25; 2007, January, 13-27

76870 **Ultrasound, scrotum and contents** ♂ Z2 Q3 80
3.73 3.73 Global Days XXX

76872 **Ultrasound, transrectal;** Z2 S 80
Do not report with (0249T)
4.09 4.09 Global Days XXX

76873 **prostate volume study for brachytherapy treatment planning (separate procedure)** ♂ Z2 S
5.19 5.19 Global Days XXX

76881-76886 Ultrasound: Extremities

EXCLUDES *Doppler studies of the extremities (93925-93926, 93930-93931, 93970-93971)*

76881 **Ultrasound, extremity, nonvascular, real-time with image documentation; complete** Z2 S
INCLUDES Any abnormal findings
Joint
Muscles
Other soft tissue
Real time scans of a specific joint including assessment of:
Tendons
3.62 3.62 Global Days XXX

76882 **limited, anatomic specific** Z3 S
INCLUDES Limited examination of a certain anatomical structure (e.g. muscle or tendon) or for evaluation of a soft-tissue mass
1.02 1.02 Global Days XXX

76885 **Ultrasound, infant hips, real time with imaging documentation; dynamic (requiring physician manipulation)** A Z2 S 80
4.46 4.46 Global Days XXX

76886 **limited, static (not requiring physician manipulation)**
3.12 3.12 Global Days XXX

76930-76970 Imaging Guidance: Ultrasound

CMS 100-3,220.5 Ultrasound Diagnostic Procedures
CMS 100-4,3,10.4 Payment of Nonphysician Services for Inpatients

INCLUDES Required permanent documentation of ultrasound images except when diagnostic purpose is biometric measurement
Written documentation

EXCLUDES *Focused ultrasound ablation of uterine leiomyomata (0071T-0072T)*
Ultrasound exam that does not include thorough assessment of organ or site, recorded image, and written report

76930 **Ultrasonic guidance for pericardiocentesis, imaging supervision and interpretation**
2.57 2.57 Global Days XXX

76932 **Ultrasonic guidance for endomyocardial biopsy, imaging supervision and interpretation**
0.00 0.00 Global Days XXX

76936 **Ultrasound guided compression repair of arterial pseudoaneurysm or arteriovenous fistulae (includes diagnostic ultrasound evaluation, compression of lesion and imaging)**
8.92 8.92 Global Days XXX

\+ **76937** **Ultrasound guidance for vascular access requiring ultrasound evaluation of potential access sites, documentation of selected vessel patency, concurrent realtime ultrasound visualization of vascular needle entry, with permanent recording and reporting (List separately in addition to code for primary procedure)**

EXCLUDES *Extremity venous non-invasive vascular diagnostic study performed separately from venous access guidance (93965, 93970, 93971)*

Code first primary procedure

Do not report with (37191-37193, 37760-37761, 76942)

1.04 1.04 Global Days ZZZ

AMA: 2009, Jan, 7-8

76940 **Ultrasound guidance for, and monitoring of, parenchymal tissue ablation**

EXCLUDES *Ablation (32998, 47370-47382, 50592, 50593)*

Do not report with (50250, 50542, 76942, 76998)

Do not report with intraoperative ultrasonic guidance (76998)

0.00 0.00 Global Days XXX

AMA: 2007, March, 7-8

76941 **Ultrasonic guidance for intrauterine fetal transfusion or cordocentesis, imaging supervision and interpretation**

Code also surgical procedure (36460, 59012)

0.00 0.00 Global Days XXX

76942 **Ultrasonic guidance for needle placement (eg, biopsy, aspiration, injection, localization device), imaging supervision and interpretation**

EXCLUDES *Platelet rich plasma injection(s) (0232T)*

Do not report with (27096, 37760-37761, 43232, 43237, 43242, 45341-45342, 64479-64484, 64490-64495, 76975, 0228T-0232T, 0249T)

6.07 6.07 Global Days XXX

AMA: 2009, Jan, 11-31; 2009, Mar, 8-9; 2008, Jan, 10-25; 2008, Jun, 8-11; 2007, January, 13-27; 2007, May, 1-2; 2007, June, 10-11

76945 **Ultrasonic guidance for chorionic villus sampling, imaging supervision and interpretation**

Code also surgical procedure (59015)

0.00 0.00 Global Days XXX

76946 **Ultrasonic guidance for amniocentesis, imaging supervision and interpretation**
1.04 1.04 Global Days XXX

76948 **Ultrasonic guidance for aspiration of ova, imaging supervision and interpretation**
1.06 1.06 Global Days XXX

76950 **Ultrasonic guidance for placement of radiation therapy fields**

EXCLUDES *Placement of interstitial device(s) for radiation therapy guidance (31627, 32553, 49411, 55876)*

1.62 1.62 Global Days XXX

76965 **Ultrasonic guidance for interstitial radioelement application**
3.04 3.04 Global Days XXX

76970 **Ultrasound study follow-up (specify)**
3.03 3.03 Global Days XXX

76975 Endoscopic Ultrasound

CMS 100-3,220.5 Ultrasound Diagnostic Procedures
CMS 100-4,3,10.4 Payment of Nonphysician Services for Inpatients
CMS 100-4,12,30.1 Upper Gastrointestinal Endoscopy Including Endoscopic Ultrasound (EUS)

INCLUDES Required permanent documentation of ultrasound images except when diagnostic purpose is biometric measurement
Written documentation

EXCLUDES *Focused ultrasound ablation of uterine leiomyomata (0071T-0072T)*
Ultrasound exam that does not include thorough assessment of organ or site, recorded image, and written report

76975 **Gastrointestinal endoscopic ultrasound, supervision and interpretation**

Do not report with (43231, 43232, 43237, 43238, 43242, 43259, 45341, 45342, 76942)

0.00 0.00 Global Days XXX

AMA: 2009, Mar, 8-9

76977 Bone Density Measurements: Ultrasound

CMS 100-3,220.5 Ultrasound Diagnostic Procedures
CMS 100-4,13,140 Bone Mass Measurements (BMMs)

INCLUDES Required permanent documentation of ultrasound images except when diagnostic purpose is biometric measurement
Written documentation

EXCLUDES *Focused ultrasound ablation of uterine leiomyomata (0071T-0072T)*
Ultrasound exam that does not include thorough assessment of organ or site, recorded image, and written report

76977 **Ultrasound bone density measurement and interpretation, peripheral site(s), any method**
0.26 0.26 Global Days XXX

76998-76999 Imaging Guidance During Surgery: Ultrasound

INCLUDES Required permanent documentation of ultrasound images except when diagnostic purpose is biometric measurement
Written documentation

EXCLUDES *Focused ultrasound ablation of uterine leiomyomata (0071T-0072T)*
Ultrasound exam that does not include thorough assessment of organ or site, recorded image, and written report

76998 Ultrasonic guidance, intraoperative N1 N 80

EXCLUDES *Radiofrequency tissue ablation, open/laparoscopic, ultrasonic guidance (76940)*

Do not report with (36475-36479, 37760-37761, 47370-47382, 0249T)

0.00 0.00 Global Days XXX

AMA: 2007, March, 7-8

76999 Unlisted ultrasound procedure (eg, diagnostic, interventional) Z2 S 80

0.00 0.00 Global Days XXX

AMA: 2009, May, 7&10

77001-77022 Imaging Guidance Techniques

\+ **77001 Fluoroscopic guidance for central venous access device placement, replacement (catheter only or complete), or removal (includes fluoroscopic guidance for vascular access and catheter manipulation, any necessary contrast injections through access site or catheter with related venography radiologic supervision and interpretation, and radiographic documentation of final catheter position) (List separately in addition to code for primary procedure)** N1 N PQ

EXCLUDES *Formal extremity venography performed separately from venous access and interpreted separately (36005, 75820, 75822, 75825, 75827)*

Code first primary procedure

Do not report with (77002)

Do not report with procedure codes that include fluoroscopic guidance in the code descriptor

3.51 3.51 Global Days ZZZ

AMA: 2009, Jan, 11-31; 2008, Jul, 9; 2008, Jun, 8-11; 2007, March, 7-8

77002 Fluoroscopic guidance for needle placement (eg, biopsy, aspiration, injection, localization device) N1 N PQ

INCLUDES Radiographic arthrography except for supervision and interpretation of CT and MRI arthrography

EXCLUDES *Platelet rich plasma injection(s) (0232T)*

Code also surgical procedure

Do not report with (70332, 73040, 73085, 73115, 73525, 73580, 73615, 0232T)

Do not report with codes that include 77002 in the radiological supervision and interpretation (49440, 74320, 74355, 74445, 74470, 74475, 75809-75810, 75885, 75887, 75980, 75982, 75989)

Do not report with procedure codes that include fluoroscopic guidance in the code descriptor

2.30 2.30 Global Days XXX

AMA: 2009, Jan, 11-31; 2008, Jan, 10-25; 2008, Jun, 8-11; 2008, Jul, 9; 2007, March, 7-8; 2007, February, 10-11; 2007, May, 1-2; 2007, June, 10-11

▲ **77003 Fluoroscopic guidance and localization of needle or catheter tip for spine or paraspinous diagnostic or therapeutic injection procedures (epidural or subarachnoid)** N1 N PQ

EXCLUDES *Destruction of paravertebral facet joint nerve by neurolysis ([64633, 64634, 64635, 64636])*
Injection and needle/catheter placement, epidural/subarachnoid (62270-62282, 62310-62319)
Injection, paravertebral facet joint (64490-64495)
Sacroiliac joint arthrography (27096)
Subarachnoid guidance puncture for myelography (72240-72270)
Transforaminal epidural needle placement/injection (64479-64484)

Do not report with procedure codes that include fluoroscopic guidance in the code descriptor

1.90 1.90 Global Days XXX

AMA: 2009, Jan, 11-31; 2008, Jul, 9; 2008, Jun, 8-11; 2007, March, 7-8

77011 Computed tomography guidance for stereotactic localization N1 N

10.61 10.61 Global Days XXX

AMA: 2007, March, 7-8

77012 Computed tomography guidance for needle placement (eg, biopsy, aspiration, injection, localization device), radiological supervision and interpretation N1 N

EXCLUDES *Platelet rich plasma injection(s) (0232T)*

Do not report with (27096, 64479-64484, 64490-64495, [64633, 64634, 64635, 64636], 0232T)

4.32 4.32 Global Days XXX

AMA: 2007, March, 7-8; 2007, May, 1-2; 2007, June, 10-11

77013 Computed tomography guidance for, and monitoring of, parenchymal tissue ablation N1 N 80

EXCLUDES *Ablation, percutaneous radiofrequency (32998, 47382, 50592)*
Percutaneous radiofrequency ablation (32998, 47382, 50592-50593)

Do not report with (20982)

0.00 0.00 Global Days XXX

AMA: 2007, March, 7-8

77014 Computed tomography guidance for placement of radiation therapy fields N1 N

Code also placement of interstitial device(s) for radiation therapy guidance (31627, 32553, 49411, 55876)

4.22 4.22 Global Days XXX

AMA: 2007, March, 7-8

77021 Magnetic resonance guidance for needle placement (eg, for biopsy, needle aspiration, injection, or placement of localization device) radiological supervision and interpretation N1 N

EXCLUDES *Platelet rich plasma injection(s) (0232T)*
Surgical procedure

Do not report with (0232T)

12.25 12.25 Global Days XXX

AMA: 2008, Jun, 8-11; 2007, March, 7-8; 2007, May, 1-2; 2007, June, 10-11

77022 **Magnetic resonance guidance for, and monitoring of, parenchymal tissue ablation** N1 N 80

EXCLUDES *Ablation:*

Percutaneous radiofrequency (32998, 47382, 50592-50593)

Uterine leiomyomata by focused ablation (0071T, 0072T)

0.00 0.00 Global Days XXX

AMA: 2007, March, 7-8

77031-77059 Radiography: Breast

CMS 100-3,220.4 Mammograms

CMS 100-4,18,20 Mammography Services

CMS 100-4,18,20.4 FI/A/B MAC Processing Mammography Services

EXCLUDES *Mammographic guidance for needle placement into lesion (77032)*

77031 **Stereotactic localization guidance for breast biopsy or needle placement (eg, for wire localization or for injection), each lesion, radiological supervision and interpretation** N1 N

EXCLUDES *Sentinel node localization injection without lymphoscintigraphy (38792)*

Code also surgical procedure (10022, 19000-19103, 19290-19291)

4.29 4.29 Global Days XXX

AMA: 2007, March, 7-8

77032 **Mammographic guidance for needle placement, breast (eg, for wire localization or for injection), each lesion, radiological supervision and interpretation** N1 N

EXCLUDES *Sentinel node localization injection without lymphoscintigraphy (38792)*

Code also surgical procedure (10022, 19000, 19102-19103, 19290-19291)

1.59 1.59 Global Days XXX

AMA: 2007, March, 7-8

+ 77051 **Computer-aided detection (computer algorithm analysis of digital image data for lesion detection) with further physician review for interpretation, with or without digitization of film radiographic images; diagnostic mammography (List separately in addition to code for primary procedure)** A

Code first mammography (77055, 77056)

0.32 0.32 Global Days ZZZ

AMA: 2007, March, 7-8; 2007, April, 1-2

+ 77052 **screening mammography (List separately in addition to code for primary procedure)** A

Code first screening mammography (77057)

0.32 0.32 Global Days ZZZ

AMA: 2007, March, 7-8; 2007, April, 1-2

77053 **Mammary ductogram or galactogram, single duct, radiological supervision and interpretation** N1 Q2

Code also injection procedure (19030)

1.87 1.87 Global Days XXX

AMA: 2007, March, 7-8

77054 **Mammary ductogram or galactogram, multiple ducts, radiological supervision and interpretation** N1 Q2

2.55 2.55 Global Days XXX

AMA: 2007, March, 7-8

77055 **Mammography; unilateral** A

Code also computer-aided detection applied to diagnostic mammogram, if performed (77051)

2.58 2.58 Global Days XXX

AMA: 2007, March, 7-8

77056 **bilateral** A

Code also computer-aided detection applied to diagnostic mammogram, if performed (77051)

3.30 3.30 Global Days XXX

AMA: 2007, March, 7-8

77057 **Screening mammography, bilateral (2-view film study of each breast)** ♀ A PQ

EXCLUDES *Breast electrical impedance scan (76499)*

Code also computer-aided detection applied to screening mammogram, if performed (77052)

2.39 2.39 Global Days XXX

AMA: 2007, March, 7-8

77058 **Magnetic resonance imaging, breast, without and/or with contrast material(s); unilateral** B

20.65 20.65 Global Days XXX

AMA: 2007, Jul, 6-10; 2007, March, 7-8

77059 **bilateral** B

21.05 21.05 Global Days XXX

AMA: 2007, Jul, 6-10; 2007, March, 7-8

77071-77084 Additional Evaluations of Bones and Joints

77071 **Manual application of stress performed by physician for joint radiography, including contralateral joint if indicated** Z3 X 26 80

1.48 1.48 Global Days XXX

AMA: 2007, March, 7-8

77072 **Bone age studies** Z3 X 80

0.69 0.69 Global Days XXX

AMA: 2007, March, 7-8

77073 **Bone length studies (orthoroentgenogram, scanogram)** Z3 X 80

1.16 1.16 Global Days XXX

AMA: 2007, March, 7-8

77074 **Radiologic examination, osseous survey; limited (eg, for metastases)** Z3 X 80

2.08 2.08 Global Days XXX

AMA: 2007, March, 7-8

77075 **complete (axial and appendicular skeleton)** Z2 X 80

3.11 3.11 Global Days XXX

AMA: 2007, March, 7-8

77076 **Radiologic examination, osseous survey, infant** Z2 X 80

3.22 3.22 Global Days XXX

AMA: 2007, March, 7-8

77077 **Joint survey, single view, 2 or more joints (specify)** Z3 X 80

1.25 1.25 Global Days XXX

AMA: 2007, March, 7-8

77078 **Computed tomography, bone mineral density study, 1 or more sites; axial skeleton (eg, hips, pelvis, spine)** Z2 S 80

4.39 4.39 Global Days XXX

AMA: 2007, March, 7-8

~~77079~~ ~~**appendicular skeleton (peripheral) (eg, radius, wrist, heel)**~~

To report, see 77078, 77080-77081

77080 **Dual-energy X-ray absorptiometry (DXA), bone density study, 1 or more sites; axial skeleton (eg, hips, pelvis, spine)** Z3 S 80

1.67 1.67 Global Days XXX

AMA: 2007, March, 7-8

77081 **appendicular skeleton (peripheral) (eg, radius, wrist, heel)** Z3 S 80

0.85 0.85 Global Days XXX

AMA: 2007, March, 7-8

77082 **vertebral fracture assessment** Z3 X 80

EXCLUDES *Dual-energy x-ray absorptiometry [DXA] body composition study (76499)*

0.85 0.85 Global Days XXX

AMA: 2007, March, 7-8

~~77083~~ ~~**Radiographic absorptiometry (eg, photodensitometry, radiogrammetry), 1 or more sites**~~

To report, see 77080-77082

77084 **Magnetic resonance (eg, proton) imaging, bone marrow blood supply** Z2 S 80

14.45 14.45 Global Days XXX

AMA: 2007, March, 7-8

77261-77263 Therapeutic Radiology: Treatment Planning

CMS 100-2,6,10 Medical and Other Services Furnished to Inpatients

CMS 100-4,3,10.4 Payment of Nonphysician Services for Inpatients

INCLUDES Determination of:

Appropriate treatment devices

Number and size of treatment ports

Treatment method

Treatment time/dosage

Treatment volume

Interpretation of special testing

Tumor localization

77261 **Therapeutic radiology treatment planning; simple** B 26 80 PO

INCLUDES Planning for single treatment area included in a single port or simple parallel opposed ports with simple or no blocking

2.09 2.09 Global Days XXX

77262 **intermediate** B 26 80 PO

INCLUDES Planning for three or more converging ports, two separate treatment sites, multiple blocks, or special time dose constraints

3.14 3.14 Global Days XXX

77263 **complex** B 26 80 PO

INCLUDES Planning for very complex blocking, custom shielding blocks, tangential ports, special wedges or compensators, three or more separate treatment areas, rotational or special beam considerations, combination of treatment modalities

4.65 4.65 Global Days XXX

77280-77299 Radiation Therapy Simulation

CMS 100-2,6,10 Medical and Other Services Furnished to Inpatients

CMS 100-4,3,10.4 Payment of Nonphysician Services for Inpatients

CMS 100-4,4,200.3.2 Additional Billing Instructions for IMRT Planning and Delivery

INCLUDES Simulation provided on a:

Dedicated simulator

Diagnostic x-ray machine

Radiation therapy treatment unit

77280 **Therapeutic radiology simulation-aided field setting; simple** Z2 X 80

INCLUDES Simple or no blocking

Simulation of a single treatment site with either a single port or parallel opposed ports

5.51 5.51 Global Days XXX

77285 **intermediate** Z2 X 80

INCLUDES Multiple blocks

Simulation of converging ports >=3

Two different treatment areas

9.73 9.73 Global Days XXX

77290 **complex** Z2 X 80

INCLUDES Complex blocking

Contrast material

Custom shielding blocks

Hyperthermia probe verification

Rotation or arc therapy

Simulation of tangential portals

Treatment to ≥ 3 treatment areas

Verification of brachytherapy source

15.75 15.75 Global Days XXX

77295 **3-dimensional** Z3 X 80 PO

INCLUDES Computer-created 3D reconstruction of tumor and surrounding tissue from direct CT scans and/or MRI data

14.69 14.69 Global Days XXX

77299 **Unlisted procedure, therapeutic radiology clinical treatment planning** Z2 X 80

0.00 0.00 Global Days XXX

AMA: 2009, May, 8-9&11

77300-77370 Radiation Physics Services

CMS 100-4,3,10.4 Payment of Nonphysician Services for Inpatients

CMS 100-4,3,10.4 Payment of Nonphysician Services for Inpatients

CMS 100-4,4,61.2 Requirements for Specific Procedures to be Reported With Device Codes

CMS 100-4,4,200.3.1 Billing for IMRT Planning and Delivery

CMS 100-4,4,200.3.2 Additional Billing Instructions for IMRT Planning and Delivery

CMS 100-4,4,220.2 Additional Billing Instructions for IMRT Planning

77300 **Basic radiation dosimetry calculation, central axis depth dose calculation, TDF, NSD, gap calculation, off axis factor, tissue inhomogeneity factors, calculation of non-ionizing radiation surface and depth dose, as required during course of treatment, only when prescribed by the treating physician** Z3 X 80

1.99 1.99 Global Days XXX

AMA: 2009, Jan, 11-31

77301 **Intensity modulated radiotherapy plan, including dose-volume histograms for target and critical structure partial tolerance specifications** Z2 X 80

58.31 58.31 Global Days XXX

77305 **Teletherapy, isodose plan (whether hand or computer calculated); simple (1 or 2 parallel opposed unmodified ports directed to a single area of interest)** Z3 X 80

INCLUDES Normal follow-up care during and three months after treatment

1.83 1.83 Global Days XXX

77310 **intermediate (3 or more treatment ports directed to a single area of interest)** Z3 X 80

INCLUDES Normal follow-up care during and three months after treatment

2.61 2.61 Global Days XXX

77315 **complex (mantle or inverted Y, tangential ports, the use of wedges, compensators, complex blocking, rotational beam, or special beam considerations)** Z3 X 80

INCLUDES Normal follow-up care during and three months after treatment

4.04 4.04 Global Days XXX

77321 **Special teletherapy port plan, particles, hemibody, total body**
2.89 2.89 Global Days XXX

77326 **Brachytherapy isodose plan; simple (calculation made from single plane, 1 to 4 sources/ribbon application, remote afterloading brachytherapy, 1 to 8 sources)**
4.23 4.23 Global Days XXX

77327 **intermediate (multiplane dosage calculations, application involving 5 to 10 sources/ribbons, remote afterloading brachytherapy, 9 to 12 sources)**
5.95 5.95 Global Days XXX

77328 **complex (multiplane isodose plan, volume implant calculations, over 10 sources/ribbons used, special spatial reconstruction, remote afterloading brachytherapy, over 12 sources)**
7.98 7.98 Global Days XXX

77331 **Special dosimetry (eg, TLD, microdosimetry) (specify), only when prescribed by the treating physician**
1.82 1.82 Global Days XXX

77332 **Treatment devices, design and construction; simple (simple block, simple bolus)**
2.27 2.27 Global Days XXX

77333 **intermediate (multiple blocks, stents, bite blocks, special bolus)**
1.60 1.60 Global Days XXX

77334 **complex (irregular blocks, special shields, compensators, wedges, molds or casts)**
4.36 4.36 Global Days XXX

77336 **Continuing medical physics consultation, including assessment of treatment parameters, quality assurance of dose delivery, and review of patient treatment documentation in support of the radiation oncologist, reported per week of therapy**
1.37 1.37 Global Days XXX

77338 **Multi-leaf collimator (MLC) device(s) for intensity modulated radiation therapy (IMRT), design and construction per IMRT plan**
EXCLUDES *Immobilization in IMRT treatment (77332-77334)*

Do not report with (0073T)

Do not report more than once per IMRT plan

14.44 14.44 Global Days XXX

77370 **Special medical radiation physics consultation**
3.33 3.33 Global Days XXX
AMA: 2009, May, 8-9&11

77371-77399 Stereotactic Radiosurgery (SRS) Planning and Delivery

CMS 100-4,4,200.3.3 Billing Multi-Source Photon Stereotactic Radiosurgery Planning and Delivery

⊙ 77371 **Radiation treatment delivery, stereotactic radiosurgery (SRS), complete course of treatment of cranial lesion(s) consisting of 1 session; multi-source Cobalt 60 based**
0.00 0.00 Global Days XXX
AMA: 2007, March, 7-8

77372 **linear accelerator based**
EXCLUDES *Radiation treatment supervision (77432)*
24.61 24.61 Global Days XXX
AMA: 2007, March, 7-8

77373 **Stereotactic body radiation therapy, treatment delivery, per fraction to 1 or more lesions, including image guidance, entire course not to exceed 5 fractions**
EXCLUDES *Single fraction cranial lesion(s) (77371-77372)*

Do not report with (77401-77416, 77418)
46.89 46.89 Global Days XXX
AMA: 2007, March, 7-8

77399 **Unlisted procedure, medical radiation physics, dosimetry and treatment devices, and special services**
0.00 0.00 Global Days XXX

77401-77417 Radiation Treatment

CMS 100-2,6,10 Medical and Other Services Furnished to Inpatients
CMS 100-4,3,10.4 Payment of Nonphysician Services for Inpatients
CMS 100-4,4,220.1 Billing for IMRT Planning and Delivery
CMS 100-4,13,70.3 Radiation Treatment Delivery

INCLUDES Technical component and assorted energy levels

EXCLUDES *Intra-fraction localization and target tracking (0197T)*

77401 **Radiation treatment delivery, superficial and/or ortho voltage**
0.65 0.65 Global Days XXX

77402 **Radiation treatment delivery, single treatment area, single port or parallel opposed ports, simple blocks or no blocks; up to 5 MeV**
5.39 5.39 Global Days XXX

77403 **6-10 MeV**
3.93 3.93 Global Days XXX

77404 **11-19 MeV**
4.39 4.39 Global Days XXX

77406 **20 MeV or greater**
4.47 4.47 Global Days XXX

77407 **Radiation treatment delivery, 2 separate treatment areas, 3 or more ports on a single treatment area, use of multiple blocks; up to 5 MeV**
7.43 7.43 Global Days XXX

77408 **6-10 MeV**
5.38 5.38 Global Days XXX

77409 **11-19 MeV**
5.99 5.99 Global Days XXX

77411 **20 MeV or greater**
5.96 5.96 Global Days XXX

77412 **Radiation treatment delivery, 3 or more separate treatment areas, custom blocking, tangential ports, wedges, rotational beam, compensators, electron beam; up to 5 MeV**
7.15 7.15 Global Days XXX

77413 **6-10 MeV**
7.08 7.08 Global Days XXX

77414 **11-19 MeV**
7.95 7.95 Global Days XXX

77416 **20 MeV or greater**
7.98 7.98 Global Days XXX

77417 **Therapeutic radiology port film(s)**
0.42 0.42 Global Days XXX
AMA: 2009, Jan, 11-31; 2008, Jan, 10-25; 2007, January, 13-27

77418 IMRT Delivery

CMS 100-2,6,10 Medical and Other Services Furnished to Inpatients
CMS 100-4,3,10.4 Payment of Nonphysician Services for Inpatients
CMS 100-4,4,220.1 Billing for IMRT Planning and Delivery

EXCLUDES *Delivery of compensator-based beam modulation treatment (0073T)*
Intra-fraction localization and target tracking (0197T)
Treatment planning (77301)

77418 Intensity modulated treatment delivery, single or multiple fields/arcs, via narrow spatially and temporally modulated beams, binary, dynamic MLC, per treatment session Z2 S TC 80

13.98 13.98 **Global Days XXX**

AMA: 2007, May, 1-2

77421 Stereoscopic Imaging Guidance

CMS 100-2,6,10 Medical and Other Services Furnished to Inpatients
CMS 100-4,3,10.4 Payment of Nonphysician Services for Inpatients

EXCLUDES *Placement of interstitial device(s) for radiation therapy guidance (31627, 32553, 49411, 55876)*

Do not report more than one time per treatment delivery session
Do not report with (77432, 77435)

77421 Stereoscopic X-ray guidance for localization of target volume for the delivery of radiation therapy N1 N 80

2.54 2.54 **Global Days XXX**

77424-77425 [77424, 77425] Intraoperative Radiation Treatment

#● **77424 Intraoperative radiation treatment delivery, x-ray, single treatment session** N1 N

0.00 0.00 **Global Days XXX**

#● **77425 Intraoperative radiation treatment delivery, electrons, single treatment session** N1 N

0.00 0.00 **Global Days XXX**

77422-77425 Neutron Therapy

77422 High energy neutron radiation treatment delivery; single treatment area using a single port or parallel-opposed ports with no blocks or simple blocking Z2 S TC 80

7.43 7.43 **Global Days XXX**

77423 1 or more isocenter(s) with coplanar or non-coplanar geometry with blocking and/or wedge, and/or compensator(s) Z2 S TC 80

7.69 7.69 **Global Days XXX**

77424 *Resequenced Code. See code following 77421.*

77425 *Resequenced Code. See code before 77422.*

77427-77499 Radiation Therapy Management

CMS 100-4,13,70.1 Weekly Radiation Therapy Management

INCLUDES Assessment of patient for medical evaluation and management (at least one per treatment management service) that includes:
Coordination of care/treatment
Evaluation of patient's response to treatment
Review of:
Dose delivery
Dosimetry
Lab tests
Patient treatment set-up
Port film
Treatment parameters
X-rays
Units of 5 fractions or treatment sessions regardless of time. 2 or more fractions performed on the same day can be counted separately provided there is a distinct break in service between sessions and the fractions are of the character usually furnished on different days.

77427 Radiation treatment management, 5 treatments B 26 PQ

INCLUDES 3 or 4 fractions beyond a multiple of five at the end of a treatment period

5.20 5.20 **Global Days XXX**

77431 Radiation therapy management with complete course of therapy consisting of 1 or 2 fractions only B 26 80 PQ

2.86 2.86 **Global Days XXX**

77432 Stereotactic radiation treatment management of cranial lesion(s) (complete course of treatment consisting of 1 session) B 26 80 PQ

EXCLUDES *Stereotactic body radiation therapy treatment (77435)*

Do not report with stereotactic radiosurgery (61796-61800)

11.75 11.75 **Global Days XXX**

77435 Stereotactic body radiation therapy, treatment management, per treatment course, to 1 or more lesions, including image guidance, entire course not to exceed 5 fractions N1 N 26 80 PQ

Do not report with (77427-77432)

Do not report with stereotactic radiosurgery (63620, 63621)

17.62 17.89 **Global Days XXX**

AMA: 2007, March, 7-8

● **77469 Intraoperative radiation treatment management** N1 N 80

EXCLUDES *Medical evaluation and management provided outside of the intraoperative treatment management*

8.74 8.74 **Global Days XXX**

▲ **77470 Special treatment procedure (eg, total body irradiation, hemibody radiation, per oral or endocavitary irradiation)** Z3 S 80 PQ

EXCLUDES *Intraoperative radiation treatment delivery and management ([77424, 77425], 77469)*

5.10 5.10 **Global Days XXX**

77499 Unlisted procedure, therapeutic radiology treatment management B 80

0.00 0.00 **Global Days XXX**

77520-77525 Proton Therapy

CMS 100-2,6,10 Medical and Other Services Furnished to Inpatients
CMS 100-4,3,10.4 Payment of Nonphysician Services for Inpatients
EXCLUDES *High dose rate electronic brachytherapy, per fraction (0182T)*

77520 **Proton treatment delivery; simple, without compensation** Z2 S TC 80
INCLUDES Single treatment area using a single nontangential/oblique port
0.00 0.00 Global Days XXX

77522 **simple, with compensation** Z2 S TC 80
INCLUDES Single treatment area using a single nontangential/oblique port
0.00 0.00 Global Days XXX

77523 **intermediate** Z2 S TC 80
INCLUDES Proton therapy delivery to one or more treatment sites using two or more ports or one or more tangential/oblique ports, with custom blocks and compensators
0.00 0.00 Global Days XXX

77525 **complex** Z2 S TC 80
INCLUDES Proton therapy delivery to one or more treatment sites using two or more ports per treatment site with matching or patching fields and/or numerous isocenters, with custom blocks and compensators
0.00 0.00 Global Days XXX

77600-77620 Hyperthermia Treatment

CMS 100-3,110.1 Hyperthermia for Treatment of Cancer
INCLUDES Interstitial insertion of temperature sensors
Management during the course of therapy
Normal follow-up care for three months after completion
Physics planning
Use of heat generating devices
EXCLUDES *High dose rate electronic brachytherapy, per fraction (0182T)*
Preliminary consultation (99241-99255)
Radiation therapy treatment (77371-77373, 77401-77416, 77422-77423)

⊙ **77600** **Hyperthermia, externally generated; superficial (ie, heating to a depth of 4 cm or less)** Z2 S 80
12.24 12.24 Global Days XXX

⊙ **77605** **deep (ie, heating to depths greater than 4 cm)** Z2 S 80
20.71 20.71 Global Days XXX

⊙ **77610** **Hyperthermia generated by interstitial probe(s); 5 or fewer interstitial applicators** Z2 S 80
19.48 19.48 Global Days XXX

⊙ **77615** **more than 5 interstitial applicators** Z2 S 80
29.10 29.10 Global Days XXX

77620 **Hyperthermia generated by intracavitary probe(s)** Z2 S 80
16.10 16.10 Global Days XXX

77750-77799 Brachytherapy

CMS 100-4,4,61.4.1 Brachytherapy Sources - General
CMS 100-4,4,61.4.3 Brachytherapy Sources Ordered for a Specific Patient
CMS 100-4,4,61.4.4 Billing for Brachytherapy Source Supervision, Handling, and Loading Costs
CMS 100-4,13,70.4 Clinical Brachytherapy
INCLUDES Hospital admission and daily visits
EXCLUDES *High dose rate electronic brachytherapy, per fraction (0182T)*
Placement of:
Heyman capsules (58346)
Ovoids and tandems (57155)

Code also brachytherapy sources (C1716-C1719, C2616, C2634-C2643, C2698-C2699)

77750 **Infusion or instillation of radioelement solution (includes 3-month follow-up care)** Z3 S 80
EXCLUDES *Monoclonal antibody infusion (79403)*
Nonantibody radiopharmaceutical therapy infusion with follow-up care (79101)
10.29 10.29 Global Days 090

77761 **Intracavitary radiation source application; simple** Z3 S 80
INCLUDES One to four sources/ribbons
Do not report with (0182T)
10.82 10.82 Global Days 090
AMA: 2009, Jan, 11-31; 2008, Jan, 10-25; 2007, January, 13-27

77762 **intermediate** Z3 S 80
INCLUDES Five to 10 sources/ribbons
Do not report with (0182T)
14.42 14.42 Global Days 090

77763 **complex** Z3 S 80
INCLUDES More than 10 sources/ribbons
Do not report with (0182T)
20.42 20.42 Global Days 090

77776 **Interstitial radiation source application; simple** Z3 S 80 PQ
INCLUDES One to four sources/ribbons
12.26 12.26 Global Days 090
AMA: 2007, May, 1-2

77777 **intermediate** Z3 S 80 PQ
INCLUDES Five to 10 sources/ribbons
16.65 16.65 Global Days 090
AMA: 2007, May, 1-2

77778 **complex** Z3 Q3 80 PQ
INCLUDES More than 10 sources/ribbons
24.46 24.46 Global Days 090
AMA: 2007, May, 1-2

77785 **Remote afterloading high dose rate radionuclide brachytherapy; 1 channel** Z3 S 80
Do not report with (0182T)
6.86 6.86 Global Days XXX

77786 **2-12 channels** Z3 S 80
Do not report with (0182T)
16.50 16.50 Global Days XXX

77787 **over 12 channels** Z2 S 80 PQ
Do not report with (0182T)
27.36 27.36 Global Days XXX

77789 **Surface application of radiation source** Z3 S 80
3.28 3.28 Global Days 000

77790 Supervision, handling, loading of radiation source
2.67 2.67 Global Days XXX

77799 Unlisted procedure, clinical brachytherapy
0.00 0.00 Global Days XXX

78000-78320 Nuclear Radiology Procedures

CMS 100-3,220.8 Nuclear Radiology Procedure
CMS 100-3,220.12 Single Photon Emission Tomography

EXCLUDES *Diagnostic services (see appropriate sections)*
Follow-up care (see appropriate section)
Radioimmunoassays (82000-84999 [82652])

Code also radiopharmaceuticals

78000 Thyroid uptake; single determination
2.19 2.19 Global Days XXX
AMA: 2009, Jan, 11-31; 2008, Jan, 10-25; 2007, January, 13-27; 2007, January, 28-31

78001 multiple determinations
2.79 2.79 Global Days XXX
AMA: 2007, January, 28-31

78003 stimulation, suppression or discharge (not including initial uptake studies)
2.44 2.44 Global Days XXX
AMA: 2007, January, 28-31

78006 Thyroid imaging, with uptake; single determination
7.24 7.24 Global Days XXX
AMA: 2007, January, 28-31

78007 multiple determinations
6.88 6.88 Global Days XXX
AMA: 2007, January, 28-31

Hypothyroidism is the syndrome caused by a deficiency of thyroid hormone; the condition may be congenital, acquired, or iatrogenic (resulting from medical treatment)

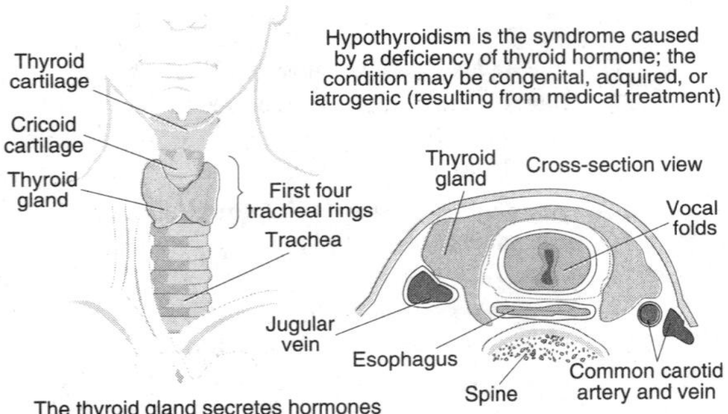

The thyroid gland secretes hormones governing the body's metabolic rate; excess levels result in hyperthyroidism; abnormal enlargement of the gland is called goiter and there are numerous forms

78010 Thyroid imaging; only
5.02 5.02 Global Days XXX
AMA: 2007, January, 28-31

78011 with vascular flow
5.37 5.37 Global Days XXX
AMA: 2007, January, 28-31

78015 Thyroid carcinoma metastases imaging; limited area (eg, neck and chest only)
6.51 6.51 Global Days XXX
AMA: 2007, January, 28-31

78016 with additional studies (eg, urinary recovery)
8.91 8.91 Global Days XXX
AMA: 2007, January, 28-31

78018 whole body
9.49 9.49 Global Days XXX
AMA: 2007, January, 28-31

\+ **78020 Thyroid carcinoma metastases uptake (List separately in addition to code for primary procedure)**
Code first (78018)
2.50 2.50 Global Days ZZZ
AMA: 2009, Jan, 11-31; 2008, Jan, 10-25; 2007, January, 13-27; 2007, January, 28-31

78070 Parathyroid imaging
4.74 4.74 Global Days XXX
AMA: 2007, January, 28-31

78075 Adrenal imaging, cortex and/or medulla
12.73 12.73 Global Days XXX
AMA: 2007, January, 28-31

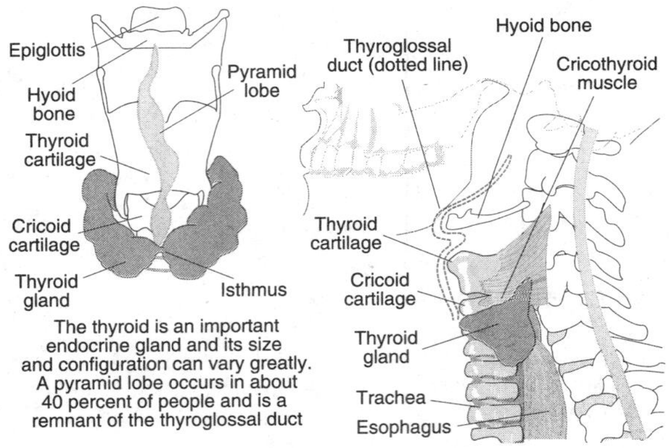

The thyroid is an important endocrine gland and its size and configuration can vary greatly. A pyramid lobe occurs in about 40 percent of people and is a remnant of the thyroglossal duct

78099 Unlisted endocrine procedure, diagnostic nuclear medicine
0.00 0.00 Global Days XXX
AMA: 2007, January, 28-31

78102 Bone marrow imaging; limited area
5.02 5.02 Global Days XXX
AMA: 2007, January, 28-31

78103 multiple areas
6.62 6.62 Global Days XXX
AMA: 2007, January, 28-31

78104 whole body
7.41 7.41 Global Days XXX
AMA: 2007, January, 28-31

78110 Plasma volume, radiopharmaceutical volume-dilution technique (separate procedure); single sampling
2.53 2.53 Global Days XXX
AMA: 2007, January, 28-31

78111 multiple samplings
2.48 2.48 Global Days XXX
AMA: 2007, January, 28-31

78120 Red cell volume determination (separate procedure); single sampling
2.61 2.61 Global Days XXX
AMA: 2007, January, 28-31

78121 multiple samplings
2.92 2.92 Global Days XXX
AMA: 2007, January, 28-31

78122 Whole blood volume determination, including separate measurement of plasma volume and red cell volume (radiopharmaceutical volume-dilution technique)
3.04 3.04 Global Days XXX
AMA: 2007, January, 28-31

78130 Red cell survival study;
4.61 4.61 Global Days XXX
AMA: 2007, January, 28-31

78135 differential organ/tissue kinetics (eg, splenic and/or hepatic sequestration)
10.75 10.75 Global Days XXX
AMA: 2007, January, 28-31

78140 Labeled red cell sequestration, differential organ/tissue (eg, splenic and/or hepatic)
4.03 4.03 Global Days XXX
AMA: 2007, January, 28-31

78185 Spleen imaging only, with or without vascular flow
EXCLUDES *Liver imaging (78215-78216)*
6.22 6.22 Global Days XXX
AMA: 2007, January, 28-31

78190 Kinetics, study of platelet survival, with or without differential organ/tissue localization
12.25 12.25 Global Days XXX
AMA: 2007, January, 28-31

78191 Platelet survival study
4.95 4.95 Global Days XXX
AMA: 2007, January, 28-31

78195 Lymphatics and lymph nodes imaging
EXCLUDES *Sentinel node identification without scintigraphy (38792)*
Sentinel node removal (38500-38542)
10.70 10.70 Global Days XXX
AMA: 2008, Sep, 5-6; 2007, January, 28-31

78199 Unlisted hematopoietic, reticuloendothelial and lymphatic procedure, diagnostic nuclear medicine
0.00 0.00 Global Days XXX
AMA: 2007, January, 28-31

78201 Liver imaging; static only
EXCLUDES *Spleen imaging only (78185)*
5.53 5.53 Global Days XXX
AMA: 2007, January, 28-31

78202 with vascular flow
EXCLUDES *Spleen imaging only (78185)*
6.15 6.15 Global Days XXX
AMA: 2007, January, 28-31

78205 Liver imaging (SPECT);
6.58 6.58 Global Days XXX
AMA: 2007, January, 28-31

78206 with vascular flow
10.37 10.37 Global Days XXX
AMA: 2007, January, 28-31

78215 Liver and spleen imaging; static only
5.80 5.80 Global Days XXX
AMA: 2007, January, 28-31

78216 with vascular flow
3.73 3.73 Global Days XXX
AMA: 2007, January, 28-31

~~78220 Liver function study with hepatobiliary agents, with serial images~~

~~78223 Hepatobiliary ductal system imaging, including gallbladder, with or without pharmacologic intervention, with or without quantitative measurement of gallbladder function~~
To report, see 78226-78227

● 78226 Hepatobiliary system imaging, including gallbladder when present;
9.65 9.65 Global Days XXX

● 78227 with pharmacologic intervention, including quantitative measurement(s) when performed
13.21 13.21 Global Days XXX

78230 Salivary gland imaging;
5.09 5.09 Global Days XXX
AMA: 2007, January, 28-31

78231 with serial images
3.76 3.76 Global Days XXX
AMA: 2007, January, 28-31

78232 Salivary gland function study
3.17 3.17 Global Days XXX
AMA: 2007, January, 28-31

78258 Esophageal motility
6.95 6.95 Global Days XXX
AMA: 2007, January, 28-31

78261 Gastric mucosa imaging
7.55 7.55 Global Days XXX
AMA: 2007, January, 28-31

78262 Gastroesophageal reflux study
7.49 7.49 Global Days XXX
AMA: 2007, January, 28-31

78264 Gastric emptying study
8.67 8.67 Global Days XXX
AMA: 2007, January, 28-31

78267 Urea breath test, C-14 (isotopic); acquisition for analysis
0.00 0.00 Global Days XXX
AMA: 2007, January, 28-31

78268 analysis
0.00 0.00 Global Days XXX
AMA: 2007, January, 28-31

78270 Vitamin B-12 absorption study (eg, Schilling test); without intrinsic factor
2.46 2.46 Global Days XXX
AMA: 2007, January, 28-31

78271 with intrinsic factor
2.64 2.64 Global Days XXX
AMA: 2007, January, 28-31

78272 Vitamin B-12 absorption studies combined, with and without intrinsic factor
2.68 2.68 Global Days XXX
AMA: 2007, January, 28-31

78278 Acute gastrointestinal blood loss imaging
10.45 10.45 Global Days XXX
AMA: 2007, January, 28-31

78282 Gastrointestinal protein loss
0.00 0.00 Global Days XXX
AMA: 2007, January, 28-31

78290 Intestine imaging (eg, ectopic gastric mucosa, Meckel's localization, volvulus)
9.90 9.90 Global Days XXX
AMA: 2007, January, 28-31

78291 Peritoneal-venous shunt patency test (eg, for LeVeen, Denver shunt)
Code also (49427)
7.60 7.60 Global Days XXX
AMA: 2007, January, 28-31

78299 Unlisted gastrointestinal procedure, diagnostic nuclear medicine
0.00 0.00 Global Days XXX
AMA: 2007, January, 28-31

78300 Bone and/or joint imaging; limited area
5.32 5.32 Global Days XXX
AMA: 2009, Jan, 11-31; 2008, Jan, 10-25; 2007, January, 13-27; 2007, January, 28-31

78305 multiple areas
7.03 7.03 Global Days XXX
AMA: 2007, January, 28-31

78306 whole body
7.56 7.56 Global Days XXX
AMA: 2009, Jan, 11-31; 2008, Jan, 10-25; 2007, January, 28-31; 2007, January, 13-27

78315 3 phase study
10.44 10.44 Global Days XXX
AMA: 2009, Jan, 11-31; 2008, Jan, 10-25; 2007, January, 28-31; 2007, January, 13-27

78320 tomographic (SPECT)
7.04 7.04 Global Days XXX
AMA: 2009, Jan, 11-31; 2008, Jan, 8-9; 2007, January, 28-31

78350-78399 Nuclear Radiology: Bone Density Studies

CMS 100-3,150.3 Bone (Mineral) Density Studies
CMS 100-3,220.8 Nuclear Radiology Procedure

Code also radiopharmaceuticals

78350 Bone density (bone mineral content) study, 1 or more sites; single photon absorptiometry
0.98 0.98 Global Days XXX
AMA: 2007, January, 28-31

78351 dual photon absorptiometry, 1 or more sites
0.44 0.43 Global Days XXX
AMA: 2007, January, 28-31

78399 Unlisted musculoskeletal procedure, diagnostic nuclear medicine
0.00 0.00 Global Days XXX
AMA: 2007, January, 28-31

78414-78499 Nuclear Radiology: Heart and Vascular

CMS 100-3,220.6 Positron Emission Tomography (PET) Scans
CMS 100-3,220.6.1 NCD for PET for Perfusion of the Heart (220.6.1)
CMS 100-3,220.6.8 PET (FDG) for Myocardial Viability
CMS 100-3,220.8 Nuclear Radiology Procedure
CMS 100-3,220.12 Single Photon Emission Tomography
CMS 100-4,13,60 Positron Emission Tomography (PET) Scans - General Information
CMS 100-4,13,60.1 Billing for PET Scans
CMS 100-4,13,60.2 Use of Gamma Cameras, Full and Partial Ring PET Scanners
CMS 100-4,13,60.3 PET Scan Qualifying Conditions
CMS 100-4,13,60.4 PET Scans for Imaging of the Perfusion of the Heart Using Rubidium 82
CMS 100-4,13,60.9 Coverage of PET Scans for Myocardial Viability
CMS 100-4,13,60.11 PET Scans for Perfusion of the Heart Using Ammonia N-13
EXCLUDES *Stress testing (93015-93018)*

Code also radiopharmaceuticals

78414 Determination of central c-v hemodynamics (non-imaging) (eg, ejection fraction with probe technique) with or without pharmacologic intervention or exercise, single or multiple determinations
0.00 0.00 Global Days XXX
AMA: 2007, January, 28-31

78428 Cardiac shunt detection
5.65 5.65 Global Days XXX
AMA: 2007, January, 28-31

78445 Non-cardiac vascular flow imaging (ie, angiography, venography)
5.19 5.19 Global Days XXX
AMA: 2007, January, 28-31

78451 Myocardial perfusion imaging, tomographic (SPECT) (including attenuation correction, qualitative or quantitative wall motion, ejection fraction by first pass or gated technique, additional quantification, when performed); single study, at rest or stress (exercise or pharmacologic)
10.60 10.60 Global Days XXX

78452 multiple studies, at rest and/or stress (exercise or pharmacologic) and/or redistribution and/or rest reinjection
14.79 14.79 Global Days XXX

78453 Myocardial perfusion imaging, planar (including qualitative or quantitative wall motion, ejection fraction by first pass or gated technique, additional quantification, when performed); single study, at rest or stress (exercise or pharmacologic)
9.13 9.13 Global Days XXX

78454 multiple studies, at rest and/or stress (exercise or pharmacologic) and/or redistribution and/or rest reinjection
13.05 13.05 Global Days XXX

78456 Acute venous thrombosis imaging, peptide
11.33 11.33 Global Days XXX
AMA: 2007, January, 28-31

78457 Venous thrombosis imaging, venogram; unilateral
6.07 6.07 Global Days XXX
AMA: 2007, January, 28-31

78458 bilateral
5.67 5.67 Global Days XXX
AMA: 2007, January, 28-31

78459 Myocardial imaging, positron emission tomography (PET), metabolic evaluation
0.00 0.00 Global Days XXX
AMA: 2007, January, 28-31

78466 Myocardial imaging, infarct avid, planar; qualitative or quantitative
5.26 5.26 Global Days XXX
AMA: 2007, January, 28-31

78468 with ejection fraction by first pass technique
6.38 6.38 Global Days XXX
AMA: 2007, January, 28-31

78469 tomographic SPECT with or without quantification
7.24 7.24 Global Days XXX
AMA: 2007, January, 28-31

78472 Cardiac blood pool imaging, gated equilibrium; planar, single study at rest or stress (exercise and/or pharmacologic), wall motion study plus ejection fraction, with or without additional quantitative processing
Do not report with (78451-78454, 78481, 78483, 78494)
7.29 7.29 Global Days XXX
AMA: 2007, January, 28-31

78473 multiple studies, wall motion study plus ejection fraction, at rest and stress (exercise and/or pharmacologic), with or without additional quantification
Do not report with (78451-78454, 78481, 78483, 78494)
9.41 9.41 Global Days XXX
AMA: 2007, January, 28-31

78481 **Cardiac blood pool imaging (planar), first pass technique; single study, at rest or with stress (exercise and/or pharmacologic), wall motion study plus ejection fraction, with or without quantification**

Do not report with (78451-78454)

5.94 5.94 Global Days XXX

AMA: 2007, January, 28-31

78483 **multiple studies, at rest and with stress (exercise and/or pharmacologic), wall motion study plus ejection fraction, with or without quantification**

EXCLUDES *Blood flow studies of the brain (78610)*

Do not report with (78451-78454)

8.09 8.09 Global Days XXX

AMA: 2007, January, 28-31

78491 **Myocardial imaging, positron emission tomography (PET), perfusion; single study at rest or stress**

0.00 0.00 Global Days XXX

AMA: 2007, January, 28-31

78492 **multiple studies at rest and/or stress**

0.00 0.00 Global Days XXX

AMA: 2007, January, 28-31

78494 **Cardiac blood pool imaging, gated equilibrium, SPECT, at rest, wall motion study plus ejection fraction, with or without quantitative processing**

7.38 7.38 Global Days XXX

AMA: 2007, January, 28-31

\+ **78496** **Cardiac blood pool imaging, gated equilibrium, single study, at rest, with right ventricular ejection fraction by first pass technique (List separately in addition to code for primary procedure)**

Code first (78472)

1.87 1.87 Global Days ZZZ

AMA: 2009, Jan, 11-31; 2008, Jan, 10-25; 2007, January, 13-27; 2007, January, 28-31

78499 **Unlisted cardiovascular procedure, diagnostic nuclear medicine**

0.00 0.00 Global Days XXX

AMA: 2007, January, 28-31

78579-78599 Nuclear Radiology: Lungs

CMS 100-2,15,80 Diagnostic Test Requirements
CMS 100-3,220.7 Xenon Scan
CMS 100-3,220.8 Nuclear Radiology Procedure
CMS 100-4,3,10.4 Payment of Nonphysician Services for Inpatients

Code also radiopharmaceuticals

● **78579** **Pulmonary ventilation imaging (eg, aerosol or gas)**

Do not report more than one time per imaging session

5.13 5.13 Global Days XXX

▲ **78580** **Pulmonary perfusion imaging (eg, particulate)**

Do not report more than one time per imaging session

6.62 6.62 Global Days XXX

AMA: 2007, January, 28-31

● **78582** **Pulmonary ventilation (eg, aerosol or gas) and perfusion imaging**

Do not report more than one time per imaging session

Do not report with (78451-78454)

9.45 9.45 Global Days XXX

~~78584~~ ~~Pulmonary perfusion imaging, particulate, with ventilation; single breath~~

To report, see 78579-78598

~~78585~~ ~~rebreathing and washout, with or without single breath~~

To report, see 78579-78598

~~78586~~ ~~Pulmonary ventilation imaging, aerosol; single projection~~

To report, see 78579, 78582, 78598

~~78587~~ ~~multiple projections (eg, anterior, posterior, lateral views)~~

To report, see 78579, 78582, 78598

~~78588~~ ~~Pulmonary perfusion imaging, particulate, with ventilation imaging, aerosol, 1 or multiple projections~~

To report, see 78579-78598

~~78591~~ ~~Pulmonary ventilation imaging, gaseous, single breath, single projection~~

To report, see 78579, 78582

~~78593~~ ~~Pulmonary ventilation imaging, gaseous, with rebreathing and washout with or without single breath; single projection~~

To report, see 78579, 78582, 78598

~~78594~~ ~~multiple projections (eg, anterior, posterior, lateral views)~~

To report, see 78579, 78582, 78598

~~78596~~ ~~Pulmonary quantitative differential function (ventilation/perfusion) study~~

To report, see 78580-78598

● **78597** **Quantitative differential pulmonary perfusion, including imaging when performed**

Do not report more than one time per imaging session

Do not report with (78451-78454)

5.78 5.78 Global Days XXX

● **78598** **Quantitative differential pulmonary perfusion and ventilation (eg, aerosol or gas), including imaging when performed**

Do not report more than one time per imaging session

Do not report with (78451-78454)

8.88 8.88 Global Days XXX

78599 **Unlisted respiratory procedure, diagnostic nuclear medicine**

0.00 0.00 Global Days XXX

AMA: 2007, January, 28-31

78600-78650 Diagnostic Imaging: Brain/Cerebrospinal Fluid

CMS 100-3,220.6.9 FDG PET for Refractory Seizures
CMS 100-3,220.8 Nuclear Radiology Procedure
Code also radiopharmaceuticals

Diagram of tomography principal (left)

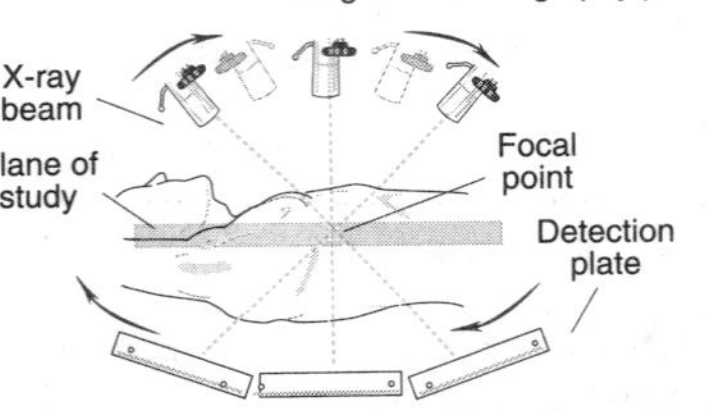

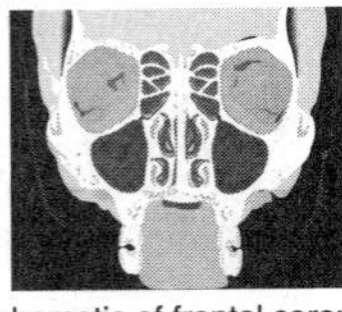

Schematic of frontal coronal CT section of skull

Tomogram is a general term for radiographic studies that focus on a single body plane, unimpeded by shadows cast by surrounding tissues and structures. The x-ray tube and the film are rotated around the patient during exposure of the focal point. Computed tomography (CT) offers a "slice" view of the study area and information is typically digitized and viewed on monitors. Magnetic resonance imaging (MRI) places a patient within the field of a powerful magnet while radio waves pass through the body; as with CT studies, views are usually of a "slice" of tissue. Ultrasound and nuclear imaging are other common radiological approaches

78600 **Brain imaging, less than 4 static views;** Z2 S 80
5.43 5.43 Global Days XXX
AMA: 2007, January, 28-31

78601 **with vascular flow** Z2 S 80
6.40 6.40 Global Days XXX
AMA: 2007, January, 28-31

78605 **Brain imaging, minimum 4 static views;** Z2 S 80
5.93 5.93 Global Days XXX
AMA: 2007, January, 28-31

78606 **with vascular flow** Z2 S 80
9.97 9.97 Global Days XXX
AMA: 2007, January, 28-31

78607 **Brain imaging, tomographic (SPECT)** Z2 S 80
10.91 10.91 Global Days XXX
AMA: 2007, January, 28-31

78608 **Brain imaging, positron emission tomography (PET); metabolic evaluation** Z2 S 80
0.00 0.00 Global Days XXX
AMA: 2007, January, 28-31

78609 **perfusion evaluation** E
2.21 2.21 Global Days XXX
AMA: 2007, January, 28-31

78610 **Brain imaging, vascular flow only** Z2 S 80
5.31 5.31 Global Days XXX
AMA: 2007, January, 28-31

78630 **Cerebrospinal fluid flow, imaging (not including introduction of material); cisternography** Z2 S 80
Code also injection procedure (61000-61070, 62270-62319)
10.27 10.27 Global Days XXX
AMA: 2007, January, 28-31

78635 **ventriculography** Z2 S 80
Code also injection procedure (61000-61070, 62270-62294)
9.98 9.98 Global Days XXX
AMA: 2007, January, 28-31

78645 **shunt evaluation** Z2 S 80
Code also injection procedure (61000-61070, 62270-62294)
9.64 9.64 Global Days XXX
AMA: 2007, January, 28-31

78647 **tomographic (SPECT)** Z2 S 80
10.31 10.31 Global Days XXX
AMA: 2007, January, 28-31

78650 **Cerebrospinal fluid leakage detection and localization** Z2 S 80
Code also injection procedure (61000-61070, 62270-62294)
9.96 9.96 Global Days XXX
AMA: 2007, January, 28-31

78660-78699 Nuclear Radiology: Lacrimal Duct System

Code also radiopharmaceuticals

78660 **Radiopharmaceutical dacryocystography** Z2 S 80
5.55 5.55 Global Days XXX
AMA: 2007, January, 28-31

78699 **Unlisted nervous system procedure, diagnostic nuclear medicine** Z2 S 80
0.00 0.00 Global Days XXX
AMA: 2007, January, 28-31

78700-78725 Nuclear Radiology: Renal Anatomy and Function

CMS 100-2,15,80 Diagnostic Test Requirements
CMS 100-3,220.8 Nuclear Radiology Procedure
CMS 100-3,220.12 Single Photon Emission Tomography
CMS 100-4,3,10.4 Payment of Nonphysician Services for Inpatients
EXCLUDES *Renal endoscopy with insertion of radioactive substances (77776-77778)*
Code also radiopharmaceuticals

78700 **Kidney imaging morphology;** Z2 S 80
5.30 5.30 Global Days XXX
AMA: 2007, March, 7-8; 2007, January, 28-31

78701 **with vascular flow** Z2 S 80
6.42 6.42 Global Days XXX
AMA: 2007, March, 7-8; 2007, January, 28-31

78707 **with vascular flow and function, single study without pharmacological intervention** Z2 S 80
7.03 7.03 Global Days XXX
AMA: 2007, March, 7-8; 2007, January, 28-31

78708 **with vascular flow and function, single study, with pharmacological intervention (eg, angiotensin converting enzyme inhibitor and/or diuretic)** Z2 S 80
5.14 5.14 Global Days XXX
AMA: 2007, March, 7-8; 2007, January, 28-31

78709 **with vascular flow and function, multiple studies, with and without pharmacological intervention (eg, angiotensin converting enzyme inhibitor and/or diuretic)** Z2 S 80
11.04 11.04 Global Days XXX
AMA: 2007, March, 7-8; 2007, January, 28-31

78710 **tomographic (SPECT)** Z2 S 80
6.37 6.37 Global Days XXX
AMA: 2007, January, 28-31; 2007, March, 7-8

78725 **Kidney function study, non-imaging radioisotopic study** Z2 S 80
3.12 3.12 Global Days XXX
AMA: 2007, January, 28-31

78730-78799 Nuclear Radiology: Urogenital

CMS 100-2,15,80 Diagnostic Test Requirements
CMS 100-3,220.8 Nuclear Radiology Procedure
CMS 100-4,3,10.4 Payment of Nonphysician Services for Inpatients
Code also radiopharmaceuticals

\+ **78730** **Urinary bladder residual study (List separately in addition to code for primary procedure)**
EXCLUDES *Measurement of postvoid residual urine and/or bladder capacity using ultrasound (51798)*
Ultrasound imaging of the bladder only with measurement of postvoid residual urine (76857)
Code first (78740)
2.30 2.30 Global Days ZZZ
AMA: 2007, March, 7-8; 2007, January, 28-31

78740 **Ureteral reflux study (radiopharmaceutical voiding cystogram)**
EXCLUDES *Catheterization (51701-51703)*
Code also urinary bladder residual study (78730)
6.90 6.90 Global Days XXX
AMA: 2007, January, 28-31

78761 **Testicular imaging with vascular flow** ♂
6.38 6.38 Global Days XXX
AMA: 2007, January, 28-31; 2007, March, 7-8

78799 **Unlisted genitourinary procedure, diagnostic nuclear medicine**
0.00 0.00 Global Days XXX
AMA: 2007, January, 28-31

78800-78804 Nuclear Radiology: Tumor Localization

CMS 100-2,15,80 Diagnostic Test Requirements
CMS 100-3,220.8 Nuclear Radiology Procedure
CMS 100-3,220.12 Single Photon Emission Tomography
CMS 100-4,3,10.4 Payment of Nonphysician Services for Inpatients
Code also radiopharmaceuticals

78800 **Radiopharmaceutical localization of tumor or distribution of radiopharmaceutical agent(s); limited area**
INCLUDES Ocular radiophosphorus tumor identification
EXCLUDES *Specific organ (see appropriate site)*
5.67 5.67 Global Days XXX
AMA: 2007, January, 28-31

78801 **multiple areas**
7.39 7.39 Global Days XXX
AMA: 2007, January, 28-31

78802 **whole body, single day imaging**
9.76 9.76 Global Days XXX
AMA: 2007, January, 28-31

78803 **tomographic (SPECT)**
10.39 10.39 Global Days XXX
AMA: 2007, January, 28-31

78804 **whole body, requiring 2 or more days imaging**
17.34 17.34 Global Days XXX
AMA: 2007, January, 28-31

78805-78807 Nuclear Radiology: Inflammation and Infection

CMS 100-2,15,80 Diagnostic Test Requirements
CMS 100-3,220.8 Nuclear Radiology Procedure
CMS 100-3,220.12 Single Photon Emission Tomography
CMS 100-4,3,10.4 Payment of Nonphysician Services for Inpatients
EXCLUDES *Brain PET scan (78608-78609)*
Imaging bone infectious or inflammatory disease with bone imaging radiopharmaceutical (78300, 78305-78306)
PET myocardial imaging (78459, 78491-78492)
Code also radiopharmaceuticals

78805 **Radiopharmaceutical localization of inflammatory process; limited area**
5.48 5.48 Global Days XXX
AMA: 2007, January, 28-31

78806 **whole body**
10.08 10.08 Global Days XXX
AMA: 2007, January, 28-31

78807 **tomographic (SPECT)**
10.41 10.41 Global Days XXX
AMA: 2007, January, 28-31

78808 Intravenous Injection for Radiopharmaceutical Localization

Code also radiopharmaceuticals

78808 **Injection procedure for radiopharmaceutical localization by non-imaging probe study, intravenous (eg, parathyroid adenoma)**
EXCLUDES *Identification of sentinel node (38792)*
1.26 1.26 Global Days XXX

78811-78999 Nuclear Radiology: Diagnosis, Staging, Restaging or Monitoring Cancer

CMS 100-4,3,10.4 Payment of Nonphysician Services for Inpatients
CMS 100-4,13,60.3 PET Scan Qualifying Conditions
CMS 100-4,13,60.3.1 Appropriate Codes for PET Scans
EXCLUDES *CT scan performed for other than attenuation correction and anatomical localization (report with the appropriate site-specific CT code)*
Ocular radiophosphorus tumor identification (78800)
Code also radiopharmaceuticals
Do not report with procedure performed more than once per session

78811 **Positron emission tomography (PET) imaging; limited area (eg, chest, head/neck)**
0.00 0.00 Global Days XXX
AMA: 2007, January, 28-31

78812 **skull base to mid-thigh**
0.00 0.00 Global Days XXX
AMA: 2007, January, 28-31

78813 **whole body**
0.00 0.00 Global Days XXX
AMA: 2007, January, 28-31

78814 **Positron emission tomography (PET) with concurrently acquired computed tomography (CT) for attenuation correction and anatomical localization imaging; limited area (eg, chest, head/neck)**
0.00 0.00 Global Days XXX
AMA: 2009, Jan, 11-31; 2008, Jan, 10-25; 2007, January, 13-27; 2007, January, 28-31

78815 **skull base to mid-thigh**
0.00 0.00 Global Days XXX
AMA: 2009, Jan, 11-31; 2008, Jan, 10-25; 2007, January, 28-31; 2007, January, 13-27

78816 **whole body** Z2 S 80
0.00 0.00 **Global Days XXX**
AMA: 2009, Jan, 11-31; 2008, Jan, 10-25; 2007, January, 13-27; 2007, January, 28-31

78999 **Unlisted miscellaneous procedure, diagnostic nuclear medicine** Z2 S 80
0.00 0.00 **Global Days XXX**
AMA: 2007, January, 28-31

79005-79999 Systemic Radiopharmaceutical Therapy

CMS 100-3,220.8 Nuclear Radiology Procedure

EXCLUDES *Imaging guidance*
Intra-arterial, intra-cavitory, intra-articular injection (see appropriate injection codes)
Radiological supervision and interpretation

79005 **Radiopharmaceutical therapy, by oral administration** Z3 S 80
EXCLUDES *Monoclonal antibody treatment (79403)*
4.03 4.03 **Global Days XXX**

79101 **Radiopharmaceutical therapy, by intravenous administration** Z3 S 80
EXCLUDES *Administration of nonantibody radioelement solution including follow-up care (77750)*
Radiolabeled monoclonal antibody IV infusion (79403)

Do not report with (36400, 36410, 79403, 96360, 96374-96375, 96409)
4.56 4.56 **Global Days XXX**

79200 **Radiopharmaceutical therapy, by intracavitary administration** Z3 S 80
4.82 4.82 **Global Days XXX**

79300 **Radiopharmaceutical therapy, by interstitial radioactive colloid administration** Z2 S 80
0.00 0.00 **Global Days XXX**

79403 **Radiopharmaceutical therapy, radiolabeled monoclonal antibody by intravenous infusion** Z3 S 80
EXCLUDES *Pretreatment imaging (78802, 78804)*

Do not report with (79101)
5.67 5.67 **Global Days XXX**

79440 **Radiopharmaceutical therapy, by intra-articular administration** Z3 S 80
4.60 4.60 **Global Days XXX**

79445 **Radiopharmaceutical therapy, by intra-arterial particulate administration** Z2 S 80
EXCLUDES *Procedural and radiological supervision and interpretation for angiographic and interventional procedures before intra-arterial radiopharmaceutical therapy*

Do not report with (96373, 96420)
0.00 0.00 **Global Days XXX**

79999 **Radiopharmaceutical therapy, unlisted procedure** Z2 S 80
0.00 0.00 **Global Days XXX**

80047-80076 Multi-test Laboratory Panels

CMS 100-2,6,10 Medical and Other Services Furnished to Inpatients
CMS 100-2,15,80 Diagnostic Test Requirements
CMS 100-4,3,10.4 Payment of Nonphysician Services for Inpatients

EXCLUDES *Test codes:*
For testing performed at a frequency greater than the number specified by panel definition
Not specified by panel definition

Do not report two or more panel codes comprising the same tests; report the panel with the highest number of tests to meet the definition of the code, and report the remaining tests individually

80047 Basic metabolic panel (Calcium, ionized)

INCLUDES Calcium, ionized (82330)
Carbon dioxide (82374)
Chloride (82435)
Creatinine (82565)
Glucose (82947)
Potassium (84132)
Sodium (84295)
Urea nitrogen (BUN) (84520)

0.00 0.00 **Global Days XXX**
AMA: 2008, Apr, 5-7

80048 Basic metabolic panel (Calcium, total)

INCLUDES Calcium, total (82310)
Carbon dioxide (82374)
Chloride (82435)
Creatinine (82565)
Glucose (82947)
Potassium (84132)
Sodium (84295)
Urea nitrogen (BUN) (84520)

0.00 0.00 **Global Days XXX**
AMA: 2008, Apr, 5-7

80050 General health panel

INCLUDES Complete blood count (CBC) automated and appropriate manual differential WBC count (85007, 85009, 85027)
Complete blood count with differential (CBC) (85004 or 85025, 85027)
Comprehensive metabolic profile OR (80053)
Thyroid stimulating hormones (84443)

0.00 0.00 **Global Days XXX**
AMA: 2009, Jan, 11-31; 2008, Jan, 10-25; 2007, January, 13-27

80051 Electrolyte panel

INCLUDES Carbon dioxide (82374)
Chloride (82435)
Potassium (84132)
Sodium (84295)

0.00 0.00 **Global Days XXX**
AMA: 2009, Jan, 11-31; 2008, Jan, 10-25; 2007, January, 13-27

80053 Comprehensive metabolic panel

INCLUDES Albumin (82040)
Bilirubin, total (82247)
Calcium, total (82310)
Carbon dioxide (bicarbonate) (82374)
Chloride (82435)
Creatinine (82565)
Glucose (82947)
Phosphatase, alkaline (84075)
Potassium (84132)
Protein, total (84155)
Sodium (84295)
Transferase, alanine amino (ALT) (SGPT) (84460)
Transferase, aspartate amino (AST) (SGOT) (84450)
Urea nitrogen (BUN) (84520)

0.00 0.00 **Global Days XXX**
AMA: 2009, Jan, 11-31; 2008, Jan, 10-25; 2008, Apr, 5-7; 2007, January, 13-27

80055 Obstetric panel

INCLUDES Blood typing, ABO and Rh (86900-86901)
CBC (85004, 85007, 85009, 85025, 85027)
Hepatitis B surface antigen (HBsAg) (87340)
RBC antibody screen, each serum technique (86850)
Rubella antibody (86762)
Syphilis test, non-treponemal antibody qualitative (86592)

Do not report panel code 80055 when syphilis screening is provided using a treponemal antibody approach (86780); report individual codes for tests performed in the OB panel instead

0.00 0.00 **Global Days XXX**
AMA: 2009, Jan, 11-31; 2008, Jan, 10-25; 2007, January, 13-27

80061 Lipid panel

INCLUDES Cholesterol, serum, total (82465)
Lipoprotein, direct measurement, high density cholesterol (HDL cholesterol) (83718)
Triglycerides (84478)

0.00 0.00 **Global Days XXX**
AMA: 2009, Jan, 11-31; 2008, Jan, 10-25; 2007, January, 13-27

80069 Renal function panel

INCLUDES Albumin (82040)
Calcium, total (82310)
Carbon dioxide (82374)
Chloride (82435)
Creatinine (82565)
Glucose (82947)
Phosphorus inorganic (84100)
Potassium (84132)
Sodium (84295)
Urea nitrogen (BUN) (84520)

0.00 0.00 **Global Days XXX**
AMA: 2009, Jan, 11-31; 2008, Jan, 10-25; 2007, January, 13-27

80074 Acute hepatitis panel

INCLUDES Hepatitis A antibody (HAAb) IgM (86709)
Hepatitis B core antibody (HBcAb), IgM (86705)
Hepatitis B surface antigen (HBsAg) (87340)
Hepatitis C antibody (86803)

0.00 0.00 **Global Days XXX**
AMA: 2009, Jan, 11-31; 2008, Jan, 10-25; 2007, January, 13-27

80076 Hepatic function panel A

INCLUDES Albumin (82040)
Bilirubin, direct (82248)
Bilirubin, total (82247)
Phosphatase, alkaline (84075)
Protein, total (84155)
Transferase, alanine amino (ALT) (SGPT) (84460)
Transferase, aspartate amino (AST) (SGOT) (84450)

0.00 0.00 Global Days XXX

AMA: 2009, Jan, 11-31; 2008, Jan, 10-25; 2007, January, 13-27

80100-80104 [80104] Drug Screening Tests

CMS 100-2,6,10 Medical and Other Services Furnished to Inpatients
CMS 100-2,15,80 Diagnostic Test Requirements
CMS 100-4,3,10.4 Payment of Nonphysician Services for Inpatients

INCLUDES Qualitative test for drugs or drug classes such as:
- Alcohols
- Amphetamines
- Barbiturates
- Benzodiazepines
- Cocaine and metabolites
- Methadones
- Opiates
- Phencyclidines
- Phenothiazines
- Propoxyphenes
- Tetrahydrocannabinoids
- Tricyclic antidepressants

Stationary and mobile chromatography

EXCLUDES *Drug quantification (80150-80299, 82000-84999 [82652])*

80100 Drug screen, qualitative; multiple drug classes chromatographic method, each procedure E

INCLUDES Each combination of mobile stage with stationary stage

EXCLUDES *Multiple drugs or drug class by multiplexed screeing ([80104])*

0.00 0.00 Global Days XXX

80101 single drug class method (eg, immunoassay, enzyme assay), each drug class E

INCLUDES Every single drug class examined and documented

EXCLUDES *Multiple drugs or drug class by multiplexed screening kit ([80104])*

0.00 0.00 Global Days XXX

AMA: 2009, Jan, 11-31; 2008, Jan, 10-25; 2007, January, 13-27

\# **80104 multiple drug classes other than chromatographic method, each procedure** E

0.00 0.00 Global Days XXX

80102 Drug confirmation, each procedure A

INCLUDES Each combination of mobile stage with stationary stage for drug verification

0.00 0.00 Global Days XXX

80103 Tissue preparation for drug analysis N

0.00 0.00 Global Days XXX

80104 Resequenced Code. See code following 80101.

80150-80299 Therapeutic Drug Levels

CMS 100-2,15,80 Diagnostic Test Requirements
CMS 100-4,3,10.4 Payment of Nonphysician Services for Inpatients

INCLUDES Tests on specimens from any source

EXCLUDES *Nonquantitative testing (80100-80103 [80104])*

80150 Amikacin A
0.00 0.00 Global Days XXX

80152 Amitriptyline A
0.00 0.00 Global Days XXX

80154 Benzodiazepines A
0.00 0.00 Global Days XXX

80156 Carbamazepine; total A
0.00 0.00 Global Days XXX

80157 free A
0.00 0.00 Global Days XXX

80158 Cyclosporine A
0.00 0.00 Global Days XXX

80160 Desipramine A
0.00 0.00 Global Days XXX

80162 Digoxin A
0.00 0.00 Global Days XXX

80164 Dipropylacetic acid (valproic acid) A
0.00 0.00 Global Days XXX

80166 Doxepin A
0.00 0.00 Global Days XXX

80168 Ethosuximide A
0.00 0.00 Global Days XXX

80170 Gentamicin A
0.00 0.00 Global Days XXX

80172 Gold A
0.00 0.00 Global Days XXX

80173 Haloperidol A
0.00 0.00 Global Days XXX

80174 Imipramine A
0.00 0.00 Global Days XXX

80176 Lidocaine A
0.00 0.00 Global Days XXX

80178 Lithium A
0.00 0.00 Global Days XXX

80182 Nortriptyline A
0.00 0.00 Global Days XXX

80184 Phenobarbital A
0.00 0.00 Global Days XXX

80185 Phenytoin; total A
0.00 0.00 Global Days XXX

80186 free A
0.00 0.00 Global Days XXX

80188 Primidone A
0.00 0.00 Global Days XXX

80190 Procainamide; A
0.00 0.00 Global Days XXX

80192 with metabolites (eg, n-acetyl procainamide) A
0.00 0.00 Global Days XXX

80194 Quinidine A
0.00 0.00 Global Days XXX

80195 Sirolimus A
0.00 0.00 Global Days XXX

80196 Salicylate A
0.00 0.00 Global Days XXX

80197 Tacrolimus [A]
0.00 0.00 Global Days XXX

80198 Theophylline [A]
0.00 0.00 Global Days XXX

80200 Tobramycin [A]
0.00 0.00 Global Days XXX

80201 Topiramate [A]
0.00 0.00 Global Days XXX

80202 Vancomycin [A]
0.00 0.00 Global Days XXX

80299 Quantitation of drug, not elsewhere specified [A]
0.00 0.00 Global Days XXX
AMA: 2009, Jan, 11-31; 2008, Jan, 10-25; 2007, January, 13-27

80400-80440 Stimulation and Suppression Test Panels

CMS 100-2,15,80 Diagnostic Test Requirements
CMS 100-4,3,10.4 Payment of Nonphysician Services for Inpatients

EXCLUDES *Administration of evocative or suppressive material (96365-96368, 96372-96376, C8957)*
Evocative or suppression test substances (99070)
Physician monitoring and attendance during the test (see Evaluation and Management codes)

80400 ACTH stimulation panel; for adrenal insufficiency [A]
INCLUDES Cortisol x 2 (82533)
0.00 0.00 Global Days XXX

80402 for 21 hydroxylase deficiency [A]
INCLUDES 17 hydroxyprogesterone X 2 (83498)
Cortisol x 2 (82533)
0.00 0.00 Global Days XXX

80406 for 3 beta-hydroxydehydrogenase deficiency [A]
INCLUDES 17 hydroxypregnenolone x 2 (84143)
Cortisol x 2 (82533)
0.00 0.00 Global Days XXX

80408 Aldosterone suppression evaluation panel (eg, saline infusion) [A]
INCLUDES Aldosterone x 2 (82088)
Renin x 2 (84244)
0.00 0.00 Global Days XXX

80410 Calcitonin stimulation panel (eg, calcium, pentagastrin) [A]
INCLUDES Calcitonin x 3 (82308)
0.00 0.00 Global Days XXX

80412 Corticotropic releasing hormone (CRH) stimulation panel [A]
INCLUDES Adrenocorticotropic hormone (ACTH) x 6 (82024)
Cortisol x 6 (82533)
0.00 0.00 Global Days XXX

80414 Chorionic gonadotropin stimulation panel; testosterone response ♀[A]
INCLUDES Testosterone x 2 on three pooled blood samples (84403)
0.00 0.00 Global Days XXX

80415 estradiol response This panel must include the following: Estradiol (82670 x 2 on 3 pooled blood samples) [A]
INCLUDES Estradiol x 2 on three pooled blood samples (82670)
0.00 0.00 Global Days XXX

80416 Renal vein renin stimulation panel (eg, captopril) [A]
INCLUDES Renin x 6 (84244)
0.00 0.00 Global Days XXX

80417 Peripheral vein renin stimulation panel (eg, captopril) [A]
INCLUDES Renin x 2 (84244)
0.00 0.00 Global Days XXX

80418 Combined rapid anterior pituitary evaluation panel [A]
INCLUDES Adrenocorticotropic hormone (ACTH) x 4 (82024)
Cortisol x 4 (82533)
Follicle stimulating hormone (FSH) x 4 (83001)
Human growth hormone x 4 (83003)
Luteinizing hormone (LH) x 4 (83002)
Prolactin x 4 (84146)
Thyroid stimulating hormone (TSH) x 4 (84443)
0.00 0.00 Global Days XXX

80420 Dexamethasone suppression panel, 48 hour [A]
INCLUDES Cortisol x 2 (82533)
Free cortisol, urine x 2 (82530)
Volume measurement for timed collection x 2 (81050)
EXCLUDES *Single dose dexamethasone (82533)*
0.00 0.00 Global Days XXX

80422 Glucagon tolerance panel; for insulinoma [A]
INCLUDES Glucose x 3 (82947)
Insulin x 3 (83525)
0.00 0.00 Global Days XXX

80424 for pheochromocytoma This panel must include the following: Catecholamines, fractionated (82384 x 2) [A]
INCLUDES Catecholamines, fractionated x 2 (82384)
0.00 0.00 Global Days XXX

80426 Gonadotropin releasing hormone stimulation panel [A]
INCLUDES Follicle stimulating hormone (FSH) x 4 (83001)
Luteinizing hormone (LH) x 4 (83002)
0.00 0.00 Global Days XXX

80428 Growth hormone stimulation panel (eg, arginine infusion, l-dopa administration) [A]
INCLUDES Human growth hormone (HGH) x 4 (83003)
0.00 0.00 Global Days XXX

80430 Growth hormone suppression panel (glucose administration) [A]
INCLUDES Glucose x 3 (82947)
Human growth hormone (HGH) x 4 (83003)
0.00 0.00 Global Days XXX

80432 Insulin-induced C-peptide suppression panel [A]
INCLUDES C-peptide x 5 (84681)
Glucose x 5 (82947)
Insulin (83525)
0.00 0.00 Global Days XXX

80434 Insulin tolerance panel; for ACTH insufficiency [A]
INCLUDES Cortisol x 5 (82533)
Glucose x 5 (82947)
0.00 0.00 Global Days XXX

80435 for growth hormone deficiency [A]
INCLUDES Glucose x 5 (82947)
Human growth hormone (HGH) x 5 (83003)
0.00 0.00 Global Days XXX

80436 **Metyrapone panel**
INCLUDES 11 deoxycortisol x 2 (82634)
Cortisol x 2 (82533)
0.00 0.00 Global Days XXX

80438 **Thyrotropin releasing hormone (TRH) stimulation panel; 1 hour**
INCLUDES Thyroid stimulating hormone (TSH) x 3 (84443)
0.00 0.00 Global Days XXX

80439 **2 hour This panel must include the following: Thyroid stimulating hormone (TSH) (84443 x 4)**
INCLUDES Thyroid stimulating hormone (TSH) x 4 (84443)
0.00 0.00 Global Days XXX

80440 **for hyperprolactinemia This panel must include the following: Prolactin (84146 x 3)**
INCLUDES Prolactin x 3 (84146)
0.00 0.00 Global Days XXX

80500-80502 Consultation By Clinical Pathologist

CMS 100-2,15,80 Diagnostic Test Requirements
CMS 100-4,3,10.4 Payment of Nonphysician Services for Inpatients
CMS 100-4,12,60 Payment for Pathology Services

INCLUDES Pharmacokinetic consultations
Written report by pathologist for tests requiring additional medical judgement

EXCLUDES *Consultations that include examination of the patient (99241-99255)*

80500 **Clinical pathology consultation; limited, without review of patient's history and medical records**
0.52 0.58 Global Days XXX

80502 **comprehensive, for a complex diagnostic problem, with review of patient's history and medical records**
1.80 1.85 Global Days XXX

81000-81099 Urine Tests

CMS 100-2,15,80 Diagnostic Test Requirements
CMS 100-4,3,10.4 Payment of Nonphysician Services for Inpatients

81000 **Urinalysis, by dip stick or tablet reagent for bilirubin, glucose, hemoglobin, ketones, leukocytes, nitrite, pH, protein, specific gravity, urobilinogen, any number of these constituents; non-automated, with microscopy**
0.00 0.00 Global Days XXX

81001 **automated, with microscopy**
0.00 0.00 Global Days XXX

81002 **non-automated, without microscopy**
INCLUDES Mosenthal test
0.00 0.00 Global Days XXX
AMA: 2007, April, 1-2

81003 **automated, without microscopy**
0.00 0.00 Global Days XXX
AMA: 2007, April, 1-2

81005 **Urinalysis; qualitative or semiquantitative, except immunoassays**
INCLUDES Benedict test for dextrose
EXCLUDES *Immunoassay, qualitative or semiquantitative (83518)*
Microalbumin (82043-82044)
Nonimmunoassay reagent strip analysis (81000, 81002)
0.00 0.00 Global Days XXX

81007 **bacteriuria screen, except by culture or dipstick**
EXCLUDES *Culture (87086-87088)*
Dipstick (81000-81002)
0.00 0.00 Global Days XXX

81015 **microscopic only**
EXCLUDES *Sperm evaluation for retrograde ejaculation (89331)*
0.00 0.00 Global Days XXX
AMA: 2008, Apr, 5-7

81020 **2 or 3 glass test**
INCLUDES Valentine's test
0.00 0.00 Global Days XXX

81025 **Urine pregnancy test, by visual color comparison methods**
0.00 0.00 Global Days XXX

81050 **Volume measurement for timed collection, each**
0.00 0.00 Global Days XXX

81099 **Unlisted urinalysis procedure**
0.00 0.00 Global Days XXX

81200-81355 Gene Analysis

INCLUDES All analytical procedures in the evaluation such as:
Amplification
Cell lysis
Detection
Digestion
Extraction
Nucleic acid stabilization
Code selection based on specific gene being reviewed
Evaluation of constitutional or somatic gene variations
Evaluation of the presence of a gene variants using the common gene variant name
Examples of proteins or diseases in the code description that are not all inclusive
Generally all the listed gene variants in the code description would be tested but lists are not all inclusive
Gene specific and genomic testing
Genes that are described using the Human Genome Organization (HUGO) approved names
Qualitative results unless otherwise stated
Tier 1 molecular pathology codes (81200-81355)

EXCLUDES *Array-based evaluation of multiple molecular probes (88384-88386)*
Codes not listed in this section for molecular methodolgy testing (83890-83914, 88384-88386)
Codes not listed in this section for Tier 2 codes (81400-81408)
Microbial identification (87149-87153, 87470-87801, 87900-87904 [87906])
Molecular diagnostics (83890-83913)
Mutation identification (83914)
Tier 1 molecular pathology codes (81370-81383)

Code also modifier 26 when only interpretation and report are performed
Code also services required before cell lysis
Do not report full gene sequencing using separately gene variant assessment codes unless it is specifically stated in the code description
Do not report other related gene variants not listed in code

● **81200** ***ASPA (aspartoacylase)*** **(eg, Canavan disease) gene analysis, common variants (eg, E285A, Y231X)**
0.00 0.00 Global Days XXX

● **81205** ***BCKDHB (branched-chain keto acid dehydrogenase E1, beta polypeptide)*** **(eg, Maple syrup urine disease) gene analysis, common variants (eg, R183P, G278S, E422X)**
0.00 0.00 Global Days XXX

● 81206 *BCR/ABL1 (t(9;22))* (eg, chronic myelogenous leukemia) translocation analysis; major breakpoint, qualitative or quantitative B
0.00 0.00 Global Days XXX

● 81207 minor breakpoint, qualitative or quantitative B
0.00 0.00 Global Days XXX

● 81208 other breakpoint, qualitative or quantitative B
0.00 0.00 Global Days XXX

● 81209 *BLM (Bloom syndrome, RecQ helicase-like)* (eg, Bloom syndrome) gene analysis, 2281del6ins7 variant B
0.00 0.00 Global Days XXX

● 81210 *BRAF (v-raf murine sarcoma viral oncogene homolog B1)* (eg, colon cancer), gene analysis, V600E variant B
0.00 0.00 Global Days XXX

● 81211 *BRCA1, BRCA2 (breast cancer 1 and 2)* (eg, hereditary breast and ovarian cancer) gene analysis; full sequence analysis and common duplication/deletion variants in BRCA1 (ie, exon 13 del 3.835kb, exon 13 dup 6kb, exon 14-20 del 26kb, exon 22 del 510bp, exon 8-9 del 7.1kb) B
0.00 0.00 Global Days XXX

● 81212 185delAG, 5385insC, 6174delT variants B
0.00 0.00 Global Days XXX

● 81213 uncommon duplication/deletion variants B
0.00 0.00 Global Days XXX

● 81214 *BRCA1 (breast cancer 1)* (eg, hereditary breast and ovarian cancer) gene analysis; full sequence analysis and common duplication/deletion variants (ie, exon 13 del 3.835kb, exon 13 dup 6kb, exon 14-20 del 26kb, exon 22 del 510bp, exon 8-9 del 7.1kb) B

EXCLUDES *BRCA1 and BRCA2 full sequence testing (81211)*

0.00 0.00 Global Days XXX

● 81215 known familial variant B
0.00 0.00 Global Days XXX

● 81216 *BRCA2 (breast cancer 2)* (eg, hereditary breast and ovarian cancer) gene analysis; full sequence analysis B

EXCLUDES *BRCA1 and BRCA2 full sequence testing (81211)*

0.00 0.00 Global Days XXX

● 81217 known familial variant B
0.00 0.00 Global Days XXX

● 81220 *CFTR (cystic fibrosis transmembrane conductance regulator)* (eg, cystic fibrosis) gene analysis; common variants (eg, ACMG/ACOG guidelines) B

Do not report these two codes together when performed on an R117H positive patient (81220, 81224)

0.00 0.00 Global Days XXX

● 81221 known familial variants B
0.00 0.00 Global Days XXX

● 81222 duplication/deletion variants B
0.00 0.00 Global Days XXX

● 81223 full gene sequence B
0.00 0.00 Global Days XXX

● 81224 intron 8 poly-T analysis (eg, male infertility) ♂ B
0.00 0.00 Global Days XXX

● 81225 *CYP2C19 (cytochrome P450, family 2, subfamily C, polypeptide 19)* (eg, drug metabolism), gene analysis, common variants (eg, *2, *3, *4, *8, *17) B
0.00 0.00 Global Days XXX

● 81226 *CYP2D6 (cytochrome P450, family 2, subfamily D, polypeptide 6)* (eg, drug metabolism), gene analysis, common variants (eg, *2, *3, *4, *5, *6, *9, *10, *17, *19, *29, *35, *41, *1XN, *2XN, *4XN) B
0.00 0.00 Global Days XXX

● 81227 *CYP2C9 (cytochrome P450, family 2, subfamily C, polypeptide 9)* (eg, drug metabolism), gene analysis, common variants (eg, *2, *3, *5, *6) B
0.00 0.00 Global Days XXX

● 81228 Cytogenomic constitutional (genome-wide) microarray analysis; interrogation of genomic regions for copy number variants (eg, Bacterial Artificial Chromosome [BAC] or oligo-based comparative genomic hybridization [CGH] microarray analysis) B

Do not report with (81229)

0.00 0.00 Global Days XXX

● 81229 interrogation of genomic regions for copy number and single nucleotide polymorphism (SNP) variants for chromosomal abnormalities B

Do not report with (81228)

0.00 0.00 Global Days XXX

● 81240 *F2 (prothrombin, coagulation factor II)* (eg, hereditary hypercoagulability) gene analysis, 20210G>A variant B
0.00 0.00 Global Days XXX

● 81241 *F5 (coagulation Factor V)* (eg, hereditary hypercoagulability) gene analysis, Leiden variant B
0.00 0.00 Global Days XXX

● 81242 *FANCC (Fanconi anemia, complementation group C)* (eg, Fanconi anemia, type C) gene analysis, common variant (eg, IVS4+4A>T) B
0.00 0.00 Global Days XXX

● 81243 *FMR1 (Fragile X mental retardation 1)* (eg, fragile X mental retardation) gene analysis; evaluation to detect abnormal (eg, expanded) alleles B

INCLUDES Testing for detection and characterization of abnormal alleles using a single assay such as PCR

Code also characterization of abnormal alleles, unless performed by a single assay technique (81244)

0.00 0.00 Global Days XXX

● 81244 characterization of alleles (eg, expanded size and methylation status) B

EXCLUDES *Testing for detection and characterization of abnormal alleles using a single assay such as PCR (81243)*

Code also characterization of abnormal alleles, unless performed by a single assay technique (81243)

0.00 0.00 Global Days XXX

● 81245 *FLT3 (fms-related tyrosine kinase 3)* (eg, acute myeloid leukemia), gene analysis, internal tandem duplication (ITD) variants (ie, exons 14, 15) B
0.00 0.00 Global Days XXX

● 81250 *G6PC (glucose-6-phosphatase, catalytic subunit)* (eg, Glycogen storage disease, Type 1a, von Gierke disease) gene analysis, common variants (eg, R83C, Q347X) B
0.00 0.00 Global Days XXX

● 81251 *GBA (glucosidase, beta, acid)* (eg, Gaucher disease) gene analysis, common variants (eg, N370S, 84GG, L444P, IVS2+1G>A) B
0.00 0.00 Global Days XXX

● 81255 *HEXA (hexosaminidase A [alpha polypeptide])* (eg, Tay-Sachs disease) gene analysis, common variants (eg, 1278insTATC, 1421+1G>C, G269S) B
0.00 0.00 Global Days XXX

● 81256 *HFE (hemochromatosis)* (eg, hereditary hemochromatosis) gene analysis, common variants (eg, C282Y, H63D) B
0.00 0.00 Global Days XXX

● 81257 *HBA1/HBA2 (alpha globin 1 and alpha globin 2)* (eg, alpha thalassemia, Hb Bart hydrops fetalis syndrome, HbH disease), gene analysis, for common deletions or variant (eg, Southeast Asian, Thai, Filipino, Mediterranean, alpha3.7, alpha4.2, alpha20.5, and Constant Spring) B
0.00 0.00 Global Days XXX

● 81260 *IKBKAP (inhibitor of kappa light polypeptide gene enhancer in B-cells, kinase complex-associated protein)* (eg, familial dysautonomia) gene analysis, common variants (eg, 2507+6T>C, R696P) B
0.00 0.00 Global Days XXX

● 81261 *IGH@ (Immunoglobulin heavy chain locus)* (eg, leukemias and lymphomas, B-cell), gene rearrangement analysis to detect abnormal clonal population(s); amplified methodology (eg, polymerase chain reaction) B
0.00 0.00 Global Days XXX

● 81262 direct probe methodology (eg, Southern blot) B
0.00 0.00 Global Days XXX

● 81263 *IGH@ (Immunoglobulin heavy chain locus)* (eg, leukemia and lymphoma, B-cell), variable region somatic mutation analysis B
0.00 0.00 Global Days XXX

● 81264 *IGK@ (Immunoglobulin kappa light chain locus)* (eg, leukemia and lymphoma, B-cell), gene rearrangement analysis, evaluation to detect abnormal clonal population(s) B

EXCLUDES *Immunoglobulin kappa deleting element (IGKDEL) testing (83890-83914)*
Immunoglobuline lambda gene (IGL@) rearrangement (83890-83914)

0.00 0.00 Global Days XXX

● 81265 Comparative analysis using Short Tandem Repeat (STR) markers; patient and comparative specimen (eg, pre-transplant recipient and donor germline testing, post-transplant non-hematopoietic recipient germline [eg, buccal swab or other germline tissue sample] and donor testing, twin zygosity testing, or maternal cell contamination of fetal cells) B

Code also the following codes for chimerism testing if comparative short tandem repeat (STR) analysis of recipient (using buccal swab or other germline tissue sample) and donor are performed after hematopoietic stem cell transplantation (81266-81268)
0.00 0.00 Global Days XXX

+ ● 81266 each additional specimen (eg, additional cord blood donor, additional fetal samples from different cultures, or additional zygosity in multiple birth pregnancies) (List separately in addition to code for primary procedure) B

Code also the following codes for chimerism testing if comparative short tandem repeat (STR) analysis of recipient (using buccal swab or other germline tissue sample) and donar are performed after hematopoietic stem cell transplantation (81265, 81267-81268)
Code first (81265)
0.00 0.00 Global Days XXX

● 81267 Chimerism (engraftment) analysis, post transplantation specimen (eg, hematopoietic stem cell), includes comparison to previously performed baseline analyses; without cell selection B

Code also the following codes for chimerism testing if comparative short tandem repeat (STR) analysis of recipient (using buccal swab or other germline tissue sample) and donor are performed after hematopoietic stem cell transplantation (81265-81266, 81268)
0.00 0.00 Global Days XXX

● 81268 with cell selection (eg, CD3, CD33), each cell type B

Code also the following codes for chimerism testing if comparative short tandem repeat (STR) analysis of recipient (using buccal swab or other germline tissue sample) and donar are performed after hematopoietic stem cell transplantation (81265-81267)
0.00 0.00 Global Days XXX

● 81270 *JAK2 (Janus kinase 2)* (eg, myeloproliferative disorder) gene analysis, p.Val617Phe (V617F) variant B
0.00 0.00 Global Days XXX

● 81275 *KRAS (v-Ki-ras2 Kirsten rat sarcoma viral oncogene)* (eg, carcinoma) gene analysis, variants in codons 12 and 13 B
0.00 0.00 Global Days XXX

● 81280 Long QT syndrome gene analyses (eg, *KCNQ1, KCNH2, SCN5A, KCNE1, KCNE2, KCNJ2, CACNA1C, CAV3, SCN4B, AKAP, SNTA1, and ANK2)*; full sequence analysis B
0.00 0.00 Global Days XXX

● 81281 known familial sequence variant B
0.00 0.00 Global Days XXX

● 81282 duplication/deletion variants B
0.00 0.00 Global Days XXX

● 81290 *MCOLN1 (mucolipin 1)* (eg, Mucolipidosis, type IV) gene analysis, common variants (eg, IVS3-2A>G, del6.4kb) B
0.00 0.00 Global Days XXX

● 81291 *MTHFR (5,10-methylenetetrahydrofolate reductase)* (eg, hereditary hypercoagulability) gene analysis, common variants (eg, 677T, 1298C) B
0.00 0.00 Global Days XXX

● 81292 *MLH1 (mutL homolog 1, colon cancer, nonpolyposis type 2)* (eg, hereditary non-polyposis colorectal cancer, Lynch syndrome) gene analysis; full sequence analysis B
0.00 0.00 Global Days XXX

● 81293 known familial variants B
0.00 0.00 Global Days XXX

● 81294 duplication/deletion variants B
0.00 0.00 Global Days XXX

● 81295 *MSH2 (mutS homolog 2, colon cancer, nonpolyposis type 1)* (eg, hereditary non-polyposis colorectal cancer, Lynch syndrome) gene analysis; full sequence analysis B
0.00 0.00 Global Days XXX

● 81296 known familial variants B
0.00 0.00 Global Days XXX

● 81297 duplication/deletion variants B
0.00 0.00 Global Days XXX

● 81298 *MSH6 (mutS homolog 6 [E. coli])* (eg, hereditary non-polyposis colorectal cancer, Lynch syndrome) gene analysis; full sequence analysis B
0.00 0.00 Global Days XXX

● 81299 known familial variants B
0.00 0.00 Global Days XXX

● 81300 duplication/deletion variants [B]
0.00 0.00 Global Days XXX

● 81301 Microsatellite instability analysis (eg, hereditary non-polyposis colorectal cancer, Lynch syndrome) of markers for mismatch repair deficiency (eg, BAT25, BAT26), includes comparison of neoplastic and normal tissue, if performed [B]
0.00 0.00 Global Days XXX

● 81302 *MECP2 (methyl CpG binding protein 2)* (eg, Rett syndrome) gene analysis; full sequence analysis [B]
0.00 0.00 Global Days XXX

● 81303 known familial variant [B]
0.00 0.00 Global Days XXX

● 81304 duplication/deletion variants [B]
0.00 0.00 Global Days XXX

● 81310 *NPM1 (nucleophosmin)* (eg, acute myeloid leukemia) gene analysis, exon 12 variants [B]
0.00 0.00 Global Days XXX

● 81315 *PML/RARalpha, (t(15;17)), (promyelocytic leukemia/retinoic acid receptor alpha)* (eg, promyelocytic leukemia) translocation analysis; common breakpoints (eg, intron 3 and intron 6), qualitative or quantitative [B]
INCLUDES Intron 3 and 6 (and exon 6 if performed) testing
0.00 0.00 Global Days XXX

● 81316 single breakpoint (eg, intron 3, intron 6 or exon 6), qualitative or quantitative [B]
EXCLUDES *Intron 3 and 6 (and exon 6 if performed) testing (81315)*

Do not report more than one unit of this code for testing intron 3 and 6 (and exon 6 if performed) (81316)
0.00 0.00 Global Days XXX

● 81317 *PMS2 (postmeiotic segregation increased 2 [S. cerevisiae])* (eg, hereditary non-polyposis colorectal cancer, Lynch syndrome) gene analysis; full sequence analysis [B]
0.00 0.00 Global Days XXX

● 81318 known familial variants [B]
0.00 0.00 Global Days XXX

● 81319 duplication/deletion variants [B]
0.00 0.00 Global Days XXX

● 81330 *SMPD1(sphingomyelin phosphodiesterase 1, acid lysosomal)* (eg, Niemann-Pick disease, Type A) gene analysis, common variants (eg, R496L, L302P, fsP330) [B]
0.00 0.00 Global Days XXX

● 81331 *SNRPN/UBE3A (small nuclear ribonucleoprotein polypeptide N and ubiquitin protein ligase E3A)* (eg, Prader-Willi syndrome and/or Angelman syndrome), methylation analysis [B]
0.00 0.00 Global Days XXX

● 81332 *SERPINA1 (serpin peptidase inhibitor, clade A, alpha-1 antiproteinase, antitrypsin, member 1)* (eg, alpha-1-antitrypsin deficiency), gene analysis, common variants (eg, *S and *Z) [B]
0.00 0.00 Global Days XXX

● 81340 *TRB@ (T cell antigen receptor, beta)* (eg, leukemia and lymphoma), gene rearrangement analysis to detect abnormal clonal population(s); using amplification methodology (eg, polymerase chain reaction) [B]
0.00 0.00 Global Days XXX

● 81341 using direct probe methodology (eg, Southern blot) [B]
0.00 0.00 Global Days XXX

● 81342 *TRG@ (T cell antigen receptor, gamma)* (eg, leukemia and lymphoma), gene rearrangement analysis, evaluation to detect abnormal clonal population(s) [B]
EXCLUDES *T cell antigen alpha [TRA@] gene arrangement testing (83890-83914)*
T cell antigen delta [TRD@] gene arrangement testing (81402)
0.00 0.00 Global Days XXX

● 81350 *UGT1A1 (UDP glucuronosyltransferase 1 family, polypeptide A1)* (eg, irinotecan metabolism), gene analysis, common variants (eg, *28, *36, *37) [B]
0.00 0.00 Global Days XXX

● 81355 *VKORC1 (vitamin K epoxide reductase complex, subunit 1)* (eg, warfarin metabolism), gene analysis, common variants (eg, -1639/3673) [B]
0.00 0.00 Global Days XXX

81370-81383 Human Leukocyte Antigen (HLA) Testing

INCLUDES Additional testing that must be performed to resolve ambiguous allele combinations for high-resolution typing
All analytical procedures in the evaluation such as:
Amplification
Cell lysis
Detection
Digestion
Extraction
Nucleic acid
Stabilization
Analysis to identify human leukocyte antigen (HLA) alleles and allele groups connected to specific deseases and individual response to drug therapy in addition to other clinical uses
Code selection based on specific gene being reviewed
Evaluation of the presence of a gene variants using the common gene variant name
Examples of proteins or diseases in the code description that are not all inclusive
Generally all the listed gene variants in the code description would be tested but lists are not all inclusive
Genes that are described using the Human Genome Organization (HUGO) approved names
High-resolution typing resolves the common well-defined (CWD) alleles and is usually identified by at least four-digits. There are some instances when high-resolution typing may include some ambiguities for rare alleles, and those may be reported as a string of alleles or an NMDP code
Histocompatibility antigen testing
Intermediate resolution HLA testing is identified by a string of alleles or a National Marrow Donor Program (NMDP) code
Low and intermediate resolution are considered low resolution for code assignment
Low-resolution HLA type reporting is identified by two-digit HLA name
Mulitple variant alleles or allele groups that can be identified by typing
One or more HLA genes in specific clinical circumstances
Qualitative results unless otherwise stated
Typing performed to determine the compatibility of recipients and potential donors undergoing solid organ or hematopoietic stem cell pretransplantation testing

EXCLUDES *Array-based evaluation of multiple molecular probes (88384-88386)*
Codes not listed in this section for molecular methodology testing (83890-83914, 88384-88386)
Codes not listed in this section for Tier 2 codes (81400-81408)
HLA antigen typing by nonmolecular pathology methods (86812-86822)
Microbial identification (87149-87153, 87470-87801, 87900-87904 [87906])
Molecular diagnostics (83890-83914, 88384-88386)
Mutation identification (83914)
Tier 1 molecular pathology codes (81200-81355)

Code also modifier 26 when only interpretation and report are performed
Code also services required before cell lysis
Do not report full gene sequencing separately using gene variant assessment codes unless it is specifically stated in the code description
Do not report other related gene variants not listed in code

● **81370** **HLA Class I and II typing, low resolution (eg, antigen equivalents); *HLA-A, -B, -C, -DRB1/3/4/5, and -DQB1*** B
0.00 0.00 Global Days XXX

● **81371** ***HLA-A, -B, and -DRB1/3/4/5*** **(eg, verification typing)** B
0.00 0.00 Global Days XXX

● **81372** **HLA Class I typing, low resolution (eg, antigen equivalents); complete *(ie, HLA-A, -B, and -C)*** B
EXCLUDES *Class I and II low-resolution HLA typing for HLA-A, -B, -C, -DRB1/3/4/5, and -DQB1 (81370)*
0.00 0.00 Global Days XXX

● **81373** **1 locus *(eg, HLA-A, -B, or -C)*, each** B
EXCLUDES *A complete Class 1 (HLA-A, -B, and -C) low-resolution typing (81372)*
Reporting the presence or absence of a single antigen equivalent using low-resolution methodology (81374)
0.00 0.00 Global Days XXX

● **81374** **1 antigen equivalent *(eg, B*27)*, each** B
EXCLUDES *Testing for the presence or absence of more than 2 antigen equivalents at a locus, use the following code for each locus test (81373)*
0.00 0.00 Global Days XXX

● **81375** **HLA Class II typing, low resolution (eg, antigen equivalents); *HLA-DRB1/3/4/5 and -DQB1*** B
EXCLUDES *Class I and II low-resolution HLA typing for HLA-A, -B, -C, -DRB 1/3/4/5, and DQB1 (81370)*
0.00 0.00 Global Days XXX

● **81376** **1 locus (eg, *HLA-DRB1/3/4/5, -DQB1, -DQA1, -DPB1, or -DPA1*), each** B
INCLUDES Low-resolution typing, HLA-DRB1/3/4/5 reported as a single locus
EXCLUDES *Low-resolution typing for HLA-DRB1/3/4/5 and -DQB1 (81375)*
0.00 0.00 Global Days XXX

● **81377** **1 antigen equivalent, each** B
EXCLUDES *Testing for presence or absence of more than two antigen equivalents at a locus (81376)*
0.00 0.00 Global Days XXX

● **81378** **HLA Class I and II typing, high resolution (ie, alleles or allele groups), *HLA-A, -B, -C, and -DRB1*** B
0.00 0.00 Global Days XXX

● **81379** **HLA Class I typing, high resolution (ie, alleles or allele groups); complete (ie, *HLA-A, -B, and -C*)** B
0.00 0.00 Global Days XXX

● **81380** **1 locus (eg, *HLA-A, -B, or -C*), each** B
EXCLUDES *Complete Class I high-resolution typing for HLA-A, -B, and -C (81379)*
Testing for presence or absence of a single allele or allele group using high-resolution methodology (81381)
0.00 0.00 Global Days XXX

● **81381** **1 allele or allele group (eg, *B*57:01P*), each** B
INCLUDES Testing for the presence or absence of more than two alleles or allele groups of locus, report the following code for each locus (81380)
0.00 0.00 Global Days XXX

● **81382** **HLA Class II typing, high resolution (ie, alleles or allele groups); one locus (eg, *HLA-DRB1, -DRB3, -DRB4, -DRB5, -DQB1, -DQA1, -DPB1, or -DPA1*), each** B
EXCLUDES *Testing for just the presence or absence of a single allele or allele group using high-resolution methodology (81383)*
0.00 0.00 Global Days XXX

● 81383 1 allele or allele group (eg, *HLA-DQB1*06:02P*), each B

EXCLUDES *For testing for the presence or absence of more than two alleles or allele groups at a locus, report the following code for each locus (81382)*

0.00 0.00 Global Days XXX

81400-81408 Molecular Pathology

INCLUDES All analytical procedures in the evaluation such as:
- Amplification
- Cell lysis
- Detection
- Digestion
- Extraction
- Nucleic acid
- Stabilization

Code selection based on specific gene being reviewed

Codes that are arranged by level of technical resources and work involved

Evaluation of the presence of a gene variant using the common gene variant name

Examples in parentheses at near the beginning of the code descriptions that are not all inclusive

Examples of proteins or diseases in the code description that are not all inclusive

Generally all the listed gene variants in the code description would be tested but lists are not all inclusive

Genes that are described using the Human Genome Organization (HUGO) approved names

Histocompatibility testing

Qualitative results unless otherwise stated

Specific analytes listed after the code description to use for selecting the appropriate molecular pathology procedure

Testing for diseases that are more rare

EXCLUDES *Codes not listed in this section, the Gene Testing section, or the HLA testing sections (83890-83914, 88384-88386)*

Microbial identification (87149-87153, 87470-87801, 87900-87904 [87906])

Tier 1 molecular pathology (81200-81383)

Code also modifier 26 when only interpretation and report are performed

Code also services required before cell lysis

Do not report full gene sequencing separately using gene variant assessment codes unless it is specifically stated in the code description

Do not report other related gene variants not listed in the code description

● **81400 Molecular pathology procedure, Level 1 (eg, identification of single germline variant [eg, SNP] by techniques such as restriction enzyme digestion or melt curve analysis)** B

INCLUDES *ACADM (acyl-CoA dehydrogenase, C-4 to C-12 straight chain, MCAD)* (eg, medium chain acyl dehydrogenase deficiency), K304E variant

ACE (angiotensin converting enzyme) (eg, hereditary blood pressure regulation), insertion/deletion variant

AGTR1 (angiotensin II receptor, type 1) (eg, essential hypertension), 1166A>C variant

CCR5 (chemokine C-C motif receptor 5) (eg, HIV resistance), 32-bp deletion mutation/794 825del32 deletion

DPYD (dihydropyrimidine dehydrogenase) (eg, 5-fluorouracil/5-FU and capecitabine drug metabolism), IVS14+1G>A variant

F2 (coagulation factor 2) (eg, hereditary hypercoagulability), 1199G>A variant

F5 (coagulation factor V) (eg, hereditary hypercoagulability), HR2 variant

F7 (coagulation factor VII [serum prothrombin conversion accelerator]) (eg, hereditary hypercoagulability), R353Q variant

F13B (coagulation factor XIII, B polypeptide) (eg, hereditary hypercoagulability), V34L variant

FGB (fibrinogen beta chain) (eg, hereditary ischemic heart disease), -455G>A variant

Human platelet antigen 1 genotyping (HPA-1), *ITGB3 (integrin, beta 3 [platelet glycoprotein IIIa], antigen CD61 [GPIIIa])* (eg, neonatal alloimmune thrombocytopenia [NAIT], post-transfusion purpura), HPA-1a/b (L33P)

Human platelet antigen 2 genotyping (HPA-2), *GP1BA (glycoprotein Ib [platelet], alpha polypeptide [GPIba])* (eg, neonatal alloimmune thrombocytopenia [NAIT], post-transfusion purpura), HPA-2a/b (T145M)

Human platelet antigen 3 genotyping (HPA-3), *ITGA2B (integrin, alpha 2b [platelet glycoprotein IIb of IIb/IIIa complex], antigen CD41 [GPIIb])* (eg, neonatal alloimmune thrombocytopenia [NAIT], post-transfusion purpura), HPA-3a/b (I843S)

Human platelet antigen 4 genotyping (HPA-4), *ITGB3 (integrin, beta 3 [platelet glycoprotein IIIa], antigen CD61 [GPIIIa])* (eg, neonatal alloimmune thrombocytopenia [NAIT], post-transfusion purpura), HPA-4a/b (R143Q)

Human platelet antigen 5 genotyping (HPA-5), *ITGA2 (integrin, alpha 2 [CD49B, alpha 2 subunit of VLA-2 receptor] [GPIa])* (eg, neonatal alloimmune thrombocytopenia [NAIT], post-transfusion purpura), HPA-5a/b (K505E)

Human platelet antigen 6 genotyping (HPA-6w), *ITGB3 (integrin, beta 3 [platelet glycoprotein IIIa, antigen CD61] [GPIIIa])* (eg, neonatal alloimmune thrombocytopenia [NAIT], post-transfusion purpura), HPA-6a/b (R489Q)

Human platelet antigen 9 genotyping (HPA-9w), *ITGA2B (integrin, alpha 2b [platelet glycoprotein IIb of IIb/IIIa complex, antigen CD41] [GPIIb])* (eg, neonatal alloimmune thrombocytopenia [NAIT], post-transfusion purpura), HPA-9a/b (V837M)

Human platelet antigen 15 genotyping (HPA-15), *CD109 (CD109 molecule)* (eg, neonatal alloimmune thrombocytopenia [NAIT], post-transfusion purpura), HPA-15a/b(S682Y)

SERPINE1 (serpine peptidase inhibitor clade E, member 1, plasminogen activator inhibitor -1, PAI-1) (eg, thrombophilia), 4G variant

0.00 0.00 Global Days XXX

● 81401 **Molecular pathology procedure, Level 2 (eg, 2-10 SNPs, 1 methylated variant, or 1 somatic variant [typically using nonsequencing target variant analysis], or detection of a dynamic mutation disorder/triplet repeat)** B

INCLUDES *ABL (c-abl oncogene 1, receptor tyrosine kinase)* (eg, acquired imatinib resistance), T315I variant
ACADM (acyl-CoA dehydrogenase, C-4 to C-12 straight chain, MCAD) (eg, medium chain acyl dehydrogenase deficiency), common variants (eg, K304E, Y42H)
ADRB2 (adrenergic beta-2 receptor surface) (eg, drug metabolism), common variants (eg, G16R, Q27E)
APOE (apolipoprotein E) (eg, hyperlipoproteinemia type III, cardiovascular disease, Alzheimer disease), common variants (eg, *2, *3, *4)
CBFB/MYH11 (inv(16)) (eg, acute myeloid leukemia), qualitative, and quantitative, if performed
CCND1/IGH (BCL1/IgH, t(11;14)) (eg, mantle cell lymphoma) translocation analysis, major breakpoint, qualitative and quantitative, if performed
CFH/ARMS2 (complement factor H/age-related maculopathy susceptibility 2) (eg, macular degeneration), common variants (eg, Y402H [CFH], A69S [ARMS2])
CYP3A4 (cytochrome P450, family 3, subfamily A, polypeptide 4) (eg, drug metabolism), common variants (eg, *2, *3, *4, *5, *6)
CYP3A5 (cytochrome P450, family 3, subfamily A, polypeptide 5) (eg, drug metabolism), common variants (eg, *2, *3, *4, *5, *6)
DMPK (dystrophia myotonica-protein kinase) (eg, myotonic dystrophy, type 1), evaluation to detect abnormal (eg, expanded) alleles
F11 (coagulation factor XI) (eg, coagulation disorder), common variants (eg, E117X [Type II], F283L [Type III], IVS14del14, and IVS14+1G>A [Type I])
FGFR3 (fibroblast growth factor receptor 3) (eg, achondroplasia), common variants (eg, 1138G>A, 1138G>C)
FIP1L1/PDGFRA (del[4q12]) (eg, imatinib-sensitive chronic eosinophilic leukemia), qualitative and quantitative, if performed
GALT (galactose-1-phosphate uridylyltransferase) (eg, galactosemia), common variants (eg, Q188R, S135L, K285N, T138M, L195P, Y209C, IVS2-2A>G, P171S, del5kb, N314D, L218L/N314D)
HBB (hemoglobin, beta) (eg, sickle cell anemia, hemoglobin C, hemoglobin E), common variants (eg, HbS, HbC, HbE)
HTT (huntingtin) (eg, Huntington disease), evaluation to detect abnormal (eg, expanded) alleles
RUNX1/RUNX1T1 (t(8;21)) (eg, acute myeloid leukemia) translocation analysis, qualitative and quantitative, if performed
SEPT9 (Septin 9) (eg, colon cancer), methylation analysis
TPMT (thiopurine S-methyltransferase) (eg, drug metabolism), common variants (eg, *2, *3)
VWF (von Willebrand factor) (eg, von Willebrand disease type 2N), common variants (eg, T791M, R816W, R854Q)

0.00 0.00 **Global Days XXX**

● 81402 **Molecular pathology procedure, Level 3 (eg, > 10 SNPs, 2-10 methylated variants, or 2-10 somatic variants [typically using non-sequencing target variant analysis], immunoglobulin and T-cell receptor gene rearrangements, duplication/deletion variants 1 exon)** B

INCLUDES *CYP21A2 (cytochrome P450, family 21, subfamily A, polypeptide 2)* (eg, congenital adrenal hyperplasia, 21-hydroxylase deficiency), common variants (eg, IVS2-13G, P30L, I172N, exon 6 mutation cluster [I235N, V236E, M238K], V281L, L307FfsX6, Q318X, R356W, P453S, G110VfsX21, 30-kb deletion variant)
ESR1/PGR (receptor 1/progesterone receptor) ratio (eg, breast cancer)
KIT (v-kit Hardy-Zuckerman 4 feline sarcoma viral oncogene homolog) (eg, mastocytosis), common variants (eg, D816V, D816Y, D816F)
MEFV (Mediterranean fever) (eg, familial Mediterranean fever), common variants (eg, E148Q, P369S, F479L, M680I, I692del, M694V, M694I, K695R, V726A, A744S, R761H)
MPL (myeloproliferative leukemia virus oncogene, thrombopoietin receptor, TPOR) (eg, myeloproliferative disorder), common variants (eg, W515A, W515K, W515L, W515R)
TRD@ (T cell antigen receptor, delta) (eg, leukemia and lymphoma), gene rearrangement analysis, evaluation to detect abnormal clonal population

0.00 0.00 **Global Days XXX**

● 81403 **Molecular pathology procedure, Level 4 (eg, analysis of single exon by DNA sequence analysis, analysis of > 10 amplicons using multiplex PCR in 2 or more independent reactions, mutation scanning or duplication/deletion variants of 2-5 exons)** B

INCLUDES *ABL1 (c-abl oncogene 1, receptor tyrosine kinase)* (eg, acquired imatinib tyrosine kinase inhibitor resistance), variants in the kinase domain

DAZ/SRY (deleted in azoospermia and sex determining region Y) (eg, male infertility), common deletions (eg, AZFa, AZFb, AZFc, AZFd)

GJB1 (gap junction protein, beta 1) (eg, Charcot-Marie-Tooth X-linked), full gene sequence

JAK2 (Janus kinase 2) (eg, myeloproliferative disorder), exon 12 sequence and exon 13 sequence, if performed

KRAS (v-Ki-ras2 Kirsten rat sarcoma viral oncogene) (eg, carcinoma), gene analysis, variant(s) in exon 2

MPL (myeloproliferative leukemia virus oncogene, thrombopoietin receptor, TPOR) (eg, myeloproliferative disorder), exon 10 sequence

VHL (von Hippel-Lindau tumor suppressor) (eg, von Hippel-Lindau familial cancer syndrome), deletion/duplication analysis

VWF (von Willebrand factor) (eg, von Willebrand disease types 2A, 2B, 2M), targeted sequence analysis (eg, exon 28)

0.00 0.00 Global Days XXX

● 81404 **Molecular pathology procedure, Level 5 (eg, analysis of 2-5 exons by DNA sequence analysis, mutation scanning or duplication/deletion variants of 6-10 exons, or characterization of a dynamic mutation disorder/triplet repeat by Southern blot analysis)** B

INCLUDES *BTD (biotinidase)* (eg, biotinidase deficiency), full gene sequence
CYP1B1 (cytochrome P450, family 1, subfamily B, polypeptide 1) (eg, primary congenital glaucoma), full gene sequence
DMPK (dystrophia myotonica-protein kinase) (eg, myotonic dystrophy type 1), characterization of abnormal (eg, expanded) alleles
EGR2 (early growth response 2) (eg, Charcot-Marie-Tooth), full gene sequence
FKRP (Fukutin related protein) (eg, congenital muscular dystrophy type 1C [MDC1C], limb-girdle muscular dystrophy [LGMD] type 2I), full gene sequence
FOXG1 (forkhead box G1) (eg, Rett syndrome), full gene sequence
FSHMD1A (facioscapulohumeral muscular dystrophy 1A) (eg, facioscapulohumeral muscular dystrophy), evaluation to detect abnormal (eg, deleted) alleles
FSHMD1A (facioscapulohumeral muscular dystrophy 1A) (eg, facioscapulohumeral muscular dystrophy), characterization of haplotype(s) (ie, chromosome 4A and 4B haplotypes)
HBB (hemoglobin, beta, beta-globin) (eg, thalassemia), full gene sequence
KIT (C-kit) (v-kit Hardy-Zuckerman 4 feline sarcoma viral oncogene homolog) (eg, GIST, acute myeloid leukemia, melanoma), targeted gene analysis (eg, exons 8, 11, 13, 17, 18)
LITAF (lipopolysaccharide-induced TNF factor) (eg, Charcot-Marie-Tooth), full gene sequence
MEFV (Mediterranean fever) (eg, familial Mediterranean fever), full gene sequence
NRAS (neuroblastoma RAS viral oncogene homolog) (eg, colorectal carcinoma), exon 1 and exon 2 sequences
PDGFRA (platelet-derived growth factor receptor alpha polypeptide) (eg, gastrointestinal stromal tumor), targeted sequence analysis (eg, exons 12, 18)
RET (RET proto-oncogene) (eg, multiple endocrine neoplasia, type 2B and familial medullary thyroid carcinoma), common variants (eg, M918T, 2647_2648delinsTT, A883F)
SDHD (succinate dehydrogenase complex, subunit D, integral membrane protein) (eg, hereditary paraganglioma), full gene sequence
VHL (von Hippel-Lindau tumor suppressor) (eg, von Hippel-Lindau familial cancer syndrome), full gene sequence
VWF (von Willebrand factor) (eg, von Willebrand disease type 1C), targeted sequence analysis (eg, exons 26, 27, 37)

0.00 0.00 Global Days XXX

● 81405 **Molecular pathology procedure, Level 6 (eg, analysis of 6-10 exons by DNA sequence analysis, mutation scanning or duplication/deletion variants of 11-25 exons)** B

INCLUDES *CYP21A2 (cytochrome P450, family 21, subfamily A, polypeptide2)* (eg, steroid 21-hydroxylase isoform, congenital adrenal hyperplasia), full gene sequence
FKTN (fukutin) (eg, limb-girdle muscular dystrophy [LGMD] type 2M or 2L), full gene sequence
MPZ (myelin protein zero) (eg, Charcot-Marie-Tooth), full gene sequence
NEFL (neurofilament, light polypeptide) (eg, Charcot-Marie-Tooth), full gene sequence
RET (RET proto-oncogene) (eg, multiple endocrine neoplasia, type 2A and familial medullary thyroid carcinoma), targeted sequence analysis (eg, exons 10, 11, 13-16)
SDHB (succinate dehydrogenase complex, subunit B, iron sulfur) (eg, hereditary paraganglioma), full gene sequence
TGFBR1 (transforming growth factor, beta receptor 1) (eg, Marfan syndrome), full gene sequence
TGFBR2 (transforming growth factor, beta receptor 2) (eg, Marfan syndrome), full gene sequence
THRB (thyroid hormone receptor, beta) (eg, thyroid hormone resistance, thyroid hormone beta receptor deficiency), full gene sequence or targeted sequence analysis of >5 exons
TP53 (tumor protein 53) (eg, Li-Fraumeni syndrome, tumor samples), full gene sequence or targeted sequence analysis of >5 exons
VWF (von Willebrand factor) (eg, von Willebrand disease type 2N), targeted sequence analysis (eg, exons 18-20, 23-25)

0.00 0.00 Global Days XXX

● 81406 **Molecular pathology procedure, Level 7 (eg, analysis of 11-25 exons by DNA sequence analysis, mutation scanning or duplication/deletion variants of 26-50 exons, cytogenomic array analysis for neoplasia)** B

INCLUDES *CAPN3 (Calpain 3)* (eg, limb-girdle muscular dystrophy [LGMD] type 2A, calpainopathy), full gene sequence

Cytogenomic microarray analysis, neoplasia (eg, interrogation of copy number, and loss of heterozygosity via single nucleotide polymorphism [SNP]-based comparative genomic hybridization [CGH] microarray analysis)

GALT (galactose-1-phosphate uridylyltransferase) (eg, galactosemia), full gene sequence

HEXA (hexosaminidase A, alpha polypeptide) (eg, Tay-Sachs disease), full gene sequence

LMNA (lamin A/C) (eg, Emery-Dreifuss muscular dystrophy [EDMD1, 2 and 3] limb-girdle muscular dystrophy [LGMD] type 1B, dilated cardiomyopathy [CMD1A], familial partial lipodystrophy [FPLD2]), full gene sequence

PAH (phenylalanine hydroxylase) (eg, phenylketonuria), full gene sequence

POLG (polymerase [DNA directed], gamma) (eg, Alpers-Huttenlocher syndrome, autosomal dominant progressive external ophthalmoplegia), full gene sequence

POMGNT1 (protein O-linked mannose beta1, 2-N acetylglucosaminyltransferase) (eg, muscle-eye-brain disease, Walker-Warburg syndrome), full gene sequence

POMT1 (protein-O-mannosyltransferase 1) (eg, limb-girdle muscular dystrophy [LGMD] type 2K, Walker-Warburg syndrome), full gene sequence

POMT2 (protein-O-mannosyltransferase 2) (eg, limb-girdle muscular dystrophy [LGMD] type 2N, Walker-Warburg syndrome), full gene sequence

RYR1 (ryanodine receptor 1, skeletal) (eg, malignant hyperthermia), targeted sequence analysis of exons with functionally confirmed mutations

VWF (von Willebrand factor) (von Willebrand disease type 2A), extended targeted sequence analysis (eg, exons 11-16, 24-26, 51, 52)

0.00 0.00 Global Days XXX

● 81407 **Molecular pathology procedure, Level 8 (eg, analysis of 26-50 exons by DNA sequence analysis, mutation scanning or duplication/deletion variants of > 50 exons, sequence analysis of multiple genes on 1 platform)** B

INCLUDES *SCN1A (sodium channel, voltage-gated, type 1, alpha subunit)* (eg, generalized epilepsy with febrile seizures), full gene sequence

0.00 0.00 Global Days XXX

● 81408 **Molecular pathology procedure, Level 9 (eg, analysis of > 50 exons in a single gene by DNA sequence analysis)** B

INCLUDES *FBN1 (fibrillin 1)* (eg, Marfan syndrome), full gene sequence

NF1 (neurofibromin 1) (eg, neurofibromatosis, type 1), full gene sequence

RYR1 (ryanodine receptor 1, skeletal) (eg, malignant hyperthermia), full gene sequence

VWF (von Willebrand factor) (eg, von Willebrand disease types 1 and 3), full gene sequence

0.00 0.00 Global Days XXX

82000-82030 Chemistry: Acetaldehyde—Adenosine

CMS 100-2,15,80 Diagnostic Test Requirements
CMS 100-4,3,10.4 Payment of Nonphysician Services for Inpatients

INCLUDES Mathematically calculated results
Quantitative analysis unless otherwise specified
Specimens from any source unless otherwise specified

EXCLUDES *Organ or disease panels (80048-80076)*
Therapeutic drug assays (80150-80299)

82000 **Acetaldehyde, blood** A
0.00 0.00 Global Days XXX

82003 **Acetaminophen** A
0.00 0.00 Global Days XXX

82009 **Acetone or other ketone bodies, serum; qualitative** A
0.00 0.00 Global Days XXX

82010 **quantitative** A ☒
0.00 0.00 Global Days XXX

82013 **Acetylcholinesterase** A
EXCLUDES *Gastric acid analysis (82930)*
0.00 0.00 Global Days XXX

82016 **Acylcarnitines; qualitative, each specimen** A
0.00 0.00 Global Days XXX

82017 **quantitative, each specimen** A
0.00 0.00 Global Days XXX

82024 **Adrenocorticotropic hormone (ACTH)** A
0.00 0.00 Global Days XXX

82030 **Adenosine, 5-monophosphate, cyclic (cyclic AMP)** A
0.00 0.00 Global Days XXX

82040-82045 Chemistry: Albumin

CMS 100-2,15,80 Diagnostic Test Requirements
CMS 100-3,190.10 Laboratory Tests--CRD Patients
CMS 100-4,3,10.4 Payment of Nonphysician Services for Inpatients

INCLUDES Mathematically calculated results
Quantitative analysis unless otherwise specified
Specimens from any other sources unless otherwise specified

EXCLUDES *Organ or disease panels (80048-80076)*
Therapeutic drug assays (80150-80299)

82040 **Albumin; serum, plasma or whole blood** A ☒
0.00 0.00 Global Days XXX

82042 **urine or other source, quantitative, each specimen** A
0.00 0.00 Global Days XXX

82043 **urine, microalbumin, quantitative** A ☒
0.00 0.00 Global Days XXX

82044 **urine, microalbumin, semiquantitative (eg, reagent strip assay)** A ✖

EXCLUDES *Prealbumin (84134)*

0.00 0.00 Global Days XXX

AMA: 2009, Jan, 11-31; 2008, Jan, 10-25; 2007, January, 13-27

82045 **ischemia modified** A

0.00 0.00 Global Days XXX

82055-82107 Chemistry: Alcohol—Alpha-fetoprotein (AFP)

CMS 100-2,15,80 Diagnostic Test Requirements

CMS 100-4,3,10.4 Payment of Nonphysician Services for Inpatients

INCLUDES Mathematically calculated results
Quantitative analysis unless otherwise specified
Specimens from any source unless otherwise specified

EXCLUDES *Organ or disease panels (80048-80076)*
Therapeutic drug assays (80150-80299)

82055 **Alcohol (ethanol); any specimen except breath** A ✖

EXCLUDES *Alcohol breath test (82075)*
Other types of alcohols, volatiles (84600)

0.00 0.00 Global Days XXX

82075 **breath** A

0.00 0.00 Global Days XXX

82085 **Aldolase** A

0.00 0.00 Global Days XXX

82088 **Aldosterone** A

0.00 0.00 Global Days XXX

82101 **Alkaloids, urine, quantitative** A

0.00 0.00 Global Days XXX

82103 **Alpha-1-antitrypsin; total** A

0.00 0.00 Global Days XXX

82104 **phenotype** A

0.00 0.00 Global Days XXX

82105 **Alpha-fetoprotein (AFP); serum** A

0.00 0.00 Global Days XXX

82106 **amniotic fluid** M ♀ A

0.00 0.00 Global Days XXX

82107 **AFP-L3 fraction isoform and total AFP (including ratio)** A

0.00 0.00 Global Days XXX

82108 Chemistry: Aluminum

CMS 100-2,15,80 Diagnostic Test Requirements

CMS 100-3,190.10 Laboratory Tests--CRD Patients

CMS 100-4,3,10.4 Payment of Nonphysician Services for Inpatients

INCLUDES Mathematically calculated results
Quantitative analysis unless otherwise specified
Specimens from any source unless otherwise specified

EXCLUDES *Organ or disease panels (80048-80076)*
Therapeutic drug assays (80150-80299)

82108 **Aluminum** A

0.00 0.00 Global Days XXX

82120-82261 Chemistry: Amines—Biotinidase

CMS 100-2,15,80 Diagnostic Test Requirements

CMS 100-4,3,10.4 Payment of Nonphysician Services for Inpatients

INCLUDES Mathematically calculated results
Quantitative analysis unless otherwise specified
Specimens from any source unless otherwise specified

EXCLUDES *Organ or disease panels (80048-80076)*
Therapeutic drug assays (80150-80299)

82120 **Amines, vaginal fluid, qualitative** ♀ A ✖

EXCLUDES *Combined pH and amines test for vaginitis (82120, 83986)*

0.00 0.00 Global Days XXX

82127 **Amino acids; single, qualitative, each specimen** A

0.00 0.00 Global Days XXX

82128 **multiple, qualitative, each specimen** A

0.00 0.00 Global Days XXX

82131 **single, quantitative, each specimen** A

INCLUDES Van Slyke method

0.00 0.00 Global Days XXX

AMA: 2009, Jan, 11-31; 2008, Jan, 10-25; 2007, January, 13-27

82135 **Aminolevulinic acid, delta (ALA)** A

0.00 0.00 Global Days XXX

82136 **Amino acids, 2 to 5 amino acids, quantitative, each specimen** A

0.00 0.00 Global Days XXX

82139 **Amino acids, 6 or more amino acids, quantitative, each specimen** A

0.00 0.00 Global Days XXX

82140 **Ammonia** A

0.00 0.00 Global Days XXX

82143 **Amniotic fluid scan (spectrophotometric)** M ♀ A

EXCLUDES *L/S ratio (83661)*

0.00 0.00 Global Days XXX

82145 **Amphetamine or methamphetamine** A

EXCLUDES *Qualitative testing (80100-80103 [80104])*

0.00 0.00 Global Days XXX

82150 **Amylase** A ✖

0.00 0.00 Global Days XXX

82154 **Androstanediol glucuronide** A

0.00 0.00 Global Days XXX

82157 **Androstenedione** A

0.00 0.00 Global Days XXX

82160 **Androsterone** A

0.00 0.00 Global Days XXX

82163 **Angiotensin II** A

0.00 0.00 Global Days XXX

82164 **Angiotensin I - converting enzyme (ACE)** A

0.00 0.00 Global Days XXX

82172 **Apolipoprotein, each** A

0.00 0.00 Global Days XXX

82175 **Arsenic** A

EXCLUDES *Heavy metal screening (83015)*

0.00 0.00 Global Days XXX

82180 **Ascorbic acid (Vitamin C), blood** A

0.00 0.00 Global Days XXX

82190 **Atomic absorption spectroscopy, each analyte** A

0.00 0.00 Global Days XXX

82205 **Barbiturates, not elsewhere specified** A

EXCLUDES *Qualitative analysis (80100-80103 [80104])*

0.00 0.00 Global Days XXX

82232 **Beta-2 microglobulin** A
0.00 0.00 Global Days XXX

82239 **Bile acids; total** A
0.00 0.00 Global Days XXX

82240 **cholylglycine** A
EXCLUDES *Bile pigments, urine (81000-81005)*
0.00 0.00 Global Days XXX

82247 **Bilirubin; total** A ☒
INCLUDES Van Den Bergh test
0.00 0.00 Global Days XXX

82248 **direct** A
0.00 0.00 Global Days XXX

82252 **feces, qualitative** A
0.00 0.00 Global Days XXX

82261 **Biotinidase, each specimen** A
0.00 0.00 Global Days XXX

82270-82274 Chemistry: Occult Blood

CMS 100-2,15,80 Diagnostic Test Requirements
CMS 100-3,190.34 Fecal Occult Blood Test (FOBT)
CMS 100-4,3,10.4 Payment of Nonphysician Services for Inpatients
CMS 100-4,18,60 Colorectal Cancer Screening
CMS 100-4,18,60.1 Payment for Colorectal Screening Services
CMS 100-4,18,60.2 Frequency and Age Requirements for Colorectal Screening
CMS 100-4,18,60.2.1 Common Working File Edits: Colorectal Screening
CMS 100-4,18,60.6 Billing for Colorectal Screening Services

INCLUDES Mathematically calculated results
Quantitative analysis unless otherwise specified
Specimens from any source unless otherwise specified

EXCLUDES *Organ or disease panels (80048-80076)*
Therapeutic drug assays (80150-80299)

82270 **Blood, occult, by peroxidase activity (eg, guaiac), qualitative; feces, consecutive collected specimens with single determination, for colorectal neoplasm screening (ie, patient was provided 3 cards or single triple card for consecutive collection)** A ☒
INCLUDES Day test
0.00 0.00 Global Days XXX
AMA: 2009, Jan, 11-31; 2008, Jan, 10-25; 2008, Apr, 5-7; 2007, January, 13-27

82271 **other sources** A ☒
0.00 0.00 Global Days XXX

82272 **Blood, occult, by peroxidase activity (eg, guaiac), qualitative, feces, 1-3 simultaneous determinations, performed for other than colorectal neoplasm screening** A ☒
0.00 0.00 Global Days XXX
AMA: 2009, Jun, 10-11; 2008, Apr, 5-7

82274 **Blood, occult, by fecal hemoglobin determination by immunoassay, qualitative, feces, 1-3 simultaneous determinations** A ☒
0.00 0.00 Global Days XXX

82286-82308 [82652] Chemistry: Bradykinin—Calcitonin

CMS 100-2,15,80 Diagnostic Test Requirements
CMS 100-4,3,10.4 Payment of Nonphysician Services for Inpatients

INCLUDES Mathematically calculated results
Quantitative analysis unless otherwise specified
Specimens from any source unless otherwise specified

EXCLUDES *Organ or disease panels (80048-80076)*
Therapeutic drug assays (80150-80299)

82286 **Bradykinin** A
0.00 0.00 Global Days XXX

82300 **Cadmium** A
0.00 0.00 Global Days XXX

82306 **Vitamin D; 25 hydroxy, includes fraction(s), if performed** A
0.00 0.00 Global Days XXX

82652 **1, 25 dihydroxy, includes fraction(s), if performed**
0.00 0.00 Global Days XXX

82308 **Calcitonin** A
0.00 0.00 Global Days XXX

82310-82373 Chemistry: Calcium, total;Carbohydrate Deficient Transferrin

CMS 100-2,15,80 Diagnostic Test Requirements
CMS 100-4,3,10.4 Payment of Nonphysician Services for Inpatients

INCLUDES Mathematically calculated results
Quantitative analysis unless otherwise specified
Specimens from any source unless otherwise specified

EXCLUDES *Organ or disease panels (80048-80076)*
Therapeutic drug assays (80150-80299)

82310 **Calcium; total** A ☒
0.00 0.00 Global Days XXX

82330 **ionized** A ☒
INCLUDES Calcium, ionized (82330)
0.00 0.00 Global Days XXX

82331 **after calcium infusion test** A
0.00 0.00 Global Days XXX

82340 **urine quantitative, timed specimen** A
0.00 0.00 Global Days XXX

82355 **Calculus; qualitative analysis** A
0.00 0.00 Global Days XXX

82360 **quantitative analysis, chemical** A
0.00 0.00 Global Days XXX

82365 **infrared spectroscopy** A
0.00 0.00 Global Days XXX

82370 **X-ray diffraction** A
0.00 0.00 Global Days XXX

82373 **Carbohydrate deficient transferrin** A
0.00 0.00 Global Days XXX

82374 Chemistry: Carbon Dioxide

CMS 100-2,15,80 Diagnostic Test Requirements
CMS 100-3,190.10 Laboratory Tests--CRD Patients
CMS 100-4,3,10.4 Payment of Nonphysician Services for Inpatients

INCLUDES Mathematically calculated results
Quantitative analysis unless otherwise specified
Specimens from any source unless otherwise specified

EXCLUDES *Organ or disease panels (80048-80076)*
Therapeutic drug assays (80150-80299)

82374 Carbon dioxide (bicarbonate) A
EXCLUDES *Blood gases (82803)*
0.00 0.00 Global Days XXX

82375-82376 Chemistry: Carboxyhemoglobin (Carbon Monoxide)

CMS 100-2,15,80 Diagnostic Test Requirements
CMS 100-4,3,10.4 Payment of Nonphysician Services for Inpatients

INCLUDES Mathematically calculated results
Specimens from any source unless otherwise specified

EXCLUDES *Organ or disease panels (80048-80076)*
Transcutaneous measurement of carboxyhemoglobin (88740)

82375 Carboxyhemoglobin; quantitative A
0.00 0.00 Global Days XXX

82376 qualitative A
EXCLUDES *Transcutaneous measurement of carboxyhemoglobin (88740)*
0.00 0.00 Global Days XXX

82378 Chemistry: Carcinoembryonic Antigen (CEA)

CMS 100-2,15,80 Diagnostic Test Requirements
CMS 100-3,190.26 Carcinoembryonic Antigen (CEA)
CMS 100-4,3,10.4 Payment of Nonphysician Services for Inpatients

82378 Carcinoembryonic antigen (CEA) A
0.00 0.00 Global Days XXX
AMA: 2009, Jan, 11-31; 2008, Jan, 10-25; 2007, January, 13-27

82379-82415 Chemistry: Carnitine—Chloramphenicol

CMS 100-2,15,80 Diagnostic Test Requirements
CMS 100-4,3,10.4 Payment of Nonphysician Services for Inpatients

INCLUDES Mathematically calculated results
Quantitative analysis unless otherwise specified
Specimens from any source unless otherwise specified

EXCLUDES *Organ or disease panels (80048-80076)*
Therapeutic drug assays (80150-80299)

82379 Carnitine (total and free), quantitative, each specimen A
EXCLUDES *Acylcarnitine (82016-82017)*
0.00 0.00 Global Days XXX

82380 Carotene A
0.00 0.00 Global Days XXX

82382 Catecholamines; total urine A
0.00 0.00 Global Days XXX

82383 blood A
0.00 0.00 Global Days XXX

82384 fractionated A
EXCLUDES *Urine metabolites (83835, 84585)*
0.00 0.00 Global Days XXX

82387 Cathepsin-D A
0.00 0.00 Global Days XXX

82390 Ceruloplasmin A
0.00 0.00 Global Days XXX

82397 Chemiluminescent assay A
0.00 0.00 Global Days XXX

82415 Chloramphenicol A
0.00 0.00 Global Days XXX

82435-82438 Chemistry: Chloride

CMS 100-2,15,80 Diagnostic Test Requirements
CMS 100-3,190.10 Laboratory Tests--CRD Patients
CMS 100-4,3,10.4 Payment of Nonphysician Services for Inpatients

INCLUDES Mathematically calculated results
Quantitative analysis unless otherwise specified
Specimens from any source unless otherwise specified

EXCLUDES *Organ or disease panels (80048-80076)*
Therapeutic drug assays (80150-80299)

82435 Chloride; blood A
0.00 0.00 Global Days XXX

82436 urine A
0.00 0.00 Global Days XXX

82438 other source A
EXCLUDES *Sweat collections by iontophoresis (89230)*
0.00 0.00 Global Days XXX

82441 Chemistry: Chlorinated Hydrocarbons

CMS 100-2,15,80 Diagnostic Test Requirements
CMS 100-4,3,10.4 Payment of Nonphysician Services for Inpatients

INCLUDES Mathematically calculated results
Quantitative analysis unless otherwise specified
Specimens from any source unless otherwise specified

82441 Chlorinated hydrocarbons, screen A
EXCLUDES *Chlorpromazine (84022)*
0.00 0.00 Global Days XXX

82465 Chemistry: Cholesterol, Total

CMS 100-2,15,80 Diagnostic Test Requirements
CMS 100-3,190.23 Lipid Testing
CMS 100-4,3,10.4 Payment of Nonphysician Services for Inpatients

INCLUDES Mathematically calculated results
Quantitative analysis unless otherwise specified

EXCLUDES *Organ or disease panels (80048-80299 [80104])*

82465 Cholesterol, serum or whole blood, total A
EXCLUDES *High density lipoprotein (HDL) (83718)*
0.00 0.00 Global Days XXX
AMA: 2009, Jan, 11-31; 2008, Jan, 10-25; 2007, January, 13-27

82480-82492 Chemistry: Cholinesterase—Chromatography

INCLUDES Mathematically calculated results
Quantitative analysis unless otherwise specified
Specimens from any source unless otherwise specified

EXCLUDES *Organ or disease panels (80048-80076)*
Therapeutic drug assays (80048-80299 [80104])

82480 Cholinesterase; serum A
0.00 0.00 Global Days XXX

82482 RBC A
0.00 0.00 Global Days XXX

82485 Chondroitin B sulfate, quantitative A
0.00 0.00 Global Days XXX

82486 Chromatography, qualitative; column (eg, gas liquid or HPLC), analyte not elsewhere specified A
0.00 0.00 Global Days XXX

82487 paper, 1-dimensional, analyte not elsewhere specified A
0.00 0.00 Global Days XXX

82488 paper, 2-dimensional, analyte not elsewhere specified A
0.00 0.00 Global Days XXX

82489 thin layer, analyte not elsewhere specified A
0.00 0.00 Global Days XXX

82491 Chromatography, quantitative, column (eg, gas liquid or HPLC); single analyte not elsewhere specified, single stationary and mobile phase A
0.00 0.00 Global Days XXX

82492 multiple analytes, single stationary and mobile phase A
0.00 0.00 Global Days XXX

82495-82520 Chemistry: Chromium—Cocaine

CMS 100-2,15,80 Diagnostic Test Requirements
CMS 100-4,3,10.4 Payment of Nonphysician Services for Inpatients

INCLUDES Mathematically calculated results
Quantitative analysis unless otherwise specified
Specimens from any source unless otherwise specified

EXCLUDES *Organ or disease panels (80048-80076)*
Therapeutic drug assays (80150-80299)

82495 Chromium A
0.00 0.00 Global Days XXX

82507 Citrate A
0.00 0.00 Global Days XXX

82520 Cocaine or metabolite A
EXCLUDES *Cocaine, qualitative testing (80100-80103 [80104])*
0.00 0.00 Global Days XXX

82523 Chemistry: Collagen Crosslinks, Any Method

CMS 100-2,15,80 Diagnostic Test Requirements
CMS 100-3,190.19 NCD for Collagen Crosslinks, Any Method
CMS 100-4,3,10.4 Payment of Nonphysician Services for Inpatients

INCLUDES Mathematically calculated results
Quantitative analysis unless otherwise specified
Specimens from any source unless otherwise specified

EXCLUDES *Organ or disease panels (80048-80076)*
Therapeutic drug assays (80150-80299)

82523 Collagen cross links, any method A
0.00 0.00 Global Days XXX

82525-82946 Chemistry: Copper—Glucagon Tolerance Test

CMS 100-2,15,80 Diagnostic Test Requirements
CMS 100-4,3,10.4 Payment of Nonphysician Services for Inpatients

INCLUDES Mathematically calculated results
Quantitative analysis unless otherwise specified
Specimens from any source unless otherwise specified

EXCLUDES *Organ or disease panels (80048-80076)*
Therapeutic drug assays (80150-80299)

82525 Copper A
0.00 0.00 Global Days XXX

82528 Corticosterone A
INCLUDES Porter-Silber test
0.00 0.00 Global Days XXX

82530 Cortisol; free A
0.00 0.00 Global Days XXX

82533 total A
0.00 0.00 Global Days XXX

82540 Creatine A
0.00 0.00 Global Days XXX

82541 Column chromatography/mass spectrometry (eg, GC/MS, or HPLC/MS), analyte not elsewhere specified; qualitative, single stationary and mobile phase A
0.00 0.00 Global Days XXX

82542 quantitative, single stationary and mobile phase A
0.00 0.00 Global Days XXX

82543 stable isotope dilution, single analyte, quantitative, single stationary and mobile phase A
0.00 0.00 Global Days XXX

82544 stable isotope dilution, multiple analytes, quantitative, single stationary and mobile phase A
0.00 0.00 Global Days XXX

82550 Creatine kinase (CK), (CPK); total A
0.00 0.00 Global Days XXX

82552 isoenzymes A
0.00 0.00 Global Days XXX

82553 MB fraction only A
0.00 0.00 Global Days XXX

82554 isoforms A
0.00 0.00 Global Days XXX

82565 Creatinine; blood A
0.00 0.00 Global Days XXX

82570 other source A
0.00 0.00 Global Days XXX

82575 clearance A
INCLUDES Holten test
0.00 0.00 Global Days XXX

82585 Cryofibrinogen A
0.00 0.00 Global Days XXX

82595 Cryoglobulin, qualitative or semi-quantitative (eg, cryocrit) A
EXCLUDES *Quantitative, cryoglobulin (82784-82785)*
0.00 0.00 Global Days XXX

82600 Cyanide A
0.00 0.00 Global Days XXX

82607 Cyanocobalamin (Vitamin B-12); A
0.00 0.00 Global Days XXX

82608 unsaturated binding capacity A
0.00 0.00 Global Days XXX

82610 Cystatin C A
0.00 0.00 Global Days XXX
AMA: 2009, Jan, 11-31; 2008, Apr, 5-7

82615 Cystine and homocystine, urine, qualitative A
0.00 0.00 Global Days XXX

82626 Dehydroepiandrosterone (DHEA) A
0.00 0.00 Global Days XXX

82627 Dehydroepiandrosterone-sulfate (DHEA-S) A
0.00 0.00 Global Days XXX

82633 Desoxycorticosterone, 11- A
0.00 0.00 Global Days XXX

82634 Deoxycortisol, 11- A
0.00 0.00 Global Days XXX

82638 Dibucaine number A
0.00 0.00 Global Days XXX

82646 **Dihydrocodeinone** A
EXCLUDES *Qualitative testing (80100-80103 [80104])*
0.00 0.00 Global Days XXX

82649 **Dihydromorphinone** A
EXCLUDES *Qualitative testing (80100-80103 [80104])*
0.00 0.00 Global Days XXX

82651 **Dihydrotestosterone (DHT)** A
0.00 0.00 Global Days XXX

82652 *Resequenced code. See code following 82306.*

82654 **Dimethadione** A
EXCLUDES *Qualitative testing (80100-80101 [80104])*
0.00 0.00 Global Days XXX

82656 **Elastase, pancreatic (EL-1), fecal, qualitative or semi-quantitative** A
0.00 0.00 Global Days XXX
AMA: 2009, Jan, 11-31; 2008, Jan, 10-25; 2007, January, 13-27

82657 **Enzyme activity in blood cells, cultured cells, or tissue, not elsewhere specified; nonradioactive substrate, each specimen** A
0.00 0.00 Global Days XXX

82658 **radioactive substrate, each specimen** A
0.00 0.00 Global Days XXX

82664 **Electrophoretic technique, not elsewhere specified** A
0.00 0.00 Global Days XXX

82666 **Epiandrosterone** A
0.00 0.00 Global Days XXX

82668 **Erythropoietin** A
0.00 0.00 Global Days XXX

82670 **Estradiol** A
0.00 0.00 Global Days XXX

82671 **Estrogens; fractionated** A
0.00 0.00 Global Days XXX

82672 **total** A
0.00 0.00 Global Days XXX

82677 **Estriol** A
0.00 0.00 Global Days XXX

82679 **Estrone** A
0.00 0.00 Global Days XXX

82690 **Ethchlorvynol** A
0.00 0.00 Global Days XXX

82693 **Ethylene glycol** A
0.00 0.00 Global Days XXX

82696 **Etiocholanolone** A
EXCLUDES *Fractionation of ketosteroids (83593)*
0.00 0.00 Global Days XXX

82705 **Fat or lipids, feces; qualitative** A
0.00 0.00 Global Days XXX

82710 **quantitative** A
0.00 0.00 Global Days XXX

82715 **Fat differential, feces, quantitative** A
0.00 0.00 Global Days XXX

82725 **Fatty acids, nonesterified** A
0.00 0.00 Global Days XXX

82726 **Very long chain fatty acids** A
EXCLUDES *Long-chain (C20-22) omega-3 fatty acids in red blood cell (RBC) membranes (0111T)*
0.00 0.00 Global Days XXX

82728 **Ferritin** A
0.00 0.00 Global Days XXX

82731 **Fetal fibronectin, cervicovaginal secretions, semi-quantitative** M ♀ A
0.00 0.00 Global Days XXX

82735 **Fluoride** A
0.00 0.00 Global Days XXX

82742 **Flurazepam** A
EXCLUDES *Qualitative testing (80100-80103 [80104])*
0.00 0.00 Global Days XXX

82746 **Folic acid; serum** A
0.00 0.00 Global Days XXX

82747 **RBC** A
0.00 0.00 Global Days XXX

82757 **Fructose, semen** ♂ A
EXCLUDES *Fructosamine (82985)*
Fructose, TLC screen (84375)
0.00 0.00 Global Days XXX

82759 **Galactokinase, RBC** A
0.00 0.00 Global Days XXX

82760 **Galactose** A
0.00 0.00 Global Days XXX

82775 **Galactose-1-phosphate uridyl transferase; quantitative** A
0.00 0.00 Global Days XXX

82776 **screen** A
0.00 0.00 Global Days XXX

82784 **Gammaglobulin (immunoglobulin); IgA, IgD, IgG, IgM, each** A
INCLUDES Farr test
0.00 0.00 Global Days XXX
AMA: 2009, Jan, 11-31; 2008, Jan, 10-25; 2007, January, 13-27

82785 **IgE** A
INCLUDES Farr test
EXCLUDES *Allergen specific, IgE (86003, 86005)*
0.00 0.00 Global Days XXX

82787 **immunoglobulin subclasses (eg, IgG1, 2, 3, or 4), each** A
EXCLUDES *Gamma-glutamyltransferase (GGT) (82977)*
0.00 0.00 Global Days XXX

82800 **Gases, blood, pH only** A
0.00 0.00 Global Days XXX

82803 **Gases, blood, any combination of pH, pCO2, pO2, CO2, HCO3 (including calculated O2 saturation);** A
INCLUDES Two or more of the listed analytes
0.00 0.00 Global Days XXX

82805 **with O2 saturation, by direct measurement, except pulse oximetry** A
0.00 0.00 Global Days XXX

82810 **Gases, blood, O2 saturation only, by direct measurement, except pulse oximetry** A
EXCLUDES *Pulse oximetry (94760)*
0.00 0.00 Global Days XXX

82820 **Hemoglobin-oxygen affinity (pO2 for 50% hemoglobin saturation with oxygen)** A
0.00 0.00 Global Days XXX

82930 **Gastric acid analysis, includes pH if performed, each specimen** A
0.00 0.00 Global Days XXX

82938 **Gastrin after secretin stimulation** A
0.00 0.00 Global Days XXX

82941 **Gastrin** A
0.00 0.00 Global Days XXX

82943 **Glucagon** A
0.00 0.00 Global Days XXX

82945 **Glucose, body fluid, other than blood**
0.00 0.00 Global Days XXX

82946 **Glucagon tolerance test** A
0.00 0.00 Global Days XXX

82947-82962 Chemistry: Glucose Testing

CMS 100-2,15,80 Diagnostic Test Requirements
CMS 100-3,190.20 Blood Glucose Testing
CMS 100-4,3,10.4 Payment of Nonphysician Services for Inpatients

INCLUDES Mathematically calculated results
Quantitative analysis unless otherwise specified
Specimens from any source unless otherwise specified

EXCLUDES *Organ or disease panels (80048-80076)*
Therapeutic drug assays (80150-80299)

Code also glucose administration injection (96374)

82947 **Glucose; quantitative, blood (except reagent strip)** A
0.00 0.00 Global Days XXX

82948 **blood, reagent strip** A
0.00 0.00 Global Days XXX
AMA: 2009, Jan, 11-31; 2008, Jan, 10-25; 2007, January, 13-27

82950 **post glucose dose (includes glucose)** A
0.00 0.00 Global Days XXX
AMA: 2009, Jan, 11-31; 2008, Jan, 10-25; 2007, January, 13-27

82951 **tolerance test (GTT), 3 specimens (includes glucose)** A
0.00 0.00 Global Days XXX
AMA: 2009, Jan, 11-31; 2008, Jan, 10-25; 2007, January, 13-27

\+ **82952** **tolerance test, each additional beyond 3 specimens (List separately in addition to code for primary procedure)** A
Code first (82951)
0.00 0.00 Global Days XXX
AMA: 2009, Jan, 11-31; 2008, Jan, 10-25; 2007, January, 13-27

82953 **tolbutamide tolerance test** A
EXCLUDES *Semiquantitative urine glucose (81000, 81002, 81005, 81099)*
0.00 0.00 Global Days XXX

82955 **Glucose-6-phosphate dehydrogenase (G6PD); quantitative** A
0.00 0.00 Global Days XXX

82960 **screen** A
Code also injection administration (96374)
0.00 0.00 Global Days XXX

82962 **Glucose, blood by glucose monitoring device(s) cleared by the FDA specifically for home use** A
0.00 0.00 Global Days XXX
AMA: 2009, Jan, 11-31; 2008, Jan, 10-25; 2007, January, 13-27

82963-83690 Chemistry: Glucosidase—Lipase

CMS 100-2,15,80 Diagnostic Test Requirements
CMS 100-4,3,10.4 Payment of Nonphysician Services for Inpatients

INCLUDES Mathematically calculated results
Quantitative analysis unless otherwise specified
Specimens from any source unless otherwise specified

EXCLUDES *Organ or disease panels (80048-80076)*
Therapeutic drug assays (80150-80299)

82963 **Glucosidase, beta** A
0.00 0.00 Global Days XXX

82965 **Glutamate dehydrogenase** A
0.00 0.00 Global Days XXX

82975 **Glutamine (glutamic acid amide)** A
0.00 0.00 Global Days XXX

82977 **Glutamyltransferase, gamma (GGT)** A
0.00 0.00 Global Days XXX

82978 **Glutathione** A
0.00 0.00 Global Days XXX

82979 **Glutathione reductase, RBC** A
0.00 0.00 Global Days XXX

82980 **Glutethimide** A
0.00 0.00 Global Days XXX

82985 **Glycated protein** A
EXCLUDES *Gonadotropin, chorionic (hCG) (84702-84703)*
0.00 0.00 Global Days XXX

83001 **Gonadotropin; follicle stimulating hormone (FSH)** A
0.00 0.00 Global Days XXX

83002 **luteinizing hormone (LH)** A
EXCLUDES *Luteinizing releasing factor (LRH) (83727)*
0.00 0.00 Global Days XXX

83003 **Growth hormone, human (HGH) (somatotropin)** A
EXCLUDES *Antibody to human growth hormone (86277)*
0.00 0.00 Global Days XXX

83008 **Guanosine monophosphate (GMP), cyclic** A
0.00 0.00 Global Days XXX

83009 **Helicobacter pylori, blood test analysis for urease activity, non-radioactive isotope (eg, C-13)** A
EXCLUDES *H. pylori, breath test analysis for urease activity (83013-83014)*
0.00 0.00 Global Days XXX

83010 **Haptoglobin; quantitative** A
0.00 0.00 Global Days XXX

83012 **phenotypes** A
0.00 0.00 Global Days XXX

83013 **Helicobacter pylori; breath test analysis for urease activity, non-radioactive isotope (eg, C-13)** A
0.00 0.00 Global Days XXX

83014 **drug administration** A
EXCLUDES *H. pylori:*
Blood test analysis for urease activity (83009)
Enzyme immunoassay (87339)
Liquid scintillation counter (78267-78268)
Stool (87338)
0.00 0.00 Global Days XXX

83015 **Heavy metal (eg, arsenic, barium, beryllium, bismuth, antimony, mercury); screen** A
INCLUDES Reinsch test
0.00 0.00 Global Days XXX

83018 **quantitative, each** A
0.00 0.00 Global Days XXX

83020 **Hemoglobin fractionation and quantitation; electrophoresis (eg, A2, S, C, and/or F)** A
0.00 0.00 Global Days XXX

83021 **chromatography (eg, A2, S, C, and/or F)** A
EXCLUDES *Glycosylated (A1c) hemoglobin analysis by chromatography in the absence of an identified hemoglobin variant (83036)*
0.00 0.00 Global Days XXX

83026 **Hemoglobin; by copper sulfate method, non-automated**
0.00 0.00 Global Days XXX

83030 **F (fetal), chemical**
0.00 0.00 Global Days XXX

83033 **F (fetal), qualitative**
0.00 0.00 Global Days XXX

83036 **glycosylated (A1C)**
EXCLUDES *Glycosylated (A1c) hemoglobin analysis by chromatography in the setting of an identified hemoglobin variant (83021)*
0.00 0.00 Global Days XXX

83037 **glycosylated (A1C) by device cleared by FDA for home use**
0.00 0.00 Global Days XXX
AMA: 2009, Jan, 11-31; 2008, Jan, 10-25; 2007, January, 13-27

83045 **methemoglobin, qualitative**
0.00 0.00 Global Days XXX

83050 **methemoglobin, quantitative**
EXCLUDES *Transcutaneous methemoglobin test (88741)*
0.00 0.00 Global Days XXX

83051 **plasma**
0.00 0.00 Global Days XXX

83055 **sulfhemoglobin, qualitative**
0.00 0.00 Global Days XXX

83060 **sulfhemoglobin, quantitative**
0.00 0.00 Global Days XXX

83065 **thermolabile**
0.00 0.00 Global Days XXX

83068 **unstable, screen**
0.00 0.00 Global Days XXX

83069 **urine**
0.00 0.00 Global Days XXX

83070 **Hemosiderin; qualitative**
0.00 0.00 Global Days XXX

83071 **quantitative**
0.00 0.00 Global Days XXX

83080 **b-Hexosaminidase, each assay**
0.00 0.00 Global Days XXX

83088 **Histamine**
0.00 0.00 Global Days XXX

83090 **Homocysteine**
0.00 0.00 Global Days XXX
AMA: 2009, Jan, 11-31; 2008, Jan, 10-25; 2007, January, 13-27

83150 **Homovanillic acid (HVA)**
0.00 0.00 Global Days XXX

83491 **Hydroxycorticosteroids, 17- (17-OHCS)**
EXCLUDES *Cortisol (82530, 82533)*
Deoxycortisol (82634)
0.00 0.00 Global Days XXX

83497 **Hydroxyindolacetic acid, 5-(HIAA)**
EXCLUDES *Urine qualitative test (81005)*
0.00 0.00 Global Days XXX

83498 **Hydroxyprogesterone, 17-d**
0.00 0.00 Global Days XXX

83499 **Hydroxyprogesterone, 20-**
0.00 0.00 Global Days XXX

83500 **Hydroxyproline; free**
0.00 0.00 Global Days XXX

83505 **total**
0.00 0.00 Global Days XXX

83516 **Immunoassay for analyte other than infectious agent antibody or infectious agent antigen; qualitative or semiquantitative, multiple step method**
0.00 0.00 Global Days XXX

83518 **qualitative or semiquantitative, single step method (eg, reagent strip)**
0.00 0.00 Global Days XXX

83519 **quantitative, by radioimmunoassay (eg, RIA)**
0.00 0.00 Global Days XXX

83520 **quantitative, not otherwise specified**
0.00 0.00 Global Days XXX

83525 **Insulin; total**
EXCLUDES *Proinsulin (84206)*
0.00 0.00 Global Days XXX

83527 **free**
0.00 0.00 Global Days XXX

83528 **Intrinsic factor**
EXCLUDES *Intrinsic factor antibodies (86340)*
0.00 0.00 Global Days XXX

83540 **Iron**
0.00 0.00 Global Days XXX

83550 **Iron binding capacity**
0.00 0.00 Global Days XXX

83570 **Isocitric dehydrogenase (IDH)**
0.00 0.00 Global Days XXX

83582 **Ketogenic steroids, fractionation**
0.00 0.00 Global Days XXX

83586 **Ketosteroids, 17- (17-KS); total**
0.00 0.00 Global Days XXX

83593 **fractionation**
0.00 0.00 Global Days XXX

83605 **Lactate (lactic acid)**
0.00 0.00 Global Days XXX

83615 **Lactate dehydrogenase (LD), (LDH);**
0.00 0.00 Global Days XXX

83625 **isoenzymes, separation and quantitation**
0.00 0.00 Global Days XXX

83630 **Lactoferrin, fecal; qualitative**
0.00 0.00 Global Days XXX

83631 **quantitative**
0.00 0.00 Global Days XXX
AMA: 2009, Jan, 11-31; 2008, Jan, 10-25; 2007, January, 28-31

83632 **Lactogen, human placental (HPL) human chorionic somatomammotropin**
0.00 0.00 Global Days XXX

83633 **Lactose, urine; qualitative**
0.00 0.00 Global Days XXX

83634 **quantitative**
EXCLUDES *Breath hydrogen test for lactase deficiency (91065)*
Glucose tolerance test (GTT) (82951-82952)
0.00 0.00 Global Days XXX

83655 **Lead**
0.00 0.00 Global Days XXX

83661 **Fetal lung maturity assessment; lecithin sphingomyelin (L/S) ratio**
0.00 0.00 Global Days XXX

83662 **foam stability test**
0.00 0.00 Global Days XXX

83663 **fluorescence polarization**
0.00 0.00 Global Days XXX

83664 **lamellar body density** M ♀ A
EXCLUDES *Phosphatidylglycerol (84081)*
0.00 0.00 Global Days XXX

83670 **Leucine aminopeptidase (LAP)** A
0.00 0.00 Global Days XXX

83690 **Lipase** A
0.00 0.00 Global Days XXX

83695-83727 Chemistry: Lipoprotein—Luteinizing Releasing Factor

CMS 100-2,15,80 Diagnostic Test Requirements
CMS 100-3,190.23 Lipid Testing
CMS 100-4,3,10.4 Payment of Nonphysician Services for Inpatients

INCLUDES Mathematically calculated results
Quantitative analysis unless otherwise specified
Specimens from any source unless otherwise specified

EXCLUDES *Organ or disease panels (80048-80076)*
Therapeutic drug assays

83695 **Lipoprotein (a)** A
0.00 0.00 Global Days XXX

83698 **Lipoprotein-associated phospholipase A2 (Lp-PLA2)** A
0.00 0.00 Global Days XXX

83700 **Lipoprotein, blood; electrophoretic separation and quantitation** A
0.00 0.00 Global Days XXX

83701 **high resolution fractionation and quantitation of lipoproteins including lipoprotein subclasses when performed (eg, electrophoresis, ultracentrifugation)** A
0.00 0.00 Global Days XXX

83704 **quantitation of lipoprotein particle numbers and lipoprotein particle subclasses (eg, by nuclear magnetic resonance spectroscopy)** A
0.00 0.00 Global Days XXX

83718 **Lipoprotein, direct measurement; high density cholesterol (HDL cholesterol)** A
0.00 0.00 Global Days XXX
AMA: 2009, Jan, 11-31; 2008, Jan, 10-25; 2007, January, 13-27

83719 **VLDL cholesterol** A
0.00 0.00 Global Days XXX
AMA: 2009, Jan, 11-31; 2008, Jan, 10-25; 2007, January, 13-27

83721 **LDL cholesterol** A
EXCLUDES *Fractionation by high resolution electrophoresis or ultracentrifugation (83701)*
Lipoprotein particle numbers and subclasses analysis by nuclear magnetic resonance spectroscopy (83704)
0.00 0.00 Global Days XXX
AMA: 2009, Jan, 11-31; 2008, Jan, 10-25; 2007, January, 13-27

83727 **Luteinizing releasing factor (LRH)** A
EXCLUDES *Qualitative analysis (80100-80103 [80104])*
0.00 0.00 Global Days XXX

83735-83887 Chemistry: Magnesium—Nicotine

CMS 100-2,15,80 Diagnostic Test Requirements
CMS 100-4,3,10.4 Payment of Nonphysician Services for Inpatients

INCLUDES Mathematically calculated results
Quantitative analysis unless otherwise specified
Specimens from any source unless otherwise specified

EXCLUDES *Organ or disease panels (80048-80076)*
Therapeutic drug assays (80150-80299)

83735 **Magnesium** A
0.00 0.00 Global Days XXX

83775 **Malate dehydrogenase** A
0.00 0.00 Global Days XXX

83785 **Manganese** A
0.00 0.00 Global Days XXX

83788 **Mass spectrometry and tandem mass spectrometry (MS, MS/MS), analyte not elsewhere specified; qualitative, each specimen** A
0.00 0.00 Global Days XXX

83789 **quantitative, each specimen** A
0.00 0.00 Global Days XXX

83805 **Meprobamate** A
EXCLUDES *Qualitative analysis (80100-80103 [80104])*
0.00 0.00 Global Days XXX

83825 **Mercury, quantitative** A
EXCLUDES *Mercury screen (83015)*
0.00 0.00 Global Days XXX

83835 **Metanephrines** A
EXCLUDES *Catecholamines (82382-82384)*
0.00 0.00 Global Days XXX

83840 **Methadone** A
EXCLUDES *Methadone qualitative analysis (80100-80103 [80104])*
0.00 0.00 Global Days XXX

83857 **Methemalbumin** A
0.00 0.00 Global Days XXX

83858 **Methsuximide** A
0.00 0.00 Global Days XXX

83861 **Microfluidic analysis utilizing an integrated collection and analysis device, tear osmolarity** A
Code also procedure performed on both eyes 83861 X 2
0.00 0.00 Global Days XXX

83864 **Mucopolysaccharides, acid; quantitative** A
0.00 0.00 Global Days XXX

83866 **screen** A
0.00 0.00 Global Days XXX

83872 **Mucin, synovial fluid (Ropes test)** A
0.00 0.00 Global Days XXX

83873 **Myelin basic protein, cerebrospinal fluid** A
EXCLUDES *Oligoclonal bands (83916)*
0.00 0.00 Global Days XXX

83874 **Myoglobin** A
0.00 0.00 Global Days XXX

83876 **Myeloperoxidase (MPO)** A
0.00 0.00 Global Days XXX

83880 **Natriuretic peptide** A
0.00 0.00 Global Days XXX

83883 **Nephelometry, each analyte not elsewhere specified** A
0.00 0.00 Global Days XXX

83885 **Nickel** A
0.00 0.00 Global Days XXX

83887 **Nicotine** A
0.00 0.00 Global Days XXX

83890-83914 Chemistry: Nucleic Acid Diagnostics

CMS 100-2,15,80 Diagnostic Test Requirements
CMS 100-4,3,10.4 Payment of Nonphysician Services for Inpatients

INCLUDES Molecular diagnostic techniques for analysis of nucleic acids
Tests reported by procedure instead of analyte

EXCLUDES *Array technology using more than 10 probes (88384-88386)*
Digestate, undigested nucleic acid, or other individually modified nucleic acid sample
Microbial identification (87149, 87152, 87470)

Do not report with or instead of (87140-87158, 87470-87801)

83890 Molecular diagnostics; molecular isolation or extraction, each nucleic acid type (ie, DNA or RNA) A CCI
0.00 0.00 Global Days XXX
AMA: 2008, Apr, 5-7

83891 isolation or extraction of highly purified nucleic acid, each nucleic acid type (ie, DNA or RNA) A CCI
0.00 0.00 Global Days XXX
AMA: 2008, Apr, 5-7

83892 enzymatic digestion, each enzyme treatment A CCI
0.00 0.00 Global Days XXX
AMA: 2008, Apr, 5-7

83893 dot/slot blot production, each nucleic acid preparation A CCI
0.00 0.00 Global Days XXX
AMA: 2008, Apr, 5-7

83894 separation by gel electrophoresis (eg, agarose, polyacrylamide), each nucleic acid preparation A CCI
0.00 0.00 Global Days XXX
AMA: 2008, Apr, 5-7

83896 nucleic acid probe, each A CCI
0.00 0.00 Global Days XXX
AMA: 2009, Jan, 11-31; 2008, Jan, 10-25; 2008, Apr, 5-7; 2007, January, 13-27

83897 nucleic acid transfer (eg, Southern, Northern), each nucleic acid preparation A CCI
0.00 0.00 Global Days XXX
AMA: 2008, Apr, 5-7

83898 amplification, target, each nucleic acid sequence A CCI
EXCLUDES *Multiple target amplification (83900-83901)*
Signal amplification (83908)
0.00 0.00 Global Days XXX
AMA: 2008, Apr, 5-7

83900 amplification, target, multiplex, first 2 nucleic acid sequences A
0.00 0.00 Global Days XXX
AMA: 2008, Apr, 5-7

+ **83901 amplification, target, multiplex, each additional nucleic acid sequence beyond 2 (List separately in addition to code for primary procedure)** A CCI
Code first (83900)
0.00 0.00 Global Days XXX
AMA: 2008, Apr, 5-7

83902 reverse transcription A CCI
0.00 0.00 Global Days XXX
AMA: 2008, Apr, 5-7

83903 mutation scanning, by physical properties (eg, single strand conformational polymorphisms [SSCP], heteroduplex, denaturing gradient gel electrophoresis [DGGE], RNA'ase A), single segment, each A CCI
0.00 0.00 Global Days XXX
AMA: 2008, Apr, 5-7

83904 mutation identification by sequencing, single segment, each segment A CCI
0.00 0.00 Global Days XXX
AMA: 2008, Apr, 5-7

83905 mutation identification by allele specific transcription, single segment, each segment A CCI
0.00 0.00 Global Days XXX
AMA: 2008, Apr, 5-7

83906 mutation identification by allele specific translation, single segment, each segment A CCI
0.00 0.00 Global Days XXX
AMA: 2008, Apr, 5-7

83907 lysis of cells prior to nucleic acid extraction (eg, stool specimens, paraffin embedded tissue), each specimen A
0.00 0.00 Global Days XXX
AMA: 2008, Apr, 5-7

83908 amplification, signal, each nucleic acid sequence A
EXCLUDES *Target amplification (83898-83901)*
0.00 0.00 Global Days XXX
AMA: 2008, Apr, 5-7

83909 separation and identification by high resolution technique (eg, capillary electrophoresis), each nucleic acid preparation A
0.00 0.00 Global Days XXX
AMA: 2008, Apr, 5-7

83912 interpretation and report A CCI
0.00 0.00 Global Days XXX
AMA: 2008, Apr, 5-7

83913 RNA stabilization A
0.00 0.00 Global Days XXX
AMA: 2008, Apr, 5-7

83914 Mutation identification by enzymatic ligation or primer extension, single segment, each segment (eg, oligonucleotide ligation assay [OLA], single base chain extension [SBCE], or allele-specific primer extension [ASPE]) A
0.00 0.00 Global Days XXX
AMA: 2008, Apr, 5-7

83915-84066 Chemistry: Nucleotidase 5'- —Phosphatase (Acid)

CMS 100-2,15,80 Diagnostic Test Requirements
CMS 100-4,3,10.4 Payment of Nonphysician Services for Inpatients

INCLUDES Mathematically calculated results
Quantitative analysis unless otherwise specified
Specimens from any source unless otherwise specified

EXCLUDES *Organ or disease panels (80048-80299 [80104])*
Therapeutic drug assays (80150-80299)

83915 Nucleotidase 5'- A
0.00 0.00 Global Days XXX

83916 Oligoclonal immune (oligoclonal bands) A CCI
0.00 0.00 Global Days XXX

83918 Organic acids; total, quantitative, each specimen A CCI
0.00 0.00 Global Days XXX
AMA: 2009, Jan, 11-31; 2008, Jan, 10-25; 2007, January, 13-27

83919 qualitative, each specimen A
0.00 0.00 Global Days XXX

83921 Organic acid, single, quantitative A CCI
0.00 0.00 Global Days XXX

83925 Opiate(s), drug and metabolites, each procedure A
0.00 0.00 Global Days XXX

83930 Osmolality; blood A
EXCLUDES *Tear osmolarity (83861)*
0.00 0.00 Global Days XXX

83935 urine A
EXCLUDES *Tear osmolarity (83861)*
0.00 0.00 Global Days XXX

83937 Osteocalcin (bone gla protein) A
0.00 0.00 Global Days XXX

83945 Oxalate A
0.00 0.00 Global Days XXX

83950 Oncoprotein; HER-2/neu A
EXCLUDES *Tissue (88342, 88365)*
0.00 0.00 Global Days XXX

83951 des-gamma-carboxy-prothrombin (DCP) A
0.00 0.00 Global Days XXX

83970 Parathormone (parathyroid hormone) A
EXCLUDES *Chlorinated hydrocarbons (82441)*
Pesticide, quantitative (see code for specific method)
0.00 0.00 Global Days XXX

83986 pH; body fluid, not otherwise specified A
EXCLUDES *Blood pH (82800, 82803)*
0.00 0.00 Global Days XXX

83987 exhaled breath condensate A
0.00 0.00 Global Days XXX

83992 Phencyclidine (PCP) A
EXCLUDES *Qualitative analysis (80100-80103 [80104])*
0.00 0.00 Global Days XXX

83993 Calprotectin, fecal A
0.00 0.00 Global Days XXX
AMA: 2008, Apr, 5-7

84022 Phenothiazine A
EXCLUDES *Qualitative analysis (80100-80101)*
0.00 0.00 Global Days XXX

84030 Phenylalanine (PKU), blood A
INCLUDES Guthrie test
EXCLUDES *Phenylalanine-tyrosine ratio (84030, 84510)*
0.00 0.00 Global Days XXX

84035 Phenylketones, qualitative A
0.00 0.00 Global Days XXX

84060 Phosphatase, acid; total A
0.00 0.00 Global Days XXX

84061 forensic examination A
0.00 0.00 Global Days XXX

84066 prostatic ♂A
0.00 0.00 Global Days XXX

84075-84080 Chemistry: Phosphatase (Alkaline)

CMS 100-2,15,80 Diagnostic Test Requirements
CMS 100-3,190.10 Laboratory Tests--CRD Patients
CMS 100-4,3,10.4 Payment of Nonphysician Services for Inpatients

INCLUDES Mathematically calculated results
Quantitative analysis unless otherwise specified
Specimens from any source unless otherwise specified

EXCLUDES *Organ or disease panels (80048-80076)*

84075 Phosphatase, alkaline; A
0.00 0.00 Global Days XXX

84078 heat stable (total not included) A
0.00 0.00 Global Days XXX

84080 isoenzymes A
0.00 0.00 Global Days XXX

84081-84150 Chemistry: Phosphatidylglycerol—Prostaglandin

CMS 100-2,15,80 Diagnostic Test Requirements
CMS 100-4,3,10.4 Payment of Nonphysician Services for Inpatients

INCLUDES Mathematically calculated results
Quantitative analysis unless otherwise specified
Specimens from any source unless otherwise specified

EXCLUDES *Organ or disease panels (80048-80076)*
Therapeutic drug assays (80150-80299)

84081 Phosphatidylglycerol A
0.00 0.00 Global Days XXX

84085 Phosphogluconate, 6-, dehydrogenase, RBC A
0.00 0.00 Global Days XXX

84087 Phosphohexose isomerase A
0.00 0.00 Global Days XXX

84100 Phosphorus inorganic (phosphate); A
0.00 0.00 Global Days XXX

84105 urine A
0.00 0.00 Global Days XXX

84106 Porphobilinogen, urine; qualitative A
0.00 0.00 Global Days XXX

84110 quantitative A
0.00 0.00 Global Days XXX

84112 Placental alpha microglobulin-1 (PAMG-1), cervicovaginal secretion, qualitative ♀A
0.00 0.00 Global Days XXX

84119 Porphyrins, urine; qualitative A
0.00 0.00 Global Days XXX

84120 quantitation and fractionation A
0.00 0.00 Global Days XXX

84126 Porphyrins, feces; quantitative A
0.00 0.00 Global Days XXX

84127 qualitative A
EXCLUDES *Porphyrin precursors (82135, 84106, 84110)*
0.00 0.00 Global Days XXX

84132 Potassium; serum, plasma or whole blood A
0.00 0.00 Global Days XXX

84133 urine A
0.00 0.00 Global Days XXX

84134 Prealbumin A
EXCLUDES *Microalbumin (82043-82044)*
0.00 0.00 Global Days XXX

84135 Pregnanediol ♀A
0.00 0.00 Global Days XXX

84138 Pregnanetriol ♀A
0.00 0.00 Global Days XXX

84140 Pregnenolone A
0.00 0.00 Global Days XXX

84143 17-hydroxypregnenolone A
0.00 0.00 Global Days XXX

84144 Progesterone A
EXCLUDES *Progesterone receptor assay (84234)*
0.00 0.00 Global Days XXX

84145 Procalcitonin (PCT) A
0.00 0.00 Global Days XXX

84146 Prolactin A
0.00 0.00 Global Days XXX

84150 Prostaglandin, each A
0.00 0.00 Global Days XXX

84152-84154 Chemistry: Prostate Specific Antigen

CMS 100-2,15,80 Diagnostic Test Requirements
CMS 100-3,190.31 Prostate Specific Antigen (PSA)
CMS 100-3,210.1 Prostate Cancer Screening Tests
CMS 100-4,3,10.4 Payment of Nonphysician Services for Inpatients

INCLUDES Mathematically calculated results
Quantitative analysis unless otherwise specified

84152 **Prostate specific antigen (PSA); complexed (direct measurement)** ♂ A
0.00 0.00 Global Days XXX

84153 **total** ♂ A
0.00 0.00 Global Days XXX
AMA: 2009, Jan, 11-31; 2008, Jan, 10-25; 2007, January, 13-27

84154 **free** ♂ A
0.00 0.00 Global Days XXX
AMA: 2009, Jan, 11-31; 2008, Jan, 10-25; 2007, January, 13-27

84155-84157 Chemistry: Protein, Total (Not by Refractometry)

CMS 100-2,15,80 Diagnostic Test Requirements
CMS 100-3,190.10 Laboratory Tests--CRD Patients
CMS 100-4,3,10.4 Payment of Nonphysician Services for Inpatients

INCLUDES Mathematically calculated results

EXCLUDES *Organ or disease panels (80048-80076)*

84155 **Protein, total, except by refractometry; serum, plasma or whole blood** A
0.00 0.00 Global Days XXX

84156 **urine** A
0.00 0.00 Global Days XXX

84157 **other source (eg, synovial fluid, cerebrospinal fluid)** A
0.00 0.00 Global Days XXX

84160-84432 Chemistry: Protein, Total (Refractometry)—Thyroglobulin

CMS 100-2,15,80 Diagnostic Test Requirements
CMS 100-4,3,10.4 Payment of Nonphysician Services for Inpatients

INCLUDES Mathematically calculated results
Quantitative analysis unless otherwise specified
Specimens from any source unless otherwise specified

EXCLUDES *Organ or disease panels (80048-80076)*
Therapeutic drug assays (80150-80299)

84160 **Protein, total, by refractometry, any source** A
EXCLUDES *Dipstick urine protein (81000-81003)*
0.00 0.00 Global Days XXX

84163 **Pregnancy-associated plasma protein-A (PAPP-A)** ♀ A
0.00 0.00 Global Days XXX

84165 **Protein; electrophoretic fractionation and quantitation, serum** A
0.00 0.00 Global Days XXX

84166 **electrophoretic fractionation and quantitation, other fluids with concentration (eg, urine, CSF)** A
0.00 0.00 Global Days XXX

84181 **Western Blot, with interpretation and report, blood or other body fluid** A
0.00 0.00 Global Days XXX

84182 **Western Blot, with interpretation and report, blood or other body fluid, immunological probe for band identification, each** A
EXCLUDES *Western Blot tissue testing (88371)*
0.00 0.00 Global Days XXX

84202 **Protoporphyrin, RBC; quantitative** A
0.00 0.00 Global Days XXX

84203 **screen** A
0.00 0.00 Global Days XXX

84206 **Proinsulin** A
0.00 0.00 Global Days XXX

84207 **Pyridoxal phosphate (Vitamin B-6)** A
0.00 0.00 Global Days XXX

84210 **Pyruvate** A
0.00 0.00 Global Days XXX

84220 **Pyruvate kinase** A
0.00 0.00 Global Days XXX

84228 **Quinine** A
0.00 0.00 Global Days XXX

84233 **Receptor assay; estrogen** A
0.00 0.00 Global Days XXX

84234 **progesterone** A
0.00 0.00 Global Days XXX

84235 **endocrine, other than estrogen or progesterone (specify hormone)** A
0.00 0.00 Global Days XXX

84238 **non-endocrine (specify receptor)** A
0.00 0.00 Global Days XXX
AMA: 2009, Jan, 11-31; 2008, Jan, 10-25; 2007, January, 13-27

84244 **Renin** A
0.00 0.00 Global Days XXX

84252 **Riboflavin (Vitamin B-2)** A
0.00 0.00 Global Days XXX

84255 **Selenium** A
0.00 0.00 Global Days XXX

84260 **Serotonin** A
EXCLUDES *Urine metabolites (HIAA) (83497)*
0.00 0.00 Global Days XXX

84270 **Sex hormone binding globulin (SHBG)** A
0.00 0.00 Global Days XXX

84275 **Sialic acid** A
0.00 0.00 Global Days XXX

84285 **Silica** A
0.00 0.00 Global Days XXX

84295 **Sodium; serum, plasma or whole blood** A
0.00 0.00 Global Days XXX

84300 **urine** A
0.00 0.00 Global Days XXX

84302 **other source** A
0.00 0.00 Global Days XXX

84305 **Somatomedin** A
0.00 0.00 Global Days XXX

84307 **Somatostatin** A
0.00 0.00 Global Days XXX

84311 **Spectrophotometry, analyte not elsewhere specified** A
0.00 0.00 Global Days XXX

84315 **Specific gravity (except urine)** A
EXCLUDES *Urine specific gravity (81000-81003)*
0.00 0.00 Global Days XXX

84375 **Sugars, chromatographic, TLC or paper chromatography** A
0.00 0.00 Global Days XXX

84376 **Sugars (mono-, di-, and oligosaccharides); single qualitative, each specimen** A
0.00 0.00 Global Days XXX

84377 **multiple qualitative, each specimen** A
0.00 0.00 Global Days XXX

84378 single quantitative, each specimen
0.00 0.00 Global Days XXX

84379 multiple quantitative, each specimen
0.00 0.00 Global Days XXX

84392 **Sulfate, urine**
0.00 0.00 Global Days XXX

84402 **Testosterone; free**
0.00 0.00 Global Days XXX

84403 total
0.00 0.00 Global Days XXX

84425 **Thiamine (Vitamin B-1)**
0.00 0.00 Global Days XXX

84430 **Thiocyanate**
0.00 0.00 Global Days XXX

84431 **Thromboxane metabolite(s), including thromboxane if performed, urine**
Code also determination of concurrent urine creatinine (82507)
0.00 0.00 Global Days XXX

84432 **Thyroglobulin**
EXCLUDES *Thyroglobulin antibody (86800)*
0.00 0.00 Global Days XXX

84436-84445 Chemistry: Thyroid Tests

CMS 100-2,15,80 Diagnostic Test Requirements
CMS 100-3,190.22 Thyroid Testing
CMS 100-4,3,10.4 Payment of Nonphysician Services for Inpatients

INCLUDES Mathematically calculated results
Quantitative analysis unless otherwise specified
Specimens from any source unless otherwise specified

EXCLUDES *Organ or disease panels (80048-80076)*
Therapeutic drug assays (80150-80299)

84436 **Thyroxine; total**
0.00 0.00 Global Days XXX

84437 requiring elution (eg, neonatal)
0.00 0.00 Global Days XXX

84439 free
0.00 0.00 Global Days XXX

84442 **Thyroxine binding globulin (TBG)**
0.00 0.00 Global Days XXX

84443 **Thyroid stimulating hormone (TSH)**
0.00 0.00 Global Days XXX

84445 **Thyroid stimulating immune globulins (TSI)**
0.00 0.00 Global Days XXX

84446-84449 Chemistry: Tocopherol Alpha—Transcortin

CMS 100-2,15,80 Diagnostic Test Requirements
CMS 100-4,3,10.4 Payment of Nonphysician Services for Inpatients

INCLUDES Mathematically calculated results
Quantitative analysis unless otherwise specified
Specimens from any source unless otherwise specified

EXCLUDES *Organ or disease panels (80048-80076)*
Therapeutic drug assays (80150-80299)

84446 **Tocopherol alpha (Vitamin E)**
0.00 0.00 Global Days XXX

84449 **Transcortin (cortisol binding globulin)**
0.00 0.00 Global Days XXX

84450-84460 Chemistry: Transferase

CMS 100-2,15,80 Diagnostic Test Requirements
CMS 100-3,190.10 Laboratory Tests--CRD Patients
CMS 100-4,3,10.4 Payment of Nonphysician Services for Inpatients

INCLUDES Mathematically calculated results
Quantitative analysis unless otherwise specified

84450 **Transferase; aspartate amino (AST) (SGOT)**
0.00 0.00 Global Days XXX

84460 alanine amino (ALT) (SGPT)
0.00 0.00 Global Days XXX

84466 Chemistry: Transferrin

CMS 100-2,15,80 Diagnostic Test Requirements
CMS 100-4,3,10.4 Payment of Nonphysician Services for Inpatients

INCLUDES Mathematically calculated results
Quantitative analysis unless otherwise specified

84466 **Transferrin**
EXCLUDES *Iron binding capacity (83550)*
0.00 0.00 Global Days XXX

84478 Chemistry: Triglycerides

CMS 100-2,15,80 Diagnostic Test Requirements
CMS 100-3,190.23 Lipid Testing
CMS 100-4,3,10.4 Payment of Nonphysician Services for Inpatients

INCLUDES Mathematically calculated results

EXCLUDES *Organ or disease panels (80048-80076)*

84478 **Triglycerides**
0.00 0.00 Global Days XXX
AMA: 2009, Jan, 11-31; 2008, Jan, 10-25; 2007, January, 13-27

84479-84482 Chemistry: Thyroid Hormone—Triiodothyronine

CMS 100-2,15,80 Diagnostic Test Requirements
CMS 100-3,190.22 Thyroid Testing
CMS 100-4,3,10.4 Payment of Nonphysician Services for Inpatients

INCLUDES Mathematically calculated results
Quantitative analysis unless otherwise specified
Specimens from any source unless otherwise specified

EXCLUDES *Organ or disease panels (80048-80076)*

84479 **Thyroid hormone (T3 or T4) uptake or thyroid hormone binding ratio (THBR)**
0.00 0.00 Global Days XXX

84480 **Triiodothyronine T3; total (TT-3)**
0.00 0.00 Global Days XXX

84481 free
0.00 0.00 Global Days XXX

84482 reverse
0.00 0.00 Global Days XXX

84484-84512 Chemistry: Troponin (Quantitative)—Troponin (Qualitative)

CMS 100-2,15,80 Diagnostic Test Requirements
CMS 100-4,3,10.4 Payment of Nonphysician Services for Inpatients

INCLUDES Mathematically calculated results
Specimens from any source unless otherwise specified

EXCLUDES *Organ or disease panels*

84484 **Troponin, quantitative**
EXCLUDES *Qualitative troponin assay (84512)*
0.00 0.00 Global Days XXX

84485 Trypsin; duodenal fluid A
0.00 0.00 Global Days XXX

84488 feces, qualitative A
0.00 0.00 Global Days XXX

84490 feces, quantitative, 24-hour collection A
0.00 0.00 Global Days XXX

84510 Tyrosine A
EXCLUDES *Urate crystal identification (89060)*
0.00 0.00 Global Days XXX

84512 Troponin, qualitative A
EXCLUDES *Quantitative tropin assay (84484)*
0.00 0.00 Global Days XXX

84520-84525 Chemistry: Urea Nitrogen (Blood)

CMS 100-2,15,80 Diagnostic Test Requirements
CMS 100-3,190.10 Laboratory Tests--CRD Patients
CMS 100-4,3,10.4 Payment of Nonphysician Services for Inpatients
INCLUDES Mathematically calculated results
EXCLUDES *Organ or disease panels (80048-80076)*

84520 Urea nitrogen; quantitative A
0.00 0.00 Global Days XXX

84525 semiquantitative (eg, reagent strip test) A
INCLUDES Patterson's test
0.00 0.00 Global Days XXX

84540-84630 Chemistry: Urea Nitrogen (Urine)—Zinc

CMS 100-2,15,80 Diagnostic Test Requirements
CMS 100-4,3,10.4 Payment of Nonphysician Services for Inpatients
INCLUDES Mathematically calculated results
Quantitative analysis unless otherwise specified
Specimens from any source unless otherwise specified
EXCLUDES *Organ or disease panels (80048-80076)*
Therapeutic drug assays (80150-80299)

84540 Urea nitrogen, urine A
0.00 0.00 Global Days XXX

84545 Urea nitrogen, clearance A
0.00 0.00 Global Days XXX

84550 Uric acid; blood A
0.00 0.00 Global Days XXX

84560 other source A
0.00 0.00 Global Days XXX

84577 Urobilinogen, feces, quantitative A
0.00 0.00 Global Days XXX

84578 Urobilinogen, urine; qualitative A
0.00 0.00 Global Days XXX

84580 quantitative, timed specimen A
0.00 0.00 Global Days XXX

84583 semiquantitative A
0.00 0.00 Global Days XXX

84585 Vanillylmandelic acid (VMA), urine A
0.00 0.00 Global Days XXX

84586 Vasoactive intestinal peptide (VIP) A
0.00 0.00 Global Days XXX

84588 Vasopressin (antidiuretic hormone, ADH) A
0.00 0.00 Global Days XXX

84590 Vitamin A A
0.00 0.00 Global Days XXX

84591 Vitamin, not otherwise specified A
0.00 0.00 Global Days XXX

84597 Vitamin K A
0.00 0.00 Global Days XXX

84600 Volatiles (eg, acetic anhydride, carbon tetrachloride, dichloroethane, dichloromethane, diethylether, isopropyl alcohol, methanol) A
EXCLUDES *Acetaldehyde (82000)*
0.00 0.00 Global Days XXX

84620 Xylose absorption test, blood and/or urine A
EXCLUDES *Administration (99070)*
0.00 0.00 Global Days XXX

84630 Zinc A
0.00 0.00 Global Days XXX

84681-84999 Other and Unlisted Chemistry Tests

CMS 100-2,15,80 Diagnostic Test Requirements
CMS 100-4,3,10.4 Payment of Nonphysician Services for Inpatients
INCLUDES Mathematically calculated results
Quantitative analysis unless otherwise specified
Specimens from any source unless otherwise specified
EXCLUDES *Organ or disease panels (80048-80076)*

84681 C-peptide A
0.00 0.00 Global Days XXX

84702 Gonadotropin, chorionic (hCG); quantitative A
0.00 0.00 Global Days XXX

84703 qualitative A
EXCLUDES *Urine pregnancy test by visual color comparison (81025)*
0.00 0.00 Global Days XXX

84704 free beta chain A
0.00 0.00 Global Days XXX
AMA: 2009, Jan, 11-31; 2008, Apr, 5-7

84830 Ovulation tests, by visual color comparison methods for human luteinizing hormone ♀ A
0.00 0.00 Global Days XXX

84999 Unlisted chemistry procedure A
0.00 0.00 Global Days XXX
AMA: 2009, Jan, 11-31; 2008, Jan, 10-25; 2007, January, 13-27

85002 Bleeding Time Test

CMS 100-2,15,80 Diagnostic Test Requirements
CMS 100-4,3,10.4 Payment of Nonphysician Services for Inpatients
EXCLUDES *Agglutinins (86000, 86156-86157)*
Antiplasmin (85410)
Antithrombin III (85300-85301)
Blood banking procedures (86850-86999)

85002 Bleeding time A
0.00 0.00 Global Days XXX

85004-85049 Blood Counts

CMS 100-2,15,80 Diagnostic Test Requirements
CMS 100-3,190.15 Blood Counts
CMS 100-4,3,10.4 Payment of Nonphysician Services for Inpatients
EXCLUDES *Agglutinins (86000, 86156-86157)*
Antiplasmin (85410)
Antithrombin III (85300-85301)
Blood banking procedures (86850-86999)

85004 Blood count; automated differential WBC count A
0.00 0.00 Global Days XXX
AMA: 2009, Jan, 11-31; 2008, Jan, 10-25; 2007, January, 13-27

85007 **blood smear, microscopic examination with manual differential WBC count** A
0.00 0.00 Global Days XXX
AMA: 2009, Jan, 11-31; 2008, Jan, 10-25; 2007, January, 13-27

85008 **blood smear, microscopic examination without manual differential WBC count** A
EXCLUDES *Cell count other fluids (eg, CSF) (89050-89051)*
0.00 0.00 Global Days XXX
AMA: 2009, Jan, 11-31; 2008, Jan, 10-25; 2007, January, 13-27

85009 **manual differential WBC count, buffy coat** A
0.00 0.00 Global Days XXX
AMA: 2009, Jan, 11-31; 2008, Jan, 10-25; 2007, January, 13-27

85013 **spun microhematocrit** A
0.00 0.00 Global Days XXX

85014 **hematocrit (Hct)** A
0.00 0.00 Global Days XXX

85018 **hemoglobin (Hgb)** A
EXCLUDES *Immunoassay, hemoglobin, fecal (82274)*
Other hemoglobin determination (83020-83069)
Transcutaneous hemoglobin measurement (88738)
0.00 0.00 Global Days XXX

85025 **complete (CBC), automated (Hgb, Hct, RBC, WBC and platelet count) and automated differential WBC count** A
0.00 0.00 Global Days XXX
AMA: 2009, Jan, 11-31; 2008, Jan, 10-25; 2007, January, 13-27

85027 **complete (CBC), automated (Hgb, Hct, RBC, WBC and platelet count)** A
0.00 0.00 Global Days XXX

85032 **manual cell count (erythrocyte, leukocyte, or platelet) each** A
0.00 0.00 Global Days XXX
AMA: 2009, Jan, 11-31; 2008, Jan, 10-25; 2007, January, 13-27

85041 **red blood cell (RBC), automated** A
Do not report with (85025, 85027)
0.00 0.00 Global Days XXX

85044 **reticulocyte, manual** A
0.00 0.00 Global Days XXX

85045 **reticulocyte, automated** A
0.00 0.00 Global Days XXX

85046 **reticulocytes, automated, including 1 or more cellular parameters (eg, reticulocyte hemoglobin content [CHr], immature reticulocyte fraction [IRF], reticulocyte volume [MRV], RNA content), direct measurement** A
0.00 0.00 Global Days XXX

85048 **leukocyte (WBC), automated** A
0.00 0.00 Global Days XXX

85049 **platelet, automated** A
0.00 0.00 Global Days XXX

85055-85705 Coagulopathy Testing

CMS 100-2,15,80 Diagnostic Test Requirements
CMS 100-4,3,10.4 Payment of Nonphysician Services for Inpatients
CMS 100-4,3,20.7.3 Payment for Blood Clotting Factor for Hemophilia Inpatients

EXCLUDES *Agglutinins (86000, 86156-86157)*
Antiplasmin (85410)
Antithrombin III (85300-85301)
Blood banking procedures (86850-86999)

85055 **Reticulated platelet assay** A
0.00 0.00 Global Days XXX

85060 **Blood smear, peripheral, interpretation by physician with written report** B 80
0.68 0.68 Global Days XXX

85097 **Bone marrow, smear interpretation** X 80
EXCLUDES *Bone biopsy (20220, 20225, 20240, 20245, 20250-20251)*
Special stains (88312-88313)
1.36 2.45 Global Days XXX
AMA: 2009, Jan, 11-31; 2008, Jan, 10-25; 2007, January, 13-27

85130 **Chromogenic substrate assay** A
0.00 0.00 Global Days XXX

85170 **Clot retraction** A
0.00 0.00 Global Days XXX

85175 **Clot lysis time, whole blood dilution** A
0.00 0.00 Global Days XXX

85210 **Clotting; factor II, prothrombin, specific** A
EXCLUDES *Prothrombin time (85610-85611)*
Russel viper venom time (85612-85613) (85612-85613)
0.00 0.00 Global Days XXX

85220 **factor V (AcG or proaccelerin), labile factor** A
0.00 0.00 Global Days XXX

85230 **factor VII (proconvertin, stable factor)** A
0.00 0.00 Global Days XXX

85240 **factor VIII (AHG), 1-stage** A
0.00 0.00 Global Days XXX

85244 **factor VIII related antigen** A
0.00 0.00 Global Days XXX

85245 **factor VIII, VW factor, ristocetin cofactor** A
0.00 0.00 Global Days XXX

85246 **factor VIII, VW factor antigen** A
0.00 0.00 Global Days XXX

85247 **factor VIII, von Willebrand factor, multimetric analysis** A
0.00 0.00 Global Days XXX

85250 **factor IX (PTC or Christmas)** A
0.00 0.00 Global Days XXX

85260 **factor X (Stuart-Prower)** A
0.00 0.00 Global Days XXX

85270 **factor XI (PTA)** A
0.00 0.00 Global Days XXX

85280 **factor XII (Hageman)** A
0.00 0.00 Global Days XXX

85290 **factor XIII (fibrin stabilizing)** A
0.00 0.00 Global Days XXX

85291 **factor XIII (fibrin stabilizing), screen solubility** A
0.00 0.00 Global Days XXX

85292 **prekallikrein assay (Fletcher factor assay)** A
0.00 0.00 Global Days XXX

85293 **high molecular weight kininogen assay (Fitzgerald factor assay)** A
0.00 0.00 Global Days XXX

85300 **Clotting inhibitors or anticoagulants; antithrombin III, activity** A
0.00 0.00 Global Days XXX

85301 **antithrombin III, antigen assay** A
0.00 0.00 Global Days XXX

85302 **protein C, antigen** A
0.00 0.00 Global Days XXX

85303 **protein C, activity** A
0.00 0.00 Global Days XXX

85305 **protein S, total** A
0.00 0.00 Global Days XXX

85306 protein S, free
0.00 0.00 Global Days XXX

85307 Activated Protein C (APC) resistance assay
0.00 0.00 Global Days XXX

85335 Factor inhibitor test
0.00 0.00 Global Days XXX

85337 Thrombomodulin
EXCLUDES *Mixing studies for inhibitors (85732)*
0.00 0.00 Global Days XXX

85345 Coagulation time; Lee and White
0.00 0.00 Global Days XXX

85347 activated
0.00 0.00 Global Days XXX

85348 other methods
0.00 0.00 Global Days XXX

85360 Euglobulin lysis
0.00 0.00 Global Days XXX

85362 Fibrin(ogen) degradation (split) products (FDP) (FSP); agglutination slide, semiquantitative
0.00 0.00 Global Days XXX

85366 paracoagulation
0.00 0.00 Global Days XXX

85370 quantitative
0.00 0.00 Global Days XXX

85378 Fibrin degradation products, D-dimer; qualitative or semiquantitative
0.00 0.00 Global Days XXX

85379 quantitative
INCLUDES Ultrasensitive and standard sensitivity quantitative D-dimer
0.00 0.00 Global Days XXX

85380 ultrasensitive (eg, for evaluation for venous thromboembolism), qualitative or semiquantitative
0.00 0.00 Global Days XXX

85384 Fibrinogen; activity
0.00 0.00 Global Days XXX

85385 antigen
0.00 0.00 Global Days XXX

85390 Fibrinolysins or coagulopathy screen, interpretation and report
0.00 0.00 Global Days XXX

85396 Coagulation/fibrinolysis assay, whole blood (eg, viscoelastic clot assessment), including use of any pharmacologic additive(s), as indicated, including interpretation and written report, per day
0.56 0.56 Global Days XXX

85397 Coagulation and fibrinolysis, functional activity, not otherwise specified (eg, ADAMTS-13), each analyte
0.00 0.00 Global Days XXX

85400 Fibrinolytic factors and inhibitors; plasmin
0.00 0.00 Global Days XXX

85410 alpha-2 antiplasmin
0.00 0.00 Global Days XXX

85415 plasminogen activator
0.00 0.00 Global Days XXX

85420 plasminogen, except antigenic assay
0.00 0.00 Global Days XXX

85421 plasminogen, antigenic assay
0.00 0.00 Global Days XXX

85441 Heinz bodies; direct
0.00 0.00 Global Days XXX

85445 induced, acetyl phenylhydrazine
0.00 0.00 Global Days XXX

85460 Hemoglobin or RBCs, fetal, for fetomaternal hemorrhage; differential lysis (Kleihauer-Betke)
EXCLUDES *Hemoglobin F (83030, 83033)*
Hemolysins (86940-86941)
0.00 0.00 Global Days XXX

85461 rosette
0.00 0.00 Global Days XXX

85475 Hemolysin, acid
INCLUDES Ham test
EXCLUDES *Hemolysins and agglutinins (86940-86941)*
0.00 0.00 Global Days XXX

85520 Heparin assay
0.00 0.00 Global Days XXX

85525 Heparin neutralization
0.00 0.00 Global Days XXX

85530 Heparin-protamine tolerance test
0.00 0.00 Global Days XXX

85536 Iron stain, peripheral blood
EXCLUDES *Iron stains on bone marrow or other tissues with physician evaluation (88313)*
0.00 0.00 Global Days XXX

85540 Leukocyte alkaline phosphatase with count
0.00 0.00 Global Days XXX

85547 Mechanical fragility, RBC
0.00 0.00 Global Days XXX

85549 Muramidase
0.00 0.00 Global Days XXX

85555 Osmotic fragility, RBC; unincubated
0.00 0.00 Global Days XXX

85557 incubated
0.00 0.00 Global Days XXX

85576 Platelet, aggregation (in vitro), each agent
EXCLUDES *Thromboxane metabolite(s), including thromboxane, when performed, in urine (84431)*
0.00 0.00 Global Days XXX
AMA: 2009, Jan, 11-31; 2008, Jan, 10-25; 2007, January, 13-27

85597 Phospholipid neutralization; platelet
0.00 0.00 Global Days XXX

85598 hexagonal phospholipid
0.00 0.00 Global Days XXX

85610 Prothrombin time;
0.00 0.00 Global Days XXX

85611 substitution, plasma fractions, each
0.00 0.00 Global Days XXX

85612 Russell viper venom time (includes venom); undiluted
0.00 0.00 Global Days XXX

85613 diluted
0.00 0.00 Global Days XXX

85635 Reptilase test
0.00 0.00 Global Days XXX

85651 Sedimentation rate, erythrocyte; non-automated
0.00 0.00 Global Days XXX

85652 automated
INCLUDES Westergren test
0.00 0.00 Global Days XXX

85660 Sickling of RBC, reduction A
EXCLUDES *Hemoglobin electrophoresis (83020)*
Smears (87207)
0.00 0.00 Global Days XXX

85670 Thrombin time; plasma A
0.00 0.00 Global Days XXX

85675 titer A
0.00 0.00 Global Days XXX

85705 Thromboplastin inhibition, tissue A
EXCLUDES *Individual clotting factors (85245-85247)*
0.00 0.00 Global Days XXX

85730-85732 Partial Thromboplastin Time (PTT)

CMS 100-2,15,80 Diagnostic Test Requirements
CMS 100-3,190.16 Partial Thromboplastin Time (PTT)
CMS 100-4,3,10.4 Payment of Nonphysician Services for Inpatients

EXCLUDES *Agglutinins (86000, 86156-86157)*
Antiplasmin (85410)
Antithrombin III (85300-85301)
Blood banking procedures (86850-86999)

85730 Thromboplastin time, partial (PTT); plasma or whole blood A
INCLUDES Hicks-Pitney test
0.00 0.00 Global Days XXX

85732 substitution, plasma fractions, each A
0.00 0.00 Global Days XXX

85810-85999 Blood Viscosity and Unlisted Hematology Procedures

CMS 100-2,15,80 Diagnostic Test Requirements
CMS 100-4,3,10.4 Payment of Nonphysician Services for Inpatients

85810 Viscosity A
0.00 0.00 Global Days XXX
AMA: 2009, Feb, 22

85999 Unlisted hematology and coagulation procedure A
0.00 0.00 Global Days XXX

86000-86063 Antibody Testing

CMS 100-2,15,80 Diagnostic Test Requirements
CMS 100-4,3,10.4 Payment of Nonphysician Services for Inpatients

86000 Agglutinins, febrile (eg, Brucella, Francisella, Murine typhus, Q fever, Rocky Mountain spotted fever, scrub typhus), each antigen A
0.00 0.00 Global Days XXX

86001 Allergen specific IgG quantitative or semiquantitative, each allergen A
0.00 0.00 Global Days XXX

86003 Allergen specific IgE; quantitative or semiquantitative, each allergen A
EXCLUDES *Total quantitative IgE (82785)*
0.00 0.00 Global Days XXX

86005 qualitative, multiallergen screen (dipstick, paddle, or disk) A
EXCLUDES *Total qualitative IgE (83518)*
0.00 0.00 Global Days XXX

86021 Antibody identification; leukocyte antibodies A
0.00 0.00 Global Days XXX

86022 platelet antibodies A
0.00 0.00 Global Days XXX

86023 platelet associated immunoglobulin assay A
0.00 0.00 Global Days XXX

86038 Antinuclear antibodies (ANA); A
0.00 0.00 Global Days XXX

86039 titer A
0.00 0.00 Global Days XXX

86060 Antistreptolysin 0; titer A
0.00 0.00 Global Days XXX

86063 screen A
0.00 0.00 Global Days XXX

86077-86079 Blood Bank Services

CMS 100-2,15,80 Diagnostic Test Requirements
CMS 100-4,3,10.4 Payment of Nonphysician Services for Inpatients
CMS 100-4,12,60 Payment for Pathology Services

86077 Blood bank physician services; difficult cross match and/or evaluation of irregular antibody(s), interpretation and written report X 80
1.40 1.50 Global Days XXX

86078 investigation of transfusion reaction including suspicion of transmissible disease, interpretation and written report X 80
1.41 1.51 Global Days XXX

86079 authorization for deviation from standard blood banking procedures (eg, use of outdated blood, transfusion of Rh incompatible units), with written report X 80
1.41 1.51 Global Days XXX

86140-86344 Diagnostic Immunology Testing

CMS 100-2,15,80 Diagnostic Test Requirements
CMS 100-4,3,10.4 Payment of Nonphysician Services for Inpatients

86140 C-reactive protein; A
0.00 0.00 Global Days XXX

86141 high sensitivity (hsCRP) A
0.00 0.00 Global Days XXX

86146 Beta 2 Glycoprotein I antibody, each A
0.00 0.00 Global Days XXX

86147 Cardiolipin (phospholipid) antibody, each Ig class A
0.00 0.00 Global Days XXX

86148 Anti-phosphatidylserine (phospholipid) antibody A
EXCLUDES *Antiprothrombin (phospholipid cofactor) antibody (0030T)*
Cell enumeration using immunologic selection and identification in fluid sample (0279T-0280T)
0.00 0.00 Global Days XXX

86155 Chemotaxis assay, specify method A
0.00 0.00 Global Days XXX

86156 Cold agglutinin; screen A
0.00 0.00 Global Days XXX

86157 titer A
0.00 0.00 Global Days XXX

86160 Complement; antigen, each component A
0.00 0.00 Global Days XXX

86161 functional activity, each component A
0.00 0.00 Global Days XXX

86162 total hemolytic (CH50) A
0.00 0.00 Global Days XXX

86171 Complement fixation tests, each antigen A
0.00 0.00 Global Days XXX

86185 Counterimmunoelectrophoresis, each antigen A
0.00 0.00 Global Days XXX

86200 Cyclic citrullinated peptide (CCP), antibody A
0.00 0.00 Global Days XXX

86215 **Deoxyribonuclease, antibody**
0.00 0.00 Global Days XXX

86225 **Deoxyribonucleic acid (DNA) antibody; native or double stranded**
EXCLUDES *Echinococcus, antibodies (see code for specific method)*
0.00 0.00 Global Days XXX

86226 **single stranded**
EXCLUDES *Anti D.S, DNA, IFA, eg, using C. lucilae (86255-86256)*
0.00 0.00 Global Days XXX

86235 **Extractable nuclear antigen, antibody to, any method (eg, nRNP, SS-A, SS-B, Sm, RNP, Sc170, J01), each antibody**
0.00 0.00 Global Days XXX

86243 **Fc receptor**
EXCLUDES *Filaria antibodies to, (see code for specific method)*
0.00 0.00 Global Days XXX

86255 **Fluorescent noninfectious agent antibody; screen, each antibody**
EXCLUDES *FTA (86780)*
0.00 0.00 Global Days XXX

86256 **titer, each antibody**
EXCLUDES *Fluorescent technique for antigen identification in tissue (88346)*
FTA (86780)
Gel (agar) diffusion tests (86331)
Indirect fluorescence (88347)
0.00 0.00 Global Days XXX

86277 **Growth hormone, human (HGH), antibody**
0.00 0.00 Global Days XXX

86280 **Hemagglutination inhibition test (HAI)**
EXCLUDES *Antibodies to infectious agents (86602-86804)*
Rubella (86762)
0.00 0.00 Global Days XXX

86294 **Immunoassay for tumor antigen, qualitative or semiquantitative (eg, bladder tumor antigen)**
EXCLUDES *Qualitative NMP22 protein (86386)*
0.00 0.00 Global Days XXX

86300 **Immunoassay for tumor antigen, quantitative; CA 15-3 (27.29)**
0.00 0.00 Global Days XXX

86301 **CA 19-9**
0.00 0.00 Global Days XXX

86304 **CA 125**
EXCLUDES *Measurement of serum HER-2/neu oncoprotein (83950)*
0.00 0.00 Global Days XXX

86305 **Human epididymis protein 4 (HE4)**
0.00 0.00 Global Days XXX

86308 **Heterophile antibodies; screening**
EXCLUDES *Antibodies to infectious agents (86602-86804)*
0.00 0.00 Global Days XXX

86309 **titer**
EXCLUDES *Antibodies to infectious agents (86602-86804)*
0.00 0.00 Global Days XXX

86310 **titers after absorption with beef cells and guinea pig kidney**
EXCLUDES *Antibodies to infectious agents (86602-86804)*
0.00 0.00 Global Days XXX

86316 **Immunoassay for tumor antigen, other antigen, quantitative (eg, CA 50, 72-4, 549), each**
0.00 0.00 Global Days XXX
AMA: 2009, Jan, 11-31; 2008, Jan, 10-25; 2007, January, 13-27

86317 **Immunoassay for infectious agent antibody, quantitative, not otherwise specified**
0.00 0.00 Global Days XXX

86318 **Immunoassay for infectious agent antibody, qualitative or semiquantitative, single step method (eg, reagent strip)**
0.00 0.00 Global Days XXX
AMA: 2009, Jan, 11-31; 2008, Jan, 10-25; 2007, March, 9-11

86320 **Immunoelectrophoresis; serum**
0.00 0.00 Global Days XXX

86325 **other fluids (eg, urine, cerebrospinal fluid) with concentration**
0.00 0.00 Global Days XXX

86327 **crossed (2-dimensional assay)**
0.00 0.00 Global Days XXX

86329 **Immunodiffusion; not elsewhere specified**
0.00 0.00 Global Days XXX
AMA: 2009, Jan, 11-31; 2008, Jan, 10-25; 2007, January, 13-27

86331 **gel diffusion, qualitative (Ouchterlony), each antigen or antibody**
0.00 0.00 Global Days XXX

86332 **Immune complex assay**
0.00 0.00 Global Days XXX

86334 **Immunofixation electrophoresis; serum**
0.00 0.00 Global Days XXX

86335 **other fluids with concentration (eg, urine, CSF)**
0.00 0.00 Global Days XXX

86336 **Inhibin A**
0.00 0.00 Global Days XXX

86337 **Insulin antibodies**
0.00 0.00 Global Days XXX

86340 **Intrinsic factor antibodies**
0.00 0.00 Global Days XXX

86341 **Islet cell antibody**
0.00 0.00 Global Days XXX

86343 **Leukocyte histamine release test (LHR)**
0.00 0.00 Global Days XXX

86344 **Leukocyte phagocytosis**
0.00 0.00 Global Days XXX

86352 Assay Cellular Function

86352 **Cellular function assay involving stimulation (eg, mitogen or antigen) and detection of biomarker (eg, ATP)**
0.00 0.00 Global Days XXX

86353 Lymphocyte Mitogen Response Assay

CMS 100-2,15,80 Diagnostic Test Requirements
CMS 100-3,190.8 Lymphocyte Mitogen Response Assays
CMS 100-4,3,10.4 Payment of Nonphysician Services for Inpatients

86353 **Lymphocyte transformation, mitogen (phytomitogen) or antigen induced blastogenesis**
EXCLUDES *Cellular function assay involving stimulation and detection of biomarker (86352)*
0.00 0.00 Global Days XXX

Pathology and Laboratory
86215 — 86353

● New Code ▲ Revised Code Maternity Age Unlisted Not Covered # Resequenced
❍ Reinstated CCI + Add-on Mod 51 Exempt Mod 63 Exempt Mod Sedation PQRS

86355-86593 Additional Diagnostic Immunology Testing

CMS 100-2,15,80 Diagnostic Test Requirements
CMS 100-4,3,10.4 Payment of Nonphysician Services for Inpatients

86355 **B cells, total count** A
Do not report with flow cytometry interpretation (88187-88189)
0.00 0.00 Global Days XXX
AMA: 2008, Apr, 5-7

86356 **Mononuclear cell antigen, quantitative (eg, flow cytometry), not otherwise specified, each antigen** A
Do not report with flow cytometry interpretation (88187-88189)
0.00 0.00 Global Days XXX
AMA: 2008, Apr, 5-7

86357 **Natural killer (NK) cells, total count** A
Do not report with flow cytometry interpretation (88187-88189)
0.00 0.00 Global Days XXX
AMA: 2008, Apr, 5-7

86359 **T cells; total count** A
Do not report with flow cytometry interpretation (88187-88189)
0.00 0.00 Global Days XXX
AMA: 2008, Apr, 5-7

86360 **absolute CD4 and CD8 count, including ratio** A
Do not report with flow cytometry interpretation (88187-88189)
0.00 0.00 Global Days XXX
AMA: 2008, Apr, 5-7; 2007, January, 28-31

86361 **absolute CD4 count** A
Do not report with flow cytometry interpretation (88187-88189)
0.00 0.00 Global Days XXX
AMA: 2008, Apr, 5-7

86367 **Stem cells (ie, CD34), total count** A
EXCLUDES *Flow cytometric immunophenotyping for the assessment of potential hematolymphoid neoplasia (88184-88189)*
Do not report with flow cytometry interpretation (88187-88189)
0.00 0.00 Global Days XXX
AMA: 2009, Jun, 3-6&11; 2008, Apr, 5-7

86376 **Microsomal antibodies (eg, thyroid or liver-kidney), each** A
0.00 0.00 Global Days XXX

86378 **Migration inhibitory factor test (MIF)** A
0.00 0.00 Global Days XXX

86382 **Neutralization test, viral** A
0.00 0.00 Global Days XXX

86384 **Nitroblue tetrazolium dye test (NTD)** A
0.00 0.00 Global Days XXX

● **86386** **Nuclear Matrix Protein 22 (NMP22), qualitative** A
0.00 0.00 Global Days XXX

86403 **Particle agglutination; screen, each antibody** A
0.00 0.00 Global Days XXX

86406 **titer, each antibody** A
EXCLUDES *Pregnancy test (84702-84703)*
Rapid plasma reagin test (RPR) (86592-86593)
0.00 0.00 Global Days XXX

86430 **Rheumatoid factor; qualitative** A
0.00 0.00 Global Days XXX

86431 **quantitative** A
0.00 0.00 Global Days XXX

86480 **Tuberculosis test, cell mediated immunity antigen response measurement; gamma interferon** A
0.00 0.00 Global Days XXX

86481 **enumeration of gamma interferon-producing T-cells in cell suspension** A
0.00 0.00 Global Days XXX

86485 **Skin test; candida** X TC 80
0.00 0.00 Global Days XXX

86486 **unlisted antigen, each** X TC 80
0.16 0.16 Global Days XXX
AMA: 2008, Apr, 5-7

86490 **coccidioidomycosis** X TC 80
0.19 0.19 Global Days XXX

86510 **histoplasmosis** X TC 80
0.19 0.19 Global Days XXX

86580 **tuberculosis, intradermal** X TC 80
INCLUDES Heaf test
Intradermal Mantoux test
EXCLUDES *Skin test for allergy (95010-95199)*
Tuberculosis test, cell mediated immunity measurement of gamma interferon antigen response (86480) (86480)
0.23 0.23 Global Days XXX

86590 **Streptokinase, antibody** A
EXCLUDES *Antibodies to infectious agents (86602-86804)*
Streptolysin O antibody (86060, 86063)
0.00 0.00 Global Days XXX

86592 **Syphilis test, non-treponemal antibody; qualitative (eg, VDRL, RPR, ART)** A
INCLUDES Wasserman test
EXCLUDES *Antibodies to infectious agents (86602-86804)*
0.00 0.00 Global Days XXX

86593 **quantitative** A
EXCLUDES *Antibodies to infectious agents (86602-86804)*
0.00 0.00 Global Days XXX

86602-86698 Testing for Antibodies to Infectious Agents: Actinomyces—Histoplasma

CMS 100-2,15,80 Diagnostic Test Requirements
CMS 100-4,3,10.4 Payment of Nonphysician Services for Inpatients

INCLUDES Qualitative or semiquantitative immunoassays performed by multiple-step methods for the detection of antibodies to infectious agents

EXCLUDES *Detection of:*
Antibodies other than those to infectious agents, see specific antibody or method (86021-86023, 86376, 86800, 86850-86870)
Infectious agent/antigen (87260-87899)
Immunoassays by single-step method (86318)

86602 **Antibody; actinomyces** A
0.00 0.00 Global Days XXX

86603 **adenovirus** A
0.00 0.00 Global Days XXX

86606 **Aspergillus** A
0.00 0.00 Global Days XXX

86609 **bacterium, not elsewhere specified** A
0.00 0.00 Global Days XXX

86611 Bartonella A
0.00 0.00 Global Days XXX

86612 Blastomyces A
0.00 0.00 Global Days XXX

86615 Bordetella A
0.00 0.00 Global Days XXX

86617 Borrelia burgdorferi (Lyme disease) confirmatory test (eg, Western Blot or immunoblot) A
0.00 0.00 Global Days XXX

86618 Borrelia burgdorferi (Lyme disease) A
0.00 0.00 Global Days XXX

86619 Borrelia (relapsing fever) A
0.00 0.00 Global Days XXX

86622 Brucella A
0.00 0.00 Global Days XXX

86625 Campylobacter A
0.00 0.00 Global Days XXX

86628 Candida A
EXCLUDES *Candida skin test (86485)*
0.00 0.00 Global Days XXX

86631 Chlamydia A
0.00 0.00 Global Days XXX

86632 Chlamydia, IgM A
EXCLUDES *Chlamydia antigen (87270, 87320)*
Fluorescent antibody technique (86255-86256)
0.00 0.00 Global Days XXX

86635 Coccidioides A
0.00 0.00 Global Days XXX

86638 Coxiella burnetii (Q fever) A
0.00 0.00 Global Days XXX

86641 Cryptococcus A
0.00 0.00 Global Days XXX

86644 cytomegalovirus (CMV) A
0.00 0.00 Global Days XXX

86645 cytomegalovirus (CMV), IgM A
0.00 0.00 Global Days XXX

86648 Diphtheria A
0.00 0.00 Global Days XXX

86651 encephalitis, California (La Crosse) A
0.00 0.00 Global Days XXX

86652 encephalitis, Eastern equine A
0.00 0.00 Global Days XXX

86653 encephalitis, St. Louis A
0.00 0.00 Global Days XXX

86654 encephalitis, Western equine A
0.00 0.00 Global Days XXX

86658 enterovirus (eg, coxsackie, echo, polio) A
0.00 0.00 Global Days XXX

86663 Epstein-Barr (EB) virus, early antigen (EA) A
0.00 0.00 Global Days XXX

86664 Epstein-Barr (EB) virus, nuclear antigen (EBNA) A
0.00 0.00 Global Days XXX

86665 Epstein-Barr (EB) virus, viral capsid (VCA) A
0.00 0.00 Global Days XXX

86666 Ehrlichia A
0.00 0.00 Global Days XXX

86668 Francisella tularensis A
0.00 0.00 Global Days XXX

86671 fungus, not elsewhere specified A
0.00 0.00 Global Days XXX

86674 Giardia lamblia A
0.00 0.00 Global Days XXX

86677 Helicobacter pylori A
0.00 0.00 Global Days XXX

86682 helminth, not elsewhere specified A
0.00 0.00 Global Days XXX

86684 Haemophilus influenza A
0.00 0.00 Global Days XXX

86687 HTLV-I A
0.00 0.00 Global Days XXX

86688 HTLV-II A
0.00 0.00 Global Days XXX

86689 HTLV or HIV antibody, confirmatory test (eg, Western Blot) A
0.00 0.00 Global Days XXX
AMA: 2008, Mar, 3&7

86692 hepatitis, delta agent A
EXCLUDES *Hepatitis delta agent, antigen (87380)*
0.00 0.00 Global Days XXX

86694 herpes simplex, non-specific type test A
0.00 0.00 Global Days XXX

86695 herpes simplex, type 1 A
0.00 0.00 Global Days XXX

86696 herpes simplex, type 2 A
0.00 0.00 Global Days XXX

86698 histoplasma A
0.00 0.00 Global Days XXX

86701-86703 Testing for HIV Antibodies

CMS 100-2,15,80 Diagnostic Test Requirements
CMS 100-3,190.9 Serologic Testing for Acquired Immunodeficiency Syndrome (AIDS)
CMS 100-3,190.14 Human Immunodeficiency Virus Testing (Diagnosis)
CMS 100-4,3,10.4 Payment of Nonphysician Services for Inpatients

INCLUDES Qualitative or semiquantitative immunoassays performed by multiple-step methods for the detection of antibodies to infectious agents

EXCLUDES *Confirmatory test for HIV antibody (86689)*
Detection of:
Antibodies other than those to infectious agents, see specific antibody or method (86021-86023, 86376, 86800, 86850-86870)
Infectious agent/antigen (87260-87899)
HIV-1 antigen (87390)
HIV-1 antigen(s) with HIV 1 and 2 antibodies, single result (87389)
HIV-2 antigen (87391)
Immunoassays by single-step method (86318)

Code also modifier 92 for test performed using a kit or transportable insrument that is all or in part consists of a single-use, disposable analytical chamber

86701 HIV-1 A
0.00 0.00 Global Days XXX
AMA: 2008, Mar, 3&7; 2008, Apr, 5-7

86702 HIV-2 A
0.00 0.00 Global Days XXX
AMA: 2008, Mar, 3&7; 2008, Apr, 5-7

▲ 86703 HIV-1 and HIV-2, single result A
0.00 0.00 Global Days XXX
AMA: 2008, Mar, 3&7; 2008, Apr, 5-7

86704-86804 Testing for Infectious Disease Antibodies: Hepatitis—Yersinia

CMS 100-2,15,80 Diagnostic Test Requirements
CMS 100-4,3,10.4 Payment of Nonphysician Services for Inpatients

INCLUDES Qualitative or semiquantitative immunoassays performed by multiple-step methods for the detection of antibodies to infectious agents

EXCLUDES *Detection of:*
Antibodies other than those to infectious agents, see specific antibody or method (86021-86023, 86376, 86800, 86850-86870)
Infectious agent/antigen
Immunoassays by single-step method (86318)

86704 Hepatitis B core antibody (HBcAb); total A
0.00 0.00 Global Days XXX

86705 IgM antibody A
0.00 0.00 Global Days XXX

86706 Hepatitis B surface antibody (HBsAb) A
0.00 0.00 Global Days XXX

86707 Hepatitis Be antibody (HBeAb) A
0.00 0.00 Global Days XXX

86708 Hepatitis A antibody (HAAb); total A
0.00 0.00 Global Days XXX
AMA: 2009, Jan, 11-31; 2008, Jan, 10-25; 2007, January, 13-27

86709 IgM antibody A
0.00 0.00 Global Days XXX
AMA: 2009, Jan, 11-31; 2008, Jan, 10-25; 2007, January, 13-27

86710 Antibody; influenza virus A
0.00 0.00 Global Days XXX
AMA: 2009, May, 6&10

86713 Legionella A
0.00 0.00 Global Days XXX

86717 Leishmania A
0.00 0.00 Global Days XXX

86720 Leptospira A
0.00 0.00 Global Days XXX

86723 Listeria monocytogenes A
0.00 0.00 Global Days XXX

86727 lymphocytic choriomeningitis A
0.00 0.00 Global Days XXX

86729 lymphogranuloma venereum A
0.00 0.00 Global Days XXX

86732 mucormycosis A
0.00 0.00 Global Days XXX

86735 mumps A
0.00 0.00 Global Days XXX
AMA: 2009, Jan, 11-31; 2008, Jan, 10-25; 2007, January, 13-27

86738 mycoplasma A
0.00 0.00 Global Days XXX

86741 Neisseria meningitidis A
0.00 0.00 Global Days XXX

86744 Nocardia A
0.00 0.00 Global Days XXX

86747 parvovirus A
0.00 0.00 Global Days XXX

86750 Plasmodium (malaria) A
0.00 0.00 Global Days XXX

86753 protozoa, not elsewhere specified A
0.00 0.00 Global Days XXX

86756 respiratory syncytial virus A
0.00 0.00 Global Days XXX

86757 Rickettsia A
0.00 0.00 Global Days XXX

86759 rotavirus A
0.00 0.00 Global Days XXX

86762 rubella A
0.00 0.00 Global Days XXX

86765 rubeola A
0.00 0.00 Global Days XXX

86768 Salmonella A
0.00 0.00 Global Days XXX

86771 Shigella A
0.00 0.00 Global Days XXX

86774 tetanus A
0.00 0.00 Global Days XXX

86777 Toxoplasma A
0.00 0.00 Global Days XXX

86778 Toxoplasma, IgM A
0.00 0.00 Global Days XXX

86780 Treponema pallidum A
EXCLUDES *Nontreponemal antibody analysis syphilis testing (86592-86593)*
0.00 0.00 Global Days XXX

86784 Trichinella A
0.00 0.00 Global Days XXX

86787 varicella-zoster A
0.00 0.00 Global Days XXX

86788 West Nile virus, IgM A
0.00 0.00 Global Days XXX

86789 West Nile virus A
0.00 0.00 Global Days XXX

86790 virus, not elsewhere specified A
0.00 0.00 Global Days XXX

86793 Yersinia A
0.00 0.00 Global Days XXX

86800 Thyroglobulin antibody A
0.00 0.00 Global Days XXX

86803 Hepatitis C antibody; A
0.00 0.00 Global Days XXX

86804 confirmatory test (eg, immunoblot) A
0.00 0.00 Global Days XXX

86805-86808 Pre-Transplant Antibody Cross Matching

CMS 100-2,15,80 Diagnostic Test Requirements
CMS 100-4,3,10.4 Payment of Nonphysician Services for Inpatients

86805 Lymphocytotoxicity assay, visual crossmatch; with titration A
0.00 0.00 Global Days XXX

86806 without titration A
0.00 0.00 Global Days XXX

86807 Serum screening for cytotoxic percent reactive antibody (PRA); standard method A
0.00 0.00 Global Days XXX
AMA: 2009, Jan, 11-31; 2008, Jan, 10-25; 2007, January, 13-27

86808 quick method A
0.00 0.00 Global Days XXX
AMA: 2009, Jan, 11-31; 2008, Jan, 10-25; 2007, January, 13-27

86812-86849 Histocompatibility Testing

CMS 100-2,15,80 Diagnostic Test Requirements
CMS 100-3,190.1 Histocompatibility Testing
CMS 100-3,190.8 Lymphocyte Mitogen Response Assays
CMS 100-4,3,10.4 Payment of Nonphysician Services for Inpatients

EXCLUDES *HLA typing by molecular pathology techniques (81370-81383)*

86812 HLA typing; A, B, or C (eg, A10, B7, B27), single antigen A
0.00 0.00 Global Days XXX
AMA: 2009, Jan, 11-31; 2008, Jan, 10-25; 2007, January, 13-27

86813 A, B, or C, multiple antigens A
0.00 0.00 Global Days XXX
AMA: 2009, Jan, 11-31; 2008, Jan, 10-25; 2007, January, 13-27

86816 DR/DQ, single antigen A
0.00 0.00 Global Days XXX
AMA: 2009, Jan, 11-31; 2008, Jan, 10-25; 2007, January, 13-27

86817 DR/DQ, multiple antigens A
0.00 0.00 Global Days XXX
AMA: 2009, Jan, 11-31; 2008, Jan, 10-25; 2007, January, 13-27

86821 lymphocyte culture, mixed (MLC) A
0.00 0.00 Global Days XXX
AMA: 2009, Jan, 11-31; 2008, Jan, 10-25; 2007, January, 13-27

86822 lymphocyte culture, primed (PLC) A
0.00 0.00 Global Days XXX
AMA: 2009, Jan, 11-31; 2008, Jan, 10-25; 2007, January, 13-27

86825 Human leukocyte antigen (HLA) crossmatch, non-cytotoxic (eg, using flow cytometry); first serum sample or dilution A

EXCLUDES *Autologous HLA crossmatch (86825-86826)*
Lymphocytotoxicity visual crossmatch (86805-86806)

Do not report with (86355, 86359, 88184-88189)
0.00 0.00 Global Days XXX

\+ **86826 each additional serum sample or sample dilution (List separately in addition to primary procedure)** A

EXCLUDES *Autologous HLA crossmatch (86825-86826)*
Lymphocytotoxicity visual crossmatch (86805-86806)

Code first (86825)
Do not report with (86355, 86359, 88184-88189)
0.00 0.00 Global Days XXX

86849 Unlisted immunology procedure A
0.00 0.00 Global Days XXX
AMA: 2009, Jan, 11-31; 2008, Jan, 10-25; 2007, January, 13-27

86850-86999 Transfusion Services

CMS 100-2,15,80 Diagnostic Test Requirements
CMS 100-3,110.5 Granulocyte Transfulsions
CMS 100-3,110.7 Blood Transfusions
CMS 100-3,110.8 Blood Platelet Transfusions
CMS 100-4,3,10.4 Payment of Nonphysician Services for Inpatients

EXCLUDES *Apheresis (36511-36512)*
Therapeutic phlebotomy (99195)

86850 Antibody screen, RBC, each serum technique X
0.00 0.00 Global Days XXX
AMA: 2008, Apr, 5-7

86860 Antibody elution (RBC), each elution X
0.00 0.00 Global Days XXX

86870 Antibody identification, RBC antibodies, each panel for each serum technique X
0.00 0.00 Global Days XXX
AMA: 2009, Jan, 11-31; 2008, Jan, 10-25; 2008, Apr, 5-7; 2007, January, 13-27

86880 Antihuman globulin test (Coombs test); direct, each antiserum X
0.00 0.00 Global Days XXX

86885 indirect, qualitative, each reagent red cell X
0.00 0.00 Global Days XXX
AMA: 2008, Apr, 5-7

86886 indirect, each antibody titer X

EXCLUDES *Indirect antihuman globulin (Coombs) test for RBC antibody identification using reagent red cell panels (86870)*
Indirect antihuman globulin (Coombs) test for RBC antibody screening (86850)

0.00 0.00 Global Days XXX
AMA: 2008, Apr, 5-7

86890 Autologous blood or component, collection processing and storage; predeposited X
0.00 0.00 Global Days XXX

86891 intra- or postoperative salvage X

EXCLUDES *Physician services to autologous donors (99201-99204)*

0.00 0.00 Global Days XXX

86900 Blood typing; ABO X
0.00 0.00 Global Days XXX

86901 Rh (D) X
0.00 0.00 Global Days XXX

86902 antigen testing of donor blood using reagent serum, each antigen test X
Code also one time for each antigen for each unit when multiple units of blood are tested for the same antigen
0.00 0.00 Global Days XXX

86904 antigen screening for compatible unit using patient serum, per unit screened X
0.00 0.00 Global Days XXX

86905 RBC antigens, other than ABO or Rh (D), each X
0.00 0.00 Global Days XXX

86906 Rh phenotyping, complete X
0.00 0.00 Global Days XXX

86910 Blood typing, for paternity testing, per individual; ABO, Rh and MN E
0.00 0.00 Global Days XXX

86911 each additional antigen system E
0.00 0.00 Global Days XXX

86920 Compatibility test each unit; immediate spin technique X
Code also each antigen for each unit (86902)
Code also same antigen on multiple units (86902)
0.00 0.00 Global Days XXX

86921 incubation technique X
0.00 0.00 Global Days XXX

86922 antiglobulin technique X
0.00 0.00 Global Days XXX

86923 electronic X
Do not report with (86920-86922)
0.00 0.00 Global Days XXX

86927 Fresh frozen plasma, thawing, each unit X
0.00 0.00 Global Days XXX

86930 **Frozen blood, each unit; freezing (includes preparation)** X
0.00 0.00 Global Days XXX

86931 **thawing** X
0.00 0.00 Global Days XXX

86932 **freezing (includes preparation) and thawing** X
0.00 0.00 Global Days XXX

86940 **Hemolysins and agglutinins; auto, screen, each** A
0.00 0.00 Global Days XXX

86941 **incubated** A
0.00 0.00 Global Days XXX

86945 **Irradiation of blood product, each unit** X
0.00 0.00 Global Days XXX
AMA: 2009, Jan, 11-31; 2007, Dec, 10-179

86950 **Leukocyte transfusion** X
EXCLUDES *Leukapheresis (36511)*
0.00 0.00 Global Days XXX

86960 **Volume reduction of blood or blood product (eg, red blood cells or platelets), each unit** X
0.00 0.00 Global Days XXX

86965 **Pooling of platelets or other blood products** X
EXCLUDES *Injection of platelet rich plasma (0232T)*
0.00 0.00 Global Days XXX

86970 **Pretreatment of RBCs for use in RBC antibody detection, identification, and/or compatibility testing; incubation with chemical agents or drugs, each** X
0.00 0.00 Global Days XXX

86971 **incubation with enzymes, each** X
0.00 0.00 Global Days XXX

86972 **by density gradient separation** X
0.00 0.00 Global Days XXX

86975 **Pretreatment of serum for use in RBC antibody identification; incubation with drugs, each** X
0.00 0.00 Global Days XXX

86976 **by dilution** X
0.00 0.00 Global Days XXX

86977 **incubation with inhibitors, each** X
0.00 0.00 Global Days XXX

86978 **by differential red cell absorption using patient RBCs or RBCs of known phenotype, each absorption** X
0.00 0.00 Global Days XXX

86985 **Splitting of blood or blood products, each unit** X
0.00 0.00 Global Days XXX

86999 **Unlisted transfusion medicine procedure** X
0.00 0.00 Global Days XXX
AMA: 2009, Mar, 10-11; 2009, Jan, 11-31; 2008, Jan, 10-25; 2007, January, 13-27

87001-87118 Identification of Microorganisms

CMS 100-2,15,80 Diagnostic Test Requirements
CMS 100-3,190.12 Urine Culture, Bacterial
CMS 100-4,3,10.4 Payment of Nonphysician Services for Inpatients

INCLUDES Bacteriology, mycology, parasitology, and virology

EXCLUDES *Additional tests using molecular probes, chromatography, nucleic acid resequencing, or immunologic techniques (87140-87158)*

Code also modifier 59 for multiple specimens or sites

Code also modifier 91 for repeat procedures performed on the same day

87001 **Animal inoculation, small animal; with observation** A
0.00 0.00 Global Days XXX

87003 **with observation and dissection** A
0.00 0.00 Global Days XXX

87015 **Concentration (any type), for infectious agents** A
Do not report with (87177)
0.00 0.00 Global Days XXX

87040 **Culture, bacterial; blood, aerobic, with isolation and presumptive identification of isolates (includes anaerobic culture, if appropriate)** A
0.00 0.00 Global Days XXX
AMA: 2009, Jan, 11-31; 2008, Jan, 10-25; 2007, January, 13-27

87045 **stool, aerobic, with isolation and preliminary examination (eg, KIA, LIA), Salmonella and Shigella species** A
0.00 0.00 Global Days XXX

87046 **stool, aerobic, additional pathogens, isolation and presumptive identification of isolates, each plate** A
0.00 0.00 Global Days XXX

87070 **any other source except urine, blood or stool, aerobic, with isolation and presumptive identification of isolates** A
EXCLUDES *Urine (87088)*
0.00 0.00 Global Days XXX
AMA: 2009, Jan, 11-31; 2008, Jan, 10-25; 2007, January, 13-27

87071 **quantitative, aerobic with isolation and presumptive identification of isolates, any source except urine, blood or stool** A
EXCLUDES *Urine (87088)*
0.00 0.00 Global Days XXX

87073 **quantitative, anaerobic with isolation and presumptive identification of isolates, any source except urine, blood or stool** A
EXCLUDES *Definitive identification of isolates (87076 or 87077)*
Typing of isolates (87140-87158)
0.00 0.00 Global Days XXX

87075 **any source, except blood, anaerobic with isolation and presumptive identification of isolates** A
0.00 0.00 Global Days XXX

87076 **anaerobic isolate, additional methods required for definitive identification, each isolate** A
0.00 0.00 Global Days XXX

87077 **aerobic isolate, additional methods required for definitive identification, each isolate** A
0.00 0.00 Global Days XXX

87081 **Culture, presumptive, pathogenic organisms, screening only;** A
0.00 0.00 Global Days XXX

87084 **with colony estimation from density chart** A
0.00 0.00 Global Days XXX

87086 **Culture, bacterial; quantitative colony count, urine** A
0.00 0.00 Global Days XXX

87088 **with isolation and presumptive identification of each isolate, urine** A
0.00 0.00 Global Days XXX

87101 **Culture, fungi (mold or yeast) isolation, with presumptive identification of isolates; skin, hair, or nail** A
0.00 0.00 Global Days XXX
AMA: 2009, Jan, 11-31; 2008, Jan, 10-25; 2007, January, 13-27

87102 **other source (except blood)** A
0.00 0.00 Global Days XXX

87103 **blood** A
0.00 0.00 Global Days XXX

87106 **Culture, fungi, definitive identification, each organism; yeast**

Code also (87101-87103)

0.00 0.00 Global Days XXX

87107 **mold**

0.00 0.00 Global Days XXX

87109 **Culture, mycoplasma, any source**

0.00 0.00 Global Days XXX

87110 **Culture, chlamydia, any source**

EXCLUDES *Immunofluorescence staining of shell vials (87140)*

0.00 0.00 Global Days XXX

87116 **Culture, tubercle or other acid-fast bacilli (eg, TB, AFB, mycobacteria) any source, with isolation and presumptive identification of isolates**

EXCLUDES *Concentration (87015)*

0.00 0.00 Global Days XXX

87118 **Culture, mycobacterial, definitive identification, each isolate**

EXCLUDES *GLC HPLC identification (87143)*
Nucleic acid probe identification (87149)

0.00 0.00 Global Days XXX

87140-87158 Additional Culture Typing Techniques

CMS 100-2,15,80 Diagnostic Test Requirements
CMS 100-4,3,10.4 Payment of Nonphysician Services for Inpatients
INCLUDES Bacteriology, mycology, parasitology, and virology

Code also definitive identification

Code also modifier 59 for multiple specimens or sites

Code also modifier 91 for repeat procedures performed on the same day

Do not report with or instead of molecular diagnosis codes (83890-83914)

87140 **Culture, typing; immunofluorescent method, each antiserum**

0.00 0.00 Global Days XXX

87143 **gas liquid chromatography (GLC) or high pressure liquid chromatography (HPLC) method**

0.00 0.00 Global Days XXX

87147 **immunologic method, other than immunofluoresence (eg, agglutination grouping), per antiserum**

0.00 0.00 Global Days XXX

AMA: 2009, Jan, 11-31; 2008, Jan, 10-25; 2007, January, 13-27

87149 **identification by nucleic acid (DNA or RNA) probe, direct probe technique, per culture or isolate, each organism probed**

Do not report with (83890-83914)

0.00 0.00 Global Days XXX

87150 **identification by nucleic acid (DNA or RNA) probe, amplified probe technique, per culture or isolate, each organism probed**

Do not report with (83890-83914)

0.00 0.00 Global Days XXX

87152 **identification by pulse field gel typing**

Do not report with (83890-83914)

0.00 0.00 Global Days XXX

87153 **identification by nucleic acid sequencing method, each isolate (eg, sequencing of the 16S rRNA gene)**

0.00 0.00 Global Days XXX

87158 **other methods**

0.00 0.00 Global Days XXX

87164-87255 Identification of Organism from Primary Source and Sensitivity Studies

CMS 100-2,15,80 Diagnostic Test Requirements
CMS 100-4,3,10.4 Payment of Nonphysician Services for Inpatients
INCLUDES Bacteriology, mycology, parasitology, and virology
EXCLUDES *Additional tests using molecular probes, chromatography, or immunologic techniques (87140-87158)*

Code also modifier 59 for multiple specimens or sites

Code also modifier 91 for repeat procedures performed on the same day

87164 **Dark field examination, any source (eg, penile, vaginal, oral, skin); includes specimen collection**

0.00 0.00 Global Days XXX

87166 **without collection**

0.00 0.00 Global Days XXX

87168 **Macroscopic examination; arthropod**

0.00 0.00 Global Days XXX

87169 **parasite**

0.00 0.00 Global Days XXX

87172 **Pinworm exam (eg, cellophane tape prep)**

0.00 0.00 Global Days XXX

87176 **Homogenization, tissue, for culture**

0.00 0.00 Global Days XXX

87177 **Ova and parasites, direct smears, concentration and identification**

EXCLUDES *Coccidia or microsporidia exam (87207)*
Complex special stain (trichrome, iron hematoxylin) (87209)
Direct smears from primary source (87207)
Nucleic acid probes in cytologic material (88365)

Do not report with (87015)

0.00 0.00 Global Days XXX

AMA: 2009, Jan, 11-31; 2008, Jan, 10-25; 2007, January, 13-27

87181 **Susceptibility studies, antimicrobial agent; agar dilution method, per agent (eg, antibiotic gradient strip)**

0.00 0.00 Global Days XXX

87184 **disk method, per plate (12 or fewer agents)**

0.00 0.00 Global Days XXX

87185 **enzyme detection (eg, beta lactamase), per enzyme**

0.00 0.00 Global Days XXX

87186 **microdilution or agar dilution (minimum inhibitory concentration [MIC] or breakpoint), each multi-antimicrobial, per plate**

0.00 0.00 Global Days XXX

+ 87187 **microdilution or agar dilution, minimum lethal concentration (MLC), each plate (List separately in addition to code for primary procedure)**

Code first (87186 or 87188)

0.00 0.00 Global Days XXX

87188 **macrobroth dilution method, each agent**

0.00 0.00 Global Days XXX

87190 **mycobacteria, proportion method, each agent**

EXCLUDES *Other mycobacterial susceptibility studies (87181, 87184, 87186 or 87188)*

0.00 0.00 Global Days XXX

87197 **Serum bactericidal titer (Schlicter test)**

0.00 0.00 Global Days XXX

87205 **Smear, primary source with interpretation; Gram or Giemsa stain for bacteria, fungi, or cell types**

0.00 0.00 Global Days XXX

87206 fluorescent and/or acid fast stain for bacteria, fungi, parasites, viruses or cell types A
0.00 0.00 Global Days XXX

87207 special stain for inclusion bodies or parasites (eg, malaria, coccidia, microsporidia, trypanosomes, herpes viruses) A
EXCLUDES *Direct smears with concentration and identification (87177)*
Fat, meat, fibers, nasal eosinophils, and starch (see miscellaneous section)
Thick smear preparation (87015)
0.00 0.00 Global Days XXX

87209 complex special stain (eg, trichrome, iron hemotoxylin) for ova and parasites A
0.00 0.00 Global Days XXX

87210 wet mount for infectious agents (eg, saline, India ink, KOH preps) A
EXCLUDES *KOH evaluation of skin, hair, or nails (87220)*
0.00 0.00 Global Days XXX

87220 Tissue examination by KOH slide of samples from skin, hair, or nails for fungi or ectoparasite ova or mites (eg, scabies) A
0.00 0.00 Global Days XXX

87230 Toxin or antitoxin assay, tissue culture (eg, Clostridium difficile toxin) A
0.00 0.00 Global Days XXX

87250 Virus isolation; inoculation of embryonated eggs, or small animal, includes observation and dissection A
0.00 0.00 Global Days XXX

87252 tissue culture inoculation, observation, and presumptive identification by cytopathic effect A
0.00 0.00 Global Days XXX

87253 tissue culture, additional studies or definitive identification (eg, hemabsorption, neutralization, immunofluoresence stain), each isolate A
EXCLUDES *Electron microscopy (88348)*
Inclusion bodies in:
Fluids (88106)
Smears (87207-87210)
Tissue sections (88304-88309)
0.00 0.00 Global Days XXX

87254 centrifuge enhanced (shell vial) technique, includes identification with immunofluorescence stain, each virus A
Code also (87252)
0.00 0.00 Global Days XXX

87255 including identification by non-immunologic method, other than by cytopathic effect (eg, virus specific enzymatic activity) A
0.00 0.00 Global Days XXX

87260-87300 Fluorescence Microscopy by Organism

CMS 100-2,15,80 Diagnostic Test Requirements
CMS 100-4,3,10.4 Payment of Nonphysician Services for Inpatients
INCLUDES Primary source code only
EXCLUDES *Comparable tests on culture material (87140-87158)*
Identification of antibodies (86602-86804)

Code also modifier 59 for different species or strains reported by the same code

Do not report with or instead of molecular diagnosis codes (83890-83914)

87260 Infectious agent antigen detection by immunofluorescent technique; adenovirus A
0.00 0.00 Global Days XXX

87265 Bordetella pertussis/parapertussis A
0.00 0.00 Global Days XXX

87267 Enterovirus, direct fluorescent antibody (DFA) A
0.00 0.00 Global Days XXX

87269 giardia A
0.00 0.00 Global Days XXX

87270 Chlamydia trachomatis A
0.00 0.00 Global Days XXX

87271 Cytomegalovirus, direct fluorescent antibody (DFA) A
0.00 0.00 Global Days XXX

87272 cryptosporidium A
0.00 0.00 Global Days XXX

87273 Herpes simplex virus type 2 A
0.00 0.00 Global Days XXX

87274 Herpes simplex virus type 1 A
0.00 0.00 Global Days XXX

87275 influenza B virus A
0.00 0.00 Global Days XXX
AMA: 2009, May, 6&10

87276 influenza A virus A
0.00 0.00 Global Days XXX
AMA: 2009, May, 6&10

87277 Legionella micdadei A
0.00 0.00 Global Days XXX

87278 Legionella pneumophila A
0.00 0.00 Global Days XXX

87279 Parainfluenza virus, each type A
0.00 0.00 Global Days XXX

87280 respiratory syncytial virus A
0.00 0.00 Global Days XXX

87281 Pneumocystis carinii A
0.00 0.00 Global Days XXX

87283 Rubeola A
0.00 0.00 Global Days XXX

87285 Treponema pallidum A
0.00 0.00 Global Days XXX

87290 Varicella zoster virus A
0.00 0.00 Global Days XXX

87299 not otherwise specified, each organism A
0.00 0.00 Global Days XXX

87300 Infectious agent antigen detection by immunofluorescent technique, polyvalent for multiple organisms, each polyvalent antiserum A
EXCLUDES *Physician evaluation of infectious disease agents by immunofluorescence (88346)*
0.00 0.00 Global Days XXX

87301-87451 Enzyme Immunoassay Technique by Organism

EXCLUDES *Nonspecific agent detection (87449-87450, 87797-87799, 87899)*

Code also modifier 59 for different species or strains reported by the same code.

Do not report with or instead of molecular diagnosis codes (83890-83914)

87301 Infectious agent antigen detection by enzyme immunoassay technique, qualitative or semiquantitative, multiple-step method; adenovirus enteric types 40/41 A
0.00 0.00 Global Days XXX

87305 Aspergillus A
0.00 0.00 Global Days XXX

87320 Chlamydia trachomatis A
0.00 0.00 Global Days XXX

87324 **Clostridium difficile toxin(s)**
0.00 0.00 Global Days XXX

87327 **Cryptococcus neoformans**
EXCLUDES *Cryptococcus latex agglutination (86403)*
0.00 0.00 Global Days XXX

87328 **cryptosporidium**
0.00 0.00 Global Days XXX

87329 **giardia**
0.00 0.00 Global Days XXX

87332 **cytomegalovirus**
0.00 0.00 Global Days XXX

87335 **Escherichia coli 0157**
EXCLUDES *Giardia antigen (87329)*
0.00 0.00 Global Days XXX

87336 **Entamoeba histolytica dispar group**
0.00 0.00 Global Days XXX

87337 **Entamoeba histolytica group**
0.00 0.00 Global Days XXX

87338 **Helicobacter pylori, stool**
0.00 0.00 Global Days XXX

87339 **Helicobacter pylori**
EXCLUDES *H. pylori:*
Breath and blood by mass spectrometry (83013-83014)
Liquid scintillation counter (78267-78268)
Stool (87338)
0.00 0.00 Global Days XXX

87340 **hepatitis B surface antigen (HBsAg)**
0.00 0.00 Global Days XXX

87341 **hepatitis B surface antigen (HBsAg) neutralization**
0.00 0.00 Global Days XXX

87350 **hepatitis Be antigen (HBeAg)**
0.00 0.00 Global Days XXX

87380 **hepatitis, delta agent**
0.00 0.00 Global Days XXX

87385 **Histoplasma capsulatum**
0.00 0.00 Global Days XXX

● 87389 **HIV-1 antigen(s), with HIV-1 and HIV-2 antibodies, single result**
Code also modifier 92 for test performed using a kit or transportable instrument that is all or in part consists of a single-use, disposable analytical chamber
0.00 0.00 Global Days XXX

87390 **HIV-1**
0.00 0.00 Global Days XXX

87391 **HIV-2**
0.00 0.00 Global Days XXX

87400 **Influenza, A or B, each**
0.00 0.00 Global Days XXX
AMA: 2009, Jan, 11-31; 2009, May, 6&10; 2008, Jan, 10-25; 2007, January, 13-27

87420 **respiratory syncytial virus**
0.00 0.00 Global Days XXX

87425 **rotavirus**
0.00 0.00 Global Days XXX

87427 **Shiga-like toxin**
0.00 0.00 Global Days XXX

87430 **Streptococcus, group A**
0.00 0.00 Global Days XXX
AMA: 2009, Jan, 11-31; 2008, Jan, 10-25; 2007, January, 13-27

87449 **Infectious agent antigen detection by enzyme immunoassay technique qualitative or semiquantitative; multiple step method, not otherwise specified, each organism**
0.00 0.00 Global Days XXX
AMA: 2009, Jan, 11-31; 2008, Jan, 10-25; 2007, January, 13-27

87450 **single step method, not otherwise specified, each organism**
0.00 0.00 Global Days XXX

87451 **multiple step method, polyvalent for multiple organisms, each polyvalent antiserum**
0.00 0.00 Global Days XXX

87470-87801 Detection Infectious Agent by Probe Techniques

87470 **Infectious agent detection by nucleic acid (DNA or RNA); Bartonella henselae and Bartonella quintana, direct probe technique**
0.00 0.00 Global Days XXX

87471 **Bartonella henselae and Bartonella quintana, amplified probe technique**
0.00 0.00 Global Days XXX

87472 **Bartonella henselae and Bartonella quintana, quantification**
0.00 0.00 Global Days XXX

87475 **Borrelia burgdorferi, direct probe technique**
0.00 0.00 Global Days XXX

87476 **Borrelia burgdorferi, amplified probe technique**
0.00 0.00 Global Days XXX

87477 **Borrelia burgdorferi, quantification**
0.00 0.00 Global Days XXX

87480 **Candida species, direct probe technique**
0.00 0.00 Global Days XXX

87481 **Candida species, amplified probe technique**
0.00 0.00 Global Days XXX

87482 **Candida species, quantification**
0.00 0.00 Global Days XXX

87485 **Chlamydia pneumoniae, direct probe technique**
0.00 0.00 Global Days XXX

87486 **Chlamydia pneumoniae, amplified probe technique**
0.00 0.00 Global Days XXX

87487 **Chlamydia pneumoniae, quantification**
0.00 0.00 Global Days XXX

87490 **Chlamydia trachomatis, direct probe technique**
0.00 0.00 Global Days XXX

87491 **Chlamydia trachomatis, amplified probe technique**
0.00 0.00 Global Days XXX

87492 **Chlamydia trachomatis, quantification**
0.00 0.00 Global Days XXX

87493 **Clostridium difficile, toxin gene(s), amplified probe technique**
0.00 0.00 Global Days XXX

87495 **cytomegalovirus, direct probe technique**
0.00 0.00 Global Days XXX

87496 **cytomegalovirus, amplified probe technique**
0.00 0.00 Global Days XXX

87497 **cytomegalovirus, quantification**
0.00 0.00 Global Days XXX

87498 **enterovirus, amplified probe technique**
0.00 0.00 Global Days XXX

87500 vancomycin resistance (eg, enterococcus species van A, van B), amplified probe technique [A]
0.00 0.00 Global Days XXX
AMA: 2008, Apr, 5-7

87501 influenza virus, reverse transcription and amplified probe technique, each type or subtype [A]
0.00 0.00 Global Days XXX

▲ 87502 influenza virus, for multiple types or sub-types, multiplex reverse transcription and amplified probe technique, first 2 types or sub-types [A]
0.00 0.00 Global Days XXX

\+ 87503 influenza virus, for multiple types or sub-types, multiplex reverse transcription and amplified probe technique, each additional influenza virus type or sub-type beyond 2 (List separately in addition to code for primary procedure) [A]
Code first (87502)
0.00 0.00 Global Days XXX

87510 Gardnerella vaginalis, direct probe technique [A]
0.00 0.00 Global Days XXX

87511 Gardnerella vaginalis, amplified probe technique [A]
0.00 0.00 Global Days XXX

87512 Gardnerella vaginalis, quantification [A]
0.00 0.00 Global Days XXX

87515 hepatitis B virus, direct probe technique [A]
0.00 0.00 Global Days XXX

87516 hepatitis B virus, amplified probe technique [A]
0.00 0.00 Global Days XXX

87517 hepatitis B virus, quantification [A]
0.00 0.00 Global Days XXX

87520 hepatitis C, direct probe technique [A]
0.00 0.00 Global Days XXX

87521 hepatitis C, amplified probe technique [A]
0.00 0.00 Global Days XXX

87522 hepatitis C, quantification [A]
0.00 0.00 Global Days XXX

87525 hepatitis G, direct probe technique [A]
0.00 0.00 Global Days XXX

87526 hepatitis G, amplified probe technique [A]
0.00 0.00 Global Days XXX

87527 hepatitis G, quantification [A]
0.00 0.00 Global Days XXX

87528 Herpes simplex virus, direct probe technique [A]
0.00 0.00 Global Days XXX

87529 Herpes simplex virus, amplified probe technique [A]
0.00 0.00 Global Days XXX

87530 Herpes simplex virus, quantification [A]
0.00 0.00 Global Days XXX

87531 Herpes virus-6, direct probe technique [A]
0.00 0.00 Global Days XXX

87532 Herpes virus-6, amplified probe technique [A]
0.00 0.00 Global Days XXX

87533 Herpes virus-6, quantification [A]
0.00 0.00 Global Days XXX

87534 HIV-1, direct probe technique [A]
0.00 0.00 Global Days XXX

87535 HIV-1, amplified probe technique [A]
0.00 0.00 Global Days XXX
AMA: 2008, Mar, 3&7

87536 HIV-1, quantification [A]
0.00 0.00 Global Days XXX

87537 HIV-2, direct probe technique [A]
0.00 0.00 Global Days XXX

87538 HIV-2, amplified probe technique [A]
0.00 0.00 Global Days XXX

87539 HIV-2, quantification [A]
0.00 0.00 Global Days XXX

87540 Legionella pneumophila, direct probe technique [A]
0.00 0.00 Global Days XXX

87541 Legionella pneumophila, amplified probe technique [A]
0.00 0.00 Global Days XXX

87542 Legionella pneumophila, quantification [A]
0.00 0.00 Global Days XXX

87550 Mycobacteria species, direct probe technique [A]
0.00 0.00 Global Days XXX

87551 Mycobacteria species, amplified probe technique [A]
0.00 0.00 Global Days XXX

87552 Mycobacteria species, quantification [A]
0.00 0.00 Global Days XXX

87555 Mycobacteria tuberculosis, direct probe technique [A]
0.00 0.00 Global Days XXX

87556 Mycobacteria tuberculosis, amplified probe technique [A]
0.00 0.00 Global Days XXX

87557 Mycobacteria tuberculosis, quantification [A]
0.00 0.00 Global Days XXX

87560 Mycobacteria avium-intracellulare, direct probe technique [A]
0.00 0.00 Global Days XXX

87561 Mycobacteria avium-intracellulare, amplified probe technique [A]
0.00 0.00 Global Days XXX

87562 Mycobacteria avium-intracellulare, quantification [A]
0.00 0.00 Global Days XXX

87580 Mycoplasma pneumoniae, direct probe technique [A]
0.00 0.00 Global Days XXX

87581 Mycoplasma pneumoniae, amplified probe technique [A]
0.00 0.00 Global Days XXX

87582 Mycoplasma pneumoniae, quantification [A]
0.00 0.00 Global Days XXX

87590 Neisseria gonorrhoeae, direct probe technique [A]
0.00 0.00 Global Days XXX

87591 Neisseria gonorrhoeae, amplified probe technique [A]
0.00 0.00 Global Days XXX

87592 Neisseria gonorrhoeae, quantification [A]
0.00 0.00 Global Days XXX

87620 papillomavirus, human, direct probe technique [A]
0.00 0.00 Global Days XXX
AMA: 2009, Jan, 11-31; 2008, Jan, 10-25; 2007, January, 13-27

87621 papillomavirus, human, amplified probe technique [A]
0.00 0.00 Global Days XXX

87622 papillomavirus, human, quantification [A]
0.00 0.00 Global Days XXX

87640 Staphylococcus aureus, amplified probe technique [A]
0.00 0.00 Global Days XXX
AMA: 2007, Aug, 7-8

87641 **Staphylococcus aureus, methicillin resistant, amplified probe technique** A
EXCLUDES *Assays that detect methicillin resistance and identify Staphylococcus aureus using a single nucleic acid sequence (87641)*
0.00 0.00 Global Days XXX
AMA: 2007, Aug, 7-8

87650 **Streptococcus, group A, direct probe technique** A
0.00 0.00 Global Days XXX

87651 **Streptococcus, group A, amplified probe technique** A
0.00 0.00 Global Days XXX
AMA: 2007, Aug, 7-8

87652 **Streptococcus, group A, quantification** A
0.00 0.00 Global Days XXX

87653 **Streptococcus, group B, amplified probe technique** A
0.00 0.00 Global Days XXX
AMA: 2007, Aug, 7-8

87660 **Trichomonas vaginalis, direct probe technique** A
0.00 0.00 Global Days XXX

87797 **Infectious agent detection by nucleic acid (DNA or RNA), not otherwise specified; direct probe technique, each organism** A
0.00 0.00 Global Days XXX

87798 **amplified probe technique, each organism** A
0.00 0.00 Global Days XXX
AMA: 2007, Aug, 7-8

87799 **quantification, each organism** A
0.00 0.00 Global Days XXX

87800 **Infectious agent detection by nucleic acid (DNA or RNA), multiple organisms; direct probe(s) technique** A
0.00 0.00 Global Days XXX

87801 **amplified probe(s) technique** A
EXCLUDES *Detection of specific infectious agents not otherwise specified (87797-87799)*
Each specific organism nucleic acid detection from a primary source (87470-87660)
0.00 0.00 Global Days XXX

87802-87899 Detection Infectious Agent by Immunoassay with Direct Optical Observation

87802 **Infectious agent antigen detection by immunoassay with direct optical observation; Streptococcus, group B** A
0.00 0.00 Global Days XXX

87803 **Clostridium difficile toxin A** A
0.00 0.00 Global Days XXX

87804 **Influenza** A
0.00 0.00 Global Days XXX
AMA: 2009, Jan, 11-31; 2009, May, 6&10; 2007, Dec, 10-179

87807 **respiratory syncytial virus** A
0.00 0.00 Global Days XXX

87808 **Trichomonas vaginalis** A
0.00 0.00 Global Days XXX

87809 **adenovirus** A
0.00 0.00 Global Days XXX
AMA: 2008, Apr, 5-7

87810 **Chlamydia trachomatis** A
0.00 0.00 Global Days XXX

87850 **Neisseria gonorrhoeae** A
0.00 0.00 Global Days XXX

87880 **Streptococcus, group A** A
0.00 0.00 Global Days XXX
AMA: 2009, Jan, 11-31; 2008, Jan, 10-25; 2007, January, 13-27

87899 **not otherwise specified** A
0.00 0.00 Global Days XXX
AMA: 2009, Jan, 11-31; 2008, Jan, 10-25; 2007, January, 13-27

87900-87999 [87906] Drug Sensitivity Genotype/Phenotype

87900 **Infectious agent drug susceptibility phenotype prediction using regularly updated genotypic bioinformatics** A
0.00 0.00 Global Days XXX

87901 **Infectious agent genotype analysis by nucleic acid (DNA or RNA); HIV-1, reverse transcriptase and protease regions** A
EXCLUDES *Infectious agent drug susceptibility phenotype prediction for HIV-1 (87900)*
0.00 0.00 Global Days XXX

\# 87906 **HIV-1, other region (eg, integrase, fusion)** A
0.00 0.00 Global Days XXX

87902 **Hepatitis C virus** A
0.00 0.00 Global Days XXX

87903 **Infectious agent phenotype analysis by nucleic acid (DNA or RNA) with drug resistance tissue culture analysis, HIV 1; first through 10 drugs tested** A
0.00 0.00 Global Days XXX

\+ 87904 **each additional drug tested (List separately in addition to code for primary procedure)** A
Code first (87903)
0.00 0.00 Global Days XXX
AMA: 2009, Jan, 11-31; 2008, Jan, 10-25; 2007, January, 13-27

87905 **Infectious agent enzymatic activity other than virus (eg, sialidase activity in vaginal fluid)** A
EXCLUDES *Isolation of a virus identified by a nonimmunologic method, and by noncytopathic effect (87255)*
0.00 0.00 Global Days XXX

87906 *Resequenced code. See code following 87901.*

87999 **Unlisted microbiology procedure** A
0.00 0.00 Global Days XXX

88000-88099 Autopsy Services

CMS 100-1,5,90.2 Laboratory Defined
CMS 100-2,15,80 Diagnostic Test Requirements
CMS 100-2,15,80.1 Payment for Clinical Laboratory Services
CMS 100-4,16,10 General Coverage: Diagnostic X-ray, Laboratory, and Other Tests
CMS 100-4,16,10.1 Laboratory Definitions
CMS 100-4,16,110.4 Carrier Contacts With Independent Clinical Laboratories

INCLUDES Services for physicians only

88000 **Necropsy (autopsy), gross examination only; without CNS** E
0.00 0.00 Global Days XXX

88005 **with brain** E
0.00 0.00 Global Days XXX

88007 **with brain and spinal cord** E
0.00 0.00 Global Days XXX

88012 **infant with brain** A E
0.00 0.00 Global Days XXX

88014 **stillborn or newborn with brain** A E
0.00 0.00 Global Days XXX

88016 **macerated stillborn** A E
0.00 0.00 Global Days XXX

88020 Necropsy (autopsy), gross and microscopic; without CNS E
0.00 0.00 Global Days XXX

88025 with brain E
0.00 0.00 Global Days XXX

88027 with brain and spinal cord E
0.00 0.00 Global Days XXX

88028 infant with brain A E
0.00 0.00 Global Days XXX

88029 stillborn or newborn with brain A E
0.00 0.00 Global Days XXX

88036 Necropsy (autopsy), limited, gross and/or microscopic; regional E
0.00 0.00 Global Days XXX

88037 single organ E
0.00 0.00 Global Days XXX

88040 Necropsy (autopsy); forensic examination E
0.00 0.00 Global Days XXX

88045 coroner's call E
0.00 0.00 Global Days XXX

88099 Unlisted necropsy (autopsy) procedure E
0.00 0.00 Global Days XXX

88104-88140 Cytopathology: Other Than Cervical/Vaginal

CMS 100-2,15,80 Diagnostic Test Requirements
CMS 100-4,3,10.4 Payment of Nonphysician Services for Inpatients
CMS 100-4,12,60 Payment for Pathology Services

88104 Cytopathology, fluids, washings or brushings, except cervical or vaginal; smears with interpretation X 80
1.99 1.99 Global Days XXX
AMA: 2009, Jan, 11-31; 2008, Jun, 14-15

88106 simple filter method with interpretation X 80
Do not report with (88104)
2.14 2.14 Global Days XXX

~~**88107** smears and simple filter preparation with interpretation~~
To report, see 88104, 88106

88108 Cytopathology, concentration technique, smears and interpretation (eg, Saccomanno technique) X 80
EXCLUDES *Cervical or vaginal smears (88150-88155)*
Gastric intubation with lavage (43754-43755)
74340
2.08 2.08 Global Days XXX

88112 Cytopathology, selective cellular enhancement technique with interpretation (eg, liquid based slide preparation method), except cervical or vaginal X 80
Do not report with (88108)
3.01 3.01 Global Days XXX

88120 Cytopathology, in situ hybridization (eg, FISH), urinary tract specimen with morphometric analysis, 3-5 molecular probes, each specimen; manual X 80
EXCLUDES *More than five probes (88399)*
Morphometric in situ hybridzation on specimens other than urinary tract (88367-88368)
13.91 13.91 Global Days XXX

88121 using computer-assisted technology X 80
EXCLUDES *More than five probes (88399)*
Morphometric in situ hybridzation on specimens other than urinary tract (88367-88368)
11.99 11.99 Global Days XXX

88125 Cytopathology, forensic (eg, sperm) X 80
0.65 0.65 Global Days XXX

88130 Sex chromatin identification; Barr bodies A
0.00 0.00 Global Days XXX

88140 peripheral blood smear, polymorphonuclear drumsticks A
EXCLUDES *Guard stain (88313)*
0.00 0.00 Global Days XXX

88141-88155 Pap Smears

CMS 100-2,15,80 Diagnostic Test Requirements
CMS 100-3,190.2 Diagnostic Pap Smears
CMS 100-3,210.2 Screening Pap Smears/Pelvic Examinations for Early Detection Cervical/Vaginal Cancer
CMS 100-4,3,10.4 Payment of Nonphysician Services for Inpatients

88141 Cytopathology, cervical or vaginal (any reporting system), requiring interpretation by physician ♀ N 26 80
Code also (88142-88154, 88164-88167, 88174-88175)
0.86 0.86 Global Days XXX
AMA: 2009, Jan, 11-31; 2008, Jan, 10-25; 2007, January, 13-27

88142 Cytopathology, cervical or vaginal (any reporting system), collected in preservative fluid, automated thin layer preparation; manual screening under physician supervision ♀ A
INCLUDES Bethesda or non-Bethesda method
0.00 0.00 Global Days XXX

88143 with manual screening and rescreening under physician supervision ♀ A
INCLUDES Bethesda or non-Bethesda method
EXCLUDES *Automated screening of automated thin layer preparation (88174-88175)*
0.00 0.00 Global Days XXX
AMA: 2009, Jan, 11-31; 2008, Jan, 10-25; 2007, January, 13-27

88147 Cytopathology smears, cervical or vaginal; screening by automated system under physician supervision ♀ A
0.00 0.00 Global Days XXX
AMA: 2009, Jan, 11-31; 2008, Jan, 10-25; 2007, January, 13-27

88148 screening by automated system with manual rescreening under physician supervision ♀ A
0.00 0.00 Global Days XXX

88150 Cytopathology, slides, cervical or vaginal; manual screening under physician supervision ♀ A
EXCLUDES *Bethesda method Pap smears (88164-88167)*
0.00 0.00 Global Days XXX

88152 with manual screening and computer-assisted rescreening under physician supervision ♀ A
EXCLUDES *Bethesda method Pap smears (88164-88167)*
0.00 0.00 Global Days XXX

88153 with manual screening and rescreening under physician supervision ♀ A
EXCLUDES *Bethesda method Pap smears (88164-88167)*
0.00 0.00 Global Days XXX
AMA: 2009, Jan, 11-31; 2008, Jan, 10-25; 2007, January, 13-27

88154 with manual screening and computer-assisted rescreening using cell selection and review under physician supervision ♀ A
EXCLUDES *Bethesda method Pap smears (88164-88167)*
0.00 0.00 Global Days XXX

\+ 88155 **Cytopathology, slides, cervical or vaginal, definitive hormonal evaluation (eg, maturation index, karyopyknotic index, estrogenic index) (List separately in addition to code[s] for other technical and interpretation services)**

Code first (88142-88154, 88164-88167, 88174-88175)

0.00 0.00 Global Days XXX

88160-88162 Cytopathology Smears (Other Than Pap)

CMS 100-2,15,80 Diagnostic Test Requirements
CMS 100-4,12,60 Payment for Pathology Services

88160 **Cytopathology, smears, any other source; screening and interpretation**

1.64 1.64 Global Days XXX

88161 **preparation, screening and interpretation**

1.68 1.68 Global Days XXX

88162 **extended study involving over 5 slides and/or multiple stains**

EXCLUDES *Aerosol collection of sputum (89220)*
Special stains (88312-88314)

2.52 2.52 Global Days XXX

88164-88167 Pap Smears: Bethesda System

CMS 100-2,15,80 Diagnostic Test Requirements
CMS 100-3,190.2 Diagnostic Pap Smears
CMS 100-3,210.2 Screening Pap Smears/Pelvic Examinations for Early Detection Cervical/Vaginal Cancer
CMS 100-4,3,10.4 Payment of Nonphysician Services for Inpatients
EXCLUDES *Non-Bethesda method (88150-88154)*

88164 **Cytopathology, slides, cervical or vaginal (the Bethesda System); manual screening under physician supervision**

0.00 0.00 Global Days XXX

88165 **with manual screening and rescreening under physician supervision**

0.00 0.00 Global Days XXX

AMA: 2009, Jan, 11-31; 2008, Jan, 10-25; 2007, January, 13-27

88166 **with manual screening and computer-assisted rescreening under physician supervision**

0.00 0.00 Global Days XXX

88167 **with manual screening and computer-assisted rescreening using cell selection and review under physician supervision**

EXCLUDES *Collection of specimen via fine needle aspiration (10021-10022)*

0.00 0.00 Global Days XXX

88172-88177 [88177] Cytopathology of Needle Biopsy

CMS 100-2,15,80 Diagnostic Test Requirements
CMS 100-4,3,10.4 Payment of Nonphysician Services for Inpatients
CMS 100-4,12,60 Payment for Pathology Services
EXCLUDES *Fine needle aspiration (10021-10022)*

88172 **Cytopathology, evaluation of fine needle aspirate; immediate cytohistologic study to determine adequacy for diagnosis, first evaluation episode, each site**

INCLUDES The submission of a complete set of cytologic material for evaluation regardless of the number of needle passes performed or slides prepared from each site

Do not report with same specimen (88333-88334)

1.55 1.55 Global Days XXX

AMA: 2009, Jan, 11-31; 2008, Jan, 10-25; 2007, January, 13-27; 2007, Aug, 15

88173 **interpretation and report**

INCLUDES The interpretation and report from each anatomical site no matter how many passes or evaluation episodes are performed during the aspiration

EXCLUDES *Fine needle aspiration (10021-10022)*

Do not report with same specimen (88333-88334)

4.08 4.08 Global Days XXX

AMA: 2009, Jan, 11-31; 2008, Jan, 10-25; 2007, January, 13-27

\+ # 88177 **immediate cytohistologic study to determine adequacy for diagnosis, each separate additional evaluation episode, same site (List separately in addition to code for primary procedure)**

Code also each additional mmediate repeat evaluation episode(s) required from the same site (e.g., previous sample is inadequate)

Code first (88172)

0.81 0.81 Global Days ZZZ

88174-88177 Pap Smears: Automated Screening

CMS 100-2,15,80 Diagnostic Test Requirements
CMS 100-3,190.2 Diagnostic Pap Smears
CMS 100-3,210.2 Screening Pap Smears/Pelvic Examinations for Early Detection Cervical/Vaginal Cancer
CMS 100-4,3,10.4 Payment of Nonphysician Services for Inpatients

88174 **Cytopathology, cervical or vaginal (any reporting system), collected in preservative fluid, automated thin layer preparation; screening by automated system, under physician supervision**

INCLUDES Bethesda or non-Bethesda method

0.00 0.00 Global Days XXX

88175 **with screening by automated system and manual rescreening or review, under physician supervision**

INCLUDES Bethesda or non-Bethesda method

EXCLUDES *Manual screening (88142-88143)*

0.00 0.00 Global Days XXX

88177 *Resequenced code, See code following 88173.*

88182-88199 Cytopathology Using the Fluorescence-Activated Cell Sorter

CMS 100-2,15,80 Diagnostic Test Requirements
CMS 100-4,3,10.4 Payment of Nonphysician Services for Inpatients
CMS 100-4,12,60 Payment for Pathology Services

88182 **Flow cytometry, cell cycle or DNA analysis**

EXCLUDES *DNA ploidy analysis by morphometric technique (88358)*

3.00 3.00 Global Days XXX

AMA: 2009, Jun, 3-6&11

88184 **Flow cytometry, cell surface, cytoplasmic, or nuclear marker, technical component only; first marker**

2.43 2.43 Global Days XXX

AMA: 2009, Jun, 3-6&11; 2007, Dec, 10-179

\+ 88185 **each additional marker (List separately in addition to code for first marker)**

Code first (88184)

1.47 1.47 Global Days ZZZ

AMA: 2009, Jan, 11-31; 2009, Jun, 3-6&11; 2007, Dec, 10-179

88187 Flow cytometry, interpretation; 2 to 8 markers
EXCLUDES *Interpretation (86355-86357, 86359-86361, 86367)*
1.96 1.96 Global Days XXX
AMA: 2009, Jun, 3-6&11; 2009, Jan, 11-31; 2008, Jan, 10-25; 2008, Apr, 5-7; 2007, January, 13-27

88188 9 to 15 markers
EXCLUDES *Interpretation (86355-86357, 86359-86361, 86367)*
2.46 2.46 Global Days XXX
AMA: 2009, Jan, 11-31; 2009, Jun, 3-6&11; 2008, Apr, 5-7; 2008, Jan, 10-25; 2007, January, 13-27

88189 16 or more markers
EXCLUDES *Interpretation (86355-86357, 86359-86361, 86367)*
Cell enumeration using immunologic selection qnd identification in fluid sample (0279T-0280T)
3.01 3.01 Global Days XXX
AMA: 2009, Jan, 11-31; 2009, Jun, 3-6&11; 2008, Apr, 5-7; 2008, Jan, 10-25; 2007, January, 13-27

88199 Unlisted cytopathology procedure
EXCLUDES *Cell enumeration using immunologic selection and identification in fluid specimen (e.g, circulation tumor cells in blood) (0279T-0280T)*
Electron microscopy (88348-88349)
0.00 0.00 Global Days XXX

88230-88299 Cytogenic Studies

CMS	100-1,5,90.2	Laboratory Defined
CMS	100-2,15,80	Diagnostic Test Requirements
CMS	100-2,15,80.1	Payment for Clinical Laboratory Services
CMS	100-3,190.3	Cytogenic Studies
CMS	100-4,3,10.4	Payment of Nonphysician Services for Inpatients
CMS	100-4,16,10	General Coverage: Diagnostic X-ray, Laboratory, and Other Tests
CMS	100-4,16,10.1	Laboratory Definitions
CMS	100-4,16,110.4	Carrier Contacts With Independent Clinical Laboratories

Code also genetic testing modifiers for oncologic or inherited disorder

88230 Tissue culture for non-neoplastic disorders; lymphocyte
0.00 0.00 Global Days XXX
AMA: 2008, May, 5-8

88233 skin or other solid tissue biopsy
0.00 0.00 Global Days XXX
AMA: 2008, May, 5-8

88235 amniotic fluid or chorionic villus cells
0.00 0.00 Global Days XXX
AMA: 2008, May, 5-8

88237 Tissue culture for neoplastic disorders; bone marrow, blood cells
0.00 0.00 Global Days XXX
AMA: 2008, May, 5-8

88239 solid tumor
0.00 0.00 Global Days XXX
AMA: 2008, May, 5-8

88240 Cryopreservation, freezing and storage of cells, each cell line
EXCLUDES *Therapeutic cryopreservation and storage (38207)*
0.00 0.00 Global Days XXX
AMA: 2009, Jun, 3-6&11

88241 Thawing and expansion of frozen cells, each aliquot
EXCLUDES *Therapeutic thawing of previous harvest (38208)*
0.00 0.00 Global Days XXX
AMA: 2009, Jun, 3-6&11

88245 Chromosome analysis for breakage syndromes; baseline Sister Chromatid Exchange (SCE), 20-25 cells
0.00 0.00 Global Days XXX
AMA: 2008, May, 5-8

88248 baseline breakage, score 50-100 cells, count 20 cells, 2 karyotypes (eg, for ataxia telangiectasia, Fanconi anemia, fragile X)
0.00 0.00 Global Days XXX
AMA: 2008, May, 5-8

88249 score 100 cells, clastogen stress (eg, diepoxybutane, mitomycin C, ionizing radiation, UV radiation)
0.00 0.00 Global Days XXX
AMA: 2008, May, 5-8

88261 Chromosome analysis; count 5 cells, 1 karyotype, with banding
0.00 0.00 Global Days XXX
AMA: 2008, May, 5-8; 2007, Dec, 10-179

88262 count 15-20 cells, 2 karyotypes, with banding
0.00 0.00 Global Days XXX
AMA: 2008, May, 5-8; 2007, Dec, 10-179

88263 count 45 cells for mosaicism, 2 karyotypes, with banding
0.00 0.00 Global Days XXX
AMA: 2008, May, 5-8

88264 analyze 20-25 cells
0.00 0.00 Global Days XXX
AMA: 2008, May, 5-8

88267 Chromosome analysis, amniotic fluid or chorionic villus, count 15 cells, 1 karyotype, with banding
0.00 0.00 Global Days XXX
AMA: 2008, May, 5-8

88269 Chromosome analysis, in situ for amniotic fluid cells, count cells from 6-12 colonies, 1 karyotype, with banding
0.00 0.00 Global Days XXX
AMA: 2008, May, 5-8

88271 Molecular cytogenetics; DNA probe, each (eg, FISH)
0.00 0.00 Global Days XXX
AMA: 2009, Jan, 11-31; 2008, May, 5-8; 2008, Jan, 10-25; 2007, January, 13-27

88272 chromosomal in situ hybridization, analyze 3-5 cells (eg, for derivatives and markers)
0.00 0.00 Global Days XXX
AMA: 2009, Jan, 11-31; 2008, Jan, 10-25; 2008, May, 5-8; 2007, January, 13-27

88273 chromosomal in situ hybridization, analyze 10-30 cells (eg, for microdeletions)
0.00 0.00 Global Days XXX
AMA: 2009, Jan, 11-31; 2008, May, 5-8; 2008, Jan, 10-25; 2007, January, 13-27

88274 interphase in situ hybridization, analyze 25-99 cells
0.00 0.00 Global Days XXX
AMA: 2009, Jan, 11-31; 2008, May, 5-8; 2008, Jan, 10-25; 2007, January, 13-27

88275 **interphase in situ hybridization, analyze 100-300 cells** A

0.00 0.00 Global Days XXX

AMA: 2009, Jan, 11-31; 2008, May, 5-8; 2008, Jan, 10-25; 2007, January, 13-27

88280 **Chromosome analysis; additional karyotypes, each study** A

0.00 0.00 Global Days XXX

AMA: 2008, May, 5-8

88283 **additional specialized banding technique (eg, NOR, C-banding)** A

0.00 0.00 Global Days XXX

AMA: 2008, May, 5-8

88285 **additional cells counted, each study** A

0.00 0.00 Global Days XXX

AMA: 2009, Jan, 11-31; 2008, May, 5-8; 2007, Dec, 10-179

88289 **additional high resolution study** A

0.00 0.00 Global Days XXX

AMA: 2008, May, 5-8

88291 **Cytogenetics and molecular cytogenetics, interpretation and report** M 26 80

0.86 0.86 Global Days XXX

AMA: 2008, May, 5-8

88299 **Unlisted cytogenetic study** X 80

0.00 0.00 Global Days XXX

88300 Evaluation of Surgical Specimen: Gross Anatomy

CMS 100-1,5,90.2 Laboratory Defined

CMS 100-4,12,60 Payment for Pathology Services

INCLUDES Attainment, examination, and reporting
Unit of service is the specimen

EXCLUDES *Additional procedures (88311-88365, 88399)*
Microscopic exam (88302-88309)

88300 **Level I - Surgical pathology, gross examination only** X 80

0.83 0.83 Global Days XXX

AMA: 2009, Jan, 11-31; 2008, Jan, 10-25; 2007, January, 13-27

88302-88309 Evaluation of Surgical Specimens: Gross and Microscopic Anatomy

CMS 100-1,5,90.2 Laboratory Defined

CMS 100-4,12,60 Payment for Pathology Services

INCLUDES Attainment, examination, and reporting
Unit of service is the specimen

EXCLUDES *Additional procedures (88311-88365, 88399)*

Do not report with Mohs surgery (17311-17315)

88302 **Level II - Surgical pathology, gross and microscopic examination** X 80

INCLUDES Appendix, incidental
Confirming identification and absence of disease
Fallopian tube, sterilization
Fingers or toes traumatic amputation
Foreskin, newborn
Hernia sac, any site
Hydrocele sac
Nerve
Skin, plastic repair
Sympathetic ganglion
Testis, castration
Vaginal mucosa, incidental
Vas deferense, sterilization

1.64 1.64 Global Days XXX

AMA: 2009, Jan, 11-31; 2008, Jan, 10-25; 2007, January, 13-27; 2007, January, 28-31

88304 Level III - Surgical pathology, gross and microscopic examination

INCLUDES Abortion, induced
Abscess
Anal tag
Aneurysm-atrial/ventricular
Appendix, other than incidental
Artery, atheromatous plaque
Bartholin's gland cyst
Bone fragment(s), other than pathologic fracture
Bursa/ synovial cyst
Carpal tunnel tissue
Cartilage, shavings
Cholesteatoma
Colon, colostomy stoma
Conjunctiva-biopsy/pterygium
Cornea
Diverticulum-esophagus/small intestine
Dupuytren's contracture tissue
Femoral head, other than fracture
Fissure/fistula
Foreskin, other than newborn
Gallbladder
Ganglion cyst
Hematoma
Hemorrhoids
Hydatid of Morgagni
Intervertebral disc
Joint, loose body
Meniscus
Mucocele, salivary
Neuroma-Morton's/traumatic
Pilonidal cyst/sinus
Polyps, inflammatory-nasal/sinusoidal
Skin-cyst/tag/debridement
Soft tissue, debridement
Soft tissue, lipoma
Spermatocele
Tendon/tendon sheath
Testicular appendage
Thrombus or embolus
Tonsil and/or adenoids
Varicocele
Vas deferens, other than sterilization
Vein, varicosity

1.82 1.82 Global Days XXX
AMA: 2009, Jan, 11-31; 2008, Jan, 10-25; 2007, January, 28-31; 2007, January, 13-27

88305 Level IV - Surgical pathology, gross and microscopic examination

INCLUDES Abortion, spontaneous/missed
Artery, biopsy
Bone exostosis
Bone marrow, biopsy
Brain/meninges, other than for tumor resection
Breast biopsy without microscopic assessment of surgical margin
Breast reduction mammoplasty
Bronchus, biopsy
Cell block, any source
Cervix, biopsy
Colon, biopsy
Duodenum, biopsy
Endocervix, curettings/biopsy
Endometrium, curettings/biopsy
Esophagus, biopsy
Extremity, amputation, traumatic
Fallopian tube, biopsy
Fallopian tube, ectopic pregnancy
Femoral head, fracture
Finger/toes, amputation, nontraumatic
Gingiva/oral mucosa, biopsy
Heart valve
Joint resection
Kidney biopsy
Larynx biopsy
Leiomyoma(s), uterine myomectomy-without uterus
Lip, biopsy/wedge resection
Lung, transbronchial biopsy
Lymph node, biopsy
Muscle, biopsy
Nasal mucosa, biopsy
Nasopharynx/oropharynx, biopsy
Nerve biopsy
Odontogenic/dental cyst
Omentum, biopsy
Ovary, biopsy/wedge resection
Ovary with or without tube, nonneoplastic
Parathyroid gland
Peritoneum, biopsy
Pituitary tumor
Placenta, other than third trimester
Pleura/pericardium-biopsy/tissue
Polyp:
- Cervical/endometrial
- Colorectal
- Stomach/small intestine

Prostate:
- Needle biopsy
- TUR

Salivary gland, biopsy
Sinus, paranasal biopsy
Skin, other than cyst/tag/debridement/plastic repair
Small intestine, biopsy
Soft tissue, other than tumor/mas/lipoma/debridement
Spleen
Stomach biopsy
Synovium
Testis, other than tumor/biopsy, castration
Thyroglossal duct/brachial cleft cyst
Tongue, biopsy
Tonsil, biopsy
Trachea biopsy
Ureter, biopsy
Urethra, biopsy
Urinary bladder, biopsy
Uterus, with or without tubes and ovaries, for prolapse
Vagina biopsy
Vulva/labial biopsy

3.11 3.11 Global Days XXX
AMA: 2009, Jan, 11-31; 2008, Jan, 10-25; 2007, January, 13-27; 2007, January, 28-31

88307 **Level V - Surgical pathology, gross and microscopic examination**

INCLUDES
Adrenal resection
Bone, biopsy/curettings
Bone fragment(s), pathologic fractures
Brain, biopsy
Brain meninges, tumor resection
Breast, excision of lesion, requiring microscopic evaluation of surgical margins
Breast, mastectomy-partial/simple
Cervix, conization
Colon, segmental resection, other than for tumor
Extremity, amputation, nontraumatic
Eye, enucleation
Kidney, partial/total nephrectomy
Larynx, partial/total resection
Liver, biopsy-needle, wedge
Lung, wedge biopsy
Lymph nodes, regional resection
Mediastinum, mass
Myocardium, biopsy
Odontogenic tumor
Ovary with or without tube, neoplastic
Pancreas, biopsy
Placenta, third trimester
Prostate, except radical resection
Salivary gland
Sentinel lymph node
Small intestine, resection, other than for tumor
Soft tissue mass (except lipoma)-biopsy/simple excision
Stomach-subtotal/total resection, other than for tumor
Testis, biopsy
Thymus, tumor
Thyroid, total/lobe
Ureter, resection
Urinary bladder, TUR
Uterus, with or without tubes and ovaries, other than neoplastic/prolapse

6.89 6.89 **Global Days XXX**

AMA: 2009, Jan, 11-31; 2008, Jan, 10-25; 2007, January, 13-27; 2007, January, 28-31

88309 **Level VI - Surgical pathology, gross and microscopic examination**

INCLUDES
Bone resection
Breast, mastectomy-with regional lymph nodes
Colon:
Segmental resection for tumor
Total resection
Esophagus, partial/total resection
Extremity, disarticulation
Fetus, with dissection
Larynx, partial/total resection-with regional lymph nodes
Lung-total/lobe/segment resection
Pancreas, total/subtotal resection
Prostate, radical resection
Small intestine, resection for tumor
Soft tissue tumor, extensive resection
Stomach, subtotal/total resection for tumor
Testis, tumor
Tongue/tonsil, resection for tumor
Urinary bladder, partial/total resection
Uterus, with or without tubes and ovaries, neoplastic
Vulva, total/subtotal resection

EXCLUDES
Evaluation of fine needle aspirate (88172-88173)
Fine needle aspiration (10021-10022)

10.44 10.44 **Global Days XXX**

AMA: 2009, Jan, 11-31; 2008, Jan, 10-25; 2007, January, 13-27; 2007, January, 28-31

88311-88399 Additional Surgical Pathology Services

CMS 100-4,12,60 Payment for Pathology Services

\+ 88311 **Decalcification procedure (List separately in addition to code for surgical pathology examination)**

Code first surgical pathology exam (88302-88309)

0.56 0.56 **Global Days XXX**

AMA: 2009, Jan, 11-31; 2008, Jan, 10-25; 2007, January, 13-27

▲ 88312 **Special stain including interpretation and report; Group I for microorganisms (eg, acid fast, methenamine silver)**

Code also this code for each special stain performed on a surgical pathology block, cytologic sample, or hematologic smear

2.75 2.75 **Global Days XXX**

AMA: 2009, Jan, 11-31; 2008, Jan, 10-25; 2007, January, 13-27

▲ 88313 **Group II, all other (eg, iron, trichrome), except stain for microorganisms, stains for enzyme constituents, or immunocytochemistry and immunohistochemistry**

EXCLUDES
Immunocytochemistry and immunohistochemistry (88342)
Immunocytochemistry and immunoperoxidase tissue studies (88342)

Code also this code for each special stain performed on a surgical pathology block, cytologic sample, or hematologic smear

1.93 1.93 **Global Days XXX**

AMA: 2009, Jan, 11-31; 2008, Jan, 10-25; 2007, January, 13-27

+ ▲ 88314 **histochemical stain on frozen tissue block (List separately in addition to code for primary procedure)**

INCLUDES Reporting one unit for each special stain on each frozen surgical pathology block

EXCLUDES *Special stain performed on frozen tissue section specimen to identify enzyme constituents (88319)*

Code also modifier 59 for nonroutine histochemical stain on frozen section during Mohs surgery

Code first (17311-17315, 88302-88309, 88331-88332)

Do not report with routine frozen section stain during Mohs surgery (17311-17315)

2.35 2.35 Global Days XXX

~~88318 Determinative histochemistry to identify chemical components (eg, copper, zinc)~~

To report, see 88313

▲ 88319 **Group III, for enzyme constituents**

INCLUDES Reporting one unit for each special stain on each frozen surgical pathology block

EXCLUDES *Detection of enzyme constituents by immunohistochemical or immunocytochemical methodology (88342)*

2.88 2.88 Global Days XXX

88321 **Consultation and report on referred slides prepared elsewhere**

2.37 2.64 Global Days XXX

AMA: 2009, Jan, 11-31; 2008, Jan, 10-25; 2007, January, 13-27

88323 **Consultation and report on referred material requiring preparation of slides**

4.03 4.03 Global Days XXX

AMA: 2009, Jan, 11-31; 2008, Jan, 10-25; 2007, January, 13-27

88325 **Consultation, comprehensive, with review of records and specimens, with report on referred material**

3.66 5.79 Global Days XXX

AMA: 2009, Jan, 11-31; 2008, Jan, 10-25; 2007, January, 13-27

88329 **Pathology consultation during surgery;**

1.01 1.56 Global Days XXX

AMA: 2009, Jan, 11-31; 2008, Jan, 10-25; 2007, January, 13-27; 2007, January, 28-31

88331 **first tissue block, with frozen section(s), single specimen**

2.72 2.72 Global Days XXX

AMA: 2007, January, 28-31

+ 88332 **each additional tissue block with frozen section(s) (List separately in addition to code for primary procedure)**

Code first (88331)

1.20 1.20 Global Days XXX

AMA: 2007, January, 28-31

88333 **cytologic examination (eg, touch prep, squash prep), initial site**

EXCLUDES *Intraprocedural cytologic evaluation of fine needle aspirate (88172)*
Nonintraoperative cytologic examination (88160-88162)

2.86 2.86 Global Days XXX

AMA: 2009, Jan, 11-31; 2008, Jun, 14-15; 2007, January, 28-31

+ 88334 **cytologic examination (eg, touch prep, squash prep), each additional site (List separately in addition to code for primary procedure)**

EXCLUDES *Intraoperative consultation on a specimen requiring both frozen section and cytologic evaluation (88331, 88334)*
Intraprocedural cytologic evaluation of fine needle aspirate (88172)
Nonintraoperative cytologic examination (88160-88162)
Percutaneous needle biopsy requiring intraprocedural cytologic examination (88333)

Code first (88331, 88333)

1.77 1.77 Global Days XXX

AMA: 2007, January, 28-31

88342 **Immunohistochemistry (including tissue immunoperoxidase), each antibody**

EXCLUDES *Quantitative or semiquantitative immunohistochemistry (88360-88361)*

Do not report with testing on the same antibody (88360-88361)

3.10 3.10 Global Days XXX

AMA: 2009, Jan, 11-31; 2008, Jan, 10-25; 2007, January, 13-27

88346 **Immunofluorescent study, each antibody; direct method**

3.04 3.04 Global Days XXX

88347 **indirect method**

2.17 2.17 Global Days XXX

88348 **Electron microscopy; diagnostic**

20.68 20.68 Global Days XXX

88349 **scanning**

11.54 11.54 Global Days XXX

88355 **Morphometric analysis; skeletal muscle**

5.70 5.70 Global Days XXX

88356 **nerve**

8.01 8.01 Global Days XXX

88358 **tumor (eg, DNA ploidy)**

Do not report with 88313 unless each procedure is for a different special stain (88313)

2.22 2.22 Global Days XXX

AMA: 2009, Jan, 11-31; 2008, Jan, 10-25; 2007, January, 13-27

88360 **Morphometric analysis, tumor immunohistochemistry (eg, Her-2/neu, estrogen receptor/progesterone receptor), quantitative or semiquantitative, each antibody; manual**

Do not report with 88342 unless each test is for different antibody (88342)

3.54 3.54 Global Days XXX

88361 **using computer-assisted technology**

EXCLUDES *Morphometric analysis using in situ hybridization techniques (88367-88368)*

Do not report with 88342 unless each test is for different antibody (88342)

4.45 4.45 Global Days XXX

88362 **Nerve teasing preparations**

8.88 8.88 Global Days XXX

88363 **Examination and selection of retrieved archival (ie, previously diagnosed) tissue(s) for molecular analysis (eg, KRAS mutational analysis)** X 80

INCLUDES Archival retrieval only

EXCLUDES *Molecular diagnostic interpretation or microdissection*

0.46 1.04 Global Days XXX

88365 **In situ hybridization (eg, FISH), each probe** X 80

Do not report with 88367-88368 for the same probe (88367-88368)

4.87 4.87 Global Days XXX

AMA: 2009, Jan, 11-31; 2008, Jan, 10-25; 2007, January, 13-27

88367 **Morphometric analysis, in situ hybridization (quantitative or semi-quantitative) each probe; using computer-assisted technology** X 80

EXCLUDES *Morphometric in situ hybridization evaluation of urinary tract cytologic specimens (88120-88121)*

7.76 7.76 Global Days XXX

AMA: 2009, Jan, 11-31; 2008, Jan, 10-25; 2007, January, 13-27

88368 **manual** X 80

EXCLUDES *Morphometric in situ hybridization evaluation of urinary tract cytologic specimens (88120-88121)*

6.50 6.50 Global Days XXX

AMA: 2009, Jan, 11-31; 2008, Jan, 10-25; 2007, January, 13-27

88371 **Protein analysis of tissue by Western Blot, with interpretation and report;** A

0.00 0.00 Global Days XXX

88372 **immunological probe for band identification, each** A

0.00 0.00 Global Days XXX

88380 **Microdissection (ie, sample preparation of microscopically identified target); laser capture** N 80

5.37 5.37 Global Days XXX

AMA: 2008, Apr, 5-7

88381 **manual** N 80

Do not report with 88381

4.74 4.74 Global Days XXX

AMA: 2008, Apr, 5-7

88384 **Array-based evaluation of multiple molecular probes; 11 through 50 probes** X 80

0.00 0.00 Global Days XXX

88385 **51 through 250 probes** X 80

16.17 16.17 Global Days XXX

AMA: 2008, May, 5-8

88386 **251 through 500 probes** X 80

EXCLUDES *Preparation and analysis of fewer than 11 probes (83890-83914)*
Preparation of array-based evaluation (83890-83892, 83898-83901)

18.31 18.31 Global Days XXX

AMA: 2009, Jan, 11-31; 2008, May, 5-8; 2008, May, 9-11

88387 **Macroscopic examination, dissection, and preparation of tissue for non-microscopic analytical studies (eg, nucleic acid-based molecular studies); each tissue preparation (eg, a single lymph node)** N 80

Do not report for tissues preparation for microbiologic cultures or flow cytometric studies

Do not report with (88329-88384, 88388)

1.02 1.02 Global Days XXX

\+ 88388 **in conjunction with a touch imprint, intraoperative consultation, or frozen section, each tissue preparation (eg, a single lymph node) (List separately in addition to code for primary procedure)** N 80

Do not report for tissue preparation for microbiologic cultures or flow cytometric studies

Code first (88329-88334)

0.90 0.90 Global Days XXX

88399 **Unlisted surgical pathology procedure** X 80

0.00 0.00 Global Days XXX

AMA: 2009, Jan, 11-31; 2008, May, 9-11

88720-88749 Transcutaneous Procedures

EXCLUDES *Transcutaneous oxyhemoglobin measurement in a leg using near infrared spectroscopy (0286T)*
Wavelength fluorescent spectroscopy of advanced glycation end products (skin) (0233T)

88720 **Bilirubin, total, transcutaneous** A

EXCLUDES *Transdermal oxygen saturation testing (94760-94762)*

0.00 0.00 Global Days XXX

88738 **Hemoglobin (Hgb), quantitative, transcutaneous** A

EXCLUDES *In vitro hemoglobin measurement (85018)*

0.00 0.00 Global Days XXX

88740 **Hemoglobin, quantitative, transcutaneous, per day; carboxyhemoglobin** A

EXCLUDES *In vitro carboxyhemoglobin measurement (82375)*

0.00 0.00 Global Days XXX

88741 **methemoglobin** A

EXCLUDES *In vitro quantitative methemoglobin measurement (83050)*

0.00 0.00 Global Days XXX

88749 **Unlisted in vivo (eg, transcutaneous) laboratory service** A

INCLUDES All in vivo measurements not specifically listed

0.00 0.00 Global Days XXX

89049-89240 Other Pathology Services

CMS 100-4,3,10.4 Payment of Nonphysician Services for Inpatients

89049 **Caffeine halothane contracture test (CHCT) for malignant hyperthermia susceptibility, including interpretation and report** X 80

1.91 7.77 Global Days XXX

AMA: 2009, Jan, 11-31; 2008, Jan, 10-25; 2007, January, 13-27

89050 **Cell count, miscellaneous body fluids (eg, cerebrospinal fluid, joint fluid), except blood;** A

0.00 0.00 Global Days XXX

89051 **with differential count** A

0.00 0.00 Global Days XXX

89055 **Leukocyte assessment, fecal, qualitative or semiquantitative** A

0.00 0.00 Global Days XXX

89060 **Crystal identification by light microscopy with or without polarizing lens analysis, tissue or any body fluid (except urine)** A

EXCLUDES *Crystal identification on paraffin embedded tissue (89060)*

0.00 0.00 Global Days XXX

89125 **Fat stain, feces, urine, or respiratory secretions** A

0.00 0.00 Global Days XXX

89160 **Meat fibers, feces** A
0.00 0.00 Global Days XXX

89190 **Nasal smear for eosinophils** A
EXCLUDES *Occult blood, feces (82270)*
Paternity tests (86910)
0.00 0.00 Global Days XXX

89220 **Sputum, obtaining specimen, aerosol induced technique (separate procedure)** X TC 80
0.48 0.48 Global Days XXX

89230 **Sweat collection by iontophoresis** X TC 80
0.08 0.08 Global Days XXX

89240 **Unlisted miscellaneous pathology test** X 80
0.00 0.00 Global Days XXX
AMA: 2009, Jan, 11-31; 2008, Jan, 10-25; 2007, January, 13-27

89250-89398 Infertility Treatment Services

CMS 100-2,1,100 Treatment for Infertility
CMS 100-4,3,10.4 Payment of Nonphysician Services for Inpatients

89250 **Culture of oocyte(s)/embryo(s), less than 4 days;** X
0.00 0.00 Global Days XXX
AMA: 2009, Jan, 11-31; 2008, Jan, 10-25; 2007, January, 13-27

89251 **with co-culture of oocyte(s)/embryos** X
EXCLUDES *Extended culture of oocyte(s)/embryo(s) (89272)*
0.00 0.00 Global Days XXX
AMA: 2009, Jan, 11-31; 2008, Jan, 10-25; 2007, January, 13-27

89253 **Assisted embryo hatching, microtechniques (any method)** X
0.00 0.00 Global Days XXX
AMA: 2009, Jan, 11-31; 2008, Jan, 10-25; 2007, January, 13-27

89254 **Oocyte identification from follicular fluid** X
0.00 0.00 Global Days XXX
AMA: 2009, Jan, 11-31; 2008, Jan, 10-25; 2007, January, 13-27

89255 **Preparation of embryo for transfer (any method)** X
0.00 0.00 Global Days XXX
AMA: 2009, Jan, 11-31; 2008, Jan, 10-25; 2007, January, 13-27

89257 **Sperm identification from aspiration (other than seminal fluid)** X
EXCLUDES *Semen analysis (89300-89320)*
Sperm identification from testis tissue (89264)
0.00 0.00 Global Days XXX
AMA: 2009, Jan, 11-31; 2008, Jan, 10-25; 2007, January, 13-27

89258 **Cryopreservation; embryo(s)** X
0.00 0.00 Global Days XXX
AMA: 2009, Jan, 11-31; 2008, Jan, 10-25; 2007, January, 13-27

89259 **sperm** X
EXCLUDES *Cryopreservation of testicular reproductive tissue (89335)*
0.00 0.00 Global Days XXX
AMA: 2009, Jan, 11-31; 2008, Jan, 10-25; 2007, January, 13-27

89260 **Sperm isolation; simple prep (eg, sperm wash and swim-up) for insemination or diagnosis with semen analysis** X
0.00 0.00 Global Days XXX
AMA: 2009, Jan, 11-31; 2008, Jan, 10-25; 2007, January, 13-27

89261 **complex prep (eg, Percoll gradient, albumin gradient) for insemination or diagnosis with semen analysis** X
EXCLUDES *Semen analysis without sperm wash or swim-up (89320)*
0.00 0.00 Global Days XXX
AMA: 2009, Jan, 11-31; 2008, Jan, 10-25; 2007, January, 13-27

89264 **Sperm identification from testis tissue, fresh or cryopreserved** ♂ X
EXCLUDES *Biopsy of testis (54500, 54505)*
Semen analysis (89300-89320)
Sperm identification from aspiration (89257)
0.00 0.00 Global Days XXX
AMA: 2009, Jan, 11-31; 2008, Jan, 10-25; 2007, January, 13-27

89268 **Insemination of oocytes** X
0.00 0.00 Global Days XXX
AMA: 2009, Jan, 11-31; 2008, Jan, 10-25; 2007, January, 13-27

89272 **Extended culture of oocyte(s)/embryo(s), 4-7 days** X
0.00 0.00 Global Days XXX
AMA: 2009, Jan, 11-31; 2008, Jan, 10-25; 2007, January, 13-27

89280 **Assisted oocyte fertilization, microtechnique; less than or equal to 10 oocytes** X
0.00 0.00 Global Days XXX
AMA: 2009, Jan, 11-31; 2008, Jan, 10-25; 2007, January, 13-27

89281 **greater than 10 oocytes** X
0.00 0.00 Global Days XXX
AMA: 2009, Jan, 11-31; 2008, Jan, 10-25; 2007, January, 13-27

89290 **Biopsy, oocyte polar body or embryo blastomere, microtechnique (for pre-implantation genetic diagnosis); less than or equal to 5 embryos** X
0.00 0.00 Global Days XXX
AMA: 2009, Jan, 11-31; 2008, Jan, 10-25; 2007, January, 13-27

89291 **greater than 5 embryos** X
0.00 0.00 Global Days XXX
AMA: 2009, Jan, 11-31; 2008, Jan, 10-25; 2007, January, 13-27

89300 **Semen analysis; presence and/or motility of sperm including Huhner test (post coital)** ♀ A
0.00 0.00 Global Days XXX
AMA: 2009, Jan, 11-31; 2008, Jan, 10-25; 2008, Apr, 5-7; 2007, January, 13-27

89310 **motility and count (not including Huhner test)** A
0.00 0.00 Global Days XXX
AMA: 2009, Jan, 11-31; 2008, Jan, 10-25; 2008, Apr, 5-7; 2007, January, 13-27

89320 **volume, count, motility, and differential** A
0.00 0.00 Global Days XXX
AMA: 2009, Jan, 11-31; 2008, Jan, 10-25; 2008, Apr, 5-7; 2007, January, 13-27

89321 **sperm presence and motility of sperm, if performed** A
EXCLUDES *Hyaluronan binding assay (HBA) (89398)*
0.00 0.00 Global Days XXX
AMA: 2009, Jan, 11-31; 2008, Jan, 10-25; 2008, Apr, 5-7; 2007, January, 13-27

89322 **volume, count, motility, and differential using strict morphologic criteria (eg, Kruger)** A
0.00 0.00 Global Days XXX
AMA: 2009, Jan, 11-31; 2008, Jan, 10-25; 2008, Apr, 5-7

89325 **Sperm antibodies** A
EXCLUDES *Medicolegal identification of sperm (88125)*
0.00 0.00 Global Days XXX
AMA: 2009, Jan, 11-31; 2008, Jan, 10-25; 2007, January, 13-27

89329 **Sperm evaluation; hamster penetration test** A
0.00 0.00 Global Days XXX
AMA: 2009, Jan, 11-31; 2008, Jan, 10-25; 2007, January, 13-27

89330 **cervical mucus penetration test, with or without spinnbarkeit test** A
0.00 0.00 Global Days XXX
AMA: 2009, Jan, 11-31; 2008, Jan, 10-25; 2007, January, 13-27

26/TC PC/TC Comp Only | CLIA Waived | ♂ Male Only | ♀ Female Only
AMA: CPT Asst | MED: Pub 100 | A-Y OPPSI | Radiology Crosswalk

89331 Sperm evaluation, for retrograde ejaculation, urine (sperm concentration, motility, and morphology, as indicated) [A]

EXCLUDES *Detection of sperm in urine (81015)*

Code also semen analysis on concurrent sperm specimen (89300-89322)

0.00 0.00 Global Days XXX

AMA: 2009, Jan, 11-31; 2008, Jan, 10-25; 2008, Apr, 5-7

89335 Cryopreservation, reproductive tissue, testicular [X]

EXCLUDES *Cryopreservation of:*

Embryo(s) (89258)

Ovarian reproductive tissue, oocytes (89240)

Sperm (89259)

0.00 0.00 Global Days XXX

AMA: 2009, Jan, 11-31; 2008, Jan, 10-25; 2007, January, 13-27

89342 Storage (per year); embryo(s) [X]

0.00 0.00 Global Days XXX

AMA: 2009, Jan, 11-31; 2008, Jan, 10-25; 2007, January, 13-27

89343 sperm/semen [X]

0.00 0.00 Global Days XXX

AMA: 2009, Jan, 11-31; 2008, Jan, 10-25; 2007, January, 13-27

89344 reproductive tissue, testicular/ovarian [X]

0.00 0.00 Global Days XXX

AMA: 2009, Jan, 11-31; 2008, Jan, 10-25; 2007, January, 13-27

89346 oocyte(s) [X]

0.00 0.00 Global Days XXX

AMA: 2009, Jan, 11-31; 2008, Jan, 10-25; 2007, January, 13-27

89352 Thawing of cryopreserved; embryo(s) [X]

0.00 0.00 Global Days XXX

AMA: 2009, Jan, 11-31; 2008, Jan, 10-25; 2007, January, 13-27

89353 sperm/semen, each aliquot [X]

0.00 0.00 Global Days XXX

AMA: 2009, Jan, 11-31; 2008, Jan, 10-25; 2007, January, 13-27

89354 reproductive tissue, testicular/ovarian [X]

0.00 0.00 Global Days XXX

AMA: 2009, Jan, 11-31; 2008, Jan, 10-25; 2007, January, 13-27

89356 oocytes, each aliquot [X]

0.00 0.00 Global Days XXX

AMA: 2009, Jan, 11-31; 2008, Jan, 10-25; 2007, January, 13-27

89398 Unlisted reproductive medicine laboratory procedure [X]

EXCLUDES *Hyaluronan binding assay (HBA) (89398)*

0.00 0.00 Global Days XXX

90281-90399 Immunoglobulin Products

CMS 100-2,15,50 Drugs and Biologicals
CMS 100-4,4,20.5 HCPCS Under OPPS

INCLUDES Immune globulin product only
Immune globulins/antioxins/various isoantibodies, and monoclonal antibodies:
Anti-infective
Broad-spectrum

Code also (96365-96368, 96372, 96374-96375)

⊘ 90281 **Immune globulin (Ig), human, for intramuscular use** E
0.00 0.00 Global Days XXX
AMA: 2009, Jan, 11-31; 2008, Jan, 10-25; 2007, January, 13-27

⊘ 90283 **Immune globulin (IgIV), human, for intravenous use** E
0.00 0.00 Global Days XXX
AMA: 2009, Jan, 11-31; 2008, Jan, 10-25

⊘ 90284 **Immune globulin (SCIg), human, for use in subcutaneous infusions, 100 mg, each** E
0.00 0.00 Global Days XXX
AMA: 2009, Jan, 11-31; 2008, Jan, 10-25

⊘ 90287 **Botulinum antitoxin, equine, any route** E
0.00 0.00 Global Days XXX
AMA: 2009, Jan, 11-31; 2008, Jan, 10-25

⊘ 90288 **Botulism immune globulin, human, for intravenous use** E
0.00 0.00 Global Days XXX
AMA: 2009, Jan, 11-31; 2008, Jan, 10-25

⊘ 90291 **Cytomegalovirus immune globulin (CMV-IgIV), human, for intravenous use** E
0.00 0.00 Global Days XXX
AMA: 2009, Jan, 11-31; 2008, Jan, 10-25

⊘ 90296 **Diphtheria antitoxin, equine, any route** E
0.00 0.00 Global Days XXX
AMA: 2009, Jan, 11-31; 2008, Jan, 10-25

⊘ 90371 **Hepatitis B immune globulin (HBIg), human, for intramuscular use** K2 K
INCLUDES Nabi-HB
0.00 0.00 Global Days XXX
AMA: 2009, Jan, 11-31; 2008, Jan, 10-25

⊘ 90375 **Rabies immune globulin (RIg), human, for intramuscular and/or subcutaneous use** K2 K
INCLUDES HyperRAB
0.00 0.00 Global Days XXX
AMA: 2009, Jan, 11-31; 2008, Jan, 10-25

⊘ 90376 **Rabies immune globulin, heat-treated (RIg-HT), human, for intramuscular and/or subcutaneous use** K2 K
0.00 0.00 Global Days XXX
AMA: 2009, Jan, 11-31; 2008, Jan, 10-25

⊘ 90378 **Respiratory syncytial virus, monoclonal antibody, recombinant, for intramuscular use, 50 mg, each** K2 K
INCLUDES Synagis
0.00 0.00 Global Days XXX
AMA: 2009, Jan, 11-31; 2008, Jan, 10-25

⊘ 90384 **Rho(D) immune globulin (RhIg), human, full-dose, for intramuscular use** E
0.00 0.00 Global Days XXX
AMA: 2009, Jan, 11-31; 2008, Jan, 10-25

⊘ 90385 **Rho(D) immune globulin (RhIg), human, mini-dose, for intramuscular use** N1 N
0.00 0.00 Global Days XXX
AMA: 2009, Jan, 11-31; 2008, Jan, 10-25

⊘ 90386 **Rho(D) immune globulin (RhIgIV), human, for intravenous use** E
0.00 0.00 Global Days XXX
AMA: 2009, Jan, 11-31; 2008, Jan, 10-25

⊘ 90389 **Tetanus immune globulin (TIg), human, for intramuscular use** E
0.00 0.00 Global Days XXX
AMA: 2009, Jan, 11-31; 2008, Jan, 10-25

⊘ 90393 **Vaccinia immune globulin, human, for intramuscular use** E
0.00 0.00 Global Days XXX
AMA: 2009, Jan, 11-31; 2008, Jan, 10-25

⊘ 90396 **Varicella-zoster immune globulin, human, for intramuscular use** K2 K
0.00 0.00 Global Days XXX
AMA: 2009, Jan, 11-31; 2008, Jan, 10-25

⊘ 90399 **Unlisted immune globulin** E
0.00 0.00 Global Days XXX
AMA: 2009, Jan, 11-31; 2008, Jan, 10-25

90460-90461 Injections Provided with Counseling

CMS 100-2,16,90 Routine Services and Appliances

INCLUDES All components of influenza vaccine, report X 1 only
Combination vaccines which comprise multiple vaccine components
Components (all antigens) in vaccines to prevent disease due to specific organisms
Counseling by physician or other qualified health care professional
Multi-valent antigens or multiple antigen serotypes against single organisms are considered one component
Patient/family face-to-face counseling by doctor or qualified health care professional for patients 18 years of age and younger

EXCLUDES *Administration of influenza and pneumococcal vaccine for Medicare patients (G0008-G0009, G9141)*
Allergy testing (95004-95075)
Bacterial/viral/fungal skin tests (86485-86580)
Vaccines provided without face-to-face counseling from a physician or qualified health care professional or to patients over the age of 18 (90471-90474)

Code also significant, separately identifiable evaluation and management service if performed (99201-99215)

Code also significant, separately identifiable preventive medicine services (99381-99429)

Code also therapeutic or diagnostic injections if performed (96372-96379)

Code also toxoid/vaccine (90476-90749 [90665])

▲ 90460 **Immunization administration through 18 years of age via any route of administration, with counseling by physician or other qualified health care professional; first or only component of each vaccine or toxoid administered** A B 80
Code also each additional component in a vaccine (e.g., A 5-year-old receives DtaP-IPV IM administration, and MMR/Varicella vaccines SQ administration. Report 90460 X 2, and 90461 X 6)
0.72 0.72 Global Days XXX

+ ▲ 90461 **each additional vaccine or toxoid component administered (List separately in addition to code for primary procedure)** A B 80
Code also each additional component in a vaccine (e.g., A 5-year-old receives DtaP-IPV IM administration, and MMR/Varicella vaccines SQ administration. Report 90460 X 2, and 90461 X 6)
Code first the initial component in each vaccine provided (90460)
0.37 0.37 Global Days ZZZ

90471-90474 Injections and Other Routes of Administration Without Physician Counseling

CMS 100-2,15,50 Drugs and Biologicals
CMS 100-2,16,90 Routine Services and Appliances
CMS 100-4,18,10.2.1 Vaccines and Administration

EXCLUDES *Administration of influenza and pneumococcal vaccine for Medicare patients (G0008-G0009, G9141)*
Administration of vaccine with counseling (90460-90461)
Allergy testing (95004-95075)
Bacterial/viral/fungal skin tests (86485-86580)
Injections, diagnostic/therapeutic (96372-96379)
Patient/family face-to-face counseling

Code also significant separately identifiable evaluation and management service if performed (99201-99215)

Code also significant, separately identifiable preventive medicine services (99381-99429)

Code also toxoid/vaccine (90476-90749 [90665])

90471 Immunization administration (includes percutaneous, intradermal, subcutaneous, or intramuscular injections); 1 vaccine (single or combination vaccine/toxoid) S 80 CCI

Do not report with intranasal/oral administration (90473)

0.71 0.71 Global Days XXX

AMA: 2009, Jan, 11-31; 2009, Jan, 3,4&9; 2009, Jul, 7; 2009, Jan, 7-8; 2008, Jan, 10-25; 2007, Jul, 12-13

\+ **90472 each additional vaccine (single or combination vaccine/toxoid) (List separately in addition to code for primary procedure)** S 80

EXCLUDES *BCG vaccine, intravesical administration (51720, 90586)*
Immune globulin administration (96365-96368, 96372-96375)
Immune globulin product (90281-90399)

Code first initial vaccine (90471, 90473)

0.35 0.35 Global Days ZZZ

AMA: 2009, Jan, 11-31; 2009, Jan, 7-8; 2009, Jul, 7; 2009, Jan, 3,4&9; 2008, Jan, 10-25; 2007, Jul, 12-13

90473 Immunization administration by intranasal or oral route; 1 vaccine (single or combination vaccine/toxoid) S 80 CCI

Do not report with percutaneous/intradermal/subcutaneous/intramuscular injections (90471)

0.65 0.65 Global Days XXX

AMA: 2009, Jan, 3,4&9; 2009, Jan, 7-8; 2009, Jul, 7

\+ **90474 each additional vaccine (single or combination vaccine/toxoid) (List separately in addition to code for primary procedure)** S 80

Code first initial vaccine (90471, 90473)

0.34 0.34 Global Days ZZZ

AMA: 2009, Jan, 7-8; 2009, Jul, 7; 2009, Jan, 3,4&9

90476-90749 [90665] Vaccination Products

CMS 100-2,15,50 Drugs and Biologicals
CMS 100-2,16,90 Routine Services and Appliances
CMS 100-4,4,20.5 HCPCS Under OPPS

INCLUDES Patient's age for coding purposes, not for product license
Vaccine product only

EXCLUDES *Immune globulins and adminstration (90281-90399, 96365, 96372-96375)*

Code also administration of vaccine (90460-90474)

Code also office/other outpatient (99201-99215)

Code also preventive medicine (99381-99429)

Code also significant separately identifiable evaluation and management service if performed

⊘ **90476 Adenovirus vaccine, type 4, live, for oral use** N1 N

0.00 0.00 Global Days XXX

AMA: 2009, Jul, 7; 2009, Jan, 11-31; 2008, Jan, 10-25; 2007, January, 13-27; 2007, February, 10-11

⊘ **90477 Adenovirus vaccine, type 7, live, for oral use** E

0.00 0.00 Global Days XXX

AMA: 2009, Jan, 11-31; 2009, Jul, 7; 2008, Jan, 10-25

⊘ ▲ **90581 Anthrax vaccine, for subcutaneous or intramuscular use** E CCI

INCLUDES BioThrax

0.00 0.00 Global Days XXX

AMA: 2009, Jul, 7; 2009, Jan, 11-31; 2008, Jan, 10-25

⊘ **90585 Bacillus Calmette-Guerin vaccine (BCG) for tuberculosis, live, for percutaneous use** K2 K CCI

INCLUDES Mycobax

0.00 0.00 Global Days XXX

AMA: 2009, Jan, 11-31; 2009, Jul, 7; 2008, Jan, 10-25

⊘ **90586 Bacillus Calmette-Guerin vaccine (BCG) for bladder cancer, live, for intravesical use** B

INCLUDES TheraCys
TICE BCG

0.00 0.00 Global Days XXX

AMA: 2009, Jan, 11-31; 2009, Jul, 7; 2008, Jan, 10-25

⊘ **90632 Hepatitis A vaccine, adult dosage, for intramuscular use** A N1 N CCI

INCLUDES HAVRIX 1440EL.U/1mL
VAQTA 50U/1mL

0.00 0.00 Global Days XXX

AMA: 2009, Jan, 11-31; 2009, Jul, 7; 2008, Jan, 10-25

⊘ **90633 Hepatitis A vaccine, pediatric/adolescent dosage-2 dose schedule, for intramuscular use** A N1 N CCI

INCLUDES HAVRIX 720EL.U/0.5mL
VAQTA 25U/0.5mL

0.00 0.00 Global Days XXX

AMA: 2009, Jul, 7; 2009, Jan, 11-31; 2008, Jan, 10-25

⊘ **90634 Hepatitis A vaccine, pediatric/adolescent dosage-3 dose schedule, for intramuscular use** N1 N CCI

0.00 0.00 Global Days XXX

AMA: 2009, Jul, 7; 2009, Jan, 11-31; 2008, Jan, 10-25

⊘ **90636 Hepatitis A and hepatitis B vaccine (HepA-HepB), adult dosage, for intramuscular use** A N1 N CCI

INCLUDES TWINRIX

0.00 0.00 Global Days XXX

AMA: 2009, Jan, 11-31; 2009, Jul, 7; 2008, Jan, 10-25

⊘ ✓▲ **90644 Meningococcal conjugate vaccine, serogroups C & Y and Hemophilus influenza B vaccine (Hib-MenCY), 4 dose schedule, when administered to children 2-15 months of age, for intramuscular use** E
0.00 0.00 Global Days XXX

⊘ **90645 Hemophilus influenza b vaccine (Hib), HbOC conjugate (4 dose schedule), for intramuscular use** N1 N
0.00 0.00 Global Days XXX
AMA: 2009, Jul, 7; 2009, Jan, 11-31; 2008, Jan, 10-25

⊘ **90646 Hemophilus influenza b vaccine (Hib), PRP-D conjugate, for booster use only, intramuscular use** N1 N
0.00 0.00 Global Days XXX
AMA: 2009, Jan, 11-31; 2009, Jul, 7; 2008, Jan, 10-25

⊘ **90647 Hemophilus influenza b vaccine (Hib), PRP-OMP conjugate (3 dose schedule), for intramuscular use** N1 N
INCLUDES PedvaxHIB
0.00 0.00 Global Days XXX
AMA: 2009, Jul, 7; 2009, Jan, 11-31; 2008, Jan, 10-25

⊘ **90648 Hemophilus influenza b vaccine (Hib), PRP-T conjugate (4 dose schedule), for intramuscular use** N1 N
INCLUDES ActHIB
Hiberix
0.00 0.00 Global Days XXX
AMA: 2009, Jan, 11-31; 2009, Jul, 7; 2008, Jan, 10-25

⊘ **90649 Human Papilloma virus (HPV) vaccine, types 6, 11, 16, 18 (quadrivalent), 3 dose schedule, for intramuscular use** M
INCLUDES GARDASIL
0.00 0.00 Global Days XXX
AMA: 2009, Jan, 11-31; 2009, Jul, 7; 2008, Jan, 10-25; 2007, Jul, 12-13

⊘ **90650 Human Papilloma virus (HPV) vaccine, types 16, 18, bivalent, 3 dose schedule, for intramuscular use** M
INCLUDES CERVARIX
0.00 0.00 Global Days XXX
AMA: 2009, Jan, 11-31; 2009, Jul, 7; 2008, Jan, 10-25

⊘ **90654 Influenza virus vaccine, split virus, preservative-free, for intradermal use** L1 L
INCLUDES Fluzone intradermal
0.00 0.00 Global Days XXX

⊘ **90655 Influenza virus vaccine, split virus, preservative free, when administered to children 6-35 months of age, for intramuscular use** A L1 L
INCLUDES Fluzone, no preservative, pediatric dose
0.00 0.00 Global Days XXX
AMA: 2009, Jan, 11-31; 2009, Jul, 7; 2008, Jan, 10-25; 2008, Apr, 8-9; 2007, April, 11-12

⊘ **90656 Influenza virus vaccine, split virus, preservative free, when administered to individuals 3 years and older, for intramuscular use** A L1 L
INCLUDES AFLURIA (prefilled syringe)
FLUARIX (prefilled syringe)
Fluvirin (prefilled syringe)
Fluzone, influenza virus vaccine, no preservative
0.00 0.00 Global Days XXX
AMA: 2009, Jan, 11-31; 2009, Jul, 7; 2008, Jan, 10-25; 2008, Apr, 8-9

⊘ **90657 Influenza virus vaccine, split virus, when administered to children 6-35 months of age, for intramuscular use** A L1 L
INCLUDES Fluzone, 0.25 mL
0.00 0.00 Global Days XXX
AMA: 2009, Jan, 11-31; 2009, Jul, 7; 2008, Jan, 10-25; 2008, Apr, 8-9; 2007, February, 10-11

⊘ **90658 Influenza virus vaccine, split virus, when administered to individuals 3 years of age and older, for intramuscular use** A E
INCLUDES AFLURIA, 0.5mL
FLULAVAL 0.5 mL
Fluvirin, 0.5mL
Fluzone, 0.5 mL
Fluzone, influenza virus vaccine (5mL vial [0.5mL dose])
0.00 0.00 Global Days XXX
AMA: 2009, Jan, 11-31; 2009, Jul, 7; 2008, Jan, 10-25; 2008, Apr, 8-9; 2007, February, 10-11; 2007, April, 11-12

⊘ **90660 Influenza virus vaccine, live, for intranasal use** L1 L
INCLUDES FluMist
0.00 0.00 Global Days XXX
AMA: 2009, Jul, 7; 2009, Jan, 11-31; 2008, Jan, 10-25; 2008, Apr, 8-9; 2007, February, 10-11

⊘ ✓ **90661 Influenza virus vaccine, derived from cell cultures, subunit, preservative and antibiotic free, for intramuscular use** E
0.00 0.00 Global Days XXX
AMA: 2009, Jan, 11-31; 2009, Jul, 7; 2008, Jan, 10-25; 2008, Apr, 8-9

⊘ **90662 Influenza virus vaccine, split virus, preservative free, enhanced immunogenicity via increased antigen content, for intramuscular use** L1 L
INCLUDES Fluzone high-dose
0.00 0.00 Global Days XXX
AMA: 2009, Jan, 11-31; 2009, Jul, 7; 2008, Jan, 10-25; 2008, Apr, 8-9

⊘ ✓ **90664 Influenza virus vaccine, pandemic formulation, live, for intranasal use** E
0.00 0.00 Global Days XXX

90665 Resequenced code, See code following 90668.

⊘ ✓ **90666 Influenza virus vaccine, pandemic formulation, split virus, preservative free, for intramuscular use** E
0.00 0.00 Global Days XXX

⊘ ✓ **90667 Influenza virus vaccine, pandemic formulation, split virus, adjuvanted, for intramuscular use** E
0.00 0.00 Global Days XXX

⊘ ✓ **90668 Influenza virus vaccine, pandemic formulation, split virus, for intramuscular use** E
0.00 0.00 Global Days XXX

⊘ # **90665 Lyme disease vaccine, adult dosage, for intramuscular use** N1 N
0.00 0.00 Global Days XXX
AMA: 2009, Jan, 11-31; 2009, Jul, 7; 2008, Jan, 10-25; 2007, February, 10-11

⊘ **90669 Pneumococcal conjugate vaccine, 7 valent, for intramuscular use** L1 L
INCLUDES Prevnar
0.00 0.00 Global Days XXX
AMA: 2009, Jan, 11-31; 2009, Jul, 7; 2008, Jan, 10-25; 2007, February, 10-11

⊘ **90670 Pneumococcal conjugate vaccine, 13 valent, for intramuscular use** L1 L
INCLUDES Prevnar 13
0.00 0.00 Global Days XXX
AMA: 2009, Jul, 7

⊘ **90675 Rabies vaccine, for intramuscular use** K2 K
INCLUDES IMOVAX
RabAvert
0.00 0.00 Global Days XXX
AMA: 2009, Jul, 7; 2009, Jan, 11-31; 2008, Jan, 10-25; 2007, February, 10-11

⊘ 90676 **Rabies vaccine, for intradermal use**
0.00 0.00 Global Days XXX
AMA: 2009, Jan, 11-31; 2009, Jul, 7; 2008, Jan, 10-25; 2007, February, 10-11

⊘ 90680 **Rotavirus vaccine, pentavalent, 3 dose schedule, live, for oral use**
INCLUDES RotaTeq
0.00 0.00 Global Days XXX
AMA: 2009, Jan, 11-31; 2009, Jul, 7; 2008, Jan, 10-25; 2007, February, 10-11

⊘ 90681 **Rotavirus vaccine, human, attenuated, 2 dose schedule, live, for oral use**
INCLUDES Rotarix
0.00 0.00 Global Days XXX
AMA: 2009, Jul, 7; 2009, Jan, 11-31; 2008, Jan, 10-25

⊘ 90690 **Typhoid vaccine, live, oral**
INCLUDES Vivotif
0.00 0.00 Global Days XXX
AMA: 2009, Jul, 7; 2009, Jan, 11-31; 2008, Jan, 10-25; 2007, February, 10-11

⊘ 90691 **Typhoid vaccine, Vi capsular polysaccharide (ViCPs), for intramuscular use**
INCLUDES Typhim Vi
0.00 0.00 Global Days XXX
AMA: 2009, Jan, 11-31; 2009, Jul, 7; 2008, Jan, 10-25; 2007, February, 10-11

⊘ 90692 **Typhoid vaccine, heat- and phenol-inactivated (H-P), for subcutaneous or intradermal use**
0.00 0.00 Global Days XXX
AMA: 2009, Jan, 11-31; 2009, Jul, 7; 2008, Jan, 10-25; 2007, February, 10-11

⊘ 90693 **Typhoid vaccine, acetone-killed, dried (AKD), for subcutaneous use (U.S. military)**
0.00 0.00 Global Days XXX
AMA: 2009, Jan, 11-31; 2009, Jul, 7; 2008, Jan, 10-25; 2007, January, 13-27; 2007, February, 10-11

⊘ 90696 **Diphtheria, tetanus toxoids, acellular pertussis vaccine and poliovirus vaccine, inactivated (DTaP-IPV), when administered to children 4 through 6 years of age, for intramuscular use**
INCLUDES KINRIX
0.00 0.00 Global Days XXX
AMA: 2009, Jan, 11-31; 2009, Jul, 7; 2008, Jan, 10-25

⊘ 90698 **Diphtheria, tetanus toxoids, acellular pertussis vaccine, haemophilus influenza Type B, and poliovirus vaccine, inactivated (DTaP - Hib - IPV), for intramuscular use**
INCLUDES Pentacel
0.00 0.00 Global Days XXX
AMA: 2009, Jan, 11-31; 2009, Jul, 7; 2008, Jan, 10-25; 2007, February, 10-11

⊘ 90700 **Diphtheria, tetanus toxoids, and acellular pertussis vaccine (DTaP), when administered to individuals younger than 7 years, for intramuscular use**
INCLUDES DAPTACEL
INFANRIX
Tripedia
0.00 0.00 Global Days XXX
AMA: 2009, Jul, 7; 2009, Jan, 11-31; 2008, Jan, 10-25; 2007, February, 10-11

⊘ 90701 **Diphtheria, tetanus toxoids, and whole cell pertussis vaccine (DTP), for intramuscular use**
0.00 0.00 Global Days XXX
AMA: 2009, Jan, 11-31; 2009, Jul, 7; 2008, Jan, 10-25; 2007, February, 10-11

⊘ 90702 **Diphtheria and tetanus toxoids (DT) adsorbed when administered to individuals younger than 7 years, for intramuscular use**
INCLUDES Diphtheria and Tetanus Toxoids Adsorbed USP (For Pediatric Use)
0.00 0.00 Global Days XXX
AMA: 2009, Jan, 11-31; 2009, Jul, 7; 2008, Jan, 10-25; 2007, February, 10-11

⊘ 90703 **Tetanus toxoid adsorbed, for intramuscular use**
INCLUDES Tetanus Toxoid Adsorbed
0.00 0.00 Global Days XXX
AMA: 2009, Jan, 11-31; 2009, Jul, 7; 2008, Jan, 10-25; 2007, February, 10-11

⊘ 90704 **Mumps virus vaccine, live, for subcutaneous use**
INCLUDES MUMPSVAX
0.00 0.00 Global Days XXX
AMA: 2009, Jan, 11-31; 2009, Jul, 7; 2008, Jan, 10-25; 2007, February, 10-11

⊘ 90705 **Measles virus vaccine, live, for subcutaneous use**
INCLUDES ATTENUVAX
0.00 0.00 Global Days XXX
AMA: 2009, Jan, 11-31; 2009, Jul, 7; 2008, Jan, 10-25; 2007, February, 10-11

⊘ 90706 **Rubella virus vaccine, live, for subcutaneous use**
INCLUDES MERUVAX II
0.00 0.00 Global Days XXX
AMA: 2009, Jan, 11-31; 2009, Jul, 7; 2008, Jan, 10-25; 2007, February, 10-11

⊘ 90707 **Measles, mumps and rubella virus vaccine (MMR), live, for subcutaneous use**
INCLUDES M-M-R II
0.00 0.00 Global Days XXX
AMA: 2009, Jan, 11-31; 2009, Jul, 7; 2008, Jan, 10-25; 2007, February, 10-11

⊘ 90708 **Measles and rubella virus vaccine, live, for subcutaneous use**
0.00 0.00 Global Days XXX
AMA: 2009, Jan, 11-31; 2009, Jul, 7; 2008, Jan, 10-25; 2007, February, 10-11

⊘ 90710 **Measles, mumps, rubella, and varicella vaccine (MMRV), live, for subcutaneous use**
INCLUDES ProQuad
0.00 0.00 Global Days XXX
AMA: 2009, Jan, 11-31; 2009, Jul, 7; 2008, Jan, 10-25; 2007, February, 10-11

⊘ 90712 **Poliovirus vaccine, (any type[s]) (OPV), live, for oral use**
0.00 0.00 Global Days XXX
AMA: 2009, Jul, 7; 2009, Jan, 11-31; 2008, Jan, 10-25; 2007, February, 10-11

⊘ 90713 **Poliovirus vaccine, inactivated (IPV), for subcutaneous or intramuscular use**
INCLUDES IPOL
0.00 0.00 Global Days XXX
AMA: 2009, Jul, 7; 2009, Jan, 11-31; 2008, Jan, 10-25; 2007, February, 10-11

⊘ **90714 Tetanus and diphtheria toxoids (Td) adsorbed, preservative free, when administered to individuals 7 years or older, for intramuscular use**
INCLUDES DECAVAC
0.00 0.00 Global Days XXX
AMA: 2009, Jan, 11-31; 2009, Jul, 7; 2008, Jan, 10-25; 2007, February, 10-11

⊘ **90715 Tetanus, diphtheria toxoids and acellular pertussis vaccine (Tdap), when administered to individuals 7 years or older, for intramuscular use**
INCLUDES Adacel
BOOSTRIX
0.00 0.00 Global Days XXX
AMA: 2009, Jan, 11-31; 2009, Jul, 7; 2008, Jan, 10-25; 2007, February, 10-11

⊘ **90716 Varicella virus vaccine, live, for subcutaneous use**
INCLUDES VARIVAX
0.00 0.00 Global Days XXX
AMA: 2009, Jan, 11-31; 2009, Jul, 7; 2008, Jan, 10-25; 2007, February, 10-11

⊘ **90717 Yellow fever vaccine, live, for subcutaneous use**
INCLUDES YF-VAX
0.00 0.00 Global Days XXX
AMA: 2009, Jan, 11-31; 2009, Jul, 7; 2008, Jan, 10-25; 2007, January, 13-27; 2007, February, 10-11

⊘ **90718 Tetanus and diphtheria toxoids (Td) adsorbed when administered to individuals 7 years or older, for intramuscular use**
INCLUDES Tetanus and Diphtheria Toxoids Adsorbed for Adult Use
0.00 0.00 Global Days XXX
AMA: 2009, Jan, 11-31; 2009, Jul, 7; 2008, Jan, 10-25; 2007, February, 10-11; 2007, January, 13-27

⊘ **90719 Diphtheria toxoid, for intramuscular use**
0.00 0.00 Global Days XXX
AMA: 2009, Jan, 11-31; 2009, Jul, 7; 2008, Jan, 10-25; 2007, January, 13-27; 2007, February, 10-11

⊘ **90720 Diphtheria, tetanus toxoids, and whole cell pertussis vaccine and Hemophilus influenza B vaccine (DTP-Hib), for intramuscular use**
0.00 0.00 Global Days XXX
AMA: 2009, Jul, 7; 2009, Jan, 11-31; 2008, Jan, 10-25; 2007, January, 13-27; 2007, February, 10-11

⊘ **90721 Diphtheria, tetanus toxoids, and acellular pertussis vaccine and Hemophilus influenza B vaccine (DtaP-Hib), for intramuscular use**
INCLUDES TriHIBit
0.00 0.00 Global Days XXX
AMA: 2009, Jan, 11-31; 2009, Jul, 7; 2008, Jan, 10-25; 2007, January, 13-27; 2007, February, 10-11

⊘ **90723 Diphtheria, tetanus toxoids, acellular pertussis vaccine, Hepatitis B, and poliovirus vaccine, inactivated (DtaP-HepB-IPV), for intramuscular use**
INCLUDES PEDIARIX
0.00 0.00 Global Days XXX
AMA: 2009, Jan, 11-31; 2009, Jul, 7; 2008, Jan, 10-25; 2007, January, 13-27; 2007, February, 10-11

⊘ **90725 Cholera vaccine for injectable use**
0.00 0.00 Global Days XXX
AMA: 2009, Jan, 11-31; 2009, Jul, 7; 2008, Jan, 10-25; 2007, January, 13-27; 2007, February, 10-11

⊘ **90727 Plague vaccine, for intramuscular use**
0.00 0.00 Global Days XXX
AMA: 2009, Jul, 7; 2009, Jan, 11-31; 2008, Jan, 10-25; 2007, January, 13-27; 2007, February, 10-11

⊘ **90732 Pneumococcal polysaccharide vaccine, 23-valent, adult or immunosuppressed patient dosage, when administered to individuals 2 years or older, for subcutaneous or intramuscular use**
INCLUDES PNEUMOVAX 23
0.00 0.00 Global Days XXX
AMA: 2009, Jan, 11-31; 2009, Jul, 7; 2008, Jan, 10-25; 2007, January, 13-27; 2007, February, 10-11

⊘ **90733 Meningococcal polysaccharide vaccine (any group(s)), for subcutaneous use**
INCLUDES Menomune-A/C/Y/W-135
0.00 0.00 Global Days XXX
AMA: 2009, Jan, 11-31; 2009, Jul, 7; 2008, Jan, 10-25; 2007, February, 10-11; 2007, January, 13-27

⊘ **90734 Meningococcal conjugate vaccine, serogroups A, C, Y and W-135 (tetravalent), for intramuscular use**
INCLUDES Menactra
Menveo
0.00 0.00 Global Days XXX
AMA: 2009, Jul, 7; 2009, Jan, 11-31; 2008, Jan, 10-25; 2007, January, 13-27; 2007, February, 10-11

⊘ **90735 Japanese encephalitis virus vaccine, for subcutaneous use**
INCLUDES JE-VAX
0.00 0.00 Global Days XXX
AMA: 2009, Jan, 11-31; 2009, Jul, 7; 2008, Jan, 10-25; 2007, January, 13-27; 2007, February, 10-11

⊘ **90736 Zoster (shingles) vaccine, live, for subcutaneous injection**
INCLUDES ZOSTAVAX
0.00 0.00 Global Days XXX
AMA: 2009, Jan, 11-31; 2009, Jul, 7; 2008, Jan, 10-25; 2007, Jul, 12-13; 2007, January, 13-27; 2007, February, 10-11

⊘ **90738 Japanese encephalitis virus vaccine, inactivated, for intramuscular use**
INCLUDES Ixiaro
0.00 0.00 Global Days XXX
AMA: 2009, Jan, 11-31; 2009, Jul, 7

⊘ **90740 Hepatitis B vaccine, dialysis or immunosuppressed patient dosage (3 dose schedule), for intramuscular use**
INCLUDES RECOMBIVAX HB 40mcg/1mL (dialysis formulation)
0.00 0.00 Global Days XXX
AMA: 2009, Jan, 11-31; 2009, Jul, 7; 2008, Jan, 10-25; 2007, January, 13-27; 2007, February, 10-11

⊘ **90743 Hepatitis B vaccine, adolescent (2 dose schedule), for intramuscular use**
INCLUDES RECOMBIVAX HB 10mcg/1mL
0.00 0.00 Global Days XXX
AMA: 2009, Jan, 11-31; 2009, Jul, 7; 2008, Jan, 10-25; 2007, January, 13-27; 2007, February, 10-11

⊘ **90744 Hepatitis B vaccine, pediatric/adolescent dosage (3 dose schedule), for intramuscular use**
INCLUDES ENGERIX-B 10mcg/0.5mL
RECOMBIVAX HB 5mcg/0.5mL
0.00 0.00 Global Days XXX
AMA: 2009, Jan, 11-31; 2009, Jul, 7; 2008, Jan, 10-25; 2007, January, 13-27; 2007, February, 10-11

⊘ **90746** **Hepatitis B vaccine, adult dosage, for intramuscular use** F

INCLUDES ENGERIX-B 20mcg/1mL
RECOMBIVAX HB 10mcg/1mL

0.00 0.00 Global Days XXX

AMA: 2009, Jan, 11-31; 2009, Jul, 7; 2008, Jan, 10-25; 2007, January, 13-27; 2007, February, 10-11

⊘ **90747** **Hepatitis B vaccine, dialysis or immunosuppressed patient dosage (4 dose schedule), for intramuscular use** F

INCLUDES ENGERIX-B 20mcg/1mL x 2 - 40mcg/2mL each dose

0.00 0.00 Global Days XXX

AMA: 2009, Jan, 11-31; 2009, Jul, 7; 2008, Jan, 10-25; 2007, January, 13-27; 2007, February, 10-11

⊘ **90748** **Hepatitis B and Hemophilus influenza b vaccine (HepB-Hib), for intramuscular use** E

INCLUDES COMVAX

0.00 0.00 Global Days XXX

AMA: 2009, Jul, 7; 2009, Jan, 11-31; 2008, Jan, 10-25; 2007, January, 13-27; 2007, February, 10-11

⊘ **90749** **Unlisted vaccine/toxoid** N1 N

0.00 0.00 Global Days XXX

AMA: 2009, Jan, 11-31; 2009, Jul, 7; 2008, Jan, 10-25; 2007, February, 10-11

90801-90802 Interactive Psychiatric Evaluation

CMS 100-4,12,110.2 Outpatient Mental Health Limitation
CMS 100-4,12,150 Clinical Social Worker (CSW) Services
CMS 100-4,12,160 Independent Psychologist Services
CMS 100-4,12,160.1 Payment for Independent Psychologists' Services
CMS 100-4,12,170 Clinical Psychologist Services
CMS 100-4,12,170.1 Payment for Clinical Psychologist Services
CMS 100-4,12,210 Outpatient Mental Health Limitation

EXCLUDES *Consultation for initial psychiatric evaluation (without psychiatric treatment) (99241-99255)*
Follow-up visits outpatient initiated by the patient or the consultant (99211-99215, 99334-99337, 99347-99350)
Further requests for advice or an opinion, documented in the medical record, that pertains to a new or existing problem from a physician or other appropriate source (99241-99255)
Transfer of care services for entire patient care management or for a specific problem or condition (99211-99215, 99334-99337, 99347-99350)

90801 **Psychiatric diagnostic interview examination** 03 80 PQ

INCLUDES Communication with family/other sources
Disposition
History
Mental status
Ordering/interpretation of lab studies
Ordering/interpretation of other medical diagnostic studies

3.52 4.48 Global Days XXX

AMA: 2007, Jul, 6-10

90802 **Interactive psychiatric diagnostic interview examination using play equipment, physical devices, language interpreter, or other mechanisms of communication** 03 80 PQ

INCLUDES Non-verbal communication
Physical aids
Services furnished to:
Children
Other individuals lacking expressive/receptive communication skills

3.79 4.88 Global Days XXX

90804-90809 Individual Outpatient Psychotherapy

CMS 100-3,130.1 Inpatient Stays for Alcoholism Treatment
CMS 100-3,130.2 Outpatient Hospital Services for Alcoholism
CMS 100-3,130.5 Treatment of Alcoholism/Drug Abuse in a Freestanding Clinic
CMS 100-3,130.6 Treatment of Drug Abuse (Chemical Dependency)
CMS 100-3,130.7 Withdrawal Treatments for Narcotic Addictions
CMS 100-4,12,110.2 Outpatient Mental Health Limitation
CMS 100-4,12,150 Clinical Social Worker (CSW) Services
CMS 100-4,12,160 Independent Psychologist Services
CMS 100-4,12,160.1 Payment for Independent Psychologists' Services
CMS 100-4,12,170 Clinical Psychologist Services
CMS 100-4,12,170.1 Payment for Clinical Psychologist Services
CMS 100-4,12,210 Outpatient Mental Health Limitation

INCLUDES Face-to-face time
Insight oriented/behavior modifying/supportive psychotherapy:
Cognitive discussion of reality
Development of insight/affective understanding
Supportive interactions
Use of behavior modification
Psychotherapy only
Psychotherapy with medical evaluation and management services includes
Face-to-face time that includes both psychotherapy and the evaluation and management services
Medical diagnostic evaluation of:
Comorbid medical conditions
Drug interactions
Drug management
Interpretation of lab/other diagnostic studies/observations
Physical examination
Physician orders
Services provided in office or other outpatient facility
Treatment for:
Behavior disturbances
Mental illiness

90804 **Individual psychotherapy, insight oriented, behavior modifying and/or supportive, in an office or outpatient facility, approximately 20 to 30 minutes face-to-face with the patient;** 03 80 PQ

1.44 1.81 Global Days XXX

AMA: 2009, Jan, 11-31; 2008, Jan, 10-25; 2007, January, 13-27

90805 **with medical evaluation and management services** 03 80 PQ

1.69 2.11 Global Days XXX

90806 **Individual psychotherapy, insight oriented, behavior modifying and/or supportive, in an office or outpatient facility, approximately 45 to 50 minutes face-to-face with the patient;** 03 80 PQ

2.20 2.41 Global Days XXX

AMA: 2009, Jan, 11-31; 2008, Jan, 10-25; 2007, January, 13-27

90807 **with medical evaluation and management services** 03 80 PQ

2.50 2.92 Global Days XXX

90808 **Individual psychotherapy, insight oriented, behavior modifying and/or supportive, in an office or outpatient facility, approximately 75 to 80 minutes face-to-face with the patient;** 03 80 PO
3.31 3.52 Global Days XXX

90809 **with medical evaluation and management services** 03 80 PO
3.69 4.07 Global Days XXX
AMA: 2009, Jul, 8-9

90810-90815 Individual Outpatient Interactive Psychotherapy

CMS 100-3,130.2 Outpatient Hospital Services for Alcoholism
CMS 100-3,130.5 Treatment of Alcoholism/Drug Abuse in a Freestanding Clinic
CMS 100-3,130.6 Treatment of Drug Abuse (Chemical Dependency)
CMS 100-3,130.7 Withdrawal Treatments for Narcotic Addictions
CMS 100-4,12,110.2 Outpatient Mental Health Limitation
CMS 100-4,12,150 Clinical Social Worker (CSW) Services
CMS 100-4,12,160 Independent Psychologist Services
CMS 100-4,12,170 Clinical Psychologist Services

INCLUDES Face-to-face time
Interactive psychotherapy:
Physical aids/non-verbal communication for individuals lacking expressive/receptive communication skills
Usually provided to children
Psychotherapy only
Psychotherapy with medical evaluation and management services
Face-to-face time that includes both psychotherapy and the evaluation and management service
Medical diagnostic evaluation:
Comorbid medical conditions
Drug interactions
Drug management
Interpretation of lab/other diagnostic studies/observations
Physical examination
Physician orders
Services provided in office or other outpatient facility
Treatment for:
Behavior disturbances
Mental illness

90810 **Individual psychotherapy, interactive, using play equipment, physical devices, language interpreter, or other mechanisms of non-verbal communication, in an office or outpatient facility, approximately 20 to 30 minutes face-to-face with the patient;** 03 80 PO
1.59 1.86 Global Days XXX

90811 **with medical evaluation and management services** 03 80 PO
1.86 2.40 Global Days XXX

90812 **Individual psychotherapy, interactive, using play equipment, physical devices, language interpreter, or other mechanisms of non-verbal communication, in an office or outpatient facility, approximately 45 to 50 minutes face-to-face with the patient;** 03 80 PO
2.34 2.64 Global Days XXX

90813 **with medical evaluation and management services** 03 80 PO
2.64 3.17 Global Days XXX

90814 **Individual psychotherapy, interactive, using play equipment, physical devices, language interpreter, or other mechanisms of non-verbal communication, in an office or outpatient facility, approximately 75 to 80 minutes face-to-face with the patient;** 03 80 PO
3.43 3.78 Global Days XXX

90815 **with medical evaluation and management services** 03 80 PO
3.84 4.36 Global Days XXX
AMA: 2009, Jul, 8-9

90816-90822 Individual Inpatient Psychotherapy

CMS 100-3,130.1 Inpatient Stays for Alcoholism Treatment
CMS 100-3,130.6 Treatment of Drug Abuse (Chemical Dependency)
CMS 100-3,130.7 Withdrawal Treatments for Narcotic Addictions
CMS 100-4,12,110.2 Outpatient Mental Health Limitation
CMS 100-4,12,150 Clinical Social Worker (CSW) Services
CMS 100-4,12,160 Independent Psychologist Services
CMS 100-4,12,160.1 Payment for Independent Psychologists' Services
CMS 100-4,12,170 Clinical Psychologist Services
CMS 100-4,12,170.1 Payment for Clinical Psychologist Services
CMS 100-4,12,210 Outpatient Mental Health Limitation

INCLUDES Face-to-face time
Insight oriented/behavior modifying/supportive psychotherapy:
Cognitive discussion of reality
Development of insight/affective understanding
Supportive interactions
Use of behavior modification
Psychotherapy only
Psychotherapy with medical evaluation and management services
Face-to-face time that includes both psychotherapy and the evaluation and management service, when provided
Medical diagnostic evaluation:
Comorbid medical conditions
Drug interactions
Drug management
Interpretation of lab/other diagnostic studies/observations
Physical examination
Physician orders
Services provided in inpatient hospital/partial hospital/residential care facility
Treatment for:
Behavior disturbances
Mental illness

90816 **Individual psychotherapy, insight oriented, behavior modifying and/or supportive, in an inpatient hospital, partial hospital or residential care setting, approximately 20 to 30 minutes face-to-face with the patient;** P 80
1.58 1.53 Global Days XXX

90817 **with medical evaluation and management services** P 80
1.86 1.84 Global Days XXX

90818 **Individual psychotherapy, insight oriented, behavior modifying and/or supportive, in an inpatient hospital, partial hospital or residential care setting, approximately 45 to 50 minutes face-to-face with the patient;** P 80
2.34 2.26 Global Days XXX

90819 **with medical evaluation and management services** P 80
2.66 2.63 Global Days XXX

90821 **Individual psychotherapy, insight oriented, behavior modifying and/or supportive, in an inpatient hospital, partial hospital or residential care setting, approximately 75 to 80 minutes face-to-face with the patient;** P 80 PO
3.46 3.34 Global Days XXX

90822 **with medical evaluation and management services** P 80 PO
3.83 3.77 Global Days XXX
AMA: 2009, Jul, 8-9

90823-90829 Inpatient Individual Psychotherapy: Interactive

CMS 100-3,130.1 Inpatient Stays for Alcoholism Treatment
CMS 100-3,130.6 Treatment of Drug Abuse (Chemical Dependency)
CMS 100-3,130.7 Withdrawal Treatments for Narcotic Addictions
CMS 100-4,12,110.2 Outpatient Mental Health Limitation
CMS 100-4,12,150 Clinical Social Worker (CSW) Services
CMS 100-4,12,160 Independent Psychologist Services
CMS 100-4,12,160.1 Payment for Independent Psychologists' Services
CMS 100-4,12,170 Clinical Psychologist Services

INCLUDES Face-to-face time
- Interactive psychotherapy:
  - Physical aids/non-verbal communication for individuals lacking expressive/receptive communication skills
  - Usually provided to children
- Psychotherapy only
- Psychotherapy with medical evaluation and management services
  - Face-to-face time that includes both psychotherapy and the evaluation and management service, when provided
  - Medical diagnostic evaluation:
    - Comorbid medical conditions
    - Drug interactions
    - Drug management
    - Interpretation of lab/other diagnostic studies/observations
    - Physical examination
    - Physician orders
- Services provided in inpatient hospital/partial hospital/residential care facility
- Treatment for:
  - Behavior disturbances
  - Mental illness

90823 **Individual psychotherapy, interactive, using play equipment, physical devices, language interpreter, or other mechanisms of non-verbal communication, in an inpatient hospital, partial hospital or residential care setting, approximately 20 to 30 minutes face-to-face with the patient;** P 80 CCI PQ
1.73 1.69 Global Days XXX

90824 **with medical evaluation and management services** P 80 CCI PQ
2.02 1.99 Global Days XXX

90826 **Individual psychotherapy, interactive, using play equipment, physical devices, language interpreter, or other mechanisms of non-verbal communication, in an inpatient hospital, partial hospital or residential care setting, approximately 45 to 50 minutes face-to-face with the patient;** P 80 CCI
2.48 2.40 Global Days XXX

90827 **with medical evaluation and management services** P 80 CCI
2.78 2.74 Global Days XXX

90828 **Individual psychotherapy, interactive, using play equipment, physical devices, language interpreter, or other mechanisms of non-verbal communication, in an inpatient hospital, partial hospital or residential care setting, approximately 75 to 80 minutes face-to-face with the patient;** P 80 CCI
3.57 3.45 Global Days XXX

90829 **with medical evaluation and management services** P 80 CCI PQ
3.96 3.90 Global Days XXX
AMA: 2009, Jul, 8-9

90845-90862 Additional Psychotherapy Services

CMS 100-2,15,160 Clinical Psychologist Services
CMS 100-3,130.1 Inpatient Stays for Alcoholism Treatment
CMS 100-3,130.2 Outpatient Hospital Services for Alcoholism
CMS 100-3,130.5 Treatment of Alcoholism/Drug Abuse in a Freestanding Clinic
CMS 100-3,130.6 Treatment of Drug Abuse (Chemical Dependency)
CMS 100-3,130.7 Withdrawal Treatments for Narcotic Addictions
CMS 100-4,12,110.2 Outpatient Mental Health Limitation
CMS 100-4,12,150 Clinical Social Worker (CSW) Services
CMS 100-4,12,160 Independent Psychologist Services
CMS 100-4,12,160.1 Payment for Independent Psychologists' Services
CMS 100-4,12,170 Clinical Psychologist Services
CMS 100-4,12,170.1 Payment for Clinical Psychologist Services

EXCLUDES *Analysis/programming of neurostimulators for vagus nerve stimulation therapy (95970, 95974-95975)*

90845 **Psychoanalysis** 03 80 CCI PQ
2.58 2.65 Global Days XXX
AMA: 2009, Jan, 11-31; 2008, Jan, 10-25; 2007, January, 13-27

90846 **Family psychotherapy (without the patient present)** 03 80 CCI
2.31 2.41 Global Days XXX

90847 **Family psychotherapy (conjoint psychotherapy) (with patient present)** 03 80 CCI
2.75 3.00 Global Days XXX

90849 **Multiple-family group psychotherapy** 03 80 CCI PQ
0.82 0.95 Global Days XXX

90853 **Group psychotherapy (other than of a multiple-family group)** 03 80 CCI PQ
0.84 0.92 Global Days XXX

90857 **Interactive group psychotherapy** 03 80 CCI PQ
0.88 1.06 Global Days XXX

90862 **Pharmacologic management, including prescription, use, and review of medication with no more than minimal medical psychotherapy** 03 80 CCI PQ
1.30 1.72 Global Days XXX

90865-90870 Other Psychiatric Treatment

CMS 100-4,12,110.2 Outpatient Mental Health Limitation
CMS 100-4,12,150 Clinical Social Worker (CSW) Services
CMS 100-4,12,160 Independent Psychologist Services
CMS 100-4,12,160.1 Payment for Independent Psychologists' Services
CMS 100-4,12,170 Clinical Psychologist Services
CMS 100-4,12,170.1 Payment for Clinical Psychologist Services
CMS 100-4,12,210 Outpatient Mental Health Limitation

EXCLUDES *Analysis/programming of neurostimulators for vagus nerve stimulation therapy (95970, 95974, 95975)*

90865 **Narcosynthesis for psychiatric diagnostic and therapeutic purposes (eg, sodium amobarbital (Amytal) interview)** 03 80 CCI
3.65 4.67 Global Days XXX

▲ 90867 **Therapeutic repetitive transcranial magnetic stimulation (TMS) treatment; initial, including cortical mapping, motor threshold determination, delivery and management** S

INCLUDES Evaluation and management services related directly to:
Cortical mapping
Delivery and management of TMS services
Motor threshold determination

EXCLUDES *Medication management (90862)*
Significant, separately identifiable evaluation and management service
Psychotherapy with and without evaluation and management service

Do not report more than one time for each course of treatment

Do not report with (90868-90869, 95928-95929)

5.10 10.19 Global Days 000

▲ 90868 **subsequent delivery and management, per session** S

INCLUDES Evaluation and management services related directly to:
Cortical mapping
Delivery and management of TMS services
Motor threshold determination

EXCLUDES *Medication management (90862)*
Significant, separately identifiable evaluation and management service
Psychotherapy with and without evaluation and management service

0.70 4.99 Global Days 000

● 90869 **subsequent motor threshold re-determination with delivery and management** S

INCLUDES Evaluation and management services related directly to:
Cortical mapping
Delivery and management of TMS services
Motor threshold determination

EXCLUDES *Medication management (90862)*
Significant, separately identifiable evaluation and management service
Psychotherapy with and without evaluation and management service

Do not report with (90867-90868)

3.40 12.42 Global Days 000

90870 **Electroconvulsive therapy (includes necessary monitoring)** S 80

3.13 4.95 Global Days 000

90875-90880 Psychiatric Therapy with Biofeedback or Hypnosis

CMS 100-3,30.1 Biofeedback Therapy
CMS 100-4,12,110.2 Outpatient Mental Health Limitation
CMS 100-4,12,150 Clinical Social Worker (CSW) Services
CMS 100-4,12,160 Independent Psychologist Services
CMS 100-4,12,160.1 Payment for Independent Psychologists' Services
CMS 100-4,12,170 Clinical Psychologist Services
CMS 100-4,12,170.1 Payment for Clinical Psychologist Services
CMS 100-4,12,210 Outpatient Mental Health Limitation

EXCLUDES *Analysis/programming of neurostimulators for vagus nerve stimulation therapy (95970, 95974, 95975)*

90875 **Individual psychophysiological therapy incorporating biofeedback training by any modality (face-to-face with the patient), with psychotherapy (eg, insight oriented, behavior modifying or supportive psychotherapy); approximately 20-30 minutes** E

1.78 2.12 Global Days XXX

AMA: 2009, Jan, 11-31; 2008, Jan, 10-25; 2007, January, 13-27

90876 **approximately 45-50 minutes** E

2.80 3.13 Global Days XXX

90880 **Hypnotherapy** 03 80

2.65 2.84 Global Days XXX

90882-90899 Psychiatric Services without Patient Face-to-Face Contact

CMS 100-1,3,30.3 Mental Health Diagnostic Services
CMS 100-4,12,110.2 Outpatient Mental Health Limitation
CMS 100-4,12,150 Clinical Social Worker (CSW) Services
CMS 100-4,12,160 Independent Psychologist Services
CMS 100-4,12,160.1 Payment for Independent Psychologists' Services
CMS 100-4,12,170 Clinical Psychologist Services
CMS 100-4,12,170.1 Payment for Clinical Psychologist Services
CMS 100-4,12,210 Outpatient Mental Health Limitation

EXCLUDES *Analysis/programming of neurostimulators for vagus nerve stimulation therapy (95970, 95974, 95975)*

90882 **Environmental intervention for medical management purposes on a psychiatric patient's behalf with agencies, employers, or institutions** E

0.00 0.00 Global Days XXX

90885 **Psychiatric evaluation of hospital records, other psychiatric reports, psychometric and/or projective tests, and other accumulated data for medical diagnostic purposes** N

1.44 1.44 Global Days XXX

AMA: 2009, Jan, 11-31; 2008, Jan, 10-25; 2007, January, 13-27

90887 **Interpretation or explanation of results of psychiatric, other medical examinations and procedures, or other accumulated data to family or other responsible persons, or advising them how to assist patient** N

2.19 2.55 Global Days XXX

AMA: 2009, Jan, 11-31; 2008, Jan, 10-25; 2007, January, 13-27

90889 **Preparation of report of patient's psychiatric status, history, treatment, or progress (other than for legal or consultative purposes) for other physicians, agencies, or insurance carriers** N

0.00 0.00 Global Days XXX

90899 **Unlisted psychiatric service or procedure** 03 80

0.00 0.00 Global Days XXX

90901-90911 Biofeedback Therapy

CMS 100-3,30.1 Biofeedback Therapy
CMS 100-3,30.1.1 Biofeedback for Urinary Incontinence
EXCLUDES *Psychophysiological therapy utilizing biofeedback training (90875, 90876)*

90901 **Biofeedback training by any modality** A 80

0.60 1.15 **Global Days 000**
AMA: 2009, Jan, 11-31; 2008, Jan, 10-25; 2007, January, 13-27

90911 **Biofeedback training, perineal muscles, anorectal or urethral sphincter, including EMG and/or manometry** T 80

EXCLUDES *Rectal sensation/tone/compliance testing (91120)*
Treatment for incontinence, pulsed magnetic neuromodulation (53899)

1.31 2.51 **Global Days 000**
AMA: 2009, Jan, 11-31; 2008, Jan, 10-25; 2007, January, 13-27

90935-90940 Hemodialysis Services: Inpatient ESRD and Outpatient Non-ESRD

CMS 100-2,1,10 Inpatient Hospital Services Covered Under Part A
CMS 100-2,11,20 Coverage of Outpatient Maintenance Dialysis
CMS 100-3,130.8 Hemodialysis for Schizophrenia
CMS 100-3,190.10 Laboratory Tests--CRD Patients
CMS 100-3,230.14 Ultrafiltration Monitor
CMS 100-4,3,100.6 Inpatient Renal Services
EXCLUDES *Blood specimen collection from partial/complete implantable venous access device (36591)*
Declotting of cannula (36831, 36833, 36860, 36861)
Hemodialysis home visit by non-physician health care professional (99512)
Physician attendance for a prolonged period of time (99354-99360)
Thrombolytic agent declotting of implanted vascular access device/catheter (36593)

Code also significant separately identifiable evaluation and management service not related to dialysis procedure or renal failure, with modifier 25

90935 **Hemodialysis procedure with single physician evaluation** S 80 PQ

INCLUDES All evaluation and management services related to the patient's renal disease rendered on a day dialysis is performed:
Inpatient ESRD and non-ESRD procedures
Only one evaluation of the patient related to hemodialysis procedure
Outpatient non-ESRD dialysis

2.14 2.14 **Global Days 000**

90937 **Hemodialysis procedure requiring repeated evaluation(s) with or without substantial revision of dialysis prescription** B 80 PQ

INCLUDES All evaluation and management services related to the patient's renal disease rendered on a day dialysis is performed:
Inpatient ESRD and non-ESRD procedures
Outpatient non-ESRD dialysis
Re-evaluation of the patient during hemodialysis procedure

3.05 3.05 **Global Days 000**

90940 **Hemodialysis access flow study to determine blood flow in grafts and arteriovenous fistulae by an indicator method** N

EXCLUDES *Hemodialysis access duplex scan (93990)*

0.00 0.00 **Global Days XXX**
AMA: 2009, Jan, 11-31; 2008, Jan, 10-25; 2007, January, 13-27

90945-90947 Dialysis Techniques Other Than Hemodialysis

CMS 100-2,1,10 Inpatient Hospital Services Covered Under Part A
CMS 100-3,110.15 Ultrafiltration, Hemoperfusion, and Hemofiltration
CMS 100-3,190.10 Laboratory Tests--CRD Patients
CMS 100-3,240.6 Transvenous (Catheter) Pulmonary Embolectomy
CMS 100-4,3,100.6 Inpatient Renal Services
CMS 100-4,4,20.5 HCPCS Under OPPS
EXCLUDES *Physician attendance for a prolonged period of time (99354-99360)*
Tunneled intraperitoneal catheter insertion
Open (49421)
Percutaneous (49418)

90945 **Dialysis procedure other than hemodialysis (eg, peritoneal dialysis, hemofiltration, or other continuous renal replacement therapies), with single physician evaluation** V 80 PQ

INCLUDES All evaluation and management services related to the patient's renal disease rendered on a day dialysis is performed:
Continuous renal replacement therapies
Hemofiltration
Only one evaluation of the patient related to the procedure
Peritoneal dialysis

EXCLUDES *Hemodialysis*
Peritoneal dialysis home infusion (99601, 99602)

Code also significant separately identifiable evaluation and management service not related to dialysis procedure or renal failure, with modifier 25

2.45 2.45 **Global Days 000**
AMA: 2009, Jan, 11-31; 2008, Jan, 10-25; 2007, January, 13-27

90947 **Dialysis procedure other than hemodialysis (eg, peritoneal dialysis, hemofiltration, or other continuous renal replacement therapies) requiring repeated physician evaluations, with or without substantial revision of dialysis prescription** B 80 PQ

INCLUDES All evaluation and management services related to the patient's renal disease rendered on a day dialysis is performed:
Continuous renal replacement therapies
Hemofiltration
Peritoneal dialysis
Re-evaluation during a procedure

EXCLUDES *Hemodialysis*

Code also significant separately identifiable evaluation and management service not related to dialysis procedure or renal failure, with modifier 25

3.61 3.61 **Global Days 000**
AMA: 2009, Jan, 11-31; 2008, Jan, 10-25; 2007, January, 13-27

90951-90962 End-stage Renal Disease Monthly Outpatient Services

CMS 100-3,190.10 Laboratory Tests--CRD Patients
CMS 100-3,230.14 Ultrafiltration Monitor

INCLUDES Establishing dialyzing cycle
Management of dialysis visits
Outpatient evaluation
Patient management
Telephone calls

EXCLUDES *Dialysis services provided during an inpatient hospitalization (90935-90937, 90945-90947)*
ESRD/non-ESRD dialysis services performed in an inpatient setting (90935-90937, 90945-90947)
Non-ESRD dialysis services performed in an outpatient setting (90935-90937, 90945-90947)
Non-ESRD related evaluation and management services that cannot be performed during the dialysis session

90951 End-stage renal disease (ESRD) related services monthly, for patients younger than 2 years of age to include monitoring for the adequacy of nutrition, assessment of growth and development, and counseling of parents; with 4 or more face-to-face physician visits per month A M 80 PQ
27.35 27.35 Global Days XXX
AMA: 2009, Jan, 3,4&9

90952 with 2-3 face-to-face physician visits per month A M 80 PQ
0.00 0.00 Global Days XXX
AMA: 2009, Jan, 3,4&9

90953 with 1 face-to-face physician visit per month A M 80 PQ
0.00 0.00 Global Days XXX
AMA: 2009, Jan, 3,4&9

90954 End-stage renal disease (ESRD) related services monthly, for patients 2-11 years of age to include monitoring for the adequacy of nutrition, assessment of growth and development, and counseling of parents; with 4 or more face-to-face physician visits per month A M 80 PQ
23.33 23.33 Global Days XXX
AMA: 2009, Jan, 3,4&9

90955 with 2-3 face-to-face physician visits per month A M 80 PQ
13.19 13.19 Global Days XXX
AMA: 2009, Jan, 3,4&9

90956 with 1 face-to-face physician visit per month A M 80 PQ
9.12 9.12 Global Days XXX
AMA: 2009, Jan, 3,4&9

90957 End-stage renal disease (ESRD) related services monthly, for patients 12-19 years of age to include monitoring for the adequacy of nutrition, assessment of growth and development, and counseling of parents; with 4 or more face-to-face physician visits per month A M 80 PQ
18.65 18.65 Global Days XXX
AMA: 2009, Jan, 3,4&9

90958 with 2-3 face-to-face physician visits per month A M 80 PQ
12.64 12.64 Global Days XXX
AMA: 2009, Jan, 3,4&9

90959 with 1 face-to-face physician visit per month A M 80 PQ
8.49 8.49 Global Days XXX
AMA: 2009, Jan, 3,4&9

90960 End-stage renal disease (ESRD) related services monthly, for patients 20 years of age and older; with 4 or more face-to-face physician visits per month A M 80 PQ
8.29 8.29 Global Days XXX
AMA: 2009, Jan, 3,4&9

90961 with 2-3 face-to-face physician visits per month A M 80 PQ
6.90 6.90 Global Days XXX
AMA: 2009, Jan, 3,4&9

90962 with 1 face-to-face physician visit per month A M 80 PQ
5.25 5.25 Global Days XXX
AMA: 2009, Jan, 3,4&9

90963-90966 End-stage Renal Disease Monthly Home Dialysis Services

INCLUDES ESRD services for home dialysis patients
Services provided for a full month services

90963 End-stage renal disease (ESRD) related services for home dialysis per full month, for patients younger than 2 years of age to include monitoring for the adequacy of nutrition, assessment of growth and development, and counseling of parents A M 80 PQ
15.82 15.82 Global Days XXX
AMA: 2009, Jan, 3,4&9

90964 End-stage renal disease (ESRD) related services for home dialysis per full month, for patients 2-11 years of age to include monitoring for the adequacy of nutrition, assessment of growth and development, and counseling of parents A M 80 PQ
13.61 13.61 Global Days XXX
AMA: 2009, Jan, 3,4&9

90965 End-stage renal disease (ESRD) related services for home dialysis per full month, for patients 12-19 years of age to include monitoring for the adequacy of nutrition, assessment of growth and development, and counseling of parents A M 80 PQ
12.98 12.98 Global Days XXX
AMA: 2009, Jan, 3,4&9

90966 End-stage renal disease (ESRD) related services for home dialysis per full month, for patients 20 years of age and older A M 80 PQ
6.87 6.87 Global Days XXX
AMA: 2009, Jan, 3,4&9

90967-90970 End-stage Renal Disease Services: Partial Month

CMS 100-3,190.10 Laboratory Tests--CRD Patients
CMS 100-3,230.14 Ultrafiltration Monitor

INCLUDES ESRD services for less than a full month, such as:
A patient who is transient, dies, recovers, or undergoes kidney transplant
Outpatient ESRD-related services initiated prior to completion of assessment
Patient spending part of the month as a hospital inpatient
Services reported on a daily basis, less the days of hospitalization

90967 End-stage renal disease (ESRD) related services for dialysis less than a full month of service, per day; for patients younger than 2 years of age A M 80
0.53 0.53 Global Days XXX
AMA: 2009, Jan, 3,4&9

90968 for patients 2-11 years of age A M 80
0.44 0.44 Global Days XXX
AMA: 2009, Jan, 3,4&9

90969 for patients 12-19 years of age A M 80 PQ
0.43 0.43 Global Days XXX
AMA: 2009, Jan, 3,4&9

90970 **for patients 20 years of age and older** A M 80 PQ
0.23 0.23 Global Days XXX
AMA: 2009, Jan, 3,4&9

90989-90993 Dialysis Training Services

90989 **Dialysis training, patient, including helper where applicable, any mode, completed course** B
0.00 0.00 Global Days XXX
AMA: 2009, Jan, 11-31; 2008, Jan, 10-25; 2007, January, 13-27

90993 **Dialysis training, patient, including helper where applicable, any mode, course not completed, per training session** B
0.00 0.00 Global Days XXX
AMA: 2009, Jan, 11-31; 2008, Jan, 10-25; 2007, January, 13-27

90997-90999 Hemoperfusion and Unlisted Dialysis Procedures

90997 **Hemoperfusion (eg, with activated charcoal or resin)** B 80
2.59 2.59 Global Days 000

90999 **Unlisted dialysis procedure, inpatient or outpatient** B 80
0.00 0.00 Global Days XXX

91010-91022 Esophageal Manometry

CMS 100-3,100.4 Esophageal Manometry

EXCLUDES *Esophagoscopy (43200-43228)*
Insertion of:
Esophageal tamponade tube (43460)
Miller-Abbott tube (44500)
Radiologic services, gastrointestinal (74210-74363)
Upper gastrointestinal endoscopy (43234-43259)

▲ 91010 **Esophageal motility (manometric study of the esophagus and/or gastroesophageal junction) study with interpretation and report;** X 80
Code also for esophageal motility studies with stimulant or perfusion (91013)
EXCLUDES *Esophageal motility studies with high-resolution esophageal pressure topography (0240T-0241T)*
5.50 5.50 Global Days 000

\+ ▲ 91013 **with stimulation or perfusion (eg, stimulant, acid or alkali perfusion) (List separately in addition to code for primary procedure)** X 80
EXCLUDES *Esophageal motility studies with high-resolution esophageal pressure topography (0240T-0241T)*
Code first (91010)
Do not report more than one time for each session
0.71 0.71 Global Days ZZZ

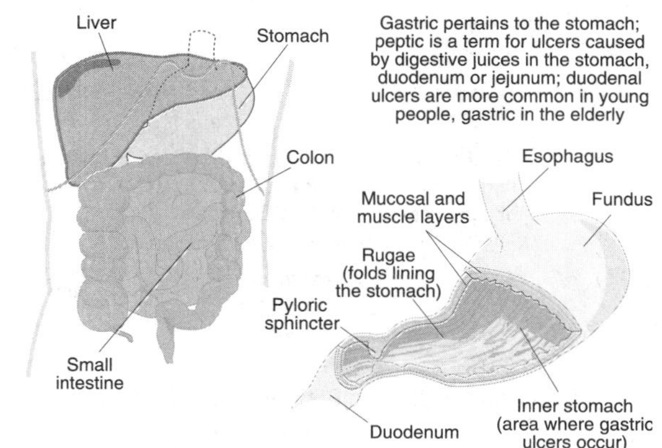

91020 **Gastric motility (manometric) studies** X 80
Do not report with (0242T)
7.21 7.21 Global Days 000

91022 **Duodenal motility (manometric) study** X 80
EXCLUDES *Fluoroscopy (76000)*
Gastric motility study (91020)
Do not report with (0242T)
5.36 5.36 Global Days 000

91030-91040 Esophageal Reflux Tests

EXCLUDES *Duodenal intubation/aspiration (43756-43757)*
Esophagoscopy (43200-43228)
Insertion of:
Esophageal tamponade tube (43460)
Miller-Abbott tube (44500)
Radiologic services, gastrointestinal (74210-74363)
Upper gastrointestinal endoscopy (43234-43259)

91030 **Esophagus, acid perfusion (Bernstein) test for esophagitis** X 80
4.23 4.23 Global Days 000

91034 **Esophagus, gastroesophageal reflux test; with nasal catheter pH electrode(s) placement, recording, analysis and interpretation** X 80
5.87 5.87 Global Days 000

91035 **with mucosal attached telemetry pH electrode placement, recording, analysis and interpretation** X 80
INCLUDES Endoscopy only to place device
EXCLUDES *Diagnostic endoscopy to look for anomalies; code also modifier 59 (43235)*
Do not report more than once even if recording is longer than 24 hours.
14.79 14.79 Global Days 000

91037 **Esophageal function test, gastroesophageal reflux test with nasal catheter intraluminal impedance electrode(s) placement, recording, analysis and interpretation;** X 80
4.94 4.94 Global Days 000

91038 **prolonged (greater than 1 hour, up to 24 hours)** X 80
11.78 11.78 Global Days 000

91040 **Esophageal balloon distension provocation study** X 80
EXCLUDES *Endoscopic balloon dilation (43220, 43249, 43456, 43458)*
9.40 9.40 Global Days 000

91065 Breath Analysis

CMS 100-3,100.5 Diagnostic Breath Analysis

EXCLUDES *H. pylori breath test analysis, radioactive (C-14) or nonradioactive (C-13) (78268 or 83013)*

91065 Breath hydrogen test (eg, for detection of lactase deficiency, fructose intolerance, bacterial overgrowth, or oro-cecal gastrointestinal transit) X 80

EXCLUDES *H. pylori breath test analysis*
Nonreactive isotope (C-13) (83013)
Radioactive isotope (C-14) (78268)

2.62 2.62 Global Days 000

91110-91299 Additional Gastrointestinal Diagnostic/Therapeutic Procedures

EXCLUDES *Abdominal paracentesis (49082-49084)*
Abdominal paracentesis with medication administration (96440, 96446)
Anoscopy (46600-46615)
Cholangiography (47500, 74320)
Colonoscopy (45355-45385)
Duodenal intubation/aspiration (43756-43757)
Esophagoscopy (43200-43228)
Proctosigmoidoscopy (45300-45321)
Radiologic services, gastrointestinal (74210-74363)
Sigmoidoscopy (45330-45339)
Small intestine/stomal endoscopy (44360-44393)
Upper gastrointestinal endoscopy (43234-43259)

91110 Gastrointestinal tract imaging, intraluminal (eg, capsule endoscopy), esophagus through ileum, with physician interpretation and report T 80

Code also modifier 52 if ileum is not visualized

Do not report with visualization of the colon separately

27.62 27.62 Global Days XXX

AMA: 2009, Jan, 11-31; 2009, May, 8-9&11; 2008, Jan, 10-25; 2007, January, 13-27

91111 Gastrointestinal tract imaging, intraluminal (eg, capsule endoscopy), esophagus with physician interpretation and report T 80

EXCLUDES *Use of wireless capsule to measure transit times or pressure in gastrointestinal tract (0242T)*

Do not report with imaging, esophagus through ileum (91110)

22.50 22.50 Global Days XXX

91117 Colon motility (manometric) study, minimum 6 hours continuous recording (including provocation tests, eg, meal, intracolonic balloon distension, pharmacologic agents, if performed), with interpretation and report T 80

EXCLUDES *Use of wireless capsule to measure transit times or pressure in gastrointestinal tract (0242T)*

Do not report more than once regardless of the number of provocations.

Do not report with (91120, 91122)

4.45 4.14 Global Days 000

91120 Rectal sensation, tone, and compliance test (ie, response to graded balloon distention) T 80

EXCLUDES *Anorectal manometry (91122)*
Biofeedback training (90911)

Do not report with (91117)

12.00 12.00 Global Days XXX

91122 Anorectal manometry T 80

Do not report with (91117)

6.66 6.66 Global Days 000

91132 Electrogastrography, diagnostic, transcutaneous; X 80

4.70 4.70 Global Days XXX

91133 with provocative testing X 80

5.46 5.46 Global Days XXX

91299 Unlisted diagnostic gastroenterology procedure X 80

0.00 0.00 Global Days XXX

92002-92014 Ophthalmic Medical Services

CMS 100-4,4,20.5 HCPCS Under OPPS
CMS 100-4,4,160 Clinic and Emergency Visits Under OPPS

INCLUDES Routine ophthalmoscopy

EXCLUDES *Surgical procedures on the eye/ocular adnexa (65091-68899)*

92002 Ophthalmological services: medical examination and evaluation with initiation of diagnostic and treatment program; intermediate, new patient V 80 PQ

INCLUDES Evaluation of new/existing condition complicated by new diagnostic or management problem
Integrated services where medical decision making cannot be separated from examination methods
Problems not related to primary diagnosis
Services provided to patients who have received no professional services from this physician or other same-specialty physicians within the same group practice within the past three years
The following for intermediate services:
- Biomicroscopy
- External ocular/adnexal examination
- General medical observation
- History
- Mydriasis
- Ophthalmoscopy
- Other diagnostic procedures
- Tonometry

1.39 2.31 Global Days XXX

AMA: 2009, Jan, 11-31; 2008, Jan, 1-3; 2008, Jan, 10-25; 2008, Sep, 7-8; 2007, January, 28-31

92004 **comprehensive, new patient, 1 or more visits** V 80 PQ

INCLUDES General evaluation of complete visual system
Integrated services where medical decision making cannot be separated from examination methods
Services provided to patients who have received no professional services from this physician or other same-specialty physicians within the same group practice within the past three years
Single service that need not be performed at one session
The following for comprehensive services:
- Basic sensorimotor examination
- Biomicroscopy
- Consultations
- Dilation (cycloplegia)
- External examinations
- General medical observation
- Gross visual fields
- History
- Initiation of diagnostic/treatment programs
- Laboratory services
- Mydriasis
- Ophthalmoscopic examinations
- Other diagnostic procedures
- Prescription of medication
- Radiological services
- Special diagnostic/treatment services
- Tonometry

2.88 4.25 Global Days XXX

AMA: 2008, Jan, 1-3; 2008, Sep, 7-8; 2007, January, 28-31

92012 **Ophthalmological services: medical examination and evaluation, with initiation or continuation of diagnostic and treatment program; intermediate, established patient** V 80 PQ

INCLUDES Evaluation of new/existing condition complicated by new diagnostic or management problem
Integrated services where medical decision making cannot be separated from examination methods
Problems not related to primary diagnosis
Services provided to patients who have received professional services from this physician or other same-specialty physicians within the same group practice within the past three years
The following for intermediate services:
- External ocular/adnexal examination
- General medical observation
- History
- Other diagnostic procedures:
  - Biomicroscopy
  - Mydriasis
  - Ophthalmoscopy
  - Tonometry

1.51 2.43 Global Days XXX

AMA: 2008, Jan, 1-3; 2008, Sep, 7-8; 2007, January, 28-31

92014 **comprehensive, established patient, 1 or more visits** V 80 PQ

INCLUDES General evaluation of complete visual system
Integrated services where medical decision making cannot be separated from examination methods
Services provided to patients who have received professional services from this physician or other same-specialty physicians within the same group practice within the past three years
Single service that need not be performed at one session
The following for comprehensive services:
- Basic sensorimotor examination
- Biomicroscopy
- Consultations
- Dilation (cycloplegia)
- External examinations
- General medical observation
- Gross visual fields
- History
- Initiation of diagnostic/treatment programs
- Laboratory services
- Mydriasis
- Ophthalmoscopic examinations
- Other diagnostic procedures
- Prescription of medication
- Radiological services
- Special diagnostic/treatment services
- Tonometry

2.30 3.52 Global Days XXX

AMA: 2009, Jan, 11-31; 2008, Jan, 10-25; 2008, Jan, 1-3; 2008, Sep, 7-8; 2007, January, 13-27; 2007, January, 28-31

92015-92140 Ophthalmic Special Services

CMS 100-2,16,90 Routine Services and Appliances
CMS 100-3,80.1 Hydrophilic Contact lens for Corneal Bandage
CMS 100-3,80.2 Photodynamic Therapy
CMS 100-3,80.4 Hydrophilic Contact Lens
CMS 100-3,80.6 Intraocular Photography
CMS 100-3,80.8 Endothelial Cell Photography
CMS 100-3,80.9 Computer Enhanced Perimetry

INCLUDES Routine ophthalmoscopy

Code also evaluation and management services, when appropriate (99201-99350 [99224, 99225, 99226])

Code also general ophthalmological services, when appropriate (92002-92014)

EXCLUDES *Surgical procedures on the eye/ocular adnexa (65091-68899)*

92015 **Determination of refractive state** E

INCLUDES Lens prescription
- Absorptive factor
- Axis
- Impact resistance
- Lens power
- Prism
- Specification of lens type:
  - Monofocal
  - Bifocal

0.57 0.68 Global Days XXX

AMA: 2009, Jan, 11-31; 2008, Jan, 10-25; 2007, January, 13-27

92018 **Ophthalmological examination and evaluation, under general anesthesia, with or without manipulation of globe for passive range of motion or other manipulation to facilitate diagnostic examination; complete** T 80

4.10 4.10 Global Days XXX

92019 limited
1.97 1.97 Global Days XXX

92020 **Gonioscopy (separate procedure)**
EXCLUDES *Gonioscopy under general anesthesia (92018)*
0.61 0.78 Global Days XXX

92025 **Computerized corneal topography, unilateral or bilateral, with interpretation and report**
EXCLUDES *Manual keratoscopy*
Do not report with (65710-65771)
1.07 1.07 Global Days XXX

92060 **Sensorimotor examination with multiple measurements of ocular deviation (eg, restrictive or paretic muscle with diplopia) with interpretation and report (separate procedure)**
1.84 1.84 Global Days XXX

92065 **Orthoptic and/or pleoptic training, with continuing medical direction and evaluation**
1.52 1.52 Global Days XXX
AMA: 2009, Jan, 11-31; 2008, Jan, 10-25; 2007, January, 13-27

~~92070 Fitting of contact lens for treatment of disease, including supply of lens~~
To report, see 92071-92072

● **92071** **Fitting of contact lens for treatment of ocular surface disease**
Code also supply of lens with appropriate supply code or (99070)
Do not report with (92072)
0.98 1.10 Global Days XXX

● **92072** **Fitting of contact lens for management of keratoconus, initial fitting**
EXCLUDES *Subsequent fittings (99211-99215, 92012-92014)*
Code also supply of lens with appropriate supply code or (99070)
Do not report with (92071)
2.81 3.51 Global Days XXX

92081 **Visual field examination, unilateral or bilateral, with interpretation and report; limited examination (eg, tangent screen, Autoplot, arc perimeter, or single stimulus level automated test, such as Octopus 3 or 7 equivalent)**
1.44 1.44 Global Days XXX

92082 **intermediate examination (eg, at least 2 isopters on Goldmann perimeter, or semiquantitative, automated suprathreshold screening program, Humphrey suprathreshold automatic diagnostic test, Octopus program 33)**
2.05 2.05 Global Days XXX

92083 **extended examination (eg, Goldmann visual fields with at least 3 isopters plotted and static determination within the central 30 degrees, or quantitative, automated threshold perimetry, Octopus program G-1, 32 or 42, Humphrey visual field analyzer full threshold programs 30-2, 24-2, or 30/60-2)**
EXCLUDES *Gross visual field testing/confrontation testing*
2.63 2.63 Global Days XXX

92100 **Serial tonometry (separate procedure) with multiple measurements of intraocular pressure over an extended time period with interpretation and report, same day (eg, diurnal curve or medical treatment of acute elevation of intraocular pressure)**
EXCLUDES *Ocular blood flow measurements (0198T)*
Single-episode tonometry (99201-99215, 92002-92004)
1.45 2.78 Global Days XXX
AMA: 2009, Jan, 11-31; 2008, Jan, 10-25; 2007, January, 13-27

~~92120 Tonography with interpretation and report, recording indentation tonometer method or perilimbal suction method~~
To report, see 92002, 92012-92014, 92100, 99211-99215

~~92130 Tonography with water provocation~~
To report, see 92002-92004, 92012-92014, 92100, 99211-99215

92132 **Scanning computerized ophthalmic diagnostic imaging, anterior segment, with interpretation and report, unilateral or bilateral**
EXCLUDES *Scanning computerized ophthalmic diagnostic imaging of optic nerve and retina (92133-92134)*
1.09 1.09 Global Days XXX

92133 **Scanning computerized ophthalmic diagnostic imaging, posterior segment, with interpretation and report, unilateral or bilateral; optic nerve**
Do not report with (92227-92228)
Do not report with scanning computerized ophthalmic imaging of retina at same visit (92134)
1.32 1.32 Global Days XXX

92134 **retina**
Do not report with (92227-92228)
Do not report with scanning computerized ophthalmic imaging of optic nerve at same visit (92133)
1.32 1.32 Global Days XXX

92136 **Ophthalmic biometry by partial coherence interferometry with intraocular lens power calculation**
2.56 2.56 Global Days XXX
AMA: 2009, Jan, 11-31; 2008, Jan, 10-25; 2007, January, 13-27

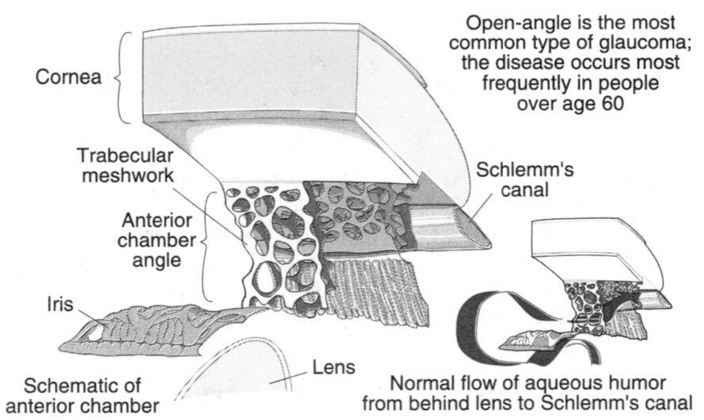

Glaucoma is caused by excessive intraocular pressure and abnormal accumulation of aqueous humor in the anterior chamber of the eye; pressure reduces blood supply to the optic nerve and causes nerve damage

92140 **Provocative tests for glaucoma, with interpretation and report, without tonography**
0.77 1.80 Global Days XXX

92225-92287 Other Ophthalmology Services

EXCLUDES *Prescription, fitting, and/or medical supervision of ocular prosthesis adaptation by physician (99201-99215, 99241-99245, 92002-92014)*

92225 **Ophthalmoscopy, extended, with retinal drawing (eg, for retinal detachment, melanoma), with interpretation and report; initial** S 80

EXCLUDES *Ophthalmoscopy under general anesthesia (92018)*

0.62 0.77 Global Days XXX

AMA: 2009, Jan, 11-31; 2008, Jan, 10-25; 2007, January, 13-27

92226 **subsequent** S 80

0.54 0.69 Global Days XXX

92227 **Remote imaging for detection of retinal disease (eg, retinopathy in a patient with diabetes) with analysis and report under physician supervision, unilateral or bilateral** X 80

Do not report with (99201-99350 [99224, 99225, 99226], 92002-92014, 92133-92134, 92228, 92250)

0.36 0.36 Global Days XXX

92228 **Remote imaging for monitoring and management of active retinal disease (eg, diabetic retinopathy) with physician review, interpretation and report, unilateral or bilateral** X 80

Do not report with (99201-99350 [99224, 99225, 99226], 92002-92014, 92133-92134, 92227, 92250)

1.01 1.01 Global Days XXX

92230 **Fluorescein angioscopy with interpretation and report** S 80

0.95 1.69 Global Days XXX

92235 **Fluorescein angiography (includes multiframe imaging) with interpretation and report** S 80

4.03 4.03 Global Days XXX

AMA: 2008, Jan, 1-3

92240 **Indocyanine-green angiography (includes multiframe imaging) with interpretation and report** S 80

7.30 7.30 Global Days XXX

AMA: 2008, Jan, 1-3

92250 **Fundus photography with interpretation and report** S 80

2.25 2.25 Global Days XXX

AMA: 2008, Jan, 1-3

92260 **Ophthalmodynamometry** S 80

EXCLUDES *Ophthalmoscopy under general anesthesia (92018)*

0.32 0.54 Global Days XXX

92265 **Needle oculoelectromyography, 1 or more extraocular muscles, 1 or both eyes, with interpretation and report** S 80

2.41 2.41 Global Days XXX

92270 **Electro-oculography with interpretation and report** S 80

2.70 2.70 Global Days XXX

AMA: 2009, Jan, 11-31; 2009, May, 8-9&11

92275 **Electroretinography with interpretation and report** S 80

EXCLUDES *Vestibular function tests/electronystagmography (92541-92548)*

76511-76529

4.45 4.45 Global Days XXX

92283 **Color vision examination, extended, eg, anomaloscope or equivalent** S 80

1.54 1.54 Global Days XXX

92284 **Dark adaptation examination with interpretation and report** S 80

1.79 1.79 Global Days XXX

92285 **External ocular photography with interpretation and report for documentation of medical progress (eg, close-up photography, slit lamp photography, goniophotography, stereo-photography)** S 80

0.73 0.73 Global Days XXX

AMA: 2009, Jan, 11-31; 2008, Jan, 10-25; 2008, Jan, 1-3; 2007, January, 13-27

92286 **Special anterior segment photography with interpretation and report; with specular endothelial microscopy and cell count** S 80

3.60 3.60 Global Days XXX

AMA: 2008, Jan, 1-3

92287 **with fluorescein angiography** S 80

1.34 3.58 Global Days XXX

92310-92326 Services Related to Contact Lenses

CMS 100-2,15,30.4 Optometrist's Services
CMS 100-2,15,120 Prosthetic Devices
CMS 100-3,80.1 Hydrophilic Contact lens for Corneal Bandage
CMS 100-3,80.4 Hydrophilic Contact Lens
CMS 100-4,4,20.5 HCPCS Under OPPS

INCLUDES Incidental revision of lens during training period
Patient training/instruction
Specification of optical/physical characteristics:
- Curvature
- Flexibility
- Gas-permeabililty
- Power
- Size

EXCLUDES *Extended wear lenses follow up (92012-92014)*
General ophthalmological services
Therapeutic/surgical use of contact lens (68340, 92071-92072)

92310 **Prescription of optical and physical characteristics of and fitting of contact lens, with medical supervision of adaptation; corneal lens, both eyes, except for aphakia** E

Code also modifier 52 for one eye

1.73 2.77 Global Days XXX

92311 **corneal lens for aphakia, 1 eye** S 80

1.65 2.93 Global Days XXX

92312 **corneal lens for aphakia, both eyes** S 80

1.87 3.34 Global Days XXX

92313 **corneoscleral lens** S 80

1.47 2.93 Global Days XXX

92314 **Prescription of optical and physical characteristics of contact lens, with medical supervision of adaptation and direction of fitting by independent technician; corneal lens, both eyes except for aphakia** E

Code also modifier 52 for one eye

1.01 2.29 Global Days XXX

92315 **corneal lens for aphakia, 1 eye** S 80

0.69 2.22 Global Days XXX

92316 **corneal lens for aphakia, both eyes** S 80

1.13 2.99 Global Days XXX

92317 **corneoscleral lens** S 80

0.62 2.16 Global Days XXX

92325 **Modification of contact lens (separate procedure), with medical supervision of adaptation** S 80

1.10 1.10 Global Days XXX

92326 Replacement of contact lens S 80
1.05 1.05 Global Days XXX

92340-92499 Services Related to Eyeglasses

CMS 100-2,15,30.4 Optometrist's Services
CMS 100-2,15,120 Prosthetic Devices
CMS 100-2,15,120 Prosthetic Devices
CMS 100-4,1,30.3.5 Effect of Assignment on Cataract Glasses from Participating Physician/Supplier
CMS 100-4,4,20.5 HCPCS Under OPPS
CMS 100-4,4,20.5 HCPCS Under OPPS

INCLUDES Anatomical facial characteristics measurement
Final adjustment of spectacles to visual axes/anatomical topography
Written laboratory specifications

EXCLUDES *Supply of materials*

92340 Fitting of spectacles, except for aphakia; monofocal E
0.55 1.04 Global Days XXX

92341 bifocal E
0.69 1.18 Global Days XXX

92342 multifocal, other than bifocal E
0.79 1.28 Global Days XXX

92352 Fitting of spectacle prosthesis for aphakia; monofocal S
0.55 1.19 Global Days XXX

92353 multifocal S
0.73 1.37 Global Days XXX

92354 Fitting of spectacle mounted low vision aid; single element system S
1.03 1.03 Global Days XXX

92355 telescopic or other compound lens system S
0.90 0.90 Global Days XXX

92358 Prosthesis service for aphakia, temporary (disposable or loan, including materials) S
0.38 0.38 Global Days XXX

92370 Repair and refitting spectacles; except for aphakia E
0.48 0.91 Global Days XXX

92371 spectacle prosthesis for aphakia S
0.36 0.36 Global Days XXX

92499 Unlisted ophthalmological service or procedure S 80
0.00 0.00 Global Days XXX

92502-92548 Special Procedures of the Ears/Nose/Throat

CMS 100-2,15,80.3 Audiology Services
CMS 100-2,15,230.3 Practice of Speech-Language Pathology

INCLUDES Diagnostic/treatment services not generally included in a comprehensive otorhinolaryngologic evaluation or office visit (92502-92700 [92558, 92618])

EXCLUDES *Laryngoscopy with stroboscopy (31579)*

Do not report anterior rhinoscopy, tuning fork testing, otoscopy, or removal of cerumen (non-impacted) separately

92502 Otolaryngologic examination under general anesthesia T 80
2.86 2.86 Global Days 000

92504 Binocular microscopy (separate diagnostic procedure) N 80
0.28 0.91 Global Days XXX
AMA: 2009, Jan, 11-31; 2008, Jan, 10-25; 2007, January, 13-27

92506 Evaluation of speech, language, voice, communication, and/or auditory processing A 80

INCLUDES Evaluation of:
- Expressive language abilities
- Receptive language
- Speech production

Examination of:
- Appropriate formulation/utterance of expressive thought
- Articulatory movements of oral musculature
- Capability of understanding the meaning/intent of written/verbal expressions
- Speech sound production

4.86 4.86 Global Days XXX
AMA: 2009, Jan, 11-31; 2009, Mar, 10-11; 2008, Jan, 10-25; 2007, January, 13-27

92507 Treatment of speech, language, voice, communication, and/or auditory processing disorder; individual A 80

EXCLUDES *Auditory rehabilitation:*
Postlingual hearing loss (92633)
Prelingual hearing loss (92630)
Programming of cochlear implant (92601-92604)

2.20 2.20 Global Days XXX

92508 group, 2 or more individuals A 80

EXCLUDES *Auditory rehabilitation:*
Postlingual hearing loss (92633)
Prelingual hearing loss (92630)
Programming of cochlear implant (92601-92604)

0.66 0.66 Global Days XXX

92511 Nasopharyngoscopy with endoscope (separate procedure) T 80
1.46 4.25 Global Days 000

92512 Nasal function studies (eg, rhinomanometry) X 80
0.83 1.82 Global Days XXX

92516 Facial nerve function studies (eg, electroneuronography) X 80
0.68 2.10 Global Days XXX

92520 Laryngeal function studies (ie, aerodynamic testing and acoustic testing) X 80

EXCLUDES *Other laryngeal function testing (92700)*
Swallowing/laryngeal sensory testing with flexible fiberoptic endoscope (92611-92617)

Code also modifier 52 for single test
1.19 2.07 Global Days XXX

92526 Treatment of swallowing dysfunction and/or oral function for feeding A 80
2.44 2.44 Global Days XXX

92531 Spontaneous nystagmus, including gaze N
Do not report with evaluation and management services
0.00 0.00 Global Days XXX

92532 Positional nystagmus test N
Do not report with evaluation and management services
0.00 0.00 Global Days XXX

92533 Caloric vestibular test, each irrigation (binaural, bithermal stimulation constitutes 4 tests) N

INCLUDES Barany caloric test

0.00 0.00 Global Days XXX

92534 **Optokinetic nystagmus test** N
0.00 0.00 Global Days XXX

92540 **Basic vestibular evaluation, includes spontaneous nystagmus test with eccentric gaze fixation nystagmus, with recording, positional nystagmus test, minimum of 4 positions, with recording, optokinetic nystagmus test, bidirectional foveal and peripheral stimulation, with recording, and oscillating tracking test, with recording** X 80

Do not report with 92541-92542, 92544-92545, (92541-92542, 92544-92545)

2.94 2.94 Global Days XXX

92541 **Spontaneous nystagmus test, including gaze and fixation nystagmus, with recording** X 80 PQ

Do not report with (92540 or 92542, 92544, 92545)

1.10 1.10 Global Days XXX

AMA: 2009, May, 8-9&11

92542 **Positional nystagmus test, minimum of 4 positions, with recording** X 80 PQ

Do not report with (92540 or 92541, 92544, 92545)

1.06 1.06 Global Days XXX

AMA: 2009, May, 8-9&11

92543 **Caloric vestibular test, each irrigation (binaural, bithermal stimulation constitutes 4 tests), with recording** X 80 PQ

0.57 0.57 Global Days XXX

AMA: 2009, Jan, 11-31; 2009, May, 8-9&11; 2008, Jan, 10-25; 2007, January, 13-27

92544 **Optokinetic nystagmus test, bidirectional, foveal or peripheral stimulation, with recording** X 80 PQ

Do not report with (92540 or 92541, 92544, 92545)

0.88 0.88 Global Days XXX

AMA: 2009, May, 8-9&11

92545 **Oscillating tracking test, with recording** X 80 PQ

Do not report with (92540 or 92541, 92542, 92544)

0.82 0.82 Global Days XXX

AMA: 2009, May, 8-9&11

92546 **Sinusoidal vertical axis rotational testing** X 80

2.98 2.98 Global Days XXX

AMA: 2009, Jan, 11-31; 2009, May, 8-9&11; 2008, Jan, 10-25; 2007, January, 13-27

\+ **92547** **Use of vertical electrodes (List separately in addition to code for primary procedure)** N TC 80 PQ

Code first (92540-92546)

0.17 0.17 Global Days ZZZ

AMA: 2009, Jan, 11-31; 2009, May, 8-9&11; 2008, Jan, 10-25; 2007, January, 13-27

92548 **Computerized dynamic posturography** X 80 PQ

3.10 3.10 Global Days XXX

92550-92596 Hearing and Speech Tests

CMS 100-2,15,230.3 Practice of Speech-Language Pathology

CMS 100-4,5,10.2 Financial Limitation for Outpatient Rehabilitation Services

CMS 100-4,12,30.3 Audiological Diagnostic Tests, Speech-Language Evaluations and Treatments

INCLUDES Diagnostic/treatment services not generally included in a comprehensive otorhinolaryngologic evaluation or office visit

Testing of both ears.

Use of calibrated electronic equipment, recording of results, and a report with interpretation

EXCLUDES *Evaluation of speech/language/hearing problems using observation/assessment of performance*

Code also modifier 52 for unilateral testing

Do not report tuning fork or whispered voice hearing tests separately

92550 **Tympanometry and reflex threshold measurements** X 80

Do not report with (92567-92568)

0.61 0.61 Global Days XXX

92551 **Screening test, pure tone, air only** E

0.35 0.35 Global Days XXX

92552 **Pure tone audiometry (threshold); air only** X TC 80 PQ

EXCLUDES *Automated test (0208T)*

0.87 0.87 Global Days XXX

92553 **air and bone** X TC 80 PQ

EXCLUDES *Automated test (0209T)*

1.06 1.06 Global Days XXX

92555 **Speech audiometry threshold;** X TC 80 PQ

EXCLUDES *Automated test (0210T)*

0.64 0.64 Global Days XXX

92556 **with speech recognition** X TC 80

EXCLUDES *Automated test (0211T)*

1.00 1.00 Global Days XXX

92557 **Comprehensive audiometry threshold evaluation and speech recognition (92553 and 92556 combined)** X 80 PQ

EXCLUDES *Automated test (0212T)*

Evaluation/selection of hearing aid (92590-92595)

1.01 1.15 Global Days XXX

92558 ***Resequenced Code. See code following 92586.***

92559 **Audiometric testing of groups** E

INCLUDES For group testing, indicate tests performed

0.00 0.00 Global Days XXX

92560 **Bekesy audiometry; screening** E

0.00 0.00 Global Days XXX

92561 **diagnostic** X TC 80 PQ

1.06 1.06 Global Days XXX

92562 **Loudness balance test, alternate binaural or monaural** X TC 80 PQ

INCLUDES ABLB test

1.14 1.14 Global Days XXX

92563 **Tone decay test** X TC 80 PQ

0.87 0.87 Global Days XXX

92564 **Short increment sensitivity index (SISI)** X TC 80 PQ

0.75 0.75 Global Days XXX

92565 **Stenger test, pure tone** X TC 80 PQ

0.46 0.46 Global Days XXX

92567 **Tympanometry (impedance testing)** X 80 PQ

0.34 0.44 Global Days XXX

92568 **Acoustic reflex testing, threshold**
0.47 0.47 Global Days XXX
AMA: 2009, Jan, 11-31; 2009, Jun, 10-11; 2008, Jan, 10-25; 2007, January, 13-27

92570 **Acoustic immittance testing, includes tympanometry (impedance testing), acoustic reflex threshold testing, and acoustic reflex decay testing**
Do not report with (92567-92568)
0.87 0.94 Global Days XXX

92571 **Filtered speech test**
0.72 0.72 Global Days XXX

92572 **Staggered spondaic word test**
0.93 0.93 Global Days XXX

92575 **Sensorineural acuity level test**
1.92 1.92 Global Days XXX

92576 **Synthetic sentence identification test**
1.00 1.00 Global Days XXX

92577 **Stenger test, speech**
0.52 0.52 Global Days XXX

92579 **Visual reinforcement audiometry (VRA)**
1.12 1.26 Global Days XXX

92582 **Conditioning play audiometry**
1.87 1.87 Global Days XXX

92583 **Select picture audiometry**
1.37 1.37 Global Days XXX

92584 **Electrocochleography**
2.09 2.09 Global Days XXX

92585 **Auditory evoked potentials for evoked response audiometry and/or testing of the central nervous system; comprehensive**
3.65 3.65 Global Days XXX

92586 **limited**
2.36 2.36 Global Days XXX

#● **92558** **Evoked otoacoustic emissions, screening (qualitative measurement of distortion product or transient evoked otoacoustic emissions), automated analysis**
0.00 0.00 Global Days XXX

▲ **92587** **Distortion product evoked otoacoustic emissions; limited evaluation (to confirm the presence or absence of hearing disorder, 3-6 frequencies) or transient evoked otoacoustic emissions, with interpretation and report**
0.83 0.83 Global Days XXX

▲ **92588** **comprehensive diagnostic evaluation (quantitative analysis of outer hair cell function by cochlear mapping, minimum of 12 frequencies), with interpretation and report**
EXCLUDES *Evaluation of central auditory function (92620, 92621)*
1.26 1.26 Global Days XXX

92590 **Hearing aid examination and selection; monaural**
0.00 0.00 Global Days XXX

92591 **binaural**
0.00 0.00 Global Days XXX

92592 **Hearing aid check; monaural**
0.00 0.00 Global Days XXX

92593 **binaural**
0.00 0.00 Global Days XXX

92594 **Electroacoustic evaluation for hearing aid; monaural**
0.00 0.00 Global Days XXX

92595 **binaural**
0.00 0.00 Global Days XXX

92596 **Ear protector attenuation measurements**
1.27 1.27 Global Days XXX

92597 Services Related to Voice Prosthesis

INCLUDES Diagnostic/treatment services not generally included in a comprehensive otorhinolaryngologic evaluation or office visit
Use of calibrated electronic equipment

92597 **Evaluation for use and/or fitting of voice prosthetic device to supplement oral speech**
EXCLUDES *Communication device services, augmentative/alternative (92605, 92607, 92608)*
2.44 2.44 Global Days XXX

92601-92609 [92618] Services Related to Hearing and Speech Devices

CMS 100-2,15,80.3 Audiology Services
CMS 100-3,50.1 Speech Generating Devices
CMS 100-3,50.2 Electronic Speech Aids
CMS 100-3,50.3 Cochlear Implantation
CMS 100-4,32,100 Billing Requirements for Cochlear Implantation

INCLUDES Diagnostic/treatment services not generally included in a comprehensive otorhinolaryngologic evaluation or office visit

92601 **Diagnostic analysis of cochlear implant, patient younger than 7 years of age; with programming**
INCLUDES Connection to cochlear implant
Postoperative analysis/fitting of previously placed external devices
Stimulator programming
EXCLUDES *Cochlear implant placement (69930)*
3.67 4.23 Global Days XXX

92602 **subsequent reprogramming**
INCLUDES Internal stimulator re-programming
Subsequent sessions for external transmitter measurements/adjustment
EXCLUDES *Aural rehabilitation services after a cochlear implant (92626-92627, 92630-92633)*
Cochlear implant placement (69930)
Do not report with 92601
2.11 2.69 Global Days XXX
AMA: 2009, Jan, 11-31; 2008, Jan, 10-25; 2007, January, 13-27

92603 **Diagnostic analysis of cochlear implant, age 7 years or older; with programming**
INCLUDES Connection to cochlear implant
Post-operative analysis/fitting of previously placed external devices
Stimulator programming
EXCLUDES *Cochlear implant placement (69930)*
3.61 4.28 Global Days XXX

92604 **subsequent reprogramming**
INCLUDES Internal stimulator re-programming
Subsequent sessions for external transmitter measurements/adjustment
EXCLUDES *Cochlear implant placement (69930)*
Do not report with 92603
2.00 2.56 Global Days XXX
AMA: 2009, Jan, 11-31; 2008, Jan, 10-25; 2007, January, 13-27

▲ **92605** **Evaluation for prescription of non-speech-generating augmentative and alternative communication device, face-to-face with the patient; first hour**
2.55 2.67 Global Days XXX

#● 92618 **each additional 30 minutes (List separately in addition to code for primary procedure)**
Code first (92605)
0.94 0.96 Global Days ZZZ

92606 **Therapeutic service(s) for the use of non-speech-generating device, including programming and modification** [A]
2.04 2.38 Global Days XXX

92607 **Evaluation for prescription for speech-generating augmentative and alternative communication device, face-to-face with the patient; first hour** [A] [80] [CCI]
EXCLUDES *Evaluation for prescription of non-speech generating device (92605)*
4.19 4.19 Global Days XXX

\+ 92608 **each additional 30 minutes (List separately in addition to code for primary procedure)** [A] [80] [CCI]
Code first initial hour (92607)
1.35 1.35 Global Days ZZZ

92609 **Therapeutic services for the use of speech-generating device, including programming and modification** [A] [80] [CCI]
EXCLUDES *Therapeutic services for use of non-speech generating device (92606)*
2.97 2.97 Global Days XXX

92610-92618 Swallowing Evaluations

CMS 100-2,15,230.3 Practice of Speech-Language Pathology
CMS 100-3,170.3 Speech-language Pathology Services for Dysphagia

92610 **Evaluation of oral and pharyngeal swallowing function** [A] [80] [CCI]
EXCLUDES *Evaluation with flexible endoscope (92612-92617)*
Motion fluoroscopic evaluation of swallowing function (92611)
1.97 2.63 Global Days XXX

92611 **Motion fluoroscopic evaluation of swallowing function by cine or video recording** [A] [80] [CCI] [PQ]
EXCLUDES *Diagnostic flexible fiberoptic laryngoscopy (31575)*
Evaluation of oral/pharyngeal swallowing function (92610)
74230
2.89 2.89 Global Days XXX

92612 **Flexible fiberoptic endoscopic evaluation of swallowing by cine or video recording;** [A] [80] [CCI]
EXCLUDES *Flexible fiberoptic endoscopic examination/testing without cine or video recording (92700)*
Do not report with diagnostic flexible fiberoptic laryngoscopy (31575)
1.98 4.99 Global Days XXX
AMA: 2009, Jan, 11-31; 2008, Jan, 10-25; 2007, January, 13-27

92613 **physician interpretation and report only** [B] [80] [CCI]
EXCLUDES *Oral/pharyngeal swallowing function examination (92610)*
Swallowing function motion fluoroscopic examination (92611)
Do not report with diagnostic flexible fiberoptic laryngoscopy (31575)
1.11 1.11 Global Days XXX

92614 **Flexible fiberoptic endoscopic evaluation, laryngeal sensory testing by cine or video recording;** [A] [80] [CCI]
EXCLUDES *Flexible fiberoptic endoscopic examination/testing without cine or video recording (92700)*
Do not report with diagnostic flexible fiberoptic laryngoscopy (31575)
2.00 4.47 Global Days XXX

92615 **physician interpretation and report only** [E] [80] [CCI]
Do not report with diagnostic flexible fiberoptic laryngoscopy (31575)
0.99 0.99 Global Days XXX

92616 **Flexible fiberoptic endoscopic evaluation of swallowing and laryngeal sensory testing by cine or video recording;** [A] [80] [CCI]
EXCLUDES *Flexible fiberoptic endoscopic examination/testing without cine or video recording (92700)*
Do not report with diagnostic flexible fiberoptic laryngoscopy (31575)
2.92 6.00 Global Days XXX

92617 **physician interpretation and report only** [E] [80] [CCI]
Do not report with diagnostic flexible fiberoptic laryngoscopy (31575)
1.22 1.22 Global Days XXX

92618 ***Resequenced Code. See code following 92605.***

92620-92700 Diagnostic Hearing Evaluations and Rehabilitation

INCLUDES Diagnostic/treatment services not generally included in a comprehensive otorhinolaryngologic evaluation or office visit

92620 **Evaluation of central auditory function, with report; initial 60 minutes** [X] [80] [CCI] [PQ]
Do not report with (92506)
2.34 2.59 Global Days XXX

\+ ▲ 92621 **each additional 15 minutes (List separately in addition to code for primary procedure)** [N] [80] [CCI] [PQ]
Code first (92620)
Do not report with (92506)
0.53 0.62 Global Days ZZZ

92625 **Assessment of tinnitus (includes pitch, loudness matching, and masking)** [X] [80] [CCI] [PQ]
Code also modifier 52 for unilateral procedure
Do not report with (92562)
1.78 1.96 Global Days XXX

92626 **Evaluation of auditory rehabilitation status; first hour** [X] [80] [PQ]
INCLUDES Face-to-face time spent with the patient or family
The ability of the patient to use residual hearing in order to identify acoustic characteristics of sounds associated with speech communication
2.25 2.58 Global Days XXX

Medicine

92618 — 92626

+ **92627** **each additional 15 minutes (List separately in addition to code for primary procedure)** N 80 PQ

INCLUDES Face-to-face time spent with the patient or family

The ability of the patient to use residual hearing in order to identify acoustic characteristics of sounds associated with speech communication

Code first initial hour (92626)

0.53 0.64 Global Days ZZZ

92630 **Auditory rehabilitation; prelingual hearing loss** E

0.00 0.00 Global Days XXX

92633 **postlingual hearing loss** E

0.00 0.00 Global Days XXX

92640 **Diagnostic analysis with programming of auditory brainstem implant, per hour** X 80 PQ

EXCLUDES *Nonprogramming services (cardiac monitoring)*

2.91 3.33 Global Days XXX

92700 **Unlisted otorhinolaryngological service or procedure** X 80

INCLUDES Lombard test

0.00 0.00 Global Days XXX

AMA: 2009, Jan, 11-31; 2008, Jan, 10-25; 2007, January, 13-27

92950-92953 Emergency Cardiac Procedures

CMS 100-4,12,30.4 Cardiovascular System

92950 **Cardiopulmonary resuscitation (eg, in cardiac arrest)** S 80

EXCLUDES *Critical care (99291, 99292)*

5.39 8.73 Global Days 000

AMA: 2009, Jan, 11-31; 2008, Jan, 10-25; 2007, January, 13-27

⊙ **92953** **Temporary transcutaneous pacing** 03 80

EXCLUDES *Physician direction of ambulance/rescue personnel outside of the hospital (99288)*

0.32 0.32 Global Days 000

AMA: 2007, Jul, 1-4; 2007, February, 10-11

92960-92961 Cardioversion

CMS 100-4,12,30.4 Cardiovascular System

⊙ **92960** **Cardioversion, elective, electrical conversion of arrhythmia; external** S 80

3.63 6.41 Global Days 000

AMA: 2009, Jan, 11-31; 2008, Jan, 10-25; 2007, January, 13-27

⊙ **92961** **internal (separate procedure)** S

Do not report with (93282-93284, 93287, 93289, 93295-93296, 93618-93624, 93631, 93640-93642, 93650-93652, 93662)

7.23 7.23 Global Days 000

92970-92971 Circulatory Assist: External/Internal

EXCLUDES *Atrial septostomy, balloon (92992)*

Catheter placement for use in circulatory assist devices (intra-aortic balloon pump) (33970)

92970 **Cardioassist-method of circulatory assist; internal** C5 C 80

5.19 5.19 Global Days 000

92971 **external** C5 C 80

2.79 2.79 Global Days 000

92973-92979 Intravascular Coronary Procedures: Insert Brachytherapy Device; Treatment of Thrombosis; Ultrasound

CMS 100-4,12,30.4 Cardiovascular System

+ ⊙ **92973** **Percutaneous transluminal coronary thrombectomy (List separately in addition to code for primary procedure)** T 80

Code first primary procedure (92980, 92982)

5.39 5.39 Global Days ZZZ

AMA: 2009, Jan, 11-31; 2008, Jan, 10-25; 2007, January, 13-27

+ ⊙ **92974** **Transcatheter placement of radiation delivery device for subsequent coronary intravascular brachytherapy (List separately in addition to code for primary procedure)** T 80

EXCLUDES *Application of intravascular radioelement (77785-77787)*

Code first primary procedure (92980, 92982, 92995, 93454-93461)

4.93 4.93 Global Days ZZZ

⊙ **92975** **Thrombolysis, coronary; by intracoronary infusion, including selective coronary angiography** C5 C 80

EXCLUDES *Thrombolysis, cerebral (37195)*

Thrombolysis other than coronary (37201, 75896)

11.92 11.92 Global Days 000

92977 **by intravenous infusion** T 80

EXCLUDES *Thrombolysis, cerebral (37195)*

Thrombolysis other than coronary (37201, 75896)

3.59 3.59 Global Days XXX

+ ⊙ **92978** **Intravascular ultrasound (coronary vessel or graft) during diagnostic evaluation and/or therapeutic intervention including imaging supervision, interpretation and report; initial vessel (List separately in addition to code for primary procedure)** N 80

Code also (C1753)

Code first primary procedure (92975, 92980, 92982, 92995, 93454-93461, 93530-93533)

0.00 0.00 Global Days ZZZ

AMA: 2009, Jan, 11-31; 2008, Jan, 10-25

+ ⊙ **92979** **each additional vessel (List separately in addition to code for primary procedure)** N 80

INCLUDES Transducer manipulations/repositioning in the vessel examined, before and after therapeutic intervention

EXCLUDES *Intravascular spectroscopy (0205T)*

Code first initial vessel (92978)

0.00 0.00 Global Days ZZZ

92980-92984 Percutaneous Transluminal Angioplasty and Stent Placement

CMS 100-3,20.7 Percutaneous Transluminal Angioplasty (PTA)
CMS 100-4,12,30.4 Cardiovascular System

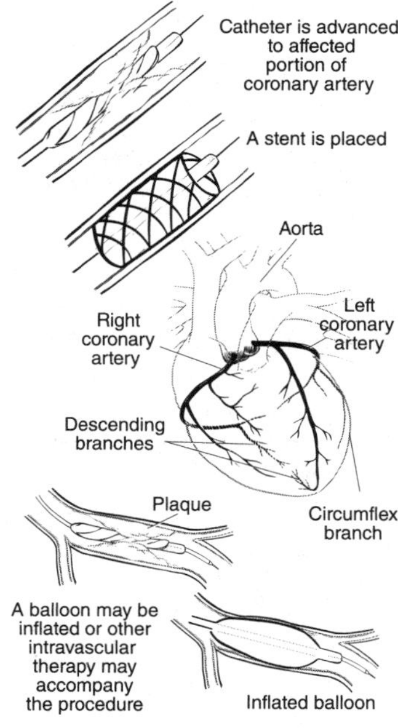

⊙ **92980** **Transcatheter placement of an intracoronary stent(s), percutaneous, with or without other therapeutic intervention, any method; single vessel** T 80 CCI PQ

EXCLUDES *Application of intravascular radioelement (77785-77787)*
Coronary brachytherapy (92974)
Intravascular ultrasound (92978, 92979)
Percutaneous transluminal coronary thrombectomy (92973)

Code also (C1874, C1875, C1876, C1877)

Do not report angioplasty or atherectomy performed in the same artery as stent placement (92982, 92984, 92995-92996)

24.61 24.61 Global Days 000

AMA: 2009, Jan, 11-31; 2008, Jan, 10-25; 2007, January, 13-27

+ ⊙ **92981** **each additional vessel (List separately in addition to code for primary procedure)** T 80 CCI

EXCLUDES *Additional vessels treated by only angioplasty or atherectomy during the same session (92984, 92996)*
Application of intravascular radioelement (77785-77787)
Transcatheter placement of radiation delivery device for coronary intravascular brachytherapy (92974)

Code also (C1874, C1875, C1876, C1877)
Code first single vessel (92980)

Do not report angioplasty or atherectomy performed in the same artery as stent placement (92982, 92984, 92995-92996)

6.84 6.84 Global Days ZZZ

AMA: 2009, Jan, 11-31; 2008, Jan, 10-25; 2007, January, 13-27

⊙ **92982** **Percutaneous transluminal coronary balloon angioplasty; single vessel** T 80 CCI PQ

Code also (C1725, C1874, C1876, C1885)

18.24 18.24 Global Days 000

AMA: 2009, Jan, 11-31; 2008, Jan, 10-25; 2007, January, 13-27

+ ⊙ **92984** **each additional vessel (List separately in addition to code for primary procedure)** T 80 CCI

EXCLUDES *Application of intravascular radioelement (77785-77787)*
Placement of stent after angioplasty/atherectomy completion (92980, 92981)
Transcatheter placement of radiation delivery device for coronary intravascular brachytherapy (92974)

Code also (C1725, C1874, C1876, C1885)
Code first single vessel (92980, 92982, 92995)

4.88 4.88 Global Days ZZZ

AMA: 2009, Jan, 11-31; 2008, Jan, 10-25; 2007, January, 13-27

92986-92993 Percutaneous Procedures of Heart Valves and Septum

CMS 100-4,12,30.4 Cardiovascular System

⊙ **92986** **Percutaneous balloon valvuloplasty; aortic valve** T 80 CCI

40.74 40.74 Global Days 090

⊙ **92987** **mitral valve** T 80 CCI

41.98 41.98 Global Days 090

92990 **pulmonary valve** T 80 CCI

32.83 32.83 Global Days 090

92992 **Atrial septectomy or septostomy; transvenous method, balloon (eg, Rashkind type) (includes cardiac catheterization)** C5 C 80 CCI

0.00 0.00 Global Days 090

AMA: 2009, Jan, 11-31; 2008, Jan, 10-25

92993 **blade method (Park septostomy) (includes cardiac catheterization)** C5 C 80 CCI

0.00 0.00 Global Days 090

92995-92996 Percutaneous Coronary Atherectomy

CMS 100-4,12,30.4 Cardiovascular System

Code also (C1714, C1724, C1885)

⊙ **92995** **Percutaneous transluminal coronary atherectomy, by mechanical or other method, with or without balloon angioplasty; single vessel** T 80 CCI PQ

Code also (C1714, C1724, C1885)

20.08 20.08 Global Days 000

+ ⊙ **92996** **each additional vessel (List separately in addition to code for primary procedure)** T 80 CCI

Code also (C1714, C1724, C1885)

EXCLUDES *Additional vessels treated by only angioplasty during the same session (92984)*
Placement of stent after angioplasty/atherectomy completion (92980, 92981)

Code first single vessel (92980, 92982, 92995)

5.36 5.36 Global Days ZZZ

92997-92998 Percutaneous Angioplasty: Pulmonary Artery

CMS 100-4,12,30.4 Cardiovascular System

92997 **Percutaneous transluminal pulmonary artery balloon angioplasty; single vessel** T 80 CCI

Code also (C1725, C1874, C1876, C1885, C2625)

19.60 19.60 Global Days 000

\+ **92998** **each additional vessel (List separately in addition to code for primary procedure)** [T] [80]
Code also (C1725, C1874, C1876, C1885, C2625)
Code first single vessel (92997)
Facility RVU 9.78 Non-Facility RVU 9.78 Global Days ZZZ

93000-93010 Electrocardiographic Services

CMS 100-3,20.15 Electrocardiographic Services
CMS 100-4,12,30.4 Cardiovascular System

INCLUDES Specific order for the service, a separate written and signed report, and documentation of medical necessity

EXCLUDES *Acoustic cardiography (0223T-0225T)*
Echocardiography (93303-93350)
EKG with 64 or more leads, graphic presentation, and analysis (0178T-0180T)
Use of these codes for the review of telemetry monitoring strips

93000 **Electrocardiogram, routine ECG with at least 12 leads; with interpretation and report** [M] [80]
EXCLUDES *ECG monitoring (99354-99360)*
Facility RVU 0.56 Non-Facility RVU 0.56 Global Days XXX
AMA: 2008, Jul, 3&14

93005 **tracing only, without interpretation and report** [S] [TC] [80]
EXCLUDES *ECG monitoring (99354-99360)*
Facility RVU 0.31 Non-Facility RVU 0.31 Global Days XXX

93010 **interpretation and report only** [B] [26] [80]
EXCLUDES *ECG monitoring (99354-99360)*
Facility RVU 0.25 Non-Facility RVU 0.25 Global Days XXX
AMA: 2007, April, 1-2

93015-93018 Stress Test

CMS 100-3,20.10 Cardiac Rehabilitation Programs
CMS 100-3,20.15 Electrocardiographic Services
CMS 100-4,12,30.4 Cardiovascular System

93015 **Cardiovascular stress test using maximal or submaximal treadmill or bicycle exercise, continuous electrocardiographic monitoring, and/or pharmacological stress; with physician supervision, with interpretation and report** [B] [80]
Facility RVU 2.60 Non-Facility RVU 2.60 Global Days XXX
AMA: 2009, Jan, 11-31; 2008, Jan, 10-25; 2008, Jul, 3&14; 2007, January, 13-27

93016 **physician supervision only, without interpretation and report** [B] [26] [80]
Facility RVU 0.65 Non-Facility RVU 0.65 Global Days XXX
AMA: 2009, Jan, 11-31; 2008, Jan, 10-25; 2008, Jul, 3&14; 2007, January, 13-27

93017 **tracing only, without interpretation and report** [X] [TC] [80]
Facility RVU 1.51 Non-Facility RVU 1.51 Global Days XXX
AMA: 2009, Jan, 11-31; 2008, Jan, 10-25; 2008, Jul, 3&14; 2007, January, 13-27

93018 **interpretation and report only** [B] [26] [80]
Facility RVU 0.44 Non-Facility RVU 0.44 Global Days XXX
AMA: 2009, Jan, 11-31; 2008, Jan, 10-25; 2008, Jul, 3&14; 2007, January, 13-27

93024 Provocation Test for Coronary Vasospasm

CMS 100-3,20.15 Electrocardiographic Services
CMS 100-4,12,30.4 Cardiovascular System

93024 **Ergonovine provocation test** [X] [80]
Facility RVU 3.36 Non-Facility RVU 3.36 Global Days XXX

93025 Microvolt T-Wave Alternans

CMS 100-3,20.30 Microvolt T-Wave Alternans (MTWA)
CMS 100-4,12,30.4 Cardiovascular System

INCLUDES Specific order for the service, a separate written and signed report, and documentation of medical necessity

EXCLUDES *Echocardiography (93303-93350)*
EKG with 64 or more leads, graphic presentation, and analysis (0178T-0180T)
Use of these codes for the review of telemetry monitoring strips

93025 **Microvolt T-wave alternans for assessment of ventricular arrhythmias** [X] [80]
Facility RVU 5.31 Non-Facility RVU 5.31 Global Days XXX

93040-93042 Rhythm Strips

CMS 100-3,20.15 Electrocardiographic Services
CMS 100-4,12,30.4 Cardiovascular System

INCLUDES Specific order for the service, a separate written and signed report, and documentation of medical necessity

EXCLUDES *Echocardiography (93303-93350)*
EKG with 64 or more leads, graphic presentation, and analysis (0178T-0180T)
Use of these codes for the review of telemetry monitoring strips

Do not report with (93279-93289, 93291-93296, 93298-93299, 0223T-0225T)

93040 **Rhythm ECG, 1-3 leads; with interpretation and report** [B] [80]
Facility RVU 0.38 Non-Facility RVU 0.38 Global Days XXX
AMA: 2009, Feb, 3-12

93041 **tracing only without interpretation and report** [X] [TC] [80]
Facility RVU 0.17 Non-Facility RVU 0.17 Global Days XXX
AMA: 2009, Feb, 3-12

93042 **interpretation and report only** [B] [26] [80]
Facility RVU 0.21 Non-Facility RVU 0.21 Global Days XXX
AMA: 2009, Feb, 3-12

93224-93227 Holter Monitor

CMS 100-3,20.15 Electrocardiographic Services
CMS 100-4,12,30.4 Cardiovascular System

INCLUDES Cardiac monitoring using in-person as well as remote technology for the assessment of electrocardiographic data
Holter monitors for up to 48 hours of recording on a continuous basis (93224-93227)

EXCLUDES *Echocardiography (93303-93352)*
EKG with 64 or more leads, graphic presentation, and analysis (0178T-0180T)
Implantable patient activated cardiac event recorders (33282, 93285, 93291, 93298)

93224 **External electrocardiographic recording up to 48 hours by continuous rhythm recording and storage; includes recording, scanning analysis with report, physician review and interpretation** [M] [80]
Code also modifier 52 when less than 12 hours of continuous recording is provided
Facility RVU 2.91 Non-Facility RVU 2.91 Global Days XXX
AMA: 2009, Mar, 5-7; 2009, Feb, 3-12; 2008, Mar, 4-5; 2007, April, 3-6

93225 **recording (includes connection, recording, and disconnection)** [S] [TC] [80]
Code also modifier 52 when less than 12 hours of continuous recording is provided
Facility RVU 0.86 Non-Facility RVU 0.86 Global Days XXX
AMA: 2009, Mar, 5-7; 2009, Feb, 3-12; 2008, Mar, 4-5; 2007, April, 3-6

93226 **scanning analysis with report** S TC 80 CCI

Code also modifier 52 when less than 12 hours of continuous recording is provided

1.27 1.27 Global Days XXX

AMA: 2009, Mar, 5-7; 2009, Feb, 3-12; 2008, Mar, 4-5; 2007, April, 3-6

93227 **physician review and interpretation** M 26 80 CCI

Code also modifier 52 when less than 12 hours of continuous recording is provided

0.78 0.78 Global Days XXX

AMA: 2009, Mar, 5-7; 2009, Feb, 3-12; 2008, Mar, 4-5; 2007, April, 3-6

93228-93229 Remote Cardiovascular Telemetry

INCLUDES Cardiac monitoring using in-person as well as remote technology for the assessment of electrocardiographic data

Mobile telemetry monitors with the capacity to:

Detect arrhythmias

Real-time data analysis for the evaluation quality of the signal

Records ECG rhythm on a continuous basis using external electrodes on the patient

Transmit a tracing at any time

Transmit data to an attended surveillance center where a technician is available to respond to device or rhythm alerts and contact the physician if needed

93228 **External mobile cardiovascular telemetry with electrocardiographic recording, concurrent computerized real time data analysis and greater than 24 hours of accessible ECG data storage (retrievable with query) with ECG triggered and patient selected events transmitted to a remote attended surveillance center for up to 30 days; physician review and interpretation with report** M 26 80

INCLUDES Reporting only once in a 30-day period

Do not report with (93224, 93227)

0.75 0.75 Global Days XXX

AMA: 2009, Mar, 5-7; 2009, Feb, 3-12

93229 **technical support for connection and patient instructions for use, attended surveillance, analysis and physician prescribed transmission of daily and emergent data reports** S TC 80

INCLUDES Reporting only once in a 30-day period

EXCLUDES *Cardiovascular monitors that do not perform automatic ECG triggered transmissions to an attended surveillance center (93224-93227, 93268-93272)*

Do not report with (93224, 93226)

20.38 20.38 Global Days XXX

AMA: 2009, Mar, 5-7; 2009, Feb, 3-12

93268-93272 Event Monitors

INCLUDES ECG rhythm derived elements, which differ from physiologic data and include rhythm of the heart, rate, ST analysis, heart rate variability, T-wave alternans, among others

Event monitors that:

Record parts of ECGs in response to patient activation or an automatic detection algorithm (or both)

Require attended surveillance

Transmit data upon request (although not immediately when activated)

Do not report with (93279-93289, 93291-93296, 93298-93299)

93268 **External patient and, when performed, auto activated electrocardiographic rhythm derived event recording with symptom-related memory loop with remote download capability up to 30 days, 24-hour attended monitoring; includes transmission, physician review and interpretation** M 80 CCI

EXCLUDES *Implanted patient activated cardiac event recording (33282, 93285, 93291, 93298)*

Do not report with (93279-93289, 93291-93296, 93298-93299)

7.00 7.00 Global Days XXX

AMA: 2009, Mar, 5-7; 2009, Feb, 3-12; 2008, Mar, 4-5; 2007, April, 3-6

93270 **recording (includes connection, recording, and disconnection)** S TC 80 CCI

Do not report with (93279-93289, 93291-93296, 93298-93299)

0.36 0.36 Global Days XXX

AMA: 2009, Mar, 5-7; 2009, Feb, 3-12; 2008, Mar, 4-5; 2007, April, 3-6

▲ 93271 **transmission and analysis** S TC 80 CCI

Do not report with (93279-93289, 93291-93296, 93298-93299)

5.91 5.91 Global Days XXX

AMA: 2009, Mar, 5-7; 2009, Feb, 3-12; 2008, Mar, 4-5; 2007, April, 3-6

93272 **physician review and interpretation** M 26 80 CCI

Do not report with (93279-93289, 93291-93296, 93298-93299)

0.73 0.73 Global Days XXX

AMA: 2009, Jan, 11-31; 2009, Mar, 5-7; 2009, Feb, 3-12; 2008, Jan, 10-25; 2008, Mar, 4-5; 2007, January, 13-27; 2007, April, 3-6

93278 Signal-averaged Electrocardiography

CMS 100-3,20.15 Electrocardiographic Services

CMS 100-4,12,30.4 Cardiovascular System

EXCLUDES *Echocardiography (93303-93352)*

EKG with 64 or more leads, graphic presentation, and analysis (0178T-0180T)

93278 **Signal-averaged electrocardiography (SAECG), with or without ECG** X 80 CCI

0.97 0.97 Global Days XXX

AMA: 2009, Mar, 5-7; 2008, Mar, 4-5

93279-93299 Monitoring of Cardiovascular Devices

INCLUDES Cardioverter-defibrillator (ICD) interrogation:
- Battery
- Capture and sensing functions
- Leads
- Presence or absence of therapy for ventricular tachyarrhythmias
- Programmed parameters
- Underlying heart rhythm

Implantable cardiovascular monitor (ICM) interrogation:
- Analysis of at least one recorded physiologic cardiovascular data element from either internal or external sensors
- Programmed parameters

Implantable loop recorder (ILR) interrogation:
- Heart rate and rhythm during recorded episodes from both patient-initiated and device detected events
- Programmed parameters

Interrogation evaluation of device

Pacemaker interrogation:
- Battery
- Capture and sensing functions
- Heart rhythm
- Leads
- Programmed parameters

Time period established by the initiation of remote monitoring or the 91st day of ICD or pacemaker monitoring or the 31st day of ILR monitoring and extends for the succeeding 30- or 90-day period

EXCLUDES *Wearable device monitoring (93224-93272)*

Do not report in-person and remote interrogation of the same device during the same period

Do not report programming and in-person interrogation on the same day by the same physician

93279 **Programming device evaluation (in person) with iterative adjustment of the implantable device to test the function of the device and select optimal permanent programmed values with physician analysis, review and report; single lead pacemaker system** S 80

Do not report with (93040-93042, 93268-93272, 93286, 93288)

Facility RVU 1.49 Non-Facility RVU 1.49 Global Days XXX

AMA: 2009, Feb, 3-12

93280 **dual lead pacemaker system** S 80

Do not report with (93040-93042, 93268-93272, 93286, 93288)

Facility RVU 1.74 Non-Facility RVU 1.74 Global Days XXX

AMA: 2009, Feb, 3-12

93281 **multiple lead pacemaker system** S 80

Do not report with (93040-93042, 93268-93272, 93286, 93288)

Facility RVU 2.01 Non-Facility RVU 2.01 Global Days XXX

AMA: 2009, Feb, 3-12

93282 **single lead implantable cardioverter-defibrillator system** S 80

Do not report with (93040-93042, 93268-93272, 93287, 93289, 93745)

Facility RVU 1.86 Non-Facility RVU 1.86 Global Days XXX

AMA: 2009, Feb, 3-12

93283 **dual lead implantable cardioverter-defibrillator system** S 80

Do not report with (93040-93042, 93268-93272, 93287, 93289)

Facility RVU 2.39 Non-Facility RVU 2.39 Global Days XXX

AMA: 2009, Feb, 3-12

93284 **multiple lead implantable cardioverter-defibrillator system** S 80

Do not report with (93040-93042, 93268-93272, 93287, 93289)

Facility RVU 2.65 Non-Facility RVU 2.65 Global Days XXX

AMA: 2009, Feb, 3-12

93285 **implantable loop recorder system** S 80

Do not report with (33282, 93040-93042, 93268-93272, 93279-93284, 93291)

Facility RVU 1.24 Non-Facility RVU 1.24 Global Days XXX

AMA: 2009, Mar, 5-7; 2009, Feb, 3-12

93286 **Peri-procedural device evaluation (in person) and programming of device system parameters before or after a surgery, procedure, or test with physician analysis, review and report; single, dual, or multiple lead pacemaker system** N 80

INCLUDES One evaluation and programming (if performed once before and once after, report as two units)

Do not report with (93040-93042, 93268-93272, 93279-93281, 93288)

Facility RVU 0.76 Non-Facility RVU 0.76 Global Days XXX

AMA: 2009, Feb, 3-12

93287 **single, dual, or multiple lead implantable cardioverter-defibrillator system** N 80

INCLUDES One evaluation and programming (if performed once before and once after, report as two units)

Do not report with (93040-93042, 93268-93272, 93282-93284, 93289)

Facility RVU 1.01 Non-Facility RVU 1.01 Global Days XXX

AMA: 2009, Feb, 3-12

93288 **Interrogation device evaluation (in person) with physician analysis, review and report, includes connection, recording and disconnection per patient encounter; single, dual, or multiple lead pacemaker system** S 80

Do not report with (93040-93042, 93268-93272, 93279-93281, 93286, 93294, 93296)

Facility RVU 1.12 Non-Facility RVU 1.12 Global Days XXX

AMA: 2009, Feb, 3-12

93289 **single, dual, or multiple lead implantable cardioverter-defibrillator system, including analysis of heart rhythm derived data elements** S 80

EXCLUDES *Monitoring physiologic cardiovascular data elements derived from an ICD (93290)*

Do not report with (93040-93042, 93268-93272, 93282-93284, 93287, 93295-93296)

Facility RVU 1.93 Non-Facility RVU 1.93 Global Days XXX

AMA: 2009, Feb, 3-12

93290 **implantable cardiovascular monitor system, including analysis of 1 or more recorded physiologic cardiovascular data elements from all internal and external sensors** X 80

EXCLUDES *Heart rhythm derived data (93289)*

Do not report with (93297, 93299)

Facility RVU 0.88 Non-Facility RVU 0.88 Global Days XXX

AMA: 2009, Feb, 3-12

93291 **implantable loop recorder system, including heart rhythm derived data analysis** S 80

Do not report with (33282, 93040-93042, 93268-93272, 93288-93290, 93298-93299)

Facility RVU 1.07 Non-Facility RVU 1.07 Global Days XXX

AMA: 2009, Mar, 5-7; 2009, Feb, 3-12

93292 **wearable defibrillator system** S 80

Do not report with (93040-93042, 93268-93272, 93745)

0.96 0.96 Global Days XXX

AMA: 2009, Feb, 3-12

93293 **Transtelephonic rhythm strip pacemaker evaluation(s) single, dual, or multiple lead pacemaker system, includes recording with and without magnet application with physician analysis, review and report(s), up to 90 days** S 80

EXCLUDES *In-person evaluation (93040-93042)*

Do not report more than once in a 90 day period

Do not report when monitoring period is less than 30 days

Do not report with (93040-93042, 93268-93272, 93288)

1.60 1.60 Global Days XXX

AMA: 2009, Feb, 3-12

93294 **Interrogation device evaluation(s) (remote), up to 90 days; single, dual, or multiple lead pacemaker system with interim physician analysis, review(s) and report(s)** M 26 80

Do not report more than once in a 90 day period

Do not report when monitoring period is less than 30 days

Do not report with (93040-93042, 93268-93272, 93288, 93293)

0.97 0.97 Global Days XXX

AMA: 2009, Feb, 3-12

93295 **single, dual, or multiple lead implantable cardioverter-defibrillator system with interim physician analysis, review(s) and report(s)** M 26 80

EXCLUDES *Remote monitoring of physiological cardiovascular ICD data (93297)*

Do not report more than once in a 90 day period

Do not report when monitoring period is less than 30 days

Do not report with (93040-93042, 93268-93272, 93289)

1.92 1.92 Global Days XXX

AMA: 2009, Feb, 3-12

93296 **single, dual, or multiple lead pacemaker system or implantable cardioverter-defibrillator system, remote data acquisition(s), receipt of transmissions and technician review, technical support and distribution of results** S TC 80

Do not report more than once in a 90 day period

Do not report with (93040-93042, 93268-93272, 93288-93289, 93299)

0.87 0.87 Global Days XXX

AMA: 2009, Feb, 3-12

93297 **Interrogation device evaluation(s), (remote) up to 30 days; implantable cardiovascular monitor system, including analysis of 1 or more recorded physiologic cardiovascular data elements from all internal and external sensors, physician analysis, review(s) and report(s)** M 26 80

EXCLUDES *Heart rhythm derived data (93295)*

Do not report more than once in a 30 day period

Do not report when monitoring period is less than 10 days

Do not report with (93290, 93298)

0.74 0.74 Global Days XXX

AMA: 2009, Feb, 3-12

93298 **implantable loop recorder system, including analysis of recorded heart rhythm data, physician analysis, review(s) and report(s)** M 26 80

Do not report more than once in a 30 day period

Do not report when monitoring period is less than 10 days

Do not report with (33282, 93040-93042, 93268-93272, 93291, 93297)

0.78 0.78 Global Days XXX

AMA: 2009, Mar, 5-7; 2009, Feb, 3-12

93299 **implantable cardiovascular monitor system or implantable loop recorder system, remote data acquisition(s), receipt of transmissions and technician review, technical support and distribution of results** S TC 80

Do not report more than once in a 30 day period

Do not report when monitoring period is less than 10 days

Do not report with (93040-93042, 93268-93272, 93290-93291, 93296)

0.00 0.00 Global Days XXX

AMA: 2009, Feb, 3-12

93303-93352 Echocardiography

CMS 100-4,4,200.7.1 Cardiac Echocardiography Without Contrast

CMS 100-4,12,30.4 Cardiovascular System

INCLUDES Interpretation and report
Obtaining ultrasonic signals from heart/great arteries
Report of study which includes:
Description of recognized abnormalities
Documentation of all clinically relevent findings which includes obtained quantitative measurements
Interpretation of all information obtained
Two-dimensional image/doppler ultrasonic signal documentation
Ultrasound exam of:
Adjacent great vessels
Cardiac chambers/valves
Pericardium

EXCLUDES *Contrast agents and/or drugs used for pharmacological stress*
Echocardiography, fetal (76825-76828)
Ultrasound without thorough examination of the organ(s) or anatomic region/documentation of the image/final written report

93303 **Transthoracic echocardiography for congenital cardiac anomalies; complete** S 80

6.11 6.11 Global Days XXX

AMA: 2009, Jan, 11-31; 2008, Mar, 4-5; 2008, Jan, 10-25; 2007, January, 13-27

93304 **follow-up or limited study** S 80

3.96 3.96 Global Days XXX

AMA: 2008, Mar, 4-5

93306 **Echocardiography, transthoracic, real-time with image documentation (2D), includes M-mode recording, when performed, complete, with spectral Doppler echocardiography, and with color flow Doppler echocardiography** S 80

INCLUDES Doppler and color flow
Two-dimensional and M-mode

EXCLUDES *Transthoracic without spectral and color doppler (93307)*

6.26 6.26 Global Days XXX

93307 **Echocardiography, transthoracic, real-time with image documentation (2D), includes M-mode recording, when performed, complete, without spectral or color Doppler echocardiography** S 80

INCLUDES Additional structures that may be viewed such as pulmonary vein or artery, pulmonic valve, inferior vena cava
Obtaining/recording appropriate measurements
Two-dimensional/selected M-mode exam of:
Adjacent portions of the aorta
Aortic/mitral/tricuspid valves
Left/right atria
Left/right ventricles
Pericardium
Using multiple views as required to obtain a complete functional/anatomic evaluation

Do not report with (93320-93321, 93325)

3.89 3.89 Global Days XXX

AMA: 2009, Jan, 11-31; 2008, Mar, 4-5; 2008, Jan, 10-25; 2007, January, 13-27

93308 **Echocardiography, transthoracic, real-time with image documentation (2D), includes M-mode recording, when performed, follow-up or limited study** S 80

INCLUDES An exam that does not evaluate/document the attempt to evaluate all the structures that comprise the complete echocardiographic exam

2.99 2.99 Global Days XXX

AMA: 2009, Jan, 11-31; 2008, Jan, 10-25; 2008, Mar, 4-5; 2007, January, 13-27

⊙ **93312** **Echocardiography, transesophageal, real-time with image documentation (2D) (with or without M-mode recording); including probe placement, image acquisition, interpretation and report** S 80

9.27 9.27 Global Days XXX

AMA: 2009, Jan, 11-31; 2008, Mar, 4-5; 2008, Jan, 10-25; 2007, January, 13-27

⊙ **93313** **placement of transesophageal probe only** S 80

1.23 1.23 Global Days XXX

AMA: 2008, Mar, 4-5

⊙ **93314** **image acquisition, interpretation and report only** N 80

8.42 8.42 Global Days XXX

AMA: 2008, Mar, 4-5

⊙ **93315** **Transesophageal echocardiography for congenital cardiac anomalies; including probe placement, image acquisition, interpretation and report** S 80

0.00 0.00 Global Days XXX

AMA: 2008, Mar, 4-5

⊙ **93316** **placement of transesophageal probe only** S 80

1.29 1.29 Global Days XXX

AMA: 2008, Mar, 4-5

⊙ **93317** **image acquisition, interpretation and report only** N 80

0.00 0.00 Global Days XXX

AMA: 2008, Mar, 4-5

⊙ **93318** **Echocardiography, transesophageal (TEE) for monitoring purposes, including probe placement, real time 2-dimensional image acquisition and interpretation leading to ongoing (continuous) assessment of (dynamically changing) cardiac pumping function and to therapeutic measures on an immediate time basis** S 80

0.00 0.00 Global Days XXX

AMA: 2008, Mar, 4-5

\+ **93320** **Doppler echocardiography, pulsed wave and/or continuous wave with spectral display (List separately in addition to codes for echocardiographic imaging); complete** N 80

Code first (93303-93304, 93312, 93314-93315, 93317, 93350-93351)

1.59 1.59 Global Days ZZZ

AMA: 2008, Mar, 4-5

\+ **93321** **follow-up or limited study (List separately in addition to codes for echocardiographic imaging)** N 80

Code first (93303-93304, 93308, 93312, 93314-93315, 93317, 93350-93351)

0.79 0.79 Global Days ZZZ

AMA: 2008, Mar, 4-5

\+ **93325** **Doppler echocardiography color flow velocity mapping (List separately in addition to codes for echocardiography)** N 80

Code first (76825-76828, 93303-93304, 93308, 93312, 93314-93315, 93317, 93350-93351)

0.83 0.83 Global Days ZZZ

AMA: 2008, Mar, 4-5

93350 **Echocardiography, transthoracic, real-time with image documentation (2D), includes M-mode recording, when performed, during rest and cardiovascular stress test using treadmill, bicycle exercise and/or pharmacologically induced stress, with interpretation and report;** S 80

Code also exercise stress testing (93016-93018)

Do not report with (93015)

6.10 6.10 Global Days XXX

AMA: 2009, Jan, 11-31; 2008, Mar, 4-5; 2008, Jan, 10-25; 2007, January, 13-27

93351 **including performance of continuous electrocardiographic monitoring, with physician supervision** S

INCLUDES Stress echocardiogram performed with a complete cardiovascular stress test

EXCLUDES *Professional only components of complete stress test and stress echocardiogram performed in a facility by same physician, report with modifier 26*

Code also components of cardiovascular stress test when professional services not performed by same physician performing stress echocardiogram (93016-93018)

Do not report 93351-26 with 93350-26

Do not report 93351-26 with (93016, 93018)

Do not report with (93015-93018, 93350)

7.13 7.13 Global Days XXX

\+ **93352** **Use of echocardiographic contrast agent during stress echocardiography (List separately in addition to code for primary procedure)** M 80

Code first (93350, 93351)

Do not report more than once for each stress echocardiogram

1.03 1.03 Global Days ZZZ

93451-93505 Heart Catheterization

CMS 100-4,12,30.4 Cardiovascular System

INCLUDES Access site imaging and placement of closure device
Catheter insertion and positioning
Contrast injection (except as listed below)
Imaging and insertion of closure device
Radiology supervision and interpretation
Roadmapping angiography

EXCLUDES *Congenital cardiac cath procedures (93530-93533)*

Code also separately identifiable:
Aortography (93567)
Noncardiac angiography (see radiology and vascular codes)
Pulmonary angiography (93568)
Right ventricular or atrial injection (93566)

⊘ ⊙ **93451 Right heart catheterization including measurement(s) of oxygen saturation and cardiac output, when performed** T 80

INCLUDES Cardiac output review
Insertion catheter into 1+ right cardiac chambers or areas
Obtaining samples for blood gas

Code also administration of medication and assessment of hemodynamic measurement (93463)
Do not report with (93453, 93456-93457, 93460-93461, 93503, 93561-93565)

Do not report with insertion of hemodynamic monitor unless done for a reason other than insertion or maintenance of hemodynamic monitoring system (0293T-0294T)

23.56 23.56 Global Days 000

⊙ **93452 Left heart catheterization including intraprocedural injection(s) for left ventriculography, imaging supervision and interpretation, when performed** T 80

INCLUDES Insertion of catheter into left cardiac chambers

Code also administration of medication and assessment of hemodynamic measurement (93463)
Code also transapical or transseptal puncture (93462)
Do not report with (93453, 93458-93461, 93503, 93561-93565)

Do not report with insertion of hemodynamic monitor unless done for a reason other than insertion or maintenance of hemodynamic monitoring system (0293T-0294T)

25.93 25.93 Global Days 000

⊙ **93453 Combined right and left heart catheterization including intraprocedural injection(s) for left ventriculography, imaging supervision and interpretation, when performed** T 80

INCLUDES Cardiac output review
Insertion catheter into 1+ right cardiac chambers or areas
Insertion of catheter into left cardiac chambers
Obtaining samples for blood gas

Code also administration of medication and assessment of hemodynamic measurement (93463)
Code also transapical or transseptal puncture (93462)
Do not report with (93451-93452, 93456-93461, 93503, 93561-93565)

Do not report with insertion of hemodynamic monitor unless done for a reason other than insertion or maintenance of hemodynamic monitoring system (0293T-0294T)

33.95 33.95 Global Days 000

⊙ **93454 Catheter placement in coronary artery(s) for coronary angiography, including intraprocedural injection(s) for coronary angiography, imaging supervision and interpretation;** T 80

Do not report with (93503, 93561-93565)

26.73 26.73 Global Days 000

⊙ **93455 with catheter placement(s) in bypass graft(s) (internal mammary, free arterial, venous grafts) including intraprocedural injection(s) for bypass graft angiography** T 80

Do not report with (93503, 93561-93565)

31.21 31.21 Global Days 000

⊘ ⊙ **93456 with right heart catheterization** T 80

INCLUDES Cardiac output review
Insertion catheter into 1+ right cardiac chambers or areas
Obtaining samples for blood gas

Code also administration of medication and assessment of hemodynamic measurement (93463)
Do not report with (93503, 93561-93565)

33.44 33.44 Global Days 000

⊙ **93457 with catheter placement(s) in bypass graft(s) (internal mammary, free arterial, venous grafts) including intraprocedural injection(s) for bypass graft angiography and right heart catheterization** T 80

INCLUDES Cardiac output review
Insertion catheter into 1+ right cardiac chambers or areas
Obtaining samples for blood gas

Code also administration of medication and assessment of hemodynamic measurement (93463)
Do not report with (93503, 93561-93565)

37.91 37.91 Global Days 000

⊙ **93458 with left heart catheterization including intraprocedural injection(s) for left ventriculography, when performed** T 80

INCLUDES Insertion of catheter into left cardiac chambers

Code also administration of medication and assessment of hemodynamic measurement
Code also transapical or transseptal puncture (93462)
Do not report with (93503, 93561-93565)

32.26 32.26 Global Days 000

⊙ 93459 **with left heart catheterization including intraprocedural injection(s) for left ventriculography, when performed, catheter placement(s) in bypass graft(s) (internal mammary, free arterial, venous grafts) with bypass graft angiography** T 80

INCLUDES Insertion of catheter into left cardiac chambers

Code also administration of medication and assessment of hemodynamic measurement

Code also transapical or transseptal puncture (93462)

Do not report with (93503, 93561-93565)

35.62 35.62 Global Days 000

⊙ 93460 **with right and left heart catheterization including intraprocedural injection(s) for left ventriculography, when performed** T 80

INCLUDES Cardiac output review
Insertion catheter into 1+ right cardiac chambers or areas
Insertion of catheter into left cardiac chambers
Obtaining samples for blood gas

Code also administration of medication and assessment of hemodynamic measurement

Code also transapical or transseptal puncture (93462)

Do not report with (93503, 93561-93565)

38.08 38.08 Global Days 000

⊙ 93461 **with right and left heart catheterization including intraprocedural injection(s) for left ventriculography, when performed, catheter placement(s) in bypass graft(s) (internal mammary, free arterial, venous grafts) with bypass graft angiography** T 80

INCLUDES Cardiac output review
Insertion catheter into 1+ right cardiac chambers or areas
Insertion of catheter into left cardiac chambers
Obtaining samples for blood gas

Code also administration of medication and assessment of hemodynamic measurement

Code also transapical or transseptal puncture (93462)

Do not report with (93503, 93561-93565)

43.68 43.68 Global Days 000

+ ⊙ 93462 **Left heart catheterization by transseptal puncture through intact septum or by transapical puncture (List separately in addition to code for primary procedure)** T 80

INCLUDES Insertion of catheter into left cardiac chambers

Code first (93452, 93453, 93458-93461, 93651, 93652)

5.92 5.92 Global Days ZZZ

+ ⊙ 93463 **Pharmacologic agent administration (eg, inhaled nitric oxide, intravenous infusion of nitroprusside, dobutamine, milrinone, or other agent) including assessing hemodynamic measurements before, during, after and repeat pharmacologic agent administration, when performed (List separately in addition to code for primary procedure)** N 80

Code first (93451-93453, 93456-93461, 93530-93533)

Do not report more than one time per catheterization

Do not report with coronary interventional procedures (92975, 92977, 92980, 92982, 92995)

3.13 3.13 Global Days ZZZ

+ ⊙ 93464 **Physiologic exercise study (eg, bicycle or arm ergometry) including assessing hemodynamic measurements before and after (List separately in addition to code for primary procedure)** N 80

EXCLUDES *Administration of pharmacologic agent (93463)*
Bundle of His recording (93600)

Code first (93451-93453, 93456-93461, 93530-93533)

Do not report more than one time per catheterization

7.84 7.84 Global Days ZZZ

⊘ 93503 **Insertion and placement of flow directed catheter (eg, Swan-Ganz) for monitoring purposes** T 80

EXCLUDES *Subsequent monitoring (99356-99357)*

Do not report with codes for diagnostic cardiac catheterization (93451-93461, 93530-93533)

3.94 3.94 Global Days 000

AMA: 2008, Mar, 4-5

⊙ 93505 **Endomyocardial biopsy** T 80

EXCLUDES *Intravascular brachytherapy radionuclide insertion (77785-77787)*
Transcatheter insertion of brachytherapy delivery device (92974)

23.77 23.77 Global Days 000

AMA: 2009, Jan, 11-31; 2008, Mar, 4-5; 2008, Jan, 10-25; 2007, January, 13-27

93530-93533 Congenital Heart Defect Catheterization

INCLUDES Access site imaging and placement of closure device
Cardiac output review
Insertion catheter into 1+ right cardiac chambers or areas
Obtaining samples for blood gas
Radiology supervision and interpretation
Roadmapping angiography

EXCLUDES *Cardiac cath on noncongenital heart (93451-93453, 93456-93461)*

Code also injection procedure (93563-93568)

Do not report with (93503)

⊙ 93530 **Right heart catheterization, for congenital cardiac anomalies** T 80

0.00 0.00 Global Days 000

AMA: 2009, Jan, 11-31; 2008, Jan, 10-25; 2008, Mar, 4-5; 2007, January, 13-27

93531 **Combined right heart catheterization and retrograde left heart catheterization, for congenital cardiac anomalies** T 80

0.00 0.00 Global Days 000

AMA: 2008, Mar, 4-5

93532 **Combined right heart catheterization and transseptal left heart catheterization through intact septum with or without retrograde left heart catheterization, for congenital cardiac anomalies** T 80

0.00 0.00 Global Days 000

AMA: 2009, Jan, 11-31; 2008, Jan, 10-25; 2008, Mar, 4-5; 2007, January, 13-27

93533 **Combined right heart catheterization and transseptal left heart catheterization through existing septal opening, with or without retrograde left heart catheterization, for congenital cardiac anomalies** T 80

0.00 0.00 Global Days 000

AMA: 2008, Mar, 4-5

93561-93568 Injections Procedures

INCLUDES Catheter repositioning
Radiology supervision and interpretation
Using automatic power injector

⊙ ▲ **93561** **Indicator dilution studies such as dye or thermodilution, including arterial and/or venous catheterization; with cardiac output measurement (separate procedure)** N 80
EXCLUDES *Cardiac output, radioisotope method (78472, 78473, 78481)*
Do not report with (93451-93462)
0.00 0.00 Global Days 000
AMA: 2009, Jan, 11-31; 2008, Jan, 10-25; 2008, Mar, 4-5; 2007, Jul, 1-4; 2007, February, 10-11

⊙ ▲ **93562** **subsequent measurement of cardiac output** N 80
EXCLUDES *Cardiac output, radioisotope method (78472, 78473, 78481)*
Code first (92987, 93460-93462, 93532, 93580-93581, 93621-93622, 93651-93652)
Do not report with (92961)
Do not report with cardiac catheterization codes
0.00 0.00 Global Days 000
AMA: 2008, Mar, 4-5; 2007, Jul, 1-4; 2007, February, 10-11

+ ⊙ **93563** **Injection procedure during cardiac catheterization including imaging supervision, interpretation, and report; for selective coronary angiography during congenital heart catheterization (List separately in addition to code for primary procedure)** N 80
Code first (93530-93533)
Do not report with (93452-93461)
1.62 1.62 Global Days ZZZ

+ ⊙ **93564** **for selective opacification of aortocoronary venous or arterial bypass graft(s) (eg, aortocoronary saphenous vein, free radial artery, or free mammary artery graft) to 1 or more coronary arteries and in situ arterial conduits (eg, internal mammary), whether native or used for bypass to 1 or more coronary arteries during congenital heart catheterization, when performed (List separately in addition to code for primary procedure)** N 80
Code first (93530-93533)
Do not report with (93452-93461)
1.66 1.66 Global Days ZZZ

+ ⊙ **93565** **for selective left ventricular or left atrial angiography (List separately in addition to code for primary procedure)** N 80
Code first (93530-93533)
Do not report with (93452-93461)
1.26 1.26 Global Days ZZZ

+ ⊙ **93566** **for selective right ventricular or right atrial angiography (List separately in addition to code for primary procedure)** N 80
Code first (93451-93461, 93530-93533)
1.25 5.28 Global Days ZZZ

+ ⊙ **93567** **for supravalvular aortography (List separately in addition to code for primary procedure)** N 80
Code first (93451-93461, 93530-93533)
1.41 4.26 Global Days ZZZ

+ ⊙ **93568** **for pulmonary angiography (List separately in addition to code for primary procedure)** N 80
Code first (93451-93461, 93530-93533)
1.29 4.78 Global Days ZZZ

93571-93572 Coronary Artery Doppler Studies

CMS 100-4,12,30.4 Cardiovascular System
INCLUDES Doppler transducer manipulations/repositioning within the vessel examined, during coronary angiography/therapeutic intervention (angioplasty)

+ ⊙ **93571** **Intravascular Doppler velocity and/or pressure derived coronary flow reserve measurement (coronary vessel or graft) during coronary angiography including pharmacologically induced stress; initial vessel (List separately in addition to code for primary procedure)** N 80
Code first primary procedure
0.00 0.00 Global Days ZZZ
AMA: 2008, Mar, 4-5

+ ⊙ **93572** **each additional vessel (List separately in addition to code for primary procedure)** N 80
Code first initial vessel (93571)
0.00 0.00 Global Days ZZZ
AMA: 2008, Mar, 4-5

93580-93581 Percutaneous Repair of Septal Defect

CMS 100-4,12,30.4 Cardiovascular System
INCLUDES Injection of contrast for atrial/ventricular angiograms
Right heart catheterization
EXCLUDES *Echocardiography (93303-93317, 93580-93581, 93662)*
Do not report with (93451-93453, 93455-93461, 93530-93533, 93564-93566)

93580 **Percutaneous transcatheter closure of congenital interatrial communication (ie, Fontan fenestration, atrial septal defect) with implant** T 80
29.88 29.88 Global Days 000
AMA: 2009, Jan, 11-31; 2008, Jan, 10-25; 2008, Mar, 4-5; 2007, January, 13-27

93581 **Percutaneous transcatheter closure of a congenital ventricular septal defect with implant** T 80
39.97 39.97 Global Days 000
AMA: 2009, Jan, 11-31; 2008, Mar, 4-5; 2008, Jan, 10-25; 2007, January, 13-27

93600-93603 Recording of Intracardiac Electrograms

CMS 100-3,20.13 HIS Bundle Study
CMS 100-4,12,30.4 Cardiovascular System
INCLUDES Unusual situations where there may be recording/pacing/attempt at arrhythmia induction from only one side of the heart

⊘ **93600** **Bundle of His recording** S 80
Code also (C1730, C1731, C1732, C1733, C1766, C1892, C1893, C1894, C2629, C2630)
0.00 0.00 Global Days 000
AMA: 2009, Jan, 11-31; 2008, Jan, 10-25; 2008, Mar, 4-5; 2007, Dec, 10-179; 2007, January, 13-27

⊘ **93602** **Intra-atrial recording** S 80
Code also (C1730, C1731, C1732, C1733, C1766, C1892, C1893, C1894, C2629, C2630)
0.00 0.00 Global Days 000
AMA: 2009, Jan, 11-31; 2008, Jan, 10-25; 2008, Mar, 4-5; 2007, January, 13-27

⊘ **93603** **Right ventricular recording** S 80
Code also (C1730, C1731, C1732, C1733, C1766, C1892, C1893, C1894, C2629, C2630)
0.00 0.00 Global Days 000
AMA: 2008, Mar, 4-5

93609-93613 Intracardiac Mapping and Pacing

CMS 100-3,20.12 Diagnostic Endocardial Electrical Stimulation (Pacing)
CMS 100-4,12,30.4 Cardiovascular System

+ ⊙ **93609** **Intraventricular and/or intra-atrial mapping of tachycardia site(s) with catheter manipulation to record from multiple sites to identify origin of tachycardia (List separately in addition to code for primary procedure)** N 80

Code also (C1730, C1731, C1733, C2629, C2630)
Code first comprehensive electrophysiologic evaluation or intracardiac catheter ablation (93620, 93651, 93652)
Do not report with (93613)
0.00 0.00 **Global Days ZZZ**
AMA: 2008, Mar, 4-5

⊘ **93610** **Intra-atrial pacing** S 80
INCLUDES Unusual situations where there may be recording/pacing/attempt at arrhythmia induction from only one side of the heart
Code also (C1730, C1731, C1732, C1733, C1766, C1892, C1893, C1894, C2629, C2630)
0.00 0.00 **Global Days 000**
AMA: 2008, Mar, 4-5

⊘ **93612** **Intraventricular pacing** S 80
INCLUDES Unusual situations where there may be recording/pacing/attempt at arrhythmia induction from only one side of the heart
Code also (C1730, C1731, C1732, C1733, C1766, C1892, C1893, C1894, C2629, C2630)
Do not report with (93620-93622)
0.00 0.00 **Global Days 000**
AMA: 2008, Mar, 4-5

+ ⊙ **93613** **Intracardiac electrophysiologic 3-dimensional mapping (List separately in addition to code for primary procedure)** N 80
Code also (C1730, C1731, C1732, C1733, C2630)
Code first comprehensive electrophysiologic evaluation or intracardiac catheter ablation (93620, 93651, 93652)
Do not report with (93609)
11.49 11.49 **Global Days ZZZ**
AMA: 2008, Mar, 4-5

93615-93616 Recording and Pacing via Esophagus

CMS 100-4,12,30.4 Cardiovascular System

⊘ ⊙ **93615** **Esophageal recording of atrial electrogram with or without ventricular electrogram(s);** S 80
Code also (C1730, C1731, C1732, C1733, C1766, C1892, C1893, C1894, C2629, C2630)
0.00 0.00 **Global Days 000**
AMA: 2008, Mar, 4-5

⊘ ⊙ **93616** **with pacing** S 80
Code also (C1730, C1731, C1732, C1733, C1756, C1766, C1892, C1893, C1894, C2629, C2630)
0.00 0.00 **Global Days 000**
AMA: 2008, Mar, 4-5

93618 Pacing to Produce an Arrhythmia

CMS 100-4,12,30.4 Cardiovascular System
INCLUDES Unusual situations where there may be recording/pacing/attempt at arrhythmia induction from only one side of the heart
EXCLUDES *Intracardiac phonocardiogram (93799)*

⊘ ⊙ **93618** **Induction of arrhythmia by electrical pacing** S 80
INCLUDES Unusual situations where there may be recording/pacing/attempt at arrhythmia induction from only one side of the heart
EXCLUDES *Intracardiac phonocardiogram (93799)*
Code also (C1730, C1731, C1732, C1733, C1766, C1892, C1893, C1894, C2629, C2630)
0.00 0.00 **Global Days 000**
AMA: 2009, Jan, 11-31; 2008, Mar, 4-5; 2008, Jan, 10-25; 2007, January, 13-27; 2007, Dec, 10-179

93619-93623 Comprehensive Electrophysiological Studies

CMS 100-3,20.12 Diagnostic Endocardial Electrical Stimulation (Pacing)
CMS 100-4,12,30.4 Cardiovascular System

⊙ **93619** **Comprehensive electrophysiologic evaluation with right atrial pacing and recording, right ventricular pacing and recording, His bundle recording, including insertion and repositioning of multiple electrode catheters, without induction or attempted induction of arrhythmia** 03 80
INCLUDES Evaluation of sinus node/atrioventricular node/His-Purkinje conduction system without arrhythmia induction
Code also (C1730, C1731, C1732, C1733, C1766, C1892, C1893, C1894, C2629, C2630)
Do not report with (93600, 93602, 93610, 93612, 93618, 93620-93622)
0.00 0.00 **Global Days 000**
AMA: 2009, Jan, 11-31; 2008, Mar, 4-5; 2008, Jan, 10-25; 2007, January, 13-27; 2007, Dec, 10-179

⊙ **93620** **Comprehensive electrophysiologic evaluation including insertion and repositioning of multiple electrode catheters with induction or attempted induction of arrhythmia; with right atrial pacing and recording, right ventricular pacing and recording, His bundle recording** 03 80
INCLUDES Recording/pacing/attempted arrhythmia induction from one or more site(s) in the heart
Code also (C1730, C1731, C1732, C1733, C1766, C1892, C1893, C1894, C2629, C2630)
Do not report with (93600, 93602, 93610, 93612, 93618, 93619)
0.00 0.00 **Global Days 000**
AMA: 2009, Jan, 11-31; 2008, Jan, 10-25; 2008, Mar, 4-5; 2008, Oct, 10-11; 2007, January, 13-27; 2007, Dec, 10-179

+ ⊙ **93621** **with left atrial pacing and recording from coronary sinus or left atrium (List separately in addition to code for primary procedure)** N 80
INCLUDES Recording/pacing/attempted arrhythmia induction from one or more site(s) in the heart
Code also (C1730, C1731, C1732, C1733, C1766, C1892, C1893, C1894, C2629, C2630)
Code first right atrial/ventricular pacing/recording (93620)
0.00 0.00 **Global Days ZZZ**
AMA: 2009, Jan, 11-31; 2008, Mar, 4-5; 2008, Jan, 10-25; 2008, Oct, 10-11; 2007, January, 13-27; 2007, Dec, 10-179

+ ⊙ **93622** **with left ventricular pacing and recording (List separately in addition to code for primary procedure)** N 80

Code also (C1730, C1731, C1732, C1733, C1766, C1892, C1893, C1894, C2629, C2630)

Code first right atrial/ventricular pacing/recording (93620)

0.00 0.00 Global Days ZZZ

AMA: 2009, Jan, 11-31; 2008, Jan, 10-25; 2008, Mar, 4-5; 2007, January, 13-27; 2007, Dec, 10-179

+ **93623** **Programmed stimulation and pacing after intravenous drug infusion (List separately in addition to code for primary procedure)** N 80

INCLUDES Recording/pacing/attempted arrhythmia induction from one or more site(s) in the heart

Code also (C1730, C1731, C1732, C1733, C1766, C1892, C1893, C1894, C2629, C2630)

Code first comprehensive eletrophysiologic evaluation (93619, 93620)

0.00 0.00 Global Days ZZZ

AMA: 2009, Jan, 11-31; 2008, Mar, 4-5; 2008, Oct, 10-11; 2007, Dec, 10-179

93624-93631 Followup and Intraoperative Electrophysiologic Studies

CMS 100-3,20.11 Intraoperative Ventricular Mapping

CMS 100-3,20.12 Diagnostic Endocardial Electrical Stimulation (Pacing)

CMS 100-4,12,30.4 Cardiovascular System

⊙ **93624** **Electrophysiologic follow-up study with pacing and recording to test effectiveness of therapy, including induction or attempted induction of arrhythmia** T 80

INCLUDES Recording/pacing/attempted arrhythmia induction from one or more site(s) in the heart

Code also (C1730, C1731, C1732, C1733, C1766, C1892, C1893, C1894)

0.00 0.00 Global Days 000

AMA: 2008, Mar, 4-5; 2007, Dec, 10-179

⊘ **93631** **Intra-operative epicardial and endocardial pacing and mapping to localize the site of tachycardia or zone of slow conduction for surgical correction** N 80

EXCLUDES *Operative ablation of an arrhythmogenic focus or pathway by a separate provider (33250-33261)*

Code also (C1730, C1731, C1732, C1733, C1766, C1892, C1893, C1894, C2629, C2630)

0.00 0.00 Global Days 000

AMA: 2008, Mar, 4-5; 2007, Dec, 10-179

93640-93642 Electrophysiologic Studies of Pacing Cardioverter-Defibrillators

CMS 100-3,20.8.2 Self-contained Pacemaker Monitors

CMS 100-3,20.12 Diagnostic Endocardial Electrical Stimulation (Pacing)

CMS 100-4,12,30.4 Cardiovascular System

INCLUDES Recording/pacing/attempted arrhythmia induction from one or more site(s) in the heart

⊙ **93640** **Electrophysiologic evaluation of single or dual chamber pacing cardioverter-defibrillator leads including defibrillation threshold evaluation (induction of arrhythmia, evaluation of sensing and pacing for arrhythmia termination) at time of initial implantation or replacement;** N 80

0.00 0.00 Global Days 000

AMA: 2008, Mar, 4-5

⊙ **93641** **with testing of single or dual chamber pacing cardioverter-defibrillator pulse generator** N 80

EXCLUDES *Single/dual chamber pacing cardioverter-defibrillators reprogramming/electronic analysis, subsequent/periodic (93282-93283, 93289, 93292, 93295, 93642)*

0.00 0.00 Global Days 000

AMA: 2008, Mar, 4-5

⊙ **93642** **Electrophysiologic evaluation of single or dual chamber pacing cardioverter-defibrillator (includes defibrillation threshold evaluation, induction of arrhythmia, evaluation of sensing and pacing for arrhythmia termination, and programming or reprogramming of sensing or therapeutic parameters)** S 80

11.81 11.81 Global Days 000

AMA: 2008, Mar, 4-5

93650-93652 Intracardiac Ablation

CMS 100-4,12,30.4 Cardiovascular System

⊙ **93650** **Intracardiac catheter ablation of atrioventricular node function, atrioventricular conduction for creation of complete heart block, with or without temporary pacemaker placement** 03 80

Code also (C1732, C1733, C1766, C1892, C1893, C1894, C2629, C2630)

17.52 17.52 Global Days 000

AMA: 2008, Mar, 4-5

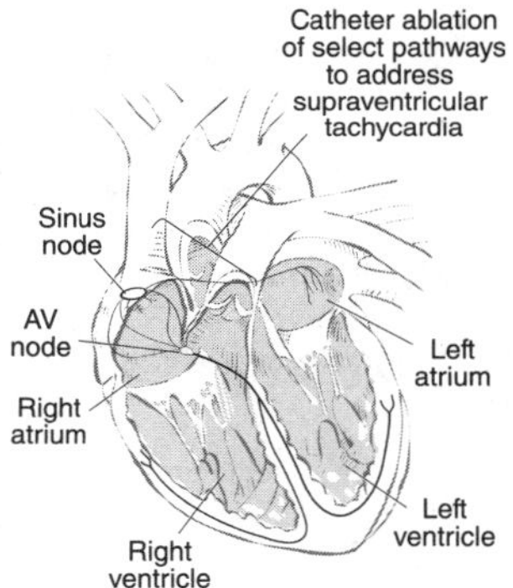

The procedure is performed to more selectively ablate electrical pathways of the heart, specifically to treat supraventricular tachycardia, excessively quick action of the atria

⊙ **93651** **Intracardiac catheter ablation of arrhythmogenic focus; for treatment of supraventricular tachycardia by ablation of fast or slow atrioventricular pathways, accessory atrioventricular connections or other atrial foci, singly or in combination** 03 80

INCLUDES Delivery of radiofrequency energy to the area to selectively destroy cardiac tissue

Services that may be performed independently on a date subsequent to or at the same time as a diagnostic electrophysiologic study/tachycardia(s) induction/mapping

Code also (C1732, C1733, C1766, C1892, C1893, C1894, C2629, C2630)

Code also transapical or transseptal puncture (93462)

26.67 26.67 Global Days 000

AMA: 2008, Mar, 4-5; 2007, Dec, 10-179

⊙ **93652** **for treatment of ventricular tachycardia** Q3 80

INCLUDES Delivery of radiofrequency energy to the area to selectively destroy cardiac tissue
Services that may be performed independently on a date subsequent to or at the same time as a diagnostic electrophysiologic study/tachycardia(s) induction/mapping

Code also (C1732, C1733, C1766, C1892, C1893, C1894, C2629, C2630)
Code also transapical or transseptal puncture (93462)
29.03 29.03 Global Days 000
AMA: 2009, Jan, 11-31; 2008, Jan, 10-25; 2008, Mar, 4-5; 2007, January, 13-27

93660-93662 Other Tests for Cardiac Function

CMS 100-4,12,30.4 Cardiovascular System

93660 **Evaluation of cardiovascular function with tilt table evaluation, with continuous ECG monitoring and intermittent blood pressure monitoring, with or without pharmacological intervention** S 80

EXCLUDES *Autonomic nervous system function testing (95921-95923)*

4.64 4.64 Global Days 000
AMA: 2008, Mar, 4-5

\+ **93662** **Intracardiac echocardiography during therapeutic/diagnostic intervention, including imaging supervision and interpretation (List separately in addition to code for primary procedure)** N 80

Code also (C1759)
Code first (92987, 93453, 93460-93462, 93532, 93580-93581, 93621-93622, 93651-93652)
Do not report with internal cardioversion (92961)
0.00 0.00 Global Days ZZZ
AMA: 2009, Jan, 11-31; 2008, Jan, 10-25; 2008, Mar, 4-5; 2007, January, 13-27

93668 Rehabilitation Services: Peripheral Arterial Disease

INCLUDES Monitoring:
Other cardiovascular limitations for adjustment of workload
Patient's claudication threshold
Motorized treadmill or track
Sessions lasting 45-60 minutes
Supervision by exercise physiologist/nurse

Code also evaulation and managment service, if appropriate

93668 **Peripheral arterial disease (PAD) rehabilitation, per session** E
0.56 0.56 Global Days XXX
AMA: 2008, Mar, 4-5

93701 Thoracic Electrical Bioimpedance

CMS 100-3,20.16 Cardiac Output Monitoring by Thoracic Electrical Bioimpedance (TEB)
CMS 100-4,12,30.4 Cardiovascular System

93701 **Bioimpedance-derived physiologic cardiovascular analysis** S TC 80

EXCLUDES *Indirect measurement of left ventricular filling pressure by computerized calibration of the arterial waveform response to Valsalva (93799)*

0.76 0.76 Global Days XXX
AMA: 2008, Mar, 4-5

93720-93722 Total Body Plethysmography

CMS 100-3,20.14 Plethysmography

~~93720~~ ~~**Plethysmography, total body; with interpretation and report**~~
To report, see 94726, 94750

~~93721~~ ~~**tracing only, without interpretation and report**~~
To report, see 94726, 94750

~~93722~~ ~~**interpretation and report only**~~
To report, see 94726, 94750

93724 Electronic Analysis of Pacemaker Function

CMS 100-3,20.8 Cardiac Pacemakers
CMS 100-3,20.8.1 Cardiac Pacemaker Evaluation Services
CMS 100-3,20.14 Plethysmography
CMS 100-4,12,30.4 Cardiovascular System

EXCLUDES *Arterial cannulization/recording of direct arterial pressure (36620)*
Chemotherapy (96409-96549)
Hemodialysis vascular cannulization (36800-36821)
Radiographic injection services (36000-36299)

93724 **Electronic analysis of antitachycardia pacemaker system (includes electrocardiographic recording, programming of device, induction and termination of tachycardia via implanted pacemaker, and interpretation of recordings)** S 80
8.23 8.23 Global Days 000
AMA: 2008, Mar, 4-5

93740 Temperature Gradient Assessment

CMS 100-4,12,30.4 Cardiovascular System

93740 **Temperature gradient studies** X
0.27 0.27 Global Days XXX

93745 Wearable Cardioverter-Defibrillator System Services

CMS 100-4,12,30.4 Cardiovascular System

EXCLUDES *Arterial cannulization/recording of direct arterial pressure (36620)*
Chemotherapy (96409-96549)
Hemodialysis vascular cannulization (36800-36821)
Radiographic injection services (36000-36299)

93745 **Initial set-up and programming by a physician of wearable cardioverter-defibrillator includes initial programming of system, establishing baseline electronic ECG, transmission of data to data repository, patient instruction in wearing system and patient reporting of problems or events** S 80

Do not report with (93282, 93292)
0.00 0.00 Global Days XXX
AMA: 2009, Mar, 5-7; 2009, Feb, 3-12

93750 Ventricular Assist Device (VAD) Interrogation

93750 **Interrogation of ventricular assist device (VAD), in person, with physician analysis of device parameters (eg, drivelines, alarms, power surges), review of device function (eg, flow and volume status, septum status, recovery), with programming, if performed, and report** S 80

Do not report with (33975-33976, 33979, 33981-33983)
1.30 1.56 Global Days XXX

93770 Peripheral Venous Blood Pressure Assessment

CMS 100-4,12,30.4 Cardiovascular System

93770 **Determination of venous pressure** N

EXCLUDES *Cannulization, central venous (36500, 36555-36556)*

0.26 0.26 **Global Days XXX**

93784-93790 Ambulatory Blood Pressure Monitoring

CMS 100-3,20.19 Ambulatory Blood Pressure Monitoring
CMS 100-4,12,30.4 Cardiovascular System
CMS 100-4,32,10.1 Ambulatory Blood Pressure Monitoring Billing Requirements

EXCLUDES *Arterial cannulization/recording of direct arterial pressure (36620)*
Chemotherapy (96409-96549)
Hemodialysis vascular cannulization (36800-36821)
Radiographic injection services (36000-36299)

93784 **Ambulatory blood pressure monitoring, utilizing a system such as magnetic tape and/or computer disk, for 24 hours or longer; including recording, scanning analysis, interpretation and report** E 80

1.73 1.73 **Global Days XXX**

93786 **recording only** S TC 80

0.92 0.92 **Global Days XXX**

93788 **scanning analysis with report** S TC 80

0.26 0.26 **Global Days XXX**

93790 **physician review with interpretation and report** M 26 80

0.55 0.55 **Global Days XXX**

93797-93799 Cardiac Rehabilitation

CMS 100-3,20.10 Cardiac Rehabilitation Programs
CMS 100-4,4,200.5 Cardiac Rehabilitation Services
CMS 100-4,12,30.4 Cardiovascular System

EXCLUDES *Arterial cannulization/recording of direct arterial pressure (36620)*
Chemotherapy (96409)
Hemodialysis vascular cannulization (36800-36821)
Radiographic injection services (36000-36299)

93797 **Physician services for outpatient cardiac rehabilitation; without continuous ECG monitoring (per session)** S 80

0.27 0.50 **Global Days 000**

93798 **with continuous ECG monitoring (per session)** S 80

0.41 0.74 **Global Days 000**

93799 **Unlisted cardiovascular service or procedure** S 80

0.00 0.00 **Global Days XXX**

AMA: 2009, Jan, 11-31; 2009, Mar, 5-7; 2008, Jan, 10-25; 2007, January, 13-27

93875-93893 Noninvasive Tests Extracranial/Intracranial Arteries

CMS 100-3,20.17 Noninvasive Tests of Carotid Function

INCLUDES Patient care required to perform/supervise studies and interpret results

Do not report for hand-held dopplers that do not provide a hard copy (See E/M codes)

Do not report for hand-held dopplers that do not permit vascular flow bidirectional analysis (see E/M codes)

~~**93875** **Noninvasive physiologic studies of extracranial arteries, complete bilateral study (eg, periorbital flow direction with arterial compression, ocular pneumoplethysmography, Doppler ultrasound spectral analysis)**~~

93880 **Duplex scan of extracranial arteries; complete bilateral study** S 80 PQ

7.41 7.41 **Global Days XXX**

93882 **unilateral or limited study** S 80 PQ

EXCLUDES *Common carotid intima-media thickness study for coronary heart disease risk factor assessment or evaluation of atherosclerotic burden (0126T)*

5.25 5.25 **Global Days XXX**

93886 **Transcranial Doppler study of the intracranial arteries; complete study** S 80

INCLUDES Complete transcranial doppler (TCD) study
Ultrasound evaluation of right/left anterior circulation territories and posterior circulation territory

10.47 10.47 **Global Days XXX**

93888 **limited study** S 80

INCLUDES Limited TCD study
Ultrasound examination of two or fewer of these territories (right/left anterior circulation, posterior circulation)

6.40 6.40 **Global Days XXX**

93890 **vasoreactivity study** S 80

Do not report with limited TCD study (93888)

8.37 8.37 **Global Days XXX**

93892 **emboli detection without intravenous microbubble injection** S 80

Do not report with limited TCD study (93888)

9.61 9.61 **Global Days XXX**

93893 **emboli detection with intravenous microbubble injection** S 80

Do not report with limited TCD study (93888)

9.70 9.70 **Global Days XXX**

93922-93971 Noninvasive Vascular Studies: Extremities

CMS 100-3,20.14 Plethysmography

INCLUDES Patient care required to perform/supervise studies and interpret results

Do not report for hand-held dopplers that do not permit vascular flow bidirectional analysis (see E/M codes)

Do not report for hand-held dopplers that do not provide a hard copy (See E/M codes)

93922 Limited bilateral noninvasive physiologic studies of upper or lower extremity arteries, (eg, for lower extremity: ankle/brachial indices at distal posterior tibial and anterior tibial/dorsalis pedis arteries plus bidirectional, Doppler waveform recording and analysis at 1-2 levels, or ankle/brachial indices at distal posterior tibial and anterior tibial/dorsalis pedis arteries plus volume plethysmography at 1-2 levels, or ankle/brachial indices at distal posterior tibial and anterior tibial/dorsalis pedis arteries with, transcutaneous oxygen tension measurement at 1-2 levels) S 80

INCLUDES Evaluation of:
- Doppler analysis of bidirectional blood flow
- Nonimaging physiologic recordings of pressure
- Oxygen tension measurements and/or plethysmography

Lower extremity (potential levels include high thigh, low thigh, calf, ankle, metatarsal and toes) limited study includes either:
- Ankle/brachial indicies at distal posterior tibial and anterior tibial/dorsalis pedis arteries plus bidirectional Doppler waveform recording and analysis as 1-2 levels; OR
- Ankle/brachial indices at distal posterior tibial and anterior tibial/dorsalis pedis arteries plus volume plethysmography at 1-2 levels; OR
- Ankle/brachial indices at distal posterior tibial and anterior tibial/dorsalis pedis arteries with transcutaneous oxygen tension measurements at 1-2 levels

Unilateral provocative functional measurement

Unilateral study of 3 or move levels

Upper extremity (potential levels include arm, forearm, wrist, and digits) limited study includes:
- Doppler-determined systolic pressures and bidirectional waveform recording with analysis at 1-2 levels; OR
- Doppler-determined systolic pressures and transcutaneous oxygen tension measurements at 1-2 levels; OR
- Doppler-determined systolic pressures and volume plethysmography at 1-2 levels

EXCLUDES *Transcutaneous oxyhemoglobin measurement in wound of lower extremity by near infrared spectroscopy (0286T)*

Code also modifier 52 for unilateral study of 1-2 levels

Code also twice with modifier 59 for upper and lower extremity study

Do not report more than once for the lower extremity

Do not report more than once for the upper extremity

3.06 3.06 Global Days XXX

93923 Complete bilateral noninvasive physiologic studies of upper or lower extremity arteries, 3 or more levels (eg, for lower extremity: ankle/brachial indices at distal posterior tibial and anterior tibial/dorsalis pedis arteries plus segmental blood pressure measurements with bidirectional Doppler waveform recording and analysis, at 3 or more levels, or ankle/brachial indices at distal posterior tibial and anterior tibial/dorsalis pedis arteries plus segmental volume plethysmography at 3 or more levels, or ankle/brachial indices at distal posterior tibial and anterior tibial/dorsalis pedis arteries plus segmental transcutaneous oxygen tension measurements at 3 or more level(s), or single level study with provocative functional maneuvers (eg, measurements with postural provocative tests, or measurements with reactive hyperemia) S 80

INCLUDES Evaluation of:
- Doppler analysis of bidirectional blood flow
- Nonimaging physiologic recordings of pressures
- Oxygen tension measurements

Lower extremity:
- Ankle/brachial indicies at distal posterior tibial and anterior tibial/dorsalis pedis arteries plus bidirectional Doppler waveform recording and analysis at 3 or more levels; OR
- Ankle/brachial indices at distal posterior tibial and anterior tibial/dorsalis pedis arteries with transcutaneous oxygen tension measurements at 3 or more levels; OR
- Ankle/brachial indices at distal posterior tibial and anterior tibial/dorsalis pedis arteries plus volume plethysmography at 3 or more levels; OR

Provocative functional maneuvers and measurement at a single level

Upper extremity complete study:
- Doppler-determined systolic pressures and bidirectional waveform recording with analysis at 3 or more levels; OR
- Doppler-determined systolic pressures and transcutaneous oxygen tension measurements at 3 or more levels; OR
- Doppler-determined systolic pressures and volume plethysmography at 3 or more levels; OR
- Provocative functional maneuvers and measurement at a single level

EXCLUDES *Transcutaneous oxyhemoglobin measurement in wound of lower extremity by near infrared spectroscopy (0286T)*
Unilateral study at 3 or more levels (93922)

Code also twice with modifier 59 for upper and lower extremity study

Do not report more than once for the lower extremity

Do not report more than once for the upper extremity

4.74 4.74 Global Days XXX

AMA: 2009, Jan, 11-31; 2008, Jan, 10-25; 2007, January, 13-27

93924 **Noninvasive physiologic studies of lower extremity arteries, at rest and following treadmill stress testing, (ie, bidirectional Doppler waveform or volume plethysmography recording and analysis at rest with ankle/brachial indices immediately after and at timed intervals following performance of a standardized protocol on a motorized treadmill plus recording of time of onset of claudication or other symptoms, maximal walking time, and time to recovery) complete bilateral study** S 80

INCLUDES Evaluation of:
- Doppler analysis of bidirectional blood flow
- Non-imaging physiologic recordings of pressures
- Oxygen tension measurements
- Plethysmography

Do not report this code for other types of exercise

Do not report with (93922-93923)

5.97 5.97 Global Days XXX

93925 **Duplex scan of lower extremity arteries or arterial bypass grafts; complete bilateral study** S 80

9.33 9.33 Global Days XXX

93926 **unilateral or limited study** S 80

6.09 6.09 Global Days XXX

93930 **Duplex scan of upper extremity arteries or arterial bypass grafts; complete bilateral study** S 80

7.45 7.45 Global Days XXX

93931 **unilateral or limited study** S 80

4.95 4.95 Global Days XXX

93965 **Noninvasive physiologic studies of extremity veins, complete bilateral study (eg, Doppler waveform analysis with responses to compression and other maneuvers, phleborheography, impedance plethysmography)** S 80

INCLUDES Evaluation of:
- Doppler analysis of bidirectional blood flow
- Nonimaging physiologic recordings of pressures
- Oxygen tension measurements
- Plethysmography

3.74 3.74 Global Days XXX

93970 **Duplex scan of extremity veins including responses to compression and other maneuvers; complete bilateral study** S 80

7.67 7.67 Global Days XXX

93971 **unilateral or limited study** S 80

4.56 4.56 Global Days XXX

AMA: 2009, Jan, 11-31; 2008, Jan, 10-25; 2007, January, 13-27

93975-93998 Noninvasive Vascular Studies: Abdomen/Pelvis/Hemodialysis Access

93975 **Duplex scan of arterial inflow and venous outflow of abdominal, pelvic, scrotal contents and/or retroperitoneal organs; complete study** S 80

11.20 11.20 Global Days XXX

AMA: 2009, Jan, 11-31; 2008, Jan, 10-25; 2007, January, 13-27

93976 **limited study** S 80

6.41 6.41 Global Days XXX

AMA: 2009, Jan, 11-31; 2008, Jan, 10-25; 2007, January, 13-27

93978 **Duplex scan of aorta, inferior vena cava, iliac vasculature, or bypass grafts; complete study** S 80

7.17 7.17 Global Days XXX

93979 **unilateral or limited study** S 80

5.00 5.00 Global Days XXX

93980 **Duplex scan of arterial inflow and venous outflow of penile vessels; complete study** ♂ S 80

5.10 5.10 Global Days XXX

93981 **follow-up or limited study** ♂ S 80

3.45 3.45 Global Days XXX

93982 **Noninvasive physiologic study of implanted wireless pressure sensor in aneurysmal sac following endovascular repair, complete study including recording, analysis of pressure and waveform tracings, interpretation and report** S 80

Do not report with (34806)

1.28 1.28 Global Days XXX

93990 **Duplex scan of hemodialysis access (including arterial inflow, body of access and venous outflow)** S 80

EXCLUDES *Hemodialysis access flow measurement by indicator method (90940)*

6.36 6.36 Global Days XXX

● 93998 **Unlisted noninvasive vascular diagnostic study** X 80

0.00 0.00 Global Days XXX

94002-94005 Ventilator Management Services

94002 **Ventilation assist and management, initiation of pressure or volume preset ventilators for assisted or controlled breathing; hospital inpatient/observation, initial day** 03 80

Do not report with (99201-99499 [99224, 99225, 99226])

2.69 2.69 Global Days XXX

AMA: 2009, Jan, 11-31; 2008, Jan, 10-25; 2007, Jul, 1-4; 2007, February, 10-11; 2007, April, 3-6; 2007, March, 9-11

94003 **hospital inpatient/observation, each subsequent day** 03 80

Do not report with (99201-99499 [99224, 99225, 99226])

1.93 1.93 Global Days XXX

AMA: 2007, Jul, 1-4; 2007, April, 3-6; 2007, February, 10-11

94004 **nursing facility, per day** B 80

Do not report with (99201-99499 [99224, 99225, 99226])

1.41 1.41 Global Days XXX

AMA: 2007, Jul, 1-4; 2007, February, 10-11; 2007, April, 3-6

94005 **Home ventilator management care plan oversight of a patient (patient not present) in home, domiciliary or rest home (eg, assisted living) requiring review of status, review of laboratories and other studies and revision of orders and respiratory care plan (as appropriate), within a calendar month, 30 minutes or more** M

Do not report with (99339-99340, 99374-99378)

2.68 2.68 Global Days XXX

AMA: 2009, Jan, 11-31; 2008, Jan, 10-25; 2007, Jul, 1-4; 2007, April, 3-6; 2007, March, 9-11

Medicine

93924 — 94005

94010-94799 Respiratory Services: Diagnostic and Therapeutic

INCLUDES Laboratory procedure(s)
Test results interpretation

EXCLUDES *Separate identifiable evaluation and management service (99201-99499 [99224, 99225, 99226])*

94010 Spirometry, including graphic record, total and timed vital capacity, expiratory flow rate measurement(s), with or without maximal voluntary ventilation

EXCLUDES *Diffusing capacity (94729)*

Do not report with (94150, 94200, 94375, 94728)

INCLUDES Measurement of expiratory airflow and volumes

1.06 1.06 Global Days XXX

AMA: 2009, Jan, 11-31; 2008, Jan, 10-25; 2008, Nov, 5-6; 2007, January, 13-27

⊙ **94011 Measurement of spirometric forced expiratory flows in an infant or child through 2 years of age**

2.95 2.95 Global Days XXX

⊙ **94012 Measurement of spirometric forced expiratory flows, before and after bronchodilator, in an infant or child through 2 years of age**

4.67 4.67 Global Days XXX

⊙ **94013 Measurement of lung volumes (ie, functional residual capacity [FRC], forced vital capacity [FVC], and expiratory reserve volume [ERV]) in an infant or child through 2 years of age**

0.97 0.97 Global Days XXX

94014 Patient-initiated spirometric recording per 30-day period of time; includes reinforced education, transmission of spirometric tracing, data capture, analysis of transmitted data, periodic recalibration and physician review and interpretation

1.39 1.39 Global Days XXX

AMA: 2008, Nov, 5-6

94015 recording (includes hook-up, reinforced education, data transmission, data capture, trend analysis, and periodic recalibration)

0.69 0.69 Global Days XXX

AMA: 2008, Nov, 5-6

94016 physician review and interpretation only

0.70 0.70 Global Days XXX

AMA: 2008, Nov, 5-6

94060 Bronchodilation responsiveness, spirometry as in 94010, pre- and post-bronchodilator administration

INCLUDES Spirometry performed prior to and after a brochodilator has been administered

EXCLUDES *Bronchospasm prolonged exercise test with pre- and post-spirometry (94620)*
Diffusing capacity (94729)

Code also bronchodilator supply with appropriate supply code or 99070

Do not report with (94150, 94200, 94375, 94728)

1.79 1.79 Global Days XXX

AMA: 2009, Jan, 11-31; 2008, Jan, 10-25; 2008, Nov, 5-6; 2007, January, 13-27

94070 Bronchospasm provocation evaluation, multiple spirometric determinations as in 94010, with administered agents (eg, antigen[s], cold air, methacholine)

EXCLUDES *Diffusing capacity (94729)*

Code also antigen(s) administration with appropriate supply code or 99070

1.79 1.79 Global Days XXX

AMA: 2008, Nov, 5-6

94150 Vital capacity, total (separate procedure)

EXCLUDES *Thoracic gas volumes (94726-94727)*

Do not report with (94010, 94060, 94728)

0.74 0.74 Global Days XXX

AMA: 2008, Nov, 5-6

94200 Maximum breathing capacity, maximal voluntary ventilation

Do not report with (94010, 94060)

0.74 0.74 Global Days XXX

AMA: 2009, Jan, 11-31; 2008, Jan, 10-25; 2008, Nov, 5-6; 2007, January, 13-27

~~94240 Functional residual capacity or residual volume: helium method, nitrogen open circuit method, or other method~~

To report, see 94726-94727

94250 Expired gas collection, quantitative, single procedure (separate procedure)

0.78 0.78 Global Days XXX

AMA: 2008, Nov, 5-6

~~94260 Thoracic gas volume~~

To report, see 94726-94727

~~94350 Determination of maldistribution of inspired gas: multiple breath nitrogen washout curve including alveolar nitrogen or helium equilibration time~~

To report, see 94726-94727

~~94360 Determination of resistance to airflow, oscillatory or plethysmographic methods~~

To report, see 94726, 94728

~~94370 Determination of airway closing volume, single breath tests~~

To report, see 94726-94727

94375 Respiratory flow volume loop

INCLUDES Identification of obstruction patterns in central or peripheral airways (inspiratory and/or expiratory)

EXCLUDES *Diffusing capacity (94729)*

Do not report with (94010, 94060, 94728)

1.15 1.15 Global Days XXX

AMA: 2008, Nov, 5-6; 2007, Jul, 1-4

94400 Breathing response to CO2 (CO2 response curve)

1.67 1.67 Global Days XXX

AMA: 2008, Nov, 5-6

94450 Breathing response to hypoxia (hypoxia response curve)

EXCLUDES *HAST - high altitude simulation test (94452, 94453)*

1.88 1.88 Global Days XXX

AMA: 2008, Nov, 5-6

94452 High altitude simulation test (HAST), with physician interpretation and report;

EXCLUDES *Obtaining arterial blood gases (36600)*

Do not report with (94453, 94760-94761)

1.71 1.71 Global Days XXX

AMA: 2008, Nov, 5-6

94453 with supplemental oxygen titration

EXCLUDES *Obtaining arterial blood gases (36600)*

Do not report with (94452, 94760-94761)

2.33 2.33 Global Days XXX

AMA: 2008, Nov, 5-6

⊘ **94610 Intrapulmonary surfactant administration by a physician through endotracheal tube**

INCLUDES Reporting once per dosing episode

EXCLUDES *Intubation, endotracheal (31500)*

Do not report with (99468-99472)

1.75 1.75 Global Days XXX

AMA: 2008, Jul, 7-8&15; 2008, Nov, 5-6; 2007, Jul, 1-4; 2007, April, 3-6

94620 Pulmonary stress testing; simple (eg, 6-minute walk test, prolonged exercise test for bronchospasm with pre- and post-spirometry and oximetry)

1.76 1.76 Global Days XXX

AMA: 2009, Jan, 11-31; 2008, Jan, 10-25; 2008, Nov, 5-6; 2007, January, 13-27; 2007, June, 10-11; 2007, April, 3-6

94621 complex (including measurements of CO2 production, O2 uptake, and electrocardiographic recordings)

4.81 4.81 Global Days XXX

AMA: 2009, Jan, 11-31; 2008, Jan, 10-25; 2008, Nov, 5-6; 2007, January, 13-27

94640 Pressurized or nonpressurized inhalation treatment for acute airway obstruction or for sputum induction for diagnostic purposes (eg, with an aerosol generator, nebulizer, metered dose inhaler or intermittent positive pressure breathing [IPPB] device)

EXCLUDES *1 hour or more of continuous inhalation treatment (94644, 94645)*

Code also modifier 76 when more than 1 inhalation treatment is performed on the same date

0.52 0.52 Global Days XXX

AMA: 2009, Jan, 11-31; 2008, Jan, 10-25; 2008, Nov, 5-6; 2007, January, 13-27; 2007, April, 3-6

94642 Aerosol inhalation of pentamidine for pneumocystis carinii pneumonia treatment or prophylaxis

0.00 0.00 Global Days XXX

AMA: 2008, Nov, 5-6

94644 Continuous inhalation treatment with aerosol medication for acute airway obstruction; first hour

EXCLUDES *Services that are less than 1 hour (94640)*

1.28 1.28 Global Days XXX

AMA: 2008, Nov, 5-6; 2007, April, 3-6

\+ **94645 each additional hour (List separately in addition to code for primary procedure)**

Code first initial hour (94644)

0.42 0.42 Global Days XXX

AMA: 2008, Nov, 5-6; 2007, April, 3-6

94660 Continuous positive airway pressure ventilation (CPAP), initiation and management

1.09 1.79 Global Days XXX

AMA: 2009, Jan, 11-31; 2008, Jan, 10-25; 2008, Nov, 5-6; 2007, Jul, 1-4; 2007, January, 13-27; 2007, February, 10-11

94662 Continuous negative pressure ventilation (CNP), initiation and management

1.06 1.06 Global Days XXX

AMA: 2009, Jan, 11-31; 2008, Jan, 10-25; 2008, Nov, 5-6; 2007, Jul, 1-4; 2007, February, 10-11; 2007, January, 13-27

94664 Demonstration and/or evaluation of patient utilization of an aerosol generator, nebulizer, metered dose inhaler or IPPB device

INCLUDES Reporting only one time per day of service

0.50 0.50 Global Days XXX

AMA: 2009, Jan, 11-31; 2008, Jan, 10-25; 2008, Nov, 5-6; 2007, January, 13-27

94667 Manipulation chest wall, such as cupping, percussing, and vibration to facilitate lung function; initial demonstration and/or evaluation

0.71 0.71 Global Days XXX

AMA: 2008, Nov, 5-6

94668 subsequent

0.70 0.70 Global Days XXX

AMA: 2008, Nov, 5-6

94680 Oxygen uptake, expired gas analysis; rest and exercise, direct, simple

1.75 1.75 Global Days XXX

AMA: 2008, Nov, 5-6

94681 including CO2 output, percentage oxygen extracted

1.59 1.59 Global Days XXX

AMA: 2008, Nov, 5-6

94690 rest, indirect (separate procedure)

EXCLUDES *Arterial puncture (36600)*

1.53 1.53 Global Days XXX

AMA: 2008, Nov, 5-6

~~94720 Carbon monoxide diffusing capacity (eg, single breath, steady state)~~

To report, see 94729

~~94725 Membrane diffusion capacity~~

To report, see 94729

● **94726 Plethysmography for determination of lung volumes and, when performed, airway resistance**

INCLUDES Airway resistance
Determination of:
Functional residual capacity
Residual volume
Total lung capacity

EXCLUDES *Bronchial provocation (94070)*
Diffusing capacity (94729)
Spirometry (94010, 94060)

Do not report with (94727-94728)

1.58 1.58 Global Days XXX

● **94727 Gas dilution or washout for determination of lung volumes and, when performed, distribution of ventilation and closing volumes**

EXCLUDES *Bronchial provocation (94070)*
Diffusing capacity (94729)
Spirometry (94010, 94060)

Do not report with (94726)

1.24 1.24 Global Days XXX

● **94728 Airway resistance by impulse oscillometry**

EXCLUDES *Diffusing capacity (94729)*
Gas dilution techniques

Do not report with (94010, 94060, 94070, 94375, 94726)

1.24 1.24 Global Days XXX

+ ● **94729** **Diffusing capacity (eg, carbon monoxide, membrane) (List separately in addition to code for primary procedure)** X 80

Code first (94010, 94060, 94070, 94375, 94726-94728)

1.57 1.57 Global Days ZZZ

94750 **Pulmonary compliance study (eg, plethysmography, volume and pressure measurements)** X 80

2.35 2.35 Global Days XXX

AMA: 2008, Nov, 5-6

94760 **Noninvasive ear or pulse oximetry for oxygen saturation; single determination** N TC 80

EXCLUDES *Blood gases (82803-82810)*

0.09 0.09 Global Days XXX

AMA: 2009, Jan, 11-31; 2008, Jan, 10-25; 2008, Nov, 5-6; 2007, Jul, 1-4; 2007, February, 10-11; 2007, January, 13-27; 2007, April, 1-2

94761 **multiple determinations (eg, during exercise)** N TC 80

0.14 0.14 Global Days XXX

AMA: 2009, Jan, 11-31; 2008, Jan, 10-25; 2008, Nov, 5-6; 2007, Jul, 1-4; 2007, January, 13-27; 2007, February, 10-11; 2007, June, 10-11; 2007, April, 1-2

94762 **by continuous overnight monitoring (separate procedure)** Q3 TC 80

0.45 0.45 Global Days XXX

AMA: 2008, Nov, 5-6; 2007, Jul, 1-4; 2007, April, 1-2; 2007, February, 10-11

94770 **Carbon dioxide, expired gas determination by infrared analyzer** X 80

EXCLUDES *Arterial catheterization/cannulation (36620)*
Arterial puncture (36600)
Bronchoscopy (31622-31656)
Flow directed catheter placement (93503)
Needle biopsy of the lung (32405)
Orotracheal/nasotracheal intubation (31500)
Placement of central venous catheter (36555-36556)
Therapeutic phlebotomy (99195)
Thoracentesis (32421)
Venipuncture (36410)

0.46 0.46 Global Days XXX

AMA: 2008, Nov, 5-6

94772 **Circadian respiratory pattern recording (pediatric pneumogram), 12-24 hour continuous recording, infant** A X 80

EXCLUDES *Separate procedure codes for electromyograms/EEG/ECG/respiration recordings*

0.00 0.00 Global Days XXX

AMA: 2008, Nov, 5-6

94774 **Pediatric home apnea monitoring event recording including respiratory rate, pattern and heart rate per 30-day period of time; includes monitor attachment, download of data, physician review, interpretation, and preparation of a report** B 80

INCLUDES Oxygen saturation monitoring

EXCLUDES *Sleep testing (95805-95811 [95800, 95801])*

Do not report with (93224-93272, 94775-94777)

0.00 0.00 Global Days YYY

AMA: 2008, Mar, 4-5; 2008, Nov, 5-6; 2007, April, 3-6

94775 **monitor attachment only (includes hook-up, initiation of recording and disconnection)** S TC 80

INCLUDES Oxygen saturation monitoring

EXCLUDES *Sleep testing (95805-95811 [95800, 95801])*

Do not report with 93224-93272

0.00 0.00 Global Days YYY

AMA: 2008, Mar, 4-5; 2008, Nov, 5-6; 2007, April, 3-6

94776 **monitoring, download of information, receipt of transmission(s) and analyses by computer only** S TC 80

INCLUDES Oxygen saturation monitoring

EXCLUDES *Sleep testing (95805-95811 [95800, 95801])*

Do not report with 93224-93272

0.00 0.00 Global Days YYY

AMA: 2008, Mar, 4-5; 2008, Nov, 5-6; 2007, April, 3-6

94777 **physician review, interpretation and preparation of report only** B 26 80

INCLUDES Oxygen saturation monitoring

EXCLUDES *Sleep testing (95805-95811 [95800, 95801])*

Do not report with (93224-93272)

0.00 0.00 Global Days YYY

AMA: 2008, Mar, 4-5; 2008, Nov, 5-6; 2007, April, 3-6

● **94780** **Car seat/bed testing for airway integrity, neonate, with continual nursing observation and continuous recording of pulse oximetry, heart rate and respiratory rate, with interpretation and report; 60 minutes** A X

Do not report for less than 60 minutes

Do not report with (99468-99472, 99477-99480, 93040-93042, 94760-94761)

0.69 1.49 Global Days XXX

+ ● **94781** **each additional full 30 minutes (List separately in addition to code for primary procedure)** A X

Code first (94780)

0.24 0.58 Global Days ZZZ

94799 **Unlisted pulmonary service or procedure** X 80

0.00 0.00 Global Days XXX

AMA: 2009, Jan, 11-31; 2008, Jan, 10-25; 2008, Nov, 5-6; 2007, January, 13-27

95004-95075 Allergy Tests

CMS 100-2,15,20.2 Physician Expense for Allergy Treatment
CMS 100-3,110.12 Challenge Ingestion Food Testing
CMS 100-3,110.13 Cytotoxic Food Tests
CMS 100-4,12,200 Allergy Testing and Immunotherapy

EXCLUDES *Intractable/severe allergic disease therapy (96365-96368, 96372, 96374-96375)*

Code also significant, separately identifiable E/M services using modifier 25

Do not report with codes for evaluation and management services when reporting test interpretation/report

95004 **Percutaneous tests (scratch, puncture, prick) with allergenic extracts, immediate type reaction, including test interpretation and report by a physician, specify number of tests** X 80

86000-86999

0.19 0.19 Global Days XXX

AMA: 2007, Dec, 9

95010 **Percutaneous tests (scratch, puncture, prick) sequential and incremental, with drugs, biologicals or venoms, immediate type reaction, including test interpretation and report by a physician, specify number of tests** X 80

86000-86999

0.16 0.36 Global Days XXX

95012 **Nitric oxide expired gas determination** X 80

86000-86999

0.60 0.60 Global Days XXX

AMA: 2009, Jan, 11-31; 2008, Jan, 10-25; 2007, April, 3-6; 2007, March, 9-11

95015 **Intracutaneous (intradermal) tests, sequential and incremental, with drugs, biologicals, or venoms, immediate type reaction, including test interpretation and report by a physician, specify number of tests** X 80

86000-86999

0.09 0.21 Global Days XXX

95024 **Intracutaneous (intradermal) tests with allergenic extracts, immediate type reaction, including test interpretation and report by a physician, specify number of tests** X 80

86000-86999

0.03 0.23 Global Days XXX

AMA: 2007, Dec, 9

95027 **Intracutaneous (intradermal) tests, sequential and incremental, with allergenic extracts for airborne allergens, immediate type reaction, including test interpretation and report by a physician, specify number of tests** X 80

86000-86999

0.15 0.15 Global Days XXX

AMA: 2009, Jan, 11-31; 2008, Jan, 10-25; 2007, January, 13-27; 2007, Dec, 9

95028 **Intracutaneous (intradermal) tests with allergenic extracts, delayed type reaction, including reading, specify number of tests** X TC 80

86000-86999

0.40 0.40 Global Days XXX

95044 **Patch or application test(s) (specify number of tests)** X 80

86000-86999

0.18 0.18 Global Days XXX

95052 **Photo patch test(s) (specify number of tests)** X 80

86000-86999

0.20 0.20 Global Days XXX

95056 **Photo tests** X 80

86000-86999

1.29 1.29 Global Days XXX

95060 **Ophthalmic mucous membrane tests** X TC 80

86000-86999

0.94 0.94 Global Days XXX

95065 **Direct nasal mucous membrane test** X TC 80

86000-86999

0.74 0.74 Global Days XXX

95070 **Inhalation bronchial challenge testing (not including necessary pulmonary function tests); with histamine, methacholine, or similar compounds** X TC 80

EXCLUDES *Pulmonary function tests (94060, 94070)*

86000-86999

1.01 1.01 Global Days XXX

95071 **with antigens or gases, specify** X TC 80

EXCLUDES *Pulmonary function tests (94060, 94070)*

86000-86999

2.00 2.00 Global Days XXX

95075 **Ingestion challenge test (sequential and incremental ingestion of test items, eg, food, drug or other substance such as metabisulfite)** X 80

86000-86999

1.36 1.85 Global Days XXX

AMA: 2009, Jan, 11-31; 2008, Jan, 10-25; 2007, January, 13-27

95115-95199 Allergy Immunotherapy

CMS 100-2,15,20.2 Physician Expense for Allergy Treatment
CMS 100-3,110.9 Antigens Prepared for Sublingual Administration
CMS 100-4,12,200 Allergy Testing and Immunotherapy

INCLUDES Allergen immunotherapy professional services

EXCLUDES *Bacterial/viral/fungal extracts skin testing (86485-86486, 95028)*
Special reports for allergy patients (99080)
The following procedures for testing (see Pathology/Immunology section or 95199):
Leukocyte histamine release (LHR)
Lymphocytic transformation test (LTT)
Mast cell degranulation test (MCDT)
Migration inhibitory factor test (MIF)
Nitroblue tetrazolium dye test (NTD)
Radioallergosorbent testing (RAST)
Rat mast cell technique (RMCT)
Transfer factor test (TFT)

Code also significantly separate identifiable evaluation and management services, if provided

95115 **Professional services for allergen immunotherapy not including provision of allergenic extracts; single injection** S 80

0.29 0.29 Global Days XXX

AMA: 2007, Dec, 9

95117 **2 or more injections** S 80

0.35 0.35 Global Days XXX

AMA: 2009, Jan, 11-31; 2008, Jan, 10-25; 2007, January, 13-27; 2007, Dec, 9

95120 **Professional services for allergen immunotherapy in prescribing physicians office or institution, including provision of allergenic extract; single injection** E

0.00 0.00 Global Days XXX

95125 **2 or more injections** E

0.00 0.00 Global Days XXX

AMA: 2009, Jan, 11-31; 2008, Jan, 10-25; 2007, January, 13-27

95130 **single stinging insect venom** E

0.00 0.00 Global Days XXX

AMA: 2009, Jan, 11-31; 2008, Jan, 10-25; 2007, January, 13-27

95131 **2 stinging insect venoms** E

0.00 0.00 Global Days XXX

AMA: 2009, Jan, 11-31; 2008, Jan, 10-25; 2007, January, 13-27

95132 **3 stinging insect venoms** E

0.00 0.00 Global Days XXX

AMA: 2009, Jan, 11-31; 2008, Jan, 10-25; 2007, January, 13-27

95133 **4 stinging insect venoms** E

0.00 0.00 Global Days XXX

AMA: 2009, Jan, 11-31; 2008, Jan, 10-25; 2007, January, 13-27

95134 **5 stinging insect venoms** E

0.00 0.00 Global Days XXX

AMA: 2009, Jan, 11-31; 2008, Jan, 10-25; 2007, January, 13-27

95144 **Professional services for the supervision of preparation and provision of antigens for allergen immunotherapy, single dose vial(s) (specify number of vials)** S 80

INCLUDES Single dose vial/single dose of antigen administered in one injection

0.09 0.37 Global Days XXX

AMA: 2009, Jan, 11-31; 2008, Jan, 10-25; 2007, January, 13-27

95145 **Professional services for the supervision of preparation and provision of antigens for allergen immunotherapy (specify number of doses); single stinging insect venom** S 80

0.09 0.60 Global Days XXX

AMA: 2009, Jan, 11-31; 2008, Jan, 10-25; 2007, January, 13-27

95146 **2 single stinging insect venoms** S 80

0.09 1.06 Global Days XXX

95147 **3 single stinging insect venoms** S 80

0.09 0.98 Global Days XXX

95148 **4 single stinging insect venoms** S 80

0.09 1.44 Global Days XXX

95149 **5 single stinging insect venoms** S 80

0.09 1.93 Global Days XXX

95165 **Professional services for the supervision of preparation and provision of antigens for allergen immunotherapy; single or multiple antigens (specify number of doses)** S 80

0.10 0.38 Global Days XXX

AMA: 2009, Jan, 11-31; 2008, Jan, 10-25; 2007, January, 13-27

95170 **whole body extract of biting insect or other arthropod (specify number of doses)** S 80

INCLUDES A dose which is the amount of antigen(s) administered in a single injection from a multiple dose vial

0.09 0.28 Global Days XXX

AMA: 2009, Jan, 11-31; 2008, Jan, 10-25; 2007, January, 13-27

95180 **Rapid desensitization procedure, each hour (eg, insulin, penicillin, equine serum)** X 80

2.99 3.99 Global Days XXX

95199 **Unlisted allergy/clinical immunologic service or procedure** X 80

0.00 0.00 Global Days XXX

95250-95251 Glucose Monitoring By Subcutaneous Device

Do not report with physiologic data collection/interpretation (99091)

95250 **Ambulatory continuous glucose monitoring of interstitial tissue fluid via a subcutaneous sensor for a minimum of 72 hours; sensor placement, hook-up, calibration of monitor, patient training, removal of sensor, and printout of recording** V TC 80

Do not report more than once per month

Do not report with (99091)

4.64 4.64 Global Days XXX

95251 **interpretation and report** B 26 80

Do not report more than once per month

Do not report with (99091)

1.23 1.23 Global Days XXX

95800-95811 [95800, 95801] Sleep Studies

CMS 100-2,6,50 Sleep Disorder Clinics

INCLUDES Assessment of sleep disorders in adults and children
- Continuous and simultaneous monitoring and recording of physiological sleep parameters of 6 hours or more
- Evaluation of patient's response to therapies
- Physician:
  - Interpretation
  - Recording
  - Report
- Recording sessions may be:
  - Attended studies that include the presence of a technologist or qualified health care professional to respond to the needs of the patient or technical issues at the bedside
  - Remote without the presence of a techologist or a qualified health professional
  - Unattended without the presence of a technologist or qualified health care professional
- Testing parameters include:
  - Actigraphy: Use of a noninvasive portable device to record gross motor movements to approximate periods of sleep and wakefulness
  - Electrooculogram (EOG): Records electrical activity associated with eye movements
  - Maintenance of wakefulness test (MWT): An attended study used to determine the patient's ability to stay awake
  - Multiple sleep latency test (MSLT): Attended study to determine the tendency of the patient to fall asleep
  - Peripheral arterial tonometry (PAT): Pulsatile volume changes in a digit are measured to determine activity in the sympathetic nervous system for respiratory analysis
  - Polysomnography: An attended continuous, simultaneous recording of physiological parameters of sleep for at least 6 hours in a sleep laboratory setting that also includes four or more of the following:
    1. Airflow-oral and/or nasal
    2. Bilateral anterior tibialis EMG
    3. Electrocardiogram (ECG)
    4. Oxyhemoglobin saturation, SpO2
    5. Respiratory effort
  - Positive airway pressure (PAP): Noninvasive devices used to treat sleep-related disorders
  - Respiratory airflow (ventilation): Assessment of air movement during inhalation and exhalation as measured by nasal pressure sensors and thermistor
  - Respiratory analysis: Assessment of components of respiration obtained by other methods such as airflow or peripheral arterial tone
  - Respiratory effort: Use of the diaphragm and/or intercostal muscle for airflow is measured using transducers to estimate thoracic and abdominal motion
  - Respiratory movement: Measures the movement of the chest and abdomen during respiration
  - Sleep latency: Pertains to the time it takes to get to sleep
  - Sleep staging: Determination of the separate levels of sleep according to physiological measurements
  - Total sleep time: Determined by the use of actigraphy and other methods
- Use of portable and in-laboratory technology

EXCLUDES *Consultation services (99241-99255)*

Evaluation and management services (99201-99499 [99224, 99225, 99226])

Code also modifier 52 for fewer than 6 hours of recording or other reduced services

95800 ***Resequenced code, See code following 95806.***

95801 ***Resequenced code. See code before 95807.***

95803 Actigraphy testing, recording, analysis, interpretation, and report (minimum of 72 hours to 14 consecutive days of recording)

Do not report more than once in any 14 day period

Do not report with (95806-95811 [95800, 95801])

4.86 4.86 Global Days XXX

95805 Multiple sleep latency or maintenance of wakefulness testing, recording, analysis and interpretation of physiological measurements of sleep during multiple trials to assess sleepiness

INCLUDES Physiological sleep parameters as measured by:
- Frontal, central, and occipital EEG leads (3 leads)
- Left and right EOG
- Submental EMG lead

EXCLUDES *Polysomnography (95808-95811)*
Sleep study, not attended (95806)

Code also modifer 52 when less than four nap opportunites are recorded

12.27 12.27 Global Days XXX

AMA: 2008, Mar, 4-5

95806 Sleep study, unattended, simultaneous recording of, heart rate, oxygen saturation, respiratory airflow, and respiratory effort (eg, thoracoabdominal movement)

EXCLUDES *Unattended sleep study with measurement of a minimum heart rate, oxygen saturation, and respiratory analysis ([95801])*
Unattended sleep study with measurement of heart rate, oxygen saturation, respiratory analysis, and sleep time ([95800])

Do not report with (93041-93229, 93268-93272, [95800, 95801])

5.40 5.40 Global Days XXX

AMA: 2009, Jan, 11-31; 2008, Jan, 10-25; 2008, Mar, 4-5; 2007, January, 13-27

\# **95800 Sleep study, unattended, simultaneous recording; heart rate, oxygen saturation, respiratory analysis (eg, by airflow or peripheral arterial tone), and sleep time**

EXCLUDES *Unattended sleep study measuring at minimum, heart rate, oxygen saturation, and respiratory analysis ([95801])*

Do not report with (93041-93229, 93268-93272, 95803, 95806, [95801])

4.73 4.73 Global Days XXX

\# **95801 minimum of heart rate, oxygen saturation, and respiratory analysis (eg, by airflow or peripheral arterial tone)**

EXCLUDES *Unattended sleep study measuring heart rate, oxygen saturation, respiratory analysis, and sleep time ([95800])*

Do not report with (93041-93229, 93268-93272, 95806, [95800])

2.54 2.54 Global Days XXX

95807 Sleep study, simultaneous recording of ventilation, respiratory effort, ECG or heart rate, and oxygen saturation, attended by a technologist

EXCLUDES *Polysomnography (95808-95811)*
Sleep study, not attended (95806)

14.64 14.64 Global Days XXX

AMA: 2008, Mar, 4-5

95808 Polysomnography; sleep staging with 1-3 additional parameters of sleep, attended by a technologist

EXCLUDES *Sleep study, not attended (95806)*

19.73 19.73 Global Days XXX

AMA: 2009, Jan, 11-31; 2008, Jan, 10-25; 2008, Mar, 4-5; 2007, January, 13-27

95810 sleep staging with 4 or more additional parameters of sleep, attended by a technologist

EXCLUDES *Sleep study, not attended (95806)*

19.47 19.47 Global Days XXX

AMA: 2008, Mar, 4-5

95811 sleep staging with 4 or more additional parameters of sleep, with initiation of continuous positive airway pressure therapy or bilevel ventilation, attended by a technologist

EXCLUDES *Sleep study, not attended (95806)*

20.76 20.76 Global Days XXX

AMA: 2008, Mar, 4-5

95812-95830 Evaluation of Brain Activity by Electroencephalogram

EXCLUDES *Clinical depression treatment by repetitive transcranial magnetic stimulation (90867-90868)*
Consultation services (99241-99255)
Evaluation and management services (99201-99499 [99224, 99225, 99226])

95812 Electroencephalogram (EEG) extended monitoring; 41-60 minutes

INCLUDES Hyperventilation
Only time when recording is taking place and data are being collected and does not include set-up and take-down
Photic stimulation
Physician interpretation
Recording of 41-60 minutes
Report

EXCLUDES *EEG digital analysis (95957)*
EEG during nonintracranial surgery (95955)
EEG monitoring, 24-hour (95950-95953, 95956)
Wada test (95958)

Code also modifier 26 for physician interpretation only

10.78 10.78 Global Days XXX

95813 greater than 1 hour

INCLUDES Hyperventilation
Only time when recording is taking place and data are being collected and does not include set-up and take-down
Photic stimulation
Physician interpretation
Recording of 61 minutes or more
Report

EXCLUDES *EEG digital analysis (95957)*
EEG during nonintracranial surgery (95955)
EEG monitoring, 24-hour (95950-95953, 95956)
Wada test (95958)

Code also modifier 26 for physician interpretation only

12.49 12.49 Global Days XXX

95816 **Electroencephalogram (EEG); including recording awake and drowsy** S 80

INCLUDES Photic stimulation
Physician interpretation
Recording of 20-40 minutes
Report

EXCLUDES *EEG digital analysis (95957)*
EEG during nonintracranial surgery (95955)
EEG monitoring, 24-hour (95950-95953, 95956)
Wada test (95958)

Code also modifier 26 for physician interpretation only
9.90 9.90 Global Days XXX
AMA: 2009, Jan, 11-31; 2008, Jan, 10-25; 2007, January, 13-27

95819 **including recording awake and asleep** S 80

INCLUDES Hyperventilation
Photic stimulation
Physician interpretation
Recording of 20-40 minutes
Report

EXCLUDES *EEG digital analysis (95957)*
EEG during nonintracranial surgery (95955)
EEG monitoring, 24-hour (95950-95953, 95956)
Wada test (95958)

Code also modifier 26 for interpretation only
11.24 11.24 Global Days XXX

95822 **recording in coma or sleep only** S 80

INCLUDES Hyperventilation
Photic stimulation
Physician interpretation
Recording of 20-40 minutes
Report

EXCLUDES *EEG digital analysis (95957)*
EEG during nonintracranial surgery (95955)
EEG monitoring, 24-hour (95950-95953, 95956)
Wada test (95958)

Code also modifier 26 for interpretation only
10.25 10.25 Global Days XXX

95824 **cerebral death evaluation only** S 80

INCLUDES Physician interpretation
Recording
Report

EXCLUDES *EEG digital analysis (95957)*
EEG during nonintracranial surgery (95955)
EEG monitoring, 24-hour (95950-95953, 95956)
Wada test (95958)

Code also modifier 26 for physician interpretation only
0.00 0.00 Global Days XXX

95827 **all night recording** S 80

INCLUDES Physician interpretation
Recording
Report

EXCLUDES *EEG digital analysis (95957)*
EEG during nonintracranial surgery (95955)
EEG monitoring, 24-hour (95950-95953, 95956)
Wada test (95958)

Code also modifier 26 for interpretation only
19.72 19.72 Global Days XXX

95829 **Electrocorticogram at surgery (separate procedure)** N 80

INCLUDES Physician interpretation
Recording
Report

Code also modifier 26 for interpretation only
49.13 49.13 Global Days XXX

95830 **Insertion by physician of sphenoidal electrodes for electroencephalographic (EEG) recording** B 80
2.54 5.91 Global Days XXX

95831-95857 Evaluation of Muscles and Range of Motion

EXCLUDES *Consultation services (99241-99255)*
Evaluation and management services (99201-99499 [99224, 99225, 99226])

95831 **Muscle testing, manual (separate procedure) with report; extremity (excluding hand) or trunk** A 80
0.43 0.83 Global Days XXX
AMA: 2009, Jan, 11-31; 2008, Jan, 10-25; 2008, May, 9-11; 2007, January, 13-27

95832 **hand, with or without comparison with normal side** A 80
0.45 0.78 Global Days XXX
AMA: 2009, Jan, 11-31; 2008, May, 9-11; 2008, Jan, 10-25; 2007, January, 13-27

95833 **total evaluation of body, excluding hands** A 80
0.63 1.09 Global Days XXX
AMA: 2008, May, 9-11

95834 **total evaluation of body, including hands** A 80
0.87 1.42 Global Days XXX
AMA: 2008, May, 9-11

95851 **Range of motion measurements and report (separate procedure); each extremity (excluding hand) or each trunk section (spine)** A 80
0.22 0.53 Global Days XXX
AMA: 2009, Jan, 11-31; 2008, Jan, 10-25; 2008, May, 9-11; 2007, January, 13-27; 2007, Dec, 10-179

95852 **hand, with or without comparison with normal side** A 80
0.17 0.47 Global Days XXX
AMA: 2008, May, 9-11

95857 **Cholinesterase inhibitor challenge test for myasthenia gravis** S 80
0.83 1.48 Global Days XXX

95860-95920 [95885, 95886, 95887] Evaluation of Nerve and Muscle Function: Electromyography/Nerve Conduction Studies

CMS 100-2,15,80 Diagnostic Test Requirements
CMS 100-3,160.10 Evoked Response Tests

INCLUDES Physician interpretation
Recording
Report

EXCLUDES *Consultation services (99241-99255)*
Evaluation and management services (99201-99499 [99224, 99225, 99226])

Code also EMG services performed with nerve conduction studies ([95885, 95886, 95887])

Do not report with nerve conduction studies on the same date of service (95860-95864, 95867-95870)

95860 Needle electromyography; 1 extremity with or without related paraspinal areas
INCLUDES Testing of five or more muscles per extremity
EXCLUDES *Dynamic electromyography during motion analysis studies (96002-96003)*
Do not report with (95873, 95874, 96000-96004)
2.82 2.82 Global Days XXX
AMA: 2009, Jan, 11-31; 2009, Jan, 7-8; 2008, Jan, 10-25; 2007, January, 13-27

95861 2 extremities with or without related paraspinal areas
INCLUDES Testing of five or more muscles per extremity
EXCLUDES *Dynamic electromyography during motion analysis studies (96002-96003)*
Do not report with (95873, 95874, 96000-96004)
4.10 4.10 Global Days XXX
AMA: 2009, Jan, 7-8; 2009, Jan, 11-31; 2008, Jan, 10-25; 2007, January, 13-27

95863 3 extremities with or without related paraspinal areas
INCLUDES Testing of five or more muscles per extremity
Do not report with (95873-95874, 96000-96004)
4.96 4.96 Global Days XXX
AMA: 2009, Jan, 11-31; 2009, Jan, 7-8; 2008, Jan, 10-25; 2007, January, 13-27

95864 4 extremities with or without related paraspinal areas
INCLUDES Testing of five or more muscles per extremity
Do not report with (95873-95874, 96000-96004)
5.37 5.37 Global Days XXX
AMA: 2009, Jan, 11-31; 2009, Jan, 7-8; 2008, Jan, 10-25; 2007, January, 13-27

95865 larynx
Code also modifier 52 for unilateral procedure
Do not report with (95873-95874, 96000-96004)
3.65 3.65 Global Days XXX
AMA: 2009, Jan, 11-31; 2009, Jan, 7-8; 2008, Jan, 10-25; 2007, Dec, 10-179; 2007, January, 13-27

95866 hemidiaphragm
Do not report with (95873-95874, 96000-96004)
3.27 3.27 Global Days XXX
AMA: 2009, Jan, 7-8; 2009, Jan, 11-31; 2008, Jan, 10-25; 2007, January, 13-27

95867 cranial nerve supplied muscle(s), unilateral
Do not report with (95873-95874, 96000-96004)
2.69 2.69 Global Days XXX
AMA: 2009, Jan, 11-31; 2009, Jan, 7-8; 2008, Jan, 10-25; 2007, Dec, 10-179; 2007, January, 13-27

95868 cranial nerve supplied muscles, bilateral
Do not report with (95873-95874, 96000-96004)
3.60 3.60 Global Days XXX
AMA: 2009, Jan, 11-31; 2009, Jan, 7-8; 2008, Jan, 10-25; 2007, January, 13-27; 2007, Dec, 10-179

95869 thoracic paraspinal muscles (excluding T1 or T12)
Do not report with (95873-95874, 96000-96004)
2.00 2.00 Global Days XXX
AMA: 2009, Jan, 11-31; 2009, Jan, 7-8; 2008, Jan, 10-25; 2007, January, 13-27

95870 limited study of muscles in 1 extremity or non-limb (axial) muscles (unilateral or bilateral), other than thoracic paraspinal, cranial nerve supplied muscles, or sphincters
INCLUDES Adson test
Testing of four or less muscles per extremity
EXCLUDES *Anal/urethral sphincter/detrusor/urethra/perineum musculature (51785-51792)*
Complete study of extremities (95860-95864)
Eye muscles (92265)
Do not report with (95873-95874, 96000-96004)
1.92 1.92 Global Days XXX
AMA: 2009, Jan, 11-31; 2009, Jan, 7-8; 2008, Jan, 10-25; 2007, January, 13-27

95872 Needle electromyography using single fiber electrode, with quantitative measurement of jitter, blocking and/or fiber density, any/all sites of each muscle studied
Do not report with motion analysis (96000-96004)
5.44 5.44 Global Days XXX
AMA: 2009, Jan, 11-31; 2009, Jan, 7-8; 2008, Jan, 10-25; 2007, January, 13-27

+ #● **95885 Needle electromyography, each extremity, with related paraspinal areas, when performed, done with nerve conduction, amplitude and latency/velocity study; limited (List separately in addition to code for primary procedure)**
INCLUDES Testing of four or less muscles per extremity
Code also complete needle electromyography test when all 4 extremities are tested ([95886])
Code first nerve conduction tests (95900-95904)
Do not report more than one time per extremity
Do not report with (95860-95864, 95870, 95905)
1.64 1.64 Global Days ZZZ

+ #● **95886 complete, 5 or more muscles studied, innervated by 3 or more nerves or 4 or more spinal levels (List separately in addition to code for primary procedure)**
INCLUDES Testing of five or more muscles in an extremity
Code also needle electromyography, limited, when all four extremities are tested ([95885])
Code first nerve conduction tests (95900-95904)
Do not report more than one time per extremity
Do not report with (95860-95864, 95870, 95905)
2.57 2.57 Global Days ZZZ

\+ #● **95887 Needle electromyography, non-extremity (cranial nerve supplied or axial) muscle(s) done with nerve conduction, amplitude and latency/velocity study (List separately in addition to code for primary procedure)** S 80

Code first nerve conduction tests (95900-95904)

Do not report with (95867-95870, 95905)

Facility RVU 2.29 Non-Facility RVU 2.29 Global Days ZZZ

\+ **95873 Electrical stimulation for guidance in conjunction with chemodenervation (List separately in addition to code for primary procedure)** N 80

Code first chemodenervation (64612-64614)

Do not report with (95860-95870, 95874, 96000-96004)

Facility RVU 1.96 Non-Facility RVU 1.96 Global Days ZZZ

AMA: 2009, Jan, 11-31; 2009, Jan, 7-8; 2008, Jan, 10-25; 2007, January, 13-27

\+ **95874 Needle electromyography for guidance in conjunction with chemodenervation (List separately in addition to code for primary procedure)** N 80

Code first chemodenervation (64612-64614)

Do not report with (95860-95870, 95873, 96000-96004)

Facility RVU 1.86 Non-Facility RVU 1.86 Global Days ZZZ

AMA: 2009, Jan, 11-31; 2009, Jan, 7-8; 2009, Jun, 10-11; 2008, Jan, 10-25; 2007, January, 13-27

95875 Ischemic limb exercise test with serial specimen(s) acquisition for muscle(s) metabolite(s) S 80

Do not report with (96000-96004)

Facility RVU 3.28 Non-Facility RVU 3.28 Global Days XXX

AMA: 2009, Jan, 11-31; 2008, Jan, 10-25; 2007, January, 13-27

95885 *Resequenced Code. See code following 95872.*

95886 *Resequenced Code. See code following 95872.*

95887 *Resequenced Code. See code before 95873.*

⊘ **95900 Nerve conduction, amplitude and latency/velocity study, each nerve; motor, without F-wave study** S 80

INCLUDES Reporting this service only once when multiple sites on the same nerve are stimulated/recorded

Facility RVU 1.89 Non-Facility RVU 1.89 Global Days XXX

AMA: 2009, Jan, 11-31; 2008, Jan, 10-25; 2008, Feb, 2; 2008, Feb, 1; 2007, January, 13-27

⊘ **95903 motor, with F-wave study** S 80

INCLUDES Reporting this service only once when multiple sites on the same nerve are stimulated/recorded

Facility RVU 2.21 Non-Facility RVU 2.21 Global Days XXX

AMA: 2009, Jan, 11-31; 2008, Jan, 10-25; 2008, Feb, 2; 2008, Feb, 1; 2007, January, 13-27

⊘ **95904 sensory** S 80

INCLUDES Reporting this service only once when multiple sites on the same nerve are stimulated/recorded

Facility RVU 1.67 Non-Facility RVU 1.67 Global Days XXX

AMA: 2009, Jan, 11-31; 2008, Jan, 10-25; 2008, Feb, 2; 2008, Feb, 1; 2007, Jul, 12-13; 2007, January, 13-27

⊘ **95905 Motor and/or sensory nerve conduction, using preconfigured electrode array(s), amplitude and latency/velocity study, each limb, includes F-wave study when performed, with interpretation and report** S 80

INCLUDES Reporting this code only once for each limb studied

Study with preconfigured electrodes that are customized to a specific body location

Do not report with ([95885, 95886], 95900-95904, 95934-95936)

Facility RVU 1.98 Non-Facility RVU 1.98 Global Days XXX

\+ **95920 Intraoperative neurophysiology testing, per hour (List separately in addition to code for primary procedure)** N 80

INCLUDES Only time when recording is taking place and data are being collected and does not include set-up and take-down

EXCLUDES *Baseline electrophysiologic study(s) (95860-95861, 95867-95868, 95870, 95900, 95904, 95928-95929)*

Electrocorticography (95829)

Interpretation of specific types of electrophysiologic procedures (92585, 95822, 95870, 95925-95930 [95938, 95939])

Intraoperative:

EEG during nonintracranial surgery (95955)

Functional cortical/subcortical mapping (95961-95962)

Neurostimulator programming/analysis (95970-95975)

Stand-by time prior to monitoring (99360)

Code also services that last past midnight using the date the service started and using the total number of hours of monitoring

Code first (92585, 95822, 95860-95861, 95867-95868, 95870, 95900, 95904, 95925-95930 [95938, 95939], 95933-95937)

Do not report this service when recording is 30 minutes or less

Facility RVU 4.89 Non-Facility RVU 4.89 Global Days ZZZ

AMA: 2009, Jan, 11-31; 2008, Jan, 10-25; 2007, January, 13-27

95921-95923 Evaluation of Autonomic Nervous System

INCLUDES Physician interpretation

Recording

Report

95921 Testing of autonomic nervous system function; cardiovagal innervation (parasympathetic function), including 2 or more of the following: heart rate response to deep breathing with recorded R-R interval, Valsalva ratio, and 30:15 ratio S 80

Facility RVU 2.47 Non-Facility RVU 2.47 Global Days XXX

AMA: 2009, Jan, 11-31; 2008, Jan, 10-25; 2007, January, 13-27

95922 vasomotor adrenergic innervation (sympathetic adrenergic function), including beat-to-beat blood pressure and R-R interval changes during Valsalva maneuver and at least 5 minutes of passive tilt S 80

Facility RVU 3.10 Non-Facility RVU 3.10 Global Days XXX

AMA: 2009, Jan, 11-31; 2008, Jan, 10-25; 2007, January, 13-27

95923 sudomotor, including 1 or more of the following: quantitative sudomotor axon reflex test (QSART), silastic sweat imprint, thermoregulatory sweat test, and changes in sympathetic skin potential S 80

Facility RVU 4.64 Non-Facility RVU 4.64 Global Days XXX

AMA: 2009, Jan, 11-31; 2008, Jan, 10-25; 2007, January, 13-27

95925-95939 [95938, 95939] Neurotransmission Studies

95925 **Short-latency somatosensory evoked potential study, stimulation of any/all peripheral nerves or skin sites, recording from the central nervous system; in upper limbs** S 80

EXCLUDES *Auditory evoked potentials (92585)*

Do not report with (95926)

4.89 4.89 Global Days XXX

95926 **in lower limbs** S 80

EXCLUDES *Auditory evoked potentials (92585)*

Code also modifier 52 for unilateral test

Do not report with (95925)

4.74 4.74 Global Days XXX

AMA: 2009, Jan, 11-31; 2008, Jan, 10-25; 2007, January, 13-27

#● 95938 **in upper and lower limbs** S 80

Do not report with (95925-95926)

8.69 8.69 Global Days XXX

95927 **in the trunk or head** S 80

EXCLUDES *Auditory evoked potentials (92585)*

Code also modifier 52 for unilateral test

4.80 4.80 Global Days XXX

95928 **Central motor evoked potential study (transcranial motor stimulation); upper limbs** S 80

Do not report with (95929)

7.49 7.49 Global Days XXX

95929 **lower limbs** S 80

Do not report with (95928)

7.61 7.61 Global Days XXX

#● 95939 **in upper and lower limbs** S 80

Do not report with (95928-95929)

13.60 13.60 Global Days XXX

95930 **Visual evoked potential (VEP) testing central nervous system, checkerboard or flash** S 80

4.44 4.44 Global Days XXX

95933 **Orbicularis oculi (blink) reflex, by electrodiagnostic testing** S 80

2.38 2.38 Global Days XXX

95934 **H-reflex, amplitude and latency study; record gastrocnemius/soleus muscle** S 80 50

1.81 1.81 Global Days XXX

AMA: 2009, Jan, 11-31; 2008, Jan, 10-25; 2007, January, 13-27

95936 **record muscle other than gastrocnemius/soleus muscle** S 80 50

1.46 1.46 Global Days XXX

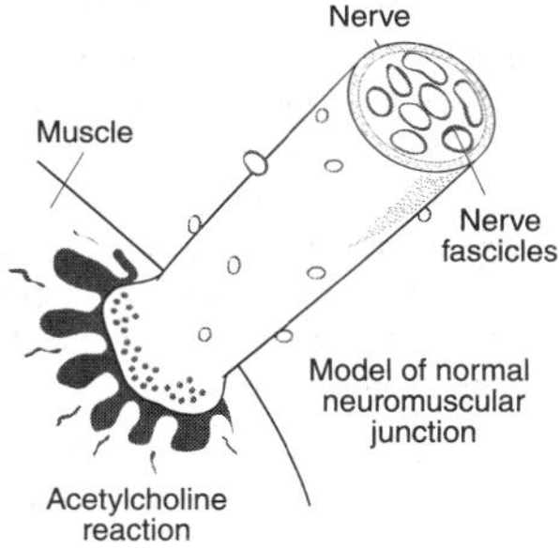

A selected neuromuscular junction is repeatedly stimulated. The test is useful to demonstrate reduced muscle action potential from fatique

95937 **Neuromuscular junction testing (repetitive stimulation, paired stimuli), each nerve, any 1 method** S 80

2.04 2.04 Global Days XXX

95938 *Resequenced Code. See code following 95926.*

95939 *Resequenced Code. See code following 95929.*

95950-95962 Electroencephalography For Seizure Monitoring/Intraoperative Use

EXCLUDES *Consultation services (99241-99255)*
Evaluation and management services (99201-99499 [99224, 99225, 99226])

95950 **Monitoring for identification and lateralization of cerebral seizure focus, electroencephalographic (eg, 8 channel EEG) recording and interpretation, each 24 hours** S 80

INCLUDES Only time when recording is taking place and data are being collected and does not include set-up and take-down
Recording for more than 12 hours up to 24 hours

Code also modifier 52 only when recording is 12 hours or less

Do not report more than once per 24 hours

8.76 8.76 Global Days XXX

95951 **Monitoring for localization of cerebral seizure focus by cable or radio, 16 or more channel telemetry, combined electroencephalographic (EEG) and video recording and interpretation (eg, for presurgical localization), each 24 hours** S 80

INCLUDES Interpretations during recording with changes to care of patient
Only time when recording is taking place and data are being collected and does not include set-up and take-down
Recording for more than 12 hours up to 24 hours

Code also modifier 52 only when recording is 12 hours or less

Do not report more than once per 24 hours

0.00 0.00 Global Days XXX

AMA: 2009, Jan, 11-31; 2008, Jan, 10-25; 2007, January, 13-27

95953 **Monitoring for localization of cerebral seizure focus by computerized portable 16 or more channel EEG, electroencephalographic (EEG) recording and interpretation, each 24 hours, unattended** S 80

INCLUDES Only time when recording is taking place and data are being collected and does not include set-up and take-down
Recording for more than 12 hours up to 24 hours

Code also modifier 52 only when recording is 12 hours or less

Do not report more than once per 24 hours

12.62 12.62 Global Days XXX

95954 **Pharmacological or physical activation requiring physician attendance during EEG recording of activation phase (eg, thiopental activation test)** S 80

11.92 11.92 Global Days XXX

95955 **Electroencephalogram (EEG) during nonintracranial surgery (eg, carotid surgery)** N 80

5.70 5.70 Global Days XXX

95956 **Monitoring for localization of cerebral seizure focus by cable or radio, 16 or more channel telemetry, electroencephalographic (EEG) recording and interpretation, each 24 hours, attended by a technologist or nurse** S 80

INCLUDES Only time when recording is taking place and data are being collected and does not include set-up and take-down

Recording for more than 12 hours up to 24 hours

Code also modifier 52 only when recording is 12 hours or less

Do not report more than once per 24 hours

34.64 34.64 Global Days XXX

95957 **Digital analysis of electroencephalogram (EEG) (eg, for epileptic spike analysis)** N 80

11.36 11.36 Global Days XXX

95958 **Wada activation test for hemispheric function, including electroencephalographic (EEG) monitoring** S 80

14.55 14.55 Global Days XXX

95961 **Functional cortical and subcortical mapping by stimulation and/or recording of electrodes on brain surface, or of depth electrodes, to provoke seizures or identify vital brain structures; initial hour of physician attendance** S 80

INCLUDES One hour of physician attendance

Code also each additional hour of physician attendance, when appropriate (95962)

Code also modifier 52 for 30 minutes or less of physician attendance

7.96 7.96 Global Days XXX

\+ **95962** **each additional hour of physician attendance (List separately in addition to code for primary procedure)** S 80

Code first initial hour (95961)

6.94 6.94 Global Days ZZZ

95965-95967 Magnetoencephalography

INCLUDES Physician interpretation

Recording

Report

EXCLUDES *Consultation services (99241-99255)*

CT provided along with magnetoencephalography (70450-70470, 70496)

Electroencephalography provided along with magnetoencephalography (95812-95827)

Evaluation and management services (99201-99499 [99224, 99225, 99226])

MRI provided along with magnetoencephalography (70551-70553)

Somatosensory evoked potentials/auditory evoked potentials/visual evoked potentials provided along with magnetic evoked field responses (92585, 95925, 95926, 95930)

95965 **Magnetoencephalography (MEG), recording and analysis; for spontaneous brain magnetic activity (eg, epileptic cerebral cortex localization)** S 80

0.00 0.00 Global Days XXX

95966 **for evoked magnetic fields, single modality (eg, sensory, motor, language, or visual cortex localization)** S 80

0.00 0.00 Global Days XXX

\+ **95967** **for evoked magnetic fields, each additional modality (eg, sensory, motor, language, or visual cortex localization) (List separately in addition to code for primary procedure)** S 80

Code first single modality (95966)

0.00 0.00 Global Days ZZZ

95970-95982 Evaluation of Implanted Neurostimulator

CMS 100-3,160.12 Neuromuscular Electrical Stimulation (NMES)

CMS 100-3,160.13 Supplies Used for Transcutaneous Electrical Nerve Stimulation and Neuromuscular Electrical Stimulation (NMES)

CMS 100-4,32,50 Deep Brain Stimulation for Essential Tremor and Parkinson's Disease

INCLUDES Simple intraoperative or subsequent programming of neurostimulator (three or less of the following); or complex neurostimulator (three or more of the following):

8 or more electrode contacts

Alternating electrode polarities

Cycling

Dose time

More than 1 clinical feature

Number of channels

Number of programs

Pulse amplitude

Pulse duration

Pulse frequency

Rate

Stimulation train duration

Train spacing

EXCLUDES *Consultation services (99241-99255)*

Electronic analysis and reprogramming of peripheral subcutaneous field stimulation pulse generator (0285T)

Evaluation and management services (99201-99499 [99224, 99225, 99226])

Neurostimulator electrodes:

Implantation (43647, 43881, 61850-61875, 63650-63655, 64553-64580)

Revision/removal (43648, 43882, 61880, 63661-63664, 64585)

Neurostimulator pulse generator/receiver:

Insertion (61885, 63685, 64590)

Revision/removal (61888, 63688, 64595)

▲ **95970** **Electronic analysis of implanted neurostimulator pulse generator system (eg, rate, pulse amplitude, pulse duration, configuration of wave form, battery status, electrode selectability, output modulation, cycling, impedance and patient compliance measurements); simple or complex brain, spinal cord, or peripheral (ie, cranial nerve, peripheral nerve, sacral nerve, neuromuscular) neurostimulator pulse generator/transmitter, without reprogramming** S 80

0.68 1.87 Global Days XXX

AMA: 2009, Jan, 11-31; 2008, Jan, 10-25; 2007, January, 13-27

▲ **95971** **simple spinal cord, or peripheral (ie, peripheral nerve, sacral nerve, neuromuscular) neurostimulator pulse generator/transmitter, with intraoperative or subsequent programming** S 80

1.17 1.69 Global Days XXX

▲ **95972** **complex spinal cord, or peripheral (ie, peripheral nerve, sacral nerve, neuromuscular) (except cranial nerve) neurostimulator pulse generator/transmitter, with intraoperative or subsequent programming, first hour** S 80

Code also modifier 52 for service less than 31 minutes

2.28 3.18 Global Days XXX

+ ▲ **95973** **complex spinal cord, or peripheral (ie, peripheral nerve, sacral nerve, neuromuscular) (except cranial nerve) neurostimulator pulse generator/transmitter, with intraoperative or subsequent programming, each additional 30 minutes after first hour (List separately in addition to code for primary procedure)** S 80

Code first initial hour (95972)

1.41 1.82 Global Days ZZZ

▲ **95974** **complex cranial nerve neurostimulator pulse generator/transmitter, with intraoperative or subsequent programming, with or without nerve interface testing, first hour** S 80

Code also modifier 52 for service less than 31 minutes

4.52 5.59 Global Days XXX

AMA: 2009, Jan, 11-31; 2008, Jan, 10-25; 2007, January, 13-27

+ ▲ **95975** **complex cranial nerve neurostimulator pulse generator/transmitter, with intraoperative or subsequent programming, each additional 30 minutes after first hour (List separately in addition to code for primary procedure)** S 80

Code first initial hour (95974)

2.56 3.01 Global Days ZZZ

AMA: 2009, Jan, 11-31; 2008, Jan, 10-25; 2007, January, 13-27

95978 **Electronic analysis of implanted neurostimulator pulse generator system (eg, rate, pulse amplitude and duration, battery status, electrode selectability and polarity, impedance and patient compliance measurements), complex deep brain neurostimulator pulse generator/transmitter, with initial or subsequent programming; first hour** S 80

Code also modifier 52 for service less than 31 minutes

5.41 6.79 Global Days XXX

+ **95979** **each additional 30 minutes after first hour (List separately in addition to code for primary procedure)** S 80

Code first initial hour (95978)

2.50 2.94 Global Days ZZZ

95980 **Electronic analysis of implanted neurostimulator pulse generator system (eg, rate, pulse amplitude and duration, configuration of wave form, battery status, electrode selectability, output modulation, cycling, impedance and patient measurements) gastric neurostimulator pulse generator/transmitter; intraoperative, with programming** N 80

INCLUDES Gastric neurostimulator of lesser curvature (95980-95982)

1.34 1.34 Global Days XXX

AMA: 2008, Jan, 8-9

95981 **subsequent, without reprogramming** S 80

0.51 0.94 Global Days XXX

AMA: 2008, Jan, 8-9

95982 **subsequent, with reprogramming** S 80

1.03 1.49 Global Days XXX

AMA: 2008, Jan, 8-9

95990-95991 Refill/Upkeep of Implanted Drug Delivery Pump to Central Nervous System

CMS 100-3,280.14 Infusion Pumps

EXCLUDES *Analysis/reprogramming of implanted pump for infusion (62367-62370)*
Consultation services (99241-99255)
Evaluation and management services (99201-99499 [99224, 99225, 99226])

Do not report with (62367-62370)

▲ **95990** **Refilling and maintenance of implantable pump or reservoir for drug delivery, spinal (intrathecal, epidural) or brain (intraventricular), includes electronic analysis of pump, when performed;** S 80

2.52 2.52 Global Days XXX

AMA: 2009, Jan, 11-31; 2008, Jan, 10-25; 2007, January, 13-27

▲ **95991** **requiring physician's skill** S 80

1.14 3.42 Global Days XXX

95992-95999 Other and Unlisted Neurological Procedures

⊘ **95992** **Canalith repositioning procedure(s) (eg, Epley maneuver, Semont maneuver), per day** A 80

Do not report with (92531-92532)

1.11 1.24 Global Days XXX

AMA: 2009, Jan, 3,4&9

95999 **Unlisted neurological or neuromuscular diagnostic procedure** S 80

0.00 0.00 Global Days XXX

AMA: 2009, Jan, 11-31; 2008, Jan, 10-25; 2007, January, 13-27; 2007, March, 4-5; 2007, April, 7-10

96000-96004 Motion Analysis Studies

CMS 100-2,15,80 Diagnostic Test Requirements

CMS 100-2,15,230.4 Services By a Physical/Occupational Therapist in Private Practice

INCLUDES Services provided as part of major therapeutic/diagnostic decision making
Services provided in a dedicated motion analysis department capable of:
3-D kinetics/dynamic electromyography
Computerized 3-D kinematics
Videotaping from the front/back/both sides

EXCLUDES *Consultation services (99241-99255)*
Evaluation and management services (99201-99499 [99224, 99225, 99226])
Gait training (97116)
Needle electromyography (95860-95875 [95885, 95886, 95887])

96000 **Comprehensive computer-based motion analysis by video-taping and 3D kinematics;** S 80

2.80 2.80 Global Days XXX

AMA: 2007, May, 3-4

96001 **with dynamic plantar pressure measurements during walking** S 80

2.89 2.89 Global Days XXX

96002 **Dynamic surface electromyography, during walking or other functional activities, 1-12 muscles** S 80

Do not report with (95860-95864, 95869-95872)

0.62 0.62 Global Days XXX

96003 **Dynamic fine wire electromyography, during walking or other functional activities, 1 muscle** S 80

Do not report with (95860-95864, 95869-95872)

0.55 0.55 Global Days XXX

● New Code ▲ Revised Code 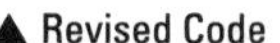 Maternity 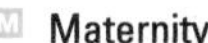 Age 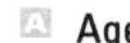 Unlisted 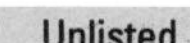 Not Covered 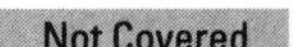 # Resequenced 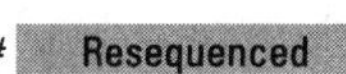
○ Reinstated CCI + Add-on ⊘ Mod 51 Exempt Mod 63 Exempt Mod Sedation PQRS

96004 **Physician review and interpretation of comprehensive computer-based motion analysis, dynamic plantar pressure measurements, dynamic surface electromyography during walking or other functional activities, and dynamic fine wire electromyography, with written report** B 26 80

3.27 3.27 Global Days XXX

96020 Neurofunctional Brain Testing

96020 **Neurofunctional testing selection and administration during noninvasive imaging functional brain mapping, with test administered entirely by a physician or psychologist, with review of test results and report** N 80

INCLUDES Selection/administration of testing of:
- Cognition
- Determination of validity of neurofunctional testing relative to separately interpreted functional magnetic resonance images
- Functional neuroimaging
- Language
- Memory
- Monitoring performance of testing
- Movement
- Other neurological functions
- Sensation

EXCLUDES *Clinical depression treatment by repetitive transcranial magnetic stimulation (90867-90868)*
Consultation services (99241-99255)

Do not report with (99201-99499 [99224, 99225, 99226], 70554, 96101-96103, 96116-96120)

70555

0.00 0.00 Global Days XXX

AMA: 2007, February, 6-7

96040 Genetic Counseling Services

INCLUDES
- Analysis for genetic risk assessment
- Counseling of patient/family
- Counseling services
- Face-to-face interviews
- Obtaining structured family genetic history
- Pedigree construction
- Review of medical data/family information
- Services provided by trained genetic counselor
- Services provided during one or more sessions
- Thirty minutes of face-to-face time and is reported one time for each 16-30 minutes of the service

EXCLUDES *Education/genetic counseling by a physician to a group (99078)*
Education/genetic counseling by a physician to an individual (99201-99499 [99224, 99225, 99226])
Education regarding genetic risks by a nonphysician to a group (98961, 98962)
Genetic counseling and/or risk factor reduction intervention from a physician, provided to patients without symptoms/diagnosis (99401-99412)

Do not report when 15 minutes or less of face-to-face time is provided

96040 **Medical genetics and genetic counseling services, each 30 minutes face-to-face with patient/family** B

INCLUDES
- Analysis for genetic risk assessment
- Counseling of patient/family
- Counseling services
- Face-to-face interviews
- Obtaining structured family genetic history
- Pedigree construction
- Review of medical data/family information
- Services provided by trained genetic counselor
- Services provided during one or more sessions

1.36 1.36 Global Days XXX

AMA: 2007, Aug, 9-12

96101-96125 Cognitive Capability Assessments

CMS 100-1,3,30 Outpatient Mental Health Treatment Limitation
CMS 100-1,3,30.1 Application of Mental Health Limitation - Status of Patient
CMS 100-1,3,30.2 Disorders Subject to Mental Health Limitation
CMS 100-2,15,80.2 Psychological and Neuropsychological Tests
CMS 100-2,15,160 Clinical Psychologist Services
CMS 100-4,12,150 Clinical Social Worker (CSW) Services
CMS 100-4,12,160 Independent Psychologist Services
CMS 100-4,12,170 Clinical Psychologist Services
CMS 100-4,12,170.1 Payment for Clinical Psychologist Services
CMS 100-4,12,210 Outpatient Mental Health Limitation

INCLUDES Cognitive function testing of the central nervous system

EXCLUDES *Cognitive skills development (97532, 97533)*
Physician conducted mini-mental status examination (99201-99499 [99224, 99225, 99226])

96101 Psychological testing (includes psychodiagnostic assessment of emotionality, intellectual abilities, personality and psychopathology, eg, MMPI, Rorschach, WAIS), per hour of the psychologist's or physician's time, both face-to-face time administering tests to the patient and time interpreting these test results and preparing the report 03 80

INCLUDES Situations when more time is needed to assimilate other clinical data sources including tests administered by a technician or computer and previously reported
Time spent face to face, interpretation, and preparing report

Do not report less than 31 minutes of time
2.24 2.40 Global Days XXX

96102 Psychological testing (includes psychodiagnostic assessment of emotionality, intellectual abilities, personality and psychopathology, eg, MMPI and WAIS), with qualified health care professional interpretation and report, administered by technician, per hour of technician time, face-to-face 03 80

Do not report less than 31 minutes of time
0.66 2.18 Global Days XXX

96103 Psychological testing (includes psychodiagnostic assessment of emotionality, intellectual abilities, personality and psychopathology, eg, MMPI), administered by a computer, with qualified health care professional interpretation and report 03 80
0.71 1.86 Global Days XXX

96105 Assessment of aphasia (includes assessment of expressive and receptive speech and language function, language comprehension, speech production ability, reading, spelling, writing, eg, by Boston Diagnostic Aphasia Examination) with interpretation and report, per hour A 80
2.99 2.99 Global Days XXX

▲ **96110 Developmental screening, with interpretation and report, per standardized instrument form** E
0.00 0.00 Global Days XXX

▲ **96111 Developmental testing, (includes assessment of motor, language, social, adaptive, and/or cognitive functioning by standardized developmental instruments) with interpretation and report** 03 80
3.49 3.65 Global Days XXX

96116 Neurobehavioral status exam (clinical assessment of thinking, reasoning and judgment, eg, acquired knowledge, attention, language, memory, planning and problem solving, and visual spatial abilities), per hour of the psychologist's or physician's time, both face-to-face time with the patient and time interpreting test results and preparing the report 03 80 PQ

Do not report less than 31 minutes of time

INCLUDES Time spent face to face, interpretation, and preparing report

2.45 2.62 Global Days XXX
AMA: 2009, Jan, 11-31; 2008, Jan, 10-25; 2007, January, 13-27

96118 Neuropsychological testing (eg, Halstead-Reitan Neuropsychological Battery, Wechsler Memory Scales and Wisconsin Card Sorting Test), per hour of the psychologist's or physician's time, both face-to-face time administering tests to the patient and time interpreting these test results and preparing the report 03 80

INCLUDES Situations when more time is needed to assimilate other clinical data sources including tests administered by a technician or computer and previously reported
Time spent face to face, interpretation, and preparing report

Do not report less than 31 minutes of time
2.22 2.73 Global Days XXX

96119 Neuropsychological testing (eg, Halstead-Reitan Neuropsychological Battery, Wechsler Memory Scales and Wisconsin Card Sorting Test), with qualified health care professional interpretation and report, administered by technician, per hour of technician time, face-to-face 03 80

Do not report less than 31 minutes of time
0.66 2.04 Global Days XXX

96120 Neuropsychological testing (eg, Wisconsin Card Sorting Test), administered by a computer, with qualified health care professional interpretation and report 03 80
0.71 2.60 Global Days XXX
AMA: 2009, Jan, 11-31; 2008, Jan, 10-25; 2007, January, 13-27

96125 Standardized cognitive performance testing (eg, Ross Information Processing Assessment) per hour of a qualified health care professional's time, both face-to-face time administering tests to the patient and time interpreting these test results and preparing the report A 80

INCLUDES Time spent face to face, interpretation, and preparing report

EXCLUDES *Psychological testing by a physician or psychologist (96101-96103)*

Do not report less than 31 minutes of time
2.91 2.91 Global Days XXX

96150-96155 Biopsychosocial Assessment/Intervention

INCLUDES Services for patients that have primary physical illnesses/diagnoses/symptoms who may benefit from assessments/interventions that focus on the biopsychosocial factors related to the patient's health status

Services used to identify the following factors which are important to the prevention/treatment/management of physical health problems:

- Behavioral
- Cognitive
- Emotional
- Psychological
- Social

EXCLUDES *Health and behavior assessment/intervention done by a physician (99201-99499 [99224, 99225, 99226])*

Preventive medicine counseling/risk factor reduction/behavioral change (99401-99412)

Do not report evaluation and management service codes on the same day
Do not report with (99401-99404, 99411-99412, 90801-90899)

96150 Health and behavior assessment (eg, health-focused clinical interview, behavioral observations, psychophysiological monitoring, health-oriented questionnaires), each 15 minutes face-to-face with the patient; initial assessment
0.59 0.60 Global Days XXX
AMA: 2009, Jan, 11-31; 2008, Jan, 10-25; 2007, January, 13-27

96151 re-assessment
0.57 0.58 Global Days XXX
AMA: 2009, Jan, 11-31; 2008, Jan, 10-25; 2007, January, 13-27

96152 Health and behavior intervention, each 15 minutes, face-to-face; individual
0.54 0.55 Global Days XXX
AMA: 2009, Jan, 11-31; 2008, Jan, 10-25; 2007, January, 13-27

96153 group (2 or more patients)
0.13 0.13 Global Days XXX
AMA: 2009, Jan, 11-31; 2008, Jan, 10-25; 2007, January, 13-27

96154 family (with the patient present)
0.53 0.54 Global Days XXX
AMA: 2009, Jan, 11-31; 2008, Jan, 10-25; 2007, January, 13-27

96155 family (without the patient present) E
0.65 0.66 Global Days XXX
AMA: 2009, Jan, 11-31; 2008, Jan, 10-25; 2007, January, 13-27

96360-96361 Intravenous Fluid Infusion for Hydration (Nonchemotherapy)

CMS 100-4,12,30.5 Payment for Injections and Infusions: Chemotherapy and Nonchemotherapy

INCLUDES Coding hierarchy rules for facility reporting only:

- Chemotherapy services are primary to diagnostic, prophylactic, and therapeutic services
- Diagnostic, prophylactic, and therapeutic services are primary to hydration services
- Infusions are primary to pushes
- Pushes are primary to injections

Direct physician supervision:

- Direction of personnel

Minimal supervision for:

- Consent
- Safety oversight
- Supervision of personnel

Physicians report the initial code for the primary reason for the visit regardless of the order in which the infusions or injections are given

Pre-packaged fluid/electrolytes

The following if done to facilitate the injection/infusion:

- Flush at the end of infusion
- Indwelling IV, subcutaneous catheter/port access
- Local anesthesia
- Start of IV
- Supplies/tubing/syringes

Treatment plan verification

EXCLUDES *Catheter/port declotting (36593)*

Drugs/other substances

Significant separately identifiable evaluation and management service if performed

Do not report a second initial service on the same date for accessing a multi-lumen catheter or restarting an IV, or when two IV lines are needed to meet an infusion rate
Do not report for physician services provided in facility settings
Do not report to keep the vein open or during other therapeutic infusions
Do not report with infusion for hydration that is 30 minutes or less

96360 Intravenous infusion, hydration; initial, 31 minutes to 1 hour S 80

Do not report hydration infusions of 31 minutes or less

Do not report if performed as a concurrent infusion

1.68 1.68 Global Days XXX
AMA: 2009, Feb, 17-21

+ **96361 each additional hour (List separately in addition to code for primary procedure)** S 80

INCLUDES Hydration infusion of more than 30 minutes beyond 1 hour

Hydration provided as a secondary or subsequent service after a different initial service via the same IV access site

Code first (96360)
0.45 0.45 Global Days ZZZ
AMA: 2009, May, 8-9&11; 2009, Feb, 17-21

96365-96371 Infusions: Diagnostic/Preventive/Therapeutic

CMS 100-4,12,30.5 Payment for Injections and Infusions: Chemotherapy and Nonchemotherapy
CMS 100-4,20,160.1 Billing for Total Parenteral Nutrition Furnished to Part B Inpatients

INCLUDES Administration of fluid
- Administration of substances/drugs
- An infusion of 15 minutes or less
- Coding heirarchy rules for facility reporting:
  - Chemotherapy services are primary to diagnostic, prophylactic, and therapeutic services
  - Diagnostic, prophylactic, and therapeutic services are primary to hydration services
  - Infusions are primary to pushes
  - Pushes are primary to injections
- Constant presence of health care professional administering the substance/drug
- Direct physician supervision:
  - Consent
  - Direction of personnel
  - Patient assessment
  - Safety oversight
  - Supervision of personnel
- The following if done to facilitate the injection/infusion:
  - Flush at the end of infusion
  - Indwelling IV, subcutaneous catheter/port access
  - Local anesthesia
  - Start of IV
  - Supplies/tubing/syringes
- Training to assess patient and monitor vital signs
- Training to prepare/dose/dispose
- Treatment plan verification

EXCLUDES *Catheter/port declotting (36593)*
Significant separately identifiable evaluation and management service if performed

Code also drugs/materials
Do not report a second initial service on the same date for accessing a multi-lumen catheter or restarting an IV, or when two IV lines are needed to meet an infusion rate
Do not report for physician services provided in facility settings
Do not report with codes for which IV push or infusion is an integral part of the procedure

96365 **Intravenous infusion, for therapy, prophylaxis, or diagnosis (specify substance or drug); initial, up to 1 hour** S 80
Code also second initial service with modifier 59 when patient's condition or drug protocol mandates the use of two IV lines
2.13 2.13 Global Days XXX
AMA: 2009, Feb, 17-21

+ **96366** **each additional hour (List separately in addition to code for primary procedure)** S 80
INCLUDES Additional hours of sequential infusion
Infusion intervals of more than 30 minutes beyond one hour
Second and subsequent infusions of the same drug or substance
Code first (96365)
0.63 0.63 Global Days ZZZ
AMA: 2009, Feb, 17-21

+ ▲ **96367** **additional sequential infusion of a new drug/substance, up to 1 hour (List separately in addition to code for primary procedure)** S 80
INCLUDES A secondary or subsequent service with a new drug or substance after a different initial service via the same IV access
Code first (96365, 96374, 96409, 96413)
Do not report more than once per sequential infusion of the same mix
0.95 0.95 Global Days ZZZ
AMA: 2009, Feb, 17-21

+ **96368** **concurrent infusion (List separately in addition to code for primary procedure)** N 80
Code first (96365, 96366, 96413, 96415, 96416)
Do not report more than one time per date of service
0.56 0.56 Global Days ZZZ
AMA: 2009, Feb, 17-21

96369 **Subcutaneous infusion for therapy or prophylaxis (specify substance or drug); initial, up to 1 hour, including pump set-up and establishment of subcutaneous infusion site(s)** S 80
EXCLUDES *Infusions of 15 minutes or less (96372)*
5.50 5.50 Global Days XXX
AMA: 2009, Feb, 17-21

+ **96370** **each additional hour (List separately in addition to code for primary procedure)** S 80
INCLUDES Infusions of more than 30 minutes beyond one hour
Code first (96369)
Do not report more than once per encounter
0.46 0.46 Global Days ZZZ
AMA: 2009, Feb, 17-21

+ **96371** **additional pump set-up with establishment of new subcutaneous infusion site(s) (List separately in addition to code for primary procedure)** S 80
Code first (96369)
Do not report more than once per encounter
2.53 2.53 Global Days ZZZ
AMA: 2009, Feb, 17-21

96372-96379 Injections: Diagnostic/Preventive/Therapeutic

CMS 100-4,12,30.5 Payment for Injections and Infusions: Chemotherapy and Nonchemotherapy

INCLUDES Administration of fluid
Administration of substances/drugs
Coding heirarchy rules for facility reporting:
Chemotherapy services are primary to diagnostic, prophylactic, and therapeutic services
Infusions are primary to pushes
Pushes are primary to injections
Constant presence of health care professional administering the substance/drug
Direct physician supervision:
Consent
Direction of personnel
Patient assessment
Safety oversight
Supervision of personnel
Infusion of 15 minutes or less
The following if done to facilitate the injection/infusion:
Flush at the end of infusion
Indwelling IV, subcutaneous catheter/port access
Local anesthesia
Start of IV
Supplies/tubing/syringes
Training to assess patient and monitor vital signs
Training to prepare/dose/dispose
Treatment plan verification

EXCLUDES *Catheter/port declotting (36593)*
Significant separately identifiable evaluation and management service if performed

Code also drugs/materials

Do not report a second initial service on the same date for accessing a multi-lumen catheter or restarting an IV, or when two IV lines are needed to meet an infusion rate

Do not report for physician services provided in facility settings

Do not report with codes for which IV push or infusion is an integral part of the procedure

96372 Therapeutic, prophylactic, or diagnostic injection (specify substance or drug); subcutaneous or intramuscular S 80

INCLUDES Direct physician supervision when reported by the physician. When reported by a hospital, physician need not be present.

EXCLUDES *Administration of vaccines/toxoids (90460-90474)*
Allergen immunotherapy injections (95115-95117)
Antineoplastic hormonal injections (96402)
Antineoplastic nonhormonal injections (96401)
Hormonal therapy injections (non-antineoplastic) (96372)

Facility RVU 0.71 Non-Facility RVU 0.71 Global Days XXX
AMA: 2009, Feb, 17-21

96373 intra-arterial S 80
Facility RVU 0.58 Non-Facility RVU 0.58 Global Days XXX
AMA: 2009, Feb, 17-21

96374 intravenous push, single or initial substance/drug S 80

Code also second initial service with modifier 59 when patient's condition or drug protocol mandates the use of two IV lines

Facility RVU 1.64 Non-Facility RVU 1.64 Global Days XXX
AMA: 2009, May, 8-9&11; 2009, Feb, 17-21

\+ **96375 each additional sequential intravenous push of a new substance/drug (List separately in addition to code for primary procedure)** S 80

INCLUDES IV push of a new substance/drug provided as a secondary or subsequent service after a different initial service via same IV access site

Code first (96365, 96374, 96409, 96413)
Facility RVU 0.66 Non-Facility RVU 0.66 Global Days ZZZ
AMA: 2009, Feb, 17-21

\+ **96376 each additional sequential intravenous push of the same substance/drug provided in a facility (List separately in addition to code for primary procedure)** N

INCLUDES Facilities only

EXCLUDES *Services performed by any provider that is not a facility*

Code first (96365, 96374, 96409, 96413)

Do not report a push performed within 30 minutes of a reported push of the same substance or drug

Facility RVU 0.00 Non-Facility RVU 0.00 Global Days ZZZ
AMA: 2009, May, 8-9&11; 2009, Feb, 17-21

96379 Unlisted therapeutic, prophylactic, or diagnostic intravenous or intra-arterial injection or infusion S 80
Facility RVU 0.00 Non-Facility RVU 0.00 Global Days XXX
AMA: 2009, Feb, 17-21

96401-96411 Chemotherapy and Other Complex Drugs, Biologicals: Injection

CMS 100-3,110.2 Certain Drugs Distributed by the National Cancer Institute
CMS 100-3,110.6 Scalp Hypothermia During Chemotherapy, to Prevent Hair Loss
CMS 100-4,4,230.2.2 Chemotherapy Drug Administration
CMS 100-4,12,30.5 Payment for Injections and Infusions: Chemotherapy and Nonchemotherapy

INCLUDES An infusion of 15 minutes or less
Constant presence of the health care professional administering the drug or substance
Highly complex services that require direct supervision for:
Consent
Patient assessment
Safety oversight
Supervision
Intravenous/intra-arterial push
More intense physician work and monitoring of clinical staff due to greater risk of severe patient reactions.
Parenteral administration of:
Anti-neoplastic agents for noncancer diagnoses
Monoclonal antibody agents
Nonradionuclide antineoplastic drugs
Other biologic response modifiers

Do not report a second initial service on the same date for accessing a multi-lumen catheter or restarting an IV, or when two IV lines are needed to meet an infusion rate

96401 Chemotherapy administration, subcutaneous or intramuscular; non-hormonal anti-neoplastic S 80 PQ

Do not report for physician services provided in facility settings

Facility RVU 2.15 Non-Facility RVU 2.15 Global Days XXX
AMA: 2009, Feb, 17-21; 2009, Jan, 11-31; 2008, Jan, 10-25; 2007, January, 13-27; 2007, May, 3-4; 2007, June, 4-6; 2007, January, 28-31

96402 **hormonal anti-neoplastic** S 80 PQ

Do not report for physician services provided in facility settings

0.99 0.99 Global Days XXX

AMA: 2009, Jan, 11-31; 2009, Feb, 17-21; 2008, Jan, 10-25; 2007, May, 3-4; 2007, June, 4-6; 2007, January, 13-27; 2007, January, 28-31

96405 **Chemotherapy administration; intralesional, up to and including 7 lesions** S PQ

0.89 2.49 Global Days 000

AMA: 2009, Jan, 11-31; 2009, Feb, 17-21; 2008, Jan, 10-25; 2007, May, 3-4; 2007, January, 13-27; 2007, June, 4-6; 2007, January, 28-31

96406 **intralesional, more than 7 lesions** S PQ

1.30 3.55 Global Days 000

AMA: 2009, Jan, 11-31; 2009, Feb, 17-21; 2008, Jan, 10-25; 2007, June, 4-6; 2007, January, 28-31; 2007, May, 3-4; 2007, January, 13-27

96409 **intravenous, push technique, single or initial substance/drug** S 80 PQ

Code also second initial service with modifier 59 when patient's condition or drug protocol mandates the use of two IV lines

Do not report for physician services provided in facility settings

Do not report with 36823

3.26 3.26 Global Days XXX

AMA: 2009, Jan, 11-31; 2009, Feb, 17-21; 2008, Jan, 10-25; 2007, January, 28-31; 2007, January, 13-27; 2007, May, 3-4; 2007, June, 4-6

+ **96411** **intravenous, push technique, each additional substance/drug (List separately in addition to code for primary procedure)** S 80 PQ

Code first initial substance/drug (96409, 96413)

Do not report for physician services provided in facility settings

Do not report with 36823

1.83 1.83 Global Days ZZZ

AMA: 2009, Jan, 11-31; 2009, Feb, 17-21; 2008, Jan, 10-25; 2007, January, 28-31; 2007, June, 4-6; 2007, January, 13-27; 2007, May, 3-4

96413-96417 Chemotherapy and Complex Drugs, Biologicals: Intravenous Infusion

CMS 100-3,110.2 Certain Drugs Distributed by the National Cancer Institute
CMS 100-3,110.6 Scalp Hypothermia During Chemotherapy, to Prevent Hair Loss
CMS 100-4,4,230.2.2 Chemotherapy Drug Administration
CMS 100-4,4,231 Coding and Payment for Drug Administration
CMS 100-4,12,30.5 Payment for Injections and Infusions: Chemotherapy and Nonchemotherapy

INCLUDES An infusion of 15 minutes or less
Constant presence of the health care professional administering the drug or substance
Highly complex services that require direct supervision for:
- Consent
- Patient assessment
- Safety oversight
- Supervision

Intravenous/intra-arterial push
More intense physician work and monitoring of clinical staff due to greater risk of severe patient reactions
Parenteral administration of:
- Anti-neoplastic agents for noncancer diagnoses
- Monoclonal antibody agents
- Nonradionuclide antineoplastic drugs
- Other biologic response modifiers

The following in the administration:
- Access to IV/catheter/port
- Drug preparation
- Flushing at the completion of the infusion
- Hydration fluid
- Routine tubing/syringe/supplies
- Starting the IV
- Use of local anesthesia

EXCLUDES *Administration of nonchemotherapy agents such as antibiotics/steriods/analgesics*
Declotting of catheter/port (36593)
Home infusion (99601-99602)

Code also drug or substance

Code also significant separately identifiable evaluation and management service, if performed

Do not report a second initial service on the same date for accessing a multi-lumen catheter or restarting an IV, or when two IV lines are needed to meet an infusion rate

Do not report for physician services provided in facility settings

Do not report with 36823

96413 **Chemotherapy administration, intravenous infusion technique; up to 1 hour, single or initial substance/drug** S 80 PQ

EXCLUDES *Hydration administered as secondary or subsequent service via same IV access site (96361)*
Therapeutic/prophylactic/diagnostic drug infusion/injection through the same intravenous access (96366, 96367, 96375)

Code also second initial service with modifier 59 when patient's condition or drug protocol mandates the use of two IV lines

4.07 4.07 Global Days XXX

AMA: 2009, Jan, 11-31; 2009, Feb, 17-21; 2008, Jan, 10-25; 2007, January, 28-31; 2007, Dec, 10-179; 2007, May, 3-4; 2007, June, 4-6; 2007, January, 13-27

+ **96415** **each additional hour (List separately in addition to code for primary procedure)**

INCLUDES Infusion intervals of more than 30 minutes past 1-hour increments

Code first initial hour (96413)

0.90 0.90 Global Days ZZZ

AMA: 2009, Jan, 11-31; 2009, Feb, 17-21; 2008, Jan, 10-25; 2007, January, 13-27; 2007, June, 4-6; 2007, Dec, 10-179; 2007, May, 3-4; 2007, January, 28-31

96416 **initiation of prolonged chemotherapy infusion (more than 8 hours), requiring use of a portable or implantable pump**

EXCLUDES *Portable or implantable infusion pump/reservoir refilling/maintenance for drug delivery (96521-96523)*

4.06 4.06 Global Days XXX

AMA: 2009, Jan, 11-31; 2009, Feb, 17-21; 2008, Jan, 10-25; 2007, January, 28-31; 2007, June, 4-6; 2007, Dec, 10-179; 2007, January, 13-27; 2007, May, 3-4

+ **96417** **each additional sequential infusion (different substance/drug), up to 1 hour (List separately in addition to code for primary procedure)**

INCLUDES Reporting only once per sequential infusion

EXCLUDES *Additional hour(s) of sequential infusion (96415)*

Code first initial substance/drug (96413)

2.09 2.09 Global Days ZZZ

AMA: 2009, Jan, 11-31; 2009, Feb, 17-21; 2008, Jan, 10-25; 2007, January, 28-31; 2007, May, 3-4; 2007, January, 13-27; 2007, June, 4-6

96420-96425 Chemotherapy and Complex Drugs, Biologicals: Intra-arterial

CMS 100-3,110.2 Certain Drugs Distributed by the National Cancer Institute
CMS 100-3,110.6 Scalp Hypothermia During Chemotherapy, to Prevent Hair Loss
CMS 100-4,4,230.2.2 Chemotherapy Drug Administration
CMS 100-4,4,231 Coding and Payment for Drug Administration
CMS 100-4,12,30.5 Payment for Injections and Infusions: Chemotherapy and Nonchemotherapy

INCLUDES Highly complex services that require direct supervision for:
- Consent
- Patient assessment
- Safety oversight
- Supervision

More intense physician work and monitoring of clinical staff due to greater risk of severe patient reactions

Parenteral administration of:
- Anti-neoplastic agents for noncancer diagnoses
- Monoclonal antibody agents
- Non-radionuclide antineoplastic drugs
- Other biologic response modifiers

The following in the administration:
- Access to IV/catheter/port
- Drug preparation
- Flushing at the completion of the infusion
- Hydration fluid
- Routine tubing/syringe/supplies
- Starting the IV
- Use of local anesthesia

EXCLUDES *Administration of non-chemotherapy agents such as antibiotics/steriods/analgesics*
Declotting of catheter/port (36593)
Home infusion (99601-99602)

Code also drug or substance

Code also significant separately identifiable evaluation and management service, if performed

Do not report a second initial service on the same date for accessing a multi-lumen catheter or restarting an IV, or when two IV lines are needed to meet an infusion rate

Do not report for physician services provided in facility settings

96420 **Chemotherapy administration, intra-arterial; push technique**

INCLUDES Regional chemotherapy perfusion

EXCLUDES *Placement of intra-arterial catheter*

Do not report with 36823

3.15 3.15 Global Days XXX

AMA: 2009, Jan, 11-31; 2009, Feb, 17-21; 2008, Jan, 10-25; 2007, January, 13-27; 2007, May, 3-4; 2007, June, 4-6; 2007, January, 28-31

96422 **infusion technique, up to 1 hour**

INCLUDES Regional chemotherapy perfusion

EXCLUDES *Placement of intra-arterial catheter*

Do not report with 36823

5.06 5.06 Global Days XXX

AMA: 2009, Jan, 11-31; 2009, Feb, 17-21; 2008, Jan, 10-25; 2007, January, 13-27; 2007, January, 28-31; 2007, May, 3-4; 2007, Dec, 10-179; 2007, June, 4-6

+ **96423** **infusion technique, each additional hour (List separately in addition to code for primary procedure)**

INCLUDES Infusion intervals of more than 30 minutes past 1-hour increments
Regional chemotherapy perfusion

EXCLUDES *Arterial/venous cannula insertion with regional chemotherapy perfusion to an extremity (36823)*
Placement of intra-arterial catheter

Code first initial hour (96422)

Do not report with 36823

2.32 2.32 Global Days ZZZ

AMA: 2009, Feb, 17-21; 2009, Jan, 11-31; 2008, Jan, 10-25; 2007, January, 28-31; 2007, June, 4-6; 2007, Dec, 10-179; 2007, January, 13-27; 2007, May, 3-4

96425 **infusion technique, initiation of prolonged infusion (more than 8 hours), requiring the use of a portable or implantable pump**

INCLUDES Regional chemotherapy perfusion

EXCLUDES *Placement of intra-arterial catheter*
Portable or implantable infusion pump/reservoir refilling/maintenance for drug delivery (96521-96523)

Do not report with 36823

5.30 5.30 Global Days XXX

AMA: 2009, Jan, 11-31; 2009, Feb, 17-21; 2008, Jan, 10-25; 2007, January, 28-31; 2007, May, 3-4; 2007, January, 13-27; 2007, June, 4-6

96440-96450 Chemotherapy Administration: Intrathecal/Peritoneal Cavity/Pleural Cavity

96440 **Chemotherapy administration into pleural cavity, requiring and including thoracentesis**

EXCLUDES *Blood specimen collection from completely implantable venous access device (36591)*

4.15 24.31 Global Days 000

AMA: 2009, Jan, 11-31; 2009, Feb, 17-21; 2008, Jan, 10-25; 2007, January, 28-31; 2007, January, 13-27; 2007, May, 3-4; 2007, June, 4-6

96446 **Chemotherapy administration into the peritoneal cavity via indwelling port or catheter**

0.62 5.65 Global Days XXX

96450 **Chemotherapy administration, into CNS (eg, intrathecal), requiring and including spinal puncture**

EXCLUDES *Blood specimen collection from completely implantable venous access device (36591)*
Chemotherapy administration, intravesical/bladder (51720)
Insertion of catheter/reservoir:
Intraventricular (61210, 61215)
Subarachnoid (62350, 62351, 62360-62362)

2.40 5.50 Global Days 000

AMA: 2009, Jan, 11-31; 2009, Feb, 17-21; 2008, Jan, 10-25; 2007, January, 13-27; 2007, May, 3-4; 2007, January, 28-31; 2007, June, 4-6

96521-96523 Refill/Upkeep of Drug Delivery Device

CMS 100-4,4,231 Coding and Payment for Drug Administration

INCLUDES Highly complex services that require direct supervision for:
Consent
Patient assessment
Safety oversight
Supervision
Parenteral administration of:
Anti-neoplastic agents for noncancer diagnoses
Monoclonal antibody agents
Non-radionuclide antineoplastic drugs
Other biologic response modifiers
The following in the administration:
Access to IV/catheter/port
Drug preparation
Flushing at the completion of the infusion
Hydration fluid
Routine tubing/syringe/supplies
Starting the IV
Use of local anesthesia
Therapeutic drugs other than chemotherapy

EXCLUDES *Administration of non-chemotherapy agents such as antibiotics/steriods/analgesics*
Blood specimen collection from completely implantable venous access device (36591)
Declotting of catheter/port (36593)
Home infusion (99601-99602)

Code also drug or substance

Code also significant separately identifiable evaluation and management service, if performed

96521 **Refilling and maintenance of portable pump**

4.02 4.02 Global Days XXX

AMA: 2009, Feb, 17-21; 2007, January, 28-31; 2007, June, 4-6; 2007, May, 3-4

96522 **Refilling and maintenance of implantable pump or reservoir for drug delivery, systemic (eg, intravenous, intra-arterial)**

EXCLUDES *Implantable infusion pump refilling/maintenance for spinal/brain drug delivery (95990-95991)*

3.26 3.26 Global Days XXX

AMA: 2009, Feb, 17-21; 2007, June, 4-6; 2007, January, 28-31; 2007, May, 3-4

96523 **Irrigation of implanted venous access device for drug delivery systems**

EXCLUDES *Blood specimen collection (36591)*
Direct physician supervision

Do not report with any other services on the same date of service.

0.74 0.74 Global Days XXX

AMA: 2009, Feb, 17-21; 2007, January, 28-31; 2007, June, 4-6; 2007, May, 3-4

96542-96549 Chemotherapy Injection Into Brain

CMS 100-3,110.2 Certain Drugs Distributed by the National Cancer Institute
CMS 100-4,4,230.2.2 Chemotherapy Drug Administration
CMS 100-4,12,30.5 Payment for Injections and Infusions: Chemotherapy and Nonchemotherapy

INCLUDES Highly complex services that require direct supervision for:
- Consent
- Patient assessment
- Safety oversight
- Supervision

Parenteral administration of:
- Anti-neoplastic agents for noncancer diagnoses
- Monoclonal antibody agents
- Non-radionuclide antineoplastic drugs
- Other biologic response modifiers

The following in the administration:
- Access to IV/catheter/port
- Drug preparation
- Flushing at the completion of the infusion
- Hydration fluid
- Routine tubing/syringe/supplies
- Starting the IV
- Use of local anesthesia

EXCLUDES *Administration of non-chemotherapy agents such as antibiotics/steriods/analgesics*
Blood specimen collection from completely implantable venous access device (36591)
Declotting of catheter/port (36593)
Home infusion (99601-99602)

Code also drug or substance
Code also significant separately identifiable evaluation and management service, if performed

96542 Chemotherapy injection, subarachnoid or intraventricular via subcutaneous reservoir, single or multiple agents S 80 PQ
79005
1.23 3.61 Global Days XXX
AMA: 2009, Feb, 17-21; 2007, January, 28-31; 2007, May, 3-4; 2007, June, 4-6

96549 Unlisted chemotherapy procedure S 80 PQ
0.00 0.00 Global Days XXX
AMA: 2009, Jan, 11-31; 2009, Feb, 17-21; 2008, Jan, 10-25; 2007, January, 28-31; 2007, May, 3-4; 2007, June, 4-6

96567-96571 Destruction of Lesions: Photodynamic Therapy

EXCLUDES *Ocular photodynamic therapy (67221)*

96567 Photodynamic therapy by external application of light to destroy premalignant and/or malignant lesions of the skin and adjacent mucosa (eg, lip) by activation of photosensitive drug(s), each phototherapy exposure session T 80
4.01 4.01 Global Days XXX

\+ **96570 Photodynamic therapy by endoscopic application of light to ablate abnormal tissue via activation of photosensitive drug(s); first 30 minutes (List separately in addition to code for endoscopy or bronchoscopy procedures of lung and gastrointestinal tract)** T
Code also for 38-52 minutes (96571)
Code also modifier 52 when services with report are less than 23 minutes
Code first (31641, 43228)
1.70 1.70 Global Days ZZZ
AMA: 2008, Oct, 6-7

\+ **96571 each additional 15 minutes (List separately in addition to code for endoscopy or bronchoscopy procedures of lung and gastrointestinal tract)** T
EXCLUDES *23-37 minutes of service (96570)*
Code first (96570)
0.78 0.78 Global Days ZZZ
AMA: 2008, Oct, 6-7

96900-96999 Diagnostic/Therapeutic Skin Procedures

CMS 100-3,190.6 Hair Analysis
CMS 100-3,250.1 Treatment of Psoriasis
CMS 100-3,250.4 Treatment of Actinic Keratosis

EXCLUDES *Consultation services (99241-99255)*
Evaluation and management services (99201-99499 [99224, 99225, 99226])
Injection, intralesional (11900-11901)

96900 Actinotherapy (ultraviolet light) S 80
EXCLUDES *Rhinophototherapy (30999)*
88160-88161
0.63 0.63 Global Days XXX
AMA: 2009, Jan, 11-31; 2008, Jan, 10-25; 2007, January, 13-27

96902 Microscopic examination of hairs plucked or clipped by the examiner (excluding hair collected by the patient) to determine telogen and anagen counts, or structural hair shaft abnormality N
88160-88161
0.61 0.63 Global Days XXX

96904 Whole body integumentary photography, for monitoring of high risk patients with dysplastic nevus syndrome or a history of dysplastic nevi, or patients with a personal or familial history of melanoma N 80
88160-88161
2.09 2.09 Global Days XXX

96910 Photochemotherapy; tar and ultraviolet B (Goeckerman treatment) or petrolatum and ultraviolet B S 80
88160-88161
2.12 2.12 Global Days XXX

96912 psoralens and ultraviolet A (PUVA) S 80
88160-88161
2.72 2.72 Global Days XXX

96913 Photochemotherapy (Goeckerman and/or PUVA) for severe photoresponsive dermatoses requiring at least 4-8 hours of care under direct supervision of the physician (includes application of medication and dressings) S 80
88160-88161
3.79 3.79 Global Days XXX

96920 Laser treatment for inflammatory skin disease (psoriasis); total area less than 250 sq cm T
EXCLUDES *Destruction by laser of:*
- *Benign lesions (17110-17111)*
- *Cutaneous vascular proliferative lesions (17106-17108)*
- *Malignant lesions (17260-17286)*
- *Premalignant lesions (17000-17004)*

88160-88161
1.96 5.15 Global Days 000

96921 **250 sq cm to 500 sq cm** T CCI

EXCLUDES *Destruction by laser of:*

Benign lesions (17110-17111)

Cutaneous vascular proliferative lesions (17106-17108)

Malignant lesions (17260-17286)

Premalignant lesions (17000-17004)

88160-88161

1.97 5.23 Global Days 000

96922 **over 500 sq cm** T CCI

EXCLUDES *Destruction by laser of:*

Benign lesions (17110-17111)

Cutaneous vascular proliferative lesions (17106-17108)

Malignant lesions (17260-17286)

Premalignant lesions (17000-17004)

88160-88161

3.54 7.37 Global Days 000

96999 **Unlisted special dermatological service or procedure** T 80

0.00 0.00 Global Days XXX

97001-97006 Physical Medicine Assessments

CMS 100-2,15,230.4 Services By a Physical/Occupational Therapist in Private Practice
CMS 100-3,20.10 Cardiac Rehabilitation Programs
CMS 100-4,5,10 Part B Outpatient Rehabilitation and Comprehensive Outpatient Rehabilitation Facility (CORF) Services - General
CMS 100-4,5,10.2 Financial Limitation for Outpatient Rehabilition Services
CMS 100-4,5,20 HCPCS Coding Requirement

EXCLUDES *EMG biofeedback training (90901)*

Muscle/range of motion testing and electromyography (95831-95904 [95885, 95886, 95887])

Transcutaneous nerve stimulation (TNS) (64550)

⊘ 97001 **Physical therapy evaluation** A 80 CCI PQ

2.16 2.16 Global Days XXX

AMA: 2009, Jan, 11-31; 2008, Jan, 10-25; 2008, May, 9-11; 2007, January, 13-27

⊘ 97002 **Physical therapy re-evaluation** A 80 CCI PQ

1.20 1.20 Global Days XXX

AMA: 2009, Jan, 11-31; 2008, May, 9-11; 2008, Jan, 10-25; 2007, January, 13-27

⊘ 97003 **Occupational therapy evaluation** A 80 CCI PQ

2.42 2.42 Global Days XXX

AMA: 2009, Jan, 11-31; 2008, May, 9-11; 2008, Jan, 10-25; 2007, January, 13-27

⊘ 97004 **Occupational therapy re-evaluation** A 80 CCI PQ

1.49 1.49 Global Days XXX

AMA: 2009, Jan, 11-31; 2008, May, 9-11; 2008, Jan, 10-25; 2007, January, 13-27

⊘ 97005 **Athletic training evaluation** E

0.00 0.00 Global Days XXX

⊘ 97006 **Athletic training re-evaluation** E

0.00 0.00 Global Days XXX

97010-97028 Physical Therapy Treatment Modalities: Supervised

CMS 100-2,15,230 Practice of Physical Therapy, Occupational Therapy, and Speech-Language Pathology
CMS 100-2,15,230.1 Practice of Physical Therapy
CMS 100-2,15,230.4 Services By a Physical/Occupational Therapist in Private Practice
CMS 100-3,20.10 Cardiac Rehabilitation Programs
CMS 100-4,5,10 Part B Outpatient Rehabilitation and Comprehensive Outpatient Rehabilitation Facility (CORF) Services - General
CMS 100-4,5,10.2 Financial Limitation for Outpatient Rehabilition Services
CMS 100-4,5,20 HCPCS Coding Requirement

EXCLUDES *Direct patient contact by the provider*

EMG biofeedback training (90901)

Muscle/range of motion testing and electromyography (95831-95904 [95885, 95886, 95887])

Transcutaneous nerve stimulation (TNS) (64550)

⊘ 97010 **Application of a modality to 1 or more areas; hot or cold packs** A

0.17 0.17 Global Days XXX

AMA: 2009, Jan, 11-31; 2008, Jan, 10-25; 2007, January, 13-27

⊘ 97012 **traction, mechanical** A 80 CCI

0.46 0.46 Global Days XXX

AMA: 2009, Jan, 11-31; 2008, Jan, 10-25; 2007, January, 13-27

⊘ 97014 **electrical stimulation (unattended)** E

EXCLUDES *Acupuncture with electrical stimulation (97813, 97814)*

0.45 0.45 Global Days XXX

AMA: 2009, Jan, 11-31; 2008, Jan, 10-25; 2007, January, 13-27

⊘ 97016 **vasopneumatic devices** A 80 CCI

0.54 0.54 Global Days XXX

⊘ 97018 **paraffin bath** A 80 CCI

0.30 0.30 Global Days XXX

⊘ 97022 **whirlpool** A 80 CCI

0.65 0.65 Global Days XXX

⊘ 97024 **diathermy (eg, microwave)** A 80 CCI

0.19 0.19 Global Days XXX

⊘ 97026 **infrared** A 80 CCI

0.17 0.17 Global Days XXX

⊘ 97028 **ultraviolet** A 80 CCI

0.21 0.21 Global Days XXX

97032-97039 Physical Therapy Treatment Modalities: Constant Attendance

CMS 100-2,15,230 Practice of Physical Therapy, Occupational Therapy, and Speech-Language Pathology
CMS 100-2,15,230.1 Practice of Physical Therapy
CMS 100-2,15,230.2 Practice of Occupational Therapy
CMS 100-2,15,230.4 Services By a Physical/Occupational Therapist in Private Practice
CMS 100-3,20.10 Cardiac Rehabilitation Programs
CMS 100-4,5,10 Part B Outpatient Rehabilitation and Comprehensive Outpatient Rehabilitation Facility (CORF) Services - General
CMS 100-4,5,10.2 Financial Limitation for Outpatient Rehabilition Services
CMS 100-4,5,20 HCPCS Coding Requirement

INCLUDES Adding incremental intervals of treatment time for the same visit to calculate the total service time
Direct patient contact by the provider

EXCLUDES *EMG biofeedback training (90901)*
Muscle/range of motion testing and electromyography (95831-95904 [95885, 95886, 95887])
Transcutaneous nerve stimulation (TNS) (64550)

⊘ **97032** **Application of a modality to 1 or more areas; electrical stimulation (manual), each 15 minutes** A 80

EXCLUDES *Transcutaneous electrical modulation pain reprocessing (TEMPR) (scrambler therapy) (0278T)*

0.54 0.54 Global Days XXX
AMA: 2009, Jan, 11-31; 2008, Jan, 10-25; 2007, January, 13-27

⊘ **97033** **iontophoresis, each 15 minutes** A 80
0.90 0.90 Global Days XXX

⊘ **97034** **contrast baths, each 15 minutes** A 80
0.50 0.50 Global Days XXX

⊘ **97035** **ultrasound, each 15 minutes** A 80
0.36 0.36 Global Days XXX
AMA: 2009, Jan, 11-31; 2008, Jan, 10-25; 2007, January, 13-27

⊘ **97036** **Hubbard tank, each 15 minutes** A 80
0.91 0.91 Global Days XXX

97039 **Unlisted modality (specify type and time if constant attendance)** A 80
0.00 0.00 Global Days XXX
AMA: 2009, Jan, 11-31; 2008, Jan, 10-25; 2007, January, 13-27

97110-97546 Other Therapeutic Techniques With Direct Patient Contact

CMS 100-2,15,230 Practice of Physical Therapy, Occupational Therapy, and Speech-Language Pathology
CMS 100-2,15,230.1 Practice of Physical Therapy
CMS 100-2,15,230.2 Practice of Occupational Therapy
CMS 100-2,15,230.4 Services By a Physical/Occupational Therapist in Private Practice
CMS 100-3,20.10 Cardiac Rehabilitation Programs
CMS 100-4,5,10 Part B Outpatient Rehabilitation and Comprehensive Outpatient Rehabilitation Facility (CORF) Services - General
CMS 100-4,5,10.2 Financial Limitation for Outpatient Rehabilition Services
CMS 100-4,5,20 HCPCS Coding Requirement

INCLUDES Application of clinical skills/services to improve function
Direct patient contact by the provider

EXCLUDES *EMG biofeedback training (90901)*
Muscle/range of motion testing and electromyography (95831-95904 [95885, 95886, 95887])
Transcutaneous nerve stimulation (TNS) (64550)

⊘ **97110** **Therapeutic procedure, 1 or more areas, each 15 minutes; therapeutic exercises to develop strength and endurance, range of motion and flexibility** A 80
0.90 0.90 Global Days XXX
AMA: 2009, Jan, 11-31; 2008, Jan, 10-25; 2008, May, 9-11; 2007, January, 13-27

⊘ **97112** **neuromuscular reeducation of movement, balance, coordination, kinesthetic sense, posture, and/or proprioception for sitting and/or standing activities** A 80
0.94 0.94 Global Days XXX
AMA: 2009, Jan, 11-31; 2008, Jan, 10-25; 2008, May, 9-11; 2007, January, 13-27

⊘ **97113** **aquatic therapy with therapeutic exercises** A 80
1.20 1.20 Global Days XXX
AMA: 2009, Jan, 11-31; 2008, Jan, 10-25; 2008, May, 9-11; 2007, January, 13-27

⊘ **97116** **gait training (includes stair climbing)** A 80

EXCLUDES *Comprehensive gait/motion analysis (96000-96003)*

0.80 0.80 Global Days XXX
AMA: 2009, Jan, 11-31; 2008, May, 9-11; 2008, Jan, 10-25; 2007, January, 13-27; 2007, February, 8-9

⊘ **97124** **massage, including effleurage, petrissage and/or tapotement (stroking, compression, percussion)** A 80

EXCLUDES *Myofascial release (97140)*

0.74 0.74 Global Days XXX
AMA: 2009, Jan, 11-31; 2008, Jan, 10-25; 2008, May, 9-11; 2007, January, 13-27

97139 **Unlisted therapeutic procedure (specify)** A 80
0.00 0.00 Global Days XXX
AMA: 2009, Jan, 11-31; 2008, May, 9-11; 2008, Jan, 10-25; 2007, January, 13-27

⊘ **97140** **Manual therapy techniques (eg, mobilization/manipulation, manual lymphatic drainage, manual traction), 1 or more regions, each 15 minutes** A 80

Do not report with (29581-29584)

0.84 0.84 Global Days XXX
AMA: 2009, Jan, 11-31; 2009, May, 8-9&11; 2008, May, 9-11; 2008, Jan, 10-25; 2007, January, 13-27

⊘ **97150 Therapeutic procedure(s), group (2 or more individuals)** A 80 CCI

INCLUDES Constant attendance by the physician/therapist
Reporting this procedure for each member of group

EXCLUDES *Osteopathic manipulative treatment (98925-98929)*

0.58 0.58 Global Days XXX
AMA: 2009, Jan, 11-31; 2008, May, 9-11; 2008, Jan, 10-25; 2007, January, 13-27

⊘ **97530 Therapeutic activities, direct (one-on-one) patient contact by the provider (use of dynamic activities to improve functional performance), each 15 minutes** A 80 CCI

0.99 0.99 Global Days XXX
AMA: 2009, Jan, 11-31; 2008, May, 9-11; 2008, Jan, 10-25; 2007, January, 13-27

⊘ **97532 Development of cognitive skills to improve attention, memory, problem solving (includes compensatory training), direct (one-on-one) patient contact by the provider, each 15 minutes** A 80 CCI PQ

0.75 0.75 Global Days XXX
AMA: 2008, May, 9-11

⊘ **97533 Sensory integrative techniques to enhance sensory processing and promote adaptive responses to environmental demands, direct (one-on-one) patient contact by the provider, each 15 minutes** A 80 CCI

0.83 0.83 Global Days XXX
AMA: 2008, May, 9-11

⊘ **97535 Self-care/home management training (eg, activities of daily living (ADL) and compensatory training, meal preparation, safety procedures, and instructions in use of assistive technology devices/adaptive equipment) direct one-on-one contact by provider, each 15 minutes** A 80 CCI

0.98 0.98 Global Days XXX
AMA: 2009, Jan, 11-31; 2008, May, 9-11; 2008, Jan, 10-25; 2007, January, 13-27

⊘ **97537 Community/work reintegration training (eg, shopping, transportation, money management, avocational activities and/or work environment/modification analysis, work task analysis, use of assistive technology device/adaptive equipment), direct one-on-one contact by provider, each 15 minutes** A 80 CCI

EXCLUDES *Wheelchair management/propulsion training (97542)*

0.85 0.85 Global Days XXX
AMA: 2008, May, 9-11

⊘ **97542 Wheelchair management (eg, assessment, fitting, training), each 15 minutes** A 80 CCI

0.87 0.87 Global Days XXX
AMA: 2008, May, 9-11

⊘ **97545 Work hardening/conditioning; initial 2 hours** A 80 CCI

0.00 0.00 Global Days XXX
AMA: 2009, Jan, 11-31; 2008, May, 9-11; 2008, Jan, 10-25; 2007, January, 13-27

\+ **97546 each additional hour (List separately in addition to code for primary procedure)** A 80

Code first initial 2 hours (97545)
0.00 0.00 Global Days ZZZ
AMA: 2009, Jan, 11-31; 2008, May, 9-11

97597-97606 Treatment of Wounds

CMS 100-2,15,230.4 Services By a Physical/Occupational Therapist in Private Practice
CMS 100-3,270.1 Electrical Stimulation and Electromagnetic Therapy for the Treatment of Wounds
CMS 100-3,270.2 Noncontact Normothermic Wound Therapy
CMS 100-3,270.3 Blood-derived Products for Chronic Nonhealing Wounds
CMS 100-3,270.4 Treatment of Decubitus
CMS 100-4,5,10 Part B Outpatient Rehabilitation and Comprehensive Outpatient Rehabilitation Facility (CORF) Services - General
CMS 100-4,5,20 HCPCS Coding Requirement

EXCLUDES *Burn wound debridement (16020-16030)*

⊘ **97597 Debridement (eg, high pressure waterjet with/without suction, sharp selective debridement with scissors, scalpel and forceps), open wound, (eg, fibrin, devitalized epidermis and/or dermis, exudate, debris, biofilm), including topical application(s), wound assessment, use of a whirlpool, when performed and instruction(s) for ongoing care, per session, total wound(s) surface area; first 20 sq cm or less** T 80 CCI

INCLUDES Direct patient contact
Removing devitalized/necrotic tissue and promoting healing

Do not report with other debridement codes for the same wound (11042-11047 [11045, 11046])

0.70 2.21 Global Days 000
AMA: 2009, Jan, 11-31; 2008, Jan, 10-25; 2007, January, 13-27

\+ **97598 each additional 20 sq cm, or part thereof (List separately in addition to code for primary procedure)** T 80 CCI

INCLUDES Direct patient contact
Removing devitalized/necrotic tissue and promoting healing

Code first (97597)

Do not report with other debridement codes for the same wound (11042-11047 [11045, 11046])

0.33 0.73 Global Days ZZZ

⊘ **97602 Removal of devitalized tissue from wound(s), non-selective debridement, without anesthesia (eg, wet-to-moist dressings, enzymatic, abrasion), including topical application(s), wound assessment, and instruction(s) for ongoing care, per session** T

INCLUDES Direct patient contact
Removing devitalized/necrotic tissue and promoting healing

Do not report with other debridement codes for the same wound (11042-11047 [11045, 11046])

0.00 0.00 Global Days XXX
AMA: 2009, Jan, 11-31; 2008, Sep, 10-11

⊘ **97605 Negative pressure wound therapy (eg, vacuum assisted drainage collection), including topical application(s), wound assessment, and instruction(s) for ongoing care, per session; total wound(s) surface area less than or equal to 50 square centimeters** T 80

INCLUDES Direct patient contact
Removing devitalized/necrotic tissue and promoting healing

0.79 1.20 Global Days XXX
AMA: 2009, Jan, 11-31; 2008, Jan, 10-25; 2007, January, 13-27

⊘ **97606 total wound(s) surface area greater than 50 square centimeters** T 80

INCLUDES Direct patient contact
Removing devitalized/necrotic tissue and promoting healing

0.87 1.28 Global Days XXX
AMA: 2009, Jan, 11-31; 2008, Jan, 10-25; 2007, January, 13-27

97750-97799 Assessments and Training

CMS 100-2,15,230 Practice of Physical Therapy, Occupational Therapy, and Speech-Language Pathology
CMS 100-2,15,230.1 Practice of Physical Therapy
CMS 100-2,15,230.2 Practice of Occupational Therapy
CMS 100-2,15,230.4 Services By a Physical/Occupational Therapist in Private Practice
CMS 100-3,20.10 Cardiac Rehabilitation Programs
CMS 100-4,5,10 Part B Outpatient Rehabilitation and Comprehensive Outpatient Rehabilitation Facility (CORF) Services - General
CMS 100-4,5,20 HCPCS Coding Requirement

⊘ 97750 **Physical performance test or measurement (eg, musculoskeletal, functional capacity), with written report, each 15 minutes** A 80

INCLUDES Direct patient contact

EXCLUDES *Muscle/range of motion testing and electromyography/nerve velocity determination (95831-95904 [95885, 95886, 95887])*

0.95 0.95 Global Days XXX
AMA: 2009, Jan, 11-31; 2008, May, 9-11; 2008, Jan, 10-25; 2007, January, 13-27; 2007, February, 10-11

⊘ 97755 **Assistive technology assessment (eg, to restore, augment or compensate for existing function, optimize functional tasks and/or maximize environmental accessibility), direct one-on-one contact by provider, with written report, each 15 minutes** A 80

INCLUDES Direct patient contact

EXCLUDES *Augmentative/alternative communication device (92605, 92607)*
Muscle/range of motion testing and electromyography/nerve velocity determination (95831-95904 [95885, 95886, 95887])

1.03 1.03 Global Days XXX

97760 **Orthotic(s) management and training (including assessment and fitting when not otherwise reported), upper extremity(s), lower extremity(s) and/or trunk, each 15 minutes** A 80

Do not report with gait training, if performed on the same extremity (97116)

1.08 1.08 Global Days XXX
AMA: 2007, February, 8-9

97761 **Prosthetic training, upper and/or lower extremity(s), each 15 minutes** A 80

0.94 0.94 Global Days XXX
AMA: 2009, Jan, 11-31; 2008, Jan, 10-25; 2007, January, 13-27; 2007, February, 8-9

97762 **Checkout for orthotic/prosthetic use, established patient, each 15 minutes** A 80

1.30 1.30 Global Days XXX
AMA: 2007, February, 8-9

97799 **Unlisted physical medicine/rehabilitation service or procedure** A 80

0.00 0.00 Global Days XXX

97802-97804 Medical Nutrition Therapy Services

CMS 100-3,40.1 Diabetes Outpatient Self-management Training
CMS 100-3,40.5 Treatment of Obesity
CMS 100-3,180.1 Medical Nutrition Therapy
CMS 100-4,4,300 Medical Nutrition Therapy Services

EXCLUDES *Physician provided medical nutrition therapy assessment/intervention (99201-99499 [99224, 99225, 99226])*

97802 **Medical nutrition therapy; initial assessment and intervention, individual, face-to-face with the patient, each 15 minutes** A 80

0.93 1.00 Global Days XXX
AMA: 2009, Feb, 13-16

97803 **re-assessment and intervention, individual, face-to-face with the patient, each 15 minutes** A 80

0.80 0.87 Global Days XXX
AMA: 2009, Feb, 13-16

97804 **group (2 or more individual(s)), each 30 minutes** A 80

0.43 0.44 Global Days XXX
AMA: 2009, Feb, 13-16

97810-97814 Acupuncture

CMS 100-3,30.3.1 Acupuncture for Fibromyalgia
CMS 100-3,30.3.2 Acupuncture for Osteoarthritis

INCLUDES 15 minute increments of face-to-face contact with the patient
Reporting only one code for each 15 minute increment

Code also evaluation and mangement time, if performed

Code also significant separately identifiable evaluation and management code (99201-99499 [99224, 99225, 99226])

97810 **Acupuncture, 1 or more needles; without electrical stimulation, initial 15 minutes of personal one-on-one contact with the patient** E

EXCLUDES *Electrical stimulation (97813-97814)*

Do not report with (97813)

0.89 1.05 Global Days XXX
AMA: 2009, Jan, 11-31; 2008, Jan, 10-25; 2007, January, 13-27

+ 97811 **without electrical stimulation, each additional 15 minutes of personal one-on-one contact with the patient, with re-insertion of needle(s) (List separately in addition to code for primary procedure)** E

EXCLUDES *Electrical stimulation (97813-97814)*

Code first initial 15 minutes (97810, 97813)

0.73 0.79 Global Days ZZZ

97813 **with electrical stimulation, initial 15 minutes of personal one-on-one contact with the patient** E

INCLUDES Electrical stimulation

Do not report with (97810)

0.96 1.12 Global Days XXX

+ 97814 **with electrical stimulation, each additional 15 minutes of personal one-on-one contact with the patient, with re-insertion of needle(s) (List separately in addition to code for primary procedure)** E

Code first initial 15 minutes (97810, 97813)

0.82 0.90 Global Days ZZZ

98925-98929 Osteopathic Manipulation

CMS 100-3,150.1 Manipulation

INCLUDES Physician applied manual treatment done to eliminate/alleviate somatic dysfunction and related disorders using a variety of techniques

The following body regions:

- Abdomen/viscera region
- Cervical region
- Head region
- Lower extremities
- Lumbar region
- Pelvic region
- Rib cage region
- Sacral region
- Thoracic region
- Upper extremities

Code also significant separately identifiable evaluation and management service (99201-99499 [99224, 99225, 99226])

98925 **Osteopathic manipulative treatment (OMT); 1-2 body regions involved** S 80
0.68 0.90 Global Days 000
AMA: 2009, Jan, 11-31; 2008, Jan, 10-25; 2007, January, 13-27

98926 **3-4 body regions involved** S 80
1.02 1.28 Global Days 000
AMA: 2009, Jan, 11-31; 2008, Jan, 10-25; 2007, January, 13-27

98927 **5-6 body regions involved** S 80
1.35 1.68 Global Days 000
AMA: 2009, Jan, 11-31; 2008, Jan, 10-25; 2007, January, 13-27

98928 **7-8 body regions involved** S 80
1.71 2.06 Global Days 000
AMA: 2009, Jan, 11-31; 2008, Jan, 10-25; 2007, January, 13-27

98929 **9-10 body regions involved** S 80
2.05 2.47 Global Days 000
AMA: 2009, Jan, 11-31; 2008, Jan, 10-25; 2007, January, 13-27

98940-98943 Chiropractic Manipulation

CMS 100-1,5,70.6 Chiropractors
CMS 100-2,15,240 Chiropractic Services - General
CMS 100-3,150.1 Manipulation

INCLUDES Form of manual treatment performed to influence joint/neurophysical function

The following five extraspinal regions:

- Abdomen
- Head, including temporomandibular joint, excluding atlanto-occipital region
- Lower extremities
- Rib cage, not including costotransverse/costovertebral joints
- Upper extremities

The following five spinal regions:

- Cervical region (atlanto-occipital joint)
- Lumbar region
- Pelvic region (sacro-iliac joint)
- Sacral region
- Thoracic region (costovertebral/costotransverse joints)

Code also signficant separately identifiable evaluation and management service (99201-99499 [99224, 99225, 99226])

98940 **Chiropractic manipulative treatment (CMT); spinal, 1-2 regions** S 80 PQ
0.61 0.76 Global Days 000
AMA: 2009, Jan, 11-31; 2008, Jan, 10-25; 2007, January, 13-27; 2007, Dec, 10-179

98941 **spinal, 3-4 regions** S 80 PQ
0.90 1.06 Global Days 000
AMA: 2009, Jan, 11-31; 2008, Jan, 10-25; 2007, January, 13-27; 2007, Dec, 10-179

98942 **spinal, 5 regions** S 80 PQ
1.19 1.35 Global Days 000
AMA: 2009, Jan, 11-31; 2008, Jan, 10-25; 2007, January, 13-27; 2007, Dec, 10-179

98943 **extraspinal, 1 or more regions** E
0.60 0.70 Global Days XXX
AMA: 2009, Jan, 11-31; 2008, Jan, 10-25; 2007, January, 13-27; 2007, Dec, 10-179

98960-98962 Self-Management Training

INCLUDES Education/training services:

- Prescribed by a physician
- Provided by a qualified nonphysician health care provider

Standardized curriculum that may be modified as necessary for:

- Clinical needs
- Cultural norms
- Health literacy

Teaching the patient how to manage the illness/delay the comorbidity(s)

EXCLUDES *Genetic counseling education services (96040)*
Health/behavior assessment (96150-96155)
Medical nutrition therapy (97802-97804)
The following services provided by physicians:
Counseling/education to a group (99078)
Counseling/education to individuals (99201-99499 [99224, 99225, 99226])
Counseling/risk factor reduction without symptoms/established disease (99401-99412)

98960 **Education and training for patient self-management by a qualified, nonphysician health care professional using a standardized curriculum, face-to-face with the patient (could include caregiver/family) each 30 minutes; individual patient** E PQ
0.80 0.80 Global Days XXX
AMA: 2009, Feb, 13-16

98961 **2-4 patients** E PQ
INCLUDES Group education regarding genetic risks
0.39 0.39 Global Days XXX
AMA: 2009, Feb, 13-16; 2007, Aug, 9-12

98962 **5-8 patients** E PQ
INCLUDES Group education regarding genetic risks
0.29 0.29 Global Days XXX
AMA: 2009, Feb, 13-16; 2007, Aug, 9-12

98966-98968 Nonphysician Telephone Services

CMS 100-1,5,70 Definition of Physician

INCLUDES Assessment and management services provided by telephone by a qualified health care professional
Episode of care initiated by an established patient or his/her guardian

EXCLUDES *Call initiated by the qualified health care professional*
Calls during the postoperative period of a procedure
Decision to see the patient at the next available urgent care appointment
Decision to see the patient within 24 hours of the call
Telephone services provided by a physician (99441-99443)
Telephone services that are considered a part of a previous or subsequent service

Do not report with 98966-98968, 98969 if performed in the seven preceding days

98966 **Telephone assessment and management service provided by a qualified nonphysician health care professional to an established patient, parent, or guardian not originating from a related assessment and management service provided within the previous 7 days nor leading to an assessment and management service or procedure within the next 24 hours or soonest available appointment; 5-10 minutes of medical discussion** E
0.36 0.40 Global Days XXX
AMA: 2008, Mar, 6-7

98967 **11-20 minutes of medical discussion** E
0.73 0.77 Global Days XXX
AMA: 2008, Mar, 6-7

98968 **21-30 minutes of medical discussion** E
1.11 1.14 Global Days XXX
AMA: 2008, Mar, 6-7

98969 Nonphysician Online Service

INCLUDES On-line assessment and management service provided by a qualified health care professional
Timely reply to the patient as well as:
Ordering laboratory services
Permanent record of the service; either hard copy or electronic
Providing a prescription
Related telephone calls

EXCLUDES *On-line evaluation service:*
Provided during the postoperative period of a procedure
Provided more than once in a seven day period
Related to a service provided in the previous seven days

Do not report with (99339-99340, 99363-99364, 99374-99380)

98969 **Online assessment and management service provided by a qualified nonphysician health care professional to an established patient, guardian, or health care provider not originating from a related assessment and management service provided within the previous 7 days, using the Internet or similar electronic communications network** E
0.00 0.00 Global Days XXX
AMA: 2009, Jul, 5-6

99000-99091 Supplemental Services and Supplies

INCLUDES Supplemental reporting for services adjunct to the basic service provided

99000 **Handling and/or conveyance of specimen for transfer from the physician's office to a laboratory** E
0.00 0.00 Global Days XXX
AMA: 2009, Jan, 11-31; 2008, Jan, 10-25; 2007, January, 28-31; 2007, January, 13-27

99001 **Handling and/or conveyance of specimen for transfer from the patient in other than a physician's office to a laboratory (distance may be indicated)** E
0.00 0.00 Global Days XXX
AMA: 2009, Jan, 11-31; 2008, Jan, 10-25; 2007, January, 28-31; 2007, January, 13-27

99002 **Handling, conveyance, and/or any other service in connection with the implementation of an order involving devices (eg, designing, fitting, packaging, handling, delivery or mailing) when devices such as orthotics, protectives, prosthetics are fabricated by an outside laboratory or shop but which items have been designed, and are to be fitted and adjusted by the attending physician** B
EXCLUDES *Venous blood routine collection (36415)*
0.00 0.00 Global Days XXX
AMA: 2009, Jan, 11-31; 2008, Jan, 10-25; 2007, January, 13-27; 2007, January, 28-31

99024 **Postoperative follow-up visit, normally included in the surgical package, to indicate that an evaluation and management service was performed during a postoperative period for a reason(s) related to the original procedure** B
0.00 0.00 Global Days XXX
AMA: 2009, Jan, 11-31; 2008, Jan, 10-25; 2007, January, 13-27; 2007, January, 28-31

99026 **Hospital mandated on call service; in-hospital, each hour** E
EXCLUDES *Physician stand-by services with prolonged physician attendance (99360)*
0.00 0.00 Global Days XXX
AMA: 2009, Jan, 11-31; 2008, Jan, 10-25; 2007, January, 13-27; 2007, January, 28-31

99027 **out-of-hospital, each hour** E
EXCLUDES *Physician stand-by services with prolonged physician attendance (99360)*
0.00 0.00 Global Days XXX
AMA: 2009, Jan, 11-31; 2008, Jan, 10-25; 2007, January, 28-31; 2007, January, 13-27

⊘ **99050** **Services provided in the office at times other than regularly scheduled office hours, or days when the office is normally closed (eg, holidays, Saturday or Sunday), in addition to basic service** B
Code first basic service provided
Code also more than one adjunct code per encounter when appropriate
0.00 0.00 Global Days XXX
AMA: 2009, Jan, 11-31; 2008, Jan, 10-25; 2007, January, 13-27; 2007, January, 28-31

⊘ **99051** **Service(s) provided in the office during regularly scheduled evening, weekend, or holiday office hours, in addition to basic service** B
Code first basic service provided
Code also more than one adjunct code per encounter when appropriate
0.00 0.00 Global Days XXX
AMA: 2009, Jan, 11-31; 2008, Jan, 10-25; 2007, January, 13-27; 2007, January, 28-31

⊘ **99053** **Service(s) provided between 10:00 PM and 8:00 AM at 24-hour facility, in addition to basic service** B
Code first basic service provided
Code also more than one adjunct code per encounter when appropriate
0.00 0.00 Global Days XXX
AMA: 2009, Jan, 11-31; 2008, Jan, 10-25; 2007, January, 28-31; 2007, January, 13-27

⊘ 99056 **Service(s) typically provided in the office, provided out of the office at request of patient, in addition to basic service** B

Code first basic service provided

Code also more than one adjunct code per encounter when appropriate

0.00 0.00 Global Days XXX

AMA: 2009, Jan, 11-31; 2008, Jan, 10-25; 2007, January, 13-27; 2007, January, 28-31

⊘ 99058 **Service(s) provided on an emergency basis in the office, which disrupts other scheduled office services, in addition to basic service** B

Code first basic service provided

Code also more than one adjunct code per encounter when appropriate

0.00 0.00 Global Days XXX

AMA: 2009, Jan, 11-31; 2008, Jan, 10-25; 2007, January, 13-27; 2007, January, 28-31

⊘ 99060 **Service(s) provided on an emergency basis, out of the office, which disrupts other scheduled office services, in addition to basic service** B

Code first basic service provided

Code also more than one adjunct code per encounter when appropriate

0.00 0.00 Global Days XXX

AMA: 2009, Jan, 11-31; 2008, Jan, 10-25; 2007, January, 13-27; 2007, January, 28-31

99070 **Supplies and materials (except spectacles), provided by the physician over and above those usually included with the office visit or other services rendered (list drugs, trays, supplies, or materials provided)** B

EXCLUDES *Spectacles supply*

0.00 0.00 Global Days XXX

AMA: 2009, Jan, 11-31; 2009, May, 8-9&11; 2008, Jan, 10-25; 2008, Sep, 10□-11; 2007, January, 28-31; 2007, January, 13-27; 2007, February, 8-9

99071 **Educational supplies, such as books, tapes, and pamphlets, provided by the physician for the patient's education at cost to physician** B

0.00 0.00 Global Days XXX

AMA: 2009, Jan, 11-31; 2008, Jan, 10-25; 2007, January, 13-27; 2007, January, 28-31

99075 **Medical testimony** E

0.00 0.00 Global Days XXX

AMA: 2009, Jan, 11-31; 2008, Jan, 10-25; 2007, January, 13-27; 2007, January, 28-31

99078 **Physician educational services rendered to patients in a group setting (eg, prenatal, obesity, or diabetic instructions)** N PQ

0.00 0.00 Global Days XXX

AMA: 2009, Jan, 11-31; 2008, Jan, 10-25; 2007, January, 28-31; 2007, Aug, 9-12; 2007, January, 13-27

99080 **Special reports such as insurance forms, more than the information conveyed in the usual medical communications or standard reporting form** B

Do not report with 99455, 99456 for completion of workmen's compensation forms

0.00 0.00 Global Days XXX

AMA: 2009, Jan, 11-31; 2008, Jan, 10-25; 2007, January, 13-27; 2007, January, 28-31

99082 **Unusual travel (eg, transportation and escort of patient)** B 80

0.00 0.00 Global Days XXX

AMA: 2009, Jan, 11-31; 2008, Jan, 10-25; 2007, January, 28-31; 2007, January, 13-27

99090 **Analysis of clinical data stored in computers (eg, ECGs, blood pressures, hematologic data)** B

EXCLUDES *Collection/interpretation by health care professional/physician of physiologic data stored/transmitted by patient or caregiver (99091)*

Do not report this service if there exists a more specific CPT code for cardiographic services, glucose monitoring, or musculoskeletal function testing (93227, 93272, 95250, 97750, 0206T)

0.00 0.00 Global Days XXX

AMA: 2009, Jan, 11-31; 2008, Jan, 10-25; 2008, Jan, 6-7; 2007, Jul, 1-4; 2007, February, 10-11; 2007, January, 13-27; 2007, January, 28-31

99091 **Collection and interpretation of physiologic data (eg, ECG, blood pressure, glucose monitoring) digitally stored and/or transmitted by the patient and/or caregiver to the physician or other qualified health care professional, requiring a minimum of 30 minutes of time** N

INCLUDES Reporting only once in a 30-day period

EXCLUDES *Transfer/interpretation of data from hospital/clinical laboratory computers*

Do not report this service if there exists a more specific CPT code for cardiographic services, glucose monitoring, or musculoskeletal function testing (93227, 93272, 95250, 97750, 0206T)

Do not report with care plan oversight services if within 30 days (99374-99380)

Do not report with evaluation and management services provided on the same date of service

1.62 1.62 Global Days XXX

AMA: 2009, Jan, 11-31; 2008, Jan, 10-25; 2007, January, 13-27; 2007, January, 28-31

99100-99140 Modifying Factors for Anesthesia Services

CMS 100-4,12,50 Anesthesia Services

CMS 100-4,12,140 Certified Registered Nurse Anesthetist Services

CMS 100-4,12,140.2 Payment for CRNA Services

CMS 100-4,12,140.3.2 Calculation of Anesthesia Time

\+ 99100 **Anesthesia for patient of extreme age, younger than 1 year and older than 70 (List separately in addition to code for primary anesthesia procedure)** A B

EXCLUDES *Services performed on infants that are less that 1 year old at the time of surgery (00326, 00561, 00834, 00836)*

Code first primary anesthesia procedure

0.00 0.00 Global Days ZZZ

AMA: 2008, Apr, 3-4

\+ 99116 **Anesthesia complicated by utilization of total body hypothermia (List separately in addition to code for primary anesthesia procedure)** B

Code first primary anesthesia procedure

0.00 0.00 Global Days ZZZ

AMA: 2008, Apr, 3-4

\+ 99135 **Anesthesia complicated by utilization of controlled hypotension (List separately in addition to code for primary anesthesia procedure)** B

Code first primary anesthesia procedure

0.00 0.00 Global Days ZZZ

AMA: 2008, Apr, 3-4

+ **99140** **Anesthesia complicated by emergency conditions (specify) (List separately in addition to code for primary anesthesia procedure)** B

INCLUDES Circumstances where a delay in treatment would lead to a significant increase in the threat to life or body part

Code first primary anesthesia procedure

0.00 0.00 Global Days ZZZ

AMA: 2009, Jan, 11-31; 2008, Jan, 10-25; 2008, Apr, 3-4; 2007, January, 13-27

99143-99150 Moderate Sedation Services

INCLUDES Administration of medication
IV access
Maintenance of sedation
Monitoring of oxygen saturation/heart rate/blood pressure
Patient assessment
Recovery (not included in intraservice time)

EXCLUDES *Minimal sedation/anxiolysis/deep sedation/monitored anesthesia care (00100-01999)*

Do not report with pulse oximetry (94760-94762)

⊘ **99143** **Moderate sedation services (other than those services described by codes 00100-01999) provided by the same physician performing the diagnostic or therapeutic service that the sedation supports, requiring the presence of an independent trained observer to assist in the monitoring of the patient's level of consciousness and physiological status; younger than 5 years of age, first 30 minutes intra-service time** N 80

0.00 0.00 Global Days XXX

AMA: 2009, Jan, 11-31; 2008, Feb, 5-6; 2008, Jan, 10-25; 2007, January, 13-27

⊘ **99144** **age 5 years or older, first 30 minutes intra-service time** A N 80

0.00 0.00 Global Days XXX

AMA: 2008, Feb, 5-6

+ **99145** **each additional 15 minutes intra-service time (List separately in addition to code for primary service)** N 80

Code first initial 30 minutes (99143, 99144)

0.00 0.00 Global Days ZZZ

AMA: 2008, Feb, 5-6

99148 **Moderate sedation services (other than those services described by codes 00100-01999), provided by a physician other than the health care professional performing the diagnostic or therapeutic service that the sedation supports; younger than 5 years of age, first 30 minutes intra-service time** A N 80

0.00 0.00 Global Days XXX

AMA: 2009, Jan, 11-31; 2008, Jan, 10-25; 2007, January, 13-27

99149 **age 5 years or older, first 30 minutes intra-service time** A N 80

0.00 0.00 Global Days XXX

+ **99150** **each additional 15 minutes intra-service time (List separately in addition to code for primary service)** N 80

Code first initial 30 minutes (99148, 99149)

0.00 0.00 Global Days ZZZ

99170 Specialized Examination of Child

99170 **Anogenital examination with colposcopic magnification in childhood for suspected trauma** A T

EXCLUDES *Conscious sedation (99143-99150)*

2.61 3.94 Global Days 000

99172-99173 Visual Acuity Screening Tests

CMS 100-2,16,90 Routine Services and Appliances

99172 **Visual function screening, automated or semi-automated bilateral quantitative determination of visual acuity, ocular alignment, color vision by pseudoisochromatic plates, and field of vision (may include all or some screening of the determination[s] for contrast sensitivity, vision under glare)** E

INCLUDES Graduated visual acuity stimuli that allow a quantitative determination of visual acuity
Ocular photoscreening

Do not report with (99173)

Do not report with evaluation and management service or general ophthalmological service (99201-99499 [99224, 99225, 99226], 92002-92014)

0.00 0.00 Global Days XXX

AMA: 2009, Jan, 11-31; 2008, Jan, 10-25; 2007, January, 13-27

99173 **Screening test of visual acuity, quantitative, bilateral** E

INCLUDES Graduated visual acuity stimuli that allow a quantitative estimate of visual acuity
Ocular photoscreening

Do not report with (99172)

0.09 0.09 Global Days XXX

99174 Screening For Amblyogenic Factors

Do not report with (92002-92014, 99172-99173)

99174 **Ocular photoscreening with interpretation and report, bilateral** E

0.85 0.85 Global Days XXX

99175 Drug Administration to Induce Vomiting

EXCLUDES *Diagnostic gastric lavage (43754-43755)*
Diagnostic intubation (43754-43755)

99175 **Ipecac or similar administration for individual emesis and continued observation until stomach adequately emptied of poison** N 80

EXCLUDES *Diagnostic gastric intubation and aspiration (43754-43755)*
Diagnostic gastric lavage (43754-43755)

0.56 0.56 Global Days XXX

99183 Hyperbaric Oxygen Therapy

CMS 100-3,20.29 Hyperbaric Oxygen Therapy

99183 **Physician attendance and supervision of hyperbaric oxygen therapy, per session** B 80

EXCLUDES *Evaluation and management services if performed*
Other procedures such as wound debridement, if performed

3.51 6.35 Global Days XXX

AMA: 2009, Jan, 11-31; 2008, Jan, 10-25; 2007, January, 13-27

99190-99192 Assemble and Manage Pump with Oxygenator/Heat Exchange

99190 **Assembly and operation of pump with oxygenator or heat exchanger (with or without ECG and/or pressure monitoring); each hour** C

0.00 0.00 Global Days XXX

99191 **45 minutes**
0.00 0.00 Global Days XXX

99192 **30 minutes**
0.00 0.00 Global Days XXX

99195-99199 Therapeutic Phlebotomy and Unlisted Procedures

99195 **Phlebotomy, therapeutic (separate procedure)**
2.74 2.74 Global Days XXX
AMA: 2009, Jan, 11-31; 2008, Jan, 10-25; 2007, January, 13-27

99199 **Unlisted special service, procedure or report**
0.00 0.00 Global Days XXX

99500-99602 Home Visit By Non-Physician Professionals

INCLUDES Services performed by non-physician providers
Services provided in patient's:
Assisted living apartment
Custodial care facility
Group home
Non-traditional private home
Residence
School

EXCLUDES *Home visits performed by physicians (99341-99350)*
Other services/procedures provided by physicians to patients at home

Code also home visit evaluation and management codes if health care provider is authorized to use (99341-99350)

Code also significant separately identifiable evaluation and management service

99500 **Home visit for prenatal monitoring and assessment to include fetal heart rate, non-stress test, uterine monitoring, and gestational diabetes monitoring**
0.00 0.00 Global Days XXX
AMA: 2009, Jan, 11-31; 2008, Jan, 10-25; 2007, January, 28-31

99501 **Home visit for postnatal assessment and follow-up care**
0.00 0.00 Global Days XXX
AMA: 2007, January, 28-31

99502 **Home visit for newborn care and assessment**
0.00 0.00 Global Days XXX
AMA: 2007, January, 28-31

99503 **Home visit for respiratory therapy care (eg, bronchodilator, oxygen therapy, respiratory assessment, apnea evaluation)**
0.00 0.00 Global Days XXX
AMA: 2007, January, 28-31

99504 **Home visit for mechanical ventilation care**
0.00 0.00 Global Days XXX
AMA: 2007, January, 28-31

99505 **Home visit for stoma care and maintenance including colostomy and cystostomy**
0.00 0.00 Global Days XXX
AMA: 2007, January, 28-31

99506 **Home visit for intramuscular injections**
0.00 0.00 Global Days XXX
AMA: 2007, January, 28-31

99507 **Home visit for care and maintenance of catheter(s) (eg, urinary, drainage, and enteral)**
0.00 0.00 Global Days XXX
AMA: 2007, January, 28-31

99509 **Home visit for assistance with activities of daily living and personal care**
EXCLUDES *Medical nutrition therapy/assessment home services (97802-97804)*
Self-care/home management training (97535)
Speech therapy home services (92507-92508)
0.00 0.00 Global Days XXX
AMA: 2007, January, 28-31

99510 **Home visit for individual, family, or marriage counseling**
0.00 0.00 Global Days XXX
AMA: 2007, January, 28-31

99511 **Home visit for fecal impaction management and enema administration**
0.00 0.00 Global Days XXX
AMA: 2007, January, 28-31

99512 **Home visit for hemodialysis**
EXCLUDES *Peritoneal dialysis home infusion (99601, 99602)*
0.00 0.00 Global Days XXX
AMA: 2007, January, 28-31

99600 **Unlisted home visit service or procedure**
0.00 0.00 Global Days XXX
AMA: 2009, Jan, 11-31; 2008, Jan, 10-25; 2007, January, 28-31

99601 **Home infusion/specialty drug administration, per visit (up to 2 hours);**
0.00 0.00 Global Days XXX

\+ 99602 **each additional hour (List separately in addition to code for primary procedure)**
Code first initial 2 hours (99601)
0.00 0.00 Global Days XXX

99605-99607 Medication Management By Pharmacist

INCLUDES Direct (face-to-face) assessment and intervention by a pharmacist for the purpose of:
Managing medication complications and/or interactions
Maximizing the patient's response to drug therapy
Documenting the following required elements:
Advice given regarding improvement of treatment compliance and outcomes
Profile of medications (prescription and nonprescription)
Review of applicable patient history

EXCLUDES *Routine tasks associated with dispensing and related activities (e.g., providing product information)*

99605 **Medication therapy management service(s) provided by a pharmacist, individual, face-to-face with patient, with assessment and intervention if provided; initial 15 minutes, new patient**
0.00 0.00 Global Days XXX

99606 **initial 15 minutes, established patient**
0.00 0.00 Global Days XXX

\+ 99607 **each additional 15 minutes (List separately in addition to code for primary service)**
Code first (99605, 99606)
0.00 0.00 Global Days XXX
AMA: 2009, Jan, 11-31

Evaluation and Management (E/M) Services Guidelines

In addition to the information presented in the Introduction, several other items unique to this section are defined or identified here.

CLASSIFICATION OF EVALUATION AND MANAGEMENT (E/M) SERVICES

The E/M section is divided into broad categories such as office visits, hospital visits, and consultations. Most of the categories are further divided into two or more subcategories of E/M services. For example, there are two subcategories of office visits (new patient and established patient) and there are two subcategories of hospital visits (initial and subsequent). The subcategories of E/M services are further classified into levels of E/M services that are identified by specific codes. This classification is important because the nature of physician work varies by type of service, place of service, and the patient's status.

The basic format of the levels of E/M services is the same for most categories. First, a unique code number is listed. The following Second, the place and/or type of service is specified, eg, office consultation. Third, the content of the service is defined, eg, comprehensive history and comprehensive examination. (See "Levels of E/M Services," for details on the content of E/M services.) Fourth, the nature of the presenting problem(s) usually associated with a given level is described. Fifth, the time typically required to provide the service is specified. (A detailed discussion of time is provided)

DEFINITIONS OF COMMONLY USED SEPARATELY TERMS

Certain key words and phrases are used throughout the E/M section. The following definitions are intended to reduce the potential for differing interpretations and to increase the consistency of reporting by physicians in differing specialties. E/M services may also be reported by other qualified health care professionals who are authorized to perform such services within the scope of their practice.

New and Established Patient

Solely for the purposes of distinguishing between new and established patients, professional services are those face-to-face services rendered by a physician and reported by a specific CPT code(s). A new patient is one who has not received any professional services from the physician or another physician of the exact same specialty and subspecialty who belongs to the same group practice, within the past three years.

An established patient is one who has received professional services from the physician or another physician of the exact same specialty and subspecialty who belongs to the same group practice, within the past three years. See Decision Tree.

In the instance where a physician is on call for or covering for another physician, the patient's encounter will be classified as it would have been by the physician who is not available.

No distinction is made between new and established patients in the emergency department. E/M services in the emergency department category may be reported for any new or established patient who presents for treatment in the emergency department.

The decision tree on the following page is provided to aid in determining whether to report the E/M service provided as a new or an established patient encounter.

Chief Complaint

A chief complaint is a concise statement describing the symptom, problem, condition, diagnosis, or other factor that is the reason for the encounter, usually stated in the patient's words.

Concurrent Care and Transfer of Care

Concurrent care is the provision of similar services (eg, hospital visits) to the same patient by more than one physician on the same day. When concurrent care is provided, no special reporting is required. Transfer of care is the process whereby a physician who is providing management for some or all of a patient's problems relinquishes this responsibility to another physician who explicitly agrees to accept this responsibility and who, from the initial encounter, is not providing consultative services. The physician transferring care is then no longer providing care for these problems though he or she may before an initial evaluation but are appropriate to report continue providing care for other conditions when if the decision to accept transfer of care cannot be made appropriate. Consultation codes should not be reported until after the initial consultation evaluation, regardless of by the physician who has agreed to accept transfer of care site of service.

Decision Tree for New vs Established Patients

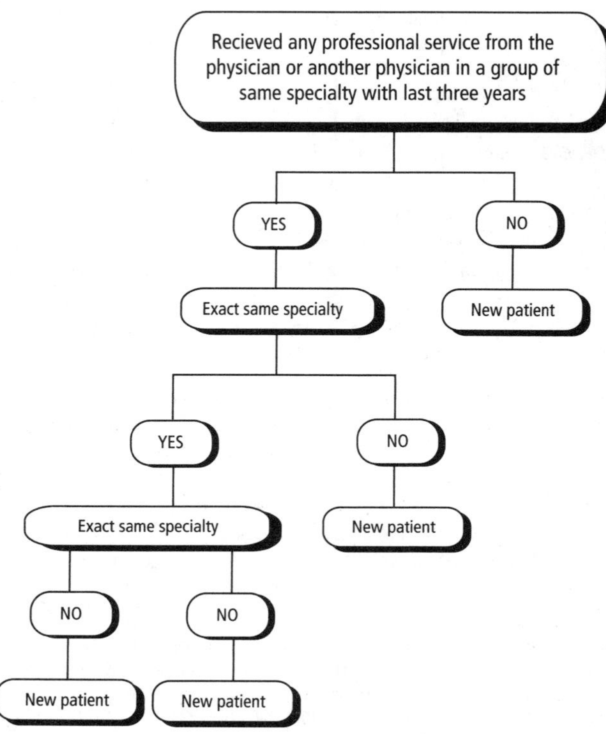

Counseling

Counseling is a discussion with a patient and/or family concerning one or more of the following areas:

- Diagnostic results, impressions, and/or recommended diagnostic studies
- Prognosis
- Risks and benefits of management (treatment) options
- Instructions for management (treatment) and/or follow-up
- Importance of compliance with chosen management (treatment) options
- Risk factor reduction
- Patient and family education

(For psychotherapy, see 90804-90857)

Family History

A review of medical events in the patient's family that includes significant information about:

- The health status or cause of death of parents, siblings, and children
- Specific diseases related to problems identified in the Chief Complaint or History of the Present Illness, and/or System Review

- Diseases of family members that may be hereditary or place the patient at risk

History of Present Illness
A chronological description of the development of the patient's present illness from the first sign and/or symptom to the present. This includes a description of location, quality, severity, timing, context, modifying factors, and associated signs and symptoms significantly related to the presenting problem(s).

Levels of E/M Services
Within each category or subcategory of E/M service, there are three to five levels of E/M services available for reporting purposes. Levels of E/M services are not interchangeable among the different categories or subcategories of service. For example, the first level of E/M services in the subcategory of office visit, new patient, does not have the same definition as the first level of E/M services in the subcategory of office visit, established patient.

The levels of E/M services include examinations, evaluations, treatments, conferences with or concerning patients, preventive pediatric and adult health supervision, and similar medical services, such as the determination of the need and/or location for appropriate care. Medical screening includes the history, examination, and medical decision-making required to determine the need and/or location for appropriate care and treatment of the patient (eg, office and other outpatient setting, emergency department, nursing facility). The levels of E/M services encompass the wide variations in skill, effort, time, responsibility, and medical knowledge required for the prevention or diagnosis and treatment of illness or injury and the promotion of optimal health. Each level of E/M services may be used by all physicians.

The descriptors for the levels of E/M services recognize seven components, six of which are used in defining the levels of E/M services. These components are:

- History
- Examination
- Medical decision making
- Counseling
- Coordination of care
- Nature of presenting problem
- Time

The first three of these components (history, examination, and medical decision making) are considered the key components in selecting a level of E/M services. (See "Determine the Extent of History Obtained)

The next three components (counseling, coordination of care, and the nature of the presenting problem) are considered contributory factors in the majority of encounters. Although the first two of these contributory factors are important E/M services, it is not required that these services be provided at every patient encounter.

Coordination of care with other providers or agencies without a patient encounter on that day is reported using the case management codes.

The final component, time, is discussed in detail seperately

Any specifically identifiable procedure (ie, identified with a specific CPT code) performed on or subsequent to the date of initial or subsequent E/M services should be reported separately.

The actual performance and/or interpretation of diagnostic tests/studies ordered during a patient encounter are not included in the levels of E/M services. Physician performance of diagnostic tests/studies for which specific CPT codes are available may be reported separately, in addition to the appropriate E/M code. The physician's interpretation of the results of diagnostic tests/ studies (ie, professional component) with preparation of a separate distinctly identifiable signed written report may also be reported separately, using the appropriate CPT code with modifier 26 appended.

The physician may need to indicate that on the day a procedure or service identified by a CPT code was performed, the patient's condition required a significant separately identifiable E/M service above and beyond other services provided or beyond the usual preservice and postservice care associated with the procedure that was performed. The E/M service may be caused or prompted by the symptoms or condition for which the procedure and/or service was provided. This circumstance may be reported by adding modifier 25 to the appropriate level of E/M service. As such, different diagnoses are not required for reporting of the procedure and the E/M services on the same date.

Nature of Presenting Problem
A presenting problem is a disease, condition, illness, injury, symptom, sign, finding, complaint, or other reason for encounter, with or without a diagnosis being established at the time of the encounter. The E/M codes recognize five types of presenting problems that are defined as follows:

Minimal: A problem that may not require the presence of the physician, but service is provided under the physician's supervision.

Self-limited or minor: A problem that runs a definite and prescribed course, is transient in nature, and is not likely to permanently alter health status OR has a good prognosis with management/compliance.

Low severity: A problem where the risk of morbidity without treatment is low; there is little to no risk of mortality without treatment; full recovery without functional impairment is expected.

Moderate severity: A problem where the risk of morbidity without treatment is moderate; there is moderate risk of mortality without treatment; uncertain prognosis OR increased probability of prolonged functional impairment.

High severity: A problem where the risk of morbidity without treatment is high to extreme; there is a moderate to high risk of mortality without treatment OR high probability of severe, prolonged functional impairment.

Past History
A review of the patient's past experiences with illnesses, injuries, and treatments that includes significant information about:

- Prior major illnesses and injuries
- Prior operations
- Prior hospitalizations
- Current medications
- Allergies (eg, drug, food)
- Age appropriate immunization status
- Age appropriate feeding/dietary status

Social History
An age appropriate review of past and current activities that includes significant information about:

- Marital status and/or living arrangements
- Current employment
- Occupational history j Use of drugs, alcohol, and tobacco
- Level of education
- Sexual history
- Other relevant social factors

System Review (Review of Systems)
An inventory of body systems obtained through a series of questions seeking to identify signs and/or symptoms that the patient may be experiencing or has experienced. For the purposes of the CPT codebook the following elements of a system review have been identified:

- Constitutional symptoms (fever, weight loss, etc)
- Eyes
- Ears, nose, mouth, throat
- Cardiovascular
- Respiratory
- Gastrointestinal
- Genitourinary
- Musculoskeletal
- Integumentary (skin and/or breast)
- Neurological
- Psychiatric
- Endocrine

- Hematologic/lymphatic
- Allergic/immunologic

The review of systems helps define the problem, clarify the differential diagnosis, identify needed testing, or serves as baseline data on other systems that might be affected by any possible management options.

Time

The inclusion of time in the definitions of levels of E/M services has been implicit in prior editions of the CPT codebook. The inclusion of time as an explicit factor beginning in CPT 1992 is done to assist physicians in selecting the most appropriate level of E/M services. It should be recognized that the specific times expressed in the visit code descriptors are averages and, therefore, represent a range of times that may be higher or lower depending on actual clinical circumstances.

Time is not a descriptive component for the emergency department levels of E/M services because emergency department services are typically provided on a variable intensity basis, often involving multiple encounters with several patients over an extended period of time. Therefore, it is often difficult for physicians to provide accurate estimates of the time spent face-to-face with the patient.

Studies to establish levels of E/M services employed surveys of practicing physicians to obtain data on the amount of time and work associated with typical E/M services. Since "work" is not easily quantifiable, the codes must rely on other objective, verifiable measures that correlate with physicians' estimates of their "work." It has been demonstrated that physicians' estimations of intraservice time (as explained on the next page), both within and across specialties, is a variable that is predictive of the "work" of E/M services. This same research has shown there is a strong relationship between intraservice time and total time for E/M services. Intraservice time, rather than total time, was chosen for inclusion with the codes because of its relative ease of measurement and because of its direct correlation with measurements of the total amount of time and work associated with typical E/M services.

Intraservice times are defined as face-to-face time for office and other outpatient visits and as unit/floor time for hospital and other inpatient visits. This distinction is necessary because most of the work of typical office visits takes place during the face-to-face time with the patient, while most of the work of typical hospital visits takes place during the time spent on the patient's floor or unit. When prolonged time occurs in either the office or the inpatient areas, the appropriate add-on code should be reported.

Face-to-face time (office and other outpatient visits and office consultations): For coding purposes, face-toface time for these services is defined as only that time that the physician spends face-to-face with the patient and/or family. This includes the time in which the physician performs such tasks as obtaining a history, performing an examination, and counseling the patient.

Physicians also spend time doing work before or after the face-to-face time with the patient, performing such tasks as reviewing records and tests, arranging for further services, and communicating further with other professionals and the patient through written reports and telephone contact.

This non-face-to-face time for office services—also called pre- and postencounter time—is not included in the time component described in the E/M codes. However, the pre- and post-non-face-to-face work associated with an encounter was included in calculating the total work of typical services in physician surveys.

Thus, the face-to-face time associated with the services described by any E/M code is a valid proxy for the total work done before, during, and after the visit.

Unit/floor time (hospital observation services, inpatient hospital care, initial inpatient hospital consultations, nursing facility): For reporting purposes, intraservice time for these services is defined as unit/floor time, which includes the time that the physician is present on the patient's hospital unit and at the bedside rendering services for that patient. This includes the time in which the physician establishes and/or reviews the patient's chart, examines the patient, writes notes, and communicates with other professionals and the patient's family.

In the hospital, pre- and post-time includes time spent off the patient's floor performing such tasks as reviewing pathology and radiology findings in another part of the hospital.

This pre- and postvisit time is not included in the time component described in these codes. However, the pre- and postwork performed during the time spent off the floor or unit was included in calculating the total work of typical services in physician surveys.

Thus, the unit/floor time associated with the services described by any code is a valid proxy for the total work done before, during, and after the visit.

UNLISTED SERVICE

An E/M service may be provided that is not listed in this section of the CPT codebook. When reporting such a service, the appropriate unlisted code may be used to indicate the service, identifying it by "Special Report," as discussed in the following paragraph. The "Unlisted Services" and accompanying codes for the E/M section are as follows:

99429 **Unlisted preventive medicine service**

99499 **Unlisted evaluation and management service**

SPECIAL REPORT

An unlisted service or one that is unusual, variable, or new may require a special report demonstrating the medical appropriateness of the service. Pertinent information should include an adequate definition or description of the nature, extent, and need for the procedure and the time, effort, and equipment necessary to provide the service. Additional items that may be included are complexity of symptoms, final diagnosis, pertinent physical findings, diagnostic and therapeutic procedures, concurrent problems, and follow-up care.

INSTRUCTIONS FOR SELECTING A LEVEL OF E/M SERVICE

Review the Reporting Instructions for the Selected Category or Subcategory

Most of the categories and many of the subcategories of service have special guidelines or instructions unique to that category or subcategory. Where these are indicated, eg, "Inpatient Hospital Care," special instructions will be presented preceding the levels of E/M services.

Review the Level of E/M Service Descriptors and Examples in the Selected Category or Subcategory

The descriptors for the levels of E/M services recognize seven components, six of which are used in defining the levels of E/M services. These components are:

- History
- Examination
- Medical decision making
- Counseling
- Coordination of care
- Nature of presenting problem
- Time

The first three of these components (ie, history, examination, and medical decision making) should be considered the key components in selecting the level of E/M services. An exception to this rule is in the case of visits that consist predominantly of counseling or coordination of care.

The nature of the presenting problem and time are provided in some levels to assist the physician in determining the appropriate level of E/M service.

Determine the Extent of History Obtained

The extent of the history is dependent upon clinical judgment and on the nature of the presenting problem(s). The levels of E/M services recognize four types of history that are defined as follows:

Problem focused: Chief complaint; brief history of present illness or problem.

Expanded problem focused: Chief complaint; brief history of present illness; problem pertinent system review.

Detailed: Chief complaint; extended history of present illness; problem pertinent system review extended to include a review of a limited number of additional systems; pertinent past, family, and/or social history directly related to the patient's problems.

Comprehensive: Chief complaint; extended history of present illness; review of systems that is directly related to the problem(s) identified in the history of the present illness plus a review of all additional body systems; complete past, family, and social history.

The comprehensive history obtained as part of the preventive medicine E/M service is not problem-oriented and does not involve a chief complaint or present illness. It does, however, include a comprehensive system review and comprehensive or interval past, family, and social history as well as a comprehensive assessment/history of pertinent risk factors.

Determine the Extent of Examination Performed

The extent of the examination performed is dependent on clinical judgment and on the nature of the presenting problem(s). The levels of E/M services recognize four types of examination that are defined as follows:

Problem focused: A limited examination of the affected body area or organ system.

Expanded problem focused: A limited examination of the affected body area or organ system and other symptomatic or related organ system(s).

Detailed: An extended examination of the affected body area(s) and other symptomatic or related organ system(s).

Comprehensive: A general multisystem examination or a complete examination of a single organ system. Note: The comprehensive examination performed as part of the preventive medicine E/M service is multisystem, but its extent is based on age and risk factors identified.

For the purposes of these CPT definitions, the following body areas are recognized:

- Head, including the face
- Neck
- Chest, including breasts and axilla
- Abdomen
- Genitalia, groin, buttocks
- Back
- Each extremity

For the purposes of these CPT definitions, the following organ systems are recognized:

- Eyes
- Ears, nose, mouth, and throat
- Cardiovascular
- Respiratory
- Gastrointestinal
- Genitourinary
- Musculoskeletal
- Skin
- Neurologic
- Psychiatric
- Hematologic/lymphatic/immunologic

Determine the Complexity of Medical Decision Making

Medical decision making refers to the complexity of establishing a diagnosis and/or selecting a management option as measured by:

- The number of possible diagnoses and/or the number of management options that must be considered
- The amount and/or complexity of medical records, diagnostic tests, and/or other information that must be obtained, reviewed, and analyzed
- The risk of significant complications, morbidity, and/or mortality, as well as comorbidities, associated with the patient's presenting problem(s), the diagnostic procedure(s), and/or the possible management options

Four types of medical decision making are recognized: straightforward, low complexity, moderate complexity, and high complexity. To qualify for a given type of decision making, two of the three elements in Table 1 must be met or exceeded.

TABLE 1

Complexity of Medical Decision Making

Number of Diagnoses or Management Options	*Amount and/or Complexity of Data to be Reviewed*	*Risk of Complications and/or Morbidity or Mortality*	*Type of Decision Making*
minimal	minimal or none	minimal	straightforward
limited	limited	low	low complexity
multiple	moderate	moderate	moderate complexity
extensive	extensive	high	high complexity

CONSULTATION CODES AND MEDICARE REIMBURSEMENT

The Centers for Medicare and Medicaid Services (CMS) no longer provides benefits for CPT consultation codes. CMS has, however, redistributed the value of the consultation codes across the other E/M codes for services which are covered by Medicare. CMS has retained codes 99241 - 99251 in the Medicare Physician Fee Schedule for those private payers that use this data for reimbursement. Note that private payers may choose to follow CMS or CPT guidelines, and the use of consultation codes should be verified with individual payers.

Comorbidities/underlying diseases, in and of themselves, are not considered in selecting a level of E/M services *unless* their presence significantly increases the complexity of the medical decision making.

Select the Appropriate Level of E/M Services Based on the Following

For the following categories/subcategories, all of the key components, ie, history, examination, and medical decision making, must meet or exceed the stated requirements to qualify for a particular level of E/M service: office, new patient; hospital observation services; initial hospital care; office consultations; initial inpatient consultations; emergency department services; initial nursing facility care; domiciliary care, new patient; and home, new patient.

For the following categories/subcategories, two of the three key components (ie, history, examination, and medical decision making) must meet or exceed the stated requirements to qualify for a particular level of E/M services: office, established patient; subsequent hospital care; subsequent nursing facility care; domiciliary care, established patient; and home, established patient.

When counseling and/or coordination of care dominates (more than 50%) the physician/patient and/or family encounter (face-to-face time in the office or other outpatient setting or floor/unit time in the hospital or nursing facility), then time shall be considered the key or controlling factor to qualify for a particular level of E/M services. This includes time spent with parties who have assumed responsibility for the care of the patient or decision making whether or not they are family members (eg, foster parents, person acting in loco parentis, legal guardian). The extent of counseling and/or coordination of care must be documented in the medical record.

Evaluation and Management (E/M) Services Guidelines

99201-99215 Outpatient and Other Visits

CMS 100-3,70.3 Physician's Offices Within an Institution--"Incident-to" Provision

CMS 100-4,12,30.6.7 Payment for Office or Other Outpatient Evaluation and Management (E/M) Visits

INCLUDES Established patients: received prior professional services from the physician or another physician in the practice of the same specialty and subspecialty in the previous three years (99211-99215)

New patients: have not received professional services from the physician or any other physician in the same practice within the exact same specialty and subspecialty in the previous three years (99201-99205)

Office visits

Outpatient services prior to formal admission to a facility

EXCLUDES *Services provided in:*

Emergency department (99281-99285)

Hospital observation (99217-99220)

Hospital observation or inpatient with same day admission and discharge (99234-99236)

99201 **Office or other outpatient visit for the evaluation and management of a new patient, which requires these 3 key components: A problem focused history; A problem focused examination; Straightforward medical decision making. Counseling and/or coordination of care with other providers or agencies are provided consistent with the nature of the problem(s) and the patient's and/or family's needs. Usually, the presenting problem(s) are self limited or minor. Physicians typically spend 10 minutes face-to-face with the patient and/or family.** V 80 PQ

0.76 1.25 Global Days XXX

AMA: 2009, Mar, 3,4&7; 2009, Jan, 11-31; 2009, Jul, 8-9; 2009, Jul, 7; 2008, Jan, 10-25; 2007, Jul, 1-4; 2007, March, 9-11; 2007, April, 11-12; 2007, January, 13-27

99202 **Office or other outpatient visit for the evaluation and management of a new patient, which requires these 3 key components: An expanded problem focused history; An expanded problem focused examination; Straightforward medical decision making. Counseling and/or coordination of care with other providers or agencies are provided consistent with the nature of the problem(s) and the patient's and/or family's needs. Usually, the presenting problem(s) are of low to moderate severity. Physicians typically spend 20 minutes face-to-face with the patient and/or family.** V 80 PQ

1.44 2.13 Global Days XXX

AMA: 2009, Jan, 11-31; 2009, Mar, 3,4&7; 2009, Jul, 7; 2009, Jul, 8-9; 2008, Jan, 10-25; 2007, Jul, 1-4; 2007, March, 9-11; 2007, January, 13-27; 2007, April, 11-12

99203 **Office or other outpatient visit for the evaluation and management of a new patient, which requires these 3 key components: A detailed history; A detailed examination; Medical decision making of low complexity. Counseling and/or coordination of care with other providers or agencies are provided consistent with the nature of the problem(s) and the patient's and/or family's needs. Usually, the presenting problem(s) are of moderate severity. Physicians typically spend 30 minutes face-to-face with the patient and/or family.** V 80 PQ

2.20 3.09 Global Days XXX

AMA: 2009, Jan, 11-31; 2009, Mar, 3,4&7; 2009, Jul, 8-9; 2009, Jul, 7; 2008, Jan, 10-25; 2007, Jul, 1-4; 2007, January, 13-27; 2007, April, 11-12; 2007, March, 9-11

99204 **Office or other outpatient visit for the evaluation and management of a new patient, which requires these 3 key components: A comprehensive history; A comprehensive examination; Medical decision making of moderate complexity. Counseling and/or coordination of care with other providers or agencies are provided consistent with the nature of the problem(s) and the patient's and/or family's needs. Usually, the presenting problem(s) are of moderate to high severity. Physicians typically spend 45 minutes face-to-face with the patient and/or family.** V 80 PQ

3.73 4.72 Global Days XXX

AMA: 2009, Mar, 3,4&7; 2009, Jul, 8-9; 2009, Jan, 11-31; 2009, Jul, 7; 2008, Jan, 10-25; 2007, Jul, 1-4; 2007, January, 13-27; 2007, April, 11-12; 2007, March, 9-11

99205 **Office or other outpatient visit for the evaluation and management of a new patient, which requires these 3 key components: A comprehensive history; A comprehensive examination; Medical decision making of high complexity. Counseling and/or coordination of care with other providers or agencies are provided consistent with the nature of the problem(s) and the patient's and/or family's needs. Usually, the presenting problem(s) are of moderate to high severity. Physicians typically spend 60 minutes face-to-face with the patient and/or family.** 03 80 PQ

4.78 5.86 Global Days XXX

AMA: 2009, Jan, 11-31; 2009, Mar, 3,4&7; 2009, Jul, 8-9; 2009, Jul, 7; 2008, Jan, 10-25; 2007, Jul, 1-4; 2007, March, 9-11; 2007, April, 11-12; 2007, January, 13-27

99211 **Office or other outpatient visit for the evaluation and management of an established patient, that may not require the presence of a physician. Usually, the presenting problem(s) are minimal. Typically, 5 minutes are spent performing or supervising these services.** V 80 PQ

0.27 0.58 Global Days XXX

AMA: 2009, Jan, 11-31; 2009, Mar, 3,4&7; 2009, Jul, 7; 2009, Jul, 8-9; 2008, Jan, 10-25; 2008, Mar, 3&7; 2007, Jul, 1-4; 2007, March, 9-11; 2007, January, 13-27; 2007, Dec, 9; 2007, April, 11-12

99212 **Office or other outpatient visit for the evaluation and management of an established patient, which requires at least 2 of these 3 key components: A problem focused history; A problem focused examination; Straightforward medical decision making. Counseling and/or coordination of care with other providers or agencies are provided consistent with the nature of the problem(s) and the patient's and/or family's needs. Usually, the presenting problem(s) are self limited or minor. Physicians typically spend 10 minutes face-to-face with the patient and/or family.** V 80 PQ

0.74 1.25 Global Days XXX

AMA: 2009, Jan, 11-31; 2009, Mar, 3,4&7; 2009, Jul, 8-9; 2009, Jul, 7; 2008, Jan, 10-25; 2008, Mar, 3&7; 2007, Jul, 1-4; 2007, January, 13-27; 2007, April, 11-12; 2007, March, 9-11

99213 **Office or other outpatient visit for the evaluation and management of an established patient, which requires at least 2 of these 3 key components: An expanded problem focused history; An expanded problem focused examination; Medical decision making of low complexity. Counseling and coordination of care with other providers or agencies are provided consistent with the nature of the problem(s) and the patient's and/or family's needs. Usually, the presenting problem(s) are of low to moderate severity. Physicians typically spend 15 minutes face-to-face with the patient and/or family.**

1.46 2.07 Global Days XXX

AMA: 2009, Jan, 11-31; 2009, Mar, 3,4&7; 2009, Jul, 8-9; 2009, Jul, 7; 2008, Jan, 10-25; 2008, Mar, 3&7; 2007, Jul, 1-4; 2007, March, 9-11; 2007, April, 11-12; 2007, January, 13-27

99214 **Office or other outpatient visit for the evaluation and management of an established patient, which requires at least 2 of these 3 key components: A detailed history; A detailed examination; Medical decision making of moderate complexity. Counseling and/or coordination of care with other providers or agencies are provided consistent with the nature of the problem(s) and the patient's and/or family's needs. Usually, the presenting problem(s) are of moderate to high severity. Physicians typically spend 25 minutes face-to-face with the patient and/or family.**

2.24 3.06 Global Days XXX

AMA: 2009, Jan, 11-31; 2009, Mar, 3,4&7; 2009, Jul, 8-9; 2009, Jul, 7; 2008, Jan, 10-25; 2008, Mar, 3&7; 2008, Jun, 12&15; 2007, Jul, 1-4; 2007, April, 11-12; 2007, January, 13-27; 2007, March, 9-11

99215 **Office or other outpatient visit for the evaluation and management of an established patient, which requires at least 2 of these 3 key components: A comprehensive history; A comprehensive examination; Medical decision making of high complexity. Counseling and/or coordination of care with other providers or agencies are provided consistent with the nature of the problem(s) and the patient's and/or family's needs. Usually, the presenting problem(s) are of moderate to high severity. Physicians typically spend 40 minutes face-to-face with the patient and/or family.**

3.15 4.11 Global Days XXX

AMA: 2009, Mar, 3,4&7; 2009, Jul, 7; 2009, Jul, 8-9; 2009, Jan, 11-31; 2008, Mar, 3&7; 2008, Jan, 10-25; 2007, Jul, 1-4; 2007, January, 13-27; 2007, March, 9-11; 2007, April, 11-12

99217-99220 Facility Observation Visits: Initial and Discharge

CMS 100-1,5,70 Definition of Physician
CMS 100-2,15,30 Physician Services
CMS 100-3,70.1 Consultations with a Beneficiary's Family and Associates
CMS 100-4,12,30.6.8 Payment for Hospital Observation Services

INCLUDES Services provided on the same date in other settings (e.g, emergency department, physician's office) associated with the observation status admission
Services provided to new and established patients admitted to a hospital specifically for observation (not required to be a designated area of the hospital)

EXCLUDES *Services provided by physicians other than the admitting physician ([99224, 99225, 99226], 99241-99245)*
Services provided to patients who are admitted and discharged from observation status on the same date (99234-99236)

99217 **Observation care discharge day management (This code is to be utilized by the physician to report all services provided to a patient on discharge from "observation status" if the discharge is on other than the initial date of "observation status." To report services to a patient designated as "observation status" or "inpatient status" and discharged on the same date, use the codes for Observation or Inpatient Care Services [including Admission and Discharge Services, 99234-99236 as appropriate.])**

INCLUDES Discussing the observation admission with the patient
Final patient evaluation
Discharge instructions
Sign off on discharge medical records

Do not report with hospital discharge day management services (99238-99239)

Do not report with observation/inpatient admission/discharge on the same date (99234-99236)

2.06 2.06 Global Days XXX

AMA: 2009, Jul, 7; 2007, Jul, 1-4; 2007, March, 9-11

▲ **99218** **Initial observation care, per day, for the evaluation and management of a patient which requires these 3 key components: A detailed or comprehensive history; A detailed or comprehensive examination; and Medical decision making that is straightforward or of low complexity. Counseling and/or coordination of care with other providers or agencies are provided consistent with the nature of the problem(s) and the patient's and/or family's needs. Usually, the problem(s) requiring admission to "observation status" are of low severity. Physicians typically spend 30 minutes at the bedside and on the patient's hospital floor or unit.**

2.77 2.77 Global Days XXX

AMA: 2009, Jan, 11-31; 2009, Jul, 7; 2008, Jan, 10-25; 2007, Jul, 1-4; 2007, January, 13-27; 2007, March, 9-11

▲ **99219** **Initial observation care, per day, for the evaluation and management of a patient, which requires these 3 key components: A comprehensive history; A comprehensive examination; and Medical decision making of moderate complexity. Counseling and/or coordination of care with other providers or agencies are provided consistent with the nature of the problem(s) and the patient's and/or family's needs. Usually, the problem(s) requiring admission to "observation status" are of moderate severity. Physicians typically spend 50 minutes at the bedside and on the patient's hospital floor or unit.** B 80 PQ

3.81 3.81 Global Days XXX

AMA: 2009, Jul, 7; 2009, Jan, 11-31; 2008, Jan, 10-25; 2007, Jul, 1-4; 2007, January, 13-27; 2007, March, 9-11

▲ **99220** **Initial observation care, per day, for the evaluation and management of a patient, which requires these 3 key components: A comprehensive history; A comprehensive examination; and Medical decision making of high complexity. Counseling and/or coordination of care with other providers or agencies are provided consistent with the nature of the problem(s) and the patient's and/or family's needs. Usually, the problem(s) requiring admission to "observation status" are of high severity. Physicians typically spend 70 minutes at the bedside and on the patient's hospital floor or unit.** B 80 PQ

5.23 5.23 Global Days XXX

AMA: 2009, Jan, 11-31; 2009, Jul, 7; 2008, Jan, 10-25; 2007, Jul, 1-4; 2007, March, 9-11; 2007, January, 13-27

99224-99226 [99224, 99225, 99226] Facility Observation Visits: Subsequent

CMS 100-4,12,30.6.8 Payment for Hospital Observation Services

INCLUDES Changes in patient's status (e.g., physical condition, history; response to medical management)
Medical record review
Review of diagnostic test results

EXCLUDES *Observation admission and discharge on the same day (99234-99236)*

\# **99224** **Subsequent observation care, per day, for the evaluation and management of a patient, which requires at least 2 of these 3 key components: Problem focused interval history; Problem focused examination; Medical decision making that is straightforward or of low complexity. Counseling and/or coordination of care with other providers or agencies are provided consistent with the nature of the problem(s) and the patient's and/or family's needs. Usually, the patient is stable, recovering, or improving. Physicians typically spend 15 minutes at the bedside and on the patient's hospital floor or unit.** B 80

1.14 1.14 Global Days XXX

\# **99225** **Subsequent observation care, per day, for the evaluation and management of a patient, which requires at least 2 of these 3 key components: An expanded problem focused interval history; An expanded problem focused examination; Medical decision making of moderate complexity. Counseling and/or coordination of care with other providers or agencies are provided consistent with the nature of the problem(s) and the patient's and/or family's needs. Usually, the patient is responding inadequately to therapy or has developed a minor complication. Physicians typically spend 25 minutes at the bedside and on the patient's hospital floor or unit.** B 80

2.06 2.06 Global Days XXX

\# **99226** **Subsequent observation care, per day, for the evaluation and management of a patient, which requires at least 2 of these 3 key components: A detailed interval history; A detailed examination; Medical decision making of high complexity. Counseling and/or coordination of care with other providers or agencies are provided consistent with the nature of the problem(s) and the patient's and/or family's needs. Usually, the patient is unstable or has developed a significant complication or a significant new problem. Physicians typically spend 35 minutes at the bedside and on the patient's hospital floor or unit.** B 80

2.96 2.96 Global Days XXX

99221-99233 Inpatient Hospital Visits: Initial and Subsequent

CMS 100-1,5,70 Definition of Physician
CMS 100-2,15,30 Physician Services
CMS 100-3,70.1 Consultations with a Beneficiary's Family and Associates
CMS 100-4,12,30.6.8 Payment for Hospital Observation Services
CMS 100-4,12,30.6.9 Hospital Visit and Critical Care on Same Day
CMS 100-4,12,30.6.9.1 Initial Hospital Care and Observation or Inpatient Care Services

INCLUDES All services provided on the date of admission in other sites of service (e.g., emergency department, physician's office, nursing facility)
Initial physician services provided to the patient in the hospital or "partial" hospital settings (99221-99223)
Physician services provided to the patient observation status on the same date as inpatient E & M service
Services provided to a new or established patient

EXCLUDES *Consultation services provided by other than the admitting physician (99231-99233, 99251-99255)*
Inpatient admission and discharge on the same date (99234-99236)
Inpatient E/M services provided by other than the admitting physician (99231-99233)

99221 **Initial hospital care, per day, for the evaluation and management of a patient, which requires these 3 key components: A detailed or comprehensive history; A detailed or comprehensive examination; and Medical decision making that is straightforward or of low complexity. Counseling and/or coordination of care with other providers or agencies are provided consistent with the nature of the problem(s) and the patient's and/or family's needs. Usually, the problem(s) requiring admission are of low severity. Physicians typically spend 30 minutes at the bedside and on the patient's hospital floor or unit.** B 80 PQ

2.89 2.89 Global Days XXX

AMA: 2009, Jul, 7; 2009, Jul, 8-9; 2009, Jan, 11-31; 2008, Jan, 10-25; 2007, Jul, 1-4; 2007, Jul, 12-13; 2007, March, 9-11; 2007, January, 13-27

99222 **Initial hospital care, per day, for the evaluation and management of a patient, which requires these 3 key components: A comprehensive history; A comprehensive examination; and Medical decision making of moderate complexity. Counseling and/or coordination of care with other providers or agencies are provided consistent with the nature of the problem(s) and the patient's and/or family's needs. Usually, the problem(s) requiring admission are of moderate severity. Physicians typically spend 50 minutes at the bedside and on the patient's hospital floor or unit.** B 80 PQ

3.91 3.91 Global Days XXX

AMA: 2009, Jul, 7; 2009, Jul, 8-9; 2009, Jan, 11-31; 2008, Jan, 10-25; 2007, Jul, 1-4; 2007, Jul, 12-13; 2007, March, 9-11; 2007, January, 13-27

99223 **Initial hospital care, per day, for the evaluation and management of a patient, which requires these 3 key components: A comprehensive history; A comprehensive examination; and Medical decision making of high complexity. Counseling and/or coordination of care with other providers or agencies are provided consistent with the nature of the problem(s) and the patient's and/or family's needs. Usually, the problem(s) requiring admission are of high severity. Physicians typically spend 70 minutes at the bedside and on the patient's hospital floor or unit.** B 80 PQ

5.74 5.74 **Global Days XXX**

AMA: 2009, Jul, 8-9; 2009, Jul, 7; 2009, Jan, 11-31; 2008, Jan, 10-25; 2007, Jul, 1-4; 2007, Jul, 12-13; 2007, March, 9-11; 2007, January, 13-27

99224 *Resequenced code, See code following 99220.*

99225 *Resequenced code, See code following 99220.*

99226 *Resequenced code, See code before 99221.*

99231 **Subsequent hospital care, per day, for the evaluation and management of a patient, which requires at least 2 of these 3 key components: A problem focused interval history; A problem focused examination; Medical decision making that is straightforward or of low complexity. Counseling and/or coordination of care with other providers or agencies are provided consistent with the nature of the problem(s) and the patient's and/or family's needs. Usually, the patient is stable, recovering or improving. Physicians typically spend 15 minutes at the bedside and on the patient's hospital floor or unit.** B 80 PQ

1.12 1.12 **Global Days XXX**

AMA: 2009, Jan, 11-31; 2009, Mar, 3,4&7; 2009, Jul, 8-9; 2009, Jul, 7; 2008, Jan, 10-25; 2007, March, 9-11; 2007, January, 13-27; 2007, Jul, 1-4

99232 **Subsequent hospital care, per day, for the evaluation and management of a patient, which requires at least 2 of these 3 key components: An expanded problem focused interval history; An expanded problem focused examination; Medical decision making of moderate complexity. Counseling and/or coordination of care with other providers or agencies are provided consistent with the nature of the problem(s) and the patient's and/or family's needs. Usually, the patient is responding inadequately to therapy or has developed a minor complication. Physicians typically spend 25 minutes at the bedside and on the patient's hospital floor or unit.** B 80 PQ

2.05 2.05 **Global Days XXX**

AMA: 2009, Jan, 11-31; 2009, Mar, 3,4&7; 2009, Jul, 8-9; 2009, Jul, 7; 2008, Jan, 10-25; 2008, Jun, 12&15; 2007, March, 9-11; 2007, January, 13-27; 2007, Jul, 1-4

99233 **Subsequent hospital care, per day, for the evaluation and management of a patient, which requires at least 2 of these 3 key components: A detailed interval history; A detailed examination; Medical decision making of high complexity. Counseling and/or coordination of care with other providers or agencies are provided consistent with the nature of the problem(s) and the patient's and/or family's needs. Usually, the patient is unstable or has developed a significant complication or a significant new problem. Physicians typically spend 35 minutes at the bedside and on the patient's hospital floor or unit.** B 80 PQ

2.94 2.94 **Global Days XXX**

AMA: 2009, Jan, 11-31; 2009, Mar, 3,4&7; 2009, Jul, 7; 2009, Jul, 8-9; 2008, Jan, 10-25; 2007, March, 9-11; 2007, Jul, 1-4

99234-99236 Observation/Inpatient Visits: Admitted/Discharged on Same Date

CMS 100-1,5,70 Definition of Physician
CMS 100-2,15,30 Physician Services
CMS 100-3,70.1 Consultations with a Beneficiary's Family and Associates
CMS 100-4,12,30.6.8 Payment for Hospital Observation Services
CMS 100-4,12,30.6.9 Hospital Visit and Critical Care on Same Day
CMS 100-4,12,30.6.9.1 Initial Hospital Care and Observation or Inpatient Care Services
CMS 100-4,12,40.2 Global Surgery Billing Requirements

INCLUDES Admission and discharge services on the same date in an observation or inpatient setting

All services provided by admitting physician on same date of service, even when initiated in another setting (e.g., emergency department, nursing facility, physician's office)

EXCLUDES *Inpatient discharge services (99238-99239)*

Inpatient initial services (99221-99223)

Inpatient subsequent care services (99231-99233)

Services provided to patients admitted to observation and discharged on a different date (99217-99220)

99234 **Observation or inpatient hospital care, for the evaluation and management of a patient including admission and discharge on the same date, which requires these 3 key components: A detailed or comprehensive history; A detailed or comprehensive examination; and Medical decision making that is straightforward or of low complexity. Counseling and/or coordination of care with other providers or agencies are provided consistent with the nature of the problem(s) and the patient's and/or family's needs. Usually the presenting problem(s) requiring admission are of low severity.** B 80 PQ

3.86 3.86 **Global Days XXX**

AMA: 2009, Jan, 11-31; 2009, Jul, 7; 2008, Jan, 10-25; 2007, Jul, 1-4; 2007, March, 9-11; 2007, January, 13-27

99235 **Observation or inpatient hospital care, for the evaluation and management of a patient including admission and discharge on the same date, which requires these 3 key components: A comprehensive history; A comprehensive examination; and Medical decision making of moderate complexity. Counseling and/or coordination of care with other providers or agencies are provided consistent with the nature of the problem(s) and the patient's and/or family's needs. Usually the presenting problem(s) requiring admission are of moderate severity.** B 80 PQ

4.84 4.84 **Global Days XXX**

AMA: 2009, Jan, 11-31; 2009, Jul, 7; 2008, Jan, 10-25; 2007, Jul, 1-4; 2007, January, 13-27; 2007, March, 9-11

99236 **Observation or inpatient hospital care, for the evaluation and management of a patient including admission and discharge on the same date, which requires these 3 key components: A comprehensive history; A comprehensive examination; and Medical decision making of high complexity. Counseling and/or coordination of care with other providers or agencies are provided consistent with the nature of the problem(s) and the patient's and/or family's needs. Usually the presenting problem(s) requiring admission are of high severity.** B 80 PQ

6.23 6.23 **Global Days XXX**

AMA: 2009, Jan, 11-31; 2009, Jul, 7; 2008, Jan, 10-25; 2007, Jul, 1-4; 2007, January, 13-27; 2007, March, 9-11

99238-99239 Inpatient Hospital Discharge Services

CMS 100-4,12,30.6.9.2 Hospital Discharge Management

INCLUDES Discharge instructions
Final preparation of the pateint's medical records
Provision of prescriptions/referrals, as needed
Review of the inpatient admission
Discharge from observation (99217)

EXCLUDES *Admission/discharge on same date (99234-99236)*
Discharge from nursing facility (99315, 99316)
Discharge services for newborns admitted and discharged the same day (99463)
Final patient evaluation
Healthy newborn evaluated and discharged on same date (99463)
Services provided by other than attending physician on date of discharge (99231-99233)

99238 Hospital discharge day management; 30 minutes or less

2.05 2.05 **Global Days XXX**

AMA: 2009, Jul, 7; 2009, Jan, 11-31; 2008, Jan, 10-25; 2007, Jul, 1-4; 2007, March, 9-11; 2007, January, 13-27

99239 more than 30 minutes

3.03 3.03 **Global Days XXX**

AMA: 2009, Jan, 11-31; 2009, Jul, 7; 2008, Jan, 10-25; 2007, Jul, 1-4; 2007, January, 13-27; 2007, March, 9-11

99241-99245 Consultations: Office and Outpatient

CMS 100-1,5,70 Definition of Physician
CMS 100-2,15,30 Physician Services
CMS 100-3,70.1 Consultations with a Beneficiary's Family and Associates
CMS 100-4,12,30.6.10 Consultation Services

INCLUDES A third-party mandated consultation
All outpatient consultations provided in the physician's office, outpatient or other ambulatory facility, domiciliary/rest home, emergency department, patient's home, and hospital observation
Documentation of a request for a consultation from an appropriate source
Documentation of the need for consultation in the patient's medical record
One consultation per consultant
Provision by a physician or qualified nonphysician practitioner whose advice, opinion, recommendation, suggestion, direction, or counsel, etc., is requested for evaluating/treating a patient since that individual's expertise in a specific medical area is beyond the scope of knowledge of the requesting physician
Provision of a written report of findings/recommendations from the consultant to the referring physician

EXCLUDES *Another appropriately requested and documented consultation pertaining to the same/new problem; repeat use of consultation codes*
Any distinctly recognizable procedure/service provided on or following the consultation
Assumption of care (all or partial); report subsequent codes as appropriate for the place of service (99211-99215, 99334-99337, 99347-99350)
Consultation prompted by the patient/family; report codes for office, domiciliary/rest home, or home visits instead (99201-99215, 99324-99337, 99341-99350)

99241 Office consultation for a new or established patient, which requires these 3 key components: A problem focused history; A problem focused examination; and Straightforward medical decision making. Counseling and/or coordination of care with other providers or agencies are provided consistent with the nature of the problem(s) and the patient's and/or family's needs. Usually, the presenting problem(s) are self limited or minor. Physicians typically spend 15 minutes face-to-face with the patient and/or family.

0.95 1.37 **Global Days XXX**

AMA: 2009, Jan, 11-31; 2009, Jul, 7; 2009, Jul, 8-9; 2008, Jan, 10-25; 2007, Jul, 1-4; 2007, January, 13-27; 2007, March, 9-11; 2007, April, 11-12

99242 Office consultation for a new or established patient, which requires these 3 key components: An expanded problem focused history; An expanded problem focused examination; and Straightforward medical decision making. Counseling and/or coordination of care with other providers or agencies are provided consistent with the nature of the problem(s) and the patient's and/or family's needs. Usually, the presenting problem(s) are of low severity. Physicians typically spend 30 minutes face-to-face with the patient and/or family.

1.99 2.58 **Global Days XXX**

AMA: 2009, Jul, 8-9; 2009, Jul, 7; 2009, Jan, 11-31; 2008, Jan, 10-25; 2007, Jul, 1-4; 2007, January, 13-27; 2007, March, 9-11; 2007, April, 11-12

99243 **Office consultation for a new or established patient, which requires these 3 key components: A detailed history; A detailed examination; and Medical decision making of low complexity. Counseling and/or coordination of care with other providers or agencies are provided consistent with the nature of the problem(s) and the patient's and/or family's needs. Usually, the presenting problem(s) are of moderate severity. Physicians typically spend 40 minutes face-to-face with the patient and/or family.**

2.77 3.52 **Global Days XXX**

AMA: 2009, Jul, 8-9; 2009, Jul, 7; 2009, Jan, 11-31; 2008, Jan, 10-25; 2007, Jul, 1-4; 2007, April, 11-12; 2007, March, 9-11; 2007, January, 13-27

99244 **Office consultation for a new or established patient, which requires these 3 key components: A comprehensive history; A comprehensive examination; and Medical decision making of moderate complexity. Counseling and/or coordination of care with other providers or agencies are provided consistent with the nature of the problem(s) and the patient's and/or family's needs. Usually, the presenting problem(s) are of moderate to high severity. Physicians typically spend 60 minutes face-to-face with the patient and/or family.**

4.38 5.20 **Global Days XXX**

AMA: 2009, Jan, 11-31; 2009, Jul, 7; 2009, Jul, 8-9; 2008, Jan, 10-25; 2007, Jul, 1-4; 2007, March, 9-11; 2007, April, 11-12; 2007, January, 13-27

99245 **Office consultation for a new or established patient, which requires these 3 key components: A comprehensive history; A comprehensive examination; and Medical decision making of high complexity. Counseling and/or coordination of care with other providers or agencies are provided consistent with the nature of the problem(s) and the patient's and/or family's needs. Usually, the presenting problem(s) are of moderate to high severity. Physicians typically spend 80 minutes face-to-face with the patient and/or family.**

5.44 6.36 **Global Days XXX**

AMA: 2009, Jul, 8-9; 2009, Jul, 7; 2009, Jan, 11-31; 2008, Jan, 10-25; 2007, Jul, 1-4; 2007, January, 13-27; 2007, March, 9-11; 2007, April, 11-12

99251-99255 Consultations: Inpatient

CMS 100-1,5,70 Definition of Physician
CMS 100-2,15,30 Physician Services
CMS 100-3,70.1 Consultations with a Beneficiary's Family and Associates
CMS 100-4,12,30.6.10 Consultation Services

INCLUDES A third-party mandated consultation
All inpatient consultations include services provided in the hospital inpatient or partial hospital settings and nursing facilities
Documentation of a request for a consultation from an appropriate source
Documentation of the need for consultation in the patient's medical record
One consultation by consultant per admission
Provision by a physician or qualified nonphysician practitioner whose advice, opinion, recommendation, suggestion, direction, or counsel, etc. is requested for evaluating/treating a patient since that individual's expertise in a specific medical area is beyond the scope of knowledge of the requesting physician
Provision of a written report of findings/recommendations from the consultant to the referring physician

EXCLUDES *Another appropriately requested and documented consultation pertaining to the same/new problem: repeat use of consultation codes*
Any distinctly recognizable procedure/service provided on or following the consultation
Assumption of care (all or partial): report subsequent codes as appropriate for the place of service (99231-99233, 99307-99310)
Consultation prompted by the patient/family: report codes for office, domiciliary/rest home, or home visits instead (99201-99215, 99324-99337, 99341-99350)

Do not report an outpatient consultation and an inpatient consutation for the same admission

99251 **Inpatient consultation for a new or established patient, which requires these 3 key components: A problem focused history; A problem focused examination; and Straightforward medical decision making. Counseling and/or coordination of care with other providers or agencies are provided consistent with the nature of the problem(s) and the patient's and/or family's needs. Usually, the presenting problem(s) are self limited or minor. Physicians typically spend 20 minutes at the bedside and on the patient's hospital floor or unit.**

1.39 1.39 **Global Days XXX**

AMA: 2009, Jan, 11-31; 2009, Jul, 7; 2009, Jul, 8-9; 2008, Jan, 10-25; 2007, Jul, 1-4; 2007, January, 13-27; 2007, March, 9-11

99252 **Inpatient consultation for a new or established patient, which requires these 3 key components: An expanded problem focused history; An expanded problem focused examination; and Straightforward medical decision making. Counseling and/or coordination of care with other providers or agencies are provided consistent with the nature of the problem(s) and the patient's and/or family's needs. Usually, the presenting problem(s) are of low severity. Physicians typically spend 40 minutes at the bedside and on the patient's hospital floor or unit.**

2.14 2.14 **Global Days XXX**

AMA: 2009, Jan, 11-31; 2009, Jul, 8-9; 2009, Jul, 7; 2008, Jan, 10-25; 2007, Jul, 1-4; 2007, January, 13-27; 2007, March, 9-11

99253 **Inpatient consultation for a new or established patient, which requires these 3 key components: A detailed history; A detailed examination; and Medical decision making of low complexity. Counseling and/or coordination of care with other providers or agencies are provided consistent with the nature of the problem(s) and the patient's and/or family's needs. Usually, the presenting problem(s) are of moderate severity. Physicians typically spend 55 minutes at the bedside and on the patient's hospital floor or unit.** E

3.26 3.26 Global Days XXX
AMA: 2009, Jul, 7; 2009, Jul, 8-9; 2009, Jan, 11-31; 2008, Jan, 10-25; 2007, Jul, 1-4; 2007, January, 13-27; 2007, March, 9-11

99254 **Inpatient consultation for a new or established patient, which requires these 3 key components: A comprehensive history; A comprehensive examination; and Medical decision making of moderate complexity. Counseling and/or coordination of care with other providers or agencies are provided consistent with the nature of the problem(s) and the patient's and/or family's needs. Usually, the presenting problem(s) are of moderate to high severity. Physicians typically spend 80 minutes at the bedside and on the patient's hospital floor or unit.** E

4.70 4.70 Global Days XXX
AMA: 2009, Jan, 11-31; 2009, Jul, 8-9; 2009, Jul, 7; 2008, Jan, 10-25; 2007, Jul, 1-4; 2007, March, 9-11; 2007, January, 13-27

99255 **Inpatient consultation for a new or established patient, which requires these 3 key components: A comprehensive history; A comprehensive examination; and Medical decision making of high complexity. Counseling and/or coordination of care with other providers or agencies are provided consistent with the nature of the problem(s) and the patient's and/or family's needs. Usually, the presenting problem(s) are of moderate to high severity. Physicians typically spend 110 minutes at the bedside and on the patient's hospital floor or unit.** E

5.68 5.68 Global Days XXX
AMA: 2009, Jul, 7; 2009, Jul, 8-9; 2009, Jan, 11-31; 2008, Jan, 10-25; 2007, Jul, 1-4; 2007, January, 13-27; 2007, March, 9-11

99281-99288 Emergency Department Visits

CMS 100-1,5,70 Definition of Physician
CMS 100-2,15,30 Physician Services
CMS 100-3,70.1 Consultations with a Beneficiary's Family and Associates
CMS 100-4,12,30.6.11 Emergency Department Visits

INCLUDES Any amount of time spent with the patient, which usually involves a series of encounters while the patient is in the emergency department
Care provided to new and established patients

EXCLUDES *Critical care services (99291-99292)*
Observation services (99217-99220, 99234-99236)

99281 **Emergency department visit for the evaluation and management of a patient, which requires these 3 key components: A problem focused history; A problem focused examination; and Straightforward medical decision making. Counseling and/or coordination of care with other providers or agencies are provided consistent with the nature of the problem(s) and the patient's and/or family's needs. Usually, the presenting problem(s) are self limited or minor.** V 80 PQ

0.60 0.60 Global Days XXX
AMA: 2009, Jan, 11-31; 2009, Jul, 7; 2008, Jan, 10-25; 2007, Jul, 1-4; 2007, January, 13-27; 2007, Dec, 10-179; 2007, March, 9-11

99282 **Emergency department visit for the evaluation and management of a patient, which requires these 3 key components: An expanded problem focused history; An expanded problem focused examination; and Medical decision making of low complexity. Counseling and/or coordination of care with other providers or agencies are provided consistent with the nature of the problem(s) and the patient's and/or family's needs. Usually, the presenting problem(s) are of low to moderate severity.** V 80 PQ

1.18 1.18 Global Days XXX
AMA: 2009, Jan, 11-31; 2009, Jul, 7; 2008, Jan, 10-25; 2007, Jul, 1-4; 2007, March, 9-11; 2007, Dec, 10-179; 2007, January, 13-27

99283 **Emergency department visit for the evaluation and management of a patient, which requires these 3 key components: An expanded problem focused history; An expanded problem focused examination; and Medical decision making of moderate complexity. Counseling and/or coordination of care with other providers or agencies are provided consistent with the nature of the problem(s) and the patient's and/or family's needs. Usually, the presenting problem(s) are of moderate severity.** V 80 PQ

1.77 1.77 Global Days XXX
AMA: 2009, Jul, 7; 2009, Jan, 11-31; 2008, Jan, 10-25; 2007, Jul, 1-4; 2007, March, 9-11; 2007, January, 13-27; 2007, Dec, 10-179

99284 **Emergency department visit for the evaluation and management of a patient, which requires these 3 key components: A detailed history; A detailed examination; and Medical decision making of moderate complexity. Counseling and/or coordination of care with other providers or agencies are provided consistent with the nature of the problem(s) and the patient's and/or family's needs. Usually, the presenting problem(s) are of high severity, and require urgent evaluation by the physician but do not pose an immediate significant threat to life or physiologic function.** Q3 80 PQ

3.37 3.37 Global Days XXX
AMA: 2009, Jan, 11-31; 2009, Jul, 7; 2008, Jan, 10-25; 2007, Jul, 1-4; 2007, Dec, 10-179; 2007, March, 9-11; 2007, January, 13-27

99285 **Emergency department visit for the evaluation and management of a patient, which requires these 3 key components within the constraints imposed by the urgency of the patient's clinical condition and/or mental status: A comprehensive history; A comprehensive examination; and Medical decision making of high complexity. Counseling and/or coordination of care with other providers or agencies are provided consistent with the nature of the problem(s) and the patient's and/or family's needs. Usually, the presenting problem(s) are of high severity and pose an immediate significant threat to life or physiologic function.** Q3 80 PQ

4.94 4.94 Global Days XXX
AMA: 2009, Jan, 11-31; 2009, Jul, 7; 2008, Jan, 10-25; 2007, Jul, 1-4; 2007, Dec, 10-179; 2007, March, 9-11; 2007, January, 13-27

99288 **Physician direction of emergency medical systems (EMS) emergency care, advanced life support** B

INCLUDES Management provided by an emergency/intensive care based physician via voice contact to ambulance/rescue staff for services such as heart monitoring and drug administration

0.00 0.00 Global Days XXX
AMA: 2009, Jul, 7; 2007, Jul, 1-4; 2007, March, 9-11

99291-99292 Critical Care Visits: Patients 72 Months of Age and Older

CMS 100-1,5,70 Definition of Physician
CMS 100-2,15,30 Physician Services
CMS 100-3,70.1 Consultations with a Beneficiary's Family and Associates
CMS 100-4,12,30.6.9 Hospital Visit and Critical Care on Same Day
CMS 100-4,12,30.6.12 Critical Care Visits

INCLUDES 30 minutes or more of direct care provided by the physician to a critically ill or injured patient, regardless of the location
All time spent exclusively with patient/family/caregivers on the nursing unit or elsewhere
For professional services for interpretation of:
Blood gases
Chest films (71010, 71015, 71020)
Measurement of cardiac output (93561-93562)
Other computer stored information (99090)
Pulse oximetry (94760-94762)
Professional services for:
Gastric intubation (43752-43753)
Transcutaneous pacing, temporary (92953)
Ventilation assistance and management, includes CPAP, CNP (94002-94004, 94660, 94662)
Venous access, arterial puncture (36000, 36410, 36415, 36591, 36600)
Includes physician presence during interfacility transfer for critically ill/injured patients over 24 months of age
Outpatient critical care provided to neonates and pediatric patients up through 71 months of age

EXCLUDES *All services that are less than 30 minutes; report appropriate E/M code*
Critical care services provided via remote real-time interactive videoconferencing (0188T, 0189T)
Inpatient critical care services provided to child 2 through 5 years of age (99475-99476)
Inpatient critical care services provided to infants 29 days through 24 months of age (99471-99472)
Inpatient critical care services provided to neonates that are age 28 days or less (99468-99469)
Other procedures not listed as included performed by the physician rendering critical care
Patients who are not critically ill but in the critical care department (report appropriate E/M code)
Physician presence during interfacility transfer for critically ill/injured patients under 24 months of age (99466, 99467)

Do not report activities performed outside of the unit or off the floor

99291 **Critical care, evaluation and management of the critically ill or critically injured patient; first 30-74 minutes** 63 80 PQ
6.38 7.85 Global Days XXX
AMA: 2009, Jan, 5&10; 2009, Jan, 11-31; 2009, Jul, 7; 2009, Mar, 3,4&7; 2008, Jan, 10-25; 2008, Jul, 7-8&15; 2007, Jul, 1-4; 2007, March, 9-11; 2007, January, 13-27

\+ **99292** **each additional 30 minutes (List separately in addition to code for primary service)** N 80
Code first (99291)
3.20 3.51 Global Days ZZZ
AMA: 2009, Jan, 11-31; 2009, Mar, 3,4&7; 2009, Jan, 5&10; 2009, Jul, 7; 2008, Jan, 10-25; 2008, Jul, 7-8&15; 2007, Jul, 1-4; 2007, March, 9-11; 2007, January, 13-27

99304-99310 Nursing Facility Visits

CMS 100-1,5,70 Definition of Physician
CMS 100-2,15,30 Physician Services
CMS 100-3,70.1 Consultations with a Beneficiary's Family and Associates
CMS 100-3,70.2 Consultation by a Podiatrist in a Skilled Nursing Facility
CMS 100-3,70.3 Physician's Offices Within an Institution--"Incident-to" Provision
CMS 100-4,12,30.6.9 Swing Bed Visits
CMS 100-4,12,30.6.13 Nursing Facility Visits

INCLUDES All E/M services provided by the admitting physican on the date of nursing facility admission in other locations (e.g, office, emergency department)
Initial care, subsequent care, discharge, and yearly assessments
Initial services include patient assessment and physician participation in developing a plan of care (99304-99306)
Services provided to new and established patients in a nursing facility (skilled, intermediate, and long-term care facilities)
Subsequent services include physician review of medical records, reassessment, review of test results (99307-99310)

EXCLUDES *Care plan oversight services (99379-99380)*

Code also hospital discharge services on the same date of admission or readmission to the nursing home (99217, 99234-99236, 99238-99239)

99304 **Initial nursing facility care, per day, for the evaluation and management of a patient, which requires these 3 key components: A detailed or comprehensive history; A detailed or comprehensive examination; and Medical decision making that is straightforward or of low complexity. Counseling and/or coordination of care with other providers or agencies are provided consistent with the nature of the problem(s) and the patient's and/or family's needs. Usually, the problem(s) requiring admission are of low severity. Physicians typically spend 25 minutes at the bedside and on the patient's facility floor or unit.** B 80 PQ
2.64 2.64 Global Days XXX
AMA: 2009, Jul, 7; 2009, Jul, 8-9; 2009, Jul, 3-4; 2007, Jul, 1-4; 2007, March, 9-11

99305 **Initial nursing facility care, per day, for the evaluation and management of a patient, which requires these 3 key components: A comprehensive history; A comprehensive examination; and Medical decision making of moderate complexity. Counseling and/or coordination of care with other providers or agencies are provided consistent with the nature of the problem(s) and the patient's and/or family's needs. Usually, the problem(s) requiring admission are of moderate severity. Physicians typically spend 35 minutes at the bedside and on the patient's facility floor or unit.** B 80 PQ
3.73 3.73 Global Days XXX
AMA: 2009, Jul, 7; 2009, Jul, 8-9; 2009, Jul, 3-4; 2007, Jul, 1-4; 2007, March, 9-11

99306 **Initial nursing facility care, per day, for the evaluation and management of a patient, which requires these 3 key components: A comprehensive history; A comprehensive examination; and Medical decision making of high complexity. Counseling and/or coordination of care with other providers or agencies are provided consistent with the nature of the problem(s) and the patient's and/or family's needs. Usually, the problem(s) requiring admission are of high severity. Physicians typically spend 45 minutes at the bedside and on the patient's facility floor or unit.** B 80 PQ
4.73 4.73 Global Days XXX
AMA: 2009, Jul, 7; 2009, Jul, 8-9; 2009, Jul, 3-4; 2007, Jul, 1-4; 2007, March, 9-11

99307 **Subsequent nursing facility care, per day, for the evaluation and management of a patient, which requires at least 2 of these 3 key components: A problem focused interval history; A problem focused examination; Straightforward medical decision making. Counseling and/or coordination of care with other providers or agencies are provided consistent with the nature of the problem(s) and the patient's and/or family's needs. Usually, the patient is stable, recovering, or improving. Physicians typically spend 10 minutes at the bedside and on the patient's facility floor or unit.** B 80 PQ

1.25 1.25 Global Days XXX

AMA: 2009, Jul, 8-9; 2009, Jul, 3-4; 2009, Jan, 11-31; 2009, Jul, 7; 2008, Jan, 10-25; 2007, March, 9-11; 2007, Jul, 1-4

99308 **Subsequent nursing facility care, per day, for the evaluation and management of a patient, which requires at least 2 of these 3 key components: An expanded problem focused interval history; An expanded problem focused examination; Medical decision making of low complexity. Counseling and/or coordination of care with other providers or agencies are provided consistent with the nature of the problem(s) and the patient's and/or family's needs. Usually, the patient is responding inadequately to therapy or has developed a minor complication. Physicians typically spend 15 minutes at the bedside and on the patient's facility floor or unit.** B 80 PQ

1.94 1.94 Global Days XXX

AMA: 2009, Jul, 8-9; 2009, Jul, 7; 2009, Jul, 3-4; 2007, Jul, 1-4; 2007, March, 9-11

99309 **Subsequent nursing facility care, per day, for the evaluation and management of a patient, which requires at least 2 of these 3 key components: A detailed interval history; A detailed examination; Medical decision making of moderate complexity. Counseling and/or coordination of care with other providers or agencies are provided consistent with the nature of the problem(s) and the patient's and/or family's needs. Usually, the patient has developed a significant complication or a significant new problem. Physicians typically spend 25 minutes at the bedside and on the patient's facility floor or unit.** B 80 PQ

2.55 2.55 Global Days XXX

AMA: 2009, Jul, 3-4; 2009, Jul, 8-9; 2009, Jul, 7; 2007, Jul, 1-4; 2007, March, 9-11

99310 **Subsequent nursing facility care, per day, for the evaluation and management of a patient, which requires at least 2 of these 3 key components: A comprehensive interval history; A comprehensive examination; Medical decision making of high complexity. Counseling and/or coordination of care with other providers or agencies are provided consistent with the nature of the problem(s) and the patient's and/or family's needs. The patient may be unstable or may have developed a significant new problem requiring immediate physician attention. Physicians typically spend 35 minutes at the bedside and on the patient's facility floor or unit.** B 80 PQ

3.79 3.79 Global Days XXX

AMA: 2009, Jan, 11-31; 2009, Jul, 7; 2009, Jul, 3-4; 2009, Jul, 8-9; 2008, Jan, 10-25; 2007, March, 9-11; 2007, Jul, 1-4

99315-99318 Nursing Home Discharge

INCLUDES Discharge services include all time spent by the physician for:
- Complete discharge records
- Discharge instructions for patient and caregivers
- Discussion regarding the stay in the facility
- Final patient examination
- Provide prescriptions and referrals as appropriate

99315 **Nursing facility discharge day management; 30 minutes or less** B 80 PQ

2.05 2.05 Global Days XXX

AMA: 2009, Jul, 3-4; 2009, Jul, 7; 2009, Jan, 11-31; 2008, Jan, 10-25; 2007, Jul, 1-4; 2007, January, 13-27; 2007, March, 9-11

99316 **more than 30 minutes** B 80 PQ

2.94 2.94 Global Days XXX

AMA: 2009, Jan, 11-31; 2009, Jul, 7; 2009, Jul, 3-4; 2008, Jan, 10-25; 2007, Jul, 1-4; 2007, January, 13-27; 2007, March, 9-11

99318 **Evaluation and management of a patient involving an annual nursing facility assessment, which requires these 3 key components: A detailed interval history; A comprehensive examination; and Medical decision making that is of low to moderate complexity. Counseling and/or coordination of care with other providers or agencies are provided consistent with the nature of the problem(s) and the patient's and/or family's needs. Usually, the patient is stable, recovering, or improving. Physicians typically spend 30 minutes at the bedside and on the patient's facility floor or unit.** B 80

Do not report with the same date of service as (99304-99316)

2.70 2.70 Global Days XXX

AMA: 2009, Jul, 7; 2009, Jul, 3-4; 2007, Jul, 1-4; 2007, March, 9-11

99324-99337 Domiciliary Care, Rest Home, Assisted Living Visits

CMS 100-3,70.1 Consultations with a Beneficiary's Family and Associates

CMS 100-4,12,30.6.14 Domiciliary Care, Rest Home, Assisted Living Visits

INCLUDES E/M services for patients residing in assisted living, domiciliary care, and rest homes where medical care is not included
Services provided to new patients or established patients (99324-99328 or 99334-99337)

EXCLUDES *Physician rest home care plan oversight services (99339-99340)*
Rest home care plan oversight services provided to a patient under the care of a home health agency (99374-99375)

99324 **Domiciliary or rest home visit for the evaluation and management of a new patient, which requires these 3 key components: A problem focused history; A problem focused examination; and Straightforward medical decision making. Counseling and/or coordination of care with other providers or agencies are provided consistent with the nature of the problem(s) and the patient's and/or family's needs. Usually, the presenting problem(s) are of low severity. Physicians typically spend 20 minutes with the patient and/or family or caregiver.** B 80 PQ

1.61 1.61 Global Days XXX

AMA: 2009, Jul, 7; 2009, Jul, 8-9; 2007, Jul, 1-4; 2007, March, 9-11

99325 Domiciliary or rest home visit for the evaluation and management of a new patient, which requires these 3 key components: An expanded problem focused history; An expanded problem focused examination; and Medical decision making of low complexity. Counseling and/or coordination of care with other providers or agencies are provided consistent with the nature of the problem(s) and the patient's and/or family's needs. Usually, the presenting problem(s) are of moderate severity. Physicians typically spend 30 minutes with the patient and/or family or caregiver. B 80 PQ

2.32 2.32 Global Days XXX

AMA: 2009, Jul, 7; 2009, Jul, 8-9; 2007, Jul, 1-4; 2007, March, 9-11

99326 Domiciliary or rest home visit for the evaluation and management of a new patient, which requires these 3 key components: A detailed history; A detailed examination; and Medical decision making of moderate complexity. Counseling and/or coordination of care with other providers or agencies are provided consistent with the nature of the problem(s) and the patient's and/or family's needs. Usually, the presenting problem(s) are of moderate to high severity. Physicians typically spend 45 minutes with the patient and/or family or caregiver. B 80 PQ

3.97 3.97 Global Days XXX

AMA: 2009, Jul, 8-9; 2009, Jul, 7; 2007, Jul, 1-4; 2007, March, 9-11

99327 Domiciliary or rest home visit for the evaluation and management of a new patient, which requires these 3 key components: A comprehensive history; A comprehensive examination; and Medical decision making of moderate complexity. Counseling and/or coordination of care with other providers or agencies are provided consistent with the nature of the problem(s) and the patient's and/or family's needs. Usually, the presenting problem(s) are of high severity. Physicians typically spend 60 minutes with the patient and/or family or caregiver. B 80 PQ

5.27 5.27 Global Days XXX

AMA: 2009, Jul, 7; 2009, Jul, 8-9; 2007, Jul, 1-4; 2007, March, 9-11

99328 Domiciliary or rest home visit for the evaluation and management of a new patient, which requires these 3 key components: A comprehensive history; A comprehensive examination; and Medical decision making of high complexity. Counseling and/or coordination of care with other providers or agencies are provided consistent with the nature of the problem(s) and the patient's and/or family's needs. Usually, the patient is unstable or has developed a significant new problem requiring immediate physician attention. Physicians typically spend 75 minutes with the patient and/or family or caregiver. B 80 PQ

6.12 6.12 Global Days XXX

AMA: 2009, Jul, 7; 2009, Jul, 8-9; 2007, Jul, 1-4; 2007, March, 9-11

99334 Domiciliary or rest home visit for the evaluation and management of an established patient, which requires at least 2 of these 3 key components: A problem focused interval history; A problem focused examination; Straightforward medical decision making. Counseling and/or coordination of care with other providers or agencies are provided consistent with the nature of the problem(s) and the patient's and/or family's needs. Usually, the presenting problem(s) are self-limited or minor. Physicians typically spend 15 minutes with the patient and/or family or caregiver. B 80 PQ

1.72 1.72 Global Days XXX

AMA: 2009, Jul, 7; 2009, Jul, 8-9; 2007, Jul, 1-4; 2007, March, 9-11

99335 Domiciliary or rest home visit for the evaluation and management of an established patient, which requires at least 2 of these 3 key components: An expanded problem focused interval history; An expanded problem focused examination; Medical decision making of low complexity. Counseling and/or coordination of care with other providers or agencies are provided consistent with the nature of the problem(s) and the patient's and/or family's needs. Usually, the presenting problem(s) are of low to moderate severity. Physicians typically spend 25 minutes with the patient and/or family or caregiver. B 80 PQ

2.68 2.68 Global Days XXX

AMA: 2009, Jul, 7; 2009, Jul, 8-9; 2007, Jul, 1-4; 2007, March, 9-11

99336 Domiciliary or rest home visit for the evaluation and management of an established patient, which requires at least 2 of these 3 key components: A detailed interval history; A detailed examination; Medical decision making of moderate complexity. Counseling and/or coordination of care with other providers or agencies are provided consistent with the nature of the problem(s) and the patient's and/or family's needs. Usually, the presenting problem(s) are of moderate to high severity. Physicians typically spend 40 minutes with the patient and/or family or caregiver. B 80 PQ

3.79 3.79 Global Days XXX

AMA: 2009, Jul, 7; 2009, Jul, 8-9; 2007, Jul, 1-4; 2007, March, 9-11

99337 Domiciliary or rest home visit for the evaluation and management of an established patient, which requires at least 2 of these 3 key components: A comprehensive interval history; A comprehensive examination; Medical decision making of moderate to high complexity. Counseling and/or coordination of care with other providers or agencies are provided consistent with the nature of the problem(s) and the patient's and/or family's needs. Usually, the presenting problem(s) are of moderate to high severity. The patient may be unstable or may have developed a significant new problem requiring immediate physician attention. Physicians typically spend 60 minutes with the patient and/or family or caregiver. B 80 PQ

5.45 5.45 Global Days XXX

AMA: 2009, Jul, 8-9; 2009, Jul, 7; 2007, Jul, 1-4; 2007, March, 9-11

99339-99340 Care Plan Oversight: Rest Home, Domiciliary Care, Assisted Living, and Home

CMS 100-4,12,30.6.14 Domiciliary Care, Rest Home, Assisted Living Visits

INCLUDES Care plan oversight for patients residing in assisted living, domiciliary care, private residences, and rest homes

EXCLUDES *Care plan oversight services furnished under a home health agency, nursing facility, or hospice (99374-99380)*

Do not report with (99441-99444, 98966-98969)

99339 **Individual physician supervision of a patient (patient not present) in home, domiciliary or rest home (eg, assisted living facility) requiring complex and multidisciplinary care modalities involving regular physician development and/or revision of care plans, review of subsequent reports of patient status, review of related laboratory and other studies, communication (including telephone calls) for purposes of assessment or care decisions with health care professional(s), family member(s), surrogate decision maker(s) (eg, legal guardian) and/or key caregiver(s) involved in patient's care, integration of new information into the medical treatment plan and/or adjustment of medical therapy, within a calendar month; 15-29 minutes** B

Do not report with time peroid reported for (99441-99444, 98966-98969)

2.23 2.23 Global Days XXX

AMA: 2009, Jul, 5-6; 2009, Jul, 7; 2009, Jul, 10; 2008, Mar, 6-7; 2008, Sep, 3-4; 2007, Jul, 1-4; 2007, April, 3-6; 2007, March, 9-11

99340 **30 minutes or more** B

Do not report with time peroid reported for (99441-99444, 98966-98969)

3.12 3.12 Global Days XXX

AMA: 2009, Jul, 5-6; 2009, Jul, 10; 2009, Jul, 7; 2008, Mar, 6-7; 2008, Sep, 3-4; 2007, Jul, 1-4; 2007, April, 3-6; 2007, March, 9-11

99341-99350 Home Visits

CMS 100-4,12,30.6.14.1 Home Visits

INCLUDES Services for a new patient or an established patient (99341-99345 or 99347-99350)

Services provided to a patient in a private home

EXCLUDES *Services provided to patients under home health agency or hospice care (99374-99378)*

99341 **Home visit for the evaluation and management of a new patient, which requires these 3 key components: A problem focused history; A problem focused examination; and Straightforward medical decision making. Counseling and/or coordination of care with other providers or agencies are provided consistent with the nature of the problem(s) and the patient's and/or family's needs. Usually, the presenting problem(s) are of low severity. Physicians typically spend 20 minutes face-to-face with the patient and/or family.** B 80 PQ

1.59 1.59 Global Days XXX

AMA: 2009, Jul, 7; 2009, Jul, 8-9; 2007, Jul, 1-4; 2007, March, 9-11; 2007, January, 28-31

99342 **Home visit for the evaluation and management of a new patient, which requires these 3 key components: An expanded problem focused history; An expanded problem focused examination; and Medical decision making of low complexity. Counseling and/or coordination of care with other providers or agencies are provided consistent with the nature of the problem(s) and the patient's and/or family's needs. Usually, the presenting problem(s) are of moderate severity. Physicians typically spend 30 minutes face-to-face with the patient and/or family.** B 80 PQ

2.31 2.31 Global Days XXX

AMA: 2009, Jul, 8-9; 2009, Jul, 7; 2007, Jul, 1-4; 2007, January, 28-31; 2007, March, 9-11

99343 **Home visit for the evaluation and management of a new patient, which requires these 3 key components: A detailed history; A detailed examination; and Medical decision making of moderate complexity. Counseling and/or coordination of care with other providers or agencies are provided consistent with the nature of the problem(s) and the patient's and/or family's needs. Usually, the presenting problem(s) are of moderate to high severity. Physicians typically spend 45 minutes face-to-face with the patient and/or family.** B 80 PQ

3.78 3.78 Global Days XXX

AMA: 2009, Jul, 7; 2009, Jul, 8-9; 2007, Jul, 1-4; 2007, March, 9-11; 2007, January, 28-31

99344 **Home visit for the evaluation and management of a new patient, which requires these 3 key components: A comprehensive history; A comprehensive examination; and Medical decision making of moderate complexity. Counseling and/or coordination of care with other providers or agencies are provided consistent with the nature of the problem(s) and the patient's and/or family's needs. Usually, the presenting problem(s) are of high severity. Physicians typically spend 60 minutes face-to-face with the patient and/or family.** B 80 PQ

5.18 5.18 Global Days XXX

AMA: 2009, Jul, 8-9; 2009, Jul, 7; 2007, Jul, 1-4; 2007, January, 28-31; 2007, March, 9-11

99345 **Home visit for the evaluation and management of a new patient, which requires these 3 key components: A comprehensive history; A comprehensive examination; and Medical decision making of high complexity. Counseling and/or coordination of care with other providers or agencies are provided consistent with the nature of the problem(s) and the patient's and/or family's needs. Usually, the patient is unstable or has developed a significant new problem requiring immediate physician attention. Physicians typically spend 75 minutes face-to-face with the patient and/or family.** B 80 PQ

6.19 6.19 Global Days XXX

AMA: 2009, Jul, 7; 2009, Jul, 8-9; 2007, Jul, 1-4; 2007, March, 9-11; 2007, January, 28-31

99347 **Home visit for the evaluation and management of an established patient, which requires at least 2 of these 3 key components: A problem focused interval history; A problem focused examination; Straightforward medical decision making. Counseling and/or coordination of care with other providers or agencies are provided consistent with the nature of the problem(s) and the patient's and/or family's needs. Usually, the presenting problem(s) are self limited or minor. Physicians typically spend 15 minutes face-to-face with the patient and/or family.** B 80 PQ

1.60 1.60 Global Days XXX

AMA: 2009, Jul, 7; 2009, Jul, 8-9; 2007, Jul, 1-4; 2007, March, 9-11; 2007, January, 28-31

99348 **Home visit for the evaluation and management of an established patient, which requires at least 2 of these 3 key components: An expanded problem focused interval history; An expanded problem focused examination; Medical decision making of low complexity. Counseling and/or coordination of care with other providers or agencies are provided consistent with the nature of the problem(s) and the patient's and/or family's needs. Usually, the presenting problem(s) are of low to moderate severity. Physicians typically spend 25 minutes face-to-face with the patient and/or family.** B 80 CCI PQ

2.41 2.41 Global Days XXX

AMA: 2009, Jul, 8-9; 2009, Jul, 7; 2007, Jul, 1-4; 2007, March, 9-11; 2007, January, 28-31

99349 **Home visit for the evaluation and management of an established patient, which requires at least 2 of these 3 key components: A detailed interval history; A detailed examination; Medical decision making of moderate complexity. Counseling and/or coordination of care with other providers or agencies are provided consistent with the nature of the problem(s) and the patient's and/or family's needs. Usually, the presenting problem(s) are moderate to high severity. Physicians typically spend 40 minutes face-to-face with the patient and/or family.** B 80 CCI PQ

3.62 3.62 Global Days XXX

AMA: 2009, Jul, 8-9; 2009, Jul, 7; 2007, Jul, 1-4; 2007, January, 28-31; 2007, March, 9-11

99350 **Home visit for the evaluation and management of an established patient, which requires at least 2 of these 3 key components: A comprehensive interval history; A comprehensive examination; Medical decision making of moderate to high complexity. Counseling and/or coordination of care with other providers or agencies are provided consistent with the nature of the problem(s) and the patient's and/or family's needs. Usually, the presenting problem(s) are of moderate to high severity. The patient may be unstable or may have developed a significant new problem requiring immediate physician attention. Physicians typically spend 60 minutes face-to-face with the patient and/or family.** B 80 CCI PQ

5.03 5.03 Global Days XXX

AMA: 2009, Jul, 7; 2009, Jul, 8-9; 2007, Jul, 1-4; 2007, January, 28-31; 2007, March, 9-11

99354-99357 Prolonged Services Direct Contact

CMS 100-1,5,70 Definition of Physician
CMS 100-2,15,30 Physician Services
CMS 100-4,12,30.6.15 Extended Services Outside Customary Services
CMS 100-4,12,30.6.15.1 Prolonged Services With Direct Face-to-Face Patient Contact

INCLUDES Personal contact with the patient by the physician or other qualified health professional (99354-99357)
Services that extend beyond the customary service provided in the inpatient or outpatient setting
Time spent providing additional indirect contact services on the floor or unit of the hospital or nursing facility during the same session as the direct contact
Time spent providing prolonged services on a date of service, even when the time is not continuous

EXCLUDES *Services provided on a different than the date of personal contact with the patient (99358, 99359)*

Do not report any service less than 30 minutes
Do not report any service that fails to extend into the next time period by 15 minutes or more

\+ ▲ **99354** **Prolonged service in the office or other outpatient setting requiring direct patient contact beyond the usual service; first hour (List separately in addition to code for office or other outpatient Evaluation and Management service)** N 80 CCI

Code first (99201-99215, 99241-99245, 99324-99337, 99341-99350, 90809, 90815)

2.63 2.83 Global Days ZZZ

AMA: 2009, Jul, 8-9; 2008, Sep, 3-4; 2008, Jun, 12&15; 2007, Jul, 1-4; 2007, March, 9-11

\+ ▲ **99355** **each additional 30 minutes (List separately in addition to code for prolonged service)** N 80 CCI

Code first (99354)

2.58 2.78 Global Days ZZZ

AMA: 2009, Jul, 8-9; 2008, Jun, 12&15; 2008, Sep, 3-4; 2007, Jul, 1-4; 2007, March, 9-11

\+ ▲ **99356** **Prolonged service in the inpatient or observation setting, requiring unit/floor time beyond the usual service; first hour (List separately in addition to code for inpatient Evaluation and Management service)** C5 C 80 CCI PQ

Code first (99218-99233 [99224, 99225, 99226], 99251-99255, 99304-99310, 90822, 90829)

2.60 2.60 Global Days ZZZ

AMA: 2009, Jul, 8-9; 2008, Sep, 3-4; 2008, Jun, 12&15; 2007, Jul, 1-4; 2007, March, 9-11

\+ ▲ **99357** **each additional 30 minutes (List separately in addition to code for prolonged service)** C5 C 80 CCI PQ

Code first (99356)

2.59 2.59 Global Days ZZZ

AMA: 2009, Jul, 8-9; 2008, Sep, 3-4; 2008, Jun, 12&15; 2007, Jul, 1-4; 2007, March, 9-11

99358-99359 Prolonged Services Indirect Contact

CMS 100-1,5,70 Definition of Physician
CMS 100-2,15,30 Physician Services
CMS 100-4,12,30.6.15 Extended Services Outside Customary Services
CMS 100-4,12,30.6.15.2 Prolonged Services Without Face to Face Service

INCLUDES Prolonged services performed in a day that are not continuous
Services provided by the physician or other qualified health care professional in relation to patient management where face-to-face services have or will occur on a different date
Time spent after direct face-to-face contact beyond the usual not necessarily on the same date of service.

EXCLUDES *Anticoagulation services*
Any additional unit or floor time in the hospital or nursing facility during the same evaluation and management session
Care plan oversight
On-line medical services
Other indirect services that have a more specific code and no upper time limit in the code
Time spent in medical team conference

Code also evaluation and management or other services provided
Code also non-face-to-face service codes that have an upper time limit
Code also the code for each additional service for the last 15-30 minutes.
Do not report services less than 15 minutes beyond the first hour
Do not report services less than 30 minutes

▲ 99358 **Prolonged evaluation and management service before and/or after direct patient care; first hour** N
3.14 3.14 Global Days XXX
AMA: 2008, Jun, 12&15; 2008, Sep, 3-4; 2007, Jul, 1-4; 2007, March, 9-11

+ ▲ 99359 **each additional 30 minutes (List separately in addition to code for prolonged service)** N
Code first (99358)
1.52 1.52 Global Days ZZZ
AMA: 2008, Jun, 12&15; 2008, Sep, 3-4; 2007, Jul, 1-4; 2007, March, 9-11

99360 Standby Services

CMS 100-4,12,30.6.15.3 Standby Services

INCLUDES Services requested by another physician that involve no direct pateint contact

EXCLUDES *History/examination of normal newborn (99460-99461, 99463)*
Less than 30 minutes of standby time
On-call services ordered by the hospital (99026, 99027)
Resuscitation of newborn (99465)

Do not report with (99464)

99360 **Physician standby service, requiring prolonged physician attendance, each 30 minutes (eg, operative standby, standby for frozen section, for cesarean/high risk delivery, for monitoring EEG)** B
EXCLUDES *Hospital mandated on call services (99026-99027)*
Code also as appropriate (99460, 99465)
Do not report with (99464)
1.77 1.77 Global Days XXX
AMA: 2009, Jan, 11-31; 2008, Jan, 10-25; 2008, Mar, 14-15; 2007, Jul, 1-4; 2007, January, 13-27; 2007, March, 9-11

99363-99364 Supervision of Warfarin Therapy

INCLUDES Services provided on an outpatient basis only
Supervision of therapy with warfarin: ordering, dosage adjustments, analysis of International Normalized Ration (INR) tests, patient discussion

EXCLUDES *Initial services provided/continued in the hospital or in observation: new period of subsequent therapy starts with discharge (99364)*
Services provided for less than 60 uninterrupted days
Services that fail to meet the required criteria (e.g., at least 8 INR tests/initial 90 days; 3 INR tests/each following 90 days
Warfarin therapy supervision accomplished online or via telephone contact (99444, 98969)

Do not report with (99217-99239 [99224, 99225, 99226], 99291-99292, 99304-99318, 99471-99480)

99363 **Anticoagulant management for an outpatient taking warfarin, physician review and interpretation of International Normalized Ratio (INR) testing, patient instructions, dosage adjustment (as needed), and ordering of additional tests; initial 90 days of therapy (must include a minimum of 8 INR measurements)** B
2.43 3.66 Global Days XXX
AMA: 2009, Jul, 5-6; 2008, Mar, 6-7; 2007, Jul, 1-4; 2007, March, 9-11

99364 **each subsequent 90 days of therapy (must include a minimum of 3 INR measurements)** B
0.93 1.24 Global Days XXX
AMA: 2009, Jul, 5-6; 2008, Mar, 6-7; 2007, Jul, 1-4; 2007, March, 9-11

99366-99368 Interdisciplinary Conferences

CMS 100-1,5,70 Definition of Physician
CMS 100-2,15,30 Physician Services
CMS 100-4,11,40.2 Independent Attending Physician Services Under Hospice

INCLUDES Documentation of participation, contribution, and recommendations of the conference
Face-to-face participation by minimum of three qualified people from different specialties or disciplines
Only participants who have performed face-to-face evaluations or direct treatment to the patient within the previous 60 days
Start of the review of an individual patient and ends at conclusion of review

EXCLUDES *Conferences of less than 30 minutes (not reportable)*
More than one individual from the same specialty at the same encounter
Time spent record keeping or writing a report.

99366 **Medical team conference with interdisciplinary team of health care professionals, face-to-face with patient and/or family, 30 minutes or more, participation by nonphysician qualified health care professional** N
INCLUDES Team conferences of 30 minutes or more
EXCLUDES *Team conferences by a physician with patient or family present (99201-99499 [99224, 99225, 99226])*
1.20 1.23 Global Days XXX
AMA: 2009, Jan, 11-31; 2008, Jun, 14-15; 2008, Sep, 3-4

99367 **Medical team conference with interdisciplinary team of health care professionals, patient and/or family not present, 30 minutes or more; participation by physician** N
INCLUDES Team conferences of 30 minutes or more
1.62 1.62 Global Days XXX
AMA: 2008, Sep, 3-4

99368 **participation by nonphysician qualified health care professional** N

INCLUDES Team conferences of 30 minutes or more

1.05 1.05 Global Days XXX

AMA: 2009, Jan, 11-31; 2008, Sep, 3-4; 2008, Jun, 14-15

99374-99380 Care Plan Oversight: Patient Under Care of HHA, Hospice, or Nursing Facility

CMS 100-4,11,40.1.3.1 CPO Services with Hospice Care
CMS 100-4,12,180 Payment of Care Plan Oversight (CPO)
CMS 100-4,12,180.1 Billing for Care Plan Oversight (CPO)

INCLUDES Analysis of reports, diagnostic tests, treatment plans
Discussions with other health care providers, outside of the practice, involved in the patient's care
Establishment of and revisions to care plans within a 30-day period
Payment to one physician per month for covered care plan oversight services (must be the same one who signed the plan of care)

EXCLUDES *Care plan oversight services provided in assisted living, domiciliary care, or private residence, not under care of a home health agency or hospice (99339, 99340)*
Routine postoperative care provided during a global surgery period
Time discussing treatment with patient and/or caregivers

Code also office/outpatient visits, hospital, home, nursing facility, domiciliary, or non-face-to-face services

Do not report with (99441-99444, 98966-98969)

99374 **Physician supervision of a patient under care of home health agency (patient not present) in home, domiciliary or equivalent environment (eg, Alzheimer's facility) requiring complex and multidisciplinary care modalities involving regular physician development and/or revision of care plans, review of subsequent reports of patient status, review of related laboratory and other studies, communication (including telephone calls) for purposes of assessment or care decisions with health care professional(s), family member(s), surrogate decision maker(s) (eg, legal guardian) and/or key caregiver(s) involved in patient's care, integration of new information into the medical treatment plan and/or adjustment of medical therapy, within a calendar month; 15-29 minutes** B

1.62 2.01 Global Days XXX

AMA: 2009, Jul, 10; 2009, Jul, 5-6; 2008, Mar, 6-7; 2008, Sep, 3-4; 2007, Jul, 1-4; 2007, March, 9-11; 2007, April, 3-6

99375 **30 minutes or more** E

2.62 3.06 Global Days XXX

AMA: 2009, Jul, 10; 2009, Jul, 5-6; 2008, Mar, 6-7; 2008, Sep, 3-4; 2007, Jul, 1-4; 2007, April, 3-6; 2007, March, 9-11

99377 **Physician supervision of a hospice patient (patient not present) requiring complex and multidisciplinary care modalities involving regular physician development and/or revision of care plans, review of subsequent reports of patient status, review of related laboratory and other studies, communication (including telephone calls) for purposes of assessment or care decisions with health care professional(s), family member(s), surrogate decision maker(s) (eg, legal guardian) and/or key caregiver(s) involved in patient's care, integration of new information into the medical treatment plan and/or adjustment of medical therapy, within a calendar month; 15-29 minutes** B

1.62 2.01 Global Days XXX

AMA: 2009, Jul, 10; 2009, Jul, 5-6; 2008, Mar, 6-7; 2008, Sep, 3-4; 2007, Jul, 1-4; 2007, April, 3-6; 2007, March, 9-11

99378 **30 minutes or more** E

2.65 3.09 Global Days XXX

AMA: 2009, Jul, 5-6; 2009, Jul, 10; 2008, Mar, 6-7; 2008, Sep, 3-4; 2007, Jul, 1-4; 2007, April, 3-6; 2007, March, 9-11

99379 **Physician supervision of a nursing facility patient (patient not present) requiring complex and multidisciplinary care modalities involving regular physician development and/or revision of care plans, review of subsequent reports of patient status, review of related laboratory and other studies, communication (including telephone calls) for purposes of assessment or care decisions with health care professional(s), family member(s), surrogate decision maker(s) (eg, legal guardian) and/or key caregiver(s) involved in patient's care, integration of new information into the medical treatment plan and/or adjustment of medical therapy, within a calendar month; 15-29 minutes** B

1.62 2.01 Global Days XXX

AMA: 2009, Jul, 5-6; 2008, Mar, 6-7; 2008, Sep, 3-4; 2007, Jul, 1-4; 2007, March, 9-11

99380 **30 minutes or more** B

2.55 3.02 Global Days XXX

AMA: 2009, Jul, 5-6; 2008, Mar, 6-7; 2008, Sep, 3-4; 2007, Jul, 1-4; 2007, March, 9-11

99381-99397 Preventive Medicine Visits

CMS 100-1,5,70 Definition of Physician
CMS 100-2,15,30 Physician Services
CMS 100-4,12,30.6.2 Medically Necessary and Preventive Medicine Service on Same Date

INCLUDES Care of a small problem or preexisting condition that requires no extra work
New patients or established patients (99381-99387 or 99391-99397)
Regular preventive care (e.g., well-child exams) for all age groups

EXCLUDES *Counseling/risk factor reduction interventions not provided with a preventive medical examination (99401-99412)*
Diagnostic tests and other procedures

Code also immunization administration and product (90460-90461, 90471-90474, 90476-90749 [90665])

Code also substantial problems that require additional work (99201-99215)

99381 **Initial comprehensive preventive medicine evaluation and management of an individual including an age and gender appropriate history, examination, counseling/anticipatory guidance/risk factor reduction interventions, and the ordering of laboratory/diagnostic procedures, new patient; infant (age younger than 1 year)** A E

2.18 3.17 Global Days XXX

AMA: 2009, Mar, 3,4&7; 2009, Jul, 7; 2009, Jan, 11-31; 2008, Jan, 10-25; 2007, Jul, 1-4; 2007, March, 9-11; 2007, January, 13-27

99382 **early childhood (age 1 through 4 years)** A E

2.32 3.31 Global Days XXX

AMA: 2009, Jul, 7; 2007, Jul, 1-4; 2007, March, 9-11

99383 **late childhood (age 5 through 11 years)** A E

2.46 3.43 Global Days XXX

AMA: 2009, Jul, 7; 2007, Jul, 1-4; 2007, March, 9-11

99384 **adolescent (age 12 through 17 years)** A E

2.90 3.87 Global Days XXX

AMA: 2009, Jul, 7; 2007, Jul, 1-4; 2007, March, 9-11

99385 **18-39 years** A E

2.80 3.77 Global Days XXX

AMA: 2009, Jul, 7; 2007, Jul, 1-4; 2007, March, 9-11

99386 **40-64 years** A E

3.39 4.37 Global Days XXX

AMA: 2009, Jul, 7; 2007, Jul, 1-4; 2007, March, 9-11

99387 65 years and older A E
3.66 4.74 Global Days XXX
AMA: 2009, Jul, 7; 2007, Jul, 1-4; 2007, March, 9-11

99391 **Periodic comprehensive preventive medicine reevaluation and management of an individual including an age and gender appropriate history, examination, counseling/anticipatory guidance/risk factor reduction interventions, and the ordering of laboratory/diagnostic procedures, established patient; infant (age younger than 1 year)** A E
1.99 2.82 Global Days XXX
AMA: 2009, Mar, 3,4&7; 2009, Jul, 7; 2007, Jul, 1-4; 2007, March, 9-11

99392 early childhood (age 1 through 4 years) A E
2.18 3.02 Global Days XXX
AMA: 2009, Jul, 7; 2007, Jul, 1-4; 2007, March, 9-11

99393 late childhood (age 5 through 11 years) A E
2.18 3.01 Global Days XXX
AMA: 2009, Jul, 7; 2007, Jul, 1-4; 2007, March, 9-11

99394 adolescent (age 12 through 17 years) A E
2.46 3.29 Global Days XXX
AMA: 2009, Jul, 7; 2007, Jul, 1-4; 2007, March, 9-11

99395 18-39 years A E
2.53 3.36 Global Days XXX
AMA: 2009, Jul, 7; 2008, Mar, 3&7; 2007, Jul, 1-4; 2007, March, 9-11

99396 40-64 years A E
2.76 3.59 Global Days XXX
AMA: 2009, Jul, 7; 2007, Jul, 1-4; 2007, March, 9-11

99397 65 years and older A E
2.93 3.88 Global Days XXX
AMA: 2009, Jan, 11-31; 2009, Jul, 7; 2008, Jan, 10-25; 2007, Jul, 1-4; 2007, January, 13-27; 2007, March, 9-11

99401-99429 Counseling Services: Risk Factor and Behavioral Change Modification

CMS 100-1,5,70 Definition of Physician
CMS 100-2,15,30 Physician Services
CMS 100-2,16,90 Routine Services and Appliances
CMS 100-3,210.4 Smoking and Tobacco-Use Cessation Counseling
CMS 100-4,4,200.6 Alcohol and/or Substance Abuse Assessment and Intervention Services
CMS 100-4,12,10 General Processing Instructions
CMS 100-4,32,12 Smoking and Tobacco-Use Cessation Counseling Services
CMS 100-4,32,12.1 Smoking And Tobacco- Use Cessation Counseling
CMS 100-4,32,12.2 Carrier Billing: Smoking and Tobacco Use Cessation Counseling
CMS 100-4,32,12.3 FI Billing: Smoking and Tobacco Use Cessation Counseling

INCLUDES Administration and analysis of a health risk assessment (99420)
Face-to-face services for new and established patients based on time increments of 15 to 60 minutes
Issues such as a healthy diet, exercise, alcohol and drug abuse
Services provided by a physician or other qualified healthcare professional for the purpose of promoting health and reducing illness and injury

EXCLUDES *Counseling and risk factor reduction interventions included in preventive medicine services (99381-99397)*
Counseling services provided to patient groups with existing symptoms or illness (99078)

Code also distinct evaluation and management services when performed in addition

Do not report with heath and behavioral services provided on the same day (96150-96155)

99401 **Preventive medicine counseling and/or risk factor reduction intervention(s) provided to an individual (separate procedure); approximately 15 minutes** E
0.71 1.05 Global Days XXX
AMA: 2007, Jul, 1-4; 2007, March, 9-11; 2007, Aug, 9-12

99402 approximately 30 minutes E
1.45 1.80 Global Days XXX
AMA: 2007, Jul, 1-4; 2007, Aug, 9-12; 2007, March, 9-11

99403 approximately 45 minutes E
2.16 2.52 Global Days XXX
AMA: 2007, Jul, 1-4; 2007, Aug, 9-12; 2007, March, 9-11

99404 approximately 60 minutes E
2.87 3.23 Global Days XXX
AMA: 2007, Jul, 1-4; 2007, Aug, 9-12; 2007, March, 9-11

99406 **Smoking and tobacco use cessation counseling visit; intermediate, greater than 3 minutes up to 10 minutes** X 80
0.34 0.40 Global Days XXX
AMA: 2008, Jan, 1-3

99407 intensive, greater than 10 minutes X 80
Do not report with (99406)
0.73 0.78 Global Days XXX
AMA: 2008, Jan, 1-3

99408 **Alcohol and/or substance (other than tobacco) abuse structured screening (eg, AUDIT, DAST), and brief intervention (SBI) services; 15 to 30 minutes** E
INCLUDES Only initial screening and brief intervention Services of 15 minutes or more

Do not report with (99420)
0.96 1.01 Global Days XXX
AMA: 2008, May, 3-4; 2008, Jul, 11-13

99409 **greater than 30 minutes** E

INCLUDES Only initial screening and brief intervention

Do not report with (99408, 99420)

1.91 1.97 Global Days XXX

AMA: 2008, Jul, 11-13; 2008, May, 3-4

99411 **Preventive medicine counseling and/or risk factor reduction intervention(s) provided to individuals in a group setting (separate procedure); approximately 30 minutes** E

0.22 0.47 Global Days XXX

AMA: 2007, Jul, 1-4; 2007, Aug, 9-12; 2007, March, 9-11

99412 **approximately 60 minutes** E

0.36 0.61 Global Days XXX

AMA: 2007, Jul, 1-4; 2007, Aug, 9-12; 2007, March, 9-11

99420 **Administration and interpretation of health risk assessment instrument (eg, health hazard appraisal)** E

0.31 0.31 Global Days XXX

AMA: 2007, Jul, 1-4; 2007, March, 9-11

99429 **Unlisted preventive medicine service** E

0.00 0.00 Global Days XXX

AMA: 2007, Jul, 1-4; 2007, March, 9-11

99441-99443 Telephone Calls for Patient Management

CMS 100-1,5,70 Definition of Physician
CMS 100-2,15,30 Physician Services
CMS 100-4,11,40.2 Independent Attending Physician Services Under Hospice
CMS 100-4,12,10 General Processing Instructions

INCLUDES Episodes of care initiated by an established patient or the patient or guardian of an established patient
Non-face-to-face evaluation and management services provided by a physician

EXCLUDES *Services provided by a qualified nonphysician healthcare professional (98966-98968)*

Do not report with anticoagulation management reported with codes: (99363-99364)
Do not report with a related evaluation and management visit within the next 24 hours or as the next available urgent visit
Do not report with a related evaluation and management service performed and reported within the previous seven days or within the postoperative period of a completed procedure
Do not report with a related evaluation and management service perfomed in the previous seven days (99441-99444)
Do not report with the same call reported with codes: (99339-99340, 99374-99380)

99441 **Telephone evaluation and management service provided by a physician to an established patient, parent, or guardian not originating from a related E/M service provided within the previous 7 days nor leading to an E/M service or procedure within the next 24 hours or soonest available appointment; 5-10 minutes of medical discussion** E

0.36 0.40 Global Days XXX

AMA: 2008, Mar, 6-7

99442 **11-20 minutes of medical discussion** E

0.73 0.77 Global Days XXX

AMA: 2008, Mar, 6-7

99443 **21-30 minutes of medical discussion** E

1.11 1.14 Global Days XXX

AMA: 2008, Mar, 6-7

99444 Online Patient Management Services

INCLUDES All related communications such as related phone calls, prescription and lab orders
Permanent electronic or hardcopy storage
Physician evaluation and management services provided via the internet in response to a patient's on-line inquiry
The physician's personal timely response

Do not report more than once per seven-day period for the same episode of care
Do not report when related to an evaluation service performed and reported within the previous seven days
Do not report when within the postoperative period of a previously completed procedure

99444 **Online evaluation and management service provided by a physician to an established patient, guardian, or health care provider not originating from a related E/M service provided within the previous 7 days, using the Internet or similar electronic communications network** E

EXCLUDES *On-line medical evaluation by a qualified nonphysician healthcare professional (98969)*

Do not report with (99339-99340, 99363-99364, 99374-99380)

0.00 0.00 Global Days XXX

AMA: 2009, Jul, 5-6

99450-99456 Life/Disability Insurance Eligibility Visits

CMS 100-1,5,70 Definition of Physician
CMS 100-2,15,30 Physician Services

INCLUDES Assessment services for insurance eligibility and work-related disability without medical management of the patient's illness/injury
Services provided to new/established patients at any site of service

EXCLUDES *Any additional E/M services or procedures performed on the same date of service: report with appropriate code*

99450 **Basic life and/or disability examination that includes: Measurement of height, weight, and blood pressure; Completion of a medical history following a life insurance pro forma; Collection of blood sample and/or urinalysis complying with "chain of custody" protocols; and Completion of necessary documentation/certificates.** E

0.00 0.00 Global Days XXX

AMA: 2007, Jul, 1-4; 2007, March, 9-11

99455 **Work related or medical disability examination by the treating physician that includes: Completion of a medical history commensurate with the patient's condition; Performance of an examination commensurate with the patient's condition; Formulation of a diagnosis, assessment of capabilities and stability, and calculation of impairment; Development of future medical treatment plan; and Completion of necessary documentation/certificates and report.** B 80 PQ

Do not report with (99080)

0.00 0.00 Global Days XXX

AMA: 2007, Jul, 1-4; 2007, March, 9-11

99456 **Work related or medical disability examination by other than the treating physician that includes: Completion of a medical history commensurate with the patient's condition; Performance of an examination commensurate with the patient's condition; Formulation of a diagnosis, assessment of capabilities and stability, and calculation of impairment; Development of future medical treatment plan; and Completion of necessary documentation/certificates and report.** B 80

Do not report with (99080)

Facility RVU 0.00 Non-Facility RVU 0.00 Global Days XXX

AMA: 2007, Jul, 1-4; 2007, March, 9-11

99460-99463 Evaluation and Management Services for Age 28 Days or Less

INCLUDES
- Family consultation
- Healthy newborn history and physical
- Medical record documentation
- Ordering of diagnostic test and treatments
- Services provied to healthy newborns age 28 days or less

EXCLUDES
- *Neonatal intensive and critical care services (99466-99469, 99477-99480)*
- *Newborn follow up services in an office or outpatient setting (99201-99215, 99381, 99391)*
- *Newborn hospital discharge sevices if provided on a date subsequent to the admission date (99238-99239)*
- *Nonroutine neonatal inpatient evaluation and management services (99221-99233)*

Code also circumcision (54150)

Code also attendance at delivery (99464)

Code also emergency resuscitation services (99465)

99460 **Initial hospital or birthing center care, per day, for evaluation and management of normal newborn infant** A V 80

Facility RVU 2.74 Non-Facility RVU 2.74 Global Days XXX

AMA: 2009, Mar, 3,4&7

99461 **Initial care, per day, for evaluation and management of normal newborn infant seen in other than hospital or birthing center** A M 80

Facility RVU 1.85 Non-Facility RVU 2.75 Global Days XXX

99462 **Subsequent hospital care, per day, for evaluation and management of normal newborn** A C 80

Facility RVU 1.23 Non-Facility RVU 1.23 Global Days XXX

99463 **Initial hospital or birthing center care, per day, for evaluation and management of normal newborn infant admitted and discharged on the same date** A V 80

EXCLUDES *Services to newborns admitted and discharged on a date other than the admission date (99238-99239)*

Facility RVU 3.24 Non-Facility RVU 3.24 Global Days XXX

AMA: 2009, Mar, 3,4&7

99464-99465 Newborn Delivery Attendance/Resuscitation

99464 **Attendance at delivery (when requested by the delivering physician) and initial stabilization of newborn** N 80

Code also (99460, 99468, 99477)

Do not report with (99465)

Facility RVU 2.11 Non-Facility RVU 2.11 Global Days XXX

AMA: 2009, Mar, 3,4&7

99465 **Delivery/birthing room resuscitation, provision of positive pressure ventilation and/or chest compressions in the presence of acute inadequate ventilation and/or cardiac output** A S 80

Code also any necessary procedures performed as part of the resuscitation

Code also as appropriate (99460, 99468, 99477)

Do not report with (99464)

Facility RVU 4.25 Non-Facility RVU 4.25 Global Days XXX

AMA: 2009, Mar, 3,4&7

99466-99467 Critical Care Transport Age 24 Months or Younger

INCLUDES The following services:
- Chest x-rays (71010, 71015, 71020)
- Data stored in computer (99090)
- Gastric intubation (43752-43753)
- Interpretation of cardiac output measurements (93562)
- Pulse oximetry (94760-94762)
- Routine monitoring (heart rate, respiratory rate, and blood pressure)
- Temporary transcutaneous pacing (92953)
- Vascular access procedures (36000, 36400, 36405-36406, 36415, 36591, 36600)
- Ventilatory management (94002-94003, 94660, 94662)

Physician presence during interfacility transfer of critically ill/injured patient 24 months of age or less

EXCLUDES
- *Neonatal hypothermia (0260T-0261T)*
- *Patient critical care transport services with personal contact with patient of less than 30 minutes*
- *Physician directed emergency care via two-way voice communication with transporting staff (99288)*

Do not report for services less than 30 minutes duration (see evaluation and management codes)

99466 **Critical care services delivered by a physician, face-to-face, during an interfacility transport of critically ill or critically injured pediatric patient, 24 months of age or younger; first 30-74 minutes of hands-on care during transport** A N 80

Facility RVU 7.82 Non-Facility RVU 7.82 Global Days XXX

AMA: 2009, Mar, 3,4&7

\+ **99467** **each additional 30 minutes (List separately in addition to code for primary service)** A N 80

Code first (99466)

Facility RVU 3.49 Non-Facility RVU 3.49 Global Days ZZZ

AMA: 2009, Mar, 3,4&7

99468-99476 Critical Care Age 5 Years or Younger

INCLUDES All services included in codes 99291-99292 as well as the following which may be reported by facilities only:
- Administration of blood/blood components (36430, 36440)
- Administration of intravenous fluids (96360-96361)
- Administration of surfactant (94610)
- Bladder aspiration, suprapubic (51100)
- Bladder catheterization (51701, 51702)
- Car seat evaluation (94780-94781)
- Catheterization umbilical artery (36660)
- Catheterization umbilical vein (36510)
- Central venous catheter, centrally inserted (36555)
- Endotracheal intubation (31500)
- Lumbar puncture (62270)
- Oral or nasogastric tube placement (43752)
- Pulmonary function testing, performed at the bedside (94375)
- Pulse or ear oximetry (94760-94762)
- Vascular access, arteries (36140, 36620)
- Vascular access, venous (36400-36406, 36420, 36600)
- Ventilatory management (94002-94004, 94660)

Initial and subsequent care provided to a critically ill infant or child

EXCLUDES *Critical care services for patients 6 years of age or older (99291-99292)*
Critical care services provided by a second physician or physician of a different specialty (99291-99292)
Critical care services to an outpatient (99291-99292)
Neonatal hypothermia (0260T-0261T)
Services provided by physician receiving a patient transferred to a lower level of care (99231-99233, 99478-99480)
Services provided by physician transferring a patient to a lower level of care (99231-99233, 99291-99292)

Do not report with remote critical care (0188T-0189T)

99468 Initial inpatient neonatal critical care, per day, for the evaluation and management of a critically ill neonate, 28 days of age or younger A C5 C 80
26.44 26.44 Global Days XXX
AMA: 2009, Jan, 5&10; 2009, Mar, 3,4&7

99469 Subsequent inpatient neonatal critical care, per day, for the evaluation and management of a critically ill neonate, 28 days of age or younger A C5 C 80
11.90 11.90 Global Days XXX
AMA: 2009, Jan, 5&10; 2009, Mar, 3,4&7

99471 Initial inpatient pediatric critical care, per day, for the evaluation and management of a critically ill infant or young child, 29 days through 24 months of age A C5 C 80
22.60 22.60 Global Days XXX
AMA: 2009, Jan, 5&10; 2009, Mar, 3,4&7

99472 Subsequent inpatient pediatric critical care, per day, for the evaluation and management of a critically ill infant or young child, 29 days through 24 months of age A C5 C 80
11.49 11.49 Global Days XXX
AMA: 2009, Jan, 5&10; 2009, Mar, 3,4&7

99475 Initial inpatient pediatric critical care, per day, for the evaluation and management of a critically ill infant or young child, 2 through 5 years of age A C5 C 80
16.07 16.07 Global Days XXX
AMA: 2009, Jan, 5&10; 2009, Jan, 3,4&9; 2009, Mar, 3,4&7

99476 Subsequent inpatient pediatric critical care, per day, for the evaluation and management of a critically ill infant or young child, 2 through 5 years of age A C5 C 80
9.75 9.75 Global Days XXX
AMA: 2009, Jan, 3,4&9; 2009, Mar, 3,4&7; 2009, Jan, 5&10

99477-99499 Initial Inpatient Neonatal Intensive Care and Other Services

INCLUDES All services included in codes 99291-99292 as well as the following that may be reported by facilities only:
- Adjustments to enteral and/or parenteral nutrition
- Airway and ventilator management (31500, 94002-94004, 94375, 94610, 94660)
- Bladder catheterization (51701-51702)
- Blood transfusion (36430, 36440)
- Car seat evaluation (94780-94781)
- Constant and/or frequent montoring of vitals signs
- Continuous observation by the healthcare team
- Heat maintenance
- Intensive cardiac or respiratory monitoring
- Oral or nasogastric tube insertion (43752)
- Oxygen saturation (94760-94762)
- Spinal puncture (62270)
- Suprapubic catherization (51100)
- Vascular access procedures (36000, 36140, 36400, 36405-36406, 36420, 36510, 36555, 36600, 36620, 36660)

EXCLUDES *Neonatal hypothermia (0260T-0261T)*
Services provided by receiving physician when patient is transferred for critical care (99469, 99472)
Services provided to patient who improves after the initial day and is transferred to a lower level of care (99231-99233)
Subsequent care of a sick neonate, under 28 days of age, more than 5000 grams, not requiring critical or intensive care services (99231-99233)

Do not report with critical care services for patient transferred after initial or subsequent intensive care is provided (99291-99292)

99477 Initial hospital care, per day, for the evaluation and management of the neonate, 28 days of age or younger, who requires intensive observation, frequent interventions, and other intensive care services A C5 C 80
EXCLUDES *Initiation of care of a critically ill neonate (99468)*
Initiation of inpatient care of a normal newborn (99460)
9.93 9.93 Global Days XXX
AMA: 2009, Mar, 3,4&7; 2008, Jan, 1-3; 2008, Jan, 8-9; 2008, Jul, 10&13

99478 Subsequent intensive care, per day, for the evaluation and management of the recovering very low birth weight infant (present body weight less than 1500 grams) A C5 C 80
3.96 3.96 Global Days XXX
AMA: 2009, Mar, 3,4&7

99479 Subsequent intensive care, per day, for the evaluation and management of the recovering low birth weight infant (present body weight of 1500-2500 grams) A C5 C 80
3.64 3.64 Global Days XXX
AMA: 2009, Mar, 3,4&7

99480 Subsequent intensive care, per day, for the evaluation and management of the recovering infant (present body weight of 2501-5000 grams) A C5 C 80
3.43 3.43 Global Days XXX
AMA: 2009, Mar, 3,4&7

99499 Unlisted evaluation and management service B 80
0.00 0.00 Global Days XXX
AMA: 2009, Jan, 11-31; 2008, Jan, 10-25; 2007, Jul, 1-4; 2007, January, 13-27; 2007, March, 9-11

0001F-0015F Quality Measures with Multiple Components

INCLUDES Several measures grouped within a single code descriptor to make possible reporting for clinical conditions when all of the components have been met

▲ **0001F** **Heart failure assessed (includes assessment of all the following components) (CAD): Blood pressure measured (2000F) Level of activity assessed (1003F) Clinical symptoms of volume overload (excess) assessed (1004F) Weight, recorded (2001F) Clinical signs of volume overload (excess) assessed (2002F)** E

INCLUDES Blood pressure measured (2000F)
Clinical signs of volume overload (excess) assessed (2002F)
Clinical symptoms of volume overload (excess) assessed (1004F)
Level of activity assessed (1003F)
Weight recorded (2001F)

0.00 0.00 Global Days XXX

0005F **Osteoarthritis assessed (OA) Includes assessment of all the following components: Osteoarthritis symptoms and functional status assessed (1006F) Use of anti-inflammatory or over-the-counter (OTC) analgesic medications assessed (1007F) Initial examination of the involved joint(s) (includes visual inspection, palpation, range of motion) (2004F)** E

INCLUDES Initial examination of the involved joint(s) (includes visual inspection/palpation/range of motion) (2004F)
Osteoarthritis symptoms and functional status assessed (1006F)
Use of anti-inflammatory or over-the-counter (OTC) analgesic medications assessed (1007F)

EXCLUDES *Tobacco use cessation intervention (4001F)*

0.00 0.00 Global Days XXX

0012F **Community-acquired bacterial pneumonia assessment (includes all of the following components) (CAP): Co-morbid conditions assessed (1026F) Vital signs recorded (2010F) Mental status assessed (2014F) Hydration status assessed (2018F)** E

INCLUDES Co-morbid conditions assessed (1026F)
Hydration status assessed (2018F)
Mental status assessed (2014F)
Vital signs recorded (2010F)

0.00 0.00 Global Days XXX

0014F **Comprehensive preoperative assessment performed for cataract surgery with intraocular lens (IOL) placement (includes assessment of all of the following components) (EC): Dilated fundus evaluation performed within 12 months prior to cataract surgery (2020F) Pre-surgical (cataract) axial length, corneal power measurement and method of intraocular lens power calculation documented (must be performed within 12 months prior to surgery) (3073F) Preoperative assessment of functional or medical indication(s) for surgery prior to the cataract surgery with intraocular lens placement (must be performed within 12 months prior to cataract surgery) (3325F)** E PQ

INCLUDES Evaluation of dilated fundus done within 12 months prior to surgery (2020F)
Preoperative assessment of functional or medical indications done within 12 months prior to sugery (3325F)
Presurgical measurement of axial length and corneal power and IOL power calculation performed within 12 months prior to sugery (3325F)

0.00 0.00 Global Days XXX
AMA: 2008, Mar, 8-12

0015F **Melanoma follow-up completed (includes assessment of all of the following components) (ML): History obtained regarding new or changing moles (1050F) Complete physical skin exam performed (2029F) Patient counseled to perform a monthly self skin examination (5005F)** E PQ

INCLUDES Complete physical skin exam (2029F)
Counseling to perform monthly skin self-examination (5005F)
History obtained of new or changing moles (1050F)

0.00 0.00 Global Days XXX
AMA: 2008, Mar, 8-12

0500F-0575F Care Provided According to Prevailing Guidelines

INCLUDES Measures of utilization or patient care provided for certain clinical purposes

0500F **Initial prenatal care visit (report at first prenatal encounter with health care professional providing obstetrical care. Report also date of visit and, in a separate field, the date of the last menstrual period [LMP]) (Prenatal)** M ♀ E

0.00 0.00 Global Days XXX

0501F **Prenatal flow sheet documented in medical record by first prenatal visit (documentation includes at minimum blood pressure, weight, urine protein, uterine size, fetal heart tones, and estimated date of delivery). Report also: date of visit and, in a separate field, the date of the last menstrual period [LMP] (Note: If reporting 0501F Prenatal flow sheet, it is not necessary to report 0500F Initial prenatal care visit) (Prenatal)** M ♀ E

0.00 0.00 Global Days XXX

0502F Subsequent prenatal care visit (Prenatal) [Excludes: patients who are seen for a condition unrelated to pregnancy or prenatal care (eg, an upper respiratory infection; patients seen for consultation only, not for continuing care)] M ♀ E

EXCLUDES *Patients seen for an unrelated pregnancy/prenatal care condition (e.g., upper respiratory infection; patients seen for consultation only, not for continuing care)*

0.00 0.00 Global Days XXX

0503F Postpartum care visit (Prenatal) M ♀ E

0.00 0.00 Global Days XXX

0505F Hemodialysis plan of care documented (ESRD, P-ESRD) E PQ

0.00 0.00 Global Days XXX

AMA: 2008, Mar, 8-12

0507F Peritoneal dialysis plan of care documented (ESRD) E PQ

0.00 0.00 Global Days XXX

AMA: 2008, Mar, 8-12

0509F Urinary incontinence plan of care documented (GER) M PQ

0.00 0.00 Global Days XXX

0513F Elevated blood pressure plan of care documented (CKD) M PQ

0.00 0.00 Global Days XXX

AMA: 2008, Mar, 8-12

0514F Plan of care for elevated hemoglobin level documented for patient receiving erythropoiesis-stimulating agent therapy (ESA) (CKD) E PQ

0.00 0.00 Global Days XXX

AMA: 2008, Mar, 8-12

0516F Anemia plan of care documented (ESRD) E

0.00 0.00 Global Days XXX

AMA: 2008, Mar, 8-12

0517F Glaucoma plan of care documented (EC) M PQ

0.00 0.00 Global Days XXX

AMA: 2008, Mar, 8-12

0518F Falls plan of care documented (GER) M PQ

0.00 0.00 Global Days XXX

AMA: 2008, Mar, 8-12

0519F Planned chemotherapy regimen, including at a minimum: drug(s) prescribed, dose, and duration, documented prior to initiation of a new treatment regimen (ONC) E

0.00 0.00 Global Days XXX

AMA: 2008, Mar, 8-12

0520F Radiation dose limits to normal tissues established prior to the initiation of a course of 3D conformal radiation for a minimum of 2 tissue/organ (ONC) M PQ

0.00 0.00 Global Days XXX

AMA: 2008, Mar, 8-12

0521F Plan of care to address pain documented (COA) (ONC) M PQ

0.00 0.00 Global Days XXX

AMA: 2008, Mar, 8-12

0525F Initial visit for episode (BkP) E

0.00 0.00 Global Days XXX

AMA: 2008, Mar, 8-12

0526F Subsequent visit for episode (BkP) M PQ

0.00 0.00 Global Days XXX

AMA: 2008, Mar, 8-12

0528F Recommended follow-up interval for repeat colonoscopy of at least 10 years documented in colonoscopy report (End/Polyp) E

0.00 0.00 Global Days XXX

0529F Interval of 3 or more years since patient's last colonoscopy, documented (End/Polyp) M PQ

0.00 0.00 Global Days XXX

0535F Dyspnea management plan of care, documented (Pall Cr) E

0.00 0.00 Global Days XXX

0540F Glucorticoid Management Plan Documented (RA) M PQ

0.00 0.00 Global Days XXX

0545F Plan for follow-up care for major depressive disorder, documented (MDD ADOL) E

0.00 0.00 Global Days XXX

● 0550F Cytopathology report on routine nongynecologic specimen finalized within 2 working days of accession date (PATH) E

0.00 0.00 Global Days XXX

● 0551F Cytopathology report on nongynecologic specimen with documentation that the specimen was nonroutine (PATH) E

0.00 0.00 Global Days XXX

● 0555F Symptom management plan of care documented (HF) E

0.00 0.00 Global Days XXX

● 0556F Plan of care to achieve lipid control documented (CAD) M

0.00 0.00 Global Days XXX

● 0557F Plan of care to manage anginal symptoms documented (CAD) M

0.00 0.00 Global Days XXX

0575F HIV RNA control plan of care, documented (HIV) M PQ

0.00 0.00 Global Days XXX

1000F-1494F Elements of History/Review of Systems

INCLUDES Measures for specific aspects of patient history or review of systems

1000F Tobacco use assessed (CAD, CAP, COPD, PV) (DM) E PQ

0.00 0.00 Global Days XXX

▲ 1002F Anginal symptoms and level of activity assessed (NMA-No Measure Associated) E PQ

0.00 0.00 Global Days XXX

▲ 1003F Level of activity assessed (NMA-No Measure Associated) E

0.00 0.00 Global Days XXX

▲ 1004F Clinical symptoms of volume overload (excess) assessed (NMA-No Measure Associated) E

0.00 0.00 Global Days XXX

▲ 1005F Asthma symptoms evaluated (includes physician documentation of numeric frequency of symptoms or patient completion of an asthma assessment tool/survey/questionnaire) (NMA-No Measure Associated) E PQ

0.00 0.00 Global Days XXX

1006F Osteoarthritis symptoms and functional status assessed (may include the use of a standardized scale or the completion of an assessment questionnaire, such as the SF-36, AAOS Hip & Knee Questionnaire) (OA) [Instructions: Report when osteoarthritis is addressed during the patient encounter] M PQ

INCLUDES Osteoarthritis when it is addressed during the patient encounter

0.00 0.00 Global Days XXX

1007F Use of anti-inflammatory or analgesic over-the-counter (OTC) medications for symptom relief assessed (OA) M PQ
0.00 0.00 Global Days XXX

1008F Gastrointestinal and renal risk factors assessed for patients on prescribed or OTC non-steroidal anti-inflammatory drug (NSAID) (OA) E
0.00 0.00 Global Days XXX

● 1010F Severity of angina assessed by level of activity (CAD) M
0.00 0.00 Global Days XXX

● 1011F Angina present (CAD) M
0.00 0.00 Global Days XXX

● 1012F Angina absent (CAD) M
0.00 0.00 Global Days XXX

1015F Chronic obstructive pulmonary disease (COPD) symptoms assessed (Includes assessment of at least 1 of the following: dyspnea, cough/sputum, wheezing), or respiratory symptom assessment tool completed (COPD) E
0.00 0.00 Global Days XXX

1018F Dyspnea assessed, not present (COPD) E
0.00 0.00 Global Days XXX

1019F Dyspnea assessed, present (COPD) E
0.00 0.00 Global Days XXX

1022F Pneumococcus immunization status assessed (CAP, COPD) E
0.00 0.00 Global Days XXX
AMA: 2008, Mar, 8-12

1026F Co-morbid conditions assessed (eg, includes assessment for presence or absence of: malignancy, liver disease, congestive heart failure, cerebrovascular disease, renal disease, chronic obstructive pulmonary disease, asthma, diabetes, other co-morbid conditions) (CAP) E
0.00 0.00 Global Days XXX

1030F Influenza immunization status assessed (CAP) E
0.00 0.00 Global Days XXX
AMA: 2008, Mar, 8-12

● 1031F Smoking status and exposure to secondhand smoke in the home assessed (Asthma) M
0.00 0.00 Global Days XXX

● 1032F Current tobacco smoker OR currently exposed to secondhand smoke (asthma) M
0.00 0.00 Global Days XXX

● 1033F Current tobacco nonsmoker AND not currently exposed to secondhand smoke (Asthma) M
0.00 0.00 Global Days XXX

1034F Current tobacco smoker (CAD, CAP, COPD, PV) (DM) E PQ
0.00 0.00 Global Days XXX
AMA: 2008, Mar, 8-12

1035F Current smokeless tobacco user (eg, chew, snuff) (PV) E PQ
0.00 0.00 Global Days XXX
AMA: 2008, Mar, 8-12

▲ 1036F Current tobacco non-user (CAD, CAP, COPD, PV) (DM) (IBD) M PQ
0.00 0.00 Global Days XXX
AMA: 2008, Mar, 8-12

1038F Persistent asthma (mild, moderate or severe) (Asthma) M PQ
0.00 0.00 Global Days XXX

1039F Intermittent asthma (Asthma) M PQ
0.00 0.00 Global Days XXX

1040F DSM-IV criteria for major depressive disorder documented at the initial evaluation (MDD, MDD ADOL) M PQ
0.00 0.00 Global Days XXX
AMA: 2008, Mar, 8-12

1050F History obtained regarding new or changing moles (ML) E
0.00 0.00 Global Days XXX
AMA: 2008, Mar, 8-12

● 1052F Type, anatomic location, and activity all assessed (IBD) M
0.00 0.00 Global Days XXX

1055F Visual functional status assessed (EC) E
0.00 0.00 Global Days XXX

1060F Documentation of permanent OR persistent OR paroxysmal atrial fibrillation (STR) E
0.00 0.00 Global Days XXX

1061F Documentation of absence of permanent AND persistent AND paroxysmal atrial fibrillation (STR) E
0.00 0.00 Global Days XXX

1065F Ischemic stroke symptom onset of less than 3 hours prior to arrival (STR) E
0.00 0.00 Global Days XXX

1066F Ischemic stroke symptom onset greater than or equal to 3 hours prior to arrival (STR) E
0.00 0.00 Global Days XXX

1070F Alarm symptoms (involuntary weight loss, dysphagia, or gastrointestinal bleeding) assessed; none present (GERD) E
0.00 0.00 Global Days XXX

1071F 1 or more present (GERD) E
0.00 0.00 Global Days XXX

1090F Presence or absence of urinary incontinence assessed (GER) M PQ
0.00 0.00 Global Days XXX

1091F Urinary incontinence characterized (eg, frequency, volume, timing, type of symptoms, how bothersome) (GER) M PQ
0.00 0.00 Global Days XXX

1100F Patient screened for future fall risk; documentation of 2 or more falls in the past year or any fall with injury in the past year (GER) M PQ
0.00 0.00 Global Days XXX
AMA: 2008, Mar, 8-12

1101F documentation of no falls in the past year or only 1 fall without injury in the past year (GER) M PQ
0.00 0.00 Global Days XXX
AMA: 2008, Mar, 8-12

1110F Patient discharged from an inpatient facility (eg, hospital, skilled nursing facility, or rehabilitation facility) within the last 60 days (GER) M PQ
0.00 0.00 Global Days XXX

1111F Discharge medications reconciled with the current medication list in outpatient medical record (COA) (GER) M PQ
0.00 0.00 Global Days XXX

1116F Auricular or periauricular pain assessed (AOE) M PQ
0.00 0.00 Global Days XXX
AMA: 2008, Mar, 8-12

1118F GERD symptoms assessed after 12 months of therapy (GERD) E
0.00 0.00 Global Days XXX
AMA: 2008, Mar, 8-12

1119F Initial evaluation for condition (HEP C) (EPI) M PQ
0.00 0.00 Global Days XXX
AMA: 2008, Mar, 8-12

1121F Subsequent evaluation for condition (HEP C) (EPI) M PQ
0.00 0.00 Global Days XXX
AMA: 2008, Mar, 8-12

▲ 1123F Advance care planning discussed and documented advance care plan or surrogate decision maker documented in the medical record (DEM) (GER, Pall Cr) M PQ
0.00 0.00 Global Days XXX
AMA: 2008, Mar, 8-12

▲ 1124F Advance care planning discussed and documented in the medical record, patient did not wish or was not able to name a surrogate decision maker or provide an advance care plan (DEM) (GER, Pall Cr) M PQ
0.00 0.00 Global Days XXX
AMA: 2008, Mar, 8-12

1125F Pain severity quantified; pain present (COA) (ONC) M PQ
0.00 0.00 Global Days XXX
AMA: 2008, Mar, 8-12

1126F no pain present (COA) (ONC) M PQ
0.00 0.00 Global Days XXX
AMA: 2008, Mar, 8-12

○ 1127F New episode for condition (NMA - No Measure Associated) E
0.00 0.00 Global Days XXX
AMA: 2008, Mar, 8-12

○ 1128F Subsequent episode for condition (NMA - No Measure Associated) E
0.00 0.00 Global Days XXX
AMA: 2008, Mar, 8-12

1130F Back pain and function assessed, including all of the following: Pain assessment AND functional status AND patient history, including notation of presence or absence of "red flags" (warning signs) AND assessment of prior treatment and response, AND employment status (BkP) M PQ
0.00 0.00 Global Days XXX
AMA: 2008, Mar, 8-12

1134F Episode of back pain lasting 6 weeks or less (BkP) E
0.00 0.00 Global Days XXX
AMA: 2008, Mar, 8-12

1135F Episode of back pain lasting longer than 6 weeks (BkP) E
0.00 0.00 Global Days XXX
AMA: 2008, Mar, 8-12

1136F Episode of back pain lasting 12 weeks or less (BkP) E
0.00 0.00 Global Days XXX
AMA: 2008, Mar, 8-12

1137F Episode of back pain lasting longer than 12 weeks (BkP) E
0.00 0.00 Global Days XXX
AMA: 2008, Mar, 8-12

1150F Documentation that a patient has a substantial risk of death within 1 year (Pall Cr) E
0.00 0.00 Global Days XXX

1151F Documentation that a patient does not have a substantial risk of death within 1 year (Pall Cr) E
0.00 0.00 Global Days XXX

1152F Documentation of advanced disease diagnosis, goals of care prioritize comfort (Pall Cr) E
0.00 0.00 Global Days XXX

1153F Documentation of advanced disease diagnosis, goals of care do not prioritize comfort (Pall Cr) E
0.00 0.00 Global Days XXX

1157F Advance care plan or similar legal document present in the medical record (COA) E
0.00 0.00 Global Days XXX

1158F Advance care planning discussion documented in the medical record (COA) M
0.00 0.00 Global Days XXX

1159F Medication list documented in medical record (COA) E
0.00 0.00 Global Days XXX

1160F Review of all medications by a prescribing practitioner or clinical pharmacist (such as, prescriptions, OTCs, herbal therapies and supplements) documented in the medical record (COA) E
0.00 0.00 Global Days XXX

1170F Functional status assessed (COA) (RA) M PQ
0.00 0.00 Global Days XXX

● 1175F Functional status for dementia assessed and results reviewed (DEM) M
0.00 0.00 Global Days XXX

1180F All specified thromboembolic risk factors assessed (AFIB) E
0.00 0.00 Global Days XXX

● 1181F Neuropsychiatric symptoms assessed and results reviewed (DEM) M
0.00 0.00 Global Days XXX

● 1182F Neuropsychiatric symptoms, 1 or more present (DEM) E
0.00 0.00 Global Days XXX

● 1183F Neuropsychiatric symptoms, absent (DEM) E
0.00 0.00 Global Days XXX

1200F Seizure type(s) and current seizure frequency(ies) documented (EPI) M
0.00 0.00 Global Days XXX

1205F Etiology of epilepsy or epilepsy syndrome(s) reviewed and documented (EPI) M
0.00 0.00 Global Days XXX

1220F Patient screened for depression (SUD) M
0.00 0.00 Global Days XXX

1400F Parkinson's disease diagnosis reviewed (Prkns) M
0.00 0.00 Global Days XXX

● 1450F Symptoms improved or remained consistent with treatment goals since last assessment (HF) E
0.00 0.00 Global Days XXX

● 1451F Symptoms demonstrated clinically important deterioration since last assessment (HF) E
0.00 0.00 Global Days XXX

● 1460F Qualifying cardiac event/diagnosis in previous 12 months (CAD) M
0.00 0.00 Global Days XXX

● 1461F No qualifying cardiac event/diagnosis in previous 12 months (CAD) M
0.00 0.00 Global Days XXX

● 1490F Dementia severity classified, mild (DEM) M
0.00 0.00 Global Days XXX

● 1491F Dementia severity classified, moderate (DEM) M
0.00 0.00 Global Days XXX

● 1493F Dementia severity classified, severe (DEM) M
0.00 0.00 Global Days XXX

● 1494F Cognition assessed and reviewed (DEM) M
0.00 0.00 Global Days XXX

2000F-2060F Elements of Examination

INCLUDES Components of clinical assessment or physical exam

▲ 2000F Blood pressure measured (CKD) (DM) M PQ
0.00 0.00 Global Days XXX
AMA: 2008, Mar, 8-12

2001F Weight recorded (HF, PAG) E
0.00 0.00 Global Days XXX

▲ 2002F Clinical signs of volume overload (excess) assessed (NMA-No Measure Associated) E
0.00 0.00 Global Days XXX

2004F Initial examination of the involved joint(s) (includes visual inspection, palpation, range of motion) (OA) [Instructions: Report only for initial osteoarthritis visit or for visits for new joint involvement] E
INCLUDES Visits for initial osteoarthritis examination or new joint involvement
0.00 0.00 Global Days XXX

2010F Vital signs (temperature, pulse, respiratory rate, and blood pressure) documented and reviewed (CAP) (EM) M PQ
0.00 0.00 Global Days XXX

2014F Mental status assessed (CAP) (EM) M PQ
0.00 0.00 Global Days XXX

● 2015F Asthma impairment assessed (Asthma) M
0.00 0.00 Global Days XXX

● 2016F Asthma risk assessed (Asthma) M
0.00 0.00 Global Days XXX

2018F Hydration status assessed (normal/mildly dehydrated/severely dehydrated) (CAP) E
0.00 0.00 Global Days XXX

2019F Dilated macular exam performed, including documentation of the presence or absence of macular thickening or hemorrhage AND the level of macular degeneration severity (EC) M PQ
0.00 0.00 Global Days XXX

2020F Dilated fundus evaluation performed within 12 months prior to cataract surgery (EC) E
0.00 0.00 Global Days XXX
AMA: 2008, Mar, 8-12

2021F Dilated macular or fundus exam performed, including documentation of the presence or absence of macular edema AND level of severity of retinopathy (EC) M PQ
0.00 0.00 Global Days XXX

2022F Dilated retinal eye exam with interpretation by an ophthalmologist or optometrist documented and reviewed (DM) M PQ
0.00 0.00 Global Days XXX
AMA: 2008, Mar, 8-12

2024F 7 standard field stereoscopic photos with interpretation by an ophthalmologist or optometrist documented and reviewed (DM) M PQ
0.00 0.00 Global Days XXX
AMA: 2008, Mar, 8-12

2026F Eye imaging validated to match diagnosis from 7 standard field stereoscopic photos results documented and reviewed (DM) M PQ
0.00 0.00 Global Days XXX
AMA: 2008, Mar, 8-12

2027F Optic nerve head evaluation performed (EC) M PQ
0.00 0.00 Global Days XXX

2028F Foot examination performed (includes examination through visual inspection, sensory exam with monofilament, and pulse exam - report when any of the 3 components are completed) (DM) M PQ
0.00 0.00 Global Days XXX

2029F Complete physical skin exam performed (ML) E
0.00 0.00 Global Days XXX
AMA: 2008, Mar, 8-12

2030F Hydration status documented, normally hydrated (PAG) E
0.00 0.00 Global Days XXX

2031F Hydration status documented, dehydrated (PAG) E
0.00 0.00 Global Days XXX

2035F Tympanic membrane mobility assessed with pneumatic otoscopy or tympanometry (OME) M PQ
0.00 0.00 Global Days XXX
AMA: 2008, Mar, 8-12

2040F Physical examination on the date of the initial visit for low back pain performed, in accordance with specifications (BkP) M PQ
0.00 0.00 Global Days XXX
AMA: 2008, Mar, 8-12

2044F Documentation of mental health assessment prior to intervention (back surgery or epidural steroid injection) or for back pain episode lasting longer than 6 weeks (BkP) E
0.00 0.00 Global Days XXX
AMA: 2008, Mar, 8-12

2050F Wound characteristics including size AND nature of wound base tissue AND amount of drainage prior to debridement documented (CWC) E
0.00 0.00 Global Days XXX

2060F Patient interviewed directly by evaluating clinician on or before date of diagnosis of major depressive disorder (MDD ADOL) E
0.00 0.00 Global Days XXX

3006F-3750F Findings from Diagnostic or Screening Tests

INCLUDES Results and medical decision making with regards to ordered tests:
Clinical laboratory tests
Other examination procedures
Radiological examinations

3006F Chest X-ray results documented and reviewed (CAP) E
0.00 0.00 Global Days XXX

3008F Body Mass Index (BMI), documented (PV) E
0.00 0.00 Global Days XXX

3011F Lipid panel results documented and reviewed (must include total cholesterol, HDL-C, triglycerides and calculated LDL-C) (CAD) E
0.00 0.00 Global Days XXX

3014F Screening mammography results documented and reviewed (PV) M PQ
0.00 0.00 Global Days XXX
AMA: 2008, Mar, 8-12

3015F Cervical cancer screening results documented and reviewed (PV) ♀ E
0.00 0.00 Global Days XXX

3016F Patient screened for unhealthy alcohol use using a systematic screening method (PV) M PQ
0.00 0.00 Global Days XXX

3017F Colorectal cancer screening results documented and reviewed (PV) M PQ
0.00 0.00 Global Days XXX
AMA: 2008, Mar, 8-12

3018F Pre-procedure risk assessment AND depth of insertion AND quality of the bowel prep AND complete description of polyp(s) found, including location of each polyp, size, number and gross morphology AND recommendations for follow-up in final colonoscopy report documented (End/Polyp) E
0.00 0.00 Global Days XXX

● 3019F Left ventricular ejection fraction (LVEF) assessment planned post discharge (HF) E
0.00 0.00 Global Days XXX

▲ 3020F Left ventricular function (LVF) assessment (eg, echocardiography, nuclear test, or ventriculography) documented in the medical record (Includes quantitative or qualitative assessment results) (NMA-No Measure Associated) E PQ
0.00 0.00 Global Days XXX

3021F Left ventricular ejection fraction (LVEF) less than 40% or documentation of moderately or severely depressed left ventricular systolic function (CAD, HF) M PQ
0.00 0.00 Global Days XXX

3022F Left ventricular ejection fraction (LVEF) greater than or equal to 40% or documentation as normal or mildly depressed left ventricular systolic function (CAD, HF) M PQ
0.00 0.00 Global Days XXX

3023F Spirometry results documented and reviewed (COPD) M PQ
0.00 0.00 Global Days XXX

3025F Spirometry test results demonstrate FEV1/FVC less than 70% with COPD symptoms (eg, dyspnea, cough/sputum, wheezing) (CAP, COPD) M PQ
0.00 0.00 Global Days XXX

3027F Spirometry test results demonstrate FEV1/FVC greater than or equal to 70% or patient does not have COPD symptoms (COPD) M PQ
0.00 0.00 Global Days XXX

3028F Oxygen saturation results documented and reviewed (includes assessment through pulse oximetry or arterial blood gas measurement) (CAP, COPD) (EM) M PQ
0.00 0.00 Global Days XXX

3035F Oxygen saturation less than or equal to 88% or a PaO2 less than or equal to 55 mm Hg (COPD) E
0.00 0.00 Global Days XXX

3037F Oxygen saturation greater than 88% or PaO2 greater than 55 mmHg (COPD) E
0.00 0.00 Global Days XXX

3038F Pulmonary function test performed within 12 months prior to surgery (Lung/Esop Cx) M
0.00 0.00 Global Days XXX

3040F Functional expiratory volume (FEV1) less than 40% of predicted value (COPD) E
0.00 0.00 Global Days XXX

3042F Functional expiratory volume (FEV1) greater than or equal to 40% of predicted value (COPD) E
0.00 0.00 Global Days XXX

3044F Most recent hemoglobin A1c (HbA1c) level less than 7.0% (DM) M PQ
0.00 0.00 Global Days XXX

3045F Most recent hemoglobin A1c (HbA1c) level 7.0-9.0% (DM) M PQ
0.00 0.00 Global Days XXX

3046F Most recent hemoglobin A1c level greater than 9.0% (DM) M PQ
0.00 0.00 Global Days XXX

▲ 3048F Most recent LDL-C less than 100 mg/dL (CAD), (DM) M PQ
0.00 0.00 Global Days XXX

▲ 3049F Most recent LDL-C 100-129 mg/dL (CAD), (DM) M PQ
0.00 0.00 Global Days XXX

▲ 3050F Most recent LDL-C greater than or equal to 130 mg/dL (CAD), (DM) M PQ
0.00 0.00 Global Days XXX

● 3055F Left ventricular ejection fraction (LVEF) less than or equal to 35% (HF) E
0.00 0.00 Global Days XXX

● 3056F Left ventricular ejection fraction (LVEF) greater than 35% or no LVEF result available (HF) E
0.00 0.00 Global Days XXX

3060F Positive microalbuminuria test result documented and reviewed (DM) M PQ
0.00 0.00 Global Days XXX

3061F Negative microalbuminuria test result documented and reviewed (DM) M PQ
0.00 0.00 Global Days XXX

3062F Positive macroalbuminuria test result documented and reviewed (DM) M PQ
0.00 0.00 Global Days XXX

3066F Documentation of treatment for nephropathy (eg, patient receiving dialysis, patient being treated for ESRD, CRF, ARF, or renal insufficiency, any visit to a nephrologist) (DM) M PQ
0.00 0.00 Global Days XXX

3072F Low risk for retinopathy (no evidence of retinopathy in the prior year) (DM) M PQ
0.00 0.00 Global Days XXX
AMA: 2008, Mar, 8-12

3073F Pre-surgical (cataract) axial length, corneal power measurement and method of intraocular lens power calculation documented within 12 months prior to surgery (EC) E
0.00 0.00 Global Days XXX
AMA: 2008, Mar, 8-12

▲ 3074F Most recent systolic blood pressure less than 130 mm Hg (DM) (HTN, CKD,CAD) M PQ
0.00 0.00 Global Days XXX
AMA: 2008, Mar, 8-12

▲ 3075F Most recent systolic blood pressure 130 - 139 mm Hg (DM) (HTN, CKD, CAD) M PQ
0.00 0.00 Global Days XXX
AMA: 2008, Mar, 8-12

▲ 3077F Most recent systolic blood pressure greater than or equal to 140 mm Hg (DM) (HTN, CKD, CAD) M PQ
0.00 0.00 Global Days XXX
AMA: 2008, Mar, 8-12

▲ 3078F Most recent diastolic blood pressure less than 80 mm Hg (DM) (HTN, CKD, CAD) M PQ
0.00 0.00 Global Days XXX
AMA: 2008, Mar, 8-12

▲ 3079F Most recent diastolic blood pressure 80-89 mm Hg (DM) (HTN, CKD, CAD) M PQ
0.00 0.00 Global Days XXX
AMA: 2008, Mar, 8-12

▲ 3080F Most recent diastolic blood pressure greater than or equal to 90 mm Hg (DM) (HTN, CKD, CAD) M PQ
0.00 0.00 Global Days XXX
AMA: 2008, Mar, 8-12

3082F Kt/V less than 1.2 (Clearance of urea [Kt]/volume [V]) (ESRD, P-ESRD) E PQ
0.00 0.00 Global Days XXX
AMA: 2008, Mar, 8-12

3083F Kt/V equal to or greater than 1.2 and less than 1.7 (Clearance of urea [Kt]/volume [V]) (ESRD, P-ESRD) E PQ
0.00 0.00 Global Days XXX
AMA: 2008, Mar, 8-12

3084F Kt/V greater than or equal to 1.7 (Clearance of urea [Kt]/volume [V]) (ESRD, P-ESRD) E PQ
0.00 0.00 Global Days XXX
AMA: 2008, Mar, 8-12

3085F Suicide risk assessed (MDD, MDD ADOL) M PQ
0.00 0.00 Global Days XXX

3088F Major depressive disorder, mild (MDD) E
0.00 0.00 Global Days XXX

3089F Major depressive disorder, moderate (MDD) E
0.00 0.00 Global Days XXX

3090F Major depressive disorder, severe without psychotic features (MDD) E
0.00 0.00 Global Days XXX

3091F Major depressive disorder, severe with psychotic features (MDD) E
0.00 0.00 Global Days XXX

3092F Major depressive disorder, in remission (MDD) M PQ
0.00 0.00 Global Days XXX

3093F Documentation of new diagnosis of initial or recurrent episode of major depressive disorder (MDD) E
0.00 0.00 Global Days XXX
AMA: 2008, Mar, 8-12

▲ 3095F Central dual-energy X-ray absorptiometry (DXA) results documented (OP) (IBD) M PQ
0.00 0.00 Global Days XXX

▲ 3096F Central dual-energy X-ray absorptiometry (DXA) ordered (OP) (IBD) M PQ
0.00 0.00 Global Days XXX

3100F Carotid imaging study report (includes direct or indirect reference to measurements of distal internal carotid diameter as the denominator for stenosis measurement) (STR, RAD) M PQ
0.00 0.00 Global Days XXX
AMA: 2008, Mar, 8-12

3110F Documentation in final CT or MRI report of presence or absence of hemorrhage and mass lesion and acute infarction (STR) M PQ
0.00 0.00 Global Days XXX

▲ 3111F CT or MRI of the brain performed in the hospital within 24 hours of arrival OR performed in an outpatient imaging center, to confirm initial diagnosis of stroke, TIA or intracranial hemorrhage (STR) M PQ
0.00 0.00 Global Days XXX

▲ 3112F CT or MRI of the brain performed greater than 24 hours after arrival to the hospital OR performed in an outpatient imaging center for purpose other than confirmation of initial diagnosis of stroke, TIA, or intracranial hemorrhage (STR) M PQ
0.00 0.00 Global Days XXX

● 3115F Quantitative results of an evaluation of current level of activity and clinical symptoms (HF) E
0.00 0.00 Global Days XXX

● 3117F Heart failure disease specific structured assessment tool completed (HF) E
0.00 0.00 Global Days XXX

● 3118F New York Heart Association (NYHA) Class documented (HF) E
0.00 0.00 Global Days XXX

● 3119F No evaluation of level of activity or clinical symptoms (HF) E
0.00 0.00 Global Days XXX

3120F 12-Lead ECG Performed (EM) M PQ
0.00 0.00 Global Days XXX

● 3125F Esophageal biopsy report with statement about dysplasia (present, absent, or indefinite) (PATH) M
0.00 0.00 Global Days XXX

3130F Upper gastrointestinal endoscopy performed (GERD) E
0.00 0.00 Global Days XXX

3132F Documentation of referral for upper gastrointestinal endoscopy (GERD) E
0.00 0.00 Global Days XXX

3140F Upper gastrointestinal endoscopy report indicates suspicion of Barrett's esophagus (GERD) E
0.00 0.00 Global Days XXX

3141F Upper gastrointestinal endoscopy report indicates no suspicion of Barrett's esophagus (GERD) E
0.00 0.00 Global Days XXX

3142F Barium swallow test ordered (GERD) E
0.00 0.00 Global Days XXX

3150F Forceps esophageal biopsy performed (GERD) E
0.00 0.00 Global Days XXX

3155F Cytogenetic testing performed on bone marrow at time of diagnosis or prior to initiating treatment (HEM) M PQ
0.00 0.00 Global Days XXX
AMA: 2008, Mar, 8-12

3160F Documentation of iron stores prior to initiating erythropoietin therapy (HEM) M PQ
0.00 0.00 Global Days XXX
AMA: 2008, Mar, 8-12

3170F Flow cytometry studies performed at time of diagnosis or prior to initiating treatment (HEM) M PQ
0.00 0.00 Global Days XXX
AMA: 2008, Mar, 8-12

3200F Barium swallow test not ordered (GERD) E
0.00 0.00 Global Days XXX

3210F Group A strep test performed (PHAR) M PQ
0.00 0.00 Global Days XXX
AMA: 2008, Mar, 8-12

3215F Patient has documented immunity to Hepatitis A (HEP-C) M PQ
0.00 0.00 Global Days XXX
AMA: 2008, Mar, 8-12

▲ 3216F Patient has documented immunity to Hepatitis B (HEP C), (IBD) M PQ
0.00 0.00 Global Days XXX
AMA: 2008, Mar, 8-12

3218F RNA testing for Hepatitis C documented as performed within 6 months prior to initiation of antiviral treatment for Hepatitis C (HEP-C) M PQ
0.00 0.00 Global Days XXX
AMA: 2008, Mar, 8-12

3220F Hepatitis C quantitative RNA testing documented as performed at 12 weeks from initiation of antiviral treatment (HEP-C) M PQ
0.00 0.00 Global Days XXX
AMA: 2008, Mar, 8-12

3230F Documentation that hearing test was performed within 6 months prior to tympanostomy tube insertion (OME) E
0.00 0.00 Global Days XXX
AMA: 2008, Mar, 8-12

3250F Specimen site other than anatomic location of primary tumor (PATH) M PQ
0.00 0.00 Global Days XXX

3260F pT category (primary tumor), pN category (regional lymph nodes), and histologic grade documented in pathology report (PATH) M PQ
0.00 0.00 Global Days XXX
AMA: 2008, Mar, 8-12

3265F Ribonucleic acid (RNA) testing for Hepatitis C viremia ordered or results documented (HEP C) M PQ
0.00 0.00 Global Days XXX
AMA: 2008, Mar, 8-12

3266F Hepatitis C genotype testing documented as performed prior to initiation of antiviral treatment for Hepatitis C (HEP C) M PQ
0.00 0.00 Global Days XXX
AMA: 2008, Mar, 8-12

● 3267F Pathology report includes pT category, pN category, Gleason score and statement about margin status (PATH) M
0.00 0.00 Global Days XXX

3268F Prostate-specific antigen (PSA), AND primary tumor (T) stage, AND Gleason score documented prior to initiation of treatment (PRCA) E
0.00 0.00 Global Days XXX
AMA: 2008, Mar, 8-12

3269F Bone scan performed prior to initiation of treatment or at any time since diagnosis of prostate cancer (PRCA) M PQ
0.00 0.00 Global Days XXX
AMA: 2008, Mar, 8-12

3270F Bone scan not performed prior to initiation of treatment nor at any time since diagnosis of prostate cancer (PRCA) M PQ
0.00 0.00 Global Days XXX
AMA: 2008, Mar, 8-12

3271F Low risk of recurrence, prostate cancer (PRCA) M PQ
0.00 0.00 Global Days XXX
AMA: 2008, Mar, 8-12

3272F Intermediate risk of recurrence, prostate cancer (PRCA) M PQ
0.00 0.00 Global Days XXX
AMA: 2008, Mar, 8-12

3273F High risk of recurrence, prostate cancer (PRCA) M PQ
0.00 0.00 Global Days XXX
AMA: 2008, Mar, 8-12

3274F Prostate cancer risk of recurrence not determined or neither low, intermediate nor high (PRCA) ♂ M PQ
0.00 0.00 Global Days XXX
AMA: 2008, Mar, 8-12

3278F Serum levels of calcium, phosphorus, intact Parathyroid Hormone (PTH) and lipid profile ordered (CKD) E PQ
0.00 0.00 Global Days XXX
AMA: 2008, Mar, 8-12

3279F Hemoglobin level greater than or equal to 13 g/dL (CKD, ESRD) E PQ
0.00 0.00 Global Days XXX
AMA: 2008, Mar, 8-12

3280F Hemoglobin level 11 g/dL to 12.9 g/dL (CKD, ESRD) E PQ
0.00 0.00 Global Days XXX
AMA: 2008, Mar, 8-12

3281F Hemoglobin level less than 11 g/dL (CKD, ESRD) E PQ
0.00 0.00 Global Days XXX
AMA: 2008, Mar, 8-12

3284F Intraocular pressure (IOP) reduced by a value of greater than or equal to 15% from the pre-intervention level (EC) M PQ
0.00 0.00 Global Days XXX
AMA: 2008, Mar, 8-12

3285F Intraocular pressure (IOP) reduced by a value less than 15% from the pre-intervention level (EC) M PQ
0.00 0.00 Global Days XXX
AMA: 2008, Mar, 8-12

3288F Falls risk assessment documented (GER) M PQ
0.00 0.00 Global Days XXX
AMA: 2008, Mar, 8-12

3290F Patient is D (Rh) negative and unsensitized (Pre-Cr) E
0.00 0.00 Global Days XXX
AMA: 2008, Mar, 8-12

3291F Patient is D (Rh) positive or sensitized (Pre-Cr) E
0.00 0.00 Global Days XXX
AMA: 2008, Mar, 8-12

3292F HIV testing ordered or documented and reviewed during the first or second prenatal visit (Pre-Cr) E
0.00 0.00 Global Days XXX

3293F ABO and Rh blood typing documented as performed (Pre-Cr) E
0.00 0.00 Global Days XXX

3294F Group B Streptococcus (GBS) screening documented as performed during week 35-37 gestation (Pre-Cr) E
0.00 0.00 Global Days XXX

3300F American Joint Committee on Cancer (AJCC) stage documented and reviewed (ONC) M PQ
0.00 0.00 Global Days XXX
AMA: 2008, Mar, 8-12

3301F Cancer stage documented in medical record as metastatic and reviewed (ONC) M PQ
0.00 0.00 Global Days XXX
AMA: 2008, Mar, 8-12

3315F Estrogen receptor (ER) or progesterone receptor (PR) positive breast cancer (ONC) M PQ
0.00 0.00 Global Days XXX
AMA: 2008, Mar, 8-12

3316F Estrogen receptor (ER) and progesterone receptor (PR) negative breast cancer (ONC) M PQ
0.00 0.00 Global Days XXX
AMA: 2008, Mar, 8-12

3317F Pathology report confirming malignancy documented in the medical record and reviewed prior to the initiation of chemotherapy (ONC) E
0.00 0.00 Global Days XXX
AMA: 2008, Mar, 8-12

3318F Pathology report confirming malignancy documented in the medical record and reviewed prior to the initiation of radiation therapy (ONC) E
0.00 0.00 Global Days XXX
AMA: 2008, Mar, 8-12

3319F 1 of the following diagnostic imaging studies ordered: chest x-ray, CT, ultrasound, MRI, PET, or nuclear medicine scans (ML) M
0.00 0.00 Global Days XXX
AMA: 2008, Mar, 8-12

3320F None of the following diagnostic imaging studies ordered: chest X-ray, CT, Ultrasound, MRI, PET, or nuclear medicine scans (ML) M
0.00 0.00 Global Days XXX
AMA: 2008, Mar, 8-12

3321F AJCC cancer Stage 0 or IA melanoma, documented (ML) M
0.00 0.00 Global Days XXX

3322F Melanoma greater than AJCC Stage 0 or IA (ML) M
0.00 0.00 Global Days XXX

3323F Clinical tumor, node and metastases (TNM) staging documented and reviewed prior to surgery (Lung/Esop Cx) M PQ
0.00 0.00 Global Days XXX

3324F MRI or CT scan ordered, reviewed or requested (EPI) E
0.00 0.00 Global Days XXX

3325F Preoperative assessment of functional or medical indication(s) for surgery prior to the cataract surgery with intraocular lens placement (must be performed within 12 months prior to cataract surgery) (EC) E
0.00 0.00 Global Days XXX
AMA: 2008, Mar, 8-12

3328F Performance status documented and reviewed within 2 weeks prior to surgery (Lung/Esop Cx) M
0.00 0.00 Global Days XXX

3330F Imaging study ordered (BkP) E
0.00 0.00 Global Days XXX
AMA: 2008, Mar, 8-12

3331F Imaging study not ordered (BkP) E
0.00 0.00 Global Days XXX
AMA: 2008, Mar, 8-12

3340F Mammogram assessment category of "incomplete: need additional imaging evaluation", documented (RAD) ♀ M PQ
0.00 0.00 Global Days XXX
AMA: 2008, Mar, 8-12

3341F Mammogram assessment category of "negative," documented (RAD) ♀ M PQ
0.00 0.00 Global Days XXX
AMA: 2008, Mar, 8-12

3342F Mammogram assessment category of "benign," documented (RAD) ♀ M PQ
0.00 0.00 Global Days XXX
AMA: 2008, Mar, 8-12

3343F Mammogram assessment category of "probably benign," documented (RAD) ♀ M PQ
0.00 0.00 Global Days XXX
AMA: 2008, Mar, 8-12

3344F Mammogram assessment category of "suspicious," documented (RAD) ♀ M PQ
0.00 0.00 Global Days XXX
AMA: 2008, Mar, 8-12

3345F Mammogram assessment category of "highly suggestive of malignancy," documented (RAD) ♀ M PQ
0.00 0.00 Global Days XXX
AMA: 2008, Mar, 8-12

3350F Mammogram assessment category of "known biopsy proven malignancy," documented (RAD) ♀ M PQ
0.00 0.00 Global Days XXX
AMA: 2008, Mar, 8-12

3351F Negative screen for depressive symptoms as categorized by using a standardized depression screening/assessment tool (MDD) E
0.00 0.00 Global Days XXX

3352F No significant depressive symptoms as categorized by using a standardized depression assessment tool (MDD) E
0.00 0.00 Global Days XXX

3353F Mild to moderate depressive symptoms as categorized by using a standardized depression screening/assessment tool (MDD) E
0.00 0.00 Global Days XXX

3354F Clinically significant depressive symptoms as categorized by using a standardized depression screening/assessment tool (MDD) E
0.00 0.00 Global Days XXX

3370F AJCC breast cancer Stage 0 documented (ONC) M PQ
0.00 0.00 Global Days XXX

3372F AJCC breast cancer Stage I: T1mic, T1a or T1b (tumor size ≤ 1 cm) documented (ONC) M PQ
0.00 0.00 Global Days XXX

3374F AJCC breast cancer Stage I: T1c (tumor size > 1 cm to 2 cm) documented (ONC) M PQ
0.00 0.00 Global Days XXX

3376F AJCC breast cancer Stage II documented (ONC) M PQ
0.00 0.00 Global Days XXX

3378F AJCC breast cancer Stage III documented (ONC) M PQ
0.00 0.00 Global Days XXX

3380F AJCC breast cancer Stage IV documented (ONC) M PQ
0.00 0.00 Global Days XXX

3382F AJCC colon cancer, Stage 0 documented (ONC) M PQ
0.00 0.00 Global Days XXX

3384F AJCC colon cancer, Stage I documented (ONC) M PQ
0.00 0.00 Global Days XXX

3386F AJCC colon cancer, Stage II documented (ONC) M PQ
0.00 0.00 Global Days XXX

3388F AJCC colon cancer, Stage III documented (ONC) M PQ
0.00 0.00 Global Days XXX

3390F AJCC colon cancer, Stage IV documented (ONC) M PQ
0.00 0.00 Global Days XXX

● 3394F Quantitative HER2 Immunohistochemistry (IHC) evaluation of breast cancer consistent with the scoring system defined in the ASCO/CAP guidelines (PATH) M
0.00 0.00 Global Days XXX

● 3395F Quantitative non-HER2 Immunohistochemistry (IHC) evaluation of breast cancer (eg, testing for estrogen or progesterone receptors [ER/PR]) performed (PATH) M
0.00 0.00 Global Days XXX

3450F Dyspnea screened, no dyspnea or mild dyspnea (Pall Cr) E
0.00 0.00 Global Days XXX

3451F Dyspnea screened, moderate or severe dyspnea (Pall Cr) E
0.00 0.00 Global Days XXX

3452F Dyspnea not screened (Pall Cr) E
0.00 0.00 Global Days XXX

▲ 3455F TB screening performed and results interpreted within 6 months prior to initiation of first-time biologic disease modifying anti-rheumatic drug therapy for RA (RA) M PQ
0.00 0.00 Global Days XXX

3470F Rheumatoid arthritis (RA) disease activity, low (RA) M PQ
0.00 0.00 Global Days XXX

3471F Rheumatoid arthritis (RA) disease activity, moderate (RA) M PQ
0.00 0.00 Global Days XXX

3472F Rheumatoid arthritis (RA) disease activity, high (RA) M PQ
0.00 0.00 Global Days XXX

3475F Disease prognosis for rheumatoid arthritis assessed, poor prognosis documented (RA) M PQ
0.00 0.00 Global Days XXX

3476F Disease prognosis for rheumatoid arthritis assessed, good prognosis documented (RA) M PQ
0.00 0.00 Global Days XXX

3490F History of AIDS-defining condition (HIV) M PQ
0.00 0.00 Global Days XXX

3491F HIV indeterminate (infants of undetermined HIV status born of HIV-infected mothers) (HIV) E
0.00 0.00 Global Days XXX

3492F History of nadir CD4+ cell count < 350 cells/mm3 (HIV) M PQ
0.00 0.00 Global Days XXX

3493F No history of nadir CD4+ cell count < 350 cells/mm3 AND no history of AIDS-defining condition (HIV) M PQ
0.00 0.00 Global Days XXX

3494F CD4+ cell count < 200 cells/mm3 (HIV) M PQ
0.00 0.00 Global Days XXX

3495F CD4+ cell count 200 - 499 cells/mm3 (HIV) M PQ
0.00 0.00 Global Days XXX

3496F CD4+ cell count ≥ 500 cells/mm3 (HIV) M PQ
0.00 0.00 Global Days XXX

▲ 3497F CD4+ cell percentage < 15% (HIV) E
0.00 0.00 Global Days XXX

3498F CD4+ cell percentage ≥ 15% (HIV) E
0.00 0.00 Global Days XXX

3500F CD4+ cell count or CD4+ cell percentage documented as performed (HIV) M PQ
0.00 0.00 Global Days XXX

3502F HIV RNA viral load below limits of quantification (HIV) M PQ
0.00 0.00 Global Days XXX

3503F HIV RNA viral load not below limits of quantification (HIV) M PQ
0.00 0.00 Global Days XXX

▲ 3510F Documentation that tuberculosis (TB) screening test performed and results interpreted (HIV) (IBD) M
0.00 0.00 Global Days XXX

3511F Chlamydia and gonorrhea screenings documented as performed (HIV) M PQ
0.00 0.00 Global Days XXX

3512F Syphilis screening documented as performed (HIV) M PQ
0.00 0.00 Global Days XXX

3513F Hepatitis B screening documented as performed (HIV) E
0.00 0.00 Global Days XXX

3514F Hepatitis C screening documented as performed (HIV) E
0.00 0.00 Global Days XXX

3515F Patient has documented immunity to Hepatitis C (HIV) E
0.00 0.00 Global Days XXX

● 3517F Hepatitis B virus (HBV) status assessed and results interpreted within 1 year prior to receiving first course of anti-TNF (tumor necrosis factor) therapy (IBD) M
0.00 0.00 Global Days XXX

● 3520F Clostridium difficile testing performed (IBD) E
0.00 0.00 Global Days XXX

3550F Low risk for thromboembolism (AFIB) E
0.00 0.00 Global Days XXX

3551F Intermediate risk for thromboembolism (AFIB) E
0.00 0.00 Global Days XXX

3552F High risk for thromboembolism (AFIB) E
0.00 0.00 Global Days XXX

3555F Patient had International Normalized Ratio (INR) measurement performed (AFIB) E
0.00 0.00 Global Days XXX

3570F Final report for bone scintigraphy study includes correlation with existing relevant imaging studies (eg, x-ray, MRI, CT) corresponding to the same anatomical region in question (NUC_MED) M PQ
0.00 0.00 Global Days XXX

3572F Patient considered to be potentially at risk for fracture in a weight-bearing site (NUC_MED) E
0.00 0.00 Global Days XXX

3573F Patient not considered to be potentially at risk for fracture in a weight-bearing site (NUC_MED) E
0.00 0.00 Global Days XXX

3650F Electroencephalogram (EEG) ordered, reviewed or requested (EPI) E
0.00 0.00 Global Days XXX

3700F Psychiatric disorders or disturbances assessed (Prkns) M
0.00 0.00 Global Days XXX

3720F Cognitive impairment or dysfunction assessed (Prkns) M
0.00 0.00 Global Days XXX

● 3725F Screening for depression performed (DEM) M
0.00 0.00 Global Days XXX

● 3750F Patient not receiving dose of corticosteroids greater than or equal to 10mg/day for 60 or greater consecutive days (IBD) M
0.00 0.00 Global Days XXX

4000F-4526F Therapies Provided (Includes Preventive Services)

INCLUDES Behavioral/pharmacologic/procedural therapies
Preventive services including patient education/counseling

▲ 4000F Tobacco use cessation intervention, counseling (COPD, CAP, CAD, Asthma)(DM)(PV) M PQ
0.00 0.00 Global Days XXX
AMA: 2008, Mar, 8-12

▲ 4001F Tobacco use cessation intervention, pharmacologic therapy (COPD, CAP,CAD, Asthma)(DM)(PV) M PQ
0.00 0.00 Global Days XXX
AMA: 2008, Mar, 8-12

~~4002F Statin therapy, prescribed (CAD)~~
To report, see 4013F

▲ 4003F Patient education, written/oral, appropriate for patients with heart failure, performed (NMA-No Measure Associated) E PQ
0.00 0.00 Global Days XXX

▲ 4004F Patient screened for tobacco use AND received tobacco cessation (intervention, counseling, pharmacotherapy, or both) if identified as a tobacco user (PV, CAD) M
0.00 0.00 Global Days XXX

▲ 4005F Pharmacologic therapy (other than minerals/vitamins) for osteoporosis prescribed (OP) (IBD) M PQ
0.00 0.00 Global Days XXX

~~4006F Beta-blocker therapy prescribed (CAD, HF)~~
To report, see 4008F

● 4008F Beta blocker therapy prescribed or currently being taken (CAD, HF) M
0.00 0.00 Global Days XXX

~~4009F Angiotensin converting enzyme (ACE) inhibitor or angiotensin receptor blocker (ARB) therapy prescribed (CKD), (DM)~~
To report, see 4010F

● **4010F Angiotensin converting enzyme (ACE) inhibitor or angiotensin receptor blocker (ARB) therapy prescribed or currently being taken (CAD, CKD, HF) (DM)** M
0.00 0.00 Global Days XXX

4011F Oral antiplatelet therapy prescribed (CAD) E PQ
0.00 0.00 Global Days XXX

▲ **4012F Warfarin therapy prescribed (NMA-No Measure Associated)** M PQ
0.00 0.00 Global Days XXX

● **4013F Statin therapy prescribed or currently being taken (CAD)** M
0.00 0.00 Global Days XXX

▲ **4014F Written discharge instructions provided to heart failure patients discharged home (Instructions include all of the following components: activity level, diet, discharge medications, follow-up appointment, weight monitoring, what to do if symptoms worsen) (NMA-No Measure Associated)** A E
EXCLUDES *Patients younger than 18 years of age*
0.00 0.00 Global Days XXX

▲ **4015F Persistent asthma, preferred long term control medication or an acceptable alternative treatment, prescribed (NMA-No Measure Associated)** E PQ
Code also modifier 2P for patient reasons for not prescribing
Do not report with modifier 1P
0.00 0.00 Global Days XXX

4016F Anti-inflammatory/analgesic agent prescribed (OA) (Use for prescribed or continued medication[s], including over-the-counter medication[s]) E
INCLUDES Over-the-counter medication(s)
Prescribed/continued medication(s)
0.00 0.00 Global Days XXX

4017F Gastrointestinal prophylaxis for NSAID use prescribed (OA) E
0.00 0.00 Global Days XXX

4018F Therapeutic exercise for the involved joint(s) instructed or physical or occupational therapy prescribed (OA) E
0.00 0.00 Global Days XXX

4019F Documentation of receipt of counseling on exercise AND either both calcium and vitamin D use or counseling regarding both calcium and vitamin D use (OP) E
0.00 0.00 Global Days XXX

4025F Inhaled bronchodilator prescribed (COPD) M PQ
0.00 0.00 Global Days XXX

4030F Long-term oxygen therapy prescribed (more than 15 hours per day) (COPD) E
0.00 0.00 Global Days XXX

4033F Pulmonary rehabilitation exercise training recommended (COPD) E
Code also dyspnea assessed, present (1019F)
0.00 0.00 Global Days XXX

▲ **4035F Influenza immunization recommended (COPD) (IBD)** M
0.00 0.00 Global Days XXX
AMA: 2008, Mar, 8-12

▲ **4037F Influenza immunization ordered or administered (COPD, PV, CKD, ESRD) (IBD)** M PQ
0.00 0.00 Global Days XXX
AMA: 2008, Mar, 8-12

▲ **4040F Pneumococcal vaccine administered or previously received (COPD), (IBD), (PV)** M PQ
0.00 0.00 Global Days XXX
AMA: 2008, Mar, 8-12

4041F Documentation of order for cefazolin OR cefuroxime for antimicrobial prophylaxis (PERI 2) M PQ
0.00 0.00 Global Days XXX

4042F Documentation that prophylactic antibiotics were neither given within 4 hours prior to surgical incision nor given intraoperatively (PERI 2) M PQ
0.00 0.00 Global Days XXX

4043F Documentation that an order was given to discontinue prophylactic antibiotics within 48 hours of surgical end time, cardiac procedures (PERI 2) M PQ
0.00 0.00 Global Days XXX

4044F Documentation that an order was given for venous thromboembolism (VTE) prophylaxis to be given within 24 hours prior to incision time or 24 hours after surgery end time (PERI 2) M PQ
0.00 0.00 Global Days XXX

4045F Appropriate empiric antibiotic prescribed (CAP), (EM) M PQ
0.00 0.00 Global Days XXX

4046F Documentation that prophylactic antibiotics were given within 4 hours prior to surgical incision or given intraoperatively (PERI 2) M PQ
0.00 0.00 Global Days XXX

4047F Documentation of order for prophylactic parenteral antibiotics to be given within 1 hour (if fluoroquinolone or vancomycin, 2 hours) prior to surgical incision (or start of procedure when no incision is required) (PERI 2) M PQ
0.00 0.00 Global Days XXX

4048F Documentation that administration of prophylactic parenteral antibiotic was initiated within 1 hour (if fluoroquinolone or vancomycin, 2 hours) prior to surgical incision (or start of procedure when no incision is required) as ordered (PERI 2) M PQ
0.00 0.00 Global Days XXX

4049F Documentation that order was given to discontinue prophylactic antibiotics within 24 hours of surgical end time, non-cardiac procedure (PERI 2) M PQ
0.00 0.00 Global Days XXX

▲ **4050F Hypertension plan of care documented as appropriate (NMA-No Measure Associated)** E
0.00 0.00 Global Days XXX

4051F Referred for an arteriovenous (AV) fistula (ESRD, CKD) E PQ
0.00 0.00 Global Days XXX
AMA: 2008, Mar, 8-12

4052F Hemodialysis via functioning arteriovenous (AV) fistula (ESRD) E
0.00 0.00 Global Days XXX
AMA: 2008, Mar, 8-12

4053F Hemodialysis via functioning arteriovenous (AV) graft (ESRD) E
0.00 0.00 Global Days XXX
AMA: 2008, Mar, 8-12

4054F Hemodialysis via catheter (ESRD) E
0.00 0.00 Global Days XXX
AMA: 2008, Mar, 8-12

4055F Patient receiving peritoneal dialysis (ESRD) E
0.00 0.00 Global Days XXX
AMA: 2008, Mar, 8-12

4056F Appropriate oral rehydration solution recommended (PAG) E
0.00 0.00 Global Days XXX

4058F Pediatric gastroenteritis education provided to caregiver (PAG) E
0.00 0.00 Global Days XXX

4060F Psychotherapy services provided (MDD, MDD ADOL) E
0.00 0.00 Global Days XXX

4062F Patient referral for psychotherapy documented (MDD, MDD ADOL) E
0.00 0.00 Global Days XXX

4063F Antidepressant pharmacotherapy considered and not prescribed (MDD ADOL) E
0.00 0.00 Global Days XXX

4064F Antidepressant pharmacotherapy prescribed (MDD, MDD ADOL) E
0.00 0.00 Global Days XXX

4065F Antipsychotic pharmacotherapy prescribed (MDD) E
0.00 0.00 Global Days XXX

4066F Electroconvulsive therapy (ECT) provided (MDD) E
0.00 0.00 Global Days XXX

4067F Patient referral for electroconvulsive therapy (ECT) documented (MDD) E
0.00 0.00 Global Days XXX

● 4069F Venous thromboembolism (VTE) prophylaxis received (IBD) E
0.00 0.00 Global Days XXX

4070F Deep vein thrombosis (DVT) prophylaxis received by end of hospital day 2 (STR) M PQ
0.00 0.00 Global Days XXX

4073F Oral antiplatelet therapy prescribed at discharge (STR) E PQ
0.00 0.00 Global Days XXX

4075F Anticoagulant therapy prescribed at discharge (STR) M PQ
0.00 0.00 Global Days XXX

4077F Documentation that tissue plasminogen activator (t-PA) administration was considered (STR) E
0.00 0.00 Global Days XXX

4079F Documentation that rehabilitation services were considered (STR) E PQ
0.00 0.00 Global Days XXX

4084F Aspirin received within 24 hours before emergency department arrival or during emergency department stay (EM) M PQ
0.00 0.00 Global Days XXX

● 4086F Aspirin or clopidogrel prescribed (CAD) M
0.00 0.00 Global Days XXX

4090F Patient receiving erythropoietin therapy (HEM) M PQ
0.00 0.00 Global Days XXX
AMA: 2008, Mar, 8-12

4095F Patient not receiving erythropoietin therapy (HEM) M PQ
0.00 0.00 Global Days XXX
AMA: 2008, Mar, 8-12

4100F Bisphosphonate therapy, intravenous, ordered or received (HEM) M PQ
0.00 0.00 Global Days XXX
AMA: 2008, Mar, 8-12

4110F Internal mammary artery graft performed for primary, isolated coronary artery bypass graft procedure (CABG) M PQ
0.00 0.00 Global Days XXX

4115F Beta blocker administered within 24 hours prior to surgical incision (CABG) M PQ
0.00 0.00 Global Days XXX

4120F Antibiotic prescribed or dispensed (URI, PHAR), (A-BRONCH) M PQ
0.00 0.00 Global Days XXX
AMA: 2008, Mar, 8-12

4124F Antibiotic neither prescribed nor dispensed (URI, PHAR), (A-BRONCH) M PQ
0.00 0.00 Global Days XXX
AMA: 2008, Mar, 8-12

4130F Topical preparations (including OTC) prescribed for acute otitis externa (AOE) M PQ
0.00 0.00 Global Days XXX
AMA: 2008, Mar, 8-12

4131F Systemic antimicrobial therapy prescribed (AOE) M PQ
0.00 0.00 Global Days XXX
AMA: 2008, Mar, 8-12

4132F Systemic antimicrobial therapy not prescribed (AOE) M PQ
0.00 0.00 Global Days XXX
AMA: 2008, Mar, 8-12

4133F Antihistamines or decongestants prescribed or recommended (OME) E
0.00 0.00 Global Days XXX
AMA: 2008, Mar, 8-12

4134F Antihistamines or decongestants neither prescribed nor recommended (OME) E
0.00 0.00 Global Days XXX
AMA: 2008, Mar, 8-12

4135F Systemic corticosteroids prescribed (OME) E
0.00 0.00 Global Days XXX
AMA: 2008, Mar, 8-12

4136F Systemic corticosteroids not prescribed (OME) E
0.00 0.00 Global Days XXX
AMA: 2008, Mar, 8-12

● 4140F Inhaled corticosteroids prescribed (Asthma) M
0.00 0.00 Global Days XXX

● 4142F Corticosteroid sparing therapy prescribed (IBD) M
0.00 0.00 Global Days XXX

● 4144F Alternative long-term control medication prescribed (Asthma) M
0.00 0.00 Global Days XXX

● 4145F Two or more anti-hypertensive agents prescribed or currently being taken (CAD, HTN) M
0.00 0.00 Global Days XXX

4148F Hepatitis A vaccine injection administered or previously received (HEP-C) M PQ
0.00 0.00 Global Days XXX

▲ 4149F Hepatitis B vaccine injection administered or previously received (HEP-C, HIV) (IBD) M PQ
0.00 0.00 Global Days XXX

4150F Patient receiving antiviral treatment for Hepatitis C (HEP-C) M PQ
0.00 0.00 Global Days XXX
AMA: 2008, Mar, 8-12

4151F Patient not receiving antiviral treatment for Hepatitis C (HEP-C) M PQ
0.00 0.00 Global Days XXX
AMA: 2008, Mar, 8-12

4153F Combination peginterferon and ribavirin therapy prescribed (HEP-C) M PQ
0.00 0.00 Global Days XXX
AMA: 2008, Mar, 8-12

4155F Hepatitis A vaccine series previously received (HEP-C) E
0.00 0.00 Global Days XXX
AMA: 2008, Mar, 8-12

4157F Hepatitis B vaccine series previously received (HEP-C) E
0.00 0.00 Global Days XXX
AMA: 2008, Mar, 8-12

4158F Patient counseled about risks of alcohol use (HEP-C) M PQ
0.00 0.00 Global Days XXX
AMA: 2008, Mar, 8-12

4159F Counseling regarding contraception received prior to initiation of antiviral treatment (HEP-C) M PQ
0.00 0.00 Global Days XXX
AMA: 2008, Mar, 8-12

4163F Patient counseling at a minimum on all of the following treatment options for clinically localized prostate cancer: active surveillance, AND interstitial prostate brachytherapy, AND external beam radiotherapy, AND radical prostatectomy, provided prior to initiation of treatment (PRCA) E
0.00 0.00 Global Days XXX
AMA: 2008, Mar, 8-12

4164F Adjuvant (ie, in combination with external beam radiotherapy to the prostate for prostate cancer) hormonal therapy (gonadotropin-releasing hormone [GnRH] agonist or antagonist) prescribed/administered (PRCA) M PQ
0.00 0.00 Global Days XXX
AMA: 2008, Mar, 8-12

4165F 3-dimensional conformal radiotherapy (3D-CRT) or intensity modulated radiation therapy (IMRT) received (PRCA) M PQ
0.00 0.00 Global Days XXX
AMA: 2008, Mar, 8-12

4167F Head of bed elevation (30-45 degrees) on first ventilator day ordered (CRIT) E
0.00 0.00 Global Days XXX
AMA: 2008, Mar, 8-12

4168F Patient receiving care in the intensive care unit (ICU) and receiving mechanical ventilation, 24 hours or less (CRIT) E
0.00 0.00 Global Days XXX
AMA: 2008, Mar, 8-12

4169F Patient either not receiving care in the intensive care unit (ICU) OR not receiving mechanical ventilation OR receiving mechanical ventilation greater than 24 hours (CRIT) E
0.00 0.00 Global Days XXX
AMA: 2008, Mar, 8-12

4171F Patient receiving erythropoiesis-stimulating agents (ESA) therapy (CKD) M PQ
0.00 0.00 Global Days XXX
AMA: 2008, Mar, 8-12

4172F Patient not receiving erythropoiesis-stimulating agents (ESA) therapy (CKD) M PQ
0.00 0.00 Global Days XXX
AMA: 2008, Mar, 8-12

4174F Counseling about the potential impact of glaucoma on visual functioning and quality of life, and importance of treatment adherence provided to patient and/or caregiver(s) (EC) E
0.00 0.00 Global Days XXX
AMA: 2008, Mar, 8-12

4175F Best-corrected visual acuity of 20/40 or better (distance or near) achieved within the 90 days following cataract surgery (EC) M PQ
0.00 0.00 Global Days XXX
AMA: 2008, Mar, 8-12

4176F Counseling about value of protection from UV light and lack of proven efficacy of nutritional supplements in prevention or progression of cataract development provided to patient and/or caregiver(s) (NMA No Measure Associated) E
0.00 0.00 Global Days XXX

4177F Counseling about the benefits and/or risks of the age-related eye disease study (AREDS) formulation for preventing progression of age-related macular degeneration (AMD) provided to patient and/or caregiver(s) (EC) M PQ
0.00 0.00 Global Days XXX
AMA: 2008, Mar, 8-12

4178F Anti-D immune globulin received between 26 and 30 weeks gestation (Pre-Cr) M ♀ E
0.00 0.00 Global Days XXX
AMA: 2008, Mar, 8-12

4179F Tamoxifen or aromatase inhibitor (AI) prescribed (ONC) M PQ
0.00 0.00 Global Days XXX
AMA: 2008, Mar, 8-12

4180F Adjuvant chemotherapy referred, prescribed, or previously received for Stage III colon cancer (ONC) M PQ
0.00 0.00 Global Days XXX
AMA: 2008, Mar, 8-12

4181F Conformal radiation therapy received (NMA-No Measure Assoc.) E
0.00 0.00 Global Days XXX

4182F Conformal radiation therapy not received (NMA-No Measure Assoc.) E
0.00 0.00 Global Days XXX

4185F Continuous (12-months) therapy with proton pump inhibitor (PPI) or histamine H2 receptor antagonist (H2RA) received (GERD) E
0.00 0.00 Global Days XXX
AMA: 2008, Mar, 8-12

4186F No continuous (12-months) therapy with either proton pump inhibitor (PPI) or histamine H2 receptor antagonist (H2RA) received (GERD) E
0.00 0.00 Global Days XXX
AMA: 2008, Mar, 8-12

4187F Disease modifying anti-rheumatic drug therapy prescribed or dispensed (RA) M PQ
0.00 0.00 Global Days XXX

4188F Appropriate angiotensin converting enzyme (ACE)/angiotensin receptor blockers (ARB) therapeutic monitoring test ordered or performed (AM) E
0.00 0.00 Global Days XXX
AMA: 2008, Mar, 8-12

4189F Appropriate digoxin therapeutic monitoring test ordered or performed (AM) E
0.00 0.00 Global Days XXX
AMA: 2008, Mar, 8-12

4190F Appropriate diuretic therapeutic monitoring test ordered or performed (AM) E
0.00 0.00 Global Days XXX
AMA: 2008, Mar, 8-12

4191F Appropriate anticonvulsant therapeutic monitoring test ordered or performed (AM) E
0.00 0.00 Global Days XXX
AMA: 2008, Mar, 8-12

4192F Patient not receiving glucocorticoid therapy (RA) M PQ
0.00 0.00 Global Days XXX

▲ 4193F Patient receiving < 10 mg daily prednisone (or equivalent), or RA activity is worsening, or glucocorticoid use is for less than 6 months (RA) M PQ
0.00 0.00 Global Days XXX

4194F Patient receiving ≥ 10 mg daily prednisone (or equivalent) for longer than 6 months, and improvement or no change in disease activity (RA) M PQ
0.00 0.00 Global Days XXX

4195F Patient receiving first-time biologic disease modifying anti-rheumatic drug therapy for rheumatoid arthritis (RA) M PQ
0.00 0.00 Global Days XXX

4196F Patient not receiving first-time biologic disease modifying anti-rheumatic drug therapy for rheumatoid arthritis (RA) M PQ
0.00 0.00 Global Days XXX

4200F External beam radiotherapy as primary therapy to prostate with or without nodal irradiation (PRCA) M PQ
0.00 0.00 Global Days XXX
AMA: 2008, Mar, 8-12

4201F External beam radiotherapy with or without nodal irradiation as adjuvant or salvage therapy for prostate cancer patient (PRCA) M PQ
0.00 0.00 Global Days XXX
AMA: 2008, Mar, 8-12

4210F Angiotensin converting enzyme (ACE) or angiotensin receptor blockers (ARB) medication therapy for 6 months or more (MM) E
0.00 0.00 Global Days XXX
AMA: 2008, Mar, 8-12

4220F Digoxin medication therapy for 6 months or more (MM) E
0.00 0.00 Global Days XXX
AMA: 2008, Mar, 8-12

4221F Diuretic medication therapy for 6 months or more (MM) E
0.00 0.00 Global Days XXX
AMA: 2008, Mar, 8-12

4230F Anticonvulsant medication therapy for 6 months or more (MM) E
0.00 0.00 Global Days XXX
AMA: 2008, Mar, 8-12

4240F Instruction in therapeutic exercise with follow-up by the physician provided to patients during episode of back pain lasting longer than 12 weeks (BkP) E
0.00 0.00 Global Days XXX
AMA: 2008, Mar, 8-12

4242F Counseling for supervised exercise program provided to patients during episode of back pain lasting longer than 12 weeks (BkP) E
0.00 0.00 Global Days XXX
AMA: 2008, Mar, 8-12

4245F Patient counseled during the initial visit to maintain or resume normal activities (BkP) M PQ
0.00 0.00 Global Days XXX
AMA: 2008, Mar, 8-12

4248F Patient counseled during the initial visit for an episode of back pain against bed rest lasting 4 days or longer (BkP) M PQ
0.00 0.00 Global Days XXX
AMA: 2008, Mar, 8-12

4250F Active warming used intraoperatively for the purpose of maintaining normothermia, OR at least 1 body temperature equal to or greater than 36 degrees Centigrade (or 96.8 degrees Fahrenheit) recorded within the 30 minutes immediately before or the 15 minutes immediately after anesthesia end time (CRIT) M PQ
0.00 0.00 Global Days XXX
AMA: 2008, Mar, 8-12

4255F Duration of general or neuraxial anesthesia 60 minutes or longer, as documented in the anesthesia record (CRIT) M PQ
0.00 0.00 Global Days XXX

4256F Duration of general or neuraxial anesthesia less than 60 minutes, as documented in the anesthesia record (CRIT) M PQ
0.00 0.00 Global Days XXX

4260F Wound surface culture technique used (CWC) M
0.00 0.00 Global Days XXX

4261F Technique other than surface culture of the wound exudate used (eg, Levine/deep swab technique, semi-quantitative or quantitative swab technique) OR wound surface culture technique not used (CWC) M
0.00 0.00 Global Days XXX

4265F Use of wet to dry dressings prescribed or recommended (CWC) M
0.00 0.00 Global Days XXX

4266F Use of wet to dry dressings neither prescribed nor recommended (CWC) M
0.00 0.00 Global Days XXX

4267F Compression therapy prescribed (CWC) M PQ
0.00 0.00 Global Days XXX

4268F Patient education regarding the need for long term compression therapy including interval replacement of compression stockings received (CWC) E
0.00 0.00 Global Days XXX

4269F Appropriate method of offloading (pressure relief) prescribed (CWC) E
0.00 0.00 Global Days XXX

4270F Patient receiving potent antiretroviral therapy for 6 months or longer (HIV) M PQ
0.00 0.00 Global Days XXX

4271F Patient receiving potent antiretroviral therapy for less than 6 months or not receiving potent antiretroviral therapy (HIV) M PQ
0.00 0.00 Global Days XXX

4274F Influenza immunization administered or previously received (HIV) (P-ESRD) E PQ
0.00 0.00 Global Days XXX

~~4275F Hepatitis B vaccine injection administered or previously received (HIV)~~
To report, see 4149F

4276F Potent antiretroviral therapy prescribed (HIV) M PQ
0.00 0.00 Global Days XXX

4279F Pneumocystis jiroveci pneumonia prophylaxis prescribed (HIV) E
0.00 0.00 Global Days XXX

4280F Pneumocystis jiroveci pneumonia prophylaxis prescribed within 3 months of low CD4+ cell count or percentage (HIV) M PQ
0.00 0.00 Global Days XXX

4290F Patient screened for injection drug use (HIV) M PQ
0.00 0.00 Global Days XXX

4293F Patient screened for high-risk sexual behavior (HIV) M PQ
0.00 0.00 Global Days XXX

4300F Patient receiving warfarin therapy for nonvalvular atrial fibrillation or atrial flutter (AFIB) E
0.00 0.00 Global Days XXX

4301F Patient not receiving warfarin therapy for nonvalvular atrial fibrillation or atrial flutter (AFIB) E
0.00 0.00 Global Days XXX

4305F Patient education regarding appropriate foot care AND daily inspection of the feet received (CWC) E
0.00 0.00 Global Days XXX

4306F Patient counseled regarding psychosocial AND pharmacologic treatment options for opioid addiction (SUD) E
0.00 0.00 Global Days XXX

4320F Patient counseled regarding psychosocial AND pharmacologic treatment options for alcohol dependence (SUD) M
0.00 0.00 Global Days XXX

● **4322F** Caregiver provided with education and referred to additional resources for support (DEM) M
0.00 0.00 Global Days XXX

4324F Patient (or caregiver) queried about Parkinson's disease medication related motor complications (Prkns) E
0.00 0.00 Global Days XXX

4325F Medical and surgical treatment options reviewed with patient (or caregiver) (Prkns) M
0.00 0.00 Global Days XXX

4326F Patient (or caregiver) queried about symptoms of autonomic dysfunction (Prkns) E
0.00 0.00 Global Days XXX

4328F Patient (or caregiver) queried about sleep disturbances (Prkns) M
0.00 0.00 Global Days XXX

4330F Counseling about epilepsy specific safety issues provided to patient (or caregiver(s)) (EPI) M
0.00 0.00 Global Days XXX

4340F Counseling for women of childbearing potential with epilepsy (EPI) M
0.00 0.00 Global Days XXX

● **4350F** Counseling provided on symptom management, end of life decision, and palliation (DEM) E
0.00 0.00 Global Days XXX

4400F Rehabilitative therapy options discussed with patient (or caregiver) (Prkns) M
0.00 0.00 Global Days XXX

● **4450F** Self-care education provided to patient (HF) E
0.00 0.00 Global Days XXX

● **4470F** Implantable cardioverter-defibrillator (ICD) counseling provided (HF) E
0.00 0.00 Global Days XXX

● **4480F** Patient receiving ACE inhibitor/ARB therapy and beta-blocker therapy for 3 months or longer (HF) E
0.00 0.00 Global Days XXX

● **4481F** Patient receiving ACE inhibitor/ARB therapy and beta-blocker therapy for less than 3 months (HF) E
0.00 0.00 Global Days XXX

● **4500F** Referred to an outpatient cardiac rehabilitation program (CAD) M
0.00 0.00 Global Days XXX

● **4510F** Previous cardiac rehabilitation for qualifying cardiac event completed (CAD) M
0.00 0.00 Global Days XXX

● **4525F** Neuropsychiatric intervention ordered (DEM) M
0.00 0.00 Global Days XXX

● **4526F** Neuropsychiatric intervention received (DEM) M
0.00 0.00 Global Days XXX

5005F-5250F Results Conveyed and Documented

INCLUDES Patient's:
- Functional status
- Morbidity/mortality
- Satisfaction/experience with care

Review/communication of test results to patients

5005F Patient counseled on self-examination for new or changing moles (ML) E
0.00 0.00 Global Days XXX
AMA: 2008, Mar, 8-12

5010F Findings of dilated macular or fundus exam communicated to the physician managing the diabetes care (EC) M PQ
0.00 0.00 Global Days XXX

5015F Documentation of communication that a fracture occurred and that the patient was or should be tested or treated for osteoporosis (OP) M PQ
0.00 0.00 Global Days XXX

5020F Treatment summary report communicated to physician(s) managing continuing care and to the patient within 1 month of completing treatment (ONC) E
0.00 0.00 Global Days XXX
AMA: 2008, Mar, 8-12

5050F Treatment plan communicated to provider(s) managing continuing care within 1 month of diagnosis (ML) M PQ
0.00 0.00 Global Days XXX
AMA: 2008, Mar, 8-12

5060F Findings from diagnostic mammogram communicated to practice managing patient's on-going care within 3 business days of exam interpretation (RAD) ♀ E
0.00 0.00 Global Days XXX
AMA: 2008, Mar, 8-12

5062F Findings from diagnostic mammogram communicated to the patient within 5 days of exam interpretation (RAD) ♀ E
0.00 0.00 Global Days XXX
AMA: 2008, Mar, 8-12

5100F Potential risk for fracture communicated to the referring physician within 24 hours of completion of the imaging study (NUC_MED) E
0.00 0.00 Global Days XXX

5200F Consideration of referral for a neurological evaluation of appropriateness for surgical therapy for intractable epilepsy within the past 3 years (EPI) E
0.00 0.00 Global Days XXX

● **5250F** Asthma discharge plan present (Asthma) E
0.00 0.00 Global Days XXX

6005F-6150F Elements Related to Patient Safety Processes

INCLUDES Patient safety practices

6005F Rationale (eg, severity of illness and safety) for level of care (eg, home, hospital) documented (CAP) E
0.00 0.00 Global Days XXX

6010F Dysphagia screening conducted prior to order for or receipt of any foods, fluids, or medication by mouth (STR) M PQ
0.00 0.00 Global Days XXX

6015F Patient receiving or eligible to receive foods, fluids, or medication by mouth (STR) M PQ
0.00 0.00 Global Days XXX

6020F NPO (nothing by mouth) ordered (STR) M PQ
0.00 0.00 Global Days XXX

6030F All elements of maximal sterile barrier technique followed including: cap AND mask AND sterile gown AND sterile gloves AND a large sterile sheet AND hand hygiene AND 2% chlorhexidine for cutaneous antisepsis (or acceptable alternative antiseptics, per current guideline) (CRIT) M PQ
0.00 0.00 Global Days XXX
AMA: 2008, Mar, 8-12

6040F Use of appropriate radiation dose reduction devices OR manual techniques for appropriate moderation of exposure, documented (RAD) E
0.00 0.00 Global Days XXX

6045F Radiation exposure or exposure time in final report for procedure using fluoroscopy, documented (RAD) M PQ
0.00 0.00 Global Days XXX
AMA: 2008, Mar, 8-12

6070F Patient queried and counseled about anti-epileptic drug (AED) side effects (EPI) M
0.00 0.00 Global Days XXX

6080F Patient (or caregiver) queried about falls (Prkns) E
0.00 0.00 Global Days XXX

6090F Patient (or caregiver) counseled about safety issues appropriate to patient's stage of disease (Prkns) M
0.00 0.00 Global Days XXX

● **6100F** Timeout to verify correct patient, correct site, and correct procedure, documented (PATH) E
0.00 0.00 Global Days XXX

● **6101F** Safety counseling for dementia provided (DEM) M
0.00 0.00 Global Days XXX

● **6102F** Safety counseling for dementia ordered (DEM) M
0.00 0.00 Global Days XXX

● **6110F** Counseling provided regarding risks of driving and the alternatives to driving (DEM) M
0.00 0.00 Global Days XXX

● **6150F** Patient not receiving a first course of anti-TNF (tumor necrosis factor) therapy (IBD) M
0.00 0.00 Global Days XXX

7010F-7025F Recall/Reminder System in Place

INCLUDES Capabilities of the provider
Measures that address the setting or system of care provided

7010F Patient information entered into a recall system that includes: target date for the next exam specified AND a process to follow up with patients regarding missed or unscheduled appointments (ML) M PQ
0.00 0.00 Global Days XXX
AMA: 2008, Mar, 8-12

7020F Mammogram assessment category (eg, Mammography Quality Standards Act [MQSA], Breast Imaging Reporting and Data System [BI-RADS], or FDA-approved equivalent categories) entered into an internal database to allow for analysis of abnormal interpretation (recall) rate (RAD) ♀ E
0.00 0.00 Global Days XXX
AMA: 2008, Mar, 8-12

7025F Patient information entered into a reminder system with a target due date for the next mammogram (RAD) ♀ M
0.00 0.00 Global Days XXX
AMA: 2008, Mar, 8-12

0019T-0042T

0019T Extracorporeal shock wave involving musculoskeletal system, not otherwise specified, low energy A 80

EXCLUDES *High energy:*
Extracorporeal shock wave (0101T)
Lateral humeral epicondyle extracorporeal shock wave (0102T)

0.00 0.00 Global Days XXX

0030T Antiprothrombin (phospholipid cofactor) antibody, each Ig class A 80

0.00 0.00 Global Days XXX

0042T Cerebral perfusion analysis using computed tomography with contrast administration, including post-processing of parametric maps with determination of cerebral blood flow, cerebral blood volume, and mean transit time N1 N 80 PQ

0.00 0.00 Global Days XXX

0048T-0053T

CMS 100-4,3,90.2.1 Artificial Hearts and Related Devices

0048T Implantation of a ventricular assist device, extracorporeal, percutaneous transseptal access, single or dual cannulation C5 C 80

EXCLUDES *Transthoracic approach (33975-33976, 33979)*

0.00 0.00 Global Days XXX

0050T Removal of a ventricular assist device, extracorporeal, percutaneous transseptal access, single or dual cannulation C5 C 80

INCLUDES Removal of the entire device and the cannulas

EXCLUDES *Replacement of ventricular assist device, extracorporeal, via percutaneous transseptal access (33999)*

0.00 0.00 Global Days XXX

0051T Implantation of a total replacement heart system (artificial heart) with recipient cardiectomy C5 C 80

EXCLUDES *Ventricular assist device implant (33975-33976)*

0.00 0.00 Global Days XXX

0052T Replacement or repair of thoracic unit of a total replacement heart system (artificial heart) C5 C 80

EXCLUDES *Exchange or repair of other artificial heart components (0053T)*

0.00 0.00 Global Days XXX

0053T Replacement or repair of implantable component or components of total replacement heart system (artificial heart), excluding thoracic unit C5 C 80

EXCLUDES *Exchange or repair of thoracic unit of artificial heart (0052T)*

0.00 0.00 Global Days XXX

0054T-0055T

\+ 0054T Computer-assisted musculoskeletal surgical navigational orthopedic procedure, with image-guidance based on fluoroscopic images (List separately in addition to code for primary procedure) N 80

Code first primary procedure

0.00 0.00 Global Days XXX

AMA: 2009, Jan, 11-31; 2007, January, 13-27

\+ 0055T Computer-assisted musculoskeletal surgical navigational orthopedic procedure, with image-guidance based on CT/MRI images (List separately in addition to code for primary procedure) N 80

INCLUDES Performance of both CT and MRI in same session (1 unit)

Code first primary procedure

0.00 0.00 Global Days XXX

AMA: 2009, Jan, 11-31; 2007, January, 13-27

0058T-0059T

0058T Cryopreservation; reproductive tissue, ovarian X 80

89258-89259, 89335

0.00 0.00 Global Days XXX

0059T oocyte(s) X 80

89258-89259, 89335

0.00 0.00 Global Days XXX

0071T-0072T

Do not report with (51702, 77022)

0071T Focused ultrasound ablation of uterine leiomyomata, including MR guidance; total leiomyomata volume less than 200 cc of tissue ♀ S 80

0.00 0.00 Global Days XXX

0072T total leiomyomata volume greater or equal to 200 cc of tissue ♀ S 80

0.00 0.00 Global Days XXX

0073T

CMS 100-4,4,220.1 Billing for IMRT Planning and Delivery

0073T Compensator-based beam modulation treatment delivery of inverse planned treatment using 3 or more high resolution (milled or cast) compensator convergent beam modulated fields, per treatment session Z2 S TC 80

EXCLUDES *Radiotherapy treatment planning (77301)*

Do not report with other treatment delivery (77401-77416, 77418)

13.98 13.98 Global Days XXX

0075T-0076T

0075T Transcatheter placement of extracranial vertebral or intrathoracic carotid artery stent(s), including radiologic supervision and interpretation, percutaneous; initial vessel C5 C 80 PQ

INCLUDES All diagnostic services for stenting
Ipsilateral extracranial vertebral or intrathoracic selective carotid when confirming the need for stenting

EXCLUDES *Selective catheterization and imaging when stenting is not required (report only slective catheteriation codes)*

0.00 0.00 Global Days XXX

\+ 0076T each additional vessel (List separately in addition to code for primary procedure) C5 C 80

Code first (0075T)

0.00 0.00 Global Days XXX

0078T-0081T

0078T **Endovascular repair using prosthesis of abdominal aortic aneurysm, pseudoaneurysm or dissection, abdominal aorta involving visceral branches (superior mesenteric, celiac and/or renal artery[s])** C5 C 80

Code also when performed outside the endoprosthesis target zone (37205-37208, 37220-37223)

Do not report with (34800-34805, 35081, 35102, 35452, 35472)

0.00 0.00 Global Days XXX

+ 0079T **Placement of visceral extension prosthesis for endovascular repair of abdominal aortic aneurysm involving visceral vessels, each visceral branch (List separately in addition to code for primary procedure)** C5 C 80

Code first (0078T)

0.00 0.00 Global Days XXX

▲ 0080T **Endovascular repair using prosthesis of abdominal aortic aneurysm, pseudoaneurysm or dissection, abdominal aorta involving visceral vessels (superior mesenteric, celiac and/or renal artery[s]), radiological supervision and interpretation** C5 C 80 PQ

Code also when performed outside the target zone for the endoprosthesis (37205-37208, 37220-37223)

Do not report with (34800-34805, 35081, 35102, 35452, 35472)

0.00 0.00 Global Days XXX

+ 0081T **Placement of visceral extension prosthesis for endovascular repair of abdominal aortic aneurysm involving visceral vessels, each visceral branch, radiological supervision and interpretation (List separately in addition to code for primary procedure)** C5 C 80

Code first (0080T)

0.00 0.00 Global Days XXX

0085T

0085T **Breath test for heart transplant rejection** E

0.00 0.00 Global Days XXX

0092T-0098T

INCLUDES Fluoroscopy

Do not report with these procedures when performed at the same level (22851, 49010)

+ 0092T **Total disc arthroplasty (artificial disc), anterior approach, including discectomy with end plate preparation (includes osteophytectomy for nerve root or spinal cord decompression and microdissection), each additional interspace, cervical (List separately in addition to code for primary procedure)** C5 C 80

EXCLUDES *Lumbar arthroplasty (0163T)*

Code first 0090T (22856)

Do not report with total disc arthroplasty (22851)

0.00 0.00 Global Days XXX

+ 0095T **Removal of total disc arthroplasty (artificial disc), anterior approach, each additional interspace, cervical (List separately in addition to code for primary procedure)** C5 C 80

EXCLUDES *Lumbar disc (0164T)*
Total disc arthroplasty removal (22865)

Code first (22864)

0.00 0.00 Global Days XXX

+ 0098T **Revision including replacement of total disc arthroplasty (artificial disc), anterior approach, each additional interspace, cervical (List separately in addition to code for primary procedure)** C5 C 80

EXCLUDES *Spinal cord decompression (63001-63048)*

Code first (22861)

Do not report with (22861, 0095T)

Do not report with instrumentation at the same level (22851)

0.00 0.00 Global Days XXX

0099T-0159T

0099T **Implantation of intrastromal corneal ring segments** R2 T 80

0.00 0.00 Global Days XXX

0100T **Placement of a subconjunctival retinal prosthesis receiver and pulse generator, and implantation of intra-ocular retinal electrode array, with vitrectomy** G2 T 80

0.00 0.00 Global Days XXX

0101T **Extracorporeal shock wave involving musculoskeletal system, not otherwise specified, high energy** G2 T 80

EXCLUDES *Low energy extracorporeal shock wave (0019T)*

0.00 0.00 Global Days XXX

0102T **Extracorporeal shock wave, high energy, performed by a physician, requiring anesthesia other than local, involving lateral humeral epicondyle** G2 T 80

EXCLUDES *Low energy extracorporeal shock wave (0019T)*

0.00 0.00 Global Days XXX

0103T **Holotranscobalamin, quantitative** A 80

0.00 0.00 Global Days XXX

0106T **Quantitative sensory testing (QST), testing and interpretation per extremity; using touch pressure stimuli to assess large diameter sensation** X 80

0.00 0.00 Global Days XXX

0107T **using vibration stimuli to assess large diameter fiber sensation** X 80

0.00 0.00 Global Days XXX

0108T **using cooling stimuli to assess small nerve fiber sensation and hyperalgesia** X 80

0.00 0.00 Global Days XXX

0109T **using heat-pain stimuli to assess small nerve fiber sensation and hyperalgesia** X 80

0.00 0.00 Global Days XXX

0110T **using other stimuli to assess sensation** X 80

0.00 0.00 Global Days XXX

0111T **Long-chain (C20-22) omega-3 fatty acids in red blood cell (RBC) membranes** A 80

EXCLUDES *Very long chain fatty acids (82726)*

0.00 0.00 Global Days XXX

0123T **Fistulization of sclera for glaucoma, through ciliary body** G2 T 80

0.00 0.00 Global Days XXX

0124T **Conjunctival incision with posterior extrascleral placement of pharmacological agent (does not include supply of medication)** R2 T 80

EXCLUDES *Suprachoroidal delivery of medication (0186T)*

Code also medication

0.00 0.00 Global Days XXX

AMA: 2008, Jan, 6-7

0126T **Common carotid intima-media thickness (IMT) study for evaluation of atherosclerotic burden or coronary heart disease risk factor assessment** 01 80
0.00 0.00 Global Days XXX

0141T ~~Pancreatic islet cell transplantation through portal vein, percutaneous~~
To report, see 48160, 48999

0142T ~~Pancreatic islet cell transplantation through portal vein, open~~
To report, see 48160, 48999

0143T ~~Laparoscopy, surgical, pancreatic islet cell transplantation through portal vein~~
To report, see 48160, 48999

0155T ~~Laparoscopy, surgical; implantation or replacement of gastric stimulation electrodes, lesser curvature (ie, morbid obesity)~~
To report, see 43659

0156T ~~revision or removal of gastric stimulation electrodes, lesser curvature (ie, morbid obesity)~~
To report, see 43659

0157T ~~Laparotomy, implantation or replacement of gastric stimulation electrodes, lesser curvature (ie, morbid obesity)~~
To report, see 43999

0158T ~~Laparotomy, revision or removal of gastric stimulation electrodes, lesser curvature (ie, morbid obesity)~~
To report, see 43999

\+ 0159T **Computer-aided detection, including computer algorithm analysis of MRI image data for lesion detection/characterization, pharmacokinetic analysis, with further physician review for interpretation, breast MRI (List separately in addition to code for primary procedure)** N 80
Code first (77058-77059)
Do not report with (76376-76377)
76376-76377, 77058-77059
0.00 0.00 Global Days ZZZ
AMA: 2007, Jul, 6-10; 2007, March, 7-8

0163T-0165T

INCLUDES Fluoroscopy

EXCLUDES *Cervical disc procedures (22856)*
Decompression (63001-63048)

Do not report with these procedures when performed at the same level (22851, 49010)

\+ 0163T **Total disc arthroplasty (artificial disc), anterior approach, including discectomy to prepare interspace (other than for decompression), each additional interspace, lumbar (List separately in addition to code for primary procedure)** C5 C 80
Code first (22857)
0.00 0.00 Global Days YYY
AMA: 2007, June, 1-3

\+ 0164T **Removal of total disc arthroplasty, (artificial disc), anterior approach, each additional interspace, lumbar (List separately in addition to code for primary procedure)** C5 C 80
Code first (22865)
0.00 0.00 Global Days YYY
AMA: 2007, June, 1-3

\+ 0165T **Revision including replacement of total disc arthroplasty (artificial disc), anterior approach, each additional interspace, lumbar (List separately in addition to code for primary procedure)** C5 C 80
Code first (22862)
0.00 0.00 Global Days YYY
AMA: 2007, June, 1-3

0166T-0167T

EXCLUDES *Percutaneous ventricular septal defect repair (93581)*

Do not report with (32551, 33210-33211)

0166T ~~Transmyocardial transcatheter closure of ventricular septal defect, with implant; without cardiopulmonary bypass~~
To report, see 33999

0167T ~~with cardiopulmonary bypass~~
To report, see 33999

0168T-0175T

0168T ~~Rhinophototherapy, intranasal application of ultraviolet and visible light, bilateral~~
To report, see 30999

0169T **Stereotactic placement of infusion catheter(s) in the brain for delivery of therapeutic agent(s), including computerized stereotactic planning and burr hole(s)** C5 C 80
Do not report with (20660, 61107, 61781-61783)
0.00 0.00 Global Days XXX
AMA: 2009, Jan, 11-31; 2008, Jul, 4; 2008, May, 9-11; 2007, Jul, 6-10

0171T **Insertion of posterior spinous process distraction device (including necessary removal of bone or ligament for insertion and imaging guidance), lumbar; single level** T 80
0.00 0.00 Global Days XXX
AMA: 2007, Jul, 6-10

\+ 0172T **each additional level (List separately in addition to code for primary procedure)** T 80
Code first (0171T)
0.00 0.00 Global Days XXX
AMA: 2007, Jul, 6-10

\+ 0173T **Monitoring of intraocular pressure during vitrectomy surgery (List separately in addition to code for primary procedure)** N 80
Code first (67036, 67039-67043, 67108, 67112-67113)
0.00 0.00 Global Days XXX
AMA: 2008, Oct, 1-5; 2007, Jul, 6-10

\+ 0174T **Computer-aided detection (CAD) (computer algorithm analysis of digital image data for lesion detection) with further physician review for interpretation and report, with or without digitization of film radiographic images, chest radiograph(s), performed concurrent with primary interpretation (List separately in addition to code for primary procedure)** N1 N 80
Code first primary procedure
71010, 71020-71022, 71030
0.00 0.00 Global Days XXX
AMA: 2007, Jul, 6-10; 2007, March, 7-8

0175T **Computer-aided detection (CAD) (computer algorithm analysis of digital image data for lesion detection) with further physician review for interpretation and report, with or without digitization of film radiographic images, chest radiograph(s), performed remote from primary interpretation** N1 N 80

Do not report with (71010, 71020-71022, 71030)

0.00 0.00 Global Days XXX

AMA: 2007, Jul, 6-10; 2007, March, 7-8

0178T-0180T

EXCLUDES *Separately performed 12-lead electrocardiogram (93000-93010)*

0178T **Electrocardiogram, 64 leads or greater, with graphic presentation and analysis; with interpretation and report** B 80

0.00 0.00 Global Days XXX

0179T **tracing and graphics only, without interpretation and report** X TC 80

0.00 0.00 Global Days XXX

0180T **interpretation and report only** B 26 80

0.00 0.00 Global Days XXX

0181T-0186T

0181T **Corneal hysteresis determination, by air impulse stimulation, bilateral, with interpretation and report** S 80

0.00 0.00 Global Days XXX

0182T **High dose rate electronic brachytherapy, per fraction** Z2 S 80

EXCLUDES *Placement or removal of an applicator into breast for radiation therapy (C9726)*

Do not report with (77761-77763, 77776-77778, 77785-77787, 77789)

0.00 0.00 Global Days XXX

0183T **Low frequency, non-contact, non-thermal ultrasound, including topical application(s), when performed, wound assessment, and instruction(s) for ongoing care, per day** T 80

0.00 0.00 Global Days XXX

0184T **Excision of rectal tumor, transanal endoscopic microsurgical approach (ie, TEMS), including muscularis propria (ie, full thickness)** T 80

INCLUDES Operating microscope (66990)

EXCLUDES *Nonendoscopic excision of rectal tumor (45160, 45171-45172)*

Do not report with (45300-45327)

0.00 0.00 Global Days XXX

AMA: 2008, Jan, 6-7

0185T **Multivariate analysis of patient-specific findings with quantifiable computer probability assessment, including report** N1 N 80

Do not report with (99090)

0.00 0.00 Global Days XXX

AMA: 2008, Jan, 6-7

0186T **Suprachoroidal delivery of pharmacologic agent (does not include supply of medication)** G2 T 80

0.00 0.00 Global Days XXX

AMA: 2008, Jan, 6-7

0188T-0189T

INCLUDES 30 minutes or more of direct medical care by a physician(s) to a critically ill or critically injured patient from an off-site location.

Additional on-site critical care services when a critically ill or injured patient requires critical care resources not available on-site

Real time ability to:

- Document the remote care services in the medical record
- Enter orders electronically
- Evaluate patients with high fidelity audio/video capabilities
- Talk to patients and family members
- Videoconference with the health care team on-site in the patient's room

Real-time access to the patient's:

- Clinical laboratory test results
- Diagnostic test results
- Medical records
- Radiographic images

Review and/or interpretation of all diagnostic information

Time spent with the patient, family, or surrogate decision makers to obtain a medical history, review the patient's condition/prognosis, or discuss treatment options from the remote site

Do not report for time spent away from the remote site without real-time capabilities

Do not report time spent for services that do not directly contribute to patient treatment

0188T **Remote real-time interactive video-conferenced critical care, evaluation and management of the critically ill or critically injured patient; first 30-74 minutes** M

INCLUDES First 30 to 74 minutes of remote critical care each day

Do not report remote critical care less than 30 minutes total duration

0.00 0.00 Global Days XXX

AMA: 2009, Jan, 5&10; 2008, Jan, 6-7

+ **0189T** **each additional 30 minutes (List separately in addition to code for primary service)** M

INCLUDES Up to 30 minutes each beyond the first 74 minutes

Code first (0188T)

0.00 0.00 Global Days XXX

AMA: 2009, Jan, 5&10; 2008, Jan, 6-7

0190T-0192T [0253T]

+ **0190T** **Placement of intraocular radiation source applicator (List separately in addition to primary procedure)** G2 T 80

EXCLUDES *Insertion of brachytherapy source by radiation oncologist (see Clinical Brachytherapy Section)*

Code first (67036)

Code also brachytherapy source

0.00 0.00 Global Days XXX

AMA: 2008, Jan, 6-7

0191T **Insertion of anterior segment aqueous drainage device, without extraocular reservoir; internal approach, into the trabecular meshwork** G2 T 80

0.00 0.00 Global Days XXX

AMA: 2008, Jan, 6-7

0253T **internal approach, into the suprachoroidal space**

0.00 0.00 Global Days YYY

0192T **external approach** G2 T 80

0.00 0.00 Global Days XXX

AMA: 2008, Jan, 6-7

0195T-0196T

Do not report with (22558, 22845, 22851, 76000, 76380, 76496, 76497)

0195T Arthrodesis, pre-sacral interbody technique, including instrumentation, imaging (when performed), and discectomy to prepare interspace, lumbar; single interspace C5 C 80
0.00 0.00 Global Days XXX

\+ **0196T each additional interspace (List separately in addition to code for primary procedure)** C5 C 80
Code first (0195T)
0.00 0.00 Global Days XXX

0197T-0199T

0197T Intra-fraction localization and tracking of target or patient motion during delivery of radiation therapy (eg, 3D positional tracking, gating, 3D surface tracking), each fraction of treatment N 80
0.00 0.00 Global Days XXX

0198T Measurement of ocular blood flow by repetitive intraocular pressure sampling, with interpretation and report S 80
0.00 0.00 Global Days XXX

0199T Physiologic recording of tremor using accelerometer(s) and/or gyroscope(s) (including frequency and amplitude), including interpretation and report S 80
0.00 0.00 Global Days XXX

0200T-0201T

EXCLUDES *Bone biopsy (20220, 20225)*

⊙ **0200T Percutaneous sacral augmentation (sacroplasty), unilateral injection(s), including the use of a balloon or mechanical device, when used, 1 or more needles** G2 T 80 50
72291-72292
0.00 0.00 Global Days XXX

⊙ **0201T Percutaneous sacral augmentation (sacroplasty), bilateral injections, including the use of a balloon or mechanical device, when used, 2 or more needles** G2 T 80
72291-72292
0.00 0.00 Global Days XXX

0202T-0207T

0202T Posterior vertebral joint(s) arthroplasty (eg, facet joint[s] replacement), including facetectomy, laminectomy, foraminotomy, and vertebral column fixation, injection of bone cement, when performed, including fluoroscopy, single level, lumbar spine C5 C 80
Do not report the following codes when performed at the same level: (22521, 22524, 22840, 22851, 22857, 63005, 63012, 63017, 63030, 63042, 63047, 63056)
0.00 0.00 Global Days XXX

\+ **0205T Intravascular catheter-based coronary vessel or graft spectroscopy (eg, infrared) during diagnostic evaluation and/or therapeutic intervention including imaging supervision, interpretation, and report, each vessel (List separately in addition to code for primary procedure)** N 80
Code first (92980, 92982, 92995, 93452-93462, 93530-93533, 93563-93564)
0.00 0.00 Global Days ZZZ

0206T Algorithmic analysis, remote, of electrocardiographic-derived data with computer probability assessment, including report 01 TC 80
Code also 12-lead ECG when performed (93000-93010)
0.00 0.00 Global Days XXX

0207T Evacuation of meibomian glands, automated, using heat and intermittent pressure, unilateral S 80
0.00 0.00 Global Days XXX

0208T-0212T

EXCLUDES *Manual audiometric testing by a qualified health care professional, using audiometers (92551-92557)*

0208T Pure tone audiometry (threshold), automated; air only X TC 80
0.00 0.00 Global Days XXX

0209T air and bone X TC 80
0.00 0.00 Global Days XXX

0210T Speech audiometry threshold, automated; X TC 80
0.00 0.00 Global Days XXX

0211T with speech recognition X TC 80
0.00 0.00 Global Days XXX

0212T Comprehensive audiometry threshold evaluation and speech recognition (0209T, 0211T combined), automated X TC 80
0.00 0.00 Global Days XXX

0213T-0215T

0213T Injection(s), diagnostic or therapeutic agent, paravertebral facet (zygapophyseal) joint (or nerves innervating that joint) with ultrasound guidance, cervical or thoracic; single level R2 T 80 50
0.00 0.00 Global Days XXX

\+ **0214T second level (List separately in addition to code for primary procedure)** R2 T 80 50
Code first (0213T)
0.00 0.00 Global Days ZZZ

\+ **0215T third and any additional level(s) (List separately in addition to code for primary procedure)** R2 T 80 50
Code first (0213T)
Do not report more than once per day.
0.00 0.00 Global Days ZZZ

0216T-0218T

EXCLUDES *Injection with CT or fluoroscopic guidance (64490-64495)*

0216T Injection(s), diagnostic or therapeutic agent, paravertebral facet (zygapophyseal) joint (or nerves innervating that joint) with ultrasound guidance, lumbar or sacral; single level R2 T 80 50
0.00 0.00 Global Days XXX

\+ **0217T second level (List separately in addition to code for primary procedure)** R2 T 80 50
Code first (0216T)
0.00 0.00 Global Days ZZZ

\+ **0218T third and any additional level(s) (List separately in addition to code for primary procedure)** R2 T 80 50
Do not report more than once a day
Code first (0216T)
0.00 0.00 Global Days ZZZ

0219T-0222T

Do not report when performed at the same level (20930-20931, 22600-22614, 22840, 22851)

Do not report with any x-ray service

0219T **Placement of a posterior intrafacet implant(s), unilateral or bilateral, including imaging and placement of bone graft(s) or synthetic device(s), single level; cervical** C5 C 80
0.00 0.00 Global Days XXX

0220T **thoracic** C5 C 80
0.00 0.00 Global Days XXX

0221T **lumbar** T 80
0.00 0.00 Global Days XXX

+ **0222T** **each additional vertebral segment (List separately in addition to code for primary procedure)** T 80
EXCLUDES *Posterior or posterolateral arthrodesis procedure (22600-22614)*
Code first (0219T-0221T)
0.00 0.00 Global Days ZZZ

0223T-0225T

INCLUDES Assessment of data including heart sounds and limited reprogramming to ensure the best hemodynamics (heart rate parameter and/or automated timing modes, including precise changes of AV/VV intervals)
Evaluation of systolic and diastolic
Rhythm strip ECG (93040-93042)

EXCLUDES *Complete programming services as separate procedure (93280-93284)*

0223T **Acoustic cardiography, including automated analysis of combined acoustic and electrical intervals; single, with interpretation and report** S 80
0.00 0.00 Global Days XXX

0224T **multiple, including serial trended analysis and limited reprogramming of device parameter, AV or VV delays only, with interpretation and report** S 80
INCLUDES Retrieving and limited reprogramming cardiac pacemaker including AV/VV intervals
EXCLUDES *Complete programming (93280-93284)*
Do not report with (93288-93289)
0.00 0.00 Global Days XXX

0225T **multiple, including serial trended analysis and limited reprogramming of device parameter, AV and VV delays, with interpretation and report** S 80
INCLUDES Retrieving and limited reprogramming cardiac pacemaker including AV/VV intervals
EXCLUDES *Complete programming (93280-93284)*
Do not report with (93288-93299)
0.00 0.00 Global Days XXX

0226T-0233T

0226T **Anoscopy, high resolution (HRA) (with magnification and chemical agent enhancement); diagnostic, including collection of specimen(s) by brushing or washing when performed** R2 X
INCLUDES Operating microscope (69990)
0.00 0.00 Global Days XXX

0227T **with biopsy(ies)** R2 T
INCLUDES Operating microscope (69990)
0.00 0.00 Global Days XXX

0228T **Injection(s), anesthetic agent and/or steroid, transforaminal epidural, with ultrasound guidance, cervical or thoracic; single level** G2 T 50
0.00 0.00 Global Days XXX

+ **0229T** **each additional level (List separately in addition to code for primary procedure)** G2 T 50
Code first (0228T)
0.00 0.00 Global Days XXX

0230T **Injection(s), anesthetic agent and/or steroid, transforaminal epidural, with ultrasound guidance, lumbar or sacral; single level** G2 T 50
0.00 0.00 Global Days XXX

+ **0231T** **each additional level (List separately in addition to code for primary procedure)** G2 T 50
EXCLUDES *Injection performed with CT or fluoroscopic guidance (64479-64484)*
Code first (0230T)
Do not report with (76942, 76998-76999)
0.00 0.00 Global Days XXX

0232T **Injection(s), platelet rich plasma, any site, including image guidance, harvesting and preparation when performed** R2 X
Do not report with (20550-20551, 20600-20610, 20926, 76942, 77002, 77012, 77021, 86965)
0.00 0.00 Global Days XXX

0233T **Skin advanced glycation endproducts (AGE) measurement by multi-wavelength fluorescent spectroscopy** A 80
0.00 0.00 Global Days XXX

0234T-0238T

INCLUDES Atherectomy by any technique in arteries above the inguinal ligaments

EXCLUDES *Accessing and catheterization of the vessel*
Atherectomy performed below the inguinal ligaments (37225, 37227, 37229, 37231, 37233, 37235)
Closure of the arteriotomy by any technique
Negotiating the lesion
Other interventions to the same or different vessels
Protection from embolism

0234T **Transluminal peripheral atherectomy, open or percutaneous, including radiological supervision and interpretation; renal artery** T 80
0.00 0.00 Global Days YYY

0235T **visceral artery (except renal), each vessel** C5 C 80
0.00 0.00 Global Days YYY

0236T **abdominal aorta** T 80
0.00 0.00 Global Days YYY

0237T **brachiocephalic trunk and branches, each vessel** T 80
0.00 0.00 Global Days YYY

0238T **iliac artery, each vessel** G2 T 80
0.00 0.00 Global Days YYY

0239T-0242T

0239T **Bioimpedance spectroscopy (BIS), measuring 100 frequencies or greater, direct measurement of extracellular fluid differences between the limbs** S 80
0.00 0.00 Global Days YYY

▲ 0240T **Esophageal motility (manometric study of the esophagus and/or gastroesophageal junction) study with interpretation and report; with high resolution esophageal pressure topography** X 80

Do not report with (91010, 91013)

0.00 0.00 Global Days YYY

+ ▲ 0241T **with stimulation or perfusion during high resolution esophageal pressure topography study (eg, stimulant, acid or alkali perfusion) (List separately in addition to code for primary procedure)** X 80

2-dimensional studies without high resolution with or without perfusion or stimulant (91010, 91013)

Code first (0240T)

Do not report more than one time each session

Do not report with (91010, 91013)

0.00 0.00 Global Days YYY

0242T **Gastrointestinal tract transit and pressure measurement, stomach through colon, wireless capsule, with interpretation and report** X 80

Do not report with (91020, 91022)

0.00 0.00 Global Days YYY

0243T-0244T

0243T **Intermittent measurement of wheeze rate for bronchodilator or bronchial-challenge diagnostic evaluation(s), with interpretation and report** S 80

Do not report intermittent measurement of wheeze rate evaluation in the same 24-hour period (0224T)

Do not report more than once in 24 hours

0.00 0.00 Global Days YYY

0244T **Continuous measurement of wheeze rate during treatment assessment or during sleep for documentation of nocturnal wheeze and cough for diagnostic evaluation 3 to 24 hours, with interpretation and report** X 80

0.00 0.00 Global Days YYY

0245T-0248T

0245T **Open treatment of rib fracture requiring internal fixation, unilateral; 1-2 ribs** T 80 50

0.00 0.00 Global Days YYY

0246T **3-4 ribs** T 80 50

0.00 0.00 Global Days YYY

0247T **5-6 ribs** T 80 50

0.00 0.00 Global Days YYY

0248T **7 or more ribs** T 80 50

0.00 0.00 Global Days YYY

0249T-0255T

0249T **Ligation, hemorrhoidal vascular bundle(s), including ultrasound guidance** G2 T 80

Do not report with (46020, 46221, [46945, 46946], 46250-46262, 46600, 76872, 76942, 76998)

0.00 0.00 Global Days YYY

+ ⊙ 0250T **Airway sizing and insertion of bronchial valve(s), each lobe (List separately in addition to code for primary procedure)** G2 T 80

Code first (31622, 31634)

0.00 0.00 Global Days YYY

⊙ 0251T **Bronchoscopy, rigid or flexible, including fluoroscopic guidance, when performed; with removal of bronchial valve(s), initial lobe** G2 T 80

Do not report with (31622-31626, 31628-31631, 31634-31636, 31638-31646)

0.00 0.00 Global Days YYY

+ ⊙ 0252T **with removal of bronchial valve(s), each additional lobe (List separately in addition to code for primary procedure)** G2 T 80

Code first (0251T)

0.00 0.00 Global Days YYY

0253T Resequenced code, See code following 0191T.

0254T **Endovascular repair of iliac artery bifurcation (eg, aneurysm, pseudoaneurysm, arteriovenous malformation, trauma) using bifurcated endoprosthesis from the common iliac artery into both the external and internal iliac artery, unilateral;** C5 C 80

0255T

0.00 0.00 Global Days YYY

0255T **radiological supervision and interpretation** C5 C 80

0.00 0.00 Global Days YYY

0256T-0259T

0256T **Implantation of catheter-delivered prosthetic aortic heart valve; endovascular approach** C5 C 80

INCLUDES Catheterization
Contrast injection
Radiologic guidance
Temporary pacing

EXCLUDES *Cardiac catheterization when performed at the same session for diagnostic purpose before aortic valve placement (93451-93572)*

Do not report with (33210-33211, 92986, 93503)

0.00 0.00 Global Days YYY

0257T **open thoracic approach (eg, transapical, transventricular)** C5 C 80

INCLUDES Catheterization
Contrast injection
Radiologic guidance
Temporary pacing

EXCLUDES *Cardiac catheterization when performed at the same session for diagnostic purpose before aortic valve placement (93451-93572)*
Transthoracic cardiac exposure (0258T-0259T)

Do not report with (33210-33211, 92986, 93503)

0.00 0.00 Global Days YYY

0258T **Transthoracic cardiac exposure (eg, sternotomy, thoracotomy, subxiphoid) for catheter-delivered aortic valve replacement; without cardiopulmonary bypass** C5 C 80

EXCLUDES *Implantation of catheter-delivered prosthetic aortic heart valve (0257T)*

Code also one aortic valve placement procedure per session

Do not report with (32100, 32551, 33210-33211, 33310, 33315, 33400-33413, 39010)

0.00 0.00 Global Days YYY

0259T **with cardiopulmonary bypass**

EXCLUDES *Implantation of catheter-delivered prosthetic aortic heart valve (0257T)*

Code also one aortic valve placement procedure per session

Do not report with (32100, 32551, 33210-33211, 33310, 33315, 33400-33413, 39010)

0.00 0.00 Global Days YYY

0260T-0261T

0260T **Total body systemic hypothermia, per day, in the neonate 28 days of age or younger**

0.00 0.00 Global Days YYY

▲ 0261T **Selective head hypothermia, per day, in the neonate 28 days of age or younger**

0.00 0.00 Global Days YYY

0262T

INCLUDES All congenital catheterization(s)
Contrast injections during procedure
Fluoroscopic radiological supervision and interpretation
Imaging guidance for for pulmonary valve procedure
Percutaneous balloon angioplasty/valvuloplasty of pulmonary valve/conduit
Stent deployment in pulmonary conduit

Code also cardiovascular stent placement performed at site separate from delivery site of the prosthetic valve (37205-37206, 75960, 92980-92981)

Code also pulmonary artery angioplasty performed at site separate from delivery site of the prosthetic valve (92997-92998)

Do not report with (76000-76001, 92990, 93530, 93563, 93566-93568)

Do not report stent placement within the pulmonary conduit separately (37205-37206, 75960, 92980-92981)

● 0262T **Implantation of catheter-delivered prosthetic pulmonary valve, endovascular approach**

0.00 0.00 Global Days YYY

0263T-0265T

● 0263T **Intramuscular autologous bone marrow cell therapy, with preparation of harvested cells, multiple injections, 1 leg, including ultrasound guidance, if performed; complete procedure including unilateral or bilateral bone marrow harvest**

Do not report with (38204-38242, 76942, 93925-93926)

0.00 0.00 Global Days XXX

● 0264T **complete procedure excluding bone marrow harvest**

Do not report with (38204-38242, 76942, 93925-93926, 0265T)

0.00 0.00 Global Days XXX

● 0265T **unilateral or bilateral bone marrow harvest only for intramuscular autologous bone marrow cell therapy**

EXCLUDES *Complete procedure (0263T)*

Do not report with (38204-38242, 0264T)

0.00 0.00 Global Days XXX

0266T-0273T

● 0266T **Implantation or replacement of carotid sinus baroreflex activation device; total system (includes generator placement, unilateral or bilateral lead placement, intra-operative interrogation, programming, and repositioning, when performed)**

0.00 0.00 Global Days YYY

● 0267T **lead only, unilateral (includes intra-operative interrogation, programming, and repositioning, when performed)**

Do not report with (0266T, 0269T-0273T)

0.00 0.00 Global Days YYY

● 0268T **pulse generator only (includes intra-operative interrogation, programming, and repositioning, when performed)**

Code also C1767, C1820, L8685-L8688 (C1767, C1820, L8685-L8688)

Do not report with (0266T, 0269T-0273T)

0.00 0.00 Global Days YYY

● 0269T **Revision or removal of carotid sinus baroreflex activation device; total system (includes generator placement, unilateral or bilateral lead placement, intra-operative interrogation, programming, and repositioning, when performed)**

Do not report with (0266T-0268T, 0270T-0273T)

0.00 0.00 Global Days XXX

● 0270T **lead only, unilateral (includes intra-operative interrogation, programming, and repositioning, when performed)**

EXCLUDES *Removal of total carotid sinus baroreflex activation device (0269T)*

Do not report with (0266T-0269T, 0271T-0273T)

0.00 0.00 Global Days XXX

● 0271T **pulse generator only (includes intra-operative interrogation, programming, and repositioning, when performed)**

EXCLUDES *Removal and replacement (0266T-0268T)*

Do not report with (0266T-0270T, 0272T-0273T)

0.00 0.00 Global Days XXX

● 0272T **Interrogation device evaluation (in person), carotid sinus baroreflex activation system, including telemetric iterative communication with the implantable device to monitor device diagnostics and programmed therapy values, with interpretation and report (eg, battery status, lead impedance, pulse amplitude, pulse width, therapy frequency, pathway mode, burst mode, therapy start/stop times each day);**

Do not report with (0266T-0271T, 0273T)

0.00 0.00 Global Days XXX

● 0273T **with programming**

Do not report with (0266T-0272T)

0.00 0.00 Global Days XXX

0274T-0275T

EXCLUDES *Laminotomy/hemilaminectomy by open and endoscopically assisted approach (63020-63035)*
Percutaneous decompression of nucleus pulposus of intervertebral disc by needle-based technique (62287)

● **0274T Percutaneous laminotomy/laminectomy (intralaminar approach) for decompression of neural elements, (with or without ligamentous resection, discectomy, facetectomy and/or foraminotomy) any method under indirect image guidance (eg, fluoroscopic, CT), with or without the use of an endoscope, single or multiple levels, unilateral or bilateral; cervical or thoracic** T 80
0.00 0.00 Global Days YYY

● **0275T lumbar** T 80
EXCLUDES *Laminotomy/hemilaminectomy by open and endoscopically assisted approach (63020-63035)*
Percutaneous decompression of nucleus pulposus of intervertebral disc by needle-based technique (62287)
0.00 0.00 Global Days YYY

0276T-0277T

⊙ ● **0276T Bronchoscopy, rigid or flexible, including fluoroscopic guidance, when performed; with bronchial thermoplasty, 1 lobe** T 80
0.00 0.00 Global Days XXX

⊙ ● **0277T with bronchial thermoplasty, 2 or more lobes** T 80
0.00 0.00 Global Days XXX

0278T-0281T

● **0278T Transcutaneous electrical modulation pain reprocessing (eg, scrambler therapy), each treatment session (includes placement of electrodes)** S 80
0.00 0.00 Global Days XXX

● **0279T Cell enumeration using immunologic selection and identification in fluid specimen (eg, circulating tumor cells in blood);** X 80
0.00 0.00 Global Days XXX

● **0280T interpretation and report** X 80
EXCLUDES *Flow cytometric immunophenotyping (88184-88189)*
Flow cytometric quantitation (86355-86357, 86359-86361, 86367)

Code also (0279T)
0.00 0.00 Global Days XXX

● **0281T Percutaneous transcatheter closure of the left atrial appendage with implant, including fluoroscopy, transseptal puncture, catheter placement(s), left atrial angiography, left atrial appendage angiography, radiological supervision and interpretation** C5 C 80

Code also for right heart catheterization separately for reasons distinct from left atrial appendage closure (93451-93461, 93530-93533)

Code also for separately performed ventriculography with transseptal approach for reasons separate from the left atrial appendage closure. (93565)

Do not report with (93462)

Do not report with the following codes unless the catheterization of the left ventricle is done by a nontransseptal approach for reasons other than the left atrial appendage repair (93452-93453, 93458-93461, 93531-93533)

Do not report with the following codes unless the complete right heart catheterization is done for reasons other than the left atrial appendage repair (93451, 93453, 93456, 93460-93461, 93530-93533)
0.00 0.00 Global Days XXX

0282T-0285T

Do not report with (64550-64595, 77002-77003, 95970-95973)

⊙ ● **0282T Percutaneous or open implantation of neurostimulator electrode array(s), subcutaneous (peripheral subcutaneous field stimulation), including imaging guidance, when performed, cervical, thoracic or lumbar; for trial, including removal at the conclusion of trial period** J8 S 80 50

Do not report with (64550-64595, 77002, 77003, 95970-95973)
0.00 0.00 Global Days XXX

⊙ ● **0283T permanent, with implantation of a pulse generator** J8 S 80 50

Do not report with (64550-64595, 77002, 77003, 95970-95973)
0.00 0.00 Global Days XXX

⊙ ● **0284T Revision or removal of pulse generator or electrodes, including imaging guidance, when performed, including addition of new electrodes, when performed** G2 T 80

Do not report with (64550-64595, 77002, 77003, 95970-95973)
0.00 0.00 Global Days XXX

● **0285T Electronic analysis of implanted peripheral subcutaneous field stimulation pulse generator, with reprogramming when performed** S 80
0.00 0.00 Global Days XXX

0286T-0287T

● **0286T Near-infrared spectroscopy studies of lower extremity wounds (eg, for oxyhemoglobin measurement)** N1 N 80
0.00 0.00 Global Days XXX

● **0287T Near-infrared guidance for vascular access requiring real-time digital visualization of subcutaneous vasculature for evaluation of potential access sites and vessel patency** N1 N 80
0.00 0.00 Global Days XXX

0288T

Do not report with (46600-46615)

● 0288T **Anoscopy, with delivery of thermal energy to the muscle of the anal canal (eg, for fecal incontinence)**

Do not report with (46600-46615)

0.00 0.00 Global Days XXX

0289T-0290T

+ ● 0289T **Corneal incisions in the donor cornea created using a laser, in preparation for penetrating or lamellar keratoplasty (List separately in addition to code for primary procedure)**

Code first (65710, 65730, 65750, 65755)

0.00 0.00 Global Days ZZZ

+ ● 0290T **Corneal incisions in the recipient cornea created using a laser, in preparation for penetrating or lamellar keratoplasty (List separately in addition to code for primary procedure)**

Code first (65710, 65730, 65750, 65755)

0.00 0.00 Global Days ZZZ

0291T-0292T

INCLUDES All manipulations and repositioning inside evaluated vessel including prior to and after the intervention

EXCLUDES *Intravascular spectroscopy (0205T)*

+ ⊙ ● 0291T **Intravascular optical coherence tomography (coronary native vessel or graft) during diagnostic evaluation and/or therapeutic intervention, including imaging supervision, interpretation, and report; initial vessel (List separately in addition to primary procedure)**

Code first cardiac catheterization (92975, 92980, 92982, 92995, 93454-93461, 93530-93533)

0.00 0.00 Global Days ZZZ

+ ⊙ ● 0292T **each additional vessel (List separately in addition to primary procedure)**

Code first cardiac catheterization (92975, 92980, 92982, 92995, 93530-93533)

0.00 0.00 Global Days ZZZ

0293T-0294T

Do not report with (93462, 93662)

Do not report with heart catheterization unless performed for separate clinical reason other than calibration or placement of left atrial hemodynamic monitoring system (93451-93453)

⊙ ● 0293T **Insertion of left atrial hemodynamic monitor; complete system, includes implanted communication module and pressure sensor lead in left atrium including transseptal access, radiological supervision and interpretation, and associated injection procedures, when performed**

0.00 0.00 Global Days XXX

+ ⊙ ● 0294T **pressure sensor lead at time of insertion of pacing cardioverter-defibrillator pulse generator including radiological supervision and interpretation and associated injection procedures, when performed (List separately in addition to code for primary procedure)**

Code first primary procedure

Do not report unless done for separate clinical reason other than placement or calibration of left atrial hemodynamic monitoring system (93451-93453)

Do not report with (93462, 93662)

0.00 0.00 Global Days ZZZ

0295T-0298T

Do not report with (93224-93272)

● 0295T **External electrocardiographic recording for more than 48 hours up to 21 days by continuous rhythm recording and storage; includes recording, scanning analysis with report, review and interpretation**

0.00 0.00 Global Days XXX

● 0296T **recording (includes connection and initial recording)**

0.00 0.00 Global Days XXX

● 0297T **scanning analysis with report**

0.00 0.00 Global Days XXX

● 0298T **review and interpretation**

0.00 0.00 Global Days XXX

0299T-0301T

● 0299T **Extracorporeal shock wave for integumentary wound healing, high energy, including topical application and dressing care; initial wound**

Code also (0300T)

0.00 0.00 Global Days XXX

+ ● 0300T **each additional wound (List separately in addition to code for primary procedure)**

Code first (0299T)

Do not report with (28890, 0101T-0102T)

0.00 0.00 Global Days ZZZ

⊙ ● 0301T **Destruction/reduction of malignant breast tumor with externally applied focused microwave, including interstitial placement of disposable catheter with combined temperature monitoring probe and microwave focusing sensocatheter under ultrasound thermotherapy guidance**

Do not report with (76645, 76942, 76998, 77600-77615)

0.00 0.00 Global Days XXX

APPENDIX A — MODIFIERS

CPT Modifiers

A modifier is a two-position alpha or numeric code appended to a CPT code to clarify the services being billed. Modifiers provide a means by which a service can be altered without changing the procedure code. They add more information, such as the anatomical site, to the code. In addition, they help to eliminate the appearance of duplicate billing and unbundling. Modifiers are used to increase accuracy in reimbursement, coding consistency, editing, and to capture payment data.

22 **Increased Procedural Services:** When the work required to provide a service is substantially greater than typically required, it may be identified by adding modifier 22 to the usual procedure code. Documentation must support the substantial additional work and the reason for the additional work (ie, increased intensity, time, technical difficulty of procedure, severity of patient's condition, physical and mental effort required).

Note: This modifier should not be appended to an E/M service.

23 **Unusual Anesthesia:** Occasionally, a procedure, which usually requires either no anesthesia or local anesthesia, because of unusual circumstances must be done under general anesthesia. This circumstance may be reported by adding modifier 23 to the procedure code of the basic service.

24 **Unrelated Evaluation and Management Service by the Same Physician During a Postoperative Period:** The physician may need to indicate that an evaluation and management service was performed during a postoperative period for a reason(s) unrelated to the original procedure. This circumstance may be reported by adding modifier 24 to the appropriate level of E/M service.

25 **Significant, Separately Identifiable Evaluation and Management Service by the Same Physician on the Same Day of the Procedure or Other Service:** It may be necessary to indicate that on the day a procedure or service identified by a CPT code was performed, the patient's condition required a significant, separately identifiable E/M service above and beyond the other service provided or beyond the usual preoperative and postoperative care associated with the procedure that was performed. A significant, separately identifiable E/M service is defined or substantiated by documentation that satisfies the relevant criteria for the respective E/M service to be reported (see Evaluation and Management Services Guidelines for instructions on determining level of E/M service). The E/M service may be prompted by the symptom or condition for which the procedure and/or service was provided. As such, different diagnoses are not required for reporting of the E/M services on the same date. This circumstance may be reported by adding modifier 25 to the appropriate level of E/M service.
Note: This modifier is not used to report an E/M service that resulted in a decision to perform surgery. See modifier 57. For significant, separately identifiable non-E/M services, see modifier 59.

26 **Professional Component:** Certain procedures are a combination of a physician component and a technical component. When the physician component is reported separately, the service may be identified by adding modifier 26 to the usual procedure number.

32 **Mandated Services:** Services related to mandated consultation and/or related services (eg, third-party payer, governmental, legislative or regulatory requirement) may be identified by adding modifier 32 to the basic procedure.

33 **Preventive Services:** When the primary purpose of the service is the delivery of an evidence-based service in accordance with a U.S. Preventive Services Task Force A or B rating in effect and other preventive services identified in preventive services mandates (legislative or regulatory), the service may be identified by adding 33 to the procedure. For separately reported services specifically identified as preventive, the modifier should not be used.

47 **Anesthesia by Surgeon:** Regional or general anesthesia provided by the surgeon may be reported by adding modifier 47 to the basic service. (This does not include local anesthesia.)
Note: Modifier 47 would not be used as a modifier for the anesthesia procedures 00100-01999.

50 **Bilateral Procedure:** Unless otherwise identified in the listings, bilateral procedures that are performed at the same session should be identified by adding modifier 50 to the appropriate 5-digit code.

51 **Multiple Procedures:** When multiple procedures, other than Evaluation and Management Services, are performed at the same session by the same provider, the primary procedure or service may be reported as listed. The additional procedure(s) or service(s) may be identified by appending modifier 51 to the additional procedure or service code(s).
Note: This modifier should not be appended to designated "add-on" codes.

52 **Reduced Services:** Under certain circumstances a service or procedure is partially reduced or eliminated at the physician's discretion. Under these circumstances the service provided can be identified by its usual procedure number and the addition of modifier 52, signifying that the service is reduced. This provides a means of reporting reduced services without disturbing the identification of the basic service.
Note: For hospital outpatient reporting of a previously scheduled procedure/service that is partially reduced or cancelled as a result of extenuating circumstances or those that threaten the well-being of the patient prior to or after administration of anesthesia, see modifiers 73 and 74 (see modifiers approved for ASC hospital outpatient use).

53 **Discontinued Procedure:** Under certain circumstances, the physician may elect to terminate a surgical or diagnostic procedure. Due to extenuating circumstances or those that threaten the well being of the patient, it may be necessary to indicate that a surgical or diagnostic procedure was started but discontinued. This circumstance may be reported by adding modifier 53 to the code reported by the physician for the discontinued procedure.
Note: This modifier is not used to report the elective cancellation of a procedure prior to the patient's anesthesia induction and/or surgical preparation in the operating suite. For outpatient hospital/ambulatory surgery center (ASC) reporting of a previously scheduled procedure/service that is partially reduced or cancelled as a result of extenuating circumstances or those that threaten the well being of the patient prior to or after administration of anesthesia, see modifiers 73 and 74 (see modifiers approved for ASC hospital outpatient use).

54 **Surgical Care Only:** When 1 physician performs a surgical procedure and another provides preoperative and/or postoperative management, surgical services may be identified by adding modifier 54 to the usual procedure number.

55 **Postoperative Management Only:** When 1 physician performs the postoperative management and another physician has performed the surgical procedure, the postoperative component may be identified by adding modifier 55 to the usual procedure number.

56 **Preoperative Management Only:** When 1 physician performs the preoperative care and evaluation and another physician performs the surgical procedure, the preoperative component may be identified by adding modifier 56 to the usual procedure number.

57 **Decision for Surgery:** An evaluation and management service that resulted in the initial decision to perform the surgery may be identified by adding modifier 57 to the appropriate level of E/M service.

58 **Staged or Related Procedure or Service by the Same Physician During the Postoperative Period:** It may be necessary to indicate that the performance of a procedure or service during the postoperative period was (a) planned or anticipated (staged); (b) more extensive than the original procedure; or (c) for therapy following a surgical procedure. This circumstance may be reported by adding modifier 58 to the staged or related procedure.
Note: For treatment of a problem that requires a return to the operating or procedure room (eg, unanticipated clinical condition), see modifier 78.

59 **Distinct Procedural Service:** Under certain circumstances, it may be necessary to indicate that a procedure or service was distinct or independent from other non-E/M services performed on the same day. Modifier 59 is used to identify procedures or services, other than E/M services, that are not normally reported together but are appropriate under the circumstances. Documentation must support a different session, different procedure or surgery, different site or organ system, separate incision or excision, separate lesion, or separate injury (or area of injury in extensive injuries) not ordinarily encountered or performed on the same day by the same individual. However, when another already established modifier is appropriate it should be used rather than modifier 59. Only if no more descriptive modifier is available and the use of modifier 59 best explains the circumstances should modifier 59 be used.

Note: Modifier 59 should not be appended to an E/M service. To report a separate and distinct E/M service with a non-E/M service performed on the same date, see modifier 25.

62 **Two Surgeons:** When 2 surgeons work together as primary surgeons performing distinct part(s) of a procedure, each surgeon should report his/her distinct operative work by adding modifier 62 to the procedure code and any associated add-on code(s) for that procedure as long as both surgeons continue to work together as primary surgeons. Each surgeon should report the co-surgery once using the same procedure code. If an additional procedure(s) (including an add-on procedure(s)) is performed during the same surgical session, a separate code(s) may be reported with the modifier 62 added.

Note: If a co-surgeon acts as an assistant in the performance of an additional procedure(s) during the same surgical session, the service(s) may be reported using a separate procedure code(s) with modifier 80 or modifier 82 added, as appropriate.

63 **Procedure Performed on Infants less than 4 kg:** Procedures performed on neonates and infants up to a present body weight of 4 kg may involve significantly increased complexity and physician work commonly associated with these patients. This circumstance may be reported by adding the modifier 63 to the procedure number.

Note: Unless otherwise designated, this modifier may only be appended to procedures/services listed in the 20000-69999 code series. Modifier 63 should not be appended to any CPT codes in the **Evaluation and Management Services, Anesthesia, Radiology, Pathology/Laboratory or Medicine** sections.

66 **Surgical Team:** Under some circumstances, highly complex procedures (requiring the concomitant services of several physicians, often of different specialties, plus other highly skilled, specially trained personnel, various types of complex equipment) are carried out under the "surgical team" concept. Such circumstances may be identified by each participating physician with the addition of modifier 66 to the basic procedure number used for reporting services.

76 **Repeat Procedure or Service by Same Physician or Other Qualified Health Care Professional:** It may be necessary to indicate that a procedure or service was repeated by the same physician or other qualified health care professional subsequent to the original procedure or service. This circumstance may be reported by adding modifier 76 to the repeated procedure or service.
Note: This modifier should not be appended to an E/M service.

77 **Repeat Procedure or Service by Another Physician or Other Qualified Health Care Professional:** It may be necessary to indicate that a basic procedure or service was repeated by another physician or other qualified health care professional subsequent to the original procedure or service. This circumstance may be reported by adding modifier 77 to the repeated procedure or service.
Note: This modifier should not be appended to an E/M service.

78 **Unplanned Return to the Operating/Procedure Room by the Same Physician or Other Qualified Health Care Professional Following Initial Procedure for a Related Procedure During the Postoperative Period:** It may be necessary to indicate that another procedure was performed during the postoperative period of the initial procedure (unplanned procedure following initial procedure). When this procedure is related to the first and requires the use of an operating/procedure room, it may be reported by adding modifier 78 to the related procedure. (For repeat procedures, see modifier 76.)

79 **Unrelated Procedure or Service by the Same Physician During the Postoperative Period:** The physician may need to indicate that the performance of a procedure or service during the postoperative period was unrelated to the original procedure. This circumstance may be reported by using modifier 79. (For repeat procedures on the same day, see modifier 76.)

80 **Assistant Surgeon:** Surgical assistant services may be identified by adding modifier 80 to the usual procedure number(s).

81 **Minimum Assistant Surgeon:** Minimum surgical assistant services are identified by adding modifier 81 to the usual procedure number.

82 **Assistant Surgeon (when qualified resident surgeon not available):** The unavailability of a qualified resident surgeon is a prerequisite for use of modifier 82 appended to the usual procedure code number(s).

90 **Reference (Outside) Laboratory:** When laboratory procedures are performed by a party other than the treating or reporting physician, the procedure may be identified by adding modifier 90 to the usual procedure number.

91 **Repeat Clinical Diagnostic Laboratory Test:** In the course of treatment of the patient, it may be necessary to repeat the same laboratory test on the same day to obtain subsequent (multiple) test results. Under these circumstances, the laboratory test performed can be identified by its usual procedure number and the addition of modifier 91.

Note: This modifier may not be used when tests are rerun to confirm initial results; due to testing problems with specimens or equipment; or for any other reason when a normal, one-time, reportable result is all that is required. This modifier may not be used when another code(s) describes a series of test results (eg, glucose tolerance tests, evocative/suppression testing). This modifier may only be used for a laboratory test(s) performed more than once on the same day on the same patient.

92 **Alternative Laboratory Platform Testing** When laboratory testing is being performed using a kit or transportable instrument that wholly or in part consists of a single use, disposable analytical chamber, the service may be identified by adding modifier 92 to the usual laboratory procedure code (HIV testing 86701-86703, and 87389). The test does not require permanent dedicated space, hence by its design may be hand carried or transported to the vicinity of the patient for immediate testing at that site, although location of the testing is not in itself determinative of the use of this modifier.

99 **Multiple Modifiers:** Under certain circumstances 2 or more modifiers may be necessary to completely delineate a service. In such situations, modifier 99 should be added to the basic procedure and other applicable modifiers may be listed as part of the description of the service.

Anesthesia Physical Status Modifiers

All anesthesia services are reported by use of the five-digit anesthesia procedure code with the appropriate physical status modifier appended.

Under certain circumstances, when other modifier(s) are appropriate, they should be reported in addition to the physical status modifier.

P1 A normal healthy patient

P2 A patient with mild systemic disease

P3 A patient with severe systemic disease

P4 A patient with severe systemic disease that is a constant threat to life

P5 A moribund patient who is not expected to survive without the operation

P6 A declared brain-dead patient whose organs are being removed for donor purposes

Modifiers Approved for Ambulatory Surgery Center (ASC) Hospital Outpatient Use

CPT Level I Modifiers

25 **Significant, Separately Identifiable Evaluation and Management Service by the Same Physician on the Same Day of the Procedure or Other Service:** It may be necessary to indicate that on the day a procedure or service identified by a CPT code was performed, the patient's condition required a significant, separately identifiable E/M service above and beyond the other service provided or beyond the usual preoperative and postoperative care associated with the procedure that was performed. A significant, separately identifiable E/M service is defined or substantiated by documentation that satisfies the relevant criteria for the respective E/M service to be reported (see **Evaluation and Management Services Guidelines** for instructions on determining level of E/M service). The E/M service may be prompted by the symptom or condition for which the procedure and/or service was provided. As such, different diagnoses are not required for reporting of the E/M services on the same date. This circumstance may be reported by adding modifier 25 to the appropriate level of E/M service.

Note: This modifier is not used to report an E/M service that resulted in a decision to perform surgery. See modifier 57. For significant, separately identifiable non-E/M services, see modifier 59.

27 Multiple Outpatient Hospital E/M Encounters on the Same Date: For hospital outpatient reporting purposes, utilization of hospital resources related to separate and distinct E/M encounters performed in multiple outpatient hospital settings on the same date may be reported by adding modifier 27 to each appropriate level outpatient and/or emergency department E/M code(s). This modifier provides a means of reporting circumstances involving evaluation and management services provided by a physician(s) in more than one (multiple) outpatient hospital setting(s) (eg, hospital emergency department, clinic).
Note: This modifier is not to be used for physician reporting of multiple E/M services performed by the same physician on the same date. For physician reporting of all outpatient evaluation and management services provided by the same physician on the same date and performed in multiple outpatient settings (eg, hospital emergency department, clinic), see **Evaluation and Management, Emergency Department, or Preventive Medicine Services** codes.

50 Bilateral Procedure: Unless otherwise identified in the listings, bilateral procedures that are performed at the same session should be identified by adding modifier 50 to the appropriate 5-digit code.

52 Reduced Services: Under certain circumstances a service or procedure is partially reduced or eliminated at the physician's discretion. Under these circumstances the service provided can be identified by its usual procedure number and the addition of modifier 52, signifying that the service is reduced. This provides a means of reporting reduced services without disturbing the identification of the basic service.
Note: For hospital outpatient reporting of a previously scheduled procedure/service that is partially reduced or cancelled as a result of extenuating circumstances or those that threaten the well-being of the patient prior to or after administration of anesthesia, see modifiers 73 and 74 (see modifiers approved for ASC hospital outpatient use).

58 Staged or Related Procedure or Service by the Same Physician During the Postoperative Period: It may be necessary to indicate that the performance of a procedure or service during the postoperative period was (a) planned or anticipated (staged); (b) more extensive than the original procedure; or (c) for therapy following a surgical procedure. This circumstance may be reported by adding modifier 58 to the staged or related procedure.

Note: For treatment of a problem that requires a return to the operating or procedure room (eg, unanticipated clinical condition), see modifier 78.

59 Distinct Procedural Service: Under certain circumstances, it may be necessary to indicate that a procedure or service was distinct or independent from other non-E/M services performed on the same day. Modifier 59 is used to identify procedures or services, other than E/M services, that are not normally reported together but are appropriate under the circumstances. Documentation must support a different session, different procedure or surgery, different site or organ system, separate incision or excision, separate lesion, or separate injury (or area of injury in extensive injuries) not ordinarily encountered or performed on the same day by the same individual. However, when another already established modifier is appropriate it should be used rather than modifier 59. Only if no more descriptive modifier is available and the use of modifier 59 best explains the circumstances should modifier 59 be used.
Note: Modifier 59 should not be appended to an E/M service. To report a separate and distinct E/M service with a non-E/M service performed on the same date, see modifier 25.

73 Discontinued Out-Patient Hospital/Ambulatory Surgery Center (ASC) Procedure Prior to the Administration of Anesthesia: Due to extenuating circumstances or those that threaten the well being of the patient, the physician may cancel a surgical or diagnostic procedure subsequent to the patient's surgical preparation (including sedation when provided, and being taken to the room where the procedure is to be performed), but prior to the administration of anesthesia (local, regional block(s), or general). Under these circumstances, the intended service that is prepared for but cancelled can be reported by its usual procedure number and the addition of modifier 73. Note: The elective cancellation of a service prior to the administration of anesthesia and/or surgical preparation of the patient should not be reported. For physician reporting of a discontinued procedure, see modifier 53.

74 Discontinued Out-Patient Hospital/Ambulatory Surgery Center (ASC) Procedure After Administration of Anesthesia: Due to extenuating circumstances or those that threaten the well being of the patient, the physician may terminate a surgical or diagnostic procedure after the administration of anesthesia (local, regional block(s), general) or after the procedure was started (incision made, intubation started, scope inserted, etc.). Under these circumstances, the procedure started but terminated can be reported by its usual procedure number and the addition of modifier 74.
Note: The elective cancellation of a service prior to the administration of anesthesia and/or surgical preparation of the patient should not be reported. For physician reporting of a discontinued procedure, see modifier 53.

76 Repeat Procedure or Service by Same Physician or Other Qualified Health Care Professional: It may be necessary to indicate that a procedure or service was repeated by the same physician or other qualified health care professional subsequent to the original procedure or service. This circumstance may be reported by adding modifier 76 to the repeated procedure or service.
Note: This modifier should not be appended to an E/M service.

77 Repeat Procedure or Service by Another Physician or Other Qualified Health Care Professional: It may be necessary to indicate that a basic procedure or service was repeated by another physician or other qualified health care professional subsequent to the original procedure or service. This circumstance may be reported by adding modifier 77 to the repeated procedure or service.
Note: This modifier should not be appended to an E/M service.

78 Unplanned Return to the Operating/Procedure Room by the Same Physician or Other Qualified Health Care Professional Following Initial Procedure for a Related Procedure During the Postoperative Period: It may be necessary to indicate that another procedure was performed during the postoperative period of the initial procedure (unplanned procedure following initial procedure). When this procedure is related to the first and requires the use of an operating/procedure room, it may be reported by adding modifier 78 to the related procedure. (For repeat procedures, see modifier 76.)

79 Unrelated Procedure or Service by the Same Physician During the Postoperative Period: The physician may need to indicate that the performance of a procedure or service during the postoperative period was unrelated to the original procedure. This circumstance may be reported by using modifier 79. (For repeat procedures on the same day, see modifier 76.)

91 Repeat Clinical Diagnostic Laboratory Test: In the course of treatment of the patient, it may be necessary to repeat the same laboratory test on the same day to obtain subsequent (multiple) test results. Under these circumstances, the laboratory test performed can be identified by its usual procedure number and the addition of modifier 91.
Note: This modifier may not be used when tests are rerun to confirm initial results; due to testing problems with specimens or equipment; or for any other reason when a normal, one-time, reportable result is all that is required. This modifier may not be used when another code(s) describe a series of test results (eg, glucose tolerance tests, evocative/suppression testing). This modifier may only be used for a laboratory test(s) performed more than once on the same day on the same patient.

Level II (HCPCS/National) Modifiers

Anatomical Modifiers

E1 Upper left, eyelid
E2 Lower left, eyelid
E3 Upper right, eyelid
E4 Lower right, eyelid
F1 Left hand, second digit
F2 Left hand, third digit
F3 Left hand, fourth digit
F4 Left hand, fifth digit
F5 Right hand, thumb
F6 Right hand, second digit
F7 Right hand, third digit
F8 Right hand, fourth digit
F9 Right hand, fifth digit
FA Left hand, thumb
LT Left side (used to identify procedures performed on the left side of the body)
RT Right side (used to identify procedures performed on the right side of the body)
T1 Left foot, second digit
T2 Left foot, third digit
T3 Left foot, fourth digit
T4 Left foot, fifth digit
T5 Right foot, great toe
T6 Right foot, second digit
T7 Right foot, third digit
T8 Right foot, fourth digit
T9 Right foot, fifth digit
TA Left foot, great toe

Anesthesia Modifiers

AA Anesthesia services performed personally by anesthesiologist
AD Medical supervision by a physician: more than four concurrent anesthesia procedures
G8 Monitored anesthesia care (MAC) for deep complex, complicated, or markedly invasive surgical procedure
G9 Monitored anesthesia care for patient who has history of severe cardiopulmonary condition
QK Medical direction of two, three, or four concurrent anesthesia procedures involving qualified individuals
QS Monitored anesthesia care service
QX CRNA service: with medical direction by a physician
QY Medical direction of one certified registered nurse anesthetist (CRNA) by an anesthesiologist
QZ CRNA service: without medical direction by a physician
P1 A normal healthy patient
P2 A patient with mild systemic disease
P3 A patient with severe systemic disease
P4 A patient with severe systemic disease that is a constant threat to life
P5 A moribund patient who is not expected to survive without the operation
P6 A declared brain-dead patient whose organs are being removed for donor purposes

Coronary Artery Modifiers

LC Left circumflex coronary artery (Hospitals use with codes 92980-92984, 92995, 92996)
LD Left anterior descending coronary artery (Hospitals use with codes 92980-92984, 92995, 92996)
RC Right coronary artery (Hospitals use with codes 92980-92984, 92995, 92996)

Ophthalmology Modifiers

AP Determination of refractive state was not performed in the course of diagnostic ophthalmological examination
LS FDA-monitored intraocular lens implant
PL Progressive addition lenses
VP Aphakic patient

Other Modifiers

AE Registered dietician
AF Specialty physician
AG Primary physician
AH Clinical psychologist
AI Principal physician of record
AJ Clinical social worker
AK Nonparticipating physician
AM Physician, team member service
AQ Physician providing a service in an unlisted health professional shortage area (HPSA)
AR Physician provider services in a physician scarcity area
AS Physician assistant, nurse practitioner, or clinical nurse specialist services for assistant at surgery
AT Acute treatment (this modifier should be used when reporting service 98940, 98941, 98942)
CA Procedure payable only in the inpatient setting when performed emergently on an outpatient who expires prior to admission
CB Service ordered by a renal dialysis facility (RDF) physician as part of the ESRD beneficiary's dialysis benefit, is not part of the composite rate, and is separately reimbursable
CC Procedure code change (use 'CC' when the procedure code submitted was changed either for administrative reasons or because an incorrect code was filed)
CG Policy criteria applied
CR Catastrophe/disaster related
CS Item or service related, in whole or in part, to an illness, injury, or condition that was caused by or exacerbated by the effects, direct or indirect, of the 2010 oil spill in the gulf of Mexico, including but not limited to subsequent clean up activities
EP Service provided as part of Medicaid early periodic screening diagnosis and treatment (EPSDT) program
ET Emergency services
EY No physician or other licensed health care provider order for this item or service
FB Item provided without cost to provider, supplier or practitioner, or full credit received for replaced device (examples, but not limited to covered under warranty, replaced due to defect, free samples)
FC Partial credit received for replacement device
FP Service provided as part of family planning program
G7 Pregnancy resulted from rape or incest or pregnancy certified by physician as life threatening
GA Waiver of liability statement issued as required by payer policy, individual case
GB Claim being resubmitted for payment because it is no longer covered under a global payment demonstration
GC This service has been performed in part by a resident under the direction of a teaching physician
GD Units of service exceeds medically unlikely edit value and represents reasonable and necessary services
GE This service has been performed by a resident without the presence of a teaching physician under the primary care exception
GF Non-physician (e.g. nurse practitioner (NP), certified registered nurse anesthetist (CRNA), certified registered nurse (CRN), clinical nurse specialist (CNS), physician assistant (PA)) services in a critical access hospital
GG Performance and payment of a screening mammogram and diagnostic mammogram on the same patient, same day

GH Diagnostic mammogram converted from screening mammogram on same day

GJ Opt out physician or practitioner emergency or urgent service

GK Reasonable and necessary item/service associated with GA or GZ modifier

GN Service delivered under an outpatient speech-language pathology plan of care

GO Service delivered an outpatient occupational therapy plan of care

GP Service delivered under an outpatient physical therapy plan of care

GQ Via asynchronous telecommunications system

GR This service was performed in whole or in part by a resident in a department of veterans affairs medical center or clinic, supervised in accordance with VA policy

GT Via interactive audio and video telecommunication systems

GU Waiver of liability statement issued as required by payer policy, routine notice

GV Attending physician not employed or paid under arrangement by the patient's hospice provider

GW Service not related to the hospice patient's terminal condition

GX Notice of liability issued, voluntary under payer policy

GY Item or service statutorily excluded, does not meet the definition of any Medicare benefit or for non-Medicare insurers, is not a contract benefit

GZ Item or service expected to be denied as not reasonable and necessary

H9 Court-ordered

HA Child/adolescent program

HB Adult program, nongeriatric

HC Adult program, geriatric

HD Pregnant/parenting women's program

HE Mental health program

HF Substance abuse program

HG Opioid addiction treatment program

HH Integrated mental health/substance abuse program

HI Integrated mental health and mental retardation/developmental disabilities program

HJ Employee assistance program

HK Specialized mental health programs for high-risk populations

HL Intern

HM Less than bachelor degree level

HN Bachelors degree level

HO Masters degree level

HP Doctoral level

HQ Group setting

HR Family/couple with client present

HS Family/couple without client present

HT Multi-disciplinary team

HU Funded by child welfare agency

HV Funded state addictions agency

HW Funded by state mental health agency

HX Funded by county/local agency

HY Funded by juvenile justice agency

HZ Funded by criminal justice agency

KB Beneficiary requested upgrade for ABN, more than four modifiers identified on claim

KX Requirements specified in the medical policy have been met

KZ New coverage not implemented by managed care

LR Laboratory round trip

M2 Medicare secondary payer (MSP)

PA Surgical or other invasive procedure on wrong body part

PB Surgical or other invasive procedure on wrong patient

PC Wrong surgery or other invasive procedure on patient

PD Diagnostic or related nondiagnostic item or service provided in a wholly owned or operated entity to a patient who is admitted as an inpatient within 3 days

PI Positron emission tomography (PET) or PET/computed tomography (CT) to inform the initial treatment strategy of tumors that are biopsy proven or strongly suspected of being cancerous based on other diagnostic testing, once per cancer diagnosis

PS Positron emission tomography (PET) or PET/computed tomography (CT) to inform the subsequent treatment strategy of cancerous tumor when the beneficiary's treating physician determines that the PET study is needed to inform subsequent anti-tumor strategy

PT Colorectal cancer screening test; converted to diagnostic test or other procedure

Q0 Investigational clinical service provided in a clinical research study that is in an approved clinical research study

Q1 Routine clinical service provided in a clinical research study that is in an approved clinical research study

Q2 HCFA/ORD demonstration project procedure/service

Q3 Live kidney donor surgery and related services

Q4 Service for ordering/referring physician qualifies as a service exemption

Q5 Service furnished by a substitute physician under a reciprocal billing arrangement

Q6 Service furnished by a locum tenens physician

Q7 One Class A finding

Q8 Two Class B findings

Q9 One Class B and two Class C findings

QC Single channel monitoring

QD Recording and storage in solid state memory by a digital recorder

QJ Services/items provided to a prisoner or patient in state or local custody, however the state or local government, as applicable, meets the requirements in 42 CRF 411.4 (B)

QP Documentation is on file showing that the laboratory test(s) was ordered individually or ordered as a CPT-recognized panel other than automated profile codes 80002-80019, G0058, G0059, and G0060

QT Recording and storage on tape by an analog tape recorder

QW CLIA waived test

RE Furnished in full compliance with FDA-mandated risk evaluation and mitigation strategy (REMS)

SA Nurse practitioner rendering service in collaboration with a physician

SB Nurse Midwife

SC Medically necessary service or supply

SD Services provided by registered nurse with specialized, highly technical home infusion training

SE State and/or federally funded programs/services

SF Second opinion ordered by a professional review organization (PRO) per section 9401, P.L.99-272 (100% reimbursement - no Medicare deductible or coinsurance)

SG Ambulatory surgical center (ASC) facility service

SH Second concurrently administered infusion therapy

SJ Third or more concurrently administered infusion therapy

SK Member of high risk population (use only with codes for immunization)

SL State supplied vaccine

SM Second surgical opinion

SN Third surgical opinion

SQ Item ordered by home health

SS Home infusion services provided in the infusion suite of the IV therapy provider

ST Related to trauma or injury

SU Procedure performed in physician's office (to denote use of facility and equipment)

SW Services provided by a certified diabetic educator

SY Persons who are in close contact with member of high-risk population (use only with codes for immunization)

TC Technical component. Under certain circumstances, a charge may be made for the technical component alone. Under those circumstances the technical component charge is identified by adding modifier 'TC' to the usual procedure number. Technical component charges are institutional charges and not billed separately by physicians. However, portable x-ray suppliers only bill for technical component and should utilize modifier TC. The charge data from portable x-ray suppliers will then be used to build customary and prevailing profiles.

TD RN

TE LPN/LVN

TF Intermediate level of care

TG Complex/high level of care

TH Obstetrical treatment/services, prenatal or postpartum

TJ Program group, child and/or adolescent

TK Extra patient or passenger, nonambulance

TL Early intervention/individualized family service plan (IFSP)

TM Individualized education program (IEP)

TN Rural/outside providers' customary service area

TR School-based individualized education program (IEP) services provided outside the public school district responsible for the student

TS Follow-up service

TT Individualized service provided to more than one patient in same setting

TU Special payment rate, overtime

TV Special payment rates, holidays/weekends

U1 Medicaid level of care 1, as defined by each state

U2 Medicaid level of care 2, as defined by each state

U3 Medicaid level of care 3, as defined by each state

U4 Medicaid level of care 4, as defined by each state

U5 Medicaid level of care 5, as defined by each state

U6 Medicaid level of care 6, as defined by each state

U7 Medicaid level of care 7, as defined by each state

U8 Medicaid level of care 8, as defined by each state

U9 Medicaid level of care 9, as defined by each state

UA Medicaid level of care 10, as defined by each state

UB Medicaid level of care 11, as defined by each state

UC Medicaid level of care 12, as defined by each state

UD Medicaid level of care 13, as defined by each state

UF Services provided in the morning

UG Services provided in the afternoon

UH Services provided in the evening

UJ Services provided at night

UK Services provided on behalf of the client to someone other than the client (collateral relationship)

UN Two patients served

UP Three patients served

UQ Four patients served

UR Five patients served

US Six or more patients served

V5 Vascular catheter (alone or with any other vascular access)

V6 Arteriovenous graft (or other vascular access not including a vascular catheter)

V7 Arteriovenous fistula only (in use with 2 needles)

V8 Infection present

V9 No infection present

Category II Modifiers

1P Performance measure exclusion modifier due to medical reasons

Includes:

- Not indicated (absence of organ/limb, already received/performed, other)
- Contraindicated (patient allergic history, potential adverse drug interaction, other)
- Other medical reasons

2P Performance measure exclusion modifier due to patient reasons

Includes:

- Patient declined
- Economic, social, or religious reasons
- Other patient reasons

3P Performance measure exclusion modifier due to system reasons

Includes:

- Resources to perform the services not available (eg, equipment, supplies)
- Insurance coverage or payer-related limitations
- Other reasons attributable to health care delivery system

8P Performance measure reporting modifier - action not performed, reason not otherwise specified

Dental Modifiers

AZ Physician providing a service in a dental health professional shortage area for the purpose of an electronic health record incentive payment

DA Oral health assessment by a licensed health professional other than a dentist

ET Emergency services (dental procedures performed in emergency situations should show the modifier ET)

ESRD Modifiers

AY Item or service furnished to an ESRD patient that is not for the treatment of ESRD

CD AMCC test has been ordered by an ESRD facility or MCP physician that is a part of the composite rate and is not separately billable

CE AMCC test has been ordered by an ESRD facility or MCP physician that is a composite rate test but is beyond the normal frequency covered under the rate and is separately reimbursable based on medically necessary

CF AMCC test has been ordered by an ESRD facility or MCP physician that is not part of the composite rate and is separately billable

G6 ESRD patient for whom less than six dialysis sessions have been provided in a month

GS Dosage of EPO or darbepoietin alfa has been reduced and maintained in response to hematocrit or hemoglobin level

Q3 Live kidney donor surgery and related services

Genetic Testing Modifiers

Neoplasia (Solid Tumor, Excluding Sarcoma and Lymphoma

0A BRCA1 (Hereditary breast/ovarian cancer)

0B BRCA2 (Hereditary breast cancer)

0C Neurofibromin (Neurofibromatosis, type 1)

0D Merlin (Neurofibromatosis, type 2)

0E c-RET (Multiple endocrine neoplasia, types 2A/B, familial medullary thyroid carcinoma)

0F VHL (Von Hippel Lindau disease, renal carcinoma)

0G SDHD (Hereditary paraganglioma)

0H SDHB (Hereditary paraganglioma)

0I ERRB2, commonly called Her-2/neu

0J MLH1 (HNPCC mismatch repair genes)

0K MSH2, MSH6, or PMS2 (HNPCC, mismatch repair genes)

0L APC (Hereditary polyposis coli)

0M Rb (Retinoblastoma)

0N TP53, commonly called p53

0O PTEN (Cowden's syndrome)

0P KIT, also called CD117 (gastrointestinal stromal tumor)

0Z Solid tumor gene, not otherwise specified

Neoplasia (Sarcoma)

1A WT1 or WT2 (Wilm's tumor)

1B PAX3, PAX7, or FOX01A (Alveolar rhabdomyosarcoma)

1C FLI1, ERG, ETV1, or EWSR1 (Ewing's sarcoma, desmoplastic round cell)

1D DDIT3 or FUS (Myxoid liposarcoma)

1E NR4A3, RBF56, or TCF12 (Myxoid chondrosarcoma)

1F SSX1, SSX2, or SYT (Synovial sarcoma)

1G MYCN (Neuroblastoma)

1H COL1A1 or PDGFB (Dermatofibrosarcoma protuberans)

1I TFE3 or ASPSCR1 (Alveolar soft parts sarcoma)

1J JAZF1 or JJAZ1 (Endometrial stromal sarcoma)

1Z Sarcoma gene, not otherwise specified

Neoplasia (Lymphoid/Hemtopoietic)

2A RUNX1 or CBFA2T1, commonly called AML1 or ETO, (genes associated with t(8;21) AML1–also ETO (Acute myelogenous leukemia)

2B BCR or ABL1, genes associated with t(9;22) (Chronic myelogenous or acute leukemia) BCR—also ABL (Chronic myeloid, acute lymphoid leukemia)

2C PBX1 or TCF3, genes associated with t(1;19) (Acute lymphoblastic leukemia) CGF1

2D CBFB or MYH11, genes associated with inv 16 (Acute myelogenous leukemia) CBF beta (leukemia)

2E MML (Acute leukemia)

2F PML or RARA, genes associated with t (15;17) (Acute promyelocytic leukemia) PML/RAR alpha (Promyelocytic leukemia)

2G ETV6, commonly called TEL, gene associated with t (12;21 (acute leukemia) TEL (Leukemia)

2H BCL2 (B cell lymphoma, follicle center cell origin) bcl-2 (Lymphoma)

2I CCND1, commonly called BCL1, cyclin D1 (Mantle cell lymphoma, myeloma) bcl-1 (Lymphoma)

2J MYC (Burkitt lymphoma) c-myc (Lymphoma)

2K IgH (Lymphoma/leukemia)

2L IGK (Lymphoma/leukemia)

2M TRB, T cell receptor beta (lymphoma/leukemia)

2N TRG, T cell receptor gamma (lymphoma/leukemia)

2O SIL or TAL1 (T cell leukemia)

2T BCL6 (B cell lymphoma)

2Q API1 or MALT1 (MALT lymphoma)

2R NPM or ALK, genes associated with t (2;5) (anaplastic large cell lymphoma)

2S FLT3 (Acute myelogenous leukemia)

2Z Lymphoid/hematopoetic neoplasia, not otherwise specified)

Non-Neoplastic Hematology/Coagulation

3A F5, commonly called Factor V (Leiden, others) (Hypercoagulable state)

3B FACC (Fanconi anemia)

3C FACD (Fanconi anemia)

3D HBB, Beta globin (Thalassemia, sickle cell anemia, other hemoglobinopathies)

3E HBA, commonly called alpha globin (thalassemia)

3F MTHFR (Elevated homocystinemia)

3G F2, commonly called prothrombin (20210, others) (Hypercoagulable state) prothrombin (Factor II, 20210A) (Hypercoagulable state)

3H F8, commonly called Factor VII (Hemophilia A/VWF)

3I F9, commonly called Factor IX (Hemophilia B)

3K F13, commonly called factor XIII (bleeding or hypercoagulable state) beta globin

3Z Non-neoplastic hematology/coagulation, not otherwise specified

Histocompatibility/Blood Typing/Identity/Microsatellite

4A HLA-A*

4B HLA-B*

4C HLA-C*

4E HLA-DRB all

#4P HLA-DRB1*

#4Q HLA-DRB3*

#4R HLA-DRB4*

#4S HLA-DRB5*

#4T HLA-DQA1*

4F HLA-DQB1 *

#4U HLA-DPA1 *

4G HLA-DPB1 *

4H Kell

4I Fingerprint for engraftment (post allogenic progenitor cell transplant)

4J Fingerprint for donor allelotype (allogeneic transplant)

4K Fingerprint for recipient allelotype (allogeneic transplant)

4L Fingerprint for leukocyte chimerism (allogeneic solid organ transplant)

4M Fingerprint for maternal versus fetal origin

4N Microsatellite instability

4O Microsatelite loss (loss of heterozygosity)

#4P *Resequenced code. See code following 4E.*

#4Q *Resequenced code. See code following 4E.*

#4R *Resequenced code. See code following 4E.*

#4S *Resequenced code. See code following 4E.*

#4T *Resequenced code. See code following 4E.*

#4U *Resequenced code. See code following 4F.*

4Z Histocompatibility typing, not otherwise specified

Neurologic, NonNeoplastic

5A ASPA, commonly called Aspartoacylase A (Canavan disease)

5B FMR-1 (Fragile X, FRAXA, syndrome)

5C FRDA, commonly called Frataxin (Freidreich's ataxia)

5D HD, commonly called Huntington (Huntington's disease)

5E GABRA5, NIPA1, UBE3A, or ANCR GABRA (Prader Willi-Angelman syndrome)

5F GJB2, commonly called Connexin-26 (Hereditary hearing loss) Connexin-26 (GJB2) (Hereditary deafness)

5G GJB1, commonly called Connexin-32 (X-linked Charcot-Marie-Tooth disease)

5H SNRPN (Prader Willi-Angelman syndrome)

5I SCA1, commonly called Ataxin-1 (Spinocerebellar ataxia, type 1)

5J SCA2, commonly called Ataxin-2 (Spinocerebellar ataxia, type 2)

5K MJD, commonly called Ataxin-3 (Spinocerebellar ataxia, type 3, Machado-Joseph disease)

5L CACNA1A (Spinocerebellar ataxia, type 6)

5M ATXN7 Ataxin-7 (Spinocerebellar ataxia, type 7)

5N PMP-22 (Charcot-Marie-Tooth disease, type 1A)

5O MECP2 (Rett syndrome)

5Z Neurologic, nonneoplastic, not otherwise specified

Muscular, NonNeoplastic

6A DMD, commonly called Dystrophin (Duchenne/Becker muscular dystrophy)

6B DMPK (Myotonic dystrophy, type 1)

6C ZNF-9 (Myotonic dystrophy, type 2)

6D SMN1/SMN2 (Autosomal recessive spinal muscular atrophy)

6E MTTK, commonly called tRNAlys (mytonic epilepsy, MERRF)

6F MTTL1, commonly called tRNAleu (mitochondrial encephalomyopathy, MELAS)

6Z Muscular, not otherwise specified

Metabolic, Other

7A APOE, commonly called Apolipoprotein E (Cardiovascular disease or Alzheimer's disease)

7B NPC1 or NPC2, commonly called sphingomyelin phosphodiesterase (Nieman-Pick disease)

7C GBA, commonly called Acid Beta Glucosidase (Gaucher disease)

7D HFE (Hemochromatosis)

7E HEXA, commonly called Hexosaminidase A (Tay-Sachs disease)

7F ACADM (medium chain acyl CoA dehydrogenase deficiency)

7Z Metabolic, other, not otherwise specified

Metabolic, Transport

8A CFTR (Cystic fibrosis)

8B PRSS1 (Hereditary pancreatitis)

8C Long QT syndrome, KCN (Jervell and Lange-Nielsen syndromes, types 1, 2, 5, and 6) and SCN (Brugada syndrome, SIDS and type 3)

8Z Metabolic, transport, not otherwise specified)

Metabolic-Pharmacogenetics

9A TPMT, commonly called (thiopurine methyltransferase) (patients on antimetabolite therapy)

9B CYP2 genes, commonly called cytochrome p450 (drug metabolism)

9C ABCB1, commonly called MDR1 or p-glycoprotein (drug transport)

9D NAT2 (drug metabolism)

9L Metabolic-pharmacogenetics, not otherwise specified

Dysmorphology

9M FGFR1 (Pfeiffer and Kallmann syndromes)

9N FGFR2 (Crouzon, Jackson-Weiss, Apert, Saethre-Chotzen syndromes)

9O FGFR3 (Achondroplasia, Hypochondroplasia, Thanatophoric dysplasia, types I and II, Crouzon syndrome with acanthosis nigricans, Muencke syndromes)

9P TWIST (Saethre-Chotzen syndrome)

9Q DCGR, commonly called CATCH-22 (DiGeorge and 22q11 deletion syndromes)

9Z Dysmorphology, not otherwise specified

APPENDIX B — NEW, CHANGED AND DELETED CODES

New Codes

15271 Application of skin substitute graft to trunk, arms, legs, total wound surface area up to 100 sq cm; first 25 sq cm or less wound surface area

15272 Application of skin substitute graft to trunk, arms, legs, total wound surface area up to 100 sq cm; each additional 25 sq cm wound surface area, or part thereof (List separately in addition to code for primary procedure)

15273 Application of skin substitute graft to trunk, arms, legs, total wound surface area greater than or equal to 100 sq cm; first 100 sq cm wound surface area, or 1% of body area of infants and children

15274 Application of skin substitute graft to trunk, arms, legs, total wound surface area greater than or equal to 100 sq cm; each additional 100 sq cm wound surface area, or part thereof, or each additional 1% of body area of infants and children, or part thereof (List separately in addition to code for primary procedure)

15275 Application of skin substitute graft to face, scalp, eyelids, mouth, neck, ears, orbits, genitalia, hands, feet, and/or multiple digits, total wound surface area up to 100 sq cm; first 25 sq cm or less wound surface area

15276 Application of skin substitute graft to face, scalp, eyelids, mouth, neck, ears, orbits, genitalia, hands, feet, and/or multiple digits, total wound surface area up to 100 sq cm; each additional 25 sq cm wound surface area, or part thereof (List separately in addition to code for primary procedure)

15277 Application of skin substitute graft to face, scalp, eyelids, mouth, neck, ears, orbits, genitalia, hands, feet, and/or multiple digits, total wound surface area greater than or equal to 100 sq cm; first 100 sq cm wound surface area, or 1% of body area of infants and children

15278 Application of skin substitute graft to face, scalp, eyelids, mouth, neck, ears, orbits, genitalia, hands, feet, and/or multiple digits, total wound surface area greater than or equal to 100 sq cm; each additional 100 sq cm wound surface area, or part thereof, or each additional 1% of body area of infants and children, or part thereof (List separately in addition to code for primary procedure)

15777 Implantation of biologic implant (eg, acellular dermal matrix) for soft tissue reinforcement (eg, breast, trunk) (List separately in addition to code for primary procedure)

20527 Injection, enzyme (eg, collagenase), palmar fascial cord (ie, Dupuytren's contracture)

22633 Arthrodesis, combined posterior or posterolateral technique with posterior interbody technique including laminectomy and/or discectomy sufficient to prepare interspace (other than for decompression), single interspace and segment; lumbar

22634 Arthrodesis, combined posterior or posterolateral technique with posterior interbody technique including laminectomy and/or discectomy sufficient to prepare interspace (other than for decompression), single interspace and segment; each additional interspace and segment (List separately in addition to code for primary procedure)

26341 Manipulation, palmar fascial cord (ie, Dupuytren's cord), post enzyme injection (eg, collagenase), single cord

29582 Application of multi-layer compression system; thigh and leg, including ankle and foot, when performed

29583 Application of multi-layer compression system; upper arm and forearm

29584 Application of multi-layer compression system; upper arm, forearm, hand, and fingers

32096 Thoracotomy, with diagnostic biopsy(ies) of lung infiltrate(s) (eg, wedge, incisional), unilateral

32097 Thoracotomy, with diagnostic biopsy(ies) of lung nodule(s) or mass(es) (eg, wedge, incisional), unilateral

32098 Thoracotomy, with biopsy(ies) of pleura

32505 Thoracotomy; with therapeutic wedge resection (eg, mass, nodule), initial

32506 Thoracotomy; with therapeutic wedge resection (eg, mass or nodule), each additional resection, ipsilateral (List separately in addition to code for primary procedure)

32507 Thoracotomy; with diagnostic wedge resection followed by anatomic lung resection (List separately in addition to code for primary procedure)

32607 Thoracoscopy; with diagnostic biopsy(ies) of lung infiltrate(s) (eg, wedge, incisional), unilateral

32608 Thoracoscopy; with diagnostic biopsy(ies) of lung nodule(s) or mass(es) (eg, wedge, incisional), unilateral

32609 Thoracoscopy; with biopsy(ies) of pleura

32666 Thoracoscopy, surgical; with therapeutic wedge resection (eg, mass, nodule), initial unilateral

32667 Thoracoscopy, surgical; with therapeutic wedge resection (eg, mass or nodule), each additional resection, ipsilateral (List separately in addition to code for primary procedure)

32668 Thoracoscopy, surgical; with diagnostic wedge resection followed by anatomic lung resection (List separately in addition to code for primary procedure)

32669 Thoracoscopy, surgical; with removal of a single lung segment (segmentectomy)

32670 Thoracoscopy, surgical; with removal of two lobes (bilobectomy)

32671 Thoracoscopy, surgical; with removal of lung (pneumonectomy)

32672 Thoracoscopy, surgical; with resection-plication for emphysematous lung (bullous or non-bullous) for lung volume reduction (LVRS), unilateral includes any pleural procedure, when performed

32673 Thoracoscopy, surgical; with resection of thymus, unilateral or bilateral

32674 Thoracoscopy, surgical; with mediastinal and regional lymphadenectomy (List separately in addition to code for primary procedure)

33221 Insertion of pacemaker pulse generator only; with existing multiple leads

33227 Removal of permanent pacemaker pulse generator with replacement of pacemaker pulse generator; single lead system

33228 Removal of permanent pacemaker pulse generator with replacement of pacemaker pulse generator; dual lead system

33229 Removal of permanent pacemaker pulse generator with replacement of pacemaker pulse generator; multiple lead system

33230 Insertion of pacing cardioverter-defibrillator pulse generator only; with existing dual leads

33231 Insertion of pacing cardioverter-defibrillator pulse generator only; with existing multiple leads

33262 Removal of pacing cardioverter-defibrillator pulse generator with replacement of pacing cardioverter-defibrillator pulse generator; single lead system

33263 Removal of pacing cardioverter-defibrillator pulse generator with replacement of pacing cardioverter-defibrillator pulse generator; dual lead system

33264 Removal of pacing cardioverter-defibrillator pulse generator with replacement of pacing cardioverter-defibrillator pulse generator; multiple lead system

36251 Selective catheter placement (first-order), main renal artery and any accessory renal artery(s) for renal angiography, including arterial puncture and catheter placement(s), fluoroscopy, contrast injection(s), image postprocessing, permanent recording of images, and radiological supervision and interpretation, including pressure gradient measurements when performed, and flush aortogram when performed; unilateral

36252 Selective catheter placement (first-order), main renal artery and any accessory renal artery(s) for renal angiography, including arterial puncture and catheter placement(s), fluoroscopy, contrast injection(s), image postprocessing, permanent recording of images, and radiological supervision and interpretation, including pressure gradient measurements when performed, and flush aortogram when performed; bilateral

36253 Superselective catheter placement (one or more second order or higher renal artery branches) renal artery and any accessory renal artery(s) for renal angiography, including arterial puncture, catheterization, fluoroscopy, contrast injection(s), image postprocessing, permanent recording of images, and radiological supervision and interpretation, including pressure gradient measurements when performed, and flush aortogram when performed; unilateral

36254 Superselective catheter placement (one or more second order or higher renal artery branches) renal artery and any accessory renal artery(s) for renal angiography, including arterial puncture, catheterization, fluoroscopy, contrast injection(s), image postprocessing, permanent recording of images, and radiological supervision and interpretation, including pressure gradient measurements when performed, and flush aortogram when performed; bilateral

37191 Insertion of intravascular vena cava filter, endovascular approach including vascular access, vessel selection, and radiological supervision and interpretation, intraprocedural roadmapping, and imaging guidance (ultrasound and fluoroscopy), when performed

37192 Repositioning of intravascular vena cava filter, endovascular approach including vascular access, vessel selection, and radiological supervision and interpretation, intraprocedural roadmapping, and imaging guidance (ultrasound and fluoroscopy), when performed

37193 Retrieval (removal) of intravascular vena cava filter, endovascular approach including vascular access, vessel selection, and radiological supervision and interpretation, intraprocedural roadmapping, and imaging guidance (ultrasound and fluoroscopy), when performed

37619 Ligation of inferior vena cava

38232 Bone marrow harvesting for transplantation; autologous

49082 Abdominal paracentesis (diagnostic or therapeutic); without imaging guidance

49083 Abdominal paracentesis (diagnostic or therapeutic); with imaging guidance

49084 Peritoneal lavage, including imaging guidance, when performed

62369 Electronic analysis of programmable, implanted pump for intrathecal or epidural drug infusion (includes evaluation of reservoir status, alarm status, drug prescription status); with reprogramming and refill

62370 Electronic analysis of programmable, implanted pump for intrathecal or epidural drug infusion (includes evaluation of reservoir status, alarm status, drug prescription status); with reprogramming and refill (requiring physician's skill)

64633 Destruction by neurolytic agent, paravertebral facet joint nerve(s), with imaging guidance (fluoroscopy or CT); cervical or thoracic, single facet joint

64634 Destruction by neurolytic agent, paravertebral facet joint nerve(s), with imaging guidance (fluoroscopy or CT); cervical or thoracic, each additional facet joint (List separately in addition to code for primary procedure)

64635 Destruction by neurolytic agent, paravertebral facet joint nerve(s), with imaging guidance (fluoroscopy or CT); lumbar or sacral, single facet joint

64636 Destruction by neurolytic agent, paravertebral facet joint nerve(s), with imaging guidance (fluoroscopy or CT); lumbar or sacral, each additional facet joint (List separately in addition to code for primary procedure)

74174 Computed tomographic angiography, abdomen and pelvis, with contrast material(s), including noncontrast images, if performed, and image postprocessing

77424 Intraoperative radiation treatment delivery, x-ray, single treatment session

77425 Intraoperative radiation treatment delivery, electrons, single treatment session

77469 Intraoperative radiation treatment management

78226 Hepatobiliary system imaging, including gallbladder when present;

78227 Hepatobiliary system imaging, including gallbladder when present; with pharmacologic intervention, including quantitative measurement(s) when performed

78579 Pulmonary ventilation imaging (eg, aerosol or gas)

78582 Pulmonary ventilation (eg, aerosol or gas) and perfusion imaging

78597 Quantitative differential pulmonary perfusion, including imaging when performed

78598 Quantitative differential pulmonary perfusion and ventilation (eg, aerosol or gas), including imaging when performed

81200 ASPA (aspartoacylase) (eg, Canavan disease) gene analysis, common variants (eg, E285A, Y231X)

81205 BCKDHB (branched-chain keto acid dehydrogenase E1, beta polypeptide) (eg, Maple syrup urine disease) gene analysis, common variants (eg, R183P, G278S, E422X)

81206 BCR/ABL1 (t(9;22)) (eg, chronic myelogenous leukemia) translocation analysis; major breakpoint, qualitative or quantitative

81207 BCR/ABL1 (t(9;22)) (eg, chronic myelogenous leukemia) translocation analysis; minor breakpoint, qualitative or quantitative

81208 BCR/ABL1 (t(9;22)) (eg, chronic myelogenous leukemia) translocation analysis; other breakpoint, qualitative or quantitative

81209 BLM (Bloom syndrome, RecQ helicase-like) (eg, Bloom syndrome) gene analysis, 2281del6ins7 variant

81210 BRAF (v-raf murine sarcoma viral oncogene homolog B1) (eg, colon cancer), gene analysis, V600E variant

81211 BRCA1, BRCA2 (breast cancer 1 and 2) (eg, hereditary breast and ovarian cancer) gene analysis; full sequence analysis and common duplication/deletion variants in BRCA1 (ie, exon 13 del 3.835kb, exon 13 dup 6kb, exon 14-20 del 26kb, exon 22 del 510bp, exon 8-9 del 7.1kb)

81212 BRCA1, BRCA2 (breast cancer 1 and 2) (eg, hereditary breast and ovarian cancer) gene analysis; 185delAG, 5385insC, 6174delT variants

81213 BRCA1, BRCA2 (breast cancer 1 and 2) (eg, hereditary breast and ovarian cancer) gene analysis; uncommon duplication/deletion variants

81214 BRCA1 (breast cancer 1) (eg, hereditary breast and ovarian cancer) gene analysis; full sequence analysis and common duplication/deletion variants (ie, exon 13 del 3.835kb, exon 13 dup 6kb, exon 14-20 del 26kb, exon 22 del 510bp, exon 8-9 del 7.1kb)

81215 BRCA1 (breast cancer 1) (eg, hereditary breast and ovarian cancer) gene analysis; known familial variant

81216 BRCA2 (breast cancer 2) (eg, hereditary breast and ovarian cancer) gene analysis; full sequence analysis

81217 BRCA2 (breast cancer 2) (eg, hereditary breast and ovarian cancer) gene analysis; known familial variant

81220 CFTR (cystic fibrosis transmembrane conductance regulator) (eg, cystic fibrosis) gene analysis; common variants (eg, ACMG/ACOG guidelines)

81221 CFTR (cystic fibrosis transmembrane conductance regulator) (eg, cystic fibrosis) gene analysis; known familial variants

81222 CFTR (cystic fibrosis transmembrane conductance regulator) (eg, cystic fibrosis) gene analysis; duplication/deletion variants

81223 CFTR (cystic fibrosis transmembrane conductance regulator) (eg, cystic fibrosis) gene analysis; full gene sequence

81224 CFTR (cystic fibrosis transmembrane conductance regulator) (eg, cystic fibrosis) gene analysis; intron 8 poly-T analysis (eg, male infertility)

81225 CYP2C19 (cytochrome P450, family 2, subfamily C, polypeptide 19) (eg, drug metabolism), gene analysis, common variants (eg, *2, *3, *4, *8, *17)

81226 CYP2D6 (cytochrome P450, family 2, subfamily D, polypeptide 6) (eg, drug metabolism), gene analysis, common variants (eg, *2, *3, *4, *5, *6, *9, *10, *17, *19, *29, *35, *41, *1XN, *2XN, *4XN)

81227 CYP2C9 (cytochrome P450, family 2, subfamily C, polypeptide 9) (eg, drug metabolism), gene analysis, common variants (eg, *2, *3, *5, *6)

81228 Cytogenomic constitutional (genome-wide) microarray analysis; interrogation of genomic regions for copy number variants (eg, Bacterial Artificial Chromosome [BAC] or oligo-based comparative genomic hybridization [CGH] microarray analysis)

81229 Cytogenomic constitutional (genome-wide) microarray analysis; interrogation of genomic regions for copy number and single nucleotide polymorphism (SNP) variants for chromosomal abnormalities

81240 F2 (prothrombin, coagulation factor II) (eg, hereditary hypercoagulability) gene analysis, 20210G>A variant

81241 F5 (coagulation Factor V) (eg, hereditary hypercoagulability) gene analysis, Leiden variant

81242 FANCC (Fanconi anemia, complementation group C) (eg, Fanconi anemia, type C) gene analysis, common variant (eg, IVS4+4A>T)

81243 FMR1 (Fragile X mental retardation 1) (eg, fragile X mental retardation) gene analysis; evaluation to detect abnormal (eg, expanded) alleles

81244 FMR1 (Fragile X mental retardation 1) (eg, fragile X mental retardation) gene analysis; characterization of alleles (eg, expanded size and methylation status)

81245 FLT3 (fms-related tyrosine kinase 3) (eg, acute myeloid leukemia), gene analysis, internal tandem duplication (ITD) variants (ie, exons 14, 15)

81250 G6PC (glucose-6-phosphatase, catalytic subunit) (eg, Glycogen storage disease, Type 1a, von Gierke disease) gene analysis, common variants (eg, R83C, Q347X)

81251 GBA (glucosidase, beta, acid) (eg, Gaucher disease) gene analysis, common variants (eg, N370S, 84GG, L444P, IVS2+1G>A)

81255 HEXA (hexosaminidase A [alpha polypeptide]) (eg, Tay-Sachs disease) gene analysis, common variants (eg, 1278insTATC, 1421+1G>C, G269S)

81256 HFE (hemochromatosis) (eg, hereditary hemochromatosis) gene analysis, common variants (eg, C282Y, H63D)

81257 HBA1/HBA2 (alpha globin 1 and alpha globin 2) (eg, alpha thalassemia, Hb Bart hydrops fetalis syndrome, HbH disease), gene analysis, for common deletions or variant (eg, Southeast Asian, Thai, Filipino, Mediterranean, alpha3.7, alpha4.2, alpha20.5, and Constant Spring)

81260 IKBKAP (inhibitor of kappa light polypeptide gene enhancer in B-cells, kinase complex-associated protein) (eg, familial dysautonomia) gene analysis, common variants (eg, 2507+6T>C, R696P)

81261 IGH@ (Immunoglobulin heavy chain locus) (eg, leukemias and lymphomas, B-cell), gene rearrangement analysis to detect abnormal clonal population(s); amplified methodology (eg, polymerase chain reaction)

81262 IGH@ (Immunoglobulin heavy chain locus) (eg, leukemias and lymphomas, B-cell), gene rearrangement analysis to detect abnormal clonal population(s); direct probe methodology (eg, Southern blot)

81263 IGH@ (Immunoglobulin heavy chain locus) (eg, leukemia and lymphoma, B-cell), variable region somatic mutation analysis

81264 IGK@ (Immunoglobulin kappa light chain locus) (eg, leukemia and lymphoma, B-cell), gene rearrangement analysis, evaluation to detect abnormal clonal population(s)

81265 Comparative analysis using Short Tandem Repeat (STR) markers; patient and comparative specimen (eg, pre-transplant recipient and donor germline testing, post-transplant non-hematopoietic recipient germline [eg, buccal swab or other germline tissue sample] and donor testing, twin zygosity testing, or maternal cell contamination of fetal cells)

81266 Comparative analysis using Short Tandem Repeat (STR) markers; each additional specimen (eg, additional cord blood donor, additional fetal samples from different cultures, or additional zygosity in multiple birth pregnancies) (List separately in addition to code for primary procedure)

81267 Chimerism (engraftment) analysis, post transplantation specimen (eg, hematopoietic stem cell), includes comparison to previously performed baseline analyses; without cell selection

81268 Chimerism (engraftment) analysis, post transplantation specimen (eg, hematopoietic stem cell), includes comparison to previously performed baseline analyses; with cell selection (eg, CD3, CD33), each cell type

81270 JAK2 (Janus kinase 2) (eg, myeloproliferative disorder) gene analysis, p.Val617Phe (V617F) variant

81275 KRAS (v-Ki-ras2 Kirsten rat sarcoma viral oncogene) (eg, carcinoma) gene analysis, variants in codons 12 and 13

81280 Long QT syndrome gene analyses (eg, KCNQ1, KCNH2, SCN5A, KCNE1, KCNE2, KCNJ2, CACNA1C, CAV3, SCN4B, AKAP, SNTA1, and ANK2); full sequence analysis

81281 Long QT syndrome gene analyses (eg, KCNQ1, KCNH2, SCN5A, KCNE1, KCNE2, KCNJ2, CACNA1C, CAV3, SCN4B, AKAP, SNTA1, and ANK2); known familial sequence variant

81282 Long QT syndrome gene analyses (eg, KCNQ1, KCNH2, SCN5A, KCNE1, KCNE2, KCNJ2, CACNA1C, CAV3, SCN4B, AKAP, SNTA1, and ANK2); duplication/deletion variants

81290 MCOLN1 (mucolipin 1) (eg, Mucolipidosis, type IV) gene analysis, common variants (eg, IVS3-2A>G, del6.4kb)

81291 MTHFR (5,10-methylenetetrahydrofolate reductase) (eg, hereditary hypercoagulability) gene analysis, common variants (eg, 677T, 1298C)

81292 MLH1 (mutL homolog 1, colon cancer, nonpolyposis type 2) (eg, hereditary non-polyposis colorectal cancer, Lynch syndrome) gene analysis; full sequence analysis

81293 MLH1 (mutL homolog 1, colon cancer, nonpolyposis type 2) (eg, hereditary non-polyposis colorectal cancer, Lynch syndrome) gene analysis; known familial variants

81294 MLH1 (mutL homolog 1, colon cancer, nonpolyposis type 2) (eg, hereditary non-polyposis colorectal cancer, Lynch syndrome) gene analysis; duplication/deletion variants

81295 MSH2 (mutS homolog 2, colon cancer, nonpolyposis type 1) (eg, hereditary non-polyposis colorectal cancer, Lynch syndrome) gene analysis; full sequence analysis

81296 MSH2 (mutS homolog 2, colon cancer, nonpolyposis type 1) (eg, hereditary non-polyposis colorectal cancer, Lynch syndrome) gene analysis; known familial variants

81297 MSH2 (mutS homolog 2, colon cancer, nonpolyposis type 1) (eg, hereditary non-polyposis colorectal cancer, Lynch syndrome) gene analysis; duplication/deletion variants

81298 MSH6 (mutS homolog 6 [E. coli]) (eg, hereditary non-polyposis colorectal cancer, Lynch syndrome) gene analysis; full sequence analysis

81299 MSH6 (mutS homolog 6 [E. coli]) (eg, hereditary non-polyposis colorectal cancer, Lynch syndrome) gene analysis; known familial variants

81300 MSH6 (mutS homolog 6 [E. coli]) (eg, hereditary non-polyposis colorectal cancer, Lynch syndrome) gene analysis; duplication/deletion variants

81301 Microsatellite instability analysis (eg, hereditary non-polyposis colorectal cancer, Lynch syndrome) of markers for mismatch repair deficiency (eg, BAT25, BAT26), includes comparison of neoplastic and normal tissue, if performed

81302 MECP2 (methyl CpG binding protein 2) (eg, Rett syndrome) gene analysis; full sequence analysis

81303 MECP2 (methyl CpG binding protein 2) (eg, Rett syndrome) gene analysis; known familial variant

81304 MECP2 (methyl CpG binding protein 2) (eg, Rett syndrome) gene analysis; duplication/deletion variants

81310 NPM1 (nucleophosmin) (eg, acute myeloid leukemia) gene analysis, exon 12 variants

81315 PML/RARalpha, (t(15;17)), (promyelocytic leukemia/retinoic acid receptor alpha) (eg, promyelocytic leukemia) translocation analysis; common breakpoints (eg, intron 3 and intron 6), qualitative or quantitative

81316 PML/RARalpha, (t(15;17)), (promyelocytic leukemia/retinoic acid receptor alpha) (eg, promyelocytic leukemia) translocation analysis; single breakpoint (eg, intron 3, intron 6 or exon 6), qualitative or quantitative

81317 PMS2 (postmeiotic segregation increased 2 [S. cerevisiae]) (eg, hereditary non-polyposis colorectal cancer, Lynch syndrome) gene analysis; full sequence analysis

81318 PMS2 (postmeiotic segregation increased 2 [S. cerevisiae]) (eg, hereditary non-polyposis colorectal cancer, Lynch syndrome) gene analysis; known familial variants

81319 PMS2 (postmeiotic segregation increased 2 [S. cerevisiae]) (eg, hereditary non-polyposis colorectal cancer, Lynch syndrome) gene analysis; duplication/deletion variants

81330 SMPD1(sphingomyelin phosphodiesterase 1, acid lysosomal) (eg, Niemann-Pick disease, Type A) gene analysis, common variants (eg, R496L, L302P, fsP330)

81331 SNRPN/UBE3A (small nuclear ribonucleoprotein polypeptide N and ubiquitin protein ligase E3A) (eg, Prader-Willi syndrome and/or Angelman syndrome), methylation analysis

81332 SERPINA1 (serpin peptidase inhibitor, clade A, alpha-1 antiproteinase, antitrypsin, member 1) (eg, alpha-1-antitrypsin deficiency), gene analysis, common variants (eg, *S and *Z)

81340 TRB@ (T cell antigen receptor, beta) (eg, leukemia and lymphoma), gene rearrangement analysis to detect abnormal clonal population(s); using amplification methodology (eg, polymerase chain reaction)

81341 TRB@ (T cell antigen receptor, beta) (eg, leukemia and lymphoma), gene rearrangement analysis to detect abnormal clonal population(s); using direct probe methodology (eg, Southern blot)

81342 TRG@ (T cell antigen receptor, gamma) (eg, leukemia and lymphoma), gene rearrangement analysis, evaluation to detect abnormal clonal population(s)

81350 UGT1A1 (UDP glucuronosyltransferase 1 family, polypeptide A1) (eg, irinotecan metabolism), gene analysis, common variants (eg, *28, *36, *37)

81355 VKORC1 (vitamin K epoxide reductase complex, subunit 1) (eg, warfarin metabolism), gene analysis, common variants (eg, -1639/3673)

81370 HLA Class I and II typing, low resolution (eg, antigen equivalents); HLA-A, -B, -C, -DRB1/3/4/5, and -DQB1

81371 HLA Class I and II typing, low resolution (eg, antigen equivalents); HLA-A, -B, and -DRB1/3/4/5 (eg, verification typing)

81372 HLA Class I typing, low resolution (eg, antigen equivalents); complete (ie, HLA-A, -B, and -C)

81373 HLA Class I typing, low resolution (eg, antigen equivalents); one locus (eg, HLA-A, -B, or -C), each

81374 HLA Class I typing, low resolution (eg, antigen equivalents); one antigen equivalent (eg, B*27), each

81375 HLA Class II typing, low resolution (eg, antigen equivalents); HLA-DRB1/3/4/5 and -DQB1

81376 HLA Class II typing, low resolution (eg, antigen equivalents); one locus (eg, HLA-DRB1/3/4/5, -DQB1, -DQA1, -DPB1, or -DPA1), each

81377 HLA Class II typing, low resolution (eg, antigen equivalents); one antigen equivalent, each

81378 HLA Class I and II typing, high resolution (ie, alleles or allele groups), HLA-A, -B, -C, and -DRB1

81379 HLA Class I typing, high resolution (ie, alleles or allele groups); complete (ie, HLA-A, -B, and -C)

81380 HLA Class I typing, high resolution (ie, alleles or allele groups); one locus (eg, HLA-A, -B, or -C), each

81381 HLA Class I typing, high resolution (ie, alleles or allele groups); one allele or allele group (eg, B*57:01P), each

81382 HLA Class II typing, high resolution (ie, alleles or allele groups); one locus (eg, HLA-DRB1, -DRB3, -DRB4, -DRB5, -DQB1, -DQA1, -DPB1, or -DPA1), each

81383 HLA Class II typing, high resolution (ie, alleles or allele groups); one allele or allele group (eg, HLA-DQB1*06:02P), each

81400 Molecular pathology procedure, Level 1 (eg, identification of single germline variant [eg, SNP] by techniques such as restriction enzyme digestion or melt curve analysis) ACADM (acyl-CoA dehydrogenase, C-4 to C-12 straight chain, MCAD) (eg, medium chain acyl dehydrogenase deficiency), K304E variant ACE (angiotensin converting enzyme) (eg, hereditary blood pressure regulation), insertion/deletion variant AGTR1 (angiotensin II receptor, type 1) (eg, essential hypertension), 1166A>C variant CCR5 (chemokine C-C motif receptor 5) (eg, HIV resistance), 32-bp deletion mutation/794 825del32 deletion DPYD (dihydropyrimidine dehydrogenase) (eg, 5-fluorouracil/5-FU and capecitabine drug metabolism), IVS14+1G>A variant F2 (coagulation factor 2) (eg, hereditary hypercoagulability), 1199G>A variant F5 (coagulation factor V) (eg, hereditary hypercoagulability), HR2 variant F7 (coagulation factor VII [serum prothrombin conversion accelerator]) (eg, hereditary hypercoagulability), R353Q variant F13B (coagulation factor XIII, B polypeptide) (eg, hereditary hypercoagulability), V34L variant FGB (fibrinogen beta chain) (eg, hereditary ischemic heart disease), -455G>A variant Human Platelet Antigen 1 genotyping (HPA-1), ITGB3 (integrin, beta 3 [platelet glycoprotein IIIa], antigen CD61 [GPIIIa]) (eg, neonatal alloimmune thrombocytopenia [NAIT], post-transfusion purpura), HPA-1a/b (L33P) Human Platelet Antigen 2 genotyping (HPA-2), GP1BA (glycoprotein Ib [platelet], alpha polypeptide [GPIba]) (eg, neonatal alloimmune thrombocytopenia [NAIT], post-transfusion purpura), HPA-2a/b (T145M) Human Platelet Antigen 3 genotyping (HPA-3), ITGA2B (integrin, alpha 2b [platelet glycoprotein IIb of IIb/IIIa complex], antigen CD41 [GPIIb]) (eg, neonatal alloimmune thrombocytopenia [NAIT], post-transfusion purpura), HPA-3a/b (I843S) Human Platelet Antigen 4 genotyping (HPA-4), ITGB3 (integrin, beta 3 [platelet glycoprotein IIIa], antigen CD61 [GPIIIa]) (eg, neonatal alloimmune thrombocytopenia [NAIT], post-transfusion purpura), HPA-4a/b (R143Q) Human Platelet Antigen 5 genotyping (HPA-5), ITGA2 (integrin, alpha 2 [CD49B, alpha 2 subunit of VLA-2 receptor] [GPIa]) (eg, neonatal alloimmune thrombocytopenia [NAIT], post-transfusion purpura), HPA-5a/b (K505E) Human Platelet Antigen 6 genotyping (HPA-6w), ITGB3 (integrin, beta 3 [platelet glycoprotein IIIa, antigen CD61] [GPIIIa]) (eg, neonatal alloimmune thrombocytopenia [NAIT], post-transfusion purpura), HPA-6a/b (R489Q) Human Platelet Antigen 9 genotyping (HPA-9w), ITGA2B (integrin, alpha 2b [platelet glycoprotein IIb of IIb/IIIa complex, antigen CD41] [GPIIb]) (eg, neonatal alloimmune thrombocytopenia [NAIT], post-transfusion purpura), HPA-9a/b (V837M) Human Platelet Antigen 15 genotyping (HPA-15), CD109 (CD109 molecule) (eg, neonatal alloimmune thrombocytopenia [NAIT], post-transfusion purpura), HPA-15a/b(S682Y) SERPINE1 (serpine peptidase inhibitor clade E, member 1, plasminogen activator inhibitor -1, PAI-1) (eg, thrombophilia), 4G variant

81401 Molecular pathology procedure, Level 2 (eg, 2-10 SNPs, 1 methylated variant, or 1 somatic variant [typically using nonsequencing target variant analysis], or detection of a dynamic mutation disorder/triplet repeat) ABL (c-abl oncogene 1, receptor tyrosine kinase) (eg, acquired imatinib resistance), T315I variant ACADM (acyl-CoA dehydrogenase, C-4 to C-12 straight chain, MCAD) (eg, medium chain acyl dehydrogenase deficiency), common variants (eg, K304E, Y42H) ADRB2 (adrenergic beta-2 receptor surface) (eg, drug metabolism), common variants (eg, G16R, Q27E) APOE (apolipoprotein E) (eg, hyperlipoproteinemia type III, cardiovascular disease, Alzheimer disease), common variants (eg, *2, *3, *4) CBFB/MYH11 (inv(16)) (eg, acute myeloid leukemia), qualitative, and quantitative, if performed CCND1/IGH (BCL1/IgH, t(11;14)) (eg, mantle cell lymphoma) translocation analysis, major breakpoint, qualitative, and quantitative, if performed CFH/ARMS2 (complement factor H/age-related maculopathy susceptibility 2) (eg, macular degeneration), common variants (eg, Y402H [CFH], A69S [ARMS2]) CYP3A4 (cytochrome P450, family 3, subfamily A, polypeptide 4) (eg, drug metabolism), common variants (eg, *2, *3, *4, *5, *6) CYP3A5 (cytochrome P450, family 3, subfamily A, polypeptide 5) (eg, drug metabolism), common variants (eg, *2, *3, *4, *5, *6) DMPK (dystrophia myotonica-protein kinase) (eg, myotonic dystrophy, type 1), evaluation to detect abnormal (eg, expanded) alleles F11 (coagulation factor XI) (eg, coagulation disorder), common variants (eg, E117X [Type II], F283L [Type III], IVS14del14, and IVS14+1G>A [Type I]) FGFR3 (fibroblast growth factor receptor 3) (eg, achondroplasia), common variants (eg, 1138G>A, 1138G>C) FIP1L1/PDGFRA (del[4q12]) (eg, imatinib-sensitive chronic eosinophilic leukemia), qualitative, and quantitative, if performed GALT (galactose-1-phosphate uridylyltransferase) (eg, galactosemia), common variants (eg, Q188R, S135L, K285N, T138M, L195P, Y209C, IVS2-2A>G, P171S, del5kb, N314D, L218L/N314D) HBB (hemoglobin, beta) (eg, sickle cell anemia, hemoglobin C, hemoglobin E), common variants (eg, HbS, HbC, HbE) HTT (huntingtin) (eg, Huntington disease), evaluation to detect abnormal (eg, expanded) alleles RUNX1/RUNX1T1 (t(8;21)) (eg, acute myeloid leukemia) translocation analysis, qualitative, and quantitative, if performed SEPT9 (Septin 9) (eg, colon cancer), methylation analysis TPMT (thiopurine S-methyltransferase) (eg, drug metabolism), common variants (eg, *2, *3) VWF (von Willebrand factor) (eg, von Willebrand disease type 2N), common variants (eg, T791M, R816W, R854Q)

81402 Molecular pathology procedure, Level 3 (eg, >10 SNPs, 2-10 methylated variants, or 2-10 somatic variants [typically using non-sequencing target variant analysis], immunoglobulin and T-cell receptor gene rearrangements, duplication/deletion variants 1 exon)

CYP21A2 (cytochrome P450, family 21, subfamily A, polypeptide 2) (eg, congenital adrenal hyperplasia, 21-hydroxylase deficiency), common variants (eg, IVS2-13G, P30L, I172N, exon 6 mutation cluster [I235N, V236E, M238K], V281L, L307FfsX6, Q318X, R356W, P453S, G110VfsX21, 30-kb deletion variant) ESR1/PGR (receptor 1/progesterone receptor) ratio (eg, breast cancer) KIT (v-kit Hardy-Zuckerman 4 feline sarcoma viral oncogene homolog) (eg, mastocytosis), common variants (eg, D816V, D816Y, D816F) MEFV (Mediterranean fever) (eg, familial Mediterranean fever), common variants (eg, E148Q, P369S, F479L, M680I, I692del, M694V, M694I, K695R, V726A, A744S, R761H) MPL (myeloproliferative leukemia virus oncogene, thrombopoietin receptor, TPOR) (eg, myeloproliferative disorder), common variants (eg, W515A, W515K, W515L, W515R) TRD@ (T cell antigen receptor, delta) (eg, leukemia and lymphoma), gene rearrangement analysis, evaluation to detect abnormal clonal population

81403 Molecular pathology procedure, Level 4 (eg, analysis of single exon by DNA sequence analysis, analysis of >10 amplicons using multiplex PCR in 2 or more independent reactions, mutation scanning or duplication/deletion variants of 2-5 exons) ABL1 (c-abl oncogene 1, receptor tyrosine kinase) (eg, acquired imatinib tyrosine kinase inhibitor resistance), variants in the kinase domain DAZ/SRY (deleted in azoospermia and sex determining region Y) (eg, male infertility), common deletions (eg, AZFa, AZFb, AZFc, AZFd) GJB1 (gap junction protein, beta 1) (eg, Charcot-Marie-Tooth X-linked), full gene sequence JAK2 (Janus kinase 2) (eg, myeloproliferative disorder), exon 12 sequence and exon 13 sequence, if performed KRAS (v-Ki-ras2 Kirsten rat sarcoma viral oncogene) (eg, carcinoma), gene analysis, variant(s) in exon 2 MPL (myeloproliferative leukemia virus oncogene, thrombopoietin receptor, TPOR) (eg, myeloproliferative disorder), exon 10 sequence VHL (von Hippel-Lindau tumor suppressor) (eg, von Hippel-Lindau familial cancer syndrome), deletion/duplication analysis VWF (von Willebrand factor) (eg, von Willebrand disease types 2A, 2B, 2M), targeted sequence analysis (eg, exon 28)

81404 Molecular pathology procedure, Level 5 (eg, analysis of 2-5 exons by DNA sequence analysis, mutation scanning or duplication/deletion variants of 6-10 exons, or characterization of a dynamic mutation disorder/triplet repeat by Southern blot analysis) BTD (biotinidase) (eg, biotinidase deficiency), full gene sequence CYP1B1 (cytochrome P450, family 1, subfamily B, polypeptide 1) (eg, primary congenital glaucoma), full gene sequence DMPK (dystrophia myotonica-protein kinase) (eg, myotonic dystrophy type 1), characterization of abnormal (eg, expanded) alleles EGR2 (early growth response 2) (eg, Charcot-Marie-Tooth), full gene sequence FKRP (Fukutin related protein) (eg, congenital muscular dystrophy type 1C [MDC1C], limb-girdle muscular dystrophy [LGMD] type 2I), full gene sequence FOXG1 (forkhead box G1) (eg, Rett syndrome), full gene sequence FSHMD1A (facioscapulohumeral muscular dystrophy 1A) (eg, facioscapulohumeral muscular dystrophy), evaluation to detect abnormal (eg, deleted) alleles FSHMD1A (facioscapulohumeral muscular dystrophy 1A) (eg, facioscapulohumeral muscular dystrophy), characterization of haplotype(s) (ie, chromosome 4A and 4B haplotypes) HBB (hemoglobin, beta, Beta-Globin) (eg, thalassemia), full gene sequence KIT (C-kit) (v-kit Hardy-Zuckerman 4 feline sarcoma viral oncogene homolog) (eg, GIST, acute myeloid leukemia, melanoma), targeted gene analysis (eg, exons 8, 11, 13, 17, 18) LITAF (lipopolysaccharide-induced TNF factor) (eg, Charcot-Marie-Tooth), full gene sequence MEFV (Mediterranean fever) (eg, familial Mediterranean fever), full gene sequence NRAS (neuroblastoma RAS viral oncogene homolog) (eg, colorectal carcinoma), exon 1 and exon 2 sequences PDGFRA (platelet-derived growth factor receptor alpha polypeptide) (eg, gastrointestinal stromal tumor), targeted sequence analysis (eg, exons 12, 18) RET (ret proto-oncogene) (eg, multiple endocrine neoplasia, type 2B and familial medullary thyroid carcinoma), common variants (eg, M918T, 2647_2648delinsTT, A883F) SDHD (succinate dehydrogenase complex, subunit D, integral membrane protein) (eg, hereditary paraganglioma), full gene sequence VHL (von Hippel-Lindau tumor suppressor) (eg, von Hippel-Lindau familial cancer syndrome), full gene sequence VWF (von Willebrand factor) (eg, von Willebrand disease type 1C), targeted sequence analysis (eg, exons 26, 27, 37)

81405 Molecular pathology procedure, Level 6 (eg, analysis of 6-10 exons by DNA sequence analysis, mutation scanning or duplication/deletion variants of 11-25 exons) CYP21A2 (cytochrome P450, family 21, subfamily A, polypeptide2) (eg, steroid 21-hydroxylase isoform, congenital adrenal hyperplasia), full gene sequence FKTN (fukutin) (eg, limb-girdle muscular dystrophy [LGMD] type 2M or 2L), full gene sequence MPZ (myelin protein zero) (eg, Charcot-Marie-Tooth), full gene sequence NEFL (neurofilament, light polypeptide) (eg, Charcot-Marie-Tooth), full gene sequence RET (ret proto-oncogene) (eg, multiple endocrine neoplasia, type 2A and familial medullary thyroid carcinoma), targeted sequence analysis (eg, exons 10, 11, 13-16) SDHB (succinate dehydrogenase complex, subunit B, iron sulfur) (eg, hereditary paraganglioma), full gene sequence TGFBR1 (transforming growth factor, beta receptor 1) (eg, Marfan syndrome), full gene sequence TGFBR2 (transforming growth factor, beta receptor 2) (eg, Marfan syndrome), full gene sequence THRB (thyroid hormone receptor, beta) (eg, thyroid hormone resistance, thyroid hormone beta receptor deficiency), full gene sequence or targeted sequence analysis of >5 exons TP53 (tumor protein 53) (eg, Li-Fraumeni syndrome, tumor samples), full gene sequence or targeted sequence analysis of >5 exons VWF (von Willebrand factor) (eg, von Willebrand disease type 2N), targeted sequence analysis (eg, exons 18-20, 23-25)

81406 Molecular pathology procedure, Level 7 (eg, analysis of 11-25 exons by DNA sequence analysis, mutation scanning or duplication/deletion variants of 26-50 exons, cytogenomic array analysis for neoplasia) CAPN3 (Calpain 3) (eg, limb-girdle muscular dystrophy [LGMD] type 2A, calpainopathy), full gene sequence Cytogenomic microarray analysis, neoplasia (eg, interrogation of copy number, and loss-of-heterozygosity via single nucleotide polymorphism [SNP]-based comparative genomic hybridization [CGH] microarray analysis) GALT (galactose-1-phosphate uridylyltransferase) (eg, galactosemia), full gene sequence HEXA (hexosaminidase A, alpha polypeptide) (eg, Tay-Sachs disease), full gene sequence LMNA (lamin A/C) (eg, Emery-Dreifuss muscular dystrophy [EDMD1, 2 and 3] limb-girdle muscular dystrophy [LGMD] type 1B, dilated cardiomyopathy [CMD1A], familial partial lipodystrophy [FPLD2]), full gene sequence PAH (phenylalanine hydroxylase) (eg, phenylketonuria), full gene sequence POLG (polymerase [DNA directed], gamma) (eg, Alpers-Huttenlocher syndrome, autosomal dominant progressive external ophthalmoplegia), full gene sequence POMGNT1 (protein O-linked mannose beta1,2-N acetylglucosaminyltransferase) (eg, muscle-eye-brain disease, Walker-Warburg syndrome), full gene sequence POMT1 (protein-O-mannosyltransferase 1) (eg, limb-girdle muscular dystrophy [LGMD] type 2K, Walker-Warburg syndrome), full gene sequence POMT2 (protein-O-mannosyltransferase 2) (eg, limb-girdle muscular dystrophy [LGMD] type 2N, Walker-Warburg syndrome), full gene sequence RYR1 (ryanodine receptor 1, skeletal) (eg, malignant hyperthermia), targeted sequence analysis of exons with functionally confirmed mutations VWF (von Willebrand factor) (von Willebrand disease type 2A), extended targeted sequence analysis (eg, exons 11-16, 24-26, 51, 52)

81407 Molecular pathology procedure, Level 8 (eg, analysis of 26-50 exons by DNA sequence analysis, mutation scanning or duplication/deletion variants of >50 exons, sequence analysis of multiple genes on one platform) SCN1A (sodium channel, voltage-gated, type 1, alpha subunit) (eg, generalized epilepsy with febrile seizures), full gene sequence

81408 Molecular pathology procedure, Level 9 (eg, analysis of >50 exons in a single gene by DNA sequence analysis) FBN1 (fibrillin 1) (eg, Marfan syndrome), full gene sequence NF1 (neurofibromin 1) (eg, neurofibromatosis, type 1), full gene sequence RYR1 (ryanodine receptor 1, skeletal) (eg, malignant hyperthermia), full gene sequence VWF (von Willebrand factor) (eg, von Willebrand disease types 1 and 3), full gene sequence

86386 Nuclear Matrix Protein 22 (NMP22), qualitative

87389 Infectious agent antigen detection by enzyme immunoassay technique, qualitative or semiquantitative, multiple-step method; HIV-1 antigen(s), with HIV-1 and HIV-2 antibodies, single result

90869 Therapeutic repetitive transcranial magnetic stimulation (TMS) treatment; subsequent motor threshold re-determination with delivery and management

92071 Fitting of contact lens for treatment of ocular surface disease

92072 Fitting of contact lens for management of keratoconus, initial fitting

92558 Evoked otoacoustic emissions, screening (qualitative measurement of distortion product or transient evoked otoacoustic emissions), automated analysis

Appendix B — New, Changed and Deleted Codes

92618 Evaluation for prescription of non-speech-generating augmentative and alternative communication device, face-to-face with the patient; each additional 30 minutes (List separately in addition to code for primary procedure)

93998 Unlisted noninvasive vascular diagnostic study

94726 Plethysmography for determination of lung volumes and, when performed, airway resistance

94727 Gas dilution or washout for determination of lung volumes and, when performed, distribution of ventilation and closing volumes

94728 Airway resistance by impulse oscillometry

94729 Diffusing capacity (eg, carbon monoxide, membrane) (List separately in addition to code for primary procedure)

94780 Car seat/bed testing for airway integrity, neonate, with continual nursing observation and continuous recording of pulse oximetry, heart rate and respiratory rate, with interpretation and report; 60 minutes

94781 Car seat/bed testing for airway integrity, neonate, with continual nursing observation and continuous recording of pulse oximetry, heart rate and respiratory rate, with interpretation and report; each additional full 30 minutes (List separately in addition to code for primary procedure)

95885 Needle electromyography, each extremity, with related paraspinal areas, when performed, done with nerve conduction, amplitude and latency/velocity study; limited (List separately in addition to code for primary procedure)

95886 Needle electromyography, each extremity, with related paraspinal areas, when performed, done with nerve conduction, amplitude and latency/velocity study; complete, five or more muscles studied, innervated by three or more nerves or four or more spinal levels (List separately in addition to code for primary procedure)

95887 Needle electromyography, non-extremity (cranial nerve supplied or axial) muscle(s) done with nerve conduction, amplitude and latency/velocity study (List separately in addition to code for primary procedure)

95938 Short-latency somatosensory evoked potential study, stimulation of any/all peripheral nerves or skin sites, recording from the central nervous system; in upper and lower limbs

95939 Central motor evoked potential study (transcranial motor stimulation); in upper and lower limbs

0262T Implantation of catheter-delivered prosthetic pulmonary valve, endovascular approach

0263T Intramuscular autologous bone marrow cell therapy, with preparation of harvested cells, multiple injections, one leg, including ultrasound guidance, if performed; complete procedure including unilateral or bilateral bone marrow harvest

0264T Intramuscular autologous bone marrow cell therapy, with preparation of harvested cells, multiple injections, 1 leg, including ultrasound guidance, if performed; complete procedure excluding bone marrow harvest

0265T Intramuscular autologous bone marrow cell therapy, with preparation of harvested cells, multiple injections, one leg, including ultrasound guidance, if performed; unilateral or bilateral bone marrow harvest only for intramuscular autologous bone marrow cell therapy

0266T Implantation or replacement of carotid sinus baroreflex activation device; total system (includes generator placement, unilateral or bilateral lead placement, intra-operative interrogation, programming, and repositioning, when performed)

0267T Implantation or replacement of carotid sinus baroreflex activation device; lead only, unilateral (includes intra-operative interrogation, programming, and repositioning, when performed)

0268T Implantation or replacement of carotid sinus baroreflex activation device; pulse generator only (includes intra-operative interrogation, programming, and repositioning, when performed)

0269T Revision or removal of carotid sinus baroreflex activation device; total system (includes generator placement, unilateral or bilateral lead placement, intra-operative interrogation, programming, and repositioning, when performed)

0270T Revision or removal of carotid sinus baroreflex activation device; lead only, unilateral (includes intra-operative interrogation, programming, and repositioning, when performed)

0271T Revision or removal of carotid sinus baroreflex activation device; pulse generator only (includes intra-operative interrogation, programming, and repositioning, when performed)

0272T Interrogation device evaluation (in person), carotid sinus baroreflex activation system, including telemetric iterative communication with the implantable device to monitor device diagnostics and programmed therapy values, with interpretation and report (eg, battery status, lead impedance, pulse amplitude, pulse width, therapy frequency, pathway mode, burst mode, therapy start/stop times each day);

0273T Interrogation device evaluation (in person), carotid sinus baroreflex activation system, including telemetric iterative communication with the implantable device to monitor device diagnostics and programmed therapy values, with interpretation and report (eg, battery status, lead impedance, pulse amplitude, pulse width, therapy frequency, pathway mode, burst mode, therapy start/stop times each day); with programming

0274T Percutaneous laminotomy/laminectomy (intralaminar approach) for decompression of neural elements, (with or without ligamentous resection, discectomy, facetectomy and/or foraminotomy) any method under indirect image guidance (eg, fluoroscopic, CT), with or without the use of an endoscope, single or multiple levels, unilateral or bilateral; cervical or thoracic

0275T Percutaneous laminotomy/laminectomy (intralaminar approach) for decompression of neural elements, (with or without ligamentous resection, discectomy, facetectomy and/or foraminotomy) any method under indirect image guidance (eg, fluoroscopic, CT), with or without the use of an endoscope, single or multiple levels, unilateral or bilateral; lumbar

0276T Bronchoscopy, rigid or flexible, including fluoroscopic guidance, when performed; with bronchial thermoplasty, 1 lobe

0277T Bronchoscopy, rigid or flexible, including fluoroscopic guidance, when performed; with bronchial thermoplasty, 2 or more lobes

0278T Transcutaneous electrical modulation pain reprocessing (eg, scrambler therapy), each treatment session (includes placement of electrodes)

0279T Cell enumeration using immunologic selection and identification in fluid specimen (eg, circulating tumor cells in blood);

0280T Cell enumeration using immunologic selection and identification in fluid specimen (eg, circulating tumor cells in blood); interpretation and report

0281T Percutaneous transcatheter closure of the left atrial appendage with implant, including fluoroscopy, transseptal puncture, catheter placement(s), left atrial angiography, left atrial appendage angiography, radiological supervision and interpretation

0282T Percutaneous or open implantation of neurostimulator electrode array(s), subcutaneous (peripheral subcutaneous field stimulation), including imaging guidance, when performed, cervical, thoracic or lumbar; for trial, including removal at the conclusion of trial period

0283T Percutaneous or open implantation of neurostimulator electrode array(s), subcutaneous (peripheral subcutaneous field stimulation), including imaging guidance, when performed, cervical, thoracic or lumbar; permanent, with implantation of a pulse generator

0284T Revision or removal of pulse generator or electrodes, including imaging guidance, when performed, including addition of new electrodes, when performed

0285T Electronic analysis of implanted peripheral subcutaneous field stimulation pulse generator, with reprogramming when performed

0286T Near-infrared spectroscopy studies of lower extremity wounds (eg, for oxyhemoglobin measurement)

0287T Near-infrared guidance for vascular access requiring real-time digital visualization of subcutaneous vasculature for evaluation of potential access sites and vessel patency

0288T Anoscopy, with delivery of thermal energy to the muscle of the anal canal (eg, for fecal incontinence)

0289T Corneal incisions in the donor cornea created using a laser, in preparation for penetrating or lamellar keratoplasty (List separately in addition to code for primary procedure)

0290T Corneal incisions in the recipient cornea created using a laser, in preparation for penetrating or lamellar keratoplasty (List separately in addition to code for primary procedure)

0291T Intravascular optical coherence tomography (coronary native vessel or graft) during diagnostic evaluation and/or therapeutic intervention, including imaging supervision, interpretation, and report; initial vessel (List separately in addition to primary procedure)

0292T Intravascular optical coherence tomography (coronary native vessel or graft) during diagnostic evaluation and/or therapeutic intervention, including imaging supervision, interpretation, and report; each additional vessel (List separately in addition to primary procedure)

0293T Insertion of left atrial hemodynamic monitor; complete system, includes implanted communication module and pressure sensor lead in left atrium including transseptal access, radiological supervision and interpretation, and associated injection procedures, when performed

0294T Insertion of left atrial hemodynamic monitor; pressure sensor lead at time of insertion of pacing cardioverter-defibrillator pulse generator including radiological supervision and interpretation and associated injection procedures, when performed (List separately in addition to code for primary procedure)

0295T External electrocardiographic recording for more than 48 hours up to 21 days by continuous rhythm recording and storage; includes recording, scanning analysis with report, review and interpretation

0296T External electrocardiographic recording for more than 48 hours up to 21 days by continuous rhythm recording and storage; recording (includes connection and initial recording)

0297T External electrocardiographic recording for more than 48 hours up to 21 days by continuous rhythm recording and storage; scanning analysis with report

0298T External electrocardiographic recording for more than 48 hours up to 21 days by continuous rhythm recording and storage; review and interpretation

0299T Extracorporeal shock wave for integumentary wound healing, high energy, including topical application and dressing care; initial wound

0300T Extracorporeal shock wave for integumentary wound healing, high energy, including topical application and dressing care; each additional wound (List separately in addition to code for primary procedure)

0301T Destruction/reduction of malignant breast tumor with externally applied focused microwave, including interstitial placement of disposable catheter with combined temperature monitoring probe and microwave focusing sensocatheter under ultrasound thermotherapy guidance

0550F Cytopathology report on routine nongynecologic specimen finalized within two working days of accession date (PATH)

0551F Cytopathology report on nongynecologic specimen with documentation that the specimen was nonroutine (PATH)

0555F Symptom management plan of care documented (HF)

0556F Plan of care to achieve lipid control documented (CAD)

0557F Plan of care to manage anginal symptoms documented (CAD)

1010F Severity of angina assessed by level of activity (CAD)

1011F Angina present (CAD)

1012F Angina absent (CAD)

1031F Smoking status and exposure to secondhand smoke in the home assessed (Asthma)

1032F Current tobacco smoker OR currently exposed to secondhand smoke (asthma)

1033F Current tobacco nonsmoker AND not currently exposed to secondhand smoke (Asthma)

1052F Type, anatomic location, and activity all assessed (IBD)

1175F Functional status for dementia assessed and results reviewed (DEM)

1181F Neuropsychiatric symptoms assessed and results reviewed (DEM)

1182F Neuropsychiatric symptoms, one or more present (DEM)

1183F Neuropsychiatric symptoms, absent (DEM)

1450F Symptoms improved or remained consistent with treatment goals since last assessment (HF)

1451F Symptoms demonstrated clinically important deterioration since last assessment (HF)

1460F Qualifying cardiac event/diagnosis in previous 12 months (CAD)

1461F No qualifying cardiac event/diagnosis in previous 12 months (CAD)

1490F Dementia severity classified, mild (DEM)

1491F Dementia severity classified, moderate (DEM)

1493F Dementia severity classified, severe (DEM)

1494F Cognition assessed and reviewed (DEM)

2015F Asthma impairment assessed (Asthma)

2016F Asthma risk assessed (Asthma)

3019F Left ventricular ejection fraction (LVEF) assessment planned post discharge (HF)

3055F Left ventricular ejection fraction (LVEF) less than or equal to 35% (HF)

3056F Left ventricular ejection fraction (LVEF) greater than 35% or no LVEF result available (HF)

3115F Quantitative results of an evaluation of current level of activity and clinical symptoms (HF)

3117F Heart failure disease specific structured assessment tool completed (HF)

3118F New York Heart Association (NYHA) Class documented (HF)

3119F No evaluation of level of activity or clinical symptoms (HF)

3125F Esophageal biopsy report with statement about dysplasia (present, absent, or indefinite) (PATH)

3267F Pathology report includes pT category, pN category, Gleason score and statement about margin status (PATH)

3394F Quantitative HER2 Immunohistochemistry (IHC) evaluation of breast cancer consistent with the scoring system defined in the ASCO/CAP guidelines (PATH)

3395F Quantitative non-HER2 Immunohistochemistry (IHC) evaluation of breast cancer (eg, testing for estrogen or progesterone receptors [ER/PR]) performed (PATH)

3517F Hepatitis B virus (HBV) status assessed and results interpreted within one year prior to receiving first course of anti-TNF (tumor necrosis factor) therapy (IBD)

3520F Clostridium difficile testing performed (IBD)

3725F Screening for depression performed (DEM)

3750F Patient not receiving dose of corticosteroids greater than or equal to 10mg/day for 60 or greater consecutive days (IBD)

4008F Beta blocker therapy prescribed or currently being taken (CAD, HF)

4010F Angiotensin converting enzyme (ACE) inhibitor or angiotensin receptor blocker (ARB) therapy prescribed or currently being taken (CAD, CKD, HF) (DM)

4013F Statin therapy prescribed or currently being taken (CAD)

4069F Venous thromboembolism (VTE) prophylaxis received (IBD)

4086F Aspirin or clopidogrel prescribed (CAD)

4140F Inhaled corticosteroids prescribed (Asthma)

4142F Corticosteroid sparing therapy prescribed (IBD)

4144F Alternative long-term control medication prescribed (Asthma)

4145F Two or more anti-hypertensive agents prescribed or currently being taken (CAD, HTN)

4322F Caregiver provided with education and referred to additional resources for support (DEM)

4350F Counseling provided on symptom management, end of life decision, and palliation (DEM)

4450F Self-care education provided to patient (HF)

4470F Implantable cardioverter-defibrillator (ICD) counseling provided (HF)

4480F Patient receiving ACE inhibitor/ARB therapy and beta-blocker therapy for 3 months or longer (HF)

4481F Patient receiving ACE inhibitor/ARB therapy and beta-blocker therapy for less than 3 months (HF)

4500F Referred to an outpatient cardiac rehabilitation program (CAD)

4510F Previous cardiac rehabilitation for qualifying cardiac event completed (CAD)

4525F Neuropsychiatric intervention ordered (DEM)

4526F Neuropsychiatric intervention received (DEM)

5250F Asthma discharge plan present (Asthma)

6100F Timeout to verify correct patient, correct site, and correct procedure, documented (PATH)

6101F Safety counseling for dementia provided (DEM)

6102F Safety counseling for dementia ordered (DEM)

6110F Counseling provided regarding risks of driving and the alternatives to driving (DEM)

6150F Patient not receiving a first course of anti-TNF (tumor necrosis factor) therapy (IBD)

Changed Codes

15150 Tissue cultured skin autograft, trunk, arms, legs; first 25 sq cm or less

15151 Tissue cultured skin autograft, trunk, arms, legs; additional 1 sq cm to 75 sq cm (List separately in addition to code for primary procedure)

15152 Tissue cultured skin autograft, trunk, arms, legs; each additional 100 sq cm, or each additional 1% of body area of infants and children, or part thereof (List separately in addition to code for primary procedure)

15155 Tissue cultured skin autograft, face, scalp, eyelids, mouth, neck, ears, orbits, genitalia, hands, feet, and/or multiple digits; first 25 sq cm or less

15156 Tissue cultured skin autograft, face, scalp, eyelids, mouth, neck, ears, orbits, genitalia, hands, feet, and/or multiple digits; additional 1 sq cm to 75 sq cm (List separately in addition to code for primary procedure)

15157 Tissue cultured skin autograft, face, scalp, eyelids, mouth, neck, ears, orbits, genitalia, hands, feet, and/or multiple digits; each additional 100 sq cm, or each additional 1% of body area of infants and children, or part thereof (List separately in addition to code for primary procedure)

22520 Percutaneous vertebroplasty (bone biopsy included when performed), 1 vertebral body, unilateral or bilateral injection; thoracic

22521 Percutaneous vertebroplasty (bone biopsy included when performed), 1 vertebral body, unilateral or bilateral injection; lumbar

22522 Percutaneous vertebroplasty (bone biopsy included when performed), 1 vertebral body, unilateral or bilateral injection; each additional thoracic or lumbar vertebral body (List separately in addition to code for primary procedure)

22610 Arthrodesis, posterior or posterolateral technique, single level; thoracic (with lateral transverse technique, when performed)

22612 Arthrodesis, posterior or posterolateral technique, single level; lumbar (with lateral transverse technique, when performed)

27096 Injection procedure for sacroiliac joint, anesthetic/steroid, with image guidance (fluoroscopy or CT) including arthrography when performed

29581 Application of multi-layer compression system; leg (below knee), including ankle and foot

29826 Arthroscopy, shoulder, surgical; decompression of subacromial space with partial acromioplasty, with coracoacromial ligament (ie, arch) release, when performed (List separately in addition to code for primary procedure)

29880 Arthroscopy, knee, surgical; with meniscectomy (medial AND lateral, including any meniscal shaving) including debridement/shaving of articular cartilage (chondroplasty), same or separate compartment(s), when performed

29881 Arthroscopy, knee, surgical; with meniscectomy (medial OR lateral, including any meniscal shaving) including debridement/shaving of articular cartilage (chondroplasty), same or separate compartment(s), when performed

32100 Thoracotomy; with exploration

32110 Thoracotomy; with control of traumatic hemorrhage and/or repair of lung tear

32120 Thoracotomy; for postoperative complications

32124 Thoracotomy; with open intrapleural pneumonolysis

32140 Thoracotomy; with cyst(s) removal, includes pleural procedure when performed

32141 Thoracotomy; with resection-plication of bullae, includes any pleural procedure when performed

32150 Thoracotomy; with removal of intrapleural foreign body or fibrin deposit

32151 Thoracotomy; with removal of intrapulmonary foreign body

32160 Thoracotomy; with cardiac massage

32440 Removal of lung, pneumonectomy;

32442 Removal of lung, pneumonectomy; with resection of segment of trachea followed by broncho-tracheal anastomosis (sleeve pneumonectomy)

32445 Removal of lung, pneumonectomy; extrapleural

32480 Removal of lung, other than pneumonectomy; single lobe (lobectomy)

32482 Removal of lung, other than pneumonectomy; 2 lobes (bilobectomy)

32484 Removal of lung, other than pneumonectomy; single segment (segmentectomy)

32486 Removal of lung, other than pneumonectomy; with circumferential resection of segment of bronchus followed by broncho-bronchial anastomosis (sleeve lobectomy)

32488 Removal of lung, other than pneumonectomy; with all remaining lung following previous removal of a portion of lung (completion pneumonectomy)

32491 Removal of lung, other than pneumonectomy; with resection-plication of emphysematous lung(s) (bullous or non-bullous) for lung volume reduction, sternal split or transthoracic approach, includes any pleural procedure, when performed

32601 Thoracoscopy, diagnostic (separate procedure); lungs, pericardial sac, mediastinal or pleural space, without biopsy

32655 Thoracoscopy, surgical; with resection-plication of bullae, includes any pleural procedure when performed

32663 Thoracoscopy, surgical; with lobectomy (single lobe)

33050 Resection of pericardial cyst or tumor

33206 Insertion of new or replacement of permanent pacemaker with transvenous electrode(s); atrial

33207 Insertion of new or replacement of permanent pacemaker with transvenous electrode(s); ventricular

33208 Insertion of new or replacement of permanent pacemaker with transvenous electrode(s); atrial and ventricular

33212 Insertion of pacemaker pulse generator only; with existing single lead

33213 Insertion of pacemaker pulse generator only; with existing dual leads

33218 Repair of single transvenous electrode, permanent pacemaker or pacing cardioverter-defibrillator

33220 Repair of 2 transvenous electrodes for permanent pacemaker or pacing cardioverter-defibrillator

33224 Insertion of pacing electrode, cardiac venous system, for left ventricular pacing, with attachment to previously placed pacemaker or pacing cardioverter-defibrillator pulse generator (including revision of pocket, removal, insertion, and/or replacement of existing generator)

33225 Insertion of pacing electrode, cardiac venous system, for left ventricular pacing, at time of insertion of pacing cardioverter-defibrillator or pacemaker pulse generator (including upgrade to dual chamber system and pocket revision) (List separately in addition to code for primary procedure)

33226 Repositioning of previously implanted cardiac venous system (left ventricular) electrode (including removal, insertion and/or replacement of existing generator)"

33233 Removal of permanent pacemaker pulse generator only

33240 Insertion of pacing cardioverter-defibrillator pulse generator only; with existing single lead

33241 Removal of pacing cardioverter-defibrillator pulse generator only

33249 Insertion or replacement of permanent pacing cardioverter-defibrillator system with transvenous lead(s), single or dual chamber

33960 Prolonged extracorporeal circulation for cardiopulmonary insufficiency; initial day

33961 Prolonged extracorporeal circulation for cardiopulmonary insufficiency; each subsequent day

38208 Transplant preparation of hematopoietic progenitor cells; thawing of previously frozen harvest, without washing, per donor

38209 Transplant preparation of hematopoietic progenitor cells; thawing of previously frozen harvest, with washing, per donor

38230 Bone marrow harvesting for transplantation; allogeneic

38746 Thoracic lymphadenectomy by thoracotomy, mediastinal and regional lymphadenectomy (List separately in addition to code for primary procedure)

38792 Injection procedure; radioactive tracer for identification of sentinel node

39200 Resection of mediastinal cyst

39220 Resection of mediastinal tumor

39400 Mediastinoscopy, includes biopsy(ies), when performed

62287 Decompression procedure, percutaneous, of nucleus pulposus of intervertebral disc, any method utilizing needle based technique to remove disc material under fluoroscopic imaging or other form of indirect visualization, with the use of an endoscope, with discography and/or epidural injection(s) at the treated level(s), when performed, single or multiple levels, lumbar

62310 Injection(s), of diagnostic or therapeutic substance(s) (including anesthetic, antispasmodic, opioid, steroid, other solution), not including neurolytic substances, including needle or catheter placement, includes contrast for localization when performed, epidural or subarachnoid; cervical or thoracic

62311 Injection(s), of diagnostic or therapeutic substance(s) (including anesthetic, antispasmodic, opioid, steroid, other solution), not including neurolytic substances, including needle or catheter placement, includes contrast for localization when performed, epidural or subarachnoid; lumbar or sacral (caudal)

62318 Injection(s), including indwelling catheter placement, continuous infusion or intermittent bolus, of diagnostic or therapeutic substance(s) (including anesthetic, antispasmodic, opioid, steroid, other solution), not including neurolytic substances, includes contrast for localization when performed, epidural or subarachnoid; cervical or thoracic

62319 Injection(s), including indwelling catheter placement, continuous infusion or intermittent bolus, of diagnostic or therapeutic substance(s) (including anesthetic, antispasmodic, opioid, steroid, other solution), not including neurolytic substances, includes contrast for localization when performed, epidural or subarachnoid; lumbar or sacral (caudal)

62367 Electronic analysis of programmable, implanted pump for intrathecal or epidural drug infusion (includes evaluation of reservoir status, alarm status, drug prescription status); without reprogramming or refill

63020 Laminotomy (hemilaminectomy), with decompression of nerve root(s), including partial facetectomy, foraminotomy and/or excision of herniated intervertebral disc; 1 interspace, cervical

63030 Laminotomy (hemilaminectomy), with decompression of nerve root(s), including partial facetectomy, foraminotomy and/or excision of herniated intervertebral disc; 1 interspace, lumbar

63035 Laminotomy (hemilaminectomy), with decompression of nerve root(s), including partial facetectomy, foraminotomy and/or excision of herniated intervertebral disc; each additional interspace, cervical or lumbar (List separately in addition to code for primary procedure)

64553 Percutaneous implantation of neurostimulator electrode array; cranial nerve

64555 Percutaneous implantation of neurostimulator electrode array; peripheral nerve (excludes sacral nerve)

64561 Percutaneous implantation of neurostimulator electrode array; sacral nerve (transforaminal placement)

64565 Percutaneous implantation of neurostimulator electrode array; neuromuscular

64575 Incision for implantation of neurostimulator electrode array; peripheral nerve (excludes sacral nerve)

64580 Incision for implantation of neurostimulator electrode array; neuromuscular

64581 Incision for implantation of neurostimulator electrode array; sacral nerve (transforaminal placement)

64585 Revision or removal of peripheral neurostimulator electrode array

70355 Orthopantogram (eg, panoramic x-ray)

72114 Radiologic examination, spine, lumbosacral; complete, including bending views, minimum of 6 views

72120 Radiologic examination, spine, lumbosacral; bending views only, 2 or 3 views

75962 Transluminal balloon angioplasty, peripheral artery other than renal, or other visceral artery, iliac or lower extremity, radiological supervision and interpretation

75964 Transluminal balloon angioplasty, each additional peripheral artery other than renal, or other visceral artery, iliac or lower extremity, radiological supervision and interpretation (List separately in addition to code for primary procedure)

77003 Fluoroscopic guidance and localization of needle or catheter tip for spine or paraspinous diagnostic or therapeutic injection procedures (epidural or subarachnoid)

77470 Special treatment procedure (eg, total body irradiation, hemibody radiation, per oral or endocavitary irradiation)

78580 Pulmonary perfusion imaging (eg, particulate)

86703 Antibody; HIV-1 and HIV-2, single result

87502 Infectious agent detection by nucleic acid (DNA or RNA); influenza virus, for multiple types or sub-types, multiplex reverse transcription and amplified probe technique, first 2 types or sub-types

88312 Special stain including interpretation and report; Group I for microorganisms (eg, acid fast, methenamine silver)

88313 Special stain including interpretation and report; Group II, all other (eg, iron, trichrome), except stain for microorganisms, stains for enzyme constituents, or immunocytochemistry and immunohistochemistry

88314 Special stain including interpretation and report; histochemical stain on frozen tissue block (List separately in addition to code for primary procedure)

88319 Special stain including interpretation and report; Group III, for enzyme constituents

90460 Immunization administration through 18 years of age via any route of administration, with counseling by physician or other qualified health care professional; first or only component of each vaccine or toxoid administered

90461 Immunization administration through 18 years of age via any route of administration, with counseling by physician or other qualified health care professional; each additional vaccine or toxoid component administered (List separately in addition to code for primary procedure)

90581 Anthrax vaccine, for subcutaneous or intramuscular use

90644 Meningococcal conjugate vaccine, serogroups C & Y and Hemophilus influenza B vaccine (Hib-MenCY), 4 dose schedule, when administered to children 2-15 months of age, for intramuscular use

90867 Therapeutic repetitive transcranial magnetic stimulation (TMS) treatment; initial, including cortical mapping, motor threshold determination, delivery and management

90868 Therapeutic repetitive transcranial magnetic stimulation (TMS) treatment; subsequent delivery and management, per session

91010 Esophageal motility (manometric study of the esophagus and/or gastroesophageal junction) study with interpretation and report;

91013 Esophageal motility (manometric study of the esophagus and/or gastroesophageal junction) study with interpretation and report; with stimulation or perfusion (eg, stimulant, acid or alkali perfusion) (List separately in addition to code for primary procedure)

92587 Distortion product evoked otoacoustic emissions; limited evaluation (to confirm the presence or absence of hearing disorder, 3-6 frequencies) or transient evoked otoacoustic emissions, with interpretation and report

92588 Distortion product evoked otoacoustic emissions; comprehensive diagnostic evaluation (quantitative analysis of outer hair cell function by cochlear mapping, minimum of 12 frequencies), with interpretation and report

92605 Evaluation for prescription of non-speech-generating augmentative and alternative communication device, face-to-face with the patient; first hour

92621 Evaluation of central auditory function, with report; each additional 15 minutes (List separately in addition to code for primary procedure)

93561 Indicator dilution studies such as dye or thermodilution, including arterial and/or venous catheterization; with cardiac output measurement (separate procedure)

93562 Indicator dilution studies such as dye or thermodilution, including arterial and/or venous catheterization; subsequent measurement of cardiac output

95970 Electronic analysis of implanted neurostimulator pulse generator system (eg, rate, pulse amplitude, pulse duration, configuration of wave form, battery status, electrode selectability, output modulation, cycling, impedance and patient compliance measurements); simple or complex brain, spinal cord, or peripheral (ie, cranial nerve, peripheral nerve, sacral nerve, neuromuscular) neurostimulator pulse generator/transmitter, without reprogramming

95971 Electronic analysis of implanted neurostimulator pulse generator system (eg, rate, pulse amplitude, pulse duration, configuration of wave form, battery status, electrode selectability, output modulation, cycling, impedance and patient compliance measurements); simple spinal cord, or peripheral (ie, peripheral nerve, sacral nerve, neuromuscular) neurostimulator pulse generator/transmitter, with intraoperative or subsequent programming

95972 Electronic analysis of implanted neurostimulator pulse generator system (eg, rate, pulse amplitude, pulse duration, configuration of wave form, battery status, electrode selectability, output modulation, cycling, impedance and patient compliance measurements); complex spinal cord, or peripheral (ie, peripheral nerve, sacral nerve, neuromuscular) (except cranial nerve) neurostimulator pulse generator/transmitter, with intraoperative or subsequent programming, first hour

95973 Electronic analysis of implanted neurostimulator pulse generator system (eg, rate, pulse amplitude, pulse duration, configuration of wave form, battery status, electrode selectability, output modulation, cycling, impedance and patient compliance measurements); complex spinal cord, or peripheral (ie, peripheral nerve, sacral nerve, neuromuscular) (except cranial nerve) neurostimulator pulse generator/transmitter, with intraoperative or subsequent programming, each additional 30 minutes after first hour (List separately in addition to code for primary procedure)

95974 Electronic analysis of implanted neurostimulator pulse generator system (eg, rate, pulse amplitude, pulse duration, configuration of wave form, battery status, electrode selectability, output modulation, cycling, impedance and patient compliance measurements); complex cranial nerve neurostimulator pulse generator/transmitter, with intraoperative or subsequent programming, with or without nerve interface testing, first hour

95975 Electronic analysis of implanted neurostimulator pulse generator system (eg, rate, pulse amplitude, pulse duration, configuration of wave form, battery status, electrode selectability, output modulation, cycling, impedance and patient compliance measurements); complex cranial nerve neurostimulator pulse generator/transmitter, with intraoperative or subsequent programming, each additional 30 minutes after first hour (List separately in addition to code for primary procedure)

95990 Refilling and maintenance of implantable pump or reservoir for drug delivery, spinal (intrathecal, epidural) or brain (intraventricular), includes electronic analysis of pump, when performed;

95991 Refilling and maintenance of implantable pump or reservoir for drug delivery, spinal (intrathecal, epidural) or brain (intraventricular), includes electronic analysis of pump, when performed; requiring physician's skill

96110 Developmental screening, with interpretation and report, per standardized instrument form

96111 Developmental testing, (includes assessment of motor, language, social, adaptive, and/or cognitive functioning by standardized developmental instruments) with interpretation and report

96367 Intravenous infusion, for therapy, prophylaxis, or diagnosis (specify substance or drug); additional sequential infusion of a new drug/substance, up to 1 hour (List separately in addition to code for primary procedure)

99218 Initial observation care, per day, for the evaluation and management of a patient which requires these 3 key components: A detailed or comprehensive history; A detailed or comprehensive examination; and Medical decision making that is straightforward or of low complexity. Counseling and/or coordination of care with other providers or agencies are provided consistent with the nature of the problem(s) and the patient's and/or family's needs. Usually, the problem(s) requiring admission to "observation status" are of low severity. Physicians typically spend 30 minutes at the bedside and on the patient's hospital floor or unit.

99219 Initial observation care, per day, for the evaluation and management of a patient, which requires these 3 key components: A comprehensive history; A comprehensive examination; and Medical decision making of moderate complexity. Counseling and/or coordination of care with other providers or agencies are provided consistent with the nature of the problem(s) and the patient's and/or family's needs. Usually, the problem(s) requiring admission to "observation status" are of moderate severity. Physicians typically spend 50 minutes at the bedside and on the patient's hospital floor or unit.

99220 Initial observation care, per day, for the evaluation and management of a patient, which requires these 3 key components: A comprehensive history; A comprehensive examination; and Medical decision making of high complexity. Counseling and/or coordination of care with other providers or agencies are provided consistent with the nature of the problem(s) and the patient's and/or family's needs. Usually, the problem(s) requiring admission to "observation status" are of high severity. Physicians typically spend 70 minutes at the bedside and on the patient's hospital floor or unit.

99354 Prolonged service in the office or other outpatient setting requiring direct patient contact beyond the usual service; first hour (List separately in addition to code for office or other outpatient Evaluation and Management service)

99355 Prolonged service in the office or other outpatient setting requiring direct patient contact beyond the usual service; each additional 30 minutes (List separately in addition to code for prolonged service)

99356 Prolonged service in the inpatient or observation setting, requiring unit/floor time beyond the usual service; first hour (List separately in addition to code for inpatient Evaluation and Management service)

99357 Prolonged service in the inpatient or observation setting, requiring unit/floor time beyond the usual service; each additional 30 minutes (List separately in addition to code for prolonged service)

99358 Prolonged evaluation and management service before and/or after direct patient care; first hour

99359 Prolonged evaluation and management service before and/or after direct patient care; each additional 30 minutes (List separately in addition to code for prolonged service)

0001F Heart failure assessed (includes assessment of all the following components) (CAD): Blood pressure measured (2000F) Level of activity assessed (1003F) Clinical symptoms of volume overload (excess) assessed (1004F) Weight, recorded (2001F) Clinical signs of volume overload (excess) assessed (2002F)

0080T Endovascular repair using prosthesis of abdominal aortic aneurysm, pseudoaneurysm or dissection, abdominal aorta involving visceral vessels (superior mesenteric, celiac and/or renal artery[s]), radiological supervision and interpretation

0240T Esophageal motility (manometric study of the esophagus and/or gastroesophageal junction) study with interpretation and report; with high resolution esophageal pressure topography

0241T Esophageal motility (manometric study of the esophagus and/or gastroesophageal junction) study with interpretation and report; with stimulation or perfusion during high resolution esophageal pressure topography study (eg, stimulant, acid or alkali perfusion) (List separately in addition to code for primary procedure)

0261T Selective head hypothermia, per day, in the neonate 28 days of age or younger

1002F Anginal symptoms and level of activity assessed (NMA-No Measure Associated)

1003F Level of activity assessed (NMA)

1004F Clinical symptoms of volume overload (excess) assessed (NMA-No Measure Associated)

1005F Asthma symptoms evaluated (includes physician documentation of numeric frequency of symptoms or patient completion of an asthma assessment tool/survey/questionnaire) (NMA-No Measure Associated)

1036F Current tobacco non-user (CAD, CAP, COPD, PV) (DM) (IBD)

1123F Advance care planning discussed and documented advance care plan or surrogate decision maker documented in the medical record (DEM) (GER, Pall Cr)

1124F Advance care planning discussed and documented in the medical record, patient did not wish or was not able to name a surrogate decision maker or provide an advance care plan (DEM) (GER, Pall Cr)

2002F Clinical signs of volume overload (excess) assessed (NMA-No Measure Associated)

3020F Left ventricular function (LVF) assessment (eg, echocardiography, nuclear test, or ventriculography) documented in the medical record (Includes quantitative or qualitative assessment results) (NMA-No Measure Associated)

3048F Most recent LDL-C less than 100 mg/dL (CAD), (DM)

3049F Most recent LDL-C 100-129 mg/dL (CAD), (DM)

3050F Most recent LDL-C greater than or equal to 130 mg/dL (CAD), (DM)

3074F Most recent systolic blood pressure less than 130 mm Hg (DM) (HTN, CKD,CAD)

3075F Most recent systolic blood pressure 130 - 139 mm Hg (DM) (HTN, CKD, CAD)

3077F Most recent systolic blood pressure greater than or equal to 140 mm Hg (DM) (HTN, CKD, CAD)

3078F Most recent diastolic blood pressure less than 80 mm Hg (DM) (HTN, CKD, CAD)

3079F Most recent diastolic blood pressure 80-89 mm Hg (DM) (HTN, CKD, CAD)

3080F Most recent diastolic blood pressure greater than or equal to 90 mm Hg (DM) (HTN, CKD, CAD)

3095F Central dual-energy X-ray absorptiometry (DXA) results documented (OP) (IBD)

3096F Central dual-energy X-ray absorptiometry (DXA) ordered (OP) (IBD)

3111F CT or MRI of the brain performed in the hospital within 24 hours of arrival OR performed in an outpatient imaging center, to confirm initial diagnosis of stroke, TIA or intracranial hemorrhage (STR)

3112F CT or MRI of the brain performed greater than 24 hours after arrival to the hospital OR performed in an outpatient imaging center for purpose other than confirmation of initial diagnosis of stroke, TIA, or intracranial hemorrhage (STR)

3216F Patient has documented immunity to Hepatitis B (HEP C), (IBD)

3510F Documentation that tuberculosis (TB) screening test performed and results interpreted (HIV) (IBD)

4000F Tobacco use cessation intervention, counseling (COPD, CAP, CAD, Asthma)(DM)(PV)

4001F Tobacco use cessation intervention, pharmacologic therapy (COPD, CAP,CAD, Asthma)(DM)(PV)

4003F Patient education, written/oral, appropriate for patients with heart failure, performed (NMA-No Measure Associated)

4004F Patient screened for tobacco use AND received tobacco cessation (intervention, counseling, pharmacotherapy, or both) if identified as a tobacco user (PV, CAD)

4005F Pharmacologic therapy (other than minerals/vitamins) for osteoporosis prescribed (OP) (IBD)

4012F Warfarin therapy prescribed (NMA-No Measure Associated)

4014F Written discharge instructions provided to heart failure patients discharged home (Instructions include all of the following components: activity level, diet, discharge medications, follow-up appointment, weight monitoring, what to do if symptoms worsen) (NMA-No Measure Associated)

4015F Persistent asthma, preferred long term control medication or an acceptable alternative treatment, prescribed (NMA-No Measure Associated)

4035F Influenza immunization recommended (COPD) (IBD)

4037F Influenza immunization ordered or administered (COPD, PV, CKD, ESRD) (IBD)

4040F Pneumococcal vaccine administered or previously received (COPD), (IBD), (PV)

4050F Hypertension plan of care documented as appropriate (NMA-No Measure Associated)

AMA Icon Changes

36200, 36245, 36246, 36247, 36248

Deleted Codes

11975	11977	15170	15171	15175	15176	15300
15301	15320	15321	15330	15331	15335	15336
15340	15341	15360	15361	15365	15366	15400
15401	15420	15421	15430	15431	32095	32402
32500	32602	32603	32605	32657	32660	35548
35549	35551	35651	37620	49080	49081	64560
64577	64622	64623	64626	64627	69802	71090
73542	75722	75724	75940	77079	77083	78220
78223	78584	78585	78586	78587	78588	78591
78593	78594	78596	88107	88318	90470	90663
92070	92120	92130	93720	93721	93722	93875
94240	94260	94350	94360	94370	94720	94725
0143T	0155T	0156T	0157T	0158T	0166T	0167T
0168T	4002F	4006F	4009F	4275F		

Code 90470 H1N1 immunization administration (intramuscular, intranasal), including counseling when performed, was deleted in 2011 with a retroactive deletion date of December 31, 2010.

APPENDIX C — CROSSWALK OF DELETED CODES

The deleted code crosswalk is meant to be used as a reference tool to find active codes that could be used in place of the deleted code. This will not always be an exact match. Please review the code descriptions and guidelines before selecting a code.

Code	Cross reference
11975	To report, see ~11981
11977	To report, see ~11976, 11981
15170	To report, see ~15271, 15273
15171	To report, see ~15272, 15274
15175	To report, see ~15275, 15277
15176	To report, see ~15276, 15278
15300	To report, see ~15271, 15273
15301	To report, see ~15272, 15274
15320	To report, see ~15275, 15277
15321	To report, see ~15276, 15278
15330	To report, see ~15271, 15273
15331	To report, see ~15272, 15274
15335	To report, see ~15275, 15277
15336	To report, see ~15276, 15278
15340	To report, see ~15271, 15273, 15275, 15277
15341	To report, see ~15272, 15274, 15276, 15278
15360	To report, see ~15271, 15273
15361	To report, see ~15272, 15274
15365	To report, see ~15275, 15277
15366	To report, see ~15276, 15278
15400	To report, see ~15271, 15273
15401	To report, see ~15272, 15274
15420	To report, see ~15275, 15277
15421	To report, see ~15276, 15278
15430	To report, see ~15271, 15273, 15275, 15277
15431	To report, see ~15272, 15274, 15276, 15278
32095	To report, see ~32096-32098
32402	To report, see ~32098
32500	To report, see ~32505-32507
32602	To report, see ~32607-32609

Code	Cross reference
32603	To report, see ~32601
32605	To report, see ~32601
32657	To report, see ~32666-32668
35548	To report, see ~35537, 35539, 35565
35549	To report, see ~35540, 35565
35551	To report, see ~35539-35540, 35556, 35583
35651	To report, see ~35646-35647, 35656
37620	To report, see ~37191, 37619
49080	To report, see ~49082-49084
49081	To report, see ~49082-49084
64622	To report, see ~64635
64623	To report, see ~64636
64626	To report, see ~64633
64627	To report, see ~64634
69802	To report, see ~69501-69511, 69601-69605, 69635-69646, 69801, 69905-69910
71090	To report, see ~33206-33249, or 76000
73542	To report, see ~27096
75722	To report, see ~36251, 36253
75724	To report, see ~36252, 36254
75940	To report, see ~37191
77079	To report, see ~77078, 77080-77081
77083	To report, see ~77080-77082
78223	To report, see ~78226-78227
78584	To report, see ~78579-78598
78585	To report, see ~78579-78598
78586	To report, see ~78579, 78582, 78598
78587	To report, see ~78579, 78582, 78598
78588	To report, see ~78579-78598
78591	To report, see ~78579, 78582
78593	To report, see ~78579, 78582, 78598
78594	To report, see ~78579, 78582, 78598

Code	Cross reference
78596	To report, see ~78580-78598
88107	To report, see ~88104, 88106
88318	To report, see ~88313
92070	To report, see ~92071-92072
92120	To report, see ~92002, 92012-92014, 92100, 99211-99215
92130	To report, see ~92002-92004, 92012-92014, 92100, 99211-99215
93720	To report, see ~94726, 94750
93721	To report, see ~94726, 94750
93722	To report, see ~94726, 94750
94240	To report, see ~94726-94727
94260	To report, see ~94726-94727
94350	To report, see ~94726-94727
94360	To report, see ~94726, 94728
94370	To report, see ~94726-94727
94720	To report, see ~94729
94725	To report, see ~94729
0141T	To report, see ~48160, 48999
0142T	To report, see ~48160, 48999
0143T	To report, see ~48160, 48999
0155T	To report, see ~43659
0156T	To report, see ~43659
0157T	To report, see ~43999
0158T	To report, see ~43999
0166T	To report, see ~33999
0167T	To report, see ~33999
0168T	To report, see ~30999
4002F	To report, see ~4013F
4006F	To report, see ~4008F
4009F	To report, see ~4010F
4275F	To report, see ~4149F

APPENDIX D: RESEQUENCED CODES

Code	Description	Reference
11045	Debridement, subcutaneous tissue (includes epidermis and dermis, if performed); each additional 20 sq cm, or part thereof (List separately in addition to code for primary procedure)	Resequenced code, See code following 11042.
11046	Debridement, muscle and/or fascia (includes epidermis, dermis, and subcutaneous tissue, if performed); each additional 20 sq cm, or part thereof (List separately in addition to code for primary procedure)	Resequenced code, See code following 11043.
21552	Excision, tumor, soft tissue of neck or anterior thorax, subcutaneous; 3 cm or greater	Resequenced code, See code following 21555.
21554	Excision, tumor, soft tissue of neck or anterior thorax, subfascial (eg, intramuscular); 5 cm or greater	Resequenced code, See code following 21556.
23071	Excision, tumor, soft tissue of shoulder area, subcutaneous; 3 cm or greater	Resequenced code, See code following 23075.
23073	Excision, tumor, soft tissue of shoulder area, subfascial (eg, intramuscular); 5 cm or greater	Resequenced code, See code following 23076.
24071	Excision, tumor, soft tissue of upper arm or elbow area, subcutaneous; 3 cm or greater	Resequenced code, See code following 24075
24073	Excision, tumor, soft tissue of upper arm or elbow area, subfascial (eg, intramuscular); 5 cm or greater	Resequenced code, See code following 24076.
25071	Excision, tumor, soft tissue of forearm and/or wrist area, subcutaneous; 3 cm or greater	Resequenced code, See code following 25075.
25073	Excision, tumor, soft tissue of forearm and/or wrist area, subfascial (eg, intramuscular); 3 cm or greater	Resequenced code, See code following 25076.
26111	Excision, tumor or vascular malformation, soft tissue of hand or finger, subcutaneous; 1.5 cm or greater	Resequenced code, See code following 26115.
26113	Excision, tumor, soft tissue, or vascular malformation, of hand or finger, subfascial (eg, intramuscular); 1.5 cm or greater	Resequenced code, See code following 26116.
27043	Excision, tumor, soft tissue of pelvis and hip area, subcutaneous; 3 cm or greater	Resequenced code, See code following 27047.
27045	Excision, tumor, soft tissue of pelvis and hip area, subfascial (eg, intramuscular); 5 cm or greater	Resequenced code, See code following 27048.
27059	Radical resection of tumor (eg, malignant neoplasm), soft tissue of pelvis and hip area; 5 cm or greater	Resequenced code, See code following 27049.
27329	Radical resection of tumor (eg, malignant neoplasm), soft tissue of thigh or knee area; less than 5 cm	Resequenced code, See code following 27360.
27337	Excision, tumor, soft tissue of thigh or knee area, subcutaneous; 3 cm or greater	Resequenced code, See code following 27327.
27339	Excision, tumor, soft tissue of thigh or knee area, subfascial (eg, intramuscular); 5 cm or greater	Resequenced code, See code following 27328.
27632	Excision, tumor, soft tissue of leg or ankle area, subcutaneous; 3 cm or greater	Resequenced code, See code following 27618.
27634	Excision, tumor, soft tissue of leg or ankle area, subfascial (eg, intramuscular); 5 cm or greater	Resequenced code, See code following 27619.
28039	Excision, tumor, soft tissue of foot or toe, subcutaneous; 1.5 cm or greater	Resequenced code, See code following 28043.
28041	Excision, tumor, soft tissue of foot or toe, subfascial (eg, intramuscular); 1.5 cm or greater	Resequenced code, See code following 28045.
29914	Arthroscopy, hip, surgical; with femoroplasty (ie, treatment of cam lesion)	Resequenced code, See code following 29863.
29915	Arthroscopy, hip, surgical; with acetabuloplasty (ie, treatment of pincer lesion)	Resequenced code, See code following 29863.
29916	Arthroscopy, hip, surgical; with labral repair	Resequenced code, See code before 29866.
33221	Insertion of pacemaker pulse generator only; with existing multiple leads	Resequenced Code. See code following 33213.
33227	Removal of permanent pacemaker pulse generator with replacement of pacemaker pulse generator; single lead system	Resequenced Code. See code following 33233.
33228	Removal of permanent pacemaker pulse generator with replacement of pacemaker pulse generator; dual lead system	Resequenced Code. See code following 33233.
33229	Removal of permanent pacemaker pulse generator with replacement of pacemaker pulse generator; multiple lead system	Resequenced Code. See code before 33234.
33230	Insertion of pacing cardioverter-defibrillator pulse generator only; with existing dual leads	Resequenced Code. See code following 33240.
33231	Insertion of pacing cardioverter-defibrillator pulse generator only; with existing multiple leads	Resequenced Code. See code before 33241.
33262	Removal of pacing cardioverter-defibrillator pulse generator with replacement of pacing cardioverter-defibrillator pulse generator; single lead system	Resequenced Code. See code following 33241.
33263	Removal of pacing cardioverter-defibrillator pulse generator with replacement of pacing cardioverter-defibrillator pulse generator; dual lead system	Resequenced Code. See code following 33241.
33264	Removal of pacing cardioverter-defibrillator pulse generator with replacement of pacing cardioverter-defibrillator pulse generator; multiple lead system	Resequenced Code. See code before 33243.
46220	Excision of single external papilla or tag, anus	Resequenced code, See code before 46230.
46320	Excision of thrombosed hemorrhoid, external	Resequenced code, See code following 46230.
46945	Hemorrhoidectomy, internal, by ligation other than rubber band; single hemorrhoid column/group	Resequenced code, See code following 46221.
46946	Hemorrhoidectomy, internal, by ligation other than rubber band; 2 or more hemorrhoid columns/groups	Resequenced code, See code following 46221.
46947	Hemorrhoidopexy (eg, for prolapsing internal hemorrhoids) by stapling	Resequenced code, See code following 46762.
51797	Voiding pressure studies, intra-abdominal (ie, rectal, gastric, intraperitoneal) (List separately in addition to code for primary procedure)	Resequenced code, See code following 51729.
64633	Destruction by neurolytic agent, paravertebral facet joint nerve(s), with imaging guidance (fluoroscopy or CT); cervical or thoracic, single facet joint	Resequenced Code. See code following 64620.
64634	Destruction by neurolytic agent, paravertebral facet joint nerve(s), with imaging guidance (fluoroscopy or CT); cervical or thoracic, each additional facet joint (List separately in addition to code for primary procedure)	Resequenced Code. See code following 64620.
64635	Destruction by neurolytic agent, paravertebral facet joint nerve(s), with imaging guidance (fluoroscopy or CT); lumbar or sacral, single facet joint	Resequenced Code. See code following 64620.
64636	Destruction by neurolytic agent, paravertebral facet joint nerve(s), with imaging guidance (fluoroscopy or CT); lumbar or sacral, each additional facet joint (List separately in addition to code for primary procedure)	Resequenced Code. See code before 64630.
77424	Intraoperative radiation treatment delivery, x-ray, single treatment session	Resequenced Code. See code following 77421.
77425	Intraoperative radiation treatment delivery, electrons, single treatment session	Resequenced Code. See code before 77422.
80104	Drug screen, qualitative; multiple drug classes other than chromatographic method, each procedure	Resequenced Code. See code following 80101.
82652	Vitamin D; 1, 25 dihydroxy, includes fraction(s), if performed	Resequenced code, See code following 82306.
87906	Infectious agent genotype analysis by nucleic acid (DNA or RNA); HIV-1, other region (eg, integrase, fusion)	Resequenced code, See code following 87901.
88177	Cytopathology, evaluation of fine needle aspirate; immediate cytohistologic study to determine adequacy for diagnosis, each separate additional evaluation episode, same site (List separately in addition to code for primary procedure)	Resequenced code, See code following 88173.
90665	Lyme disease vaccine, adult dosage, for intramuscular use	Resequenced code, See code following 90668.

Appendix D: Resequenced Codes

Code	Description	Reference
92558	Evoked otoacoustic emissions, screening (qualitative measurement of distortion product or transient evoked otoacoustic emissions), automated analysis	Resequenced Code. See code following 92586.
92618	Evaluation for prescription of non-speech-generating augmentative and alternative communication device, face-to-face with the patient; each additional 30 minutes (List separately in addition to code for primary procedure)	Resequenced Code. See code following 92605.
95800	Sleep study, unattended, simultaneous recording; heart rate, oxygen saturation, respiratory analysis (eg, by airflow or peripheral arterial tone), and sleep time	Resequenced code, See code following 95806.
95801	Sleep study, unattended, simultaneous recording; minimum of heart rate, oxygen saturation, and respiratory analysis (eg, by airflow or peripheral arterial tone)	Resequenced code, See code before 95807.
95885	Needle electromyography, each extremity, with related paraspinal areas, when performed, done with nerve conduction, amplitude and latency/velocity study; limited (List separately in addition to code for primary procedure)	Resequenced Code. See code following 95872.
95886	Needle electromyography, each extremity, with related paraspinal areas, when performed, done with nerve conduction, amplitude and latency/velocity study; complete, five or more muscles studied, innervated by three or more nerves or four or more spinal levels (List separately in addition to code for primary procedure)	Resequenced Code. See code following 95872.
95887	Needle electromyography, non-extremity (cranial nerve supplied or axial) muscle(s) done with nerve conduction, amplitude and latency/velocity study (List separately in addition to code for primary procedure)	Resequenced Code. See code before 95873.
95938	Short-latency somatosensory evoked potential study, stimulation of any/all peripheral nerves or skin sites, recording from the central nervous system; in upper and lower limbs	Resequenced Code. See code following 95926.
95939	Central motor evoked potential study (transcranial motor stimulation); in upper and lower limbs	Resequenced Code. See code following 95929.
99224	Subsequent observation care, per day, for the evaluation and management of a patient, which requires at least 2 of these 3 key components: Problem focused interval history; Problem focused examination; Medical decision making that is straightforward or of low complexity. Counseling and/or coordination of care with other providers or agencies are provided consistent with the nature of the problem(s) and the patient's and/or family's needs. Usually, the patient is stable, recovering, or improving. Physicians typically spend 15 minutes at the bedside and on the patient's hospital floor or unit.	Resequenced code, See code following 99220.
99225	Subsequent observation care, per day, for the evaluation and management of a patient, which requires at least 2 of these 3 key components: An expanded problem focused interval history; An expanded problem focused examination; Medical decision making of moderate complexity. Counseling and/or coordination of care with other providers or agencies are provided consistent with the nature of the problem(s) and the patient's and/or family's needs. Usually, the patient is responding inadequately to therapy or has developed a minor complication. Physicians typically spend 25 minutes at the bedside and on the patient's hospital floor or unit.	Resequenced code, See code following 99220.
99226	Subsequent observation care, per day, for the evaluation and management of a patient, which requires at least 2 of these 3 key components: A detailed interval history; A detailed examination; Medical decision making of high complexity. Counseling and/or coordination of care with other providers or agencies are provided consistent with the nature of the problem(s) and the patient's and/or family's needs. Usually, the patient is unstable or has developed a significant complication or a significant new problem. Physicians typically spend 35 minutes at the bedside and on the patient's hospital floor or unit.	Resequenced code, See code before 99221.
0253T	Insertion of anterior segment aqueous drainage device, without extraocular reservoir; internal approach, into the suprachoroidal space	Resequenced code, See code following 0191T.

APPENDIX E: ADD-ON CODES, MODIFIER 51, 63, AND MODERATE SEDATION CODES

Codes specified as add-on, exempt from modifier 51 and 63, and include conscious sedation are listed. The lists are designed to be read left to right rather than vertically.

Add-on codes

01953 01968 01969 11001 11008 11045 11046
11047 11101 11201 11732 11922 13102 13122
13133 13153 14302 15003 15005 15101 15111
15116 15121 15131 15136 15151 15152 15156
15157 15201 15221 15241 15261 15272 15274
15276 15278 15777 15787 15847 16036 17003
17312 17314 17315 19001 19126 19291 19295
19297 20930 20931 20936 20937 20938 20985
22103 22116 22208 22216 22226 22328 22522
22525 22527 22534 22552 22585 22614 22632
22634 22840 22841 22842 22843 22844 22845
22846 22847 22848 22851 26125 26861 26863
27358 27692 29826 31620 31627 31632 31633
31637 32501 32506 32507 32667 32668 32674
33141 33225 33257 33258 33259 33508 33517
33518 33519 33521 33522 33523 33530 33572
33768 33884 33924 34806 34808 34813 34826
35306 35390 35400 35500 35572 35600 35681
35682 35683 35685 35686 35697 35700 36148
36218 36248 36476 36479 37185 37186 37206
37208 37222 37223 37232 37233 37234 37235
37250 37251 38102 38746 38747 38900 43273
43283 43338 43635 44015 44121 44128 44139
44203 44213 44701 44955 47001 47550 48400
49326 49327 49412 49435 49568 49905 51797
56606 57267 58110 58611 59525 60512 61316
61517 61609 61610 61611 61612 61641 61642
61781 61782 61783 61797 61799 61800 61864
61868 62148 62160 63035 63043 63044 63048
63057 63066 63076 63078 63082 63086 63088
63091 63103 63295 63308 63621 64480 64484
64491 64492 64494 64495 64634 64636 64727
64778 64783 64787 64832 64837 64859 64872
64874 64876 64901 64902 65757 66990 67225
67320 67331 67332 67334 67335 67340 69990
74301 75565 75774 75946 75964 75968 76125
76802 76810 76812 76814 76937 77001 77051
77052 78020 78496 78730 81266 82952 83901
86826 87187 87503 87904 88155 88177 88185
88311 88314 88332 88334 88388 90461 90472
90474 91013 92547 92608 92618 92621 92627
92973 92974 92978 92979 92981 92984 92996
92998 93320 93321 93325 93352 93462 93463
93464 93563 93564 93565 93566 93567 93568
93571 93572 93609 93613 93621 93622 93623
93662 94645 94729 94781 95873 95874 95885
95886 95887 95920 95962 95967 95973 95975
95979 96361 96366 96367 96368 96370 96371
96375 96376 96411 96415 96417 96423 96570
96571 97546 97598 97811 97814 99100 99116
99135 99140 99145 99150 99292 99354 99355
99356 99357 99359 99467 99602 99607 0054T
0055T 0076T 0079T 0081T 0092T 0095T 0098T
0159T 0163T 0164T 0165T 0172T 0173T 0174T
0189T 0190T 0196T 0205T 0214T 0215T 0217T
0218T 0222T 0229T 0231T 0241T 0250T 0252T
0289T 0290T 0291T 0292T 0294T 0300T

Modifier 51 Exempt Codes

17004 20697 20974 20975 31500 33961 36620
44500 61107 90281 90283 90284 90287 90288
90291 90296 90371 90375 90376 90378 90384
90385 90386 90389 90393 90396 90399 90476
90477 90581 90585 90586 90632 90633 90634
90636 90644 90645 90646 90647 90648 90649
90650 90654 90655 90656 90657 90658 90660
90661 90662 90664 90665 90666 90667 90668
90669 90670 90675 90676 90680 90681 90690
90691 90692 90693 90696 90698 90700 90701
90702 90703 90704 90705 90706 90707 90708
90710 90712 90713 90714 90715 90716 90717
90718 90719 90720 90721 90723 90725 90727
90732 90733 90734 90735 90736 90738 90740
90743 90744 90746 90747 90748 90749 93451
93456 93503 93600 93602 93603 93610 93612
93615 93616 93618 93631 94610 95900 95903
95904 95905 95992 99050 99051 99053 99056
99058 99060 99143 99144

Modifier 63 Exempt Codes

30540 30545 31520 33401 33403 33470 33472
33502 33503 33505 33506 33610 33611 33619
33647 33670 33690 33694 33730 33732 33735
33736 33750 33755 33762 33778 33786 33922
33960 33961 36415 36420 36450 36460 36510
36660 39503 43313 43314 43520 43831 44055
44126 44127 44128 46070 46705 46715 46716
46730 46735 46740 46742 46744 47700 47701
49215 49491 49492 49495 49496 49600 49605
49606 49610 49611 53025 54000 54150 54160
63700 63702 63704 63706 65820

Moderate Sedation Codes

19298 20982 22520 22521 22526 22527 31615
31620 31622 31623 31624 31625 31626 31627
31628 31629 31634 31635 31645 31646 31656
31725 32201 32405 32550 32551 32553 33010
33011 33206 33207 33208 33210 33211 33212
33213 33214 33216 33217 33218 33220 33221
33222 33223 33227 33228 33229 33230 33231
33233 33234 33235 33240 33241 33244 33249
33262 33263 33264 35471 35472 35475 35476
36147 36148 36200 36245 36246 36247 36248
36251 36252 36253 36254 36481 36555 36557
36558 36560 36561 36563 36565 36566 36568
36570 36571 36576 36578 36581 36582 36583
36585 36590 36870 37183 37184 37185 37186
37187 37188 37191 37192 37193 37203 37210
37215 37216 37220 37221 37222 37223 37224
37225 37226 37227 37228 37229 37230 37231
37232 37233 37234 37235 43200 43201 43202
43204 43205 43215 43216 43217 43219 43220
43226 43227 43228 43231 43232 43234 43235
43236 43237 43238 43239 43240 43241 43242
43243 43244 43245 43246 43247 43248 43249
43250 43251 43255 43256 43257 43258 43259
43260 43261 43262 43263 43264 43265 43267
43268 43269 43271 43272 43273 43453 43456
43458 44360 44361 44363 44364 44365 44366
44369 44370 44372 44373 44376 44377 44378
44379 44380 44382 44383 44385 44386 44388
44389 44390 44391 44392 44393 44394 44397
44500 44901 45303 45305 45307 45308 45309
45315 45317 45320 45321 45327 45332 45333
45334 45335 45337 45338 45339 45340 45341
45342 45345 45355 45378 45379 45380 45381
45382 45383 45384 45385 45386 45387 45391
45392 47000 47011 47382 47525 48511 49021
49041 49061 49411 49418 49440 49441 49442
49446 50021 50200 50382 50384 50385 50386
50387 50592 50593 57155 58823 66720 69300
77371 77600 77605 77610 77615 92953 92960
92961 92973 92974 92975 92978 92979 92980
92981 92982 92984 92986 92987 92995 92996
93312 93313 93314 93315 93316 93317 93318
93451 93452 93453 93454 93455 93456 93457
93458 93459 93460 93461 93462 93463 93464
93505 93530 93561 93562 93563 93564 93565
93566 93567 93568 93571 93572 93609 93613
93615 93616 93618 93619 93620 93621 93622
93624 93640 93641 93642 93650 93651 93652
94011 94012 94013 0200T 0201T 0250T 0251T
0252T 0276T 0277T 0282T 0283T 0284T 0291T
0292T 0293T 0294T 0301T

Appendix E: Add-on Codes, Modifier 51, 63, and Moderate Sedation Codes

APPENDIX F — PLACE OF SERVICE AND TYPE OF SERVICE

Place-of-Service Codes for Professional Claims

Listed below are place of service codes and descriptions. These codes should be used on professional claims to specify the entity where service(s) were rendered. Check with individual payers (e.g., Medicare, Medicaid, other private insurance) for reimbursement policies regarding these codes. To comment on a code(s) or description(s), please send your request to posinfo@cms.gov.

Code	Name	Description
01	Pharmacy	A facility or location where drugs and other medically related items and services are sold, dispensed, or otherwise provided directly to patients.
02	Unassigned	N/A
03	School	A facility whose primary purpose is education.
04	Homeless shelter	A facility or location whose primary purpose is to provide temporary housing to homeless individuals (e.g., emergency shelters, individual or family shelters).
05	Indian Health Service freestanding facility	A facility or location, owned and operated by the Indian Health Service, which provides diagnostic, therapeutic (surgical and non-surgical), and rehabilitation services to American Indians and Alaska natives who do not require hospitalization.
06	Indian Health Service provider-based facility	A facility or location, owned and operated by the Indian Health Service, which provides diagnostic, therapeutic (surgical and nonsurgical), and rehabilitation services rendered by, or under the supervision of, physicians to American Indians and Alaska natives admitted as inpatients or outpatients.
07	Tribal 638 freestanding facility	A facility or location owned and operated by a federally recognized American Indian or Alaska native tribe or tribal organization under a 638 agreement, which provides diagnostic, therapeutic (surgical and nonsurgical), and rehabilitation services to tribal members who do not require hospitalization.
08	Tribal 638 Provider-based Facility	A facility or location owned and operated by a federally recognized American Indian or Alaska native tribe or tribal organization under a 638 agreement, which provides diagnostic, therapeutic (surgical and nonsurgical), and rehabilitation services to tribal members admitted as inpatients or outpatients.
09	Prison/correctional facility	A prison, jail, reformatory, work farm, detention center, or any other similar facility maintained by either federal, state or local authorities for the purpose of confinement or rehabilitation of adult or juvenile criminal offenders.
10	Unassigned	N/A
11	Office	Location, other than a hospital, skilled nursing facility (SNF), military treatment facility, community health center, State or local public health clinic, or intermediate care facility (ICF), where the health professional routinely provides health examinations, diagnosis, and treatment of illness or injury on an ambulatory basis.
12	Home	Location, other than a hospital or other facility, where the patient receives care in a private residence.
13	Assisted living facility	Congregate residential facility with self-contained living units providing assessment of each resident's needs and on-site support 24 hours a day, 7 days a week, with the capacity to deliver or arrange for services including some health care and other services.
14	Group home	A residence, with shared living areas, where clients receive supervision and other services such as social and/or behavioral services, custodial service, and minimal services (e.g., medication administration).
15	Mobile unit	A facility/unit that moves from place-to-place equipped to provide preventive, screening, diagnostic, and/or treatment services.
16	Temporary lodging	A short-term accommodation such as a hotel, campground, hostel, cruise ship or resort where the patient receives care, and which is not identified by any other POS code.
17	Walk-in retail health clinic	A walk-in health clinic, other than an office, urgent care facility, pharmacy, or independent clinic and not described by any other place of service code, that is located within a retail operation and provides preventive and primary care services on an ambulatory basis.
18-19	Unassigned	N/A
20	Urgent care facility	Location, distinct from a hospital emergency room, an office, or a clinic, whose purpose is to diagnose and treat illness or injury for unscheduled, ambulatory patients seeking immediate medical attention.
21	Inpatient hospital	A facility, other than psychiatric, which primarily provides diagnostic, therapeutic (both surgical and nonsurgical), and rehabilitation services by, or under, the supervision of physicians to patients admitted for a variety of medical conditions.
22	Outpatient hospital	A portion of a hospital which provides diagnostic, therapeutic (both surgical and nonsurgical), and rehabilitation services to sick or injured persons who do not require hospitalization or institutionalization.
23	Emergency room—hospital	A portion of a hospital where emergency diagnosis and treatment of illness or injury is provided.
24	Ambulatory surgical center	A freestanding facility, other than a physician's office, where surgical and diagnostic services are provided on an ambulatory basis.
25	Birthing center	A facility, other than a hospital's maternity facilities or a physician's office, which provides a setting for labor, delivery, and immediate post-partum care as well as immediate care of new born infants.
26	Military treatment facility	A medical facility operated by one or more of the uniformed services. Military treatment facility (MTF) also refers to certain former U.S. Public Health Service (USPHS) facilities now designated as uniformed service treatment facilities (USTF).
27-30	Unassigned	N/A

31	Skilled nursing facility	A facility which primarily provides inpatient skilled nursing care and related services to patients who require medical, nursing, or rehabilitative services but does not provide the level of care or treatment available in a hospital.
32	Nursing facility	A facility which primarily provides to residents skilled nursing care and related services for the rehabilitation of injured, disabled, or sick persons, or, on a regular basis, health-related care services above the level of custodial care to other than mentally retarded individuals.
33	Custodial care facility	A facility which provides room, board, and other personal assistance services, generally on a long-term basis, and which does not include a medical component.
34	Hospice	A facility, other than a patient's home, in which palliative and supportive care for terminally ill patients and their families are provided.
35-40	Unassigned	N/A
41	Ambulance—land	A land vehicle specifically designed, equipped and staffed for lifesaving and transporting the sick or injured.
42	Ambulance—air or water	An air or water vehicle specifically designed, equipped and staffed for lifesaving and transporting the sick or injured.
43-48	Unassigned	N/A
49	Independent clinic	A location, not part of a hospital and not described by any other place-of-service code, that is organized and operated to provide preventive, diagnostic, therapeutic, rehabilitative, or palliative services to outpatients only.
50	Federally qualified health center	A facility located in a medically underserved area that provides Medicare beneficiaries preventive primary medical care under the general direction of a physician.
51	Inpatient psychiatric facility	A facility that provides inpatient psychiatric services for the diagnosis and treatment of mental illness on a 24-hour basis, by or under the supervision of a physician.
52	Psychiatric facility-partial hospitalization	A facility for the diagnosis and treatment of mental illness that provides a planned therapeutic program for patients who do not require full time hospitalization, but who need broader programs than are possible from outpatient visits to a hospital-based or hospital-affiliated facility.
53	Community mental health center	A facility that provides the following services: outpatient services, including specialized outpatient services for children, the elderly, individuals who are chronically ill, and residents of the CMHC's mental health services area who have been discharged from inpatient treatment at a mental health facility; 24 hour a day emergency care services; day treatment, other partial hospitalization services, or psychosocial rehabilitation services; screening for patients being considered for admission to state mental health facilities to determine the appropriateness of such admission; and consultation and education services.
54	Intermediate care facility/mentally retarded	A facility which primarily provides health-related care and services above the level of custodial care to mentally retarded individuals but does not provide the level of care or treatment available in a hospital or SNF.
55	Residential substance abuse treatment facility	A facility which provides treatment for substance (alcohol and drug) abuse to live-in residents who do not require acute medical care. Services include individual and group therapy and counseling, family counseling, laboratory tests, drugs and supplies, psychological testing, and room and board.
56	Psychiatric residential treatment center	A facility or distinct part of a facility for psychiatric care which provides a total 24-hour therapeutically planned and professionally staffed group living and learning environment.
57	Non-residential substance abuse treatment facility	A location which provides treatment for substance (alcohol and drug) abuse on an ambulatory basis. Services include individual and group therapy and counseling, family counseling, laboratory tests, drugs and supplies, and psychological testing.
58-59	Unassigned	N/A
60	Mass immunization center	A location where providers administer pneumococcal pneumonia and influenza virus vaccinations and submit these services as electronic media claims, paper claims, or using the roster billing method. This generally takes place in a mass immunization setting, such as, a public health center, pharmacy, or mall but may include a physician office setting.
61	Comprehensive inpatient rehabilitation facility	A facility that provides comprehensive rehabilitation services under the supervision of a physician to inpatients with physical disabilities. Services include physical therapy, occupational therapy, speech pathology, social or psychological services, and orthotics and prosthetics services.
62	Comprehensive outpatient rehabilitation facility	A facility that provides comprehensive rehabilitation services under the supervision of a physician to outpatients with physical disabilities. Services include physical therapy, occupational therapy, and speech pathology services.
63-64	Unassigned	N/A
65	End-stage renal disease treatment facility	A facility other than a hospital, which provides dialysis treatment, maintenance, and/or training to patients or caregivers on an ambulatory or home-care basis.
66-70	Unassigned	N/A
71	State or local public health clinic	A facility maintained by either state or local health departments that provides ambulatory primary medical care under the general direction of a physician.
72	Rural health clinic	A certified facility which is located in a rural medically underserved area that provides ambulatory primary medical care under the general direction of a physician.
73-80	Unassigned	N/A
81	Independent laboratory	A laboratory certified to perform diagnostic and/or clinical tests independent of an institution or a physician's office.
82-98	Unassigned	N/A
99	Other place of service	Other place of service not identified above.

Type of Service

Common Working File Type of Service (TOS) Indicators

For submitting a claim to the Common Working File (CWF), use the following table to assign the proper TOS. Some procedures may have more than one applicable TOS. CWF will reject alerts on codes with incorrect TOS designations. CWF will produce alerts on codes with incorrect TOS designations.

The only exceptions to this table are:

- Surgical services billed for dates of service through December 31, 2007, containing the ASC facility service modifier SG must be reported as TOS F. Effective for services on or after January 1, 2008, the SG modifier is no longer applicable for Medicare services. ASC providers should discontinue applying the SG modifier on ASC facility claims. The indicator F does not appear in the TOS table because its use depends upon claims submitted with POS 24 (ASC facility) from an ASC (specialty 49). This became effective for dates of service January 1, 2008, or after.
- Surgical services billed with an assistant-at-surgery modifier (80-82, AS,) must be reported with TOS 8. The 8 indicator does not appear on the TOS table because its use is dependent upon the use of the appropriate modifier. (See Pub. 100-4 *Medicare Claims Processing Manual*, chapter 12, "Physician/Practitioner Billing," for instructions on when assistant-at-surgery is allowable.)
- Psychiatric treatment services that are subject to the outpatient mental health treatment limitation should be reported with TOS T.
- TOS H appears in the list of descriptors. However, it does not appear in the table. In CWF, "H" is used only as an indicator for hospice. The carrier should not submit TOS H to CWF at this time.
- For outpatient services, when a transfusion medicine code appears on a claim that also contains a blood product, the service is paid under reasonable charge at 80 percent; coinsurance and deductible apply. When transfusion medicine codes are paid under the clinical laboratory fee schedule they are paid at 100 percent; coinsurance and deductible do not apply.

Note: For injection codes with more than one possible TOS designation, use the following guidelines when assigning the TOS:

When the choice is L or 1:

- Use TOS L when the drug is used related to ESRD; or
- Use TOS 1 when the drug is not related to ESRD and is administered in the office.

When the choice is G or 1:

- Use TOS G when the drug is an immunosuppressive drug; or
- Use TOS 1 when the drug is used for other than immunosuppression.

When the choice is P or 1:

- Use TOS P if the drug is administered through durable medical equipment (DME); or
- Use TOS 1 if the drug is administered in the office.

The place of service or diagnosis may be considered when determining the appropriate TOS. The descriptors for each of the TOS codes listed in the following table are:

0 Whole blood
1 Medical care
2 Surgery
3 Consultation
4 Diagnostic radiology
5 Diagnostic laboratory
6 Therapeutic radiology
7 Anesthesia
8 Assistant at surgery
9 Other medical items or services
A Used DME
B High risk screening mammography
C Low risk screening mammography
D Ambulance
E Enteral/parenteral nutrients/supplies
F Ambulatory surgical center (facility usage for surgical services)
G Immunosuppressive drugs
H Hospice
J Diabetic shoes
K Hearing items and services
L ESRD supplies
M Monthly capitation payment for dialysis
N Kidney donor
P Lump sum purchase of DME, prosthetics, orthotics
Q Vision items or services
R Rental of DME
S Surgical dressings or other medical supplies
T Outpatient mental health treatment limitation
U Occupational therapy
V Pneumococcal/flu vaccine
W Physical therapy

Berenson-Eggers Type of Service (BETOS) Codes

The BETOS coding system was developed primarily for analyzing the growth in Medicare expenditures. The coding system covers all HCPCS codes; assigns a HCPCS code to only one BETOS code; consists of readily understood clinical categories (as opposed to statistical or financial categories); consists of categories that permit objective assignment; is stable over time; and is relatively immune to minor changes in technology or practice patterns.

BETOS Codes and Descriptions:

1. Evaluation and Management

1. M1A Office visits—new
2. M1B Office visits—established
3. M2A Hospital visit—initial
4. M2B Hospital visit—subsequent
5. M2C Hospital visit—critical care
6. M3 Emergency room visit
7. M4A Home visit
8. M4B Nursing home visit
9. M5A Specialist—pathology
10. M5B Specialist—psychiatry
11. M5C Specialist—ophthalmology
12. M5D Specialist—other
13. M6 Consultations

2. Procedures

1. P0 Anesthesia
2. P1A Major procedure—breast
3. P1B Major procedure—colectomy
4. P1C Major procedure—cholecystectomy
5. P1D Major procedure—TURP
6. P1E Major procedure—hysterectomy
7. P1F Major procedure—explor/decompr/excis disc
8. P1G Major procedure—other
9. P2A Major procedure, cardiovascular—CABG
10. P2B Major procedure, cardiovascular—aneurysm repair
11. P2C Major procedure, cardiovascular—thromboendarterectomy
12. P2D Major procedure, cardiovascular—coronary angioplasty (PTCA)
13. P2E Major procedure, cardiovascular—pacemaker insertion
14. P2F Major procedure, cardiovascular—other

15. P3A Major procedure, orthopedic—hip fracture repair
16. P3B Major procedure, orthopedic—hip replacement
17. P3C Major procedure, orthopedic—knee replacement
18. P3D Major procedure, orthopedic—other
19. P4A Eye procedure—corneal transplant
20. P4B Eye procedure—cataract removal/lens insertion
21. P4C Eye procedure—retinal detachment
22. P4D Eye procedure—treatment of retinal lesions
23. P4E Eye procedure—other
24. P5A Ambulatory procedures—skin
25. P5B Ambulatory procedures—musculoskeletal
26. P5C Ambulatory procedures—groin hernia repair
27. P5D Ambulatory procedures—lithotripsy
28. P5E Ambulatory procedures—other
29. P6A Minor procedures—skin
30. P6B Minor procedures—musculoskeletal
31. P6C Minor procedures—other (Medicare fee schedule)
32. P6D Minor procedures—other (non-Medicare fee schedule)
33. P7A Oncology—radiation therapy
34. P7B Oncology—other
35. P8A Endoscopy—arthroscopy
36. P8B Endoscopy—upper gastrointestinal
37. P8C Endoscopy—sigmoidoscopy
38. P8D Endoscopy—colonoscopy
39. P8E Endoscopy—cystoscopy
40. P8F Endoscopy—bronchoscopy
41. P8G Endoscopy—laparoscopic cholecystectomy
42. P8H Endoscopy—laryngoscopy
43. P8I Endoscopy—other
44. P9A Dialysis services (Medicare fee schedule)
45. P9B Dialysis services (non-Medicare fee schedule)

3. Imaging

1. I1A Standard imaging—chest
2. I1B Standard imaging—musculoskeletal
3. I1C Standard imaging—breast
4. I1D Standard imaging—contrast gastrointestinal
5. I1E Standard imaging—nuclear medicine
6. I1F Standard imaging—other
7. I2A Advanced imaging—CAT/CT/CTA; brain/head/neck
8. I2B Advanced imaging—CAT/CT/CTA; other
9. I2C Advanced imaging—MRI/MRA; brain/head/neck
10. I2D Advanced imaging—MRI/MRA; other
11. I3A Echography/ultrasoundography—eye
12. I3B Echography/ultrasoundography—abdomen/pelvis
13. I3C Echography/ultrasoundography—heart
14. I3D Echography/ultrasoundography—carotid arteries
15. I3E Echography/ultrasoundography—prostate, transrectal
16. I3F Echography/ultrasoundography—other
17. I4A Imaging/procedure—heart, including cardiac catheterization
18. I4B Imaging/procedure—other

4. Tests

1. T1A Lab tests—routine venipuncture (non-Medicare fee schedule)
2. T1B Lab tests—automated general profiles
3. T1C Lab tests—urinalysis
4. T1D Lab tests—blood counts
5. T1E Lab tests—glucose
6. T1F Lab tests—bacterial cultures
7. T1G Lab tests—other (Medicare fee schedule)
8. T1H Lab tests—other (non-Medicare fee schedule)
9. T2A Other tests—electrocardiograms
10. T2B Other tests—cardiovascular stress tests
11. T2C Other tests—EKG monitoring
12. T2D Other tests—other

5. Durable Medical Equipment

1. D1A Medical/surgical supplies
2. D1B Hospital beds
3. D1C Oxygen and supplies
4. D1D Wheelchairs
5. D1E Other DME
6. D1F Prosthetic/orthotic devices
7. D1G Drugs administered through DME

6. Other

1. O1A Ambulance
2. O1B Chiropractic
3. O1C Enteral and parenteral
4. O1D Chemotherapy
5. O1E Other drugs
6. O1F Hearing and speech services
7. O1G Immunizations/vaccinations

7. Exceptions/Unclassified

1. Y1 Other—Medicare fee schedule
2. Y2 Other—Non-Medicare fee schedule
3. Z1 Local codes
4. Z2 Undefined codes

APPENDIX G — PUB 100 REFERENCES

The Centers for Medicare and Medicaid Services restructured its paper-based manual system as a web-based system on October 1, 2003. Called the online CMS manual system, it combines all of the various program instructions into internet-only manuals (IOMs), which are used by all CMS programs and contractors. In many instances, the references from the online manuals in appendix E contain a mention of the old paper manuals from which the current information was obtained when the manuals were converted. This information is shown in the header of the text, in the following format, when applicable, as A3-3101, HO-210, and B3-2049. Complete versions of all of the manuals can be found at http://www.cms.gov/manuals.

Effective with implementation of the IOMs, the former method of publishing program memoranda (PMs) to communicate program instructions was replaced by the following four templates:

- One-time notification
- Manual revisions
- Business requirements
- Confidential requirements

The web-based system has been organized by functional area (e.g., eligibility, entitlement, claims processing, benefit policy, program integrity) in an effort to eliminate redundancy within the manuals, simplify updating, and make CMS program instructions available more quickly. The web-based system contains the functional areas included below:

Pub. 100	Introduction
Pub. 100-1	Medicare General Information, Eligibility, and Entitlement Manual
Pub. 100-2	Medicare Benefit Policy Manual
Pub. 100-3	Medicare National Coverage Determinations (NCD) Manual
Pub. 100-4	Medicare Claims Processing Manual
Pub. 100-5	Medicare Secondary Payer Manual
Pub. 100-6	Medicare Financial Management Manual
Pub. 100-7	State Operations Manual
Pub. 100-8	Medicare Program Integrity Manual
Pub. 100-9	Medicare Contractor Beneficiary and Provider Communications Manual
Pub. 100-10	Quality Improvement Organization Manual
Pub. 100-11	Programs of All-Inclusive Care for the Elderly (PACE) Manual
Pub. 100-12	State Medicaid Manual (under development)
Pub. 100-13	Medicaid State Children's Health Insurance Program (under development)
Pub. 100-14	Medicare ESRD Network Organizations Manual
Pub. 100-15	Medicaid Integrity Program (MIP)
Pub. 100-16	Medicare Managed Care Manual
Pub. 100-17	CMS/Business Partners Systems Security Manual
Pub. 100-18	Medicare Prescription Drug Benefit Manual
Pub. 100-19	Demonstrations
Pub. 100-20	One-Time Notification
Pub. 100-21	Recurring Update Notification
Pub. 100-22	Medicare Quality Reporting Incentive Programs Manual
Pub. 100-24	State Buy-In Manual
Pub. 100-25	Information Security Acceptable Risk Safeguards Manual

A brief description of the Medicare manuals primarily used for *CPC Expert* follows:

The ***National Coverage Determinations Manual*** (NCD), is organized according to categories such as diagnostic services, supplies, and medical procedures. The table of contents lists each category and subject within that category. Revision transmittals identify any new or background material, recap the changes, and provide an effective date for the change.

When complete, the manual will contain two chapters. Chapter 1 currently includes a description of CMS's national coverage determinations. When available, chapter 2 will contain a list of HCPCS codes related to each coverage determination. The manual is organized in accordance with CPT category sequences.

The ***Medicare Benefit Policy Manual*** contains Medicare general coverage instructions that are not national coverage determinations. As a general rule, in the past these instructions have been found in chapter II of the ***Medicare Carriers Manual,*** the ***Medicare Intermediary Manual***, other provider manuals, and program memoranda.

The ***Medicare Claims Processing Manual*** contains instructions for processing claims for contractors and providers.

The ***Medicare Program Integrity Manual*** communicates the priorities and standards for the Medicare integrity programs.

Medicare IOM references

100-1, 3, 20.5

Blood Deductibles (Part A and Part B)

Program payment may not be made for the first 3 pints of whole blood or equivalent units of packed red cells received under Part A and Part B combined in a calendar year. However, blood processing (e.g., administration, storage) is not subject to the deductible.

The blood deductibles are in addition to any other applicable deductible and coinsurance amounts for which the patient is responsible.

The deductible applies only to the first 3 pints of blood furnished in a calendar year, even if more than one provider furnished blood.

100-1, 3, 20.5.2

Part B Blood Deductible

Blood is furnished on an outpatient basis or is subject to the Part B blood deductible and is counted toward the combined limit. It should be noted that payment for blood may be made to the hospital under Part B only for blood furnished in an outpatient setting. Blood is not covered for inpatient Part B services.

100-1, 3, 20.5.3

Items Subject to Blood Deductibles

The blood deductibles apply only to whole blood and packed red cells. The term whole blood means human blood from which none of the liquid or cellular components have been removed. Where packed red cells are furnished, a unit of packed red cells is considered equivalent to a pint of whole blood. Other components of blood such as platelets, fibrinogen, plasma, gamma globulin, and serum albumin are not subject to the blood deductible. However, these components of blood are covered as biologicals.

Refer to Pub. 100-04, Medicare Claims Processing Manual, chapter 4, Sec.231 regarding billing for blood and blood products under the Hospital Outpatient Prospective Payment System (OPPS).

100-1, 3, 30

Outpatient Mental Health Treatment Limitation

Regardless of the actual expenses a beneficiary incurs for treatment of mental, psychoneurotic, and personality disorders while the beneficiary is not an inpatient of a hospital at the time such expenses are incurred, the amount of those expenses that may be recognized for Part B deductible and payment purposes is limited to 62.5 percent of the Medicare allowed amount for these services. The limitation is called the outpatient mental health treatment limitation. Since Part B deductible also applies the program pays for about half of the allowed amount recognized for mental health therapy services.

Expenses for diagnostic services (e.g., psychiatric testing and evaluation to diagnose the patient's illness) are not subject to this limitation. This limitation applies only to therapeutic services and to services performed to evaluate the progress of a course of treatment for a diagnosed condition.

100-1, 3, 30.1

Application of Mental Health Limitation - Status of Patient

The limitation is applicable to expenses incurred in connection with the treatment of an individual who is not an inpatient of a hospital. Thus, the limitation applies to mental health services furnished to a person in a physician's office, in the patient's home, in a skilled nursing facility, as an outpatient, and so forth. The term "hospital" in this context means an institution which is primarily engaged in providing to inpatients, by or under the supervision of a physician(s):

- Diagnostic and therapeutic services for medical diagnosis, and treatment, and care of injured, disabled, or sick persons;
- Rehabilitation services for injured, disabled, or sick persons; or
- Psychiatric services for the diagnosis and treatment of mentally ill patients.

100-1, 3, 30.2

Disorders Subject to Mental Health Limitation

The term "mental, psychoneurotic, and personality disorders" is defined as the specific psychiatric conditions described in the American Psychiatric Association's Diagnostic and Statistical Manual of Mental Disorders, Third Edition - Revised (DSM-III-R).

If the treatment services rendered are for both a psychiatric condition and one or more nonpsychiatric conditions, the charges are separated to apply the limitation only to the mental health charge. Normally HCPCS code and diagnoses are used. Where HCPCS code is not available on the claim, revenue code is used.

If the service is primarily on the basis of a diagnosis of Alzheimer's Disease (coded 331.0 in the International Classification of Diseases, 9th Revision) or Alzheimer's or other disorders (coded 290.XX in DSM-III-R), treatment typically represents medical management of the patient's condition (rather than psychiatric treatment) and is not subject to the limitation.

100-1, 3, 30.3

Diagnostic Services

The mental health limitation does not apply to tests and evaluations performed to establish or confirm the patient's diagnosis. Diagnostic services include psychiatric or psychological tests and interpretations, diagnostic consultations, and initial evaluations. However, testing services performed to evaluate a patient's progress during treatment are considered part of treatment and are subject to the limitation.

100-1, 5, 70

Physician Defined

Physician means doctor of medicine, doctor of osteopathy (including osteopathic practitioner), doctor of dental surgery or dental medicine (within the limitations in subsection Sec.70.2), doctor of podiatric medicine (within the limitations in subsection Sec.70.3), or doctor of optometry (within the limitations of subsection Sec.70.5), and, with respect to certain specified treatment, a doctor of chiropractic legally authorized to practice by a State in which he/she performs this function. The services performed by a physician within these definitions are subject to any limitations imposed by the State on the scope of practice. The issuance by a State of a license to practice medicine constitutes legal authorization. Temporary State licenses also constitute legal authorization to practice medicine. If State law authorizes local political subdivisions to establish higher standards for medical practitioners than those set by the State licensing board, the local standards determine whether a particular physician has legal authorization. If State licensing law limits the scope of practice of a particular type of medical practitioner, only the services within the limitations are covered. The issuance by a State of a license to practice medicine constitutes legal authorization. Temporary State licenses also constitute legal authorization to practice medicine. If State law authorizes local political subdivisions to establish higher standards for medical practitioners than those set by the State licensing board, the local standards determine whether a particular physician has legal authorization. If State licensing law limits the scope of practice of a particular type of medical practitioner, only the services within the limitations are covered. NOTE:The term physician does not include such practitioners as a Christian Science practitioner or naturopath.

100-1, 5 , 70.6

Chiropractors

A. General

A licensed chiropractor who meets uniform minimum standards (see subsection C) is a physician for specified services. Coverage extends only to treatment by means of manual manipulation of the spine to correct a subluxation demonstrated by X-ray, provided such treatment is legal in the State where performed. All other services furnished or ordered by chiropractors are not covered. An X-ray obtained by a chiropractor for his or her own diagnostic purposes before commencing treatment may suffice for claims documentation purposes. This means that if a chiropractor orders, takes, or interprets an X-ray to demonstrate a subluxation of the spine, the X-ray can be used for claims processing purposes. However, there is no coverage or payment for these services or for any other diagnostic or therapeutic service ordered or furnished by the chiropractor. In addition, in performing manual manipulation of the spine, some chiropractors use manual devices that are hand-held with the thrust of the force of the device being controlled manually. While such manual manipulation may be covered, there is no separate payment permitted for use of this device.

B. Licensure and Authorization to Practice

A chiropractor must be licensed or legally authorized to furnish chiropractic services by the State or jurisdiction in which the services are furnished.

C. Uniform Minimum Standards

I. Prior to July 1, 1974, Chiropractors licensed or authorized to practice prior to July 1, 1974, and those individuals who commenced their studies in a chiropractic college before that date must meet all of the following minimum standards to render payable services under the program:

   a. Preliminary education equal to the requirements for graduation from an accredited high school or other secondary school;

   b. Graduation from a college of chiropractic approved by the State's chiropractic examiners that included the completion of a course of study covering a period of not less than 3 school years of 6 months each year in actual continuous attendance covering adequate course of study in the subjects of anatomy, physiology, symptomatology and diagnosis, hygiene and sanitation, chemistry, histology, pathology, and principles and practice of chiropractic, including clinical instruction in vertebral palpation, nerve tracing and adjusting; and

   c. Passage of an examination prescribed by the State's chiropractic examiners covering the subjects listed in subsection b.

2. After June 30, 1974 - Individuals commencing their studies in a chiropractic college after June 30, 1974, must meet all of the following additional requirements:

   a. Satisfactory completion of 2 years of pre-chiropractic study at the college level;

   b. Satisfactory completion of a 4-year course of 8 months each year (instead of a 3-year course of 6 months each year) at a college or school of chiropractic that includes not less than 4,000 hours in the scientific and chiropractic courses specified in subsection 1.b, plus courses in the use and effect of X-ray and chiropractic analysis; and

   c. The practitioner must be over 21 years of age.

100-1, 5, 90.2

Laboratory Defined

Laboratory means a facility for the biological, microbiological, serological, chemical, immuno-hematological, hematological, biophysical, cytological, pathological, or other examination of materials derived from the human body for the purpose of providing information for the diagnosis, prevention, or treatment of any disease or impairment of, or the assessment of the health of, human beings. These examinations also include procedures to determine, measure, or otherwise describe the presence or absence of various substances or organisms in the body. Facilities only collecting or preparing specimens (or both) or only serving as a mailing service and not performing testing are not considered laboratories.

100-2, 1, 10

Covered Inpatient Hospital Services Covered Under Part A

A3-3101, HO-210

Patients covered under hospital insurance are entitled to have payment made on their behalf for inpatient hospital services. (Inpatient hospital services do not include extended care services provided by hospitals pursuant to swing bed approvals. See Pub. 100-1, Chapter 8, Sec.10.1, "Hospital Providers of Extended Care Services."). However, both inpatient hospital and inpatient SNF benefits are provided under Part A - Hospital Insurance Benefits for the Aged and Disabled, of Title XVIII).

Additional information concerning the following topics can be found in the following manual chapters:

- Benefit periods is found in Chapter 3, "Duration of Covered Inpatient Services";
- Copayment days is found in Chapter 2, "Duration of Covered Inpatient Services";
- Lifetime reserve days is found in Chapter 5, "Lifetime Reserve Days";
- Related payment information is housed in the Provider Reimbursement Manual.

Blood must be furnished on a day which counts as a day of inpatient hospital services to be covered as a Part A service and to count toward the blood deductible. Thus, blood is not covered under Part A and does not count toward the Part A blood deductible when furnished to an inpatient after the inpatient has exhausted all benefit days in a benefit period, or where the individual has elected not to use lifetime reserve days. However, where the patient is discharged on their first day of entitlement or on the hospital's first day of participation, the hospital is permitted to submit a billing form with no accommodation charge, but with ancillary charges including blood.

The records for all Medicare hospital inpatient discharges are maintained in CMS for statistical analysis and use in determining future PPS DRG classifications and rates.

Non-PPS hospitals do not pay for noncovered services generally excluded from coverage in the Medicare Program. This may result in denial of a part of the billed charges or in denial of the entire admission, depending upon circumstance. In PPS hospitals, the following are also possible:

1. In appropriately admitted cases where a noncovered procedure was performed, denied services may result in payment of a different DRG (i.e., one which excludes payment for the noncovered procedure); or
2. In appropriately admitted cases that become cost outlier cases, denied services may lead to denial of some or all of an outlier payment.

The following examples illustrate this principle. If care is noncovered because a patient does not need to be hospitalized, the intermediary denies the admission and makes no Part A (i.e., PPS) payment unless paid under limitation on liability. Under limitation on liability, Medicare payment may be made when the provider and the beneficiary were not aware the services were not necessary and could not reasonably be expected to know that he services were not necessary. For detailed instructions, see the Medicare Claims Processing Manual, Chapter 30,"Limitation on Liability." If a patient is appropriately hospitalized but receives (beyond routine services) only noncovered care, the admission is denied.

NOTE: The intermediary does not deny an admission that includes covered care, even if noncovered care was also rendered. Under PPS, Medicare assumes that it is paying for only the covered care rendered whenever covered services needed to treat and/or diagnose the illness were in fact provided.

If a noncovered procedure is provided along with covered nonroutine care, a DRG change rather than an admission denial might occur. If noncovered procedures are elevating costs into the cost outlier category, outlier payment is denied in whole or in part.

When the hospital is included in PPS, most of the subsequent discussion regarding coverage of inpatient hospital services is relevant only in the context of determining the appropriateness of admissions, which DRG, if any, to pay, and the appropriateness of payment for any outlier cases.

If a patient receives items or services in excess of, or more expensive than, those for which payment can be made, payment is made only for the covered items or services or for only the appropriate prospective payment amount. This provision applies not only to inpatient services, but also to all hospital services under Parts A and B of the program. If the items or services were requested by the patient, the hospital may charge him the difference between the amount customarily charged for the services requested and the amount customarily charged for covered services.

An inpatient is a person who has been admitted to a hospital for bed occupancy for purposes of receiving inpatient hospital services. Generally, a patient is considered an inpatient if formally admitted as inpatient with the expectation that he or she will remain at least overnight and occupy a bed even though it later develops that the patient can be discharged or transferred to another hospital and not actually use a hospital bed overnight.

The physician or other practitioner responsible for a patient's care at the hospital is also responsible for deciding whether the patient should be admitted as an inpatient. Physicians should use a 24-hour period as a benchmark, i.e., they should order admission for patients who are expected to need hospital care for 24 hours or more, and treat other patients on an outpatient basis. However, the decision to admit a patient is a complex medical judgment which can be made only after the physician has considered a number of factors, including the patient's medical history and current medical needs, the types of facilities available to inpatients and to outpatients, the hospital's by-laws and admissions policies, and the relative appropriateness of treatment in each setting. Factors to be considered when making the decision to admit include such things as:

- The severity of the signs and symptoms exhibited by the patient;
- The medical predictability of something adverse happening to the patient;
- The need for diagnostic studies that appropriately are outpatient services (i.e., their performance does not ordinarily require the patient to remain at the hospital for 24 hours or more) to assist in assessing whether the patient should be admitted; and
- The availability of diagnostic procedures at the time when and at the location where the patient presents.

Admissions of particular patients are not covered or noncovered solely on the basis of the length of time the patient actually spends in the hospital. In certain specific situations coverage of services on an inpatient or outpatient basis is determined by the following rules:

Minor Surgery or Other Treatment - When patients with known diagnoses enter a hospital for a specific minor surgical procedure or other treatment that is expected to keep them in the hospital for only a few hours (less than 24), they are considered outpatients for coverage purposes regardless of: the hour they came to the hospital, whether they used a bed, and whether they remained in the hospital past midnight.

Renal Dialysis - Renal dialysis treatments are usually covered only as outpatient services but may under certain circumstances be covered as inpatient services depending on the patient's condition. Patients staying at home, who are ambulatory, whose conditions are stable and who come to the hospital for routine chronic dialysis treatments, and not for a diagnostic workup or a change in therapy, are considered outpatients. On the other hand, patients undergoing short-term dialysis until their kidneys recover from an acute illness (acute dialysis), or persons with borderline renal failure who develop acute renal failure every time they have an illness and require dialysis (episodic dialysis) are usually inpatients. A patient may begin dialysis as an inpatient and then progress to an outpatient status.

Under original Medicare, the Quality Improvement Organization (QIO), for each hospital is responsible for deciding, during review of inpatient admissions on a case-by-case basis, whether the admission was medically necessary. Medicare law authorizes the QIO to make these judgments, and the judgments are binding for purposes of Medicare coverage. In making these judgments, however, QIOs consider only the medical evidence which was available to the physician at the time an admission decision had to be made. They do not take into account other information (e.g., test results) which became available only after admission, except in cases where considering the post-admission information would support a finding that an admission was medically necessary.

Refer to Parts 4 and 7 of the QIO Manual with regard to initial determinations for these services. The QIO will review the swing bed services in these PPS hospitals as well.

NOTE: When patients requiring extended care services are admitted to beds in a hospital, they are considered inpatients of the hospital. In such cases, the services furnished in the hospital will not be considered extended care services, and payment may not be made under the program for such services unless the services are extended care services furnished pursuant to a swing bed agreement granted to the hospital by the Secretary of Health and Human Services.

100-2, 1, 90

Termination of Pregnancy

B3-4276.1,.2

Effective for services furnished on or after October 1, 1998, Medicare will cover abortions procedures in the following situations:

1. If the pregnancy is the result of an act or rape or incest; or
2. In the case where a woman suffers from a physical disorder, physical injury, or physical illness, including a life-endangering physical condition caused by the pregnancy itself that would, as certified by a physician, place the woman in danger of death unless an abortion is performed.

NOTE: The "G7" modifier must be used with the following CPT codes in order for these services to be covered when the pregnancy resulted from rape or incest, or the pregnancy is certified by a physician as life threatening to the mother:

59840, 59841, 59850, 59851, 59852, 59855, 59856, 59857, 59866

100-2, 1, 100

Treatment for Infertility

A3-3101.13

Effective for services rendered on or after January 15, 1980, reasonable and necessary services associated with treatment for infertility are covered under Medicare. Like pregnancy (see Sec. 80 above), infertility is a condition sufficiently at variance with the usual state of health to make it appropriate for a person who normally would be expected to be fertile to seek medical consultation and treatment. Contractors should coordinate with QIOs to see that utilization guidelines are established for this treatment if inappropriate utilization or abuse is suspected.

100-2 , 6, 10

Medical and Other Health Services Furnished to Inpatients of Participating Hospitals

Payment may be made under Part B for physician services and for the nonphysician medical and other health services listed below when furnished by a participating hospital (either directly or under arrangements) to an inpatient of the hospital, but only if payment for these services cannot be made under Part A.

In PPS hospitals, this means that Part B payment could be made for these services if:

- No Part A prospective payment is made at all for the hospital stay because of patient exhaustion of benefit days before admission;
- The admission was disapproved as not reasonable and necessary (and waiver of liability payment was not made);
- The day or days of the otherwise covered stay during which the services were provided were not reasonable and necessary (and no payment was made under waiver of liability);
- The patient was not otherwise eligible for or entitled to coverage under Part A (See the Medicare Benefit Policy Manual, Chapter 1, Sec.150, for services received as a result of noncovered services); or
- No Part A day outlier payment is made (for discharges before October 1997) for one or more outlier days due to patient exhaustion of benefit days after admission but before the case's arrival at outlier status, or because outlier days are otherwise not covered and waiver of liability payment is not made.

However, if only day outlier payment is denied under Part A (discharges before October 1997), Part B payment may be made for only the services covered under Part B and furnished on the denied outlier days.

In non-PPS hospitals, Part B payment may be made for services on any day for which Part A payment is denied (i.e., benefit days are exhausted; services are not at the hospital level of care; or patient is not otherwise eligible or entitled to payment under Part A).

Services payable are:

- Diagnostic x-ray tests, diagnostic laboratory tests, and other diagnostic tests;
- X-ray, radium, and radioactive isotope therapy, including materials and services of technicians;
- Surgical dressings, and splints, casts, and other devices used for reduction of fractures and dislocations;
- Prosthetic devices (other than dental) which replace all or part of an internal body organ (including contiguous tissue), or all or part of the function of a permanently inoperative or malfunctioning internal body organ, including replacement or repairs of such devices;
- Leg, arm, back, and neck braces, trusses, and artificial legs, arms, and eyes including adjustments, repairs, and replacements required because of breakage, wear, loss, or a change in the patient's physical condition;
- Outpatient physical therapy, outpatient speech-language pathology services, and outpatient occupational therapy (see the Medicare Benefit Policy Manual, Chapter 15, "Covered Medical and Other Health Services," Sec.Sec.220 and 230);
- Screening mammography services;
- Screening pap smears;
- Influenza, pneumococcal pneumonia, and hepatitis B vaccines;
- Colorectal screening;
- Bone mass measurements;
- Diabetes self-management;
- Prostate screening;
- Ambulance services;
- Hemophilia clotting factors for hemophilia patients competent to use these factors without supervision);
- Immunosuppressive drugs;
- Oral anti-cancer drugs;
- Oral drug prescribed for use as an acute anti-emetic used as part of an anti-cancer chemotherapeutic regimen; and Epoetin Alfa (EPO).

Coverage rules for these services are described in the Medicare Benefit Policy Manual, Chapters: 11, "End Stage Renal Disease (ESRD);" 14, "Medical Devices;" or 15, "Medical and Other Health Services."

For services to be covered under Part A or Part B, a hospital must furnish nonphysician services to its inpatients directly or under arrangements. A nonphysician service is one which does not meet the criteria defining physicians' services specifically provided for in regulation at 42 CFR 415.102. Services "incident to" physicians' services (except for the services of nurse anesthetists employed by anesthesiologists) are nonphysician services for purposes of this provision. This provision is applicable to all hospitals participating in Medicare, including those paid under alternative arrangements such as State cost control systems, and to emergency hospital services furnished by nonparticipating hospitals.

In all hospitals, every service provided to a hospital inpatient other than those listed in the next paragraph must be treated as an inpatient hospital service to be paid for under Part A, if Part A coverage is available and the beneficiary is entitled to Part A. This is because every hospital must provide directly or arrange for any nonphysician service rendered to its inpatients, and a hospital can be paid under Part B for a service provided in this manner only if Part A coverage does not exist.

These services, when provided to a hospital inpatient, may be covered under Part B, even though the patient has Part A coverage for the hospital stay. This is because these services are covered under Part B and not covered under Part A. They are:

- Physicians' services (including the services of residents and interns in unapproved teaching programs);
- Influenza vaccine;
- Pneumoccocal vaccine and its administration;
- Hepatitis B vaccine and its administration;
- Screening mammography services;
- Screening pap smears and pelvic exams;
- Colorectal screening;
- Bone mass measurements;
- Diabetes self management training services; and
- Prostate screening.

However, note that in order to have any Medicare coverage at all (Part A or Part B), any nonphysician service rendered to a hospital inpatient must be provided directly or arranged for by the hospital.

100-2, 6, 50

Sleep Disorder Clinics

A3-3112.5

Sleep disorder clinics are facilities in which certain conditions are diagnosed through the study of sleep. Such clinics are for diagnosis, therapy, and research. Sleep disorder clinics may provide some diagnostic or therapeutic services that are covered under Medicare. These clinics may be affiliated either with a hospital or a freestanding facility. Whether a clinic is hospital-affiliated or freestanding, coverage for diagnostic services under some circumstances is covered under provisions of the law different from those for coverage of therapeutic services.

100-2, 11, 20

Coverage of Outpatient Maintenance Dialysis

A3-3167, B3-2230.2, RDF-202, SOM-2272, RDF-317.1, PM AB-03-001

Medicare covers maintenance dialysis treatments when they are provided to ESRD patients by an approved hospital-based dialysis facility, an independent dialysis facility, or a special purpose dialysis facility. Outpatient dialysis treatments are covered in various settings: hospital outpatient facility, independent dialysis facility, or the patient's home. Dialysis treatments at dialysis facilities differ according to the types of patients being treated, the types of equipment and supplies used, the preferences of the treating physician, and the capability and makeup of the staff. Although not all facilities provide an identical range of services, the most common elements of a dialysis treatment are:

a. Personnel services;

b. Equipment and supplies - dialysis machine and its maintenance;

c. Administrative services;

d. Overhead costs;

e. Monitoring access and related declotting the access or referring the patient;

f. ESRD related laboratory tests; and

g. Biologicals.

Direct nursing services include registered nurses, licensed practical nurses, technicians, social workers, and dietitians. Facilities with self-dialysis units must meet specific health and safety requirements. Certain standards applicable to staff assisted dialysis have been adjusted for self-dialysis units in consideration of the differences in the two modalities. Before participating in self-dialysis, patients must have completed an appropriate training program in emergency procedures and have a safe storage area for their supplies. Access to the self-dialysis unit is limited to patients for whom the facility maintains patient care plans in order to exclude transient patients who might not be familiar with the facility's equipment or emergency procedures. The self-dialysis unit need not be physically separate from the rest of the facility nor operate on a separate shift.

100-2, 12, 40.11

Vaccines

A CORF may provide pneumococcal pneumonia, influenza virus, and hepatitis B vaccines to its patients. While not included as a service under the CORF benefit, Medicare will make payment to the CORF for certain vaccines and their administration provided to CORF patients (CY 2008 PFS Rule 72 FR 66293).

The following three vaccinations are covered in a CORF if a physician who is a doctor of medicine or osteopathy orders it for a CORF patient: Pneumococcal pneumonia vaccine and its administration;

Hepatitis B vaccine and its administration furnished to a beneficiary who is at high or intermediate risk of contracting hepatitis B; and

Influenza virus vaccine and its administration

Payment for covered pneumococcal pneumonia, influenza virus, and hepatitis B vaccines provided in the CORF setting is based on 95 percent of the average wholesale price. The CORF registered nurse provides administration of any of these vaccines using HCPCS codes G0008, G0009 or G0010 with payment based on CPT code 90471.

100-2, 13, 30

Rural Health Clinic and Federally Qualified Health Center Service Defined

Payments for covered RHC/FQHC services furnished to Medicare beneficiaries are made on the basis of an all-inclusive rate per covered visit (except for pneumococcal and influenza vaccines and their administration, which is paid at 100 percent of reasonable cost). The term "visit" is defined as a face-to-face encounter between the patient and a physician, physician assistant, nurse practitioner, certified nurse midwife, visiting nurse, clinical psychologist, or clinical social worker during which an RHC/FQHC service is rendered. As a result of section 5114 of the Deficit Reduction Act of 2005 (DRA), the FQHC definition of a face-to-face encounter is expanded to include encounters with qualified practitioners of Outpatient Diabetes Self-Management Training Services (DSMT) and medical nutrition therapy (MNT) services when the FQHC meets all relevant program requirements for the provision of such services.

Encounters with (1) more than one health professional; and (2) multiple encounters with the same health professional which take place on the same day and at a single location, constitute a single visit. An exception occurs in cases in which the patient, subsequent to the first encounter, suffers an illness or injury requiring additional diagnosis or treatment.

100-2, 15, 20.1

Physician Expense for Surgery, Childbirth, and Treatment for Infertility

B3-2005.I

A. Surgery and Childbirth

Skilled medical management is covered throughout the events of pregnancy, beginning with diagnosis, continuing through delivery and ending after the necessary postnatal care. Similarly, in the event of termination of pregnancy, regardless of whether terminated spontaneously or for therapeutic reasons (i.e., where the life of the mother would be endangered if the fetus were brought to term), the need for skilled medical management and/or medical services is equally important as in those cases carried to full term. After the infant is delivered and is a separate individual, items and services furnished to the infant are not covered on the basis of the mother's eligibility.

Most surgeons and obstetricians bill patients an all-inclusive package charge intended to cover all services associated with the surgical procedure or delivery of the child. All expenses for surgical and obstetrical care, including preoperative/prenatal examinations and tests and post-operative/postnatal services, are considered incurred on the date of surgery or delivery, as appropriate. This policy applies whether the physician bills on a package charge basis, or itemizes the bill separately for these items.

Occasionally, a physician's bill may include charges for additional services not directly related to the surgical procedure or the delivery. Such charges are considered incurred on the date the additional services are furnished.

The above policy applies only where the charges are imposed by one physician or by a clinic on behalf of a group of physicians. Where more than one physician imposes charges for surgical or obstetrical services, all preoperative/prenatal and post-operative/postnatal services performed by the physician who performed the surgery or delivery are considered incurred on the date of the surgery or delivery. Expenses for services rendered by other physicians are considered incurred on the date they were performed.

B. Treatment for Infertility

Reasonable and necessary services associated with treatment for infertility are covered under Medicare. Infertility is a condition sufficiently at variance with the usual state of health to make it appropriate for a person who normally is expected to be fertile to seek medical consultation and treatment.

100-2, 15, 20.2

Physician Expense for Allergy Treatment

B3-2005.2, B3-4145 Allergists commonly bill separately for the initial diagnostic workup and for the treatment (See Sec.60.2). Where it is necessary to provide treatment over an extended period, the allergist may submit a single bill for all of the treatments, or may bill periodically. In either case the Form CMS-1500 claim shows the Healthcare Common Procedure Coding System (HCPCS) codes and from and through dates of service, or the Form CMS-1450 outpatient claim shows the HCPCS code and date of service (except for critical access hospital (CAH) claims).

100-2, 15, 20.3

Artificial Limbs, Braces, and Other Custom Made Items Ordered But Not Furnished

B3-2005.3

A. Date of Incurred Expense

If a custom-made item was ordered but not furnished to a beneficiary because the individual died or because the order was canceled by the beneficiary or because the beneficiary's condition changed and the item was no longer reasonable and necessary or appropriate, payment can be made based on the supplier's expenses. (See subsection B for determination of the allowed amount.) In such cases, the expense is considered incurred on the date the beneficiary died or the date the supplier learned of the cancellation or that the item was no longer reasonable and necessary or appropriate for the beneficiary's condition. If the beneficiary died or the beneficiary's condition changed and the item was no longer reasonable and necessary or appropriate, payment can be made on either an assigned or unassigned claim. If the beneficiary, for any other reason, canceled the order, payment can be made to the supplier only.

B. Determination of Allowed Amount
The allowed amount is based on the services furnished and materials used, up to the date the supplier learned of the beneficiary's death or of the cancellation of the order or that the item was no longer reasonable and necessary or appropriate. The Durable Medical Equipment Regional Carrier (DMERC), carrier or intermediary, as appropriate, determines the services performed and the allowable amount appropriate in the particular situation. It takes into account any salvage value of the device to the supplier. Where a supplier breaches an agreement to make a prosthesis, brace, or other custom-made device for a Medicare beneficiary, e.g., an unexcused failure to provide the article within the time specified in the contract, payment may not be made for any work or material expended on the item. Whether a particular supplier has lived up to its agreement, of course, depends on the facts in the individual case.

100-2, 15, 30

Physician Services

A. General
Physician services are the professional services performed by a physician or physicians for a patient including diagnosis, therapy, surgery, consultation, and care plan oversight.

The physician must render the service for the service to be covered. (See Pub. 100-01, Medicare General Information, Eligibility, and Entitlement Manual, Chapter 5, §70, for definition of physician.) A service may be considered to be a physician's service where the physician either examines the patient in person or is able to visualize some aspect of the patient's condition without the interposition of a third person's judgment. Direct visualization would be possible by means of x-rays, electrocardiogram and electroencephalogram tapes, tissue samples, etc.

For example, the interpretation by a physician of an actual electrocardiogram or electroencephalogram reading that has been transmitted via telephone (i.e., electronically rather than by means of a verbal description) is a covered service.

Professional services of the physician are covered if provided within the United States, and may be performed in a home, office, institution, or at the scene of an accident. A patient's home, for this purpose, is anywhere the patient makes his or her residence, e.g., home for the aged, a nursing home, a relative's home.

B. Telephone Services
Services by means of a telephone call between a physician and a beneficiary, or between a physician and a member of a beneficiary's family, are covered under Medicare, but carriers may not make separate payment for these services under the program. The physician work resulting from telephone calls is considered to be an integral part of the prework and postwork of other physician services, and the fee schedule amount for the latter services already includes payment for the telephone calls. See §270 of this manual for coverage of telehealth services.

C. Consultations
As of January 1, 2010, CMS no longer recognizes consultation codes for Medicare payment, except for inpatient telehealth consultation HCPCS G-codes. Instead, physicians and qualified nonphysician practitioners are instructed to bill a new or established patient office/outpatient visit CPT code or appropriate hospital or nursing facility care code. For further detail regarding reporting services that would otherwise be described by the CPT consultation codes (99241-99245 and 99251-99255), see Pub. 100-04, Medicare Claims Processing Manual, chapter 12, section 30.6. For detailed instructions regarding reporting telehealth consultation services and other telehealth services, see Pub. 100-04, chapter 12, section 190.3.

D. Patient-Initiated Second Opinions
Patient-initiated second opinions that relate to the medical need for surgery or for major nonsurgical diagnostic and therapeutic procedures (e.g., invasive diagnostic techniques such as cardiac catheterization and gastroscopy) are covered under Medicare. In the event that the recommendation of the first and second physician differs regarding the need for surgery (or other major procedure), a third opinion is also covered. Second and third opinions are covered even though the surgery or other procedure, if performed, is determined not covered. Payment may be made for the history and examination of the patient, and for other covered diagnostic services required to properly evaluate the patient's need for a procedure and to render a professional opinion. In some cases, the results of tests done by the first physician may be available to the second physician.

E. Concurrent Care
Concurrent care exists where more than one physician renders services more extensive than consultative services during a period of time. The reasonable and necessary services of each physician rendering concurrent care could be covered where each is required to play an active role in the patient's treatment, for example, because of the existence of more than one medical condition requiring diverse specialized medical services.

In order to determine whether concurrent physicians' services are reasonable and necessary, the carrier must decide the following:

1. Whether the patient's condition warrants the services of more than one physician on an attending (rather than consultative) basis, and
2. Whether the individual services provided by each physician are reasonable and necessary.

In resolving the first question, the carrier should consider the specialties of the physicians as well as the patient's diagnosis, as concurrent care is usually (although not always) initiated because of the existence of more than one medical condition requiring diverse specialized medical or surgical services. The specialties of the physicians are an indication of the necessity for concurrent services, but the patient's condition and the inherent reasonableness and necessity of the services, as determined by the carrier's medical staff in accordance with locality norms, must also be considered. For example, although cardiology is a sub-specialty of internal medicine, the treatment of both diabetes and of a serious heart condition might require the concurrent services of two physicians, each practicing in internal medicine but specializing in different sub-specialties.

While it would not be highly unusual for concurrent care performed by physicians in different specialties (e.g., a surgeon and an internist) or by physicians in different subspecialties of the same specialty (e.g., an allergist and a cardiologist) to be found medically necessary, the need for such care by physicians in the same specialty or

subspecialty (e.g., two internists or two cardiologists) would occur infrequently since in most cases both physicians would possess the skills and knowledge necessary to treat the patient. However, circumstances could arise which would necessitate such care. For example, a patient may require the services of two physicians in the same specialty or sub-specialty when one physician has further limited his or her practice to some unusual aspect of that specialty, e.g., tropical medicine. Similarly, concurrent services provided by a family physician and an internist may or may not be found to be reasonable and necessary, depending on the circumstances of the specific case. If it is determined that the services of one of the physicians are not warranted by the patient's condition, payment may be made only for the other physician's (or physicians') services.

Once it is determined that the patient requires the active services of more than one physician, the individual services must be examined for medical necessity, just as where a single physician provides the care. For example, even if it is determined that the patient requires the concurrent services of both a cardiologist and a surgeon, payment may not be made for any services rendered by either physician which, for that condition, exceed normal frequency or duration unless there are special circumstances requiring the additional care.

The carrier must also assure that the services of one physician do not duplicate those provided by another, e.g., where the family physician visits during the post-operative period primarily as a courtesy to the patient.

Hospital admission services performed by two physicians for the same beneficiary on the same day could represent reasonable and necessary services, provided, as stated above, that the patient's condition necessitates treatment by both physicians. The level of difficulty of the service provided may vary between the physicians, depending on the severity of the complaint each one is treating and that physician's prior contact with the patient. For example, the admission services performed by a physician who has been treating a patient over a period of time for a chronic condition would not be as involved as the services performed by a physician who has had no prior contact with the patient and who has been called in to diagnose and treat a major acute condition.

Carriers should have sufficient means for identifying concurrent care situations. A correct coverage determination can be made on a concurrent care case only where the claim is sufficiently documented for the carrier to determine the role each physician played in the patient's care (i.e., the condition or conditions for which the physician treated the patient). If, in any case, the role of each physician involved is not clear, the carrier should request clarification.

F. Completion of Claims Forms
Separate charges for the services of a physician in completing a Form CMS-1500, a statement in lieu of a Form CMS-1500, or an itemized bill are not covered. Payment for completion of the Form CMS-1500 claim form is considered included in the fee schedule amount.

G. Care Plan Oversight Services
Care plan oversight is supervision of patients under care of home health agencies or hospices that require complex and multidisciplinary care modalities involving regular physician development and/or revision of care plans, review of subsequent reports of patient status, review of laboratory and other studies, communication with other health professionals not employed in the same practice who are involved in the patient's care, integration of new information into the care plan, and/or adjustment of medical therapy.

Such services are covered for home health and hospice patients, but are not covered for patients of skilled nursing facilities (SNFs), nursing home facilities, or hospitals.

These services are covered only if all the following requirements are met:

1. The beneficiary must require complex or multi-disciplinary care modalities requiring ongoing physician involvement in the patient's plan of care;
2. The care plan oversight (CPO) services should be furnished during the period in which the beneficiary was receiving Medicare covered HHA or hospice services;
3. The physician who bills CPO must be the same physician who signed the home health or hospice plan of care;
4. The physician furnished at least 30 minutes of care plan oversight within the calendar month for which payment is claimed. Time spent by a physician's nurse or the time spent consulting with one's nurse is not countable toward the 30-minute threshold. Low-intensity services included as part of other evaluation and management services are not included as part of the 30 minutes required for coverage;
5. The work included in hospital discharge day management (codes 99238-99239) and discharge from observation (code 99217) is not countable toward the 30 minutes per month required for work on the same day as discharge but only for those services separately documented as occurring after the patient is actually physically discharged from the hospital;
6. The physician provided a covered physician service that required a face-to-face encounter with the beneficiary within the 6 months immediately preceding the first care plan oversight service. Only evaluation and management services are acceptable prerequisite face-to-face encounters for CPO. EKG, lab, and surgical services are not sufficient face-to-face services for CPO;
7. The care plan oversight billed by the physician was not routine post-operative care provided in the global surgical period of a surgical procedure billed by the physician;
8. If the beneficiary is receiving home health agency services, the physician did not have a significant financial or contractual interest in the home health agency. A physician who is an employee of a hospice, including a volunteer medical director, should not bill CPO services. Payment for the services of a physician employed by the hospice is included in the payment to the hospice;

9. The physician who bills the care plan oversight services is the physician who furnished them;
10. Services provided incident to a physician's service do not qualify as CPO and do not count toward the 30-minute requirement;
11. The physician is not billing for the Medicare end stage renal disease (ESRD) capitation payment for the same beneficiary during the same month; and
12. The physician billing for CPO must document in the patient's record the services furnished and the date and length of time associated with those services

100-2, 15, 30.4

Optometrist's Services

B3-2020.25

Effective April 1, 1987, a doctor of optometry is considered a physician with respect to all services the optometrist is authorized to perform under State law or regulation. To be covered under Medicare, the services must be medically reasonable and necessary for the diagnosis or treatment of illness or injury, and must meet all applicable coverage requirements. See the Medicare Benefit Policy Manual, Chapter 16, "General Exclusions from Coverage," for exclusions from coverage that apply to vision care services, and the Medicare Claims Processing Manual, Chapter 12, "Physician/Practitioner Billing," for information dealing with payment for items and services furnished by optometrists.

A. FDA Monitored Studies of Intraocular Lenses

Special coverage rules apply to situations in which an ophthalmologist is involved in a Food and Drug Administration (FDA) monitored study of the safety and efficacy of an investigational Intraocular Lens (IOL). The investigation process for IOLs is unique in that there is a core period and an adjunct period. The core study is a traditional, well-controlled clinical investigation with full record keeping and reporting requirements. The adjunct study is essentially an extended distribution phase for lenses in which only limited safety data are compiled. Depending on the lens being evaluated, the adjunct study may be an extension of the core study or may be the only type of investigation to which the lens may be subject.

All eye care services related to the investigation of the IOL must be provided by the investigator (i.e., the implanting ophthalmologist) or another practitioner (including a doctor of optometry) who provides services at the direction or under the supervision of the investigator and who has an agreement with the investigator that information on the patient is given to the investigator so that he or she may report on the patient to the IOL manufacturer. Eye care services furnished by anyone other than the investigator (or a practitioner who assists the investigator, as described in the preceding paragraph) are not covered during the period the IOL is being investigated, unless the services are not related to the investigation.

B. Concurrent Care

Where more than one practitioner furnishes concurrent care, services furnished to a beneficiary by both an ophthalmologist and another physician (including an optometrist) may be recognized for payment if it is determined that each practitioner's services were reasonable and necessary. (See Sec.30.E

100-2, 15, 30.5

Chiropractor's Services

B3-2020.26

A chiropractor must be licensed or legally authorized to furnish chiropractic services by the State or jurisdiction in which the services are furnished. In addition, a licensed chiropractor must meet the following uniform minimum standards to be considered a physician for Medicare coverage. Coverage extends only to treatment by means of manual manipulation of the spine to correct a subluxation provided such treatment is legal in the State where performed. All other services furnished or ordered by chiropractors are not covered. If a chiropractor orders, takes, or interprets an x-ray or other diagnostic procedure to demonstrate a subluxation of the spine, the x-ray can be used for documentation. However, there is no coverage or payment for these services or for any other diagnostic or therapeutic service ordered or furnished by the chiropractor. For detailed information on using x-rays to determine subluxation, see Sec.240.1.2. In addition, in performing manual manipulation of the spine, some chiropractors use manual devices that are hand-held with the thrust of the force of the device being controlled manually. While such manual manipulation may be covered, there is no separate payment permitted for use of this device.

A. Uniform Minimum Standards

Prior to July 1, 1974 Chiropractors licensed or authorized to practice prior to July 1, 1974, and those individuals who commenced their studies in a chiropractic college before that date must meet all of the following three minimum standards to render payable services under the program:

Preliminary education equal to the requirements for graduation from an accredited high school or other secondary school;Graduation from a college of chiropractic approved by the State's chiropractic examiners that included the completion of a course of study covering a period of not less than 3 school years of 6 months each year in actual continuous attendance covering adequate course of study in the subjects of anatomy, physiology, symptomatology and diagnosis, hygiene and sanitation, chemistry, histology, pathology, and principles and practice of chiropractic, including clinical instruction in vertebral palpation, nerve tracing, and adjusting; andPassage of an examination prescribed by the State's chiropractic examiners covering the subjects listed above.

After June 30, 1974Individuals commencing their studies in a chiropractic college after June 30, 1974, must meet all of the above three standards and all of the following additional requirements:Satisfactory completion of 2 years of pre-chiropractic study at the college level;Satisfactory completion of a 4-year course of 8 months each year (instead of a 3-year course of 6 months each year) at a college or school of chiropractic that includes not less than 4,000 hours in the scientific and chiropractic courses specified in the second bullet under "Prior to July 1, 1974" above, plus courses in the use and effect of x-ray and chiropractic analysis; andThe practitioner must be over 21 years of age.

B. Maintenance Therapy

Under the Medicare program, Chiropractic maintenance therapy is not considered to be medically reasonable or necessary, and is therefore not payable. Maintenance therapy is defined as a treatment plan that seeks to prevent disease, promote health, and prolong and enhance the quality of life; or therapy that is performed to maintain or prevent deterioration of a chronic condition. When further clinical improvement cannot reasonably be expected from continuous ongoing care, and the chiropractic treatment becomes supportive rather than corrective in nature, the treatment is then considered maintenance therapy. For information on how to indicate on a claim a treatment is or is not maintenance, see Sec.240.1.

100-2, 15, 50

Drugs and Biologicals

B3-2049, A3-3112.4.B, HO-230.4.B

The Medicare program provides limited benefits for outpatient drugs. The program covers drugs that are furnished "incident to" a physician's service provided that the drugs are not usually self-administered by the patients who take them. Generally, drugs and biologicals are covered only if all of the following requirements are met:

- They meet the definition of drugs or biologicals (see Sec.50.1);
- They are of the type that are not usually self-administered. (see Sec.50.2);
- They meet all the general requirements for coverage of items as incident to a physician's services (see Sec.Sec.50.1 and 50.3);
- They are reasonable and necessary for the diagnosis or treatment of the illness or injury for which they are administered according to accepted standards of medical practice (see Sec.50.4);
- They are not excluded as noncovered immunizations (see Sec.50.4.4.2); and
- They have not been determined by the FDA to be less than effective. (See Sec.Sec.50.4.4).

Medicare Part B does generally not cover drugs that can be self-administered, such as those in pill form, or are used for self-injection. However, the statute provides for the coverage of some self-administered drugs. Examples of self-administered drugs that are covered include blood-clotting factors, drugs used in immunosuppressive therapy, erythropoietin for dialysis patients, osteoporosis drugs for certain homebound patients, and certain oral cancer drugs. (See Sec.110.3 for coverage of drugs, which are necessary to the effective use of Durable Medical Equipment (DME) or prosthetic devices.)

100-2, 15, 50.4.4.2

100-2, 15, 50.4.4.2

Immunizations

Vaccinations or inoculations are excluded as immunizations unless they are directly related to the treatment of an injury or direct exposure to a disease or condition, such as anti-rabies treatment, tetanus antitoxin or booster vaccine, botulin antitoxin, antivenin sera, or immune globulin. In the absence of injury or direct exposure, preventive immunization (vaccination or inoculation) against such diseases as smallpox, polio, diphtheria, etc., is not covered. However, pneumococcal, hepatitis B, and influenza virus vaccines are exceptions to this rule. (See items A, B, and C below.) In cases where a vaccination or inoculation is excluded from coverage, related charges are also not covered.

A. Pneumococcal Pneumonia Vaccinations

Effective for services furnished on or after May 1, 1981, the Medicare Part B program covers pneumococcal pneumonia vaccine and its administration when furnished in compliance with any applicable State law by any provider of services or any entity or individual with a supplier number. This includes revaccination of patients at highest risk of pneumococcal infection. Typically, these vaccines are administered once in a lifetime except for persons at highest risk. Effective July 1, 2000, Medicare does not require for coverage purposes that a doctor of medicine or osteopathy order the vaccine. Therefore, the beneficiary may receive the vaccine upon request without a physician's order and without physician supervision.

An initial vaccine may be administered only to persons at high risk (see below) of pneumococcal disease. Revaccination may be administered only to persons at highest risk of serious pneumococcal infection and those likely to have a rapid decline in pneumococcal antibody levels, provided that at least 5 years have passed since the previous dose of pneumococcal vaccine.

Persons at high risk for whom an initial vaccine may be administered include all people age 65 and older; immunocompetent adults who are at increased risk of pneumococcal disease or its complications because of chronic illness (e.g., cardiovascular disease, pulmonary disease, diabetes mellitus, alcoholism, cirrhosis, or cerebrospinal fluid leaks); and individuals with compromised immune

(e.g., splenic dysfunction or anatomic asplenia, Hodgkin's disease, lymphoma, multiple myeloma, chronic renal failure, HIV infection, nephrotic syndrome, sickle cell disease, or organ transplantation).

Persons at highest risk and those most likely to have rapid declines in antibody levels are those for whom revaccination may be appropriate. This group includes persons with functional or anatomic asplenia (e.g., sickle cell disease, splenectomy), HIV infection, leukemia, lymphoma, Hodgkin's disease, multiple myeloma, generalized malignancy, chronic renal failure, nephrotic syndrome, or other conditions associated with immunosuppression such as organ or bone marrow transplantation, and those receiving immunosuppressive chemotherapy. It is not appropriate for routine revaccination of people age 65 or older that are not at highest risk.

Those administering the vaccine should not require the patient to present an immunization record prior to administering the pneumococcal vaccine, nor should they feel compelled to review the patient's complete medical record if it is not available. Instead, provided that the patient is competent, it is acceptable to rely on the patient's verbal history to determine prior vaccination status. If the patient is uncertain about his or her vaccination history in the past 5 years, the vaccine should be given. However, if the patient is certain he/she was were vaccinated in the last 5 years, the vaccine should not be given. If the patient is certain that the vaccine was given more than 5 years ago, revaccination is covered only if the patient is at high risk.

B. Hepatitis B Vaccine
Effective for services furnished on or after September 1, 1984, P.L. 98-369 provides coverage under Part B for hepatitis B vaccine and its administration, furnished to a Medicare beneficiary who is at high or intermediate risk of contracting hepatitis B. This coverage is effective for services furnished on or after September 1, 1984. High-risk groups currently identified include (see exception below):

- ESRD patients;
- Hemophiliacs who receive Factor VIII or IX concentrates;
- Clients of institutions for the mentally retarded;
- Persons who live in the same household as a Hepatitis B Virus (HBV) carrier;
- Homosexual men; and
- Illicit injectable drug abusers.
- Intermediate risk groups currently identified include:
- Staff in institutions for the mentally retarded; and
- Workers in health care professions who have frequent contact with blood or blood-derived body fluids during routine work.

EXCEPTION: Persons in both of the above-listed groups in paragraph B, would not be considered at high or intermediate risk of contracting hepatitis B, however, if there were laboratory evidence positive for antibodies to hepatitis B. (ESRD patients are routinely tested for hepatitis B antibodies as part of their continuing monitoring and therapy.)

For Medicare program purposes, the vaccine may be administered upon the order of a doctor of medicine or osteopathy, by a doctor of medicine or osteopathy, or by home health agencies, skilled nursing facilities, ESRD facilities, hospital outpatient departments, and persons recognized under the incident to physicians' services provision of law.

A charge separate from the ESRD composite rate will be recognized and paid for administration of the vaccine to ESRD patients.

C. Influenza Virus Vaccine
Effective for services furnished on or after May 1, 1993, the Medicare Part B program covers influenza virus vaccine and its administration when furnished in compliance with any applicable State law by any provider of services or any entity or individual with a supplier number. Typically, these vaccines are administered once a flu season. Medicare does not require, for coverage purposes, that a doctor of medicine or osteopathy order the vaccine. Therefore, the beneficiary may receive the vaccine upon request without a physician's order and without physician supervision

100-2, 15, 50.5

Self-Administered Drugs and Biologicals

B3-2049.5 Medicare Part B does not cover drugs that are usually self-administered by the patient unless the statute provides for such coverage. The statute explicitly provides coverage, for blood clotting factors, drugs used in immunosuppressive therapy, erythropoietin for dialysis patients, certain oral anti-cancer drugs and anti-emetics used in certain situations.

100-2, 15, 60.3

Incident to Physician's Service in Clinic

B3-2050.3

Services and supplies incident to a physician's service in a physician directed clinic or group association are generally the same as those described above.

A physician directed clinic is one where:

1. A physician (or a number of physicians) is present to perform medical (rather than administrative) services at all times the clinic is open;
2. Each patient is under the care of a clinic physician; and
3. The nonphysician services are under medical supervision.

In highly organized clinics, particularly those that are departmentalized, direct physician supervision may be the responsibility of several physicians as opposed to an individual attending physician. In this situation, medical management of all services provided in the clinic is assured. The physician ordering a particular service need not be the physician who is supervising the service. Therefore, services performed by auxiliary personnel and other aides are covered even though they are performed in another department of the clinic. Supplies provided by the clinic during the course of treatment are also covered. When the auxiliary personnel perform services outside the clinic premises, the services are covered only if performed under the direct supervision of a clinic physician. If the clinic refers a patient for auxiliary services performed by personnel who are not supervised by clinic physicians, such services are not incident to a physician's service.

100-2, 15, 70

Sleep Disorder Clinics

B3-2055

Sleep disorder clinics are facilities in which certain conditions are diagnosed through the study of sleep. Such clinics are for diagnosis, therapy, and research. Sleep disorder clinics may provide some diagnostic or therapeutic services which are covered under Medicare. These clinics may be affiliated either with a hospital or a freestanding facility. Whether a clinic is hospital-affiliated or freestanding, coverage for diagnostic services under some circumstances is covered under provisions of the law different from those for coverage of therapeutic services.

A. Criteria for Coverage of Diagnostic Tests

- All reasonable and necessary diagnostic tests given for the medical conditions listed in subsection B are covered when the following criteria are met:
- The clinic is either affiliated with a hospital or is under the direction and control of physicians. Diagnostic testing routinely performed in sleep disorder clinics may be covered even in the absence of direct supervision by a physician;
- Patients are referred to the sleep disorder clinic by their attending physicians, and the clinic maintains a record of the attending physician's orders; and
- The need for diagnostic testing is confirmed by medical evidence, e.g., physician examinations and laboratory tests. Diagnostic testing that is duplicative of previous testing done by the attending physician to the extent the results are still pertinent is not covered because it is not reasonable and necessary under §1862(a)(1)(A) of the Act.

B. Medical Conditions for Which Testing is Covered
Diagnostic testing is covered only if the patient has the symptoms or complaints of one of the conditions listed below. Most of the patients who undergo the diagnostic testing are not considered inpatients, although they may come to the facility in the evening for testing and then leave after testing is over. The overnight stay is considered an integral part of these tests.

1. Narcolepsy - This term refers to a syndrome that is characterized by abnormal sleep tendencies, e.g., excessive daytime sleepiness or disturbed nocturnal sleep. Related diagnostic testing is covered if the patient has inappropriate sleep episodes or attacks (e.g., while driving, in the middle of a meal, in the middle of a conversation), amnesiac episodes, or continuous disabling drowsiness. The sleep disorder clinic must submit documentation that this condition is severe enough to interfere with the patient's well being and health before Medicare benefits may be provided for diagnostic testing. Ordinarily, a diagnosis of narcolepsy can be confirmed by three sleep naps. If more than three sleep naps are claimed, the carrier will require persuasive medical evidence justifying the medical necessity for the additional test(s). It will use HCPCS procedure codes 95828 and 95805.
2. Sleep Apnea - This is a potentially lethal condition where the patient stops breathing during sleep. Three types of sleep apnea have been described (central, obstructive, and mixed). The nature of the apnea episodes can be documented by appropriate diagnostic testing. Ordinarily, a single polysomnogram and electroencephalogram (EEG) can diagnose sleep apnea. If more than one such testing session is claimed, the carrier will require persuasive medical evidence justifying the medical necessity for the additional tests. It will use HCPCS procedure codes 95807, 95810, and 95822.
3. Impotence - Diagnostic nocturnal penile tumescence testing may be covered, under limited circumstances, to determine whether erectile impotence in men is organic or psychogenic. Although impotence is not a sleep disorder, the nature of the testing requires that it be performed during sleep. The tests ordinarily are covered only where necessary to confirm the treatment to be given (surgical, medical, or psychotherapeutic). Ordinarily, a diagnosis may be determined by two nights of diagnostic testing. If more than two nights of testing are claimed, the carrier will require persuasive medical evidence justifying the medical necessity for the additional tests. It will have its medical staff review questionable cases to ensure that the tests are reasonable and necessary for the individual. It will use HCPCS procedure code 54250. (See the Medicare National Coverage Determinations Manual, Chapter 1, for policy on coverage of diagnosis and treatment of impotence.)
4. Parasomnia- Parasomnias are a group of conditions that represent undesirable or unpleasant occurrences during sleep. Behavior during these times can often lead to damage to the surroundings and injury to the patient or to others. Parasomnia may include conditions such as sleepwalking, sleep terrors, and rapid eye movement (REM) sleep behavior disorders. In many of these cases, the nature of these conditions may be established by careful clinical evaluation. Suspected seizure disorders as possible cause of the parasomnia are appropriately evaluated by standard or prolonged sleep EEG studies. In cases where seizure disorders have been ruled out and in cases that present a history of repeated violent or injurious episodes during sleep, polysomnography may be useful in providing a diagnostic classification or prognosis. The carrier must use HCPCS procedure codes 95807, 95810, and/or 95822.

C. Polysomnography for Chronic Insomnia Is Not Covered. Evidence at the present time is not convincing that polysomnography in a sleep disorder clinic for chronic insomnia provides definitive diagnostic data or that such information is useful in patient treatment or is associated with improved clinical outcome. The use of polysomnography for diagnosis of patients with chronic insomnia is not covered under Medicare because it is not reasonable and necessary under §1862(a)(1)(A) of the Act.

D. Coverage of Therapeutic Services. Sleep disorder clinics may at times render therapeutic as well as diagnostic services. Therapeutic services may be covered in a hospital outpatient setting or in a freestanding facility provided they meet the pertinent requirements for the particular type of services and are reasonable and necessary for the patient, and are performed under the direct supervision of a physician.

100-2, 15, 80

Requirements for Diagnostic X-Ray, Diagnostic Laboratory, and Other Diagnostic Tests

This section describes the levels of physician supervision required for furnishing the technical component of diagnostic tests for a Medicare beneficiary who is not a hospital inpatient. For hospital outpatient diagnostic services, the supervision levels assigned to each CPT or Level II HCPCS code in the Medicare Physician Fee Schedule Relative Value File that is updated quarterly, apply as described below. For more information, see Chapter 6 (Hospital Services Covered Under Part B), Sec.20.4 (Outpatient Diagnostic Services).

Section 410.32(b) of the Code of Federal Regulations (CFR) requires that diagnostic tests covered under Sec.1861(s)(3) of the Act and payable under the physician fee schedule, with certain exceptions listed in the regulation, have to be performed under the supervision of an individual meeting the definition of a physician (Sec.1861(r) of the Act) to be considered reasonable and necessary and, therefore, covered under Medicare. The regulation defines these levels of physician supervision for diagnostic tests as follows:

General Supervision - means the procedure is furnished under the physician's overall direction and control, but the physician's presence is not required during the performance of the procedure. Under general supervision, the training of the nonphysician personnel who actually performs the diagnostic procedure and the maintenance of the necessary equipment and supplies are the continuing responsibility of the physician.

Direct Supervision - in the office setting means the physician must be present in the office suite and immediately available to furnish assistance and direction throughout the performance of the procedure. It does not mean that the physician must be present in the room when the procedure is performed.

Personal Supervision - means a physician must be in attendance in the room during the performance of the procedure.

One of the following numerical levels is assigned to each CPT or HCPCS code in the Medicare Physician Fee Schedule Database:

- 0 Procedure is not a diagnostic test or procedure is a diagnostic test which is not subject to the physician supervision policy.
- 1 Procedure must be performed under the general supervision of a physician.
- 2 Procedure must be performed under the direct supervision of a physician.
- 3 Procedure must be performed under the personal supervision of a physician.
- 4 Physician supervision policy does not apply when procedure is furnished by a qualified, independent psychologist or a clinical psychologist or furnished under the general supervision of a clinical psychologist; otherwise must be performed under the general supervision of a physician.
- 5 Physician supervision policy does not apply when procedure is furnished by a qualified audiologist; otherwise must be performed under the general supervision of a physician.
- 6 Procedure must be performed by a physician or by a physical therapist (PT) who is certified by the American Board of Physical Therapy Specialties (ABPTS) as a qualified electrophysiologic clinical specialist and is permitted to provide the procedure under State law.
- 6a Supervision standards for level 66 apply; in addition, the PT with ABPTS certification may supervise another PT but only the PT with ABPTS certification may bill.
- 7a Supervision standards for level 77 apply; in addition, the PT with ABPTS certification may supervise another PT but only the PT with ABPTS certification may bill.
- 9 Concept does not apply.
- 21 Procedure must be performed by a technician with certification under general supervision of a physician; otherwise must be performed under direct supervision of a physician.
- 22 Procedure may be performed by a technician with on-line real-time contact with physician.
- 66 Procedure must be performed by a physician or by a PT with ABPTS certification and certification in this specific procedure.
- 77 Procedure must be performed by a PT with ABPTS certification or by a PT without certification under direct supervision of a physician, or by a technician with certification under general supervision of a physician.

Nurse practitioners, clinical nurse specialists, and physician assistants are not defined as physicians under Sec.1861(r) of the Act. Therefore, they may not function as supervisory physicians under the diagnostic tests benefit (Sec.1861(s)(3) of the Act). However, when these practitioners personally perform diagnostic tests as provided under Sec.1861(s)(2)(K) of the Act, Sec.1861(s)(3) does not apply and they may perform diagnostic tests pursuant to State scope of practice laws and under the applicable State requirements for physician supervision or collaboration.

Because the diagnostic tests benefit set forth in Sec.1861(s)(3) of the Act is separate and distinct from the incident to benefit set forth in Sec.1861(s)(2) of the Act, diagnostic tests need not meet the incident to requirements. Diagnostic tests may be furnished under situations that meet the incident to requirements but this is not required. However, carriers must not scrutinize claims for diagnostic tests utilizing the incident to requirements.

100-2, 15, 80.1

Clinical Laboratory Services

Section 1833 and 1861 of the Act provides for payment of clinical laboratory services under Medicare Part B. Clinical laboratory services involve the biological, microbiological, serological, chemical, immunohematological, hematological, biophysical, cytological, pathological, or other examination of materials derived from the human body for the diagnosis, prevention, or treatment of a disease or assessment of a medical condition. Laboratory services must meet all applicable requirements of the Clinical Laboratory Improvement Amendments of 1988 (CLIA), as set forth at 42 CFR part 493. Section 1862(a)(1)(A) of the Act provides that Medicare payment may not be made for services that are not reasonable and necessary. Clinical laboratory services must be ordered and used promptly by the physician who is treating the beneficiary as described in 42 CFR 410.32(a), or by a qualified nonphysician practitioner, as described in 42 CFR 410.32(a)(3).

See section 80.6 of this manual for related physician ordering instructions.

See the Medicare Claims Processing Manual Chapter 16 for related claims processing instructions.

100-2, 15, 80.2

Psychological Tests and Neuropsychological Tests

Medicare Part B coverage of psychological tests and neuropsychological tests is authorized under section 1861(s)(3) of the Social Security Act. Payment for psychological and neuropsychological tests is authorized under section 1842(b)(2)(A) of the Social Security Act. The payment amounts for the new psychological and neuropsychological tests (CPT codes 96102, 96103, 96119 and 96120) that are effective January 1, 2006, and are billed for tests administered by a technician or a computer reflect a site of service payment differential for the facility and non-facility settings.

Additionally, there is no authorization for payment for diagnostic tests when performed on an "incident to" basis.

Under the diagnostic tests provision, all diagnostic tests are assigned a certain level of supervision. Generally, regulations governing the diagnostic tests provision require that only physicians can provide the assigned level of supervision for diagnostic tests.

However, there is a regulatory exception to the supervision requirement for diagnostic psychological and neuropsychological tests in terms of who can provide the supervision.

That is, regulations allow a clinical psychologist (CP) or a physician to perform the general supervision assigned to diagnostic psychological and neuropsychological tests.

In addition, nonphysician practitioners such as nurse practitioners (NPs), clinical nurse specialists (CNSs) and physician assistants (PAs) who personally perform diagnostic psychological and neuropsychological tests are excluded from having to perform these tests under the general supervision of a physician or a CP. Rather, NPs and CNSs must perform such tests under the requirements of their respective benefit instead of the requirements for diagnostic psychological and neuropsychological tests. Accordingly, NPs and CNSs must perform tests in collaboration (as defined under Medicare law at section 1861(aa)(6) of the Act) with a physician. PAs perform tests under the general supervision of a physician as required for services furnished under the PA benefit.

Furthermore, physical therapists (PTs), occupational therapists (OTs) and speech language pathologists (SLPs) are authorized to bill three test codes as "sometimes therapy" codes. Specifically, CPT codes 96105, 96110 and 96111 may be performed by these therapists. However, when PTs, OTs and SLPs perform these three tests, they must be performed under the general supervision of a physician or a CP.

Who May Bill for Diagnostic Psychological and Neuropsychological Tests

- CPs - see qualifications under chapter 15, section 160 of the Benefits Policy Manual, Pub. 100-02.
- NPs -to the extent authorized under State scope of practice. See qualifications under chapter 15, section 200 of the Benefits Policy Manual, Pub. 100-02.
- CNSs -to the extent authorized under State scope of practice. See qualifications under chapter 15, section 210 of the Benefits Policy Manual, Pub. 100-02.
- PAs - to the extent authorized under State scope of practice. See qualifications under chapter 15, section 190 of the Benefits Policy Manual, Pub. 100-02.
- Independently Practicing Psychologists (IPPs)
- PTs, OTs and SLPs - see qualifications under chapter 15, sections 220-230.6 of the Benefits Policy Manual, Pub. 100-02.

Psychological and neuropsychological tests performed by a psychologist (who is not a CP) practicing independently of an institution, agency, or physician's office are covered when a physician orders such tests. An IPP is any psychologist who is licensed or certified to practice psychology in the State or jurisdiction where furnishing services or, if the jurisdiction does not issue licenses, if provided by any practicing psychologist. (It is CMS' understanding that all States, the District of Columbia, and Puerto Rico license psychologists, but that some trust territories do not. Examples of psychologists, other than CPs, whose psychological and neuropsychological tests are covered under the diagnostic tests provision include, but are not limited to, educational psychologists and counseling psychologists.)

The carrier must secure from the appropriate State agency a current listing of psychologists holding the required credentials to determine whether the tests of a particular IPP are covered under Part B in States that have statutory licensure or certification. In States or territories that lack statutory licensing or certification, the carrier checks individual qualifications before provider numbers are issued. Possible reference sources are the national directory of membership of the American Psychological Association, which provides data about the educational background of individuals and indicates which members are board-certified, the records and directories of the State or territorial psychological association, and the National Register of Health Service Providers. If qualification is dependent on a doctoral degree from a currently accredited program, the carrier verifies the date of accreditation of the school involved, since such accreditation is not retroactive. If the listed reference sources do not provide enough information (e.g., the psychologist is not a member of one of these sources), the carrier contacts the psychologist personally for the required information. Generally, carriers maintain a continuing list of psychologists whose qualifications have been verified.

NOTE: When diagnostic psychological tests are performed by a psychologist who is not practicing independently, but is on the staff of an institution, agency, or clinic, that entity bills for the psychological tests.

The carrier considers psychologists as practicing independently when:

- They render services on their own responsibility, free of the administrative and professional control of an employer such as a physician, institution or agency;
- The persons they treat are their own patients; and
- They have the right to bill directly, collect and retain the fee for their services.

A psychologist practicing in an office located in an institution may be considered an independently practicing psychologist when both of the following conditions exist:

- The office is confined to a separately-identified part of the facility which is used solely as the psychologist's office and cannot be construed as extending throughout the entire institution; and
- The psychologist conducts a private practice, i.e., services are rendered to patients from outside the institution as well as to institutional patients.

Payment for Diagnostic Psychological and Neuropsychological Tests
Expenses for diagnostic psychological and neuropsychological tests are not subject to the outpatient mental health treatment limitation, that is, the payment limitation on treatment services for mental, psychoneurotic and personality disorders as authorized under Section 1833(c) of the Act. The payment amount for the new psychological and neuropsychological tests (CPT codes 96102, 96103, 96119 and 96120) that are billed for tests performed by a technician or a computer reflect a site of service payment differential for the facility and non-facility settings. CPs, NPs, CNSs and PAs are required by law to accept assigned payment for psychological and neuropsychological tests. However, while IPPs are not required by law to accept assigned payment for these tests, they must report the name and address of the physician who ordered the test on the claim form when billing for tests.

CPT Codes for Diagnostic Psychological and Neuropsychological Tests
The range of CPT codes used to report psychological and neuropsychological tests is 96101-96120. CPT codes 96101, 96102, 96103, 96105, 96110, and 96111 are appropriate for use when billing for psychological tests. CPT codes 96116, 96118, 96119 and 96120 are appropriate for use when billing for neuropsychological tests.

All of the tests under this CPT code range 96101-96120 are indicated as active codes under the physician fee schedule database and are covered if medically necessary.

Payment and Billing Guidelines for Psychological and Neuropsychological Tests The technician and computer CPT codes for psychological and neuropsychological tests include practice expense, malpractice expense and professional work relative value units.

Accordingly, CPT psychological test code 96101 should not be paid when billed for the same tests or services performed under psychological test codes 96102 or 96103. CPT neuropsychological test code 96118 should not be paid when billed for the same tests or services performed under neuropsychological test codes 96119 or 96120. However, CPT codes 96101 and 96118 can be paid separately on the rare occasion when billed on the same date of service for different and separate tests from 96102, 96103, 96119 and 96120.

Under the physician fee schedule, there is no payment for services performed by students or trainees. Accordingly, Medicare does not pay for services represented by CPT codes 96102 and 96119 when performed by a student or a trainee. However, the presence of a student or a trainee while the test is being administered does not prevent a physician, CP, IPP, NP, CNS or PA from performing and being paid for the psychological test under 96102 or the neuropsychological test under 96119.

100-2, 15, 80.3

Audiology Services

References.

1861(ll)(3) of the Social Security Act for the definition of audiology services.

1861(ll)(4)(B) of the Social Security Act for qualifications of audiologists.

42 CFR 410.32(b) for the physician supervision requirements for diagnostic tests.

Pub. 100-04, chapter 12, section 30.3 for coding and billing information related to audiological services and aural rehabilitation.

Pub. 100-02, chapter 15, sections 220 and 230 for the physical therapy and speech-language pathology policies relative to aural rehabilitation and balance, section 60 for services incident to a physician's service, and section 80.6 for policies relevant to ordering for diagnostic tests.

Pub. 100-02, chapter 16, section 100 for hearing aid policies.

A list of audiology service codes is found at: http://www.cms.gov/PhysicianFeeSched/50_Audiology.asp.

A. Benefit.
Hearing and balance assessment services are generally covered as "other diagnostic tests" under section 1861(s)(3) of the Social Security Act. Hearing and balance assessment services furnished to an outpatient of a hospital are covered as "diagnostic services" under section 1861(s)(2)(C).

As defined in the Social Security Act, section 1861(ll)(3), the term "audiology services" specifically means such hearing and balance assessment services furnished by a qualified audiologist as the audiologist is legally authorized to perform under State law (or the State regulatory mechanism provided by State law), as would otherwise be covered if furnished by a physician.

Herein after in this section, hearing and balance assessment services are termed "audiology services," regardless of whether they are furnished by an audiologist, physician, nonphysician practitioner (NPP), or hospital.

Because audiology services are diagnostic tests, when furnished by a physician in an office or hospital outpatient department, they must be furnished under the appropriate level of supervision of a physician as established in 42 CFR 410.32(b)(1) and 410.28(e). However, as specified in 42 CFR 410.32(b)(2)(ii) or (v), respectively, they are excepted from physician supervision when they are personally furnished by a qualified audiologist

or performed by a nurse practitioner or clinical nurse specialist authorized to perform the tests under applicable State laws.

Audiological diagnostic testing refers to tests of the audiological and vestibular systems, e.g., hearing, balance, auditory processing, tinnitus and diagnostic programming of certain prosthetic devices, performed by qualified audiologists.

Audiological diagnostic tests are not covered under the benefit for services incident to a physician's service (described in Pub. 100-02, chapter 15, section 60), because they have their own benefit as "other diagnostic tests". See Pub. 100-04, chapter 13 for general diagnostic test policies.

Audiology services, like all other services, should be reported under the most specific HCPCS code that describes the service that was furnished and in accordance with all CPT guidance and Medicare national and local contractor instructions.

B. Orders.
Audiology tests are covered as "other diagnostic tests" under section 1861(s)(3) or 1861(s)(2)(C) of the Act in the physician's office or hospital outpatient settings, respectively, when a physician (or an NPP, as applicable) orders such testing for the purpose of obtaining information necessary for the physician's diagnostic medical evaluation or to determine the appropriate medical or surgical treatment of a hearing deficit or related medical problem. See section 80.6 of this chapter for policies regarding the ordering of diagnostic tests.

If a beneficiary undergoes diagnostic testing performed by an audiologist without a physician order, the tests are not covered even if the audiologist discovers a pathologic condition.

When a qualified physician orders a qualified technician (see definition in subsection D of this section) to furnish an appropriate audiology service, that order must specify which test is to be furnished by the technician under the direct supervision of a physician. Only that test may be provided on that order by the technician.

When the qualified physician or NPP orders diagnostic audiology services furnished by an audiologist without naming specific tests, the audiologist may select the appropriate battery of tests.

C. Coverage and Payment for Audiology Services.
Diagnostic services furnished by a qualified audiologist meeting the requirements in section 80.3.1 of this chapter or physicians and NPPs as described in section 80.6 are covered and payable under the MPFS as "other diagnostic tests."

Services furnished in a hospital outpatient department are covered and payable under the hospital Outpatient Prospective Payment System (OPPS) or other payment methodology applicable to the provider furnishing the services.

Coverage and, therefore, payment for audiological diagnostic tests is determined by the reason the tests were performed, rather than by the diagnosis or the patient's condition.

Under any Medicare payment system, payment for audiological diagnostic tests is not allowed by virtue of their exclusion from coverage in section 1862(a)(7) of the Social Security Act when:

The type and severity of the current hearing, tinnitus or balance status needed to determine the appropriate medical or surgical treatment is known to the physician before the test; or

The test was ordered for the specific purpose of fitting or modifying a hearing aid.

Payment of audiological diagnostic tests is allowed for other reasons and is not limited, for example, by:

- Any information resulting from the test, for example:
- Confirmation of a prior diagnosis;
- Post-evaluation diagnoses; or
- Treatment provided after diagnosis, including hearing aids, or
- The type of evaluation or treatment the physician anticipates before the diagnostic test; or
- Timing of reevaluation. Reevaluation is appropriate at a schedule dictated by the ordering physician when the information provided by the diagnostic test is required, for example, to determine changes in hearing, to evaluate the appropriate medical or surgical treatment or to evaluate the results of treatment. For example, reevaluation may be appropriate, even when the evaluation was recent, in cases where the hearing loss, balance, or tinnitus may be progressive or fluctuating, the patient or caregiver complains of new symptoms, or treatment (such as medication or surgery) may have changed the patient's audiological condition with or without awareness by the patient.

Examples of appropriate reasons for ordering audiological diagnostic tests that could be covered include, but are not limited to:

- Evaluation of suspected change in hearing, tinnitus, or balance; Evaluation of the cause of disorders of hearing, tinnitus, or balance;
- Determination of the effect of medication, surgery, or other treatment; Reevaluation to follow-up changes in hearing, tinnitus, or balance that may be caused by established diagnoses that place the patient at probable risk for a change in status including, but not limited to: otosclerosis, atelectatic tympanic membrane, tympanosclerosis, cholesteatoma, resolving middle ear infection, MeniÐ©re's disease, sudden idiopathic sensorineural hearing loss, autoimmune inner ear disease, acoustic neuroma, demyelinating diseases, ototoxicity secondary to medications, or genetic vascular and viral conditions; Failure of a screening test (although the screening test is not covered);
- Diagnostic analysis of cochlear or brainstem implant and programming; and
- Audiology diagnostic tests before and periodically after implantation of auditory prosthetic devices.

If a physician refers a beneficiary to an audiologist for testing related to signs or symptoms associated with hearing loss, balance disorder, tinnitus, ear disease, or ear injury, the audiologist's diagnostic testing services should be covered even if the only outcome is the prescription of a hearing aid.

D. Individuals Who Furnish Audiology Tests.

1. Qualified Professionals. See section 80.3.1 of this chapter for the qualifications of audiologists. See section 80.6 of this chapter for the qualifications of physicians and NPPs who may furnish diagnostic tests.
2. Qualified Technicians or Other Qualified Staff. References to technicians in this section include other qualified clinical staff. The qualifications for technicians vary locally and may also depend on the type of test, the patient, and the level of participation of the physician who is directly supervising the test. Therefore, an individual must meet qualifications appropriate to the service furnished as determined by the contractor to whom the claim is billed. If it is necessary to determine whether the individual who furnished the labor for appropriate audiology services is qualified, contractors may request verification of any relevant education and training that has been completed by the technician, which shall be available in the records of the clinic or facility.

Depending on the qualifications determined by the contractor, individuals who are also hearing instrument specialists, students of audiology, or other health care professionals may furnish the labor for appropriate audiology services under direct physician supervision when these services are billed by physicians or hospital outpatient departments.

E. Documentation for Audiology Services.

1. Documentation for Orders (Reasons for Tests).

   The reason for the test should be documented either on the order, on the audiological evaluation report, or in the patient's medical record. (See subsection C. of this section concerning reasons for tests.)
2. Documenting skilled services. When the medical record is subject to medical review, it is necessary that the record contains sufficient information so that the contractor may determine that the service qualifies for payment. For example, documentation should indicate that the test was ordered, that the reason for the test results in coverage, and that the test was furnished to the patient by a qualified individual.

   Records that support the appropriate provision of an audiological diagnostic test shall be made available to the contractor on request.

F. Audiological Treatment.

There is no provision in the law for Medicare to pay audiologists for therapeutic services. For example, vestibular treatment, auditory rehabilitation treatment, auditory processing treatment, and canalith repositioning, while they are generally within the scope of practice of audiologists, are not those hearing and balance assessment services that are defined as audiology services in 1861(ll)(3) of the Social Security Act and, therefore, shall not be billed by audiologists to Medicare. Services for the purpose of hearing aid evaluation and fitting are not covered regardless of how they are billed. Services identified as "always" therapy in Pub. 100-04, chapter 5, section 20 may not be billed by hospitals, physicians, NPPs, or audiologists when provided by audiologists. (See also Pub. 100-04, chapter 12, section 30.3.)

Treatment related to hearing may be covered under the speech-language pathology benefit when the services are provided by speech-language pathologists. Treatment related to balance (e.g., services described by "always therapy" codes 97001-97004, 97110, 97112, 97116, and 97750) may be covered under the physical therapy or occupational therapy benefit when the services are provided by therapists or their assistants, where appropriate. Covered therapy services incident to a physician's service must conform to policies in sections 60, 220, and 230 of this chapter. Audiological treatment provided under the benefits for physical therapy and speech-language pathology services may also be personally provided and billed by physicians and NPPs when the services are within their scope of practice and consistent with State and local laws.

For example, aural rehabilitation and signed communication training may be payable according to the benefit for speech-language pathology services or as speech-language pathology services incident to a physician's or NPP's service. Treatment for balance disorders may be payable according to the benefit for physical therapy services or as a

physical therapy service incident to the services of a physician or NPP. See the policies in this chapter, sections 220 and 230, for details.

G. Assignment.

Nonhospital entities billing for the audiologist's services may accept assignment under the usual procedure or, if not accepting assignment, may charge the patient and submit a nonassigned claim on their behalf.

H. Opt Out and Mandatory Claims Submissions.

The opt out law does not define "physician" or "practitioner" to include audiologists; therefore, they may not opt out of Medicare and provide services under private contracts. See section 40.4 of this chapter for details.

When a physician or supplier furnishes a service that is covered by Medicare, then it is subject to the mandatory claim submission provisions of section 1848(g)(4) of the Social Security Act. Therefore, if an audiologist charges or attempts to charge a beneficiary any remuneration for a service that is covered by Medicare, then the audiologist must submit a claim to Medicare.

I. Non-Audiology Services Furnished by Audiologists.

Audiologists may be qualified to furnish all or part of some diagnostic tests or treatments that are not defined as audiology services under the MPFS, such as non-auditory evoked potentials or cerumen removal. Audiologists may not bill Medicare for services that are not audiology services according to Medicare's definition (see list at: http://www.cms.gov/PhysicianFeeSched/50_Audiology.asp). However, the labor for the Technical Component (TC) of certain other diagnostic tests or treatment services may qualify to be billed when furnished by audiologists under physician supervision when all the appropriate policies are followed.

When furnishing services that are not on the Medicare list of audiology services, the audiologist may or may not be working within the scope of practice of an audiologist according to State law. The audiologist furnishing the service must have the qualifications that are ordinarily required of any person providing that service. Consult the following policies for details:

Policies for physical therapy, occupational therapy, and speech-language pathology services are in sections 220 and 230 of this chapter and in Pub. 100-04, chapter 5, sections 10 and 20. Policies for services furnished incident to physicians' services in the physician's office are in section 60 of this chapter.

Policies for therapeutic services furnished incident to physicians' services in the hospital outpatient setting are in chapter 6, section 20.5, of this manual. Policies for diagnostic tests in the physician's office are in section 80 of this chapter. Policies for diagnostic tests furnished in the hospital outpatient setting are in chapter 6, section 20.4, of this manual. Therapeutic or treatment services that are not audiology services and are not "always" therapy (according to the policy in Pub.100-04, chapter 5, section 20) and are furnished by audiologists may be billed incident to the services of a physician when all other appropriate requirements are met.

In addition, the TC or facility services for diagnostic tests that are not audiology services may be billed by physicians or hospital outpatient departments when provided by qualified personnel (who may be audiologists), and physicians and hospital outpatient departments may bill for these diagnostic tests when provided by those qualified personnel under the specified level of physician supervision for the diagnostic test

100-2, 15, 80.5.4

Conditions for Coverage

Medicare covers BMM under the following conditions:

1. Is ordered by the physician or qualified nonphysician practitioner who is treating the beneficiary following an evaluation of the need for a BMM and determination of the appropriate BMM to be used. A physician or qualified nonphysician practitioner treating the beneficiary for purposes of this provision is one who furnishes a consultation or treats a beneficiary for a specific medical problem, and who uses the results in the management of the patient. For the purposes of the BMM benefit, qualified nonphysician practitioners include physician assistants, nurse practitioners, clinical nurse specialists, and certified nurse midwives.
2. Is performed under the appropriate level of physician supervision as defined in 42 CFR 410.32(b).
3. Is reasonable and necessary for diagnosing and treating the condition of a beneficiary who meets the conditions described in Sec.80.5.6.
4. In the case of an individual being monitored to assess the response to or efficacy of an FDA-approved osteoporosis drug therapy, is performed with a dual-energy x-ray absorptiometry system (axial skeleton).
5. In the case of any individual who meets the conditions of 80.5.6 and who has a confirmatory BMM, is performed by a dual-energy x-ray absorptiometry system (axial skeleton) if the initial BMM was not performed by a dual-energy x-ray absorptiometry system (axial skeleton). A confirmatory baseline BMM is not covered if the initial BMM was performed by a dual-energy x-ray absorptiometry system (axial skeleton).

100-2, 15, 80.5.5

Frequency Standards

Medicare pays for a screening BMM once every 2 years (at least 23 months have passed since the month the last covered BMM was performed).

When medically necessary, Medicare may pay for more frequent BMMs. Examples include, but are not limited to, the following medical circumstances: Monitoring beneficiaries on long-term glucocorticoid (steroid) therapy of more than 3 months.

Confirming baseline BMMs to permit monitoring of beneficiaries in the future.

100-2, 15, 80.5.6

Beneficiaries Who May be Covered

To be covered, a beneficiary must meet at least one of the five conditions listed below:

1. A woman who has been determined by the physician or qualified nonphysician practitioner treating her to be estrogen-deficient and at clinical risk for osteoporosis, based on her medical history and other findings.

   NOTE: Since not every woman who has been prescribed estrogen replacement therapy (ERT) may be receiving an "adequate" dose of the therapy, the fact that a woman is receiving ERT should not preclude her treating physician or other qualified treating nonphysician practitioner from ordering a bone mass measurement for her. If a BMM is ordered for a woman following a careful evaluation of her medical need, however, it is expected that the ordering treating physician (or other qualified treating nonphysician practitioner) will document in her medical record why he or she believes that the woman is estrogen-deficient and at clinical risk for osteoporosis.
2. An individual with vertebral abnormalities as demonstrated by an x-ray to be indicative of osteoporosis, osteopenia, or vertebral fracture.
3. An individual receiving (or expecting to receive) glucocorticoid (steroid) therapy equivalent to an average of 5.0 mg of prednisone, or greater, per day, for more than 3 months.
4. An individual with primary hyperparathyroidism.
5. An individual being monitored to assess the response to or efficacy of an FDAapproved osteoporosis drug therapy.

100-2, 15, 100

Surgical Dressings, Splints, Casts, and Other Devices Used for Reductions of Fractures and Dislocations

B3-2079, A3-3110.3, HO-228.3

Surgical dressings are limited to primary and secondary dressings required for the treatment of a wound caused by, or treated by, a surgical procedure that has been performed by a physician or other health care professional to the extent permissible under State law. In addition, surgical dressings required after debridement of a wound are also covered, irrespective of the type of debridement, as long as the debridement was reasonable and necessary and was performed by a health care professional acting within the scope of his/her legal authority when performing this function. Surgical dressings are covered for as long as they are medically necessary.

Primary dressings are therapeutic or protective coverings applied directly to wounds or lesions either on the skin or caused by an opening to the skin. Secondary dressing materials that serve a therapeutic or protective function and that are needed to secure a primary dressing are also covered. Items such as adhesive tape, roll gauze, bandages, and disposable compression material are examples of secondary dressings. Elastic stockings, support hose, foot coverings, leotards, knee supports, surgical leggings, gauntlets, and pressure garments for the arms and hands are examples of items that are not ordinarily covered as surgical dressings. Some items, such as transparent film, may be used as a primary or secondary dressing.

If a physician, certified nurse midwife, physician assistant, nurse practitioner, or clinical nurse specialist applies surgical dressings as part of a professional service that is billed to Medicare, the surgical dressings are considered incident to the professional services of the health care practitioner. (See Sec. 60.1, 180, 190, 200, and 210.) When surgical dressings are not covered incident to the services of a health care practitioner and are obtained by the patient from a supplier (e.g., a drugstore, physician, or other health care practitioner that qualifies as a supplier) on an order from a physician or other health care professional authorized under State law or regulation to make such an order, the surgical dressings are covered separately under Part B.

Splints and casts, and other devices used for reductions of fractures and dislocations are covered under Part B of Medicare. This includes dental splints.

100-2, 15, 120

Prosthetic Devices

B3-2130, A3-3110.4, HO-228.4, A3-3111, HO-229

A. General

Prosthetic devices (other than dental) which replace all or part of an internal body organ (including contiguous tissue), or replace all or part of the function of a permanently inoperative or malfunctioning internal body organ are covered when furnished on a physician's order. This does not require a determination that there is no possibility that the patient's condition may improve sometime in the future. If the medical record, including the judgment of the attending physician, indicates the condition is of long and indefinite duration, the test of permanence is considered met. (Such a device may also be covered under Sec.60.l as a supply when furnished incident to a physician's service.)

Examples of prosthetic devices include artificial limbs, parenteral and enteral (PEN) nutrition, cardiac pacemakers, prosthetic lenses (see subsection B), breast prostheses (including a surgical brassiere) for postmastectomy patients, maxillofacial devices, and devices which replace all or part of the ear or nose. A urinary collection and retention system with or without a tube is a prosthetic device replacing bladder function in case of permanent urinary incontinence. The foley catheter is also considered a prosthetic device when ordered for a patient with permanent urinary incontinence. However, chucks, diapers, rubber sheets, etc., are supplies that are not covered under this provision. Although hemodialysis equipment is a prosthetic device, payment for the rental or purchase of such equipment in the home is made only for use under the provisions for payment applicable to durable medical equipment.

An exception is that if payment cannot be made on an inpatient's behalf under Part A, hemodialysis equipment, supplies, and services required by such patient could be covered under Part B as a prosthetic device, which replaces the function of a kidney. See the Medicare Benefit Policy Manual, Chapter 11, "End Stage Renal Disease," for payment for hemodialysis equipment used in the home. See the Medicare Benefit Policy Manual, Chapter 1, "Inpatient Hospital Services," Sec.10, for additional instructions on hospitalization for renal dialysis.

NOTE: Medicare does not cover a prosthetic device dispensed to a patient prior to the time at which the patient undergoes the procedure that makes necessary the use of the device. For example, the carrier does not make a separate Part B payment for an intraocular lens (IOL) or pacemaker that a physician, during an office visit prior to the actual surgery, dispenses to the patient for his or her use. Dispensing a prosthetic device in this manner raises health and safety issues. Moreover, the need for the device cannot be clearly established until the procedure that makes its use possible is successfully performed. Therefore, dispensing a prosthetic device in this manner is not considered reasonable and necessary for the treatment of the patient's condition.

Colostomy (and other ostomy) bags and necessary accouterments required for attachment are covered as prosthetic devices. This coverage also includes irrigation and flushing equipment and other items and supplies directly related to ostomy care, whether the attachment of a bag is required. Accessories and/or supplies which are used directly with an enteral or parenteral device to achieve the therapeutic benefit of the prosthesis or to assure the proper functioning of the device may also be covered under the prosthetic device benefit subject to the additional guidelines in the Medicare National Coverage Determinations Manual.

Covered items include catheters, filters, extension tubing, infusion bottles, pumps (either food or infusion), intravenous (I.V.) pole, needles, syringes, dressings, tape, Heparin Sodium (parenteral only), volumetric monitors (parenteral only), and parenteral and enteral nutrient solutions. Baby food and other regular grocery products that can be blenderized and used with the enteral system are not covered. Note that some of these items, e.g., a food pump and an I.V. pole, qualify as DME. Although coverage of the enteral and parenteral nutritional therapy systems is provided on the basis of the prosthetic device benefit, the payment rules relating to lump sum or monthly payment for DME apply to such items.

The coverage of prosthetic devices includes replacement of and repairs to such devices as explained in subsection D.

Finally, the Benefits Improvement and Protection Act of 2000 amended Sec.1834(h)(1) of the Act by adding a provision (1834 (h)(1)(G)(i)) that requires Medicare payment to be made for the replacement of prosthetic devices which are artificial limbs, or for the replacement of any part of such devices, without regard to continuous use or useful lifetime restrictions if an ordering physician determines that the replacement device, or replacement part of such a device, is necessary.

Payment may be made for the replacement of a prosthetic device that is an artificial limb, or replacement part of a device if the ordering physician determines that the replacement device or part is necessary because of any of the following:

1. A change in the physiological condition of the patient;
2. An irreparable change in the condition of the device, or in a part of the device; or
3. The condition of the device, or the part of the device, requires repairs and the cost of such repairs would be more than 60 percent of the cost of a replacement device, or, as the case may be, of the part being replaced.

This provision is effective for items replaced on or after April 1, 2001. It supersedes any rule that that provided a 5-year or other replacement rule with regard to prosthetic devices.

B. Prosthetic Lenses

The term "internal body organ" includes the lens of an eye. Prostheses replacing the lens of an eye include post-surgical lenses customarily used during convalescence from eye surgery in which the lens of the eye was removed. In addition, permanent lenses are also covered when required by an individual lacking the organic lens of the eye because of surgical removal or congenital absence. Prosthetic lenses obtained on or after the beneficiary's date of entitlement to supplementary medical insurance benefits may be covered even though the surgical removal of the crystalline lens occurred before entitlement.

1. Prosthetic Cataract Lenses
   One of the following prosthetic lenses or combinations of prosthetic lenses furnished by a physician (see Sec.30.4 for coverage of prosthetic lenses prescribed by a doctor of optometry) may be covered when determined to be reasonable and necessary to restore essentially the vision provided by the crystalline lens of the eye:
   - Prosthetic bifocal lenses in frames;
   - Prosthetic lenses in frames for far vision, and prosthetic lenses in frames for near vision; or
   - When a prosthetic contact lens(es) for far vision is prescribed (including cases of binocular and monocular aphakia), make payment for the contact lens(es) and prosthetic lenses in frames for near vision to be worn at the same time as the contact lens(es), and prosthetic lenses in frames to be worn when the contacts have been removed.

   Lenses which have ultraviolet absorbing or reflecting properties may be covered, in lieu of payment for regular (untinted) lenses, if it has been determined that such lenses are medically reasonable and necessary for the individual patient.

   Medicare does not cover cataract sunglasses obtained in addition to the regular (untinted) prosthetic lenses since the sunglasses duplicate the restoration of vision function performed by the regular prosthetic lenses.
2. Payment for Intraocular Lenses (IOLs) Furnished in Ambulatory Surgical Centers (ASCs)
   Effective for services furnished on or after March 12, 1990, payment for intraocular lenses (IOLs) inserted during or subsequent to cataract surgery in a Medicare certified ASC is included with the payment for facility services that are furnished in connection with the covered surgery.

   Refer to the Medicare Claims Processing Manual, Chapter 14, "Ambulatory Surgical Centers," for more information.
3. Limitation on Coverage of Conventional Lenses One pair of conventional eyeglasses or conventional contact lenses furnished after each cataract surgery with insertion of an IOL is covered.

C. Dentures

Dentures are excluded from coverage. However, when a denture or a portion of the denture is an integral part (built-in) of a covered prosthesis (e.g., an obturator to fill an opening in the palate), it is covered as part of that prosthesis.

D. Supplies, Repairs, Adjustments, and Replacement

Supplies are covered that are necessary for the effective use of a prosthetic device (e.g., the batteries needed to operate an artificial larynx). Adjustment of prosthetic devices required by wear or by a change in the patient's condition is covered when ordered by a physician. General provisions relating to the repair and replacement of durable medical equipment in Sec.110.2 for the repair and replacement of prosthetic devices are applicable. (See the Medicare Benefit Policy Manual, Chapter 16, "General Exclusions from Coverage," Sec.40.4, for payment for devices replaced under a warranty.) Replacement of conventional eyeglasses or contact lenses furnished in accordance with Sec.120.B.3 is not covered. Necessary supplies, adjustments, repairs, and replacements are covered even when the device had been in use before the user enrolled in Part B of the program, so long as the device continues to be medically required.

100-2, 15, 150

Dental Services

B3-2136

As indicated under the general exclusions from coverage, items and services in connection with the care, treatment, filling, removal, or replacement of teeth or structures directly supporting the teeth are not covered. "Structures directly supporting the teeth" means the periodontium, which includes the gingivae, dentogingival junction, periodontal membrane, cementum of the teeth, and alveolar process.

In addition to the following, see Pub 100-01, the Medicare General Information, Eligibility, and Entitlement Manual, Chapter 5, Definitions and Pub 3, the Medicare National Coverage Determinations Manual for specific services which may be covered when furnished by a dentist. If an otherwise noncovered procedure or service is performed by a dentist as incident to and as an integral part of a covered procedure or service performed by the dentist, the total service performed by the dentist on such an occasion is covered.

EXAMPLE 1: The reconstruction of a ridge performed primarily to prepare the mouth for dentures is a noncovered procedure. However, when the reconstruction of a ridge is performed as a result of and at the same time as the surgical removal of a tumor (for other than dental purposes), the totality of surgical procedures is a covered service.

EXAMPLE 2: Medicare makes payment for the wiring of teeth when this is done in connection with the reduction of a jaw fracture.

The extraction of teeth to prepare the jaw for radiation treatment of neoplastic disease is also covered. This is an exception to the requirement that to be covered, a noncovered procedure or service performed by a dentist must be an incident to and an integral part of a covered procedure or service performed by the dentist. Ordinarily, the dentist extracts the patient's teeth, but another physician, e.g., a radiologist, administers the radiation treatments.

When an excluded service is the primary procedure involved, it is not covered, regardless of its complexity or difficulty. For example, the extraction of an impacted tooth is not covered. Similarly, an alveoplasty (the surgical improvement of the shape and condition of the alveolar process) and a frenectomy are excluded from coverage when either of these procedures is performed in connection with an excluded service, e.g., the preparation of the mouth for dentures. In a like manner, the removal of a torus palatinus (a bony protuberance of the hard palate) may be a covered service. However, with rare exception, this surgery is performed in connection with an excluded service, i.e., the preparation of the mouth for dentures. Under such circumstances, Medicare does not pay for this procedure.

Dental splints used to treat a dental condition are excluded from coverage under 1862(a)(12) of the Act. On the other hand, if the treatment is determined to be a covered medical condition (i.e., dislocated upper/lower jaw joints), then the splint can be covered.

Whether such services as the administration of anesthesia, diagnostic x-rays, and other related procedures are covered depends upon whether the primary procedure being performed by the dentist is itself covered. Thus, an x-ray taken in connection with the reduction of a fracture of the jaw or facial bone is covered. However, a single x-ray or x-ray survey taken in connection with the care or treatment of teeth or the periodontium is not covered.

Medicare makes payment for a covered dental procedure no matter where the service is performed. The hospitalization or nonhospitalization of a patient has no direct bearing on the coverage or exclusion of a given dental procedure.

Payment may also be made for services and supplies furnished incident to covered dental services. For example, the services of a dental technician or nurse who is under the direct supervision of the dentist or physician are covered if the services are included in the dentist's or physician's bill.

100-2, 15, 160

Clinical Psychologist Services

A. Clinical Psychologist (CP) Defined

To qualify as a clinical psychologist (CP), a practitioner must meet the following requirements:

- Hold a doctoral degree in psychology;
- Be licensed or certified, on the basis of the doctoral degree in psychology, by the State in which he or she practices, at the independent practice level of psychology to furnish diagnostic, assessment, preventive, and therapeutic services directly to individuals.

B. Qualified Clinical Psychologist Services Defined

Effective July 1, 1990, the diagnostic and therapeutic services of CPs and services and supplies furnished incident to such services are covered as the services furnished by a physician or as incident to physician's services are covered. However, the CP must be legally authorized to perform the services under applicable licensure laws of the State in which they are furnished.

C. Types of Clinical Psychologist Services That May Be Covered

Diagnostic and therapeutic services that the CP is legally authorized to perform in accordance with State law and/or regulation. Carriers pay all qualified CPs based on the physician fee schedule for the diagnostic and therapeutic services. (Psychological tests by practitioners who do not meet the requirements for a CP may be covered under the provisions for diagnostic tests as described in Sec.80.2.

Services and supplies furnished incident to a CP's services are covered if the requirements that apply to services incident to a physician's services, as described in Sec.60 are met. These services must be:

- Mental health services that are commonly furnished in CPs' offices;
- An integral, although incidental, part of professional services performed by the CP;
- Performed under the direct personal supervision of the CP; i.e., the CP must be physically present and immediately available;
- Furnished without charge or included in the CP's bill; and
- Performed by an employee of the CP (or an employee of the legal entity that employs the supervising CP) under the common law control test of the Act, as set forth in 20 CFR 404.1007 and Sec.RS 2101.020 of the Retirement and Survivors Insurance part of the Social Security Program Operations Manual System.
- Diagnostic psychological testing services when furnished under the general supervision of a CP.

Carriers are required to familiarize themselves with appropriate State laws and/or regulations governing a CP's scope of practice.

D. Noncovered Services

The services of CPs are not covered if the service is otherwise excluded from Medicare coverage even though a clinical psychologist is authorized by State law to perform them.

For example, Sec.1862(a)(1)(A) of the Act excludes from coverage services that are not "reasonable and necessary for the diagnosis or treatment of an illness or injury or to improve the functioning of a malformed body member." Therefore, even though the services are authorized by State law, the services of a CP that are determined to be not reasonable and necessary are not covered. Additionally, any therapeutic services that are billed by CPs under CPT psychotherapy codes that include medical evaluation and management services are not covered.

E. Requirement for Consultation

When applying for a Medicare provider number, a CP must submit to the carrier a signed Medicare provider/supplier enrollment form that indicates an agreement to the effect that, contingent upon the patient's consent, the CP will attempt to consult with the patient's attending or primary care physician in accordance with accepted professional ethical norms, taking into consideration patient confidentiality.

If the patient assents to the consultation, the CP must attempt to consult with the patient's physician within a reasonable time after receiving the consent. If the CP's attempts to consult directly with the physician are not successful, the CP must notify the physician within a reasonable time that he or she is furnishing services to the patient. Additionally, the CP must document, in the patient's medical record, the date the patient consented or declined consent to consultations, the date of consultation, or, if attempts to consult did not succeed, that date and manner of notification to the physician.

The only exception to the consultation requirement for CPs is in cases where the patient's primary care or attending physician refers the patient to the CP. Also, neither a CP nor a primary care nor attending physician may bill Medicare or the patient for this required consultation.

F. Outpatient Mental Health Services Limitation

All covered therapeutic services furnished by qualified CPs are subject to the outpatient mental health services limitation in Pub 100-01, Medicare General Information, Eligibility, and Entitlement Manual, Chapter 3, "Deductibles, Coinsurance Amounts, and Payment Limitations," Sec.30, (i.e., only 62 1/2 percent of expenses for these services are considered incurred expenses for Medicare purposes). The limitation does not apply to diagnostic services.

G. Assignment Requirement

Assignment Sec. required.

100-2, 15, 170

Clinical Social Worker (CSW) Services

B3-2152

See the Medicare Claims Processing Manual Chapter 12, Physician/Nonphysician Practitioners, Sec.150, "Clinical Social Worker Services," for payment requirements.

A. Clinical Social Worker Defined

Section 1861(hh) of the Act defines a "clinical social worker" as an individual who:

- Possesses a master's or doctor's degree in social work;
- Has performed at least two years of supervised clinical social work; and
- Is licensed or certified as a clinical social worker by the State in which the services are performed; or
- In the case of an individual in a State that does not provide for licensure or certification, has completed at least 2 years or 3,000 hours of post master's degree supervised clinical social work practice under the supervision of a master's level social worker in an appropriate setting such as a hospital, SNF, or clinic.

B. Clinical Social Worker Services Defined

Section 1861(hh)(2) of the Act defines "clinical social worker services" as those services that the CSW is legally authorized to perform under State law (or the State regulatory mechanism provided by State law) of the State in which such services are performed for the diagnosis and treatment of mental illnesses. Services furnished to an inpatient of a hospital or an inpatient of a SNF that the SNF is required to provide as a requirement for participation are not included. The services that are covered are those that are otherwise covered if furnished by a physician or as incident to a physician's professional service.

C. Covered Services

Coverage is limited to the services a CSW is legally authorized to perform in accordance with State law (or State regulatory mechanism established by State law). The services of a CSW may be covered under Part B if they are: The type of services that are otherwise covered if furnished by a physician, or as incident to a physician's service. (See Sec.30 for a description of physicians' services and Sec.70 of Pub 100-1, the Medicare General Information, Eligibility, and Entitlement Manual, Chapter 5, for the definition of a physician.); Performed by a person who meets the definition of a CSW (See subsection A.); and Not otherwise excluded from coverage. Carriers should become familiar with the State law or regulatory mechanism governing a CSW's scope of practice in their service area.

D. Noncovered Services

Services of a CSW are not covered when furnished to inpatients of a hospital or to inpatients of a SNF if the services furnished in the SNF are those that the SNF is required to furnish as a condition of participation in Medicare. In addition, CSW services are not covered if they are otherwise excluded from Medicare coverage even though a CSW is authorized by State law to perform them. For example, the Medicare law excludes from coverage services that are not "reasonable and necessary for the diagnosis or treatment of an illness or injury or to improve the functioning of a malformed body member."

E. Outpatient Mental Health Services
Limitation All covered therapeutic services furnished by qualified CSWs are subject to the outpatient psychiatric services limitation in Pub 100-01, Medicare General Information, Eligibility, and Entitlement Manual, Chapter 3, "Deductibles, Coinsurance Amounts, and Payment Limitations," Sec.30, (i.e., only 62 1/2 percent of expenses for these services are considered incurred expenses for Medicare purposes). The limitation does not apply to diagnostic services.

F. Assignment Requirement
Assignment is required.

100-2, 15, 180

Nurse-Midwife (CNM) Services

B3-2154

A. General
Effective on or after July 1, 1988, the services provided by a certified nurse-midwife or incident to the certified nurse-midwife's services are covered. Payment is made under assignment only. See the Medicare Claims Processing Manual, Chapter 12, "Physician and Nonphysician Practitioners," Sec.130, for payment methodology for nurse midwife services.

B. Certified Nurse-Midwife Defined
A certified nurse-midwife is a registered nurse who has successfully completed a program of study and clinical experience in nurse-midwifery, meeting guidelines prescribed by the Secretary, or who has been certified by an organization recognized by the Secretary. The Secretary has recognized certification by the American College of Nurse-Midwives and State qualifying requirements in those States that specify a program of education and clinical experience for nurse-midwives for these purposes. A nurse-midwife must:

- Be currently licensed to practice in the State as a registered professional nurse; and
- Meet one of the following requirements:
    1. Be legally authorized under State law or regulations to practice as a nurse-midwife and have completed a program of study and clinical experience for nurse-midwives, as specified by the State; or
    2. If the State does not specify a program of study and clinical experience that nurse-midwives must complete to practice in that State, the nurse-midwife must:
        a. Be currently certified as a nurse-midwife by the American College of Nurse-Midwives;
        b. Have satisfactorily completed a formal education program (of at least one academic year) that, upon completion, qualifies the nurse to take the certification examination offered by the American College of Nurse-Midwives; or
        c. Have successfully completed a formal education program for preparing registered nurses to furnish gynecological and obstetrical care to women during pregnancy, delivery, and the postpartum period, and care to normal newborns, and have practiced as a nurse-midwife for a total of 12 months during any 18-month period from August 8, 1976, to July 16, 1982.

C. Covered Services

1. General - Effective January 1, 1988, through December 31, 1993, the coverage of nurse-midwife services was restricted to the maternity cycle. The maternity cycle is a period that includes pregnancy, labor, and the immediate postpartum period.

   Beginning with services furnished on or after January 1, 1994, coverage is no longer limited to the maternity cycle. Coverage is available for services furnished by a nurse-midwife that he or she is legally authorized to perform in the State in which the services are furnished and that would otherwise be covered if furnished by a physician, including obstetrical and gynecological services.

2. Incident To- Services and supplies furnished incident to a nurse midwife's service are covered if they would have been covered when furnished incident to the services of a doctor of medicine or osteopathy, as described in Sec.60.

D. Noncovered Services
The services of nurse-midwives are not covered if they are otherwise excluded from Medicare coverage even though a nurse-midwife is authorized by State law to perform them. For example, the Medicare program excludes from coverage routine physical checkups and services that are not reasonable and necessary for the diagnosis or treatment of an illness or injury or to improve the functioning of a malformed body member. Coverage of service to the newborn continues only to the point that the newborn is or would normally be treated medically as a separate individual. Items and services furnished the newborn from that point are not covered on the basis of the mother's eligibility.

E. Relationship With Physician
Most States have licensure and other requirements applicable to nurse-midwives. For example, some require that the nurse-midwife have an arrangement with a physician for the referral of the patient in the event a problem develops that requires medical attention. Others may require that the nurse-midwife function under the general supervision of a physician. Although these and similar State requirements must be met in order for the nurse-midwife to provide Medicare covered care, they have no effect on the nurse-midwife's right to personally bill for and receive direct Medicare payment. That is, billing does not have to flow through a physician or facility. See Sec.60.2 for coverage of services performed by nurse-midwives incident to the service of physicians.

F. Place of Service
There is no restriction on place of service. Therefore, nurse-midwife services are covered if provided in the nurse-midwife's office, in the patient's home, or in a hospital or other facility, such as a clinic or birthing center owned or operated by a nurse-midwife.

G. Assignment Requirement
Assignment is required.

100-2, 15, 230

Practice of Physical Therapy, Occupational Therapy, and Speech-Language Pathology

A. Group Therapy Services.
Contractors pay for outpatient physical therapy services (which includes outpatient speech-language pathology services) and outpatient occupational therapy services provided simultaneously to two or more individuals by a practitioner as group therapy services (97150). The individuals can be, but need not be performing the same activity. The physician or therapist involved in group therapy services must be in constant attendance, but one-on-one patient contact is not required.

B. Therapy Students

1. General

   Only the services of the therapist can be billed and paid under Medicare Part B. The services performed by a student are not reimbursed even if provided under "line of sight" supervision of the therapist; however, the presence of the student "in the room" does not make the service unbillable. Pay for the direct (one-to-one) patient contact services of the physician or therapist provided to Medicare Part B patients. Group therapy services performed by a therapist or physician may be billed when a student is also present "in the room".

   EXAMPLES:

   Therapists may bill and be paid for the provision of services in the following scenarios:

   - The qualified practitioner is present and in the room for the entire session. The student participates in the delivery of services when the qualified practitioner is directing the service, making the skilled judgment, and is responsible for the assessment and treatment.
   - The qualified practitioner is present in the room guiding the student in service delivery when the therapy student and the therapy assistant student are participating in the provision of services, and the practitioner is not engaged in treating another patient or doing other tasks at the same time
   - The qualified practitioner is responsible for the services and as such, signs all documentation. (A student may, of course, also sign but it is not necessary since the Part B payment is for the clinician's service, not for the student's services).

2. Therapy Assistants as Clinical Instructors

   Physical therapist assistants and occupational therapy assistants are not precluded from serving as clinical instructors for therapy students, while providing services within their scope of work and performed under the direction and supervision of a licensed physical or occupational therapist to a Medicare beneficiary.

3. Services Provided Under Part A and Part B

   The payment methodologies for Part A and B therapy services rendered by a student are different. Under the MPFS (Medicare Part B), Medicare pays for services provided by physicians and practitioners that are specifically authorized by statute. Students do not meet the definition of practitioners under Medicare Part B. Under SNF PPS, payments are based upon the case mix or Resource Utilization Group (RUG) category that describes the patient. In the rehabilitation groups, the number of therapy minutes delivered to the patient determines the RUG category. Payment levels for each category are based upon the costs of caring for patients in each group rather than providing pecific payment for each therapy service as is done in Medicare Part B.

100-2, 15, 230.1

Practice of Physical Therapy

A. General
Physical therapy services are those services provided within the scope of practice of physical therapists and necessary for the diagnosis and treatment of impairments, functional limitations, disabilities or changes in physical function and health status. (See Pub. 100-03, the Medicare National Coverage Determinations Manual, for specific conditions or services.) For descriptions of aquatic therapy in a community center pool see section 220C of this chapter.

B. Qualified Physical Therapist Defined
Reference: 42CFR484.4

The new personnel qualifications for physical therapists were discussed in the 2008 Physician Fee Schedule. See the Federal Register of November 27, 2007, for the full text. See also the correction notice for this rule, published in the Federal Register on January 15, 2008.

The regulation provides that a qualified physical therapist (PT) is a person who is licensed, if applicable, as a PT by the state in which he or she is practicing unless licensure does not apply, has graduated from an accredited PT education program and passed a national examination approved by the state in which PT services are provided. The phrase, "by the state in which practicing" includes any authorization to practice provided by the same state in which the service is provided, including temporary licensure, regardless of the location of the entity billing the services. The curriculum accreditation is provided by the Commission on Accreditation in Physical Therapy Education (CAPTE) or, for those who graduated before CAPTE, curriculum approval was provided by the American Physical Therapy Association (APTA). For internationally educated PTs, curricula are approved by a credentials evaluation organization either approved by the APTA or identified in 8 CFR 212.15(e) as it relates to PTs. For example, in 2007, 8 CFR 212.15(e) approved the credentials evaluation provided by the Federation of State Boards of Physical Therapy (FSBPT) and the Foreign Credentialing Commission on Physical Therapy (FCCPT). The requirements above apply to all PTs effective January 1, 2010, if they have not met any of the following requirements prior to January 1, 2010.

Physical therapists whose current license was obtained on or prior to December 31, 2009, qualify to provide PT services to Medicare beneficiaries if they:

- graduated from a CAPTE approved program in PT on or before December 31, 2009 (examination is not required); or,
- graduated on or before December 31, 2009, from a PT program outside the U.S. that is determined to be substantially equivalent to a U.S. program by a credentials evaluating organization approved by either the APTA or identified in 8 CFR 212.15(e) and also passed an examination for PTs approved by the state in which practicing.

Or, PTs whose current license was obtained before January 1, 2008, may meet the requirements in place on that date (i.e., graduation from a curriculum approved by either the APTA, the Committee on Allied Health Education and Accreditation of the American Medical Association, or both).

Or, PTs meet the requirements who are currently licensed and were licensed or qualified as a PT on or before December 31, 1977, and had 2 years appropriate experience as a PT, and passed a proficiency examination conducted, approved, or sponsored by the U.S. Public Health Service.

Or, PTs meet the requirements if they are currently licensed and before January 1, 1966, they were:

- admitted to membership by the APTA; or
- admitted to registration by the American Registry of Physical Therapists; or
- graduated from a 4-year PT curriculum approved by a State Department of Education; or
- licensed or registered and prior to January 1, 1970, they had 15 years of fulltime experience in PT under the order and direction of attending and referring doctors of medicine or osteopathy.

Or, PTs meet requirements if they are currently licensed and they were trained outside the U.S. before January 1, 2008, and after 1928 graduated from a PT curriculum approved in the country in which the curriculum was located, if that country had an organization that was a member of the World Confederation for Physical Therapy, and that PT qualified as a member of the organization.

For outpatient PT services that are provided incident to the services of physicians/NPPs, the requirement for PT licensure does not apply; all other personnel qualifications do apply. The qualified personnel providing PT services incident to the services of a physician/NPP must be trained in an accredited PT curriculum. For example, a person who, on or before December 31, 2009, graduated from a PT curriculum accredited by CAPTE, but who has not passed the national examination or obtained a license, could provide Medicare outpatient PT therapy services incident to the services of a physician/NPP if the physician assumes responsibility for the services according to the incident to policies. On or after January 1, 2010, although licensure does not apply, both education and examination requirements that are effective January 1, 2010, apply to qualified personnel who provide PT services incident to the services of a physician/NPP.

C. Services of Physical Therapy Support Personnel

Reference: 42CFR 484.4

Personnel Qualifications. The new personnel qualifications for physical therapist assistants (PTA) were discussed in the 2008 Physician Fee Schedule. See the Federal Register of November 27, 2007, for the full text. See also the correction notice for this rule, published in the Federal Register on January 15, 2008.

The regulation provides that a qualified PTA is a person who is licensed as a PTA unless licensure does not apply, is registered or certified, if applicable, as a PTA by the state in which practicing, and graduated from an approved curriculum for PTAs, and passed a national examination for PTAs. The phrase, "by the state in which practicing" includes any authorization to practice provided by the same state in which the service is provided, including temporary licensure, regardless of the location or the entity billing for the services. Approval for the curriculum is provided by CAPTE or, if internationally or military trained PTAs apply, approval will be through a credentialing body for the curriculum for PTAs identified by either the American Physical Therapy Association or identified in 8 CFR 212.15(e). A national examination for PTAs is, for example the one furnished by the Federation of State Boards of Physical Therapy. These requirements above apply to all PTAs effective January 1, 2010, if they have not met any of the following requirements prior to January 1, 2010.

Those PTAs also qualify who, on or before December 31, 2009, are licensed, registered or certified as a PTA and met one of the two following requirements:

1. Is licensed or otherwise regulated in the state in which practicing; or
2. In states that have no licensure or other regulations, or where licensure does not apply, PTAs have:
   - graduated on or before December 31, 2009, from a 2-year college-level program approved by the APTA or CAPTE; and
   - effective January 1, 2010, those PTAs must have both graduated from a CAPTE approved curriculum and passed a national examination for PTAs; or

   PTAs may also qualify if they are licensed, registered or certified as a PTA, if applicable and meet requirements in effect before January 1, 2008, that is,
     - they have graduated before January 1, 2008, from a 2 year college level program approved by the APTA; or
     - on or before December 31, 1977, they were licensed or qualified as a PTA and passed a proficiency examination conducted, approved, or sponsored by the U.S. Public Health Service.

Services. The services of PTAs used when providing covered therapy benefits are included as part of the covered service. These services are billed by the supervising physical therapist. PTAs may not provide evaluation services, make clinical judgments or decisions or take responsibility for the service. They act at the direction and under the supervision of the treating physical therapist and in accordance with state laws.

A physical therapist must supervise PTAs. The level and frequency of supervision differs by setting (and by state or local law). General supervision is required for PTAs in all settings except private practice (which requires direct supervision) unless state practice requirements are more stringent, in which case state or local requirements must be followed. See specific settings for details. For example, in clinics, rehabilitation services, either on or off the organization's premises, those services are supervised by a qualified physical therapist who makes an onsite supervisory visit at least once every 30 days or more frequently if required by state or local laws or regulation.

The services of a PTA shall not be billed as services incident to a physician/NPP's service, because they do not meet the qualifications of a therapist.

The cost of supplies (e.g., theraband, hand putty, electrodes) used in furnishing covered therapy care is included in the payment for the HCPCS codes billed by the physical therapist, and are, therefore, not separately billable. Separate coverage and billing provisions apply to items that meet the definition of brace in Sec.130.

Services provided by aides, even if under the supervision of a therapist, are not therapy services and are not covered by Medicare. Although an aide may help the therapist by providing unskilled services, those services that are unskilled are not covered by Medicare and shall be denied as not reasonable and necessary if they are billed as therapy services.

D. Application of Medicare Guidelines to PT Services
This subsection will be used in the future to illustrate the application of the above guidelines to some of the physical therapy modalities and procedures utilized in the treatment of patient

100-2, 15, 230.2

Practice of Occupational Therapy

(Rev. 88, Issued: 05-07-08, Effective: 01-01-08, Implementation: 06-09-08)

A. General
Occupational therapy services are those services provided within the scope of practice of occupational therapists and necessary for the diagnosis and treatment of impairments, functional disabilities or changes in physical function and health status. (See Pub. 100- 03, the Medicare National Coverage Determinations Manual, for specific conditions or services.)

Occupational therapy is medically prescribed treatment concerned with improving or restoring functions which have been impaired by illness or injury or, where function has been permanently lost or reduced by illness or injury, to improve the individual's ability to perform those tasks required for independent functioning. Such therapy may involve:

The evaluation, and reevaluation as required, of a patient's level of function by administering diagnostic and prognostic tests;

The selection and teaching of task-oriented therapeutic activities designed to restore physical function; e.g., use of woodworking activities on an inclined table to restore shoulder, elbow, and wrist range of motion lost as a result of burns;

The planning, implementing, and supervising of individualized therapeutic activity programs as part of an overall "active treatment" program for a patient with a diagnosed psychiatric illness; e.g., the use of sewing activities which require following a pattern to reduce confusion and restore reality orientation in a schizophrenic patient;

The planning and implementing of therapeutic tasks and activities to restore sensoryintegrative function; e.g., providing motor and tactile activities to increase sensory input and improve response for a stroke patient with functional loss resulting in a distorted body image;

The teaching of compensatory technique to improve the level of independence in the activities of daily living, for example:

- Teaching a patient who has lost the use of an arm how to pare potatoes and chop vegetables with one hand;
- Teaching an upper extremity amputee how to functionally utilize a prosthesis;
- Teaching a stroke patient new techniques to enable the patient to perform feeding, dressing, and other activities as independently as possible; or
- Teaching a patient with a hip fracture/hip replacement techniques of standing tolerance and balance to enable the patient to perform such functional activities as dressing and homemaking tasks.

The designing, fabricating, and fitting of orthotics and self-help devices; e.g., making a hand splint for a patient with rheumatoid arthritis to maintain the hand in a functional position or constructing a device which would enable an individual to hold a utensil and feed independently; or Vocational and prevocational assessment and training, subject to the limitations specified in item B below.

Only a qualified occupational therapist has the knowledge, training, and experience required to evaluate and, as necessary, reevaluate a patient's level of function, determine whether an occupational therapy program could reasonably be expected to improve, restore, or compensate for lost function and, where appropriate, recommend to the physician/NPP a plan of treatment.

B. Qualified Occupational Therapist Defined
Reference: 42CFR484.4 The new personnel qualifications for occupational therapists (OT) were discussed in the 2008 Physician Fee Schedule. See the Federal Register of November 27, 2007, for the full text. See also the correction notice for this rule, published in the Federal Register on January 15, 2008.

The regulation provides that a qualified OT is an individual who is licensed, if licensure applies, or otherwise regulated, if applicable, as an OT by the state in which practicing, and graduated from an accredited education program for OTs, and is eligible to take or has passed the examination for OTs administered by the National Board for Certification in Occupational Therapy, Inc. (NBCOT). The phrase, "by the state in which practicing" includes any authorization to practice provided by the same state in which the service is provided, including temporary licensure, regardless of the location of the entity billing the services. The education program for U.S. trained OTs is accredited by the Accreditation Council for Occupational Therapy Education (ACOTE). The requirements above apply to all OTs effective January 1, 2010, if they have not met any of the following requirements prior to January 1, 2010.

The OTs may also qualify if on or before December 31, 2009:

- they are licensed or otherwise regulated as an OT in the state in which practicing (regardless of the qualifications they met to obtain that licensure or regulation); or
- when licensure or other regulation does not apply, OTs have graduated from an OT education program accredited by ACOTE and are eligible to take, or have successfully completed the NBCOT examination for OTs.

Also, those OTs who met the Medicare requirements for OTs that were in 42CFR484.4 prior to January 1, 2008, qualify to provide OT services for Medicare beneficiaries if:

- on or before January 1, 2008, they graduated an OT program approved jointly by the American Medical Association and the AOTA, or
- they are eligible for the National Registration Examination of AOTA or the National Board for Certification in OT.

Also, they qualify who on or before December 31, 1977, had 2 years of appropriate experience as an occupational therapist, and had achieved a satisfactory grade on a proficiency examination conducted, approved, or sponsored by the U.S. Public Health Service.

Those educated outside the U.S. may meet the same qualifications for domestic trained OTs. For example, they qualify if they were licensed or otherwise regulated by the state in which practicing on or before December 31, 2009. Or they are qualified if they:

- graduated from an OT education program accredited as substantially equivalent to a U.S. OT education program by ACOTE, the World Federation of Occupational Therapists, or a credentialing body approved by AOTA; and
- passed the NBCOT examination for OT; and
- Effective January 1, 2010, are licensed or otherwise regulated, if applicable as an OT by the state in which practicing.

For outpatient OT services that are provided incident to the services of physicians/NPPs, the requirement for OT licensure does not apply; all other personnel qualifications do apply. The qualified personnel providing OT services incident to the services of a physician/NPP must be trained in an accredited OT curriculum. For example, a person who, on or before December 31, 2009, graduated from an OT curriculum accredited by ACOTE and is eligible to take or has successfully completed the entry-level certification examination for OTs developed and administered by NBCOT, could provide Medicare outpatient OT services incident to the services of a physician/NPP if the physician assumes responsibility for the services according to the incident to policies. On or after January 1, 2010, although licensure does not apply, both education and examination requirements that are effective January 1, 2010, apply to qualified personnel who provide OT services incident to the services of a physician/NPP.

C. Services of Occupational Therapy Support Personnel
Reference: 42CFR 484.4

The new personnel qualifications for occupational therapy assistants were discussed in the 2008 Physician Fee Schedule. See the Federal Register of November 27, 2007, for the full text. See also the correction notice for this rule, published in the Federal Register on January 15, 2008.

The regulation provides that an occupational therapy assistant is a person who is licensed, unless licensure does not apply, or otherwise regulated, if applicable, as an OTA by the state in which practicing, and graduated from an OTA education program accredited by ACOTE and is eligible to take or has successfully completed the NBCOT examination for OTAs. The phrase, "by the state in which practicing" includes any authorization to practice provided by the same state in which the service is provided, including temporary licensure, regardless of the location of the entity billing the services.

If the requirements above are not met, an OTA may qualify if, on or before December 31, 2009, the OTA is licensed or otherwise regulated as an OTA, if applicable, by the state in which practicing, or meets any qualifications defined by the state in which practicing.

Or, where licensure or other state regulation does not apply, OTAs may qualify if they have, on or before December 31, 2009:

- completed certification requirements to practice as an OTA established by a credentialing organization approved by AOTA; and
- after January 1, 2010, they have also completed an education program accredited by ACOTE and passed the NBCOT examination for OTAs.

OTAs who qualified under the policies in effect prior to January 1, 2008, continue to qualify to provide OT directed and supervised OTA services to Medicare beneficiaries.

Therefore, OTAs qualify who after December 31, 1977, and on or before December 31, 2007:

- completed certification requirements to practice as an OTA established by a credentialing organization approved by AOTA; or
- completed the requirements to practice as an OTA applicable in the state in which practicing.

Those OTAs who were educated outside the U.S. may meet the same requirements as domestically trained OTAs. Or, if educated outside the U.S. on or after January 1, 2008, they must have graduated from an OTA program accredited as substantially equivalent to OTA entry level education in the U.S. by ACOTE, its successor organization, or the World Federation of Occupational Therapists or a credentialing body approved by AOTA. In addition, they must have passed an exam for OTAs administered by NBCOT.

Services. The services of OTAs used when providing covered therapy benefits are included as part of the covered service. These services are billed by the supervising occupational therapist. OTAs may not provide evaluation services, make clinical judgments or decisions or take responsibility for the service. They act at the direction and under the supervision of the treating occupational therapist and in accordance with state laws.

An occupational therapist must supervise OTAs. The level and frequency of supervision differs by setting (and by state or local law). General supervision is required for OTAs in all settings except private practice (which requires direct supervision) unless state practice requirements are more stringent, in which case state or local requirements must be followed. See specific settings for details. For example, in clinics, rehabilitation agencies, and public health agencies, 42CFR485.713 indicates that when an OTA provides services, either on or off the organization's premises, those services are supervised by a qualified occupational therapist who makes an onsite supervisory visit at least once every 30 days or more frequently if required by state or local laws or regulation.

The services of an OTA shall not be billed as services incident to a physician/NPP's service, because they do not meet the qualifications of a therapist.

The cost of supplies (e.g., looms, ceramic tiles, or leather) used in furnishing covered therapy care is included in the payment for the HCPCS codes billed by the occupational therapist and are, therefore, not separately billable. Separate coverage and billing provisions apply to items that meet the definition of brace in Sec.130 of this manual.

Services provided by aides, even if under the supervision of a therapist, are not therapy services in the outpatient setting and are not covered by Medicare. Although an aide may help the therapist by providing unskilled services, those services that are unskilled are not covered by Medicare and shall be denied as not reasonable and necessary if they are billed as therapy services.

D. Application of Medicare Guidelines to Occupational Therapy Services
Occupational therapy may be required for a patient with a specific diagnosed psychiatric illness. If such services are required, they are covered assuming the coverage criteria are met. However, where an individual's motivational needs are not related to a specific diagnosed psychiatric illness, the meeting of such needs does not usually require an individualized therapeutic program. Such needs can be met through general activity programs or the efforts of other professional personnel involved in the care of the patient. Patient motivation is an appropriate and inherent function of all health disciplines, which is interwoven with other functions performed by such personnel for the patient. Accordingly, since the special skills of an occupational therapist are not required, an occupational therapy program for individuals who do not have a specific diagnosed psychiatric illness is not to be considered reasonable and necessary for the treatment of an illness or injury. Services furnished under such a program are not covered.

Occupational therapy may include vocational and prevocational assessment and training. When services provided by an occupational therapist are related solely to specific employment opportunities, work skills, or work settings, they are not reasonable or necessary for the diagnosis or treatment of an illness or injury and are not covered. However, carriers and intermediaries exercise care in applying this exclusion, because the assessment of level of function and the teaching of compensatory techniques to improve the level of function, especially in activities of daily living, are services which occupational therapists provide for both vocational and nonvocational purposes. For example, an assessment of sitting and standing tolerance might be nonvocational for a mother of young children or a retired individual living alone, but could also be a vocational test for a sales clerk. Training an amputee in the use of prosthesis for telephoning is necessary for everyday activities as well as for employment purposes. Major changes in life style may be mandatory for an individual with a substantial disability. The techniques of adjustment cannot be considered exclusively vocational or nonvocational.

100-2, 15, 230.3

Practice of Speech-Language Pathology

A. General
Speech-language pathology services are those services provided within the scope of practice of speech-language pathologists and necessary for the diagnosis and treatment of speech and language disorders, which result in communication disabilities and for the diagnosis and treatment of swallowing disorders (dysphagia), regardless of the presence of a communication disability. (See Pub. 100-03, chapter 1, Sec.170.3)

B. Qualified Speech-Language Pathologist Defined
A qualified speech-language pathologist for program coverage purposes meets one of the following requirements:

- The education and experience requirements for a Certificate of Clinical Competence in (speech-language pathology) granted by the American Speech- Language Hearing Association; or
- Meets the educational requirements for certification and is in the process of accumulating the supervised experience required for certification.

For outpatient speech-language pathology services that are provided incident to the services of physicians/NPPs, the requirement for speech-language pathology licensure does not apply; all other personnel qualifications do apply. Therefore, qualified personnel providing speech-language pathology services incident to the services of a physician/NPP must meet the above qualifications.

C. Services of Speech-Language Pathology Support Personnel
Services of speech-language pathology assistants are not recognized for Medicare coverage. Services provided by speech-language pathology assistants, even if they are licensed to provide services in their states, will be considered unskilled services and denied as not reasonable and necessary if they are billed as therapy services.

Services provided by aides, even if under the supervision of a therapist, are not therapy services and are not covered by Medicare. Although an aide may help the therapist by providing unskilled services, those services are not covered by Medicare and shall be denied as not reasonable and necessary if they are billed as therapy services.

D. Application of Medicare Guidelines to Speech-Language Pathology Services

1. Evaluation Services
   Speech-language pathology evaluation services are covered if they are reasonable and necessary and not excluded as routine screening by Sec.1862(a)(7) of the Act. The speechlanguage pathologist employs a variety of formal and informal speech, language, and dysphagia assessment tests to ascertain the type, causal factor(s), and severity of the speech and language or swallowing disorders. Reevaluation of patients for whom speech, language and swallowing were previously contraindicated is covered only if the patient exhibits a change in medical condition. However, monthly reevaluations; e.g., a Western Aphasia Battery, for a patient undergoing a rehabilitative speech-language pathology program, are considered a part of the treatment session and shall not be covered as a separate evaluation for billing purposes. Although hearing screening by the speechlanguage pathologist may be part of an evaluation, it is not billable as a separate service.
2. Therapeutic Services
   The following are examples of common medical disorders and resulting communication deficits, which may necessitate active rehabilitative therapy. This list is not all-inclusive:
   - Cerebrovascular disease such as cerebral vascular accidents presenting with dysphagia, aphasia/dysphasia, apraxia, and dysarthria;
   - Neurological disease such as Parkinsonism or
   - Multiple Sclerosis with dysarthria, dysphagia, inadequate respiratory volume/control, or voice disorder; or
   - Laryngeal carcinoma requiring laryngectomy resulting in aphonia.
3. Impairments of the Auditory System
   The terms, aural rehabilitation, auditory rehabilitation, auditory processing, lipreading and speech reading are among the terms used to describe covered services related to perception and comprehension of sound through the auditory system. See Pub. 100-04, chapter 12, section 30.3 for billing instructions. For example:
   - Auditory processing evaluation and treatment may be covered and medically necessary. Examples include but are not limited to services for certain neurological impairments or the absence of natural auditory stimulation that results in impaired ability to process sound. Certain auditory processing disorders require diagnostic audiological tests in addition to speech-language pathology evaluation and treatment.
   - Evaluation and treatment for disorders of the auditory system may be covered and medically necessary, for example, when it has been determined by a speechlanguage pathologist in collaboration with an audiologist that the hearing impaired beneficiary's current amplification options (hearing aid, other amplification device or cochlear implant) will not sufficiently meet the patient's functional communication needs. Audiologists and speech-language pathologists both evaluate beneficiaries for disorders of the auditory system using different skills and techniques, but only speech-language pathologists may provide treatment.

Assessment for the need for rehabilitation of the auditory system (but not the vestibular system) may be done by a speech language pathologist. Examples include but are not limited to: evaluation of comprehension and production of language in oral, signed or written modalities, speech and voice production, listening skills, speech reading, communications strategies, and the impact of the hearing loss on the patient/client and family.

Examples of rehabilitation include but are not limited to treatment that focuses on comprehension, and production of language in oral, signed or written modalities; speech and voice production, auditory training, speech reading, multimodal (e.g., visual, auditory-visual, and tactile) training, communication strategies, education and counseling. In determining the necessity for treatment, the beneficiary's performance in both clinical and natural environment should be considered.

4. Dysphagia
Dysphagia, or difficulty in swallowing, can cause food to enter the airway, resulting in coughing, choking, pulmonary problems, aspiration or inadequate nutrition and hydration with resultant weight loss, failure to thrive, pneumonia and death. It is most often due to complex neurological and/or structural impairments including head and neck trauma, cerebrovascular accident, neuromuscular degenerative diseases, head and neck cancer, dementias, and encephalopathies. For these reasons, it is important that only qualified professionals with specific training and experience in this disorder provide evaluation and treatment.

The speech-language pathologist performs clinical and instrumental assessments and analyzes and integrates the diagnostic information to determine candidacy for intervention as well as appropriate compensations and rehabilitative therapy techniques.

The equipment that is used in the examination may be fixed, mobile or portable.

Professional guidelines recommend that the service be provided in a team setting with a physician/NPP who provides supervision of the radiological examination and interpretation of medical conditions revealed in it.

Swallowing assessment and rehabilitation are highly specialized services. The professional rendering care must have education, experience and demonstrated competencies. Competencies include but are not limited to: identifying abnormal upper aerodigestive tract structure and function; conducting an oral, pharyngeal, laryngeal and respiratory function examination as it relates to the functional assessment of swallowing; recommending methods of oral intake and risk precautions; and developing a treatment plan employing appropriate compensations and therapy techniques.

100-2, 15, 230.4

Services Furnished by a Physical or Occupational Therapist in Private Practice

A. General
In order to qualify to bill Medicare directly as a therapist, each individual must be enrolled as a private practitioner and employed in one of the following practice types: an unincorporated solo practice, unincorporated partnership, unincorporated group practice, physician/NPP group or groups that are not professional corporations, if allowed by state and local law. Physician/NPP group practices may employ physical therapists in private practice (PTPP) and/or occupational therapists in private practice (OTPP) if state and local law permits this employee relationship.

For purposes of this provision, a physician/NPP group practice is defined as one or more physicians/NPPs enrolled with Medicare who may bill as one entity. For further details on issues concerning enrollment, see the provider enrollment Web site at www.cms.hhs.gov/providers/enrollment.

Private practice also includes therapists who are practicing therapy as employees of another supplier, of a professional corporation or other incorporated therapy practice. Private practice does not include individuals when they are working as employees of an institutional provider.

Services should be furnished in the therapist's or group's office or in the patient's home. The office is defined as the location(s) where the practice is operated, in the state(s) where the therapist (and practice, if applicable) is legally authorized to furnish services, during the hours that the therapist engages in the practice at that location. If services are furnished in a private practice office space, that space shall be owned, leased, or rented by the practice and used for the exclusive purpose of operating the practice. For descriptions of aquatic therapy in a community center pool see section 220C of this chapter.

Therapists in private practice must be approved as meeting certain requirements, but do not execute a formal provider agreement with the Secretary.

If therapists who have their own Medicare Personal Identification number (PIN) or National Provider Identifier (NPI) are employed by therapist groups, physician/NPP groups, or groups that are not professional organizations, the requirement that therapy space be owned, leased, or rented may be satisfied by the group that employs the therapist. Each physical or occupational therapist employed by a group should enroll as a PT or OT in private practice.

When therapists with a Medicare PIN/NPI provide services in the physician's/NPP's office in which they are employed, and bill using their PIN/NPI for each therapy service, then the direct supervision requirement for PTAs and OTAs apply.

When the PT or OT who has a Medicare PIN/ NPI is employed in a physician's/NPP's office the services are ordinarily billed as services of the PT or OT, with the PT or OT identified on the claim as the supplier of services. However, services of the PT or OT who has a Medicare PIN/NPI may also be billed by the physician/NPP as services incident to the physician's/NPP's service. (See Sec.230.5 for rules related to PTA and OTA services incident to a physician.) In that case, the physician/NPP is the supplier of service, the Unique Provider Identification Number (UPIN) or NPI of the physician/NPP (ordering or supervising, as indicated) is reported on the claim with the service and all the rules for incident to services (Sec.230.5) must be followed.

B. Private Practice Defined
Reference: Federal Register November, 1998, pages 58863-58869; 42CFR 410.38(b)

The carrier considers a therapist to be in private practice if the therapist maintains office space at his or her own expense and furnishes services only in that space or the patient's home. Or, a therapist is employed by another supplier and furnishes services in facilities provided at the expense of that supplier.

The therapist need not be in full-time private practice but must be engaged in private practice on a regular basis; i.e., the therapist is recognized as a private practitioner and for that purpose has access to the necessary equipment to provide an adequate program of therapy.

The physical or occupational therapy services must be provided either by or under the direct supervision of the therapist in private practice. Each physical or occupational therapist in a practice should be enrolled as a Medicare provider. If a physical or occupational therapist is not enrolled, the services of that therapist must be directly supervised by an enrolled physical or occupational therapist. Direct supervision requires that the supervising private practice therapist be present in the office suite at the time the service is performed. These direct supervision requirements apply only in the private practice setting and only for physical therapists and occupational therapists and their assistants. In other outpatient settings, supervision rules differ. The services of support personnel must be included in the therapist's bill. The supporting personnel, including other therapists, must be W-2 or 1099 employees of the therapist in private practice or other qualified employer.

Coverage of outpatient physical therapy and occupational therapy under Part B includes the services of a qualified therapist in private practice when furnished in the therapist's office or the beneficiary's home. For this purpose, "home" includes an institution that is used as a home, but not a hospital, CAH or SNF, (Federal Register Nov. 2, 1998, pg 58869). Place of Service (POS) includes:

- 03/School, only if residential,
- 04/Homeless Shelter,
- 12/Home, other than a facility that is a private residence,
- 14/Group Home, 33/Custodial Care Facility.

C. Assignment
Reference: Nov. 2, 1998 Federal Register, pg. 58863

See also Pub. 100-04 chapter 1, Sec.30.2.

When physicians, NPPs, PTPPs or OTPPs obtain provider numbers, they have the option of accepting assignment (participating) or not accepting assignment (nonparticipating). In contrast, providers, such as outpatient hospitals, SNFs, rehabilitation agencies, and CORFs, do not have the option. For these providers, assignment is mandatory.

If physicians/NPPs, PTPPs or OTPPs accept assignment (are participating), they must accept the Medicare Physician Fee Schedule amount as payment. Medicare pays 80% and the patient is responsible for 20%. In contrast, if they do not accept assignment, Medicare will only pay 95% of the fee schedule amount. However, when these services are not furnished on an assignment-related basis, the limiting charge applies. (See Sec.1848(g)(2)(c) of the Act.)

NOTE: Services furnished by a therapist in the therapist's office under arrangements with hospitals in rural communities and public health agencies (or services provided in the beneficiary's home under arrangements with a provider of outpatient physical or occupational therapy services) are not covered under this provision. See section 230.6.

100-2, 15, 232

Cardiac Rehabilitation (CR) and Intensive Cardiac Rehabilitation (ICR) Services Furnished On or After January 1, 2010

Cardiac rehabilitation (CR) services mean a physician-supervised program that furnishes physician prescribed exercise, cardiac risk factor modification, including education, counseling, and behavioral intervention; psychosocial assessment, outcomes assessment, and other items/services as determined by the Secretary under certain conditions. Intensive cardiac rehabilitation (ICR) services mean a physician-supervised program that furnishes the same items/services under the same conditions as a CR program but must also demonstrate, as shown in peer-reviewed published research, that it improves patients' cardiovascular disease through specific outcome measurements described in 42 CFR 410.49(c). Effective January 1, 2010, Medicare Part B pays for CR/ICR programs and related items/services if specific criteria is met by the Medicare beneficiary, the CR/ICR program itself, the setting in which is it administered, and the physician administering the program, as outlined below:

CR/ICR Program Beneficiary Requirements:

Medicare covers CR/ICR program services for beneficiaries who have experienced one or more of the following:

Acute myocardial infarction within the preceding 12 months;

Coronary artery bypass surgery;

Current stable angina pectoris;

Heart valve repair or replacement;

Percutaneous transluminal coronary angioplasty (PTCA) or coronary stenting;

Heart or heart-lung transplant.

For CR only, other cardiac conditions as specified through a national coverage determination (NCD).

CR/ICR Program Component Requirements:
Physician-prescribed exercise. This physical activity includes aerobic exercise combined with other types of exercise (i.e., strengthening, stretching) as determined to be appropriate for individual patients by a physician each day CR/ICR items/services are furnished.

Cardiac risk factor modification. This includes education, counseling, and behavioral intervention, tailored to the patients' individual needs.

Psychosocial assessment. This assessment means an evaluation of an individual's mental and emotional functioning as it relates to the individual's rehabilitation. It should include: (1) an assessment of those aspects of the individual's family and home situation that affects the individual's rehabilitation treatment, and, (2) a psychosocial evaluation of the individual's response to, and rate of progress under, the treatment plan.

Outcomes assessment. These should include: (i) minimally, assessments from the commencement and conclusion of CR/ICR, based on patient-centered outcomes which must be measured by the physician immediately at the beginning and end of the program, and, (ii) objective clinical measures of the effectiveness of the CR/ICR program for the individual patient, including exercise performance and self-reported measures of exertion and behavior.

Individualized treatment plan. This plan should be written and tailored to each individual patient and include (i) a description of the individual's diagnosis; (ii) the type, amount, frequency, and duration of the CR/ICR items/services furnished; and (iii) the goals set for the individual under the plan. The individualized treatment plan must be established, reviewed, and signed by a physician every 30 days.

As specified at 42 CFR 410.49(f)(1), CR sessions are limited to a maximum of 2 1-hour sessions per day for up to 36 sessions over up to 36 weeks with the option for an additional 36 sessions over an extended period of time if approved by the contractor under section 1862(a)(1)(A) of the Act. ICR sessions are limited to 72 1-hour sessions (as defined in section 1848(b)(5) of the Act), up to 6 sessions per day, over a period of up to 18 weeks.

CR/ICR Program Setting Requirements:
CR/ICR services must be furnished in a physician's office or a hospital outpatient setting (for ICR, the hospital outpatient setting must provide ICR using an approved ICR program). All settings must have a physician immediately available and accessible for medical consultations and emergencies at all times when items/services are being furnished under the program. This provision is satisfied if the physician meets the requirements for direct supervision of physician office services as specified at 42 CFR 410.26, and for hospital outpatient services as specified at 42 CFR 410.27.

ICR Program Approval Requirements:
All prospective ICR programs must be approved through the national coverage determination (NCD) process. To be approved as an ICR program, it must demonstrate through peer-reviewed, published research that it has accomplished one or more of the following for its patients: (i) positively affected the progression of coronary heart disease, (ii) reduced the need for coronary bypass surgery, or, (iii) reduced the need for percutaneous coronary interventions.

An ICR program must also demonstrate through peer-reviewed, published research that it accomplished a statistically significant reduction in five or more of the following measures for patients from their levels before CR services to after CR services: (i) low density lipoprotein, (ii) triglycerides, (iii) body mass index, (iv) systolic blood pressure, (v) diastolic blood pressure, and (vi) the need for cholesterol, blood pressure, and diabetes medications.

A list of approved ICR programs, identified through the NCD process, will be posted to the CMS Web site and listed in the Federal Register.

Once an ICR program is approved through the NCD process, all prospective ICR sites wishing to furnish ICR items/services via an approved ICR program may enroll with their local contractor to become an ICR program supplier using the designated forms as specified at 42 CFR 424.510, and report specialty code 31 to be identified as an enrolled ICR supplier. For purposes of appealing an adverse determination concerning site approval, an ICR site is considered a supplier (or prospective supplier) as defined in 42 CFR 498.2.

CR/ICR Program Physician Requirements:
Physicians responsible for CR/ICR programs are identified as medical directors who oversee or supervise the CR/ICR program at a particular site. The medical director, in consultation with staff, is involved in directing the progress of individuals in the program. The medical director, as well as physicians acting as the supervising physician, must possess all of the following: (1) expertise in the management of individuals with cardiac pathophysiology, (2) cardiopulmonary training in basic life support or advanced cardiac life support, and (3) licensed to practice medicine in the state in which the CR/ICR program is offered. Direct physician supervision may be provided by a supervising physician or the medical director.

(See Pub. 100-04, Medicare Claims Processing Manual, chapter 32, section 140.2, for specific claims processing, coding, and billing requirements for CR/ICR program services.)

100-2, 15, 240

Chiropractic Services - General

B3-2250, B3-4118

The term "physician" under Part B includes a chiropractor who meets the specified qualifying requirements set forth in Sec.30.5 but only for treatment by means of manual manipulation of the spine to correct a subluxation.

Effective for claims with dates of services on or after January 1, 2000, an x-ray is not required to demonstrate the subluxation.

Implementation of the chiropractic benefit requires an appreciation of the differences between chiropractic theory and experience and traditional medicine due to fundamental differences regarding etiology and theories of the pathogenesis of disease. Judgments about the reasonableness of chiropractic treatment must be based on the application of chiropractic principles. So that Medicare beneficiaries receive equitable adjudication of claims based on such principles and are not deprived of the benefits intended by the law, carriers may use chiropractic consultation in carrier review of Medicare chiropractic claims.

Payment is based on the physician fee schedule and made to the beneficiary or, on assignment, to the chiropractor.

A. Verification of Chiropractor's Qualifications
Carriers must establish a reference file of chiropractors eligible for payment as physicians under the criteria in Sec.30.1. They pay only chiropractors on file. Information needed to establish such files is furnished by the CMS RO.

The RO is notified by the appropriate State agency which chiropractors are licensed and whether each meets the national uniform standards.

100-2, 15, 240.1.1

Manual Manipulation

Coverage of chiropractic service is specifically limited to treatment by means of manual manipulation, i.e., by use of the hands. Additionally, manual devices (i.e., those that are hand-held with the thrust of the force of the device being controlled manually) may be used by chiropractors in performing manual manipulation of the spine. However, no additional payment is available for use of the device, nor does Medicare recognize an extra charge for the device itself.

No other diagnostic or therapeutic service furnished by a chiropractor or under the chiropractor's order is covered. This means that if a chiropractor orders, takes, or interprets an x-ray, or any other diagnostic test, the x-ray or other diagnostic test, can be used for claims processing purposes, but Medicare coverage and payment are not available for those services. This prohibition does not affect the coverage of x-rays or other diagnostic tests furnished by other practitioners under the program. For example, an x-ray or any diagnostic test taken for the purpose of determining or demonstrating the existence of a subluxation of the spine is a diagnostic x-ray test covered under §1861(s)(3) of the Act if ordered, taken, and interpreted by a physician who is a doctor of medicine or osteopathy.

Manual devices (i.e., those that are hand-held with the thrust of the force of the device being controlled manually) may be used by chiropractors in performing manual manipulation of the spine. However, no additional payment is available for use of the device, nor does Medicare recognize an extra charge for the device itself.

Effective for claims with dates of service on or after January 1, 2000, an x-ray is not required to demonstrate the subluxation. However, an x-ray may be used for this purpose if the chiropractor so chooses.

The word "correction" may be used in lieu of "treatment." Also, a number of different terms composed of the following words may be used to describe manual manipulation as defined above:

- Spine or spinal adjustment by manual means;
- Spine or spinal manipulation;
- Manual adjustment; and

- Vertebral manipulation or adjustment.

In any case in which the term(s) used to describe the service performed suggests that it may not have been treatment by means of manual manipulation, the carrier analyst refers the claim for professional review and interpretation.

100-2, 15, 240.1.3

Necessity for Treatment

The patient must have a significant health problem in the form of a neuromusculoskeletal condition necessitating treatment, and the manipulative services rendered must have a direct therapeutic relationship to the patient's condition and provide reasonable expectation of recovery or improvement of function. The patient must have a subluxation of the spine as demonstrated by x-ray or physical exam, as described above.

Most spinal joint problems fall into the following categories:

- Acute subluxation-A patient's condition is considered acute when the patient is being treated for a new injury, identified by x-ray or physical exam as specified above. The result of chiropractic manipulation is expected to be an improvement in, or arrest of progression, of the patient's condition.
- Chronic subluxation-A patient's condition is considered chronic when it is not expected to significantly improve or be resolved with further treatment (as is the case with an acute condition), but where the continued therapy can be expected to result in some functional improvement. Once the clinical status has remained stable for a given condition, without expectation of additional objective clinical improvements, further manipulative treatment is considered maintenance therapy and is not covered.

For Medicare purposes, a chiropractor must place an AT modifier on a claim when providing active/corrective treatment to treat acute or chronic subluxation. However the presence of the AT modifier may not in all instances indicate that the service is reasonable and necessary. As always, contractors may deny if appropriate after medical review.

A. Maintenance Therapy

Maintenance therapy includes services that seek to prevent disease, promote health and prolong and enhance the quality of life, or maintain or prevent deterioration of a chronic condition. When further clinical improvement cannot reasonably be expected from continuous ongoing care, and the chiropractic treatment becomes supportive rather than corrective in nature, the treatment is then considered maintenance therapy. The AT modifier must not be placed on the claim when maintenance therapy has been provided. Claims without the AT modifier will be considered as maintenance therapy and denied. Chiropractors who give or receive from beneficiaries an ABN shall follow the instructions in Pub. 100-04, Medicare Claims Processing Manual, chapter 23, section 20.9.1.1 and include a GA (or in rare instances a GZ) modifier on the claim.

B. Contraindications

Dynamic thrust is the therapeutic force or maneuver delivered by the physician during manipulation in the anatomic region of involvement. A relative contraindication is a condition that adds significant risk of injury to the patient from dynamic thrust, but does not rule out the use of dynamic thrust. The doctor should discuss this risk with the patient and record this in the chart. The following are relative contraindications to dynamic thrust:

Articular hyper mobility and circumstances where the stability of the joint is uncertain;

Severe demineralization of bone;

Benign bone tumors (spine);

Bleeding disorders and anticoagulant therapy; and

Radiculopathy with progressive neurological signs.

Dynamic thrust is absolutely contraindicated near the site of demonstrated subluxation and proposed manipulation in the following:

Acute arthropathies characterized by acute inflammation and ligamentous laxity and anatomic subluxation or dislocation; including acute rheumatoid arthritis and ankylosing spondylitis;

Acute fractures and dislocations or healed fractures and dislocations with signs of instability;

An unstable os odontoideum;

Malignancies that involve the vertebral column;

Infection of bones or joints of the vertebral column;

Signs and symptoms of myelopathy or cauda equina syndrome;

For cervical spinal manipulations, vertebrobasilar insufficiency syndrome; and

A significant major artery aneurysm near the proposed manipulation.

100-2, 15, 260

Ambulatory Surgical Center Services

Facility services furnished by ambulatory surgical centers (ASCs) in connection with certain surgical procedures are covered under Part B. To receive coverage of and payment for its services under this provision, a facility must be certified as meeting the requirements for an ASC and enter into a written agreement with CMS. Medicare periodically updates the list of covered procedures and related payment amounts through release of regulations and Program Memoranda. The ASC must accept Medicare's payment for such procedures as payment in full with respect to those services defined as ASC facility services.

Where services are performed in an ASC, the physician and others who perform covered services may also be paid for his/her professional services; however, the "professional" rate is then adjusted since the ASC incurs the facility costs.

100-2, 15, 270

Telehealth Services

Background

Section 223 of the Medicare, Medicaid and SCHIP Benefits Improvement and Protection Act of 2000 (BIPA) - Revision of Medicare Reimbursement for Telehealth Services amended §1834 of the Act to provide for an expansion of Medicare payment for telehealth services.

Effective October 1, 2001, coverage and payment for Medicare telehealth includes consultation, office visits, individual psychotherapy, and pharmacologic management delivered via a telecommunications system. Eligible geographic areas include rural health professional shortage areas (HPSA) and counties not classified as a metropolitan statistical area (MSA). Additionally, Federal telemedicine demonstration projects as of December 31, 2000, may serve as the originating site regardless of geographic location.

An interactive telecommunications system is required as a condition of payment; however, BIPA does allow the use of asynchronous "store and forward" technology in delivering these services when the originating site is a Federal telemedicine demonstration program in Alaska or Hawaii. BIPA does not require that a practitioner present the patient for interactive telehealth services.

With regard to payment amount, BIPA specified that payment for the professional service performed by the distant site practitioner (i.e., where the expert physician or practitioner is physically located at time of telemedicine encounter) is equal to what would have been paid without the use of telemedicine. Distant site practitioners include only a physician as described in §1861(r) of the Act and a medical practitioner as described in §1842(b)(18)(C) of the Act. BIPA also expanded payment under Medicare to include a $20 originating site facility fee (location of beneficiary).

Previously, the Balanced Budget Act of 1997 (BBA) limited the scope of Medicare telehealth coverage to consultation services and the implementing regulation prohibited the use of an asynchronous 'store and forward' telecommunications system. The BBA of 1997 also required the professional fee to be shared between the referring and consulting practitioners, and prohibited Medicare payment for facility fees and line charges associated with the telemedicine encounter.

The BIPA required that Medicare Part B (Supplementary Medical Insurance) pay for this expansion of telehealth services beginning with services furnished on October 1, 2001.

Section 149 of the Medicare Improvements for Patients and Providers Act of 2008 (MIPPA) amended §1834(m) of the Act to add certain entities as originating sites for payment of telehealth services. Effective for services furnished on or after January 1, 2009, eligible originating sites include a hospital-based or critical access hospital-based renal dialysis center (including satellites); a skilled nursing facility (as defined in §1819(a) of the Act); and a community mental health center (as defined in §1861(ff)(3)(B) of the Act). MIPPA also amended§1888(e)(2)(A)(ii) of the Act to exclude telehealth services furnished under §1834(m)(4)(C)(ii)(VII) from the consolidated billing provisions of the skilled nursing facility prospective payment system (SNF PPS).

NOTE: MIPPA did not add independent renal dialysis facilities as originating sites for payment of telehealth services.

The telehealth provisions authorized by §1834(m) of the Act are implemented in 42 CFR 410.78 and 414.65.

100-2, 15, 270.2

List of Medicare Telehealth Services

The use of a telecommunications system may substitute for an in-person encounter for professional consultations, office visits, office psychiatry services, and a limited number of other physician fee schedule (PFS) services. These services are listed below.

- Consultations (Effective October 1, 2001- December 31, 2009)
- Initial inpatient telehealth consultations (Effective January 1, 2010)
- Follow-up inpatient telehealth consultations (Effective January 1, 2009)
- Office or other outpatient visits
- Subsequent hospital care services (with the limitation of one telehealth visit every 3 days) (Effective January 1, 2011)
- Subsequent nursing facility care services (with the limitation of one telehealth visit every 30 days) (Effective January 1, 2011)
- Individual psychotherapy
- Pharmacologic management
- Psychiatric diagnostic interview examination (Effective March 1, 2003)
- End stage renal disease related services (Effective January 1, 2005)
- Individual and group medical nutrition therapy (Individual effective January 1, 2006; group effective January 1, 2011)
- Neurobehavioral status exam (Effective January 1, 2008)
- Individual and group health and behavior assessment and intervention (Individual effective January 1, 2010; group effective January 1, 2011)
- Individual and group kidney disease education (KDE) services (Effective January 1, 2011)
- Individual and group diabetes self-management training (DSMT) services (with a minimum of 1 hour of in-person instruction to be furnished in the initial year training period to ensure effective injection training) (Effective January 1, 2011)

NOTE: Beginning January 1, 2010, CMS eliminated the use of all consultation codes, except for inpatient telehealth consultation G-codes. CMS no longer recognizes office/outpatient or inpatient consultation CPT codes for payment of office/outpatient or inpatient visits. Instead, physicians and practitioners are instructed to bill a new or established patient office/outpatient visit CPT code or appropriate hospital or nursing facility care code, as appropriate to the particular patient, for all office/outpatient or inpatient visits. For detailed instructions regarding reporting these and other telehealth services, see Pub. 100-04, Medicare Claims Processing Manual, chapter 12, section 190.3.

The conditions of payment for Medicare telehealth services, including qualifying originating sites and the types of telecommunications systems recognized by Medicare, are subject to the provisions of 42 CFR 410.78. Payment for these services is subject to the provisions of 42 CFR 414.65.

100-2, 15, 270.4

The term "distant site" means the site where the physician or practitioner providing the professional service is located at the time the service is provided via a telecommunications system.

The payment amount for the professional service provided via a telecommunications system by the physician or practitioner at the distant site is equal to the current physician fee schedule amount for the service. Payment for telehealth services (see section 270.2 of this chapter) should be made at the same amount as when these services are furnished without the use of a telecommunications system. For Medicare payment to occur, the service must be within a practitioner's scope of practice under State law. The beneficiary is responsible for any unmet deductible amount and applicable coinsurance.

Medicare Practitioners Who May Receive Payment at the Distant Site (i.e., at a Site Other Than Where the Beneficiary is Located)

As a condition of Medicare Part B payment for telehealth services, the physician or practitioner at the distant site must be licensed to provide the service under State law. When the physician or practitioner at the distant site is licensed under State law to provide a covered telehealth service (see section 270.2 of this chapter) then he or she may bill for and receive payment for this service when delivered via a telecommunications system.

Medicare practitioners who may bill for a covered telehealth service are listed below (subject to State law):

- Physician;
- Nurse practitioner;
- Physician assistant;
- Nurse midwife;
- Clinical nurse specialist;
- Clinical psychologist;
- Clinical social worker; and
- Registered dietitian or nutrition professional.

* Clinical psychologists and clinical social workers cannot bill for psychotherapy services that include medical evaluation and management services under Medicare. These practitioners may not bill or receive payment for the following CPT codes: 90805, 90807, and 90809.

100-2, 15, 270.4.2

Payment for Subsequent Hospital Care Services and Subsequent Nursing Facility Care Services as Telehealth Services

Subsequent hospital care services are limited to one telehealth visit every 3 days. The frequency limit of the benefit is not intended to apply to consulting physicians or practitioners, who should continue to report initial or follow-up inpatient telehealth consultations using the applicable HCPCS G-codes.

Similarly, subsequent nursing facility care services are limited to one telehealth visit every 30 days. Furthermore, subsequent nursing facility care services reported for a Federally-mandated periodic visit under 42 CFR 483.40(c) may not be furnished through telehealth. The frequency limit of the benefit is not intended to apply to consulting physicians or practitioners, who should continue to report initial or follow-up inpatient telehealth consultations using the applicable HCPCS G-codes.

Inpatient telehealth consultations are furnished to beneficiaries in hospitals or skilled nursing facilities via telehealth at the request of the physician of record, the attending physician, or another appropriate source. The physician or practitioner who furnishes the initial inpatient consultation via telehealth cannot be the physician or practitioner of record or the attending physician or practitioner, and the initial inpatient telehealth consultation would be distinct from the care provided by the physician or practitioner of record or the attending physician or practitioner. Counseling and coordination of care with other providers or agencies is included as well, consistent with the nature of the problem(s) and the patient's needs. Initial and follow-up inpatient telehealth consultations are subject to the criteria for inpatient telehealth consultation services, as described in Pub. 100-04, Medicare Claims Processing Manual, chapter 12, section 190.3.

100-2, 15, 290

Foot Care

A. Treatment of Subluxation of Foot

Subluxations of the foot are defined as partial dislocations or displacements of joint surfaces, tendons ligaments, or muscles of the foot. Surgical or nonsurgical treatments undertaken for the sole purpose of correcting a subluxated structure in the foot as an isolated entity are not covered.

However, medical or surgical treatment of subluxation of the ankle joint (talo-crural joint) is covered. In addition, reasonable and necessary medical or surgical services, diagnosis, or treatment for medical conditions that have resulted from or are associated with partial displacement of structures is covered. For example, if a patient has osteoarthritis that has resulted in a partial displacement of joints in the foot, and the primary treatment is for the osteoarthritis, coverage is provided.

B. Exclusions from Coverage

The following foot care services are generally excluded from coverage under both Part A and Part B. (See Sec.290.F and Sec.290.G for instructions on applying foot care exclusions.)

1. Treatment of Flat Foot

   The term "flat foot" is defined as a condition in which one or more arches of the foot have flattened out. Services or devices directed toward the care or correction of such conditions, including the prescription of supportive devices, are not covered.

2. Routine Foot Care

   Except as provided above, routine foot care is excluded from coverage. Services that normally are considered routine and not covered by Medicare include the following:

   - The cutting or removal of corns and calluses;
   - The trimming, cutting, clipping, or debriding of nails; and
   - Other hygienic and preventive maintenance care, such as cleaning and soaking the feet, the use of skin creams to maintain skin tone of either ambulatory or bedfast patients, and any other service performed in the absence of localized illness, injury, or symptoms involving the foot.

3. Supportive Devices for Feet

   Orthopedic shoes and other supportive devices for the feet generally are not covered. However, this exclusion does not apply to such a shoe if it is an integral part of a leg brace, and its expense is included as part of the cost of the brace. Also, this exclusion does not apply to therapeutic shoes furnished to diabetics.

C. Exceptions to Routine Foot Care Exclusion

1. Necessary and Integral Part of Otherwise Covered Services

   In certain circumstances, services ordinarily considered to be routine may be covered if they are performed as a necessary and integral part of otherwise covered services, such as diagnosis and treatment of ulcers, wounds, or infections.

2. Treatment of Warts on Foot

   The treatment of warts (including plantar warts) on the foot is covered to the same extent as services provided for the treatment of warts located elsewhere on the body.

3. Presence of Systemic Condition

   The presence of a systemic condition such as metabolic, neurologic, or peripheral vascular disease may require scrupulous foot care by a professional that in the absence of such condition(s) would be considered routine (and, therefore, excluded from coverage). Accordingly, foot care that would otherwise be considered routine may be covered when systemic condition(s) result in severe circulatory embarrassment or areas of diminished sensation in the individual's legs or feet. (See subsection A.)

   In these instances, certain foot care procedures that otherwise are considered routine (e.g., cutting or removing corns and calluses, or trimming, cutting, clipping, or debriding nails) may pose a hazard when performed by a nonprofessional person on patients with such systemic conditions. (See Sec.290.G for procedural instructions.)

4. Mycotic Nails

   In the absence of a systemic condition, treatment of mycotic nails may be covered.

   The treatment of mycotic nails for an ambulatory patient is covered only when the physician attending the patient's mycotic condition documents that (1) there is clinical evidence of mycosis of the toenail, and (2) the patient has marked limitation of ambulation, pain, or secondary infection resulting from the thickening and dystrophy of the infected toenail plate.

   The treatment of mycotic nails for a nonambulatory patient is covered only when the physician attending the patient's mycotic condition documents that (1) there is clinical evidence of mycosis of the toenail, and (2) the patient suffers from pain or secondary infection resulting from the thickening and dystrophy of the infected toenail plate.

   For the purpose of these requirements, documentation means any written information that is required by the carrier in order for services to be covered. Thus, the information submitted with claims must be substantiated by information found in the patient's medical record. Any information, including that contained in a form letter, used for documentation purposes is subject to carrier verification in order to ensure that the information adequately justifies coverage of the treatment of mycotic nails.

D. Systemic Conditions That Might Justify Coverage

Although not intended as a comprehensive list, the following metabolic, neurologic, and peripheral vascular diseases (with synonyms in parentheses) most commonly represent the underlying conditions that might justify coverage for routine foot care.

- Diabetes mellitus *
- Arteriosclerosis obliterans (A.S.O., arteriosclerosis of the extremities, occlusive peripheral arteriosclerosis)
- Buerger's disease (thromboangiitis obliterans)
- Chronic thrombophlebitis *
- Peripheral neuropathies involving the feet -

  Associated with malnutrition and vitamin deficiency *

  - Malnutrition (general, pellagra)
  - Alcoholism
  - Malabsorption (celiac disease, tropical sprue)
  - Pernicious anemia

  Associated with carcinoma *

  Associated with diabetes mellitus *

Associated with drugs and toxins *

Associated with multiple sclerosis *

Associated with uremia (chronic renal disease) *

Associated with traumatic injury

Associated with leprosy or neurosyphilis

Associated with hereditary disorders

- Hereditary sensory radicular neuropathy
- Angiokeratoma corporis diffusum (Fabry's)
- Amyloid neuropathy

When the patient's condition is one of those designated by an asterisk (*), routine procedures are covered only if the patient is under the active care of a doctor of medicine or osteopathy who documents the condition.

E. Supportive Devices for Feet
Orthopedic shoes and other supportive devices for the feet generally are not covered. However, this exclusion does not apply to such a shoe if it is an integral part of a leg brace, and its expense is included as part of the cost of the brace. Also, this exclusion does not apply to therapeutic shoes furnished to diabetics.

F. Presumption of Coverage
In evaluating whether the routine services can be reimbursed, a presumption of coverage may be made where the evidence available discloses certain physical and/or clinical findings consistent with the diagnosis and indicative of severe peripheral involvement. For purposes of applying this presumption the following findings are pertinent:

Class A Findings

- Nontraumatic amputation of foot or integral skeletal portion thereof.

Class B Findings

- Absent posterior tibial pulse;
- Advanced trophic changes as: hair growth (decrease or absence) nail changes (thickening) pigmentary changes (discoloration) skin texture (thin, shiny) skin color (rubor or redness) (Three required); and
- Absent dorsalis pedis pulse.

Class C Findings

- Claudication;
- Temperature changes (e.g., cold feet);
- Edema;
- Paresthesias (abnormal spontaneous sensations in the feet); and
- Burning.

The presumption of coverage may be applied when the physician rendering the routine foot care has identified:

1. A Class A finding;
2. Two of the Class B findings; or
3. One Class B and two Class C findings.

Cases evidencing findings falling short of these alternatives may involve podiatric treatment that may constitute covered care and should be reviewed by the intermediary's medical staff and developed as necessary.

For purposes of applying the coverage presumption where the routine services have been rendered by a podiatrist, the contractor may deem the active care requirement met if the claim or other evidence available discloses that the patient has seen an M.D. or D.O. for treatment and/or evaluation of the complicating disease process during the 6-month period prior to the rendition of the routine-type services. The intermediary may also accept the podiatrist's statement that the diagnosing and treating M.D. or D.O. also concurs with the podiatrist's findings as to the severity of the peripheral involvement indicated.

Services ordinarily considered routine might also be covered if they are performed as a necessary and integral part of otherwise covered services, such as diagnosis and treatment of diabetic ulcers, wounds, and infections.

G. Application of Foot Care Exclusions to Physician's Services
The exclusion of foot care is determined by the nature of the service. Thus, payment for an excluded service should be denied whether performed by a podiatrist, osteopath, or a doctor of medicine, and without regard to the difficulty or complexity of the procedure.

When an itemized bill shows both covered services and noncovered services not integrally related to the covered service, the portion of charges attributable to the noncovered services should be denied. (For example, if an itemized bill shows surgery for an ingrown toenail and also removal of calluses not necessary for the performance of toe surgery, any additional charge attributable to removal of the calluses should be denied.)

In reviewing claims involving foot care, the carrier should be alert to the following exceptional situations:

1. Payment may be made for incidental noncovered services performed as a necessary and integral part of, and secondary to, a covered procedure. For example, if trimming of toenails is required for application of a cast to a fractured foot, the carrier need not allocate and deny a portion of the charge for the trimming of the nails. However, a separately itemized charge for such excluded service should be disallowed. When the primary procedure is covered the administration of anesthesia necessary for the performance of such procedure is also covered.
2. Payment may be made for initial diagnostic services performed in connection with a specific symptom or complaint if it seems likely that its treatment would be covered even though the resulting diagnosis may be one requiring only noncovered care.

The name of the M.D. or D.O. who diagnosed the complicating condition must be submitted with the claim. In those cases, where active care is required, the approximate date the beneficiary was last seen by such physician must also be indicated.

NOTE: Section 939 of P.L. 96-499 removed "warts" from the routine foot care exclusion effective July 1, 1981.

Relatively few claims for routine-type care are anticipated considering the severity of conditions contemplated as the basis for this exception. Claims for this type of foot care should not be paid in the absence of convincing evidence that nonprofessional performance of the service would have been hazardous for the beneficiary because of an underlying systemic disease. The mere statement of a diagnosis such as those mentioned in Sec.D above does not of itself indicate the severity of the condition. Where development is indicated to verify diagnosis and/or severity the carrier should follow existing claims processing practices which may include review of carrier's history and medical consultation as well as physician contacts.

The rules in Sec.290.F concerning presumption of coverage also apply.

Codes and policies for routine foot care and supportive devices for the feet are not exclusively for the use of podiatrists. These codes must be used to report foot care services regardless of the specialty of the physician who furnishes the services. Carriers must instruct physicians to use the most appropriate code available when billing for routine foot care.

100-2, 16, 10

General Exclusions From Coverage

A3-3150, HO-260, HHA-232, B3-2300

No payment can be made under either the hospital insurance or supplementary medical insurance program for certain items and services, when the following conditions exist:

- Not reasonable and necessary (Sec.20);
- No legal obligation to pay for or provide (Sec.40);
- Paid for by a governmental entity (Sec.50);
- Not provided within United States (Sec.60);
- Resulting from war (Sec.70);
- Personal comfort (Sec.80);
- Routine services and appliances (Sec.90);
- Custodial care (Sec.110);
- Cosmetic surgery (Sec.120);
- Charges by immediate relatives or members of household (Sec.130);
- Dental services (Sec.140);
- Paid or expected to be paid under workers' compensation (Sec.150);
- Nonphysician services provided to a hospital inpatient that were not provided directly or arranged for by the hospital (Sec.170);
- Services Related to and Required as a Result of Services Which are not Covered Under Medicare (Sec.180);
- Excluded foot care services and supportive devices for feet (Sec.30); or
- Excluded investigational devices (See Chapter 14, Sec.30).

100-2, 16, 20

Services Not Reasonable and Necessary

A3-3151, HO-260.1, B3-2303, AB-00-52 - 6/00

Items and services which are not reasonable and necessary for the diagnosis or treatment of illness or injury or to improve the functioning of a malformed body member are not covered, e.g., payment cannot be made for the rental of a special hospital bed to be used by the patient in their home unless it was a reasonable and necessary part of the patient's treatment. See also Sec.80.

A health care item or service for the purpose of causing, or assisting to cause, the death of any individual (assisted suicide) is not covered. This prohibition does not apply to the provision of an item or service for the purpose of alleviating pain or discomfort, even if such use may increase the risk of death, so long as the item or service is not furnished for the specific purpose of causing death.

100-2, 16, 90

Routine Services and Appliances

A3-3157, HO-260.7, B3-2320, R-1797A3 - 5/00

Routine physical checkups; eyeglasses, contact lenses, and eye examinations for the purpose of prescribing, fitting, or changing eyeglasses; eye refractions by whatever practitioner and for whatever purpose performed; hearing aids and examinations for hearing aids; and immunizations are not covered.

The routine physical checkup exclusion applies to (a) examinations performed without relationship to treatment or diagnosis for a specific illness, symptom, complaint, or injury; and (b) examinations required by third parties such as insurance companies business establishments, or Government agencies.

If the claim is for a diagnostic test or examination performed solely for the purpose of establishing a claim under title IV of Public Law 91-173, "Black Lung Benefits," the service is not covered under Medicare and the claimant should be advised to contact their Social Security office regarding the filing of a claim for reimbursement under the "Black Lung" program.

The exclusions apply to eyeglasses or contact lenses, and eye examinations for the purpose of prescribing, fitting, or changing eyeglasses or contact lenses for refractive errors. The exclusions do not apply to physicians' services (and services incident to a physicians' service) performed in conjunction with an eye disease, as for example, glaucoma or cataracts, or to post-surgical prosthetic lenses which are customarily used during convalescence from eye surgery in which the lens of the eye was removed, or to permanent prosthetic lenses required by an individual lacking the organic lens of the eye whether by surgical removal or congenital disease. Such prosthetic lens is a replacement for an internal body organ - the lens of the eye. (See the Medicare Benefit Policy Manual, Chapter 15, "Covered Medical and Other Health Services," Sec.120). Expenses for all refractive procedures, whether performed by an ophthalmologist (or any other physician) or an optometrist and without regard to the reason for performance of the refraction, are excluded from coverage.

A. Immunizations
Vaccinations or inoculations are excluded as immunizations unless they are either

- Directly related to the treatment of an injury or direct exposure to a disease or condition, such as antirabies treatment, tetanus antitoxin or booster vaccine, botulin antitoxin, antivenin sera, or immune globulin. (In the absence of injury or direct exposure, preventive immunization (vaccination or inoculation) against such diseases as smallpox, polio, diphtheria, etc., is not covered.); or
- Specifically covered by statute, as described in the Medicare Benefit Policy Manual, Chapter 15, "Covered Medical and Other Health Services," Sec.50.

B. Antigens
Prior to the Omnibus Reconciliation Act of 1980, a physician who prepared an antigen for a patient could not be reimbursed for that service unless the physician also administered the antigen to the patient. Effective January 1, 1981, payment may be made for a reasonable supply of antigens that have been prepared for a particular patient even though they have not been administered to the patient by the same physician who prepared them if:

- The antigens are prepared by a physician who is a doctor of medicine or osteopathy, and
- The physician who prepared the antigens has examined the patient and has determined a plan of treatment and a dosage regimen.

A reasonable supply of antigens is considered to be not more than a 12-week supply of antigens that has been prepared for a particular patient at any one time. The purpose of the reasonable supply limitation is to assure that the antigens retain their potency and effectiveness over the period in which they are to be administered to the patient. (See the Medicare Benefit Policy Manual, Chapter 15, "Covered Medical and Other Health Services," Sec.50.4.4.2)

100-2, 16, 100

Hearing Aids and Auditory Implants

Section 1862(a)(7) of the Social Security Act states that no payment may be made under part A or part B for any expenses incurred for items or services "where such expenses are for . . . hearing aids or examinations therefore. . . ." This policy is further reiterated at 42 CFR 411.15(d) which specifically states that "hearing aids or examination for the purpose of prescribing, fitting, or changing hearing aids" are excluded from coverage.

Hearing aids are amplifying devices that compensate for impaired hearing. Hearing aids include air conduction devices that provide acoustic energy to the cochlea via stimulation of the tympanic membrane with amplified sound. They also include bone conduction devices that provide mechanical energy to the cochlea via stimulation of the scalp with amplified mechanical vibration or by direct contact with the tympanic membrane or middle ear ossicles.

Certain devices that produce perception of sound by replacing the function of the middle ear, cochlea or auditory nerve are payable by Medicare as prosthetic devices. These devices are indicated only when hearing aids are medically inappropriate or cannot be utilized due to congenital malformations, chronic disease, severe sensorineural hearing loss or surgery. The following are prosthetic devices:

- Cochlear implants and auditory brainstem implants, i.e., devices that replace the function of cochlear structures or auditory nerve and provide electrical energy to auditory nerve fibers and other neural tissue via implanted electrode arrays.
- Osseointegrated implants, i.e., devices implanted in the skull that replace the function of the middle ear and provide mechanical energy to the cochlea via a mechanical transducer.

Medicare contractors deny payment for an item or service that is associated with any hearing aid as defined above. See Sec.180 for policy for the medically necessary treatment of complications of implantable hearing aids, such as medically necessary removals of implantable hearing aids due to infection.

100-2, 16, 120

Cosmetic Surgery

A3-3160, HO-260.11, B3-2329

Cosmetic surgery or expenses incurred in connection with such surgery is not covered. Cosmetic surgery includes any surgical procedure directed at improving appearance, except when required for the prompt (i.e., as soon as medically feasible) repair of accidental injury or for the improvement of the functioning of a malformed body member. For example, this exclusion does not apply to surgery in connection with treatment of severe burns or repair of the face following a serious automobile accident, or to surgery for therapeutic purposes which coincidentally also serves some cosmetic purpose.

100-2, 16, 180

Services Related to and Required as a Result of Services Which Are Not Covered Under Medicare

B3-2300.1, A3-3101.14, HO-210.12

Medical and hospital services are sometimes required to treat a condition that arises as a result of services that are not covered because they are determined to be not reasonable and necessary or because they are excluded from coverage for other reasons. Services "related to" noncovered services (e.g., cosmetic surgery, noncovered organ transplants, noncovered artificial organ implants, etc.), including services related to follow-up care and complications of noncovered services which require treatment during a hospital stay in which the noncovered service was performed, are not covered services under Medicare. Services "not related to" noncovered services are covered under Medicare.

Following are examples of services "related to" and "not related to" noncovered services while the beneficiary is an inpatient:

- A beneficiary was hospitalized for a noncovered service and broke a leg while in the hospital. Services related to care of the broken leg during this stay is a clear example of "not related to" services and are covered under Medicare.
- A beneficiary was admitted to the hospital for covered services, but during the course of hospitalization became a candidate for a noncovered transplant or implant and actually received the transplant or implant during that hospital stay. When the original admission was entirely unrelated to the diagnosis that led to a recommendation for a noncovered transplant or implant, the services related to the admitting condition would be covered.
- A beneficiary was admitted to the hospital for covered services related to a condition which ultimately led to identification of a need for transplant and receipt of a transplant during the same hospital stay. If, on the basis of the nature of the services and a comparison of the date they are received with the date on which the beneficiary is identified as a transplant candidate, the services could reasonably be attributed to preparation for the noncovered transplant, the services would be "related to" noncovered services and would also be noncovered.

Following is an example of services received subsequent to a noncovered inpatient stay:

- After a beneficiary has been discharged from the hospital stay in which the beneficiary received noncovered services, medical and hospital services required to treat a condition or complication that arises as a result of the prior noncovered services may be covered when they are reasonable and necessary in all other respects. Thus, coverage could be provided for subsequent inpatient stays or outpatient treatment ordinarily covered by Medicare, even if the need for treatment arose because of a previous noncovered procedure. Some examples of services that may be found to be covered under this policy are the reversal of intestinal bypass surgery for obesity, repair of complications from transsexual surgery or from cosmetic surgery, removal of a noncovered bladder stimulator, or treatment of any infection at the surgical site of a noncovered transplant that occurred following discharge from the hospital.

However, any subsequent services that could be expected to have been incorporated into a global fee are considered to have been paid in the global fee, and may not be paid again. Thus, where a patient undergoes cosmetic surgery and the treatment regimen calls for a series of postoperative visits to the surgeon for evaluating the patient's progress, these visits are not paid.

100-3, 10.1

Use of Visual Tests Prior to and General Anesthesia during Cataract Surgery

A - Pre-Surgery Evaluations
Cataract surgery with an intraocular lens (IOL) implant is a high volume Medicare procedure. Along with the surgery, a substantial number of preoperative tests are available to the surgeon. In most cases, a comprehensive eye examination (ocular history and ocular examination) and a single scan to determine the appropriate pseudophakic power of the IOL are sufficient. In most cases involving a simple cataract, a diagnostic ultrasound A-scan is used. For patients with a dense cataract, an ultrasound B-scan may be used.

Accordingly, where the only diagnosis is cataract(s), Medicare does not routinely cover testing other than one comprehensive eye examination (or a combination of a brief/intermediate examination not to exceed the charge of a comprehensive examination) and an A-scan or, if medically justified, a B-scan. Claims for additional tests are denied as not reasonable and necessary unless there is an additional diagnosis and the medical need for the additional tests is fully documented.

Because cataract surgery is an elective procedure, the patient may decide not to have the surgery until later, or to have the surgery performed by a physician other than the diagnosing physician. In these situations, it may be medically appropriate for the operating physician to conduct another examination. To the extent the additional tests are considered reasonable and necessary by the carrier's medical staff, they are covered.

B - General Anesthesia
The use of general anesthesia in cataract surgery may be considered reasonable and necessary if, for particular medical indications, it is the accepted procedure among ophthalmologists in the local community to use general anesthesia

100-3, 10.2

NCD for Transcutaneous Electrical Nerve Stimulation (TENS) for Acute Post-Operative Pain (10.2)

The use of TENS for the relief of acute post-operative pain is covered under Medicare. TENS may be covered whether used as an adjunct to the use of drugs, or as an alternative to drugs, in the treatment of acute pain resulting from surgery.

TENS devices, whether durable or disposable, may be used in furnishing this service. When used for the purpose of treating acute post-operative pain, TENS devices are considered supplies. As such they may be hospital supplies furnished inpatients covered under Part A, or supplies incident to a physician's service when furnished in connection with surgery done on an outpatient basis, and covered under Part B.

It is expected that TENS, when used for acute post-operative pain, will be necessary for relatively short periods of time, usually 30 days or less. In cases when TENS is used for longer periods, contractors should attempt to ascertain whether TENS is no longer being used for acute pain but rather for chronic pain, in which case the TENS device may be covered as durable medical equipment as described in 280.13.

100-3,10.3

NCD for Inpatient Hospital Pain Rehabilitation Programs (10.3)

Since pain rehabilitation programs of a lesser scope than that described above would raise a question as to whether the program could be provided in a less intensive setting than on an inpatient hospital basis, carefully evaluate such programs to determine whether the program does, in fact, necessitate a hospital level of care. Some pain rehabilitation programs may utilize services and devices which are excluded from coverage, e.g., acupuncture (see 35-8), biofeedback (see 35-27), dorsal column stimulator (see 65-8), and family counseling services (see 35-14). In determining whether the scope of a pain program does necessitate inpatient hospital care, evaluate only those services and devices which are covered. Although diagnostic tests may be an appropriate part of pain rehabilitation programs, such tests would be covered in an individual case only where they can be reasonably related to a patient's illness, complaint, symptom, or injury and where they do not represent an unnecessary duplication of tests previously performed.

An inpatient program of 4 weeks' duration is generally required to modify pain behavior. After this period it would be expected that any additional rehabilitation services which might be required could be effectively provided on an outpatient basis under an outpatient pain rehabilitation program (see 10.4 of the NCD Manual) or other outpatient program. The first 7-10 days of such an inpatient program constitute, in effect, an evaluation period. If a patient is unable to adjust to the program within this period, it is generally concluded that it is unlikely that the program will be effective and the patient is discharged from the program. On occasions a program longer than 4 weeks may be required in a particular case. In such a case there should be documentation to substantiate that inpatient care beyond a 4-week period was reasonable and necessary. Similarly, where it appears that a patient participating in a program is being granted frequent outside passes, a question would exist as to whether an inpatient program is reasonable and necessary for the treatment of the patient's condition.

An inpatient hospital stay for the purpose of participating in a pain rehabilitation program would be covered as reasonable and necessary to the treatment of a patient's condition where the pain is attributable to a physical cause, the usual methods of treatment have not been successful in alleviating it, and a significant loss of ability to function independently has resulted from the pain. Chronic pain patients often have psychological problems which accompany or stem from the physical pain and it is appropriate to include psychological treatment in the multidisciplinary approach. However, patients whose pain symptoms result from a mental condition, rather than from any physical cause, generally cannot be succesfully treated in a pain rehabilitation program.

100-3,10.4

NCD for Outpatient Hospital Pain Rehabilitation Programs (10.4)

Coverage of services furnished under outpatient hospital pain rehabilitation programs, including services furnished in group settings under individualized plans of treatment, is available if the patient's pain is attributable to a physical cause, the usual methods of treatment have not been successful in alleviating it, and a significant loss of ability by the patient to function independently has resulted from the pain. If a patient meets these conditions and the program provides services of the types discussed in 10.3 of the NCD Manual, the services provided under the program may be covered. Noncovered services (e.g., vocational counseling, meals for outpatients, or acupuncture) continue to be excluded from coverage, and intermediaries would not be precluded from finding, in the case of particular patients, that the pain rehabilitation program is not reasonable and necessary under 1862(a)(1) of the Act for the treatment of their conditions.

100-3,10.5

NCD for Autogenous Epidural Blood Graft (10.5)

Autogenous epidural blood grafts are considered a safe and effective remedy for severe headaches that may occur after performance of spinal anesthesia, spinal taps or myelograms, and are covered.

100-3, 10.6

The use of general or monitored anesthesia during transvenous cardiac pacemaker surgery may be reasonable and necessary and therefore covered under Medicare only if adequate documentation of medical necessity is provided on a case-by-case basis. The contractor obtains advice from its medical consultants or from appropriate specialty physicians or groups in its locality regarding the adequacy of documentation before deciding whether a particular claim should be covered.

A second type of pacemaker surgery that is sometimes performed involves the use of the thoracic method of implantation which requires open surgery. Where the thoracic method is employed, general anesthesia is always used and should not require special medical documentation.

100-3, 20.1

NCD for Vertebral Artery Surgery (20.1)

- These procedures can be medically reasonable and necessary, but only if each of the following conditions is met:
- Symptoms of vertebral artery obstruction exist;
- Other causes have been considered and ruled out;
- There is radiographic evidence of a valid vertebral artery obstruction; and
- Contraindications to the procedure do not exist, such as coexistent obstructions of multiple cerebral vessels.

Angiograms documenting a valid obstruction should show not only the aortic arch with the vessels off the arch, but also show the vessels in the neck and head (providing biplane views of the carotid and vertebral vascular system). In addition, serial views are needed to diagnose "subclavian steal," the condition in which subclavian artery obstruction causes the symptoms of vertebral artery obstruction. Because the symptoms are not specific for vertebral artery obstruction, other causes must be considered. In addition to vertebral artery obstruction, the differential diagnosis should include various degenerative disorders of the brain, orthostatic hypotension, acoustic neuroma, labyrinthitis, diabetes mellitus and hypoglycemia related disorders.

Obstructions which can cause symptoms of blocked vertebral artery blood flow and which can be documented by an angiogram include:

- Intravascular obstructions - arteriosclerotic lesions within the vertebral artery or in other arteries.
- Extravascular obstructions.
- Bony tissue or osteophytes, located laterally in the C6(C7)-C2 cervical vertebral area course of the vertebral artery, most commonly at C5 -C6.
- Anatomical variations - Anomalous location of the origin of the vertebral artery, a congenital aberration, and tortuosity and kinks of the vertebral artery.
- Fibrous tissue - Tissue changed as a result of manipulation of the neck for neck pain or injury associated with hematoma; external bands, tendinous slings, and fibrous bands.

The most controversial obstructions include vertebral artery tortuosity and kinks and connective tissue along the course of the vertebral artery, and variously called external bands, tendinous slings and fibrous bands. In the absence of symptoms of vertebral artery obstruction, vascular surgeons feel such abnormalities are insignificant. Vascular surgery experts, however, agree that these abnormalities in very rare cases do cause symptoms of vertebral artery obstruction and do necessitate surgical correction.

Vertebral artery construction and vertebral artery surgery are phrases which most physicians interpret to include only surgical cleaning (endarterectomy) and bypass (resection) procedures. However, some physicians who use these terms mean all operative manipulations which remove vertebral artery blood flow obstructions. Also, some physicians use general terms of vascular surgery, such as endarterectomy when vertebral artery related surgery is performed. Use of the above terminology specifies neither the surgical procedure performed nor its relationship to the vertebral artery. Therefore, in developing claims for this type of procedure, require specific identification of the obstruction in question and the surgical procedure performed. Also, in view of the specific coverage criteria given, develop all claims for vertebral artery surgery on a case-by-case basis.

Make payment for a surgical procedure listed above if: (1) it is reasonable and necessary for the individual patient to have the surgery performed to remove or relieve an obstruction to vertebral artery flow, and (2) the four conditions noted are met.

In all other cases, these procedures cannot be considered reasonable and necessary within the meaning of Sec.1862(a)(1) of the Act and are not reimbursable under the program.

100-3, 20.3

NCD for Thoracic Duct Drainage (TDD) in Renal Transplants (20.3)

TDD is performed on an inpatient basis, and the inpatient stay is covered for patients admitted for treatment in advance of a kidney transplant as well as for those receiving it post-transplant. TDD is a covered technique when furnished to a kidney transplant recipient or an individual approved to receive kidney transplantation in a hospital approved to perform kidney transplantation.

100-3, 20.4

NCD for Implantable Automatic Defibrillators (20.4)

A. General

The implantable automatic defibrillator is an electronic device designed to detect and treat life-threatening tachyarrhythmias. The device consists of a pulse generator and electrodes for sensing and defibrillating.

B. Covered Indications

1. Documented episode of cardiac arrest due to ventricular fibrillation (VF), not due to a transient or reversible cause (effective July 1, 1991).
2. Documented sustained ventricular tachyarrhythmia (VT), either spontaneous or induced by an electrophysiology (EP) study, not associated with an acute myocardial infarction (MI) and not due to a transient or reversible cause (effective July 1, 1999).
3. Documented familial or inherited conditions with a high risk of life-threatening VT, such as long QT syndrome or hypertrophic cardiomyopathy (effective July 1, 1999).

   Additional indications effective for services performed on or after October 1, 2003:
4. Coronary artery disease with a documented prior MI, a measured left ventricular ejection fraction (LVEF) <0.35, and inducible, sustained VT or VF at EP study. (The MI must have occurred more than 40 days prior to defibrillator insertion. The EP test must be performed more than 4 weeks after the qualifying MI.)
5. Documented prior MI and a measured LVEF <0.30 and a QRS duration of >120 milliseconds (the QRS restriction does not apply to services performed on or after January 27, 2005). Patients must not have:

a. New York Heart Association (NYHC) classification IV;

b. Cardiogenic shock or symptomatic hypotension while in a stable baseline rhythm;

c. Had a coronary artery bypass graft (CABG) or percutaneous transluminal coronary angioplasty (PTCA) within past 3 months;

d. Had an enzyme positive MI within past month (Effective for services on or after January 27, 2005, patients must not have an acute MI in the past 40 days);

e. Clinical symptoms or findings that would make them a candidate for coronary revascularization; or

f. Any disease, other than cardiac disease (e.g., cancer, uremia, liver failure), associated with a likelihood of survival less than 1 year.

Additional indications effective for services performed on or after January 27, 2005:

6. Patients with ischemic dilated cardiomyopathy (IDCM), documented prior MI, NYHA Class II and III heart failure, and measured LVEF <35%;

7. Patients with non-ischemic dilated cardiomyopathy (NIDCM) >9 months, NYHA Class II and III heart failure, and measured LVEF <35%;

8. Patients who meet all current Centers for Medicare & Medicaid Services (CMS) coverage requirements for a cardiac resynchronization therapy (CRT) device and have NYHA Class IV heart failure;

All indications must meet the following criteria:

a. Patients must not have irreversible brain damage from preexisting cerebral disease;

b. MIs must be documented and defined according to the consensus document of the Joint European Society of Cardiology/American College of Cardiology Committee for the Redefinition of Myocardial Infarction[1];

Either one of the following criteria satisfies the diagnosis for an acute, evolving or recent MI:

1. Typical rise and gradual fall (troponin) or more rapid rise and fall (CK-MB) of biochemical markers of myocardial necrosis with at least one of the following:

   a. ischemic symptoms;

   b. development of pathologic Q waves on the ECG;

   c. ECG changes indicative of ischemia (ST segment elevation or depression); or

   d. coronary artery intervention (e.g., coronary angioplasty).

2. Pathologic findings of an acute MI.

   Criteria for established MI.

   Any one of the following criteria satisfies the diagnosis for established MI:

   Indications 3-8 (primary prevention of sudden cardiac death) must also meet the following critera:

   a. Patients must be able to give informed consent;

   b. Patients must have:

      - Cardiogenic shock or symptomatic hypotension while in a stable baseline rhythm;
      - Had a CABG or PTCA within the past 3 months;
      - Had an acute MI within the past 40 days;
      - Clinical symptoms or findings that would make them a candidate for coronary revascularization;
      - Any disease, other than cardiac disease (e.g., cancer, uremia, liver failure), associated with a likelihood of survival less than 1 year;

   c. Ejection fractions must be measured by angiography, radionuclide scanning, or echocardiography;

   d. The beneficiary receiving the defibrillator implantation for primary prevention is enrolled in either a Food and Drug Administration (FDA)-approved category B investigational device exemption (IDE) clinical trial (42 CFR Sec.405.201), a trial under the CMS Clinical Trial Policy (National Coverage Determination (NCD) Manual Sec.310.1) or a qualifying data collection system including approved clinical trials and registries. Initially, an implantable cardiac defibrillator (ICD) database will be maintained using a data submission mechanism that is already in use by Medicare participating hospitals to submit data to the Iowa Foundation for Medical Care (IFMC)--a Quality Improvement Organization (QIO) contractor--for determination of reasonable and necessary and quality improvement. Initial hypothesis and data elements are specified in this decision (Appendix VI) and are the minimum necessary to ensure that the device is reasonable and necessary. Data collection will be completed using the ICDA (ICD Abstraction Tool) and transmitted via QNet (Quality Network Exchange) to the IFMC who will collect and maintain the database. Additional stakeholder-developed data collection systems to augment or replace the initial QNet system, addressing at a minimum the hypotheses specified in this decision, must meet the following basic criteria:

      - Written protocol on file;

        1) Development of new pathologic Q waves on serial ECGs. The patient may or may not remember previous symptoms. Biochemical markers of myocardial necrosis may have normalized, depending on the length of time that has passed since the infarct developed.

        2) Pathologic findings of a healed or healing MI.

      - Institutional review board review and approval;
      - Scientific review and approval by two or more qualified individuals who are not part of the research team;
      - Certification that investigators have not been disqualified.

   e. For purposes of this coverage decision, CMS will determine whether specific registries or clinical trials meet these criteria.

   f. Providers must be able to justify the medical necessity of devices other than single lead devices. This justification should be available in the patient's medical record.

9. Patients with NIDCM >3 months, NYHA Class II or III heart failure, and measured LVEF = 35%, only if the following additional criteria are also met:

   a. Patients must be able to give informed consent;

   b. Patients must not have:

      - Cardiogenic shock or symptomatic hypotension while in a stable baseline rhythm;
      - Had a CABG or PTCA within the past 3 months;
      - Had an acute MI within the past 40 days;
      - Clinical symptoms or findings that would make them a candidate for coronary revascularization;
      - Irreversible brain damage from preexisting cerebral disease;
      - Any disease, other than cardiac disease (e.g. cancer, uremia, liver failure), associated with a likelihood of survival less than 1 year;

   c. Ejection fractions must be measured by angiography, radionuclide scanning, or echocardiography;

   d. MIs must be documented and defined according to the consensus document of the Joint European Society of Cardiology/American College of Cardiology Committee for the Redefinition of Myocardial Infarction;[2]

   e. The beneficiary receiving the defibrillator implantation for this indication is enrolled in either an FDA-approved category B IDE clinical trial (42 CFR §405.201), a trial under the CMS Clinical Trial Policy (NCD Manual §310.1), or a prospective data collection system meeting the following basic criteria:

      - Written protocol on file;
      - Institutional Review Board review and approval;
      - Scientific review and approval by two or more qualified individuals who are not part of the research team;
      - Certification that investigators have not been disqualified.

For purposes of this coverage decision, CMS will determine whether specific registries or clinical trials meet these criteria.

d. Providers must be able to justify the medical necessity of devices other than single lead devices. This justification should be available in the patient's medical record.

C. Other Indications
All other indications for implantable automatic defibrillators not currently covered in accordance with this decision will continue to be covered under Category B IDE trials (42 CFR §405.201) and the CMS routine clinical trials policy (NCD §310.1).

(This NCD last reviewed February 2005.)

100-3, 20.5

NCD for Extracorporeal Immunoadsorption (ECI) Using Protein A Columns (20.5)

For claims with dates of service on or after January 1, 2001, Medicare covers the use of Protein A columns for the treatment of ITP. In addition, Medicare will cover Protein A columns for the treatment of rheumatoid arthritis (RA) under the following conditions:

- Patient has severe RA. Patient disease is active, having >5 swollen joints, >20 tender joints, and morning stiffness >60 minutes.
- Patient has failed an adequate course of a minimum of 3 Disease Modifying Anti-Rheumatic Drugs (DMARDs). Failure does not include intolerance.

Other uses of these columns are currently considered to be investigational and, therefore, not reasonable and necessary under the Medicare law. (See Sec.1862(a)(1)(A) of the Act.)

100-3, 20.6

NCD for Transmyocardial Revascularization (TMR) (20.6)

CMS therefore covers TMR as a late or last resort for patients with severe (Canadian Cardiovascular Society classification Classes III or IV) angina (stable or unstable), which has been found refractory to standard medical therapy, including drug therapy at the maximum tolerated or maximum safe dosages. In addition, the angina symptoms must be caused by areas of the heart not amenable to surgical therapies such as percutaneous transluminal coronary angioplasty, stenting, coronary atherectomy or coronary bypass. Coverage is further limited to those uses of the laser used in performing the procedure which have been approved by the Food and Drug Administration for the purpose for which they are being used.

1. Alpert and Thygesen et al., 2000. Criteria for acute, evolving or recent MI.

2. Ibid.

Patients would have to meet the following additional selection guidelines:

- An ejection fraction of 25% or greater;
- Have areas of viable ischemic myocardium (as demonstrated by diagnostic study) which are not capable of being revascularized by direct coronary intervention; and
- Have been stabilized, or have had maximal efforts to stabilize acute conditions such as severe ventricular arrhythmias, decompensated congestive heart failure or acute myocardial infarction.

Coverage is limited to physicians who have been properly trained in the procedure. Providers of this service is performed must also document that all ancillary personnel, including physicians, nurses, operating room personnel and technicians, are trained in the procedure and the proper use of the equipment involved. Coverage is further limited to providers which have dedicated cardiac care units, including the diagnostic and support services necessary for care of patients undergoing this therapy. In addition, these providers must conform to the standards for laser safety set by the American National Standards Institute, ANSIZ1363.

100-3, 20.7

NCD for Percutaneous Transluminal Angioplasty (PTA) (20.7)

A. General

This procedure involves inserting a balloon catheter into a narrow or occluded blood vessel to recanalize and dilate the vessel by inflating the balloon. The objective of PTA is to improve the blood flow through the diseased segment of a vessel so that vessel patency is increased and embolization is decreased. With the development and use of balloon angioplasty for treatment of atherosclerotic and other vascular stenoses, PTA (with and without the placement of a stent) is a widely used technique for dilating lesions of peripheral, renal, and coronary arteries.

Indications and Limitations of Coverage

B. Nationally Covered Indications

The PTA is covered when used under the following conditions:

1. Treatment of Atherosclerotic Obstructive Lesions

- In the lower extremities, i.e., the iliac, femoral, and popliteal arteries, or in the upper extremities, i.e., the innominate, subclavian, axillary, and brachial arteries. The upper extremities do not include head or neck vessels.
- Of a single coronary artery for patients for whom the likely alternative treatment is coronary bypass surgery and who exhibit the following characteristics:

  Angina refractory to optimal medical management;

  Objective evidence of myocardial ischemia; and

  Lesions amenable to angioplasty.
- Of the renal arteries for patients in whom there is an inadequate response to a thorough medical management of symptoms and for whom surgery is the likely alternative. PTA for this group of patients is an alternative to surgery, not simply an addition to medical management.
- Of arteriovenous dialysis fistulas and grafts when performed through either a venous or arterial approach.

2. Concurrent with Carotid Stent Placement in Food and Drug Administration (FDA)-Approved Category B Investigational Device Exemption (IDE) Clinical Trials

Effective July 1, 2001, Medicare covers PTA of the carotid artery concurrent with carotid stent placement when furnished in accordance with the FDA-approved protocols governing Category B IDE clinical trials. PTA of the carotid artery, when provided solely for the purpose of carotid

artery dilation concurrent with carotid stent placement, is considered to be a reasonable and necessary service when provided in the context of such a clinical trial.

3. Concurrent with Carotid Stent Placement in FDA-Approved Post-Approval Studies
Effective October 12, 2004, Medicare covers PTA of the carotid artery concurrent with the placement of an FDA-approved carotid stent and an FDA-approved or -cleared embolic protection device (effective December 9, 2009) for an FDA-approved indication when furnished in accordance with FDA-approved protocols governing post-approval studies. CMS determines that coverage of PTA of the carotid artery is reasonable and necessary in these circumstances.

4. Concurrent with Carotid Stent Placement in Patients at High Risk for Carotid Endarterectomy (CEA)
Effective March 17, 2005, Medicare covers PTA of the carotid artery concurrent with the placement of an FDA-approved carotid stent with embolic protection for the following:

Patients who are at high risk for CEA and who also have symptomatic carotid artery stenosis >=70%. Coverage is limited to procedures performed using FDA-approved carotid artery stenting systems and FDA-approved or -cleared (effective December 9, 2009) embolic protection devices. If deployment of the embolic protection device is not technically possible, and not performed, then the procedure is not covered by Medicare (effective December 9, 2009);

Patients who are at high risk for CEA and have symptomatic carotid artery stenosis between 50% and 70%, in accordance with the Category B IDE clinical trials regulation (42 CFR 405.201), as a routine cost under the clinical trials policy (Medicare NCD Manual 310.1), or in accordance with the NCD on carotid artery stenting (CAS) post-approval studies (Medicare NCD Manual 20.7);

Patients who are at high risk for CEA and have asymptomatic carotid artery stenosis >=80%, in accordance with the Category B IDE clinical trials regulation (42 CFR 405.201), as a routine cost under the clinical trials policy (Medicare NCD Manual 310.1), or in accordance with the NCD on CAS post-approval studies (Medicare NCD Manual 20.7).

Coverage is limited to procedures performed using FDA-approved carotid artery stents and FDA-approved or -cleared embolic protection devices.

The use of an FDA-approved or cleared embolic protection device is required. If deployment of the embolic protection device is not technically possible, and not performed, then the procedure is not covered by Medicare.

Patients at high risk for CEA are defined as having significant comorbidities and/or anatomic risk factors (i.e., recurrent stenosis and/or previous radical neck dissection), and would be poor candidates for CEA. Significant comorbid conditions include but are not limited to:

Congestive heart failure (CHF) class III/IV;

Left ventricular ejection fraction (LVEF) <30%;

Unstable angina;

Contralateral carotid occlusion;

Recent myocardial infarction (MI);

Previous CEA with recurrent stenosis;

Prior radiation treatment to the neck; and

Other conditions that were used to determine patients at high risk for CEA in the prior carotid artery stenting trials and studies, such as ARCHER, CABERNET, SAPPHIRE, BEACH, and MAVERIC II.

Symptoms of carotid artery stenosis include carotid transient ischemic attack (distinct focal neurological dysfunction persisting less than 24 hours), focal cerebral ischemia producing a non-disabling stroke (modified Rankin scale <3 with symptoms for 24 hours or more), and transient monocular blindness (amaurosis fugax). Patients who have had a disabling stroke (modified Rankin scale >=3) shall be excluded from coverage.

The determination that a patient is at high risk for CEA and the patient's symptoms of carotid artery stenosis shall be available in the patient medical records prior to performing any procedure.

The degree of carotid artery stenosis shall be measured by duplex Doppler ultrasound or carotid artery angiography and recorded in the patient's medical records. If the stenosis is measured by ultrasound prior to the procedure, then the degree of stenosis must be confirmed by angiography at the start of the procedure. If the stenosis is determined to be <70% by angiography, then CAS should not proceed.

In addition, CMS has determined that CAS with embolic protection is reasonable and necessary only if performed in facilities that have been determined to be competent in performing the evaluation, procedure and follow-up necessary to ensure optimal patient outcomes. Standards to determine competency include specific physician training standards, facility support requirements and data collection to evaluate outcomes during a required reevaluation.

The CMS has created a list of minimum standards modeled in part on professional society statements on competency. All facilities must at least meet CMS's standards in order to receive coverage for carotid artery stenting for high-risk patients.

Facilities must have necessary imaging equipment, device inventory, staffing, and infrastructure to support a dedicated carotid stent program. Specifically, high-quality x-ray imaging equipment is a critical component of any carotid interventional suite, such as high-resolution digital imaging systems with the capability of subtraction, magnification, road mapping, and orthogonal angulation.

Advanced physiologic monitoring must be available in the interventional suite. This includes real time and archived physiologic, hemodynamic, and cardiac rhythm monitoring equipment, as well as support staff who are capable of interpreting the findings and responding appropriately.

Emergency management equipment and systems must be readily available in the interventional suite such as resuscitation equipment, a defibrillator, vasoactive and antiarrhythmic drugs, endotracheal intubation capability, and anesthesia support.

Each institution shall have a clearly delineated program for granting carotid stent privileges and for monitoring the quality of the individual interventionalists and the program as a whole. The oversight committee for this program shall be empowered to identify the minimum case volume for an operator to maintain privileges, as well as the (risk-adjusted) threshold for complications that the institution will allow before suspending privileges or instituting measures for remediation. Committees are encouraged to apply published standards from national specialty societies recognized by the American Board of Medical Specialties to determine appropriate physician qualifications. Examples of standards and clinical competence guidelines include those published in the December 2004 edition of the American Journal of Neuroradiology, and those published in the August 18, 2004, Journal of the American College of Cardiology.

To continue to receive Medicare payment for CAS under this decision, the facility or a contractor to the facility must collect data on all CAS procedures done at that particular facility. This data must be analyzed routinely to ensure patient safety. This data must be made available to CMS upon request. The interval for data analysis will be determined by the facility but shall not be less frequent than every 6 months.

Since there currently is no recognized entity that evaluates CAS facilities, CMS has established a mechanism for evaluating facilities. Facilities must provide written documentation to CMS that the facility meets one of the following:

1. The facility was an FDA-approved site that enrolled patients in prior CAS IDE trials, such as SAPPHIRE, and ARCHER;

2. The facility is an FDA-approved site that is participating and enrolling patients in ongoing CAS IDE trials, such as CREST;
3. The facility is an FDA-approved site for one or more FDA post approval studies; or
4. The facility has provided a written affidavit to CMS attesting that the facility has met the minimum facility standards. This should be sent to:

   Director, Coverage and Analysis Group
   7500 Security Boulevard, Mailstop C1-09-06
   Baltimore, MD 21244

   The letter must include the following information:

   Facility's name and complete address;

   Facility's national provider identifier (formerly referred to as the Medicare provider number);

   Point-of-contact for questions with telephone number;

   Discussion of how each standard has been met by the hospital;

   Mechanism of data collection of CAS procedures; and

   Signature of a senior facility administrative official.

   A list of certified facilities will be made available and viewable at: http://www.cms.hhs.gov/coverage/carotid-stent-facilities.asp.

   In addition, CMS will publish a list of approved facilities in the Federal Register.

   Facilities must recertify every two (2) years in order to maintain Medicare coverage of CAS procedures. Recertification will occur when the facility documents that and describes how it continues to meet the CMS standards.

The process for recertification is as follows:

1. At 23 months after initial certification:

   Submission of a letter to CMS stating how the facility continues to meet the minimum facility standards as listed above.

2. At 27 months after initial certification:

   Submission of required data elements for all CAS procedures performed on patients during the previous two (2) years of certification.

   Data elements:

   a. Patients' Medicare identification number if a Medicare beneficiary;

   b. Patients' date of birth;

   c. Date of procedure;

   d. Does the patient meet high surgical risk criteria (defined below)?

   - Age >=80;
   - Recent (<30 days) Myocardial Infarction (MI);
   - Left Ventricle Ejection Fraction (LVEF) <30%;
   - Contralateral carotid occlusion;
   - New York Heart Association (NYHA) Class III or IV congestive heart failure;
   - Unstable angina: Canadian Cardiovascular Society (CCS) Class III/IV;
   - Renal failure: end stage renal disease on dialysis;
   - Common Carotid Artery (CCA) lesion(s) below clavicle;
   - Severe chronic lung disease;
   - Previous neck radiation;
   - High cervical Internal Carotid Artery (ICA) lesion(s);
   - Restenosis of prior carotid endarterectomy (CEA);
   - Tracheostomy;
   - Contralateral laryngeal nerve palsy.

   e. Is the patient symptomatic (defined below)?

   - Carotid Transient Ischemic Attack (TIA) persisting less than 24 hours;
   - Non-disabling stroke: Modified Rankin Scale
   - Transient monocular blindness:amaurosis fugax.

   f. Modified Rankin Scale score if the patient experienced a stroke.

   g. Percent of stenosis of stented lesion(s) by angiography.

   h. Was embolic protection used?

   i. Were there any complications during hospitalization (defined below)?

   - All stroke: an ischemic neurologic deficit that persisted more than 24 hours;
   - MI;
   - All death.

Recertification is effective for two (2) additional years during which facilities will be required to submit the requested data every April 1 and October 1.

The CMS will consider the approval of national CAS registries that provide CMS with a comprehensive overview of the registry and its capabilities, and the manner in which the registry meets CMS data collection and evaluation requirements. Specific standards for CMS approval are listed below. Facilities enrolled in a CMS-approved national CAS registry will automatically meet the data collection standards required for initial and continued facility certification. Hospitals' contracts with an approved registry may include authority for the registry to submit required data to CMS for the hospital. A list of approved registries will be available on the CMS Coverage Web site.

National Registries

As noted above, CMS will approve national registries developed by professional societies and other organizations and allow these entities to collect and submit data to CMS on behalf of participating facilities to meet facility certification and recertification requirements. To be eligible to perform these functions and become a CMS-approved registry, the national registry, at a minimum, must be able to:

1. Enroll facilities in every U.S. state and territory;
2. Assure data confidentiality and compliance with HIPPA;
3. Collect the required CMS data elements as listed in the above section;
4. Assure data quality and data completeness;
5. Address deficiencies in the facility data collection, quality, and submission;
6. Validate the data submitted by facilities as needed;
7. Track long term outcomes such as stroke and death;
8. Conduct data analyses and produce facility specific data reports and summaries;
9. Submit data to CMS on behalf of the individual facilities; and
10. Provide quarterly reports to CMS on facilities that do not meet or no longer meet the CMS facility certification and recertification requirements pertaining to data collection and analysis.

Registries wishing to receive this designation from CMS must submit evidence that they meet or exceed our standards. Though the registry requirements pertain to CAS, CMS strongly encourages all national registries to establish a similar mechanism to collect comparable data on CEA. Having both CAS and CEA data will help answer questions about carotid revascularization, in general, in the Medicare population.

The CAS for patients who are not at high risk for CEA remains covered only in FDA-approved Category B IDE clinical trials under 42 CFR 405.201.

The CMS has determined that PTA of the carotid artery concurrent with the placement of an FDA-approved carotid stent and an FDA-approved or -cleared embolic protection device is not reasonable and necessary for all other patients.

5. Concurrent with Intracranial Stent Placement in FDA-Approved Category B IDE Clinical Trials

   Effective November 6, 2006, Medicare covers PTA and stenting of intracranial arteries for the treatment of cerebral artery stenosis >=50% in patients with intracranial atherosclerotic disease when furnished in accordance with the FDA-approved protocols governing Category B IDE clinical trials. CMS determines that coverage of intracranial PTA and stenting is reasonable and necessary under these circumstances.

C. Nationally Non-Covered Indications

All other indications for PTA with or without stenting to treat obstructive lesions of the vertebral and cerebral arteries remain non-covered. The safety and efficacy of these procedures are not established.

All other indications for PTA without stenting for which CMS has not specifically indicated coverage remain non-covered.

D. Other

Coverage of PTA with stenting not specifically addressed or discussed in this NCD is at local Medicare contractor discretion.

(This NCD last reviewed December 2009.)

100-3, 20.8

NCD for Cardiac Pacemakers (20.8)

Cardiac pacemakers are self-contained, battery-operated units that send electrical stimulation to the heart. They are generally implanted to alleviate symptoms of decreased cardiac output related to abnormal heart rate and/or rhythm. Pacemakers are generally used for persistent, symptomatic second- or third-degree atrioventricular (AV) block and symptomatic sinus bradycardia.

Cardiac pacemakers are covered as prosthetic devices under the Medicare program, subject to the following conditions and limitations. While cardiac pacemakers have been covered under Medicare for many years, there were no specific guidelines for their use other than the general Medicare requirement that covered services be reasonable and necessary for the treatment of the condition. Services rendered for cardiac pacing on or after the effective dates of this instruction are subject to these guidelines, which are based on certain assumptions regarding the clinical goals of cardiac pacing. While some uses of pacemakers are relatively certain or unambiguous, many other uses require considerable expertise and judgment.

Consequently, the medical necessity for permanent cardiac pacing must be viewed in the context of overall patient management. The appropriateness of such pacing may be conditional on other diagnostic or therapeutic modalities having been undertaken. Although significant complications and adverse side effects of pacemaker use are relatively rare, they cannot be ignored when considering the use of pacemakers for dubious medical conditions, or marginal clinical benefit.

These guidelines represent current concepts regarding medical circumstances in which permanent cardiac pacing may be appropriate or necessary. As with other areas of medicine, advances in knowledge and techniques in cardiology are expected. Consequently, judgments about the medical necessity and acceptability of new uses for cardiac pacing in new classes of patients may change as more more conclusive evidence becomes available. This instruction applies only to permanent cardiac pacemakers, and does not address the use of temporary, non-implanted pacemakers.

The two groups of conditions outlined below deal with the necessity for cardiac pacing for patients in general. These are intended as guidelines in assessing the medical necessity for pacing therapies, taking into account the particular circumstances in each case. However, as a general rule, the two groups of current medical concepts may be viewed as representing:

Group I: Single-Chamber Cardiac Pacemakers – a) conditions under which single chamber pacemaker claims may be considered covered without further claims development; and b) conditions under which single-chamber pacemaker claims would be denied unless further claims development shows that they fall into the covered category, or special medical circumstances exist of the sufficiency to convince the contractor that the claim should be paid.

Group II: Dual-Chamber Cardiac Pacemakers - a) conditions under which dual-chamber pacemaker claims may be considered covered without further claims development, and b) conditions under which dual-chamber pacemaker claims would be denied unless further claims development shows that they fall into the covered categories for single- and dual-chamber pacemakers, or special medical circumstances exist sufficient to convince the contractor that the claim should be paid.

The CMS opened the NCD on Cardiac Pacemakers to afford the public an opportunity to comment on the proposal to revise the language contained in the instruction. The revisions transfer the focus of the NCD from the actual pacemaker implantation procedure itself to the reasonable and necessary medical indications that justify cardiac

pacing. This is consistent with our findings that pacemaker implantation is no longer considered routinely harmful or an experimental procedure.

Group I: Single-Chamber Cardiac Pacemakers (Effective March 16, 1983)

A. Nationally Covered Indications

Conditions under which cardiac pacing is generally considered acceptable or necessary, provided that the conditions are chronic or recurrent and not due to transient causes such as acute myocardial infarction, drug toxicity, or electrolyte imbalance. (In cases where there is a rhythm disturbance, if the rhythm disturbance is chronic or recurrent, a single episode of a symptom such as syncope or seizure is adequate to establish medical necessity.)

1. Acquired complete (also referred to as third-degree) AV heart block.
2. Congenital complete heart block with severe bradycardia (in relation to age), or significant physiological deficits or significant symptoms due to the bradycardia.
3. Second-degree AV heart block of Type II (i.e., no progressive prolongation of P-R interval prior to each blocked beat. P-R interval indicates the time taken for an impulse to travel from the atria to the ventricles on an electrocardiogram).
4. Second-degree AV heart block of Type I (i.e., progressive prolongation of P-R interval prior to each blocked beat) with significant symptoms due to hemodynamic instability associated with the heart block.
5. Sinus bradycardia associated with major symptoms (e.g., syncope, seizures, congestive heart failure); or substantial sinus bradycardia (heart rate less than 50) associated with dizziness or confusion. The correlation between symptoms and bradycardia must be documented, or the symptoms must be clearly attributable to the bradycardia rather than to some other cause.
6. In selected and few patients, sinus bradycardia of lesser severity (heart rate 50-59) with dizziness or confusion. The correlation between symptoms and bradycardia must be documented, or the symptoms must be clearly attributable to the bradycardia rather than to some other cause.
7. Sinus bradycardia is the consequence of long-term necessary drug treatment for which there is no acceptable alternative when accompanied by significant symptoms (e.g., syncope, seizures, congestive heart failure, dizziness or confusion). The correlation between symptoms and bradycardia must be documented, or the symptoms must be clearly attributable to the bradycardia rather than to some other cause.
8. Sinus node dysfunction with or without tachyarrhythmias or AV conduction block (i.e., the bradycardia-tachycardia syndrome, sino-atrial block, sinus arrest) when accompanied by significant symptoms (e.g., syncope, seizures, congestive heart failure, dizziness or confusion).
9. Sinus node dysfunction with or without symptoms when there are potentially life-threatening ventricular arrhythmias or tachycardia secondary to the bradycardia (e.g., numerous premature ventricular contractions, couplets, runs of premature ventricular contractions, or ventricular tachycardia).
10. Bradycardia associated with supraventricular tachycardia (e.g., atrial fibrillation, atrial flutter, or paroxysmal atrial tachycardia) with high-degree AV block which is unresponsive to appropriate pharmacological management and when the bradycardia is associated with significant symptoms (e.g., syncope, seizures, congestive heart failure, dizziness or confusion).
11. The occasional patient with hypersensitive carotid sinus syndrome with syncope due to bradycardia and unresponsive to prophylactic medical measures.
12. Bifascicular or trifascicular block accompanied by syncope which is attributed to transient complete heart block after other plausible causes of syncope have been reasonably excluded.
13. Prophylactic pacemaker use following recovery from acute myocardial infarction during which there was temporary complete (third-degree) and/or Mobitz Type II second-degree AV block in association with bundle branch block.
14. In patients with recurrent and refractory ventricular tachycardia, "overdrive pacing" (pacing above the basal rate) to prevent ventricular tachycardia.

    (Effective May 9, 1985)
15. Second-degree AV heart block of Type I with the QRS complexes prolonged.

B. Nationally Noncovered Indications

Conditions which, although used by some physicians as a basis for permanent cardiac pacing, are considered unsupported by adequate evidence of benefit and therefore should not generally be considered appropriate uses for single-chamber pacemakers in the absence of the above indications. Contractors should review claims for pacemakers with these indications to determine the need for further claims development prior to denying the claim, since additional claims development may be required. The object of such further development is to establish whether the particular claim actually meets the conditions in a) above. In claims where this is not the case or where such an event appears unlikely, the contractor may deny the claim

1. Syncope of undetermined cause.
2. Sinus bradycardia without significant symptoms.
3. Sino-atrial block or sinus arrest without significant symptoms.
4. Prolonged P-R intervals with atrial fibrillation (without third-degree AV block) or with other causes of transient ventricular pause.
5. Bradycardia during sleep.
6. Right bundle branch block with left axis deviation (and other forms of fascicular or bundle branch block) without syncope or other symptoms of intermittent AV block).
7. Asymptomatic second-degree AV block of Type I unless the QRS complexes are prolonged or electrophysiological studies have demonstrated that the block is at or beyond the level of the His bundle (a component of the electrical conduction system of the heart).

    Effective October 1, 2001
8. Asymptomatic bradycardia in post-mycardial infarction patients about to initiate long-term beta-blocker drug therapy.

C. Other

All other indications for single-chamber cardiac pacing for which CMS has not specifically indicated coverage remain nationally noncovered, except for Category B Investigational Device Exemption (IDE) clinical trials, or as routine costs of single-chamber cardiac pacing associated with clinical trials, in accordance with section 310.1 of the NCD Manual.

Group II: Dual-Chamber Cardiac Pacemakers – (Effective May 9, 1985)

A. Nationally Covered Indications

Conditions under dual-chamber cardiac pacing are considered acceptable or necessary in the general medical community unless conditions 1 and 2 under Group II. B., are present:

1. Patients in who single-chamber (ventricular pacing) at the time of pacemaker insertion elicits a definite drop in blood pressure, retrograde conduction, or discomfort.
2. Patients in whom the pacemaker syndrome (atrial ventricular asynchrony), with significant symptoms, has already been experienced with a pacemaker that is being replaced.
3. Patients in whom even a relatively small increase in cardiac efficiency will importantly improve the quality of life, e.g., patients with congestive heart failure despite adequate other medical measures.
4. Patients in whom the pacemaker syndrome can be anticipated, e.g., in young and active people, etc.

Dual-chamber pacemakers may also be covered for the conditions, as listed in Group I. A., if the medical necessity is sufficiently justified through adequate claims development. Expert physicians differ in their judgments about what constitutes appropriate criteria for dual-chamber pacemaker use. The judgment that such a pacemaker is warranted in the patient meeting accepted criteria must be based upon the individual needs and characteristics of that patient, weighing the magnitude and likelihood of anticipated benefits against the magnitude and likelihood of disadvantages to the patient.

B. Nationally Noncovered Indications

Whenever the following conditions (which represent overriding contraindications) are present, dual-chamber pacemakers are not covered:

1. Ineffective atrial contractions (e.g., chronic atrial fibrillation or flutter, or giant left atrium.
2. Frequent or persistent supraventricular tachycardias, except where the pacemaker is specifically for the control of the tachycardia.
3. A clinical condition in which pacing takes place only intermittently and briefly, and which is not associated with a reasonable likelihood that pacing needs will become prolonged, e.g., the occasional patient with hypersensitive carotid sinus syndrome with syncope due to bradycardia and unresponsive to prophylactic medical measures.
4. Prophylactic pacemaker use following recovery from acute myocardial infarction during which there was temporary complete (third-degree) and/or Type II second-degree AV block in association with bundle branch block.

C. Other

All other indications for dual-chamber cardiac pacing for which CMS has not specifically indicated coverage remain nationally noncovered, except for Category B IDE clinical trials, or as routine costs of dual-chamber cardiac pacing associated with clinical trials, in accordance with section 310.1 of the NCD Manual.

(This NCD last reviewed June 2004.)

100-3, 20.8.1

NCD for Cardiac Pacemaker Evaluation Services (20.8.1)

Medicare covers a variety of services for the post-implant follow-up and evaluation of implanted cardiac pacemakers. The following guidelines are designed to assist contractors in identifying and processing claims for such services.

NOTE: These new guidelines are limited to lithium battery-powered pacemakers, because mercury-zinc battery-powered pacemakers are no longer being manufactured and virtually all have been replaced by lithium units. Contractors still receiving claims for monitoring such units should continue to apply the guidelines published in 1980 to those units until they are replaced.

One fact of which contractors should be aware is that many dual-chamber units may be programmed to pace only the ventricles; this may be done either at the time the pacemaker is implanted or at some time afterward. In such cases, a dual-chamber unit, when programmed or reprogrammed for ventricular pacing, should be treated as a single-chamber pacemaker in applying screening guidelines.

The decision as to how often any patient's pacemaker should be monitored is the responsibility of the patient's physician who is best able to take into account the condition and circumstances of the individual patient. These may vary over time, requiring modifications of the frequency with which the patient should be monitored. In cases where monitoring is done by some entity other than the patient's physician, such as a commercial monitoring service or hospital outpatient department, the physician's prescription for monitoring is required and should be periodically renewed (at least annually) to assure that the frequency of monitoring is proper for the patient. When a patient is monitered both during clinica visits and transtelephonically, the contractor should be sure to include frequency data on both ypes of monitoring in evaluating the reasonableness of the frequency of monitoring services received by the patient.

Since there are over 200 pacemaker models in service at any given point, and a variety of patient conditions that give rise to the need for pacemakers, the question of the appropriate frequency of monitorings is a complex one. Nevertheless, it is possible to develop guidelines within which the vast majority of pacemaker monitorings will fall and contractors should do this, using their own data and experience, as well as the frequency guidelines which follow, in order to limit extensive claims development to those cases requiring special attention.

100-3, 20.8.2

NCD for Self-Contained Pacemaker Monitors (20.8.2)

Self-contained pacemaker monitors are accepted devices for monitoring cardiac pacemakers. Accordingly, program payment may be made for the rental or purchase of either of the following pacemaker monitors when it is prescribed by a physician for a patient with a cardiac pacemaker:

A. Digital Electronic Pacemaker Monitor.
This device provides the patient with an instantaneous digital readout of his pacemaker pulse rate. Use of this device does not involve professional services until there has been a change of five pulses (or more) per minute above or below the initial rate of the pacemaker; when such change occurs, the patient contacts his physician.

B. Audible/Visible Signal Pacemaker Monitor.
This device produces an audible and visible signal which indicates the pacemaker rate. Use of this device does not involve professional services until a change occurs in these signals; at such time, the patient contacts his physician.

NOTE: The design of the self-contained pacemaker monitor makes it possible for the patient to monitor his pacemaker periodically and minimizes the need for regular visits to the outpatient department of the provider.

Therefore, documentation of the medical necessity for pacemaker evaluation in the outpatient department of the provider should be obtained where such evaluation is employed in addition to the self-contained pacemaker monitor used by the patient in his home.

100-3, 20.10

NCD for Cardiac Rehabilitation Programs (20.10)

A. General
Phase II cardiac rehabilitation, as described by the U.S. Public Health Service, is a comprehensive, long-term program including medical evaluation, prescribed exercise, cardiac risk factor modification, education, and counseling. Phase II refers to outpatient, medically supervised programs that are typically initiated 1-3 weeks after hospital discharge and provide appropriate electrocardiographic monitoring.

B. Nationally Covered Indications
Effective for services performed on or after March 22, 2006, Medicare coverage of cardiac rehabilitation programs is considered reasonable and necessary only for patients who: (1) have a documented diagnosis of acute myocardial infarction within the preceding 12 months; or (2) have had coronary bypass surgery; or (3) have stable angina pectoris; or (4) have had heart valve repair/replacement; or (5) have had percutaneous transluminal coronary angioplasty (PTCA) or coronary stenting; or (6) have had a heart or heart-lung transplant.

1. Program Requirements
   a. Duration

      Services provided in connection with a cardiac rehabilitation exercise program may be considered reasonable and necessary for up to 36 sessions. Patients generally receive 2 to 3 sessions per week for 12 to 18 weeks. Coverage of additional sessions is discussed in section D below.

   b. Components

      Cardiac rehabilitation programs must be comprehensive and to be comprehensive they must include a medical evaluation, a program to modify cardiac risk factors (e.g., nutritional counseling), prescribed exercise, education, and counseling.

   c. Facility

      The facility must have available for immediate use the necessary cardio-pulmonary, emergency, diagnostic, and therapeutic life-saving equipment accepted by the medical community as medically necessary, e.g., oxygen, cardiopulmonary resuscitation equipment, or defibrillator.

   d. Staff

      The program must be staffed by personnel necessary to conduct the program safely and effectively, who are trained in both basic and advanced life support techniques and in exercise therapy for coronary disease. The program must be under the direct supervision of a physician, as defined in 42 CFR Sec.410.26(a)(2) (defined through cross reference to 42 CFR Sec.410.32(b)(3)(ii), or 42 CFR Sec.410.27(f)).

C. Nationally Non-Covered Indications
Except as provided in section D., all other indications are not covered.

D. Other
The contractor has the discretion to cover cardiac rehabilitation services beyond 18 weeks. Coverage must not exceed a total of 72 sessions for 36 weeks.

(This NCD last reviewed March 2006.)

100-3, 20.11

NCD for Intraoperative Ventricular Mapping (20.11)

Intraoperative ventricular mapping is the technique of recording cardiac electrical activity directly from the heart. The recording sites are usually identified from an anatomical grid and may consist of epicardial, intramural, and endocardial sites. A probe with electrodes is used to explore these surfaces and generate a map that displays the sequence of electrical activation. This information is used by the surgeon to locate precisely the site of an operative intervention.

The intraoperative ventricular mapping procedure is covered under Medicare only for the uses and medical conditions described below:

- Localize accessory pathways associated with the Wolff-Parkinson-White (WPW) and other preexcitation syndromes;
- Map the sequence of atrial and ventricular activation for drug-resistant supraventricular tachycardias;
- Delineate the anatomical course of His bundle and/or bundle branches during corrective cardiac surgery for congenital heart diseases; and
- Direct the surgical treatment of patients with refractory ventricular tachyarrhythmias.

100-3, 20.12

NCD for Diagnostic Endocardial Electrical Stimulation (Pacing) (20.12)

Diagnostic endocardial electrical stimulation (EES), also called programmed electrical stimulation of the heart, is covered under Medicare when used for patients with severe cardiac arrhythmias.

100-3, 20.13

NCD for HIS Bundle Study (20.13)

Medicare coverage of the procedure would be limited to selected patients: those with complex ongoing acute arrhythmias, those with intermittent or permanent heart block in whom pacemaker implantation is being considered, and those patients who have recently developed heart block secondary to a myocardial infarction. When heart catheterization and the HIS Bundle Study are performed at the same time, the program will cover only one catheterization and a small additional charge for the study.

When a HIS bundle cardiogram is obtained as part of a diagnostic endocardial electrical stimulation, no separate charge will be recognized for the His bundle study.

100-3, 20.14

NCD for Plethysmography (20.14)

Medicare coverage is extended to those procedures listed in Category I below when used for the accepted medical indications mentioned above. The procedures in Category II are still considered experimental and are not covered at this time. Denial of claims becuase a noncovered procedure was used or because there was no medical indication for plethysmographic evaluation of any type should be based on Sec.1862(a)(1) of the Act.

Category I - Covered
Segmental Plethysmography - Included under this procedure are services performed with a regional plethysmograph, differential plethysmograph, recording oscillometer, and a pulse volume recorder.

Electrical Impedance Plethysmography

Ultrasonic Measurement of Blood Flow (Doppler) - While not strictly a plethysmographic method, this is also a useful tool in the evaluation of suspected peripheral vascular disease or preoperative screening of podiatric patients with suspected peripheral vascular compromise. (See Sec.50-7 for the applicable coverage policy on this procedure.)

Oculoplethysmography - See NCD on Noninvasive Tests of Carotid Function, Sec.20.17.

Strain Gauge Plethysmography - This test is based on recording the non-pulsatile aspects of inflowing blood at various points on an extremity by a mercury-in-silastic strain gauge sensor. The instrument consists of a chart recorder, an automatic cuff inflation and deflation system, and a recording manometer.

Category II - Experimental
The following methods have not yet reached a level of development such as to allow their routine use in the evaluation of suspected peripheral vascular disease.

Inductance Plethysmography - This method is considered experimental and does not provide reproducible results.

Capacitance Plethysmography - This method is considered experimental and does not provide reproducible results.

Mechanical Oscillometry - This is a non-standardized method which offers poor sensitivity and is not considered superior to the simple measurement of peripheral blood pressure.

Photoelectric Plethysmography - This method is considered useful only in determining whether or not a pulse is present and does not provide reproducible measurements of blood flow.

Differential plethysmography, on the other hand, is a system which uses an impedance technique to compare pulse pressures at various points along a limb, with a reference pressure at the mid-brachial or wrist level. It is not clear whether this technique, as usually performed in the physician's office, meets the definition of plethysmography because quantitative measurements of blood flow are usually not made. It has been concluded, in any event, that the differential plethysmography system is a blood pulse recorder of undetermined value, which has the potential for significant overutilization. Therefore, reimbursement for studies done by techniques other than venous occlusive pneumoplethysmography should be denied, at least until additional data on these devices, including controlled clinical studies, become available.

100-3, 20.15

NCD for Electrocardiographic (EKG) Services (20.15)

Nationally Covered Indications

1. The following indications are covered nationally unless otherwise indicated:
2. Computer analysis of EKGs when furnished in a setting and under the circumstances required for coverage of other EKG services.
3. EKG services rendered by an independent diagnostic testing facility (IDTF), including physician review and interpretation. Separate physician services are not covered unless he/she is the patient's attending or consulting physician.
4. Emergency EKGs (i.e., when the patient is or may be experiencing a lifethreatening event) performed as a laboratory or diagnostic service by a portable x-ray supplier only when a physician is in attendance at the time the service is performed or immediately thereafter.
5. Home EKG services with documentation of medical necessity.
6. Trans-telephonic EKG transmissions (effective March 1, 1980) as a diagnostic service for the indications described below, when performed with equipment meeting the standards described below, subject to the limitations and conditions specified below. Coverage is further limited to the amounts payable with respect to the physician's service in interpreting the results of such transmissions, including charges for rental of the equipment. The device used by the beneficiary is part of a total diagnostic system and is not considered DME separately. Covered uses are to:
   a. Detect, characterize, and document symptomatic transient arrhythmias;
   b. Initiate, revise, or discontinue arrhythmic drug therapy; or,
   c. Carry out early post-hospital monitoring of patients discharged after myocardial infarction (MI); (only if 24-hour coverage is provided, see C.5. below).

   Certain uses other than those specified above may be covered if, in the judgment of the local contractor, such use is medically necessary.

   Additionally, the transmitting devices must meet at least the following criteria:
   a. They must be capable of transmitting EKG Leads, I, II, or III; and,
   b. The tracing must be sufficiently comparable to a conventional EKG.

24-hour attended coverage used as early post-hospital monitoring of patients discharged after MI is only covered if provision is made for such 24-hour attended coverage in the manner described below:

24-hour attended coverage means there must be, at a monitoring site or central data center, an EKG technician or other non-physician, receiving calls and/or EKG data; tape recording devices do not meet this requirement. Further, such technicians should have immediate, 24-hour access to a physician to review transmitted data and make clinical decisions regarding the patient. The technician should also be instructed as to when and how to contact available facilities to assist the patient in case of emergencies.

Nationally Non-covered Indications

The following indications are non-covered nationally unless otherwise specified below:

1. The time-sampling mode of operation of ambulatory EKG cardiac event monitoring/recording.
2. Separate physician services other than those rendered by an IDTF unless rendered by the patient's attending or consulting physician.
3. Home EKG services without documentation of medical necessity.
4. Emergency EKG services by a portable x-ray supplier without a physician in attendance at the time of service or immediately thereafter.
5. 24-hour attended coverage used as early post-hospital monitoring of patients discharged after MI unless provision is made for such 24-hour attended coverage in the manner described in section B.5. above.
6. Any marketed Food and Drug Administration (FDA)-approved ambulatory cardiac monitoring device or service that cannot be categorized according to the framework below.

Other

Ambulatory cardiac monitoring performed with a marketed, FDA-approved device, is eligible for coverage if it can be categorized according to the framework below. Unless there is a specific NCD for that device or service, determination as to whether a device or service that fits into the framework is reasonable and necessary is according to local contractor discretion.

Electrocardiographic Services Framework

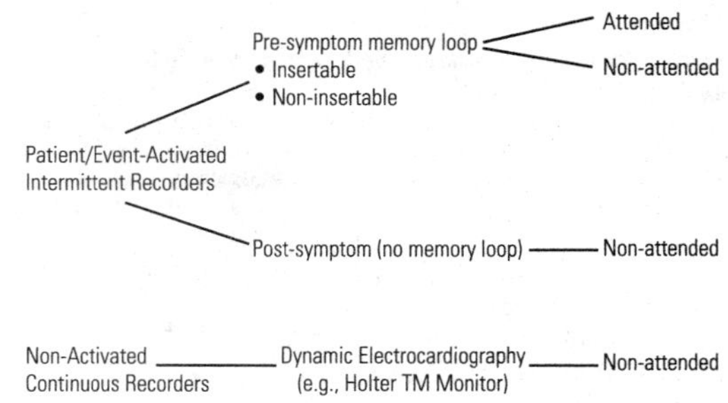

100-3, 20.16

NCD for Cardiac Output Monitoring by Thoracic Electrical Bioimpedance (TEB) (20.16)

Indications and Limitations of Coverage

B. Nationally Covered Indications

Effective for services performed on and after January 23, 2004, TEB is covered for the following uses:

1. Differentiation of cardiogenic from pulmonary causes of acute dyspnea when medical history, physical examination, and standard assessment tools provide insufficient information, and the treating physician has determined that TEB hemodynamic data are necessary for appropriate management of the patient.
2. Optimization of atrioventricular (A/V) interval for patients with A/V sequential cardiac pacemakers when medical history, physical examination, and standard assessment tools provide insufficient information, and the treating physician has determined that TEB hemodynamic data are necessary for appropriate management of the patient.
3. Monitoring of continuous inotropic therapy for patients with terminal congestive heart failure, when those patients have chosen to die with comfort at home, or for patients waiting at home for a heart transplant.
4. Evaluation for rejection in patients with a heart transplant as a predetermined alternative to a myocardial biopsy. Medical necessity must be documented should a biopsy be performed after TEB.
5. Optimization of fluid management in patients with congestive heart failure when medical history, physical examination, and standard assessment tools provide insufficient information, and the treating physician has determined that TEB hemodynamic data are necessary for appropriate management of the patient.

C. Nationally Non-Covered Indications

1. TEB is non-covered when used for patients:
   - With proven or suspected disease involving severe regurgitation of the aorta;
   - With minute ventilation (MV) sensor function pacemakers, since the device may adversely affect the functioning of that type of pacemaker;
   - During cardiac bypass surgery; or,
   - In the management of all forms of hypertension (with the exception of drug-resistant hypertension as outlined below).
2. All other uses of TEB not otherwise specified remain non-covered.

D. Other

Contractors have discretion to determine whether the use of TEB for the management of drug-resistant hypertension is reasonable and necessary. Drug resistant hypertension is defined as failure to achieve goal blood pressure in patients who are adhering to full doses of an appropriate 3-drug regimen that includes a diuretic. Effective November 24, 2006, after reconsideration of Medicare policy, CMS will continue current Medicare policy for TEB.

(This NCD last reviewed November 2006.)

100-3, 20.17

NCD for Noninvasive Tests of Carotid Function (20.17)

It is important to note that the names of these tests are not standardized. Following are some of the acceptable tests, recognizing that this list is not inclusive and that local medical consultants should make determinations:

Direct Tests

- Carotid Phonoangiography
- Direct Bruit Analysis
- Spectral Bruit Analysis
- Doppler Flow Velocity
- Ultrasound Imaging including Real Time
- B-Scan and Doppler Devices

Indirect Tests

- Periorbital Directional Doppler Ultrasonography
- Oculoplethysmography

- Ophthalmodynamometry

100-3, 20.18

NCD for Carotid Body Resection/Carotid Body Denervation (20.18)

Carotid body resection is occasionally used to relieve pulmonary symptoms, including asthma, but has been shown to lack general acceptance of the professional medical community. In addition, controlled clinical studies establishing the safety and effectiveness of this procedure are needed. Therefore, all carotid body resections to relieve pulmonary symptoms must be considered investigational and cannot be considered reasonable and necessary within the meaning of section 1862(a)(l) of the law. No program reimbursement may be made in such cases.

There is, however, one instance where carotid body resection has been accepted by the medical community as effective. That instance is when evidence of a mass in the carotid body,with or without symptoms, indicates the need for surgery to remove the carotid body tumor.

Denervation of a carotid sinus to treat hypersensitive carotid sinus reflex is another procedure performed in the area of the carotid body. In the case of hypersensitive carotid sinus, light pressure on the upper part of the neck (such as might be experienced when turning or raising one's head) results in symptoms such as dizziness or syncope due to hypotension and slowed heart rate. Failure of medical therapy and continued deterioration in the condition of the patient in such cases may indicate need for surgery. Denervation of the carotid sinus is rarely performed, but when elected as the therapy of choice with the above indications, this procedure may be considered reasonable and necessary.

100-3, 20.19

NCD for Ambulatory Blood Pressure Monitoring (20.19)

ABPM must be performed for at least 24 hours to meet coverage criteria.

ABPM is only covered for those patients with suspected white coat hypertension. Suspected white coat hypertension is defined as

1) office blood pressure >140/90 mm Hg on at least three separate clinic/office visits with two separate measurements made at each visit;
2) at least two documented blood pressure measurements taken outside the office which are <140/90 mm Hg; and
3) no evidence of end-organ damage.

The information obtained by ABPM is necessary in order to determine the appropriate management of the patient. ABPM is not covered for any other uses. In the rare circumstance that ABPM needs to be performed more than once in a patient, the qualifying criteria described above must be met for each subsequent ABPM test.

For those patients that undergo ABPM and have an ambulatory blood pressure of <135/85 with no evidence of end-organ damage, it is likely that their cardiovascular risk is similar to that of normotensives. They should be followed over time. Patients for which ABPM demonstrates a blood pressure of >135/85 may be at increased cardiovascular risk, and a physician may wish to consider antihypertensive therapy.

100-3, 20.23

NCD for Fabric Wrapping of Abdominal Aneurysms (20.23)

Fabric wrapping of abdominal aneurysms is not a covered Medicare procedure. This is a treatment for abdominal aneurysms which involves wrapping aneurysms with cellophane or fascia lata. This procedure has not been shown to prevent eventual rupture. In extremely rare instances, external wall reinforcement may be indicated when the current accepted treatment (excision of the aneurysm and reconstruction with synthetic materials) is not a viable alternative, but external wall reinforcement is not fabric wrapping. Accordingly, fabric wrapping of abdominal aneurysms is not considered reasonable and necessary within the meaning of Sec.1862(a)(1) of the Act.

100-3, 20.25

NCD for Cardiac Catheterization Performed in Other than a Hospital Setting (20.25)

(Effective January 12, 2006 - Repealed)

100-3, 20.26

NCD for Partial Ventriculectomy (20.26)

Since the mortality rate is high and there are no published scientific articles or clinical studies regarding partial ventriculectomy, this procedure cannot be considered reasonable and necessary within the meaning of Sec.1862(a)(1) of the Act. Therefore, partial ventriculectomy is not covered by Medicare.

100-3, 20.28

NCD for Therapeutic Embolization (20.28)

Therapeutic embolization is covered when done for hemorrhage, and for other conditions amenable to treatment by the procedure, when reasonable and necessary for the individual patient. Renal embolization for the treatment of renal adenocarcinoma continues to be covered, effective December 15, 1978, as one type of therapeutic embolization, to:

- Reduce tumor vascularity preoperatively;
- Reduce tumor bulk in inoperable cases; or
- Palliate specific symptoms.

100-3, 20.29

NCD for Hyperbaric Oxygen Therapy (20.29)

A. Covered Conditions

Program reimbursement for HBO therapy will be limited to that which is administered in a chamber (including the one man unit) and is limited to the following conditions:

1. Acute carbon monoxide intoxication,
2. Decompression illness,
3. Gas embolism,
4. Gas gangrene,
5. Acute traumatic peripheral ischemia. HBO therapy is a valuable adjunctive treatment to be used in combination with accepted standard therapeutic measures when loss of function, limb, or life is threatened.
6. Crush injuries and suturing of severed limbs. As in the previous conditions, HBO therapy would be an adjunctive treatment when loss of function, limb, or life is threatened.
7. Progressive necrotizing infections (necrotizing fasciitis),
8. Acute peripheral arterial insufficiency,
9. Preparation and preservation of compromised skin grafts (not for primary management of wounds),
10. Chronic refractory osteomyelitis, unresponsive to conventional medical and surgical management,
11. Osteoradionecrosis as an adjunct to conventional treatment,
12. Soft tissue radionecrosis as an adjunct to conventional treatment,
13. Cyanide poisoning,
14. Actinomycosis, only as an adjunct to conventional therapy when the disease process is refractory to antibiotics and surgical treatment,
15. Diabetic wounds of the lower extremities in patients who meet the following three criteria:
    a. Patient has type I or type II diabetes and has a lower extremity wound that is due to diabetes;
    b. Patient has a wound classified as Wagner grade III or higher; and
    c. Patient has failed an adequate course of standard wound therapy.

The use of HBO therapy is covered as adjunctive therapy only after there are no measurable signs of healing for at least 30 -days of treatment with standard wound therapy and must be used in addition to standard wound care. Standard wound care in patients with diabetic wounds includes: assessment of a patient's vascular status and correction of any vascular problems in the affected limb if possible, optimization of nutritional status, optimization of glucose control, debridement by any means to remove devitalized tissue, maintenance of a clean, moist bed of granulation tissue with appropriate moist dressings, appropriate off-loading, and necessary treatment to resolve any infection that might be present. Failure to respond to standard wound care occurs when there are no measurable signs of healing for at least 30 consecutive days. Wounds must be evaluated at least every 30 days during administration of HBO therapy. Continued treatment with HBO therapy is not covered if measurable signs of healing have not been demonstrated within any 30-day period of treatment.

B. Noncovered Conditions

All other indications not specified under Sec.270.4(A) are not covered under the Medicare program. No program payment may be made for any conditions other than those listed in Sec.270.4(A).

No program payment may be made for HBO in the treatment of the following conditions:

1. Cutaneous, decubitus, and stasis ulcers.
2. Chronic peripheral vascular insufficiency.
3. Anaerobic septicemia and infection other than clostridial.
4. Skin burns (thermal).
5. Senility.
6. Myocardial infarction.
7. Cardiogenic shock.
8. Sickle cell anemia.
9. Acute thermal and chemical pulmonary damage, i.e., smoke inhalation with pulmonary insufficiency.
10. Acute or chronic cerebral vascular insufficiency.
11. Hepatic necrosis.
12. Aerobic septicemia.
13. Nonvascular causes of chronic brain syndrome (Pick's disease, Alzheimer's disease, Korsakoff's disease).
14. Tetanus.
15. Systemic aerobic infection.
16. Organ transplantation.
17. Organ storage.
18. Pulmonary emphysema.
19. Exceptional blood loss anemia.
20. Multiple Sclerosis.
21. Arthritic Diseases.
22. Acute cerebral edema.

C. Topical Application of Oxygen

This method of administering oxygen does not meet the definition of HBO therapy as stated above. Also, its clinical efficacy has not been established. Therefore, no Medicare reimbursement may be made for the topical application of oxygen.

100-3, 20.30

NCD for Microvolt T-Wave Alternans (MTWA) (20.30)

B. Nationally Covered Indications

Microvolt T-wave Alternans diagnostic testing is covered for the evaluation of patients at risk for SCD, only when the spectral analysis method is used.

C. Nationally Non-Covered Indications

Microvolt T-wave Alternans diagnostic test is non-covered for the evaluation of patients at risk for SCD if measurement is not performed employing the spectral analysis.

D. Other

N/A

100-3, 30.1

NCD for Biofeedback Therapy (30.1)

Biofeedback therapy is covered under Medicare only when it is reasonable and necessary for the individual patient for muscle re-education of specific muscle groups or for treating pathological muscle abnormalities of spasticity, incapacitating muscle spasm, or weakness, and more conventional treatments (heat, cold, massage, exercise, support) have not been successful. This therapy is not covered for treatment of ordinary muscle tension states or for psychosomatic conditions. (See the Medicare Benefit Policy Manual, Chapter 15, for general coverage requirements about physical therapy requirements.)

100-3, 30.1.1

NCD for Biofeedback Therapy for the Treatment of Urinary Incontinence (30.1.1)

This policy applies to biofeedback therapy rendered by a practitioner in an office or other facility setting.

Biofeedback is covered for the treatment of stress and/or urge incontinence in cognitively intact patients who have failed a documented trial of pelvic muscle exercise (PME)training. Biofeedback is not a treatment, per se, but a tool to help patients learn how to perform PME. Biofeedback-assisted PME incorporates the use of an electronic or mechanical device to relay visual and/or auditory evidence of pelvic floor muscle tone, in order to improve awareness of pelvic floor musculature and to assist patients in the performance of PME.

A failed trial of PME training is defined as no clinically significant improvement in urinary incontinence after completing 4 weeks of an ordered plan of pelvic muscle exercises to increase periurethral muscle strength.

Contractors may decide whether or not to cover biofeedback as an initial treatment modality.

Home use of biofeedback therapy is not covered.

100-3, 30.3

NCD for Acupuncture (30.3)

Although acupuncture has been used for thousands of years in China and for decades in parts of Europe, it is a new agent of unknown use and efficacy in the United States. Even in those areas of the world where it has been widely used, its mechanism is not known. Three units of the National Institutes of Health, the National Institute of General Medical Sciences, National Institute of Neurological Diseases and Stroke, and Fogarty International Center have been designed to assess and identify specific opportunities and needs for research attending the use of acupuncture for surgical anesthesia and relief of chronic pain. Until the pending scientific assessment of the technique has been completed and its efficacy has been established, Medicare reimbursement for acupuncture, as an anesthetic or as an analgesic or for other therapeutic purposes, may not be made. Accordingly, acupuncture is not considered reasonable and necessary within the meaning of §1862(a)(1) of the Act.

100-3, 30.5

NCD for Transcendental Meditation (TM) (30.5)

After review of this issue, CMS has concluded that the evidence concerning the medical efficacy of TM is incomplete at best and does not demonstrate effectiveness and that a professional level of skill is not required for the training of patients to engage in TM.

Although many articles have been written about application of TM for patients with certain forms of hypertension and anxiety, there are no rigorous scientific studies that demonstrate the effectiveness of TM for use as an adjunct medical therapy for such conditions. Accordingly, neither TM nor the training of patients for its use are covered under the Medicare program.

100-3, 30.6

NCD for Intravenous Histamine Therapy (30.6)

However, there is no scientifically valid clinical evidence that histamine therapy is effective for any condition regardless of the method of administration, nor is it accepted or widely used by the medical profession. Therefore, histamine therapy cannot be considered reasonable and necessary, and program payment for such therapy is not made.

100-3, 40.1

NCD for Diabetes Outpatient Self-Management Training (40.1)

Please refer to 42 CFR 410.140 - 410.146 for conditions that must be met for Medicare coverage.

100-3, 40.5

NCD for Treatment of Obesity (40.5)

B. Nationally Covered Indications

Certain designated surgical services for the treatment of obesity are covered for Medicare beneficiaries who have a BMI >=35, have at least one co-morbidity related to obesity and have been previously unsuccessful with the medical treatment of obesity. See Sec.100.1.

C. Nationally Noncovered Indications

1. Treatments for obesity alone remain non-covered.
2. Supplemented fasting is not covered under the Medicare program as a general treatment for obesity (see section D. below for discretionary local coverage).

D. Other

Where weight loss is necessary before surgery in order to ameliorate the complications posed by obesity when it coexists with pathological conditions such as cardiac and respiratory diseases, diabetes, or hypertension (and other more conservative techniques to achieve this end are not regarded as appropriate), supplemented fasting with adequate monitoring of the patient is eligible for coverage on a case-by-case basis or pursuant to a local coverage determination. The risks associated with the achievement of rapid weight loss must be carefully balanced against the risk posed by the condition requiring surgical treatment.

(This NCD last reviewed February 2006.)

100-3, 50.1

NCD for Speech Generating Devices (50.1)

Effective January 1, 2001, augmentative and alternative communication devices or communicators, which are hereafter referred to as "speech generating devices" are now considered to fall within the DME benefit category established by Sec.1861(n) of the Act. They may be covered if the contractor's medical staff determines that the patient suffers from a severe speech impairment and that the medical condition warrants the use of a device based on the definitions above.

100-3, 50.2

NCD for Electronic Speech Aids (50.2)

Electronic speech aids are covered under Part B as prosthetic devices when the patient has had a laryngectomy or his larynx is permanently inoperative.

100-3, 50.3

NCD for Cochlear Implantation (50.3)

B. Nationally Covered Indications

1. Effective for services performed on or after April 4, 2005, cochlear implantation may be covered for treatment of bilateral pre- or-post-linguistic, sensorineural, moderate-to-profound hearing loss in individuals who demonstrate limited benefit from amplification. Limited benefit from amplification is defined by test scores of less than or equal to 40% correct in the best-aided listening condition on tape-recorded tests of open-set sentence cognition. Medicare coverage is provided only for those patients who meet all of the following selection guidelines.
   - Diagnosis of bilateral moderate-to-profound sensorineural hearing impairment with limited benefit from appropriate hearing (or vibrotactile) aids;
   - Cognitive ability to use auditory clues and a willingness to undergo an extended program of rehabilitation;
   - Freedom from middle ear infection, an accessible cochlear lumen that is structurally suited to implantation, and freedom from lesions in the auditory nerve and acoustic areas of the central nervous system;
   - No contraindications to surgery; and
   - The device must be used in accordance with Food and Drug Administration (FDA)-approved labeling.
2. Effective for services performed on or after April 4, 2005, cochlear implantation may be covered for individuals meeting the selection guidelines above and with hearing test scores of greater than 40% and less than or equal to 60% only when the provider is participating in, and patients are enrolled in, either an FDA-approved category B investigational device exemption clinical trial as defined at 42 CFR 405.201, a trial under the Centers for Medicare & Medicaid (CMS) Clinical Trial Policy as defined at section 310.1 of the National Coverage Determinations Manual, or a prospective, controlled comparative trial approved by CMS as consistent with the evidentiary requirements for National Coverage Analyses and meeting specific quality standards.

C. Nationally Noncovered Indications

Medicare beneficiaries not meeting all of the coverage criteria for cochlear implantation listed are deemed not eligible for Medicare coverage under section 1862(a)(1)(A) of the Social Security Act.

D. Other

All other indications for cochlear implantation not otherwise indicated as nationally covered or non-covered above remain at local contractor discretion.

(This NCD last reviewed May 2005.)

100-3, 70.1

NCD for Consultations with a Beneficiary's Family and Associates (70.1)

In certain types of medical conditions, including when a patient is withdrawn and uncommunicative due to a mental disorder or comatose, the physician may contact relatives and close associates to secure background information to assist in diagnosis and treatment planning. When a physician contacts his patient's relatives or associates for this purpose, expenses of such interviews are properly chargeable as physician's services to the patient on whose behalf the information was secured. If the beneficiary is not an inpatient of a hospital, Part B reimbursement for such an interview is subject to the special limitation on payments for physicians' services in connection with mental, psychoneurotic, and personality disorders.

A physician may also have contacts with a patient's family and associates for purposes other than securing background information. In some cases, the physician will provide counseling to members of the household. Family counseling services are covered only where the primary purpose of such counseling is the treatment of the patient's condition. For example, two situations where family counseling services would be appropriate are as follows: (1) where there is a need to observe the patient's interaction with family members; and/or (2) where there is a need to assess the capability of and assist the family members in aiding in the management of the patient. Counseling principally concerned with the effects of the patient's condition on the individual being interviewed would not be reimbursable as part of the physician's personal services to the patient. While to a limited degree, the counseling described in the second situation may be used to modify the behavior of the family members, such services nevertheless are covered because they relate primarily to the management of the patient's problems and not to the treatment of the family member's problems.

100-3, 70.2

NCD for Consultation Services Rendered by a Podiatrist in a Skilled Nursing Facility (70.2)

Consultation services rendered by a podiatrist in a skilled nursing facility are covered if the services are reasonable and necessary and do not come within any of the specific statutory exclusions. Section 1862(a)(13) of the Act excludes payment for the treatment of flat foot conditions, the treatment of subluxations of the foot, and routine foot care. To determine whether the consultation comes within the foot care exclusions, apply the same rule as for initial diagnostic examinations, i.e., where services are performed in connection with specific symptoms or complaints which suggest the need for covered services, the services are covered regardless of the resulting diagnosis. The exclusion of routine physician examinations is also pertinent and would generally exclude podiatric consultation performed on all patients in a skilled nursing facility on a routine basis for screening purposes, except in those cases where a specific foot ailment is involved. Section 1862(a)(7) of the Act excludes payment for routine physical checkups.

100-3, 70.2.1

NCD for Services Provided for the Diagnosis and Treatment of Diabetic Sensory Neuropathy with Loss of Protective Sensation (AKA Diabetic Peripheral Neuropathy) (70.2.1)

Diabetic sensory neuropathy with LOPS is a localized illness of the feet and falls within the regulation's exception to the general exclusionary rule (see 42 CFR Sec.411.15(l)(1)(i)). Foot exams for people with diabetic sensory neuropathy with LOPS are reasonable and necessary to allow for early intervention in serious complications that typically afflict diabetics with the disease.

Effective for services furnished on or after July 1, 2002, Medicare covers, as a physician service, an evaluation (examination and treatment) of the feet no more often than every six months for individuals with a documented diagnosis of diabetic sensory neuropathy and LOPS, as long as the beneficiary has not seen a foot care specialist for some other reason in the interim. LOPS shall be diagnosed through sensory testing with the 5.07 monofilament using established guidelines, such as those developed by the National Institute of Diabetes and Digestive and Kidney Diseases guidelines. Five sites should be tested on the plantar surface of each foot, according to the National Institute of Diabetes and Digestive and Kidney Diseases guidelines. The areas must be tested randomly since the loss of protective sensation may be patchy in distribution, and the patient may get clues if the test is done rhythmically. Heavily callused areas should be avoided. As suggested by the American Podiatric Medicine Association, an absence of sensation at two or more sites out of 5 tested on either foot when tested with the 5.07 Semmes-Weinstein monofilament must be present and documented to diagnose peripheral neuropathy with loss of protective sensation.

The examination includes:

1. A patient history.
2. A physical examination that must consist of at least the following elements:
   - Visual inspection of forefoot and hindfoot (including toe web spaces).
   - Evaluation of protective sensation.
   - Evaluation of foot structure and biomechanics.
   - Evaluation of vascular status and skin integrity.
   - Evaluation of the need for special footwear.
3. Patient education.

A. Treatment includes, but is not limited to:

- Local care of superficial wounds.
- Debridement of corns and calluses.
- Trimming and debridement of nails.

The diagnosis of diabetic sensory neuropathy with LOPS should be established and documented prior to coverage of foot care. Other causes of peripheral neuropathy should be considered and investigated by the primary care physician prior to initiating or referring for foot care for persons with LOPS.

100-3, 80.1

NCD for Hydrophilic Contact Lens For Corneal Bandage (80.1)

Payment may be made under Sec.1861(s)(2) of the Act for a hydrophilic contact les approved by the Food and Drug Administration (FDA) and used as a supply incident to a pphysician's service. Payment for the lens is included in the payment for the physician's service to which the lens is incident. Contractors are authorized to accept an FDA letter of approval or other FDA published material as evidence of FDA approval. (See Sec.80.4 of the NCD Manual for coverage of a hydrophilic contact lens as prosthetic device.)

100-3, 80.2

Photodynamic Therapy

(Rev. 1, 10-03-03)

CIM 35-100

Photodynamic therapy is a medical procedure which involves the infusion of a photosensitive (light-activated) drug with a very specific absorption peak. This drug is chemically designed to have a unique affinity for the diseased tissue intended for treatment. Once introduced to the body, the drug accumulates and is retained in diseased tissue to a greater degree than in normal tissue. Infusion is followed by the targeted irradiation of this tissue with a non-thermal laser, calibrated to emit light at a wavelength that corresponds to the drug's absorption peak. The drug then becomes active and locally treats the diseased tissue.

Ocular photodynamic therapy (OPT)

The OPT is used in the treatment of ophthalmologic diseases. OPT is only covered when used in conjunction with verteporfin (see §80.3, "Photosensitive Drugs").

- Classic Subfoveal Choroidal Neovascular (CNV) Lesions - OPT is covered with a diagnosis of neovascular age-related macular degeneration (AMD) with predominately classic subfoveal choroidal neovascular (CNV) lesions (where the area of classic CNV occupies . 50 percent of the area of the entire lesion) at the initial visit as determined by a fluorescein angiogram. Subsequent follow-up visits will require a fluorescein angiogram prior to treatment. There are no requirements regarding visual acuity, lesion size, and number of re-treatments.
- Occult Subfoveal Choroidal Neovascular (CNV) Lesions - OPT is noncovered for patients with a diagnosis of age-related macular degeneration (AMD) with occult and no classic CNV lesions.
- Other Conditions - Use of OPT with verteporfin for other types of AMD (e.g., patients with minimally classic CNV lesions, atrophic, or dry AMD) is noncovered. OPT with verteporfin for other ocular indications such as pathologic myopia or presumed ocular histoplasmosis syndrome, is eligible for coverage through individual contractor discretion.

100-3, 80.4

NCD for Hydrophilic Contact Lenses (80.4)

Hydrophilic contact lenses are eyeglasses within the meaning of the exclusion in Sec.1862(a)(7) of the Act and are not covered when used in the treatment of nondiseased eyes with spherical ametrophia, refractive astigmatism, and/or corneal astigmatism. Payment may be made under the prosthetic device benefit, however, for hydrophilic contact lenses when prescribed for an aphakic patient.

Contractors are authorized to accept an FDA letter of approval or other FDA published material as evidence of FDA approval. (See Sec.80.1 of the NCD Manual for coverage of a hydrophilic lens as a corneal bandage.)

100-3, 80.6

NCD for Intraocular Photography (80.6)

Intraocular photography is covered when used for the diagnosis of such conditions as macular degeneration, retinal neoplasms, choroid disturbances and diabetic retinopathy, or to identify glaucoma, multiple sclerosis and other central nervous system abnormalities. Make Medicare payment for the use of this procedure by an opthalmologist in these situations when it is reasonable and necessary for the individual patient to receive these services.

100-3, 80.7

NCD for Refractive Keratoplasty (80.7)

The correction of common refractive errors by eyeglasses, contact lenses or other prosthetic devices is specifically excluded from coverage. The use of radial keratotomy and/or keratoplasty for the purpose of refractive error compensation is considered a substitute or alternative to eye glasses or contact lenses, which are specifically excluded by Sec.1862(a)(7) of the Act (except in certain cases in connection with cataract surgery). In addition, many in the medical community consider such procedures cosmetic surgery, which is excluded by section Sec.1862(a)(10) of the Act. Therefore, radial keratotomy and keratoplasty to treat refractive defects are not covered.

Keratoplasty that treats specific lesions of the cornea, such as phototherapeutic keratectomy that removes scar tissue from the visual field, deals with an abnormality of the eye and is not cosmetic surgery. Such cases may be covered under Sec.1862(a)(1)(A) of the Act.

The use of lasers to treat ophthalmic disease constitutes opthalmalogic surgery. Coverage is restricted to practitioners who have completed an approved training program in ophthalmologic surgery.

100-3, 80.8

NCD for Endothelial Cell Photography (80.8)

Endothelial cell photography is a covered procedure under Medicare when reasonable and necessary for patients who meet one or more of the following criteria:

- Have slit lamp evidence of endothelial dystrophy (cornea guttata),
- Have slit lamp evidence of corneal edema (unilateral or bilateral),
- Are about to undergo a secondary intraocular lens implantation,

- Have had previous intraocular surgery and require cataract surgery,
- Are about to undergo a surgical procedure associated with a higher risk to corneal endothelium; i.e., phacoemulsification, or refractive surgery (see Sec.80.7 for excluded refractive procedures),
- With evidence of posterior polymorphous dystrophy of the cornea or irido-corneal-endothelium syndrome, or
- Are about to be fitted with extended wear contact lenses after intraocular surgery.

When a pre-surgical examination for cataract surgery is performed and the conditions of this section are met, if the only visual problem is cataracts, endothelial cell photography is covered as part of the presurgical comprehensive eye examination or combination brief/intermediate examination provided prior to cataract surgery, and not in addition to it. (See Sec.10.1.)

100-3, 80.9

NCD for Computer Enhanced Perimetry (80.9)

It is a covered service when used in assessing visual fields in patients with glaucoma or other neuropathologic defects.

100-3, 80.10

NCD for Phaco-Emulsification procedure - cataract extraction (80.10)

In view of recommendations of authoritative sources in the field of ophthalmology, the subject technique is viewed as an accepted procedure for removal of cataracts. Accordingly, program reimbursement may be made for necessary services furnished in connection with cataract extraction utilizing the phaco-emulsification procedure.

100-3, 80.11

NCD for Vitrectomy (80.11)

Vitrectomy may be considered reasonable and necessary for the following conditions: vitreous loss incident to cataract surgery, vitreous opacities due to vitreous hemorrhage or other causes, retinal detachments secondary to vitreous strands, proliferative retinopathy, and vitreous retraction. See Chapter 23 of the Medicare Claims Manual for how to determine payment for physician vitrectomy services and Chapter 14 Sec.40 for how to determine payment for ASC facility vitrectomy services. Also, see Chapter 23 Sec.20.9 to identify when, for Medicare payment purposes, certain vitrectomy codes are included in other codes or when codes for other services include vitrectomy codes.

100-3, 80.12

NCD for Intraocular Lenses (IOLs) (80.12)

Intraocular lens implantation services, as well as the lens itself, may be covered if reasonable and necessary for the individual. Implantation services may include hospital, surgical, and other medical services, including pre-implantation ultrasound (A-scan) eye measurement of one or both eyes.

100-3,100.1

NCD for Bariatric Surgery for Treatment of Morbid Obesity (100.1)

A. General

Bariatric surgery procedures are performed to treat comorbid conditions associated with morbid obesity. Two types of surgical procedures are employed. Malabsorptive procedures divert food from the stomach to a lower part of the digestive tract where the normal mixing of digestive fluids and absorption of nutrients cannot occur. Restrictive procedures restrict the size of the stomach and decrease intake. Surgery can combine both types of procedures.

The following are descriptions of bariatric surgery procedures:

1. Roux-en-Y Gastric Bypass (RYGBP)

   The RYGBP achieves weight loss by gastric restriction and malabsorption. Reduction of the stomach to a small gastric pouch (30 cc) results in feelings of satiety following even small meals. This small pouch is connected to a segment of the jejunum, bypassing the duodenum and very proximal small intestine, thereby reducing absorption. RYGBP procedures can be open or laparoscopic.

2. Biliopancreatic Diversion with Duodenal Switch (BPD/DS)

   The BPD achieves weight loss by gastric restriction and malabsorption. The stomach is partially resected, but the remaining capacity is generous compared to that achieved with RYGBP. As such, patients eat relatively normal-sized meals and do not need to restrict intake radically, since the most proximal areas of the small intestine (i.e., the duodenum and jejunum) are bypassed, and substantial malabsorption occurs. The partial BPD/DS is a variant of the BPD procedure. It involves resection of the greater curvature of the stomach, preservation of the pyloric sphincter, and transection of the duodenum above the ampulla of Vater with a duodeno-ileal anastomosis and a lower ileo-ileal anastomosis. BPD/DS procedures can be open or laparoscopic.

3. Adjustable Gastric Banding (AGB)

   The AGB achieves weight loss by gastric restriction only. A band creating a gastric pouch with a capacity of approximately 15 to 30 cc's encircles the uppermost portion of the stomach. The band is an inflatable doughnut-shaped balloon, the diameter of which can be adjusted in the clinic by adding or removing saline via a port that is positioned beneath the skin. The bands are adjustable, allowing the size of the gastric outlet to be modified as needed, depending on the rate of a patient's weight loss. AGB procedures are laparoscopic only.

4. Sleeve Gastrectomy

   Sleeve gastrectomy is a 70%-80% greater curvature gastrectomy (sleeve resection of the stomach) with continuity of the gastric lesser curve being maintained while simultaneously reducing stomach volume. It may be the first step in a two-stage procedure when performing RYGBP. Sleeve gastrectomy procedures can be open or laparoscopic.

5. Vertical Gastric Banding (VGB)

   The VGB achieves weight loss by gastric restriction only. The upper part of the stomach is stapled, creating a narrow gastric inlet or pouch that remains connected with the remainder of the stomach. In addition, a non-adjustable band is placed around this new inlet in an attempt to prevent future enlargement of the stoma (opening). As a result, patients experience a sense of fullness after eating small meals. Weight loss from this procedure results entirely from eating less. VGB procedures are essentially no longer performed.

B. Nationally Covered Indications

Effective for services performed on and after February 21, 2006, Open and laparoscopic Roux-en-Y gastric bypass (RYGBP), open and laparoscopic Biliopancreatic Diversion with Duodenal Switch (BPD/DS), and laparoscopic adjustable gastric banding (LAGB) are covered for Medicare beneficiaries who have a body-mass index > 35, have at least one co-morbidity related to obesity, and have been previously unsuccessful with medical treatment for obesity. These procedures are only covered when performed at facilities that are: (1) certified by the American College of Surgeons as a Level 1 Bariatric Surgery Center (program standards and requirements in effect on February 15, 2006); or (2) certified by the American Society for Bariatric Surgery as a Bariatric Surgery Center of Excellence (program standards and requirements in effect on February 15, 2006).

Effective for services performed on and after February 12, 2009, the Centers for Medicare & Medicaid Services (CMS) determines that Type 2 diabetes mellitus is a co-morbidity for purposes of this NCD.

A list of approved facilities and their approval dates are listed and maintained on the CMS Coverage Web site at http://www.cms.hhs.gov/center/coverage.asp, and published in the Federal Register.

C. Nationally Non-Covered Indications

The following bariatric surgery procedures are non-covered for all Medicare beneficiaries:

- Open adjustable gastric banding;
- Open and laparoscopic sleeve gastrectomy; and,
- Open and laparoscopic vertical banded gastroplasty.

The two previous non-coverage determinations remain unchanged - Gastric Balloon (Section 100.11) and Intestinal Bypass (Section 100.8).

D. Other

N/A

100-3, 100.2

NCD for Endoscopy (100.2)

Endoscopic procedures are covered when reasonable and necessary for the individual patient.

100-3, 100.4

NCD for Esophageal Manometry (100.4)

Esophageal manometry is covered under Medicare where it is determined to be reasonable and necessary for the individual patient.

100-3, 100.5

NCD for Diagnostic Breath Analyses (100.5)

The Following Breath Test is Covered:

- Lactose breath hydrogen to detect lactose malabsorption .

The Following Breath Tests are Excluded from Coverage;

- Lactulose breath hydrogen for diagnosing small bowel bacterial overgrowth and measuring small bowel transit time.
- CO2 for diagnosing bile acid malabsorption.
- CO2 for diagnosing fat malabsorption.

100-3, 100.8

NCD for Intestinal By-Pass Surgery (100.8)

The safety of intestinal bypass surgery for treatment of obesity has not been demonstrated. Severe adverse reactions such as steatorrhea, electrolyte depletion, liver failure, arthralgia, hypoplasia of bone marrow, and avitaminosis have sometimes occurred as a result of this procedure. It does not meet the reasonable and necessary provisions of Sec.1862(a)(1) of the Act and is not a covered Medicare procedure.

100-3, 100.9

NCD for Implantation of Anti-Gastroesophageal Reflux Device (100.9)

The implantation of this device may be considered reasonable and necessary in specific clinical situations where a conventional valvuloplasty procedure is contraindicated. The implantation of an anti-gastroesophageal reflux device is covered only for patients with documented severe or life threatening gastroesophageal reflux disease whose conditions have been resistant to medical treatment and who also:

- have esophageal involvement with progressive systemic sclerosis; or
- have foreshortening of the esophagus such that insufficient tissue exists to permit a valve reconstruction; or
- are poor surgical risks for a valvuloplasty procedure; or
- have failed previous attempts at surgical treatment with valvuloplasty procedures.

100-3, 100.10

NCD for Injection Sclerotherapy for Esophageal Variceal Bleeding (100.10)

Injection sclerotherapy is a technique involving insertion of a flexible fiberoptic endoscope into the esophagus, and the injection of a sclerosing agent or solution into the varicosities to control bleeding. This procedure is covered under Medicare.

100-3, 100.12

NCD for Gastrophotography (100.12)

Gastrophotography is an accepted procedure for diagnosis and treatment of gastrointestinal disorders. The photographic record provided by this procedure is often necessary for consultation and/or followup purposes and when required for such purposes, is more valuable than a conventional gastroscopic examination. Such a record facilitates the documentation and evaluation (healing or worsening) of lesions such as the gastric ulcer, facilitates consultation between physicians concerning difficult-to-interpret lesions, provides preoperative characterization for the surgeon, and permits better diagnosis of postoperative gastric bleeding to help determine whether there is a need for reoperation. Therefore, program reimbursement may be made for this procedure.

100-3, 100.13

NCD for Laparoscopic Cholecystectomy (100.13)

Laparoscopic cholecystectomy is a covered surgical procedure in which a diseased gall bladder is removed through the use of instruments introduced via cannulae, with vision of the operative field maintained by use of a high-resolution television camera-monitor system (video laparoscope). For inpatient claims, use ICD-9-CM code 51.23, Laparoscopic cholecystectomy. For all other claims, use CPT codes 49310 for laparoscopy, surgical; cholecystectomy (any method), and 49311 for laparoscopy, surgical: cholecystectomy with cholangiography.

100-3, 110.1

NCD for Hyperthermia for Treatment of Cancer (110.1)

Local hyperthermia is covered under Medicare when used in connection with radiation therapy for the treatment of primary or metastatic cutaneous or subcutaneous superficial malignancies. It is not covered when used alone or in connection with chemotherapy.

100-3,110.2

NCD for Certain Drugs Distributed by the National Cancer Institute (110.2)

A physician is eligible to receive Group C drugs from the Division of Cancer Treatment only if the following requirements are met:

A physician must be registered with the NCI as an investigator by having completed an FD-Form 1573;

A written request for the drug, indicating the disease to be treated, must be submitted to the NCI;

The use of the drug must be limited to indications outlined in the NCI's guidelines; and

All adverse reactions must be reported to the Investigational Drug Branch of the Division of Cancer Treatment.

In view of these NCI controls on distribution and use of Group C drugs, intermediaries may assume, in the absence of evidence to the contrary, that a Group C drug and the related hospital stay are covered if all other applicable coverage requirements are satisfied.

If there is reason to question coverage in a particular case, the matter should be resolved with the assistance of the Quality improvemetn organization (QIO), or if there is none, the assistance of your medical consultants.

Information regarding those drugs which are classified as Group C drugs may be obtained from:

Office of the Chief, Investigational Drug Branch
Division of Cancer Treatment, CTEP, Landow Building
Room 4C09, National Cancer Institute
Bethesda, Maryland 20205

100-3, 110.3

NCD for Anti-Inhibitor Coagulant Complex (AICC) (110.3)

Anti-inhibitor coagulant complex, AICC, is a drug used to treat hemophilia in patients with factor VIII inhibitor antibodies. AICC has been shown to be safe and effective and has Medicare coverage when furnished to patients with hemophilia A and inhibitor antibodies to factor VIII who have major bleeding episodes and who fail to respond to other, less expensive therapies.

100-3, 110.4

NCD for Extracorporeal Photopheresis (110.4)

B. Nationally Covered Indications

The CMS has determined that extracorporeal photopheresis is reasonable and necessary under Sec.1862(a)(1)(A) of the Social Security Act under the following circumstances:

1. Effective April 8, 1988, Medicare provides coverage for:

   Palliative treatment of skin manifestations of CTCL that has not responded to other therapy.

2. Effective December 19, 2006, Medicare also provides coverage for:

   Patients with acute cardiac allograft rejection whose disease is refractory to standard immunosuppressive drug treatment; and

   Patients with chronic graft versus host disease whose disease is refractory to standard immunosuppressive drug treatment.

C. Nationally Noncovered Indications

All other indications for extracorporeal photopheresis remain noncovered.

D. Other

Claims processing instructions can be found in chapter 32, section 190 of the Medicare Claims Processing Manual.

(This NCD last reviewed December 2006.)

100-3, 110.5

NCD for Granulocyte Transfusions (110.5)

Granulocyte transfusions to patients suffering from severe infection and granulocytopenia are a covered service under Medicare. Granulocytopenia is usually identified as fewer than 500 granulocytes/mm 3 whole blood. Accepted indications for granulocyte transfusions include:

Granulocytopenia with evidence of gram negative sepsis; and

Granulocytopenia in febrile patients with local progressive infections unresponsive to appropriate antibiotic therapy, thought to be due to gram negative organisms.

100-3, 110.6

NCD for Scalp Hypothermia During Chemotherapy, to Prevent Hair Loss (110.6)

While ice-filled bags or bandages or other devices used for scalp hypothermia during chemotherapy may be covered as supplies of the kind commonly furnished without a separate charge, no separate charge for them would be recognized.

100-3, 110.7

NCD for Blood Transfusions (110.7)

B. Policy Governing Transfusions

For Medicare coverage purposes, it is important to distinguish between a transfusion itself and preoperative blood services; e.g., collection, processing, storage. Medically necessary transfusion of blood, regardless of the type, may generally be a covered service under both Part A and Part B of Medicare. Coverage does not make a distinction between the transfusion of homologous, autologous, or donor-directed blood. With respect to the coverage of the services associated with the preoperative collection, processing, and storage of autologous and donor-directed blood, the following policies apply.

1. Hospital Part A and B Coverage and Payment

   Under Sec.1862(a)(14) of the Act, non-physician services furnished to hospital patients are covered and paid for as hospital services. As provided in Sec.1886 of the Act, under the prospective [payment system (PPS), the diganosis related group (DRG) payment to the hospital includes all covered blood and blood processing expenses, whether or not the blood is eventually used.

   Under its provider agreement, a hospital is required to furnish or arrange for all covered services furnished to hospital patients. medicare payment is made to the hospital, under PPS or cost reimbursement, for covered inpatient services, and it is intended to reflect payment for all costs of furnishing those services.

2. Nonhospital Part B Coverage

   Under Part B, to be eligible for separate coverage, a service must fit the definition of one of the services authorized by Sec.1832 of the Act. These services are defined in 42 CFR 410.10 and do not include a separate category for a supplier's services associated with blood donation services, either autologous or donor-directed. That is, the collection, processing, and storage of blood for later transfusion into the beneficiary is not recognized as a separate service under Part B. Therefore, there is no avenue through which a blood supplier can receive direct payment under Part B for blood donation services.

C.Perioperative Blood Salvage

When the perioperative blood salvage process is used in surgery on a hospital patient, payment made to the hospital (under PPS or through cost reimbursement) for the procedure in which that process is used is intended to encompass payment for all costs relating to that process.

100-3, 110.8

NCD for Blood Platelet Transfusions (110.8)

Blood platelet transplants are safe and effective for the correction of thrombocytopenia and other blood defects. It is covered under Medicare when treatment is reasonable and necessary for the individual patient.

100-3, 110.8.1

NCD for Stem Cell Transplantation (110.8.1)

A. General

Stem cell transplantation is a process in which stem cells are harvested from either a patient's (autologous) or donor's (allogeneic) bone marrow or peripheral blood for intravenous infusion. Autologous stem cell transplants (AuSCT) must be used to effect hematopoietic reconstitution following severely myelotoxic doses of chemotherapy (HDCT) and/or radiotherapy used to treat various malignancies. Allogeneic stem cell transplants may be used to restore function in recipients having an inherited or acquired deficiency or defect. Hematopoietic stem cells are multi-potent stem cells that give rise to all the blood cell types; these stem cells form blood and immune cells. A hematopoietic stem cell is a cell isolated from blood or bone marrow that can renew itself, differentiate to a variety of specialized cells, can mobilize out of the bone marrow into circulating blood, and can undergo programmed cell death, called apoptosis - a process by which cells that are unneeded or detrimental self destruct.

The Centers for Medicare & Medicaid Services (CMS) is clarifying that bone marrow and peripheral blood stem cell transplantation is a process which includes mobilization, harvesting, and transplant of bone marrow or peripheral blood stem cells and the administration of high dose chemotherapy or radiotherapy prior to the actual transplant. When bone marrow or peripheral blood stem cell transplantation is covered, all necessary steps are included in coverage. When bone marrow or peripheral blood stem cell transplantation is non-covered, none of the steps are covered.

1. Allogeneic Hematopoietic Stem Cell Transplantation (HSCT)

   Allogeneic hematopoietic stem cell transplantation (HSCT) is a procedure in which a portion of a healthy donor's stem cell or bone marrow is obtained and prepared for intravenous infusion.

   a. Nationally Covered Indications

      The following uses of allogeneic HSCT are covered under Medicare:

      i. Effective for services performed on or after August 1, 1978, for the treatment of leukemia, leukemia in remission, or aplastic anemia when it is reasonable and necessary,

      ii. Effective for services performed on or after June 3, 1985, for the treatment of severe combined immunodeficiency disease (SCID) and for the treatment of Wiskott-Aldrich syndrome.

      iii. Effective for services performed on or after August 4, 2010, for the treatment of Myelodysplastic Syndromes (MDS) pursuant to Coverage with Evidence Development (CED) in the context of a Medicare-approved, prospective clinical study.

The MDS refers to a group of diverse blood disorders in which the bone marrow does not produce enough healthy, functioning blood cells. These disorders are varied with regard to clinical characteristics, cytologic and pathologic features, and cytogenetics. The abnormal production of blood cells in the bone marrow leads to low blood cell counts, referred to as cytopenias, which are a hallmark feature of MDS along with a dysplastic and hypercellular-appearing bone marrow.

Medicare payment for these beneficiaries will be restricted to patients enrolled in an approved clinical study. In accordance with the Stem Cell Therapeutic and Research Act of 2005 (US Public Law 109-129) a standard dataset is collected for all allogeneic transplant patients in the United States by the Center for International Blood and Marrow Transplant Research. The elements in this dataset, comprised of two mandatory forms plus one additional form, encompass the information we require for a study under CED.

A prospective clinical study seeking Medicare payment for treating a beneficiary with allogeneic HSCT for MDS pursuant to CED must meet one or more aspects of the following questions:

- Prospectively, compared to Medicare beneficiaries with MDS who do not receive HSCT, do Medicare beneficiaries with MDS who receive HSCT have improved outcomes as indicated by:
  - Relapse-free mortality,
  - progression free survival,
  - relapse, and
  - overall survival?
- Prospectively, in Medicare beneficiaries with MDS who receive HSCT, how do International Prognostic Scoring System (IPSS) score, patient age, cytopenias and comorbidities predict the following outcomes:
  - Relapse-free mortality,
  - progression free survival,
  - relapse, and
  - overall survival?
- Prospectively, in Medicare beneficiaries with MDS who receive HSCT, what treatment facility characteristics predict meaningful clinical improvement in the following outcomes:
  - Relapse-free mortality,
  - progression free survival,
  - relapse, and
  - overall survival?

In addition, the clinical study must adhere to the following standards of scientific integrity and relevance to the Medicare population:

a. The principal purpose of the research study is to test whether a particular intervention potentially improves the participants' health outcomes.

b. The research study is well supported by available scientific and medical information or it is intended to clarify or establish the health outcomes of interventions already in common clinical use.

c. The research study does not unjustifiably duplicate existing studies.

d. The research study design is appropriate to answer the research question being asked in the study.

e. The research study is sponsored by an organization or individual capable of executing the proposed study successfully.

f. The research study is in compliance with all applicable Federal regulations concerning the protection of human subjects found at 45 CFR Part 46.

g. All aspects of the research study are conducted according to appropriate standards of scientific integrity (see http://www.icmje.org).

h. The research study has a written protocol that clearly addresses, or incorporates by reference, the standards listed here as Medicare requirements for CED coverage.

i. The clinical research study is not designed to exclusively test toxicity or disease pathophysiology in healthy individuals. Trials of all medical technologies measuring therapeutic outcomes as one of the objectives meet this standard only if the disease or condition being studied is life threatening as defined in 21 CFR §312.81(a) and the patient has no other viable treatment options.

j. The clinical research study is registered on the ClinicalTrials.gov Web site by the principal sponsor/investigator prior to the enrollment of the first study subject.

k. The research study protocol specifies the method and timing of public release of all pre-specified outcomes to be measured including release of outcomes if outcomes are negative or study is terminated early. The results must be made public within 24 months of the end of data collection. If a report is planned to be published in a peer-reviewed journal, then that initial release may be an abstract that meets the requirements of the International Committee of Medical Journal Editors (http://www.icmje.org). However a full report of the outcomes must be made public no later than 3 years after the end of data collection.

l. The research study protocol must explicitly discuss subpopulations affected by the treatment under investigation, particularly traditionally underrepresented groups in clinical studies, how the inclusion and exclusion criteria effect enrollment of these populations, and a plan for the retention and reporting of said populations on the trial. If the inclusion and exclusion criteria are expected to have a negative effect on the recruitment or retention of underrepresented populations, the protocol must discuss why these criteria are necessary.

m. The research study protocol explicitly discusses how the results are or are not expected to be generalizable to the Medicare population to infer whether Medicare patients may benefit from the intervention. Separate discussions in the protocol may be necessary for populations eligible for Medicare due to age, disability or Medicaid eligibility. Consistent with section 1142 of the Social Security Act, the Agency for Health Research and Quality (AHRQ) supports clinical research studies that CMS determines meet the above-listed standards and address the above-listed research questions.

The clinical research study should also have the following features:

- It should be a prospective, longitudinal study with clinical information from the period before HSCT and short- and long-term follow-up information.
- Outcomes should be measured and compared among pre-specified subgroups within the cohort.
- The study should be powered to make inferences in subgroup analyses.
- Risk stratification methods should be used to control for selection bias. Data elements to be used in risk stratification models should include:

Patient selection:

- Patient Age at diagnosis of MDS and at transplantation
- Date of onset of MDS
- Disease classification (specific MDS subtype at diagnosis prior to preparative/conditioning regimen using World Health Organization (WHO) classifications). Include presence/absence of refractory cytopenias
- Comorbid conditions
- IPSS score (and WHO-adapted Prognostic Scoring System (WPSS) score, if applicable) at diagnosis and prior to transplantation
- Score immediately prior to transplantation and one year post-transplantation Disease assessment at diagnosis at start of preparative regimen and last assessment prior to preparative regimen Subtype of MDS (refractory anemia with or without blasts, degree of blasts, etc.)

Type of preparative/conditioning regimen administered (myeloabalative, non-myeloablative, reduced–intensity conditioning)

- Donor type
- Cell Source
- IPSS Score at diagnosis Facilities must submit the required transplant essential data to the Stem Cell Therapeutics Outcomes Database.

b. Nationally Non-Covered Indications

Effective for services performed on or after May 24, 1996, allogeneic HSCT is not covered as treatment for multiple myeloma.

2. Autologous Stem Cell Transplantation (AuSCT)

Autologous stem cell transplantation (AuSCT) is a technique for restoring stem cells using the patient's own previously stored cells.

a. Nationally Covered Indications

   i. Effective for services performed on or after April 28, 1989, AuSCT is considered reasonable and necessary under §l862(a)(1)(A) of the Social Security Act (the Act) for the following conditions and is covered under Medicare for patients with:

      - Acute leukemia in remission who have a high probability of relapse and who have no human leucocyte antigens (HLA)-matched;
      - Resistant non-Hodgkin's lymphomas or those presenting with poor prognostic features following an initial response;
      - Recurrent or refractory neuroblastoma; or
      - Advanced Hodgkin's disease who have failed conventional therapy and have no HLA-matched donor.

   ii. Effective October 1, 2000, single AuSCT is only covered for Durie-Salmon Stage II or III patients that fit the following requirements:

      - Newly diagnosed or responsive multiple myeloma. This includes those patients with previously untreated disease, those with at least a partial response to prior chemotherapy (defined as a 50% decrease either in measurable paraprotein [serum and/or urine] or in bone marrow infiltration, sustained for at least 1 month), and those in responsive relapse; and,

- Adequate cardiac, renal, pulmonary, and hepatic function.

iii. Effective for services performed on or after March 15, 2005, when recognized clinical risk factors are employed to select patients for transplantation, high dose melphalan (HDM) together with AuSCT is reasonable and necessary for Medicare beneficiaries of any age group with primary amyloid light chain (AL) amyloidosis who meet the following criteria:

- Amyloid deposition in 2 or fewer organs; and,
- Cardiac left ventricular ejection fraction (EF) greater than 45%.

b. Nationally Non-Covered Indications

Insufficient data exist to establish definite conclusions regarding the efficacy of AuSCT for the following conditions:

- Acute leukemia not in remission;
- Chronic granulocytic leukemia;
- Solid tumors (other than neuroblastoma);
- Up to October 1, 2000, multiple myeloma;
- Tandem transplantation (multiple rounds of AuSCT) for patients with multiple myeloma;
- Effective October 1, 2000, non primary AL amyloidosis; and,
- Effective October 1, 2000, thru March 14, 2005, primary AL amyloidosis for Medicare beneficiaries age 64 or older.

In these cases, AuSCT is not considered reasonable and necessary within the meaning of §l862(a)(1)(A) of the Act and is not covered under Medicare.

B. Other
All other indications for stem cell transplantation not otherwise noted above as covered or non-covered nationally remain at local contractor discretion.

(This NCD last reviewed August 2010.)

100-3, 110.9

NCD for Antigens Prepared for Sublingual Administration (110.9)

For antigens provided to patients on or after November 17, 1996, Medicare does not cover such antigens if they are to be administered sublingually, i.e., by placing drops under the patient's tongue. This kind of allergy therapy has not been proven to be safe and effective. Antigens are covered only if they are administered by injection.

100-3, 110.10

NCD for Intravenous Iron Therapy (110.10)

Effective December 1, 2000, Medicare covers sodium ferric gluconate complex in sucrose injection as a first line treatment of iron deficiency anemia when furnished intravenously to patients undergoing chronic hemodialysis who are receiving supplemental erythropoeitin therapy.

Effective October 1, 2001, Medicare also covers iron sucrose injection as a first line treatment of iron deficiency anemia when furnished intravenously to patients undergoing chronic hemodialysis who are receiving supplemental erythropoeitin therapy.

100-3, 110.12

NCD for Challenge Ingestion Food Testing (110.12)

This procedure is covered when it is used on an outpatient basis if it is reasonable and necessary for the individual patient.

Challenge ingestion food testing has not been proven to be effective in the diagnosis of rheumatoid arthritis, depression, or respiratory disorders. Accordingly, its use in the diagnosis of these conditions is not reasonable and necessary within the meaning of section 1862(a)(1) of the Medicare law, and no program payment is made for this procedure when it is so used.

100-3, 110.14

NCD for Apheresis (Therapeutic Pheresis) (110.14)

B. Indications
Apheresis is covered for the following indications:

- Plasma exchange for acquired myasthenia gravis;
- Leukapheresis in the treatment of leukemekia
- Plasmapheresis in the treatment of primary macroglobulinemia (Waldenstrom);
- Treatment of hyperglobulinemias, including (but not limited to) multiple myelomas, cryoglobulinemia and hyperviscosity syndromes;
- Plasmapheresis or plasma exchange as a last resort treatment of thromobotic thrombocytopenic purpura (TTP);
- Plasmapheresis or plasma exchange in the last resort treatment of life threatening rheumatoid vasculitis;
- Plasma perfusion of charcoal filters for treatment of pruritis of cholestatic liver disease;
- Plasma exchange in the treatment of Goodpasture's Syndrome;
- Plasma exchange in the treatment of glomerulonephritis associated with antiglomerular basement membrane antibodies and advancing renal failure or pulmonary hemorrhage;
- Treatment of chronic relapsing polyneuropathy for patients with severe or life threatening symptoms who have failed to respond to conventional therapy;
- Treatment of life threatening scleroderma and polymyositis when the patient is unresponsive to conventional therapy;
- Treatment of Guillain-Barre Syndrome; and
- Treatment of last resort for life threatening systemic lupus erythematosus (SLE) when conventional therapy has failed to prevent clinical deterioration.

C. Settings
Apheresis is covered only when performed in a hospital setting (either inpatient or outpatient). or in a nonhospital setting. e.g. physician directed clinic when the following conditions are met:

- A physician (or a number of physicians) is present to perform medical services and to respond to medical emergencies at all times during patient care hours;
- Each patient is under the care of a physician; and
- All nonphysician services are furnished under the direct, personal supervision of a physician.

100-3, 110.15

NCD for Ultrafiltration, Hemoperfusion and Hemofiltration (110.15)

A. Ultrafiltration.
This is a process for removing excess fluid from the blood through the dialysis membrane by means of pressure. It is not a substitute for dialysis. Ultrafiltration is utilized in cases where excess fluid cannot be removed easily during the regular course of hemodialysis. When it is performed, it is commonly done during the first hour or two of each hemodialysis on patients who, e.g., have refractory edema. Ultrafiltration is a covered procedure under the Medicare program (effective for services performed on and after 9/1/79).

Predialysis Ultrafiltration.--While this procedure requires additional staff care, the facility dialysis rate is intended to cover the full range of complicated and uncomplicated nonacute dialysis treatments. Therefore, no additional facility charge is recognized for predialysis ultrafiltration. The physician's role in ultrafiltration varies with the stability of the patient's condition. In unstable patients, the physician may need to be present at the initiation of dialysis, and available either in- house or in close proximity to monitor the patient carefully. In patients who are relatively stable, but who seem to accumulate excessive weight gain, the procedure requires only a modest increase in physician involvement over routine outpatient hemodialysis.

Occasionally, medical complications may occur which require that ultrafiltration be performed separate from the dialysis treatment, and in these cases an additional charge can be recognized. However, the claim must be documented as to why the ultrafiltration could not have been performed at the same time as the dialysis.

B. Hemoperfusion.
This is a process which removes substances from the blood using a charcoal or resin artificial kidney. When used in the treatment of life threatening drug overdose, hemoperfusion is a covered service for patients with or without renal failure (effective for services performed on and after 9/1/79). Hemoperfusion generally requires a physician to be present to initiate treatment and to be present in the hospital or an adjacent medical office during the entire procedure, as changes may be sudden. Special staff training and equipment are required.

Develop charges for hemoperfusion in the same manner as for any new or unusual service. One or two treatments are usually all that is necessary to remove the toxic compound; document additional treatments. Hemoperfusion may be performed concurrently with dialysis, and in those cases payment for the hemoperfusion reflects only the additional care rendered over and above the care given with dialysis.

The effects of using hemoperfusion to improve the results of chronic hemodialysis are not known. Therefore, hemoperfusion is not a covered service when used to improve the results of hemodialysis. In addition, it has not been demonstrated that the use of hemoperfusion in conjunction with deferoxamine (DFO), in treating symptomatic patients with iron overload, is efficacious. There is also a paucity of data regarding its efficacy in treating asymptomatic patients with iron overload. Therefore, hemoperfusion used in conjunction with DFO in treating patients with iron overload is not a covered service; i.e., it is not considered reasonable and necessary within the meaning of Sec.1862(a)(1) of the Act.

However, the use of hemoperfusion in conjunction with DFO for the treatment of patients with aluminum toxicity has been demonstrated to be clinically efficacious and is therefore regarded as a covered service.

C. Hemofiltration.
This is a process which removes fluid, electrolytes and other low molecular weight toxic substances from the blood by filtration through hollow artificial membranes and may be routinely performed in 3 weekly sessions. Hemofiltration (which is also known as diafiltration) is a covered procedure under Medicare and is a safe and effective technique for the treatment of ESRD patients and an alternative to peritoneal dialysis and hemodialysis (effective for services performed on and after August 20, 1987). In contrast to both hemodialysis and peritoneal dialysis treatments, which eliminate dissolved substances via diffusion across semipermeable membranes, hemofiltration mimics the filtration process of the normal kidney. The technique requires an arteriovenous access. Hemofiltration may be performed either in facility or at home.

The procedure is most advantageous when applied to high-risk unstable patients, such as older patients with cardiovascular diseases or diabetes, because there are fewer side effects such as hypotension, hypertension or volume overload.

100-3, 110.16

NCD for Nonselective (Random) Transfusions and Living Related Donor Specific Transfusions (DST) in Kidney Transplantation (110.16)

These pretransplant transfusions are covered under Medicare without a specific limitation on the number of transfusions, subject to the normal Medicare blood deductible provisions. Where blood is given directly to the transplant patient; e.g., in the case of donor specific transfusions, the blood is considered replaced for purposes of the blood deductible provisions.

100-3, 130.1

NCD for Inpatient Hospital Stays for the Treatment of Alcoholism (130.1)

A. Inpatient Hospital Stay for Alcohol Detoxification

Many hospitals provide detoxification services during the more acute stages of alcoholism or alcohol withdrawal. When the high probability or occurrence of medical complications (e.g., delirium, confusion, trauma, or unconsciousness) during detoxification for acute alcoholism or alcohol withdrawal necessitates the constant availability of physicians and/or complex medical equipment found only in the hospital setting, inpatient hospital care during this period is considered reasonable and necessary and is therefore covered under the program. Generally, detoxification can be accomplished within 2-3 days with an occasional need for up to 5 days where the patient's condition dictates. This limit (5 days) may be extended in an individual case where there is a need for a longer period for detoxification for a particular patient. In such cases, however, there should be documentation by a physician which substantiates that a longer period of detoxification was reasonable and necessary. When the detoxification needs of an individual no longer require an inpatient hospital setting, coverage should be denied on the basis that inpatient hospital care is not reasonable and necessary as required by section l862(a)(l) of the Act. Following detoxification a patient may be transferred to an inpatient rehabilitation unit or discharged to a residential treatment program or outpatient treatment setting.

B. Inpatient Hospital Stay for Alcohol Rehabilitation

Hospitals may also provide structured inpatient alcohol rehabilitation programs to the chronic alcoholic. These programs are composed primarily of coordinated educational and psychotherapeutic services provided on a group basis. Depending on the subject matter, a series of lectures, discussions, films, and group therapy sessions are led by either physicians, psychologists, or alcoholism counselors from the hospital or various outside organizations. In addition, individual psychotherapy and family counseling (see Sec.70.1 of the NCD Manual) may be provided in selected cases. These programs are conducted under the supervision and direction of a physician. Patients may directly enter an inpatient hospital rehabilitation program after having undergone detoxification in the same hospital or in another hospital or may enter an inpatient hospital rehabilitation program without prior hospitalization for detoxification.

Alcohol rehabilitation can be provided in a variety of settings other than the hospital setting. In order for an inpatient hospital stay for alcohol rehabilitation to be covered under Medicare it must be medically necessary for the care to be provided in the inpatient hospital setting rather than in a less costly facility or on an outpatient basis. Inpatient hospital care for receipt of an alcohol rehabilitation program would generally be medically necessary where either (l) there is documentation by the physician that recent alcohol rehabilitation services in a less intensive setting or on an outpatient basis have proven unsuccessful and, as a consequence, the patient requires the supervision and intensity of services which can only be found in the controlled environment of the hospital, or (2) only the hospital environment can assure the medical management or control of the patient's concomitant conditions during the course of alcohol rehabilitation. (However, a patient's concomitant condition may make the use of certain alcohol treatment modalities medically inappropriate.) In addition, the "active treatment" criteria (see the Medicare Benefit Policy Manual, Chapter 2, "Inpatient Psychiatric Hospital Services," Sec.20) should be applied to psychiatric care in the general hospital as well as to psychiatric care in a psychiatric hospital. Since alcoholism is classifiable as a psychiatric condition the "active treatment" criteria must also be met in order for alcohol rehabilitation services to be covered under Medicare. (Thus, it is the combined need for "active treatment" and for covered care which can only be provided in the inpatient hospital setting, rather than the fact that rehabilitation immediately follows a period of detoxification, which provides the basis for coverage of inpatient hospital alcohol rehabilitation programs.) Generally 16-19 days of rehabilitation services are sufficient to bring a patient to a point where care could be continued in other than an inpatient hospital setting. An inpatient hospital stay for alcohol rehabilitation may be extended beyond this limit in an individual case where a longer period of alcohol rehabilitation is medically necessary. In such cases, however, there should be documentation by a physician which substantiates the need for such care. Where the rehabilitation needs of an individual no longer require an inpatient hospital setting, coverage should be denied on the basis that inpatient hospital care is not reasonable and necessary as required by section l862(a)(l) of the Act.

Subsequent admissions to the inpatient hospital setting for alcohol rehabilitation followup, reinforcement, or "recap" treatments are considered to be readmissions (rather than an extension of the original stay) and must meet the requirements of this section for coverage under Medicare. Prior admissions to the inpatient hospital setting--either in the same hospital or in a different hospital--may be an indication that the "active treatment" requirements are not met (i.e., there is no reasonable expectation of improvement) and the stay should not be covered. Accordingly, there should be documentation to establish that "readmission" to the hospital setting for alcohol rehabilitation services can reasonably be expected to result in improvement of the patient's condition. For example, the documentation should indicate what changes in the patient's medical condition, social or emotional status, or treatment plan make improvement likely, or why the patient's initial hospital treatment was not sufficient.

C. Combined Alcohol Detoxification/Rehabilitation Programs.

iscal intermediaries should apply the guidelines in A. and B. above to both phases of a combined inpatient hospital alcohol detoxification/rehabilitation program. Not all patients who require the inpatient hospital setting for detoxification also need the inpatient hospital setting for rehabilitation. (See Sec.130.1 of the NCD Manual for coverage of outpatient hospital alcohol rehabilitation services.) Where the inpatient hospital setting is medically necessary for both alcohol detoxification and rehabilitation, generally a 3-week period is reasonable and necessary to bring the patient to the point where care can be continued in other than an inpatient hospital setting.

Decisions regarding reasonableness and necessity of treatment, the need for an inpatient hospital level of care, and length of treatment should be made by intermediaries based on accepted medical practice with the advice of their medical consultant. (In hospitals under PSRO review, PSRO determinations of medical necessity of services and appropriateness of the level of care at which services are provided are binding on the title XVIII fiscal intermediaries for purposes of adjudicating claims for payment.)

100-3, 130.2

NCD for Outpatient Hospital Services for Treatment of Alcoholism (130.2)

Coverage is available for both diagnostic and therapeutic services furnished for the treatment of alcoholism by the hospital to outpatients subject to the same rules applicable to outpatient hospital services in general. While there is no coverage for day hospitalization programs, per se, individual services which meet the requirements in the Medicare Benefit Policy Manual, Chapter 6, Sec.20 may be covered. (Meals, transportation and recreational and social activities do not fall within the scope of covered outpatient hospital services under Medicare.)

All services must be reasonable and necessary for diagnosis or treatment of the patient's condition (see the Medicare Benefit Policy Manual, chapter 16 Sec.20). Thus, educational services and family counseling would only be covered where they are directly related to treatment of the patient's condition. The frequency of treatment and period of time over which it occurs must also be reasonable and necessary.

100-3, 130.3

NCD for Chemical Aversion Therapy for Treatment of Alcoholism (130.3)

Available evidence indicates that chemical aversion therapy may be an effective component of certain alcoholism treatment programs, particularly as part of multimodality treatment programs which include other behavioral techniques and therapies, such as psychotherapy. Based on this evidence, CMS's medical consultants have recommended that chemical aversion therapy be covered under Medicare. However, since chemical aversion therapy is a demanding therapy which may not be appropriate for all Medicare beneficiaries needing treatment for alcoholism, a physician should certify to the appropriateness of chemical aversion therapy in the individual case. Therefore, if chemical aversion therapy for treatment of alcoholism is determined to be reasonable and necessary for an individual patient, it is covered under Medicare.

When it is medically necessary for a patient to receive chemical aversion therapy as a hospital inpatient, coverage for care in that setting is available. (See Sec.130.1 regarding coverage of multimodality treatment programs.) Followup treatments for chemical aversion therapy can generally be provided on an outpatient basis. Thus, where a patient is admitted as an inpatient for receipt of chemical aversion therapy, there must be documentation by the physician of the need in the individual case for the inpatient hospital admission.

Decisions regarding reasonableness and necessity of treatment and the need for an inpatient hospital level of care should be made by intermediaries based on accepted medical practice with the advice of their medical consultant. (In hospitals under QIO review, QIO determinations of medical necessity of services and appropriateness of the level of care at which services are provided are binding on the title XVIII fiscal intermediaries for purposes of adjudicating claims for payment.)

100-3, 130.4

NCD for Electrical Aversion Therapy for Treatment of Alcoholism (130.4)

Electrical aversion therapy has not been shown to be safe and effective and therefore is excluded from coverage.

100-3, 130.5

NCD for Treatment of Alcoholism and Drug Abuse in a Freestanding Clinic (130.5)

Coverage is available for alcoholism or drug abuse treatment services (such as drug therapy, psychotherapy, and patient education) that are provided incident to a physician's professional service in a freestanding clinic to patients who, for example, have been discharged from an inpatient hospital stay for the treatment of alcoholism or drug abuse or to individuals who are not in the acute stages of alcoholism or drug abuse but require treatment. The coverage available for these services is subject to the same rules generally applicable to the coverage of clinic services. Of course, the services also must be reasonable and necessary for the diagnosis or treatment of the individual's alcoholism or drug abuse. The Part B psychiatric limitation would apply to alcoholism or drug abuse treatment services furnished by physicians to individuals who are not hospital inpatients.

100-3, 130.6

NCD for Treatment of Drug Abuse (Chemical Dependency) (130.6)

Accordingly, when it is medically necessary for a patient to receive detoxification and/or rehabilitation for drug substance abuse as a hospital inpatient, coverage for care in that setting is available. Coverage is also available for treatment services that are provided in the outpatient department of a hospital to patients who, for example, have been discharged from an inpatient stay for the treatment of drug substance abuse or who require treatment but do not require the availability and intensity of services found only in the inpatient hospital setting. The coverage available for these services is subject to the same rules generally applicable to the coverage of outpatient hospital services. The services must also be reasonable and necessary for treatment of the individual's condition. Decisions regarding reasonableness and necessity of treatment, the need for an inpatient hospital level of care, and length of treatment should be made by intermediaries based on accepted medical practice with the advice of their medical consultant. (In hospitals under QIO review, QIO determinations of medical necessity of services and appropriateness of the level of care at which services are provided are binding on the title XVIII fiscal intermediaries for purposes of adjudicating claims for payment.)

100-3, 130.7

NCD for Withdrawal Treatments for Narcotic Addictions (130.7)

Withdrawal is an accepted treatment for narcotic addiction, and Part B payment can be made for these services if they are provided by the physician directly or under his personal supervision and if they are reasonable and necessary. In reviewing claims, reasonableness and necessity are determined with the aid of the contractor's medical staff.

Drugs that the physician provides in connection with this treatment are also covered if they cannot be self-administered and meet all other statutory requirements.

100-3, 130.8

NCD for Hemodialysis for Treatment of Schizophrenia (130.8)

Scientific evidence supporting use of hemodialysis as a safe and effective means of treatment for schizophrenia is inconclusive at this time. Accordingly, Medicare does not cover hemodialysis for treatment of schizophrenia.

100-3, 140.1

NCD for Abortion (140.1)

Abortions are not covered Medicare procedures except:

1. If the pregnancy is the result of an act of rape or incest; or
2. In the case where a woman suffers from a physical disorder, physical injury, or physical illness, including a life-endangering physical condition caused by or arising from the pregnancy itself, that would, as certified by a physician, place the woman in danger of death unless an abortion is performed.

100-3, 140.2

NCD for Breast Reconstruction Following Mastectomy (140.2)

Reconstruction of the affected and the contralateral unaffected breast following a medically necessary mastectomy is considered a relatively safe and effective noncosmetic procedure. Accordingly, program payment may be made for breast reconstruction surgery following removal of a breast for any medical reason.

Program payment may not be made for breast reconstruction for cosmetic reasons. (Cosmetic surgery is excluded from coverage under Sec.l862(a)(l0) of the Social Security Act.)

100-3, 140.3

NCD for Transsexual Surgery (140.3)

Transsexual surgery for sex reassignment of transsexuals is controversial. Because of the lack of well controlled, long term studies of the safety and effectiveness of the surgical procedures and attendant therapies for transsexualism, the treatment is considered experimental. Moreover, there is a high rate of serious complications for these surgical procedures. For these reasons, transsexual surgery is not covered.

100-3, 140.4

NCD for Plastic Surgery to Correct "Moon Face" (140.4)

The cosmetic surgery exclusion precludes payment for any surgical procedure directed at improving appearance. The condition giving rise to the patient's preoperative appearance is generally not a consideration. The only exception to the exclusion is surgery for the prompt repair of an accidental injury or for the improvement of a malformed body member which coincidentally serves some cosmetic purpose. Since surgery to correct a condition of "moon face" which developed as a side effect of cortisone therapy does not meet the exception to the exclusion, it is not covered under Medicare (Sec.1862(a)(10) of the Act).

100-3, 140.5

NCD for Laser Procedures (140.5)

Medicare recognizes the use of lasers for many medical indications. Procedures performed with lasers are sometimes used in place of more conventional techniques. In the absence of a specific noncoverage instruction, and where a laser has been approved for marketing by the Food and Drug Administration, contractor discretion may be used to determine whether a procedure performed with a laser is reasonable and necessary and, therefore, covered.

The determination of coverage for a procedure performed using a laser is made on the basis that the use of lasers to alter, revise, or destroy tissue is a surgical procedure. Therefore, coverage of laser procedures is restricted to practitioners with training in the surgical management of the disease or condition being treated.

100-3, 150.1

NCD for Manipulation (150.1)

A. Manipulation of the Rib Cage.
Manual manipulation of the rib cage contributes to the treatment of respiratory conditions such as bronchitis, emphysema, and asthma as part of a regimen which includes other elements of therapy, and is covered only under such circumstances.

B. Manipulation of the Head.
Manipulation of the occipitocervical or temporomandibular regions of the head when indicated for conditions affecting those portions of the head and neck is a covered service.

100-3, 150.2

NCD for Osteogenic Stimulators (150.2)

Electrical Osteogenic Stimulators

B. Nationally Covered Indications

1. Noninvasive Stimulator.

   The noninvasive stimulator device is covered only for the following indications:

   - Nonunion of long bone fractures;
   - Failed fusion, where a minimum of nine months has elapsed since the last surgery;
   - Congenital pseudarthroses; and
   - Effective July 1, 1996, as an adjunct to spinal fusion surgery for patients at high risk of pseudarthrosis due to previously failed spinal fusion at the same site or for those undergoing multiple level fusion. A multiple level fusion involves 3 or more vertebrae (e.g., L3-L5, L4-S1, etc).
   - Effective September 15, 1980, nonunion of long bone fractures is considered to exist only after 6 or more months have elapsed without healing of the fracture.
   - Effective April 1, 2000, nonunion of long bone fractures is considered to exist only when serial radiographs have confirmed that fracture healing has ceased for 3 or more months prior to starting treatment with the electrical osteogenic stimulator. Serial radiographs must include a minimum of 2 sets of radiographs, each including multiple views of the fracture site, separated by a minimum of 90 days.

2. Invasive (Implantable) Stimulator.

   The invasive stimulator device is covered only for the following indications:

   - Nonunion of long bone fractures
   - Effective July 1, 1996, as an adjunct to spinal fusion surgery for patients at high risk of pseudarthrosis due to previously failsed spinal fusion at the same site or for those undergoing multiple level fusion. A multiple level fusion involves 3 or more vertebrae (e.g., L3-5, L4-S1, etc.)
   - Effective September 15, 1980, nonunion of long bone fractures is considered to exist only after 6 or more months have elapsed without healing of the fracture.
   - Effective April 1, 2000, non union of long bone fractures is considered to exist only when serial radiographs have confirmed that fracture healing has ceased for 3 or more months prior to starting treatment with the electrical osteogenic stimulator. Serial radiographs must include a minimum of 2 sets of radiographs, each including multiple views of the fracture site, separated by a minimum of 90 days.
   - Effective for services performed on or after January 1, 2001, ultrasonic osteogenic stimulators are covered as medically reasonable and necessary for the treatment of non-union fractures. In demonstrating nonunion of fractures, we would expect:
   - A minimum of two sets of radiographs obtained prior to starting treatment with the osteogenic stimulator, separated by a minimum of 90 days. Each radiograph must include multiple views of the fracture site accompanied with a written interpretation by a physician stating that there has been no clinically significant evidence of fracture healing between the two sets of radiographs.
   - Indications that the patient failed at least one surgical intervention for the treatment of the fracture.
   - Effective April 27, 2005, upon the recommendation of the ultrasound stimulation for nonunion fracture healing, CMS determins that the evidence is adequate to condlude that noninvasive ultrasound stimulation for the treatment of nonunion bone fractures prior to surfical intervention is reasonable and necessary. In demonstrating non-union fracturs, CMS expects:
   - A minimum of 2 sets of radiographs, obtained prior to starting treating with the osteogenic stimulator, separated by a minimum of 90 days. Each radiograph set must include multiple views of the fracture site accompanied with a written interpretation by a physician stating that there has been no clinically significant evidence of fracture healing between the 2 sets of radiographs.

C. Nationally Non-Covered Indications
Nonunion fractures of the skull, vertebrae and those that are tumor-related are excluded from coverage.

Ultrasonic osteogenic stimulators may not be used concurrently with other non-invasive osteogenic devices.

Ultrasonic osteogenic stimulators for fresh fracturs and delayed unions remain non-covered.

(This NCD last reviewed June 2005)

100-3, 150.3

NCD for Bone (Mineral) Density Studies (150.3)

Conditions for coverage of bone mass measurements are now contained in chapter 15, section 80.5 of Pub. 100-02, Medicare Benefit Policy Manual . Claims processing instructions can be found in chapter 13, section 140 of Pub. 100-04, Medicare Claims Processing Manual .

100-3, 150.5

NCD for Diathermy Treatment (150.5)

High energy pulsed wave diathermy machines have been found to produce some degree of therapeutic benefit for essentially the same conditions and to the same extent as standard diathermy. Accordingly, where the contractor's medical staff has determined that the pulsed wave diathermy apparatus used is one which is considered therapeutically effective, the treatments are considered a covered service, but only for those conditions for which standard diathermy is medically indicated and only when rendered by a physician or incident to a physician's professional services.

100-3, 150.6

NCD for Vitamin B12 Injections to Strengthen Tendons, Ligaments, etc., of the Foot (150.6)

Vitamin B12 injections to strengthen tendons, ligaments, etc., of the foot are not covered under Medicare because (1) there is no evidence that vitamin B12 injections are effective for the purpose of strengthening weakened tendons and ligaments, and (2) this is nonsurgical treatment under the subluxation exclusion. Accordingly, vitamin B12 injections are not considered reasonable and necessary within the meaning of Sec.1862(a)(1) of the Act.

100-3, 150.7

NCD for Prolotherapy, Joint Sclerotherapy, and Ligamentous Injections with Sclerosing Agents (150.7)

The medical effectiveness of the above therapies has not been verified by scientifically controlled studies. Accordingly, reimbursement for these modalities should be denied on the ground that they are not reasonable and necessary as required by Sec.1862(a)(1) of the Act.

100-3, 150.10

NCD for Lumbar Artificial Disc Replacement (LADR) (150.10)

B. Nationally Covered Indications
N/A

C. Nationally Non-Covered Indications
Effective for services performed from May 16, 2006 through August 13, 2007, the Centers for Medicare and Medicaid Services (CMS) has found that LADR with the Charite TM lumbar artificial disc is not reasonable and necessary for the Medicare population over 60 years of age; therefore, LADR with the Charite TM lumbar artificial disc is non-covered for Medicare beneficiaries over 60 years of age.

Effective for services performed on or after August 14, 2007, CMS has found that LADR is not reasonable and necessary for the Medicare population over 60 years of age; therefore, LADR is non-covered for Medicare beneficiaries over 60 years of age.

D. Other
For Medicare beneficiaries 60 years of age and younger, there is no national coverage determination for LADR, leaving such determinations to continue to be made by the local contractors.

For dates of service May 16, 2006 through August 13, 2007, Medicare coverage under the investigational device exemption (IDE) for LADR with a disc other than the Charite TM lumbar disc in eligible clinical trials is not impacted.

(This NCD last reviewed August 2007.)

100-3, 150.11

Thermal Intradiscal Procedures (TIPs)

A. General
Percutaneous thermal intradiscal procedures (TIPs) involve the insertion of a catheter(s)/probe(s) in the spinal disc under fluoroscopic guidance for the purpose of producing or applying heat and/or disruption within the disc to relieve low back pain.

The scope of this national coverage determination on TIPs includes percutaneous intradiscal techniques that employ the use of a radiofrequency energy source or electrothermal energy to apply or create heat and/or disruption within the disc for coagulation and/or decompression of disc material to treat symptomatic patients with annular disruption of a contained herniated disc, to seal annular tears or fissures, or destroy nociceptors for the purpose of relieving pain. This includes techniques that use single or multiple probe(s)/catheter(s), which utilize a resistance coil or other delivery system technology, are flexible or rigid, and are placed within the nucleus, the nuclear-annular junction, or the annulus. Although not intended to be an all inclusive list, TIPs are commonly identified as intradiscal electrothermal therapy (IDET), intradiscal thermal annuloplasty (IDTA), percutaneous intradiscal radiofrequency thermocoagulation (PIRFT), radiofrequency annuloplasty (RA), intradiscal biacuplasty (IDB), percutaneous (or plasma) disc decompression (PDD) or coblation, or targeted disc decompression (TDD). At times, TIPs are identified or labeled based on the name of the catheter/probe that is used (e.g., SpineCath, discTRODE, SpineWand, Accutherm, or TransDiscal electrodes). Each technique or device has it own protocol for application of the therapy. Percutaneous disc decompression or nucleoplasty procedures that do not utilize a radiofrequency energy source or electrothermal energy (such as the disc decompressor procedure or laser procedure) are not within the scope of this NCD.

B. Nationally Covered Indications
N/A

C. Nationally Non-Covered Indications
Effective for services performed on or after September 29, 2008, the Centers for Medicare and Medicaid Services has determined that TIPs are not reasonable and necessary for the treatment of low back pain. Therefore, TIPs, which include procedures that employ the use of a radiofrequency energy source or electrothermal energy to apply or create heat and/or disruption within the disc for the treatment of low back pain, are noncovered.

D. Other
N/A

(This NCD last reviewed September 2008.)

100-3, 150.12

Collagen Meniscus Implant (Effective May 25, 2010)

A. General
The knee menisci are wedge-shaped, semi-lunar discs of fibrous tissue located in the knee joint between the ends of the femur and the tibia and fibula. There is a lateral and medial meniscus in each knee. It is known now that the menisci provide mechanical support, localized pressure distribution, and lubrication of the knee joint. Initially, meniscal tears were treated with total meniscectomy; however, as knowledge of the function of the menisci and the potential long term effects of total meniscectomy on the knee joint evolved, treatment of symptomatic meniscal tears gravitated to repair of the tear, when possible, or partial meniscectomy.

The collagen meniscus implant (also referred to as collagen scaffold (CS), CMI or MenaflexTM meniscus implant throughout the published literature) is used to fill meniscal defects that result from partial meniscectomy. The collagen meniscus implant is not intended to replace the entire meniscus at it requires a meniscal rim for attachment. The literature describes the placement of the collagen meniscus implant through an arthroscopic procedure with an additional incision for capture of the repair needles and tying of the sutures. After debridement of the damaged meniscus, the implant is trimmed to the size of meniscal defect and sutured into place. The collagen meniscus implant is described as a tissue engineered scaffold to support the generation of new meniscus-like tissue. The collagen meniscus implant is manufactured from bovine collagen and should not be confused with the meniscus transplant which involves the replacement of the meniscus with a transplant meniscus from a cadaver donor. The meniscus transplant is not addressed under this national coverage determination.

B. Nationally Covered Indications
N/A

C. Nationally Non-Covered Indications
Effective for claims with dates of service performed on or after May 25, 2010, the Centers for Medicare & Medicaid Services has determined that the evidence is adequate to conclude that the collagen meniscus implant does not improve health outcomes and, therefore, is not reasonable and necessary for the treatment of meniscal injury/tear under section 1862(a)(1)(A) of the Social Security Act. Thus, the collagen meniscus implant is non-covered by Medicare.

D. Other
N/A

(This NCD last reviewed May 2010.)

100-3, 160.1

NCD for Induced Lesions of Nerve Tracts (160.1)

Accordingly, program payment may be made for these denervation procedures when used in selected cases (concurred in by contractor's medical staff) to treat chronic pain.

100-3, 160.2

NCD for Treatment of Motor Function Disorders with Electric Nerve Stimulation (160.2)

Where electric nerve stimulation is employed to treat motor function disorders, no reimbursement may be made for the stimulator or for the services related to its implantation since this treatment cannot be considered reasonable and necessary.

Note: For Medicare coverage of deep brain stimulation for essential tremor and Parkinson's disease, see Sec.160.24 of the NCD Manual.

100-3, 160.4

NCD for Stereotactic Cingulotomy as a Means of Psychosurgery (160.4)

Stereotactic cingulotomy is not covered under Medicare because the procedure is considered to be investigational.

100-3, 160.5

NCD for Stereotaxic Depth Electrode Implantation (160.5)

Stereotaxic depth electrode implantation prior to surgical treatment of focal epilepsy for patients who are unresponsive to anticonvulsant medications has been found both safe and effective for diagnosing resectable seizure foci that may go undetected by conventional scalp electroencephalographs (EEGs).

100-3, 160.6

NCD for Carotid Sinus Nerve Stimulator (160.6)

Implantation of the carotid sinus nerve stimulator is indicated for relief of angina pectoris in carefully selected patients who are refractory to medical therapy and who after undergoing coronary angiography study either are poor candidates for or refuse to have coronary bypass surgery. In such cases, Medicare reimbursement may be made for this device and for the related services required for its implantation.

However, the use of the carotid sinus nerve stimulator in the treatment of paroxysmal supraventricular tachycardia is considered investigational and is not in common use by the medical community. The device and related services in such cases cannot be considered as reasonable and necessary for the treatment of an illness or injury or to improve the functioning of a malformed body member as required by Sec.1862(a)(1) of the Act.

100-3, 160.7

NCD for Electrical Nerve Stimulators (160.7)

Two general classifications of electrical nerve stimulators are employed to treat chronic intractable pain: peripheral nerve stimulators and central nervous system stimulators.

A. Implanted Peripheral Nerve Stimulators
Payment may be made under the prosthetic device benefit for implanted peripheral nerve stimulators. Use of this stimulator involves implantation of electrodes around a selected peripheral nerve. The stimulating electrode is connected by an insulated lead to a receiver unit which is implanted under the skin at a depth not greater than 1/2 inch. Stimulation is induced by a generator connected to an antenna unit which is attached to the skin surface over the receiver unit. Implantation of electrodes requires surgery and usually necessitates an operating room.

Note: Peripheral nerve stimulators may also be employed to assess a patient's suitability for continued treatment with an electric nerve stimulator. As explained in Sec.160.7.1, such use of the stimulator is covered as part of the total diagnostic service furnished to the beneficiary rather than as a prosthesis.

B. Central Nervous System Stimulators (Dorsal Column and Depth Brain Stimulators)
The implantation of central nervous system stimulators may be covered as therapies for the relief of chronic intractable pain, subject to the following conditions:

1. Types of Implantations

   There are two types of implantations covered by this instruction:

   Dorsal Column (Spinal Cord) Neurostimulation - The surgical implantation of neurostimulator electrodes within the dura mater (endodural) or the percutaneous insertion of electrodes in the epidural space is covered.

   Depth Brain Neurostimulation - The stereotactic implantation of electrodes in the deep brain (e.g., thalamus and periaqueductal gray matter) is covered.

2. Conditions for Coverage

   No payment may be made for the implantation of dorsal column or depth brain stimulators or services and supplies related to such implantation, unless all of the conditions listed below have been met:

   The implantation of the stimulator is used only as a late resort (if not a last resort) for patients with chronic intractable pain;

   With respect to item a, other treatment modalities (pharmacological, surgical, physical, or psychological therapies) have been tried and did not prove satisfactory, or are judged to be unsuitable or contraindicated for the given patient;

   Patients have undergone careful screening, evaluation and diagnosis by a multidisciplinary team prior to implantation. (Such screening must include psychological, as well as physical evaluation);

   All the facilities, equipment, and professional and support personnel required for the proper diagnosis, treatment training, and followup of the patient (including that required to satisfy item c) must be available; and

   Demonstration of pain relief with a temporarily implanted electrode precedes permanent implantation.

   Contractors may find it helpful to work with QIOs to obtain the information needed to apply these conditions to claims.

100-3, 160.7.1

NCD for Assessing Patient's Suitability for Electrical Nerve Stimulation Therapy (160.7.1)

Indications and Limitations of Coverage

CIM 35-46

Electrical nerve stimulation is an accepted modality for assessing a patient's suitability for ongoing treatment with a transcutaneous or an implanted nerve stimulator.

Accordingly, program payment may be made for the following techniques when used to determine the potential therapeutic usefulness of an electrical nerve stimulator:

A. Transcutaneous Electrical Nerve Stimulation(TENS)
This technique involves attachment of a transcutaneous nerve stimulator to the surface of the skin over the peripheral nerve to be stimulated. It is used by the patient on a trial basis and its effectiveness in modulating pain is monitored by the physician, or physical therapist. Generally, the physician or physical therapist is able to determine whether the patient is likely to derive a significant therapeutic benefit from continuous use of a transcutaneous stimulator within a trial period of 1 month; in a few cases this determination may take longer to make. Document the medical necessity for such services which are furnished beyond the first month. (See Sec.160.13 for an explanation of coverage of medically necessary supplies for the effective use of TENS.)

If TENS significantly alleviates pain, it may be considered as primary treatment; if it produces no relief or greater discomfort than the original pain electrical nerve stimulation therapy is ruled out. However, where TENS produces incomplete relief, further evaluation with percutaneous electrical nerve stimulation may be considered to determine whether an implanted peripheral nerve stimulator would provide significant relief from pain.

Usually, the physician or physical therapist providing the services will furnish the equipment necessary for assessment. Where the physician or physical therapist advises the patient to rent the TENS from a supplier during the trial period rather than supplying it himself/herself, program payment may be made for rental of the TENS as well as for the services of the physician or physical therapist who is evaluating its use. However, the combined program payment which is made for the physician's or physical therapist's services and the rental of the stimulator from a supplier should not exceed the amount which would be payable for the total service, including the stimulator, furnished by the physician or physical therapist alone.

B. Percutaneous Electrical Nerve Stimulation (PENS)
This diagnostic procedure which involves stimulation of peripheral nerves by a needle electrode inserted through the skin is performed only in a physician's office, clinic, or hospital outpatient department. Therefore, it is covered only when performed by a physician or incident to physician's service. If pain is effectively controlled by percutaneous stimulation, implantation of electrodes is warranted.

As in the case of TENS (described in subsection A), generally the physician should be able to determine whether the patient is likely to derive a significant therapeutic benefit from continuing use of an implanted nerve stimulator within a trial period of 1 month. In a few cases, this determination may take longer to make. The medical necessity for such diagnostic services which are furnished beyond the first month must be documented.

NOTE: Electrical nerve stimulators do not prevent pain but only alleviate pain as it occurs. A patient can be taught how to employ the stimulator, and once this is done, can use it safely and effectively without direct physician supervision. Consequently, it is inappropriate for a patient to visit his/her physician, physical therapist, or an outpatient clinic on a continuing basis for treatment of pain with electrical nerve stimulation. Once it is determined that electrical nerve stimulation should be continued as therapy and the patient has been trained to use the stimulator, it is expected that a stimulator will be implanted or the patient will employ the TENS on a continual basis in his/her home. Electrical nerve stimulation treatments furnished by a physician in his/her office, by a physical therapist or outpatient clinic are excluded from coverage by Sec.1862(a)(1) of the Act. (See Sec.160.7 for an explanation of coverage of the therapeutic use of implanted peripheral nerve stimulators under the prosthetic devices benefit. See Sec.280.13 for an explanation of coverage of the therapeutic use of TENS under the durable medical equipment benefit.)

100-3, 160.8

NCD for Electroencephalographic (EEG) Monitoring During Surgical Procedures Involving the Cerebral Vasculature (160.8)

CIM 35-57

Electroencephalographic (EEG) monitoring is a safe and reliable technique for the assessment of gross cerebral blood flow during general anesthesia and is covered under Medicare. Very characteristic changes in the EEG occur when cerebral perfusion is inadequate for ce rebral function. EEG monitoring as an indirect measure of cerebral perfusion requires the expertise of an electroencephalographer, a neurologist trained in EEG, or an advanced EEG technician for its proper interpretation.

The EEG monitoring may be covered routinely in carotid endarterectomies and in other neurological procedures where cerebral perfusion could be reduced. Such other procedures might include aneurysm surgery where hypotensive anesthesia is used or other cerebral vascular procedures where cerebral blood flow may be interrupted.

100-3, 160.9

NCD for Electronecephalographic (EEG) Monitoring during Open-Heart Surgery (160.9)

The value of EEG monitoring during open heart surgery and in the immediate post-operative period is debatable because there are little published data based on well designed studies regarding its clinical effectiveness. The procedure is not frequently used and does not enjoy widespread acceptance of benefit.

Accordingly, Medicare does not cover EEG monitoring during open heart surgery and during the immediate post-operative period.

100-3, 160.10

NCD for Evoked Response Tests (160.10)

Evoked response tests, including brain stem evoked response and visual evoked response tests, are generally accepted as safe and effective diagnostic tools. Program payment may be made for these procedures.

100-3, 160.12

NCD for Neuromuscular Electrical Stimulaton (NMES) (160.12)

Indications and Limitations of Coverage

Treatment of Muscle Atrophy
Coverage of NMES to treat muscle atrophy is limited to the treatment of disuse atrophy where nerve supply to the muscle is intact, including brain, spinal cord and peripheral nerves, and other non-neurological reasons for disuse atrophy. Some examples would be casting or splinting of a limb, contracture due to scarring of soft tissue as in burn lesions, and hip replacement surgery (until orthotic training begins). (See Sec.160.13 of the NCD Manual for an explanation of coverage of medically necessary supplies for the effective use of NMES.)

Use for Walking in Patients with Spinal Cord Injury (SCI)
The type of NMES that is use to enhance the ability to walk of SCI patients is commonly referred to as functional electrical stimulation (FES). These devices are surface units that use electrical impulses to activate paralyzed or weak muscles in precise sequence. Coverage for the use of NMES/FES is limited to SCI patients for walking, who have completed a training program which consists of at least 32 physical therapy sessions with the device over a period of three months. The trial period of physical therapy will enable the physician treating the patient for his or her spinal cord injury to properly evaluate the person's ability to use these devices frequently and for the long term. Physical therapy necessary to perform this training must be directly performed by the physical therapist as part of a one-on-one training program.

The goal of physical therapy must be to train SCI patients on the use of NMES/FES devices to achieve walking, not to reverse or retard muscle atrophy.

Coverage for NMES/FES for walking will be covered in SCI patients with all of the following characteristics:

- Persons with intact lower motor unite (L1 and below) (both muscle and peripheral nerve);
- Persons with muscle and joint stability for weight bearing at upper and lower extremities that can demonstrate balance and control to maintain an upright support posture independently;
- Persons that demonstrate brisk muscle contraction to NMES and have sensory perception electrical stimulation sufficient for muscle contraction;
- Persons that possess high motivation, commitment and cognitive ability to use such devices for walking;
- Persons that can transfer independently and can demonstrate independent standing tolerance for at least 3 minutes;
- Persons that can demonstrate hand and finger function to manipulate controls;
- Persons with at least 6-month post recovery spinal cord injury and restorative surgery;
- Persons with hip and knee degenerative disease and no history of long bone fracture secondary to osteoporosis; and

- Persons who have demonstrated a willingness to use the device long-term.

NMES/FES for walking will not be covered in SCI patient with any of the following:

- Persons with cardiac pacemakers;
- Severe scoliosis or severe osteoporosis;
- Skin disease or cancer at area of stimulation;
- Irreversible contracture; or
- Autonomic dysflexia.

The only settings where therapists with the sufficient skills to provide these services are employed, are inpatient hospitals; outpatient hospitals; comprehensive outpatient rehabilitation facilities; and outpatient rehabilitation facilities. The physical therapy necessary to perform this training must be part of a one-on-one training program.

Additional therapy after the purchase of the DME would be limited by our general policies in converge of skilled physical therapy.

100-3, 160.13

NCD for Supplies Used in the Delivery of Transcutaneous Electrical Nerve Stimulation (TENS) and Neuromuscular Electrical Stimulation (NMES) (160.13)

A form-fitting conductive garment (and medically necessary related supplies) may be covered under the program only when:

1. It has received permission or approval for marketing by the Food and Drug Administration;
2. It has been prescribed by a physician for use in delivering covered TENS or NMES treatment; and
3. One of the medical indications outlined below is met:
   - The patient cannot manage without the conductive garment because there is such a large area or so many sites to be stimulated and the stimulation would have to be delivered so frequently that it is not feasible to use conventional electrodes, adhesive tapes and lead wires;
   - The patient cannot manage without the conductive garment for the treatment of chronic intractable pain because the areas or sites to be stimulated are inaccessible with the use of conventional electrodes, adhesive tapes and lead wires;
   - The patient has a documented medical condition such as skin problems that preclude the application of conventional electrodes, adhesive tapes and lead wires;
   - The patient requires electrical stimulation beneath a cast either to treat disuse atrophy, where the nerve supply to the muscle is intact, or to treat chronic intractable pain; or
   - The patient has a medical need for rehabilitation strengthening (pursuant to a written plan of rehabilitation) following an injury where the nerve supply to the muscle is intact.

   A conductive garment is not covered for use with a TENS device during the trial period specified in Sec.160.3 unless:

   - The patient has a documented skin problem prior to the start of the trial period; and
   - The carrier's medical consultants are satisfied that use of such an item is medically necessary for the patient.

100-3, 160.15

NCD for Electrotherapy for Treatment of Facial Nerve Paralysis (Bell's Palsy) (160.15)

Electrotherapy for the treatment of facial nerve paralysis, commonly known as Bell's Palsy, is not covered under Medicare because its clinical effectiveness has not been established.

100-3, 160.17

NCD for L-DOPA (160.17)

A - Part A Payment for L-Dopa and Associated Inpatient Hospital Services

A hospital stay and related ancillary services for the administration of L-Dopa are covered if medically required for this purpose. Whether a drug represents an allowable inpatient hospital cost during such stay depends on whether it meets the definition of a drug in Sec.1861(t) of the Act; i.e., on its inclusion in the compendia named in the Act or approval by the hospital's pharmacy and drug therapeutics (P&DT) or equivalent committee. (Levodopa (L-Dopa) has been favorably evaluated for the treatment of Parkinsonism by A.M.A. Drug Evaluations, First Edition 1971, the replacement compendia for "New Drugs.")

Inpatient hospital services are frequently not required in many cases when L-Dopa therapy is initiated. Therefore, determine the medical need for inpatient hospital services on the basis of medical facts in the individual case. It is not necessary to hospitalize the typical, well-functioning, ambulatory Parkinsonian patient who has no concurrent disease at the start of L-Dopa treatment. It is reasonable to provide inpatient hospital services for Parkinsonian patients with concurrent diseases, particularly of the cardiovascular, gastrointestinal, and neuropsychiatric systems. Although many patients require hospitalization for a period of under 2 weeks, a 4-week period of inpatient care is not unreasonable.

Laboratory tests in connection with the administration of L-Dopa - The tests medically warranted in connection with the achievement of optimal dosage and the control of the side effects of L-Dopa include a complete blood count, liver function tests such as SGOT, SGPT, and/or alkaline phosphatase, BUN or creatinine and urinalysis, blood sugar, and electrocardiogram.

Whether or not the patient is hospitalized, laboratory tests in certain cases are reasonable at weekly intervals although some physicians prefer to perform the tests much less frequently.

Physical therapy furnished in connection with administration of L-Dopa - Where, following administration of the drug, the patient experiences a reduction of rigidity which permits the reestablishment of a restorative goal for him/her, physical therapy services required to enable him/her to achieve this goal are payable provided they require the skills of a qualified physical therapist and are furnished by or under the supervision of such a therapist. However, once the individual's restoration potential has been achieved, the services required to maintain him/her at this level do not generally require the skills of a qualified physical therapist. In such situations, the role of the therapist is to evaluate the patient's needs in consultation with his/her physician and design a program of exercise appropriate to the capacity and tolerance of the patient and treatment objectives of the physician, leaving to others the actual carrying out of the program. While the evaluative services rendered by a qualified physical therapist are payable as physical therapy, services furnished by others in connection with the carrying out of the maintenance program established by the therapist are not.

B - Part A Reimbursement for L-Dopa Therapy in SNFs

Initiation of L-Dopa therapy can be appropriately carried out in the SNF setting, applying the same guidelines used for initiation of L-Dopa therapy in the hospital, including the types of patients who should be covered for inpatient services, the role of physical therapy, and the use of laboratory tests. (See subsection A.) Where inpatient care is required and L-Dopa therapy is initiated in the SNF, limit the stay to a maximum of 4 weeks; but in many cases the need may be no longer than 1 or 2 weeks, depending upon the patient's condition. However, where L-Dopa therapy is begun in the hospital and the patient is transferred to an SNF for continuation of the therapy, a combined length of stay in hospital and SNF of no longer than 4 weeks is reasonable (i.e., 1 week hospital stay followed by 3 weeks SNF stay; or 2 weeks hospital stay followed by 2 weeks SNF stay; etc.). Medical need must be demonstrated in cases where the combined length of stay in hospital and SNF is longer than 4 weeks. The choice of hospital or SNF, and the decision regarding the relative length of time spent in each, should be left to the medical judgment of the treating physician.

C - L-Dopa Coverage Under Part B

Part B reimbursement may not be made for the drug L-Dopa since it is a self-administrable drug. However, physician services rendered in connection with its administration and control of its side effects are covered if determined to be reasonable and necessary. Initiation of L-Dopa therapy on an outpatient basis is possible in most cases. Visit frequency ranging from every week to every 2 or 3 months is acceptable. However, after half a year of therapy, visits more frequent than every month would usually not be reasonable.

100-3, 160.18

NCD for Vagus Nerve Stimulation for Treatment of Seizures (160.18)

B. Nationally Covered Indications

Effective for services performed on or after July 1, 1999, VNS is reasonable and necessary for patients with medically refractory partial onset seizures for whom surgery is not recommended or for whom surgery has failed.

C. Nationally Non-Covered Indications

Effective for services performed on or after July 1, 1999, VNS is not reasonable and necessary for all other types of seizure disorders which are medically refractory and for whom surgery is not recommended or for whom surgery has failed.

Effective for services performed on or after May 4, 2007, VNS is not reasonable and necessary for resistant depression. (Information on the national coverage analysis leading to this determination can be found at: http://www.cms.hhs.gov/mcd/viewnca.asp?where= index&nca_id= 195.)

D. Other

Also see Sec.160, "Electrical Nerve Stimulators."

(This NCD last reviewed May 2007.)

100-3, 160.20

NCD for Transfer Factor for Treatment of Multiple Sclerosis (160.20)

Transfer factor is the dialysate of an extract from sensitized leukocytes which increases cellular immune activity in the recipient. It is not covered as a treatment for multiple sclerosis because its use for the purpose is still experimental.

100-3, 160.21

NCD for Telephone Transmission of Electroencephalograms (EEGs) (160.21)

Telephone transmission of electroencephalograms (EEGs) is covered as a physician's service or as incident to a physician's service when reasonable and necessary for the individual patient, under appropriate circumstances. The service is safe, and may save time and cost in sending EEGs from remote areas without special competence in neurology, neurosurgery, and electroencephalography, by avoiding the need to transport patients to large medical centers for standard EEG testing.

100-3, 160.22

NCD for Ambulatory EEG Monitoring (160.22)

Ambulatory EEG monitoring is a diagnostic procedure for patients in whom a seizure diathesis is suspected but not defined by history, physical or resting EEG. Ambulatory EEG can be utilized in the differential diagnosis of syncope and transient ischemic attacks if not elucidated by conventional studies. Ambulatory EEG should always be preceded by a resting EEG.

Ambulatory EEG monitoring is considered an established technique and covered under Medicare for the above purposes.

100-3, 170.3

NCD for Speech Pathology Services for the Treatment of Dysphagia (170.3)

Speech -language pathology services are covered under Medicare for the treatment of dysphagia, regardless of the presence of a communication disability.

100-3, 180.1

NCD for Medical Nutrition Therapy (180.1)

Effective October 1, 2002, basic coverage of MNT for the first year a beneficiary receives MNT with either a diagnosis of renal disease or diabetes as defined at 42 CFR Sec.410.130 is 3 hours. Also effective October 1, 2002, basic coverage in subsequent years for renal disease or diabetes is 2 hours. The dietitian/nutritionist may choose how many units are performed per day as long as all of the other requirements in this NCD and 42 CFR Secs.410.130-410.134 are met. Pursuant to the exception at 42 CFR Sec.410.132(b)(5), additional hours are considered to be medically necessary and covered if the treating physician determines that there is a change in medical condition, diagnosis, or treatment regimen that requires a change in MNT and orders additional hours during that episode of care.

Effective October 1, 2002, if the treating physician determines that receipt of both MNT and DSMT is medically necessary in the same episode of care, Medicare will cover both DSMT and MNT initial and subsequent years without decreasing either benefit as long as DSMT and MNT are not provided on the same date of service. The dietitian/nutritionist may choose how many units are performed per day as long as all of the other requirements in the NCD and 42 CFR Secs.410.130-410.134 are met. Pursuant to the exception at 42 CFR 410.132(b)(5), additional hours are considered to be medically necessary and covered if the treating physician determines that there is a change in medical condition, diagnosis, or treatment regimen that requires a change in MNT and orders additional hours during that episode of care.

100-3, 190.1

NCD for Histocompatibility Testing (190.1)

This testing is safe and effective when it is performed on patients:

- In preparation for a kidney transplant;
- In preparation for bone marrow transplantation;
- In preparation for blood platelet transfusions (particularly where multiple infusions are involved); or
- Who are suspected of having ankylosing spondylitis.

This testing is covered under Medicare when used for any of the indications listed in A, B, and C and if it is reasonable and necessary for the patient.

It is covered for ankylosing spondylitis in cases where other methods of diagnosis would not be appropriate or have yielded inconclusive results. Request documentation supporting the medical necessity of the test from the physician in all cases where ankylosing spondylitis is indicated as the reason for the test.

100-3, 190.2

NCD for Diagnostic Pap Smears (190.2)

CIM 50-20, CIM 50-20.1

A diagnostic pap smear and related medically necessary services are covered under Medicare Part B when ordered by a physician under one of the following conditions:

- Previous cancer of the cervix, uterus, or vagina that has been or is presently being treated;
- Previous abnormal pap smear;
- Any abnormal findings of the vagina, cervix, uterus, ovaries, or adnexa;
- Any significant complaint by the patient referable to the female reproductive system; or
- Any signs or symptoms that might in the physician's judgment reasonably be related to a gynecologic disorder.

Screening Pap Smears and Pelvic Examinations for Early Detection of Cervical or Vaginal Cancer. (See section 210.2.)

100-3, 190.3

NCD for Cytogenetic Studies (190.3)

Medicare covers these tests when they are reasonable and necessary for the diagnosis or treatment of the following conditions:

Genetic disorders (e.g., mongolism) in a fetus (See Medicare Benefit Policy Manual, Chapter 15, "Covered medical and Other health Services," Sec.20.1)

Failure of sexual development;

Chronic myelogenous leukemia;

Acute leukemias lymphoid (FAB L1-L3), myeloid (FAB M0-M7), and unclassified; or

Mylodysplasia

100-3, 190.4

NCD for Electron Microscope (190.4)

The electron microscope has been used in the examination of biopsies for years; its efficacy, and therefore its Medicare coverage, is not being questioned. However, there are less expensive methods for examining biopsies which are normally adequate. The additional expense for the electron microscope is normally warranted only when distinguishing different types of nephritis from renal needle biopsies or when there is an uncertain diagnosis from the pathologist. When an uncertain diagnosis from the pathologists results from a less expensive method of examination and an electron microscope examination is therefore necessary, both biopsy examinations are covered. Where the additional expense for an electron microscope examination is not warranted, payment is based upon the less costly methods of examining biopsies.

100-3, 190.5

NCD for Sweat Test (190.5)

Indications and Limitations of Coverage

The sweat test is an important diagnostic tool in cystic fibrosis and may be covered when used for that purpose. Usage of the sweat test as a predictor of efficacy of sympathectomy in peripheral vascular disease is unproven and, therefore, is not covered.

100-3, 190.6

NCD for Hair Analysis (190.6)

Indications and Limitations of Coverage

Hair analysis to detect mineral traces as an aid in diagnosing human disease is not a covered service under Medicare.

The correlation of hair analysis to the chemical state of the whole body is not possible at this time, and therefore this diagnostic procedure cannot be considered to be reasonable and necessary under Sec.1862(a)(1) of the Act.

100-3, 190.8

NCD for Lymphocyte Mitogen Response Assays (190.8)

It is a covered test under Medicare when it is medically necessary to assess lymphocytic function in diagnosed immunodeficiency diseases and to monitor immunotherapy.

It is not covered when it is used to monitor the treatment of cancer, because its use for that purpose is experimental.

100-3, 190.9

NCD for Serologic Testing for Acquired Immunodeficiency Syndrome (AIDS) (190.9)

These tests may be covered when performed to help determine a diagnosis for symptomaticpatients. They are not covered when furnished as part of a screening program for asymptomatic persons.

Note: Two enzyme-linked immunosorbent assay (ELISA) tests that were conducted on the same specimen must both be positive before Medicare will cover the Western blot test.

100-3, 190.10

NCD for Laboratory Tests - CRD Patients (190.10)

Laboratory tests are essential to monitor the progress of CRD patients. The following list and frequencies of tests constitute the level and types of routine laboratory tests that are covered. Bills for other types of tests are considered nonroutine. Routine tests at greater frequencies must include medical justification. Nonroutine tests generally are justified by the diagnosis.

The routinely covered regimen includes the following tests:

Per Dialysis

- All hematocrit or hemoglobin and clotting time tests furnished incident to dialysis treatments.

Per Week

- Prothrombin time for patients on anticoagulant therapy
- Serum Creatinine

Per Week or Thirteen Per Quarter

- BUN

Monthly

- CBC
- Serum Calcium
- Serum Potassium
- Serum Chloride
- Serum Bicarbonate
- Serum Phosphorous
- Total Protein
- Serum Albumin
- Alkaline Phospatase
- AST, SGOT
- LDH

Guidelines for tests other than those routinely performed include:

- Serum Aluminum - one every 3 months
- Serum Ferritin - one every 3 months

The following tests for hepatitis B are covered when patients first enter a dialysis facility:

- Hepatitis B surface antigen (HBsAg)
- Anti-HBs

Coverage of future testing in these patients depends on their serologic status and on whether they have been successfully immunized against hepatitis B virus. The following table summarizes the frequency of serologic surveillance for hepatitis B. Tests furnished according to this table do not require additional documentation and are paid separately because payment for maintenance dialysis treatments does not take them into account.

Frequency of Screening

	Vaccination and Serologic Status	HbsAg Patients	Anti-HBs Patients
Unvaccinated	Susceptible	Monthly	Semiannually
Unvaccinated	HBsAg Carrier	Annually	None
Unvaccinated	Anti-HBs-Positive (1)	None	Annually
Vaccinated	Anti-HBs-Positive (1)	None	Annually
Vaccinated	Low Level or No Anti-HBs	Monthly	Semiannually

(1) At least 10 sample ration units by radioimmunoassay or positive by enzyme immunoassay.

Patients who are in the process of receiving hepatitis B vaccines, but have not received the complete series, should continue to be routinely screened as susceptible. Between one and six months after the third dose, all vaccines should be tested for anti-HBs to confirm their response to the vaccine. Patients who have a level of anti-HBs of at least 10 sample ratio units (SRUs) by radioimmunoassay (RIA) or who are positive by enzyme immunoassay (EIA) are considered adequate responders to vaccine and need only be tested for anti-HBs annually to verify their immune status. If anti-HBs drops below 10 SRUs by RIA or is negative by EIA, a booster dose of hepatitis B vaccine should be given.

Laboratory tests are subject to the normal coverage requirements. If the laboratory services are performed by a free-standing facility, be sure it meets the conditions of coverage for independent laboratories.

100-3, 190.11

NCD for Home Prothrombin Time International Normalized Ratio (INR) Monitoring for Anticoagulation Management (190.11)

A. General

Use of the International Normalized Ratio (INR) or prothrombin time (PT) - standard measurement for reporting the blood's clotting time) - allows physicians to determine the level of anticoagulation in a patient independent of the laboratory reagents used. The INR is the ratio of the patient's PT (extrinsic or tissue-factor dependent coagulation pathway) compared to the mean PT for a group of normal individuals. Maintaining patients within his/her prescribed therapeutic range minimizes adverse events associated with inadequate or excessive anticoagulation such as serious bleeding or thromboembolic events. Patient self-testing and self-management through the use of a home INR monitor may be used to improve the time in therapeutic rate (TTR) for select groups of patients. Increased TTR leads to improved clinical outcomes and reductions in thromboembolic and hemorrhagic events.

Warfarin (also prescribed under other trade names, e.g., Coumadin(R)) is a self-administered, oral anticoagulant (blood thinner) medication that affects the vitamin K- dependent clotting factors II, VII, IX and X. It is widely used for various medical conditions, and has a narrow therapeutic index, meaning it is a drug with less than a 2-fold difference between median lethal dose and median effective dose. For this reason, since October 4, 2006, it falls under the category of a Food and Drug dministration (FDA) "black-box" drug whose dosage must be closely monitored to avoid serious complications. A PT/INR monitoring system is a portable testing device that includes a finger-stick and an FDA-cleared meter that measures the time it takes for a person's blood plasma to clot.

B. Nationally Covered Indications

For services furnished on or after March 19, 2008, Medicare will cover the use of home PT/INR monitoring for chronic, oral anticoagulation management for patients with mechanical heart valves, chronic atrial fibrillation, or venous thromboembolism (inclusive of deep venous thrombosis and pulmonary embolism) on warfarin. The monitor and the home testing must be prescribed by a treating physician as provided at 42 CFR 410.32(a), and all of the following requirements must be met:

1. The patient must have been anticoagulated for at least 3 months prior to use of the home INR device; and,
2. The patient must undergo a face-to-face educational program on anticoagulation anagement and must have demonstrated the correct use of the device prior to its use in the home; and,
3. The patient continues to correctly use the device in the context of the management of the anticoagulation therapy following the initiation of home monitoring; and,
4. Self-testing with the device should not occur more frequently than once a week.

C. Nationally Non-Covered Indications

N/A

D. Other

1. All other indications for home PT/INR monitoring not indicated as nationally covered above remain at local Medicare contractor discretion.
2. This national coverage determination (NCD) is distinct from, and makes no changes to, the PT clinical laboratory NCD at section 190.17 of Publication 100-03 of the NCD Manual.

100-3, 190.12

NCD for Urine Culture, Bacterial (190.12)

Indications

1. A patient's urinalysis is abnormal suggesting urinary tract infection, for example, abnormal microscopic (hematuria, pyuria, bacteriuria); abnormal biochemical urinalysis (positive leukocyte esterase, nitrite, protein, blood); a Gram's stain positive for microorganisms; positive bacteriuria screen by a non?culture technique; or other significant abnormality of a urinalysis. While it is not essential to evaluate a urine specimen by one of these methods before a urine culture is performed, certain clinical presentations with highly suggestive signs and symptoms may lend themselves to an antecedent urinalysis procedure where follow-up culture depends upon an initial positive or abnormal test result.
2. A patient has clinical signs and symptoms indicative of a possible urinary tract infection (UTI). Acute lower UTI may present with urgency, frequency, nocturia, dysuria, discharge or incontinence. These findings may also be noted in upper UTI with additional systemic symptoms (for example, fever, chills, lethargy); or pain in the costovertebral, abdominal, or pelvic areas. Signs and symptoms may overlap considerably with other inflammatory conditions of the genitourinary tract (for example, prostatitis, urethritis, vaginitis, or cervicitis). Elderly or immunocompromised patients, or patients with neurologic disorders may present atypically (for example, general debility, acute mental status changes, declining functional status).
3. The patient is being evaluated for suspected urosepsis, fever of unknown origin, or other systemic manifestations of infection but without a known source. Signs and symptoms used to define sepsis have been well established.
4. A test-of cure is generally not indicated in an uncomplicated infection. However, it may be indicated if the patient is being evaluated for response to therapy and there is a complicating co-existing urinary abnormality including structural or functional abnormalities, calculi, foreign bodies, or ureteral/renal stents or there is clinical or laboratory evidence of failure to respond as described in Indications 1 and 2.
5. In surgical procedures involving major manipulations of the genitourinary tract, preoperative examination to detect occult infection may be indicated in selected cases (for example, prior to renal transplantation, manipulation or removal of kidney stones, or transurethral surgery of the bladder or prostate).
6. Urine culture may be indicated to detect occult infection in renal transplant recipients on immunosuppressive therapy.

Limitations

1. CPT 87086 may be used one time per encounter.
2. Colony count restrictions on coverage of CPT 87088 do not apply as they may be highly variable according to syndrome or other clinical circumstances (for example, antecedent therapy, collection time, degree of hydration).
3. CPT 87088, 87184, and 87186 may be used multiple times in association with or independent of 87086, as urinary tract infections may be polymicrobial.
4. Testing for asymptomatic bacteriuria as part of a prenatal evaluation may be medically appropriate but is considered screening and, therefore, not covered by Medicare. The US Preventive Services Task Force has concluded that screening for asymptomatic bacteriuria outside of the narrow indication for pregnant women is generally not indicated. There are insufficient data to recommend screening in ambulatory elderly patients including those with diabetes. Testing may be clinically indicated on other grounds including likelihood of recurrence or potential adverse effects of antibiotics, but is considered screening in the absence of clinical or laboratory evidence of infection.

100-3, 190.13

NCD for Human Immunodeficiency Virus (HIV) Testing (Prognosis Including Monitoring) (190.13)

Indications

1. A plasma HIV RNA baseline level may be medically necessary in any patient with confirmed HIV infection.
2. Regular periodic measurement of plasma HIV RNA levels may be medically necessary to determine risk for disease progression in an HIV-infected individual and to determine when to initiate or modify antiretroviral treatment regimens.
3. In clinical situations where the risk of HIV infection is significant and initiation of therapy is anticipated, a baseline HIV quantification may be performed. These situations include:
    a. Persistence of borderline or equivocal serologic reactivity in an at-risk individual.
    b. Signs and symptoms of acute retroviral syndrome characterized by fever, malaise, lymphadenopathy and rash in an at-risk individual.

Limitations

1. Viral quantification may be appropriate for prognostic use including baseline determination, periodic monitoring, and monitoring of response to therapy. Use as a diagnostic test method is not indicated.
2. Measurement of plasma HIV RNA levels should be performed at the time of establishment of an HIV infection diagnosis. For an accurate baseline, 2 specimens in a 2-week period are appropriate.
3. For prognosis including anti-retroviral therapy monitoring, regular, periodic measurements are appropriate. The frequency of viral load testing should be consistent with the most current Centers for Disease Control and Prevention guidelines for use of anti-retroviral agents in adults and adolescents or pediatrics.
4. Because differences in absolute HIV copy number are known to occur using different assays, plasma HIV RNA levels should be measured by the same analytical method. A change in assay method may necessitate re-establishment of a baseline.
5. Nucleic acid quantification techniques are representative of rapidly emerging and evolving new technologies. As such, users are advised to remain current on FDA-approval status.

100-3, 190.14

NCD for Human Immunodeficiency Virus (HIV) Testing (Diagnosis) (190.14)

Indications and Limitations of Coverage

Indications

Diagnostic testing to establish HIV infection may be indicated when there is a strong clinical suspicion supported by one or more of the following clinical findings:

The patient has a documented, otherwise unexplained, AIDS-defining or AIDS-associated opportunistic infection.

The patient has another documented sexually transmitted disease which identifies significant risk of exposure to HIV and the potential for an early or subclinical infection.

The patient has documented acute or chronic hepatitis B or C infection that identifies a significant risk of exposure to HIV and the potential for an early or subclinical infection.

The patient has a documented AIDS-defining or AIDS-associated neoplasm.

The patient has a documented AIDS-associated neurologic disorder or otherwise unexplained dementia.

The patient has another documented AIDS-defining clinical condition, or a history of other severe, recurrent, or persistent conditions which suggest an underlying immune deficiency (for example, cutaneous or mucosal disorders).

The patient has otherwise unexplained generalized signs and symptoms suggestive of a chronic process with an underlying immune deficiency (for example, fever, weight loss, malaise, fatigue, chronic diarrhea, failure to thrive, chronic cough, hemoptysis, shortness of breath, or lymphadenopathy).

The patient has otherwise unexplained laboratory evidence of a chronic disease process with an underlying immune deficiency (for example, anemia, leukopenia, pancytopenia, lymphopenia, or low CD4+ lymphocyte count).

The patient has signs and symptoms of acute retroviral syndrome with fever, malaise, lymphadenopathy, and skin rash.

The patient has documented exposure to blood or body fluids known to be capable of transmitting HIV (for example, needlesticks and other significant blood exposures) and antiviral therapy is initiated or anticipated to be initiated.

The patient is undergoing treatment for rape. (HIV testing is a part of the rape treatment protocol.)

Limitations

HIV antibody testing in the United States is usually performed using HIV-1 or HIV-½ combination tests. HIV-2 testing is indicated if clinical circumstances suggest HIV-2 is likely (that is, compatible clinical findings and HIV-1 test negative). HIV-2 testing may also be indicated in areas of the country where there is greater prevalence of HIV-2 infections.

The Western Blot test should be performed only after documentation that the initial EIA tests are repeatedly positive or equivocal on a single sample.

The HIV antigen tests currently have no defined diagnostic usage.

Direct viral RNA detection may be performed in those situations where serologic

testing does not establish a diagnosis but strong clinical suspicion persists (for example, acute retroviral syndrome, nonspecific serologic evidence of HIV, or perinatal HIV infection).

If initial serologic tests confirm an HIV infection, repeat testing is not indicated.

If initial serologic tests are HIV EIA negative and there is no indication for confirmation of infection by viral RNA detection, the interval prior to retesting is 3-6 months.

Testing for evidence of HIV infection using serologic methods may be medically appropriate in situations where there is a risk of exposure to HIV. However, in the absence of a documented AIDS defining or HIV- associated disease, an HIV associated sign or symptom, or documented exposure to a known HIV-infected source, the testing is considered by Medicare to be screening and thus is not covered by Medicare (for example, history of multiple blood component transfusions, exposure to blood or body fluids not resulting in consideration of therapy, history of transplant, history of illicit drug use, multiple sexual partners, same-sex encounters, prostitution, or contact with prostitutes).

The CPT Editorial Panel has issued a number of codes for infectious agent detection by direct antigen or nucleic acid probe techniques that have not yet been developed or are only being used on an investigational basis. Laboratory providers are advised to remain current on FDA-approval status for these tests.

100-3, 190.15

NCD for Blood Counts (190.15)

Indications

Indications for a CBC or hemogram include red cell, platelet, and white cell disorders. Examples of these indications are enumerated individually below.

1. Indications for a CBC generally include the evaluation of bone marrow dysfunction as a result of neoplasms, therapeutic agents, exposure to toxic substances, or pregnancy. The CBC is also useful in assessing peripheral destruction of blood cells, suspected bone marrow failure or bone marrow infiltrate, suspected myeloproliferative, myelodysplastic, or lymphoproliferative processes, and immune disorders.
2. Indications for hemogram or CBC related to red cell (RBC) parameters of the hemogram include signs, symptoms, test results, illness, or disease that can be associated with anemia or other red blood cell disorder (e.g., pallor, weakness, fatigue, weight loss, bleeding, acute injury associated with blood loss or suspected blood loss, abnormal menstrual bleeding, hematuria, hematemesis, hematochezia, positive fecal occult blood test, malnutrition, vitamin deficiency, malabsorption, neuropathy, known malignancy, presence of acute or chronic disease that may have associated anemia, coagulation or hemostatic disorders, postural dizziness, syncope, abdominal pain, change in bowel habits, chronic marrow hypoplasia or decreased RBC production, tachycardia, systolic heart murmur, congestive heart failure, dyspnea, angina, nailbed deformities, growth retardation, jaundice, hepatomegaly, splenomegaly, lymphadenopathy, ulcers on the lower extremities).
3. Indications for hemogram or CBC related to red cell (RBC) parameters of the hemogram include signs, symptoms, test results, illness, or disease that can be associated with polycythemia (for example, fever, chills, ruddy skin, conjunctival redness, cough, wheezing, cyanosis, clubbing of the fingers, orthopnea, heart murmur, headache, vague cognitive changes including memory changes, sleep apnea, weakness, pruritus, dizziness, excessive sweating, visual symptoms, weight loss, massive obesity, gastrointestinal bleeding, paresthesias, dyspnea, joint symptoms, epigastric distress, pain and erythema of the fingers or toes, venous or arterial thrombosis, thromboembolism, myocardial infarction, stroke, transient ischemic attacks, congenital heart disease, chronic obstructive pulmonary disease, increased erythropoietin production associated with neoplastic, renal or hepatic disorders, androgen or diuretic use, splenomegaly, hepatomegaly, diastolic hypertension.)
4. Specific indications for CBC with differential count related to the WBC include signs, symptoms, test results, illness, or disease associated with leukemia, infections or inflammatory processes, suspected bone marrow failure or bone marrow infiltrate, suspected myeloproliferative, myelodysplastic or lymphoproliferative disorder, use of drugs that may cause leukopenia, and immune disorders (e.g., fever, chills, sweats, shock, fatigue, malaise, tachycardia, tachypnea, heart murmur, seizures, alterations of consciousness, meningismus, pain such as headache, abdominal pain, arthralgia, odynophagia, or dysuria, redness or swelling of skin, soft tissue bone, or joint, ulcers of the skin or mucous membranes, gangrene, mucous membrane discharge, bleeding, thrombosis, respiratory failure, pulmonary infiltrate, jaundice, diarrhea, vomiting, hepatomegaly, splenomegaly, lymphadenopathy, opportunistic infection such as oral candidiasis.)
5. Specific indications for CBC related to the platelet count include signs, symptoms, test results, illness, or disease associated with increased or decreased platelet production and destruction, or platelet dysfunction (e.g., gastrointestinal bleeding, genitourinary tract bleeding, bilateral epistaxis, thrombosis, ecchymosis, purpura, jaundice, petechiae, fever, heparin therapy, suspected DIC, shock, pre-eclampsia, neonate with maternal ITP, massive transfusion, recent platelet transfusion, cardiopulmonary bypass, hemolytic uremic syndrome, renal diseases, lymphadenopathy, hepatomegaly, splenomegaly, hypersplenism, neurologic abnormalities, viral or other infection, myeloproliferative, myelodysplastic, or lymphoproliferative disorder, thrombosis, exposure to toxic agents, excessive alcohol ingestion, autoimmune disorders (SLE, RA and other).
6. Indications for hemogram or CBC related to red cell (RBC) parameters of the hemogram include, in addition to those already listed, thalassemia, suspected hemoglobinopathy, lead poisoning, arsenic poisoning, and spherocytosis.
7. Specific indications for CBC with differential count related to the WBC include, in addition to those already listed, storage diseases; mucopolysaccharidoses, and use of drugs that cause leukocytosis such as G-CSF or GM-CSF
8. Specific indications for CBC related to platelet count include, in addition to those already listed, May-Hegglin syndrome and Wiskott-Aldrich syndrome.

Limitations

1. Testing of patients who are asymptomatic, or who do not have a condition that could be expected to result in a hematological abnormality, is screening and is not a covered service.
2. In some circumstances it may be appropriate to perform only a hemoglobin or hematocrit to assess the oxygen carrying capacity of the blood. When the ordering provider requests only a hemoglobin or hematocrit, the remaining components of the CBC are not covered.
3. When a blood count is performed for an end-stage renal disease (ESRD) patient, and is billed outside the ESRD rate, documentation of the medical necessity for the blood count must be submitted with the claim.
4. In some patients presenting with certain signs, symptoms or diseases, a single CBC may be appropriate. Repeat testing may not be indicated unless abnormal results are found, or unless there is a change in clinical condition. If repeat testing is performed, a more descriptive diagnosis code (e.g., anemia) should be reported to support medical necessity. However, repeat testing may be indicated where results are normal in patients with conditions where there is a continued risk for the development of hematologic abnormality.

100-3, 190.16

NCD for Partial Thromboplastin Time (PTT) (190.16)

Indications and Limitations of Coverage

Indications

1. The PTT is most commonly used to quantitate the effect of therapeutic unfractionated heparin and to regulate its dosing. Except during transitions between heparin and warfarin therapy, in general both the PTT and PT are not necessary together to assess the effect of anticoagulation therapy. PT and PTT must be justified separately.
2. A PTT may be used to assess patients with signs or symptoms of hemorrhage or thrombosis. For example: abnormal bleeding, hemorrhage or hematoma petechiae or other signs of thrombocytopenia that could be due to disseminated intravascular coagulation; swollen extremity with or without prior trauma.
3. A PTT may be useful in evaluating patients who have a history of a condition known to be associated with the risk of hemorrhage or thrombosis that is related to the intrinsic coagulation pathway. Such abnormalities may be genetic or acquired. For example: dysfibrinogenemia; afibrinogenemia (complete); acute or chronic liver dysfunction or failure, including Wilson's disease; hemophilia; liver disease and failure; infectious processes; bleeding disorders; disseminated intravascular coagulation; lupus erythematosus or other

conditions associated with circulating inhibitors, e.g., Factor VIII Inhibitor, lupus-like anticoagulant, etc.; sepsis; von Willebrand's disease; arterial and venous thrombosis, including the evaluation of hypercoagulable states; clinical conditions associated with nephrosis or renal failure; other acquired and congenital coagulopathies as well as thrombotic states.

4. A PTT may be used to assess the risk of thrombosis or hemorrhage in patients who are going to have a medical intervention known to be associated with increased risk of bleeding or thrombosis. An example is as follows: evaluation prior to invasive procedures or operations of patients with personal or family history of bleeding or who are on heparin therapy.

Limitations

1. The PTT is not useful in monitoring the effects of warfarin on a patient's coagulation routinely. However, a PTT may be ordered on a patient being treated with warfarin as heparin therapy is being discontinued. A PTT may also be indicated when the PT is markedly prolonged due to warfarin toxicity.
2. The need to repeat this test is determined by changes in the underlying medical condition and/or the dosing of heparin.
3. Testing prior to any medical intervention associated with a risk of bleeding and thrombosis (other than thrombolytic therapy) will generally be considered medically necessary only where there are signs or symptoms of a bleeding or thrombotic abnormality or a personal history of bleeding, thrombosis or a condition associated with a coagulopathy. Hospital/clinic-specific policies, protocols, etc., in and of themselves, cannot alone justify coverage.

100-3, 190.17

NCD for Prothrombin Time (PT) (190.17)

Indications

1. A PT may be used to assess patients taking warfarin. The prothrombin time is generally not useful in monitoring patients receiving heparin who are not taking warfarin.
2. A PT may be used to assess patients with signs or symptoms of abnormal bleeding or thrombosis. For example: swollen extremity with or without prior trauma; unexplained bruising; abnormal bleeding, hemorrhage or hematoma; petechiae or other signs of thrombocytopenia that could be due to disseminated intravascular coagulation.
3. A PT may be useful in evaluating patients who have a history of a condition known to be associated with the risk of bleeding or thrombosis that is related to the extrinsic coagulation pathway. Such abnormalities may be genetic or acquired. For example: dysfibrinogenemia; afibrinogenemia (complete); acute or chronic liver dysfunction or failure, including Wilson's disease and Hemochromatosis; disseminated intravascular coagulation (DIC); congenital and acquired deficiencies of factors II, V, VII, X; vitamin K deficiency; lupus erythematosus; hypercoagulable state; paraproteinemia; lymphoma; amyloidosis; acute and chronic leukemias; plasma cell dyscrasia; HIV infection; malignant neoplasms; hemorrhagic fever; salicylate poisoning; obstructive jaundice; intestinal fistula; malabsorption syndrome; colitis; chronic diarrhea; presence of peripheral venous or arterial thrombosis or pulmonary emboli or myocardial infarction; patients with bleeding or clotting tendencies; organ transplantation; presence of circulating coagulation inhibitors.
4. A PT may be used to assess the risk of hemorrhage or thrombosis in patients who are going to have a medical intervention known to be associated with increased risk of bleeding or thrombosis. For example: evaluation prior to invasive procedures or operations of patients with personal history of bleeding or a condition associated with coagulopathy prior to the use of thrombolytic medication.

Limitations

1. When an ESRD patient is tested for PT, testing more frequently than weekly requires documentation of medical necessity, e.g., other than chronic renal failure or renal failure, unspecified.
2. The need to repeat this test is determined by changes in the underlying medical condition and/or the dosing of warfarin. In a patient on stable warfarin therapy, it is ordinarily not necessary to repeat testing more than every two to three weeks. When testing is performed to evaluate a patient with signs or symptoms of abnormal bleeding or thrombosis and the initial test result is normal, it is ordinarily not necessary to repeat testing unless there is a change in the patient's medical status.
3. Since the INR is a calculation, it will not be paid in addition to the PT when expressed in seconds, and is considered part of the conventional prothrombin time.
4. Testing prior to any medical intervention associated with a risk of bleeding and thrombosis (other than thrombolytic therapy) will generally be considered medically necessary only where there are signs or symptoms of a bleeding or thrombotic abnormality or a personal history of bleeding, thrombosis or a condition associated with a coagulopathy. Hospital/clinic-specific policies, protocols, etc., in and of themselves, cannot alone justify coverage.

100-3, 190.18

100-3, 190.18

Indications

1. Ferritin (82728), iron (83540) and either iron binding capacity (83550) or transferrin (84466) are useful in the differential diagnosis of iron deficiency, anemia, and for iron overload conditions.
   a. The following presentations are examples that may support the use of these studies for evaluating iron deficiency:
      - Certain abnormal blood count values (i.e., decreased mean corpuscular volume (MCV), decreased hemoglobin/hematocrit when the MCV is low or normal, or increased red cell distribution width (RDW) and low or normal MCV);
      - Abnormal appetite (pica);
      - Acute or chronic gastrointestinal blood loss;
      - Hematuria;
      - Menorrhagia;
      - Malabsorption;
      - Status post-gastrectomy;
      - Status post-gastrojejunostomy;
      - Malnutrition;
      - Preoperative autologous blood collection(s);
      - Malignant, chronic inflammatory and infectious conditions associated with anemia which may present in a similar manner to iron deficiency anemia;
      - Following a significant surgical procedure where blood loss had occurred and had not been repaired with adequate iron replacement.

   b. The following presentations are examples that may support the use of these studies for evaluating iron overload:
      - Chronic Hepatitis;
      - Diabetes;
      - Hyperpigmentation of skin;
      - Arthropathy;
      - Cirrhosis;
      - Hypogonadism;
      - Hypopituitarism;
      - Impaired porphyrin metabolism;
      - Heart failure;
      - Multiple transfusions;
      - Sideroblastic anemia;
      - Thalassemia major;
      - Cardiomyopathy, cardiac dysrhythmias and conduction disturbances.
2. Follow-up testing may be appropriate to monitor response to therapy, e.g., oral or parenteral iron, ascorbic acid, and erythropoietin.
3. Iron studies may be appropriate in patients after treatment for other nutritional deficiency anemias, such as folate and vitamin B12, because iron deficiency may not be revealed until such a nutritional deficiency is treated.
4. Serum ferritin may be appropriate for monitoring iron status in patients with chronic renal disease with or without dialysis.
5. Serum iron may also be indicated for evaluation of toxic effects of iron and other metals (e.g., nickel, cadmium, aluminum, lead) whether due to accidental, intentional exposure or metabolic causes.

Limitations

1. Iron studies should be used to diagnose and manage iron deficiency or iron overload states. These tests are not to be used solely to assess acute phase reactants where disease management will be unchanged. For example, infections and malignancies are associated with elevations in acute phase reactants such as ferritin, and decreases in serum iron concentration, but iron studies would only be medically necessary if results of iron studies might alter the management of the primary diagnosis or might warrant direct treatment of an iron disorder or condition.
2. If a normal serum ferritin level is documented, repeat testing would not ordinarily be medically necessary unless there is a change in the patient's condition, and ferritin assessment is needed for the ongoing management of the patient. For example, a patient presents with new onset insulin-dependent diabetes mellitus and has a serum ferritin level performed for the suspicion of hemochromatosis. If the ferritin level is normal, the repeat ferritin for diabetes mellitus would not be medically necessary.
3. When an End Stage Renal Disease (ESRD) patient is tested for ferritin, testing more frequently than every three months (the frequency authorized by 3167.3, Fiscal Intermediary manual) requires documentation of medical necessity [e.g., other than "Chronic Renal Failure" (ICD-9-CM 585) or "Renal Failure, Unspecified" (ICD-9-CM 586)].
4. It is ordinarily not necessary to measure both transferrin and TIBC at the same time because TIBC is an indirect measure of transferrin. When transferrin is ordered as part of the nutritional assessment for evaluating malnutrition, it is not necessary to order other iron studies unless iron deficiency or iron overload is suspected as well.
5. It is not ordinarily necessary to measure both iron/TIBC (or transferrin) and ferritin in initial patient testing. If clinically indicated after evaluation of the initial iron studies, it may be appropriate to perform additional iron studies either on the initial specimen or on a subsequently obtained specimen. After a diagnosis of iron deficiency or iron overload is established, either iron/TIBC (or transferrin) or ferritin may be medically necessary for monitoring, but not both.
6. It would not ordinarily be considered medically necessary to do a ferritin as a preoperative test except in the presence of anemia or recent autologous blood collections prior to the surgery.

100-3, 190.19

Collagen Crosslinks, Any Method

Indications

Generally speaking, collagen crosslink testing is useful mostly in "fast losers" of bone. The age when these bone markers can help direct therapy is often pre-Medicare. By the time a fast loser of bone reaches age 65, she will most likely have been stabilized by appropriate therapy or have lost so much bone mass that further testing is useless. Coverage for bone marker assays may be established, however, for younger Medicare beneficiaries and for those men and women who might become fast losers because of some other therapy such as glucocorticoids. Safeguards should be incorporated to prevent excessive use of tests in patients for whom they have no clinical relevance.

Collagen crosslinks testing is used to:

1. Identify individuals with elevated bone resorption, who have osteoporosis in whom response to treatment is being monitored;
2. Predict response (as assessed by bone mass measurements) to FDA approved antiresorptive therapy in postmenopausal women; and
3. Assess response to treatment of patients with osteoporosis, Paget's disease of the bone, or risk for osteoporosis where treatment may include FDA approved antiresorptive agents, anti-estrogens or selective estrogen receptor moderators.

Limitations

Because of significant specimen to specimen collagen crosslink physiologic variability (15-20%), current recommendations for appropriate utilization include: one or two base-line assays from specified urine collections on separate days; followed by a repeat assay about three months after starting anti-resorptive therapy; followed by a repeat assay in 12 months after the three-month assay; and thereafter not more than annually, unless there is a change in therapy in which circumstance an additional test may be indicated three months after the initiation of new therapy.

Some collagen crosslink assays may not be appropriate for use in some disorders, according to FDA labeling restrictions.

100-3, 190.20

NCD for Blood Glucose Testing (190.20)

Indications

Blood glucose values are often necessary for the management of patients with diabetes mellitus, where hyperglycemia and hypoglycemia are often present. They are also critical in the determination of control of blood glucose levels in the patient with impaired fasting glucose (FPG 110-125 mg/dL), the patient with insulin resistance syndrome and/or carbohydrate intolerance (excessive rise in glucose following ingestion of glucose or glucose sources of food), in the patient with a hypoglycemia disorder such as nesidioblastosis or insulinoma, and in patients with a catabolic or malnutrition state. In addition to those conditions already listed, glucose testing may be medically necessary in patients with tuberculosis, unexplained chronic or recurrent infections, alcoholism, coronary artery disease (especially in women), or unexplained skin conditions (including pruritis, local skin infections, ulceration and gangrene without an established cause).

Many medical conditions may be a consequence of a sustained elevated or depressed glucose level. These include comas, seizures or epilepsy, confusion, abnormal hunger, abnormal weight loss or gain, and loss of sensation. Evaluation of glucose may also be indicated in patients on medications known to affect carbohydrate metabolism.

Effective January 1, 2005, the Medicare law expanded coverage to diabetic screening services. Some forms of blood glucode testing covered under this national coverage determination may be covered for screening purposes subject to specified frequencies. See 42 CFR 410.18 and section 90, chapter 18 of the Claims Processing Manual, for a full description of this screening benefit.

Limitations

Frequent home blood glucose testing by diabetic patients should be encouraged. In stable, non-hospitalized patients who are unable or unwilling to do home monitoring, it may be reasonable and necessary to measure quantitative blood glucose up to four times annually.

Depending upon the age of the patient, type of diabetes, degree of control, complications of diabetes, and other co-morbid conditions, more frequent testing than four times annually may be reasonable and necessary.

In some patients presenting with nonspecific signs, symptoms, or diseases not normally associated with disturbances in glucose metabolism, a single blood glucose test may be medically necessary. Repeat testing may not be indicated unless abnormal results are found or unless there is a change in clinical condition. If repeat testing is performed, a specific diagnosis code (e.g., diabetes) should be reported to support medical necessity. However, repeat testing may be indicated where results are normal in patients with conditions where there is a confirmed continuing risk of glucose metabolism abnormality (e.g., monitoring glucocorticoid therapy).

100-3, 190.21

NCD for Glycated Hemoglobin/Glycated Protein (190.21)

Indications

Glycated hemoglobin/protein testing is widely accepted as medically necessary for the management and control of diabetes. It is also valuable to assess hyperglycemia, a history of hyperglycemia or dangerous hypoglycemia. Glycated protein testing may be used in place of glycated hemoglobin in the management of diabetic patients, and is particularly useful in patients who have abnormalities of erythrocytes such as hemolytic anemia or hemoglobinopathies.

Limitations

It is not considered reasonable and necessary to perform glycated hemoglobin tests more often than every three months on a controlled diabetic patient to determine whether the patient's metabolic control has been on average within the target range. It is not considered reasonable and necessary for these tests to be performed more frequently than once a month for diabetic pregnant women. Testing for uncontrolled type one or two diabetes mellitus may require testing more than four times a year. The above Description Section provides the clinical basis for those situations in which testing more frequently than four times per annum is indicated, and medical necessity documentation must support such testing in excess of the above guidelines.

Many methods for the analysis of glycated hemoglobin show significant interference from elevated levels of fetal hemoglobin or by variant hemoglobin molecules. When the glycated hemoglobin assay is initially performed in these patients, the laboratory may inform the ordering physician of a possible analytical interference. Alternative testing, including glycated protein, for example, fructosamine, may be indicated for the monitoring of the degree of glycemic control in this situation. It is therefore conceivable that a patient will have both a glycated hemoglobin and glycated protein ordered on the same day. This should be limited to the initial assay of glycated hemoglobin, with subsequent exclusive use of glycated protein. These tests are not considered to be medically necessary for the diagnosis of diabetes.

100-3, 190.22

NCD for Thyroid Testing (190.22)

Indications

Thyroid function tests are used to define hyper function, euthyroidism, or hypofunction of thyroid disease. Thyroid testing may be reasonable and necessary to:

- Distinguish between primary and secondary hypothyroidism;
- Confirm or rule out primary hypothyroidism;
- Monitor thyroid hormone levels (for example, patients with goiter, thyroid nodules, or thyroid cancer);
- Monitor drug therapy in patients with primary hypothyroidism;
- Confirm or rule out primary hyperthyroidism; and
- Monitor therapy in patients with hyperthyroidism.

Thyroid function testing may be medically necessary in patients with disease or neoplasm of the thyroid and other endocrine glands. Thyroid function testing may also be medically necessary in patients with metabolic disorders; malnutrition; hyperlipidemia; certain types of anemia; psychosis and non-psychotic personality disorders; unexplained depression; ophthalmologic disorders; various cardiac arrhythmias; disorders of menstruation; skin conditions; myalgias; and a wide array of signs and symptoms, including alterations in consciousness; malaise; hypothermia; symptoms of the nervous and musculoskeletal system; skin and integumentary system; nutrition and metabolism; cardiovascular; and gastrointestinal system.

It may be medically necessary to do follow-up thyroid testing in patients with a personal history of malignant neoplasm of the endocrine system and in patients on long-term thyroid drug therapy.

Limitations

Testing may be covered up to two times a year in clinically stable patients; more frequent testing may be reasonable and necessary for patients whose thyroid therapy has been altered or in whom symptoms or signs of hyperthyroidism or hypothyroidism are noted.

100-3, 190.23

NCD for Lipid Testing (190.23)

Indications and Limitations of Coverage

Indications

The medical community recognizes lipid testing as appropriate for evaluating atherosclerotic cardiovascular disease. Conditions in which lipid testing may be indicated include:

- Assessment of patients with atherosclerotic cardiovascular disease.
- Evaluation of primary dyslipidemia.
- Any form of atherosclerotic disease, or any disease leading to the formation of atherosclerotic disease.
- Diagnostic evaluation of diseases associated with altered lipid metabolism, such as: nephrotic syndrome, pancreatitis, hepatic disease, and hypo and hyperthyroidism.
- Secondary dyslipidemia, including diabetes mellitus, disorders of gastrointestinal absorption, chronic renal failure.
- Signs or symptoms of dyslipidemias, such as skin lesions.
- As follow-up to the initial screen for coronary heart disease (total cholesterol + HDL cholesterol) when total cholesterol is determined to be high (>240 mg/dL), or borderline-high (200-240 mg/dL) plus two or more coronary heart disease risk factors, or an HDL cholesterol, <35 mg/dl.

To monitor the progress of patients on anti-lipid dietary management and pharmacologic therapy for the treatment of elevated blood lipid disorders, total cholesterol, HDL cholesterol and LDL cholesterol may be used. Triglycerides may be obtained if this lipid fraction is also elevated or if the patient is put on drugs (for example, thiazide diuretics, beta blockers, estrogens, glucocorticoids, and tamoxifen) which may raise the triglyceride level.

When monitoring long term anti-lipid dietary or pharmacologic therapy and when following patients with borderline high total or LDL cholesterol levels, it may be reasonable to perform the lipid panel annually. A lipid panel at a yearly interval will usually be adequate while measurement of the serum total cholesterol or a measured LDL should suffice for interim visits if the patient does not have hypertriglyceridemia.

Any one component of the panel or a measured LDL may be reasonable and necessary up to six times the first year for monitoring dietary or pharmacologic therapy. More frequent total cholesterol HDL cholesterol, LDL cholesterol and triglyceride testing may be indicated for marked elevations or for changes to anti-lipid therapy due to inadequate initial patient response to dietary or pharmacologic therapy. The LDL cholesterol or total cholesterol may be measured three times yearly after treatment goals have been achieved.

Electrophoretic or other quantitation of lipoproteins may be indicated if the patient has a primary disorder of lipoid metabolism.

Effective January 1, 2005, the Medicare law expanded coverage to cardiovascular screening services. Several of the procedures included in this NCD may be covered for screening purposes subject to specified frequencies. See 42 CFR 410.17 and section 100, chapter 18, of the Claims Processing Manual, for a full description of this benefit.Limitations

Limitations
Lipid panel and hepatic panel testing may be used for patients with severe psoriasis which has not responded to conventional therapy and for which the retinoid etretinate has been prescribed and who have developed hyperlipidemia or hepatic toxicity. Specific examples include erythrodermia and generalized pustular type and psoriasis associated with arthritis.

Routine screening and prophylactic testing for lipid disorder are not covered by Medicare. While lipid screening may be medically appropriate, Medicare by statute does not pay for it. Lipid testing in asymptomatic individuals is considered to be screening regardless of the presence of other risk factors such as family history, tobacco use, etc.

Once a diagnosis is established, one or several specific tests are usually adequate for monitoring the course of the disease. Less specific diagnoses (for example, other chest pain) alone do not support medical necessity of these tests.

When monitoring long term anti-lipid dietary or pharmacologic therapy and when following patients with borderline high total or LDL cholesterol levels, it is reasonable to perform the lipid panel annually. A lipid panel at a yearly interval will usually be adequate while measurement of the serum total cholesterol or a measured LDL should suffice for interim visits if the patient does not have hypertriglyceridemia.

Any one component of the panel or a measured LDL may be medically necessary up to six times the first year for monitoring dietary or pharmacologic therapy. More frequent total cholesterol HDL cholesterol, LDL cholesterol and triglyceride testing may be indicated for marked elevations or for changes to anti-lipid therapy due to inadequate initial patient response to dietary or pharmacologic therapy. The LDL cholesterol or total cholesterol may be measured three times yearly after treatment goals have been achieved.

If no dietary or pharmacological therapy is advised, monitoring is not necessary.

When evaluating non-specific chronic abnormalities of the liver (for example, elevations of transaminase, alkaline phosphatase, abnormal imaging studies, etc.), a lipid panel would generally not be indicated more than twice per year

100-3, 190.24

NCD for Digoxin Therapeutic Drug Assay (190.24)

Indications and Limitations of Coverage

Indications
Digoxin levels may be performed to monitor drug levels of individuals receiving digoxin therapy because the margin of safety between side effects and toxicity is narrow or because the blood level may not be high enough to achieve the desired clinical effect.

Clinical indications may include individuals on digoxin:

- With symptoms, signs or electrocardiogram (ECG) suggestive of digoxin toxicity.
- Taking medications that influence absorption, bioavailability, distribution, and/or elimination of digoxin.
- With impaired renal, hepatic, gastrointestinal, or thyroid function.
- With pH and/or electrolyte abnormalities.
- With unstable cardiovascular status, including myocarditis.
- Requiring monitoring of patient compliance.

Clinical indications may include individuals:

- Suspected of accidental or intended overdose.
- Who have an acceptable cardiac diagnosis (as listed) and for whom an accurate history of use of digoxin is unobtainable.

The value of obtaining regular serum digoxin levels is uncertain, but it may be reasonable to check levels once yearly after a steady state is achieved. In addition, it may be reasonable to check the level if:

- Heart failure status worsens.
- Renal function deteriorates.
- Additional medications are added that could affect the digoxin level.
- Signs or symptoms of toxicity develop.

Steady state will be reached in approximately 1 week in patients with normal renal function, although 2?3 weeks may be needed in patients with renal impairment. After changes in dosages or the addition of a medication that could affect the digoxin level, it is reasonable to check the digoxin level one week after the change or addition. Based on the clinical situation, in cases of digoxin toxicity, testing may need to be done more than once a week.

Digoxin is indicated for the treatment of patients with heart failure due to systolic dysfunction and for reduction of the ventricular response in patients with atrial fibrillation or flutter. Digoxin may also be indicated for the treatment of other supraventricular arrhythmias, particularly in the presence of heart failure.

Limitations
This test is not appropriate for patients on digitoxin or treated with digoxin FAB (fragment antigen binding) antibody.

100-3, 190.25

NCD for Alpha-fetoprotein (AFP) (190.25)

Indications and Limitations of Coverage
AFP is useful for the diagnosis of hepatocellular carcinoma in high-risk patients (such as alcoholic cirrhosis, cirrhosis of viral etiology, hemochromatosis, and alpha 1-antitrypsin deficiency) and in separating patients with benign hepatocellular neoplasms or metastases from those with hepatocellular carcinoma and, as a non-specific tumor associated antigen, serves in marking germ cell neoplasms of the testis, ovary, retro peritoneum, and mediastinum.

100-3, 190.26

NCD for Carcinoembryonic Antigen (CEA) (190.26)

Indications
CEA may be medically necessary for follow-up of patients with colorectal carcinoma. It would however only be medically necessary at treatment decision?making points. In some clinical situations (e.g. adenocarcinoma of the lung, small cell carcinoma of the lung, and some gastrointestinal carcinomas) when a more specific marker is not expressed by the tumor, CEA may be a medically necessary alternative marker for monitoring. Preoperative CEA may also be helpful in determining the post?operative adequacy of surgical resection and subsequent medical management. In general, a single tumor marker will suffice in following patients with colorectal carcinoma or other malignancies that express such tumor markers.

In following patients who have had treatment for colorectal carcinoma, ASCO guideline suggests that if resection of liver metastasis would be indicated, it is recommended that post-operative CEA testing be performed every two to three months in patients with initial stage II or stage III disease for at least two years after diagnosis.

For patients with metastatic solid tumors which express CEA, CEA may be measured at the start of the treatment and with subsequent treatment cycles to assess the tumor's response to therapy.

Limitations
Serum CEA determinations are generally not indicated more frequently than once per chemotherapy treatment cycle for patients with metastatic solid tumors which express CEA or every two months post-surgical treatment for patients who have had colorectal carcinoma. However, it may be proper to order the test more frequently in certain situations, for example, when there has been a significant change from prior CEA level or a significant change in patient status which could reflect disease progression or recurrence.

Testing with a diagnosis of an in situ carcinoma is not reasonably done more frequently than once, unless the result is abnormal, in which case the test may be repeated once.

100-3, 190.27

NCD for Human Chorionic Gonadotropin (hCG) (190.27)

Indications and Limitations of Coverage

Indications
hCG is useful for monitoring and diagnosis of germ cell neoplasms of the ovary, testis, mediastinum, retroperitoneum, and central nervous system. In addition, hCG is useful for monitoring pregnant patients with vaginal bleeding, hypertension and/or suspected fetal loss.

Limitations
It is not reasonable and necessary to perform hCG testing more than once per month for diagnostic purposes. It may be performed as needed for monitoring of patient progress and treatment. Qualitative hCG assays are not appropriate for medically managing patients with known or suspected germ cell neoplasms.

100-3, 190.28

NCD for Tumor Antigen by Immunoassay - CA125 (190.28)

Indications
CA 125 is a high molecular weight serum tumor marker elevated in 80% of patients who present with epithelial ovarian carcinoma. It is also elevated in carcinomas of the fallopian tube, endometrium, and endocervix. An elevated level may also be associated with the presence of a malignant mesothelioma or primary peritoneal carcinoma.

A CA125 level may be obtained as part of the initial pre-operative work-up for women presenting with a suspicious pelvic mass to be used as a baseline for purposes of post-operative monitoring. Initial declines in CA 125 after initial surgery and/or chemotherapy for ovarian carcinoma are also measured by obtaining three serum levels during the first month post treatment to determine the patient's CA 125 half-life, which has significant prognostic implications.

The CA 125 levels are again obtained at the completion of chemotherapy as an index of residual disease. Surveillance CA125 measurements are generally obtained every 3 months for 2 years, every 6 months for the next 3 years, and yearly thereafter. CA 125 levels are also an important indicator of a patient's response to therapy in the presence of advanced or recurrent disease. In this setting, CA 125 levels may be obtained prior to each treatment cycle.

Limitations
These services are not covered for the evaluation of patients with signs or symptoms suggestive of malignancy. The service may be ordered at times necessary to assess either the presence of recurrent disease or the patient's response to treatment with subsequent treatment cycles.

The CA 125 is specifically not covered for aiding in the differential diagnosis of patients with a pelvic mass as the sensitivity and specificity of the test is not sufficient. In general, a single "tumor marker" will suffice in following a patient with one of these malignancies.

100-3, 190.29

NCD for Tumor Antigen by Immunoassay CA 15-3/CA 27.29 (190.29)

Indications

Multiple tumor markers are available for monitoring the response of certain malignancies to therapy and assessing whether residual tumor exists post-surgical therapy.

CA 15-3 is often medically necessary to aid in the management of patients with breast cancer. Serial testing must be used in conjunction with other clinical methods for monitoring breast cancer. For monitoring, if medically necessary, use consistently either CA 15-3 or CA 27.29, not both.

CA 27.29 is equivalent to CA 15-3 in its usage in management of patients with breast cancer.

Limitations

These services are not covered for the evaluation of patients with signs or symptoms suggestive of malignancy. The service may be ordered at times necessary to assess either the presence of recurrent disease or the patient's response to treatment with subsequent treatment cycles.

100-3, 190.30

NCD for Tumor Antigen by Immunoassay CA 19-9 (190.30)

Indications

Multiple tumor markers are available for monitoring the response of certain malignancies to therapy and assessing whether residual tumor exists post-surgical therapy.

Levels are useful in following the course of patients with established diagnosis of pancreatic and biliary ductal carcinoma. The test is not indicated for diagnosing these two diseases.

Limitations

These services are not covered for the evaluation of patients with signs or symptoms suggestive of malignancy. The service may be ordered at times necessary to assess either the presence of recurrent disease or the patient's response to treatment with subsequent treatment cycles.

100-3, 190.31

NCD for Prostate Specific Antigen (PSA) (190.31)

Indications

PSA is of proven value in differentiating benign from malignant disease in men with lower urinary tract signs and symptoms (e.g., hematuria, slow urine stream, hesitancy, urgency, frequency, nocturia and incontinence) as well as with patients with palpably abnormal prostate glands on physician exam, and in patients with other laboratory or imaging studies that suggest the possibility of a malignant prostate disorder. PSA is also a marker used to follow the progress of prostate cancer once a diagnosis has been established, such as in detecting metastatic or persistent disease in patients who may require additional treatment. PSA testing may also be useful in the differential diagnosis of men presenting with as yet undiagnosed disseminated metastatic disease.

Limitations

Generally, for patients with lower urinary tract signs or symptoms, the test is performed only once per year unless there is a change in the patient's medical condition.

Testing with a diagnosis of in situ carcinoma is not reasonably done more frequently than once, unless the result is abnormal, in which case the test may be repeated once.

100-3, 190.32

NCD for Gamma Glutamyl Transferase (GGT) (190.32)

Indications

1. To provide information about known or suspected hepatobiliary disease, for example:
   a. Following chronic alcohol or drug ingestion.
   b. Following exposure to hepatotoxins.
   c. When using medication known to have a potential for causing liver toxicity (e.g., following the drug manufacturer's recommendations).
   d. Following infection (e.g., viral hepatitis and other specific infections such as amoebiasis, tuberculosis, psittacosis, and similar infections).
2. To assess liver injury/function following diagnosis of primary or secondary malignant neoplasms.
3. To assess liver injury/function in a wide variety of disorders and diseases known to cause liver involvement (e.g., diabetes mellitus, malnutrition, disorders of iron and mineral metabolism, sarcoidosis, amyloidosis, lupus, and hypertension).
4. To assess liver function related to gastrointestinal disease.
5. To assess liver function related to pancreatic disease.
6. To assess liver function in patients subsequent to liver transplantation.
7. To differentiate between the different sources of elevated alkaline phosphatase activity.

Limitations

When used to assess liver dysfunction secondary to existing non-hepatobiliary disease with no change in signs, symptoms, or treatment, it is generally not necessary to repeat a GGT determination after a normal result has been obtained unless new indications are present.

If the GGT is the only "liver" enzyme abnormally high, it is generally not necessary to pursue further evaluation for liver disease for this specific indication.

When used to determine if other abnormal enzyme tests reflect liver abnormality rather than other tissue, it generally is not necessary to repeat a GGT more than one time per week.

Because of the extreme sensitivity of GGT as a marker for cytochrome oxidase induction or cell membrane permeability, it is generally not useful in monitoring patients with known liver disease.

100-3, 190.33

NCD for Hepatitis Panel/Acute Hepatitis Panel (190.33)

Indications

1. To detect viral hepatitis infection when there are abnormal liver function test results, with or without signs or symptoms of hepatitis.
2. Prior to and subsequent to liver transplantation.

Limitations

After a hepatitis diagnosis has been established, only individual tests, rather than the entire panel, are needed.

100-3, 190.34

NCD for Fecal Occult Blood Test (FOBT) (190.34)

NCD for Fecal Occult Blood Test (FOBT) (190.34)

Indications

1. To evaluate known or suspected alimentary tract conditions that might cause bleeding into the intestinal tract.
2. To evaluate unexpected anemia.
3. To evaluate abnormal signs, symptoms, or complaints that might be associated with loss of blood.
4. To evaluate patient complaints of black or red-tinged stools.

Limitations

1. The FOBT is reported once for the testing of up to three separate specimens (comprising either one or two tests per specimen).
2. In patients who are taking non-steroidal anti-inflammatory drugs and have a history of gastrointestinal bleeding but no other signs, symptoms, or complaints associated with gastrointestinal blood loss, testing for occult blood may generally be appropriate no more than once every three months.

When testing is done for the purpose of screening for colorectal cancer in the absence of signs, symptoms, conditions, or complaints associated with gastrointestinal blood loss, report the HCPCS code for colorectal cancer screening; fecal-occult blood test, 1-3 simultaneous determinations should be used.

100-3, 210.1

NCD for Prostate Cancer Screening Tests (210.1)

Indications and Limitations of Coverage

CIM 50-55

Covered

A. General

Section 4103 of the Balanced Budget Act of 1997 provides for coverage of certain prostate cancer screening tests subject to certain coverage, frequency, and payment limitations. Medicare will cover prostate cancer screening tests/procedures for the early detection of prostate cancer. Coverage of prostate cancer screening tests includes the following procedures furnished to an individual for the early detection of prostate cancer:

- Screening digital rectal examination; and
- Screening prostate specific antigen blood test

B. Screening Digital Rectal Examinations

Screening digital rectal examinations are covered at a frequency of once every 12 months for men who have attained age 50 (at least 11 months have passed following the month in which the last Medicare-covered screening digital rectal examination was performed). Screening digital rectal examination means a clinical examination of an individual's prostate for nodules or other abnormalities of the prostate. This screening must be performed by a doctor of medicine or osteopathy (as defined in §1861(r)(1) of the Act), or by a physician assistant, nurse practitioner, clinical nurse specialist, or certified nurse midwife (as defined in §1861(aa) and §1861(gg) of the Act) who is authorized under State law to perform the examination, fully knowledgeable about the beneficiary's medical condition, and would be responsible for using the results of any examination performed in the overall management of the beneficiary's specific medical problem.

C. Screening Prostate Specific Antigen Tests

Screening prostate specific antigen tests are covered at a frequency of once every 12 months for men who have attained age 50 (at least 11 months have passed following the month in which the last Medicare-covered screening prostate specific antigen test was performed). Screening prostate specific antigen tests (PSA) means a test to detect the marker for adenocarcinoma of prostate. PSA is a reliable immunocytochemical marker for primary and metastatic adenocarcinoma of prostate. This screening must be ordered by the beneficiary's physician or by the beneficiary's physician assistant, nurse practitioner, clinical nurse specialist, or certified nurse midwife (the term "attending physician" is defined in §1861(r)(1) of the Act to mean a doctor of medicine or osteopathy and the terms "physician assistant, nurse practitioner, clinical nurse specialist, or certified nurse midwife" are defined in §1861(aa) and §1861(gg) of the Act) who is fully knowledgeable about the beneficiary's medical condition, and who would be responsible for using the results of any examination (test) performed in the overall management of the beneficiary's specific medica

100-3, 210.2

NCD for Screening Pap Smears and Pelvic Examinations for Early Detection of Cervical or Vaginal Cancer (210.2)

Indications and Limitations of Coverage

CIM 50-20.1

Screening Pap Smear

A screening pap smear and related medically necessary services provided to a woman for the early detection of cervical cancer (including collection of the sample of cells and a physician's interpretation of the test results) and pelvic examination (including clinical breast examination) are covered under Medicare Part B when ordered by a physician (or authorized practitioner) under one of the following conditions:

- She has not had such a test during the preceding two years or is a woman of childbearing age (§1861(nn) of the Act).
- There is evidence (on the basis of her medical history or other findings) that she is at high risk of developing cervical cancer and her physician (or authorized practitioner) recommends that she have the test performed more frequently than every two years.

High risk factors for cervical and vaginal cancer are:

- Early onset of sexual activity (under 16 years of age).
- Multiple sexual partners (five or more in a lifetime).
- History of sexually transmitted disease (including HIV infection).
- Fewer than three negative or any pap smears within the previous 7 years.; and
- DES (diethylstilbestrol) - exposed daughters of women who took DES during pregnancy.

NOTE: Claims for pap smears must indicate the beneficiary's low or high risk status by including the appropriate ICD-9-CM on the line item (Item 24E of the Form CMS-1500).

Definitions

- A woman as described in §1861(nn) of the Act is a woman who is of childbearing age and has had a pap smear test during any of the preceding three years that indicated the presence of cervical or vaginal cancer or other abnormality, or is at high risk of developing cervical or vaginal cancer.
- A woman of childbearing age is one who is premenopausal and has been determined by a physician or other qualified practitioner to be of childbearing age, based upon the medical history or other findings.
- Other qualified practitioner, as defined in 42 CFR 410.56(a) includes a certified nurse midwife (as defined in §1861(gg) of the Act), or a physician assistant, nurse practitioner, or clinical nurse specialist (as defined in §1861(aa) of the Act) who is authorized under State law to perform the examination.

Screening Pelvic Examination

Section 4102 of the Balanced Budget Act of 1997 provides for coverage of screening pelvic examinations (including a clinical breast examination) for all female beneficiaries, subject to certain frequency and other limitations. A screening pelvic examination (including a clinical breast examination) should include at least seven of the following eleven elements:

- Inspection and palpation of breasts for masses or lumps, tenderness, symmetry, or nipple discharge.
- Digital rectal examination including sphincter tone, presence of hemorrhoids, and rectal masses. Pelvic examination (with or without specimen collection for smears and cultures) including:
- External genitalia (for example, general appearance, hair distribution, or lesions).
- Urethral maetus (for example, size, location, lesions, or prolapse).
- Urethra (for example, masses, tenderness, or scarring).
- Bladder (for example, fullness, masses, or tenderness).
- Vagina (for example, general appearance, estrogen effect, discharge lesions, pelvic support, cystocele, or rectocele).
- Cervix (for example, general appearance, lesions, or discharge).
- Uterus (for example, size, contour, position, mobility, tenderness, consistency, descent, or support).
- Adnexa/parametria (for example, masses, tenderness, organomegaly, or nodularity).
- Anus and perineum.

This description is from Documentation Guidelines for Evaluation and Management Services, published in May 1997 and was developed by the Centers for Medicare and Medicaid

100-3, 210.3

Colorectal Cancer Screening Tests

A. General

Section 4104 of the Balanced Budget Act of 1997 provides for coverage of screening colorectal cancer procedures under Medicare Part B. Medicare currently covers: (1) annual fecal occult blood tests (FOBTs); (2) flexible sigmoidoscopy over 4 years; (3) screening colonoscopy for persons at average risk for colorectal cancer every 10 years, or for persons at high risk for colorectal cancer every 2 years; (4) barium enema every 4 years as an alternative to flexible sigmoidoscopy, or every 2 years as an alternative to colonoscopy for persons at high risk for colorectal cancer; and, (5) other procedures the Secretary finds appropriate based on consultation with appropriate experts and organizations.

Coverage of the above screening examinations was implemented in regulations through a final rule that was published on October 31, 1997 (62 FR 59079), and was effective January 1, 1998. At that time, based on consultation with appropriate experts and organizations, the definition of the term "FOBT" was defined in 42 CFR Sec.410.37(a)(2) of the regulation to mean a "guaiac-based test for peroxidase activity, testing two samples from each of three consecutive stools."

In the 2003 Physician Fee Schedule Final Rule (67 FR 79966) effective March 1, 2003, the Centers for Medicare & Medicaid Services (CMS) amended the FOBT screening test regulation definition to provide that it could include either: (1) a guaiac-based FOBT, or, (2) other tests determined by the Secretary through a national coverage determination.

B. Nationally Covered Indications

Fecal Occult Blood Tests (FOBT) (effective for services performed on or after January 1, 2004)

1. History

   The FOBTs are generally divided into two types: immunoassay and guaiac types. Immunoassay (or immunochemical) fecal occult blood tests (iFOBT) use "antibodies directed against human globin epitopes. While most iFOBTs use spatulas to collect stool samples, some use a brush to collect toilet water surrounding the stool. Most iFOBTs require laboratory processing.

   Guaiac fecal occult blood tests (gFOBT) use a peroxidase reaction to indicate presence of the heme portion of hemoglobin. Guaiac turns blue after oxidation by oxidants or peroxidases in the presence of an oxygen donor such as hydrogen peroxide. Most FOBTs use sticks to collect stool samples and may be developed in a physician's office or a laboratory. In 1998, Medicare began reimbursement for guaiac FOBTs, but not immunoassay type tests for colorectal cancer screening. Since the fundamental process is similar for other iFOBTs, CMS evaluated colorectal cancer screening using immunoassay FOBTs in general.

2. Expanded Coverage

   Medicare covers one screening FOBT per annum for the early detection of colorectal cancer. This means that Medicare will cover one guaiac-based (gFOBT) or one immunoassay-based (iFOBT) at a frequency of every 12 months; i.e., at least 11 months have passed following the month in which the last covered screening FOBT was performed, for beneficiaries aged 50 years and older. The beneficiary completes the existing gFOBT by taking samples from two different sites of three consecutive stools; the beneficiary completes the iFOBT by taking the appropriate number of stool samples according to the specific manufacturer's instructions. This screening requires a written order from the beneficiary's attending physician. ("Attending physician means a doctor of medicine or osteopathy (as defined in Sec.1861(r)(1) of the Social Security Act) who is fully knowledgeable about the beneficiary's medical condition, and who would be responsible for using the results of any examination performed in the overall management of the beneficiary's specific medical problem.)

C. Nationally Non-Covered Indications

All other indications for colorectal cancer screening not otherwise specified above remain non-covered. Non-coverage specifically includes:

1. Screening DNA (Deoxyribonucleic acid) stool tests, effective April 28, 2008, and,
2. Screening computed tomographic colonography (CTC), effective May 12, 2009.

D. Other

N/A

(This NCD last reviewed May 2009.)

100-3, 220.1

NCD for Computerized Tomography (220.1)

A. General

Diagnostic examinations of the head (head scans) and of other parts of the body (body scans) performed by computerized tomography (CT) scanners are covered if you find that the medical and scientific literature and opinion support the effective use of a scan for the condition, and the scan is: (1) reasonable and necessary for the individual patient; and (2) performed on a model of CT equipment that meets the criteria in C below.

CT scans have become the primary diagnostic tool for many conditions and symptoms. CT scanning used as the primary diagnostic tool can be cost effective because it can eliminate the need for a series of other tests, is non-invasive and thus virtually eliminates complications, and does not require hospitalization.

B. Determining Whether a CT Scan Is Reasonable and Necessary

Sufficient information must be provided with claims to differentiate CT scans from other radiology services and to make coverage determinations. Carefully review claims to insure that a scan is reasonable and necessary for the individual patient; i.e., the use must be found to be medically appropriate considering the patient's symptoms and preliminary diagnosis.

There is no general rule that requires other diagnostic tests to be tried before CT scanning is used. However, in an individual case the contractor's medical staff may determine that use of a CT scan as the initial diagnostic test was not reasonable and necessary because it was not supported by the patient's symptoms or complaints stated on the claim form; e.g., "periodic headaches."

Claims for CT scans are reviewed for evidence of abuse which might include the absence of reasonable indications for the scans, an excessive number of scans or unnecessarily expensive types of scans considering the facts in the particular cases.

C-Approved Models of CT Equipment

1. Criteria for Approval

   In the absence of evidence to the contrary, you may assume that a CT scan for which payment is requested has been performed on equipment that meets the following criteria:

   a. The model must be known to the Food and Drug Administration, and
   b. Must be in the full market release phase of development.

Should it be necessary to confirm that those criteria are met, ask the manufacturer to submit the information in subsection C.2. If manufacturers inquire about obtaining Medicare approval for their equipment, inform them of the foregoing criteria.

2. Evidence of Approval

   a. The letter sent by the Bureau of Radiological Health, Food and Drug Administration (FDA), to the manufacturer acknowledging the FDA's receipt of information on the specific CT scanner system model submitted as required under Public Law 90-602, "The Radiation Control for Health and Safety Act of 1968."

   b. A letter signed by the chief executive officer or other officer acting in a similar capacity for the manufacturer which:

      1) Furnishes the CT scanner system model number, all names that hospitals and physicians' offices may use to refer to the CT scanner system on claims, and the accession number assigned by FDA to the specific model; \

      2) Specifies whether the scanner performs head scans only, body scans only (i.e., scans of parts of the body other than the head), or head and body scans;

      3) States that the company or corporation is satisfied with the results of the developmental stages that preceded the full market release phase of the equipment, that the equipment is in the full market release phase, and the date on which it was decided to put the product into the full market release phase.

D-Mobile Ct Equipment

CT scans performed on mobile units are subject to the same Medicare coverage requirements applicable to scans performed on stationary units, as well as certain health and safety requirements recommended by PHS. As with scans performed on stationary units, the scans must be determined medically necessary for the individual patient. The scans must be performed on types of CT scanning equipment that have been approved for use as stationary units (see C above), and must be in compliance with applicable State laws and regulations for control of radiation.

1. Hospital Setting

   The hospital must assume responsibility for the quality of the scan furnished to inpatients and outpatients and must assure that a radiologist or other qualified physician is in charge of the procedure. The radiologist or other physician (i.e., one who is with the mobile unit) who is responsible for the procedure must be approved by the hospital for similar privileges.

2. Ambulatory Setting

   If mobile CT scan services are furnished at an ambulatory health care facility other than a hospital-based facility, e.g., a freestanding physician-directed clinic, the diagnostic procedure must be performed by or under the direct personal supervision of a radiologist or other qualified physician. In addition, the facility must maintain a record of the attending physician's order for a scan performed on a mobile unit.

3. Billing for Mobile CT Scans

   Hospitals, hospital-associated radiologists, ambulatory health care facilities, and physician owner/operators of mobile units may bill for mobile scans as they would for scans performed on stationary equipment.

4. Claims Review

   Evidence of compliance with applicable State laws and regulations for control of radiation should be requested from owners of mobile CT scan units upon receipt of the first claims. All mobile scan claims should be reviewed very carefully in accordance with instructions applicable to scans performed on fixed units, with particular emphasis on the medical necessity for scans performed in an ambulatory setting.

E-Multi-Planar Diagnostic Imaging (MPDI)

In usual computerized tomography (CT) scanning procedures, a series of transverse or axial images are reproduced. These transverse images are routinely translated into coronal and/or sagittal views. Multiplanar diagnostic imaging (MPDI) is a process which further translates the data produced by CT scanning by providing reconstructed oblique images which can contribute to diagnostic information. MPDI, also known as planar image reconstruction or reformatted imaging, is covered under Medicare when provided as a service to an entity performing a covered CT scan.

NCD for Magnetic Resonance Imaging (220.2)

A. General

1. Method of Operation

   Magnetic Resonance Imaging (MRI), formerly called nuclear magnetic resonance (NMR), is a non-invasive method of graphically representing the distribution of water and other hydrogen-rich molecules in the human body. In contrast to conventional radiographs or computed tomography (CT) scans, in which the image is produced by x-ray beam attenuation by an object, MRI is capable of producing images by several techniques. In fact, various combinations of MRI image production methods may be employed to emphasize particular characteristics of the tissue or body part being examined. The basic elements by which MRI produces an image are the density of hydrogen nuclei in the object being examined, their motion, and the relaxation times, and the period of time required for the nuclei to return to their original states in the main, static magnetic field after being subjected to a brief additional magnetic field. These relaxation times reflect the physical-chemical properties of tissue and the molecular environment of its hydrogen nuclei. Only hydrogen atoms are present in human tissues in sufficient concentration for current use in clinical MRI.

   Magnetic Resonance Angiography (MRA) is a non-invasive diagnostic test that is an application of MRI. By analyzing the amount of energy released from tissues exposed to a strong magnetic field, MRA provides images of normal and diseased blood vessels, as well as visualization and quantification of blood flow through these vessels.

2. General Clinical Utility

   Overall, MRI is a useful diagnostic imaging modality that is capable of demonstrating a wide variety of soft-tissue lesions with contrast resolution equal or superior to CT scanning in various parts of the body.

   Among the advantages of MRI are the absence of ionizing radiation and the ability to achieve high levels of tissue contrast resolution without injected iodinated radiological contrast agents. Recent advances in technology have resulted in development and Food and Drug Administration (FDA) approval of new paramagnetic contrast agents for MRI which allow even better visualization in some instances. Multislice imaging and the ability to image in multiple planes, especially sagittal and coronal, have provided flexibility not easily available with other modalities. Because cortical (outer layer) bone and metallic prostheses do not cause distortion of MR images, it has been possible to visualize certain lesions and body regions with greater certainty than has been possible with CT. The use of MRI on certain soft tissue structures for the purpose of detecting disruptive, neoplastic, degenerative, or inflammatory lesions has now become established in medical practice.

   Phase contrast (PC) and time-of-flight (TOF) are some of the available MRA techniques at the time these instructions are being issued. PC measures the difference between the phases of proton spins in tissue and blood and measures both the venous and arterial blood flow at any point in the cardiac cycle. TOF measures the difference between the amount of magnetization of tissue and blood and provides information on the structure of blood vessels, thus indirectly indicating blood flow. Two-dimensional (2D) and three-dimensional (3D) images can be obtained using each method.

   Contrast-enhanced MRA (CE-MRA) involves blood flow imaging after the patient receives an intravenous injection of a contrast agent. Gadolinium, a non-ionic element, is the foundation of all contrast agents currently in use. Gadolinium affects the way in which tissues respond to magnetization, resulting in better visualization of structures when compared to un-enhanced studies. Unlike ionic (i.e., iodine-based) contrast agents used in conventional contrast angiography (CA), allergic reactions to gadolinium are extremely rare. Additionally, gadolinium does not cause the kidney failure occasionally seen with ionic contrast agents. Digital subtraction angiography (DSA) is a computer-augmented form of CA that obtains digital blood flow images as contrast agent courses through a blood vessel. The computer ‚Äúsubtracts‚Äù bone and other tissue from the image, thereby improving visualization of blood vessels. Physicians elect to use a specific MRA or CA technique based upon clinical information from each patient.

B. Nationally Covered MRI and MRA Indications

1. MRI

   Although several uses of MRI are still considered investigational and some uses are clearly contraindicated (see subsection C), MRI is considered medically efficacious for a number of uses. Use the following descriptions as general guidelines or examples of what may be considered covered rather than as a restrictive list of specific covered indications. Coverage is limited to MRI units that have received FDA premarket approval, and such units must be operated within the parameters specified by the approval. In addition, the services must be reasonable and necessary for the diagnosis or treatment of the specific patient involved.

   a. Effective November 22, 1985, MRI is useful in examining the head, central nervous system, and spine. Multiple sclerosis can be diagnosed with MRI and the contents of the posterior fossa are visible. The inherent tissue contrast resolution of MRI makes it an appropriate standard diagnostic modality for general neuroradiology.

   b. Effective November 22, 1985, MRI can assist in the differential diagnosis of mediastinal and retroperitoneal masses, including abnormalities of the large vessels such as aneurysms and dissection. When a clinical need exists to visualize the parenchyma of solid organs to detect anatomic disruption or neoplasia, this can be accomplished in the liver, urogenital system, adrenals, and pelvic organs without the use of radiological contrast materials. When MRI is considered reasonable and necessary, the use of paramagnetic contrast materials may be covered as part of the study. MRI may also be used to detect and stage pelvic and retroperitoneal neoplasms and to evaluate disorders of cancellous bone and soft tissues. It may also be used in the detection of pericardial thickening. Primary and secondary bone neoplasm and aseptic necrosis can be detected at an early stage and monitored with MRI. Patients with metallic prostheses, especially of the hip, can be imaged in order to detect the early stages of infection of the bone to which the prosthesis is attached.

   c. Effective March 22, 1994, MRI may also be covered to diagnose disc disease without regard to whether radiological imaging has been tried first to diagnose the problem.

   d. Effective March 4, 1991, MRI with gating devices and surface coils, and gating devices that eliminate distorted images caused by cardiac and respiratory movement cycles are now considered state of the art techniques and may be covered. Surface and other specialty coils may also be covered, as they are used routinely for high resolution imaging where small limited regions of the body are studied. They produce high signal-to-noise ratios resulting in images of enhanced anatomic detail.

2. MRA (MRI for Blood Flow)

   Currently covered indications include using MRA for specific conditions to evaluate flow in internal carotid vessels of the head and neck, peripheral arteries of lower extremities, abdomen and pelvis, and the chest. Coverage is limited to MRA units that have received FDA premarket approval, and such units must be operated within the parameters specified by the approval. In addition, the services must be reasonable and necessary for the diagnosis or treatment of the specific patient involved.

   a. Head and Neck

      Effective April 15, 2003, studies have proven that MRA is effective for evaluating flow in internal carotid vessels of the head and neck. However, not all potential applications of MRA have been shown to be reasonable and necessary. All of the following criteria must apply in order for Medicare to provide coverage for MRA of the head and neck:

MRA is used to evaluate the carotid arteries, the circle of Willis, the anterior, middle or posterior cerebral arteries, the vertebral or basilar arteries or the venous sinuses;

MRA is performed on patients with conditions of the head and neck for which surgery is anticipated and may be found to be appropriate based on the MRA. These conditions include, but are not limited to, tumor, aneurysms, vascular malformations, vascular occlusion or thrombosis. Within this broad category of disorders, medical necessity is the underlying determinant of the need for an MRA in specific diseases. The medical records should clearly justify and demonstrate the existence of medical necessity; and

MRA and CA are not expected to be performed on the same patient for diagnostic purposes prior to the application of anticipated therapy. Only one of these tests will be covered routinely unless the physician can demonstrate the medical need to perform both tests.

b. Peripheral Arteries of Lower Extremities

Effective April 15, 2003, studies have proven that MRA of peripheral arteries is useful in determining the presence and extent of peripheral vascular disease in lower extremities. This procedure is non-invasive and has been shown to find occult vessels in some patients for which those vessels were not apparent when CA was performed. Medicare will cover either MRA or CA to evaluate peripheral arteries of the lower extremities. However, both MRA and CA may be useful in some cases, such as:

A patient has had CA and this test was unable to identify a viable run-off vessel for bypass. When exploratory surgery is not believed to be a reasonable medical course of action for this patient, MRA may be performed to identify the viable runoff vessel; or

A patient has had MRA, but the results are inconclusive.

c. Abdomen and Pelvis

i. Pre-operative Evaluation of Patients Undergoing Elective Abdominal Aortic Aneurysm (AAA) Repair

Effective July 1, 1999, MRA is covered for pre-operative evaluation of patients undergoing elective AAA repair if the scientific evidence reveals MRA is considered comparable to CA in determining the extent of AAA, as well as in evaluating aortoiliac occlusion disease and renal artery pathology that may be necessary in the surgical planning of AAA repair. These studies also reveal that MRA could provide a net benefit to the patient. If preoperative CA is avoided, then patients are not exposed to the risks associated with invasive procedures, contrast media, end-organ damage, or arterial injury.

ii. Imaging the Renal Arteries and the Aortoiliac Arteries in the Absence of AAA or Aortic Dissection

Effective July 1, 2003, MRA coverage is expanded to include imaging the renal arteries and the aortoiliac arteries in the absence of AAA or aortic dissection. MRA should be obtained in those circumstances in which using MRA is expected to avoid obtaining CA, when physician history, physical examination, and standard assessment tools provide insufficient information for patient management, and obtaining an MRA has a high probability of positively affecting patient management. However, CA may be ordered after obtaining the results of an MRA in those rare instances where medical necessity is demonstrated.

d. Chest

i. Diagnosis of Pulmonary Embolism

Current scientific data has shown that diagnostic pulmonary MRAs are improving due to recent developments such as faster imaging capabilities and gadolinium-enhancement. However, these advances in MRA are not significant enough to warrant replacement of pulmonary angiography in the diagnosis of pulmonary embolism for patients who have no contraindication to receiving intravenous iodinated contrast material. Patients who are allergic to iodinated contrast material face a high risk of developing complications if they undergo pulmonary angiography or computed tomography angiography. Therefore, Medicare will cover MRA of the chest for diagnosing a suspected pulmonary embolism when it is contraindicated for the patient to receive intravascular iodinated contrast material.

ii. Evaluation of Thoracic Aortic Dissection and Aneurysm

Studies have shown that MRA of the chest has a high level of diagnostic accuracy for pre-operative and post-operative evaluation of aortic dissection of aneurysm. Depending on the clinical presentation, MRA may be used as an alternative to other non-invasive imaging technologies, such as transesophageal echocardiography and CT. Generally, Medicare will provide coverage only for MRA or for CA when used as a diagnostic test. However, if both MRA and CA of the chest are used, the physician must demonstrate the medical need for performing these tests.

While the intent of this policy is to provide reimbursement for either MRA or CA, CMS is also allowing flexibility for physicians to make appropriate decisions concerning the use of these tests based on the needs of individual patients. CMS anticipates, however, low utilization of the combined use of MRA and CA. As a result, CMS encourages contractors to monitor the use of these tests and, where indicated, require evidence of the need to perform both MRA and CA.

C. Contraindications and Nationally Non-Covered Indications

1. Contraindications

The MRI is not covered when the following patient-specific contraindications are present:

MRI is not covered for patients with cardiac pacemakers or with metallic clips on vascular aneurysms unless the Medicare beneficiary meets the provisions of the following exceptions:

Effective July 7, 2011, the contraindications will not apply to pacemakers when used according to the FDA-approved labeling in an MRI environment, or

Effective February 24, 2011, CMS believes that the evidence is promising although not yet convincing that MRI will improve patient health outcomes if certain safeguards are in place to ensure that the exposure of the device to an MRI environment adversely affects neither the interpretation of the MRI result nor the proper functioning of the implanted device itself. We believe that specific precautions (as listed below) could maximize benefits of MRI exposure for beneficiaries enrolled in clinical trials designed to assess the utility and safety of MRI exposure. Therefore, CMS determines that MRI will be covered by Medicare when provided in a clinical study under section 1862(a)(1)(E) (consistent with section 1142 of the Act) through the Coverage with Study Participation (CSP) form of Coverage with Evidence Development (CED) if the study meets the criteria in each of the three paragraphs below:

The approved prospective clinical study of MRI must, with appropriate methodology, address one or more aspects of the following questions:

1. Do results of MRI in implanted permanent pacemaker (PM)/implantable cardioverter defibrillator (ICD) beneficiaries with implanted cardiac devices affect physician decision making related to: a. Clinical management strategy (e.g., in oncology, toward palliative or curative care)?

   b. Planning of treatment interventions?; or

   c. Prevention of unneeded diagnostic studies or interventions, or preventable exposures?

2. Do results of MRI in PM/ICD beneficiaries with implanted cardiac devices affect patient outcomes related to:

   a. Survival?

   b. Quality of life?; or

   c. Adverse events during and after MR scanning?

In addition, the prospective clinical study of MRI must include safety criteria for all participants. Such required safety measures for such studies, as further explained in guidance documents from professional societies must include, but are not limited to:

1. MRI should be done on a case-by-case and site-by-site basis.
2. MRI scan sequences, field intensity, and field(s) of exposure should be selected to minimize risk to the patient while gaining needed diagnostic information for diagnosis or for managing therapy.
3. MRI scanning should be done only if the site is staffed with individuals with the appropriate radiology and cardiology knowledge and expertise on hand.
4. Implanted device patients who are candidates for recruitment for an MRI clinical study should be advised that life-threatening arrhythmias might occur during MRI and serious device malfunction might occur, requiring replacement of the device.
5. Radiology and cardiology personnel and a fully stocked crash cart should be readily available throughout the procedure in case a significant arrhythmia develops during the examination that does not terminate with the cessation of the MRI study. The cardiologist should be familiar with the patient's arrhythmia history and the implanted device. A programmer that can be used to adjust the device as necessary should be readily available.
6. All such patients should be actively monitored for cardiac and respiratory function throughout the examination. At a minimum, ECG and pulse oximetry should be used. Visual and verbal contact with the patient must be maintained throughout the MRI scan. The patient should be instructed to alert the MRI staff on hand to any unusual sensations, pains, or to any problems.
7. At the conclusion of the examination, the cardiologist should examine the device to confirm that the function is consistent with its pre-examination state.
8. Follow-up should include a check of the patient's device at a time remote (1,Äì6 weeks) after the scan to confirm appropriate function.
9. If the implanted device manufacturer has indicated additional safety precautions appropriate for safe MRI performance, these must be included in the study protocol.

   The clinical study must adhere to the following standards of scientific integrity and relevance to the Medicare population:

   a. The principal purpose of the research study is to test whether a particular intervention potentially improves the participants' health outcomes.

   b. The research study is well supported by available scientific and medical information or it is intended to clarify or establish the health outcomes of interventions already in common clinical use.

   c. The research study does not unjustifiably duplicate existing studies.

   d. The research study design is appropriate to answer the research question being asked in the study.

   e. The research study is sponsored by an organization or individual capable of executing the proposed study successfully.

   f. The research study is in compliance with all applicable Federal regulations concerning the protection of human subjects found at 45 CFR Part 46. If a study is regulated by the FDA, it must be in compliance with 21 CFR Parts 50 and 56.

   g. All aspects of the research study are conducted according to appropriate standards of scientific integrity (see http://www.icmje.org).

h. The research study has a written protocol that clearly addresses, or incorporates by reference, the standards listed here as Medicare requirements for CED coverage.

i. The clinical research study is not designed to exclusively test toxicity or disease pathophysiology in healthy individuals. Trials of all medical technologies measuring therapeutic outcomes as one of the objectives meet this standard only if the disease or condition being studied is life threatening as defined in 21 CFR § 312.81(a) and the patient has no other viable treatment options.

j. The clinical research study is registered on the ClinicalTrials.gov website by the principal sponsor/investigator prior to the enrollment of the first study subject.

k. The research study protocol specifies the method and timing of public release of all pre-specified outcomes to be measured, including release of outcomes if outcomes are negative or study is terminated early. The results must be made public within 24 months of the end of data collection. If a report is planned to be published in a peer reviewed journal, then that initial release may be an abstract that meets the requirements of the International Committee of Medical Journal Editors (http://www.icmje.org). However, a full report of the outcomes must be made public no later than three (3) years after the end of data collection.

l. The research study protocol must explicitly discuss subpopulations affected by the treatment under investigation, particularly traditionally underrepresented groups in clinical studies, how the inclusion and exclusion criteria effect enrollment of these populations, and a plan for the retention and reporting of said populations in the trial. If the inclusion and exclusion criteria are expected to have a negative effect on the recruitment or retention of underrepresented populations, the protocol must discuss why these criteria are necessary.

m. The research study protocol explicitly discusses how the results are or are not expected to be generalizable to the Medicare population to infer whether Medicare patients may benefit from the intervention. Separate discussions in the protocol may be necessary for populations eligible for Medicare due to age, disability, or Medicaid eligibility.

Consistent with section 1142 of the Act, the Agency for Healthcare Research and Quality (AHRQ) supports clinical research studies that CMS determines meet the above-listed standards and address the above-listed research questions.

- MRI during a viable pregnancy is also contraindicated at this time.
- The danger inherent in bringing ferromagnetic materials within range of MRI units generally constrains the use of MRI on acutely ill patients requiring life support systems and monitoring devices that employ ferromagnetic materials.
- In addition, the long imaging time and the enclosed position of the patient may result in claustrophobia, making patients who have a history of claustrophobia unsuitable candidates for MRI procedures.

2. Nationally Non-Covered Indications

   CMS has determined that MRI of cortical bone and calcifications, and procedures involving spatial resolution of bone and calcifications, are not considered reasonable and necessary indications within the meaning of section 1862(a)(1)(A) of the Act, and are therefore non-covered.

D. Other
Effective June 3, 2010, all other uses of MRI or MRA for which CMS has not specifically indicated coverage or non-coverage continue to be eligible for coverage through individual local contractor discretion.

(This NCD last reviewed July 2011.)

100-3, 220.3

NCD for Magnetic Resonance Angiography (MRA) (220.3)

B. Nationally Covered Indications

1. Head and Neck
   Studies have proven that MRA is effective for evaluating flow in internal carotid vessels of the head and neck. However, not all potential applications of MRA have been shown to be reasonable and necessary. All of the following criteria must apply in order for Medicare to provide coverage for MRA of the head and neck:

   a. MRA is used to evaluate the carotid arteries, the circle of Willis, the anterior, middle or posterior cerebral arteries, the vertebral or basilar arteries or the venous sinuses;

   b. MRA is performed on patients with conditions of the head and neck for which surgery is anticipated and may be found to be appropriate based on the MRA. These conditions include, but are not limited to, tumor, aneurysms, vascular malformations, vascular occlusion or thrombosis. Within this broad category of disorders, medical necessity is the underlying determinant of the need for an MRA in specific diseases. The medical records should clearly justify and demonstrate the existence of medical necessity; and

   c. MRA and contrast angiography (CA) are not expected to be performed on the same patient for diagnostic purposes prior to the application of anticipated therapy. Only one of these tests will be covered routinely unless the physician can demonstrate the medical need to perform both tests.

2. Peripheral Arteries of Lower Extremities
   Studies have proven that MRA of peripheral arteries is useful in determining the presence and extent of peripheral vascular disease in lower extremities. This procedure is non-invasive and has been shown to find occult vessels in some patients for which those vessels were not apparent when CA was performed. Medicare will cover either MRA or CA to evaluate peripheral arteries of the lower extremities. However, both MRA and CA may be useful is some cases, such as:

   a. A patient has had CA and this test was unable to identify a viable run-off vessel for bypass. When exploratory surgery is not believed to be a reasonable medical course of action for this patient, MRA may be performed to identify the viable runoff vessel; or

   b. A patient has had MRA, but the results are inconclusive.

3. Abdomen and Pelvis

   a. Pre-operative Evaluation of Patients Undergoing Elective Abdominal Aortic Aneurysm (AAA) Repair (Effective July 1, 1999)

      The MRA is covered for pre-operative evaluation of patients undergoing elective AAA repair if the scientific evidence reveals MRA is considered comparable to CA in determining the extent of AAA, as well as in evaluating aortoiliac occlusion disease and renal artery pathology that may be necessary in the surgical planning of AAA repair. These studies also reveal that MRA could provide a net benefit to the patient. If preoperative CA is avoided, then patients are not exposed to the risks associated with invasive procedures, contrast media, end-organ damage, or arterial injury.

   b. Imaging the Renal Arteries and the Aortoiliac Arteries in the Absence of AAA or Aortic Dissection (Effective July 1, 2003)

      The MRA coverage is expanded to include imaging the renal arteries and the aortoiliac arteries in the absence of AAA or aortic dissection. MRA should be obtained in those circumstances in which using MRA is expected to avoid obtaining CA, when physician history, physical examination, and standard assessment tools provide insufficient information for patient management, and obtaining an MRA has a high probability of positively affecting patient management. However, CA may be ordered after obtaining the results of an MRA in those rare instances where medical necessity is demonstrated.

4. Chest

   a. Diagnosis of Pulmonary Embolism

      Current scientific data has shown that diagnostic pulmonary MRAs are improving due to recent developments such as faster imaging capabilities and gadolinium-enhancement. However, these advances in MRA are not significant enough to warrant replacement of pulmonary angiography in the diagnosis of pulmonary embolism for patients who have no contraindication to receiving intravenous iodinated contrast material. Patients who are allergic to iodinated contrast material face a high risk of developing complications if they undergo pulmonary angiography or computed tomography angiography. Therefore, Medicare will cover MRA of the chest for diagnosing a suspected pulmonary embolism when it is contraindicated for the patient to receive intravascular iodinated contrast material.

   b. Evaluation of Thoracic Aortic Dissection and Aneurysm

      Studies have shown that MRA of the chest has a high level of diagnostic accuracy for pre-operative and post-operative evaluation of aortic dissection of aneurysm. Depending on the clinical presentation, MRA may be used as an alternative to other non-invasive imaging technologies, such as transesophageal echocardiography and CT. Generally, Medicare will provide coverage only for MRA or for CA when used as a diagnostic test. However, if both MRA and CA of the chest are used, the physician must demonstrate the medical need for performing these tests.

      While the intent of this policy is to provide reimbursement for either MRA or CA, CMS is also allowing flexibility for physicians to make appropriate decisions concerning the use of these tests based on the needs of individual patients. CMS anticipates, however, low utilization of the combined use of MRA and CA. As a result, CMS encourages contractors to monitor the use of these tests and, where indicated, requires evidence of the need to perform both MRA and CA.

C. Nationally Noncovered Indications
All other uses of MRA for which CMS has not specifically indicated coverage continue to be noncovered.

D. Other
Not applicable.

(This NCD last reviewe

100-3, 220.5

NCD for Ultrasound Diagnostic Procedures (220.5)

A. General
Ultrasound diagnostic procedures utilizing low energy sound waves are being widely employed to determine the composition and contours of nearly all body tissues except bone and air-filled spaces. This technique permits noninvasive visualization of even the deepest structures in the body. The use of the ultrasound technique is sufficiently developed that it can be considered essential to good patient care in diagnosing a wide variety of conditions.

Ultrasound diagnostic procedures are listed below and are divided into two categories. Medicare coverage is extended to the procedures listed in Category I. Periodic claims review by the intermediary's medical consultants should be conducted to ensure that the techniques are medically appropriate and the general indications specified in these categories are met. Techniques in Category II are considered experimental and should not be covered at this time.

Indications and Limitations of Coverage

B. Nationally Covered Indications
Category I - (Clinically effective, usually part of initial patient evaluation, may be an adjunct to radiologic and nuclear medicine diagnostic technique)

- Echoencephalography, (Diencephalic Midline) (A-Mode).
- Echoencephalography, Complete (Diencephalic Midline and Ventricular Size).
- Ocular and Orbital Echography (A-Mode).

- Covered procedures include efforts to determine the suitability of aphakic patients for implantation of an artificial lens (pseudophakoi) following cataract surgery.
- Ocular and Orbital Sonography (B-Mode).
- Echocardiography, Pericardial Effusion (M-Mode).
- Pericardiocentesis, by Ultrasonic Guidance.
- Echocardiography, Cardiac Valve(s) (M-Mode).
- Echocardiography, Complete (M-Mode).
- Echocardiography, limited (e.g., follow-up or limited study) (M-Mode).
- Pleural Effusion Echography.
- Thoracentesis, by Ultrasonic Guidance.
- Abdominal Sonography, complete survey study (B-Scan).
- Abdominal Sonography, limited (e.g., follow-up or limited study) (B-Scan).
- Abdominal Sonography is not synonymous with ultrasound examination of individual organs.
- Renal Cyst Aspiration, by Ultrasonic Guidance.
- Renal Biopsy, by Ultrasonic Guidance.
- Pancreas Sonography (B-Scan).
- Pancreatic Sonography has proven effective in diagnosing pseudocysts.
- Spleen Sonography (B-Scan).
- Abdominal Aorta Echography (A-Mode).
- Abdominal Aorta Sonography (B-Scan).
- Retroperitoneal Sonography (B-Scan).
- Retroperitoneal Sonography does not include planning of fields for radiation therapy.
- Urinary Bladder Sonography (B-Scan).
- Urinary bladder Sonography does not include staging of bladder tumors.
- Pregnancy Diagnosis Sonography (B-Scan).
- Fetal Age Determination (Biparietal Diameter) Sonography (B-Scan).
- Fetal Growth Rate Sonography (B-Scan).
- Placenta Localization Sonography (B-Scan).
- Pregnancy Sonography, Complete (B-Scan).
- Molar Pregnancy Diagnosis Sonography (B-Scan).
- Ectopic Pregnancy Diagnosis Sonography (B-Scan).
- Passive Testing (Antepartum Monitoring of Fetal Heart Rate In the Resting Fetus).
- Intrauterine Contraceptive Device Sonography (B-Scan).
- Pelvic Mass Diagnosis Sonography (B-Scan).
- Amniocentesis, by Ultrasonic Guidance.
- Arterial Flow Study, Peripheral (Doppler).
- Venous Flow Study, Peripheral (Doppler).
- Arterial Aneurysm, Peripheral (B-Scan).
- Radiation Therapy Planning Sonography (B-Scan).
- Thyroid Echography (A-Mode).
- Thyroid Sonography (B-Scan).
- Breast Echography (A-Mode).
- Breast Sonography (B-Scan).
- Hepatic Sonography (B-Scan).
- Gallbladder Sonography.
- Renal Sonography.
- Two-Dimensional Echocardiography (B-Mode).
- Monitoring of cardiac output(Esophageal Doppler) for ventilated patients in the ICU and operative patients with a need for intra-operative fluid optimization

C. Nationally Non-Covered Indications
Category II - (Clinical reliability and efficacy not proven):

- B-Scan for atherosclerotic narrowing of peripheral arteries.

D. Other
Uses for ultrasound diagnostic procedures not listed in Category I or II above are left to local contractor discretion. In view of the rapid changes in the field of ultrasound diagnosis, uses for ultrasound diagnostic procedures other than those listed under Categories I and II should be carefully reviewed before payment. Medical justification may be required.

(This NCD last reviewed June 2007.)

100-3, 220.6

NCD for Positron Emission Tomography (PET) Scans (220.6)

Item/Service Description Positron Emission Tomography (PET) is a minimally invasive diagnostic imaging procedure used to evaluate metabolism in normal tissue as well as in diseased tissues in conditions such as cancer, ischemic heart disease, and some neurologic disorders. A radiopharmaceutical is injected into the patient that gives off sub-atomic particles, known as positrons, as it decays. PET uses a positron camera (tomograph) to measure the decay of the radiopharmaceutical. The rate of decay provides biochemical information on the metabolism of the tissue being studied. (This NCD last reviewed March 2009.)

100-3, 220.6.1

NCD for PET for Perfusion of the Heart (220.6.1)

Indications and Limitations of Coverage

1. Rubidium 82 (Effective March 14, 1995)
   Effective for services performed on or after March 14, 1995, PET scans performed at rest or with pharmacological stress used for noninvasive imaging of the perfusion of the heart for the diagnosis and management of patients with known or suspected coronary artery disease using the FDA-approved radiopharmaceutical Rubidium 82 (Rb 82) are covered, provided the requirements below are met:

   The PET scan, whether at rest alone, or rest with stress, is performed in place of, but not in addition to, a single photon emission computed tomography (SPECT); or

   The PET scan, whether at rest alone or rest with stress, is used following a SPECT that was found to be inconclusive. In these cases, the PET scan must have been considered necessary in order to determine what medical or surgical intervention is required to treat the patient. (For purposes of this requirement, an inconclusive test is a test(s) whose results are equivocal, technically uninterpretable, or discordant with a patient's other clinical data and must be documented in the beneficiary's file.)

   For any PET scan for which Medicare payment is claimed for dates of services prior to July 1, 2001, the claimant must submit additional specified information on the claim form (including proper codes and/or modifiers), to indicate the results of the PET scan. The claimant must also include information on whether the PET scan was performed after an inconclusive noninvasive cardiac test. The information submitted with respect to the previous noninvasive cardiac test must specify the type of test performed prior to the PET scan and whether it was inconclusive or unsatisfactory. These explanations are in the form of special G codes used for billing PET scans using Rb 82. Beginning July 1, 2001, claims should be submitted with the appropriate codes.
2. Ammonia N-13 (Effective October 1, 2003)
   Effective for services performed on or after October 1, 2003, PET scans performed at rest or with pharmacological stress used for noninvasive imaging of the perfusion of the heart for the diagnosis and management of patients with known or suspected coronary artery disease using the FDA-approved radiopharmaceutical ammonia N-13 are covered, provided the requirements below are met:

   The PET scan, whether at rest alone, or rest with stress, is performed in place of, but not in addition to, a SPECT; or

   The PET scan, whether at rest alone or rest with stress, is used following a SPECT that was found to be inconclusive. In these cases, the PET scan must have been considered necessary in order to determine what medical or surgical intervention is required to treat the patient. (For purposes of this requirement, an inconclusive test is a test whose results are equivocal, technically uninterpretable, or discordant with a patient's other clinical data and must be documented in the beneficiary's file.)

   (This NCD last reviewed March 2005.)

100-3, 220.6.2

NCD for PET (FDG) for Lung Cancer (220.6.2)

220.6.2 - FDG PET for Lung Cancer (Replaced with Section 220.6.17)

100-3, 220.6.3

NCD for PET (FDG) for Esophageal Cancer (220.6.3)

220.6.3 - FDG PET for Esophageal Cancer (Replaced with Section 220.6.17)

100-3, 220.6.4

NCD for PET (FDG) for Colorectal Cancer (220.6.4)

220.6.4 - FDG PET for Colorectal Cancer (Replaced with Section 220.6.17

100-3, 220.6.5

NCD for PET (FDG) for Lymphoma (220.6.5)

220.6.5 - FDG PET for Lymphoma (Replaced with Section 220.6.17)

100-3, 220.6.6

NCD for PET (FDG) for Melanoma (220.6.6)

220.6.6 - FDG PET for Melanoma (Replaced with Section 220.6.17)

100-3, 220.6.7

NCD for PET (FDG) for Head and Neck Cancers (220.6.7)

220.6.7 - FDG PET for Head and Neck Cancers (Replaced with Section 220.6.17)

100-3, 220.6.8

NCD for PET (FDG) for Myocardial Viability (220.6.8)

1. FDG PET is covered for the determination of myocardial viability following an inconclusive single photon emission computed tomography (SPECT) test from July 1, 2001, through September 30, 2002. Only full ring PET scanners are covered from July 1, 2001, through

December 31, 2001. However, as of January 1, 2002, full and partial ring scanners are covered.

2. Beginning October 1, 2002, Medicare covers FDG PET for the determination of myocardial viability as a primary or initial diagnostic study prior to revascularization, or following an inconclusive SPECT. Studies performed by full and partial ring scanners are covered.

Limitations
In the event a patient receives a SPECT test with inconclusive results, a PET scan may be covered. However, if a patient receives a FDG PET study with inconclusive results, a follow up SPECT test is not covered.

Documentation that these conditions are met should be maintained by the referring physician in the beneficiary's medical record, as is normal business practice.

(This NCD last reviewed September 2002.)

100-3, 220.6.9

FDG PET for Refractory Seizures (Effective July 1, 2001)

Beginning July 1, 2001, Medicare covers FDG PET for pre-surgical evaluation for the purpose of localization of a focus of refractory seizure activity.

Limitations: Covered only for pre-surgical evaluation.

Documentation that these conditions are met should be maintained by the referring physician in the beneficiary's medical record, as is normal business practice.

(This NCD last reviewed June 2001.)

100-3, 220.6.10

NCD for PET (FDG) for Breast Cancer (220.6.10)

220.6.10 - FDG PET for Breast Cancer (Effective October 1, 2002) (Replaced with Section 220.6.17)

100-3, 220.6.11

NCD for PET (FDG) for Thyroid Cancer (220.6.11)

220.6.11 - FDG PET for Thyroid Cancer (Various Effective Dates Below) (Replaced with Section 220.6.17)

100-3, 220.6.12

NCD for PET (FDG) for Soft Tissue Sarcoma (220.6.12)

220.6.12 - FDG PET for Soft Tissue Sarcoma (Various Effective Dates Below) (Replaced with Section 220.6.17)

100-3, 220.6.13

NCD for PET (FDG) for Dementia and Neurodegenerative Diseases (220.6.13)

A. General
Medicare covers FDG PET scans for either the differential diagnosis of fronto-temporal dementia (FTD) and Alzheimer's disease (AD) under specific requirements; OR, its use in a Centers for Medicare & Medicaid Services (CMS)-approved practical clinical trial focused on the utility of FDG PET in the diagnosis or treatment of dementing neurodegenerative diseases. Specific requirements for each indication are clarified below:

B. Nationally Covered Indications
1. FDG PET Requirements for Coverage in the Differential Diagnosis of AD and FTD

An FDG PET scan is considered reasonable and necessary in patients with a recent diagnosis of dementia and documented cognitive decline of at least 6 months, who meet diagnostic criteria for both AD and FTD. These patients have been evaluated for specific alternate neurodegenerative diseases or other causative factors, but the cause of the clinical symptoms remains uncertain.

The following additional conditions must be met before an FDG PET scan will be covered:

a. The patient's onset, clinical presentation, or course of cognitive impairment is such that FTD is suspected as an alternative neurodegenerative cause of the cognitive decline. Specifically, symptoms such as social disinhibition, awkwardness, difficulties with language, or loss of executive function are more prominent early in the course of FTD than the memory loss typical of AD;

b. The patient has had a comprehensive clinical evaluation (as defined by the American Academy of Neurology (AAN)) encompassing a medical history from the patient and a well-acquainted informant (including assessment of activities of daily living), physical and mental status examination (including formal documentation of cognitive decline occurring over at least 6 months) aided by cognitive scales or neuropsychological testing, laboratory tests, and structural imaging such as magnetic resonance imaging (MRI) or computed tomography (CT);

c. The evaluation of the patient has been conducted by a physician experienced in the diagnosis and assessment of dementia;

d. The evaluation of the patient did not clearly determine a specific neurodegenerative disease or other cause for the clinical symptoms, and information available through FDG PET is reasonably expected to help clarify the diagnosis between FTD and AD and help guide future treatment;

e. The FDG PET scan is performed in a facility that has all the accreditation necessary to operate nuclear medicine equipment. The reading of the scan should be done by an expert in nuclear medicine, radiology, neurology, or psychiatry, with experience interpreting such scans in the presence of dementia;

f. A brain single photon emission computed tomography (SPECT) or FDG PET scan has not been obtained for the same indication. (The indication can be considered to be different in patients who exhibit important changes in scope or severity of cognitive decline, and meet all other qualifying criteria listed above and below (including the judgment that the likely diagnosis remains uncertain). The results of a prior SPECT or FDG PET scan must have been inconclusive or, in the case of SPECT, difficult to interpret due to immature or inadequate technology. In these instances, an FDG PET scan may be covered after 1 year has passed from the time the first SPECT or FDG PET scan was performed.)

g The referring and billing provider(s) have documented the appropriate evaluation of the Medicare beneficiary. Providers should establish the medical necessity of an FDG PET scan by ensuring that the following information has been collected and is maintained in the beneficiary medical record:

- Date of onset of symptoms;
- Diagnosis of clinical syndrome (normal aging; mild cognitive impairment (MCI); mild, moderate or severe dementia);
- Mini mental status exam (MMSE) or similar test score;
- Presumptive cause (possible, probable, uncertain AD);
- Any neuropsychological testing performed;
- Results of any structural imaging (MRI or CT) performed;
- Relevant laboratory tests (B12, thyroid hormone); and,
- Number and name of prescribed medications.

The billing provider must furnish a copy of the FDG PET scan result for use by CMS and its contractors upon request. These verification requirements are consistent with federal requirements set forth in 42 Code of Federal Regulations section 410.32 generally for diagnostic x-ray tests, diagnostic laboratory tests, and other tests. In summary, section 410.32 requires the billing physician and the referring physician to maintain information in the medical record of each patient to demonstrate medical necessity [410.32(d) (2)] and submit the information demonstrating medical necessity to CMS and/or its agents upon request [410.32(d)(3)(I)] (OMB number 0938-0685).

2. FDG PET Requirements for Coverage in the Context of a CMS-approved Practical Clinical Trial Utilizing a Specific Protocol to Demonstrate the Utility of FDG PET in the Diagnosis, and Treatment of Neurodegenerative Dementing Diseases An FDG PET scan is considered reasonable and necessary in patients with MCI or early dementia (in clinical circumstances other than those specified in subparagraph 1) only in the context of an approved clinical trial that contains patient safeguards and protections to ensure proper administration, use and evaluation of the FDG PET scan.

   The clinical trial must compare patients who do and do not receive an FDG PET scan and have as its goal to monitor, evaluate, and improve clinical outcomes. In addition, it must meet the following basic criteria:

   a. Written protocol on file;

   b. Institutional Review Board review and approval;

   c. Scientific review and approval by two or more qualified individuals who are not part of the research team; and,

   d. Certification that investigators have not been disqualified.

C. Nationally Non-Covered Indications
All other uses of FDG PET for patients with a presumptive diagnosis of dementia-causing neurodegenerative disease (e.g., possible or probable AD, clinically typical FTD, dementia of Lewy bodies, or Creutzfeld-Jacob disease) for which CMS has not specifically indicated coverage continue to be non-covered.

D. Other
Not applicable.

(This NCD last reviewed September 2004.)

100-3, 220.6.14

NCD for PET (FDG) for Brain, Cervical, Ovarian, Pancreatic, Small Cell Lung, and Testicular Cancers (220.6.14)

See section 220.6.17

100-3, 220.6.17

Positron Emission Tomography (PET) (FDG) for Oncologic Conditions - (Various Effective Dates)

General
The Centers for Medicare and Medicaid Services (CMS) was asked to reconsider section 220.6, of the National Coverage Determinations (NCD) Manual, to end the prospective data collection requirements across all oncologic indications of FDG PET except for monitoring response to treatment. Section 220.6 of the NCD Manual, establishes the requirement for prospective data collection for FDG PET used in the diagnosis, staging, restaging, and monitoring response to treatment for brain, cervical, ovarian, pancreatic, small cell lung and testicular cancers, as well as for cancer indications not previously specified in section 220.6 in its entirety.

The CMS received public input indicating that the current coverage framework, which required cancer-by-cancer consideration of diagnosis, staging, restaging, and monitoring response to treatment should be replaced by a more omnibus consideration. Thus, CMS broadened the scope of this review through an announcement on the Web site and solicited additional public comment on the use of FDG PET imaging for solid tumors so that it could transparently consider this possibility.

1. Framework
   Effective for claims with dates of service on and after April 3, 2009, CMS is adopting a coverage framework that replaces the four-part diagnosis, staging, restaging and monitoring

response to treatment categories with a two-part framework that differentiates FDG PET imaging used to inform the initial antitumor treatment strategy from other uses related to guiding subsequent antitumor treatment strategies after the completion of initial treatment. CMS is making this change for all NCDs that address coverage of FDG PET for the specific oncologic conditions addressed in this decision.

2. Initial Anti-tumor Treatment Strategy
Effective for claims with dates of service on and after April 3, 2009, CMS has determined that the evidence is adequate to determine that the results of FDG PET imaging are useful in determining the appropriate initial treatment strategy for beneficiaries with suspected solid tumors and myeloma and improve health outcomes and thus are reasonable and necessary under Sec.1862(a)(1)(A) of the Social Security Act (the Act).

Therefore, CMS will cover only one FDG PET study for beneficiaries who have solid tumors that are biopsy proven or strongly suspected based on other diagnostic testing when the beneficiary's treating physician determines that the FDG PET study is needed to determine the location and/or extent of the tumor for the following therapeutic purposes related to the initial treatment strategy:

To determine whether or not the beneficiary is an appropriate candidate for an invasive diagnostic or therapeutic procedure; or

To determine the optimal anatomic location for an invasive procedure; or

To determine the anatomic extent of tumor when the recommended anti-tumor treatment reasonably depends on the extent of the tumor.

As exceptions to the April 3, 2009, initial treatment strategy section above:

a. The CMS has reviewed evidence on the use of FDG PET imaging to determine initial anti-tumor treatment in patients with adenocarcinoma of the prostate. CMS has determined that the available evidence does not demonstrate that FDG PET imaging improves physician decision making in the determination of initial anti-tumor treatment strategy in Medicare beneficiaries who have adenocarcinoma of the prostate, does not improve health outcomes and is thus not reasonable and necessary under Sec.1862(a)(1)(A) of the Act. Therefore, FDG PET is nationally non-covered for this indication of this tumor type.

b. The CMS received no new evidence demonstrating a change was warranted with respect to the use of FDG PET imaging to determine initial anti-tumor treatment in breast cancer; thus CMS is not making any change to the current coverage policy for FDG PET in breast cancer. CMS is continuing to cover FDG PET imaging for the initial treatment strategy for male and female breast cancer only when used in staging distant metastasis. FDG PET imaging for diagnosis and initial staging of axillary nodes will remain non-covered.

c. The CMS received no new evidence demonstrating a change was warranted with respect to use of FDG PET imaging of regional lymph nodes in melanoma; thus CMS is not changing the current NCD for FDG PET in melanoma. CMS will continue non-coverage of FDG PET for the evaluation of regional lymph nodes in melanoma. Other uses to determine initial treatment strategy remain covered.

d. The CMS received no new evidence demonstrating a change was warranted with respect to use of FDG PET imaging in the initial treatment strategy for cervical cancer. CMS is continuing to cover FDG PET imaging as an adjunct test for the detection of pre-treatment metastasis (i.e., staging) in newly diagnosed cervical cancers following conventional imaging that is negative for extra-pelvic metastasis. All other uses of FDG PET for the initial treatment strategy for beneficiaries diagnosed with cervical cancer will continue to only be covered as research under Sec.1862(a)(1)(E) of the Act through Coverage with Evidence Development (CED). Therefore, CMS will cover one initial FDG PET study for newly diagnosed cervical cancer when not used as an adjunct test for the detection of pre-treatment metastases following conventional imaging that is negative for extra-pelvic metastasis only when the beneficiary's treating physician determines that the FDG PET study is needed to inform the initial anti-tumor treatment strategy and the beneficiary is enrolled in, and the FDG PET provider is participating in, the specific type of prospective clinical study outlined under subsequent treatment strategy below.

e. Effective November 10, 2009, as a result of a reconsideration request, CMS ended the prospective data collection requirements, or coverage with evidence development, for the use of FDG PET imaging in the initial staging of cervical cancer related to initial treatment strategy.

CMS is continuing to cover FDG PET imaging as an adjunct test for the detection of pre-treatment metastasis (i.e., staging) in newly diagnosed cervical cancers following conventional imaging that is negative for extra-pelvic metastasis.

Therefore, CMS will cover one initial FDG PET study for staging in beneficiaries who have biopsy-proven cervical cancer when the beneficiary's treating physician determines that the FDG PET study is needed to determine the location and/or extent of the tumor for the following therapeutic purposes related to initial treatment strategy: To determine whether or not the beneficiary is an appropriate candidate for an invasive diagnostic or therapeutic procedure; or

To determine the optimal anatomic location for an invasive procedure; or

To determine the anatomic extent of the tumor when the recommended anti-tumor treatment reasonably depends on the extent of the tumor.

Additionally, effective November 10, 2009, following a reconsideration request, CMS determines that there is no credible evidence that the results of FDG PET imaging are useful to make the initial diagnoses of cervical cancer, does not improve health outcomes, and is not reasonable and necessary under section 1862(a)(1)(A) of the Social Security Act. Therefore, CMS will non-cover FDG PET imaging for initial diagnosis of cervical cancer related to initial treatment strategy.

3. Subsequent Anti-tumor Treatment Strategy

As part of its April 3, 2009, NCD, the CMS reviewed evidence on the use of FDG PET in the subsequent treatment strategy for patients with tumor types other than those seven indications currently covered without exception (breast, colorectal, esophagus, head and neck (non-CNS/thyroid), lymphoma, melanoma, and non-small cell lung).

As a result, CMS determined that the available evidence is adequate to determine that FDG PET imaging also improves physician decision making in the determination of subsequent treatment strategy in Medicare beneficiaries who have ovarian cancer, cervical cancer, and myeloma, improves health outcomes, and is thus reasonable and necessary under Sec.1862(a)(1)(A) of the Act.

Therefore, effective for claims with dates of service on and after April 3, 2009, for tumor types other than breast, colorectal, esophagus, head and neck (non-CNS/thyroid), lymphoma, melanoma, non-small cell lung, ovarian, cervical, and myeloma, CMS has determined that the available evidence is not adequate to determine that FDG PET imaging improves physician decision making in the determination of subsequent anti-tumor treatment strategy or improves health outcomes in Medicare beneficiaries and thus is not reasonable and necessary under Sec.1862(a)(1)(A) of the Act.

However, CMS has determined that the available evidence is sufficient to determine that FDG PET imaging for subsequent anti-tumor treatment strategy for all other tumor types other than the 10 indications noted above may be covered as research under Sec.1862(a)(1)(E) of the Act through CED. Therefore, CMS will cover a subsequent FDG PET study for all other tumor types other than the 10 indications noted above, when the beneficiary's treating physician determines that the FDG PET study is needed to inform the subsequent anti-tumor treatment strategy and the beneficiary is enrolled in, and the FDG PET provider is participating in, the following type of prospective clinical study:

An FDG PET clinical study that is designed to collect additional information at the time of the scan to assist in patient management. Qualifying clinical studies must ensure that specific hypotheses are addressed; appropriate data elements are collected; hospitals and providers are qualified to provide the FDG PET scan and interpret the results; participating hospitals and providers accurately report data on all enrolled patients not included in other qualifying trials through adequate auditing mechanisms; and all patient confidentiality, privacy, and other Federal laws must be followed.

The clinical studies for which CMS will provide coverage must answer one or more of the following three questions:

Prospectively, in Medicare beneficiaries whose treating physician determines that the FDG PET study is needed to inform the subsequent anti-tumor treatment strategy, does the addition of FDG PET imaging lead to:

A change in the likelihood of appropriate referrals for palliative care;

Improved quality of life; or,

Improved survival?

The study must adhere to the following standards of scientific integrity and relevance to the Medicare population:

a. The principal purpose of the research study is to test whether a particular intervention potentially improves the participants' health outcomes.

b. The research study is well-supported by available scientific and medical information or it is intended to clarify or establish the health outcomes of interventions already in common clinical use.

c. The research study does not unjustifiably duplicate existing studies.

d. The research study design is appropriate to answer the research question being asked in the study.

e. The research study is sponsored by an organization or individual capable of executing the proposed study successfully.

f. The research study is in compliance with all applicable Federal regulations concerning the protection of human subjects found in the Code of Federal Regulations (CFR) at 45 CFR Part 46.

   If a study is regulated by the Food and Drug Administration (FDA), it also must be in compliance with 21 CFR Parts 50 and 56.

g. All aspects of the research study are conducted according to the appropriate standards of scientific integrity.

h. The research study has a written protocol that clearly addresses, or incorporates by reference, the Medicare standards.

i. The clinical research study is not designed to exclusively test toxicity or disease pathophysiology in healthy individuals. Trials of all medical technologies measuring therapeutic outcomes as one of the objectives meet this standard only if the disease or condition being studied is life-threatening as defined in 21 CFR 312.81(a) and the patient has no other viable treatment options.

j. The clinical research study is registered on the www.ClinicalTrials.gov Web site by the principal sponsor/investigator prior to the enrollment of the first study subject.

k. The research study protocol specifies the method and timing of public release of all pre-specified outcomes to be measured including release of outcomes if outcomes are negative or study is terminated early. The results must be made public within 24 months of the end of data collection. If a report is planned to be published in a peer-reviewed journal, then that initial release may be an abstract that meets the requirements of the International Committee of Medical Journal Editors. However, a full report of the outcomes must be made public no later than 3 years after the end of data collection.

l. The research study protocol must explicitly discuss subpopulations affected by the treatment under investigation, particularly traditionally underrepresented groups in clinical studies, how the inclusion and exclusion criteria affect enrollment of these populations, and a plan for the retention and reporting of said populations on the trial. If the inclusion and exclusion criteria are expected to have a negative effect on the recruitment or retention of underrepresented populations, the protocol must discuss why these criteria are necessary.

m. The research study protocol explicitly discusses how the results are or are not expected to be generalizable to the Medicare population to infer whether Medicare patients may benefit from the intervention. Separate discussions in the protocol may be necessary for populations eligible for Medicare due to age, disability or Medicaid eligibility.

Consistent with section 1142 of the Act, the Agency for Healthcare Research and Quality (AHRQ) supports clinical research studies that CMS determines meet the above-listed standards and address the above-listed research questions.

4. Synopsis of New Framework

Effective for claims with dates of service on and after April 3, 2009, the CMS transitioned the prior framework-diagnosis, staging, restaging, and monitoring response to treatment-into the initial treatment strategy and subsequent treatment strategy framework. The chart below summarizes FDG PET coverage as of November 10, 2009:

FDG PET Coverage for Solid Tumors and Myeloma Tumor Type	***Initial Treatment Strategy (formerly "diagnosis" & "staging")***	***Subsequent Treatment Strategy (formerly "restaging" & "monitoring response to treatment")***
Colorectal	Cover	Cover
Esophagus	Cover	Cover
Head & Neck (not Thyroid, CNS)	Cover	Cover
Lymphoma	Cover	Cover
Non-Small Cell Lung	Cover	Cover
Ovary	Cover	Cover
Brain	Cover	CED
Cervix	Cover w/exception*	Cover
Small Cell Lung	Cover	CED
Soft Tissue Sarcoma	Cover	CED
Pancreas	Cover	CED
Testes	Cover	CED
Breast (female and male)	Cover w/exception*	Cover
Melanoma	Cover w/exception*	Cover
Prostate	Non-Cover	CED
Thyroid	Cover	Cover w/exception or CED*
All Other Solid Tumors	Cover	CED
Myeloma	Cover	Cover
All other cancers not listed	CED	CED

*Cervix: Non-covered for the initial diagnosis of cervical cancer related to initial treatment strategy. All other indications for initial treatment strategy are covered.

*Breast: Non-covered for initial diagnosis and/or staging of axillary lymph nodes. Covered for initial staging of metastatic disease. All other indications for initial treatment strategy are covered.

*Melanoma: Non-covered for initial staging of regional lymph nodes. All other indications for initial treatment strategy are covered.

*Thyroid: Covered for subsequent treatment strategy of recurrent or residual thyroid cancer of follicular cell origin previously treated by thyroidectomy and radioiodine ablation and have a serum thyroglobulin >10ng/ml and have a negative I-131 whole body scan. All other indications for subsequent treatment strategy are CED.

(This NCD last reviewed November 2009.)

100-3, 220.6.19

Positron Emission Tomography NaF-18 (NaF-18 PET) to Identify Bone Metastasis of Cancer (Effective February 26, 2010)

A. General

Positron Emission Tomography (PET) is a non-invasive, diagnostic imaging procedure that assesses the level of metabolic activity and perfusion in various organ systems of the body. A positron camera (tomograph) is used to produce cross-sectional tomographic images, which are obtained from positron-emitting radioactive tracer substances (radiopharmaceuticals) such as

F-18 sodium fluoride. NaF-18 PET has been recognized as an excellent technique for imaging areas of altered osteogenic activity in bone. The clinical value of detecting and assessing the initial extent of metastatic cancer in bone is attested by a number of professional guidelines for oncology. Imaging to detect bone metastases is also recommended when a patient, following completion of initial treatment, is symptomatic with bone pain suspicious for metastases from a known primary tumor.

B. Nationally Covered Indications

Effective February 26, 2010, the Centers for Medicare & Medicaid Services (CMS) will cover NaF-18 PET imaging when the beneficiary's treating physician determines that the NaF-18 PET study is needed to inform to inform the initial antitumor treatment strategy or to guide subsequent antitumor treatment strategy after the completion of initial treatment, and when the beneficiary is enrolled in, and the NaF-18 PET provider is participating in, the following type of prospective clinical study:

A NaF-18 PET clinical study that is designed to collect additional information at the time of the scan to assist in initial antitumor treatment planning or to guide subsequent treatment strategy by the identification, location and quantification of bone metastases in beneficiaries in whom bone metastases are strongly suspected based on clinical symptoms or the results of other diagnostic studies. Qualifying clinical studies must ensure that specific hypotheses are addressed; appropriate data elements are collected; hospitals and providers are qualified to provide the PET scan and interpret the results; participating hospitals and providers accurately report data on all enrolled patients not included in other qualifying trials through adequate auditing mechanisms; and all patient confidentiality, privacy, and other Federal laws must be followed.

The clinical studies for which Medicare will provide coverage must answer one or more of the following questions:

Prospectively, in Medicare beneficiaries whose treating physician determines that the NaF-18 PET study results are needed to inform the initial antitumor treatment strategy or to guide subsequent antitumor treatment strategy after the completion of initial treatment, does the addition of NaF-18 PET imaging lead to:

A change in patient management to more appropriate palliative care; or A change in patient management to more appropriate curative care; or Improved quality of life; or Improved survival?

The study must adhere to the following standards of scientific integrity and relevance to the Medicare population:

a. The principal purpose of the research study is to test whether a particular intervention potentially improves the participants' health outcomes.

b. The research study is well-supported by available scientific and medical information or it is intended to clarify or establish the health outcomes of interventions already in common clinical use.

c. The research study does not unjustifiably duplicate existing studies.

d. The research study design is appropriate to answer the research question being asked in the study.

e. The research study is sponsored by an organization or individual capable of executing the proposed study successfully.

f. The research study is in compliance with all applicable Federal regulations concerning the protection of human subjects found in the Code of Federal Regulations (CFR) at 45 CFR Part 46. If a study is regulated by the Food and Drug Administration (FDA), it also must be in compliance with 21 CFR Parts 50 and 56.

g. All aspects of the research study are conducted according to the appropriate standards of scientific integrity.

h. The research study has a written protocol that clearly addresses, or incorporates by reference, the Medicare standards.

i. The clinical research study is not designed to exclusively test toxicity or disease pathophysiology in healthy individuals. Trials of all medical technologies measuring therapeutic outcomes as one of the objectives meet this standard only if the disease or condition being studied is life-threatening as defined in 21 CFR Sec.312.81(a) and the patient has no other viable treatment options.

j. The clinical research study is registered on the www.ClinicalTrials.gov Web site by the principal sponsor/investigator prior to the enrollment of the first study subject.

k. The research study protocol specifies the method and timing of public release of all pre-specified outcomes to be measured including release of outcomes if outcomes are negative or study is terminated early. The results must be made public within 24 months of the end of data collection. If a report is planned to be published in a peer-reviewed journal, then that initial release may be an abstract that meets the requirements of the International Committee of Medical Journal Editors. However, a full report of the outcomes must be made public no later than three (3) years after the end of data collection.

l. The research study protocol must explicitly discuss subpopulations affected by the treatment under investigation, particularly traditionally underrepresented groups in clinical studies, how the inclusion and exclusion criteria affect enrollment of these populations, and a plan for the retention and reporting of said populations on the trial. If the inclusion and exclusion criteria are expected to have a negative effect on the recruitment or retention of underrepresented populations, the protocol must discuss why these criteria are necessary.

m. The research study protocol explicitly discusses how the results are or are not expected to be generalizable to the Medicare population to infer whether Medicare patients may benefit from the intervention. Separate discussions in the protocol may be necessary for populations eligible for Medicare due to age, disability or Medicaid eligibility.

Consistent with section 1142 of the Social Security Act (the Act), the Agency for Healthcare Research and Quality (AHRQ) supports clinical research studies that the Centers for Medicare and Medicaid Services (CMS) determines meet the above-listed standards and address the above-listed research questions.

C. Nationally Non-Covered Indications
Effective February 26, 2010, CMS determines that the evidence is not sufficient to determine that the results of NaF-18 PET imaging to identify bone metastases improve health outcomes of beneficiaries with cancer and is not reasonable and necessary under Sec.1862(a)(1)(A) of the Act unless it is to inform initial antitumor treatment strategy or to guide subsequent antitumor treatment strategy after completion of initial treatment, and then only under CED. All other uses and clinical indications of NaF-18 PET are nationally non-covered.

D. Other
The only radiopharmaceutical diagnostic imaging agents covered by Medicare for PET cancer imaging are 2-[F-18] Fluoro-D-Glucose (FDG) and NaF-18 (sodium fluoride-18). All other PET radiopharmaceutical diagnostic imaging agents are non-covered for this indication.

(This NCD was last reviewed in February 2010.)

100-3, 220.7

NCD for Xenon Scan (220.7)

Program payment may be made for this diagnostic procedure which involves perfusion lung imaging with 133 xenon. However, review for evidence of abuse which might include absence of reasonable indications, inappropriate sequence, or excessive number or kinds of procedures used in the care of individual patients.

100-3, 220.8

NCD for Nuclear Radiology Procedure (220.8)

Nuclear radiology procedures, including nuclear examinations performed with mobile radiological equipment, are covered if reasonable and necessary for the individual patient. Although these procedures may not be widely used, they are generally accepted. Review claims for these procedures for evidence of abuse which might absence of reasonable indications, inappropriate sequence, or excessive number or kinds of procedures used in the care of individual patients.

100-3, 220.12

NCD for Single Photon Emission Computed Tomography (SPECT) (220.12)

Frequency limitations: Contractor discretion.

In the case of myocardial viability, FDG PET may be used following a SPECT that was found to be inconclusive. However, SPECT may not be used following an inconclusive FDG PET performed to evaluate myocardial viability.

100-3, 220.13

NCD for Percutaneous Image-Guided Breast Biopsy (220.13)

The Breast Imaging Reporting and Data System (or BIRADS system) employed by the American College of Radiology provides a standardized lexicon with which radiologists may report their interpretation of a mammogram. The BIRADS grading of mammograms is as follows: Grade I-Negative, Grade II-Benign finding, Grade III-Probably benign, Grade IV-Suspicious abnormality, and Grade V-Highly suggestive of malignant neoplasm.

A. Nonpalpable Breast Lesions.
Effective January 1, 2003, Medicare covers percutaneous image-guided breast biopsy using stereotactic or ultrasound imaging for a radiographic abnormality that is nonpalpable and is graded as a BIRADS III, IV, or V.

B. Palpable Breast Lesions.
Effective January 1, 2003, Medicare covers percutaneous image guided breast biopsy using stereotactic or ultrasound imaging for palpable lesions that are difficult to biopsy using palpation alone. Contractors have the discretion to decide what types of palpable lesions are difficult to biopsy using palpation.

100-3, 230.1

NCD for Treatment of Kidney Stones (230.1)

In addition to the traditional surgical/endoscopic techniques for the treatment of kidney stones, the following lithotripsy techniques are also covered for services rendered on or after March l5, l985.

Extracorporeal Shock Wave Lithotripsy.--Extracorporeal Shock Wave Lithotripsy (ESWL) is a non-invasive method of treating kidney stones using a device called a lithotriptor. The lithotriptor uses shock waves generated outside of the body to break up upper urinary tract stones. It focuses the shock waves specifically on stones under X-ray visualization, pulverizing them by repeated shocks. ESWL is covered under Medicare for use in the treatment of upper urinary tract kidney stones.

Percutaneous Lithotripsy.--Percutaneous lithotripsy (or nephrolithotomy) is an invasive method of treating kidney stones by using ultrasound, electrohydraulic or mechanical lithotripsy. A probe is inserted through an incision in the skin directly over the kidney and applied to the stone. A form of lithotripsy is then used to fragment the stone. Mechanical or electrohydraulic lithotripsy may be used as an alternative or adjunct to ultrasonic lithotripsy. Percutaneous lithotripsy of kidney stones by ultrasound or by the related techniques of electrohydraulic or mechanical lithotripsy is covered under Medicare.

The following is covered for services rendered on or after January 16, 1988.

Transurethral Ureteroscopic Lithotripsy.--Transurethral ureteroscopic lithotripsy is a method of fragmenting and removing ureteral and renal stones through a cystoscope. The cystoscope is inserted through the urethra into the bladder. Catheters are passed through the scope into the opening where the ureters enter the bladder. Instruments passed through this opening into the ureters are used to manipulate and ultimately disintegrate stones, using either mechanical crushing, transcystoscopic electrohydraulic shock waves, ultrasound or laser. Transurethral ureteroscopic lithotripsy for the treatment of urinary tract stones of the kidney or ureter is covered under Medicare.

100-3, 230.2

NCD for Uroflowmetric Evaluations (230.2)

Uroflowmetric evaluations (also referred to as urodynamic voiding or urodynamic flow studies) are covered under Medicare for diagnosing various urological dysfunctions, including bladder outlet obstructions.

100-3, 230.3

NCD for Sterilization (230.3)

Payment may be made only where sterilization is a necessary part of the treatment of an illness or injury, e.g., removal of a uterus because of a tumor, removal of diseased ovaries (bilateral oophorectomy), or bilateral orchidectomy in a case of cancer of the prostate. Deny claims when the pathological evidence of the necessity to perform any such procedures to treat an illness or injury is absent; and

Sterilization of a mentally retarded beneficiary is covered if it is a necessary part of the treatment of an illness or injury.

Monitor such surgeries closely and obtain the information needed to determine whether in fact the surgery was performed as a means of treating an illness or injury or only to achieve sterilization.

B - Noncovered Conditions
Elective hysterectomy, tubal ligation, and vasectomy, if the stated reason for these procedures is sterilization;

A sterilization that is performed because a physician believes another pregnancy would endanger the overall general health of the woman is not considered to be reasonable and necessary for the diagnosis or treatment of illness or injury within the meaning of Sec.1862(a)(1) of the Act. The same conclusion would apply where the sterilization is performed only as a measure to prevent the possible development of, or effect on, a mental condition should the individual become pregnant; and

Sterilization of a mentally retarded person where the purpose is to prevent conception, rather than the treatment of an illness or injury.

100-3, 230.4

NCD for Diagnosis and Treatment of Impotence (230.4)

Program payment may be made for diagnosis and treatment of sexual impotence.¬

100-3, 230.6

NCD for Vabra Aspirator (230.6)

Program payment cannot be made for the aspirator or the related diagnostic services when furnished in connection with the examination of an asymptomatic patient. Payment for routine physical checkups is precluded under the statute (Sec.1862(a)(7) of the Act).

100-3, 230.9

NCD for Cryosurgery of Prostate (230.9)

Cryosurgery of the prostate as a salvage therapy is not covered for any services performed prior to June 30, 2001.

Salvage Cryosurgery of Prostate After Radiation Failure. Salvage cryosurgery of the prostate for recurrent cancer is medically necessary and appropriate only for those patients with localized disease who:

1. Have failed a trial of radiation therapy as their primary treatment; and
2. Meet one of the following conditions: Stage T2B or below, Gleason score <9, PSA <8 ng/mL.

Cryosurgery as salvage therapy is therefore not covered under Medicare after failure of other therapies as the primary treatment. Cryosurgery as salvage is only covered after the failure of a trial of radiation therapy, under the conditions noted above.

100-3, 230.10

NCD for Incontinence Control Devices (230.10)

A - Mechanical/Hydraulic Incontinence Control Devices
Mechanical/hydraulic incontinence control devices are accepted as safe and effective in the management of urinary incontinence in patients with permanent anatomic and neurologic dysfunctions of the bladder. This class of devices achieves control of urination by compression of the urethra. The materials used and the success rate may vary somewhat from device to device. Such a device is covered when its use is reasonable and necessary for the individual patient.

B - Collagen Implant
A collagen implant, which is injected into the submucosal tissues of the urethra and/or the bladder neck and into tissues adjacent to the urethra, is a prosthetic device used in the treatment of stress urinary incontinence resulting from intrinsic sphincter deficiency (ISD). ISD is a cause of stress urinary incontinence in which the urethral sphincter is unable to contract and generate sufficient resistance in the bladder, especially during stress maneuvers.

Prior to collagen implant therapy, a skin test for collagen sensitivity must be administered and evaluated over a 4 week period.

In male patients, the evaluation must include a complete history and physical examination and a simple cystometrogram to determine that the bladder fills and stores properly. The patient then is asked to stand upright with a full bladder and to cough or otherwise exert abdominal pressure on his bladder. If the patient leaks, the diagnosis of ISD is established.

In female patients, the evaluation must include a complete history and physical examination (including a pelvic exam) and a simple cystometrogram to rule out abnormalities of bladder compliance and abnormalities of urethral support. Following that determination, an abdominal leak point pressure (ALLP) test is performed. Leak point pressure, stated in cm H2O, is defined as the intra-abdominal pressure at which leakage occurs from the bladder (around a catheter) when the bladder has been filled with a minimum of 150 cc fluid. If the patient has an ALLP of less than 100 cm H2O, the diagnosis of ISD is established.

To use a collagen implant, physicians must have urology training in the use of a cystoscope and must complete a collagen implant training program.

Coverage of a collagen implant, and the procedure to inject it, is limited to the following types of patients with stress urinary incontinence due to ISD:

- Male or female patients with congenital sphincter weakness secondary to conditions such as myelomeningocele or epispadias;
- Male or female patients with acquired sphincter weakness secondary to spinal cord lesions;
- Male patients following trauma, including prostatectomy and/or radiation; and
- Female patients without urethral hypermobility and with abdominal leak point pressures of 100 cm H2O or less.

Patients whose incontinence does not improve with 5 injection procedures (5 separate treatment sessions) are considered treatment failures, and no further treatment of urinary incontinence by collagen implant is covered. Patients who have a reoccurrence of incontinence following successful treatment with collagen implants in the past (e.g., 6-12 months previously) may benefit from additional treatment sessions. Coverage of additional sessions may be allowed but must be supported by medical justification.

100-3, 230.12

NCD for Dimethyl Sulfoxide (DMSO) (230.12)

The Food and Drug Administration has determined that the only purpose for which DMSO is safe and effective for humans is in the treatment of the bladder condition, interstitial cystitis. Therefore, the use of DMSO for all other indications is not considered to be reasonable and necessary. Payment may be made for its use only when reasonable and necessary for a patient in the treatment of interstitial cystitis.

100-3, 230.14

NCD for Ultrafiltration Monitor (230.14)

Covered:

Ultrafiltration and ultrafiltration monitoring as a component of hemodialysis has an established and critical role in maintaining the well-being of ESRD patients and is a covered service. The Ultrafiltration Monitor is covered under the Medicare program when it is used to calculate fluid rates for those recipients who present difficult fluid management problems. Determine the medical necessity of this device on a case-by-case basis.

Not Covered:

Ultrafiltration, independent of conventional dialysis, is considered experimental, and technology exclusively designed for this purpose is not covered under Medicare.

100-3, 240.3

NCD for Heat Treatment, including the Use of Diathermy and Ultrasound for Pulmonary Conditions (240.3)

There is no physiological rationale or valid scientific documentation of effectiveness of diathermy or ultrasound heat treatments for asthma, bronchitis, or any other pulmonary condition and for such purpose this treatment cannot be considered reasonable and necessary within the meaning of section 1862(a)(1) of the Act.

100-3, 240.4.1

Sleep Testing for Obstructive Sleep Apnea (OSA) (Effective March 3, 2009)

A. General
Obstructive sleep apnea (OSA) is the collapse of the oropharyngeal walls and the obstruction of airflow occurring during sleep. Diagnostic tests for OSA have historically been classified into four types. The most comprehensive is designated Type I attended facility based polysomnography (PSG), which is considered the reference standard for diagnosing OSA. Attended facility based polysomnogram is a comprehensive diagnostic sleep test including at least electroencephalography (EEG), electro-oculography (EOG), electromyography (EMG), heart rate or electrocardiography (ECG), airflow, breathing/respiratory effort, and arterial oxygen saturation (SaO2) furnished in a sleep laboratory facility in which a technologist supervises the recording during sleep time and has the ability to intervene if needed. Overnight PSG is the conventional diagnostic test for OSA. The American Thoracic Society and the American Academy of Sleep Medicine have recommended supervised PSG in the sleep laboratory over 2 nights for the diagnosis of OSA and the initiation of continuous positive airway pressure (CPAP).

Three categories of portable monitors (used both in attended and unattended settings) have been developed for the diagnosis of OSA. Type II monitors have a minimum of 7 channels (e.g., EEG, EOG, EMG, ECG-heart rate, airflow, breathing/respiratory effort, SaO2)-this type of device monitors sleep staging, so AHI can be calculated). Type III monitors have a minimum of 4 monitored channels including ventilation or airflow (at least two channels of respiratory movement or respiratory movement and airflow), heart rate or ECG, and oxygen saturation. Type IV devices may measure one, two, three or more parameters but do not meet all the criteria of a higher category device. Some monitors use an actigraphy algorithm to identify periods of sleep and wakefulness.

B. Nationally Covered Indications
Effective for claims with dates of service on and after March 3, 2009, the Centers for Medicare & Medicaid Services finds that the evidence is sufficient to determine that the results of the sleep tests identified below can be used by a beneficiary's treating physician to diagnose OSA, that the use of such sleep testing technologies demonstrates improved health outcomes in Medicare beneficiaries who have OSA and receive the appropriate treatment, and that these tests are thus reasonable and necessary under section 1862(a)(1)(A) of the Social Security Act.

1. Type I PSG is covered when used to aid the diagnosis of OSA in beneficiaries who have clinical signs and symptoms indicative of OSA if performed attended in a sleep lab facility.
2. Type II or Type III sleep testing devices are covered when used to aid the diagnosis of OSA in beneficiaries who have clinical signs and symptoms indicative of OSA if performed unattended in or out of a sleep lab facility or attended in a sleep lab facility.
3. Type IV sleep testing devices measuring three or more channels, one of which is airflow, are covered when used to aid the diagnosis of OSA in beneficiaries who have signs and symptoms indicative of OSA if performed unattended in or out of a sleep lab facility or attended in a sleep lab facility.
4. Sleep testing devices measuring three or more channels that include actigraphy, oximetry, and peripheral arterial tone, are covered when used to aid the diagnosis of OSA in beneficiaries who have signs and symptoms indicative of OSA if performed unattended in or out of a sleep lab facility or attended in a sleep lab facility.

C. Nationally Non-Covered Indications
Effective for claims with dates of services on and after March 3, 2009, other diagnostic sleep tests for the diagnosis of OSA, other than those noted above for prescribing CPAP, are not sufficient for the coverage of CPAP and are not covered.

D. Other
N/A

(This NCD last reviewed March 2009.)

100-3, 240.6

NCD for Transvenous (Catheter) Pulmonary Embolectomy (240.6)

It is not covered under Medicare because it is still experimental.

100-3, 240.7

NCD for Postural Drainage Procedures and Pulmonary Exercises (240.7)

In most cases, postural drainage procedures and pulmonary exercises can be carried out safely and effectively by nursing personnel. However, in some cases patients may have acute or severe pulmonary conditions involving complex situations in which these procedures or exercises require the knowledge and skills of a physical therapist or a respiratory therapist. Therefore, if the attending physician determines as part of his/her plan of treatment that for the safe and effective administration of such services the procedures or exercises in question need to be performed by a physical therapist, the services of such a therapist constitute covered physical therapy when provided as an inpatient hospital service, extended care service, home health service, or outpatient physical therapy service.

NOTE: Physical therapy furnished in the outpatient department of a hospital is covered under the outpatient physical therapy benefit.

If the attending physician determines that the services should be performed by a respiratory therapist, the services of such a therapist constitute covered respiratory therapy when provided as an inpatient hospital service, outpatient hospital service, or extended care service, assuming that such services are furnished to the skilled nursing facility by a hospital with which the facility has a transfer agreement. Since the services of a respiratory therapist are not covered under the home health benefit, payment may not be made under the home health benefit for visits by a respiratory therapist to a patient's home to provide such services. Postural drainage procedures and pulmonary exercises are also covered when furnished by a physical therapist or a respiratory therapist as incident to a physician's professional service.

100-3, 250.1

NCD for Treatment of Psoriasis (250.1)

Psoriasis is a chronic skin disease, for which several conventional methods of treatment have been recognized as covered. These include topical application of steroids or other drugs; ultraviolet light (actinotherapy); and coal tar alone or in combination with ultraviolet B light (Goeckerman treatment).

A newer treatment for psoriasis uses a psoralen derivative drug in combination with ultraviolet A light, known as PUVA. PUVA therapy is covered for treatment of intractable, disabling psoriasis, but only after the psoriasis has not responded to more conventional treatment. The contractor should document this before paying for PUVA therapy.

In addition, reimbursement for PUVA therapy should be limited to amounts paid for other types of photochemotherapy; ordinarily, payment should not be allowed for more than 30 days of treatment, unless improvement is documented.

100-3, 250.3

NCD for Intravenous Immune Globulin for the Treatment of Autoimmune Mucocutaneous Blistering Diseases (250.3)

Effective October 1, 2002, IVIg is covered for the treatment of biopsy-proven (1) Pemphigus Vulgaris, (2) Pemphigus Foliaceus, (3) Bullous Pemphigoid, (4) Mucous Membrane Pemphigoid (a.k.a., Cicatricial Pemphigoid), and (5) Epidermolysis Bullosa Acquisita for the following patient subpopulations:

- Patients who have failed conventional therapy. Contractors have the discretion to define what constitutes failure of conventional therapy;
- Patients in whom conventional therapy is otherwise contraindicated. Contractors have the discretion to define what constitutes contraindications to conventional therapy; or
- Patients with rapidly progressive disease in whom a clinical response could not be affected quickly enough using conventional agents. In such situations IVIg therapy would be given along with conventional treatment(s) and the IVIg would be used only until the conventional therapy could take effect.

In addition, IVIg for the treatment of autoimmune mucocutaneous blistering diseases must be used only for short-term therapy and not as a maintenance therapy. Contractors have the discretion to decide what constitutes short-term therapy.

100-3, 250.4

NCD for Treatment of Actinic Keratosis (AKs) (250.4)

Actinic keratoses (AKs), also known as solar keratoses, are common, sun-induced skin lesions that are confined to the epidermis and have the potential to become a skin cancer.

Various options exist for treating AKs. Clinicians should select an appropriate treatment based on the patient's medical history, the lesion's characteristics, and on the patient's preference for a specific treatment. Commonly performed treatments for AKs include cryosurgery with liquid nitrogen, topical drug therapy, and curettage. Less commonly performed treatments for AK include dermabrasion, excision, chemical peels, laser therapy, and photodynamic therapy (PDT). An alternative approach to treating AKs is to observe the lesions over time and remove them only if they exhibit specific clinical features suggesting possible transformation to invasive squamous cell carcinoma (SCC).

Effective for services performed on and after November 26, 2001, Medicare covers the destruction of actinic keratoses without restrictions based on lesion or patient characteristics.

100-3, 260.1

NCD for Adult Liver Transplantation (260.1)

A - General

Effective July 15, 1996, adult liver transplantation when performed on beneficiaries with end stage liver disease other than hepatitis B or malignancies is covered under Medicare when performed in a facility which is approved by CMS as meeting institutional coverage criteria.

Effective December 10, 1999, adult liver transplantation when performed on beneficiaries with end stage liver disease other than malignancies is covered under Medicare when performed in a facility which is approved by CMS as meeting institutional coverage criteria.

Effective September 1, 2001, Medicare covers adult liver transplantation for hepatocellular carcinoma when the following conditions are met:

- The patient is not a candidate for subtotal liver resection;
- The patient's tumor(s) is less than or equal to 5 cm in diameter;
- There is no macrovascular involvement;
- There is no identifiable extrahepatic spread of tumor to surrounding lymph nodes, lungs, abdominal organs or bone; and
- The transplant is furnished in a facility which is approved by CMS as meeting institutional coverage criteria for liver transplants (See 65 FR 15006).

Adult liver transplantation for other malignancies remains excluded from coverage.

Coverage of adult liver transplantation is effective as of the date of the facility's approval, but for applications received before July 13, 1991, can be effective as early as March 8, 1990. (See "Federal Register" 56 FR 15006 dated April 12, 1991.)

B - Follow-up Care

Follow-up care or retransplantation (ICD-9-M 996.82, Complications of Transplanted Organ, Liver required as a result of a covered liver transplant is covered, provided such services are otherwise reasonable and necessary. Follow-up care is also covered for patients who have been discharged from a hospital after receiving noncoverd liver transplant. Coverage for follow-up care is for items and services that are reasonable and necessary as determined by Medicare guidelines.

C - Immunosuppressive Drugs

See the Medicare Benefit Policy Manual, Chapter 15, "Covered Medical and Other Health Services," Sec.50.5.1 and the Medicare Claims Processing Manual, Chapter 17, "Drugs and Biologicals," Sec.80.3.

100-3, 260.2

NCD for Pediatric Liver Transplantation (260.2)

Liver transplantation is covered for children (under age 18) with extrahepatic biliary atresia or any other form of end stage liver disease, except that coverage is not provided for children with a malignancy extending beyond the margins of the liver or those with persistent viremia.

Liver transplantation is covered for Medicare beneficiaries when performed in a pediatric hospital that performs pediatric liver transplants if the hospital submits an application which CMS approves documenting that:

The hospital's pediatric liver transplant program is operated jointly by the hospital and another facility that has been found by CMS to meet the institutional coverage criteria in the "Federal Register" notice of April 12, 1991;

- The unified program shares the same transplant surgeons and quality assurance program (including oversight committee, patient protocol, and patient selection criteria); and
- The hospital is able to provide the specialized facilities, services, and personnel that are required by pediatric liver transplant patients.

100-3, 260.3

NCD for Pancreas Transplants (260.3)

B. Nationally Covered Indications

Effective for services performed on or after July 1, 1999, whole organ pancreas transplantation is nationally covered by Medicare when performed simultaneous with or after a kidney transplant. If the pancreas transplant occurs after the kidney transplant, immunosuppressive therapy begins with the date of discharge from the inpatient stay for the pancreas transplant.

Effective for services performed on or after April 26, 2006, pancreas transplants alone (PA) are reasonable and necessary for Medicare beneficiaries in the following limited circumstances:

1. PA will be limited to those facilities that are Medicare-approved for kidney transplantation. (Approved centers can be found at http://www.cms.hhs.gov/ESRDGeneralInformation/02_Data.asp#TopOfPage
2. Patients must have a diagnosis of type I diabetes: ul.mylist2 li{list-style-type : circle}
   - Patient with diabetes must be beta cell autoantibody positive; or
   - Patient must demonstrate insulinopenia defined as a fasting C-peptide level that is less than or equal to 110% of the lower limit of normal of the laboratory's measurement method. Fasting C-peptide levels will only be considered valid with a concurrently obtained fasting glucose <225 mg/dL;
3. Patients must have a history of medically-uncontrollable labile (brittle) insulin-dependent diabetes mellitus with documented recurrent, severe, acutely life-threatening metabolic complications that require hospitalization. Aforementioned complications include frequent hypoglycemia unawareness or recurring severe ketoacidosis, or recurring severe hypoglycemic attacks;
4. Patients must have been optimally and intensively managed by an endocrinologist for at least 12 months with the most medically-recognized advanced insulin formulations and delivery systems;
5. Patients must have the emotional and mental capacity to understand the significant risks associated with surgery and to effectively manage the lifelong need for immunosuppression; and,
6. Patients must otherwise be a suitable candidate for transplantation.

C. Nationally Non-Covered Indications

The following procedure is not considered reasonable and necessary within the meaning of section 1862(a)(1)(A) of the Social Security Act:

1. Transplantation of partial pancreatic tissue or islet cells (except in the context of a clinical trial (see section 260.3.1 of the National Coverage Determinations Manual).

D. Other

Not applicable.

(This NCD last reviewed April 2006.)

100-3, 260.7

NCD for Lymphocyte Immune Globulin, Anti-Thymocyte Globulin (Equine) (260.7)

The FDA has approved one lymphocyte immune globulin preparation for marketing, lymphocyte immune globulin, anti-thymocyte globulin (equine). This drug is indicated for the management of allograft rejection episodes in renal transplantation. It is covered under Medicare when used for this purpose. Other forms of lymphocyte globulin preparation which the FDA approves for this indication in the future may be covered under Medicare.

100-3, 260.9

NCD for Heart Transplants (260.9)

A - General

Cardiac transplantation is covered under Medicare when performed in a facility which is approved by Medicare as meeting institutional coverage criteria. (See CMS Ruling 87-1.)

B - Exceptions

In certain limited cases, exceptions to the criteria may be warranted if there is justification and if the facility ensures our objectives of safety and efficacy. Under no circumstances will exceptions be made for facilities whose transplant programs have been in existence for less than two years, and applications from consortia will not be approved.

Although consortium arrangements will not be approved for payment of Medicare heart transplants, consideration will be given to applications from heart transplant facilities that consist of more than one hospital where all of the following conditions exist:

The hospitals are under the common control or have a formal affiliation arrangement with each other under the auspices of an organization such as a university or a legally-constituted medical research institute; and

The hospitals share resources by routinely using the same personnel or services in their transplant programs. The sharing of resources must be supported by the submission of operative notes or other information that documents the routine use of the same personnel and services in all of the individual hospitals. At a minimum, shared resources means:

The individual members of the transplant team, consisting of the cardiac transplant surgeons, cardiologists and pathologists, must practice in all the hospitals and it can be documented that they otherwise function as members of the transplant team;

The same organ procurement organization, immunology, and tissue-typing services must be used by all the hospitals;

The hospitals submit, in the manner required (Kaplan-Meier method) their individual and pooled experience and survival data; and

The hospitals otherwise meet the remaining Medicare criteria for heart transplant facilities; that is, the criteria regarding patient selection, patient management, program commitment, etc.

C - Pediatric Hospitals
Cardiac transplantation is covered for Medicare beneficiaries when performed in a pediatric hospital that performs pediatric heart transplants if the hospital submits an application which CMS approves as documenting that:

The hospital's pediatric heart transplant program is operated jointly by the hospital and another facility that has been found by CMS to meet the institutional coverage criteria in CMS Ruling 87-1;

The unified program shares the same transplant surgeons and quality assurance program (including oversight committee, patient protocol, and patient selection criteria); and

The hospital is able to provide the specialized facilities, services, and personnel that are required by pediatric heart transplant patients.

D - Follow-Up Care
Follow-up care required as a result of a covered heart transplant is covered, provided such services are otherwise reasonable and necessary. Follow-up care is also covered for patients who have been discharged from a hospital after receiving a noncovered heart transplant. Coverage for follow-up care would be for items and services that are reasonable and necessary, as determined by Medicare guidelines. (See the Medicare Benefit Policy Manual, Chapter 16, "General Exclusions from Coverage," Sec.180.)

E - Immunosuppressive Drugs
See the Medicare Claims Processing Manual, Chapter 17, "Drugs and Biologicals," Sec.80.3.1, and Chapter 8, "Outpatient ESRD Hospital, Independent Facility, and Physician/Supplier Claims," Sec.120.1.

F - Artificial Hearts
Medicare does not cover the use of artificial hearts as a permanent replacement for a human heart or as a temporary life-support system until a human heart becomes available for transplant (often referred to as a "bridge to transplant"). Medicare does cover a ventricular assist device (VAD) when used in conjunction with specific criteria listed in Sec.20.9 of the NCD Manual.

100-3, 270.1

NCD for Electrical Stimulation (ES) and Electromagnetic Therapy for the Treatment of Wounds (270.1)

A. Nationally Covered Indications
The use of ES and electromagnetic therapy for the treatment of wounds are considered adjunctive therapies, and will only be covered for chronic Stage III or Stage IV pressure ulcers, arterial ulcers, diabetic ulcers, and venous stasis ulcers. Chronic ulcers are defined as ulcers that have not healed within 30 days of occurrence. ES or electromagnetic therapy will be covered only after appropriate standard wound therapy has been tried for at least 30 days and there are no measurable signs of improved healing. This 30-day period may begin while the wound is acute.

Standard wound care includes: optimization of nutritional status, debridement by any means to remove devitalized tissue, maintenance of a clean, moist bed of granulation tissue with appropriate moist dressings, and necessary treatment to resolve any infection that may be present. Standard wound care based on the specific type of wound includes: frequent repositioning of a patient with pressure ulcers (usually every 2 hours), offloading of pressure and good glucose control for diabetic ulcers, establishment of adequate circulation for arterial ulcers, and the use of a compression system for patients with venous ulcers.

Measurable signs of improved healing include: a decrease in wound size (either surface area or volume), decrease in amount of exudates, and decrease in amount of necrotic tissue. ES or electromagnetic therapy must be discontinued when the wound demonstrates 100% epitheliliazed wound bed.

ES and electromagnetic therapy services can only be covered when performed by a physician, physical therapist, or incident to a physician service. Evaluation of the wound is an integral part of wound therapy. When a physician, physical therapist, or a clinician incident to a physician, performs ES or electromagnetic therapy, the practitioner must evaluate the wound and contact the treating physician if the wound worsens. If ES or electromagnetic therapy is being used, wounds must be evaluated at least monthly by the treating physician.

B. Nationally Noncovered Indications

1. ES and electromagnetic therapy will not be covered as an initial treatment modality.
2. Continued treatment with ES or electromagnetic therapy is not covered if measurable signs of healing have not been demonstrated within any 30-day period of treatment.
3. Unsupervised use of ES or electromagnetic therapy for wound therapy will not be covered, as this use has not been found to be medically reasonable and necessary.

C. Other
All other uses of ES and electromagnetic therapy not otherwise specified for the treatment of wounds remain at local contractor discretion.

(This NCD last reviewed March 2004.)

100-3, 270.2

NCD for Noncontact Normothermic Wound Therapy (NNWT) (270.2)

There is insufficient scientific or clinical evidence to consider this device as reasonable and necessary for the treatment of wounds within the meaning of Sec.1862(a)(1)(A) of the Social Security Act and will not be covered by Medicare.

100-3, 270.4

NCD for Treatment of Decubitus Ulcers (270.4)

An accepted procedure for healing decubitus ulcers is to remove dead tissue from the lesions and to keep them clean to promote the growth of new tissue. This may be accomplished by hydrotherapy (whirlpool) treatments. Hydrotherapy (whirlpool) treatment for decubitus ulcers is a covered service under Medicare for patients when treatment is reasonable and necessary. Some other methods of treating decubitus ulcers, the safety and effectiveness of which have not been established, are not covered under the Medicare program. Some examples of these types of treatments are: ultraviolet light, low intensity direct current, topical application of oxygen, and topical dressings with Balsam of Peru in castor oil.

100-3, 270.5

NCD for Porcine Skin and Gradient Pressure Dressings (270.5)

Porcine (pig) skin dressings are covered, if reasonable and necessary for the individual patient as an occlusive dressing for burns, donor sites of a homograft, and decubiti and other ulcers.

100-3, 280.13

NCD for Transcutaneous Electrical Nerve Stimulators (TENS) (280.13)

(Rev. 1, 10-03-03)

CIM 60-20

The TENS is a type of electrical nerve stimulator that is employed to treat chronic intractable pain. This stimulator is attached to the surface of the patient's skin over the peripheral nerve to be stimulated. It may be applied in a variety of settings (in the patient's home, a physician's office, or in an outpatient clinic). Payment for TENS may be made under the durable medical equipment benefit. (See §160.13 for an explanation of coverage of medically necessary supplies for the effective use of TENS and §10.2 for an explanation of coverage of TENS for acute post-operative pain.)

100-3, 280.14

NCD for Infusion Pumps (280.14)

B. Nationally Covered Indications

The following indications for treatment using infusion pumps are covered under Medicare:

1. External Infusion Pumps
   a. Iron Poisoning (Effective for Services Performed On or After September 26, 1984)

      When used in the administration of deferoxamine for the treatment of acute iron poisoning and iron overload, only external infusion pumps are covered.

   b. Thromboembolic Disease (Effective for Services Performed On or After September 26, 1984)

      When used in the administration of heparin for the treatment of thromboembolic disease and/or pulmonary embolism, only external infusion pumps used in an institutional setting are covered.

   c. Chemotherapy for Liver Cancer (Effective for Services Performed On or After January 29, 1985)

      The external chemotherapy infusion pump is covered when used in the treatment of primary hepatocellular carcinoma or colorectal cancer where this disease is unresectable; OR, where the patient refuses surgical excision of the tumor.

   d. Morphine for Intractable Cancer Pain (Effective for Services Performed On or After April 22, 1985)

      Morphine infusion via an external infusion pump is covered when used in the treatment of intractable pain caused by cancer (in either an inpatient or outpatient setting, including a hospice).

   e. Continuous Subcutaneous Insulin Infusion (CSII) Pumps (Effective for Services Performed On or after December 17, 2004)

      Continuous subcutaneous insulin infusion (CSII) and related drugs/supplies are covered as medically reasonable and necessary in the home setting for the treatment of diabetic patients who: (1) either meet the updated fasting C-Peptide testing requirement, or, are beta cell autoantibody positive; and, (2) satisfy the remaining criteria for insulin pump therapy as described below. Patients must meet either Criterion A or B as follows:

      Criterion A: The patient has completed a comprehensive diabetes education program, and has been on a program of multiple daily injections of insulin (i.e., at least 3 injections per day), with frequent self-adjustments of insulin doses for at least 6 months prior to initiation of the insulin pump, and has documented frequency of glucose self-testing an average of at least 4 times per day during the 2 months prior to initiation of the insulin pump, and meets one or more of the following criteria while on the multiple daily injection regimen:

      - Glycosylated hemoglobin level (HbAlc) > 7.0 percent;
      - History of recurring hypoglycemia;
      - Wide fluctuations in blood glucose before mealtime;
      - Dawn phenomenon with fasting blood sugars frequently exceeding 200 mg/dl; or,

- History of severe glycemic excursions.

Criterion B: The patient with diabetes has been on a pump prior to enrollment in Medicare and has documented frequency of glucose self-testing an average of at least 4 times per day during the month prior to Medicare enrollment.

General CSII Criteria

In addition to meeting Criterion A or B above, the following general requirements must be met:

The patient with diabetes must be insulinopenic per the updated fasting C-peptide testing requirement, or, as an alternative, must be beta cell autoantibody positive.

Updated fasting C-peptide testing requirement:

- Insulinopenia is defined as a fasting C-peptide level that is less than or equal to 110% of the lower limit of normal of the laboratory's measurement method.
- For patients with renal insufficiency and creatinine clearance (actual or calculated from age, gender, weight, and serum creatinine) <50 ml/minute, insulinopenia is defined as a fasting C-peptide level that is less than or equal to 200% of the lower limit of normal of the laboratory's measurement method.
- Fasting C-peptide levels will only be considered valid with a concurrently obtained fasting glucose <225 mg/dL.
- Levels only need to be documented once in the medical records.

Continued coverage of the insulin pump would require that the patient be seen and evaluated by the treating physician at least every 3 months.

The pump must be ordered by and follow-up care of the patient must be managed by a physician who manages multiple patients with CSII and who works closely with a team including nurses, diabetes educators, and dietitians who are knowledgeable in the use of CSII.

Other Uses of CSII

The CMS will continue to allow coverage of all other uses of CSII in accordance with the Category B investigational device exemption (IDE) clinical trials regulation (42 CFR 405.201) or as a routine cost under the clinical trials policy (Medicare National Coverage Determinations (NCD) Manual 310.1).

f. Other Uses

Other uses of external infusion pumps are covered if the contractor's medical staff verifies the appropriateness of the therapy and the prescribed pump for the individual patient.

NOTE: Payment may also be made for drugs necessary for the effective use of a covered external infusion pump as long as the drug being used with the pump is itself reasonable and necessary for the patient's treatment.

2. Implantable Infusion Pumps

a. Chemotherapy for Liver Cancer (Effective for Services Performed On or After September 26, 1984)

The implantable infusion pump is covered for intra-arterial infusion of 5-FUdR for the treatment of liver cancer for patients with primary hepatocellular carcinoma or Duke's Class D colorectal cancer, in whom the metastases are limited to the liver, and where: (1) the disease is unresectable, or (2) the patient refuses surgical excision of the tumor.

b. Anti-Spasmodic Drugs for Severe Spasticity

An implantable infusion pump is covered when used to administer anti-spasmodic drugs intrathecally (e.g., baclofen) to treat chronic intractable spasticity in patients who have proven unresponsive to less invasive medical therapy as determined by the following criteria:

As indicated by at least a 6-week trial, the patient cannot be maintained on noninvasive methods of spasm control, such as oral anti-spasmodic drugs, either because these methods fail to control adequately the spasticity or produce intolerable side effects, and prior to pump implantation, the patient must have responded favorably to a trial intrathecal dose of the anti-spasmodic drug.

c. Opioid Drugs for Treatment of Chronic Intractable Pain

An implantable infusion pump is covered when used to administer opioid drugs (e.g., morphine) intrathecally or epidurally for treatment of severe chronic intractable pain of malignant or nonmalignant origin in patients who have a life expectancy of at least 3 months, and who have proven unresponsive to less invasive medical therapy as determined by the following criteria:

The patient's history must indicate that he/she would not respond adequately to noninvasive methods of pain control, such as systemic opioids (including attempts to eliminate physical and behavioral abnormalities which may cause an exaggerated reaction to pain); and a preliminary trial of intraspinal opioid drug administration must be undertaken with a temporary intrathecal/epidural catheter to substantiate adequately acceptable pain relief and degree of side effects (including effects on the activities of daily living) and patient acceptance.

d. Coverage of Other Uses of Implanted Infusion Pumps

Determinations may be made on coverage of other uses of implanted infusion pumps if the contractor's medical staff verifies that:

- The drug is reasonable and necessary for the treatment of the individual patient;
- It is medically necessary that the drug be administered by an implanted infusion pump; and,
- The Food and Drug Administration (FDA)-approved labeling for the pump must specify that the drug being administered and the purpose for which it is administered is an indicated use for the pump.

e. Implantation of Infusion Pump Is Contraindicated

The implantation of an infusion pump is contraindicated in the following patients:

- With a known allergy or hypersensitivity to the drug being used (e.g., oral baclofen, morphine, etc.);
- Who have an infection;
- Whose body size is insufficient to support the weight and bulk of the device; and,
- With other implanted programmable devices since crosstalk between devices may inadvertently change the prescription.

NOTE: Payment may also be made for drugs necessary for the effective use of an implantable infusion pump as long as the drug being used with the pump is itself reasonable and necessary for the patient's treatment.

C. Nationally Noncovered Indications

The following indications for treatment using infusion pumps are not covered under Medicare:

1. External Infusion Pumps

a. Vancomycin (Effective for Services Beginning On or After September 1, 1996)

Medicare coverage of vancomycin as a durable medical equipment infusion pump benefit is not covered. There is insufficient evidence to support the necessity of using an external infusion pump, instead of a disposable elastomeric pump or the gravity drip method, to administer vancomycin in a safe and appropriate manner.

2. Implantable Infusion Pump

a. Thromboembolic Disease (Effective for Services Performed On or After September 26, 1984)

According to the Public Health Service, there is insufficient published clinical data to support the safety and effectiveness of the heparin implantable pump. Therefore, the use of an implantable infusion pump for infusion of heparin in the treatment of recurrent thromboembolic disease is not covered.

b. Diabetes

An implanted infusion pump for the infusion of insulin to treat diabetes is not covered. The data does not demonstrate that the pump provides effective administration of insulin.

D. Other

Not applicable.

(This NCD last reviewed January 2005.)

100-3, 300.1

NCD for Obsolete or Unreliable Diagnostic Tests (300.1)

CIM 50-34

A. Diagnostic Tests

Do not routinely pay for the following diagnostic tests because they are obsolete and have been replaced by more advanced procedures. The listed tests may be paid for only if the medical need for the procedure is satisfactorily justified by the physician who performs it. When the services are subject to the Quality Improvement Organization (QIO) Review, the QIO is responsible for determining that satisfactory medical justification exists. When the services are not subject to QIO review, the intermediary or carrier is responsible for determining that satisfactory medical justification exists. This includes:

- Amylase, blood isoenzymes, electrophoretic,
- Chromium, blood,
- Guanase, blood,
- Zinc sulphate turbidity, blood,
- Skin test, cat scratch fever,
- Skin test, lymphopathia venereum,
- Circulation time, one test,
- Cephalin flocculation,
- Congo red, blood,
- Hormones, adrenocorticotropin quantitative animal tests,
- Hormones, adrenocorticotropin quantitative bioassay,
- Thymol turbidity, blood,
- Skin test, actinomycosis,
- Skin test, brucellosis,
- Skin test, psittacosis,
- Skin test, trichinosis,
- Calcium, feces, 24-hour quantitative,
- Starch, feces, screening,
- Chymotrypsin, duodenal contents,

- Gastric analysis, pepsin,
- Gastric analysis, tubeless,
- Calcium saturation clotting time,
- Capillary fragility test (Rumpel-Leede),
- Colloidal gold,
- Bendien's test for cancer and tuberculosis,
- Bolen's test for cancer,
- Rehfuss test for gastric acidity, and
- Serum seromucoid assay for cancer and other diseases.

B. Cardiovascular Tests
Do not pay for the following phonocardiography and vectorcardiography diagnostic tests because they have been determined to be outmoded and of little clinical value. They include:

- Phonocardiogram with or without ECG lead; with supervision during recording with interpretation and report (when equipment is supplied by the physician),
- Phonocardiogram; tracing only, without interpretation and report (e.g., when equipment is supplied by the hospital, clinic),
- Phonocardiogram; interpretation and report,
- Phonocardiogram with ECG lead, with indirect carotid artery and/or jugular vein tracing, and/or apex cardiogram; with interpretation and report,
- Phonocardiogram; without interpretation and report,
- Phonocardiogram; interpretation and report only,
- Intracardiac,
- Vectorcardiogram (VCG), with or without ECG; with interpretation and report,
- Vectorcardiogram; tracing only, without interpretation and report, and
- Vectorcardiogram; interpretation and report only.

100-4, 1, 30.3.5

Effect of Assignment Upon Purchase of Cataract Glasses FromParticipating Physician or Supplier on Claims Submitted to Carriers

B3-3045.4

A pair of cataract glasses is comprised of two distinct products: a professional product (the prescribed lenses) and a retail commercial product (the frames). The frames serve not only as a holder of lenses but also as an article of personal apparel. As such, they are usually selected on the basis of personal taste and style. Although Medicare will pay only for standard frames, most patients want deluxe frames. Participating physicians and suppliers cannot profitably furnish such deluxe frames unless they can make an extra (noncovered) charge for the frames even though they accept assignment.

Therefore, a participating physician or supplier (whether an ophthalmologist, optometrist, or optician) who accepts assignment on cataract glasses with deluxe frames may charge the Medicare patient the difference between his/her usual charge to private pay patients for glasses with standard frames and his/her usual charge to such patients for glasses with deluxe frames, in addition to the applicable deductible and coinsurance on glasses with standard frames, if all of the following requirements are met:

A. The participating physician or supplier has standard frames available, offers them for saleto the patient, and issues and ABN to the patient that explains the price and other differences between standard and deluxe frames. Refer to Chapter 30.

B. The participating physician or supplier obtains from the patient (or his/her representative) and keeps on file the following signed and dated statement:

Name of Patient Medicare Claim Number

Having been informed that an extra charge is being made by the physician or supplier for deluxe frames, that this extra charge is not covered by Medicare, and that standard frames are available for purchase from the physician or supplier at no extra charge, I have chosen to purchase deluxe frames.

Signature Date

C. The participating physician or supplier itemizes on his/her claim his/her actual charge for the lenses, his/her actual charge for the standard frames, and his/her actual extra charge for the deluxe frames (charge differential). Once the assigned claim for deluxe frames has been processed, the carrier will follow the ABN instructions as described in Sec.60.

100-4, 3, 10.4

Payment of Nonphysician Services for Inpatients

All items and nonphysician services furnished to inpatients must be furnished directly by the hospital or billed through the hospital under arrangements. This provision applies to all hospitals, regardless of whether they are subject to PPS.

Other Medical Items, Supplies, and Services the following medical items, supplies, and services furnished to inpatients are covered under Part A. Consequently, they are covered by the prospective payment rate or reimbursed as reasonable costs under Part A to hospitals excluded from PPS.

- Laboratory services (excluding anatomic pathology services and certain clinical pathology services);
- Pacemakers and other prosthetic devices including lenses, and artificial limbs, knees, and hips;
- Radiology services including computed tomography (CT) scans furnished to inpatients by a physician's office, other hospital, or radiology clinic;
- Total parenteral nutrition (TPN) services; and
- Transportation, including transportation by ambulance, to and from another hospital or freestanding facility to receive specialized diagnostic or therapeutic services not available at the facility where the patient is an inpatient.

The hospital must include the cost of these services in the appropriate ancillary service cost center, i.e., in the cost of the diagnostic or therapeutic service. It must not show them separately under revenue code 0540.

EXCEPTIONS

- Pneumococcal Vaccine -is payable under Part B only and is billed by the hospital on the Form CMS-1450.
- Ambulance Service For purposes of this section "hospital inpatient" means beneficiary who has been formally admitted it does not include a beneficiary who is in the process of being transferred from one hospital to another. Where the patient is transferred from one hospital to another, and is admitted as an inpatient to the second, the ambulance service is payable under only Part B. If transportation is by a hospital owned and operated ambulance, the hospital bills separately on Form CMS-1450 as appropriate. Similarly, if the hospital arranges for the ambulance transportation with an ambulance operator, including paying the ambulance operator, it bills separately. However, if the hospital does not assume any financial responsibility, the billing is to the carrier by the ambulance operator or beneficiary, as appropriate, if an ambulance is used for the transportation of a hospital inpatient to another facility for diagnostic tests or special treatment the ambulance trip is considered part of the DRG, and not separately billable, if the resident hospital is under PPS.
- Part B Inpatient Services Where Part A benefits are not payable, payment maybe made to the hospital under Part B for certain medical and other health services. See Chapter 4 for a description of Part B inpatient services.
- Anesthetist Services "Incident to" Physician Services-If a physician's practice was to employ anesthetists and to bill on a reasonable charge basis for these services and that practice was in effect as of the last day of the hospital's most recent 12-month cost reporting period ending before September 30, 1983, the physician may continue that practice through cost reporting periods beginning October 1, 1984. However, if the physician chooses to continue this practice, the hospital may not add costs of the anesthetist's service to its base period costs for purposes of its transition payment rates. If it is the existing or new practice of the physician to employ certified registered nurse anesthetists (CRNAs) and other qualified anesthetists and include charges for their services in the physician bills for anesthesiology services for the hospital's cost report periods beginning on or after October 1, 1984, and before October 1, 1987, the physician may continue to do so.

B. Exceptions/Waivers
These provisions were waived before cost reporting periods beginning on or after October1, 1986, under certain circumstances. The basic criteria for waiver was that services furnished by outside suppliers are so extensive that a sudden change in billing practices would threaten the stability of patient care. Specific criteria for waiver and processing procedures are in Sec.2804 of the Provider Reimbursement Manual (CMS Pub. 15-1).

100-4, 3, 20.1.2.8

Special Outlier Payments for Burn Cases

For discharges occurring on or after April 1, 1988, the additional payment amount for the DRGs related to burn cases, which are identified in the most recent annual notice of prospective payment rates is computed using the same methodology (as stated above in section 20.1.2.3) except that the payment is made using a marginal cost factor of 90 percent instead of 80 percent.

100-4, 3, 20.2.1

Medicare Code Editor (MCE)

A. General
The MCE edits claims to detect incorrect billing data. In determining the appropriate DRG for a Medicare patient, the age, sex, discharge status, principal diagnosis, secondary diagnosis, and procedures performed must be reported accurately to the Grouper program. The logic of the Grouper software assumes that this information is accurate and the Grouper does not make any attempt to edit the data for accuracy. Only where extreme inconsistencies occur in the patient information will a patient not be assigned to a DRG. Therefore, the MCE is used to improve the quality of information given to Grouper.

The MCE addresses three basic types of edits which will support the DRG assignment:

- Code Edits - Examines a record for the correct use of ICD-9-CM codes that describe a patient's diagnoses and procedures. They include basic consistency checks on the interrelationship among a patient's age, sex, and diagnoses and procedures.
- Coverage Edits - Examines the type of patient and procedures performed to determine if the services where covered.
- Clinical Edits - Examines the clinical consistency of the diagnostic and procedural information on the medical claim to determine if they are clinically reasonable and, therefore, should be paid.

B. Implementation Requirements
The FI processes all inpatient Part A discharge/transfer bills for both PPS and non-PPS facilities (including waiver States, long-term care hospitals, and excluded units) through the MCE. It processes claims that have been reviewed by the QIO prior to billing through the MCE only for edit types 1, 2, 3, 4, 7, and 12. It does not process the following kinds of bills through the MCE:

- Where no Medicare payment is due (amounts reported by value codes 12, 13, 14, 15, or 16 equal or exceed charges).
- Where no Medicare payment is being made. Where partial payment is made, editing is required.
- Where QIO reviewed prior to billing (code C1 or C3 in FL 24-30). It may process these exceptions through the program and ignore development codes or bypass the program.

The MCE software contains multiple versions. The version of the MCE accessed by the program depends upon the patient discharge date entered on the claim.

C. Bill System/MCE Interface
The FI installs the MCE online, if possible, so that prepayment edit requirements identified in subsection C can be directed to hospitals without clerical handling.

The MCE needs the following data elements to analyze the bill:

- Age;
- Sex;
- Discharge status;
- Diagnosis (9 maximum - principal diagnosis and up to 8 additional diagnoses);
- Procedures (6 maximum); and
- Discharge date.

The MCE provides the FI an analysis of "errors" on the bill as described in subsection D. The FI develops its own interface program to provide data to MCE and receive data from it.

The MCE Installation Manual describes the installation and operation of the program, including data base formats and locations.

D. Processing Requirements
The hospital must follow the procedure described below for each error code. For bills returned to the provider, the FI considers the bill improperly completed for control and processing time purposes. (See chapter 1.)

1. Invalid Diagnosis or Procedure Code
   The MCE checks each diagnosis code, including the admitting diagnosis, and each procedure code against a table of valid ICD-9-CM codes. An admitting diagnosis, a principle diagnosis, and up to eight additional diagnoses may be reported. Up to six total procedure codes may be reported on an inpatient claim. If the recorded code is not in this table, the code is invalid, and the FI returns the bill to the provider.

   For a list of all valid ICD-9-CM codes see "International Classification of Diseases, 9th Revision, Clinical Modification (ICD-9-CM), January 1979, Volume I (Diseases)" and "Volume 3 (Procedures)," and the "Addendum/Errata" and new codes furnished by the FI. The hospital must review the medical record and/or face sheet and enter the correct diagnosis/procedure codes before returning the bill.
2. Invalid Fourth or Fifth Digit
   The MCE identifies any diagnosis code, including the admitting diagnosis or any procedure that requires a fourth or fifth digit, which is either missing or not valid for the code in question.

   For a list of all valid fourth and fifth digit ICD-9-CM codes see "International Classification of Diseases, 9th Revision, Clinical Modification (ICD-9-CM), January 1979, Volume 1 (Diseases)" and "Volume 3 (Procedures)," and "Addendum/Errata" and new codes furnished by the FI. The FI returns claims edited for this reason to the hospital. The hospital must review the medical record and/or face sheet and enter the correct diagnosis/procedure before returning the bill.
3. E-Code as Principal Diagnosis
   E-codes describe the circumstances that caused an injury, not the nature of the injury, and therefore are not recognized by the Grouper program as acceptable principal diagnoses. E-codes are all ICD-9-CM diagnosis codes that begin with the letter E. For a list of all E-codes, see "International Classification of Diseases, 9th Revision, Clinical Modification (ICD-9-CM), January 1979, Volume I (Diseases)." The hospital must review the medical record and/or face sheet and enter the correct diagnosis before returning the bill.
4. Duplicate of PDX
   Any secondary diagnosis that is the same code as the principal diagnosis is identified as a duplicate of the principal diagnoses. This is unacceptable because the secondary diagnosis may cause an erroneous assignment to a higher severity MS-DRG. Hospitals may not repeat a diagnosis code. The FI will delete the duplicate secondary diagnosis and process the bill.
5. Age Conflict
   The MCE detects inconsistencies between a patient's age and any diagnosis on the patient's record. Examples are:

   - A 5-year-old patient with benign prostatic hypertrophy.
   - A 78-year-old delivery.

   In the above cases, the diagnosis is clinically impossible in a patient of the stated age. Therefore, either the diagnosis or age is presumed to be incorrect. Four age code categories are described below.

   - A subset of diagnoses is intended only for newborns and neonates. These are "Newborn" diagnoses. For "Newborn" diagnoses, the patient's age must be 0 years.
   - Certain diagnoses are considered reasonable only for children between the ages of 0 and 17. These are "Pediatric" diagnoses.
   - Diagnoses identified as "Maternity" are coded only for patients between the ages of I2 and 55 years.
   - A subset of diagnoses is considered valid only for patients over the age of 14. These are "Adult" diagnoses. For "Adult" diagnoses the age range is 15 through 124.

   The diagnoses described in the Medicare Code Editor, posted on the CMS Webpage at: http://www.cms.hhs.gov/AcuteInpatientPPS/FFD/itemdetail.asp?filterType=none&filterByDID=-99&sortByDID=2&sortOrder=ascending&itemID=CMS1206058&intNumPerPage=10 are acceptable only for the age categories shown. If the FI edits online, it will return such bills for a proper diagnosis or correction of age as applicable. If the FI edits in batch operations after receipt of the admission query response, it uses the age based on CMS records and returns bills that fail this edit. The hospital must review the medical record and/or face sheet and enter the proper diagnosis or patient's age before returning the bill.
6. Sex Conflict
   The MCE detects inconsistencies between a patient's sex and a diagnosis or procedure on the patient's record. Examples are:

   - Male patient with cervical cancer (diagnosis).
   - Male patient with a hysterectomy (procedure).

   In both instances, the indicated diagnosis or the procedure conflicts with the stated sex of the patient. Therefore, either the patient's diagnosis, procedure or sex is incorrect.

   The Medicare Code Editor contains listings of male and female related ICD-9-CM diagnosis and procedure codes and the corresponding English descriptions. The hospital should review the medical record and/or face sheet and enter the proper sex, diagnosis, and procedure before returning the bill.
7. Manifestation Code As Principal Diagnosis
   A manifestation code describes the manifestation of an underlying disease, not the disease itself, and therefore, cannot be a principal diagnosis. The Medicare Code Editor contains listings of ICD-9-CM diagnoses identified as manifestation codes. The hospital should review the medical record and/or face sheet and enter the proper diagnosis before returning the bill.
8. Nonspecific Principal Diagnosis
   Effective October 1, 2007 (FY 2008), the non-specific principal diagnosis edit was discontinued and will appear for claims processed using MCE version 2.0-23.0 only.
9. Questionable Admission
   There are some diagnoses which are not usually sufficient justification for admission to an acute care hospital. For example, if a patient is given a principal diagnosis of:

   4011 - Benign Hypertension

   then this patient would have a questionable admission, since benign hypertension is not normally sufficient justification for admission.

   The Medicare Code Editor contains a listing of ICD-9-CM diagnosis codes identified as "Questionable Admission" when used as principal diagnosis.

   The A/B MACs or the FIs may review on a post-payment basis all questionable admission cases. Where the A/B MACs or the FIs determines the denial rate is sufficiently high to warrant, it may review the claim before payment.
10. Unacceptable Principal Diagnosis
    There are selected codes that describe a circumstance which influences an individual's health status but is not a current illness or injury; therefore, they are unacceptable as a principal diagnosis. For example, VI73 (Family History of Ischemic Heart Disease) is an unacceptable principal diagnosis.

    In a few cases, there are codes that are acceptable if a secondary diagnosis is coded. If no secondary diagnosis is present for them, MCE returns the message "requires secondary dx." The A/B MAC or the FI may review claims with diagnosis V571, V5721, V5722, V573, V5789, and V579 and a secondary diagnosis. A/B MACs or FIs may choose to review as a principal diagnosis if data analysis deems it a priority.

    If these codes are identified without a secondary diagnosis, the FI returns the bill to the hospital and requests a secondary diagnosis that describes the origin of the impairment. Also, bills containing other "unacceptable principal diagnosis" codes are returned.

    The hospital reviews the medical record and/or face sheet and enters the principal diagnosis that describes the illness or injury before returning the bill.
11. Nonspecific O.R. Procedures
    Effective October 1, 2007 (FY 2008), the non-specific O.R. procedure edit was discontinued and will appear for claims processed using MCE version 2.0-23.0 only.
12. Noncovered O.R. Procedures
    There are some O.R. procedures for which Medicare does not provide payment. The FI will return the bill requesting either:

    - A no pay bill, or
    - A correction in the procedure code.
    - A bill indicating the covered and noncovered procedures.

    If the hospital indicates that there are covered and noncovered procedures, the FI refers the bill to the QIO for prepayment review. Upon receipt of the QIOs response, it either deletes the noncovered procedures and charges or requires the hospital to delete them. It does not process the noncovered procedures through Grouper or the noncovered charges through Pricer.
13. Open Biopsy Check
    Biopsies can be performed as open (i.e., a body cavity is entered surgically), percutaneously, or endoscopically. The DRG Grouper logic assign a patient to different DRGs depending upon whether or not the biopsy was open. In general, for most organ systems, open biopsies are performed infrequently.

    Effective October 1, 1987, there are revised biopsy codes that distinguish between open and closed biopsies. To make sure that hospitals are using ICD-9-CM codes correctly, the FI requests O.R. reports on a sample of 10 percent of claims with open biopsy procedures for review on a post payment basis.

If the O.R. report reveals that the biopsy was closed (performed percutaneously, endoscopically, etc.) the FI changes the procedure code on the bill to the closed biopsy code and processes an adjustment bill. Some biopsy codes (3328 and 5634) have two related closed biopsy codes, one for closed endoscopic and for closed percutaneous biopsies. The FI assigns the appropriate closed biopsy code after reviewing the medical information.

14. Medicare as Secondary Payer - MSP Alert
The MCE identifies situations that may involve automobile medical, no-fault or liability insurance. The hospital must develop other insurance coverage as provided in the Medicare Secondary Payer Manuals, before billing Medicare.

15. Bilateral Procedure
There are codes that do not accurately reflect performed procedures in one admission on two or more different bilateral joints of the lower extremities. A combination of these codes show a bilateral procedure when, in fact, they could be single joint procedures (i.e., duplicate procedures).

If two more of these procedures are coded, and the principal diagnosis is in MDC 8, the claim is flagged for post-pay development. The FI processes the bill as coded but requests an O.R. report. If the report substantiates bilateral surgery, no further action is necessary. If the O.R. report does not substantiate bilateral surgery, an adjustment bill is processed.

If the error rate for any provider is sufficiently high, the FI may develop claims prior to payment on a provider-specific basis.

16. Invalid Age
If the hospital reports an age over I24, the FI requests the hospital to determine if it made a bill preparation error. If the beneficiary's age is established at over I24, the hospital enters 123.

17. Invalid Sex
A patient's sex is sometimes necessary for appropriate DRG determination. Usually the FI can resolve the issue without hospital assistance. The sex code reported must be either 1 (male) or 2 (female).

18. Invalid Discharge Status
A patient's discharge status is sometimes necessary for appropriate DRG determination. Discharge status must be coded according to the Form CMS-1450 conventions. See Chapter 25.

19. Invalid Discharge Date
An invalid discharge date is a discharge date that does not fall into the acceptable range of numbers to represent, either the month, day or year (e.g., 13/03/01, 12/32/01). If no discharge date is entered, it is also invalid. MCE reports when an invalid discharge date is entered.

20. Limited Coverage
Effective October 1, 2003, for certain procedures whose medical complexity and serious nature incur extraordinary associated costs, Medicare limits coverage. The edit message indicates the type of limited coverage (e.g., LVRS, heart transplant, etc). The procedures receiving limited coverage edits previously were listed as non-covered procedures, but were covered under Medicare in certain circumstances. The FIs will handle these procedures as they had previously.

100-4, 3, 20.7.3

Payment for Blood Clotting Factor Administered to Hemophilia Patients

Section 6011 of Public Law (P.L.) 101-239 amended Sec.1886(a)(4) of the Social Security Act (the Act) to provide that prospective payment system (PPS) hospitals receive anadditional payment for the costs of administering blood clotting factor to Medicare hemophiliacs who are hospital inpatients. Section 6011(b) of P.L. 101.239 specified that the payment be based on a predetermined price per unit of clotting factor multiplied by the number of units provided. This add-on payment originally was effective for blood clotting factors furnished on or after June 19, 1990, and before December 19, 1991. Section 13505 of P. L. 103-66 amended Sec.6011 (d) of P.L. 101-239 to extend the period covered by the add-on payment for blood clotting factors administered to Medicare inpatients with hemophilia through September 30, 1994. Section 4452 of P.L. 105-33 amended Sec.6011(d) of P.L. 101-239 to reinstate the add-on payment for the costs of administering blood clotting factor to Medicare beneficiaries who have hemophilia and who are hospital inpatients for discharges occurring on or after October 1, 1998.

Local carriers shall process non-institutional blood clotting factor claims.

The FIs shall process institutional blood clotting factor claims payable under either Part A or Part B.

A. Inpatient Bills
Under the Inpatient Prospective Payment System (PPS), hospitals receive a special add-on payment for the costs of furnishing blood clotting factors to Medicare beneficiaries with hemophilia, admitted as inpatients of PPS hospitals. The clotting factor add-on payment is calculated using the number of units (as defined in the HCPCS code long descriptor) billed by the provider under special instructions for units of service.

The PPS Pricer software does not calculate the payment amount. The Fiscal Intermediary Standard System (FISS) calculates the payment amount and subtracts the charges from those submitted to Pricer so that the clotting factor charges are not included in cost outlier computations.

Blood clotting factors not paid on a cost or PPS basis are priced as a drug/biological under the Medicare Part B Drug Pricing File effective for the specific date of service. As of January 1, 2005, the average sales price (ASP) plus 6 percent shall be used.

If a beneficiary is in a covered Part A stay in a PPS hospital, the clotting factors are paid in addition to the DRG/HIPPS payment (For FY 2004, this payment is based on 95 percent of average wholesale price.) For a SNF subject to SNF/PPS, the payment is bundled into the SNF/PPS rate.

For SNF inpatient Part A, there is no add-on payment for blood clotting factors.

The codes for blood-clotting factors are found on the Medicare Part B Drug Pricing File. This file is distributed on a quarterly basis.

For discharges occurring on or after October 1, 2000, and before December 31, 2005, report HCPCS Q0187 based on 1 billing unit per 1.2 mg. Effective January 1, 2006, HCPCS code J7189 replaces Q0187 and is defined as 1 billing unit per 1 microgram (mcg).

The examples below include the HCPCS code and indicate the dosage amount specified in the descriptor of that code. Facilities use the units field as a multiplier to arrive at the dosage amount.

EXAMPLE 1

HCPCS	**Drug**	**Dosage**
J7189	Factor VIIa	1 mcg

Actual dosage: 13,365 mcg

On the bill, the facility shows J7189 and 13,365 in the units field (13,365 mcg divided by 1 mcg = 13,365 units).

NOTE: The process for dealing with one international unit (IU) is the same as the process of dealing with one microgram.

EXAMPLE 2

HCPCS	**Drug**	**Dosage**
J9355	Trastuzumab	10 mg

Actual dosage: 140 mg

On the bill, the facility shows J9355 and 14 in the units field (140 mg divided by 10mg = 14 units).

When the dosage amount is greater than the amount indicated for the HCPCS code, the facility rounds up to determine units. When the dosage amount is less than the amount indicated for the HCPCS code, use 1 as the unit of measure.

EXAMPLE 3

HCPCS	Drug	Dosage
J3100	Tenecteplase	50 mg

Actual Dosage: 40 mg

The provider would bill for 1 unit, even though less than 1 full unit was furnished.

At times, the facility provides less than the amount provided in a single use vial and there is waste, i.e.; some drugs may be available only in packaged amounts that exceed the needs of an individual patient. Once the drug is reconstituted in the hospital's pharmacy, it may have a limited shelf life. Since an individual patient may receive less than the fully reconstituted amount, we encourage hospitals to schedule patients in such a way that the hospital can use the drug most efficiently. However, if the hospital must discard the remainder of a vial after administering part of it to a Medicare patient, the provider may bill for the amount of drug discarded plus the amount administered.

Example 1:

Drug X is available only in a 100-unit size. A hospital schedules three Medicare patients to receive drug X on the same day within the designated shelf life of the product. An appropriate hospital staff member administers 30 units to each patient. The remaining 10 units are billed to Medicare on the account of the last patient. Therefore, 30 units are billed on behalf of the first patient seen and 30 units are billed on behalf of the second patient seen. Forty units are billed on behalf of the last patient seen because the hospital had to discard 10 units at that point.

Example 2:

An appropriate hospital staff member must administer 30 units of drug X to a Medicare patient, and it is not practical to schedule another patient who requires the same drug. For example, the hospital has only one patient who requires drug X, or the hospital sees the patient for the first time and did not know the patient's condition. The hospital bills for 100 units on behalf of the patient, and Medicare pays for 100 units.

When the number of units of blood clotting factor administered to hemophiliac inpatients exceeds 99,999, the hospital reports the excess as a second line for revenue code 0636 and repeats the HCPCS code. One hundred thousand fifty (100,050) units are reported on one line as 99,999, and another line shows 1,051.

Revenue Code 0636 is used. It requires HCPCS. Some other inpatient drugs continue to be billed without HCPCS codes under pharmacy.

No changes in beneficiary notices are required. Coverage is applicable to hospital Part A claims only. Coverage is also applicable to inpatient Part B services in SNFs and all types of hospitals, including CAHs. Separate payment is not made to SNFs for beneficiaries in an inpatient Part A stay.

B. FI Action

The FI is responsible for the following:

- It accepts HCPCS codes for inpatient services;

- It edits to require HCPCS codes with Revenue Code 0636. Multiple iterations of the revenue code are possible with the same or different HCPCS codes. It does not edit units except to ensure a numeric value;
- It reduces charges forwarded to Pricer by the charges for hemophilia clotting factors in revenue code 0636. It retains the charges and revenue and HCPCS codes for CWF; and
- It modifies data entry screens to accept HCPCS codes for hospital (including CAH) swing bed, and SNF inpatient claims (bill types 11X, 12X, 18x, 21x and, 22x).

The September 1, 1993, IPPS final rule (58 FR 46304) states that payment will be made for the blood clotting factor only if an ICD-9-CM diagnosis code for hemophilia is included on the bill.

Since inpatient blood-clotting factors are covered only for beneficiaries with hemophilia, the FI must ensure that one of the following hemophilia diagnosis codes is listed on the bill before payment is made:

286.0 Congenital factor VIII disorder

286.1 Congenital factor IX disorder

286.2 Congenital factor IX disorder

286.3 Congenital deficiency of other clotting factor

286.4 von Willebrands' disease

Effective for discharges on or after August 1, 2001, payment may also be made if one of the following diagnosis codes is reported:

286.5 Hemorrhagic disorder due to circulating anticoagulants

286.7 Acquired coagulation factor deficiency

C. Part A Remittance Advice

1. X12.835 Ver. 003030M
   For remittance reporting PIP and/or non-PIP payments, the Hemophilia Add on will be reported in a claims level 2-090-CAS segment (CAS is the element identifier) exhibiting an "OA" Group Code and adjustment reason code "97" (payment is included in the allowance for the basic service/ procedure) followed by the associated dollar amount (POSITIVE) and units of service. For this version of the 835, "OA" group coded line level CAS segments are informational and are not included in the balancing routine. The Hemophilia Add On amount will always be included in the 2-010-CLP04 Claim Payment Amount.

   For remittance reporting PIP payments, the Hemophilia Add On will also be reported in the provider level adjustment (element identifier PLB) segment with the provider level adjustment reason code "CA" (Manual claims adjustment) followed by the associated dollar amount (NEGATIVE).

   NOTE: A data maintenance request will be submitted to ANSI ASC X12 for a new PLB adjustment reason code specifically for PIP payment Hemophilia Add On situations for future use. However, continue to use adjustment reason code "CA" until further notice.

   The FIs enter MA103 (Hemophilia Add On) in an open MIA (element identifier) remark code data element. This will alert the provider that the reason code 97 and PLB code "CA" adjustments are related to the Hemophilia Add On.
2. X12.835 Ver. 003051
   For remittances reporting PIP and/or non-PIP payments, Hemophilia Add On information will be reported in the claim level 2-062-AMT and 2-064-QTY segments. The 2-062-AMT01 element will carry a "ZK" (Federal Medicare claim MANDATE - Category 1) qualifier code followed by the total claim level Hemophilia Add On amount (POSITIVE). The 2-064QTY01 element will carry a "FL" (Units) qualifier code followed by the number of units approved for the Hemophilia Add On for the claim. The Hemophilia Add On amount will always be included in the 2-010-CLP04 Claim Payment Amount.

   NOTE: A data maintenance request will be submitted to ANSI ASC X12 for a new AMT qualifier code specifically for the Hemophilia Add On for future use. However, continue to use adjustment reason code "ZK" until further notice.

   For remittances reporting PIP payments, the Hemophilia Add On will be reported in the provider level adjustment PLB segment with the provider level adjustment reason "ZZ" followed by the associated dollar amount (NEGATIVE).

   NOTE: A data maintenance request will be submitted to ANSI ASC X12 for a new PLB, adjustment reason code specifically for the Hemophilia Add On for future use. However, continue to use PLB adjustment reason code "ZZ" until further notice. The FIs enter MA103 (Hemophilia Add On) in an open MIA remark code data element. This will alert the provider that the ZK, FL and ZZ entries are related to the Hemophilia Add On. (Effective with version 4010 of the 835, report ZK in lieu of FL in the QTY segment.)
3. Standard Hard Copy Remittance Advice
   For paper remittances reporting non-PIP payments involving Hemophilia Add On, add a "Hemophilia Add On" category to the end of the "Pass Thru Amounts" listings in the "Summary" section of the paper remittance. Enter the total of the Hemophilia Add On amounts due for the claims covered by this remittance next to the Hemophilia Add On heading.

   The FIs add the Remark Code "MA103" (Hemophilia Add On) to the remittance advice under the REM column for those claims that qualify for Hemophilia Add On payments.

   This will be the full extent of Hemophilia Add On reporting on paper remittance notices; providers wishing more detailed information must subscribe to the Medicare Part A specifications for the ANSI ASC X12N 835, where additional information is available.

   See chapter 22, for detailed instructions and definitions.

100-4, 3, 40.2.2

Charges to Beneficiaries for Part A Services

The hospital submits a bill even where the patient is responsible for a deductible which covers the entire amount of the charges for non-PPS hospitals, or in PPS hospitals, where the DRG payment amount will be less than the deductible.

A hospital receiving payment for a covered hospital stay (or PPS hospital that includes at least one covered day, or one treated as covered under guarantee of payment or limitation on liability) may charge the beneficiary, or other person, for items and services furnished during the stay only as described in subsections A through H. If limitation of liability applies, a beneficiary's liability for payment is governed by the limitation on liability notification rules in Chapter 30 of this manual. For related notices for inpatient hospitals, see CMS Transmittal 594, Change Request3903, dated June 24, 2005.

A. Deductible and Coinsurance
The hospital may charge the beneficiary or other person for applicable deductible and coinsurance amounts. The deductible is satisfied only by charges for covered services. The FI deducts the deductible and coinsurance first from the PPS payment. Where the deductible exceeds the PPS amount, the excess will be applied to a subsequent payment to the hospital. (See Chapter 3 of the Medicare General Information, Eligibility, and Entitlement Manual for specific policies.)

B. Blood Deductible
The Part A blood deductible provision applies to whole blood and red blood cells, and reporting of the number of pints is applicable to both PPS and non-PPS hospitals. (See Chapter 3 of the Medicare General Information, Eligibility, and Entitlement Manual for specific policies.) Hospitals shall report charges for red blood cells using revenue code 381, and charges for whole blood using revenue code 382.

C. Inpatient Care No Longer Required
The hospital may charge for services that are not reasonable and necessary or that constitute custodial care. Notification may be required under limitation of liability. See CMS Transmittal 594, Change Request3903, dated June 24, 2005, section V. of the attachment, for specific notification requirements. Note this transmittal will be placed in Chapter 30 of this manual at a future point. Chapter 1, section 150 of this manual also contains related billing information in addition to that provided below.

In general, after proper notification has occurred, and assuming an expedited decision is received from a Quality Improvement Organization (QIO), the following entries are required on the bill the hospital prepares:

- Occurrence code 3l (and date) to indicate the date the hospital notified the patient in accordance with the first bullet above;
- Occurrence span code 76 (and dates) to indicate the period of noncovered care for which it is charging the beneficiary;
- Occurrence span code 77 (and dates) to indicate the period of noncovered care for which the provider is liable, when it is aware of this prior to billing; and
- Value code 3l (and amount) to indicate the amount of charges it may bill the beneficiary for days for which inpatient care was no longer required. They are included as noncovered charges on the bill.

D. Change in the Beneficiary's Condition
If the beneficiary remains in the hospital after receiving notice as described in subsection C, and the hospital, the physician who concurred in the hospital's determination, or the QIO, subsequently determines that the beneficiary again requires inpatient hospital care, the hospital may not charge the beneficiary or other person for services furnished after the beneficiary again required inpatient hospital care until proper notification occurs (see subsection C).

If a patient who needs only a SNF level of care remains in the hospital after the SNF bed becomes available, and the bed ceases to be available, the hospital may continue to charge the beneficiary. It need not provide the beneficiary with another notice when the patient chose not to be discharged to the SNF bed.

E. Admission Denied
If the entire hospital admission is determined to be not reasonable or necessary, limitation of liability may apply. See 2005 CMS transmittal 594, section V. of the attachment, for specific notification requirements.

NOTE: This transmittal will be placed in Chapter 30 of this manual at a future point.

In such cases the following entries are required on the bill:

- Occurrence code 3l (and date) to indicate the date the hospital notified the beneficiary.
- Occurrence span code 76 (and dates) to indicate the period of noncovered care for which the hospital is charging the beneficiary.
- Occurrence span code 77 (and dates) to indicate any period of noncovered care for which the provider is liable (e.g., the period between issuing the notice and the time it may charge the beneficiary) when the provider is aware of this prior to billing.
- Value code 3l (and amount) to indicate the amount of charges the hospital may bill the beneficiary for hospitalization that was not necessary or reasonable. They are included as noncovered charges on the bill.

F. Procedures, Studies and Courses of Treatment That Are Not Reasonable or Necessary
If diagnostic procedures, studies, therapeutic studies and courses of treatment are excluded from coverage as not reasonable and necessary (even though the beneficiary requires inpatient hospital care) the hospital may charge the beneficiary or other person for the services or care according the procedures given in CMS Transmittal 594, Change Request3903, dated June 24, 2005.

The following bill entries apply to these circumstances:

- Occurrence code 32 (and date) to indicate the date the hospital provided the notice to the beneficiary.
- Value code 3I (and amount) to indicate the amount of such charges to be billed to the beneficiary. They are included as noncovered charges on the bill.

G. Nonentitlement Days and Days after Benefits Exhausted
If a hospital stay exceeds the day outlier threshold, the hospital may charge for some, or all, of the days on which the patient is not entitled to Medicare Part A, or after the Part A benefits are exhausted (i.e., the hospital may charge its customary charges for services furnished on those days). It may charge the beneficiary for the lesser of:

- The number of days on which the patient was not entitled to benefits or after the benefits were exhausted; or
- The number of outlier days. (Day outliers were discontinued at the end of FY 1997.)

If the number of outlier days exceeds the number of days on which the patient was not entitled to benefits, or after benefits were exhausted, the hospital may charge for all days on which the patient was not entitled to benefits or after benefits were exhausted. If the number of days on which the beneficiary was not entitled to benefits, or after benefits were exhausted, exceeds the number of outlier days, the hospital determines the days for which it may charge by starting with the last day of the stay (i.e., the day before the day of discharge) and identifying and counting off in reverse order, days on which the patient was not entitled to benefits or after the benefits were exhausted, until the number of days counted off equals the number of outlier days. The days counted off are the days for which the hospital may charge.

H. Contractual Exclusions
In addition to receiving the basic prospective payment, the hospital may charge the beneficiary for any services that are excluded from coverage for reasons other than, or in addition to, absence of medical necessity, provision of custodial care, non-entitlement to Part A, or exhaustion of benefits. For example, it may charge for most cosmetic and dental surgery.

I. Private Room Care
Payment for medically necessary private room care is included in the prospective payment. Where the beneficiary requests private room accommodations, the hospital must inform the beneficiary of the additional charge. (See the Medicare Benefit Policy Manual, Chapter 1.) When the beneficiary accepts the liability, the hospital will supply the service, and bill the beneficiary directly. If the beneficiary believes the private room was medically necessary, the beneficiary has a right to a determination and may initiate a Part A appeal.

J. Deluxe Item or Service
Where a beneficiary requests a deluxe item or service, i.e., an item or service which is more expensive than is medically required for the beneficiary's condition, the hospital may collect the additional charge if it informs the beneficiary of the additional charge. That charge is the difference between the customary charge for the item or service most commonly furnished by the hospital to private pay patients with the beneficiary's condition, and the charge for the more expensive item or service requested. If the beneficiary believes that the more expensive item or service was medically necessary, the beneficiary has a right to a determination and may initiate a Part A appeal.

K. Inpatient Acute Care Hospital Admission Followed By a Death or Discharge Prior To Room Assignment
A patient of an acute care hospital is considered an inpatient upon issuance of written doctor's orders to that effect. If a patient either dies or is discharged prior to being assigned and/or occupying a room, a hospital may enter an appropriate room and board charge on the claim. If a patient leaves of their own volition prior to being assigned and/or occupying a room, a hospital may enter an appropriate room and board charge on the claim as well as a patient status code 07 which indicates they left against medical advice. A hospital is not required to enter a room and board charge, but failure to do so may have a minimal impact on future DRG weight calculations.

100-4, 3, 40.3

Outpatient Services Treated as Inpatient Services

A3-3610.3, HO-415.6, HO-400D, A-03-008, A-03-013, A-03-054

A Outpatient Services Followed by Admission Before Midnight of the Following Day
(Effective For Services Furnished Before October 1, 1991)

When a beneficiary receives outpatient hospital services during the day immediately preceding the hospital admission, the outpatient hospital services are treated as inpatient services if the beneficiary has Part A coverage. Hospitals and FIs apply this provision only when the beneficiary is admitted to the hospital before midnight of the day following receipt of outpatient services. The day on which the patient is formally admitted as an inpatient is counted as the first inpatient day.

When this provision applies, services are included in the applicable PPS payment and not billed separately. When this provision applies to hospitals and units excluded from the hospital PPS, services are shown on the bill and included in the Part A payment. See Chapter 1 for FI requirements for detecting duplicate claims in such cases.

B Preadmission Diagnostic Services
(Effective for Services Furnished On or After January 1, 1991)

Diagnostic services (including clinical diagnostic laboratory tests) provided to a beneficiary by the admitting hospital, or by an entity wholly owned or wholly operated by the admitting hospital (or by another entity under arrangements with the admitting hospital), within 3 days prior to and including the date of the beneficiary's admission are deemed to be inpatient services and included in the inpatient payment, unless there is no Part A coverage. For example, if a patient is admitted on a Wednesday, outpatient services provided by the hospital on Sunday, Monday, Tuesday, or Wednesday are included in the inpatient Part A payment.

This provision does not apply to ambulance services and maintenance renal dialysis services (see the Medicare Benefit Policy Manual, Chapters 10 and 11, respectively). Additionally, Part A services furnished by skilled nursing facilities, home health agencies, and hospices are excluded from the payment window provisions.

For services provided before October 31, 1994, this provision applies to both hospitals subject to the hospital inpatient prospective payment system (IPPS) as well as those hospitals and units excluded from IPPS.

For services provided on or after October 31, 1994, for hospitals and units excluded from IPPS, this provision applies only to services furnished within one day prior to and including the date of the beneficiary's admission. The hospitals and units that are excluded from IPPS are: psychiatric hospitals and units; inpatient rehabilitation facilities (IRF) and units; long-term care hospitals (LTCH); children's hospitals; and cancer hospitals.

Critical access hospitals (CAHs) are not subject to the 3-day (nor 1-day) DRG payment window.

An entity is considered to be "wholly owned or operated" by the hospital if the hospital is the sole owner or operator. A hospital need not exercise administrative control over a facility in order to operate it. A hospital is considered the sole operator of the facility if the hospital has exclusive responsibility for implementing facility policies (i.e., conducting or overseeing the facility's routine operations), regardless of whether it also has the authority to make the policies.

For this provision, diagnostic services are defined by the presence on the bill of the following revenue and/or CPT codes:

0254 -	Drugs incident to other diagnostic services
0255 -	Drugs incident to radiology
030X -	Laboratory
031X -	Laboratory pathological
032X -	Radiology diagnostic
0341, 0343 -	Nuclear medicine, diagnostic/Diagnostic Radiopharmaceuticals
035X -	CT scan
0371 -	Anesthesia incident to Radiology
0372 -	Anesthesia incident to other diagnostic services
040X -	Other imaging services
046X -	Pulmonary function
0471 -	Audiology diagnostic
0481, 0489-	Cardiology, Cardiac Catheter Lab/Other Cardiology with CPT codes 93501, 93503, 93505, 93508, 93510, 93526, 93541, 93542, 93543, 93544, 93556, 93561, or 93562 diagnostic
0482-	Cardiology, Stress Test
0483-	Cardiology, Echocardiology
053X -	Osteopathic services
061X -	MRT
062X -	Medical/surgical supplies, incident to radiology or other diagnostic services
073X -	EKG/ECG
074X -	EEG
0918-	Testing- Behavioral Health
092X -	Other diagnostic services

The CWF rejects services furnished January 1, 1991, or later when outpatient bills for diagnostic services with through dates or last date of service (occurrence span code 72) fall on the day of admission or any of the 3 days immediately prior to admission to an IPPS or IPPS-excluded hospital. This reject applies to the bill in process, regardless of whether the outpatient or inpatient bill is processed first. Hospitals must analyze the two bills and report appropriate corrections. For services on or after October 31, 1994, for hospitals and units excluded from IPPS, CWF will reject outpatient diagnostic bills that occur on the day of or one day before admission. For IPPS hospitals, CWF will continue to reject outpatient diagnostic bills for services that occur on the day of or any of the 3 days prior to admission. Effective for dates of service on or after July 1, 2008, CWF will reject diagnostic services when the line item date of service (LIDOS) falls on the day of admission or any of the 3 days immediately prior to an admission to an IPPS hospital or on the day of admission or one day prior to admission for hospitals excluded from IPPS.

Hospitals in Maryland that are under the jurisdiction of the Health Services Cost Review Commission are subject to the 3-day payment window.

C Other Preadmission Services
(Effective for Services Furnished On or After October 1, 1991)

Nondiagnostic outpatient services that are related to a patient's hospital admission and that are provided by the hospital, or by an entity wholly owned or wholly operated by the admitting hospital (or by another entity under arrangements with the admitting hospital), to the patient during the 3 days immediately preceding and including the date of the patient's admission are deemed to be inpatient services and are included in the inpatient payment. Effective March 13, 1998, we defined nondiagnostic preadmission services as being related to the admission only when there is an exact match (for all digits) between the ICD-9-CM principal diagnosis code assigned for both the preadmission services and the inpatient stay. Thus, whenever Part A covers an admission, the hospital may bill nondiagnostic preadmission services to Part B as outpatient services only if they are not related to the admission. The FI shall assume, in the absence of evidence to the contrary, that such bills are not admission related and, therefore, are not deemed to be inpatient (Part A) services. If there are both diagnostic and nondiagnostic preadmission services and the nondiagnostic services are unrelated to the admission, the hospital may separately bill the nondiagnostic preadmission services to Part B. This provision applies only when the patient has Part A coverage. This provision does not apply to ambulance services and maintenance renal dialysis. Additionally, Part A services furnished by skilled nursing facilities, home health agencies, and hospices are excluded from the payment window provisions.

For services provided before October 31, 1994, this provision applies to both hospitals subject to IPPS as well as those hospitals and units excluded from IPPS (see section B above).

For services provided on or after October 31, 1994, for hospitals and units excluded from IPPS, this provision applies only to services furnished within one day prior to and including the date of the beneficiary's admission.

Critical access hospitals (CAHs) are not subject to the 3-day (nor 1-day) DRG payment window.

Hospitals in Maryland that are under the jurisdiction of the Health Services Cost Review Commission are subject to the 3-day payment window.

Effective for dates of service on or after July 1, 2008, CWF will reject therapeutic services when the line item date of service (LIDOS) falls on the day of admission or any of the 3 days immediately prior to an admission to an IPPS hospital or on the day of admission or one day prior to admission for hospitals excluded from IPPS.

100-4, 3, 90.1

Kidney Transplant - General

A3-3612, HO-E414

A major treatment for patients with ESRD is kidney transplantation. This involves removing a kidney, usually from a living relative of the patient or from an unrelated person who has died, and surgically placing the kidney into the patient. After the beneficiary receives a kidney transplant, Medicare pays the transplant hospital for the transplant and appropriate standard acquisition charges. Special provisions apply to payment. For the list of approved Medicare certified transplant facilities, refer to the following Web site: http://www.cms.hhs.gov/CertificationandComplianc/20_Transplant.asp#TopOfPage

A transplant hospital may acquire cadaver kidneys by:

- Excising kidneys from cadavers in its own hospital; and
- Arrangements with a freestanding organ procurement organization (OPO) that provides cadaver kidneys to any transplant hospital or by a hospital based OPO.

A transplant hospital that is also a certified organ procurement organization may acquire cadaver kidneys by:

- Having its organ procurement team excise kidneys from cadavers in other hospitals;
- Arrangements with participating community hospitals, whether they excise kidneys on a regular or irregular basis; and
- Arrangements with an organ procurement organization that services the transplant hospital as a member of a network.

When the transplant hospital also excises the cadaver kidney, the cost of the procedure is included in its kidney acquisition costs and is considered in arriving at its standard cadaver kidney acquisition charge. When the transplant hospital excises a kidney to provide another hospital, it may use its standard cadaver kidney acquisition charge or its standard detailed departmental charges to bill that hospital.

When the excising hospital is not a transplant hospital, it bills its customary charges for services used in excising the cadaver kidney to the transplant hospital or organ procurement agency.

If the transplanting hospital's organ procurement team excises the cadaver kidney at another hospital, the cost of operating such a team is included in the transplanting hospital's kidney acquisition costs, along with the reasonable charges billed by the other hospital of its services.

100-4, 3, 90.1.1

The Standard Kidney Acquisition Charge

A3-3612.1, A3-3612.3, HO-E417, HO-406, HO-E408, HO-E410, HO-E412, HO-E416,HO-E418, HO-E420

There are two basic standard charges that must be developed by transplant hospitals fromcosts expected to be incurred in the acquisition of kidneys:

- The standard charge for acquiring a live donor kidney; and
- The standard charge for acquiring a cadaver kidney.

The standard charge is not a charge representing the acquisition cost of a specific kidney;rather, it is a charge that reflects the average cost associated with each type of kidney acquisition.When the transplant hospital bills the program for the transplant, it shows its standard kidney acquisition charge on a separate line on the billing form.Acquisition services are billed from the excising hospital to the transplant hospital. A billing form is not submitted from the excising hospital to the FI. The transplant hospital keeps an itemized statement that identifies the services furnished, the charges, the person receiving the service (donor/recipient), and whether this is a potential transplant donor orrecipient. These charges are reflected in the transplant hospital's kidney acquisition costcenter and are used in determining the hospital's standard charge for acquiring a live donor's kidney or a cadaver's kidney. The standard charge is not a charge representing theacquisition cost of a specific kidney. Rather, it is a charge that reflects the average costassociated with each type of kidney acquisition. Also, it is an all-inclusive charge for allservices required in acquisition of a kidney, i.e., tissue typing, post-operative evaluation.

A. Billing For Blood And Tissue Typing of the Transplant Recipient Whether or NotMedicare Entitlement Is Established

Tissue typing and pre-transplant evaluation can be reflected only through the kidney acquisition charge of the hospital where the transplant will take place. The transplant hospital includes in its kidney acquisition cost center the reasonable charges it pays to the independent laboratory or other hospital which typed the potential transplant recipient,either before or after his entitlement. It also includes reasonable charges paid for physician tissue typing services, applicable to live donors and recipients (during the preentitlement period and after entitlement, but prior to hospital admission for transplantation).

B. Billing for Blood and Tissue Typing and Other Pre-Transplant Evaluation of LiveDonors

The entitlement date of the beneficiary who will receive the transplant is not aconsideration in reimbursing for the services to donors, since no bill is submitted directly to Medicare. All charges for services to donors prior to admission into the hospital fo rexcision are "billed" indirectly to Medicare through the live donor acquisition charge oftransplanting hospitals.

C. Billing Donor And Recipient Pre-Transplant Services (Performed by Transplant Hospitals or Other Providers) to the Kidney Acquisition Cost Center

The transplant hospital prepares an itemized statement of the services rendered for submittal to its cost accounting department. Regular Medicare billing forms are not necessary for this purpose, since no bills are submitted to the FI at this point.The itemized statement should contain information that identifies the person receiving theservice (donor/recipient), the health care insurance number, the service rendered and the charge for the service, as well as a statement as to whether this is a potential transplantdonor or recipient. If it is a potential donor, the provider must identify the prospective recipient.

EXAMPLE:

Mary Jones
Health care insurance number
200 Adams St.
Anywhere, MS

Transplant donor evaluation services for recipient:

John Jones
Health care insurance number
200 Adams St.
Anywhere, MS

Services performed in a hospital other than the potential transplant hospital or by an independent laboratory are billed by that facility to the potential transplant hospital. This holds true regardless of where in the United States the service is performed. For example, if the donor services are performed in a Florida hospital and the transplant is to take place in a California hospital, the Florida hospital bills the California hospital (as described inabove). The Florida hospital is paid by the California hospital, which recoups the monies through the kidney acquisition cost center.

D. Billing for Cadaveric Donor Services

Normally, various tests are performed to determine the type and suitability of a cadaver kidney. Such tests may be performed by the excising hospital (which may also be a transplant hospital) or an independent laboratory. When the excising-only hospital performs the tests, it includes the related charges on its bill to the transplant hospital or tothe organ procurement agency.When the tests are performed by the transplant hospital, it uses the related costs in establishing the standard charge for acquiring the cadaver kidney. The transplant hospitalincludes the costs and charges in the appropriate departments for final cost settlementpurposes.When the tests are performed by an independent laboratory for the excising-only hospital or the transplant hospital, the laboratory bills the hospital that engages its services or the organ procurement agency. The excising-only hospital includes such charges in itscharges to the transplant hospital, which then includes the charges in developing its standard charge for acquiring the cadaver kidney. It is the transplant hospitals'responsibility to assure that the independent laboratory does not bill both hospitals.The cost of these services cannot be billed directly to the program, since such tests andother procedures performed on a cadaver are not identifiable to a specific patient.

E. Billing For Physicians' Services Prior to Transplantation

Physicians' services applicable to kidney excisions involving live donors and recipients (during the pre-entitlement period and after entitlement, but prior to entrance into the hospital for transplantation) as well as all physicians' services applicable to cadavers are considered Part A hospital services (kidney acquisition costs).

F. Billing for Physicians' Services After Transplantation

All physicians' services rendered to the living donor and all physicians' services renderedto the transplant recipient are billed to the Medicare program in the same manner as all Medicare Part B services are billed. All donor physicians' services must be billed to the account of the recipient (i.e., the recipient's Medicare number).

G. Billing For Physicians' Renal Transplantation Services

To ensure proper payment when submitting a Part B bill for the renal surgeon's services to the recipient, the appropriate HCPCS codes must be submitted, including HCPCS codes for concurrent surgery, as applicable.The bill must include all living donor physicians' services, e.g., Revenue Center code 081X.

100-4, 3, 90.1.2

Billing for Kidney Transplant and Acquisition Services

Applicable standard kidney acquisition charges are identified separately in FL 42 by revenue code 0811 (Living Donor Kidney Acquisition) or 0812 (Cadaver Donor Kidney Acquisition). Where interim bills are submitted, the standard acquisition charge appears on the billing form for the period during which the transplant took place. This charge is in addition to the hospital's charges for services rendered directly to the Medicare recipient.

The contractor deducts kidney acquisition charges for PPS hospitals for processing through Pricer. These costs, incurred by approved kidney transplant hospitals, are not included in the prospective payment DRG 302 (kidney transplant). They are paid on a reasonable cost basis. Interim payment is paid as a "pass through" item. (See the Provider Reimbursement Manual, Part 1, Sec.2802 B.8.) The contractor includes kidney acquisition charges under the appropriate revenue code in CWF.

Bill Review Procedures
The Medicare Code Editor (MCE) creates a Limited Coverage edit for procedure code 55.69 (kidney transplant). Where this procedure code is identified by MCE, the contractor checks the provider number to determine if the provider is an approved transplant center, and checks the effective approval date. The contractor shall also determine if the facility is certified for adults and/or pediatric transplants dependent upon the patient's age. If payment is appropriate (i.e., the center is approved and the service is on or after the approval date) it overrides the limited coverage edit.

100-4, 3, 90.2

Heart Transplants

A3-3613, HO-416

Cardiac transplantation is covered under Medicare when performed in a facility which is approved by Medicare as meeting institutional coverage criteria. On April 6, 1987, CMS Ruling 87-1, "Criteria for Medicare Coverage of Heart Transplants" was published in the "Federal Register." For Medicare coverage purposes, heart transplants are medically reasonable and necessary when performed in facilities that meet these criteria. If a hospital wishes to bill Medicare for heart transplants, it must submit an application and documentation, showing its ongoing compliance with each criterion.

If a contractor has any questions concerning the effective or approval dates of its hospitals, it should contact its RO.

For a complete list of approved transplant centers, visit:
http://www.cms.hhs.gov/CertificationandComplianc/20_Transplant.asp#TopOfPage

A. Effective Dates
The effective date of coverage for heart transplants performed at facilities applying after July 6, 1987, is the date the facility receives approval as a heart transplant facility. Coverage is effective for discharges October 17, 1986 for facilities that would have qualified and that applied by July 6, 1987. All transplant hospitals will be recertified under the final rule, Federal Register / Vol. 72, No. 61 / Friday, March 30, 2007, / Rules and Regulations.

The CMS informs each hospital of its effective date in an approval letter.

B. Drugs
Medicare Part B covers immunosuppressive drugs following a covered transplant in an approved facility.

C. Noncovered Transplants
Medicare will not cover transplants or re-transplants in facilities that have not been approved as meeting the facility criteria. If a beneficiary is admitted for and receives a heart transplant from a hospital that is not approved, physicians' services, and inpatient services associated with the transplantation procedure are not covered.

If a beneficiary received a heart transplant from a hospital while it was not an approved facility and later requires services as a result of the noncovered transplant, the services are covered when they are reasonable and necessary in all other respects.

D. Charges for Heart Acquisition Services
The excising hospital bills the OPO, who in turn bills the transplant (implant) hospital for applicable services. It should not submit a bill to its contractor. The transplant hospital must keep an itemized statement that identifies the services rendered, the charges, the person receiving the service (donor/recipient), and whether this person is a potential transplant donor or recipient. These charges are reflected in the transplant hospital's heart acquisition cost center and are used in determining its standard charge for acquiring a donor's heart. The standard charge is not a charge representing the acquisition cost of a specific heart; rather, it reflects the average cost associated with each type of heart acquisition. Also, it is an all inclusive charge for all services required in acquisition of a heart, i.e., tissue typing, post-operative evaluation, etc.

E. Bill Review Procedures
The contractor takes the following actions to process heart transplant bills. It may accomplish them manually or modify its MCE and Grouper interface programs to handle the processing.

1. Change in MCE Interface
   The MCE creates a Limited Coverage edit for procedure code 37.51 (heart transplant). Where this procedure code is identified by MCE, the contractor checks the provider number to determine if the provider is an approved transplant center, and checks the effective approval date. The contractor shall also determine if the facility is certified for adults and/or pediatric transplants dependent upon the patient's age. If payment is appropriate (i.e., the center is approved and the service is on or after the approval date) it overrides the limited coverage edit.
2. Handling Heart Transplant Billings From Nonapproved Hospitals
   Where a heart transplant and covered services are provided by a nonapproved hospital, the bill data processed through Grouper and Pricer must exclude transplant procedure codes and related charges.

100-4, 3, 90.2.1

Artificial Hearts and Related Devices

Effective for discharges before May 1, 2008, Medicare does not cover the use of artificial hearts, either as a permanent replacement for a human heart or as a temporary life-support system until a human heart becomes available for transplant (often referred to a "bridge to transplant").

Medicare does cover a Ventricular Assist Device (VAD). A VAD is used to assist a damaged or weakened heart in pumping blood. VADs are used as a bridge to a heart transplant, for support of blood circulation postcardiotomy or destination therapy. Refer to the NCD Manual, section 20.9 for coverage criteria.

The MCE creates a Limited Coverage edit for procedure code 37.66. This procedure code has limited coverage due to the stringent conditions that must be met by hospitals. Where this procedure code is identified by MCE, the FI shall determine if coverage criteria is met and override the MCE if appropriate.

Effective for discharges on or after May 1, 2008, the use of artificial hearts will be covered by Medicare under Coverage with Evidence Development when beneficiaries are enrolled in a clinical study that meets all of the criteria listed in Pub. 100-03, Medicare NCD Manual, section 20.9.

100-4, 3, 90.3

Stem Cell Transplantation

Stem cell transplantation is a process in which stem cells are harvested from either a patient's or donor's bone marrow or peripheral blood for intravenous infusion. Autologous stem cell transplants (AuSCT) must be used to effect hematopoietic reconstitution following severely myelotoxic doses of chemotherapy (HDCT) and/or radiotherapy used to treat various malignancies. Allogeneic stem cell transplant may also be used to restore function in recipients having an inherited or acquired deficiency or defect.

Bone marrow and peripheral blood stem cell transplantation is a process which includes mobilization, harvesting, and transplant of bone marrow or peripheral blood stem cells and the administration of high dose chemotherapy or radiotherapy prior to the actual transplant. When bone marrow or peripheral blood stem cell transplantation is covered, all necessary steps are included in coverage. When bone marrow or peripheral blood stem cell transplantation is non-covered, none of the steps are covered.

Allogeneic and autologous stem cell transplants are covered under Medicare for specific diagnoses. Effective October 1, 1990, these cases were assigned to MS-DRG 009, Bone Marrow Transplant.

The FI's Medicare Code Editor (MCE) will edit stem cell transplant procedure codes 4101, 4102, 4103, 4104, 4105, 4107, 4108, and 4109 against diagnosis codes to determine which cases meet specified coverage criteria. Cases with a diagnosis code for a covered condition will pass (as covered) the MCE noncovered procedure edit. When a stem cell transplant case is selected for review based on the random selection of beneficiaries, the QIO will review the case on a post-payment basis to assure proper coverage decisions.

Procedure code 41.00 (bone marrow transplant, not otherwise specified) will be classified as noncovered and the claim will be returned to the hospital for a more specific procedure code.

The A/B MACs or the FI may choose to review if data analysis deems it a priority.

100-4, 3, 90.3.1

Allogeneic Stem Cell Transplantation

A. General
Allogeneic stem cell transplantation (ICD-9-CM Procedure Codes 41.02, 41.03, 41.05, and 41.08, CPT-4 Code 38240) is a procedure in which a portion of a healthy donor's stem cells are obtained and prepared for intravenous infusion to restore normal hematopoietic function in recipients having an inherited or acquired hematopoietic deficiency or defect. See Pub. 100-03, National Coverage Determinations Manual, chapter 1, section 110.8.1, for more information.

Expenses incurred by a donor are a covered benefit to the recipient/beneficiary but, except for physician services, are not paid separately. Services to the donor include physician services, hospital care in connection with screening the stem cell, and ordinary follow-up care.

B. Covered Conditions

1. Effective for services performed on or after August 1, 1978:
   - For the treatment of leukemia, leukemia in remission (ICD-9-CM codes 204.00 through 208.91), or aplastic anemia (ICD-9-CM codes 284.0 through 284.9) when it is reasonable and necessary; and
2. Effective for services performed on or after June 3, 1985:
   - For the treatment of severe combined immunodeficiency disease (SCID) (ICD-9-CM code 279.2), and for the treatment of Wiskott-Aldrich syndrome (ICD-9-CM 279.12).

C. Non-Covered Conditions

3. Effective for services performed on or after May 24, 1996:
   - Allogeneic stem cell transplantation is not covered as treatment for multiple myeloma (ICD-9-CM codes 203.00 and 203.01).
4. Effective for services performed on or after August 4, 2010:

The Centers for Medicare & Medicaid Services (CMS) issued an NCD stating that it believes the evidence does not demonstrate that the use of allogeneic hematopoietic stem cell transplantation (HSCT) improves health outcomes in Medicare beneficiaries with Myelodysplastic Syndrome (MDS). Therefore, allogeneic HSCT for MDS is not reasonable and necessary under §1862(a)(1)(A) of the Social Security Act (the Act).

However, allogeneic HSCT for MDS is reasonable and necessary under §1862(a)(1)(E) of the Act and therefore covered by Medicare ONLY if provided pursuant to a Medicare-approved clinical study under Coverage with Evidence Development (CED). These services are covered in both the inpatient and outpatient hospital setting. Refer to Pub. 100-03, NCD Manual, chapter 1, section 110.8.1, for further information about this policy, and Pub. 100-04, MCP Manual, chapter 32, section 90.6, for information on CED.

NOTE: Coverage for conditions other than these specifically designated as covered or non-covered in the CP or NCD Manuals are left to local Medicare contractor discretion.

100-4, 3, 90.3.2

Billing for Stem Cell Transplantation

A. Billing for Allogeneic Stem Cell Transplants

1. Definition of Acquisition Charges for Allogeneic Stem Cell Transplants

   Acquisition charges for allogeneic stem cell transplants include, but are not limited to, charges for the costs of the following services:

   National Marrow Donor Program fees, if applicable, for stem cells from an unrelated donor;

   Tissue typing of donor and recipient;

   Donor evaluation;

   Physician pre-admission/pre-procedure donor evaluation services;

   Costs associated with harvesting procedure (e.g., general routine and special care services, procedure/operating room and other ancillary services, apheresis services, etc.);

   Post-operative/post-procedure evaluation of donor; and

   Preparation and processing of stem cells.

   Payment for these acquisition services is included in the MS-DRG payment for the allogeneic stem cell transplant when the transplant occurs in the inpatient setting, and in the OPPS APC payment for the allogeneic stem cell transplant when the transplant occurs in the outpatient setting. The Medicare contractor does not make separate payment for these acquisition services, because hospitals may bill and receive payment only for services provided to the Medicare beneficiary who is the recipient of the stem cell transplant and whose illness is being treated with the stem cell transplant. Unlike the acquisition costs of solid organs for transplant (e.g., hearts and kidneys), which are paid on a reasonable cost basis, acquisition costs for allogeneic stem cells are included in prospective payment.

   Acquisition charges for stem cell transplants apply only to allogeneic transplants, for which stem cells are obtained from a donor (other than the recipient himself or herself). Acquisition charges

   do not apply to autologous transplants (transplanted stem cells are obtained from the recipient himself or herself), because autologous transplants involve services provided to the beneficiary only (and not to a donor), for which the hospital may bill and receive payment (see Pub. 100-04, chapter 4, Sec.231.10 and paragraph B of this section for information regarding billing for autologous stem cell transplants).

2. Billing for Acquisition Services

   The hospital bills and shows acquisition charges for allogeneic stem cell transplants based on the status of the patient (i.e., inpatient or outpatient) when the transplant is furnished. See Pub. 100-04, chapter 4, Sec.231.11 for instructions regarding billing for acquisition services for allogeneic stem cell transplants that are performed in the outpatient setting.

   When the allogeneic stem cell transplant occurs in the inpatient setting, the hospital identifies stem cell acquisition charges for allogeneic bone marrow/stem cell transplants separately in FL 42 of Form CMS-1450 (or electronic equivalent) by using revenue code 0819 (Other Organ Acquisition). Revenue code 0819 charges should include all services required to acquire stem cells from a donor, as defined above.

   On the recipient's transplant bill, the hospital reports the acquisition charges, cost report days, and utilization days for the donor's hospital stay (if applicable) and/or charges for other encounters in which the stem cells were obtained from the donor. The donor is covered for medically necessary inpatient hospital days of care or outpatient care provided in connection with the allogeneic stem cell transplant under Part A. Expenses incurred for complications are paid only if they are directly and immediately attributable to the stem cell donation procedure. The hospital reports the acquisition charges on the billing form for the recipient, as described in the first paragraph of this section. It does not charge the donor's days of care against the recipient's utilization record. For cost reporting purposes, it includes the covered donor days and charges as Medicare days and charges.

   The transplant hospital keeps an itemized statement that identifies the services furnished, the charges, the person receiving the service (donor/recipient), and whether this is a potential transplant donor or recipient. These charges will be reflected in the transplant hospital's stem cell/bone marrow acquisition cost center. For allogeneic stem cell acquisition services in cases that do not result in transplant, due to death of the intended recipient or other causes, hospitals include the costs associated with the acquisition services on the Medicare cost report.

   The hospital shows charges for the transplant itself in revenue center code 0362 or another appropriate cost center. Selection of the cost center is up to the hospital.

B. Billing for Autologous Stem Cell Transplants

The hospital bills and shows all charges for autologous stem cell harvesting, processing, and transplant procedures based on the status of the patient (i.e., inpatient or outpatient) when the services are furnished. It shows charges for the actual transplant, described by the appropriate

ICD-9-CM procedure or CPT codes, in revenue center code 0362 or another appropriate cost center.

The CPT codes describing autologous stem cell harvesting procedures may be billed and are separately payable under the OPPS when provided in the hospital outpatient setting of care. Autologous harvesting procedures are distinct from the acquisition services described in Pub. 100-04, chapter 4, Sec.231.11 and section A. above for allogeneic stem cell transplants, which include services provided when stem cells are obtained from a donor and not from the patient undergoing the stem cell transplant. The CPT codes describing autologous stem cell processing procedures also may be billed and are separately payable under the OPPS when provided to hospital outpatients.

Payment for autologous stem cell harvesting procedures performed in the hospital inpatient setting of care, with transplant also occurring in the inpatient setting of care, is included in the MS-DRG payment for the autologous stem cell transplant.

Billing for Stem Cell Transplantation

A. Billing for Allogeneic Stem Cell Transplants

1. Definition of Acquisition Charges for Allogeneic Stem Cell Transplants

   Acquisition charges for allogeneic stem cell transplants include, but are not limited to, charges for the costs of the following services:

   National Marrow Donor Program fees, if applicable, for stem cells from an unrelated donor;

   Tissue typing of donor and recipient;

   Donor evaluation;

   Physician pre-admission/pre-procedure donor evaluation services;

   Costs associated with harvesting procedure (e.g., general routine and special care services, procedure/operating room and other ancillary services, apheresis services, etc.);

   Post-operative/post-procedure evaluation of donor; and

   Preparation and processing of stem cells.

   Payment for these acquisition services is included in the MS-DRG payment for the allogeneic stem cell transplant when the transplant occurs in the inpatient setting, and in the OPPS APC payment for the allogeneic stem cell transplant when the transplant occurs in the outpatient setting. The Medicare contractor does not make separate payment for these acquisition services, because hospitals may bill and receive payment only for services provided to the Medicare beneficiary who is the recipient of the stem cell transplant and whose illness is being treated with the stem cell transplant. Unlike the acquisition costs of solid organs for transplant (e.g., hearts and kidneys), which are paid on a reasonable cost basis, acquisition costs for allogeneic stem cells are included in prospective payment.

   Acquisition charges for stem cell transplants apply only to allogeneic transplants, for which stem cells are obtained from a donor (other than the recipient himself or herself). Acquisition charges

   do not apply to autologous transplants (transplanted stem cells are obtained from the recipient himself or herself), because autologous transplants involve services provided to the beneficiary only (and not to a donor), for which the hospital may bill and receive payment (see Pub. 100-04, chapter 4, Sec.231.10 and paragraph B of this section for information regarding billing for autologous stem cell transplants).

2. Billing for Acquisition Services

   The hospital bills and shows acquisition charges for allogeneic stem cell transplants based on the status of the patient (i.e., inpatient or outpatient) when the transplant is furnished. See Pub. 100-04, chapter 4, Sec.231.11 for instructions regarding billing for acquisition services for allogeneic stem cell transplants that are performed in the outpatient setting.

   When the allogeneic stem cell transplant occurs in the inpatient setting, the hospital identifies stem cell acquisition charges for allogeneic bone marrow/stem cell transplants separately in FL 42 of Form CMS-1450 (or electronic equivalent) by using revenue code 0819 (Other Organ Acquisition). Revenue code 0819 charges should include all services required to acquire stem cells from a donor, as defined above.

   On the recipient's transplant bill, the hospital reports the acquisition charges, cost report days, and utilization days for the donor's hospital stay (if applicable) and/or charges for other encounters in which the stem cells were obtained from the donor. The donor is covered for medically necessary inpatient hospital days of care or outpatient care provided in connection with the allogeneic stem cell transplant under Part A. Expenses incurred for complications are paid only if they are directly and immediately attributable to the stem cell donation procedure. The hospital reports the acquisition charges on the billing form for the recipient, as described in the first paragraph of this section. It does not charge the donor's days of care against the recipient's utilization record. For cost reporting purposes, it includes the covered donor days and charges as Medicare days and charges.

   The transplant hospital keeps an itemized statement that identifies the services furnished, the charges, the person receiving the service (donor/recipient), and whether this is a potential transplant donor or recipient. These charges will be reflected in the transplant hospital's stem cell/bone marrow acquisition cost center. For allogeneic stem cell acquisition services in cases that do not result in transplant, due to death of the intended recipient or other causes, hospitals include the costs associated with the acquisition services on the Medicare cost report.

   The hospital shows charges for the transplant itself in revenue center code 0362 or another appropriate cost center. Selection of the cost center is up to the hospital.

B. Billing for Autologous Stem Cell Transplants

The hospital bills and shows all charges for autologous stem cell harvesting, processing, and transplant procedures based on the status of the patient (i.e., inpatient or outpatient) when the services are furnished. It shows charges for the actual transplant, described by the appropriate

ICD-9-CM procedure or CPT codes, in revenue center code 0362 or another appropriate cost center.

The CPT codes describing autologous stem cell harvesting procedures may be billed and are separately payable under the OPPS when provided in the hospital outpatient setting of care. Autologous harvesting procedures are distinct from the acquisition services described in Pub. 100-04, chapter 4, Sec.231.11 and section A. above for allogeneic stem cell transplants, which include services provided when stem cells are obtained from a donor and not from the patient undergoing the stem cell transplant. The CPT codes describing autologous stem cell processing procedures also may be billed and are separately payable under the OPPS when provided to hospital outpatients.

Payment for autologous stem cell harvesting procedures performed in the hospital inpatient setting of care, with transplant also occurring in the inpatient setting of care, is included in the MS-DRG payment for the autologous stem cell transplant.

100-4, 3, 90.4

Liver Transplants

A. Background
For Medicare coverage purposes, liver transplants are considered medically reasonable and necessary for specified conditions when performed in facilities that meet specific criteria.

To review the current list of approved Liver Transplant Centers, see http://www.cms.hhs.gov/CertificationandComplianc/20_Transplant.asp#TopOfPage

100-4, 3, 90.4.1

Standard Liver Acquisition Charge

A3-3615.1, A3-3615.3

Each transplant facility must develop a standard charge for acquiring a cadaver liver from costs it expects to incur in the acquisition of livers.

This standard charge is not a charge that represents the acquisition cost of a specific liver. Rather, it is a charge that reflects the average cost associated with a liver acquisition.

Services associated with liver acquisition are billed from the organ procurement organization or, in some cases, the excising hospital to the transplant hospital. The excising hospital does not submit a billing form to the FI. The transplant hospital keeps an itemized statement that identifies the services furnished, the charges, the person receiving the service (donor/recipient), and the potential transplant donor. These charges are reflected in the transplant hospital's liver acquisition cost center and are used in determining the hospital's standard charge for acquiring a cadaver's liver. The standard charge is not a charge representing the acquisition cost of a specific liver. Rather, it is a charge that reflects the average cost associated with liver acquisition. Also, it is an all inclusive charge for all services required in acquisition of a liver, e.g., tissue typing, transportation of organ, and surgeons' retrieval fees.

100-4, 3, 90.4.2

Billing for Liver Transplant and Acquisition Services

Form CMS-1450 or its electronic equivalent is completed in accordance with instructions in chapter 25 for the beneficiary who receives a covered liver transplant. Applicable standard liver acquisition charges are identified separately in FL 42 by revenue code 0817 (Donor-Liver). Where interim bills are submitted, the standard acquisition charge appears on the billing form for the period during which the transplant took place. This charge is in addition to the hospital's charge for services furnished directly to the Medicare recipient.

The contractor deducts liver acquisition charges for IPPS hospitals prior to processing through Pricer. Costs of liver acquisition incurred by approved liver transplant facilities are not included in prospective payment DRG 480 (Liver Transplant). They are paid on a reasonable cost basis. This item is a "pass-through" cost for which interim payments are made. (See the Provider Reimbursement Manual, Part 1, Sec.2802 B.8.) The contractor includes liver acquisition charges under revenue code 0817 in the HUIP record that it sends to CWF and the QIO.

A. Bill Review Procedures
The contractor takes the following actions to process liver transplant bills.

1. Operative Report
   The contractor requires the operative report with all claims for liver transplants, or sends a development request to the hospital for each liver transplant with a diagnosis code for a covered condition.

2. MCE Interface
   Code 50.51 (Auxiliary liver transplant) is always a non-covered procedure. However, the MCE contains a limited coverage edit for procedure code 50.59 (liver transplant). Where procedure code 50.59 is identified by the MCE, the contractor shall check the provider number and effective date to determine if the provider is an approved liver transplant facility at the time of the transplant, and the contractor shall also determine if the facility is certified for adults and/or pediatric transplants dependent upon the patient's age. If yes, the claim is suspended for review of the operative report to determine whether the beneficiary has at least one of the covered conditions when the diagnosis code is for a covered condition. If payment is appropriate (i.e., the facility is approved, the service is furnished on or after the approval date, and the beneficiary has a covered condition), the contractor sends the claim to Grouper and Pricer.

   If none of the diagnoses codes are for a covered condition, or if the provider is not an approved liver transplant facility, the contractor denies the claim.

   NOTE: Some non-covered conditions are included in the covered diagnostic codes. (The diagnostic codes are broader than the covered conditions. For example, primary biliary cirrhosis is a covered condition, secondary biliary cirrhosis is not a covered condition. Both primary and secondary biliary cirrhosis have the same diagnosis code ICD 9 571.6) Do not pay for noncovered conditions.

3. Grouper
   If the bill shows a discharge date before March 8, 1990, the liver transplant procedure is not covered. If the discharge date is March 8, 1990 or later, the contractor processes the bill through Grouper and Pricer. If the discharge date is after March 7, 1990, and before October 1, 1990, Grouper assigned CMS DRG 191 or 192. The contractor sent the bill to Pricer with review code 08. Pricer would then overlay CMS DRG 191 or 192 with CMS DRG 480 and the weights and thresholds for CMS DRG 480 to price the bill. If the discharge date is after September 30, 1990, Grouper assigns CMS DRG 480 and Pricer is able to price without using review code 08. If the discharge date is after September 30, 2007, Grouper assigns MS-DRG 005 or 006 (Liver transplant with MCC or Intestinal Transplant or Liver transplant without MCC, respectively) and Pricer is able to price without using review code 08.

4. Liver Transplant Billing From Non-approved Hospitals
   Where a liver transplant and covered services are provided by a non-approved hospital, the bill data processed through Grouper and Pricer must exclude transplant procedure codes and related charges.

   When CMS approves a hospital to furnish liver transplant services, it informs the hospital of the effective date in the approval letter. The contractor will receive a copy of the letter.

100-4, 3, 90.5

Pancreas Transplants Kidney Transplants

A. Background
Effective July 1, 1999, Medicare covered pancreas transplantation when performed simultaneously with or following a kidney transplant (ICD-9-CM procedure code 55.69). Pancreas transplantation is performed to induce an insulin independent, euglycemic state in diabetic patients. The procedure is generally limited to those patients with severe secondary complications of diabetes including kidney failure. However, pancreas transplantation is sometimes performed on patients with labile diabetes and hypoglycemic unawareness.

Medicare has had a policy of not covering pancreas transplantation. The Office of Health Technology Assessment performed an assessment on pancreas-kidney transplantation in 1994. They found reasonable graft survival outcomes for patients receiving either simultaneous pancreas-kidney (SPK) transplantation or pancreas after kidney (PAK) transplantation. For a list of facilities approved to perform SPK or PAK, refer to the following Web site: http://www.cms.hhs.gov/CertificationandComplianc/20_Transplant.asp#TopOfPage

B. Billing for Pancreas Transplants
There are no special provisions related to managed care participants. Managed care plans are required to provide all Medicare covered services. Medicare does not restrict which hospitals or physicians may perform pancreas transplantation.

The transplant procedure and revenue code 0360 for the operating room are paid under these codes. Procedures must be reported using the current ICD-9-CM procedure codes for pancreas and kidney transplants. Providers must place at least one of the following transplant procedure codes on the claim:

52.80 Transplant of pancreas

52.82 Homotransplant of pancreas

The Medicare Code Editor (MCE) has been updated to include 52.80 and 52.82 as limited coverage procedures. The contractor must determine if the facility is approved for the transplant and certified for either pediatric or adult transplants dependent upon the age of the patient.

Effective October 1, 2000, ICD-9-CM code 52.83 was moved in the MCE to non-covered. The contractor must override any deny edit on claims that came in with 52.82 prior to October 1, 2000 and adjust, as 52.82 is the correct code.

If the discharge date is July 1, 1999, or later: the contractor processes the bill through Grouper and Pricer.

Pancreas transplantation is reasonable and necessary for the following diagnosis codes. However, since this is not an all-inclusive list, the contractor is permitted to determine if any additional diagnosis codes will be covered for this procedure.

Diabetes Diagnosis Codes

250.00 Diabetes mellitus without mention of complication, type II (non-insulin dependent) (NIDDM) (adult onset) or unspecified type, not stated as uncontrolled.

250.01 Diabetes mellitus without mention of complication, type I (insulin dependent) (IDDM) (juvenile), not stated as uncontrolled.

250.02 Diabetes mellitus without mention of complication, type II (non-insulin dependent) (NIDDM) (adult onset) or unspecified type, uncontrolled.

250.03 Diabetes mellitus without mention of complication, type I (insulin dependent) (IDDM) (juvenile), uncontrolled.

250.1X Diabetes with ketoacidosis

250.2X Diabetes with hyperosmolarity

250.3X Diabetes with coma

250.4X Diabetes with renal manifestations

250.5X Diabetes with ophthalmic manifestations

250.6X Diabetes with neurological manifestations

250.7X Diabetes with peripheral circulatory disorders

250.8X Diabetes with other specified manifestations

250.9X Diabetes with unspecified complication

NOTE: X=0-3

Hypertensive Renal Diagnosis Codes:

403.01 Malignant hypertensive renal disease, with renal failure

403.11 Benign hypertensive renal disease, with renal failure

403.91 Unspecified hypertensive renal disease, with renal failure

404.02 Malignant hypertensive heart and renal disease, with renal failure

404.03 Malignant hypertensive heart and renal disease, with congestive heart failure or renal failure

404.12 Benign hypertensive heart and renal disease, with renal failure

404.13 Benign hypertensive heart and renal disease, with congestive heart failure or renal failure

404.92 Unspecified hypertensive heart and renal disease, with renal failure

404.93 Unspecified hypertensive heart and renal disease, with congestive heart failure or renal failure

585.1-585.6, 585.9Chronic Renal Failure Code

NOTE: If a patient had a kidney transplant that was successful, the patient no longer has chronic kidney failure, therefore it would be inappropriate for the provider to bill 585.1 - 585.6, 585.9 on such a patient. In these cases one of the following V-codes should be present on the claim or in the beneficiary's history.

The provider uses the following V-codes only when a kidney transplant was performed before the pancreas transplant:

V42.0 Organ or tissue replaced by transplant kidney

V43.89 Organ tissue replaced by other means, kidney or pancreas

NOTE: If a kidney and pancreas transplants are performed simultaneously, the claim should contain a diabetes diagnosis code and a renal failure code or one of the hypertensive renal failure diagnosis codes. The claim should also contain two transplant procedure codes. If the claim is for a pancreas transplant only, the claim should contain a diabetes diagnosis code and a V-code to indicate a previous kidney transplant. If the V-code is not on the claim for the pancreas transplant, the contractor will search the beneficiary's claim history for a V-code.

C. Drugs
If the pancreas transplant occurs after the kidney transplant, immunosuppressive therapy will begin with the date of discharge from the inpatient stay for the pancreas transplant.

D. Charges for Pancreas Acquisition Services
A separate organ acquisition cost center has been established for pancreas transplantation. The Medicare cost report will include a separate line to account for pancreas transplantation costs. The 42 CFR 412.2(e)(4) was changed to include pancreas in the list of organ acquisition costs that are paid on a reasonable cost basis.

Acquisition costs for pancreas transplantation as well as kidney transplants will occur in Revenue Center 081X. The contractor overrides any claims that suspend due to repetition of revenue code 081X on the same claim if the patient had a simultaneous kidney/pancreas transplant. It pays for acquisition costs for both kidney and pancreas organs if transplants are performed simultaneously. It will not pay for more than two organ acquisitions on the same claim.

E. Medicare Summary Notices (MSN) and Remittance Advice Messages
If the provider submits a claim for simultaneous pancreas kidney transplantation or pancreas transplantation following a kidney transplant, and omits one of the appropriate diagnosis/procedure codes, the contractor rejects the claim, using the following MSN:

- MSN 16.32, "Medicare does not pay separately for this service."
- Use the following Remittance Advice Message:
- Claim adjustment reason code B15, "Claim/service denied/reduced because this procedure or service is not paid separately."
- If a claim is denied because no evidence of a prior kidney transplant is presented, use the following MSN message:
- MSN 15.4, "The information provided does not support the need for this service or item."

The contractor uses the following Remittance Advice Message:

- Claim adjustment reason code 50, "These are non-covered services because this is not deemed a 'medical necessity' by the payer."

To further clarify the situation, the contractor should also use new claim level remark code MA 126, "Pancreas transplant not covered unless kidney transplant performed."

100-4, 3, 90.6

Intestinal and Multi-Visceral Transplants

A. Background
Effective for services on or after April 1, 2001, Medicare covers intestinal and multi-visceral transplantation for the purpose of restoring intestinal function in patients with irreversible intestinal failure. Intestinal failure is defined as the loss of absorptive capacity of the small bowel secondary to severe primary gastrointestinal disease or surgically induced short bowel syndrome. Intestinal failure prevents oral nutrition and may be associated with both mortality and profound morbidity. Multi-Visceral transplantation includes organs in the digestive system (stomach, duodenum, liver, and intestine). See Sec.260.5 of the National Coverage Determinations Manual for further information.

B. Approved Transplant Facilities
Medicare will cover intestinal transplantation if performed in an approved facility. The approved facilities are located at:
http://www.cms.hhs.gov/CertificationandComplianc/20_Transplant.asp#TopOfPage

C. Billing
ICD-9-CM procedure code 46.97 is effective for discharges on or after April 1, 2001. The Medicare Code Editor (MCE) lists this code as a limited coverage procedure. The contractor shall override the MCE when this procedure code is listed and the coverage criteria are met in an approved transplant facility, and also determine if the facility is certified for adults and/or pediatric transplants dependent upon the patient's age.

For this procedure where the provider is approved as transplant facility and certified for the adult and/or pediatric population, and the service is performed on or after the transplant approval date, the contractor must suspend the claim for clerical review of the operative report to determine whether the beneficiary has at least one of the covered conditions listed when the diagnosis code is for a covered condition.

This review is not part of the contractor's medical review workload. Instead, the contractor should complete this review as part of its claims processing workload.

Charges for ICD-9-CM procedure code 46.97 should be billed under revenue code 0360, Operating Room Services.

For discharge dates on or after October 1, 2001, acquisition charges are billed under revenue code 081X, Organ Acquisition. For discharge dates between April 1, 2001, and September 30, 2001, hospitals were to report the acquisition charges on the claim, but there was no interim pass-through payment made for these costs.

Bill the procedure used to obtain the donor's organ on the same claim, using appropriate ICD-9-CM procedure codes.

The 11X bill type should be used when billing for intestinal transplants.

Immunosuppressive therapy for intestinal transplantation is covered and should be billed consistent with other organ transplants under the current rules.

There is no specific ICD-9-CM diagnosis code for intestinal failure. Diagnosis codes exist to capture the causes of intestinal failure. Some examples of intestinal failure include, but are not limited to:

- Volvulus 560.2,
- Volvulus gastroschisis 756.79, other [congenital] anomalies of abdominal wall,
- Volvulus gastroschisis 569.89, other specified disorders of intestine,
- Necrotizing enterocolitis 777.5, necrotizing enterocolitis in fetus or newborn,
- Necrotizing enterocolitis 014.8, other tuberculosis of intestines, peritoneum, and mesenteric,
- Necrotizing enterocolitis and splanchnic vascular thrombosis 557.0, acute vascular insufficiency of intestine,
- Inflammatory bowel disease 569.9, unspecified disorder of intestine,
- Radiation enteritis 777.5, necrotizing enterocolitis in fetus or newborn, and
- Radiation enteritis 558.1.

D. Acquisition Costs
A separate organ acquisition cost center was established for acquisition costs incurred on or after October 1, 2001. The Medicare Cost Report will include a separate line to account for these transplantation costs. For intestinal and multi-visceral transplants performed between April 1, 2001, and October 1, 2001, the DRG payment was payment in full for all hospital services related to this procedure.

E. Medicare Summary Notices (MSN), Remittance Advice Messages, and Notice of Utilization Notices (NOU)
If an intestinal transplant is billed by an unapproved facility after April 1, 2001, the contractor shall deny the claim and use MSN message 21.6, "This item or service is not covered when performed, referred, or ordered by this provider;" 21.18, "This item or service is not covered when performed or ordered by this provider;" or, 16.2, "This service cannot be paid when provided in this location/facility;" and Remittance Advice Message, Claim Adjustment Reason Code 52, "The referring/prescribing/rendering provider is not eligible to refer/prescribe/order/perform the service billed."

100-4, 3, 100.1

Billing for Abortion Services

A3-3652

Effective October 1, 1998,abortions are not covered under the Medicare program except for instances where the pregnancy is a result of an act of rape or incest; or the woman suffers from a physical disorder, physical injury, or physical illness, including a life endangering physical condition caused by the pregnancy itself that would, as certified by a physician, place the woman in danger of death unless an abortion is performed.

A. "G" Modifier
The "G7" modifier is defined as "the pregnancy resulted from rape or incest, or pregnancy certified by physician as life threatening."

Beginning July 1, 1999, providers should bill for abortion services using the new Modifier G7. This modifier can be used on claims with dates of services October 1, 1998, and after. CWF will be able to recognize the modifier beginning July 1, 1999.

B. FI Billing Instructions

1. Hospital Inpatient Billing
   Hospitals will bill the FI on Form CMS-1450 using bill type 11X. Medicare will pay only when condition code A7 or A8 is used in FLs 24-30 of UB92 along with an appropriate ICD-9-CM principal diagnosis code that will group to DRG 380 or with an appropriate ICD-9-CM principal diagnosis code and one of the four appropriate ICD-9-CM operating room procedure codes listed below that will group to DRG 381.

69.01 69.02 69.51 74.91

Providers must use ICD-9-CM codes 69.01 and 69.02 to describe exactly the procedure or service performed.

The FI must manually review claims with the above ICD-9-CM procedure codes to verify that all of the above conditions are met.

2. Outpatient Billing
Hospitals will bill the FI on Form CMS-1450 using bill type 13X, 83X and 85X.

Medicare will pay only if one of the following CPT codes is used with the "G7" modifier.

59840 59851 59856

59841 59852 59857

59850 59855 59866

C. Common Working File (CWF) Edits
For hospital outpatient claims, CWF will bypass its edits for a managed care beneficiary who is having an abortion outside their plan and the claim is submitted with the "G7" modifier and one of the above CPT codes.

For hospital inpatient claims, CWF will bypass its edits for a managed care beneficiary who is having an abortion outside their plan and the claim is submitted with one of the above ICD-9-CM procedure codes.

D. Medicare Summary Notices (MSN)/Explanation of Your Medicare Benefits
Remittance Advice Message

If a claim is submitted with one of the above CPT procedure codes but no "G7" modifier, the claim is denied. The FI states on the MSN the following message:

This service was denied because Medicare covers this service only under certain circumstances." (MSN Message 21.21).

For the remittance advice the FI uses existing American National Standard Institute (ANSI) X12-835 claim adjustment reason code B5, "Claim/service denied/reduced because coverage guidelines were not met or were exceeded."

100-4, 3, 100.2

Payment for CRNA or AA Services

A3-3660.9

Anesthesia services furnished on or after January 1, 1990, at a qualified rural hospital by a hospital employed or contracted CRNA or AA can be paid on a reasonable cost basis. The FI determines the hospital's qualification using the following criteria.

The hospital must be located in a rural area (as defined for PPS purposes) to be considered. A rural hospital that qualified and was paid on a reasonable cost basis for CRNA or AA services during calendar year 1989 could continue to be paid on a reasonable cost basis for these services furnished during calendar year 1990 if it could establish before January 1, 1990, that it did not provide more than 500 surgical procedures, both inpatient and outpatient, requiring anesthesia services during 1989.

A rural hospital that was not paid on a reasonable cost basis for CRNA or AA services during calendar year 1989 could be paid on a reasonable cost basis for these services furnished during calendar year 1990 if it established before January 1, 1990, that:

As of January 1, 1988, it employed or contracted with a CRNA or AA (but not more than one full-time equivalent CRNA or AA); and

In both 1987 and 1989, it had a volume of 500 or fewer surgical procedures, including inpatient and outpatient procedures, requiring anesthesia services.

Each CRNA or AA employed by, or under contract with the hospital, must agree in writing not to bill on a fee schedule basis for services furnished at the hospital. A rural hospital can qualify and continue to be paid on a reasonable cost basis for qualified CRNA or AA services for a calendar year beyond 1990 if it could establish before January 1 of that year that it did not provide more than 500 surgical procedures, both inpatient and outpatient, requiring anesthesia services during the preceding year. For a calendar year beyond 1990, it must make its election after September 30, but before January 1. The FI determines the number of anesthetics by annualizing the number of surgical procedures for the 9-month period ending September 30.

A rural hospital that first elects reasonable cost payment for CRNA services for a calendar year after 1990 must demonstrate that:

It had a volume of 500 or fewer surgical procedures, including inpatient and outpatient, requiring anesthesia services in the preceding year; and

It meets the criteria that would have been met by a rural hospital first electing reasonable cost in calendar year 1990.

To prevent duplicate payments, the FI informs carriers of the names of CRNAs or AAs, the hospitals with which they have agreements, and the effective dates of the agreements. If the CRNA or AA bills Part B for anesthesia services furnished prior to the hospital's election of reasonable cost payments, the carrier must recover the overpayment from the CRNA or AA.

100-4, 3, 100.6

Inpatient Renal Services

HO-E400

Section 405.103I of Subpart J of Regulation 5 stipulates that only approved hospitals may bill for ESRD services. Hence, to allow hospitals to bill and be reimbursed for inpatient dialysis services furnished under arrangements, both facilities participating in the arrangement must meet the conditions of 405.2120 and 405.2160 of Subpart U of Regulation 5. In order for renal dialysis facilities to have a written arrangement with each other to provide inpatient dialysis care both facilities must meet the minimum utilization rate requirement, i.e., two dialysis stations with a performance capacity of at least four dialysis treatments per week.

Dialysis may be billed by an SNF as a service if: (a) it is provided by a hospital with which the facility has a transfer agreement in effect, and that hospital is approved to provide staff-assisted dialysis for the Medicare program; or (b) it is furnished directly by an SNF meeting all nonhospital maintenance dialysis facility requirements, including minimum utilization requirements. (See 1861(h)(6), 1861(h)(7), title XVIII.)

100-4, 3, 100.7

Lung Volume Reduction Surgery (LVRS) (also known as reduction pneumoplasty, lung shaving, or lung contouring) is an invasive surgical procedure to reduce the volume of a hyperinflated lung in order to allow the underlying compressed lung to expand, and thus, establish improved respiratory function.

Effective for discharges on or after January 1, 2004, Medicare will cover LVRS under certain conditions as described in 240 of Pub. 100-03, "National Coverage Determinations".

The Medicare Code Editor (MCE) creates a Limited Coverage edit for procedure code 32.22. This procedure code has limited coverage due to the stringent conditions that must be met by hospitals. Where this procedure code is identified by MCE, the FI shall determine if coverage criteria is met and override the MCE if appropriate.

The LVRS can only be performed in the facilities listed on the following Web site: www.cms.hhs.gov/coverage/lvrsfacility.pdf

Medicare previously only covered LVRS as part of the National Emphysema Treatment Trial (NETT). The study was limited to 18 hospitals, and patients were randomized into two arms, either medical management and LVRS or medical management. The study was conducted by The National Heart, Lung, and Blood Institute of the National Institutes of Health and coordinated by Johns Hopkins University (JHU). Hospital claims for patients in the NETT were identified by the presence of Condition Code EY. The JHU instructed hospitals of the correct billing procedures for billing claims under the NETT.

100-4,4,10.4

Packaging

Under the OPPS, packaged services are items and services that are considered to be an integral part of another service that is paid under the OPPS. No separate payment is made for packaged services, because the cost of these items and services is included in the APC payment for the service of which they are an integral part. For example, routine supplies, anesthesia, recovery room use, and most drugs are considered to be an integral part of a surgical procedure so payment for these items is packaged into the APC payment for the surgical procedure.

A. Packaging for Claims Resulting in APC Payments
If a claim contains services that result in an APC payment but also contains packaged services, separate payment for the packaged services is not made since payment is included in the APC. However, charges related to the packaged services are used for outlier and Transitional Corridor Payments (TOPs) as well as for future rate setting.

Therefore, it is extremely important that hospitals report all HCPCS codes and all charges for all services they furnish, whether payment for the services is made separately paid or is packaged.

B. Packaging for Claims Resulting in No APC Payments
If the claim contains only services payable under cost reimbursement, such as corneal tissue, and services that would be packaged services if an APC were payable, then the packaged services are not separately payable. In addition, these charges for the packaged services are not used to calculate TOPs.

If the claim contains only services payable under a fee schedule, such as clinical diagnostic laboratory tests, and also contains services that would be packaged services if an APC were payable, the packaged services are not separately payable. In addition, the charges are not used to calculate TOPs.

If a claim contains services payable under cost reimbursement, services payable under a fee schedule, and services that would be packaged services if an APC were payable, the packaged services are not separately payable. In addition, the charges are not used to calculate TOPs payments.

C. Packaging Types Under the OPPS

1. Unconditionally packaged services are services for which separate payment is never made because the payment for the service is always packaged into the payment for other services. Unconditionally packaged services are identified in the OPPS Addendum B with status indictor of N. See the OPPS Web site at http://www.cms.hhs.gov/HospitalOutpatientPPS/ for the most recent Addendum B (HCPCS codes with status indicators). In general, the charges for unconditionally packaged services are used to calculate outlier and TOPS payments when they appear on a claim with a service that is separately paid under the OPPS because the packaged service is considered to be part of the package of services for which payment is being made through the APC payment for the separately paid service.
2. STVX-packaged services are services for which separate payment is made only if there is no service with status indicator S, T, V or X reported with the same date of service on the same claim. If a claim includes a service that is assigned status indicator S, T, V, or X reported on the same date of service as the STVXpackaged service, the payment for the STVX-packaged service is packaged into the payment for the service(s) with status indicator S, T, V or X and no separate payment is made for the STVX-packaged service. STVX-packaged services are assigned status indicator Q. See the OPPS Webpage at http://www.cms.hhs.gov/HospitalOutpatientPPS/ for identification of STVXpackaged codes.

3. T-packaged services are services for which separate payment is made only if there is no service with status indicator T reported with the same date of service on the same claim. When there is a claim that includes a service that is assigned status indicator T reported on the same date of service as the T-packaged service, the payment for the T-packaged service is packaged into the payment for the service(s) with status indicator T and no separate payment is made for the T-packaged service. T-packaged services are assigned status indicator Q. See the OPPS Web site at http://www.cms.hhs.gov/HospitalOutpatientPPS/ for identification of T-packaged codes.
4. A service that is assigned to a composite APC is a major component of a single episode of care. The hospital receives one payment through a composite APC for multiple major separately identifiable services. Services mapped to composite APCs are assigned status indicator Q. See the discussion of composite APCs in section 10.2.1.

100-4, 4, 10.5

Discounting

- Fifty percent of the full OPPS amount is paid if a procedure for which anesthesia is planned is discontinued after the patient is prepared and taken to the room where the procedure is to be performed but before anesthesia is provided.
- Fifty percent of the full OPPS amount is paid if a procedure for which anesthesia is not planned is discontinued after the patient is prepared and taken to the room where the procedure is to be performed.
- Multiple surgical procedures furnished during the same operative session are discounted.
  - The full amount is paid for the surgical procedure with the highest weight;
  - Fifty percent is paid for any other surgical procedure(s) performed at the same time;
  - Similar discounting occurs now under the physician fee schedule and the payment system for ASCs;
- When multiple surgical procedures are performed during the same operative session, beneficiary coinsurance is discounted in proportion to the APC payment.

100-4, 4, 10.10

Biweekly Interim Payments for Certain Hospital Outpatient Items and Services Paid on a Cost Basis, and Direct Medical Education Payments, Not Included in the Hospital OPPS

A-01-32

For hospitals subject to the OPPS, payment for certain items that are not paid under the OPPS, but which are reimbursable in addition to OPPS, are made through biweekly interim payments subject to retrospective adjustment based on a settled cost report.

These payments include:

Direct medical education payments;

Costs of nursing and allied health programs;

Costs associated with interns and residents not in an approved teaching program as described in 42 CFR 415.202;

Teaching physicians costs attributable to Part B services for hospitals that elect cost-based reimbursement for teaching physicians under 42 CFR 415.160;

CRNA services;

For hospitals that meet the requirements under 42 CFR 412.113(c), the reasonable costs of anesthesia services furnished to hospital outpatients by qualified nonphysician anesthetists (i.e., certified registered nurse anesthetists and anesthesiologists' assistants) employed by the hospital or obtained under arrangements;

Bad debts for uncollectible deductibles and coinsurance;

Organ acquisition costs paid under Part B.

For hospitals that are paid under the OPPS, interim payments for these items attributable to both hospital outpatients, as well as inpatients whose services are paid under Part B of the Medicare program are made on a biweekly basis. The FI determines the amount of the biweekly payment by estimating a hospital's reimbursement amount for these items for the cost reporting period by using:

Medicare principles of cost reimbursement for cost-based items; and

Medicare rules for determining payment for graduate medical education for direct medical education, and dividing the total annual estimated amount for these items into 26 equal biweekly payments.

The estimated annual amount is based on the most current data available. Biweekly interim payments are reviewed and, if necessary, adjusted at least twice during the reporting period, with final settlement based on a submitted cost report. Because hospitals subject to the OPPS have not received payment for these items attributable to services furnished on or after August 1, 2000, the date the OPPS was implemented, the first payment to each hospital included all the payments due to the hospital retroactive to August 1, 2000. Thereafter, FIs continue to make payment on a biweekly basis. Each payment is made two weeks after the end of a biweekly period of services. The FI was required to make retroactive payments and begin making biweekly interim payments to all hospitals that are due these payments no later than 60 days after March 8, 2001.

These biweekly payments may be combined with the inpatient biweekly payments that the FI makes under Sec.2405.2 of the Medicare Provider Reimbursement Manual (CMS Pub.15-I). However, if a single payment is made, for purposes of final cost report settlement, they must maintain records to separately identify the amount of the hospital's combined payment that is paid out of the Part A or Part B trust fund.

100-4, 4, 61.4.1

Billing for Brachytherapy Sources - General

Brachytherapy sources (e.g., brachytherapy devices or seeds, solutions) are paid separately from the services to administer and deliver brachytherapy in the OPPS, per section 1833(t)(2)(H) of the Act, reflecting the number, isotope, and radioactive intensity of devices furnished, as well as stranded versus non-stranded configurations of sources. Therefore, providers must bill for brachytherapy sources in addition to the brachytherapy services with which the sources are applied, in order to receive payment for the sources. The list of separately payable sources is found in Addendum B of the most recent OPPS annual update published in the Federal Register, as well as in the recurring update notifications of the current year for billing purposes. New sources meeting the OPPS definition of a brachytherapy source may be added for payment beginning any quarter, and the new source codes and descriptors are announced in the recurring update notifications. Each unit of a billable source is identified by the unit measurement in the respective source's long descriptor. Seed-like sources are generally billed and paid "per source" based on the number of units of the source HCPCS code reported, including the billing of the number of sources within a stranded configuration of sources. Providers therefore must bill the number of units of a source used with the brachytherapy service rendered.

100-4, 4, 61.4.2

Definition of Brachytherapy Source for Separate Payment

Brachytherapy sources eligible for separate billing and payment must be radioactive sources, meaning that the source contains a radioactive isotope. Separate brachytherapy source payments reflect the number, isotope, and radioactive intensity of sources furnished to patients, as well as stranded and non-stranded configurations.

100-4, 4, 61.4.3

Billing of Brachytherapy Sources Ordered for a Specific Patient

A hospital may report and charge Medicare and the Medicare beneficiary for all brachytherapy sources that are ordered by the physician for a specific patient, acquired by the hospital, and used in the care of the patient. Specifically, brachytherapy sources prescribed by the physician in accordance with high quality clinical care, acquired by the hospital, and actually implanted in the patient may be reported and charged. In the case where most, but not all, prescribed sources are implanted in the patient, CMS will consider the relatively few brachytherapy sources that were ordered but not implanted due to specific clinical considerations to be used in the care of the patient and billable to Medicare under the following circumstances. The hospital may charge for all sources if they were specifically acquired by the hospital for the particular patient according to a physician's prescription for the sources that was consistent with standard clinical practice and high quality brachytherapy treatment, in order to ensure that the clinically appropriate number of sources was available for the implantation procedure, and they were not implanted in any other patient. Those sources that were not implanted must have been disposed of in accordance with all appropriate requirements for their handling.

In general, the number of sources used in the care of the patient but not implanted would not be expected to constitute more than a small fraction of the sources actually implanted in the patient. Under these circumstances, the beneficiary is liable for the copayment for all the sources billed to Medicare.

100-4, 4, 61.4.4

Billing for Brachytherapy Source Supervision, Handling and Loading Costs

Providers should report charges related to supervision, handling, and loading of radiation sources, including brachytherapy sources, in one of two ways:

1. Report the charge separately using CPT code 77790 (Supervision, handling, loading of radiation source), in addition to reporting the associated HCPCS procedure code(s) for application of the radiation source;
2. Include the supervision, handling, and/or loading charges as part of the charge reported with the HCPCS procedure code(s) for application of the radiation source.

Do not bill a separate charge for brachytherapy source storage costs. These costs are treated as part of the department's overhead costs.

100-4, 4, 160

Clinic and Emergency Visits

CMS has acknowledged from the beginning of the OPPS that CMS believes that CPT Evaluation and Management (E/M) codes were designed to reflect the activities of physicians and do not describe well the range and mix of services provided by hospitals during visits of clinic and emergency department patients. While awaiting the development of a national set of facility-specific codes and guidelines, providers should continue to apply their current internal guidelines to the existing CPT codes. Each hospital's internal guidelines should follow the intent of the CPT code descriptors, in that the guidelines should be designed to reasonably relate the intensity of hospital resources to the different levels of effort represented by the codes. Hospitals should ensure that their guidelines accurately reflect resource distinctions between the five levels of codes.

Effective January 1, 2007, CMS is distinguishing between two types of emergency departments: Type A emergency departments and Type B emergency departments.

A Type A emergency department is defined as an emergency department that is available 24 hours a day, 7 days a week and is either licensed by the State in which it is located under applicable State law as an emergency room or emergency department or it is held out to the public (by name, posted signs, advertising, or other means) as a place that provides care for emergency medical conditions on an urgent basis without requiring a previously scheduled appointment.

A Type B emergency department is defined as an emergency department that meets the definition of a "dedicated emergency department" as defined in 42 CFR 489.24 under the EMTALA regulations. It must meet at least one of the following requirements:

(1) It is licensed by the State in which it is located under applicable State law as an emergency room or emergency department;

(2) It is held out to the public (by name, posted signs, advertising, or other means) as a place that provides care for emergency medical conditions on an urgent basis without requiring a previously scheduled appointment; or

(3) During the calendar year immediately preceding the calendar year in which a determination under 42 CFR 489.24 is being made, based on a representative sample of patient visits that occurred during that calendar year, it provides at least one-third of all of its outpatient visits for the treatment of emergency medical conditions on an urgent basis without requiring a previously scheduled appointment.

Hospitals must bill for visits provided in Type A emergency departments using CPT emergency department E/M codes. Hospitals must bill for visits provided in Type B emergency departments using the G-codes that describe visits provided in Type B emergency departments.

Hospitals that will be billing the new Type B ED visit codes may need to update their internal guidelines to report these codes.

Emergency department and clinic visits are paid in some cases separately and in other cases as part of a composite APC payment. See section 10.2.1 of this chapter for further details.

100-4, 4, 160.1

Critical Care Services

Beginning January 1, 2007, critical care services will be paid at two levels, depending on the presence or absence of trauma activation. Providers will receive one payment rate for critical care without trauma activation and will receive additional payment when critical care is associated with trauma activation.

To determine whether trauma activation occurs, follow the National Uniform Billing Committee (NUBC) guidelines in the Claims Processing Manual, Pub 100-04, Chapter 25, Sec.75.4 related to the reporting of the trauma revenue codes in the 68x series. The revenue code series 68x can be used only by trauma centers/hospitals as licensed or designated by the state or local government authority authorized to do so, or as verified by the American College of Surgeons. Different subcategory revenue codes are reported by designated Level 1-4 hospital trauma centers. Only patients for whom there has been prehospital notification based on triage information from prehospital caregivers, who meet either local, state or American College of Surgeons field triage criteria, or are delivered by inter-hospital transfers, and are given the appropriate team response can be billed a trauma activation charge.

When critical care services are provided without trauma activation, the hospital may bill CPT code 99291, Critical care, evaluation and management of the critically ill or critically injured patient; first 30-74 minutes (and 99292, if appropriate). If trauma activation occurs under the circumstances described by the NUBC guidelines that would permit reporting a charge under 68x, the hospital may also bill one unit of code G0390, which describes trauma activation associated with hospital critical care services. Revenue code 68x must be reported on the same date of service. The OCE will edit to ensure that G0390 appears with revenue code 68x on the same date of service and that only one unit of G0390 is billed. CMS believes that trauma activation is a one-time occurrence in association with critical care services, and therefore, CMS will only pay for one unit of G0390 per day.

The CPT code 99291 is defined by CPT as the first 30-74 minutes of critical care. This 30 minute minimum has always applied under the OPPS. The CPT code 99292, Critical care, evaluation and management of the critically ill or critically injured patient; each additional 30 minutes, remains a packaged service under the OPPS, so that hospitals do not have the ongoing administrative burden of reporting precisely the time for each critical service provided. As the CPT guidelines indicate, hospitals that provide less than 30 minutes of critical care should bill for a visit, typically an emergency department visit, at a level consistent with their own internal guidelines.

Under the OPPS, the time that can be reported as critical care is the time spent by a physician and/or hospital staff engaged in active face-to-face critical care of a critically ill or critically injured patient. If the physician and hospital staff or multiple hospital staff members are simultaneously engaged in this active face-to-face care, the time involved can only be counted once.

- In CY 2007 hospitals may continue to report a charge with RC 68x without any HCPCS code when trauma team activation occurs. In order to receive additional payment when critical care services are associated with trauma activation, the hospital must report G0390 on the same date of service as RC 68x, in addition to CPT code 99291 (or 99292, if appropriate.)

In CY 2007 hospitals should continue to report 99291 (and 99292 as appropriate) for critical care services furnished without trauma team activation. CPT 99291 maps to APC 0617 (Critical Care). (CPT 99292 is packaged and not paid separately, but should be reported if provided.)

Critical care services are paid in some cases separately and in other cases as part of a composite APC payment. See Section 10.2.1 of this chapter for further details.

100-4, 4, 180.3

Unlisted Service or Procedure

This section does not apply to OPPS hospitals.

There may be services or procedures performed that are not found in HCPCS. These are typically services that are rarely provided, unusual, variable, or new. A number of specific code numbers have been designated for reporting unlisted procedures. When an unlisted procedure code is used, a report describing the service is submitted with the claim. Pertinent information includes a definition or description of the nature, extent, and need for the procedure and the time, effort, and equipment necessary to provide the service.

When an FI receives a claim with an unlisted procedure code, it reviews it to verify that there is no existing code that adequately describes the procedure. If it determines that an adequately descriptive code is contained in HCPCS, it advises the hospital of the proper code and processes the claim. If it determines that no existing code is sufficiently descriptive, it pays the claim using the unlisted procedure code. If the frequency of the procedure warrants assignment of a local code, the FI forwards a copy and the operative report to the RO HCPCS coordinator for a code determination. When it receives a determination, the FI informs the hospital of the correct code for future reporting. Local codes are not accepted under OPPS and line items for local codes are no longer paid on cost.

NOTE:If the claim is submitted via EMC or identified after the bill has been processed, an operative report, the provider number, revenue codes, and charges are sufficient.

The "Unlisted Procedures" and codes for surgery are:

HCPCS code	Unlisted Procedure
15999	Unlisted procedure, excision pressure ulcer
17999	Unlisted procedure, skin, mucous membrane and subcutaneous tissue
19499	Unlisted procedure, breast
20999	Unlisted procedure, musculoskeletal system, general
21299	Unlisted craniofacial and maxillofacial procedures
21499	Unlisted orthopedic procedure, head
21899	Unlisted procedure, neck or thorax
22899	Unlisted procedure, spine
22999	Unlisted procedure, abdomen, musculoskeletal system
23929	Unlisted procedure, shoulder
24999	Unlisted procedure, humerus or elbow
25999	Unlisted procedure, forearm or wrist
26989	Unlisted procedure, hands or fingers
27299	Unlisted procedure, pelvis or hip joint
27599	Unlisted procedure, femur or knee
27899	Unlisted procedure, leg or ankle
28899	Unlisted procedure, foot or toes
29799	Unlisted procedure, casting or strapping
29909	Unlisted procedure, arthroscopy
30999	Unlisted procedure, nose
31299	Unlisted procedure, accessory sinuses
31599	Unlisted procedure, larynx
31899	Unlisted procedure, trachea, bronchi
32999	Unlisted procedure, lungs, and pleura
33999	Unlisted procedure, cardiac surgery
36299	Unlisted procedure, vascular injection
37799	Unlisted procedure, vascular surgery
38999	Unlisted procedure, hemic or lymphatic system
39499	Unlisted procedure, mediastinum
39599	Unlisted procedure, diaphragm
40799	Unlisted procedure, lips
40899	Unlisted procedure, vestibule of mouth
41599	Unlisted procedure, tongue, floor of mouth
41899	Unlisted procedure, dentoalveolar structures
42299	Unlisted procedure, palate, uvula
42699	Unlisted procedure, salivary glands or ducts
42999	Unlisted procedure, pharynx, adenoids, or tonsils
43499	Unlisted procedure, esophag
43999	Unlisted procedure, stomach
44799	Unlisted procedure, intestine
44899	Unlisted procedure, Meckel's diverticulum and the mesentery
45999	Unlisted procedure, rectum
46999	Unlisted procedure, anus
47399	Unlisted procedure, liver
47999	Unlisted procedure, biliary tract
48999	Unlisted procedure, pancreas
49999	Unlisted procedure, abdomen, peritoneum, and omentum
53899	Unlisted procedure, urinary system
55899	Unlisted procedure, male genital system
56399	Unlisted procedure, laparoscopy, hysteroscopy
58999	Unlisted procedure, female genital system non-obstetrical
59899	Unlisted procedure, maternity care and delivery
60699	Unlisted procedure, endocrine system
64999	Unlisted procedure, nervous system
66999	Unlisted procedure, anterior segment of eye

HCPCS code	Unlisted Procedure
67299	Unlisted procedure, posterior segment
67399	Unlisted procedure, ocular muscle
67599	Unlisted procedure, orbit
67999	Unlisted procedure, eyelids
68399	Unlisted procedure, conjunctiva
68899	Unlisted procedure, lacrimal system
69399	Unlisted procedure, external ear
69799	Unlisted procedure, middle ear
69949	Unlisted procedure, inner ear
69979	Unlisted procedure, temporal bone, middle fossa approach

100-4, 4, 200.3.1

Billing for IMRT Planning and Delivery

Effective for services furnished on or after April 1, 2002, HCPCS codes G0174 (IMRT delivery) and G0178 (IMRT planning) are no longer valid codes. HCPCS code G0174 has been replaced with CPT codes 77418 and 0073T for IMRT delivery and HCPCS code G0178 with CPT code 77301. Therefore, hospitals must use CPT codes 77418 or 0073T for IMRT delivery and CPT code 77301 for IMRT planning. Any of the CPT codes 77401 through 77416 or 77418 may be reported on the same day as long as the services are furnished at separate treatment sessions. In these cases, modifier -59 must be appended to the appropriate codes. Additionally, in the context of billing 77301, regardless of the same or different dates of service, CPT codes 77014, 77280-77295, 77305-77321, 77331, 77336, and 77370 may only be billed in addition to 77301 if they are not provided as part of developing the IMRT treatment plan.

7730 Intensity modulated radiotherapy plan, including dose-volume histograms for target and critical structure partial tolerance specifications

77418 Intensity modulated treatment delivery, single or multiple fields/arcs, via narrow spatially and temporally modulated beams, binary, dynamic MLC, per treatment session

0073T Compensator-based beam modulation treatment delivery of inverse planned treatment using three or more high resolution (milled or cast) compensator convergent beam modulated fields, per treatment session

100-4, 4, 200.3.2

Additional Billing Instructions for IMRT Planning

Payment for the services identified by CPT codes 77014, 77280-77295, 77305-77321, 77331, 77336, and 77370 is included in the APC payment for IMRT planning when these services are performed as part of developing an IMRT plan that is reported using CPT code 77301. Under those circumstances, these codes should not be billed in addition to CPT code 77301 for IMRT planning.

100-4, 4, 200.3.3

Billing for Multi-Source Photon (Cobalt 60-Based) Stereotactic

Radiosurgery (SRS) Planning and Delivery

Effective for services furnished on or after January 1, 2006, hospitals must bill for multisource photon (cobalt 60-based) SRS planning using existing CPT codes that most accurately describe the service furnished, and HCPCS code G0243 for the delivery. For CY 2007, HCPCS code G0243 is no longer be reportable under the hospital OPPS because the code has been deleted and replaced with CPT code 77371, effective January 1, 2007.

77371 Radiation treatment delivery, stereotactic radiosurgery (SRS) (complete course of treatment of cerebral lesion[s] consisting of 1 session); multisource Cobalt 60 based.

Payment for CPT code 20660 is included in CPT code 77371; therefore, hospitals should not report 20660 separately.

100-4, 4, 200.4

Billing for Amniotic Membrane

Hospitals should report HCPCS code V2790 (Amniotic membrane for surgical reconstruction, per procedure) to report amniotic membrane tissue when the tissue is used. A specific procedure code associated with use of amniotic membrane tissue is CPT code 65780 (Ocular surface reconstruction; amniotic membrane transplantation).

Payment for the amniotic membrane tissue is packaged into payment for CPT code 65780 or other procedures with which the amniotic membrane is used.

100-4, 4, 200.5

Billing and Payment for Cardiac Rehabilitation Services

The National Coverage Determination for cardiac rehabilitation programs requires that programs must be comprehensive and to be comprehensive they must include a medical evaluation, a program to modify cardiac risk factors (e.g., nutritional counseling), prescribed exercise, education, and counseling. See the National Coverage Determination (NCD) Manual, Pub. 100-03, section 20.10, for more information. A cardiac rehabilitation session may include more than one aspect of the comprehensive program. For CY 2008, hospitals will continue to use CPT code 93797 (Physician services for outpatient cardiac rehabilitation, without continuous ECG monitoring (per session)) and CPT code 93798 (Physician services for outpatient cardiac rehabilitation, with continuous ECG monitoring (per session)) to report cardiac rehabilitation services.

However, effective for dates of service on or after January 1, 2008, hospitals may report more than one unit of HCPCS code 93797 or 97398 for a date of service if more than one cardiac rehabilitation session lasting at least 1 hour each is provided on the same day.

In order to report more than one session for a given date of service, each session must last a minimum of 60 minutes. For example, if the cardiac rehabilitation services provided on a given day total 1 hour and 50 minutes, then only one session should be billed to report the cardiac rehabilitation services provided on that day.

100-4, 4, 200.6

Billing and Payment for Alcohol and/or Substance Abuse Assessment and Intervention Services

For CY 2008, the CPT Editorial Panel has created two new Category I CPT codes for reporting alcohol and/or substance abuse screening and intervention services. They are CPT code 99408 (Alcohol and/or substance (other than tobacco) abuse structured screening (e.g., AUDIT, DAST), and brief intervention (SBI) services; 15 to 30 minutes); and CPT code 99409 (Alcohol and/or substance (other than tobacco) abuse structured screening (e.g., AUDIT, DAST), and brief intervention (SBI) services; greater than 30 minutes). However, screening services are not covered by Medicare without specific statutory authority, such as has been provided for mammography, diabetes, and colorectal cancer screening. Therefore, beginning January 1, 2008, the OPPS recognizes two parallel G-codes (HCPCS codes G0396 and G0397) to allow for appropriate reporting and payment of alcohol and substance abuse structured assessment and intervention services that are not provided as screening services, but that are performed in the context of the diagnosis or treatment of illness or injury.

Contractors shall make payment under the OPPS for HCPCS code G0396 (Alcohol and/or substance (other than tobacco) abuse structured assessment (e.g., AUDIT, DAST) and brief intervention, 15 to 30 minutes) and HCPCS code G0397, (Alcohol and/or substance(other than tobacco) abuse structured assessment (e.g., AUDIT, DAST) and intervention greater than 30 minutes), only when reasonable and necessary (i.e., when the service is provided to evaluate patients with signs/symptoms of illness or injury) as per section 1862(a)(1)(A) of the Act.

HCPCS codes G0396 and G0397 are to be used for structured alcohol and/or substance (other than tobacco) abuse assessment and intervention services that are distinct from other clinic and emergency department visit services performed during the same encounter. Hospital resources expended performing services described by HCPCS codes G0396 and G0397 may not be counted as resources for determining the level of a visit service and vice versa (i.e., hospitals may not double count the same facility resources in order to reach a higher level clinic or emergency department visit). However, alcohol and/or substance structured assessment or intervention services lasting less than 15 minutes should not be reported using these HCPCS codes, but the hospital resources expended should be included in determining the level of the visit service reported.

100-4, 4, 200.7.1

Cardiac Echocardiography Without Contrast

Hospitals are instructed to bill for echocardiograms without contrast in accordance with the CPT code descriptors and guidelines associated with the applicable Level I CPT code(s) (93303-93350).

Billing for "Sometimes Therapy" Services that May be Paid as Non-Therapy Services for Hospital Outpatients

Section 1834(k) of the Act, as added by Section 4541 of the BBA, allows payment at 80 percent of the lesser of the actual charge for the services or the applicable fee schedule amount for all outpatient therapy services; that is, physical therapy services, speech-language pathology services, and occupational therapy services. As provided under Section 1834(k)(5) of the Act, a therapy code list was created based on a uniform coding system (that is, the HCPCS) to identify and track these outpatient therapy services paid under the Medicare Physician Fee Schedule (MPFS).

The list of therapy codes, along with their respective designation, can be found on the CMS Website, specifically at http://www.cms.hhs.gov/TherapyServices/05_Annual_Therapy_Update.asp#TopOfPage. Two of the designations that are used for therapy services are: "always therapy" and "sometimes therapy." An "always therapy" service must be performed by a qualified therapist under a certified therapy plan of care, and a "sometimes therapy" service may be performed by an individual outside of a certified therapy plan of care.

Under the OPPS, separate payment is provided for certain services designated as "sometimes therapy" services if these services are furnished to hospital outpatients as a non-therapy service, that is, without a certified therapy plan of care. Specifically, to be paid under the OPPS for a non-therapy service, hospitals SHOULD NOT append the therapy modifier GP (physical therapy), GO (occupational therapy), or GN (speech language pathology), or report a therapy revenue code 042x, 043x, or 044x in association with the "sometimes therapy" codes listed in the table below.

To receive payment under the MPFS, when "sometimes therapy" services are performed by a qualified therapist under a certified therapy plan of care, providers should append the appropriate therapy modifier GP, GO, or GN, and report the charges under an appropriate therapy revenue code, specifically 042x, 043x, or 044x. This instruction does not apply to claims for "sometimes therapy" codes furnished as therapy services in the hospital outpatient department and paid under the MPFS.

Effective January 1, 2010, CPT code 92520 (Laryngeal function studies (i.e., aerodynamic testing and acoustic testing)), is newly designated as a "sometimes therapy" service under the MPFS. CPT code 92520 is not a new code, however, its "sometimes therapy" designation is new and effective January 1, 2010. Under the OPPS, hospitals will receive separate payment when they bill CPT code 92520 as a non-therapy service.

The list of HCPCS codes designated as "sometimes therapy" services that may be paid as non-therapy services when furnished to hospital outpatients as of January 1, 2010, is displayed in the table below.

Services Designated as "Sometimes Therapy" that May be Paid as Non-Therapy Services for Hospital Outpatients as of January 1, 2010

HCPCS Code	Long Descriptor
92520	Laryngeal function studies (i.e., aerodynamic testing and acoustic testing)
97597	Removal of devitalized tissue from wound(s), selective debridement, without anesthesia (e.g., high pressure waterjet with/without suction, sharp selective debridement with scissors, scalpel and forceps), with or without topical application(s), wound assessment, and instruction(s) for ongoing care, may include use of a whirlpool, per session; total wound(s) surface area less than or equal to 20 square centimeters
97598	Removal of devitalized tissue from wound(s), selective debridement, without anesthesia (e.g., high pressure waterjet with/without suction, sharp selective debridement with scissors, scalpel and forceps), with or without topical application(s), wound assessment, and instruction(s) for ongoing care, may include use of a whirlpool, per session; total wound(s) surface area greater than 20 square centimeters
97602	Removal of devitalized tissue from wound(s), non-selective debridement, without anesthesia (e.g., wet-to-moist dressings, enzymatic, abrasion), including topical application(s), wound assessment, and instruction(s) for ongoing care, per session
97605	Negative pressure wound therapy (e.g., vacuum assisted drainage collection), including topical application(s), wound assessment, and instruction(s) for ongoing care, per session; total wound(s) surface area less than or equal to 50 square centimeters
97606	Negative pressure wound therapy (eg., vacuum assisted drainage collection), including topical application(s), wound assessment, and instruction(s) for ongoing care, per session; total wound(s) surface area greater than 50 square centimeters
0183T	Low frequency, non-contact, non-thermal ultrasound, including topical application(s), when performed, wound assessment, and instruction(s) for ongoing care, per day

100-4, 4, 230.2

Coding and Payment for Drug Administration

A. Overview
Drug administration services furnished under the Hospital Outpatient Prospective Payment System (OPPS) during CY 2005 were reported using CPT codes 90780, 90781, and 96400-96459.

Effective January 1, 2006, some of these CPT codes were replaced with more detailed CPT codes incorporating specific procedural concepts, as defined and described by the CPT manual, such as initial, concurrent, and sequential.

Hospitals are instructed to use the full set of CPT codes, including those codes referencing concepts of initial, concurrent, and sequential, to bill for drug administration services furnished in the hospital outpatient department beginning January 1, 2007. In addition, hospitals are instructed to continue billing the HCPCS codes that most accurately describe the service(s) provided.

Hospitals are reminded to bill a separate Evaluation and Management code (with modifier 25) only if a significant, separately identifiable E/M service is performed in the same encounter with OPPS drug administration services.

B. Billing for Infusions and Injections
Beginning in CY 2007, hospitals were instructed to use the full set of drug administration CPT codes (90760-90779; 96401-96549), (96413-96523 beginning in CY 2008) (96360-96549 beginning in CY 2009) when billing for drug administration services provided in the hospital outpatient department. In addition, hospitals are to continue to bill HCPCS code C8957 (Intravenous infusion for therapy/diagnosis; initiation of prolonged infusion (more than 8 hours), requiring use of portable or implantable pump) when appropriate. Hospitals are expected to report all drug administration CPT codes in a manner consistent with their descriptors, CPT instructions, and correct coding principles. Hospitals should note the conceptual changes between CY 2006 drug administration codes effective under the OPPS and the CPT codes in effect beginning January 1, 2007, in order to ensure accurate billing under the OPPS. Hospitals should report all HCPCS codes that describe the drug administration services provided, regardless of whether or not those services are separately paid or their payment is packaged.

Medicare's general policy regarding physician supervision within hospital outpatient departments meets the physician supervision requirements for use of CPT codes 90760-90779, 96401-96549, (96413-96523 beginning in CY 2008). (Reference: Pub.100-02, Medicare Benefit Policy Manual, Chapter 6, §20.4.)

Drug administration services are to be reported with a line item date of service on the day they are provided. In addition, only one initial drug administration service is to be reported per vascular access site per encounter, including during an encounter where observation services span more than 1 calendar day.

C. Payments For Drug Administration Services
For CY 2007, OPPS drug administration APCs were restructured, resulting in a six-level hierarchy where active HCPCS codes have been assigned according to their clinical coherence and resource use. Contrary to the CY 2006 payment structure that bundled payment for several instances of a type of service (non-chemotherapy, chemotherapy by infusion, non-infusion chemotherapy) into a per-encounter APC payment, structure introduced in CY 2007 provides a separate APC payment for each reported unit of a separately payable HCPCS code.

Hospitals should note that the transition to the full set of CPT drug administration codes provides for conceptual differences when reporting, such as those noted below.

- In CY 2006, hospitals were instructed to bill for the first hour (and any additional hours) by each type of infusion service (non-chemotherapy, chemotherapy by infusion, non-infusion chemotherapy). Beginning in CY 2007, the first hour concept no longer exists. CPT codes in CY 2007 and beyond allow for only one initial service per encounter, for each vascular access site, no matter how many types of infusion services are provided; however, hospitals will receive an APC payment for the initial service and separate APC payment(s) for additional hours of infusion or other drug administration services provided that are separately payable.
- In CY 2006, hospitals providing infusion services of different types (non-chemotherapy, chemotherapy by infusion, non-infusion chemotherapy) received payment for the associated per-encounter infusion APC even if these infusions occurred during the same time period. Beginning in CY 2007, hospitals should report only one initial drug administration service, including infusion services, per encounter for each distinct vascular access site, with other services through the same vascular access site being reported via the sequential, concurrent or additional hour codes. Although new CPT guidance has been issued for reporting initial drug administration services, Medicare contractors shall continue to follow the guidance given in this manual.

(**NOTE:** This list above provides a brief overview of a limited number of the conceptual changes between CY 2006 OPPS drug administration codes and CY 2007 OPPS drug administration codes - this list is not comprehensive and does not include all items hospitals will need to consider during this transition)

For APC payment rates, refer to the most current quarterly version of Addendum B on the CMS Web site at http://www.cms.hhs.gov/HospitalOutpatientPPS/.

D. Infusions Started Outside the Hospital
Hospitals may receive Medicare beneficiaries for outpatient services who are in the process of receiving an infusion at their time of arrival at the hospital (e.g., a patient who arrives via ambulance with an ongoing intravenous infusion initiated by paramedics during transport). Hospitals are reminded to bill for all services provided using the HCPCS code(s) that most accurately describe the service(s) they provided. This includes hospitals reporting an initial hour of infusion, even if the hospital did not initiate the infusion, and additional HCPCS codes for additional or sequential infusion services if needed.

100-4, 4, 231

Coding and Payment for Drug Administration

A. Overview
Drug administration services furnished under the Hospital Outpatient Prospective Payment System (OPPS) during CY 2005 were reported using CPT codes 90780, 90781, and 96400-96459.

Effective January 1, 2006, some of these CPT codes were replaced with more detailed CPT codes incorporating specific procedural concepts, as defined and described by the CPT manual, such as initial, concurrent, and sequential.

Hospitals are instructed to use the full set of CPT codes, including those codes referencing concepts of initial, concurrent, and sequential, to bill for drug administration services furnished in the hospital outpatient department beginning January 1, 2007. In addition, hospitals are instructed to continue billing the HCPCS codes that most accurately describe the service(s) provided.

Hospitals are reminded to bill a separate Evaluation and Management code (with modifier 25) only if a significant, separately identifiable E/M service is performed in the same encounter with OPPS drug administration services.

B. Billing for Infusions and Injections
In CY 2007, hospitals are instructed to use the full set of drug administration CPT codes (90760-90779; 96401-96549) when billing for drug administration services provided in the hospital outpatient department. In addition, hospitals are to continue to bill HCPCS code C8957 (Intravenous infusion for therapy/diagnosis; initiation of prolonged infusion (more than 8 hours), requiring use of portable or implantable pump) when appropriate.

Hospitals are expected to report all drug administration CPT codes in a manner consistent with their descriptors, CPT instructions, and correct coding principles. Hospitals should note the conceptual changes between CY 2006 drug administration codes effective under the OPPS and the CY 2007 CPT codes in order to ensure accurate billing under the OPPS.

Medicare's general policy regarding physician supervision within hospital outpatient departments meets the physician supervision requirements for use of CPT codes 90760- 90779, 96401-96549. (Reference: Medicare Benefit Policy Manual, Pub.100-02, Chapter 6, Sec.20.4.1.) C. Payments For Drug Administration Services For CY 2007, OPPS drug administration APCs have been restructured resulting in a sixlevel hierarchy where active HCPCS codes have been assigned according to their clinical coherence and resource use. Contrary to the CY 2006 payment structure that bundled payment for several instances of a type of service (non-chemotherapy, chemotherapy by infusion, non-infusion chemotherapy) into a per-encounter APC payment, the CY 2007 structure provides a separate APC payment for each reported unit of a separately payable HCPCS code.

Hospitals should note that the transition to the full set of CPT drug administration codes provides for conceptual differences when reporting, such as those noted below.

In CY 2006, hospitals were instructed to bill for the first hour (and any additional hours) by each type of infusion service (non-chemotherapy, chemotherapy by infusion, non-infusion chemotherapy). In CY 2007, the first hour concept no longer exists. CY 2007 CPT codes allow for only one initial service per encounter, for each vascular access site, no matter how many types of infusion services are provided; however, hospitals will receive an APC payment for the initial service and separate APC payment(s) for additional hours of infusion or other drug administration services provided that are separately payable .

In CY 2006, hospitals providing infusion services of different types (nonchemotherapy, chemotherapy by infusion, non-infusion chemotherapy) received payment for the associated per-encounter infusion APC even if these infusions occurred during the same time period. In CY 2007, CPT instructions allow reporting of only one initial drug administration service, including infusion services, per encounter for each distinct vascular access site, with other services through the same vascular access site being reported via the sequential, concurrent or additional hour codes.

NOTE: This list provides a brief overview of a limited number of the conceptual changes between CY 2006 OPPS drug administration codes and CY 2007 OPPS drug administration codes - this list is not comprehensive and does not include all items hospitals will need to consider during this transition) For CY 2007 APC payment rates, refer to Addendum B on the CMS Web site at http://www.cms.hhs.gov/HospitalOutpatientPPS/.

D. Infusions Started Outside the Hospital

Hospitals may receive Medicare beneficiaries for outpatient services who are in the process of receiving an infusion at their time of arrival at the hospital (e.g. a patient who arrives via ambulance with an ongoing intravenous infusion initiated by paramedics during transport). Hospitals are reminded to bill for all services provided using the HCPCS code(s) that most accurately describe the service(s) they provided. This includes hospitals reporting an initial hour of infusion, even if the hospital did not initiate the infusion, and additional HCPCS codes for additional or sequential infusion services if needed.

100-4, 4, 231.4

Billing for Split Unit of Blood

HCPCS code P9011 was created to identify situations where one unit of blood or a blood product is split and some portion of the unit is transfused to one patient and the other portions are transfused to other patients or to the same patient at other times. When a patient receives a transfusion of a split unit of blood or blood product, OPPS providers should bill P9011 for the blood product transfused, as well as CPT 86985 (Splitting, blood products) for each splitting procedure performed to prepare the blood product for a specific patient.

Providers should bill split units of packed red cells and whole blood using Revenue Code 389 (Other blood), and should not use Revenue Codes 381 (Packed red cells) or 382 (Whole blood). Providers should bill split units of other blood products using the applicable revenue codes for the blood product type, such as 383 (Plasma) or 384 (Platelets), rather than 389. Reporting revenue codes according to these specifications will ensure the Medicare beneficiary's blood deductible is applied correctly.

EXAMPLE: OPPS provider splits off a 100cc aliquot from a 250 cc unit of leukocytereduced red blood cells for a transfusion to Patient X. The hospital then splits off an 80cc aliquot of the remaining unit for a transfusion to Patient Y. At a later time, the remaining 70cc from the unit is transfused to Patient Z.

In billing for the services for Patient X and Patient Y, the OPPS provider should report the charges by billing P9011 and 86985 in addition to the CPT code for the transfusion service, because a specific splitting service was required to prepare a split unit for transfusion to each of those patients. However, the OPPS provider should report only P9011 and the CPT code for the transfusion service for Patient Z because no additional splitting was necessary to prepare the split unit for transfusion to Patient Z. The OPPS provider should bill Revenue Code 0389 for each split unit of the leukocyte-reduced red blood cells that was transfused.

100-4, 4, 231.9

Billing for Pheresis and Apheresis Services

Apheresis/pheresis services are billed on a per visit basis and not on a per unit basis. OPPS providers should report the charge for an Evaluation and Management (E&M) visit only if there is a separately identifiable E&M service performed which extends beyond the evaluation and management portion of a typical apheresis/pheresis service. If the OPPS provider is billing an E&M visit code in addition to the apheresis/pheresis service, it may be appropriate to use the HCPCS modifier -25.

100-4, 4, 231.11

Billing for Allogeneic Stem Cell Transplants

1. Definition of Acquisition Charges for Allogeneic Stem Cell Transplants

Acquisition charges for allogeneic stem cell transplants include, but are not limited to, charges for the costs of the following services:

National Marrow Donor Program fees, if applicable, for stem cells from an unrelated donor;

Tissue typing of donor and recipient;

Donor evaluation;

Physician pre-procedure donor evaluation services;

Costs associated with harvesting procedure (e.g., general routine and special care services, procedure/operating room and other ancillary services, apheresis services, etc.);

Post-operative/post-procedure evaluation of donor; and

Preparation and processing of stem cells.

Payment for these acquisition services is included in the OPPS APC payment for the allogeneic stem cell transplant when the transplant occurs in the hospital outpatient setting, and in the MS-DRG payment for the allogeneic stem cell transplant when the transplant occurs in the inpatient setting. The Medicare contractor does not make separate payment for these acquisition services, because hospitals may bill and receive payment only for services provided to the Medicare beneficiary who is the recipient of the stem cell transplant and whose illness is being treated with the stem cell transplant. Unlike the acquisition costs of solid organs for transplant (e.g., hearts and kidneys), which are paid on a reasonable cost basis, acquisition costs for allogeneic stem cells are included in prospective payment. Recurring update notifications describing changes to and billing instructions for various payment policies implemented in the OPPS are issues annually.

Acquisition charges for stem cell transplants apply only to allogeneic transplants, for which stem cells are obtained from a donor (other than the recipient himself or herself). Acquisition charges do not apply to autologous transplants (transplanted stem cells are obtained from the recipient himself or herself), because autologous transplants involve services provided to the beneficiary only (and not to a donor), for which the hospital may bill and receive payment (see Pub. 100-04, chapter 3, Sec.90.3.3 and Sec.231.10 of this chapter for information regarding billing for autologous stem cell transplants).

2. Billing for Acquisition Services

The hospital bills and shows acquisition charges for allogeneic stem cell transplants based on the status of the patient (i.e., inpatient or outpatient) when the transplant is furnished. See Pub. 100-04, chapter 3, Sec.90.3.3 for instructions regarding billing for acquisition services for allogeneic stem cell transplants that are performed in the inpatient setting.

When the allogeneic stem cell transplant occurs in the outpatient setting, the hospital identifies stem cell acquisition charges for allogeneic bone marrow/stem cell transplants separately in FL 42 of Form CMS-1450 (or electronic equivalent) by using revenue code 0819 (Other Organ Acquisition). Revenue code 0819 charges should include all services required to acquire stem cells from a donor, as defined above, and should be reported on the same date of service as the transplant procedure in order to be appropriately packaged for payment purposes.

The transplant hospital keeps an itemized statement that identifies the services furnished, the charges, the person receiving the service (donor/recipient), and whether this is a potential transplant donor or recipient. These charges will be reflected in the transplant hospital's stem cell/bone marrow acquisition cost center. For allogeneic stem cell acquisition services in cases that do not result in transplant, due to death of the intended recipient or other causes, hospitals include the costs associated with the acquisition services on the Medicare cost report.

In the case of an allogeneic transplant in the hospital outpatient setting, the hospital reports the transplant itself with the appropriate CPT code, and a charge under revenue center code 0362 or another appropriate cost center. Selection of the cost center is up to the hospital.

100-4, 4, 240

Inpatient Part B Hospital Services

Inpatient Part B services which are paid under OPPS include:

- Diagnostic x-ray tests, and other diagnostic tests (excluding clinical diagnostic laboratory tests);
- X-ray, radium, and radioactive isotope therapy, including materials and services of technicians;
- Surgical dressings applied during an encounter at the hospital and splints, casts, and other devices used for reduction of fractures and dislocations (splints and casts, etc., include dental splints);
- Implantable prosthetic devices;
- Hepatitis B vaccine and its administration, and certain preventive screening services (pelvic exams, screening sigmoidoscopies, screening colonoscopies, bone mass measurements, and prostate screening.)
- Bone Mass measurements;
- Prostate screening;
- Immunosuppressive drugs;
- Oral anti-cancer drugs;
- Oral drug prescribed for use as an acute anti-emetic used as part of an anti-cancer chemotherapeutic regimen; and
- Epoetin Alfa (EPO)

When a hospital that is not paid under the OPPS furnishes an implantable prosthetic device that meets the criteria for coverage in Medicare Benefits Policy Manual, Pub.100-02, Chapter 6, Sec.10 to an inpatient who has coverage under Part B, payment for the implantable prosthetic device is made under the payment mechanism that applies to other hospital outpatient services (e.g. reasonable cost, all inclusive rate, waiver).

When a hospital that is paid under the OPPS furnishes an implantable prosthetic device to an inpatient who has coverage under Part B, but who does not have coverage of inpatient services on the date that the implanted prosthetic device is furnished, the hospital should report new HCPCS code, C9899, Implanted Prosthetic Device, Payable Only for Inpatients who do not Have Inpatient Coverage, that will be effective for services furnished on or after January 1, 2009. This code may be reported only on claims with TOB 12X when the prosthetic device is implanted on a day on which the beneficiary does not have coverage of the hospital inpatient services he or she is receiving. The line containing this new code will be rejected if it is reported on a claim that is not a TOB 12X or if it is reported with a line item date of service on which the beneficiary has coverage of inpatient hospital services. By reporting C9899, the hospital is reporting that all of the criteria for payment under Part B are met as specified in the Medicare Benefits Policy Manual, Pub.100-02, Chapter 6, Sec.10, and that the item meets all Medicare criteria for coverage as an implantable prosthetic device as defined in that section.

Medicare contractors shall first determine that the item furnished meets the Medicare criteria for coverage as an implantable prosthetic device as specified in the Medicare Benefits Policy Manual, Pub. 100-02, Chapter 6, Sec.10. If the item does not meet the criteria for coverage as an implantable prosthetic device, the contractor shall deny payment on the basis that the item is outside the scope of the benefits for which there is coverage for Part B inpatients. The beneficiary is liable for the charges for the noncovered item when the item does not meet the criteria for coverage as an implanted prosthetic device as specified in the Medicare Benefits Policy Manual, Pub.100-02, Chapter 6, Sec.10.

If the contractor determines that the device is covered, the contractor shall determine if the device has pass through status under the OPPS. If so, the contractor shall establish the payment amount for the device at the product of the charge for the device and the hospital specific cost to charge ratio. Where the device does not have pass through status under the OPPS, the contractor shall establish the payment amount for the device at the amount for a comparable device in the DMEPOS fee schedule where there is such an amount. Payment under the DMEPOS fee schedule is made at the lesser of charges or the fee schedule amount and therefore if there is a fee for the specific item on the DMEPOS fee schedule, the payment amount for the item will be set at the lesser of the actual charges or the DMEPOS fee schedule amount. Where the item does not have pass through payment status and where there is no amount for a comparable device in the DMEPOS fee schedule, the contractor shall establish a payment amount that is specific to the particular implanted prosthetic device for the applicable calendar year. This amount (less applicable unpaid deductible and coinsurance) will be paid for that specific device for services furnished in the applicable calendar year unless the actual charge for the item is less than the established amount). Where the actual charge is less than the established amount, the contractor will pay the actual charge for the item (less applicable unpaid deductible and coinsurance).

In setting a contractor established payment rate for the specific device, the contractor takes into account the cost information available at the time the payment rate is established. This information may include, but is not limited to, the amount of device cost that would be removed from an applicable APC payment for implantation of the device if the provider received a device without cost or a full credit for the cost of the device.

If the contractor chooses to use this amount, see www.cms.hhs.gov/HospitalOutpatientPPS/ for the amount of reduction to the APC payment that would apply in these cases. From the OPPS webpage, select "Device, Radiolabeled Product, and Procedure Edits" from the list on the left side of the page. Open the file "Procedure to Device edits" to determine the HCPCS code that best describes the procedure in which the device would be used. Then identify the APC to which that procedure code maps from the most recent Addenda B on the OPPS webpage and open the file "FB/FC Modifier Procedures and Devices". Select the applicable year's file of APCs subject to full and partial credit reductions (for example: CY 2008 APCs Subject to Full and Partial Credit Reduction Policy"). Select the "Full offset reduction amount" that pertains to the APC that is most applicable to the device described by C9899. It would be reasonable to set this amount as a payment for a device furnished to a Part B inpatient.

For example, if C9899 is reporting insertion of a single chamber pacemaker (C1786 or equivalent narrative description on the claim in "remarks") the file of procedure to device edits shows that a single chamber pacemaker is the dominant device for APC 0090 (APC 0089 is for insertion of both pacemaker and electrodes and therefore would not apply if electrodes are not also billed). The table of offset reduction amounts for CY 2008 shows that the estimated cost of a single chamber pacemaker for APC 0090 is $4881.77. It would therefore be reasonable for the contractor/MAC to set the payment rate for a single chamber pacemaker furnished to a Part B inpatient to $4881.77. In this case the coinsurance would be $936.75 (20 percent of $4881.77, which is less than the inpatient deductible).

The beneficiary coinsurance is 20 percent of the payment amount for the device (i.e. the pass through payment amount, the DMEPOS fee schedule amount, the contractor established amount, or the actual charge if less than the DMEPOS fee schedule amount or the contractor established amount for the specific device), not to exceed the Medicare inpatient deductible that is applicable to the year in which the implanted prosthetic device is furnished.

Inpatient Part B services paid under other payment methods include:

- Clinical diagnostic laboratory tests, prosthetic devices other than implantable ones and other than dental which replace all or part of an internal body organ (including contiguous tissue), or all or part of the function of a permanently inoperative or malfunctioning internal body organ, including replacement or repairs of such devices;
- Leg, arm, back and neck braces; trusses and artificial legs; arms and eyes including adjustments, repairs, and replacements required because of breakage, wear, loss, or a change in the patient's physical condition; take home surgical dressings; outpatient physical therapy; outpatient occupational therapy; and outpatient speech-language pathology services;
- Ambulance services;
- Screening pap smears, screening colorectal tests, and screening mammography;
- Influenza virus vaccine and its administration, pneumococcal vaccine and its administration;
- Diabetes self-management training;
- Hemophilia clotting factors for hemophilia patients competent to use these factors without supervision).

See Chapter 6 of the Medicare Benefit Policy Manual for a discussion of the circumstances under which the above services may be covered as Part B Inpatient services.

100-4, 4, 250.3.2

Physician Rendering Anesthesia in a Hospital Outpatient Setting

When a medically necessary anesthesia service is furnished within a HPSA area by a physician, a HPSA bonus is payable. In addition to using the PC/TC indicator on the CORF extract of the MPFS Summary File to identify HPSA services, pay physicians the HPSA bonus when CPT codes 00100 through 01999 are billed with the following modifiers: QY, QK, AA, or GC and "QB" or "QU" in revenue code 963. Modifier QB or QU must be submitted to receive payment of the HPSA bonus for claims with dates of service prior to January 01, 2006. Effective for claims with dates of service on or after January 01, 2006, the modifier AQ, physician providing a service in a health professional shortage area, may be required to receive the HPSA bonus. Refer to 250.2.2 of this chapter for more information on when modifier AQ is required.

The modifiers signify that a physician performed an anesthesia service. Using the Anesthesia File (See Section above) the physician service will be 115 percent times the payment amount to be paid to a CAH on Method II payment plus 10 percent HPSA bonus payment.

Anesthesiology modifiers:

AA = anesthesia services performed personally by anesthesiologist.

GC =service performed, in part, by a resident under the direction of a teaching physician.

QK = medical direction of two, three, or four concurrent anesthesia procedures involving qualified individuals.

QY = medical direction of one CRNA by an anesthesiologist.

Modifiers AA and GC result in physician payment at 80% of the allowed amount. Modifiers QK and QY result in physician payment at 50% of the allowed amount.

Data elements needed to calculate payment:

HCPCS plus Modifier,

Base Units,

Time units, based on standard 15 minute intervals,

Locality specific anesthesia Conversion factor, and

Allowed amount minus applicable deductions and coinsurance amount.

Formula 1: Calculate payment for a physician performing anesthesia alone

HCPCS = xxxxx
Modifier = AA
Base Units = 4

Anesthesia Time is 60 minutes. Anesthesia time units = 4 (60/15)
Sum of Base Units plus Time Units = 4 + 4 = 8
Locality specific Anesthesia conversion factor = $17.00 (varies by localities)
Coinsurance = 20%

Example 1: Physician personally performs the anesthesia case

Base Units plus time units - 4+4=8
Total units multiplied by the anesthesia conversion factor times .80
8 x $17= ($136.00 - (deductible*) x .80 = $108.80

Payment amount times 115 percent for the CAH method II payment.

$108.80 x 1.15 = $125.12 (Payment amount)

$125.12 x .10 = $12.51 (HPSA bonus payment)

*Assume the Part B deductible has already been met for the calendar year

Formula 2: Calculate the payment for the physician's medical direction service when the physician directs two concurrent cases involving CRNAs. The medical direction allowance is 50% of the allowance for the anesthesia service personally performed by the physician.

HCPCS = xxxxx
Modifier = QK
Base Units = 4
Time Units 60/15=4

Sum of base units plus time units = 8
Locality specific anesthesia conversion factor = $17(varies by localities)
Coinsurance = 20 %

(Allowed amount adjusted for applicable deductions and coinsurance and to reflect payment percentage for medical direction).

Example 2: Physician medically directs two concurrent cases involving CRNAs

Base units plus time - 4+4=8
Total units multiplied by the anesthesia conversion factor times. 50 equal allowed amount minus any remaining deductible
8 x $17 = $136 x .50 = $68.00 -(deductible*) = $68.00

Allowed amount Times 80 percent times 1.15
$68.00 x .80 = $54.40 x 1.15 = 62.56 (Payment amount)
$62.56 x .10 = $6.26 (HPSA bonus payment)

*Assume the deductible has already been met for the calendar year.

100-4, 4, 250.3.3.1

Payment for CRNA Pass-Through Services

If a CAH that meets the criteria for a pass-through exemption is interested in selecting the Method II option, it can choose this option for all outpatient professionals except the CRNA's and still retain the approved CRNAs exemption for both inpatient and outpatient professional services of CRNAs. The CAH, with an approved exemption, can choose to give up its exemption for both inpatient and outpatient professional services of CRNAs in order to include its CRNA outpatient professional services along with those of all other professional services under the Method II option. By choosing to include the CRNAs under the Method II for outpatient services, it loses its CRNA pass-through exemption for not only the outpatient CRNA services, but also the inpatient CRNA services. In this case the CAH would have to bill the Part B carrier for the CRNA inpatient professional services.

All intermediary payments for CRNA services are subject to cost settlement.

If a CAH that meets the criteria for a pass-through exemption is not interested in selecting the Method II option, the CAH can still receive the CRNA pass-through under the Standard Option (Method I). Below are the billing requirements for Method I.

Provider Billing Requirements for Method I
TOBs = 85X and 11X

Revenue Code 037X for CRNA technical services
Revenue Code 0964 for Professional services
HCPCS Code = Anesthesia HCPCS code (00100 through 01999 HCPCS range)

Units = Anesthesia
Reimbursement
Revenue Code 37X, CRNA technical service = Cost Reimbursement

Revenue Code 0964, CRNA professional service = Cost Reimbursement for both inpatient and outpatient

Deductible and coinsurance apply.

100-4, 4, 290.5.1

Billing and Payment for Observation Services Beginning January 1, 2008

Observation services are reported using HCPCS code G0378 (Hospital observation service, per hour). Beginning January 1, 2008, HCPCS code G0378 for hourly observation services is assigned status indicator N, signifying that its payment is always packaged. No separate payment is made for observation services reported with HCPCS code G0378, and APC 0339 is deleted as of January 1, 2008. In most circumstances, observation services are supportive and ancillary to the other services provided to a patient. In certain circumstances when observation care is billed in conjunction with a high level clinic visit (Level 5), high level Type A emergency department visit (Level 4 or 5), high level Type B emergency department visit (Level 5), critical care services, or a direct referral as an integral part of a patient's extended encounter of care, payment may be made for the entire extended care encounter through one of two composite APCs when certain criteria are met. For information about payment for extended assessment and management composite APCs, see Sec.10.2.1 (Composite APCs) of this chapter.

APC 8002 (Level I Extended Assessment and Management Composite) describes an encounter for care provided to a patient that includes a high level (Level 5) clinic visit or direct referral for observation in conjunction with observation services of substantial duration (8 or more hours). APC 8003 (Level II Extended Assessment and Management Composite) describes an encounter for care provided to a patient that includes a high level (Level 4 or 5) emergency department visit or critical care services in conjunction with observation services of substantial duration. Beginning January 1, 2009, APC 8003 also includes high level (Level 5) Type B emergency department visits. There is no limitation on diagnosis for payment of these composite APCs; however, composite APC payment will not be made when observation services are reported in association with a surgical procedure (T status procedure) or the hours of observation care reported are less than 8. The I/OCE evaluates every claim received to determine if payment through a composite APC is appropriate. If payment through a composite APC is inappropriate, the I/OCE, in conjunction with the Pricer, determines the appropriate status indicator, APC, and payment for every code on a claim.

All of the following requirements must be met in order for a hospital to receive an APC payment for an extended assessment and management composite APC:

1. Observation Time
   a. Observation time must be documented in the medical record.
   b. Hospital billing for observation services begins at the clock time documented in the patient's medical record, which coincides with the time that observation services are initiated in accordance with a physician's order for observation services.
   c. A beneficiary's time receiving observation services (and hospital billing) ends when all clinical or medical interventions have been completed, including follow-up care furnished by hospital staff and physicians that may take place after a physician has ordered the patient be released or admitted as an inpatient.
   d. The number of units reported with HCPCS code G0378 must equal or exceed 8 hours.
2. Additional Hospital Services
   a. The claim for observation services must include one of the following services in addition to the reported observation services. The additional services listed below must have a line item date of service on the same day or the day before the date reported for observation:
      - A Type A or B emergency department visit (CPT codes 99284 or 99285 or HCPCS code G0384); or
      - A clinic visit (CPT code 99205 or 99215); or
      - Critical care (CPT code 99291); or
      - Direct referral for observation care reported with HCPCS code G0379 (APC 0604) must be reported on the same date of service as the date reported for observation services.
   b. No procedure with a T status indicator can be reported on the same day or day before observation care is provided.
3. Physician Evaluation
   a. The beneficiary must be in the care of a physician during the period of observation, as documented in the medical record by outpatient registration, discharge, and other appropriate progress notes that are timed, written, and signed by the physician.
   b. he medical record must include documentation that the physician explicitly assessed patient risk to determine that the beneficiary would benefit from observation care.

Criteria 1 and 3 related to observation care beginning and ending time and physician evaluation apply regardless of whether the hospital believes that the criteria will be met for payment of the extended encounter through extended assessment and management composite payment.

Only visits, critical care and observation services that are billed on a 13X bill type may be considered for a composite APC payment.

Non-repetitive services provided on the same day as either direct referral for observation care or observation services must be reported on the same claim because the OCE claim-by-claim logic cannot function properly unless all services related to the episode of observation care, including hospital clinic visits, emergency department visits, critical care services, and T status procedures, are reported on the same claim. Additional guidance can be found in chapter 1, section 50.2.2 of this manual.

If a claim for services provided during an extended assessment and management encounter including observation care does not meet all of the requirements listed above, then the usual APC logic will apply to separately payable items and services on the claim; the special logic for direct admission will apply, and payment for the observation care will be packaged into payments for other separately payable services provided to the beneficiary in the same encounter.

100-4, 4, 300

Medical Nutrition Therapy (MNT) Services

Section 105 of the Medicare, Medicaid, and SCHIP Benefits Improvement and Protection Act of 2000 (BIPA) permits Medicare coverage of Medical Nutrition Therapy (MNT) services when furnished by a registered dietitian or nutrition professional meeting certain requirements. The benefit is available for beneficiaries with diabetes or renal disease, when referral is made by a physician as defined in §1861(r)(l) of the Act. It also allows registered dietitians and nutrition professionals to receive direct Medicare reimbursement for the first time. The effective date of this provision is January 1, 2002.

The benefit consists of an initial visit for an assessment; follow-up visits for interventions; and reassessments as necessary during the 12-month period beginning with the initial assessment ("episode of care") to assure compliance with the dietary plan. Effective October 1, 2002, basic coverage of MNT for the first year a beneficiary receives MNT with either a diagnosis of renal disease or diabetes as defined at 42 CFR, 410.130 is 3 hours. Also effective October 1, 2002, basic coverage in subsequent years for renal disease is 2 hours.

For the purposes of this benefit, renal disease means chronic renal insufficiency or the medical condition of a beneficiary who has been discharged from the hospital after a successful renal transplant within the last 36 months. Chronic renal insufficiency means a reduction in renal function not severe enough to require dialysis or transplantation (glomerular filtration rate (GFR) 13-50 ml/min/1.73m^2). Effective January 1, 2004, CMS updated the definition of diabetes to be as follows: Diabetes is defined as diabetes mellitus, a condition of abnormal glucose metabolism diagnosed using the following criteria: a fasting blood sugar greater than or equal to 126 mg/dL on two different occasions; a 2 hour post-glucose challenge greater than or equal to 200 mg/dL on 2 different occasions; or a random glucose test over 200 mg/dL for a person with symptoms of uncontrolled diabetes.

The MNT benefit is a completely separate benefit from the diabetes self-management training (DSMT) benefit. CMS had originally planned to limit how much of both benefits a beneficiary might receive in the same time period. However, the national coverage decision, published May 1, 2002, allows a beneficiary to receive the full amount of both benefits in the same period. Therefore, a beneficiary can receive the full 10 hours of initial DSMT and the full 3 hours of MNT. However, providers are not allowed to bill for both DSMT and MNT on the same date of service for the same beneficiary.

100-4, 4, 300.6

Common Working File (CWF) Edits

The CWF edit will allow 3 hours of therapy for MNT in the initial calendar year. The edit will allow more than 3 hours of therapy if there is a change in the beneficiary's medical condition, diagnosis, or treatment regimen and this change must be documented in the beneficiary's medical record. Two new G codes have been created for use when a beneficiary receives a second referral in a calendar year that allows the beneficiary to receive more than 3 hours of therapy. Another edit will allow 2 hours of follow up MNT with another referral in subsequent years.

Advance Beneficiary Notice (ABN)

The beneficiary is liable for services denied over the limited number of hours with referrals for MNT. An ABN should be issued in these situations. In absence of evidence of a valid ABN, the provider will be held liable.

An ABN should not be issued for Medicare-covered services such as those provided by hospital dietitians or nutrition professionals who are qualified to render the service in their state but who have not obtained Medicare provider numbers.

Duplicate Edits

Although beneficiaries are allowed to receive training and therapy during the same time period Diabetes Self-Management and Training (DSMT) and Medical Nutrition Therapy (MNT) services may not be provided on the same day to the same beneficiary. Effective April 1, 2010 CWF shall implement a new duplicate crossover edit to identify and prevent claims for DSMT/MNT services from being billed with the same dates of services for the same beneficiaries submitted from institutional providers and from a professional provider.

100-4, 4, 320.1

HCPCS Coding for OIVIT

HCPCS code G9147, effective with the April IOCE and MPFSDB updates, is to be used on claims with dates of service on and after December 23, 2009, billing for non-covered OIVIT and any services comprising an OIVIT regimen.

NOTE: HCPCS codes 99199 or 94681(with or without diabetes related conditions 250.00-250.93) are not to be used on claims billing for non-covered OIVIT and any services comprising an OIVIT regimen when furnished pursuant to an OIVIT regimen. Claims billing for HCPCS codes 99199 and 94681 for non-covered OIVIT are to be returned to provider/returned as unprocessable.

100-4, 4, 320.2

Outpatient Intravenous Insulin Treatment (OIVIT)

Effective for claims with dates of service on and after December 23, 2009, the Centers for Medicare and Medicaid Services (CMS) determines that the evidence does not support a conclusion that OIVIT improves health outcomes in Medicare beneficiaries. Therefore, CMS has determined that OIVIT is not reasonable and necessary for any indication under section 1862(a)(1)(A) of the Social Security Act. Services comprising an OIVIT regimen are nationally non-covered under Medicare when furnished pursuant to an OIVIT regimen.

See Pub. 100-03, Medicare National Coverage Determinations Manual, Section 40.7, Outpatient Intravenous Insulin Treatment (Effective December 23, 2009), for general information and coverage indications.

100-4, 5, 10

Part B Outpatient Rehabilitation and Comprehensive Outpatient Rehabilitation Facility (CORF) Services - General

Language in this section is defined or described in Pub. 100-02, chapter 15, sections 220 and 230.

Section 4541(a)(2) of the Balanced Budget Act (BBA) (P.L. 105-33), which added §1834(k)(5) to the Social Security Act (the Act), required that all claims for outpatient rehabilitation services and comprehensive outpatient rehabilitation facility (CORF) services, be reported using a uniform coding system. The CMS chose HCPCS (Healthcare Common Procedure Coding System) as the coding system to be used for the reporting of these services. This coding requirement is effective for all claims for outpatient rehabilitation services and CORF services submitted on or after April 1, 1998.

The BBA also required payment under a prospective payment system for outpatient rehabilitation services including CORF services. Effective for claims with dates of service on or after January 1, 1999, the Medicare Physician Fee Schedule (MPFS) became the method of payment for outpatient therapy services furnished by:

- Comprehensive outpatient rehabilitation facilities (CORFs);
- Outpatient physical therapy providers (OPTs);
- Other rehabilitation facilities (ORFs);
- Hospitals (to outpatients and inpatients who are not in a covered Part A stay);
- Skilled nursing facilities (SNFs) (to residents not in a covered Part A stay and to nonresidents who receive outpatient rehabilitation services from the SNF); and
- Home health agencies (HHAs) (to individuals who are not homebound or otherwise are not receiving services under a home health plan of care (POC)).

NOTE: No provider or supplier other than the SNF will be paid for therapy services during the time the beneficiary is in a covered SNF Part A stay. For information regarding SNF consolidated billing see chapter 6, section 10 of this manual.

Similarly, under the HH prospective payment system, HHAs are responsible to provide, either directly or under arrangements, all outpatient rehabilitation therapy services to beneficiaries receiving services under a home health POC. No other provider or supplier will be paid for these services during the time the beneficiary is in a covered Part A stay. For information regarding HH consolidated billing see chapter10, section 20 of this manual.

Section 143 of the Medicare Improvements for Patients and Provider's Act of 2008 (MIPPA) authorizes the Centers for Medicare & Medicaid Services (CMS) to enroll speech-language pathologists (SLP) as suppliers of Medicare services and for SLPs to begin billing Medicare for outpatient speech-language pathology services furnished in private practice beginning July 1, 2009. Enrollment will allow SLPs in private practice to bill Medicare and receive direct payment for their services. Previously, the Medicare program could only pay SLP services if an institution, physician or nonphysician practitioner billed them.

In Chapter 23, as part of the CY 2009 Medicare Physician Fee Schedule Database, the descriptor for PC/TC indicator "7", as applied to certain HCPCS/CPT codes, is described as specific to the services of privately practicing therapists. Payment may not be made if the service is provided to either a hospital outpatient or a hospital inpatient by a physical therapist, occupational therapist, or speech-language pathologist in private practice.

The MPFS is used as a method of payment for outpatient rehabilitation services furnished under arrangement with any of these providers.

In addition, the MPFS is used as the payment system for CORF services identified by the HCPCS codes in §20. Assignment is mandatory.

The Medicare allowed charge for the services is the lower of the actual charge or the MPFS amount. The Medicare payment for the services is 80 percent of the allowed charge after the Part B deductible is met. Coinsurance is made at 20 percent of the lower of the actual charge or the MPFS amount. The general coinsurance rule (20 percent of the actual charges) does not apply when making payment under the MPFS. This is a final payment.

The MPFS does not apply to outpatient rehabilitation services furnished by critical access hospitals (CAHs). CAHs are to be paid on a reasonable cost basis.

Contractors process outpatient rehabilitation claims from hospitals, including CAHs, SNFs, HHAs, CORFs, outpatient rehabilitation agencies, and outpatient physical therapy providers for which they have received a tie in notice from the RO. These provider types submit their claims to the contractors using the 837 Institutional electronic claim format or the UB-04 paper form when permissible. Contractors also process claims from physicians, certain nonphysician practitioners (NPPs), therapists in private practices (TPPs), (which are limited to physical and occupational therapists, and speech-language pathologists in private practices), and physician-directed clinics that bill for services furnished incident to a physician's service (see Pub. 100-02, Medicare Benefit Policy Manual, chapter 15, for a definition of "incident to"). These provider types submit their claims to the contractor using the 837 Professional electronic claim format or the CMS-1500 paper form when permissible.

There are different fee rates for nonfacility and facility services. Chapter 23 describes the differences in these two rates. (See fields 28 and 29 of the record therein described). Facility rates apply to professional services performed in a facility other than the professional's office. Nonfacility rates apply when the service is performed in the professional's office. The nonfacility rate (that is paid when the provider performs the services in its own facility) accommodates overhead and indirect expenses the provider incurs by operating its own facility. Thus it is somewhat higher than the facility rate.

Contractors pay the nonfacility rate on institutional claims for services performed in the provider's facility. Contractors may pay professional claims using the facility or nonfacility rate depending upon where the service is performed (place of service on the claim), and the provider specialty.

Contractors pay the codes in §20 under the MPFS on professional claims regardless of whether they may be considered rehabilitation services. However, contractors must use this list for institutional claims to determine whether to pay under outpatient rehabilitation rules or whether payment rules for other types of service may apply, e.g., OPPS for hospitals, reasonable costs for CAHs.

Note that because a service is considered an outpatient rehabilitation service does not automatically imply payment for that service. Additional criteria, including coverage, plan of care and physician certification must also be met. These criteria are described in Pub. 100-02, Medicare Benefit Policy Manual, chapters 1 and 15.

Payment for rehabilitation services provided to Part A inpatients of hospitals or SNFs is included in the respective PPS rate. Also, for SNFs (but not hospitals), if the beneficiary has Part B, but not Part A coverage (e.g., Part A benefits are exhausted), the SNF must bill for any rehabilitation service.

Payment for rehabilitation therapy services provided by home health agencies under a home health plan of care is included in the home health PPS rate. HHAs may submit bill type 34X and be paid under the MPFS if there are no home health services billed under a home health plan of care at the same time, and there is a valid rehabilitation POC (e.g., the patient is not homebound).

An institutional employer (other than a SNF) of the TPPs, or physician performing outpatient services, (e.g., hospital, CORF, etc.), or a clinic billing on behalf of the physician or therapist may bill the contractor on a professional claim.

The MPFS is the basis of payment for outpatient rehabilitation services furnished by TPPs, physicians, and certain nonphysician practitioners or for diagnostic tests provided incident to the services of such physicians or nonphysician practitioners. (See Pub. 100-02, Medicare Benefit Policy Manual, chapter 15, for a definition of "incident to, therapist, therapy and related instructions.") Such services are billed to the contractor on the professional claim format. Assignment is mandatory.

The following table identifies the provider and supplier types, and identifies which claim format they may use to submit bills to the contractor. "Provider/Supplier Service" Type

Format	*Bill Type*	*Comment*
Inpatient hospital Part A Institutional	11X	Included in PPS
Inpatient SNF Part A Institutional	21X	Included in PPS
Inpatient hospital Part B Institutional	12X	Hospitals may obtain services under arrangements and bill, or rendering provider may bill.
Inpatient SNF Part B (audiology tests are not included) Institutional	22X	SNF must provide and bill, or obtain under arrangements and bill.
Outpatient hospital Institutional	13X	Hospital may provide and bill or obtain under arrangements and bill, or rendering provider may bill.

Format	*Bill Type*	*Comment*
Outpatient SNF Institutional	23X	SNF must provide and bill or obtain under arrangements and bill.
HHA billing for services rendered under a Part A or Part B home health plan of care. Institutional	32X	Service is included in PPS rate. CMS determines whether payment is from Part A or Part B trust fund.
HHA billing for services not rendered under a Part A or Part B home health plan of care, but rendered under a therapy plan of care. Institutional	34X	Service not under home health plan of care.
Other Rehabilitation Facility (ORF) Institutional	74X	Paid MPFS for outpatient rehabilitation services effective January 1, 1999, and all other services except drugs effective July 1, 2000. Starting April 1, 2002, drugs are paid 95% of the AWP. For claims with dates of service on or after July 1, 2003, drugs and biologicals do not apply in an OPT setting. Therefore, FIs are to advise their OPTs not to bill for them.
Comprehensive Outpatient Rehabilitation Facility (CORF) Institutional	75X	Paid MPFS for outpatient rehabilitation services effective January 1, 1999, and all other services except drugs effective July 1, 2000. Starting April 1, 2002, drugs are paid 95% of the AWP.
Physician, NPPs, TPPs, (service in hospital or SNF) Professional	See Chapter 26 for place of service, and type of service coding.	Payment may not be made for therapy services to Part A inpatients of hospitals or SNFs, or for Part B SNF residents. Otherwise, suppliers bill to the contractor using the professional claim format. Note that services of a physician/ NPP/TPP employee of a facility may be billed by the facility to a contractor.
Physician/NPP/TPPs office, independent clinic or patient's home Professional	See Chapter 26 for place of service, and type of service coding.	Paid via Physician fee schedule.
Critical Access Hospital - inpatient Part A Institutional	11X	Rehabilitation services are paid at cost.
Critical Access Hospital - inpatient Part B Institutional	85X	Rehabilitation services are paid at cost.
Critical Access Hospital – outpatient Part B Institutional	85X	Rehabilitation services are paid at cost.

Complete Claim form completion requirements are contained in chapters 25 and 26.

For a list of the outpatient rehabilitation HCPCS codes see §20.

If a contractor receives an institutional claim for one of these HCPCS codes with dates of service on or after July 1, 2003, that does not appear on the supplemental file it currently uses to pay the therapy claims, it contacts its professional claims area to obtain the non-facility price in order to pay the claim.

NOTE: The list of codes in §20 contains commonly utilized codes for outpatient rehabilitation services. Contractors may consider other codes on institutional claims for payment under the MPFS as outpatient rehabilitation services to the extent that such codes are determined to be medically reasonable and necessary and could be performed within the scope of practice of the therapist providing the service.

100-4, 5, 10.2

The Financial Limitation

A. Financial Limitation Prior to the Balanced Budget Refinement Act (BBRA)

Section 4541(a)(2) of the Balanced Budget Act (BBA) (P.L. 105-33) of 1997, which added Sec.1834(k)(5) to the Act, required payment under a prospective payment system for outpatient rehabilitation services (except those furnished by or under arrangements with a hospital). Outpatient rehabilitation services include the following services: Physical therapy (which includes outpatient speech-language pathology); and Occupational therapy.

Section 4541(c) of the BBA required application of a financial limitation to all outpatient rehabilitation services (except those furnished by or under arrangements with a hospital). In 1999, an annual per beneficiary limit of $1,500 applied to all outpatient physical therapy services (including speech-language pathology services). A separate limit applied to all occupational therapy services. The limit is based on incurred expenses and includes applicable deductible and coinsurance. The BBA provided that the limits be indexed by the Medicare Economic Index (MEI) each year beginning in 2002.

The limitation is based on therapy services the Medicare beneficiary receives, not the type of practitioner who provides the service. Physical therapists, speech-language pathologists, occupational therapists as well as physicians and certain nonphysician practitioners could render a therapy service.

As a transitional measure, effective in 1999, providers/suppliers were instructed to keep track of the allowed incurred expenses. This process was put in place to assure providers/suppliers did not bill Medicare for patients who exceeded the annual limitations for physical therapy, and for occupational therapy services rendered by individual providers/suppliers. In 2003 and later, the limitation was applied through CMS systems.

B. Moratoria and Exceptions for Therapy Claims

Section 221 of the BBRA of 1999 placed a 2-year moratorium on the application of the financial limitation for claims for therapy services with dates of service January 1, 2000, through December 31, 2001.

Section 421 of the Medicare, Medicaid, and SCHIP Benefits Improvement and Protection Act (BIPA) of 2000, extended the moratorium on application of the financial limitation to claims for outpatient rehabilitation services with dates of service January 1, 2002, through December 31, 2002. Therefore, the moratorium was for a 3-year period and applied to outpatient rehabilitation claims with dates of service January 1, 2000, through December 31, 2002.

In 2003, there was not a moratorium on therapy caps. Implementation was delayed until September 1, 2003. Therapy caps were in effect for services rendered on September 1, 2003 through December 7, 2003.

Congress re-enacted a moratorium on financial limitations on outpatient therapy services on December 8, 2003 that extended through December 31, 2005. Caps were implemented again on January 1, 2006 and policies were modified to allow exceptions as directed by the Deficit Reduction Act of 2005 only for calendar year 2006. The Tax Relief and Health Care Act of 2006 extended the cap exceptions process through calendar year 2007. The Medicare, Medicaid, and SCHIP Extension Act of 2007 extended the cap exceptions process for services furnished through June 30, 2008. The Medicare Improvements for Patients and Providers Act of 2008 extended the exceptions process from July 1, 2008 through December 31, 2009.

Future exceptions. The cap exception for therapy services billed by outpatient hospitals was part of the original legislation and applies as long as caps are in effect. Exceptions to caps based on the medical necessity of the service are in effect only when Congress legislates the exceptions, as noted above.

References to the exceptions process in subsection C of this section apply only when the exceptions are in effect.

C. Application of Financial Limitations

Financial limitations on outpatient therapy services, as described above, began for therapy services rendered on or after on January 1, 2006. See C 1 to C 7 of this section when exceptions to therapy caps apply. The limits were $1740 in 2006 and $1780 in 2007, $1810 for 2008, and $1840 for 2009. For 2010, the annual limit on the allowed amount for outpatient physical therapy and speech-language pathology combined is $1860; the limit for occupational therapy is $1860. Limits apply to outpatient Part B therapy services from all settings except outpatient hospital and hospital emergency room. These excluded hospital services are reported on types of bill 12x or 13x, or 85x.

Contractors apply the financial limitations to the Medicare Physician Fee Schedule (MPFS) amount (or the amount charged if it is smaller) for therapy services for each beneficiary.

As with any Medicare payment, beneficiaries pay the coinsurance (20 percent) and any deductible that may apply. Medicare will pay the remaining 80 percent of the limit after the deductible is met. These amounts will change each calendar year. Medicare Contractors shall publish the financial limitation amount in educational articles. It is also available at 1-800-Medicare.

Medicare shall apply these financial limitations in order, according to the dates when the claims were received. When limitations apply, the Common Working File (CWF) tracks the limits. Shared system maintainers are not responsible for tracking the dollar amounts of incurred expenses of rehabilitation services for each therapy limit.

In processing claims where Medicare is the secondary payer, the shared system takes the lowest secondary payment amount from MSPPAY and sends this amount on to CWF as the amount applied to therapy limits.

1. Exceptions to Therapy Caps

   General The Deficit Reduction Act of 2005 directed CMS to develop exceptions to therapy caps for calendar year 2006 and those exceptions have been extended several times by subsequent legislation. The following policies concerning exceptions to caps due to medical necessity apply only when the exceptions process is in effect. With the exception of the use of the KX modifier, the guidance in this section concerning medical necessity applies as well to services provided before caps are reached.

Instructions for contractors to manage automatic process for exceptions will be found in the Program Integrity Manual, chapter 3, section 3.4.1.2. Provider and supplier information concerning exceptions is in this manual and in IOM Pub. 100-02, chapter 15, section 220.3. Exceptions shall be identified by a modifier on the claim and supported by documentation.

Since the providers and suppliers will take an active role in obtaining an exception for a beneficiary, this manual section is written to address them as well as Medicare contractors.

The beneficiary may qualify for use of the cap exceptions at any time during the episode when documented medically necessary services exceed caps. All covered and medically necessary services qualify for exceptions to caps.

In 2006, the Exception Processes fell into two categories, Automatic Process Exceptions, and Manual Process Exceptions. Beginning January 1, 2007, there is no manual process for exceptions. All services that require exceptions to caps shall be processed using the automatic process. All requests for exception are in the form of a KX modifier added to claim lines. (See subsection C6 for use of the KX modifier.) Use of the automatic process for exceptions increases the responsibility of the provider/supplier for determining and documenting that services are appropriate.

Also, use of the automatic process for exception does not exempt services from manual or other medical review processes as described in Pub. 100-08, chapter 3, section 3.4.1.1.1. Rather, atypical use of the automatic exception process may invite contractor scrutiny. Particular care should be taken to document improvement and avoid billing for services that do not meet the requirements for skilled services, or for services which are maintenance rather than rehabilitative treatment (See Pub. 100-02, chapter 15, sections 220.2, 220.3, and 230).

The KX modifier, described in subsection C6, is added to claim lines to indicate that the clinician attests that services are medically necessary and justification is documented in the medical record.

2. Automatic Process Exceptions
The term "automatic process exceptions" indicates that the claims processing for the exception is automatic, and not that the exception is automatic. An exception may be made when the patient's condition is justified by documentation indicating that the beneficiary requires continued skilled therapy, i.e., therapy beyond the amount payable under the therapy cap, to achieve their prior functional status or maximum expected functional status within a reasonable amount of time.

No special documentation is submitted to the contractor for automatic process exceptions. The clinician is responsible for consulting guidance in the Medicare manuals and in the professional literature to determine if the beneficiary may qualify for the automatic process exception because documentation justifies medically necessary services above the caps. The clinician's opinion is not binding on the Medicare contractor who makes the final determination concerning whether the claim is payable.

Documentation justifying the services shall be submitted in response to any Additional Documentation Request (ADR) for claims that are selected for medical review. Follow the documentation requirements in Pub. 100-02, chapter 15, section 220.3. If medical records are requested for review, clinicians may include, at their discretion, a summary that specifically addresses the justification for therapy cap exception.

In making a decision about whether to utilize the automatic process exception, clinicians shall consider, for example, whether services are appropriate to-- The patient's condition including the diagnosis, complexities and severity (A list of the excepted evaluation codes are in C.2.a. A list of the ICD-9 codes for conditions and complexities that might qualify a beneficiary for exception to caps is in 10.2 C3. The list is a guideline and neither assures that services on the list will be excepted nor limits provision of covered and medically necessary services for conditions not on the list); The services provided including their type, frequency and duration; The interaction of current active conditions and complexities that directly and significantly influence the treatment such that it causes services to exceed caps.

In addition, the following should be considered before using the automatic exception process: a. Exceptions for Services Evaluation. The CMS will except therapy evaluations from caps after the therapy caps are reached when evaluation is necessary, e.g., to determine if the current status of the beneficiary requires therapy services.

For example, the following evaluation procedures may be appropriate: 92506, 92597, 92607, 92608, 92610, 92611, 92612, 92614, 92616, 96105, 97001, 97002, 97003, 97004.

These codes will continue to be reported as outpatient therapy procedures as described in the Claims Processing Manual, Chapter 5, Section 20(B) "Applicable Outpatient Rehabilitation HCPCS Codes." They are not diagnostic tests. Definition of evaluations and documentation is found in Pub. 100-02, sections 220 and 230.

Other Services. There are a number of sources that suggest the amount of certain services that may be typical, either per service, per episode, per condition, or per discipline. For example, see the CSC - Therapy Cap Report, 3/21/2008, and CSC - Therapy Edits Tables 4/14/2008 at www.cms.hhs.gov/TherapyServices (Studies and Reports). Professional literature and guidelines from professional associations also provide a basis on which to estimate whether the type, frequency and intensity of services are appropriate to an individual. Clinicians and contractors should utilize available evidence related to the patient's condition to justify provision of medically necessary services to individual beneficiaries, especially when they exceed caps. Contractors shall not limit medically necessary services that are justified by scientific research applicable to the beneficiary. Neither contractors nor clinicians shall utilize professional literature and scientific reports to justify payment for continued services after an individual's goals have been met earlier than is typical. Conversely, professional literature and scientific reports shall not be used as justification to deny payment to patients whose needs are greater than is typical or when the patient's condition is not represented by the literature.

b. Exceptions for Conditions or Complexities Identified by ICD-9 codes.
Clinicians may utilize the automatic process for exception for any diagnosis for which they can justify services exceeding the cap. Based upon analysis of claims data, research and evidence based practice guidelines, CMS has identified conditions and complexities represented by ICD-9 codes that may be more likely than others to require therapy services that exceed therapy caps. This list appears in 10.2 C3.

Clinicians may use the automatic process of exception for beneficiaries who do not have a condition or complexity on this list when they justify the provision of therapy services that exceed caps for that patient's condition.

Not all patients who have a condition or complexity on the list are "automatically" excepted from therapy caps. See Pub. 100-02, chapter 15, section 230.3 for documenting the patient's condition and complexities. Contractors may scrutinize claims from providers whose services exceed caps more frequently than is typical.

Regardless of the condition, the patient must also meet other requirements for coverage. For example, the patient must require skilled treatment for a covered, medically necessary service; the services must be appropriate in type, frequency and duration for the patient's condition and service must be documented appropriately. Guidelines for utilization of therapy services may be found in Medicare manuals, local coverage determinations of Medicare contractors, and professional guidelines issued by associations and states.

Bill the most relevant diagnosis. As always, when billing for therapy services, the ICD-9 code that best relates to the reason for the treatment shall be on the claim, unless there is a compelling reason. For example, when a patient with diabetes is being treated for gait training due to amputation, the preferred diagnosis is abnormality of gait (which characterizes the treatment). Where it is possible in accordance with State and local laws and the contractors local coverage determinations, avoid using vague or general diagnoses. When a claim includes several types of services, or where the physician/NPP must supply the diagnosis, it may not be possible to use the most relevant therapy code in the primary position. In that case, the relevant code should, if possible, be on the claim in another position.

Codes representing the medical condition that caused the treatment are used when there is no code representing the treatment. Complicating conditions are preferably used in non-primary positions on the claim and are billed in the primary position only in the rare circumstance that there is no more relevant code.

The condition or complexity that caused treatment to exceed caps must be related to the therapy goals and must either be the condition that is being treated or a complexity that directly and significantly impacts the rate of recovery of the condition being treated such that it is appropriate to exceed the caps. Codes marked as complexities represented by ICD-9 codes on the list below are unlikely to require therapy services that would exceed the caps unless they occur in a patient who also has another condition (either listed or not listed). Therefore, documentation for an exception should indicate how the complexity (or combination of complexities) directly and significantly affects treatment for a therapy condition. For example, if the condition underlying the reason for therapy is V43.64, hip replacement, the treatment may have a goal to ambulate 60' with stand-by assistance and a KX modifier may be appropriate for gait training (assuming the severity of the patient is such that the services exceed the cap). Alternatively, it would not be appropriate to use the KX modifier for a patient who recovered from hip replacement last year and is being treated this year for a sprain of a severity which does not justify extensive therapy exceeding caps.

3. ICD-9 Codes That are More Likely to Qualify for the Automatic Process Therapy Cap Exception Based Upon Clinical Condition or Complexity When using this table, refer to the ICD-9 code book for coding instructions. Some contractors' local coverage determinations do not allow the use of some of the codes on this list in the primary diagnosis position on a claim. If the contractor has determined that these codes do not characterize patients who require medically necessary services, providers/suppliers may not use these codes, but must utilize a billable diagnosis code allowed by their contractor to describe the patient's condition. Contractors shall not apply therapy caps to services based on the patient's condition, but only on the medical necessity of the service for the condition. If a service would be payable before the cap is reached and is still medically necessary after the cap is reached, that service is excepted. This list is illustrative and not exclusive.

Providers/suppliers may use the automatic process for exception for medically necessary services when the patient has a billable condition that is not on the list below. The diagnosis on the list below may be put in a secondary position on the claim and/or in the medical records, as the contractor directs.

When two codes are listed in the left cell in a row, all the codes between them are also eligible for exception. If one code is in the cell, only that one code is likely to qualify for exception. The descriptions in the table are not always identical to those in the ICD-9 code book, but may be summaries.

Contact your contractor for interpretation if you are not sure that a condition or complexity is applicable for automatic process exception.

It is very important to recognize that most of the conditions on this list would not ordinarily result in services exceeding the cap. Use the KX modifier only in cases where the condition of the individual patient is such that services are APPROPRIATELY provided in an episode that exceeds the cap. In most cases, the severity of the condition, comorbidities, or complexities will contribute to the necessity of services exceeding the cap, and these should be documented. Routine use of the KX modifier for all patients with these conditions will likely show up on data analysis as aberrant and invite inquiry. Be sure that documentation is sufficiently detailed to support the use of the modifier.

The following ICD-9 codes describe the conditions (etiology or underlying medical conditions) that may result in excepted conditions (marked X) and complexities (marked *) that MIGHT cause medically necessary therapy services to qualify for the automatic process exception for each discipline separately.

When the field corresponding to the therapy discipline treating and the diagnosis code is marked with a dash (-) services by that discipline are not appropriate for that diagnosis and, therefore, services do not qualify for exception to caps.

These codes are grouped only to facilitate reference to them. The codes may be used only when the code is applicable to the condition being actively treated. For example, an exception should not be claimed for a diagnosis of hip replacement when the service provided is for an unrelated dysphagia.

ICD-9 Cluster	ICD-9 (Cluster) Description	PT	OT	SLP
V43.61-V43.69	Joint Replacement	X	X	--
V45.4	Arthrodesis Status	*	*	--
V45.81-V45.82 and V45.89	Other Postprocedural Status	*	*	--
V49.61-V49.67	Upper Limb Amputation Status	X	X	--
V49.71-V49.77	Lower Limb Amputation Status	X	X	--
V54.10-V54.29	Aftercare for Healing Traumatic or Pathologic Fracture	X	X	--
V58.71-V58.78	Aftercare Following Surgery to Specified Body Systems, Not Elsewhere Classified	*	*	*
244.0-244.9	Acquired Hypothyroidism	*	*	*
250.00-251.9	Diabetes Mellitus and Other Disorders of Pancreatic Internal Secretion	*	*	*
276.0-276.9	Disorders of Fluid, Electrolyte, and Acid- Base Balance	*	*	*
278.00-278.01	Obesity and Morbid Obesity	*	*	*
280.0-289.9	Diseases of the blood and blood-forming organs	*	*	*
290.0-290.43	Dementias	*	*	*
294.0-294.9	Persistent Mental Disorders due to Conditions Classified Elsewhere	*	*	*
295.00-299.91	Other Psychoses	*	*	*
300.00-300.9	Anxiety, Disassociative and Somatoform Disorders	*	*	*
310.0-310.9	Specific Nonpsychotic Mental Disorders due to Brain Damage	*	*	*
311	Depressive Disorder, Not Elsewhere Classified	*	*	*
315.00-315.9	Specific delays in Development	*	*	*
317	Mild Mental Retardation	*	*	*
320.0-326	Inflammatory Diseases of the Central Nervous System	*	*	*
330.0-337.9	Hereditary and Degenerative Diseases of the Central Nervous System	X	X	X
340-345.91 and 348.0-349.9	Other Disorders of the Central Nervous System	X	X	X
353.0-359.9	Disorders of the Peripheral Nervous system	X	X	--
365.00-365.9	Glaucoma	*	*	*
369.00-369.9	Blindness and Low Vision	*	*	*
386.00-386.9	Vertiginous Syndromes and Other Disorders of Vestibular System	*	*	*
389.00-389.9	Hearing Loss	*	*	*
401.0-405.99	Hypertensive Disease	*	*	*
410.00-414.9	Ischemic Heart Disease	*	*	*
415.0-417.9	Diseases of Pulmonary Circulation	*	*	*
420.0-429.9	Other Forms of Heart Disease	*	*	*
430-438.9	Cerebrovascular Disease	X	X	X
440.0-448.9	Diseases of Arteries, Arterioles, and Capillaries	*	*	*
451.0-453.9 and 456.0-459.9	Diseases of Veins and Lymphatics, and Other Diseases of Circulatory System	*	*	*
465.0-466.19	Acute Respiratory Infections	*	*	*
478.30-478.5	Paralysis, Polyps, or Other Diseases of Vocal Cords	*	*	*
480.0-486	Pneumonia	*	*	*
490-496	Chronic Obstructive Pulmonary Disease and Allied Conditions	*	*	*
507.0-507.8	Pneumonitis due to solids and liquids	*	*	*

X Automatic (only ICD-9 needed on claim)
* Complexity (requires another ICD-9 on claim)
-- Does not serve as qualifying ICD-9 on claim

ICD-9 Cluster	ICD-9 (Cluster) Description	PT	OT	SLP
510.0-519.9	Other Diseases of Respiratory System	*	*	*
560.0-560.9	Intestinal Obstruction Without Mention of Hernia	*	*	*
578.0-578.9	Gastrointestinal Hemorrhage	*	*	*
584.5-586	Renal Failure and Chronic Kidney Disease	*	*	*
590.00-599.9	Other Diseases of Urinary System	*	*	*
682.0-682.8	Other Cellulitis and Abscess	*	*	--
707.00-707.9	Chronic Ulcer of Skin	*	*	--
710.0-710.9	Diffuse Diseases of Connective Tissue	*	*	*
711.00-711.99	Arthropathy Associated with Infections	*	*	--
712.10-713.8	Crystal Arthropathies and Arthropathy Associated with Other Disorders Classified Elsewhere	*	*	--
714.0-714.9	Rheumatoid Arthritis and Other Inflammatory Polyarthropathies	*	*	--
715.00-715.98	Osteoarthrosis and Allied Disorders (Complexity except as listed below)	*	*	--
715.09	Osteoarthritis and allied disorders, multiple sites	X	X	--
715.11	Osteoarthritis, localized, primary, shoulder region	X	X	--
715.15	Osteoarthritis, localized, primary, pelvic region and thigh	X	X	--
715.16	Osteoarthritis, localized, primary, lower leg	X	X	--
715.91	Osteoarthritis, unspecified id gen. or local, shoulder	X	X	--
715.96	Osteoarthritis, unspecified if gen. or local, lower leg	X	X	--
716.00-716.99	Other and Unspecified Arthropathies	*	*	--
717.0-717.9	Internal Derangement of Knee	*	*	--
718.00-718.99	Other Derangement of Joint (Complexity except as listed below)	*	*	--
718.49	Contracture of Joint, Multiple Sites	X	X -	-
719.00-719.99	Other and Unspecified Disorders of Joint (Complexity except as listed below)	*	*	--
719.7	Difficulty Walking	X	X	--
720.0-724.9	Dorsopathies	*	*	--
725-729.9	Rheumatism, Excluding Back (Complexity except as listed below)	*	*	--
726.10-726.19	Rotator Cuff Disorder and Allied Syndromes	X	X	--
727.61-727.62	Rupture of Tendon, Nontraumatic	X	X	--
730.00-739.9	Osteopathies, Chondropathies, and Acquired Musculoskeletal Deformities (Complexity except as listed below)	*	*	--
733.00	Osteoporosis	X	X	--
741.00-742.9 and 745.0-748.9 and 754.0-756.9	Congenital Anomalies	*	*	*
780.31-780.39	Convulsions	*	*	*
780.71-780.79	Malaise and Fatigue	*	*	*
780.93	Memory Loss	*	*	*
781.0-781.99	Symptoms Involving Nervous and Musculoskeletal System (Complexity except as listed below)	*	*	*
781.2	Abnormality of Gait	X	X	--
781.3	Lack of Coordination	X	X	--
783.0-783.9	Symptoms Concerning Nutrition, Metabolism, and Development	*	*	*
784.3-784.69	Aphasia, Voice and Other Speech Disturbance, Other Symbolic Dysfunction	*	*	X
785.4	Gangrene	*	*	--

X Automatic (only ICD-9 needed on claim)
* Complexity (requires another ICD-9 on claim)
-- Does not serve as qualifying ICD-9 on claim

ICD-9 Cluster	ICD-9 (Cluster) Description	PT	OT	SLP
786.00-786.9	Symptoms involving Respiratory System and Other Chest Symptoms	*	*	*
787.2	Dysphagia	*	*	X
800.00-828.1	Fractures (Complexity except as listed below)	*	*	--
806.00-806.9	Fracture of Vertebral Column With Spinal Cord Injury	X	X	--
810.11-810.13	Fracture of Clavicle	X	X	--
811.00-811.19	Fracture of Scapula	X	X	--
812.00-812.59	Fracture of Humerus	X	X	--
813.00-813.93	Fracture of Radius and Ulna	X	X	--
820.00-820.9	Fracture of Neck of Femur	X	X	--
821.00-821.39	Fracture of Other and Unspecified Parts of Femur	X	X -	-
828.0-828.1	Multiple Fractures Involving Both Lower Limbs, Lower with Upper Limb, and Lower Limb(s) with Rib(s) and Sternum	X	X	--
830.0-839.9	Dislocations	X	X	--
840.0-848.8	Sprains and Strains of Joints and Adjacent Muscles	*	*	--
851.00-854.19	Intracranial Injury, excluding those With Skull Fracture	X	X	X
880.00-884.2	Open Wound of Upper Limb	*	*	--
885.0-887.7	Traumatic Amputation, Thumb(s), Finger(s), Arm and Hand (complete)(partial)	X	X	--
890.0-894.2	Open Wound Lower Limb	*	*	--
895.0-897.7	Traumatic Amputation, Toe(s), Foot/Feet, Leg(s) (complete)(partial)	X	X	--
905.0-905.9	Late Effects of Musculoskeletal and Connective Tissue Injuries	*	*	*
907.0-907.9	Late Effects of Injuries to the Nervous System	*	*	*
941.00-949.5	Burns	*	*	*
952.00-952.9	Spinal Cord Injury Without Evidence of Spinal Bone Injury	X	X	X
953.0-953.8	Injury to Nerve Roots and Spinal Plexus	X	X	*
959.01	Head Injury, Unspecified	X	X	X

X Automatic (only ICD-9 needed on claim)
* Complexity (requires another ICD-9 on claim)
-- Does not serve as qualifying ICD-9 on claim

4. Additional Considerations for Exceptions In justifying exceptions for therapy caps, clinicians and contractors should not only consider the medical diagnoses and medical complications that might directly and significantly influence the amount of treatment required. Other variables (such as the availability of a caregiver at home) that affect appropriate treatment shall also be considered. Factors that influence the need for treatment should be supportable by published research, clinical guidelines from professional sources, and/or clinical/common sense. See Pub. 100-02, chapter 15, section 230.3 subsections related to documentation of the evaluation, and section 220.2 on medical necessity for some factors that complicate treatment.

Note that the patient's lack of access to outpatient hospital therapy services alone does not justify excepted services. Residents of skilled nursing facilities prevented by consolidated billing from accessing hospital services, debilitated patients for whom transportation to the hospital is a physical hardship or lack of therapy services at hospitals in the beneficiary's county may or may not qualify for continued services above the caps. The patient's condition and complexities might justify extended services, but their location does not.

5. Appeals Related to Disapproval of Cap Exceptions Disapproval of Exception from Caps.

The DRA allows that certain services that would not be covered due to caps, but are medically necessary, may be covered. Therefore, when a service beyond the cap is determined to be medically necessary, it is covered and payable. But, when a service provided beyond the cap (outside the benefit) is determined to be NOT medically necessary, it is denied as a benefit category denial. Contractors may review claims with KX modifiers to determine whether the services are medically necessary, or for other reasons. Services that exceed therapy caps but do not meet Medicare criteria for medically necessary services are not payable even when clinicians recommend and furnish and these services.

Services without a Medicare benefit may be billed to Medicare with a GY modifier for the purpose of obtaining a denial that can be used with other insurers. See Pub. 100-04, chapter 1, section 60 for appropriate use of modifiers.

APPEALS -If a beneficiary whose excepted services do not meet the Medicare criteria for medical necessity elects to receive such services and a claim is submitted for such services, the resulting determination would be subject to the administrative appeals process. Further details concerning appeals are found in Pub. 100-04, chapter 29.

6. Use of the KX Modifier for Therapy Cap Exceptions

When exceptions are in effect and when the beneficiary qualifies for a therapy cap exception, the provider shall add a KX modifier to the therapy HCPCS subject to the cap limits The KX modifier shall not be added to any line of service that is not a medically necessary service; this applies to services that, according to a Local Coverage Determination by the contractor, are not medically necessary services.

The codes subject to the therapy cap tracking requirements are listed in a table in the Claims Processing Manual, Pub. 100-04, chapter 5, section 20(B), "Applicable Outpatient Rehabilitation HCPCS Codes." The GN, GO, or GP therapy modifiers are currently required. In addition to the KX modifier, the GN, GP and GO modifiers shall continue to be used. Providers may report the modifiers on claims in any order.

If there is insufficient room on a claim line for multiple modifiers, additional modifiers may be reported in the remarks field. Follow the routine procedure for placing HCPCS modifiers on a claim as described below.

For professional claims, sent to the carrier or A/B Mac, refer to: o Pub.100-04, Medicare Claims Processing Manual, chapter 26, for more detail regarding completing the CMS- Form 1500 claim form, including the placement of HCPCS modifiers. Note that the CMS-Form1500 claim form currently has space for providing two modifiers in block 24D, but, if you have more than two to report, you can do so by placing the -99 modifier (which indicates multiple modifiers) in block 24D and placing the additional modifiers in block 19.

You may access the Medicare Claims Processing Manual at this web address http://www.cms.hhs.gov/Manuals/ From this site, click the links to Internet-Only Manuals (IOMs), then Pub. 100-04, to reach the Medicare Claims Processing Manual.

- The ASC X12N 837 Health Care Claim: Professional Implementation Guide, Version 4010A1, for more detail regarding how to electronically submit a health care claim transaction, including the placement of HCPCS modifiers. The ASC X12N 837 implementation guides are the standards adopted under the Health Insurance Portability and Accountability Act of 1996 (HIPAA) for submitting health care claims electronically. The 837 professional transaction currently permits the placement of up to four modifiers, in the 2400 loop, SV1 segment, data elements SV101-3, SV101-4, SV101-5, and SV101-6. You may obtain copies of the ASC X12N 837 implementation guides from the Washington Publishing Company.
- For claims paid to carrier or A/B Mac, it is only appropriate to use a KX for a service that reasonably may exceed the cap. Use of the KX modifier when there is no indication that the cap is likely to be exceeded is abusive. For example, use of the KX modifier for low cost services early in an episode when there is no evidence of a previous episode that might have exceeded the cap is inappropriate.

For institutional claims, sent to the FI: When the cap is exceeded by at least one line on the claim, use the KX modifier on all of the lines on that institutional claim that refer to the same therapy cap (PT/SLP or, OT,) regardless of whether the other services exceed the cap. For example, if one PT service line exceeds the cap, use the KX on all the PT and SLP service lines (also identified with the GP or GN modifier) for that claim. (When the PT/SLP cap is exceeded by PT services, the SLP lines on the claim may meet the requirements for an exception due to the complexity of two episodes of service. Use the KX on either all or none of the SLP lines on the claim, as appropriate.) In contrast, if all the OT lines on the claim are below the cap, do not use the KX modifier on any of the OT lines, even when the KX is appropriately used on all of the PT lines.

Refer to Pub.100-04 Medicare Claims Processing Manual, chapter 25, for more detail .

You may access the Medicare Claims Processing Manual at this web address http://www.cms.hhs.gov/Manuals/. From this site, click the links to Internet-Only Manuals (IOMs), then Pub. 100-04 to reach the Medicare Claims Processing Manual.

By attaching the KX modifier, the provider is attesting that the services billed: Are reasonable and necessary services that require the skills of a therapist; (See Pub. 100- 02, chapter 15, section 220.2); and Are justified by appropriate documentation in the medical record, (See Pub. 100-02, chapter 15, section 220.3); and Qualify for an exception using the automatic process exception.

If this attestation is determined to be inaccurate, the provider/supplier is subject to sanctions resulting from providing inaccurate information on a claim.

When the KX modifier is attached to a therapy HCPCS, the contractor will override the CWF system reject for services that exceed the caps and pay the claim if it is otherwise payable.

Providers and suppliers shall continue to attach correct coding initiative (CCI) HCPCS modifiers under current instructions.

If a claim is submitted without KX modifiers and the cap is exceeded, those services will be denied. In cases where the KX would have been appropriate, contractors may reopen and/or adjust the claim, if it is brought to their attention.

Services billed after the cap has been exceeded which are not eligible for exceptions may be billed for the purpose of obtaining a denial using condition code 21.

D. MSN Messages Existing

MSN message 38.18 shall continue to appear on all Medicare MSN forms. It has been updated to the following: ALERT: Coverage by Medicare is limited to $1840 for 2009 and $1860 for 2010 for outpatient physical therapy and speech-language pathology combined. Occupational therapy services have the same limits. Medicare pays up to 80 percent of the limits after the deductible has been met. Exceptions to these limits apply to therapy billed by hospital outpatient departments and may also apply to medically necessary services.

Spanish Translation: ALERTA: La cobertura de Medicare se limita a $1,840 en el 2009 y a $1860 en el 2010 para los servicios combinados de terapia física ambulatoria y terapia de patología del habla. Los servicios de terapia ocupacional tienen los mismos límites. Medicare paga hasta 80 por ciento de los límites despues de que se haya pagado el deducible. Estos límites no se aplican a terapia que usted obtenga en los departamentos de hospital para paciente ambulatorio, y pueden tambien aplicarse a los servicios medicamente necesarios.

Existing MSN messages 17.13, 17.18 and 17.19 shall be issued on all claims containing outpatient rehabilitation services as noted in this manual. Add applied amount for individual beneficiaries and the generic limit amount (e.g., $1740 in 2006, $1780 in 2007, $1810 in 2008, $1840 in 2009, and $1860 in 2010) to all MSN that require them.

17.13 - Medicare approves a limited dollar amount each year for physical therapy and speechlanguage pathology services and a separate limit each year for occupational therapy services when billed by providers, physical and occupational therapists, physicians, and other non-physician practitioners.

Medically necessary therapy over these limits is covered when received at a hospital outpatient department or when approved by Medicare.

Spanish Translation 17.13 Cada año, Medicare aprueba una cantidad límite por servicios de terapia física y patología del lenguaje. Anualmente tambien aprueba otra cantidad límite por servicios de terapia ocupacional cuando son facturados por proveedores, terapistas físicos y ocupacionales, medicos y otros practicantes no medicos. La terapia que es medicamente necesaria y que sobrepasa estas cantidades límites esta cubierta cuando se recibe en una unidad de hospital ambulatorio o cuando esta aprobada por Medicare.

17.18 - ($) has been applied during this calendar year (CCYY) towards the ($) limit on outpatient physical therapy and speech-language pathology benefits.

Spanish Translation 17.18 - En este año (CCYY), ($) han sido deducidos de la cantidad límite de ($) por los beneficios de terapia física ambulatoria y de patología del lenguage hablado.

17.19 ($) has been applied during this calendar year (CCYY) towards the ($) limit on outpatient occupational therapy benefits.

Spanish Translation 17.19 - En este año (CCYY), ($) han sido deducidos de la cantidad límite de ($) por los beneficios de terapia ocupacional ambulatoria.

Contractors shall use the existing Medicare Summary Notice message 17.6 to inform the beneficiaries that they have reached the financial limitation. Apply this message at the line level: 17.6 - Full payment was not made for this service because the yearly limit has been met.

Spanish Translation 17.6 - Debido a que usted alcanzó su límite anual por este servicio, no se hara un pago completo.

E. FI Requirements

1. General Requirements Regardless of financial limits on therapy services, CMS requires modifiers (See Sec. 20.1 of this chapter) on specific codes for the purpose of data analysis. Edit to ensure that the therapy modifiers are present on a claim based on the presence of revenue codes 042X, 043X, or 044X. Claims containing revenue codes 042X, 043X, or 044X without a therapy modifier GN, GP, or GO should be returned to the provider.

Beneficiaries may not be simultaneously covered by Medicare as an outpatient of a hospital and as a patient in another facility. They must be discharged from the other setting and registered as a hospital outpatient in order to receive payment for outpatient rehabilitation services in a hospital outpatient setting after the limitation has been reached.

A hospital may bill for services of a facility as hospital outpatient services if that facility meets the requirements of a department of the provider (hospital) under 42 CFR 413.65. Facilities that do not meet those requirements are not considered to be part of the hospital and may not bill under the hospital's provider number, even if they are owned by the hospital. For example, services of a Comprehensive Outpatient Rehabilitation Facility (CORF) must be billed as CORF services and not a hospital outpatient services, even if the CORF is owned by the hospital. Only services billed by the hospital as bill type 12X or 13X are exempt from limitations on therapy services.

2. When Financial Limits Are in Effect
The CWF applies the financial limitation to the following bill types 22X, 23X, 34X, 74X and 75X using the MPFS allowed amount (before adjustment for beneficiary liability).

For SNFs, the financial limitation does apply to rehabilitation services furnished to those SNF residents in noncovered stays (bill type 22X) who are in a Medicare-certified section of the facility-i.e., one that is either certified by Medicare alone, or is dually certified (by Medicare as a SNF and by Medicaid as a nursing facility (NF). For SNF residents, consolidated billing requires all outpatient rehabilitation services be billed to Part B by the SNF. If a resident has reached the financial limitation, and remains in the Medicare-certified section of the SNF, no further payment will be made to the SNF or any other entity. Therefore, SNF residents who are subject to consolidated billing may not obtain services from an outpatient hospital after the cap has been exceeded.

Once the financial limitation has been reached, SNF residents who are in a non-Medicare certified section of the facility-i.e., one that is certified only by Medicaid as a NF or that is not certified at all by either program-FIs use bill type 23X. For SNF residents in non-Medicare certified portions of the facility and SNF nonresidents who go to the SNF for outpatient treatment (bill type 23X), medically necessary outpatient therapy may be covered at an outpatient hospital facility after the financial limitation has been exceeded.

Limitations do not apply for SNF residents in a covered Part A stay, including swing beds. Rehabilitation services are included within the global Part A per diem payment that the SNF receives under the PPS for the covered stay. Also, limitations do not apply to any therapy services billed under PPS Home Health, or inpatient hospitals including critical access hospitals.

F. Carrier or A/B Mac Requirements when Financial Limits are in Effect
Claims containing any of the "Applicable Outpatient Rehabilitation HCPCS Codes" in section 20 below marked "always therapy" (underlined) codes should contain one of the therapy modifiers (GN, GO, GP).

All claims submitted for codes underlined but without a therapy modifier shall be returned as unprocessable.

When any code on the list of "Applicable Outpatient Rehabilitation HCPCS Codes" codes are submitted with specialty codes "65" (physical therapist in private practice), and "67" (occupational therapist in private practice), they always represent therapy services, because they are provided by therapists. Carrier or A/B Mac shall return claims for these services when they do not contain therapy modifiers for the applicable HCPCS codes.

The "Applicable Outpatient Rehabilitation HCPCS Codes in section 20 of this chapter that are marked (+) are sometimes therapy codes. Claims from physicians (all specialty codes) and nonphysician practitioners, including specialty codes "50," "89," and "97" may be processed without therapy modifiers.

On review of these claims, services that are not accompanied by a therapy modifier must be documented, reasonable and necessary, and payable as physician or nonphysician practitioner services, and not services that the contractor interprets as therapy services.

The CWF will capture the amount and apply it to the limitation whenever a service is billed using the GN, GO, or GP modifier.

G. FI Action Based on CWF Trailer During the Time Therapy Limits are in Effect
Upon receipt of the CWF error code/trailer, FIs are responsible for assuring that payment does not exceed the financial limitations, when the limits are in effect, except as noted below.

In cases where a claim line partially exceeds the limit, the FI must adjust the line based on information contained in the CWF trailer. For example, where the MPFS allowed amount is greater than the financial limitation available, always report the MPFS allowed amount in the "Financial Limitation" field of the CWF record and include the CWF override code. See example below for situations where the claim contains multiple lines that exceed the limit.

EXAMPLE: Based on the 2009 limit of $1840 for a beneficiary who has paid the deductible and the coinsurance: Services received to date $1825 ($15 under the limit) Incoming claim: Line 1 MPFS allowed amount is $50.

Line 2 MPFS allowed amount is $25.

Line 3, MPFS allowed amount is $30.

Based on this example, lines 1 and 3 are denied and line 2 is paid. The FI reports in the "Financial Limitation" field of the CWF record "$25.00 along with the CWF override code. The FI always applies the amount that would least exceed the limit. Since the FI systems cannot split the payment on a line, CWF will allow payment on the line that least exceeds the limit and deny other lines.

H. Additional Information for Contractors During the Time Financial Limits Are in Effect With or Without Exceptions
Once the limit is reached, if a claim is submitted, CWF returns an error code stating the financial limitation has been met. Over applied lines will be identified at the line level. The outpatient rehabilitation therapy services that exceed the limit should be denied. The contractors use group code PR and claim adjustment reason code 119 - Benefit maximum for this time period or occurrence has been reached- in the provider remittance advice to establish the reason for denial.

In situations where a beneficiary is close to reaching the financial limitation and a particular claim might exceed the limitation, the provider/supplier should bill the usual and customary charges for the services furnished even though such charges might exceed the limit. The CWF will return an error code/trailer that will identify the line that exceeds the limitation.

Because CWF applies the financial limitation according to the date when the claim was received (when the date of service is within the effective date range for the limitation), it is possible that the financial limitation will have been met before the date of service of a given claim. Such claims will prompt the CWF error code and subsequent contractor denial.

When the provider/supplier knows that the limit has been reached, further billing should not occur. The provider/supplier should inform the beneficiary of the limit and their option of receiving further covered services from an outpatient hospital (unless consolidated billing rules prevent the use of the outpatient hospital setting). If the beneficiary chooses to continue treatment at a setting other than the outpatient hospital where me dically necessary services may be covered, the services may be billed at the rate the provider/supplier determines. Services provided in a capped setting after the limitation has been reached are not Medicare benefits and are not governed by Medicare policies.

If a beneficiary elects to receive services that exceed the cap limitation and a claim is submitted for such services, the resulting determination is subject to the administrative appeals process as described in subsection C.6 of this section and Pub. 100-04, chapter 29.

I. Provider Notification for Beneficiaries Exceeding Therapy Limits
Contractors will advise providers/suppliers to notify beneficiaries of the therapy financial limitations at their first therapy encounter with the beneficiary. Providers/suppliers should inform beneficiaries that beneficiaries are responsible for 100 percent of the costs of therapy services above each respective therapy limit, unless this outpatient care is furnished directly or under arrangements by a hospital.

Patients who are residents in a Medicare certified part of a SNF may not utilize outpatient hospital services for therapy services over the financial limits, because consolidated billing rules require all services to be billed by the SNF. However, when therapy cap exceptions apply, SNF residents may qualify for exceptions that allow billing within the consolidated billing rules.

It is the provider's responsibility to present each beneficiary with accurate information about the therapy limits, and that, where necessary, appropriate care above the limits can be obtained at a hospital outpatient therapy department. Medicare contractors shall advise providers/suppliers to use a form of their own design to inform beneficiaries of the therapy financial limitation and the cap exclusion process.

Prior to March 1, 2009, providers could use the Notice of Exclusion from Medicare Benefits (NEMB Form No. CMS 20007) to inform a beneficiary of financial liability for therapy above the cap, where no exception applies; however, the NEMB form has been discontinued. In its place, providers may now use a form of their own design, or the Advanced Beneficiary Notice of Noncoverage (ABN, Form CMS-R-131) may be used as a voluntary notice. When using the ABN form as a voluntary notice, the form requirements specified for its mandatory use do not apply.

The beneficiary should not be asked to choose an option or sign the form. The provider should include the beneficiary's name on the form and the reason that Medicare may not pay in the space provided within the form's table. Insertion of the following reason is suggested: "Services do not qualify for exception to therapy caps. Medicare will not pay for physical therapy and speech-language pathology services over (add the dollar amount of the cap and the year or the dates of service to which it applies, e.g., $1860 in 2010) unless the beneficiary qualifies for a cap exception." Providers are to supply this same information for occupational therapy services over the limit for the same time period, if appropriate. A cost estimate for the services may be included but is not required.

After the cap is exceeded, voluntary notice via a provider's own form or the ABN is appropriate, even when services are excepted from the cap. The ABN is also used BEFORE the cap is exceeded when notice about noncovered services is mandatory. For example, whenever the treating clinician determines that the services being provided are no longer expected to be covered because they do not satisfy Medicare's medical necessity requirements, an ABN must be issued before the beneficiary receives that service. At the time the clinician determines that skilled services are not necessary, the clinical goals have been met, or that there is no longer potential for the rehabilitation of health and/or function in a reasonable time, the beneficiary should be informed. If the beneficiary requests further services, inform the beneficiary that Medicare most likely will not provide additional coverage, and issue the ABN prior to delivering any services. The ABN informs the beneficiary of his/her potential financial obligation to the provider and provides guidance regarding appeal rights. When the ABN is used as a mandatory notice, providers must adhere to the form requirements set forth in this manual in chapter 30, section 50.6.3.

The ABN can be found at: http://www.cms.hhs.gov/BNI/Downloads/ABNFormInstructions.zip Access to Accrued Amount All providers and contractors may access the accrued amount of therapy services from the ELGA screen inquiries into CWF. Provider/suppliers may access

100-4, 5, 20

HCPCS Coding Requirement

A. Uniform Coding

Section 1834(k)(5) of the Act requires that all claims for outpatient rehabilitation therapy services and all comprehensive outpatient rehabilitation facility (CORF) services be reported using a uniform coding system. The current Healthcare Common Procedure Coding System/Current Procedural Terminology is used for the reporting of these services. The uniform coding requirement in the Act is specific to payment for all CORF services and outpatient rehabilitation therapy services - including physical therapy, occupational therapy, and speech-language pathology - that is provided and billed to carriers and fiscal intermediaries (FIs). The Medicare physician fee schedule (MPFS) is used to make payment for these therapy services at the nonfacility rate.

Effective for claims submitted on or after April 1, 1998, providers that had not previously reported HCPCS/CPT for outpatient rehabilitation and CORF services began using HCPCS to report these services. This requirement does not apply to outpatient rehabilitation services provided by:

- Critical access hospitals, which are paid on a cost basis, not MPFS;
- RHCs, and FQHCs for which therapy is included in the all-inclusive rate; or
- Providers that do not furnish therapy services.

The following "providers of services" must bill the FI for outpatient rehabilitation services using HCPCS codes:

- Hospitals (to outpatients and inpatients who are not in a covered Part A1 stay);
- Skilled nursing facilities (SNFs) (to residents not in a covered Part A1 stay and to nonresidents who receive outpatient rehabilitation services from the SNF);
- Home health agencies (HHAs) (to individuals who are not homebound or otherwise are not receiving services under a home health plan of care2 (POC);
- Comprehensive outpatient rehabilitation facilities (CORFs); and
- Providers of outpatient physical therapy and speech-language pathology services (OPTs), also known as rehabilitation agencies (previously termed outpatient physical therapy facilities in this instruction).

Note 1. The requirements for hospitals and SNFs apply to inpatient Part B and outpatient services only. Inpatient Part A services are bundled into the respective prospective payment system payment; no separate payment is made.

Note 2. For HHAs, HCPCS/CPT coding for outpatient rehabilitation services is required only when the HHA provides such service to individuals that are not homebound and, therefore, not under a home health plan of care.

The following practitioners must bill the carriers for outpatient rehabilitation therapy services using HCPCS/CPT codes:

- Physical therapists in private practice (PTPPs),
- Occupational therapists in private practice (OTPPs),
- Physicians, including MDs, DOs, podiatrists and optometrists, and
- Certain nonphysician practitioners (NPPs), acting within their State scope of practice, e.g., nurse practitioners and clinical nurse specialists.

Providers billing to intermediaries shall report:

- The date the therapy plan of care was either established or last reviewed (see Sec.220.1.3B) in Occurrence Code 17, 29, or 30.
- The first day of treatment in Occurrence Code 35, 44, or 45.

B. Applicable Outpatient Rehabilitation HCPCS Codes

The CMS identifies the following codes as therapy services, regardless of the presence of a financial limitation. Therapy services include only physical therapy, occupational therapy and speech-language pathology services. Therapist means only a physical therapist, occupational therapist or speech-language pathologist. Therapy modifiers are GP for physical therapy, GO for occupational therapy, and GN for speech-language pathology. Check the notes below the chart for details about each code.

When in effect, any financial limitation will also apply to services represented by the following codes, except as noted below.

NOTE: Listing of the following codes does not imply that services are covered or applicable to all provider settings.

64550+	90901+	92506¿	92507¿	92508	92526
92597	92605****	92606****	92607	92608	92609
92610+	92611+	92612+	92614+	92616+	95831+
95832+	95833+	95834+	95851+	95852+	95992****
96105+	96110+				

100-4, 5, 20.2

Reporting of Service Units With HCPCS

A. General

Effective with claims submitted on or after April 1, 1998, providers billing on Form CMS-1450 were required to report the number of units for outpatient rehabilitation services based on the procedure or service, e.g., based on the HCPCS code reported instead of the revenue code. This was already in effect for billing on the Form CMS-1500, and CORFs were required to report their full range of CORF services on the Form CMS-1450. These unit-reporting requirements continue with the standards required for electronically submitting health care claims under the Health Insurance Portability and Accountability Act of 1996 (HIPAA) - the currently adopted version of the ASC X12 837 transaction standards and implementation guides. The Administrative Simplification Compliance Act mandates that claims be sent to Medicare electronically unless certain exceptions are met.

B. Timed and Untimed Codes

When reporting service units for HCPCS codes where the procedure is not defined by a specific timeframe ("untimed" HCPCS), the provider enters "1" in the field labeled units. For untimed codes, units are reported based on the number of times the procedure is performed, as described in the HCPCS code definition (often once per day).

EXAMPLE: A beneficiary received a speech-language pathology evaluation represented by HCPCS "untimed" code 92506. Regardless of the number of minutes spent providing this service only one unit of service is appropriately billed on the same day.

Several CPT codes used for therapy modalities, procedures, and tests and measurements specify that the direct (one on one) time spent in patient contact is 15 minutes. Providers report procedure codes for services delivered on any single calendar day using CPT codes and the appropriate number of 15 minute units of service.

EXAMPLE: A beneficiary received occupational therapy (HCPCS "timed" code 97530 which is defined in 15 minute units) for a total of 60 minutes. The provider would then report revenue code 043X and 4 units.

C. Counting Minutes for Timed Codes in 15 Minute Units

When only one service is provided in a day, providers should not bill for services performed for less than 8 minutes. For any single timed CPT code in the same day measured in 15 minute units, providers bill a single 15-minute unit for treatment greater than or equal to 8 minutes through and including 22 minutes. If the duration of a single modality or procedure in a day is greater than or equal to 23 minutes through and including 37 minutes, then 2 units should be billed. Time intervals for 1 through 8 units are as follows:

Units	Number of Minutes
1 unit:	≥ 8 minutes through 22 minutes
2 units:	≥ 23 minutes through 37 minutes
3 units:	≥ 38 minutes through 52 minutes
4 units:	≥ 53 minutes through 67 minutes
5 units:	≥ 68 minutes through 82 minutes
6 units:	≥ 83 minutes through 97 minutes
7 units:	≥ 98 minutes through 112 minutes
8 units:	≥ 113 minutes through 127 minutes

The pattern remains the same for treatment times in excess of 2 hours.

If a service represented by a 15 minute timed code is performed in a single day for at least 15 minutes, that service shall be billed for at least one unit. If the service is performed for at least 30 minutes, that service shall be billed for at least two units, etc. It is not appropriate to count all minutes of treatment in a day toward the units for one code if other services were performed for more than 15 minutes. See examples 2 and 3 below.

When more than one service represented by 15 minute timed codes is performed in a single day, the total number of minutes of service (as noted on the chart above) determines the number of timed units billed. See example 1 below.

If any 15 minute timed service that is performed for 7 minutes or less than 7 minutes on the same day as another 15 minute timed service that was also performed for 7 minutes or less and the total time of the two is 8 minutes or greater than 8 minutes, then bill one unit for the service performed for the most minutes. This is correct because the total time is greater than the minimum time for one unit. The same logic is applied when three or more different services are provided for 7 minutes or less than 7 minutes. See example 5 below.

The expectation (based on the work values for these codes) is that a provider's direct patient contact time for each unit will average 15 minutes in length. If a provider has a consistent practice of billing less than 15 minutes for a unit, these situations should be highlighted for review.

If more than one 15 minute timed CPT code is billed during a single calendar day, then the total number of timed units that can be billed is constrained by the total treatment minutes for that day. See all examples below.

Pub. 100-02, Medicare Benefit Policy Manual, Chapter 15, Section 220.3B, Documentation Requirements for Therapy Services, indicates that the amount of time for each specific intervention/modality provided to the patient is not required to be documented in the Treatment Note. However, the total number of timed minutes must be documented. These examples indicate how to count the appropriate number of units for the total therapy minutes provided.

Example 1–

24 minutes of neuromuscular reeducation, code 97112,

23 minutes of therapeutic exercise, code 97110,

Total timed code treatment time was 47 minutes.

See the chart above. The 47 minutes falls within the range for 3 units = 38 to 52 minutes.

Appropriate billing for 47 minutes is only 3 timed units. Each of the codes is performed for more than 15 minutes, so each shall be billed for at least 1 unit. The correct coding is 2 units of code 97112 and one unit of code 97110, assigning more timed units to the service that took the most time.

Example 2–

20 minutes of neuromuscular reeducation (97112)

20 minutes therapeutic exercise (97110),

40 Total timed code minutes.

Appropriate billing for 40 minutes is 3 units. Each service was done at least 15 minutes and should be billed for at least one unit, but the total allows 3 units. Since the time for each service is the same, choose either code for 2 units and bill the other for 1 unit. Do not bill 3 units for either one of the codes.

Example 3–

33 minutes of therapeutic exercise (97110),

7 minutes of manual therapy (97140),

40 Total timed minutes

Appropriate billing for 40 minutes is for 3 units. Bill 2 units of 97110 and 1 unit of 97140. Count the first 30 minutes of 97110 as two full units. Compare the remaining time for 97110 (33-30 = 3 minutes) to the time spent on 97140 (7 minutes) and bill the larger, which is 97140.

Example 4–

18 minutes of therapeutic exercise (97110),

13 minutes of manual therapy (97140),

10 minutes of gait training (97116),

8 minutes of ultrasound (97035),

49 Total timed minutes

Appropriate billing is for 3 units. Bill the procedures you spent the most time providing. Bill 1 unit each of 97110, 97116, and 97140. You are unable to bill for the ultrasound because the total time of timed units that can be billed is constrained by the total timed code treatment minutes (i.e., you may not bill 4 units for less than 53 minutes regardless of how many services were performed). You would still document the ultrasound in the treatment notes.

Example 5–

7 minutes of neuromuscular reeducation (97112)

7 minutes therapeutic exercise (97110)

7 minutes manual therapy (97140)

21 Total timed minutes

Appropriate billing is for one unit. The qualified professional (See definition in Pub. 100-02, chapter 15, section 220) shall select one appropriate CPT code (97112, 97110, 97140) to bill since each unit was performed for the same amount of time and only one unit is allowed.

NOTE: The above schedule of times is intended to provide assistance in rounding time into 15-minute increments. It does not imply that any minute until the eighth should be excluded from the total count. The total minutes of active treatment counted for all 15 minute timed codes includes all direct treatment time for the timed codes. Total treatment minutes-- including minutes spent providing services represented by untimed codes,Äî are also documented. For documentation in the medical record of the services provided see Pub. 100-02, chapter 15, section 220.3.

D. Specific Limits for HCPCS

The Deficit Reduction Act of 2005, section 5107 requires the implementation of clinically appropriate code edits to eliminate improper payments for outpatient therapy services. The following codes may be billed, when covered, only at or below the number of units indicated on the chart per treatment day. When higher amounts of units are billed than those indicated in the table below, the units on the claim line that exceed the limit shall be denied as medically unnecessary (according to 1862(a)(1)(A)). Denied claims may be appealed and an ABN is appropriate to notify the beneficiary of liability.

This chart does not include all of the codes identified as therapy codes; refer to section 20 of this chapter for further detail on these and other therapy codes. For example, therapy codes called "always therapy" must always be accompanied by therapy modifiers identifying the type of therapy plan of care under which the service is provided.

Use the chart in the following manner:

The codes that are allowed one unit for "Allowed Units" in the chart below may be billed no more than once per provider, per discipline, per date of service, per patient.

The codes allowed 0 units in the column for "Allowed Units", may not be billed under a plan of care indicated by the discipline in that column. Some codes may be billed by one discipline (e.g., PT) and not by others (e.g., OT or SLP).

When physicians/NPPs bill ‚Äìalways therapy codes they must follow the policies of the type of therapy they are providing e.g., utilize a plan of care, bill with the appropriate therapy modifier (GP, GO, GN), bill the allowed units on the chart below for PT, OT or SLP depending on the plan. A physician/NPP shall not bill an "always therapy" code unless the service is provided under a therapy plan of care. Therefore, NA stands for "Not Applicable" in the chart below.

When a ‚Äìsometimes therapy,Äñ code is billed by a physician/NPP, but as a medical service, and not under a therapy plan of care, the therapy modifier shall not be used, but the number of units billed must not exceed the number of units indicated in the chart below per patient, per provider/supplier, per day.

HCPCS	Code Description and Claim Line Outlier/Edit Details	Timed or Untimed	'PT Allowed units	OT Allowed units	SLP Allowed units	Physician/NPP NOT under Therapy POC
92506	Speech/hearing evaluation	Untimed	0	0	1	NA
92597	Oral speech device eval	Untimed	0	1	1	NA
92607	Ex for speech device rx, 1hr	Timed	0	1	1	NA
92611	Motion fluroscopy/swallow	Untimed	0	1	1	1
92612	Endoscope swallow test (fees)	Untimed	0	1	1	1
92614	Laryngoscopic sensory test	Untimed	0	1	1	1
92616	Fees w/laryngeal sense test	Untimed	0	1	1	1
95833	Limb muscle testing, manual	Untimed	1	1	0	1
95834	Limb muscle	Untimed	1	1	0	1

100-4, 5, 20.4

Coding Guidance for Certain CPT Codes - All Claims

The following provides guidance about the use of codes 96105, 97026, 97150, 97545, 97546, and G0128.

CPT Codes 96105, 97545, and 97546.

Providers report code 96105, assessment of aphasia with interpretation and report in 1-hour units. This code represents formal evaluation of aphasia with an instrument such as the Boston Diagnostic Aphasia Examination. If this formal assessment is performed during treatment, it is typically performed only once during treatment and its medical necessity should be documented.

If the test is repeated during treatment, the medical necessity of the repeat administration of the test must also be documented. It is common practice for regular assessment of a patient's progress in therapy to be documented in the chart, and this may be done using test items taken from the formal examinations. This is considered to be part of the treatment and should not be billed as 96105 unless a full, formal assessment is completed.

Other timed physical medicine codes are 97545 and 97546. The interval for code 97545 is 2 hours and for code 97546, 1 hour. These are specialized codes to be used in the context of rehabilitating a worker to return to a job. The expectation is that the entire time period specified in the codes 97545 or 97546 would be the treatment period, since a shorter period of treatment could be coded with another code such as codes 97110, 97112, or 97537. (Codes 97545 and 97546 were developed for reporting services to persons in the worker's compensation program, thus we do not expect to see them reported for Medicare patients except under very unusual circumstances. Further, we would not expect to see code 97546 without also seeing code 97545 on the same claim. Code 97546, when used, is used in conjunction with 97545.) CPT Code 97026 Effective for services performed on or after October 24, 2006, the Centers for Medicare & Medicaid Services announce a NCD stating the use of infrared and/or near-infrared light and/or heat, including monochromatic infrared energy (MIRE), is non-covered for the treatment, including symptoms such as pain arising from these conditions, of diabetic and/or non-diabetic peripheral sensory neuropathy, wounds and/or ulcers of the skin and/or subcutaneous tissues in Medicare beneficiaries. Further coverage guidelines can be found in the National Coverage Determination Manual (Publication 100-03), section 270.6.

Contractors shall deny claims with CPT 97026 (infrared therapy incident to or as a PT/OT benefit) and HCPCS E0221 or A4639, if the claim contains any of the following ICD-9 codes: 250.60-250.63 354.4, 354.5, 354.9 355.1-355.4 355.6-355.9 356.0, 356.2-356.4, 356.8-356.9 357.0-357.7 674.10, 674.12, 674.14, 674.20, 674.22, 674.24 707.00-707.07, 707.09-707.15, 707.19 870.0-879.9 880.00-887.7 890.0-897.7 998.31-998.32 Contractors can use the following messages when denying the service: Medicare Summary Notice # 21.11 "This service was not covered by Medicare at the time you received it." Reason Claim Adjustment Code #50 "These are noncovered services because this is not deemed a medical necessity by the payer." Advanced Beneficiary Notice (ABN): Physicians, physical therapists, occupational therapists, outpatient rehabilitation facilities (ORFs), comprehensive outpatient rehabilitation facilities (CORFs), home health agencies (HHA), and hospital outpatient departments are liable if the service is performed, unless the beneficiary signs an ABN.

Similarly, DME suppliers and HHA are liable for the devices when they are supplied, unless the beneficiary signs an ABN.

100-4, 5, 100.10

Group Therapy Services (Code 97150)

Policies for group therapy services for CORF are the same as group therapy services for other Part B outpatient services. See Pub 100-02, chapter 15, section 230.

100-4, 8, 50.9

Coding for Adequacy of Dialysis, Vascular Access and Infection

A. Reporting the Urea Reduction Ratio(URR) for ESRD Hemodialysis Claims
All hemodialysis claims must indicate the most recent Urea Reduction Ratio (URR) for the dialysis patient. Code all claims using HCPCS code 90999 along with the appropriate G modifier listed in section B.

Claims for dialysis treatments must include the adequacy of hemodialysis data as measured by URR. Dialysis facilities must monitor the adequacy of dialysis treatments monthly for facility patients. Home hemodialysis and peritoneal dialysis patients may be monitored less frequently, but not less than quarterly. If a home hemodialysis patient is not monitored during a month, the last, most recent URR for the dialysis patient must be reported.

HCPCS code 90999 (unlisted dialysis procedure, inpatient or outpatient) must be reported in field location 44 for all bill types 72X. The appropriate G-modifier in field location 44 (HCPCS/RATES) is used, for patients that received seven or more dialysis treatments in a month. Continue to report revenue codes 0820, 0821, 0825, and 0829 in field location 43.

G1 - Most recent URR of less than 60%

G2 - Most recent URR of 60% to 64.9%

G3 - Most recent URR of 65% to 69.9%

G4 - Most recent URR of 70% to 74.9%

G5 - Most recent URR of 75% or greater

For patients that have received dialysis 6 days or less in a month, facilities use the following modifier:

G6 - ESRD patient for whom less than seven dialysis sessions have been provided in a month.

For services beginning January 1, 2003, and after, if the modifier is not present, FIs must return the claim to the provider for the appropriate modifier. Effective April, 2007 due to the requirement of line item billing, at least one revenue code line for hemodialysis on the claim must contain one of the URR modifiers shown above. The URR modifier is not required on every hemodialysis line on the claim.

The techniques to be used to draw the pre- and post-dialysis blood urea Nitrogen samples are listed in the National Kidney Foundation Dialysis Outcomes Quality Initiative Clinical Practice Guidelines for Hemodialysis Adequacy, Guideline 8, Acceptable Methods for BUN sampling, New York, National Kidney Foundation, 2000, pp.53-60.

B. Reporting the Vascular Access for ESRD Hemodialysis Claims
ESRD claims for hemodialysis with dates of service on or after July 1, 2010 must indicate the type of vascular access used for the delivery of the hemodialysis at the last hemodialysis session of the month. One of the following codes is required to be reported on the latest line item date of service billing for hemodialysis revenue code 0821. It may be reported on all revenue code 0821 lines at the discretion of the provider.

Modifier V5: Vascular Catheter

Modifier V6: Arteriovenous Graft

Modifier V7: Arteriovenous Fistula

C. Reporting the Kt/V for ALL ESRD Claims
All ESRD claims with dates of service on or after July 1, 2010 must indicate the applicable Kt/V reading for the dialysis patient. The reading result and the date of the reading must be reported on the claim using the following claim codes:

Value Code D5–Result of last Kt/V reading. For in-center hemodialysis patients this is the last reading taken during the billing period. For peritoneal dialysis patients and home hemodialysis this may be before the current billing period but should be within 4 months of the claim date of service.

- Hemodialysis: For in-center and home-hemodialysis patients prescribed for three or fewer treatments per week the Kt/V must be reported for the last dialysis session covered by the claim, each month. Facilities must report single pool Kt/V using the preferred National Quality Forum (NQF) endorsed methods for deriving the single pool Kt/V value: Daugirdas 2or Urea Kinetic Modeling (UKM).

For patients routinely prescribed four or more hemodialysis treatments per week a value of 8.88 should be entered on the claim. The 8.88 value should not be used for patients who are receiving "extra" treatments for temporary clinical need.

- Peritoneal Dialysis: When measured the delivered weekly total Kt/V (dialytic and residual) should be reported.

This code is effective and required on all ESRD claims with dates of service on or after July 1, 2010. In the event that no Kt/V reading was performed providers must report the D5 with a value of 9.99.

Occurrence Code 51–Date of last Kt/V reading. For in-center hemodialysis patients, this is the date of the last reading taken during the billing period. For peritoneal dialysis patients and home hemodialysis patients, this date may be before the current billing period but should be within 4 months of the claim date of service. This code is effective for ESRD claims with dates of service on or after July 1, 2010. If no Kt/V reading was performed do not report this code.

D. Reporting of Infection for ALL ESRD Claims
All ESRD claims with dates of service on or after July 1, 2010 must indicate on the claim if an infection was present at the time of treatment. Claims must report on each dialysis revenue code line one of the following codes:

Modifier V8: Infection present

Modifier V9: No infection present

100-4, 8, 60.6

Vaccines Furnished to ESRD Patients

The Medicare program covers hepatitis B, influenza virus and Pneumococcal pneumonia virus (PPV) vaccines and their administration when furnished to eligible beneficiaries in accordance with coverage rules. Payment may be made for both the vaccine and the administration. The costs associated with the syringe and supplies are included in the administration fee: HCPCS code A4657 should not be billed for these vaccines.

Vaccines and their administration are reported using separate codes. See Chapter 18 of this manual for the codes required for billing vaccines and the administration of the vaccine.

Payment for vaccine administration (PPV, Influenza Virus, and Hepatitis B Virus) to freestanding RDFs is based on the Medicare Physician Fee Schedule (MPFS) according to the rate in the MPFS associated with code 90782 for services provided prior to March 1, 2003 and code 90471 for services provided March 1, 2005 and later and on reasonable cost for provider-based RDFs.

Vaccines remain separately payable under the ESRD PPS.

100-4, 8, 140

Monthly Capitation Payment Method for Physicians' Services Furnished to Patients on Maintenance Dialysis

Physicians and practitioners managing patients on dialysis (center based) are paid a monthly capitation payment (MCP) for most outpatient dialysis-related physician services furnished to a Medicare end stage renal disease (ESRD) beneficiary. The payment amount varies based on the number of visits provided within each month and the age of the ESRD beneficiary. Physicians and practitioners managing ESRD patients who dialyze at home are paid a single monthly rate based on the age of the ESRD beneficiary, regardless of the number of face-to-face physician or practitioner visits. The MCP is reported once per month for services performed in an outpatient setting that are related to the patients' ESRD.

Physicians and practitioners may receive payment for managing patients on dialysis for less than a full month of care in specific circumstances as discussed in section 140.2. Payment for ESRD related services, less than a full month, is made on a per diem bases.

Payment for ESRD-related services is made at 80 percent of the Medicare approved amount (lesser of the actual charge or applicable Medicare fee schedule amount) after the beneficiary's Part B deductible is met. The beneficiary is responsible for the Part B deductible and the 20 percent coinsurance for physician and practitioner ESRD-related services.

A. Services Included in Monthly Capitation Payment
The following physician services are included in the MCP:

- Assessment of the need for a specified diet and the need for nutritional supplementation for the control of chronic renal failure. Specification of the quantity of total protein, high biologic protein, sodium, potassium, and amount of fluids to be allowed during a given time period. For diabetic patients with chronic renal failure, the prescription usually specifies the number of calories in the diet.
- Assessment of which mode(s) of chronic dialysis (types of hemodialysis or peritoneal dialysis) are suitable for a given patient and recommendation of the type(s) of therapy for a given patient.
- Assessment and determination of which type of dialysis access is best suited for a given patient and arrangement for creation of dialysis access.
- Assessment of whether the patient meets preliminary criteria as a renal transplant candidate and presentation of this assessment to the patient and family.
- Prescription of the parameters of intradialytic management. For chronic hemodialysis therapies, this includes the type of dialysis access, the type and amount of anticoagulant to be employed, blood flow rates, dialysate flow rate, ultrafiltration rate, dialysate temperature, type of dialysate (acetate versus bicarbonate) and composition of the electrolytes in the dialysate, size of hemodialyzer (surface area) and composition of the dialyzer membrane (conventional versus high flux), duration and frequency of treatments, the type and frequency of measuring indices of clearance, and intradialytic medications to be

administered. For chronic peritoneal dialysis therapies, this includes the type of peritoneal dialysis, the volume of dialysate, concentration of dextrose in the dialysate, electrolyte composition of the dialysate, duration of each exchange, and addition of medication to the dialysate, such as heparin, and the type and frequency of measuring indices of clearance. For diabetics, the quantity of insulin to be added to each exchange is prescribed.

- Assessment of whether the patient has significant renal failure-related anemia, determination of the etiology(ies) for the anemia based on diagnostic tests, and prescription of therapy for correction of the anemia, such as vitamins, oral or parenteral iron, and hormonal therapy such as erythropoietin.
- Assessment of whether the patient has hyperparathyroidism and/or renal osteodystrophy secondary to chronic renal failure and prescription of appropriate therapy, such as calcium and phosphate binders for control of hyperphosphatemia. Based upon assessment of parahormone levels, serum calcium levels, and evaluation for the presence of metabolic bone disease, the physician determines whether oral or parenteral therapy with vitamin D or its analogs is indicated and prescribes the appropriate therapy. Based upon assessment and diagnosis of bone disease, the physician may prescribe specific chelation therapy with deferoxamine and the use of hemoperfusion for removal of aluminum and the chelation.
- Assessment of whether the patient has dialysis-related arthropathy or neuropathy and adjustment of the patient's prescription accordingly. Referral of the patient for any additional needed specialist evaluation and management of these endorgan problems.
- Assessment of whether the patient has fluid overload resulting from renal failure and establishment of an estimated "ideal (dry) weight." The physician determines the need for fluid removal independent of the dialysis prescription and implements these measures when indicated.
- Determination of the need for and prescription of antihypertensive medications and their timing relative to dialysis when the patient is hypertensive in spite of correction of fluid overload.
- Periodic review of the dialysis records to ascertain whether the patient is receiving the prescribed amount of dialysis and ordering of indices of clearance, such as urea kinetics, in order to ascertain whether the dialysis prescription is producing adequate dialysis. If the indices of clearance suggest that the prescription requires alteration, the physician orders changes in the hemodialysis prescription, such as blood flow rate, dialyzer surface area, dialysis frequency, and/or dialysis duration (length of treatment). For peritoneal dialysis patients, the physician may order changes in the volume of dialysate, dextrose concentration of the dialysate, and duration of the exchanges.
- Periodic visits (at least one per month) to the patient during dialysis to ascertain whether the dialysis is working well and whether the patient is tolerating the procedure well (physiologically and psychologically). During these visits, the physician determines whether alteration in any aspect of a given patient's prescription is indicated, such as changes in the estimate of the patient's dry weight. Review of the treatment with the nurse or technician performing the therapy is also included. The frequency of these visits will vary depending upon the patient's medical status, complicating conditions, and other determinants.
- Performance of periodic physical assessments, based upon the patient's clinical stability, in order to determine the necessity for alterations in various aspects of the patient's prescription. Similarly, the physician reviews the results of periodic laboratory testing in order to determine the need for alterations in the patient's prescription, such as changes in the amount and timing of phosphate binders or dose of erythropoietin.
- Periodic assessment of the adequacy and function of the patient's dialysis access appropriate tests and antibiotic therapy.
- Interpretations of the following tests:
  - Bone mineral density studies (CPT codes 76070, 76075, 78350, and 78351);
  - Noninvasive vascular diagnostic studies of hemodialysis access (CPT codes 93925, 93926, 93930, 93931, and 93990);
  - Nerve conduction studies (CPT codes 95900, 95903, 95904, 95925, 95926, 95927, 95934, 95935, and 95936);
  - Electromyography studies (CPT codes 95860, 95861, 95863, 95864, 95867, 95867, 95869, and 95872).
- Periodic review and update of the patient's short-term and long-term care plans with staff.
- Coordination and direction of the care of patients by other professional staff, such as dieticians and social workers.
- Certification of the need for items and services such as durable medical equipment and home health care services. Care plan oversight services described by CPT code 99375 are included in the MCP and may not be separately reported.

B. Services Excluded from Monthly Capitation Payment

The following physician services furnished to the physician's ESRD patients are excluded from the MCP and should be paid in accordance with the physician fee schedule:

1. Administration of hepatitis B vaccine.
2. Surgical services such as:
   - Temporary or permanent hemodialysis catheter placement;
   - Temporary or permanent peritoneal dialysis catheter placement;
   - Repair of existing dialysis accesses;
   - Placement of catheter(s) for thrombolytic therapy;
   - Thrombolytic therapy (systemic, regional, or access catheter only; hemodialysis or peritoneal dialysis);
   - Thrombectomy of clotted cannula;
   - Arthrocentesis;
   - Bone marrow aspiration; and
   - Bone marrow biopsy.
3. Interpretation of tests that have a professional component such as:
   - Electrocardiograms (12 lead, Holter monitor, stress tests, etc.);
   - Echocardiograms;
   - 24-hour blood pressure monitor;
   - Biopsies; and
   - Spirometry and complete pulmonary function tests.
4. Complete evaluation for renal transplantation. While the physician assessment of whether the patient meets preliminary criteria as a renal transplant candidate is included under the MCP, the complete evaluation for renal transplantation is excluded from the MCP
5. Evaluation of potential living transplant donors.
6. The training of patients to perform home hemodialysis, self hemodialysis, and the various forms of self peritoneal dialysis.
7. Non-renal related physician's services. These services may be furnished by the physician providing renal care or by another physician. They may not be incidental to services furnished during a dialysis session or office visit necessitated by the renal condition. The physician must provide documentation that the illness is not related to the renal condition and that the added visits are required. The contractor's medical staff determines whether additional reimbursement is warranted for treatment of the unrelated illness. For example, the medical management of diabetes mellitus that is not related to the dialysis or furnished during a dialysis session is excluded.
8. Covered physician services furnished to hospital inpatients.
9. All physician services that antedate the initiation of outpatient dialysis.
10. Covered physician services furnished by another physician when the patient is not available to receive the outpatient services as usual; for example, when the patient is traveling out of tow

100-4, 8, 140.1

Payment for ESRD-Related Services Under the Monthly Capitation Payment (Center Based Patients)

Physicians and practitioners managing center based patients on dialysis are paid a monthly rate for most outpatient dialysis-related physician services furnished to a Medicare ESRD beneficiary. The payment amount varies based on the number of visits provided within each month and the age of the ESRD beneficiary. Under this methodology, separate codes are billed for providing one visit per month, two to three visits per month and four or more visits per month. The lowest payment amount applies when a physician provides one visit per month; a higher payment is provided for two to three visits per month. To receive the highest payment amount, a physician or practitioner would have to provide at least four ESRD-related visits per month. The MCP is reported once per month for services performed in an outpatient setting that are related to the patients' ESRD.

The physician or practitioner who provides the complete assessment, establishes the patient's plan of care, and provides the ongoing management is the physician or practitioner who submits the bill for the monthly service.

a Month defined.

For purposes of billing for physician and practitioner ESRD related services, the term 'month' means a calendar month. The first month the beneficiary begins dialysis treatments is the date the dialysis treatments begin through the end of the calendar month. Thereafter, the term 'month' refers to a calendar month.

b. Determination of the age of beneficiary.

The beneficiary's age at the end of the month is the age of the patient for determining the appropriate age related ESRD-related services code.

c. Qualifying Visits Under the MCP

General policy.

Visits must be furnished face-to-face by a physician, clinical nurse specialist, nurse practitioner, or physician's assistant.

Visits furnished by another physician or practitioner (who is not the MCP physician or practitioner).

The MCP physician or practitioner may use other physicians or qualified nonphysician practitioners to provide some of the visits during the month. The MCP physician or practitioner does not have to be present when these other physicians or practitioners provide visits. In this instance, the rules are consistent with the requirements for hospital split/shared evaluation and management visits. The non-MCP physician or practitioner must be a partner, an employee of the same group practice, or an employee of the MCP physician or practitioner. For example, the physician or practitioner furnishing visits under the MCP may be either a W-2 employee or 1099 independent contractor.

When another physician is used to furnish some of the visits during the month, the physician who provides the complete assessment, establishes the patient's plan of care, and provides the ongoing management should bill for the MCP service.

If the nonphysician practitioner is the practitioner who performs the complete assessment and establishes the plan of care, then the MCP service should be billed under the PIN of the clinical nurse specialist, nurse practitioner, or physician assistant.

Residents, interns and fellows.

Patient visits by residents, interns and fellows enrolled in an approved Medicare graduate medical education (GME) program may be counted towards the MCP visits if the teaching MCP physician is present during the visit.

Patients designated/admitted as hospital observation status.

ESRD-related visits furnished to patients in hospital observation status that occur on or after January 1, 2005, should be counted for purposes of billing the MCP codes. Visits furnished to patients in hospital observation status are included when submitting MCP claims for ESRD-related services.

ESRD-related visits furnished to beneficiaries residing in a SNF.

ESRD-related visits furnished to beneficiaries residing in a SNF should be counted for purposes of billing the MCP codes.

SNF residents admitted as an inpatient.

Inpatient visits are not counted for purposes of the MCP service. If the beneficiary residing in a SNF is admitted to the hospital as an inpatient, the appropriate inpatient visit code should be billed.

ESRD Related Visits as a Telehealth Service

ESRD-related services with 2 or 3 visits per month and ESRD-related services with 4 or more visits per month may be furnished as a telehealth service. However, at least one visit per month is required in person to examine the vascular access site. A clinical examination of the vascular access site must be furnished face-to-face (not as a telehealth service) by a physician, nurse practitioner or physician's assistant. For more information on how ESRD-related visits may be furnished as a Medicare telehealth service and for general Medicare telehealth policy see Pub. 100-02, Medicare Benefit Policy manual, chapter 15, section 270. For claims processing instructions see Pub. 100-04, Medicare Claims Processing manual chapter 12, section 190.

100-4, 8, 140.1.1

Payment for Managing Patients on Home Dialysis

Physicians and practitioners managing ESRD patients who dialyze at home are paid a single monthly rate based on the age of the beneficiary. The MCP physician (or practitioner) must furnish at least one face-to-face patient visit per month for the home dialysis MCP service. Documentation by the MCP physician (or practitioner) should support at least one face-to-face encounter per month with the home dialysis patient. Medicare contractors may waive the requirement for a monthly face-to-face visit for the home dialysis MCP service on a case by case basis, for example, when the nephrologist's notes indicate that the physician actively and adequately managed the care of the home dialysis patient throughout the month. The management of home dialysis patients who remain a home dialysis patient the entire month should be coded using the ESRD-related services for home dialysis patients HCPCS codes.

When another physician is used to furnish some of the visits during the month, the physician who provides the complete assessment, establishes the patient's plan of care, and provides the ongoing management should bill for the MCP service.

If the nonphysician practitioner is the practitioner who performs the complete assessment and establishes the plan of care, then the MCP service should be billed under the PIN of the clinical nurse specialist, nurse practitioner, or physician assistant.

Residents, interns and fellows. Patient visits by residents, interns and fellows enrolled in an approved Medicare graduate medical education (GME) program may be counted towards the MCP visits if the teaching MCP physician is present during the visit.

a. Month defined.

For purposes of billing for physician and practitioner ESRD related services, the term 'month' means a calendar month. The first month the beneficiary begins dialysis treatments is the date the dialysis treatments begin through the end of the calendar month. Thereafter, the term 'month' refers to a calendar month.

b. Qualifying Visits under the MCP

General policy. Visits must be furnished face-to-face by a physician, clinical nurse specialist, nurse practitioner, or physician's assistant.

Visits furnished by another physician or practitioner (who is not the MCP physician or practitioner). The MCP physician or practitioner may use other physicians or qualified nonphysician practitioners to provide the visit(s) during the month. The MCP physician or practitioner does not have to be present when these other physicians or practitioners provide visit(s). The non-MCP physician or practitioner must be a partner, an employee of the same group practice, or an employee of the MCP physician or practitioner. For example, the physician or practitioner furnishing visits under the MCP may be either a W-2 employee or 1099 independent contractor.

100-4, 9, 182

Medical Nutrition Therapy (MNT) Services

A - FQHCs

Previously, MNT type services were considered incident to services under the FQHC benefit, if all relevant program requirements were met. Therefore, separate all-inclusive encounter rate payment could not be made for the provision of MNT services. With passage of DRA, effective January 1, 2006, FQHCs are eligible for a separate payment under Part B for these services provided they meet all program requirements. Payment is made at the all-inclusive encounter rate to the FQHC. This payment can be in addition to payment for any other qualifying visit on the same date of service as the beneficiary received qualifying MNT services.

For FQHCs to qualify for a separate visit payment for MNT services, the services must be a one-on-one face-to-face encounter. Group sessions don't constitute a billable visit for any FQHC services. Rather, the cost of group sessions is included in the calculation of the all-inclusive FQHC visit rate. To receive payment for MNT services, the MNT services must be billed on TOB 73X with the appropriate individual MNT HCPCS code (codes 97802, 97803, or G0270) and with the appropriate site of service revenue code in the 052X revenue code series. This payment can be in addition to payment for any other qualifying visit on the same date of service as the beneficiary received qualifying MNT services as long as the claim for MNT services contain the appropriate coding specified above.

NOTE: MNT is not a qualifying visit on the same day that DSMT is provided.

Additional information on MNT can be found in Chapter 4, section 300 of this manual.

Group services (HCPCS 97804 or G0271) do not meet the criteria for a separate qualifying encounter. All line items billed on TOB 73x with HCPCS code 97804 or G0271 will be denied.

B - RHCs

Separate payment to RHCs for these practitioners/services continues to be precluded as these services are not within the scope of Medicare-covered RHC benefits. All line items billed on TOB 71x with HCPCS codes for MNT services will be denied.

100-4, 11, 10

Overview

Medicare beneficiaries entitled to hospital insurance (Part A) who have terminal illnesses and a life expectancy of six months or less have the option of electing hospice benefits in lieu of standard Medicare coverage for treatment and management of their terminal condition. Only care provided by a Medicare certified hospice is covered under the hospice benefit provisions.

Hospice care is available for two 90-day periods and an unlimited number of 60-day periods during the remainder of the hospice patient's lifetime. However, a beneficiary may voluntarily terminate his hospice election period. Election/termination dates are retained on CWF.

When hospice coverage is elected, the beneficiary waives all rights to Medicare Part B payments for services that are related to the treatment and management of his/her terminal illness during any period his/her hospice benefit election is in force, except for professional services of an attending physician, which may include a nurse practitioner. If the attending physician, who may be a nurse practitioner, is an employee of the designated hospice, he or she may not receive compensation from the hospice for those services under Part B. These physician professional services are billed to Medicare Part A by the hospice.

To be covered, hospice services must be reasonable and necessary for the palliation or management of the terminal illness and related conditions. The individual must elect hospice care and a certification that the individual is terminally ill must be completed by the patient's attending physician (if there is one), and the Medical Director (or the physician member of the Interdisciplinary Group (IDG)). Nurse practitioners serving as the attending physician may not certify or re-certify the terminal illness. A plan of care must be established before services are provided. To be covered, services must be consistent with the plan of care. Certification of terminal illness is based on the physician's or medical director's clinical judgment regarding the normal course of an individual's illness. It should be noted that predicting life expectancy is not always exact.

See the Medicare Benefit Policy Manual, Chapter 9, for additional general information about the Hospice benefit.

See Chapter 29 of this manual for information on the appeals process that should be followed when an entity is dissatisfied with the determination made on a claim.

See Chapter 9 of the Medicare Benefit Policy Manual for hospice eligibility requirements and election of hospice care.

100-4, 11, 10.1

Hospice Pre-Election Evaluation and Counseling Services

Effective January 1, 2005, Medicare allows payment to a hospice for specified hospice pre-election evaluation and counseling services when furnished by a physician who is either the medical director of or employee of the hospice.

Medicare covers a one- time only payment on behalf of a beneficiary who is terminally ill, (defined as having a prognosis of 6 months or less if the disease follows its normal course), has no previous hospice elections, and has not previously received hospice pre-election evaluation and counseling services.

HCPCS code G0337 "Hospice Pre-Election Evaluation and Counseling Services" is used to designate that these services have been provided by the medical director or a physician employed by the hospice. Hospice agencies bill their Medicare contractor with home health and hospice jurisdiction directly using HCPCS G0337 with Revenue Code 0657. No other revenue codes may appear on the claim.

Claims for "Hospice Pre-Election and Counseling Services", HCPCS code G0337, are not subject to the editing usually required on hospice claims to match the claim to an established hospice period. Further, contractors do not apply payments for hospice pre-election evaluation and counseling consultation services to the overall hospice cap amount.

Medicare must ensure that this counseling service occurs only one time per beneficiary by imposing safeguards to detect and prevent duplicate billing for similar services. If "new patient" physician services (HCPCS codes 99201-99205) are submitted by a Medicare contractor to CWF for payment authorization but HCPCS code G0337 (Hospice Pre-Election Evaluation and Counseling Services) has already been approved for a hospice claim for the same beneficiary, for the same date of service, by the same physician, the physician service will be rejected by CWF and the service shall be denied as a duplicate. Medicare contractors use the following messages in this case:

MSN messages: 16.8: "Payment is included in another service received on the same day" and

16.45: "You cannot be billed separately for this item or service. You do not have to pay this amount."

Claim adjustment reason code (CARC) 97: "The benefit for this service is included in the payment/allowance for another service/procedure that has already been adjudicated."

Remittance advice remark code (RARC) M86:

Likewise, if a "new patient" claim for HCPCS codes 99201-99205 has been approved and subsequently, a hospice claim is submitted to CWF for payment authorization for HCPCS code G0337, (for same beneficiary, same date of service, same physician), CWF shall reject the claim and the contractor shall deny the bill and use the messages above.

HCPCS code G0337 is only payable when billed on a hospice claim. Contractors shall not make payment for HCPCS code G0337 on professional claims. Contractors shall deny line items on professional claims for HCPCS code G0337 and use the following messages:

MSN message 17.9: "Medicare (Part A/Part B) pays for this service. The provider must bill the correct Medicare contractor."

CARC 109: "Claim not covered by this payer/contractor. You must send the claim to the correct payer/contractor ."

100-4, 11, 40.1.3

Independent Attending Physician Services

When hospice coverage is elected, the beneficiary waives all rights to Medicare Part B payments for professional services that are related to the treatment and management of his/her terminal illness during any period his/her hospice benefit election is in force, except for professional services of an independent attending physician, who is not an employee of the designated hospice nor receives compensation from the hospice for those services. For purposes of administering the hospice benefit provisions, an "attending physician" means an individual who:

Is a doctor of medicine or osteopathy or

A nurse practitioner (for professional services related to the terminal illness that are furnished on or after December 8, 2003); and

Is identified by the individual, at the time he/she elects hospice coverage, as having the most significant role in the determination and delivery of their medical care.

Hospices should reiterate with patients that they must not see independent physicians for care related to their terminal illness other than their independent attending physician unless the hospice arranges it.

Even though a beneficiary elects hospice coverage, he/she may designate and use an independent attending physician, who is not employed by nor receives compensation from the hospice for professional services furnished, in addition to the services of hospice-employed physicians. The professional services of an independent attending physician, who may be a nurse practitioner as defined in Chapter 9, that are reasonable and necessary for the treatment and management of a hospice patient's terminal illness are not considered Medicare Part A hospice services.

Where the service is related to the hospice patient's terminal illness but was furnished by someone other than the designated "attending physician" [or a physician substituting for the attending physician]) the physician or other provider must look to the hospice for payment.

Professional services related to the hospice patient's terminal condition that were furnished by an independent attending physician, who may be a nurse practitioner, are billed to the Medicare contractor through Medicare Part B. When the independent attending physician furnishes a terminal illness related service that includes both a professional and technical component (e.g., x-rays), he/she bills the professional component of such services to the carrier and looks to the hospice for payment for the technical component. Likewise, the independent attending physician, who may be a nurse practitioner, would look to the hospice for payment for terminal illness related services furnished that have no professional component (e.g., clinical lab tests). The remainder of this section explains this in greater detail.

When a Medicare beneficiary elects hospice coverage he/she may designate an attending physician, who may be a nurse practitioner, not employed by the hospice, in addition to receiving care from hospice-employed physicians. The professional services of a non-hospice affiliated attending physician for the treatment and management of a hospice patient's terminal illness are not considered Medicare Part A "hospice services." These independent attending physician services are billed through Medicare Part B to the Medicare contractor, provided they were not furnished under a payment arrangement with the hospice. The independent attending physician codes services with the GV modifier "Attending physician not employed or paid under agreement by the patient's hospice provider" when billing his/her professional services furnished for the treatment and management of a hospice patient's terminal condition. The Medicare contractor makes payment to the independent attending physician or beneficiary, as appropriate, based on the payment and deductible rules applicable to each covered service.

Payments for the services of an independent attending physician are not counted in determining whether the hospice cap amount has been exceeded because Part B services provided by an independent attending physician are not part of the hospice's care.

Services provided by an independent attending physician who may be a nurse practitioner must be coordinated with any direct care services provided by hospice physicians.

Only the direct professional services of an independent attending physician, who may be a nurse practitioner, to a patient may be billed; the costs for services such as lab or x-rays are not to be included in the bill.

If another physician covers for a hospice patient's designated attending physician, the services of the substituting physician are billed by the designated attending physician under the reciprocal or locum tenens billing instructions. In such instances, the attending physician bills using the GV modifier in conjunction with either the Q5 or Q6 modifier.

When services related to a hospice patient's terminal condition are furnished under a payment arrangement with the hospice by the designated attending physician who may be a nurse practitioner (i.e., by a non-independent physician/nurse practitioner), the physician must look to the hospice for payment. In this situation the physicians' services are Part A hospice services and are billed by the hospice to its Medicare contractor.

Medicare contractors must process and pay for covered, medically necessary Part B services that physicians furnish to patients after their hospice benefits are revoked even if the patient remains under the care of the hospice. Such services are billed without the GV or GW modifiers. Make payment based on applicable Medicare payment and deductible rules for each covered service even if the beneficiary continues to be treated by the hospice after hospice benefits are revoked.

The CWF response contains the periods of hospice entitlement. This information is a permanent part of the notice and is furnished on all CWF replies and automatic notices. Medicare contractor use the CWF reply for validating dates of hospice coverage and to research, examine and adjudicate services coded with the GV or GW modifiers.

100-4, 11, 40.1.3.1

Care Plan Oversight

Care plan oversight (CPO) exists where there is physician supervision of patients under care of hospices that require complex and multidisciplinary care modalities involving regular physician development and/or revision of care plans. Implicit in the concept of CPO is the expectation that the physician has coordinated an aspect of the patient's care with the hospice during the month for which CPO services were billed.

For a physician or NP employed by or under arrangement with a hospice agency, CPO functions are incorporated and are part of the hospice per diem payment and as such may not be separately billed.

For information on separately billable CPO services by the attending physician or nurse practitioner see Chapter 12, 180 of this manual.

100-4, 11, 40.2

Independent Attending Physician Services

Professional services of attending physicians, who may be nurse practitioners, furnished to hospice beneficiaries are coded with modifier GV. Attending physician not employed or paid under arrangement by the patient's hospice provider. This modifier must be retained and reported to CWF.

Local Part B carriers shall presume that hospice benefits are not involved unless the biller codes services on the claim to indicate that the patient is a hospice enrollee (e.g. the GV modifier is billed by the attending physician, who may be a nurse practitioner, or the GW modifier is billed for services unrelated to the terminal illness) or the trailer information on the CWF reply shows a hospice election. The carrier shall use the hospice enrollment trailer information on the CWF reply to examine and validate the claim information.

For beneficiaries enrolled in hospice, carriers shall deny any services furnished on or after January 1, 2002, that are submitted without either the GV or GW modifier. For services furnished to a hospice patient prior to January 1, 2002, the attending physician is to include an attestation statement that is the written equivalent of the GV modifier and carriers are responsible for determining whether or not a service is related to the patient's terminal condition.

Deny claims for all other services related to the terminal illness furnished by individuals or entities other than the designated attending physician, who may be a nurse practitioner.

Such claims include bills for any DME, supplies or independently practicing speech-language pathologists or physical therapists that are related to the terminal condition.

These services are included in the hospice rate and paid through the FI.

See §110 for MSN and Remittance Advice (RA) coding.

100-4, 12, 30

Correct Coding Policy

B3-15068

The Correct Coding Initiative was developed to promote national correct coding methodologies and to control improper coding leading to inappropriate payment in Part B claims. Refer to Chapter 23 for additional information on the initiative.

The principles for the correct coding policy are:

The service represents the standard of care in accomplishing the overall procedure;

The service is necessary to successfully accomplish the comprehensive procedure.

Failure to perform the service may compromise the success of the procedure; and

The service does not represent a separately identifiable procedure unrelated to the comprehensive procedure planned.

For a detailed description of the correct coding policy, refer to http://www.cms.hhs.gov/medlearn/ncci.asp.

The CMS as well as many third party payers have adopted the HCPCS/CPT coding system for use by physicians and others to describe services rendered. The system contains three levels of codes. Level I contains the American Medical Association's Current Procedural Terminology (CPT) numeric codes. Level II contains alpha-numeric codes primarily for items and services not included in CPT. Level III contains carrier specific codes that are not included in either Level I or Level II. For a list of CPT and HCPCS codes refer to the CMS Web site.

The following general coding policies encompass coding principles that are to be applied in the review of Medicare claims. They are the basis for the correct coding edits that are installed in the claims processing systems effective January 1, 1996.

A. Coding Based on Standards of Medical/Surgical Practice
All services integral to accomplishing a procedure are considered bundled into that procedure and, therefore, are considered a component part of the comprehensive code. Many of these generic activities are common to virtually all procedures and, on other occasions, some are integral to only a certain group of procedures, but are still essential to accomplish these particular procedures. Accordingly, it is inappropriate to separately report these services based on standard medical and surgical principles.

Because many services are unique to individual CPT coding sections, the rationale for rebundling is described in that particular section of the detailed coding narratives that are transmitted to carriers periodically.

B. CPT Procedure Code Definition
The format of the CPT manual includes descriptions of procedures, which are, in order to conserve space, not listed in their entirety for all procedures. The partial description is indented under the main entry. The main entry then encompasses the portion of the description preceding the semicolon. The main entry applies to and is a part of all indented entries, which follow with their codes.

In the course of other procedure descriptions, the code definition specifies other procedures that are included in this comprehensive code. In addition, a code description may define a rebundling relationship where one code is a part of another based on the language used in the descriptor.

C. CPT Coding Manual Instruction/Guideline
Each of the six major subsections include guidelines that are unique to that section.

These directions are not all inclusive of nor limited to, definitions of terms, modifiers, unlisted procedures or services, special or written reports, details about reporting separate, and multiple or starred procedures and qualifying circumstances.

D. Coding Services Supplemental to Principal Procedure (Add-On Codes) Code
Generally, these are identified with the statement "list separately in addition to code for primary procedure" in parentheses, and other times the supplemental code is used only with certain primary codes, which are parenthetically identified. The reason for these CPT codes is to enable physicians and others to separately identify a service that is performed in certain situations as an additional service. Incidental services that are necessary to accomplish the primary procedure (e.g., lysis of adhesions in the course of an open cholecystectomy) are not separately billed.

E. Separate Procedures
The narrative for many CPT codes includes a parenthetical statement that the procedure represents a "separate procedure."

The inclusion of this statement indicates that the procedure, while possible to perform separately, is generally included in a more comprehensive procedure, and the service is not to be billed when a related, more comprehensive, service is performed. The "separate procedure" designation is used with codes in the surgery (CPT codes 10000-69999), radiology (CPT codes 70000-79999), and medicine (CPT codes 90000-99199) sections.

When a related procedure from the same section, subsection, category, or subcategory is performed, a code with the designation of "separate procedure" is not to be billed with the primary procedure.

F. Designation of Sex
Many procedure codes have a sex designation within their narrative. These codes are not billed with codes having an opposite sex designation because this would reflect a conflict in sex classification either by the definition of the code descriptions themselves, or by the fact that the performance of these procedures on the same beneficiary would be anatomically impossible.

G. Family of Codes
In a family of codes, there are two or more component codes that are not billed separately because they are included in a more comprehensive code as members of the code family.

Comprehensive codes include certain services that are separately identifiable by other component codes. The component codes as members of the comprehensive code family represent parts of the procedure that should not be listed separately when the complete procedure is done. However, the component codes are considered individually if performed independently of the complete procedure and if not all the services listed in the comprehensive codes were rendered to make up the total service.

H. Most Extensive Procedures
When procedures are performed together that are basically the same or performed on the same site but are qualified by an increased level of complexity, the less extensive procedure is bundled into the more extensive procedure.

I. Sequential Procedures
An initial approach to a procedure may be followed at the same encounter by a second, usually more invasive approach. There may be separate CPT codes describing each service. The second procedure is usually performed because the initial approach was unsuccessful in accomplishing the medically necessary service. These procedures are considered "sequential procedures." Only the CPT code for one of the services, generally the more invasive service, should be billed.

J. With/Without Procedures
In the CPT manual, there are various procedures that have been separated into two codes with the definitional difference being "with" versus "without" (e.g., with and without contrast). Both procedure codes cannot be billed. When done together, the "without" procedure is bundled into the "with" procedure.

K. Laboratory Panels
When components of a specific organ or disease oriented laboratory panel (e.g., codes 80061 and 80059) or automated multi-channel tests (e.g., codes 80002 - 80019) are billed separately, they must be bundled into the comprehensive panel or automated multichannel test code as appropriate that includes the multiple component tests. The individual tests that make up a panel or can be performed on an automated multi-channel test analyzer are not to be separately billed.

L Mutually Exclusive Procedures
There are numerous procedure codes that are not billed together because they are mutually exclusive of each other. Mutually exclusive codes are those codes that cannot reasonably be done in the same session.

An example of a mutually exclusive situation is when the repair of the organ can be performed by two different methods. One repair method must be chosen to repair the organ and must be billed. Another example is the billing of an "initial" service and a subsequent" service. It is contradictory for a service to be classified as an initial and a subsequent service at the same time.

CPT codes which are mutually exclusive of one another based either on the CPT definition or the medical impossibility/improbability that the procedures could be performed at the same session can be identified as code pairs. These codes are not necessarily linked to one another with one code narrative describing a more comprehensive procedure compared to the component code, but can be identified as code pairs which should not be billed together.

M. Use of Modifiers
When certain component codes or mutually exclusive codes are appropriately furnished, such as later on the same day or on a different digit or limb, it is appropriate that these services be reported using a HCPCS code modifier. Such modifiers are modifiers E1 -E4, FA, F1 - F9, TA, T1 - T9, LT, RT, LC, LD, RC, -58, -78, -79, and -94.

Modifier -59 is not appropriate to use with weekly radiation therapy management codes (77427) or with evaluation and management services codes (99201 - 99499).

Application of these modifiers prevent erroneous denials of claims for several procedures performed on different anatomical sites, on different sides of the body, or at different sessions on the same date of service. The medical record must reflect that the modifier is being used appropriately to describe separate services.

100-4, 12, 30.1

Digestive System (Codes 40000 - 49999)

B3-15100

A. Upper Gastrointestinal Endoscopy Including Endoscopic Ultrasound (EUS) (Code 43259)
If the person performing the original diagnostic endoscopy has access to the EUS and the clinical situation requires an EUS, the EUS may be done at the same time. The procedure, diagnostic and EUS, is reported under the same code, CPT 43259. This code conforms to CPT guidelines for the indented codes. The service represented by the indented code, in this case code 43259 for EUS, includes the service represented by the unintended code preceding the list of indented codes. Therefore, when a diagnostic examination of the upper gastrointestinal tract "including esophagus, stomach, and either the duodenum or jejunum as appropriate," includes the use of endoscopic ultrasonography, the service is reported by a single code, namely 43259.

Interpretation, whether by a radiologist or endoscopist, is reported under CPT code 76975-26. These codes may both be reported on the same day.

B. Incomplete Colonoscopies (Codes 45330 and 45378)
An incomplete colonoscopy, e.g., the inability to extend beyond the splenic flexure, is billed and paid using colonoscopy code 45378 with modifier "-53." The Medicare physician fee schedule database has specific values for code 45378-53. These values are the same as for code 45330, sigmoidoscopy, as failure to extend beyond the splenic flexure means that a sigmoidoscopy rather than a colonoscopy has been performed.

However, code 45378-53 should be used when an incomplete colonoscopy has been done because other MPFSDB indicators are different for codes 45378 and 45330.

100-4, 12, 30.2

Urinary and Male Genital Systems (Codes 50010 - 55899)

B3-15200

A. Cystourethroscopy With Ureteral Catheterization (Code 52005)
Code 52005 has a zero in the bilateral field (payment adjustment for bilateral procedure does not apply) because the basic procedure is an examination of the bladder and urethra (cystourethroscopy), which are not paired organs. The work RVUs assigned take into account that it may be necessary to examine and catheterize one or both ureters. No additional payment is made when the procedure is billed with bilateral modifier "-50." Neither is any additional payment made when both ureters are examined and code 52005 is billed with multiple surgery modifier "-51." It is inappropriate to bill code 52005 twice, once by itself and once with modifier "-51," when both ureters are examined.

B. Cystourethroscopy With Fulgration and/or Resection of Tumors (Codes 52234, 52235, and 52240)
The descriptors for codes 52234 through 52240 include the language "tumor(s)." This means that regardless of the number of tumors removed, only one unit of a single code can be billed on a given date of service. It is inconsistent to allow payment for removal of a small (code 52234) and a large (code 52240) tumor using two codes when only one code is allowed for the removal of more than one large tumor. For these three codes only one unit may be billed for any of these codes, only one of the codes may be billed, and the billed code reflects the size of the largest tumor removed.

100-4, 12, 30.3

Audiology Services

Section 1861(ll)(3)of the Social Security Act (the Act) defines "audiology services" as such hearing and balance assessment services furnished by a qualified audiologist as the audiologist is legally authorized to perform under State law (or the State regulatory mechanism provided by State law), as would otherwise by covered if furnished by a physician. In this section, these hearing and balance assessment services are termed "audiology services," regardless of whether they are furnished by an audiologist, physician, nonphysician practitioner (NPP), or hospital.

Because audiology services are diagnostic tests, when furnished in an office or hospital outpatient department, they must be furnished by or under the appropriate level of supervision of a physician as established in 42 CFR 410.32(b)(1) and 410.28(e). If not personally furnished by a physician, audiologist, or NPP, audiology services must be performed under direct physician supervision. As specified in 42 CFR 410.32(b)(2)(ii) or (v), respectively, these services are excepted from physician supervision when they are personally furnished by a qualified audiologist or performed by a nurse practitioner or clinical nurse specialist authorized to perform the tests under applicable State laws.

References to technicians apply also to other qualified clinical staff. See Pub. 100-02, chapter 15, section 80.3.D.

A - Correct Reporting

1. General. Contact the contractor for guidance if the CPT codebook changes the description of codes mentioned in this section.

   Other policies concerning audiological services are found in Pub. 100-02, chapter 15, section 80.3.

   See chapter 26 of this manual for place of service and type of service coding.

   Section 4541(a)(2) of the Balanced Budget Act (BBA) (P.L. 105-33), which added section 1834(k)(5) to (the Act), required that all claims for certain audiology services be reported using a uniform coding system. CMS chose HCPCS (Healthcare Common Procedure Coding System) as the coding system for the reporting of these services. This coding requirement is effective for all claims for audiology services submitted on or after April 1, 1998.

   The BBA also required payment under a prospective payment system for audiology services. Effective for claims with dates of service on or after January 1, 1999, the Medicare Physician Fee Schedule (MPFS) became the method of payment for audiology services furnished in the office setting and for the associated professional services furnished in physician's office and hospital outpatient settings.

   2. Use of the NPI. For audiologists who are enrolled and bill independently for services they render, the audiologist's NPI is required on all claims they submit. For example, in offices and private practice settings, an enrolled audiologist shall use his or her own NPI in the rendering loop to bill under the MPFS for the services the audiologist furnished. If an enrolled audiologist furnishing services to hospital outpatients reassigns his/her benefits to the hospital, the hospital may bill the carrier or Medicare administrative contractor for the professional services of the audiologist under the MPFS using the NPI of the audiologist. If an audiologist is employed by a hospital but is not enrolled in Medicare, the only payment for a hospital outpatient audiology service that can be made is the payment to the hospital for its facility services under the hospital Outpatient Prospective Payment System (OPPS) or other applicable hospital payment system. No payment can be made under the MPFS for professional services of an audiologist who is not enrolled.

   Audiologists must be enrolled and use their NPI on claims for services they render in office settings on or after October 1, 2008 (for additional information about enrollment, refer to Pub. 100-08, Medicare Program Integrity Manual, chapter 15). Before October 1, 2008, the services of audiologists who were not yet enrolled in Medicare were billed by a physician or group who employed the audiologist. Audiologists shall use the billing instructions in the Medicare manuals; for example, see this manual, chapter 1, section 30.

   See the most recent MPFS for pricing and physician supervision levels for audiology services: http://www.cms.hhs.gov/PFSlookup/01_Overview.asp#TopOfPage. The NPI of the supervising physician shall be used to bill audiology services when supervision is appropriate.

The most recent OPPS pricing for audiology services is available in Addendum B at: http://www.cms.gov/HospitalOutpatientPPS/AU/list.asp#TopOfPage.

B. Billing for Audiology Services

See the CMS Web site at http://www.cms.gov/PhysicianFeeSched/50_Audiology.asp

for a listing of all CPT codes for audiology services. For information concerning codes that are not on the list, and which codes may be billed when furnished by technicians, contractors shall provide guidance. The Physician Fee Schedule at http://www.cms.gov/PFSlookup/01_Overview.asp#TopOfPage allows you to search pricing amounts, various payment policy indicators, RVUs, and GPCIs.

Audiology services may not be billed when the place of service is a comprehensive outpatient rehabilitation facility (CORF) or a rehabilitation agency.

Audiology services may be furnished and billed by audiologists and, when these services are furnished by an audiologist, no physician supervision is required.

The interpretation and report shall be written in the medical record by the audiologist, physician, or NPP who personally furnished any audiology service, or by the physician who supervised the service. Technicians shall not interpret audiology services, but may record objective test results of those services they may furnish under direct physician supervision.

Payment for the interpretation and report of the services is included in payment for all audiology services, and specifically in the professional component if the audiology service has a professional component/technical component split.

1. Billing under the MPFS for Audiology Services Outside the Facility Setting

   The individuals who furnish audiology services in all settings must be qualified to furnish those services. The qualifications of the individual performing the services must be consistent with the number, type and complexity of the tests, the abilities of the individual, and the patient's ability to interact to produce valid and reliable results. The physician who supervises and bills for the service is responsible for assuring the qualifications of the technician, if applicable are appropriate to the test.

   a. Professional Skills.

      When a professional personally furnishes an audiology service, that individual must interact with the patient to provide professional skills and be directly involved in decision-making and clinical judgment during the test.

      The skills required when professionals furnish audiology services for payment under the MPFS are masters or doctoral level skills that involve clinical judgment or assessment and specialized knowledge and ability including, but not limited to, knowledge of anatomy and physiology, neurology, psychology, physics, psychometrics, and interpersonal communication. The interactions of these knowledge bases are required to attain the clinical expertise for audiology tests. Also required are skills to administer valid and reliable tests safely, especially when they involve stimulating the auditory nerve and testing complex brain functions.

      Diagnostic audiology services also require skills and judgment to administer and modify tests, to make informed interpretations about the causes and implications of the test results in the context of the history and presenting complaints, and to provide both objective results and professional knowledge to the patient and to the ordering physician.

      Examples include, but are not limited to:

      Comparison or consideration of the anatomical or physiological implications of test results or patient responsiveness to stimuli during the test; Development and modification of the test battery and test protocols; Clinical judgment, assessment, evaluation, and decision-making; Interpretation and reporting observations, in addition to the objective data, that may influence interpretation of the test outcomes; Tests related to implantation of auditory prosthetic devices, central auditory processing, contralateral masking; and/or

      Tests to identify central auditory processing disorders, tinnitus, or nonorganic hearing loss. Audiology codes may be billed under the MPFS by audiologists, physicians, and NPPs using their own NPI in the rendering loop when those professionals personally furnish the test. Physicians and NPPs may not bill for these codes when an audiologist has furnished the service.

   b. Technician Skills.

      There may be subtests, or parts of a battery of tests, that may be appropriately furnished by an educated and experienced technician using a specific protocol under the direction of a supervising physician. These services are identified by local contractor determination as services that do not require professional skills. They may be furnished by a qualified technician under the direct supervision of a physician, but not under the supervision of an audiologist or an NPP. The supervising physician is responsible for rendering and documenting all clinical judgment and for the appropriate provision of the service by the technician.

      A technician may not perform any part of a service that requires professional skills. A technician also may not perform a global service. For example, a technician may not interpret test results or engage in clinical decision-making.

   c. Professional Component (PC)/Technical Component (TC) Split Codes.

      The PC of a PC/TC split code may be billed by the audiologist, physician, or NPP who personally furnishes the service. (Note this is also true in the facility setting.) A physician or NPP may bill for the PC when the physician or NPP furnish the PC and an (unsupervised) audiologist furnishes and bills for the TC. The PC may not be billed if a technician furnishes the service. A physician or NPP may not bill for a PC service furnished by an audiologist. The TC of a PC/TC split code may be billed by the audiologist, physician, or NPP who personally furnishes the service. Physicians may bill the TC for services furnished by technicians when the technician furnishes the service under the direct supervision of that physician. Audiologists and NPPs may not bill for the TC of the service when a technician furnishes the service, even if the technician is supervised by the NPP or audiologist. The "global" service is billed when both the PC and TC of a service are personally furnished by the same audiologist, physician, or NPP. The global service may also be billed by a physician, but not an audiologist or NPP, when a technician furnishes the TC of the service under direct physician supervision and that physician furnishes the PC, including the interpretation and report. d. Tests that are Not Described by Specific CPT Codes. Tests that have no appropriate CPT code may be reported under CPT code 92700 (Unlisted otorhinolaryngological service or procedure).

   e. Tests that are Contractor-Priced. For codes valued by contractors, the contractor determines whether and how much, if applicable, to pay for the service. The contractor sets the requirements for personnel furnishing the tests.

2. Billing for Audiology Services Furnished to Hospital Outpatients.

   All codes may be reported for audiology services furnished in the hospital outpatient setting and, in such cases, the code represents the facility service for the diagnostic test. All audiology services furnished to hospital outpatients must be billed and paid to the hospital under the OPPS or other applicable hospital payment system. The hospital bills its fiscal intermediary or Medicare administrative contractor (A/B MAC) and is paid for the facility resources required to furnish the services, regardless of whether the service is furnished by a physician, NPP, audiologist, or technician.

Physicians, NPPs, and audiologists cannot bill and be paid for the TC of PC/TC split codes when these services are furnished to hospital outpatients. The associated professional services (represented by the PC or the CPT code for the audiology test which has no PC/TC split) of an enrolled audiologist, physician, or NPP who has reassigned benefits may be billed by the hospital to the carrier or A/B MAC, as appropriate. Alternatively, if the physician, NPP, or audiologist has not assigned benefits, the professional would bill his/her carrier or A/B MAC for the professional services furnished.

The appropriate revenue code for reporting audiology services is 0470 (Audiology; General Classification). Providers are required to report a line-item date of service per revenue code line for audiology services.

3. Billing for Audiology Services Furnished to Skilled Nursing Facility (SNF) Patients.

Payment for the facility resources (including the TC of PC/TC split codes) of audiology services provided to Part A inpatients of SNFs is included in the PPS rate. For SNFs, if the beneficiary has Part B but not Part A coverage (e.g., Part A benefits are exhausted), the SNF may elect to bill for audiology services but is not required to do so. As explained in Pub. 100-04, chapter 7, section 40.1, since audiology services furnished during a noncovered SNF stay are not bundled with speech-language pathology services, payment can be made either to the SNF or to the audiology service provider/supplier.

Audiologists, physicians, and NPPs enrolled in Medicare may bill directly for services rendered to Medicare beneficiaries who are in a SNF stay that is not covered by Part A but who have Part B eligibility. Payment is made based on the MPFS, whether on an institutional or professional claim. For beneficiaries in a noncovered SNF stay, audiology services are payable under Part B when billed by the SNF on an institutional claim as type of bill 22X, or when billed directly by the provider or supplier of the service (the audiologist, physician, or NPP who personally

furnishes the test) on a professional claim. For PC/TC split codes, the SNF may elect to bill for the TC of the test on an institutional claim but is not required to bill for the service.

C - Implant Processing

Payment for diagnostic testing of implants, such as cochlear, osseointegrated or brainstem implants, including programming or reprogramming following implantation surgery is not included in the global fee for the surgery.

The diagnostic analysis of a cochlear implant shall be billed using CPT codes 92601 through 92604.

Osseointegrated prosthetic devices should be billed and paid for under provisions of the applicable payment system. For example, payment may differ depending upon whether the device is furnished on an inpatient or outpatient basis, and by a hospital subject to the OPPS, or by a Critical Access Hospital, physician's clinic, or a Federally Qualified Health Center.

D - Aural Rehabilitation Services

General policy for evaluation and treatment of conditions related to the auditory system.

For evaluation of auditory processing disorders and speech-reading or lip-reading by a speech-language pathologist, use the untimed code 92506 with "1" as the unit of service, regardless of the duration of the service on a given day. This "always therapy" evaluation code must be provided by speech-language pathologists according to the policies in Pub. 100-02, chapter 15, sections 220 and 230. The codes 92620 and 92621 are diagnostic audiological tests and may not be used for SLP services.

For treatment of auditory processing disorders or auditory rehabilitation/auditory training (including speech-reading or lip-reading), 92507, and 92508 are used to report a single encounter with "1" as the unit of service, regardless of the duration of the service on a given day. These codes always represent SLP services. See Pub. 100-02, chapter 15, sections 220 and 230 for SLP policies. These SLP evaluation and treatment services are not covered when performed or billed by audiologists, even if they are supervised by physicians or qualified NPPs.

For evaluation of auditory rehabilitation to instruct the use of residual hearing provided by an implant or hearing aid related to hearing loss, the timed codes 92626 and 92627 are used. These are not "always therapy" codes. Evaluation of auditory rehabilitation shall be appropriately provided and billed by an audiologist or speech-language pathologist. Also, these services may be provided incident to a physician's or qualified NPP's service by a speech-language pathologist, or personally by a physician or qualified NPP within their scope of practice. Evaluation of auditory rehabilitation is a covered diagnostic test when performed and billed by an audiologist and is an SLP evaluation service covered under the SLP benefit when performed by a speech-language pathologist.

General policies for post implant services.

The services of a speech-language pathologist may be covered for SLP services provided after implantation of auditory devices. For example, a speech-language pathologist may provide evaluation and treatment of speech, language, cognition, voice, and auditory processing using code 92506 and 92507. Use 92626 and 92627 for auditory (aural) rehabilitation evaluation following cochlear implantation or for other hearing impairments.

For diagnostic testing of cochlear implants, audiologists use codes 92601, 92602, 92603 and 92604. These services may not be provided by speech-language pathologists or others, with the exception of physicians and NPPs who may personally provide the services that are within their scope of practice.

100-4, 12, 30.4

Cardiovascular System (Codes 92950-93799)

A. Echocardiography Contrast Agents

Effective October 1, 2000, physicians may separately bill for contrast agents used in echocardiography. Physicians should use HCPCS Code A9700 (Supply of Injectable Contrast Material for Use in Echocardiography, per study). The type of service code is 9. This code will be carrier-priced.

B. Electronic Analyses of Implantable Cardioverter-defibrillators and Pacemakers

The CPT codes 93731, 93734, 93741 and 93743 are used to report electronic analyses of single or dual chamber pacemakers and single or dual chamber implantable cardioverterdefibrillators. In the office, a physician uses a device called a programmer to obtain information about the status and performance of the device and to evaluate the patient's cardiac rhythm and response to the implanted device.

Advances in information technology now enable physicians to evaluate patients with implanted cardiac devices without requiring the patient to be present in the physician's office. Using a manufacturer's specific monitor/transmitter, a patient can send complete device data and specific cardiac data to a distant receiving station or secure Internet server. The electronic analysis of cardiac device data that is remotely obtained provides immediate and long-term data on the device and clinical data on the patient's cardiac functioning equivalent to that obtained during an in-office evaluation. Physicians should report the electronic analysis of an implanted cardiac device using remotely obtained data as described above with CPT code 93731, 93734, 93741 or 93743, depending on the type of cardiac device implanted in the patient.

100-4, 12, 30.5

Payment for Codes for Chemotherapy Administration and Nonchemotherapy Injections and Infusions

A. General

Codes for Chemotherapy administration and nonchemotherapy injections and infusions include the following three categories of codes in the American Medical Association's Current Procedural Terminology (CPT):

1. Hydration;
2. Therapeutic, prophylactic, and diagnostic injections and infusions (excluding chemotherapy); and
3. Chemotherapy administration.

Physician work related to hydration, injection, and infusion services involves the affirmation of the treatment plan and the supervision (pursuant to incident to requirements) of nonphysician clinical staff.

B. Hydration

The hydration codes are used to report a hydration IV infusion which consists of a prepackaged fluid and /or electrolytes (e.g. normal saline, D5-1/2 normal saline +30 mg EqKC1/liter) but are not used to report infusion of drugs or other substances.

C. Therapeutic, prophylactic, and diagnostic injections and infusions (excluding chemotherapy)

A therapeutic, prophylactic, or diagnostic IV infusion or injection, other than hydration, is for the administration of substances/drugs. The fluid used to administer the drug (s) is incidental hydration and is not separately payable.

If performed to facilitate the infusion or injection or hydration, the following services and items are included and are not separately billable:

1. Use of local anesthesia;
2. IV start;
3. Access to indwelling IV, subcutaneous catheter or port;
4. Flush at conclusion of infusion; and
5. Standard tubing, syringes and supplies.

Payment for the above is included in the payment for the chemotherapy administration or nonchemotherapy injection and infusion service.

If a significant separately identifiable evaluation and management service is performed, the appropriate E & M code should be reported utilizing modifier 25 in addition to the chemotherapy administration or nonchemotherapy injection and infusion service. For an evaluation and management service provided on the same day, a different diagnosis is not required.

The CPT 2006 includes a parenthetical remark immediately following CPT code 90772 (Therapeutic, prophylactic or diagnostic injection; (specify substance or drug); subcutaneous or intramuscular.) It states, "Do not report 90772 for injections given without direct supervision. To report, use 99211." This coding guideline does not apply to Medicare patients. If the RN, LPN or other auxiliary personnel furnishes the injection in the office and the physician is not present in the office to meet the supervision requirement, which is one of the requirements for coverage of an incident to service, then the injection is not covered. The physician would also not report 99211 as this would not be covered as an incident to service.

D. Chemotherapy Administration

Chemotherapy administration codes apply to parenteral administration of nonradionuclide anti-neoplastic drugs; and also to anti-neoplastic agents provided for treatment of noncancer diagnoses (e.g., cyclophosphamide for auto-immune conditions) or to substances such as monoclonal antibody agents, and other biologic response modifiers. The following drugs are commonly considered to fall under the category of monoclonal antibodies: infliximab, rituximab, alemtuzumb, gemtuzumab, and trastuzumab. Drugs commonly considered to fall under the category of hormonal antineoplastics include leuprolide acetate and goserelin acetate. The drugs cited are not intended to be a complete list of drugs that may be administered using the chemotherapy administration codes. Local carriers may provide additional guidance as to which drugs may be considered to be chemotherapy drugs under Medicare.

The administration of anti-anemia drugs and anti-emetic drugs by injection or infusion for cancer patients is not considered chemotherapy administration.

If performed to facilitate the chemotherapy infusion or injection, the following services and items are included and are not separately billable:

1. Use of local anesthesia;
2. IV access;

3. Access to indwelling IV, subcutaneous catheter or port;
4. Flush at conclusion of infusion;
5. Standard tubing, syringes and supplies; and
6. Preparation of chemotherapy agent(s).

Payment for the above is included in the payment for the chemotherapy administration service.

If a significant separately identifiable evaluation and management service is performed, the appropriate E & M code should be reported utilizing modifier 25 in addition to the chemotherapy code. For an evaluation and management service provided on the same day, a different diagnosis is not required.

E. Coding Rules for Chemotherapy Administration and Nonchemotherapy Injections and Infusion Services
Instruct physicians to follow the CPT coding instructions to report chemotherapy administration and nonchemotherapy injections and infusion services with the exception listed in subsection C for CPT code 90772. The physician should be aware of the following specific rules.

When administering multiple infusions, injections or combinations, the physician should report only one "initial" service code unless protocol requires that two separate IV sites must be used. The initial code is the code that best describes the key or primary reason for the encounter and should always be reported irrespective of the order in which the infusions or injections occur. If an injection or infusion is of a subsequent or concurrent nature, even if it is the first such service within that group of services, then a subsequent or concurrent code should be reported. For example, the first IV push given subsequent to an initial one-hour infusion is reported using a subsequent IV push code.

If more than one "initial" service code is billed per day, the carrier shall deny the second initial service code unless the patient has to come back for a separately identifiable service on the same day or has two IV lines per protocol. For these separately identifiable services, instruct the physician to report with modifier 59.

The CPT includes a code for a concurrent infusion in addition to an intravenous infusion for therapy, prophylaxis or diagnosis. Allow only one concurrent infusion per patient per encounter. Do not allow payment for the concurrent infusion billed with modifier 59 unless it is provided during a second encounter on the same day with the patient and is documented in the medical record.

For chemotherapy administration and therapeutic, prophylactic and diagnostic injections and infusions, an intravenous or intra-arterial push is defined as: 1.) an injection in which the healthcare professional is continuously present to administer the substance/drug and observe the patient; or 2.) an infusion of 15 minutes or less.

The physician may report the infusion code for "each additional hour" only if the infusion interval is greater than 30 minutes beyond the 1 hour increment. For example if the patient receives an infusion of a single drug that lasts 1 hour and 45 minutes, the physician would report the "initial" code up to 1 hour and the add-on code for the additional 45 minutes.

Several chemotherapy administration and nonchemotherapy injection and infusion service codes have the following parenthetical descriptor included as a part of the CPT code, "List separately in addition to code for primary procedure." Each of these codes has a physician fee schedule indicator of "ZZZ" meaning this service is allowed if billed with another chemotherapy administration or nonchemotherapy injection and infusion service code.

Do not interpret this parenthetical descriptor to mean that the add-on code can be billed only if it is listed with another drug administration primary code. For example, code 90761 will be ordinarily billed with code 90760. However, there may be instances when only the add-on code, 90761, is billed because an "initial" code from another section in the drug administration codes, instead of 90760, is billed as the primary code.

Pay for code 96523, "Irrigation of implanted venous access device for drug delivery systems," if it is the only service provided that day. If there is a visit or other chemotherapy administration or nonchemotherapy injection or infusion service provided on the same day, payment for 96523 is included in the payment for the other service.

F. Chemotherapy Administration (or Nonchemotherapy Injection and Infusion) and Evaluation and Management Services Furnished on the Same Day
For services furnished on or after January 1, 2004, do not allow payment for CPT code 99211, with or without modifier 25, if it is billed with a nonchemotherapy drug infusion code or a chemotherapy administration code. Apply this policy to code 99211 when it is billed with a diagnostic or therapeutic injection code on or after January 1, 2005.

Physicians providing a chemotherapy administration service or a nonchemotherapy drug infusion service and evaluation and management services, other than CPT code 99211, on the same day must bill in accordance with 30.6.6 using modifier 25. The carriers pay for evaluation and management services provided on the same day as the chemotherapy administration services or a nonchemotherapy injection or infusion service if the evaluation and management service meets the requirements of section 30.6.6 even though the underlying codes do not have global periods. If a chemotherapy service and a significant separately identifiable evaluation and management service are provided on the same day, a different diagnosis is not required.

In 2005, the Medicare physician fee schedule status database indicators for therapeutic and diagnostic injections were changed from T to A. Thus, beginning in 2005, the policy on evaluation and management services, other than 99211, that is applicable to a chemotherapy or a nonchemotherapy injection or infusion service applies equally to these codes.

100-4, 12, 30.6.1

Selection of Level of Evaluation and Management Service

A. Use of CPT Codes
Advise physicians to use CPT codes (level 1 of HCPCS) to code physician services, including evaluation and management services. Medicare will pay for E/M services for specific non-physician practitioners (i.e., nurse practitioner (NP), clinical nurse specialist (CNS) and certified nurse midwife (CNM)) whose Medicare benefit permits them to bill these services. A physician assistant (PA) may also provide a physician service, however, the physician collaboration and general supervision rules as well as all billing rules apply to all the above non-physician practitioners. The service provided must be medically necessary and the service must be within the scope of practice for a non-physician practitioner in the State in which he/she practices. Do not pay for CPT evaluation and management codes billed by physical therapists in independent practice or by occupational therapists in independent practice.

Medical necessity of a service is the overarching criterion for payment in addition to the individual requirements of a CPT code. It would not be medically necessary or appropriate to bill a higher level of evaluation and management service when a lower level of service is warranted. The volume of documentation should not be the primary influence upon which a specific level of service is billed. Documentation should support the level of service reported. The service should be documented during, or as soon as practicable after it is provided in order to maintain an accurate medical record.

B. Selection of Level Of Evaluation and Management Service
Instruct physicians to select the code for the service based upon the content of the service. The duration of the visit is an ancillary factor and does not control the level of the service to be billed unless more than 50 percent of the face-to-face time (for non-inpatient services) or more than 50 percent of the floor time (for inpatient services) is spent providing counseling or coordination of care as described in subsection C.

Any physician or non-physician practitioner (NPP) authorized to bill Medicare services will be paid by the carrier at the appropriate physician fee schedule amount based on the rendering UPIN/PIN.

"Incident to" Medicare Part B payment policy is applicable for office visits when the requirements for "incident to" are met (refer to sections 60.1, 60.2, and 60.3, chapter 15 in IOM 100-02).

SPLIT/SHARED E/M SERVICE

Office/Clinic Setting
In the office/clinic setting when the physician performs the E/M service the service must be reported using the physician's UPIN/PIN. When an E/M service is a shared/split encounter between a physician and a non-physician practitioner (NP, PA, CNS or CNM), the service is considered to have been performed "incident to" if the requirements for "incident to" are met and the patient is an established patient. If "incident to" requirements are not met for the shared/split E/M service, the service must be billed under the NPP's UPIN/PIN, and payment will be made at the appropriate physician fee schedule payment.

Hospital Inpatient/Outpatient/Emergency Department Setting

When a hospital inpatient/hospital outpatient or emergency department E/M is shared between a physician and an NPP from the same group practice and the physician provides any face-to-face

portion of the E/M encounter with the patient, the service may be billed under either the physician's or the NPP's UPIN/PIN number. However, if there was no face-to-face encounter between the patient and the physician (e.g., even if the physician participated in the service by only reviewing the patient's medical record) then the service may only be billed under the NPP's UPIN/PIN. Payment will be made at the appropriate physician fee schedule rate based on the UPIN/PIN entered on the claim.

EXAMPLES OF SHARED VISITS

1. If the NPP sees a hospital inpatient in the morning and the physician follows with a later face-to-face visit with the patient on the same day, the physician or the NPP may report the service.
2. In an office setting the NPP performs a portion of an E/M encounter and the physician completes the E/M service. If the "incident to" requirements are met, the physician reports the service. If the "incident to" requirements are not met, the service must be reported using the NPP's UPIN/PIN.

In the rare circumstance when a physician (or NPP) provides a service that does not reflect a CPT code description, the service must be reported as an unlisted service with CPT code 99499. A description of the service provided must accompany the claim. The carrier has the discretion to value the service when the service does not meet the full terms of a CPT code description (e.g., only a history is performed). The carrier also determines the payment based on the applicable percentage of the physician fee schedule depending on whether the claim is paid at the physician rate or the non-physician practitioner rate. CPT modifier -52 (reduced services) must not be used with an evaluation and management service. Medicare does not recognize modifier -52 for this purpose.

C. Selection Of Level Of Evaluation and Management Service Based On Duration Of Coordination Of Care and/or Counseling
Advise physicians that when counseling and/or coordination of care dominates (more than 50 percent) the face-to-face physician/patient encounter or the floor time (in the case of inpatient services), time is the key or controlling factor in selecting the level of service. In general, to bill an E/M code, the physician must complete at least 2 out of 3 criteria applicable to the type/level of service provided. However, the physician may document time spent with the patient in conjunction with the medical decision-making involved and a description of the coordination of care or counseling provided. Documentation must be in sufficient detail to support the claim.

Appendix G — Pub 100 References

EXAMPLE: A cancer patient has had all preliminary studies completed and a medical decision to implement chemotherapy. At an office visit the physician discusses the treatment options and subsequent lifestyle effects of treatment the patient may encounter or is experiencing. The physician need not complete a history and physical examination in order to select the level of service. The time spent in counseling/coordination of care and medical decision-making will determine the level of service billed.

The code selection is based on the total time of the face-to-face encounter or floor time, not just the counseling time. The medical record must be documented in sufficient detail to justify the selection of the specific code if time is the basis for selection of the code.

In the office and other outpatient setting, counseling and/or coordination of care must be provided in the presence of the patient if the time spent providing those services is used to determine the level of service reported. Face-to-face time refers to the time with the physician only. Counseling by other staff is not considered to be part of the face-to-face physician/patient encounter time. Therefore, the time spent by the other staff is not considered in selecting the appropriate level of service. The code used depends upon the physician service provided.

In an inpatient setting, the counseling and/or coordination of care must be provided at the bedside or on the patient's hospital floor or unit that is associated with an individual patient. Time spent counseling the patient or coordinating the patient's care after the patient has left the office or the physician has left the patient's floor or begun to care for another patient on the floor is not considered when selecting the level of service to be reported.

The duration of counseling or coordination of care that is provided face-to-face or on the floor may be estimated but that estimate, along with the total duration of the visit, must be recorded when time is used for the selection of the level of a service that involves predominantly coordination of care or counseling.

D. Use of Highest Levels of Evaluation and Management Codes
Contractors must advise physicians that to bill the highest levels of visit codes, the services furnished must meet the definition of the code (e.g., to bill a Level 5 new patient visit, the history must meet CPT's definition of a comprehensive history).

The comprehensive history must include a review of all the systems and a complete past (medical and surgical) family and social history obtained at that visit. In the case of an established patient, it is acceptable for a physician to review the existing record and update it to reflect only changes in the patient's medical, family, and social history from the last encounter, but the physician must review the entire history for it to be considered a comprehensive history.

The comprehensive examination may be a complete single system exam such as cardiac, respiratory, psychiatric, or a complete multi-system examination.

100-4, 12, 30.6.1.1

Initial Preventive Physical Examination (IPPE) and Annual Wellness Visit (AWV)

A. Definitions

1. Initial Preventive Physical Examination (IPPE)

   The initial preventive physical examination (IPPE), or "Welcome to Medicare Visit" (WMV) is a preventive evaluation and management service (E/M), allowed by Section 611 of the Medicare Prescription Drug Improvement and Modernization Act (MMA) of 2003, that includes:

   (1) review of the individual's medical and social history with attention to modifiable risk factors for disease detection,

   (2) review of the individual's potential (risk factors) for depression or other mood disorders,

   (3) review of the individual's functional ability and level of safety,

   (4) a physical examination to include measurement of the individual's height, weight, blood pressure, a visual acuity screen, and other factors as deemed appropriate by the examining physician or qualified nonphysician practitioner (NPP),

   (5) performance and interpretation of an electrocardiogram (EKG),

   (6) education, counseling, and referral, as deemed appropriate, based on the results of the review and evaluation services described in the previous 5 elements, and,

   (7) education, counseling, and referral including a brief written plan (e.g., a checklist or alternative) provided to the individual for obtaining the appropriate screening and other preventive services.

   Effective January 1, 2007, Section 5112 of the Deficit Reduction Act of 2005 allows for one ultrasound screening for Abdominal Aortic Aneurysm (AAA), HCPCS code G0389, as a result of a referral from an IPPE. This service is not subject to the Part B annual deductible. For AAA physician/practitioner billing, correct coding, and payment policy, refer to chapter 18, §110, of this manual.

   Effective January 1, 2009, Section 101 (b) of the Medicare Improvement for Patients and Providers Act (MIPPA) of 2008 requires the addition of the measurement of an individual's body mass index and, upon an individual's consent, end-of-life planning, to the IPPE. Also, effective January 1, 2009, MIPPA removes the screening electrocardiogram (EKG) as a mandatory service of the IPPE. MIPPA requires that there be education, counseling, and referral for an EKG, as appropriate. This is a once-in-a-lifetime screening EKG as a result of a referral from an IPPE.

   The MIPPA of 2008 allows for possible future payment for additional preventive services not otherwise described in Title XVIII of the Social Security Act (the Act) that identify medical conditions or risk factors for eligible individuals if the Secretary determines through the national coverage determination (NCD) process (as defined in Section 1869(f)(1)(B) of the Act) that they are: (1) reasonable and necessary for the prevention or early detection of illness or disability, (2) recommended with a grade of A or B by the United States Preventive Services Task Force (USPSTF), and, (3) appropriate for individuals entitled to benefits under Part A or enrolled under Part B, or both. MIPPA requires that there be education, counseling, and referral for additional preventive services, as appropriate, under the IPPE, if the Secretary determines in the future that such services are covered.

2. Annual Wellness Visit (AWV)

   Effective January 1, 2011, Section 4103 of the Affordable Care Act (ACA), allows for a preventive physical examination, called the annual wellness visit (AWV), and includes personal prevention plan services (PPPS). The AWV is a new annual Medicare preventive physical examination, available for eligible beneficiaries, and identified by new HCPCS codes G0438 (Annual wellness visit, including PPPS, first visit) and G0439 (Annual wellness visit, including PPPS, subsequent visit). Definitions relative to the AWV are included at Pub. 100-02, Medicare Benefit Policy Manual, chapter 15, section 280.5.

   First AWV services providing PPPS (HCPCS G0438) are a 'one time' allowed Medicare benefit and include the following key elements furnished to an eligible beneficiary by a health professional:

   - ,Establishment of the individual's medical/family history,
   - Measurement of the individual's height, weight, body mass index (or waist circumference, if appropriate), blood pressure (BP), and other routine measurements as deemed appropriate, based on the individual's medical and family history,
   - Establishment of a list of current providers and suppliers that are regularly involved in providing medical care to the individual,
   - Detection of any cognitive impairment that the individual may have,
   - Review of an individual's potential risk factors for depression , including current or past experiences with depression or other mood disorders, based on the use of an appropriate screening instrument for persons without a current diagnosis of depression, which the health professional may select from various available standardized screening tests designed for this purpose and recognized by national professional medical organizations,
   - Review of the individual's functional ability and level of safety, based on direct observation of the individual, or the use of appropriate screening questions or a screening questionnaire, which the health professional may select from various available screening questions or standardized questionnaires designed for this purpose and recognized by national professional medical organizations,
   - Establishment of a written screening schedule for the individual, such as a checklist for the next 5 to 10 years, as appropriate, based on recommendations of the USPSTF and Advisory Committee of Immunizations Practices (ACIP), the individual's health status, screening history, and age-appropriate preventive services covered by Medicare,
   - Establishment of a list of risk factors and conditions of which primary, secondary, or tertiary interventions are recommended or underway for the individual, including any mental health conditions or any such risk factors or conditions that have been identified through an IPPE, and a list of treatment options and their associated risks and benefits,
   - Provision of personalized health advice to the individual and a referral, as appropriate, to health education or preventive counseling services or programs aimed at reducing identified risk factors and improving self-management or community-based lifestyle interventions to reduce health risks and promote self-management and wellness, including weight loss, physical activity, smoking cessation, fall prevention, and nutrition, and,
   - Any other element(s) determined appropriate by the Secretary through the NCD process.

Subsequent AWV services providing PPPS (HCPCS G0439) include the following key elements furnished to an eligible beneficiary by a health professional:

- Update to the individual's medical /family history,
- Measurements of an individual's weight (or waist circumference), BP, and other routine measurements as deemed appropriate, based on the individual's medical and family history,
- Update to the list of the individual's current medical providers and suppliers that are regularly involved in providing medical care to the individual as that list was developed for the first AWV providing PPPS,
- Detection of any cognitive impairment that the individual may have,
- Update to the individual's written screening schedule as developed at the first AWV providing PPPS,
- Update to the individual's list of risk factors and conditions for which primary, secondary, or tertiary interventions are recommended or are underway for the individual, as that list was developed at the first AWV providing PPPS,
- Furnish appropriate personalized health advice to the individual and a referral, as appropriate, to health education or preventive counseling services or programs, and,
- Any other element determined appropriate by the Secretary through the NCD process.

Preventive services are separately covered under Medicare Part B. See chapter 18 of this manual.

B. Who May Perform

The IPPE and the AWV may be performed by a doctor of medicine or osteopathy as defined in Section 1861(r) (1) of the Act, by a qualified NPP (nurse practitioner, physician assistant or clinical nurse specialist), or for the AWV, by a health professional (a medical professional including a health educator, registered dietitian, nutrition professional, or other licensed practitioner) or a team of such medical professionals who are working under the direct supervision of a physician. The contractor pays the appropriate physician fee schedule amount based on the rendering National Provider Identification (NPI) number.

C. Eligibility

1. IPPE

   As a result of the MMA 2003, Medicare will pay for one IPPE per beneficiary per lifetime. A beneficiary is eligible when he/she first enrolls in Medicare Part B. For beneficiaries enrolled on or after January 1, 2005, beneficiaries must have received their IPPE within the first 6 months of Medicare coverage. The MIPPA extends the eligibility period for an IPPE to 12 months effective January 1, 2009.

   Beneficiaries in their first 12 months of Part B coverage will continue to be eligible for only the IPPE. Medicare continues to pay for only one IPPE per beneficiary per lifetime.

2. AWV

   As a result of the ACA, effective January 1, 2011, Medicare will pay for an AWV for a beneficiary who is no longer within 12 months after the effective date of his/her first Medicare Part B coverage period, and he/she has not received either an IPPE or an

   AWV providing PPPS within the past 12 months. Medicare pays for only one first AWV (HCPCS G0438), per beneficiary per lifetime, and all subsequent wellness visits must be billed as a subsequent AWV (HCPCS G0439).

   Beneficiaries in their first 12 months of Part B coverage will continue to be eligible for only the IPPE (see 30.6.1.1.A.1).

D. Deductible and Coinsurance

1. IPPE

   The Medicare deductible and coinsurance apply for the IPPE provided before January 1, 2009.

   The Medicare deductible is waived effective for the IPPE provided on or after January 1, 2009. However, the applicable coinsurance continues to apply for the IPPE provided on or after January 1, 2009.

   As a result of the ACA, effective for the IPPE provided on or after January 1, 2011, the Medicare deductible and coinsurance (for HCPCS code G0402 only) are waived.

2. AWV

   As a result of the ACA, effective January 1, 2011, the Medicare deductible and coinsurance for the AWV (HCPCS G0438 and G0439) are waived.

E. The EKG Component of the IPPE

Under the MMA of 2003, if the physician or qualified NPP is not able to perform both the examination and the screening EKG, an arrangement may be made to ensure that another physician or entity performs the screening EKG and reports the EKG separately using the appropriate HCPCS G code(s) identified in F.1. of this section. When the screening EKG is performed, the primary physician or qualified NPP shall document the results of the screening EKG into the beneficiary's medical record to complete and bill for the IPPE benefit.

NOTE: Both components of the IPPE (the examination and the screening EKG) must be performed before the claims can be submitted by the physician, qualified NPP, and/or entity.

MIPPA 2008 changes the once-in-a-lifetime screening EKG from a mandated service to a service that may be performed, as appropriate, with a referral from an IPPE. When an EKG is furnished with the IPPE, the deductible and coinsurance will continue to apply for EKG services only.

F. HCPCS Codes Used to Bill the IPPE or AWV

1. HCPCS Codes Used to Bill the IPPE

   For IPPE and EKG services provided prior to January 1, 2009, the physician or qualified NPP shall bill HCPCS code G0344 for the physical examination performed face-to-face, and HCPCS code G0366 for performing a screening EKG that includes both the interpretation and report. If the primary physician or qualified NPP performs only the examination, he/she shall bill HCPCS code G0344 only. The physician or entity that performs the screening EKG that includes both the interpretation and report shall bill HCPCS code G0366. The physician or entity that performs the screening EKG tracing only (without interpretation and report) shall bill HCPCS code G0367. The physician or entity that performs the interpretation and report only (without the EKG tracing) shall bill HCPCS code G0368. Medicare will pay for a screening EKG only as part of the IPPE. HCPCS codes G0344, G0366, G0367 and G0368 will not be billable codes effective on or after January 1, 2009.

   Effective for a beneficiary who has the IPPE on or after January 1, 2009, and within his/her 12-month enrollment period of Medicare Part B, the IPPE and screening EKG services are billable with the appropriate HCPCS G code(s).

   The physician or qualified NPP shall bill HCPCS code G0402 for the physical examination performed face-to-face with the patient.

   The physician or entity shall bill HCPCS code G0403 for performing the complete screening EKG that includes the tracing, interpretation and report.

   The physician or entity that performs the screening EKG tracing only (without interpretation and report) shall bill HCPCS code G0404.

   The physician or entity that performs the screening EKG interpretation and report only, (without the EKG tracing) shall bill HCPCS code G0405.

2. HCPCS Codes Used to Bill the AWV

   For the first AWV provided on or after January 1, 2011, the health professional shall bill HCPCS G0438 (Annual wellness visit, including PPPS, first visit). This is a once per beneficiary per lifetime allowable Medicare benefit.

   All subsequent AWVs shall be billed with HCPCS G0439 (Annual Wellness Visit, including PPPS, subsequent visit). In the event that a beneficiary selects a new health professional to complete a subsequent AWV, the new health professional will continue to bill the subsequent AWV with HCPCS G0439.

NOTE: For an IPPE or AWV performed during the global period of surgery refer to chapter 12, §30.6.6 of this manual for reporting instructions.

G. Documentation for the IPPE or AWV

The physician and qualified NPP, or for AWV the health professional, shall use the appropriate screening tools typically used in routine physician practice. Physicians, qualified NPPs, and medical professionals are required to use the 1995 and 1997 E/M documentation guidelines to document the medical record with the appropriate clinical information. (http://www.cms.hhs.gov/MLNEdWebGuide/25_EMDOC.asp). All referrals and a written medical plan must be included in this documentation.

H. Reporting a Medically Necessary E/M Service Furnished During the Same Encounter as an IPPE or AWV

When the physician or qualified NPP, or for AWV the health professional, provides a significant, separately identifiable medically necessary E/M service in addition to the IPPE or an AWV, CPT codes 99201–99215 may be reported depending on the clinical appropriateness of the circumstances. CPT Modifier ‚Äì25 shall be appended to the medically necessary E/M service identifying this service as a significant, separately identifiable service from the IPPE or AWV code reported (HCPCS code G0344 or G0402, whichever applies based on the date the IPPE is performed, or HCPCS code G0438 or G0439 whichever AWV code applies).

NOTE: Some of the components of a medically necessary E/M service (e.g., a portion of history or physical exam portion) may have been part of the IPPE or AWV and should not be included when determining the most appropriate level of E/M service to be billed for the medically necessary, separately identifiable, E/M service.

100-4, 12, 30.6.2

Billing for Medically Necessary Visit on Same Occasion as Preventive Medicine Service

See Chapter 18 for payment for covered preventive services.

When a physician furnishes a Medicare beneficiary a covered visit at the same place and on the same occasion as a noncovered preventive medicine service (CPT codes 99381- 99397), consider the covered visit to be provided in lieu of a part of the preventive medicine service of equal value to the visit. A preventive medicine service (CPT codes 99381-99397) is a noncovered service. The physician may charge the beneficiary, as a charge for the noncovered remainder of the service, the amount by which the physician's current established charge for the preventive medicine service exceeds his/her current established charge for the covered visit. Pay for the covered visit based on the lesser of the fee schedule amount or the physician's actual charge for the visit. The physician is not required to give the beneficiary written advance notice of noncoverage of the part of the visit that constitutes a routine preventive visit. However, the physician is responsible for notifying the patient in advance of his/her liability for the charges for services that are not medically necessary to treat the illness or injury.

There could be covered and noncovered procedures performed during this encounter (e.g., screening x-ray, EKG, lab tests.). These are considered individually. Those procedures which are for screening for asymptomatic conditions are considered noncovered and, therefore, no payment is made. Those procedures ordered to diagnose or monitor a symptom, medical condition, or treatment are evaluated for medical necessity and, if covered, are paid.

100-4, 12, 30.6.4

Evaluation and Management (E/M) Services Furnished Incident to Physician's Service by Nonphysician Practitioners

When evaluation and management services are furnished incident to a physician's service by a nonphysician practitioner, the physician may bill the CPT code that describes the evaluation and management service furnished.

When evaluation and management services are furnished incident to a physician's service by a nonphysician employee of the physician, not as part of a physician service, the physician bills code 99211 for the service.

A physician is not precluded from billing under the "incident to" provision for services provided by employees whose services cannot be paid for directly under the Medicare program. Employees of the physician may provide services incident to the physician's service, but the physician alone is permitted to bill Medicare.

Services provided by employees as "incident to" are covered when they meet all the requirements for incident to and are medically necessary for the individual needs of the patien

100-4, 12, 30.6.7

Payment for Office or Other Outpatient Evaluation and Management (E/M) Visits (Codes 99201 - 99215)

A Definition of New Patient for Selection of E/M Visit Code

Interpret the phrase "new patient" to mean a patient who has not received any professional services, i.e., E/M service or other face-to-face service (e.g., surgical procedure) from the physician or physician group practice (same physician specialty) within the previous 3 years. For example, if a professional component of a previous procedure is billed in a 3 year time period, e.g., a lab interpretation is billed and no E/M service or other face-to-face service with the patient is performed, then this patient remains a new patient for the initial visit. An interpretation of a diagnostic test, reading an x-ray or EKG etc., in the absence of an E/M service or other face-to-face service with the patient does not affect the designation of a new patient.

B. Office/Outpatient E/M Visits Provided on Same Day for Unrelated Problems
As for all other E/M services except where specifically noted, carriers may not pay two E/M office visits billed by a physician (or physician of the same specialty from the same group practice) for the same beneficiary on the same day unless the physician documents that the visits were for unrelated problems in the office or outpatient setting which could not be provided during the same encounter (e.g., office visit for blood pressure medication evaluation, followed five hours later by a visit for evaluation of leg pain following an accident).

C. Office/Outpatient or Emergency Department E/M Visit on Day of Admission to Nursing Facility
Carriers may not pay a physician for an emergency department visit or an office visit and a comprehensive nursing facility assessment on the same day. Bundle E/M visits on the same date provided in sites other than the nursing facility into the initial nursing facility care code when performed on the same date as the nursing facility admission by the same physician.

D. Drug Administration Services and E/M Visits Billed on Same Day of Service
Carriers must advise physicians that CPT code 99211 cannot be paid if it is billed with a drug administration service such as a chemotherapy or nonchemotherapy drug infusion code (effective January 1, 2004). This drug administration policy was expanded in the Physician Fee Schedule Final Rule, November 15, 2004, to also include a therapeutic or diagnostic injection code (effective January 1, 2005). Therefore, when a medically necessary, significant and separately identifiable E/M service (which meets a higher complexity level than CPT code 99211) is performed, in addition to one of these drug administration services, the appropriate E/M CPT code should be reported with modifier -25. Documentation should support the level of E/M service billed. For an E/M service provided on the same day, a different diagnosis is not required.

100-4, 12, 30.6.8

Payment for Hospital Observation Services (Codes 99217-99220) and Observation or Inpatient Care Services (Including Admission and Discharge Services – (Codes 99234-99236))

A. Who May Bill Observation Care Codes
Observation care is a well-defined set of specific, clinically appropriate services, which include ongoing short term treatment, assessment, and reassessment, that are furnished while a decision is being made regarding whether patients will require further treatment as hospital inpatients or if they are able to be discharged from the hospital. Observation services are commonly ordered for patients who present to the emergency department and who then require a significant period of treatment or monitoring in order to make a decision concerning their admission or discharge.

In only rare and exceptional cases do reasonable and necessary outpatient observation services span more than 48 hours. In the majority of cases, the decision whether to discharge a patient from the hospital following resolution of the reason for the observation care or to admit the patient as an inpatient can be made in less than 48 hours, usually in less than 24 hours.

Contractors pay for initial observation care billed by only the physician who ordered hospital outpatient observation services and was responsible for the patient during his/her observation care. A physician who does not have inpatient admitting privileges but who is authorized to furnish hospital outpatient observation services may bill these codes.

For a physician to bill observation care codes, there must be a medical observation record for the patient which contains dated and timed physician's orders regarding the observation services the patient is to receive, nursing notes, and progress notes prepared by the physician while the patient received observation services. This record must be in addition to any record prepared as a result of an emergency department or outpatient clinic encounter.

Payment for an initial observation care code is for all the care rendered by the ordering physician on the date the patient's observation services began. All other physicians who furnish consultations or additional evaluations or services while the patient is receiving hospital outpatient observation services must bill the appropriate outpatient service codes.

For example, if an internist orders observation services and asks another physician to additionally evaluate the patient, only the internist may bill the initial and subsequent observation care codes. The other physician who evaluates the patient must bill the new or established office or other outpatient visit codes as appropriate.

For information regarding hospital billing of observation services, see Chapter 4, §290.

B. Physician Billing for Observation Care Following Initiation of Observation Services
Similar to initial observation codes, payment for a subsequent observation care code is for all the care rendered by the treating physician on the day(s) other than the initial or discharge date. All other physicians who furnish consultations or additional evaluations or services while the patient is receiving hospital outpatient observation services must bill the appropriate outpatient service codes.

When a patient receives observation care for less than 8 hours on the same calendar date, the Initial Observation Care, from CPT code range 99218–99220, shall be reported by the physician. The Observation Care Discharge Service, CPT code 99217, shall not be reported for this scenario.

When a patient is admitted for observation care and then is discharged on a different calendar date, the physician shall report Initial Observation Care, from CPT code range 99218–99220, and CPT observation care discharge CPT code 99217. On the rare occasion when a patient remains in observation care for 3 days, the physician shall report an initial observation care code (99218-99220) for the first day of observation care, a subsequent observation care code (99224-99226) for the second day of observation care, and an observation care discharge CPT code 99217 for the observation care on the discharge date. When observation care continues beyond 3 days, the physician shall report a subsequent observation care code (99224-99226) for each day between the first day of observation care and the discharge date.

When a patient receives observation care for a minimum of 8 hours, but less than 24 hours, and is discharged on the same calendar date, Observation or Inpatient Care Services (Including Admission and Discharge Services) from CPT code range 99234–99236 shall be reported. The observation discharge, CPT code 99217, cannot also be reported for this scenario.

C. Documentation Requirements for Billing Observation or Inpatient Care Services (Including Admission and Discharge Services)
The physician shall satisfy the E/M documentation guidelines for furnishing observation care or inpatient hospital care. In addition to meeting the documentation requirements for history, examination, and medical decision making, documentation in the medical record shall include:

- Documentation stating the stay for observation care or inpatient hospital care involves 8 hours, but less than 24 hours;
- Documentation identifying the billing physician was present and personally performed the services; and
- Documentation identifying the order for observation services, progress notes, and discharge notes were written by the billing physician.

In the rare circumstance when a patient receives observation services for more than 2 calendar dates, the physician shall bill observation services furnished on day(s) other than the initial or discharge date using subsequent observation care codes. The physician may not use the subsequent hospital care codes since the patient is not an inpatient of the hospital.

D. Admission to Inpatient Status Following Observation Care
If the same physician who ordered hospital outpatient observation services also admits the patient to inpatient status before the end of the date on which the patient began receiving hospital outpatient observation services, pay only an initial hospital visit for the evaluation and management services provided on that date. Medicare payment for the initial hospital visit includes all services provided to the patient on the date of admission by that physician, regardless of the site of service. The physician may not bill an initial or subsequent observation care code for services on the date that he or she admits the patient to inpatient status. If the patient is admitted to inpatient status from hospital outpatient observation care subsequent to the date of initiation of observation services, the physician must bill an initial hospital visit for the services provided on that date. The physician may not bill the hospital observation discharge management code (code 99217) or an outpatient/office visit for the care provided while the patient received hospital outpatient observation services on the date of admission to inpatient status.

E. Hospital Observation Services During Global Surgical Period
The global surgical fee includes payment for hospital observation (codes 99217, 99218, 99219, 99220, 99224, 99225, 99226, 99234, 99235, and 99236) services unless the criteria for use of CPT modifiers "-24," "-25," or "-57" are met. Contractors must pay for these services in addition to the global surgical fee only if both of the following requirements are met:

- The hospital observation service meets the criteria needed to justify billing it with CPT modifiers "-24," "-25," or "-57" (decision for major surgery); and
- The hospital observation service furnished by the surgeon meets all of the criteria for the hospital observation code billed.

Examples of the decision for surgery during a hospital observation period are:

- An emergency department physician orders hospital outpatient observation services for a patient with a head injury. A neurosurgeon is called in to evaluate the need for surgery while the patient is receiving observation services and decides that the patient requires surgery. The surgeon would bill a new or established office or other outpatient visit code as appropriate with the "-57" modifier to indicate that the decision for surgery was made during the evaluation. The surgeon must bill the office or other outpatient visit code because the patient receiving hospital outpatient observation services is not an inpatient of the hospital. Only the physician who ordered hospital outpatient observation services may bill for observation care.
- A neurosurgeon orders hospital outpatient observation services for a patient with a head injury. During the observation period, the surgeon makes the decision for surgery. The surgeon would bill the appropriate level of hospital observation code with the "-57" modifier to indicate that the decision for surgery was made while the surgeon was providing hospital observation care.

Examples of hospital observation services during the postoperative period of a surgery are:

- A surgeon orders hospital outpatient observation services for a patient with abdominal pain from a kidney stone on the 80th day following a TURP (performed by that surgeon). The surgeon decides that the patient does not require surgery. The surgeon would bill the observation code with CPT modifier "-24" and documentation to support that the observation services are unrelated to the surgery.
- A surgeon orders hospital outpatient observation services for a patient with abdominal pain on the 80th day following a TURP (performed by that surgeon). While the patient is receiving hospital outpatient observation services, the surgeon decides that the patient requires kidney surgery. The surgeon would bill the observation code with HCPCS modifier "-57" to indicate that the decision for surgery was made while the patient was receiving hospital outpatient observation services. The subsequent surgical procedure would be reported with modifier "-79."
- A surgeon orders hospital outpatient observation services for a patient with abdominal pain on the 20th day following a resection of the colon (performed by that surgeon). The surgeon determines that the patient requires no further colon surgery and discharges the patient. The surgeon may not bill for the observation services furnished during the global period because they were related to the previous surgery.

An example of a billable hospital observation service on the same day as a procedure is when a physician repairs a laceration of the scalp in the emergency department for a patient with a head injury and then subsequently orders hospital outpatient observation services for that patient. The physician would bill the observation code with a CPT modifier 25 and the procedure code.

100-4, 12, 30.6.9

Payment for Inpatient Hospital Visits - General (Codes 99221 - 99239)

A. Hospital Visit and Critical Care on Same Day
When a hospital inpatient or office/outpatient evaluation and management service (E/M) are furnished on a calendar date at which time the patient does not require critical care and the patient subsequently requires critical care both the critical Care Services (CPT codes 99291 and 99292) and the previous E/M service may be paid on the same date of service. Hospital emergency department services are not paid for the same date as critical care services when provided by the same physician to the same patient.

During critical care management of a patient those services that do not meet the level of critical care shall be reported using an inpatient hospital care service with CPT Subsequent Hospital Care using a code from CPT code range 99231–99233.

Both Initial Hospital Care (CPT codes 99221–99223) and Subsequent Hospital Care codes are "per diem" services and may be reported only once per day by the same physician or physicians of the same specialty from the same group practice.

Physicians and qualified nonphysician practitioners (NPPs) are advised to retain documentation for discretionary contractor review should claims be questioned for both hospital care and critical care claims. The retained documentation shall support claims for critical care when the same physician or physicians of the same specialty in a group practice report critical care services for the same patient on the same calendar date as other E/M services.

B. Two Hospital Visits Same Day
Contractors pay a physician for only one hospital visit per day for the same patient, whether the problems seen during the encounters are related or not. The inpatient hospital visit descriptors contain the phrase "per day" which means that the code and the payment established for the code represent all services provided on that date. The physician should select a code that reflects all services provided during the date of the service.

C. Hospital Visits Same Day But by Different Physicians
In a hospital inpatient situation involving one physician covering for another, if physician A sees the patient in the morning and physician B, who is covering for A, sees the same patient in the evening, contractors do not pay physician B for the second visit. The hospital visit descriptors include the phrase "per day" meaning care for the day.

If the physicians are each responsible for a different aspect of the patient's care, pay both visits if the physicians are in different specialties and the visits are billed with different diagnoses. There are circumstances where concurrent care may be billed by physicians of the same specialty.

D. Visits to Patients in Swing Beds
If the inpatient care is being billed by the hospital as inpatient hospital care, the hospital care codes apply. If the inpatient care is being billed by the hospital as nursing facility care, then the nursing facility codes apply.

100-4, 12, 30.6.9.1

Payment for Initial Hospital Care Services (Codes 99221–99223 and Observation or Inpatient Care Services (Including Admission and Discharge Services) (Codes 99234–99236)

A. Initial Hospital Care From Emergency Room
Contractors pay for an initial hospital care service if a physician sees a patient in the emergency room and decides to admit the person to the hospital. They do not pay for both E/M services. Also, they do not pay for an emergency department visit by the same physician on the same date of service. When the patient is admitted to the hospital via another site of service (e.g., hospital emergency department, physician's office, nursing facility), all services provided by the physician in conjunction with that admission are considered part of the initial hospital care when performed on the same date as the admission.

B. Initial Hospital Care on Day Following Visit
Contractors pay both visits if a patient is seen in the office on one date and admitted to the hospital on the next date, even if fewer than 24 hours has elapsed between the visit and the admission.

C. Initial Hospital Care and Discharge on Same Day
When the patient is admitted to inpatient hospital care for less than 8 hours on the same date, then Initial Hospital Care, from CPT code range 99221–99223, shall be reported by the physician. The Hospital Discharge Day Management service, CPT codes 99238 or 99239, shall not be reported for this scenario.

When a patient is admitted to inpatient initial hospital care and then discharged on a different calendar date, the physician shall report an Initial Hospital Care from CPT code range 99221–99223 and a Hospital Discharge Day Management service, CPT code 99238 or 99239.

When a patient has been admitted to inpatient hospital care for a minimum of 8 hours but less than 24 hours and discharged on the same calendar date, Observation or Inpatient Hospital Care Services (Including Admission and Discharge Services), from CPT code range 99234–99236, shall be reported.

D. Documentation Requirements for Billing Observation or Inpatient Care Services (Including Admission and Discharge Services)
The physician shall satisfy the E/M documentation guidelines for admission to and discharge from inpatient observation or hospital care. In addition to meeting the documentation requirements for history, examination and medical decision making documentation in the medical record shall include:

- Documentation stating the stay for hospital treatment or observation care status involves 8 hours but less than 24 hours;
- Documentation identifying the billing physician was present and personally performed the services; and
- Documentation identifying the admission and discharge notes were written by the billing physician.

E. Physician Services Involving Transfer From One Hospital to Another; Transfer Within Facility to Prospective Payment System (PPS) Exempt Unit of Hospital; Transfer From One Facility to Another Separate Entity Under Same Ownership and/or Part of Same Complex; or Transfer From One Department to Another Within Single Facility
Physicians may bill both the hospital discharge management code and an initial hospital care code when the discharge and admission do not occur on the same day if the transfer is between:

- Different hospitals;
- Different facilities under common ownership which do not have merged records; or
- Between the acute care hospital and a PPS exempt unit within the same hospital when there are no merged records.

In all other transfer circumstances, the physician should bill only the appropriate level of subsequent hospital care for the date of transfer.

F. Initial Hospital Care Service History and Physical That Is Less Than Comprehensive
When a physician performs a visit that meets the definition of a Level 5 office visit several days prior to an admission and on the day of admission performs less than a comprehensive history and physical, he or she should report the office visit that reflects the services furnished and also report the lowest level initial hospital care code (i.e., code 99221) for the initial hospital admission. Contractors pay the office visit as billed and the Level 1 initial hospital care code.

Physicians who provide an initial visit to a patient during inpatient hospital care that meets the minimum key component work and/or medical necessity requirements shall report an initial hospital care code (99221-99223). The principal physician of record shall append modifier "-AI" (Principal Physician of Record) to the claim for the initial hospital care code. This modifier will identify the physician who oversees the patient's care from all other physicians who may be furnishing specialty care.

Physicians may bill initial hospital care service codes (99221-99223), for services that were reported with CPT consultation codes (99241–99255) prior to January 1, 2010, when the furnished service and documentation meet the minimum key component work and/or medical necessity requirements. Physicians must meet all the requirements of the initial hospital care codes, including "a detailed or comprehensive history" and "a detailed or comprehensive examination" to report CPT code 99221, which are greater than the requirements for consultation codes 99251 and 99252.

Subsequent hospital care CPT codes 99231 and 99232, respectively, require "a problem focused interval history" and "an expanded problem focused interval history." An E/M service that could be described by CPT consultation code 99251 or 99252 could potentially meet the component work and medical necessity requirements to report 99231 or 99232. Physicians may report a subsequent hospital care CPT code for services that were reported as CPT consultation codes (99241–99255) prior to January 1, 2010, where the medical record appropriately demonstrates that the work and medical necessity requirements are met for reporting a subsequent hospital care code (under the level selected), even though the reported code is for the provider's first E/M service to the inpatient during the hospital stay.

Reporting CPT code 99499 (Unlisted evaluation and management service) should be limited to cases where there is no other specific E/M code payable by Medicare that describes that service.

Reporting CPT code 99499 requires submission of medical records and contractor manual medical review of the service prior to payment. Contractors shall expect reporting under these circumstances to be unusual.

G. Initial Hospital Care Visits by Two Different M.D.s or D.O.s When They Are Involved in Same Admission
In the inpatient hospital setting all physicians (and qualified nonphysician practitioners where permitted) who perform an initial evaluation may bill the initial hospital care codes (99221–99223) or nursing facility care codes (99304–99306). Contractors consider only one M.D. or D.O. to be the principal physician of record (sometimes referred to as the admitting physician.) The principal physician of record is identified in Medicare as the physician who oversees the patient's care from other physicians who may be furnishing specialty care. Only the principal physician of record shall append modifier "-AI" (Principal Physician of Record) in addition to the E/M code. Follow-up visits in the facility setting shall be billed as subsequent hospital care visits and subsequent nursing facility care visits.

100-4, 12, 30.6.9.2

Subsequent Hospital Visit and Hospital Discharge Day Management (Codes 99231 - 99239)

A. Subsequent Hospital Visits During the Global Surgery Period
(Refer to Secs.40-40.4 on global surgery)

The Medicare physician fee schedule payment amount for surgical procedures includes all services (e.g., evaluation and management visits) that are part of the global surgery payment; therefore, contractors shall not pay more than that amount when a bill is fragmented for staged procedures.

B. Hospital Discharge Day Management Service
Hospital Discharge Day Management Services, CPT code 99238 or 99239 is a face-to-face evaluation and management (E/M) service between the attending physician and the patient. The E/M discharge day management visit shall be reported for the date of the actual visit by the physician or qualified nonphysician practitioner even if the patient is discharged from the facility on a different calendar date. Only one hospital discharge day management service is payable per patient per hospital stay.

Only the attending physician of record reports the discharge day management service. Physicians or qualified nonphysician practitioners, other than the attending physician, who have been managing concurrent health care problems not primarily managed by the attending physician, and who are not acting on behalf of the attending physician, shall use Subsequent Hospital Care (CPT code range 99231 - 99233) for a final visit.

Medicare pays for the paperwork of patient discharge day management through the pre- and post- service work of an E/M service.

C. Subsequent Hospital Visit and Discharge Management on Same Day
Pay only the hospital discharge management code on the day of discharge (unless it is also the day of admission, in which case, refer to Sec.30.6.9.1 C for the policy on Observation or Inpatient Care Services (Including Admission and Discharge Services CPT Codes 99234 - 99236). Contractors do not pay both a subsequent hospital visit in addition to hospital discharge day management service on the same day by the same physician. Instruct physicians that they may not bill for both a hospital visit and hospital discharge management for the same date of service.

D. Hospital Discharge Management (CPT Codes 99238 and 99239) and Nursing Facility Admission Code When Patient Is Discharged From Hospital and Admitted to Nursing Facility on Same Day
Contractors pay the hospital discharge code (codes 99238 or 99239) in addition to a nursing facility admission code when they are billed by the same physician with the same date of service.

If a surgeon is admitting the patient to the nursing facility due to a condition that is not as a result of the surgery during the postoperative period of a service with the global surgical period, he/she bills for the nursing facility admission and care with a modifier "-24" and provides documentation that the service is unrelated to the surgery (e.g., return of an elderly patient to the nursing facility in which he/she has resided for five years following discharge from the hospital for cholecystectomy).

Contractors do not pay for a nursing facility admission by a surgeon in the postoperative period of a procedure with a global surgical period if the patient's admission to the nursing facility is to receive post operative care related to the surgery (e.g., admission to a nursing facility to receive physical therapy following a hip replacement). Payment for the nursing facility admission and subsequent nursing facility services are included in the global fee and cannot be paid separately.

E. Hospital Discharge Management and Death Pronouncement
Only the physician who personally performs the pronouncement of death shall bill for the face-to-face Hospital Discharge Day Management Service, CPT code 99238 or 99239. The date of the pronouncement shall reflect the calendar date of service on the day it was performed even if the paperwork is delayed to a subsequent date.

100-4, 12, 30.6.10

Consultation Services

Consultation Services versus Other Evaluation and Management (E/M) Visits
Effective January 1, 2010, the consultation codes are no longer recognized for Medicare Part B payment. Physicians shall code patient evaluation and management visits with E/M codes that represent where the visit occurs and that identify the complexity of the visit performed.

In the inpatient hospital setting and the nursing facility setting, physicians (and qualified nonphysician practitioners where permitted) may bill the most appropriate initial hospital care code (99221-99223), subsequent hospital care code (99231 and 99232), initial nursing facility care code (99304-99306), or subsequent nursing facility care code (99307-99310) that reflects the services the physician or practitioner furnished. Subsequent hospital care codes could potentially meet the component work and medical necessity requirements to be reported for an E/M service that could be described by CPT consultation code 99251 or 99252. Contractors shall not find fault in cases where the medical record appropriately demonstrates that the work and medical necessity requirements are met for reporting a subsequent hospital care code (under the level selected), even though the reported code is for the provider's first E/M service to the inpatient during the hospital stay. Unlisted evaluation and management service (code 99499) shall only be reported for consultation services when an E/M service that could be described by codes 99251 or 99252 is furnished, and there is no other specific E/M code payable by Medicare that describes that service. Reporting code 99499 requires submission of medical records and contractor manual medical review of the service prior to payment. CMS expects reporting under these circumstances to be unusual. T he principal physician of record is identified in Medicare as the physician who oversees the patient's care from other physicians who may be furnishing specialty care. The principal physician of record shall append modifier "-AI" (Principal Physician of Record), in addition to the E/M code. Follow-up visits in the facility setting shall be billed as subsequent hospital care visits and subsequent nursing facility care visits.

In the CAH setting, those CAHs that use method II shall bill the appropriate new or established visit code for those physician and non-physician practitioners who have reassigned their billing rights, depending on the relationship status between the physician and patient.

In the office or other outpatient setting where an evaluation is performed, physicians and qualified nonphysician practitioners shall use the CPT codes (99201–99215) depending on the complexity of the visit and whether the patient is a new or established patient to that physician. All physicians and qualified nonphysician practitioners shall follow the E/M documentation guidelines for all E/M services. These rules are applicable for Medicare secondary payer claims as well as for claims in which Medicare is the primary payer.

100-4, 12, 30.6.11

Emergency Department Visits (Codes 99281 - 99288)

A. Use of Emergency Department Codes by Physicians Not Assigned to Emergency Department
Any physician seeing a patient registered in the emergency department may use emergency department visit codes (for services matching the code description). It is not required that the physician be assigned to the emergency department.

B. Use of Emergency Department Codes In Office
Emergency department coding is not appropriate if the site of service is an office or outpatient setting or any sight of service other than an emergency department. The emergency department codes should only be used if the patient is seen in the emergency department and the services described by the HCPCS code definition are provided. The emergency department is defined as an organized hospital-based facility for the provision of unscheduled or episodic services to patients who present for immediate medical attention.

C. Use of Emergency Department Codes to Bill Nonemergency Services
Services in the emergency department may not be emergencies. However the codes (99281 - 99288) are payable if the described services are provided.

However, if the physician asks the patient to meet him or her in the emergency department as an alternative to the physician's office and the patient is not registered as a patient in the emergency department, the physician should bill the appropriate office/outpatient visit codes. Normally a lower level emergency department code would be reported for a nonemergency condition.

D. Emergency Department or Office/Outpatient Visits on Same Day As Nursing Facility Admission
Emergency department visit provided on the same day as a comprehensive nursing facility assessment are not paid. Payment for evaluation and management services on the same date provided in sites other than the nursing facility are included in the payment for initial nursing facility care when performed on the same date as the nursing facility admission.

E. Physician Billing for Emergency Department Services Provided to Patient by Both Patient's Personal Physician and Emergency Department Physician
If a physician advises his/her own patient to go to an emergency department (ED) of a hospital for care and the physician subsequently is asked by the ED physician to come to the hospital to evaluate the patient and to advise the ED physician as to whether the patient should be admitted to the hospital or be sent home, the physicians should bill as follows:

If the patient is admitted to the hospital by the patient's personal physician, then the patient's regular physician should bill only the appropriate level of the initial hospital care (codes 99221 - 99223) because all evaluation and management services provided by that physician in conjunction with that admission are considered part of the initial hospital care when performed on the same date as the admission. The ED physician who saw the patient in the emergency department should bill the appropriate level of the ED codes.

If the ED physician, based on the advice of the patient's personal physician who came to the emergency department to see the patient, sends the patient home, then the ED physician should bill the appropriate level of emergency department service. The patient's personal physician should also bill the level of emergency department code that describes the service he or she provided in the emergency department. If the patient's personal physician does not come to the hospital to see the patient, but only advises the emergency department physician by telephone, then the patient's personal physician may not bill.

F. Emergency Department Physician Requests Another Physician to See the Patient in Emergency Department or Office/Outpatient Setting

If the emergency department physician requests that another physician evaluate a given patient, the other physician should bill an emergency department visit code. If the patient is admitted to the hospital by the second physician performing the evaluation, he or she should bill an initial hospital care code and not an emergency department visit code.

100-4, 12, 30.6.12

Critical Care Visits and Neonatal Intensive Care (Codes 99291 - 99292)

CRITICAL CARE SERVICES (CODES 99291-99292)

A. Use of Critical Care Codes
Pay for services reported with CPT codes 99291 and 99292 when all the criteria for critical care and critical care services are met. Critical care is defined as the direct delivery by a physician(s) medical care for a critically ill or critically injured patient. A critical illness or injury acutely impairs one or more vital organ systems such that there is a high probability of imminent or life threatening deterioration in the patient's condition.

Critical care involves high complexity decision making to assess, manipulate, and support vital system functions(s) to treat single or multiple vital organ system failure and/or to prevent further life threatening deterioration of the patient's condition.

Examples of vital organ system failure include, but are not limited to: central nervous system failure, circulatory failure, shock, renal, hepatic, metabolic, and/or respiratory failure. Although critical care typically requires interpretation of multiple physiologic parameters and/or application of advanced technology(s), critical care may be provided in life threatening situations when these elements are not present.

Providing medical care to a critically ill, injured, or post-operative patient qualifies as a critical care service only if both the illness or injury and the treatment being provided meet the above requirements.

Critical care is usually, but not always, given in a critical care area such as a coronary care unit, intensive care unit, respiratory care unit, or the emergency department. However, payment may be made for critical care services provided in any location as long as the care provided meets the definition of critical care.

Consult the American Medical Association (AMA) CPT Manual for the applicable codes and guidance for critical care services provided to neonates, infants and children.

B. Critical Care Services and Medical Necessity
Critical care services must be medically necessary and reasonable. Services provided that do not meet critical care services or services provided for a patient who is not critically ill or injured in accordance with the above definitions and criteria but who happens to be in a critical care, intensive care, or other specialized care unit should be reported using another appropriate E/M code (e.g., subsequent hospital care, CPT codes 99231 - 99233).

As described in Section A, critical care services encompass both treatment of "vital organ failure" and "prevention of further life threatening deterioration of the patient's condition." Therefore, although critical care may be delivered in a moment of crisis or upon being called to the patient's bedside emergently, this is not a requirement for providing critical care service. The treatment and management of the patient's condition, while not necessarily emergent, shall be required, based on the threat of imminent deterioration (i.e., the patient shall be critically ill or injured at the time of the physician's visit).

Chronic Illness and Critical Care:

Examples of patients whose medical condition may not warrant critical care services:

1. Daily management of a patient on chronic ventilator therapy does not meet the criteria for critical care unless the critical care is separately identifiable from the chronic long term management of the ventilator dependence.
2. Management of dialysis or care related to dialysis for a patient receiving ESRD hemodialysis does not meet the criteria for critical care unless the critical care is separately identifiable from the chronic long term management of the dialysis dependence (refer to Chapter 8, Sec.160.4). When a separately identifiable condition (e.g., management of seizures or pericardial tamponade related to renal failure) is being managed, it may be billed as critical care if critical care requirements are met. Modifier -25 should be appended to the critical care code when applicable in this situation.

Examples of patients whose medical condition may warrant critical care services:

1. An 81 year old male patient is admitted to the intensive care unit following abdominal aortic aneurysm resection. Two days after surgery he requires fluids and pressors to maintain adequate perfusion and arterial pressures. He remains ventilator dependent.
2. A 67 year old female patient is 3 days status post mitral valve repair. She develops petechiae, hypotension and hypoxia requiring respiratory and circulatory support.
3. A 70 year old admitted for right lower lobe pneumococcal pneumonia with a history of COPD becomes hypoxic and hypotensive 2 days after admission.
4. A 68 year old admitted for an acute anterior wall myocardial infarction continues to have symptomatic ventricular tachycardia that is marginally responsive to antiarrhythmic therapy.

Examples of patients who may not satisfy Medicare medical necessity criteria, or do not meet critical care criteria or who do not have a critical care illness or injury and therefore not eligible for critical care payment:

1. Patients admitted to a critical care unit because no other hospital beds were available;
2. Patients admitted to a critical care unit for close nursing observation and/or frequent monitoring of vital signs (e.g., drug toxicity or overdose); and
3. Patients admitted to a critical care unit because hospital rules require certain treatments (e.g., insulin infusions) to be administered in the critical care unit.

Providing medical care to a critically ill patient should not be automatically deemed to be a critical care service for the sole reason that the patient is critically ill or injured. While more than one physician may provide critical care services to a patient during the critical care episode of an illness or injury each physician must be managing one or more critical illness(es) or injury(ies) in whole or in part.

EXAMPLE: A dermatologist evaluates and treats a rash on an ICU patient who is maintained on a ventilator and nitroglycerine infusion that are being managed by an intensivist. The dermatologist should not report a service for critical care.

C. Critical Care Services and Full Attention of the Physician

The duration of critical care services to be reported is the time the physician spent evaluating, providing care and managing the critically ill or injured patient's care. That time must be spent at the immediate bedside or elsewhere on the floor or unit so long as the physician is immediately available to the patient.

For example, time spent reviewing laboratory test results or discussing the critically ill patient's care with other medical staff in the unit or at the nursing station on the floor may be reported as critical care, even when it does not occur at the bedside, if this time represents the physician's full attention to the management of the critically ill/injured patient.

For any given period of time spent providing critical care services, the physician must devote his or her full attention to the patient and, therefore, cannot provide services to any other patient during the same period of time. D. Critical Care Services and Qualified Non-Physician Practitioners (NPP) Critical care services may be provided by qualified NPPs and reported for payment under the NPP's National Provider Identifier (NPI) when the services meet the definition and requirements of critical care services in Sections A and B. The provision of critical care services must be within the scope of practice and licensure requirements for the State in which the qualified NPP practices and provides the service(s). Collaboration, physician supervision and billing requirements must also be met. A physician assistant shall meet the general physician supervision requirements.

E. Critical Care Services and Physician Time

Critical care is a time- based service, and for each date and encounter entry, the physician's progress note(s) shall document the total time that critical care services were provided. More than one physician can provide critical care at another time and be paid if the service meets critical care, is medically necessary and is not duplicative care. Concurrent care by more than one physician (generally representing different physician specialties) is payable if these requirements are met (refer to the Medicare Benefit Policy Manual, Pub. 100-02, Chapter 15, Sec.30 for concurrent care policy discussion).

The CPT critical care codes 99291 and 99292 are used to report the total duration of time spent by a physician providing critical care services to a critically ill or critically injured patient, even if the time spent by the physician on that date is not continuous. Non-continuous time for medically necessary critical care services may be aggregated. Reporting CPT code 99291 is a prerequisite to reporting CPT code 99292. Physicians of the same specialty within the same group practice bill and are paid as though they were a single physician (Sec.30.6.5).

1. Off the Unit/Floor
   Time spent in activities (excluding those identified previously in Section C) that occur outside of the unit or off the floor (i.e., telephone calls, whether taken at home, in the office, or elsewhere in the hospital) may not be reported as critical care because the physician is not immediately available to the patient. This time is regarded as pre- and post service work bundled in evaluation and management services.
2. Split/Shared Service
   A split/shared E/M service performed by a physician and a qualified NPP of the same group practice (or employed by the same employer) cannot be reported as a critical care service. Critical care services are reflective of the care and management of a critically ill or critically injured patient by an individual physician or qualified non-physician practitioner for the specified reportable period of time.

   Unlike other E/M services where a split/shared service is allowed the critical care service reported shall reflect the evaluation, treatment and management of a patient by an individual physician or qualified non-physician practitioner and shall not be representative of a combined service between a physician and a qualified NPP.

   When CPT code time requirements for both 99291 and 99292 and critical care criteria are met for a medically necessary visit by a qualified NPP the service shall be billed using the appropriate individual NPI number. Medically necessary visit(s) that do not meet these requirements shall be reported as subsequent hospital care services.
3. Unbundled Procedures
   Time involved performing procedures that are not bundled into critical care (i.e., billed and paid separately) may not be included and counted toward critical care time. The physician's progress note(s) in the medical record should document that time involved in the performance of separately billable procedures was not counted toward critical care time.
4. Family Counseling/Discussions
   Critical care CPT codes 99291 and 99292 include pre and post service work. Routine daily updates or reports to family members and or surrogates are considered part of this service. However, time involved with family members or other surrogate decision makers, whether to obtain a history or to discuss treatment options (as described in CPT), may be counted toward critical care time when these specific criteria are met:

   a) The patient is unable or incompetent to participate in giving a history and/or making treatment decisions, and

   b) The discussion is necessary for determining treatment decisions.

   For family discussions, the physician should document:

   a. The patient is unable or incompetent to participate in giving history and/or making treatment decisions

   b. The necessity to have the discussion (e.g., "no other source was available to obtain a history" or "because the patient was deteriorating so rapidly I needed to immediately discuss treatment options with the family",

   c. Medically necessary treatment decisions for which the discussion was needed, and

   d. A summary in the medical record that supports the medical necessity of the discussion All other family discussions, no matter how lengthy, may not be additionally counted towards critical care. Telephone calls to family members and or surrogate decision-makers may be counted towards critical care time, but only if they meet the same criteria as described in the aforementioned paragraph.
5. Inappropriate Use of Time for Payment of Critical Care Services.
   Time involved in activities that do not directly contribute to the treatment of the critically ill or injured patient may not be counted towards the critical care time, even when they are performed in the critical care unit at a patient's bedside (e.g., review of literature, and teaching sessions with physician residents whether conducted on hospital rounds or in other venues).

F. Hours and Days of Critical Care that May Be Billed

Critical care service is a time-based service provided on an hourly or fraction of an hour basis. Payment should not be restricted to a fixed number of hours, a fixed number of physicians, or a fixed number of days, on a per patient basis, for medically necessary critical care services. Time counted towards critical care services may be continuous or intermittent and aggregated in time increments (e.g., 50 minutes of continuous clock time or (5) 10 minute blocks of time spread over a given calendar date). Only one physician may bill for critical care services during any one single period of time even if more than one physician is providing care to a critically ill patient.

For Medicare Part B physician services paid under the physician fee schedule, critical care is not a service that is paid on a "shift" basis or a "per day" basis. Documentation may be requested for any claim to determine medical necessity. Examples of critical care billing that may require further review could include: claims from several physicians submitting multiple units of critical care for a single patient, and submitting claims for more than 12 hours of critical care time by a physician for one or more patients on the same given calendar date. Physicians assigned to a critical care unit (e.g., hospitalist, intensivist, etc.) may not report critical care for patients based on a "per shift" basis.

The CPT code 99291 is used to report the first 30 - 74 minutes of critical care on a given calendar date of service. It should only be used once per calendar date per patient by the same physician or physician group of the same specialty. CPT code 99292 is used to report additional block(s) of time, of up to 30 minutes each beyond the first 74 minutes of critical care (See table below). Critical care of less than 30 minutes total duration on a given calendar date is not reported separately using the critical care codes. This service should be reported using another appropriate E/M code such as subsequent hospital care.

Clinical Example of Correct Billing of Time:

A patient arrives in the emergency department in cardiac arrest. The emergency department physician provides 40 minutes of critical care services. A cardiologist is called to the ED and assumes responsibility for the patient, providing 35 minutes of critical care services. The patient

Appendix G — Pub 100 References

stabilizes and is transferred to the CCU. In this instance, the ED physician provided 40 minutes of critical care services and reports only the critical care code (CPT code 99291) and not also emergency department services. The cardiologist may report the 35 minutes of critical care services (also CPT code 99291) provided in the ED. Additional critical care services by the cardiologist in the CCU may be reported on the same calendar date using 99292 or another appropriate E/M code depending on the clock time involved.

G. Counting of Units of Critical Care Services
The CPT code 99291 (critical care, first hour) is used to report the services of a physician providing full attention to a critically ill or critically injured patient from 30-74 minutes on a given date. Only one unit of CPT code 99291 may be billed by a physician for a patient on a given date. Physicians of the same specialty within the same group practice bill and are paid as though they were a single physician and would not each report CPT 99291on the same date of service.

The following illustrates the correct reporting of critical care services:

Total Duration of Critical Care	Code(s)
Less than 30 minutes	99232 or 99233 or other appropriate E/M code
30-74 minutes	99291 x 1
75-104 minutes	99291 x 1 and 99292 x 1
105-134 minutes	99291 x 1 and 99292 x 2
135-164 minutes	99291 x 1 and 99292 x 3
165-194 minutes	99291 x 1 and 99292 x 4
194 minutes or longer	99291 - 99292 as appropriate (per the above illustrations)

H. Critical Care Services and Other Evaluation and Management Services Provided on Same Day
When critical care services are required upon the patient's presentation to the hospital emergency department, only critical care codes 99291 - 99292 may be reported. An emergency department visit code may not also be reported.

When critical care services are provided on a date where an inpatient hospital or office/outpatient evaluation and management service was furnished earlier on the same date at which time the patient did not require critical care, both the critical care and the previous evaluation and management service may be paid. Hospital emergency department services are not payable for the same calendar date as critical care services when provided by the same physician to the same patient.

Physicians are advised to submit documentation to support a claim when critical care is additionally reported on the same calendar date as when other evaluation and management services are provided to a patient by the same physician or physicians of the same specialty in a group practice.

I. Critical Care Services Provided by Physicians in Group Practice(s)
Medically necessary critical care services provided on the same calendar date to the same patient by physicians representing different medical specialties that are not duplicative services are payable. The medical specialists may be from the same group practice or from different group practices.

Critically ill or critically injured patients may require the care of more than one physician medical specialty. Concurrent critical care services provided by each physician must be medically necessary and not provided during the same instance of time. Medical record documentation must support the medical necessity of critical care services provided by each physician (or qualified NPP). Each physician must accurately report the service(s) he/she provided to the patient in accordance with any applicable global surgery rules or concurrent care rules. (Refer to Medicare Claims Processing Manual, Pub. 100-04, Chapter 12, Sec.40, and the Medicare Benefit Policy Manual, Pub. 100-02, Chapter 15, Sec.30.)

CPT Code 99291
The initial critical care time, billed as CPT code 99291, must be met by a single physician or qualified NPP. This may be performed in a single period of time or be cumulative by the same physician on the same calendar date. A history or physical exam performed by one group partner for another group partner in order for the second group partner to make a medical decision would not represent critical care services.

CPT Code 99292
Subsequent critical care visits performed on the same calendar date are reported using CPT code 99292. The service may represent aggregate time met by a single physician or physicians in the same group practice with the same medical specialty in order to meet the duration of minutes required for CPT code 99292. The aggregated critical care visits must be medically necessary and each aggregated visit must meet the definition of critical care in order to combine the times.

Physicians in the same group practice who have the same specialty may not each report CPT initial critical care code 99291 for critical care services to the same patient on the same calendar date. Medicare payment policy states that physicians in the same group practice who are in the same specialty must bill and be paid as though each were the single physician. (Refer to the Medicare Claims Processing Manual, Pub. 100-04, Chapter 12, Sec.30.6.) Physician specialty means the designated primary specialty by which the physician bills Medicare and is known to the contractor that adjudicates the claims. Physicians in the same group practice who have different medical specialties may bill and be paid without regard to their membership in the same group. For example, if a cardiologist and an endocrinologist are group partners and the critical care services of each are medically necessary and not duplicative, the critical care services may be reported by each regardless of their group practice relationship.

Two or more physicians in the same group practice who have different specialties and who provide critical care to a critically ill or critically injured patient may not in all cases each report the initial critical care code (CPT 99291) on the same date. When the group physicians are providing care that is unique to his/her individual medical specialty and managing at least one of the patient's critical illness(es) or critical injury(ies) then the initial critical care service may be payable to each.

However, if a physician or qualified NPP within a group provides "staff coverage" or "follow-up" for each other after the first hour of critical care services was provided on the same calendar date by the previous group clinician (physician or qualified NPP), the subsequent visits by the "covering" physician or qualified NPP in the group shall be billed using CPT critical care add-on code 99292. The appropriate individual NPI number shall be reported on the claim. The services will be paid at the specific physician fee schedule rate for the individual clinician (physician or qualified NPP) billing the service.

Clinical Examples of Critical Care Services

1. Drs. Smith and Jones, pulmonary specialists, share a group practice. On Tuesday Dr. Smith provides critical care services to Mrs. Benson who is comatose and has been in the intensive care unit for 4 days following a motor vehicle accident. She has multiple organ dysfunction including cerebral hematoma, flail chest and pulmonary contusion. Later on the same calendar date Dr. Jones covers for Dr. Smith and provides critical care services. Medically necessary critical care services provided at the different time periods may be reported by both Drs. Smith and Jones. Dr. Smith would report CPT code 99291 for the initial visit and Dr. Jones, as part of the same group practice would report CPT code 99292 on the same calendar date if the appropriate time requirements are met.
2. Mr. Marks, a 79 year old comes to the emergency room with vague joint pains and lethargy. The ED physician evaluates Mr. Marks and phones his primary care physician to discuss his medical evaluation. His primary care physician visits the ER and admits Mr. Marks to the observation unit for monitoring, and diagnostic and laboratory tests. In observation Mr. Marks has a cardiac arrest. His primary care physician provides 50 minutes of critical care services. Mr. Marks' is admitted to the intensive care unit. On the same calendar day Mr. Marks' condition deteriorates and he requires intermittent critical care services. In this scenario the ED physician should report an emergency department visit and the primary care physician should report both an initial hospital visit and critical care services.

J. Critical Care Services and Other Procedures Provided on the Same Day by the Same Physician as Critical Care Codes 99291- 99292
The following services when performed on the day a physician bills for critical care are included in the critical care service and should not be reported separately:

- The interpretation of cardiac output measurements (CPT 93561, 93562);
- Chest x-rays, professional component (CPT 71010, 71015, 71020);
- Blood draw for specimen (CPT 36415);
- Blood gases, and information data stored in computers (e.g., ECGs, blood pressures, hematologic data-CPT 99090);
- Gastric intubation (CPT 43752, 91105);
- Pulse oximetry (CPT 94760, 94761, 94762);
- Temporary transcutaneous pacing (CPT 92953);
- Ventilator management (CPT 94002 - 94004, 94660, 94662); and
- Vascular access procedures (CPT 36000, 36410, 36415, 36591, 36600).

No other procedure codes are bundled into the critical care services. Therefore, other medically necessary procedure codes may be billed separately.

K. Global Surgery
Critical care services shall not be paid on the same calendar date the physician also reports a procedure code with a global surgical period unless the critical care is billed with CPT modifier -25 to indicate that the critical care is a significant, separately identifiable evaluation and management service that is above and beyond the usual pre and post operative care associated with the procedure that is performed.

Services such as endotracheal intubation (CPT code 31500) and the insertion and placement of a flow directed catheter e.g., Swan-Ganz (CPT code 93503) are not bundled into the critical care codes. Therefore, separate payment may be made for critical care in addition to these services if the critical care was a significant, separately identifiable service and it was reported with modifier -25. The time spent performing the pre, intra, and post procedure work of these unbundled services, e.g., endotracheal intubation, shall be excluded from the determination of the time spent providing critical care.

This policy applies to any procedure with a 0, 10 or 90 day global period including cardiopulmonary resuscitation (CPT code 92950). CPR has a global period of 0 days and is not bundled into critical care codes. Therefore, critical care may be billed in addition to CPR if critical care was a significant, separately identifiable service and it was reported with modifier -25. The time spent performing CPR shall be excluded from the determination of the time spent providing critical care. In this instance it must be the physician who performs the resuscitation who bills for this service. Members of a code team must not each bill Medicare Part B for this service.

When postoperative critical care services (for procedures with a global surgical period) are provided by a physician other than the surgeon, no modifier is required unless all surgical postoperative care has been officially transferred from the surgeon to the physician performing the critical care services. In this situation, CPT modifiers "-54" (surgical care only) and "-55"(postoperative management only) must be used by the surgeon and intensivist who are submitting claims. Medical record documentation by the surgeon and the physician who assumes a transfer (e.g., intensivist) is required to support claims for services when CPT modifiers -54 and -55 are used indicating the transfer of care from the surgeon to the intensivist. Critical care services must meet all the conditions previously described in this manual section.

L. Critical Care Services Provided During Preoperative Portion and Postoperative Portion of Global Period of Procedure with 90 Day Global Period in Trauma and Burn Cases

Preoperative

Preoperative critical care may be paid in addition to a global fee if the patient is critically ill and requires the full attention of the physician, and the critical care is unrelated to the specific anatomic injury or general surgical procedure performed. Such patients may meet the definition of being critically ill and criteria for conditions where there is a high probability of imminent or life threatening deterioration in the patient's condition.

Preoperatively, in order for these services to be paid, two reporting requirements must be met. Codes 99291 - 99292 and modifier -25 (significant, separately identifiable evaluation and management services by the same physician on the day of the procedure) must be used, and documentation identifying that the critical care was unrelated to the specific anatomic injury or general surgical procedure performed shall be submitted. An ICD-9-CM code in the range 800.0 through 959.9 (except 930.0 - 939.9), which clearly indicates that the critical care was unrelated to the surgery, is acceptable documentation.

Postoperative

Postoperatively, in order for critical care services to be paid, two reporting requirements must be met. Codes 99291 - 99292 and modifier -24 (unrelated evaluation and management service by the same physician during a postoperative period) must be used, and documentation that the critical care was unrelated to the specific anatomic injury or general surgical procedure performed must be submitted. An ICD-9-CM code in the range 800.0 through 959.9 (except 930.0 - 939.9), which clearly indicates that the critical care was unrelated to the surgery, is acceptable documentation.

Medicare policy allows separate payment to the surgeon for postoperative critical care services during the surgical global period when the patient has suffered trauma or burns. When the surgeon provides critical care services during the global period, for reasons unrelated to the surgery, these are separately payable as well.

M. Teaching Physician Criteria

In order for the teaching physician to bill for critical care services the teaching physician must meet the requirements for critical care described in the preceding sections. For CPT codes determined on the basis of time, such as critical care, the teaching physician must be present for the entire period of time for which the claim is submitted. For example, payment will be made for 35 minutes of critical care services only if the teaching physician is present for the full 35 minutes. (See IOM, Pub 100-04, Chapter12, Sec. 100.1.4)

1. Teaching
   Time spent teaching may not be counted towards critical care time. Time spent by the resident, in the absence of the teaching physician, cannot be billed by the teaching physician as critical care or other time-based services. Only time spent by the resident and teaching physician together with the patient or the teaching physician alone with the patient can be counted toward critical care time.
2. Documentation
   A combination of the teaching physician's documentation and the resident's documentation may support critical care services. Provided that all requirements for critical care services are met, the teaching physician documentation may tie into the resident's documentation. The teaching physician may refer to the resident's documentation for specific patient history, physical findings and medical assessment. However, the teaching physician medical record documentation must provide substantive information including: (1) the time the teaching physician spent providing critical care, (2) that the patient was critically ill during the time the teaching physician saw the patient, (3) what made the patient critically ill, and (4) the nature of the treatment and management provided by the teaching physician. The medical review criteria are the same for the teaching physician as for all physicians. (See the Medicare Claims Processing, Pub. 100-04, Chapter 12, Sec.100.1.1 for teaching physician documentation guidance.)

Unacceptable Example of Documentation:

"I came and saw (the patient) and agree with (the resident)".

Acceptable Example of Documentation:

"Patient developed hypotension and hypoxia; I spent 45 minutes while the patient was in this condition, providing fluids, pressor drugs, and oxygen. I reviewed the resident's documentation and I agree with the resident's assessment and plan of care."

N. Ventilator Management

Medicare recognizes the ventilator codes (CPT codes 94002 - 94004, 94660 and 94662) as physician services payable under the physician fee schedule. Medicare Part B under the physician fee schedule does not pay for ventilator management services in addition to an evaluation and management service (e.g., critical care services, CPT codes 99291 - 99292) on the same day for the patient even when the evaluation and management service is billed with CPT modifier -2

100-4, 12, 30.6.13

Nursing Facility Services

A. Visits to Perform the Initial Comprehensive Assessment and Annual Assessments

The distinction made between the delegation of physician visits and tasks in a skilled nursing facility (SNF) and in a nursing facility (NF) is based on the Medicare Statute. Section 1819 (b) (6) (A) of the Social Security Act (the Act) governs SNFs while section 1919 (b) (6) (A) of the Act governs NFs. For further information refer to Medlearn Matters article number SE0418 at www.cms.hhs.gov/medlearn/matters.

The federally mandated visits in a SNF and NF must be performed by the physician except as otherwise permitted (42 CFR 483.40 (c) (4) and (f)). The principal physician of record must append the modifier "-AI", (Principal Physician of Record), to the initial nursing facility care code. This modifier will identify the physician who oversees the patient's care from other physicians who may be furnishing specialty care. All other physicians or qualified NPPs who perform an initial evaluation in the NF or SNF may bill the initial nursing facility care code. The initial federally mandated visit is defined in S&C-04-08 (see www.cms.hhs.gov/medlearn/matters) as the initial comprehensive visit during which the physician completes a thorough assessment, develops a plan of care, and writes or verifies admitting orders for the nursing facility resident. For Survey and Certification requirements, a visit must occur no later than 30 days after admission.

Further, per the Long Term Care regulations at 42 CFR 483.40 (c) (4) and (e) (2), in a SNF the physician may not delegate a task that the physician must personally perform. Therefore, as stated in S&C-04-08 the physician may not delegate the initial federally mandated comprehensive visit in a SNF.

The only exception, as to who performs the initial visit, relates to the NF setting. In the NF setting, a qualified NPP (i.e., a nurse practitioner (NP), physician assistant (PA), or a clinical nurse specialist (CNS)), who is not employed by the facility, may perform the initial visit when the State law permits. The evaluation and management (E/M) visit shall be within the State scope of practice and licensure requirements where the E/M visit is performed and the requirements for physician collaboration and physician supervision shall be met.

Under Medicare Part B payment policy, other medically necessary E/M visits may be performed and reported prior to and after the initial visit, if the medical needs of the patient require an E/M visit. A qualified NPP may perform medically necessary E/M visits prior to and after the initial visit if all the requirements for collaboration, general physician supervision, licensure, and billing are met.

The CPT Nursing Facility Services codes shall be used with place of service (POS) 31 (SNF) if the patient is in a Part A SNF stay. They shall be used with POS 32 (nursing facility) if the patient does not have Part A SNF benefits or if the patient is in a NF or in a non-covered SNF stay (e.g., there was no preceding 3-day hospital stay). The CPT Nursing Facility code definition also includes POS 54 (Intermediate Care Facility/Mentally Retarded) and POS 56 (Psychiatric Residential Treatment Center). For further guidance on POS codes and associated CPT codes refer to §30.6.14.

Effective January 1, 2006, the Initial Nursing Facility Care codes 99301,Äì 99303 are deleted.

Beginning January 1, 2006, the new CPT codes, Initial Nursing Facility Care, per day, (99304–99306) shall be used to report the initial federally mandated visit. Only a physician may report these codes for an initial federally mandated visit performed in a SNF or NF (with the exception of the qualified NPP in the NF setting who is not employed by the facility and when State law permits, as explained above).

A readmission to a SNF or NF shall have the same payment policy requirements as an initial admission in both the SNF and NF settings.

A physician who is employed by the SNF/NF may perform the E/M visits and bill independently to Medicare Part B for payment. An NPP who is employed by the SNF or NF may perform and bill Medicare Part B directly for those services where it is permitted as discussed above. The employer of the PA shall always report the visits performed by the PA. A physician, NP or CNS has the option to bill Medicare directly or to reassign payment for his/her professional service to the facility.

As with all E/M visits for Medicare Part B payment policy, the E/M documentation guidelines apply.

Medically Necessary Visits

Qualified NPPs may perform medically necessary E/M visits prior to and after the physician's initial federally mandated visit in both the SNF and NF. Medically necessary E/M visits for the diagnosis or treatment of an illness or injury or to improve the functioning of a malformed body member are payable under the physician fee schedule under Medicare Part B. A physician or NPP may bill the most appropriate initial nursing facility care code (CPT codes 99304-99306) or subsequent nursing facility care code (CPT codes 99307-99310), even if the E/M service is provided prior to the initial federally mandated visit.

SNF Setting--Place of Service Code 31

Following the initial federally mandated visit by the physician, the physician may delegate alternate federally mandated physician visits to a qualified NPP who meets collaboration and physician supervision requirements and is licensed as such by the State and performing within the scope of practice in that State.

NF Setting--Place of Service Code 32

Per the regulations at 42 CFR 483.40 (f), a qualified NPP, who meets the collaboration and physician supervision requirements, the State scope of practice and licensure requirements, and who is not employed by the NF, may at the option of the State, perform the initial federally mandated visit in a NF, and may perform any other federally mandated physician visit in a NF in addition to performing other medically necessary E/M visits.

Questions pertaining to writing orders or certification and recertification issues in the SNF and NF settings shall be addressed to the appropriate State Survey and Certification Agency departments for clarification.

B. Visits to Comply With Federal Regulations (42 CFR 483.40 (c) (1)) in the SNF and NF

Payment is made under the physician fee schedule by Medicare Part B for federally mandated visits. Following the initial federally mandated visit by the physician or qualified NPP where permitted, payment shall be made for federally mandated visits that monitor and evaluate residents at least once every 30 days for the first 90 days after admission and at least once every 60 days thereafter.

Effective January 1, 2006, the Subsequent Nursing Facility Care, per day, codes 99311,Äì 99313 are deleted.

Beginning January 1, 2006, the new CPT codes, Subsequent Nursing Facility Care, per day, (99307–99310) shall be used to report federally mandated physician E/M visits and medically necessary E/M visits.

Carriers shall not pay for more than one E/M visit performed by the physician or qualified NPP for the same patient on the same date of service. The Nursing Facility Services codes represent a "per day" service.

The federally mandated E/M visit may serve also as a medically necessary E/M visit if the situation arises (i.e., the patient has health problems that need attention on the day the scheduled mandated physician E/M visit occurs). The physician/qualified NPP shall bill only one E/M visit.

Beginning January 1, 2006, the new CPT code, Other Nursing Facility Service (99318), may be used to report an annual nursing facility assessment visit on the required schedule of visits on an annual basis. For Medicare Part B payment policy, an annual nursing facility assessment visit code may substitute as meeting one of the federally mandated physician visits if the code requirements for CPT code 99318 are fully met and in lieu of reporting a Subsequent Nursing Facility Care, per day, service (codes 99307–99310). It shall not be performed in addition to the required number of federally mandated physician visits. The new CPT annual assessment code does not represent a new benefit service for Medicare Part B physician services.

Qualified NPPs, whether employed or not by the SNF, may perform alternating federally mandated physician visits, at the option of the physician, after the initial federally mandated visit by the physician in a SNF.

Qualified NPPs in the NF setting, who are not employed by the NF and who are working in collaboration with a physician, may perform federally mandated physician visits, at the option of the State.

Medicare Part B payment policy does not pay for additional E/M visits that may be required by State law for a facility admission or for other additional visits to satisfy facility or other administrative purposes. E/M visits, prior to and after the initial federally mandated physician visit, that are reasonable and medically necessary to meet the medical needs of the individual patient (unrelated to any State requirement or administrative purpose) are payable under Medicare Part B.

C. Visits by Qualified Nonphysician Practitioners
All E/M visits shall be within the State scope of practice and licensure requirements where the visit is performed and all the requirements for physician collaboration and physician supervision shall be met when performed and reported by qualified NPPs. General physician supervision and employer billing requirements shall be met for PA services in addition to the PA meeting the State scope of practice and licensure requirements where the E/M visit is performed.

Medically Necessary Visits
Qualified NPPs may perform medically necessary E/M visits prior to and after the physician's initial visit in both the SNF and NF. Medically necessary E/M visits for the diagnosis or treatment of an illness or injury or to improve the functioning of a malformed body member are payable under the physician fee schedule under Medicare Part B. A physician or NPP may bill the most appropriate initial nursing facility care code (CPT codes 99304-99306) or subsequent nursing facility care code (CPT codes 99307-99310), even if the E/M service is provided prior to the initial federally mandated visit.

SNF Setting--Place of Service Code 31
Following the initial federally mandated visit by the physician, the physician may delegate alternate federally mandated physician visits to a qualified NPP who meets collaboration and physician supervision requirements and is licensed as such by the State and performing within the scope of practice in that State.

NF Setting--Place of Service Code 32
Per the regulations at 42 CFR 483.40 (f), a qualified NPP, who meets the collaboration and physician supervision requirements, the State scope of practice and licensure requirements, and who is not employed by the NF, may at the option of the State, perform the initial federally mandated visit in a NF, and may perform any other federally mandated physician visit in a NF in addition to performing other medically necessary E/M visits.

Questions pertaining to writing orders or certification and recertification issues in the SNF and NF settings shall be addressed to the appropriate State Survey and Certification Agency departments for clarification.

D. Medically Complex Care
Payment is made for E/M visits to patients in a SNF who are receiving services for medically complex care upon discharge from an acute care facility when the visits are reasonable and medically necessary and documented in the medical record. Physicians and qualified NPPs shall report initial nursing facility care codes for their first visit with the patient. The principal physician of record must append the modifier "-AI" (Principal Physician of Record), to the initial nursing facility care code when billed to identify the physician who oversees the patient's care from other physicians who may be furnishing specialty care. Follow-up visits shall be billed as subsequent nursing facility care visits.

E. Incident to Services
Where a physician establishes an office in a SNF/NF, the "incident to" services and requirements are confined to this discrete part of the facility designated as his/her office. "Incident to" E/M visits, provided in a facility setting, are not payable under the Physician Fee Schedule for Medicare Part B. Thus, visits performed outside the designated "office" area in the SNF/NF would be subject to the coverage and payment rules applicable to the SNF/NF setting and shall not be reported using the CPT codes for office or other outpatient visits or use place of service code 11.

F. Use of the Prolonged Services Codes and Other Time-Related Services
Beginning January 1, 2008, typical/average time units for E/M visits in the SNF/NF settings are reestablished. Medically necessary prolonged services for E/M visits (codes 99356 and 99357) in a SNF or NF may be billed with the Nursing Facility Services in the code ranges (99304–99306, 99307–99310 and 99318).

Counseling and Coordination of Care Visits
With the reestablishment of typical/average time units, medically necessary E/M visits for counseling and coordination of care, for Nursing Facility Services in the code ranges (99304–99306, 99307–99310 and 99318) that are time-based services, may be billed with the appropriate prolonged services codes (99356 and 99357).

G. Multiple Visits
The complexity level of an E/M visit and the CPT code billed must be a covered and medically necessary visit for each patient (refer to §§1862 (a)(1)(A) of the Act). Claims for an unreasonable number of daily E/M visits by the same physician to multiple patients at a facility within a 24-hour period may result in medical review to determine medical necessity for the visits. The E/M visit (Nursing Facility Services) represents a "per day" service per patient as defined by the CPT code. The medical record must be personally documented by the physician or qualified NPP who performed the E/M visit and the documentation shall support the specific level of E/M visit to each individual patient.

H. Split/Shared E/M Visit
A split/shared E/M visit cannot be reported in the SNF/NF setting. A split/shared E/M visit is defined by Medicare Part B payment policy as a medically necessary encounter with a patient where the physician and a qualified NPP each personally perform a substantive portion of an E/M visit face-to-face with the same patient on the same date of service. A substantive portion of an E/M visit involves all or some portion of the history, exam or medical decision making key components of an E/M service. The physician and the qualified NPP must be in the same group practice or be employed by the same employer. The split/shared E/M visit applies only to selected E/M visits and settings (i.e., hospital inpatient, hospital outpatient, hospital observation, emergency department, hospital discharge, office and non facility clinic visits, and prolonged visits associated with these E/M visit codes). The split/shared E/M policy does not apply to critical care services or procedures.

I. SNF/NF Discharge Day Management Service
Medicare Part B payment policy requires a face-to-face visit with the patient provided by the physician or the qualified NPP to meet the SNF/NF discharge day management service as defined by the CPT code. The E/M discharge day management visit shall be reported for the date of the actual visit by the physician or qualified NPP even if the patient is discharged from the facility on a different calendar date. The CPT codes 99315–99316 shall be reported for this visit. The Discharge Day Management Service may be reported using CPT code 99315 or 99316, depending on the code requirement, for a patient who has expired, but only if the physician or qualified NPP personally performed the death pronouncement.

100-4, 12, 30.6.14

Home Care and Domiciliary Care Visits (Codes 99324- 99350)

Physician Visits to Patients Residing in Various Places of Service
The American Medical Association's Current Procedural Terminology (CPT) 2006 new patient codes 99324 - 99328 and established patient codes 99334 - 99337(new codes beginning January 2006), for Domiciliary, Rest Home (e.g., Boarding Home), or Custodial Care Services, are used to report evaluation and management (E/M) services to residents residing in a facility which provides room, board, and other personal assistance services, generally on a long-term basis. These CPT codes are used to report E/M services in facilities assigned places of service (POS) codes 13 (Assisted Living Facility), 14 (Group Home), 33 (Custodial Care Facility) and 55 (Residential Substance Abuse Facility). Assisted living facilities may also be known as adult living facilities.

Physicians and qualified nonphysician practitioners (NPPs) furnishing E/M services to residents in a living arrangement described by one of the POS listed above must use the level of service code in the CPT code range 99324 - 99337 to report the service they provide. The CPT codes 99321 - 99333 for Domiciliary, Rest Home (e.g., Boarding Home), or Custodial Care Services are deleted beginning January, 2006.

Beginning in 2006, reasonable and medically necessary, face-to-face, prolonged services, represented by CPT codes 99354 - 99355, may be reported with the appropriate companion E/M codes when a physician or qualified NPP, provides a prolonged service involving direct (face-to-face) patient contact that is beyond the usual E/M visit service for a Domiciliary, Rest Home (e.g., Boarding Home) or Custodial Care Service. All the requirements for prolonged services at Sec.30.6.15.1 must be met.

The CPT codes 99341 through 99350, Home Services codes, are used to report E/M services furnished to a patient residing in his or her own private residence (e.g., private home, apartment, town home) and not residing in any type of congregate/shared facility living arrangement including assisted living facilities and group homes. The Home Services codes apply only to the specific 2-digit POS 12 (Home). Home Services codes may not be used for billing E/M services provided in settings other than in the private residence of an individual as described above.

Beginning in 2006, E/M services provided to patients residing in a Skilled Nursing Facility (SNF) or a Nursing Facility (NF) must be reported using the appropriate CPT level of service code within the range identified for Initial Nursing Facility Care (new CPT codes 99304 - 99306) and Subsequent Nursing Facility Care (new CPT codes 99307 - 99310). Use the CPT code, Other Nursing Facility Services (new CPT code 99318), for an annual nursing facility assessment. Use CPT codes 99315 - 99316 for SNF/NF discharge services. The CPT codes 99301 - 99303 and 99311 - 99313 are deleted beginning January, 2006. The Home Services codes should not be used for these places of service.

The CPT SNF/NF code definition includes intermediate care facilities (ICFs) and long term care facilities (LTCFs). These codes are limited to the specific 2-digit POS 31 (SNF), 32 (Nursing Facility), 54 (Intermediate Care Facility/Mentally Retarded) and 56 (Psychiatric Residential Treatment Center).

The CPT nursing facility codes should be used with POS 31 (SNF) if the patient is in a Part A SNF stay and POS 32 (nursing facility) if the patient does not have Part A SNF benefits. There is no longer a different payment amount for a Part A or Part B benefit period in these POS settings.

100-4, 12, 30.6.14.1

Home Services (Codes 99341 - 99350)

B3-15515, B3-15066

A. Requirement for Physician Presence

Home services codes 99341-99350 are paid when they are billed to report evaluation and management services provided in a private residence. A home visit cannot be billed by a physician unless the physician was actually present in the beneficiary's home.

B. Homebound Status

Under the home health benefit the beneficiary must be confined to the home for services to be covered. For home services provided by a physician using these codes, the beneficiary does not need to be confined to the home. The medical record must document the medical necessity of the home visit made in lieu of an office or outpatient visit.

C. Fee Schedule Payment for Services to Homebound Patients under General Supervision

Payment may be made in some medically underserved areas where there is a lack of medical personnel and home health services for injections, EKGs, and venipunctures that are performed for homebound patients under general physician supervision by nurses and paramedical employees of physicians or physician-directed clinics. Section 10 provides additional information on the provision of services to homebound Medicare patients.

100-4, 12, 30.6.15.1

Prolonged Services With Direct Face-to-Face Patient Contact Service (Codes 99354-99357) (ZZZ codes)

A. Definition

Prolonged physician services (CPT code 99354) in the office or other outpatient setting with direct face-to-face patient contact which require 1 hour beyond the usual service are payable when billed on the same day by the same physician or qualified nonphysician practitioner (NPP) as the companion evaluation and management codes. The time for usual service refers to the typical/average time units associated with the companion evaluation and management service as noted in the CPT code. Each additional 30 minutes of direct face-to-face patient contact following the first hour of prolonged services may be reported by CPT code 99355.

Prolonged physician services (code 99356) in the inpatient setting, with direct face-to-face patient contact which require 1 hour beyond the usual service are payable when they are billed on the same day by the same physician or qualified NPP as the companion evaluation and management codes. Each additional 30 minutes of direct face-to-face patient contact following the first hour of prolonged services may be reported by CPT code 99357.

Prolonged service of less than 30 minutes total duration on a given date is not separately reported because the work involved is included in the total work of the evaluation and management codes.

Code 99355 or 99357 may be used to report each additional 30 minutes beyond the first hour of prolonged services, based on the place of service. These codes may be used to report the final 15–30 minutes of prolonged service on a given date, if not otherwise billed. Prolonged service of less than 15 minutes beyond the first hour or less than 15 minutes beyond the final 30 minutes is not reported separately.

B. Required Companion Codes

The companion evaluation and management codes for 99354 are the Office or Other Outpatient visit codes (99201 - 99205, 99212–99215), the Domiciliary, Rest Home, or Custodial Care Services codes (99324–99328, 99334–99337), the Home Services codes (99341 - 99345, 99347–99350);

The companion codes for 99355 are 99354 and one of the evaluation and management codes required for 99354 to be used;

The companion evaluation and management codes for 99356 are the Initial Hospital Care codes and Subsequent Hospital Care codes (99221 - 99223, 99231–99233); Nursing Facility Services codes (99304 -99318); or

The companion codes for 99357 are 99356 and one of the evaluation and management codes required for 99356 to be used.

Prolonged services codes 99354–99357 are not paid unless they are accompanied by the companion codes as indicated.

C. Requirement for Physician Presence

Physicians may count only the duration of direct face-to-face contact between the physician and the patient (whether the service was continuous or not) beyond the typical/average time of the visit code billed to determine whether prolonged services can be billed and to determine the prolonged services codes that are allowable. In the case of prolonged office services, time spent by office staff with the patient, or time the patient remains unaccompanied in the office cannot be billed. In the case of prolonged hospital services, time spent reviewing charts or discussion of a patient with house medical staff and not with direct face-to-face contact with the patient, or waiting for test results, for changes in the patient's condition, for end of a therapy, or for use of facilities cannot be billed as prolonged services.

D. Documentation

Documentation is not required to accompany the bill for prolonged services unless the physician has been selected for medical review. Documentation is required in the medical record about the duration and content of the medically necessary evaluation and management service and prolonged services billed. The medical record must be appropriately and sufficiently documented by the physician or qualified NPP to show that the physician or qualified NPP personally furnished the direct face-to-face time with the patient specified in the CPT code definitions. The start and end times of the visit shall be documented in the medical record along with the date of service.

E. Use of the Codes

Prolonged services codes can be billed only if the total duration of the physician or qualified NPP direct face-to-face service (including the visit) equals or exceeds the threshold time for the evaluation and management service the physician or qualified NPP provided (typical/average time associated with the CPT E/M code plus 30 minutes). If the total duration of direct face-to-face time does not equal or exceed the threshold time for the level of evaluation and management service the physician or qualified NPP provided, the physician or qualified NPP may not bill for prolonged services.

F. Threshold Times for Codes 99354 and 99355 (Office or Other Outpatient Setting)

If the total direct face-to-face time equals or exceeds the threshold time for code 99354, but is less than the threshold time for code 99355, the physician should bill the evaluation and management visit code and code 99354. No more than one unit of 99354 is acceptable. If the total direct face-to-face time equals or exceeds the threshold time for code 99355 by no more than 29 minutes, the physician should bill the visit code 99354 and one unit of code 99355. One additional unit of code 99355 is billed for each additional increment of 30 minutes extended duration. Contractors use the following threshold times to determine if the prolonged services codes 99354 and/or 99355 can be billed with the office or other outpatient settings including domiciliary, rest home, or custodial care services and home services codes.

Threshold Time for Prolonged Visit Codes 99354 and/or 99355 Billed with Office/Outpatient and Consultation Codes

Code	*Typical Time for Code*	*Threshold Time to Bill Code 99354*	*Threshold Time to Bill Codes 99354 and 99355*
99201	10	40	85
99202	20	50	95
99203	30	60	105
99204	45	75	120
99205	60	90	135
99212	10	40	85
99213	15	45	90
99214	25	55	100
99215	40	70	115
99324	20	50	95
99325	30	60	105
99326	45	75	120
99327	60	90	135
99328	75	105	150
99334	15	45	90
99335	25	55	100
99336	40	70	115
99337	60	90	135
99341	20	50	95
99342	30	60	105
99343	45	75	120
99344	60	90	135
99345	75	105	150
99347	15	45	90
99348	25	55	100
99349	40	70	115
99350	60	90	135

G. Threshold Times for Codes 99356 and 99357

(Inpatient Setting) If the total direct face-to-face time equals or exceeds the threshold time for code 99356, but is less than the threshold time for code 99357, the physician should bill the visit and code 99356. Contractors do not accept more than one unit of code 99356. If the total direct face-to-face time equals or exceeds the threshold time for code 99356 by no more than 29 minutes, the physician bills the visit code 99356 and one unit of code 99357. One additional unit of code 99357 is billed for each additional increment of 30 minutes extended duration. Contractors use the following threshold times to determine if the prolonged services codes 99356 and/or 99357 can be billed with the inpatient setting codes.

Threshold Time for Prolonged Visit Codes 99356 and/or 99357 Billed with Inpatient Setting Codes

Code	*Typical Time for Code*	*Threshold Time to Bill Code 99356*	*Threshold Time to Bill Codes 99356 and 99357*
99221	30	60	105
99222	50	80	125
99223	70	100	145
99231	15	45	90
99232	25	55	100
99233	35	65	110
99304	25	55	100
99305	35	65	110
99306	45	75	120

Code	Typical Time for Code	Threshold Time to Bill Code 99356	Threshold Time to Bill Codes 99356 and 99357
99307	10	40	85
99308	15	45	90
99309	25	55	100
99310	35	65	110
99318	30	60	10

Add 30 minutes to the threshold time for billing codes 99356 and 99357 to get the threshold time for billing code 99356 and two units of 99357.

H. Prolonged Services Associated With Evaluation and Management Services Based on Counseling and/or Coordination of Care (Time-Based)
When an evaluation and management service is dominated by counseling and/or coordination of care (the counseling and/or coordination of care represents more than 50% of the total time with the patient) in a face-to-face encounter between the physician or qualified NPP and the patient in the office/clinic or the floor time (in the scenario of an inpatient service), then the evaluation and management code is selected based on the typical/average time associated with the code levels. The time approximation must meet or exceed the specific CPT code billed (determined by the typical/average time associated with the evaluation and management code) and should not be "rounded" to the next higher level.

In those evaluation and management services in which the code level is selected based on time, prolonged services may only be reported with the highest code level in that family of codes as the companion code.

I. Examples of Billable Prolonged Services

EXAMPLE 1
A physician performed a visit that met the definition of an office visit code 99213 and the total duration of the direct face-to-face services (including the visit) was 65 minutes. The physician bills code 99213 and one unit of code 99354.

EXAMPLE 2
A physician performed a visit that met the definition of a domiciliary, rest home care visit code 99327 and the total duration of the direct face-to-face contact (including the visit) was 140 minutes. The physician bills codes 99327, 99354, and one unit of code 99355.

EXAMPLE 3
A physician performed an office visit to an established patient that was predominantly counseling, spending 75 minutes (direct face-to-face) with the patient. The physician should report CPT code 99215 and one unit of code 99354.

J. Examples of Nonbillable Prolonged Services

EXAMPLE 1
A physician performed a visit that met the definition of visit code 99212 and the total duration of the direct face-to-face contact (including the visit) was 35 minutes. The physician cannot bill prolonged services because the total duration of direct face-to-face service did not meet the threshold time for billing prolonged services.

EXAMPLE 2
A physician performed a visit that met the definition of code 99213 and, while the patient was in the office receiving treatment for 4 hours, the total duration of the direct face-to-face service of the physician was 40 minutes. The physician cannot bill prolonged services because the total duration of direct face-to-face service did not meet the threshold time for billing prolonged services.

EXAMPLE 3
A physician provided a subsequent office visit that was predominantly counseling, spending 60 minutes (face-to-face) with the patient. The physician cannot code 99214, which has a typical time of 25 minutes, and one unit of code 99354. The physician must bill the highest level code in the code family (99215 which has 40 minutes typical/average time units associated with it). The additional time spent beyond this code is 20 minutes and does not meet the threshold time for billing prolonged services.

100-4,1 2, 30.6.15.2

Prolonged Services Without Face to Face Service (Codes 99358 - 99359)

Contractors may not pay prolonged services codes 99358 and 99359, which do not require any direct patient face-to-face contact (e.g., telephone calls). Payment for these services is included in the payment for direct face-to-face services that physicians bill. The physician cannot bill the patient for these services since they are Medicare covered services and payment is included in the payment for other billable services.

100-4, 12, 30.6.15.3

Physician Standby Service (Code 99360)

Standby services are not payable to physicians. Physicians may not bill Medicare or beneficiaries for standby services. Payment for standby services is included in the Part A payment to the facility. Such services are a part of hospital costs to provide quality care.

If hospitals pay physicians for standby services, such services are part of hospital costs to provide quality care.

100-4, 12, 30.6.16

Case Management Services (Codes 99362 and 99371 - 99373)

A. Team Conferences
Team conferences (codes 99361-99362) may not be paid separately. Payment for these services is included in the payment for the services to which they relate.

B. Telephone Calls
Telephone calls (codes 99371-99373) may not be paid separately. Payment for telephone calls is included in payment for billable services (e.g., visit, surgery, diagnostic procedure results).

100-4, 12, 40.2

Billing Requirements for Global Surgeries

To ensure the proper identification of services that are, or are not, included in the global package, the following procedures apply.

A. Procedure Codes and Modifiers
Use of the modifiers in this section apply to both major procedures with a 90-day postoperative period and minor procedures with a 10-day postoperative period (and/or a zero day postoperative period in the case of modifiers "-22" and "-25").

1. Physicians Who Furnish the Entire Global Surgical Package
   Physicians who perform the surgery and furnish all of the usual pre-and postoperative work bill for the global package by entering the appropriate CPT code for the surgical procedure only. Billing is not allowed for visits or other services that are included in the global package.
2. Physicians in Group Practice
   When different physicians in a group practice participate in the care of the patient, the group bills for the entire global package if the physicians reassign benefits to the group. The physician who performs the surgery is shown as the performing physician. (For dates of service prior to January 1, 1994, however, where a new physician furnishes the entire postoperative care, the group billed for the surgical care and the postoperative care as separate line items with the appropriate modifiers.)
3. Physicians Who Furnish Part of a Global Surgical Package
   Where physicians agree on the transfer of care during the global period, the following modifiers are used:
   - "-54" for surgical care only; or
   - "-55" for postoperative management only.

   Both the bill for the surgical care only and the bill for the postoperative care only, will contain the same date of service and the same surgical procedure code, with the services distinguished by the use of the appropriate modifier.

   Providers need not specify on the claim that care has been transferred. However, the date on which care was relinquished or assumed, as applicable, must be shown on the claim. This should be indicated in the remarks field/free text segment on the claim form/format. Both the surgeon and the physician providing the postoperative care must keep a copy of the written transfer agreement in the beneficiary's medical record.

   Where a transfer of postoperative care occurs, the receiving physician cannot bill for any part of the global services until he/she has provided at least one service. Once the physician has seen the patient, that physician may bill for the period beginning with the date on which he/she assumes care of the patient.

   EXCEPTIONS:
   - Where a transfer of care does not occur, occasional post-discharge services of a physician other than the surgeon are reported by the appropriate evaluation and management code. No modifiers are necessary on the claim.
   - If the transfer of care occurs immediately after surgery, the physician other than the surgeon who provides the in-hospital postoperative care bills using subsequent hospital care codes for the inpatient hospital care and the surgical code with the "-55" modifier for the post-discharge care. The surgeon bills the surgery code with the "-54" modifier.
   - Physicians who provide follow-up services for minor procedures performed in emergency departments bill the appropriate level of office visit code. The physician who performs the emergency room service bills for the surgical procedure without a modifier.
   - If the services of a physician other than the surgeon are required during a postoperative period for an underlying condition or medical complication, the other physician reports the appropriate evaluation and management code. No modifiers are necessary on the claim. An example is a cardiologist who manages underlying cardiovascular conditions of a patient.
4. Evaluation and Management Service Resulting in the Initial Decision to Perform Surgery
   Evaluation and management services on the day before major surgery or on the day of major surgery that result in the initial decision to perform the surgery are not included in the global surgery payment for the major surgery and, therefore, may be billed and paid separately.

   In addition to the CPT evaluation and management code, modifier "-57" (decision for surgery) is used to identify a visit which results in the initial decision to perform surgery. (Modifier "-QI" was used for dates of service prior to January 1, 1994.)

   If evaluation and management services occur on the day of surgery, the physician bills using modifier "-57," not "-25." The "-57" modifier is not used with minor surgeries because the global period for minor surgeries does not include the day prior to the surgery. Moreover, where the decision to perform the minor procedure is typically done immediately before the service, it is considered a routine preoperative service and a visit or consultation is not billed in addition to the procedure.
5. Return Trips to the Operating Room During the Postoperative Period
   When treatment for complications requires a return trip to the operating room, physicians must bill the CPT code that describes the procedure(s) performed during the return trip. If no such code exists, use the unspecified procedure code in the correct series, i.e., 47999 or 64999. The procedure code for the original surgery is not used except when the identical procedure is repeated.

   In addition to the CPT code, physicians use CPT modifier "-78" for these return trips (return to the operating room for a related procedure during a postoperative period.)

The physician may also need to indicate that another procedure was performed during the postoperative period of the initial procedure. When this subsequent procedure is related to the first procedure and requires the use of the operating room, this circumstance may be reported by adding the modifier "-78" to the related procedure.

NOTE: The CPT definition for this modifier does not limit its use to treatment for complications.

6. Staged or Related Procedures
Modifier "-58" was established to facilitate billing of staged or related surgical procedures done during the postoperative period of the first procedure. This modifier is not used to report the treatment of a problem that requires a return to the operating room.

The physician may need to indicate that the performance of a procedure or service during the postoperative period was:

a. Planned prospectively or at the time of the original procedure;

b. More extensive than the original procedure; or

c. For therapy following a diagnostic surgical procedure.

These circumstances may be reported by adding modifier "-58" to the staged procedure. A new postoperative period begins when the next procedure in the series is billed.

7. Unrelated Procedures or Visits During the Postoperative Period
Two CPT modifiers were established to simplify billing for visits and other procedures which are furnished during the postoperative period of a surgical procedure, but which are not included in the payment for the surgical procedure.

Modifier "-79": Reports an unrelated procedure by the same physician during a postoperative period. The physician may need to indicate that the performance of a procedure or service during a postoperative period was unrelated to the original procedure.

A new postoperative period begins when the unrelated procedure is billed.

Modifier "-24": Reports an unrelated evaluation and management service by same physician during a postoperative period. The physician may need to indicate that an evaluation and management service was performed during the postoperative period of an unrelated procedure. This circumstance is reported by adding the modifier "-24" to the appropriate level of evaluation and management service.

Services submitted with the "-24" modifier must be sufficiently documented to establish that the visit was unrelated to the surgery. An ICD-9-CM code that clearly indicates that the reason for the encounter was unrelated to the surgery is acceptable documentation.

A physician who is responsible for postoperative care and has reported and been paid using modifier "-55" also uses modifier "-24" to report any unrelated visits.

8. Significant Evaluation and Management on the Day of a Procedure
Modifier "-25" is used to facilitate billing of evaluation and management services on the day of a procedure for which separate payment may be made.

It is used to report a significant, separately identifiable evaluation and management service by same physician on the day of a procedure. The physician may need to indicate that on the day a procedure or service that is identified with a CPT code was performed, the patient's condition required a significant, separately identifiable evaluation and management service above and beyond the usual preoperative and postoperative care associated with the procedure or service that was performed. This circumstance may be reported by adding the modifier "-25" to the appropriate level of evaluation and management service.

Claims containing evaluation and management codes with modifier "-25" are not subject to prepayment review except in the following situations:

- Effective January 1, 1995, all evaluation and management services provided on the same day as inpatient dialysis are denied without review with the exception of CPT Codes 99221-9223, 99251-99255, and 99238. These codes may be billed with modifier "-25" and reviewed for possible allowance if the evaluation and management service is unrelated to the treatment of ESRD and was not, and could not, have been provided during the dialysis treatment;
- When preoperative critical care codes are being billed for within a global surgical period; and
- When carriers have conducted a specific medical review process and determined, after reviewing the data, that an individual or group have high statistics in terms of the use of modifier "-25," have done a case-by-case review of the records to verify that the use of modifier "-25" was inappropriate, and have educated the individual or group as to the proper use of this modifier.

9. Critical Care
Critical care services provided during a global surgical period for a seriously injured or burned patient are not considered related to a surgical procedure and may be paid separately under the following circumstances.

Preoperative and postoperative critical care may be paid in addition to a global fee if:

- The patient is critically ill and requires the constant attendance of the physician; and
- The critical care is above and beyond, and, in most instances, unrelated to the specific anatomic injury or general surgical procedure performed.

Such patients are potentially unstable or have conditions that could pose a significant threat to life or risk of prolonged impairment.

In order for these services to be paid, two reporting requirements must be met:

- Codes 99291/99292 and modifier "-25" (for preoperative care) or "-24" (for postoperative care) must be used; and
- Documentation that the critical care was unrelated to the specific anatomic injury or general surgical procedure performed must be submitted. An ICD-9-CM code in the range 800.0 through 959.9 (except 930-939), which clearly indicates that the critical care was unrelated to the surgery, is acceptable documentation.

10. Unusual Circumstances
Surgeries for which services performed are significantly greater than usually required may be billed with the "-22" modifier added to the CPT code for the procedure. Surgeries for which services performed are significantly less than usually required may be billed with the "-52" modifier. The biller must provide:

- A concise statement about how the service differs from the usual; and
- An operative report with the claim.

Modifier "-22" should only be reported with procedure codes that have a global period of 0, 10, or 90 days. There is no such restriction on the use of modifier "-52."

B. Date(s) of Service
Physicians, who bill for the entire global surgical package or for only a portion of the care, must enter the date on which the surgical procedure was performed in the "From/To" date of service field. This will enable carriers to relate all appropriate billings to the correct surgery. Physicians who share postoperative management with another physician must submit additional information showing when they assumed and relinquished responsibility for the postoperative care. If the physician who performed the surgery relinquishes care at the time of discharge, he or she need only show the date of surgery when billing with modifier "-54."

However, if the surgeon also cares for the patient for some period following discharge, the surgeon must show the date of surgery and the date on which postoperative care was relinquished to another physician. The physician providing the remaining postoperative care must show the date care was assumed. This information should be shown in Item 19 on the paper Form CMS-1500, in the narrative portion of the HA0 record on the National Standard Format, and in the NTE segment for ANSI X12N electronic claims.

C. Care Provided in Different Payment Localities
If portions of the global period are provided in different payment localities, the services should be billed to the carriers servicing each applicable payment locality. For example, if the surgery is performed in one state and the postoperative care is provided in another state, the surgery is billed with modifier "-54" to the carrier servicing the payment locality where the surgery was performed and the postoperative care is billed with modifier "-55" to the carrier servicing the payment locality where the postoperative care was performed. This is true whether the services were performed by the same physician/group or different physicians/groups.

D. Health Professional Shortage Area (HPSA) Payments for Services Which are Subject to the Global Surgery Rules
HPSA bonus payments may be made for global surgeries when the services are provided in HPSAs. The following are guidelines for the appropriate billing procedures:

- If the entire global package is provided in a HPSA, physicians should bill for the appropriate global surgical code with the applicable HPSA modifier.
- If only a portion of the global package is provided in a HPSA, the physician should bill using a HPSA modifier for the portion which is provided in the HPSA.

EXAMPLE

The surgical portion of the global service is provided in a non-HPSA and the postoperative portion is provided in a HPSA. The surgical portion should be billed with the "-54" modifier and no HPSA modifier. The postoperative portion should be billed with the "-55" modifier and the appropriate HPSA modifier. The 10 percent bonus will be paid on the appropriate postoperative portion only. If a claim is submitted with a global surgical code and a HPSA modifier, the carrier assumes that the entire global service was provided in a HPSA in the absence of evidence otherwise.

NOTE: The sum of the payments made for the surgical and postoperative services provided in different localities will not equal the global amount in either of the localities because of geographic adjustments made through the Geographic Practice Cost Indices.

100-4, 12, 40.6

Claims for Multiple Surgeries

B3-4826, B3-15038, B3-15056

A. General
Multiple surgeries are separate procedures performed by a single physician or physicians in the same group practice on the same patient at the same operative session or on the same day for which separate payment may be allowed. Co-surgeons, surgical teams, or assistants-at-surgery may participate in performing multiple surgeries on the same patient on the same day.

Multiple surgeries are distinguished from procedures that are components of or incidental to a primary procedure. These intra-operative services, incidental surgeries, or components of more major surgeries are not separately billable. See Chapter 23 for a description of mandatory edits to prevent separate payment for those procedures. Major surgical procedures are determined based on the MFSDB approved amount and not on the submitted amount from the providers. The major surgery, as based on the MFSDB, may or may not be the one with the larger submitted amount.

Also, see subsection D below for a description of the standard payment policy on multiple surgeries. However, these standard payment rules are not appropriate for certain procedures. Field 21 of the MFSDB indicates whether the standard payment policy rules apply to a multiple surgery, or whether special payment rules apply. Site of service payment adjustments (codes with an indicator of "1" in Field 27 of the MFSDB) should be applied before multiple surgery payment adjustments.

B. Billing Instructions
The following procedures apply when billing for multiple surgeries by the same physician on the same day.

- Report the more major surgical procedure without the multiple procedures modifier "-51."

- Report additional surgical procedures performed by the surgeon on the same day with modifier "-51."

There may be instances in which two or more physicians each perform distinctly different, unrelated surgeries on the same patient on the same day (e.g., in some multiple trauma cases). When this occurs, the payment adjustment rules for multiple surgeries may not be appropriate. In such cases, the physician does not use modifier "-51" unless one of the surgeons individually performs multiple surgeries.

C. Carrier Claims Processing System Requirements
Carriers must be able to:

1. Identify multiple surgeries by both of the following methods:
   - The presence on the claim form or electronic submission of the "-51" modifier; and
   - The billing of more than one separately payable surgical procedure by the same physician performed on the same patient on the same day, whether on different lines or with a number greater than 1 in the units column on the claim form or inappropriately billed with modifier "-78" (i.e., after the global period has expired);
2. Access Field 34 of the MFSDB to determine the Medicare fee schedule payment amount for each surgery;
3. Access Field 21 for each procedure of the MFSDB to determine if the payment rules for multiple surgeries apply to any of the multiple surgeries billed on the same day;
4. If Field 21 for any of the multiple procedures contains an indicator of "0," the multiple surgery rules do not apply to that procedure. Base payment on the lower of the billed amount or the fee schedule amount (Field 34 or 35) for each code unless other payment adjustment rules apply;
5. For dates of service prior to January 1, 1995, if Field 21 contains an indicator of "1," the standard rules for pricing multiple surgeries apply (see items 6-8 below);
6. Rank the surgeries subject to the standard multiple surgery rules (indicator "1") in descending order by the Medicare fee schedule amount;
7. Base payment for each ranked procedure on the lower of the billed amount, or:
   - 100 percent of the fee schedule amount (Field 34 or 35) for the highest valued procedure;
   - 50 percent of the fee schedule amount for the second highest valued procedure; and
   - 25 percent of the fee schedule amount for the third through the fifth highest valued procedures;
8. If more than five procedures are billed, pay for the first five according to the rules listed in 5, 6, and 7 above and suspend the sixth and subsequent procedures for manual review and payment, if appropriate, "by report." Payment determined on a "by report" basis for these codes should never be lower than 25 percent of the full payment amount;
9. For dates of service on or after January 1, 1995, new standard rules for pricing multiple surgeries apply. If Field 21 contains an indicator of "2," these new standard rules apply (see items 10-12 below);
10. Rank the surgeries subject to the multiple surgery rules (indicator "2") in descending order by the Medicare fee schedule amount;
11. Base payment for each ranked procedure (indicator "2") on the lower of the billed amount:
    - 100 percent of the fee schedule amount (Field 34 or 35) for the highest valued procedure; and
    - 50 percent of the fee schedule amount for the second through the fifth highest valued procedures; or
12. If more than five procedures with an indicator of "2" are billed, pay for the first five according to the rules listed in 9, 10, and 11 above and suspend the sixth and subsequent procedures for manual review and payment, if appropriate, "by report." Payment determined on a "by report" basis for these codes should never be lower than 50 percent of the full payment amount. Pay by the unit for services that are already reduced (e.g., 17003). Pay for 17340 only once per session, regardless of how many lesions were destroyed;

    NOTE: For dates of service prior to January 1, 1995, the multiple surgery indicator of "2" indicated that special dermatology rules applied. The payment rules for these codes have not changed. The rules were expanded, however, to all codes that previously had a multiple surgery indicator of "1." For dates of service prior to January 1, 1995, if a dermatological procedure with an indicator of "2" was billed with the "-51" modifier with other procedures that are not dermatological procedures (procedures with an indicator of "1" in Field 21), the standard multiple surgery rules applied. Pay no less than 50 percent for the dermatological procedures with an indicator of "2." See 40.6.C.6-8 for required actions.
13. If Field 21 contains an indicator of "3," and multiple endoscopies are billed, the special rules for multiple endoscopic procedures apply. Pay the full value of the highest valued endoscopy, plus the difference between the next highest and the base endoscopy. Access Field 31A of the MFSDB to determine the base endoscopy.

    EXAMPLE

    In the course of performing a fiber optic colonoscopy (CPT code 45378), a physician performs a biopsy on a lesion (code 45380) and removes a polyp (code 45385) from a different part of the colon. The physician bills for codes 45380 and 45385. The value of codes 45380 and 45385 have the value of the diagnostic colonoscopy (45378) built in.

    Rather than paying 100 percent for the highest valued procedure (45385) and 50 percent for the next (45380), pay the full value of the higher valued endoscopy (45385), plus the difference between the next highest endoscopy (45380) and the base endoscopy (45378).

    Carriers assume the following fee schedule amounts for these codes:

    45378 - $255.40

    45380 - $285.98

    45385 - $374.56

    Pay the full value of 45385 ($374.56), plus the difference between 45380 and 45378 ($30.58), for a total of $405.14.

    NOTE: If an endoscopic procedure with an indicator of "3" is billed with the "-51" modifier with other procedures that are not endoscopies (procedures with an indicator of "1" in Field 21), the standard multiple surgery rules apply. See 40.6.C.6-8 for required actions.
14. Apply the following rules where endoscopies are performed on the same day as unrelated endoscopies or other surgical procedures:
    - Two unrelated endoscopies (e.g., 46606 and 43217): Apply the usual multiple surgery rules;
    - Two sets of unrelated endoscopies (e.g., 43202 and 43217; 46606 and 46608): Apply the special endoscopy rules to each series and then apply the multiple surgery rules. Consider the total payment for each set of endoscopies as one service;
    - Two related endoscopies and a third, unrelated procedure: Apply the special endoscopic rules to the related endoscopies, and, then apply the multiple surgery rules. Consider the total payment for the related endoscopies as one service and the unrelated endoscopy as another service.
15. If two or more multiple surgeries are of equal value, rank them in descending dollar order billed and base payment on the percentages listed above (i.e., 100 percent for the first billed procedure, 50 percent for the second, etc.);
16. If any of the multiple surgeries are bilateral surgeries, consider the bilateral procedure at 150 percent as one payment amount, rank this with the remaining procedures, and apply the appropriate multiple surgery reductions. See 40.7 for bilateral surgery payment instructions.);
17. Round all adjusted payment amounts to the nearest cent;
18. If some of the surgeries are subject to special rules while others are subject to the standard rules, automate pricing to the extent possible. If necessary, price manually;
19. In cases of multiple interventional radiological procedures, both the radiology code and the primary surgical code are paid at 100 percent of the fee schedule amount. The subsequent surgical procedures are paid at the standard multiple surgical percentages (50 percent, 50 percent, 50 percent and 50 percent);
20. Apply the requirements in 40 on global surgeries to multiple surgeries;
21. Retain the "-51" modifier in history for any multiple surgeries paid at less than the full global amount; and
22. Follow the instructions on adjudicating surgery claims submitted with the "-22" modifier. Review documentation to determine if full payment should be made for those distinctly different, unrelated surgeries performed by different physicians on the same day.

D. Ranking of Same Day Multiple Surgeries When One Surgery Has a "-22" Modifier and Additional Payment is Allowed

B3-4826

If the patient returns to the operating room after the initial operative session on the same day as a result of complications from the original surgery, the complications rules apply to each procedure required to treat the complications from the original surgery. The multiple surgery rules would not apply.

However, if the patient is returned to the operating room during the postoperative period of the original surgery, not on the same day of the original surgery, for multiple procedures that are required as a result of complications from the original surgery, the complications rules would apply. The multiple surgery rules would also not apply.

Multiple surgeries are defined as separate procedures performed by a single physician or physicians in the same group practice on the same patient at the same operative session or on the same day for which separate payment may be allowed. Co-surgeons, surgical teams, or assistants-at-surgery may participate in performing multiple surgeries on the same patient on the same day.

Multiple surgeries are distinguished from procedures that are components of or incidental to a primary procedure. These intra-operative services, incidental surgeries, or components of more major surgeries are not separately billable. See Chapter 23 for a description of mandatory edits to prevent separate payment for those procedures.

100-4, 12, 40.7

Claims for Bilateral Surgeries

B3-4827, B3-15040

A. General
Bilateral surgeries are procedures performed on both sides of the body during the same operative session or on the same day.

The terminology for some procedure codes includes the terms "bilateral" (e.g., code 27395; Lengthening of the hamstring tendon; multiple, bilateral.) or "unilateral or bilateral" (e.g., code 52290; cystourethroscopy; with ureteral meatotomy, unilateral or bilateral). The payment adjustment rules for bilateral surgeries do not apply to procedures identified by CPT as "bilateral" or "unilateral or bilateral" since the fee schedule reflects any additional work required for bilateral surgeries.

Field 22 of the MFSDB indicates whether the payment adjustment rules apply to a surgical procedure.

B. Billing Instructions for Bilateral Surgeries

If a procedure is not identified by its terminology as a bilateral procedure (or unilateral or bilateral), physicians must report the procedure with modifier "-50." They report such procedures as a single line item. (NOTE: This differs from the CPT coding guidelines which indicate that bilateral procedures should be billed as two line items.)

If a procedure is identified by the terminology as bilateral (or unilateral or bilateral), as in codes 27395 and 52290, physicians do not report the procedure with modifier "-50."

C. Claims Processing System Requirements

Carriers must be able to:

1. Identify bilateral surgeries by the presence on the claim form or electronic submission of the "-50" modifier or of the same code on separate lines reported once with modifier "-LT" and once with modifier "-RT";
2. Access Field 34 or 35 of the MFSDB to determine the Medicare payment amount;
3. Access Field 22 of the MFSDB:
   - If Field 22 contains an indicator of "0," "2," or "3," the payment adjustment rules for bilateral surgeries do not apply. Base payment on the lower of the billed amount or 100 percent of the fee schedule amount (Field 34 or 35) unless other payment adjustment rules apply.

     NOTE: Some codes which have a bilateral indicator of "0" in the MFSDB may be performed more than once on a given day. These are services that would never be considered bilateral and thus should not be billed with modifier "-50." Where such a code is billed on multiple line tems or with more than 1 in the units field and carriers have determined that the code may be reported more than once, bypass the "0" bilateral indicator and refer to the multiple surgery field for pricing;
   - If Field 22 contains an indicator of "1," the standard adjustment rules apply. Base payment on the lower of the billed amount or 150 percent of the fee schedule amount (Field 34 or 35). (Multiply the payment amount in Field 34 or 35 for the surgery by 150 percent and round to the nearest cent.)
4. Apply the requirements 40 - 40.4 on global surgeries to bilateral surgeries; and
5. Retain the "-50" modifier in history for any bilateral surgeries paid at the adjusted amount.

   (NOTE: The "-50" modifier is not retained for surgeries which are bilateral by definition such as code 27395.)

100-4, 12, 40.8

Claims for Co-Surgeons and Team Surgeons

B3-4828, B3-15046

A. General

Under some circumstances, the individual skills of two or more surgeons are required to perform surgery on the same patient during the same operative session. This may be required because of the complex nature of the procedure(s) and/or the patient's condition.

In these cases, the additional physicians are not acting as assistants-at-surgery.

B. Billing Instructions

The following billing procedures apply when billing for a surgical procedure or procedures that required the use of two surgeons or a team of surgeons:

- If two surgeons (each in a different specialty) are required to perform a specific procedure, each surgeon bills for the procedure with a modifier "-62. " Co-surgery also refers to surgical procedures involving two surgeons performing the parts of the procedure simultaneously, i.e., heart transplant or bilateral knee replacements. Documentation of the medical necessity for two surgeons is required for certain services identified in the MFSDB. (See 40.8.C.5.);
- If a team of surgeons (more than 2 surgeons of different specialties) is required to perform a specific procedure, each surgeon bills for the procedure with a modifier "-66." Field 25 of the MFSDB identifies certain services submitted with a "-66" modifier which must be sufficiently documented to establish that a team was medically necessary. All claims for team surgeons must contain sufficient information to allow pricing "by report."
- If surgeons of different specialties are each performing a different procedure (with specific CPT codes), neither co-surgery nor multiple surgery rules apply (even if the procedures are performed through the same incision). If one of the surgeons performs multiple procedures, the multiple procedure rules apply to that surgeon's services. (See 40.6 for multiple surgery payment rules.)

For co-surgeons (modifier 62), the fee schedule amount applicable to the payment for each co-surgeon is 62.5 percent of the global surgery fee schedule amount. Team surgery (modifier 66) is paid for on a "By Report" basis.

C. Claims Processing System Requirements

Carriers must be able to:

1. Identify a surgical procedure performed by two surgeons or a team of surgeons by the presence on the claim form or electronic submission of the "-62" or "-66" modifier;
2. Access Field 34 or 35 of the MFSDB to determine the fee schedule payment amount for the surgery;
3. Access Field 24 or 25, as appropriate, of the MFSDB. These fields provide guidance on whether two or team surgeons are generally required for the surgical procedure;
4. If the surgery is billed with a "-62" or "-66" modifier and Field 24 or 25 contains an indicator of "0," payment adjustment rules for two or team surgeons do not apply:
   - Carriers pay the first bill submitted, and base payment on the lower of the billed amount or 100 percent of the fee schedule amount (Field 34 or 35) unless other payment adjustment rules apply;
   - Carriers deny bills received subsequently from other physicians and use the appropriate MSN message in 40.8.D. As these are medical necessity denials, the instructions in the Program Integrity Manual regarding denial of unassigned claims for medical necessity are applied;
5. If the surgery is billed with a "-62" modifier and Field 24 contains an indicator of "1," suspend the claim for manual review of any documentation submitted with the claim. If the documentation supports the need for co-surgeons, base payment for each physician on the lower of the billed amount or 62.5 percent of the fee schedule amount (Field 34 or 35);
6. If the surgery is billed with a "-62" modifier and Field 24 contains an indicator of "2," payment rules for two surgeons apply. Carriers base payment for each physician on the lower of the billed amount or 62.5 percent of the fee schedule amount (Field 34 or 35);
7. If the surgery is billed with a "-66" modifier and Field 25 contains an indicator of "1," carriers suspend the claim for manual review. If carriers determine that team surgeons were medically necessary, each physician is paid on a "by report" basis;
8. If the surgery is billed with a "-66" modifier and Field 25 contains an indicator of "2," carriers pay "by report";

   NOTE: A Medicare fee may have been established for some surgical procedures that are billed with the "-66" modifier. In these cases, all physicians on the team must agree on the percentage of the Medicare payment amount each is to receive.If carriers receive a bill with a "-66" modifier after carriers have paid one surgeon the full Medicare payment amount (on a bill without the modifier), deny the subsequent claim.
9. Apply the rules global surgical packages to each of the physicians participating in a co- or team surgery; and
10. Retain the "-62" and "-66" modifiers in history for any co- or team surgeries.

D. Beneficiary Liability on Denied Claims for Assistant, Co- surgeon and Team Surgeons

MSN message 23.10 which states "Medicare does not pay for a surgical assistant for this kind of surgery," was established for denial of claims for assistant surgeons. Where such payment is denied because the procedure is subject to the statutory restriction against payment for assistants-at-surgery. Carriers include the following statement in the MSN:

"You cannot be charged for this service." (Unnumbered add-on message.)

Carriers use Group Code CO on the remittance advice to the physician to signify that the beneficiary may not be billed for the denied service and that the physician could be subject to penalties if a bill is issued to the beneficiary.

If Field 23 of the MFSDB contains an indicator of "0" or "1" (assistant-at-surgery may not be paid) for procedures CMS has determined that an assistant surgeon is not generally medically necessary.

For those procedures with an indicator of "0," the limitation on liability provisions described in Chapter 30 apply to assigned claims. Therefore, carriers include the appropriate limitation of liability language from Chapter 21. For unassigned claims, apply the rules in the Program Integrity Manual concerning denial for medical necessity.

Where payment may not be made for a co- or team surgeon, use the following MSN message (MSN message number 15.13):

Medicare does not pay for team surgeons for this procedure.

Where payment may not be made for a two surgeons, use the following MSN message (MSN message number 15.12):

Medicare does not pay for two surgeons for this procedure.

Also see limitation of liability remittance notice REF remark codes M25, M26, and M27.

Use the following message on the remittance notice:

Multiple physicians/assistants are not covered in this case. (Reason code 54.)

100-4,12,50

Payment for Anesthesiology Services

A. General Payment Rule

The fee schedule amount for physician anesthesia services furnished on or after January 1, 1992 is, with the exceptions noted, based on allowable base and time units multiplied by an anesthesia conversion factor specific to that locality. The base unit for each anesthesia procedure is communicated to the Part B Contractors by means of the HCPCS file released annually. The public can access the base units on the CMS homepage through the anesthesiologist's center. The way in which time units are calculated is described in Sec.50.G. CMS releases the conversion factor annually.

B. Payment at Personally Performed Rate

The Part B Contractor must determine the fee schedule payment, recognizing the base unit for the anesthesia code and one time unit per 15 minutes of anesthesia time if: The physician personally performed the entire anesthesia service alone; The physician is involved with one anesthesia case with a resident, the physician is a teaching physician as defined in Sec.100, and the service is furnished on or after January 1, 1996; The physician is involved in the training of physician residents in a single anesthesia case, two concurrent anesthesia cases involving residents or a single anesthesia case involving a resident that is concurrent to another case paid under the medical direction rules. The physician meets the teaching physician criteria in Sec.100.1.4 and the service is furnished on or after January 1, 2010; The physician is continuously involved in a single case involving a student nurse anesthetist; The physician is continuously involved in one anesthesia case involving a CRNA (or AA) and the service was furnished prior to January 1, 1998. If the physician is involved with a single case with a CRNA (or AA) and the service was furnished on or after January 1, 1998, carriers may pay the physician service and the CRNA (or AA) service in accordance with the medical direction payment policy; or The physician and the CRNA (or AA) are involved in one anesthesia case and the services of each are found to be medically necessary. Documentation must be submitted by both the CRNA and the physician to support payment of the full fee for each of the two providers. The physician reports the "AA" modifier and the CRNA reports the "QZ" modifier for a nonmedically directed case.

C. Payment at the Medically Directed Rate
The Part B Contractor determines payment for the physician's medical direction service furnished on or after January 1, 1998, on the basis of 50 percent of the allowance for the service performed by the physician alone. Medical direction occurs if the physician medically directs qualified individuals in two, three, or four concurrent cases and the physician performs the following activities.

Performs a pre-anesthetic examination and evaluation; Prescribes the anesthesia plan; Personally participates in the most demanding procedures in the anesthesia plan, including induction and emergence; Ensures that any procedures in the anesthesia plan that he or she does not perform are performed by a qualified anesthetist; Monitors the course of anesthesia administration at frequent intervals; Remains physically present and available for immediate diagnosis and treatment of emergencies; and Provides indicated-post-anesthesia care.

Prior to January 1, 1999, the physician was required to participate in the most demanding procedures of the anesthesia plan, including induction and emergence.

For medical direction services furnished on or after January 1, 1999, the physician must participate only in the most demanding procedures of the anesthesia plan, including, if applicable, induction and emergence. Also for medical direction services furnished on or after January 1, 1999, the physician must document in the medical record that he or she performed the pre-anesthetic examination and evaluation. Physicians must also document that they provided indicated post-anesthesia care, were present during some portion of the anesthesia monitoring, and were present during the most demanding procedures, including induction and emergence, where indicated.

For services furnished on or after January 1, 1994, the physician can medically direct two, three, or four concurrent procedures involving qualified individuals, all of whom could be CRNAs, AAs, interns, residents or combinations of these individuals. The medical direction rules apply to cases involving student nurse anesthetists if the physician directs two concurrent cases, each of which involves a student nurse anesthetist, or the physician directs one case involving a student nurse anesthetist and another involving a CRNA, AA, intern or resident.

For services furnished on or after January 1, 2010, the medical direction rules do not apply to a single resident case that is concurrent to another anesthesia case paid under the medical direction rules or to two concurrent anesthesia cases involving residents.

If anesthesiologists are in a group practice, one physician member may provide the pre-anesthesia examination and evaluation while another fulfills the other criteria. Similarly, one physician member of the group may provide post-anesthesia care while another member of the group furnishes the other component parts of the anesthesia service. However, the medical record must indicate that the services were furnished by physicians and identify the physicians who furnished them.

A physician who is concurrently directing the administration of anesthesia to not more than four surgical patients cannot ordinarily be involved in furnishing additional services to other patients. However, addressing an emergency of short duration in the immediate area, administering an epidural or caudal anesthetic to ease labor pain, or periodic, rather than continuous, monitoring of an obstetrical patient does not substantially diminish the scope of control exercised by the physician in directing the administration of anesthesia to surgical patients. It does not constitute a separate service for the purpose of determining whether the medical direction criteria are met. Further, while directing concurrent anesthesia procedures, a physician may receive patients entering the operating suite for the next surgery, check or discharge patients in the recovery room, or handle scheduling matters without affecting fee schedule payment.

However, if the physician leaves the immediate area of the operating suite for other than short durations or devotes extensive time to an emergency case or is otherwise not available to respond to the immediate needs of the surgical patients, the physician's services to the surgical patients are supervisory in nature. Carriers may not make payment under the fee schedule.

See Sec.50.J for a definition of concurrent anesthesia procedures.

D. Payment at Medically Supervised Rate
The Part B Contractor may allow only three base units per procedure when the anesthesiologist is involved in furnishing more than four procedures concurrently or is performing other services while directing the concurrent procedures. An additional time unit may be recognized if the physician can document he or she was present at induction.

E. Billing and Payment for Multiple Anesthesia Procedures
Physicians bill for the anesthesia services associated with multiple bilateral surgeries by reporting the anesthesia procedure with the highest base unit value with the multiple procedure modifier "-51." They report the total time for all procedures in the line item with the highest base unit value.

If the same anesthesia CPT code applies to two or more of the surgical procedures, billers enter the anesthesia code with the "-51" modifier and the number of surgeries to which the modified CPT code applies.

Payment can be made under the fee schedule for anesthesia services associated with multiple surgical procedures or multiple bilateral procedures. Payment is determined based on the base unit of the anesthesia procedure with the highest base unit value and time units based on the actual anesthesia time of the multiple procedures. See Sec.Sec.40.6-40.7 for a definition and appropriate billing and claims processing instructions for multiple and bilateral surgeries. F.

F. Payment for Medical and Surgical Services Furnished in Addition to Anesthesia Procedure Payment may be made under the fee schedule for specific medical and surgical services furnished by the anesthesiologist as long as these services are reasonable and medically necessary or provided that other rebundling provisions (see Sec.30 and Chapter 23) do not preclude separate payment. These services may be furnished in conjunction with the anesthesia procedure to the patient or may be furnished as single services, e.g., during the day of or the day before the anesthesia service. These services include the insertion of a Swan Ganz catheter, the insertion of central venous pressure lines, emergency intubation, and critical care visits.

G. Anesthesia Time and Calculation of Anesthesia Time Units
Anesthesia time is defined as the period during which an anesthesia practitioner is present with the patient. It starts when the anesthesia practitioner begins to prepare the patient for anesthesia services in the operating room or an equivalent area and ends when the anesthesia practitioner is no longer furnishing anesthesia services to the patient, that is, when the patient may be placed safely under postoperative care. Anesthesia time is a continuous time period from the start of anesthesia to the end of an anesthesia service. In counting anesthesia time for services furnished on or after January 1, 2000, the anesthesia practitioner can add blocks of time around an interruption in anesthesia time as long as the anesthesia practitioner is furnishing continuous anesthesia care within the time periods around the interruption.

Actual anesthesia time in minutes is reported on the claim. For anesthesia services furnished on or after January 1, 1994, the A/B MAC computes time units by dividing reported anesthesia time by 15 minutes. Round the time unit to one decimal place. The A/B MAC does not recognize time units for CPT codes 01995 or 01996.

For purposes of this section, anesthesia practitioner means a physician who performs the anesthesia service alone, a CRNA who is not medically directed, or a CRNA or AA, who is medically directed. The physician who medically directs the CRNA or AA would ordinarily report the same time as the CRNA or AA reports for the CRNA service.

H. Base Unit Reduction for Concurrent Medically Directed Procedures
If the physician medically directs concurrent medically directed procedures prior to January 1, 1994, reduce the number of base units for each concurrent procedure as follows.

For two concurrent procedures, the base unit on each procedure is reduced 10 percent.

For three concurrent procedures, the base unit on each procedure is reduced 25 percent.

For four concurrent procedures, the base on each concurrent procedure is reduced 40 percent.

If the physician medically directs concurrent procedures prior to January 1, 1994, and any of the concurrent procedures are cataract or iridectomy anesthesia, reduce the base units for each cataract or iridectomy procedure by 10 percent.

I. Monitored Anesthesia Care
The Part B Contractor pays for reasonable and medically necessary monitored anesthesia care services on the same basis as other anesthesia services. Anesthesiologists use modifier QS to report monitored anesthesia care cases. Monitored anesthesia care involves the intra-operative monitoring by a physician or qualified individual under the medical direction of a physician or of the patient's vital physiological signs in anticipation of the need for administration of general anesthesia or of the development of adverse physiological patient reaction to the surgical procedure. It also includes the performance of a pre-anesthetic examination and evaluation, prescription of the anesthesia care required, administration of any necessary oral or parenteral medications (e.g., atropine, demerol, valium) and provision of indicated postoperative anesthesia care.

Payment is made under the fee schedule using the payment rules in subsection B if the physician personally performs the monitored anesthesia care case or under the rules in subsection C if the physician medically directs four or fewer concurrent cases and monitored anesthesia care represents one or more of these concurrent cases.

J. Definition of Concurrent Medically Directed Anesthesia Procedures
Concurrency is defined with regard to the maximum number of procedures that the physician is medically directing within the context of a single procedure and whether these other procedures overlap each other. Concurrency is not dependent on each of the cases involving a Medicare patient. For example, if an anesthesiologist directs three concurrent procedures, two of which involve non-Medicare patients and the remaining a Medicare patient, this represents three concurrent cases. The following example illustrates this concept and guides physicians in determining how many procedures they are directing.

EXAMPLE Procedures A through E are medically directed procedures involving CRNAs and furnished between January 1, 1992 and December 31, 1997 (1998 concurrent instructions can be found in subsection C.) The starting and ending times for each procedure represent the periods during which anesthesia time is counted. Assume that none of the procedures were cataract or iridectomy anesthesia.

Procedure A begins at 8:00 a.m. and lasts until 8:20 a.m.

Procedure B begins at 8:10 a.m. and lasts until 8:45 a.m.

Procedure C begins at 8:30 a.m. and lasts until 9:15 a.m.

Procedure D begins at 9:00 a.m. and lasts until 12:00 noon.

Procedure E begins at 9:10 a.m. and lasts until 9:55 a.m.

Procedure	***Number of Concurrent Medically Directed Procedures***	***Base Unit Reduction Percentage***
A	2	10%
B	2	0%
C	3	25%
D	3	25%
E	3	25%

From 8:00 a.m. to 8:20 a.m., the length of procedure A, the anesthesiologist medically directed two concurrent procedures, A and B.

From 8:10 a.m. to 8:45 a.m., the length of procedure B, the anesthesiologist medically directed two concurrent procedures. From 8:10 to 8:20 a.m., the anesthesiologist medically directed procedures A and B. From 8:20 to 8:30 a.m., the anesthesiologist medically directed only procedure B. From 8:30 to 8:45 a.m., the anesthesiologist medically directed procedures B and C. Thus, during procedure B, the anesthesiologist medically directed, at most, two concurrent procedures.

From 8:30 a.m. to 9:15 a.m., the length of procedure C, the anesthesiologist medically directed three concurrent procedures. From 8:30 to 8:45 a.m., the anesthesiologist medically directed procedures B and C. From 8:45 to 9:00 a.m., the anesthesiologist medically directed procedure C. From 9:00 to 9:10 a.m., the anesthesiologist medically directed procedures C and D. From 9:10 to 9:15 a.m., the anesthesiologist medically directed procedures C, D and E. Thus, during procedure C, the anesthesiologist medically directed, at most, three concurrent procedures.

The same analysis shows that during procedure D or E, the anesthesiologist medically directed, at most, three concurrent procedures.

K. Anesthesia Claims Modifiers
Physicians report the appropriate anesthesia modifier to denote whether the service was personally performed, medically directed, or medically supervised.

Specific anesthesia modifiers include:

AA - Anesthesia Services performed personally by the anesthesiologist;
AD - Medical Supervision by a physician; more than 4 concurrent anesthesia procedures;
G8 - Monitored anesthesia care (MAC) for deep complex complicated, or markedly invasive surgical procedures;
G9 - Monitored anesthesia care for patient who has a history of severe cardio-pulmonary condition;
QK - Medical direction of two, three or four concurrent anesthesia procedures involving qualified individuals;
QS - Monitored anesthesia care service;
QX - CRNA service; with medical direction by a physician;
QY - Medical direction of one certified registered nurse anesthetist by an anesthesiologist;
QZ - CRNA service: without medical direction by a physician; and
GC - these services have been performed by a resident under the direction of a teaching physician.

The GC modifier is reported by the teaching physician to indicate he/she rendered the service in compliance with the teaching physician requirements in Sec.100.1.2. One of the payment modifiers must be used in conjunction with the GC modifier.

The QS modifier is for informational purposes. Providers must report actual anesthesia time on the claim.

The Part B Contractor must determine payment for anesthesia in accordance with these instructions. They must be able to determine the uniform base unit that is assigned to the anesthesia code and apply the appropriate reduction where the anesthesia procedure is medically directed. They must also be able to determine the number of anesthesia time units from actual anesthesia time reported on the claim. The Part B Contractor must multiply allowable units by the anesthesia-specific conversion factor used to determine fee schedule payment for the payment area.

L. Anesthesia and Medical/Surgical Service Provided by the Same Physician
Anesthesia services range in complexity. The continuum of anesthesia services, from least intense to most intense in complexity is as follows: local or topical anesthesia, moderate (conscious) sedation, regional anesthesia and general anesthesia. Prior to 2006, Medicare did not recognize separate payment if the same physician provided the medical or surgical procedure and the anesthesia needed for the procedure.

Moderate sedation is a drug induced depression of consciousness during which the patient responds purposefully to verbal commands, either alone or accompanied by light tactile stimulation. Moderate sedation does not include minimal sedation, deep sedation or monitored anesthesia care. In 2006, the CPT added new codes 99143 to 99150 for moderate or conscious sedation. The moderate (conscious) sedation codes are carrier priced under the Medicare physician fee schedule.

The CPT codes 99143 to 99145 describe moderate sedation provided by the same physician performing the diagnostic or therapeutic service that the sedation supports, requiring the presence of an independent trained observer to assist in the monitoring of the patient's level of consciousness and physiological status. The physician can bill the conscious sedation codes 99143 to 99145 as long as the procedure with it is billed is not listed in Appendix G of CPT. CPT codes 99148 to 99150 describe moderate sedation provided by a physician other than the health care professional performing the diagnostic or therapeutic service that the sedation supports.

The CPT includes Appendix G, Summary of CPT Codes That Include Moderate (Conscious) Sedation. This appendix lists those procedures for which moderate (conscious) sedation is an inherent part of the procedure itself. CPT coding guidelines instruct practices not to report CPT codes 99143 to 99145 in conjunction with codes listed in Appendix G. The National Correct Coding Initiative has established edits that bundle CPT codes 99143 and 99144 into the procedures listed in Appendix G.

In the unusual event when a second physician other than the health care professional performing the diagnostic or therapeutic services provides moderate sedation in the facility setting for the procedures listed in Appendix G, the second physician can bill 99148 to 99150. The term, facility, includes those places of service listed in Chapter 23 Addendum -- field 29. However, when these services are performed by the second physician in the nonfacility setting, CPT codes 99148 to 99150 are not to be reported.

If the anesthesiologist or CRNA provides anesthesia for diagnostic or therapeutic nerve blocks or injections and a different provider performs the block or injection, then the anesthesiologist or CRNA may report the anesthesia service using CPT code 01991. The service must meet the criteria for monitored anesthesia care. If the anesthesiologist or CRNA provides both the anesthesia service and the block or injection, then the anesthesiologist or CRNA may report the anesthesia service using the conscious sedation code and the injection or block. However, the anesthesia service must meet the requirements for conscious sedation and if a lower level complexity anesthesia service is provided, then the conscious sedation code should not be reported.

If the physician performing the medical or surgical procedure also provides a level of anesthesia lower in intensity than moderate or conscious sedation, such as a local or topical anesthesia, then the conscious sedation code should not be reported and no payment should be allowed by the carrier. There is no CPT code for the performance of local anesthesia and as payment for this service is considered in the payment for the underlying medical or surgical service.

100-4, 12, 60

Payment for Pathology Services

B3-15020, AB-01-47 (CR1499)

A. General Payment Rule
Payment may be made under the fee schedule for the professional component of physician laboratory or physician pathology services furnished to hospital inpatients or outpatients by hospital physicians or by independent laboratories, if they qualify as the reassignee for the physician service.. Payment may be made under the fee schedule, as noted below, for the technical component (TC) of pathology services furnished by an independent laboratory to hospital inpatients or outpatients. Payment may be made under the fee schedule for the technical component of physician pathology services furnished by an independent laboratory, or a hospital if it is acting as an independent laboratory, to non-hospital patients. The Medicare physician fee schedule identifies those physician laboratory or physician pathology services that have a technical component service.

CMS published a final regulation in 1999 that would no longer allow independent laboratories to bill under the physician fee schedule for the TC of physician pathology services. The implementation of this regulation was delayed by Section 542 of the Benefits and Improvement and Protection Act of 2000 (BIPA). Section 542 allows the Medicare carrier to continue to pay for the TC of physician pathology services when an independent laboratory furnishes this service to an inpatient or outpatient of a covered hospital. This provision is applicable to TC services furnished in 2001, 2002, 2003, 2004, 2005 or 2006.

For this provision, a covered hospital is a hospital that had an arrangement with an independent laboratory that was in effect as of July 22, 1999, under which a laboratory furnished the TC of physician pathology services to fee-for-service Medicare beneficiaries who were hospital inpatients or outpatients, and submitted claims for payment for the TC to a carrier. The TC could have been submitted separately or combined with the professional component and reported as a combined service.

The term, fee-for-service Medicare beneficiary, means an individual who:

Is entitled to benefits under Part A or enrolled under Part B of title XVIII or both; and

Is not enrolled in any of the following: A Medicare + Choice plan under Part C of such title; a plan offered by an eligible organization under 1876 of the Social Security Act; a program of all-inclusive care for the elderly under 1894; or a social health maintenance organization demonstration project established under Section 4108 of the Omnibus Budget Reconciliation Act of 1987.

In implementing Section 542, the carriers should consider as independent laboratories those entities that it has previously recognized as independent laboratories. An independent laboratory that has acquired another independent laboratory that had an arrangement of July 22, 1999, with a covered hospital, can bill the TC of physician pathology services for that hospital's inpatients and outpatients under the physician fee schedule.

An independent laboratory that furnishes the TC of physician pathology services to inpatients or outpatients of a hospital that is not a covered hospital may not bill the carrier for the TC of physician pathology services during the time 542 is in effect.

If the arrangement between the independent laboratory and the covered hospital limited the provision of TC physician pathology services to certain situations or at particular times, then the independent laboratory can bill the carrier only for these limited services.

The carrier shall require independent laboratories that had an arrangement, on or prior to July 22, 1999 with a covered hospital, to bill for the technical component of physician pathology services to provide a copy of this agreement, or other documentation substantiating that an arrangement was in effect between the hospital and the independent laboratory as of this date. The independent laboratory must submit this documentation for each covered hospital that the independent laboratory services.

See Chapter 16 for additional instruction on laboratory services including clinical diagnostic laboratory services.

Physician laboratory and pathology services are limited to:

- Surgical pathology services;
- Specific cytopathology, hematology and blood banking services that have been identified to require performance by a physician and are listed below;
- Clinical consultation services that meet the requirements in subsection D below;
- and
- Clinical laboratory interpretation services that meet the requirements and which are specifically listed in subsection E below.

B. Surgical Pathology Services
Surgical pathology services include the gross and microscopic examination of organ tissue performed by a physician, except for autopsies, which are not covered by Medicare. Surgical pathology services paid under the physician fee schedule are reported under the following CPT codes:

88300, 88302, 88304, 88305, 88307, 88309, 88311, 88312, 88313, 88314, 88318, 88319, 88321, 88323, 88325, 88329, 88331, 88332, 88342, 88346, 88347, 88348, 88349, 88355, 88356, 88358, 88361, 88362, 88365, 88380.

Depending upon circumstances and the billing entity, the carriers may pay professional component, technical component or both.

C. Specific Hematology, Cytopathology and Blood Banking Services
Cytopathology services include the examination of cells from fluids, washings, brushings or smears, but generally excluding hematology. Examining cervical and vaginal smears are the most common service in cytopathology. Cervical and vaginal smears do not require interpretation by a physician unless the results are or appear to be abnormal. In such cases, a physician personally conducts a separate microscopic evaluation to determine the nature of an abnormality. This microscopic evaluation ordinarily does require performance by a physician. When medically necessary and when furnished by a physician, it is paid under the fee schedule.

These codes include 88104, 88106, 88107, 88108, 88112, 88125, 88141, 88160, 88161, 88162, 88172, 88173, 88180, 88182.

For services furnished prior to January 1, 1999, carriers pay separately under the physician fee schedule for the interpretation of an abnormal pap smear furnished to a hospital inpatient by a physician. They must pay under the clinical laboratory fee schedule for pap smears furnished in all other situations. This policy also applies to screening pap smears requiring a physician interpretation. For services furnished on or after January 1, 1999, carriers allow separate payment for a physician's interpretation of a pap smear to any patient (i.e., hospital or non-hospital) as long as: (1) the laboratory's screening personnel suspect an abnormality; and (2) the physician reviews and interprets the pap smear.

This policy also applies to screening pap smears requiring a physician interpretation and described in the National Coverage Determination Manual and Chapter 18. These services are reported under codes P3000 or P3001.

Physician hematology services include microscopic evaluation of bone marrow aspirations and biopsies. It also includes those limited number of peripheral blood smears which need to be referred to a physician to evaluate the nature of an apparent abnormality identified by the technologist. These codes include 85060, 38220, 85097, and 38221.

Carriers pay the professional component for the interpretation of an abnormal blood smear (code 85060) furnished to a hospital inpatient by a hospital physician or an independent laboratory.

For the other listed hematology codes, payment may be made for the professional component if the service is furnished to a patient by a hospital physician or independent laboratory. In addition, payment may be made for these services furnished to patients by an independent laboratory.

Codes 38220 and 85097 represent professional-only component services and have no technical component values.

Blood banking services of hematologists and pathologists are paid under the physician fee schedule when analyses are performed on donor and/or patient blood to determine compatible donor units for transfusion where cross matching is difficult or where contamination with transmissible disease of donor is suspected.

The blood banking codes are 86077, 86078, and 86079 and represent professional component only services. These codes do not have a technical component.

D. Clinical Consultation Services
Clinical consultations are paid under the physician fee schedule only if they:

- Are requested by the patient's attending physician;
- Relate to a test result that lies outside the clinically significant normal or expected range in view of the condition of the patient;
- Result in a written narrative report included in the patient's medical record; and
- Require the exercise of medical judgment by the consultant physician.

Clinical consultations are professional component services only. There is no technical component. The clinical consultation codes are 80500 and 80502.

Routine conversations held between a laboratory director and an attending physician about test orders or results do not qualify as consultations unless all four requirements are met. Laboratory personnel, including the director, may from time to time contact attending physicians to report test results or to suggest additional testing or be contacted by attending physicians on similar matters. These contacts do not constitute clinical consultations. However, if in the course of such a contact, the attending physician requests a consultation from the pathologist, and if that consultation meets the other criteria and is properly documented, it is paid under the fee schedule.

EXAMPLE: A pathologist telephones a surgeon about a patient's suitability for surgery based on the results of clinical laboratory test results. During the course of their conversation, the surgeon ask the pathologist whether, based on test results, patient history and medical records, the patient is a candidate for surgery. The surgeon's request requires the pathologist to render a medical judgment and provide a consultation. The athologist follows up his/her oral advice with a written report and the surgeon notes in the patient's medical record that he/she requested a consultation. This consultation is paid under the fee schedule.

In any case, if the information could ordinarily be furnished by a nonphysician laboratory specialist, the service of the physician is not a consultation payable under the fee schedule.

See the Program Integrity Manual for guidelines for related data analysis to identify inappropriate patterns of billing for consultations.

E. Clinical Laboratory Interpretation Services
Only clinical laboratory interpretation services listed below and which meet the criteria in subsections D.1, D.3, and D.4 for clinical consultations and, as a result, are billable under the fee schedule. These services are reported under the clinical laboratory code with modifier 26. These services can be paid under the physician fee schedule if they are furnished to a patient by a hospital pathologist or an independent laboratory. Note that a hospital's standing order policy can be used as a substitute for the individual request by the patient's attending physician. Carriers are not allowed to revise CMS's list to accommodate local medical practice. The CMS periodically reviews this list and adds or deletes clinical laboratory codes as warranted.

Clinical Laboratory Interpretation Services

Code	Definition
83020	Hemoglobin; electrophoresis
83912	Nucleic acid probe, with electrophoresis, with examination and report
84165	Protein, total, serum; electrophoretic fractionation and quantitation
84181	Protein; Western Blot with interpretation and report, blood or other body fluid
84182	Protein; Western Blot, with interpretation and report, blood or other body fluid, immunological probe for band identification; each
85390	Fibrinolysin; screening
85576	Platelet; aggregation (in vitro), any agent
86255	Fluorescent antibody; screen
86256	Fluorescent antibody; titer
86320	Immunoelectrophoresis; serum, each specimen
86325	Immunoelectrophoresis; other fluids (e.g.urine) with concentration, each specimen
86327	Immunoelectrophoresis; crossed (2 dimensional assay)
86334	Immunofixation electrophoresis
87164	Dark field examination, any source (e.g. penile, vaginal, oral, skin); includes specimen collection
87207	Smear, primary source, with interpretation; special stain for inclusion bodies or intracellular parasites (e.g. malaria, kala azar, herpes)
88371	Protein analysis of tissue by Western Blot, with interpretation and report.
88372	Protein analysis of tissue by Western Blot, immunological probe for band identification, each
89060	Crystal identification by light microscopy with or without polarizing lens analysis, any body fluid (except urine)

100-4, 12, 80.3

Unusual Travel (CPT Code 99082)

B3-15026 In general, travel has been incorporated in the MPFSDB individual fees and is thus not separately payable. Carriers must pay separately for unusual travel (CPT code 99082) only when the physician submits documentation to demonstrate that the travel was very unusual.

100-4, 12, 90.3

Physicians' Services Performed in Ambulatory Surgical Centers (ASC)

B3-2265, B3-2265.4

See Chapter 14, for a description of services that may be billed by an ASC and services separately billed by physicians.

The ASC payment does not include the professional services of the physician. These are billed separately by the physician. Physicians' services include the services of anesthesiologists administering or supervising the administration of anesthesia to ASC patients and the patients' recovery from the anesthesia. The term physicians' services also includes any routine pre- or postoperative services, such as office visits, consultations, diagnostic tests, removal of stitches, changing of dressings, and other services which the individual physician usually performs.

The physician must enter the place of service code (POS) 24 on the claim to show that the procedure was performed in an ASC.

The carrier pays the "facility" fee from the MPFSDB to the physician. The facility fee is for services done in a facility other than the physician's office and is less then the nonfacility fee for services performed in the physician's office.

100-4, 12, 100

Teaching Physician Services

Definitions
For purposes of this section, the following definitions apply.

Resident -An individual who participates in an approved graduate medical education (GME) program or a physician who is not in an approved GME program but who is authorized to practice only in a hospital setting. The term includes interns and fellows in GME programs recognized as approved for purposes of direct GME payments made by the FI. Receiving a staff or faculty appointment or participating in a fellowship does not by itself alter the status of "resident". Additionally, this status remains unaffected regardless of whether a hospital includes the physician in its full time equivalency count of residents.

Student- An individual who participates in an accredited educational program (e.g., a medical school) that is not an approved GME program. A student is never considered to be an intern or a resident. Medicare does not pay for any service furnished by a student. See 100.1.1B for a discussion concerning E/M service documentation performed by students.

Teaching Physician -A physician (other than another resident) who involves residents in the care of his or her patients.

Direct Medical and Surgical Services -Services to individual beneficiaries that are either personally furnished by a physician or furnished by a resident under the supervision of a physician in a teaching hospital making the reasonable cost election for physician services furnished in teaching hospitals. All payments for such services are made by the FI for the hospital.

Teaching Hospital -A hospital engaged in an approved GME residency program in medicine, osteopathy, dentistry, or podiatry.

Teaching Setting -Any provider, hospital-based provider, or nonprovider setting in which Medicare payment for the services of residents is made by the FI under the direct graduate medical education payment methodology or freestanding SNF or HHA in which such payments are made on a reasonable cost basis.

Critical or Key Portion- That part (or parts) of a service that the teaching physician determines is (are) a critical or key portion(s). For purposes of this section, these terms are interchangeable.

Documentation- Notes recorded in the patient's medical records by a resident, and/or teaching physician or others as outlined in the specific situations below regarding the service furnished. Documentation may be dictated and typed or hand-written, or computer-generated and typed or handwritten. Documentation must be dated and include a legible signature or identity. Pursuant to 42 CFR 415.172 (b), documentation must identify, at a minimum, the service furnished, the participation of the teaching physician in providing the service, and whether the teaching physician was physically present. In the context of an electronic medical record, the term 'macro' means a command in a computer or dictation application that automatically generates predetermined text that is not edited by the user.

When using an electronic medical record, it is acceptable for the teaching physician to use a macro as the required personal documentation if the teaching physician adds it personally in a secured (password protected) system. In addition to the teaching physician's macro, either the resident or the teaching physician must provide customized information that is sufficient to support a medical necessity determination. The note in the electronic medical record must sufficiently describe the specific services furnished to the specific patient on the specific date. It is insufficient documentation if both the resident and the teaching physician use macros only.

Physically Present- The teaching physician is located in the same room (or partitioned or curtained area, if the room is subdivided to accommodate multiple patients) as the patient and/or performs a face-to-face service.

100-4, 12, 100.1.1

Evaluation and Management (E/M) Services

A. General Documentation Instructions and Common Scenarios

Evaluation and Management (E/M) Services -- For a given encounter, the selection of the appropriate level of E/M service should be determined according to the code definitions in the American Medical Association's Current Procedural Terminology (CPT) and any applicable documentation guidelines.

For purposes of payment, E/M services billed by teaching physicians require that they personally document at least the following:

- That they performed the service or were physically present during the key or critical portions of the service when performed by the resident; and
- The participation of the teaching physician in the management of the patient.

When assigning codes to services billed by teaching physicians, reviewers will combine the documentation of both the resident and the teaching physician.

Documentation by the resident of the presence and participation of the teaching physician is not sufficient to establish the presence and participation of the teaching physician.

On medical review, the combined entries into the medical record by the teaching physician and the resident constitute the documentation for the service and together must support the medical necessity of the service.

Following are four common scenarios for teaching physicians providing E/M services:

Scenario 1:

The teaching physician personally performs all the required elements of an E/M service without a resident. In this scenario the resident may or may not have performed the E/M service independently.

In the absence of a note by a resident, the teaching physician must document as he/she would document an E/M service in a nonteaching setting.

Where a resident has written notes, the teaching physician's note may reference the resident's note. The teaching physician must document that he/she performed the critical or key portion(s) of the service, and that he/she was directly involved in the management of the patient. For payment, the composite of the teaching physician's entry and the resident's entry together must support the medical necessity of the billed service and the level of the service billed by the teaching physician.

Scenario 2:

The resident performs the elements required for an E/M service in the presence of, or jointly with, the teaching physician and the resident documents the service. In this case, the teaching physician must document that he/she was present during the performance of the critical or key portion(s) of the service and that he/she was directly involved in the management of the patient. The teaching physician's note should reference the resident's note. For payment, the composite of the teaching physician's entry and the resident's entry together must support the medical necessity and the level of the service billed by the teaching physician.

Scenario 3:

The resident performs some or all of the required elements of the service in the absence of the teaching physician and documents his/her service. The teaching physician independently performs the critical or key portion(s) of the service with or without the resident present and, as appropriate, discusses the case with the resident. In this instance, the teaching physician must document that he/she personally saw the patient, personally performed critical or key portions of the service, and participated in the management of the patient. The teaching physician's note should reference the resident's note. For payment, the composite of the teaching physician's entry and the resident's entry together must support the medical necessity of the billed service and the level of the service billed by the teaching physician.

Scenario 4:

When a medical resident admits a patient to a hospital late at night and the teaching physician does not see the patient until later, including the next calendar day:

- The teaching physician must document that he/she personally saw the patient and participated in the management of the patient. The teaching physician may reference the resident's note in lieu of re-documenting the history of present illness, exam, medical decision-making, review of systems and/or past family/social history provided that the patient's condition has not changed, and the teaching physician agrees with the resident's note.
- The teaching physician's note must reflect changes in the patient's condition and clinical course that require that the resident's note be amended with further information to address the patient's condition and course at the time the patient is seen personally by the teaching physician.
- The teaching physician's bill must reflect the date of service he/she saw the patient and his/her personal work of obtaining a history, performing a physical, and participating in medical decision-making regardless of whether the combination of the teaching physician's and resident's documentation satisfies criteria for a higher level of service. For payment, the composite of the teaching physician's entry and the resident's entry together must support the medical necessity of the billed service and the level of the service billed by the teaching physician.

Following are examples of minimally acceptable documentation for each of these scenarios:

Scenario 1:

Admitting Note: "I performed a history and physical examination of the patient and discussed his management with the resident. I reviewed the resident's note and agree with the documented findings and plan of care."

Follow-up Visit: "Hospital Day #3. I saw and evaluated the patient. I agree with the findings and the plan of care as documented in the resident's note."

Follow-up Visit: "Hospital Day #5. I saw and examined the patient. I agree with the resident's note except the heart murmur is louder, so I will obtain an echo to evaluate."

(**NOTE:** In this scenario if there are no resident notes, the teaching physician must document as he/she would document an E/M service in a non-teaching setting.)

Scenario 2:

Initial or Follow-up Visit: "I was present with the resident during the history and exam. I discussed the case with the resident and agree with the findings and plan as documented in the resident's note."

Follow-up Visit: "I saw the patient with the resident and agree with the resident's findings and plan."

Scenarios 3 and 4:

Initial Visit: "I saw and evaluated the patient. I reviewed the resident's note and agree, except that picture is more consistent with pericarditis than myocardial ischemia. Will begin NSAIDs."

Initial or Follow-up Visit: "I saw and evaluated the patient. Discussed with resident and agree with resident's findings and plan as documented in the resident's note."

Follow-up Visit: "See resident's note for details. I saw and evaluated the patient and agree with the resident's finding and plans as written."

Follow-up Visit: "I saw and evaluated the patient. Agree with resident's note but lower extremities are weaker, now 3/5; MRI of L/S Spine today."

Following are examples of unacceptable documentation:

"Agree with above.", followed by legible countersignature or identity;

"Rounded, Reviewed, Agree.", followed by legible countersignature or identity;

"Discussed with resident. Agree.", followed by legible countersignature or identity;

"Seen and agree.", followed by legible countersignature or identity;

"Patient seen and evaluated.", followed by legible countersignature or identity; and

A legible countersignature or identity alone.

Such documentation is not acceptable, because the documentation does not make it possible to determine whether the teaching physician was present, evaluated the patient, and/or had any involvement with the plan of care.

B. E/M Service Documentation Provided By Students
Any contribution and participation of a student to the performance of a billable service (other than the review of systems and/or past family/social history which are not separately billable, but are taken as part of an E/M service) must be performed in the physical presence of a teaching physician or physical presence of a resident in a service meeting the requirements set forth in this section for teaching physician billing.

Students may document services in the medical record. However, the documentation of an E/M service by a student that may be referred to by the teaching physician is limited to documentation related to the review of systems and/or past family/social history. The teaching physician may not refer to a student's documentation of physical exam findings or medical decision making in his or her personal note. If the medical student documents E/M services, the teaching physician must verify and redocument the history of present illness as well as perform and redocument the physical exam and medical decision making activities of the service.

C. Exception for E/M Services Furnished in Certain Primary Care Centers
Teaching physicians providing E/M services with a GME program granted a primary care exception may bill Medicare for lower and mid-level E/M services provided by residents. For the E/M codes listed below, teaching physicians may submit claims for services furnished by residents in the absence of a teaching physician:

New Patient	Established Patient
99201	99211
99202	99212
99203	99213

Effective January 1, 2005, the following code is included under the primary care exception: HCPCS code G0402 (Initial preventive physical examination; face-to-face visit services limited to new beneficiary during the first 12 months of Medicare enrollment).

Effective January 1, 2011, the following codes are included under the primary care exception: HCPCS codes G0438 (Annual wellness visit, including personal preventive plan service, first visit) and G0439 (Annual wellness visit, including personal preventive plan service, subsequent visit).

If a service other than those listed above needs to be furnished, then the general teaching physician policy set forth in §100.1 applies. For this exception to apply, a center must attest in writing that all the following conditions are met for a particular residency program. Prior approval is not necessary, but centers exercising the primary care exception must maintain records demonstrating that they qualify for the exception.

The services must be furnished in a center located in the outpatient department of a hospital or another ambulatory care entity in which the time spent by residents in patient care activities is included in determining direct GME payments to a teaching hospital by the hospital's FI. This requirement is not met when the resident is assigned to a physician's office away from the center or makes home visits. In the case of a nonhospital entity, verify with the FI that the entity meets the requirements of a written agreement between the hospital and the entity set forth at 42 CFR 413.78(e)(3)(ii).

Under this exception, residents providing the billable patient care service without the physical presence of a teaching physician must have completed at least 6 months of a

GME approved residency program. Centers must maintain information under the provisions at 42 CFR 413.79(a)(6).

Teaching physicians submitting claims under this exception may not supervise more than four residents at any given time and must direct the care from such proximity as to constitute immediate availability. Teaching physicians may include residents with less than 6 months in a GME approved residency program in the mix of four residents under the teaching physician's supervision. However, the teaching physician must be physically present for the critical or key portions of services furnished by the residents with less than 6 months in a GME approved residency program. That is, the primary care exception does not apply in the case of residents with less than 6 months in a GME approved residency program.

Teaching physicians submitting claims under this exception must:

- Not have other responsibilities (including the supervision of other personnel) at the time the service was provided by the resident;
- Have the primary medical responsibility for patients cared for by the residents;
- Ensure that the care provided was reasonable and necessary;
- Review the care provided by the resident during or immediately after each visit. This must include a review of the patient's medical history, the resident's findings on physical examination, the patient's diagnosis, and treatment plan (i.e., record of tests and therapies); and
- Document the extent of his/her own participation in the review and direction of the services furnished to each patient.

Patients under this exception should consider the center to be their primary location for health care services. The residents must be expected to generally provide care to the same group of established patients during their residency training. The types of services furnished by residents under this exception include:

- Acute care for undifferentiated problems or chronic care for ongoing conditions including chronic mental illness;
- Coordination of care furnished by other physicians and providers; and,
- Comprehensive care not limited by organ system or diagnosis.

Residency programs most likely qualifying for this exception include family practice, general internal medicine, geriatric medicine, pediatrics, and obstetrics/gynecology.

Certain GME programs in psychiatry may qualify in special situations such as when the program furnishes comprehensive care for chronically mentally ill patients. These would be centers in which the range of services the residents are trained to furnish, and actually do furnish, include comprehensive medical care as well as psychiatric care. For example, antibiotics are being prescribed as well as psychotropic drugs.

100-4, 12, 110.2

Outpatient Mental Health Limitation

B3-4112, B3-2472.4 The carrier must apply the outpatient mental health limitation to all covered mental health therapeutic services furnished by PAs. The reduction is 62.5 percent applied after the 85 percent.

Refer to 210 below for a complete discussion of the outpatient mental health limitation.

100-4, 12, 140

Certified Registered Nurse Anesthetist (CRNA) Services

B3-16003, B3-16003 A, B3-3040.4, B3-4172 Section 9320 of OBRA 1986 provides for payment under a fee schedule to certified registered nurse anesthetists (CRNAs) and anesthesia assistants (AAs). CRNAs and AAs may bill Medicare directly for their services or have payment made to an employer or an entity under which they have a contract. This could be a hospital, physician or ASC. This provision is effective for services rendered on or after January 1, 1989. Anesthesia services are subject to the usual Part B coinsurance and deductible and when furnished on or after January 1, 1992 by a qualified nurse anesthetist and are paid at the lesser of the actual charge, the physician fee schedule, or the CRNA fee schedule. Payment for CRNA services is made only on an assignment basis.

100-4, 12, 140.2

Entity or Individual to Whom CRNA Fee Schedule is Payable

B3-16003.C, B3-4830.A

Payment for the services of a CRNA may be made to the CRNA who furnished the anesthesia services or to a hospital, physician, group practice, or ASC with which the CRNA has an employment or contractual relationship.

100-4, 12, 140.3.2

Anesthesia Time and Calculation of Anesthesia Time Units

B3-15018.G Anesthesia time means the time during which a CRNA is present with the patient. It starts when the CRNA begins to prepare the patient for anesthesia services in the operating room or an equivalent area and ends when the CRNA is no longer furnishing anesthesia services to the patient, that is, when the patient may be placed safely under postoperative care. Anesthesia time is a continuous time period from the start of anesthesia to the end of an anesthesia service. In counting anesthesia time for services furnished on or after January 1, 2000, the CRNA can add blocks of time around an interruption in anesthesia time as long as the CRNA is furnishing continuous anesthesia care within the time periods around the interruption.

100-4, 12, 150

Clinical Social Worker (CSW) Services

B3-2152, B3-17000 See Medicare Benefit Policy Manual, Chapter 15, for coverage requirements.

Assignment of benefits is required.

Payment is at 75 percent of the physician fee schedule.

CSWs are identified on the provider file by specialty code 80 and provider type 56.

Medicare applies the outpatient mental health limitation to all covered therapeutic services furnished by qualified CSWs. Refer to 210, below, for a discussion of the outpatient mental health limitation. The modifier "AJ" must be applied on CSN services.

100-4, 12, 160

Independent Psychologist Services

B3-2150, B3-2070.2 See the Medicare Benefit Policy Manual, Chapter 15, for coverage requirements.

There are a number of types of psychologists. Educational psychologists engage in identifying and treating education-related issues. In contrast, counseling psychologists provide services that include a broader realm including phobias, familial issues, etc.

Psychometrists are psychologists who have been trained to administer and interpret tests.

However, clinical psychologists are defined as a provider of diagnostic and therapeutic services. Because of the differences in services provided, services provided by psychologists who do not provide clinical services are subject to different billing guidelines. One service often provided by nonclinical psychologist is diagnostic testing.

NOTE:Diagnostic psychological testing services performed by persons who meet these requirements are covered as other diagnostic tests. When, however, the psychologist is not practicing independently, but is on the staff of an institution, agency, or clinic, that entity bills for the diagnostic services.

Expenses for such testing are not subject to the payment limitation on treatment for mental, psychoneurotic, and personality disorders. Independent psychologists are not required by law to accept assignment when performing psychological tests. However, regardless of whether the psychologist accepts assignment, he or she must report on the claim form the name and address of the physician who ordered the test.

100-4, 12, 160.1

Payment

Diagnostic testing services are not subject to the outpatient mental health limitation. Refer to §210, below, for a discussion of the outpatient mental health limitation.

The diagnostic testing services performed by a psychologist (who is not a clinical psychologist) practicing independently of an institution, agency, or physician's office are covered as other diagnostic tests if a physician orders such testing. Medicare covers this type of testing as an outpatient service if furnished by any psychologist who is licensed or certified to practice psychology in the State or jurisdiction where he or she is furnishing services or, if the jurisdiction does not issue licenses, if provided by any practicing psychologist. (It is CMS' understanding that all States, the District of Columbia, and Puerto Ricolicense psychologists, but that some trust territories do not. Examples of psychologists, other than clinical psychologists, whose services are covered under this provision include, but are not limited to, educational psychologists and counseling psychologists.)

To determine whether the diagnostic psychological testing services of a particular independent psychologist are covered under Part B in States which have statutory licensure or certification, carriers must secure from the appropriate State agency a current listing of psychologists holding the required credentials. In States or territories which lack statutory licensing and certification, carriers must check individual qualifications as claims are submitted. Possible reference sources are the national directory of membership of the American Psychological Association, which provides data about the educational background of individuals and indicates which members are board-certified, and records and directories of the State or territorial psychological association. If qualification is dependent on a doctoral degree from a currently accredited program, carriers must verify the date of accreditation of the school involved, since such accreditation is not retroactive. If the reference sources listed above do not provide enough information (e.g., the psychologist is not a member of the association), carriers must contact the psychologist personally for the required information. Carriers may wish to maintain a continuing list of psychologists whose qualifications have been verified.

Medicare excludes expenses for diagnostic testing from the payment limitation on treatment for mental/psychoneurotic/personality disorders.

Carriers must identify the independent psychologist's choice whether or not to accept assignment when performing psychological tests.

Carriers must accept an independent psychologist claim only if the psychologist reports the name/UPIN of the physician who ordered a test.

Carriers pay nonparticipating independent psychologists at 95 percent of the physician fee schedule allowed amount. Carriers pay participating independent psychologists at 100 percent of the physician fee schedule allowed amount.

Independent psychologists are identified on the provider file by specialty code 62 and provider type 35.

100-4, 12, 170

Clinical Psychologist Services

B3-2150 See Medicare Benefit Policy Manual, Chapter 15, for general coverage requirements.

Direct payment may be made under Part B for professional services. However, services furnished incident to the professional services of CPs to hospital patients remain bundled.

Therefore, payment must continue to be made to the hospital (by the FI) for such "incident to" services.

100-4, 12, 170.1

Payment

B3-2150, B3-17001.1 All covered therapeutic services furnished by qualified CPs are subject to the outpatient mental health services limitation (i.e., only 62 1/2 percent of expenses for these services are considered incurred expenses for Medicare purposes). The limitation does not apply to diagnostic services. Refer to 210 below for a discussion of the outpatient mental health limitation.

Payment for the services of CPs is made on the basis of a fee schedule or the actual charge, whichever is less, and only on the basis of assignment.

CPs are identified by specialty code 68 and provider type 27. Modifier "AH" is required on CP services.

100-4, 12, 180

Care Plan Oversight Services

The Medicare Benefit Policy Manual, Chapter 15, contains requirements for coverage for medical and other health services including those of physicians and non-physician practitioners.

Care plan oversight (CPO) is the physician supervision of a patient receiving complex and/or multidisciplinary care as part of Medicare-covered services provided by a participating home health agency or Medicare approved hospice.

CPO services require complex or multidisciplinary care modalities involving:

- Regular physician development and/or revision of care plans;
- Review of subsequent reports of patient status;
- Review of related laboratory and other studies;
- Communication with other health professionals not employed in the same practice who are involved in the patient's care;
- Integration of new information into the medical treatment plan; and/or
- Adjustment of medical therapy.

The CPO services require recurrent physician supervision of a patient involving 30 or more minutes of the physician's time per month. Services not countable toward the 30 minutes threshold that must be provided in order to bill for CPO include, but are not limited to:

- Time associated with discussions with the patient, his or her family or friends to adjust medication or treatment;
- Time spent by staff getting or filing charts;
- Travel time; and/or
- Physician's time spent telephoning prescriptions into the pharmacist unless the telephone conversation involves discussions of pharmaceutical therapies.

Implicit in the concept of CPO is the expectation that the physician has coordinated an aspect of the patient's care with the home health agency or hospice during the month for which CPO services were billed. The physician who bills for CPO must be the same physician who signs the plan of care.

Nurse practitioners, physician assistants, and clinical nurse specialists, practicing within the scope of State law, may bill for care plan oversight. These non-physician practitioners must have been providing ongoing care for the beneficiary through evaluation and management services. These non-physician practitioners may not bill for CPO if they have been involved only with the delivery of the Medicare-covered home health or hospice service.

A. Home Health CPO

Non-physician practitioners can perform CPO only if the physician signing the plan of care provides regular ongoing care under the same plan of care as does the NPP billing for CPO and either:

- The physician and NPP are part of the same group practice; or
- If the NPP is a nurse practitioner or clinical nurse specialist, the physician signing the plan of care also has a collaborative agreement with the NPP; or
- If the NPP is a physician assistant, the physician signing the plan of care is also the physician who provides general supervision of physician assistant services for the practice.

Billing may be made for care plan oversight services furnished by an NPP when:

- The NPP providing the care plan oversight has seen and examined the patient;
- The NPP providing care plan oversight is not functioning as a consultant whose participation is limited to a single medical condition rather than multidisciplinary coordination of care; and
- The NPP providing care plan oversight integrates his or her care with that of the physician who signed the plan of care.

NPPs may not certify the beneficiary for home health care.

B. Hospice CPO

The attending physician or nurse practitioner (who has been designated as the attending physician) may bill for hospice CPO when they are acting as an "attending physician".

An "attending physician" is one who has been identified by the individual, at the time he/she elects hospice coverage, as having the most significant role in the determination and delivery of their medical care. They are not employed nor paid by the hospice. The care plan oversight services are billed using Form CMS-1500 or electronic equivalent.

For additional information on hospice CPO, see Chapter 11, 40.1.3.1 of this manual.

100-4, 12, 180.1

Care Plan Oversight Billing Requirements

A. Codes for Which Separate Payment May Be Made

Effective January 1, 1995, separate payment may be made for CPO oversight services for 30 minutes or more if the requirements specified in the Medicare Benefits Policy Manual, Chapter 15 are met.

Providers billing for CPO must submit the claim with no other services billed on that claim and may bill only after the end of the month in which the CPO services were rendered. CPO services may not be billed across calendar months and should be submitted (and paid) only for one unit of service.

Physicians may bill and be paid separately for CPO services only if all the criteria in the Medicare Benefit Policy Manual, Chapter 15 are met.

B. Physician Certification and Recertification of Home Health Plans of Care

Effective 2001, two new HCPCS codes for the certification and recertification and development of plans of care for Medicare-covered home health services were created.

See the Medicare General Information, Eligibility, and Entitlement Manual, Pub. 100-01, Chapter 4, "Physician Certification and Recertification of Services," 10-60, and the Medicare Benefit Policy Manual, Pub. 100-02, Chapter 7, "Home Health Services", 30.

The home health agency certification code can be billed only when the patient has not received Medicare-covered home health services for at least 60 days. The home health agency recertification code is used after a patient has received services for at least 60 days (or one certification period) when the physician signs the certification after the initial certification period. The home health agency recertification code will be reported only once every 60 days, except in the rare situation when the patient starts a new episode before 60 days elapses and requires a new plan of care to start a new episode.

C. Provider Number of Home Health Agency (HHA) or Hospice

For claims for CPO submitted on or after January 1, 1997, physicians must enter on the Medicare claim form the 6-character Medicare provider number of the HHA or hospice providing Medicare-covered services to the beneficiary for the period during which CPO services was furnished and for which the physician signed the plan of care. Physicians are responsible for obtaining the HHA or hospice Medicare provider numbers.

Additionally, physicians should provide their UPIN to the HHA or hospice furnishing services to their patient.

NOTE: There is currently no place on the HIPAA standard ASC X12N 837 professional format to specifically include the HHA or hospice provider number required for a care plan oversight claim. For this reason, the requirement to include the HHA or hospice provider number on a care plan oversight claim is temporarily waived until a new version of this electronic standard format is adopted under HIPAA and includes a place to provide the HHA and hospice provider numbers for care plan oversight claims.

100-4, 12, 190.3

List of Medicare Telehealth Services

The use of a telecommunications system may substitute for an in-person encounter for professional consultations, office visits, office psychiatry services, and a limited number of other physician fee schedule (PFS) services. The various services and corresponding current procedure terminology (CPT) or Healthcare Common Procedure Coding System (HCPCS) codes are listed below.

- Consultations (CPT codes 99241 - 99275) - Effective October 1, 2001–December 31, 2005;
- Consultations (CPT codes 99241 - 99255) - Effective January 1, 2006–December 31, 2009;
- Initial inpatient telehealth consultations (HCPCS codes G0425–G0427) - Effective January 1, 2010;
- Follow-up inpatient telehealth consultations (HCPCS codes G0406, G0407, and G0408) - Effective January 1, 2009;
- Office or other outpatient visits (CPT codes 99201 - 99215);
- Subsequent hospital care services, with the limitation of one telehealth visit every 3 days (CPT codes 99231, 99232, and 99233)–Effective January 1, 2011;
- Subsequent nursing facility care services, with the limitation of one telehealth visit every 30 days (CPT codes 99307, 99308, 99309, and 99310)–Effective January 1, 2011;
- Pharmacologic management (CPT code 90862);
- Individual psychotherapy (CPT codes 90804 - 90809); Psychiatric diagnostic interview examination (CPT code 90801)–Effective March 1, 2003;
- Neurobehavioral status exam (CPT code 96116) - Effective January 1, 2008;
- End Stage Renal Disease (ESRD) related services (HCPCS codes G0308, G0309, G0311, G0312, G0314, G0315, G0317, and G0318)–Effective January 1, 2005–December 31, 2008;
- End Stage Renal Disease (ESRD) related services (CPT codes 90951, 90952, 90954, 90955, 90957, 90958, 90960, and 90961)–Effective January 1, 2009;
- Individual and group medical nutrition therapy (HCPCS codes G0270, 97802, 97803, and 97804)–Individual effective January 1, 2006; group effective January 1, 2011;
- Individual and group health and behavior assessment and intervention (CPT codes 96150–96154)–Individual effective January 1, 2010; group effective January 1, 2011.
- Individual and group kidney disease education (KDE) services (HCPCS codes G0420 and G0421)–Effective January 1, 2011; and
- Individual and group diabetes self-management training (DSMT) services, with a minimum of 1 hour of in-person instruction to be furnished in the initial year training period to ensure effective injection training (HCPCS codes G0108 and G0109) - Effective January 1, 2011.

NOTE: Beginning January 1, 2010, CMS eliminated the use of all consultation codes, except for inpatient telehealth consultation G-codes. CMS no longer recognizes office/outpatient or inpatient consultation CPT codes for payment of office/outpatient or inpatient visits. Instead, physicians and practitioners are instructed to bill a new or established patient office/outpatient visit CPT code or appropriate hospital or nursing facility care code, as appropriate to the particular patient, for all office/outpatient or inpatient visits.

100-4, 12, 190.7

Contractor Editing of Telehealth Claims

Medicare telehealth services (as listed in section 190.3) are billed with either the "GT" or "GQ" modifier. The contractor shall approve covered telehealth services if the physician or practitioner is licensed under State law to provide the service. Contractors must familiarize themselves with licensure provisions of States for which they process claims and disallow telehealth services furnished by physicians or practitioners who are not authorized to furnish the applicable telehealth service under State law. For example, if a nurse practitioner is not licensed to provide individual psychotherapy under State law, he or she would not be permitted to receive payment for individual psychotherapy under Medicare. The contractor shall install edits to ensure that only properly licensed physicians and practitioners are paid for covered telehealth services.

If a contractor receives claims for professional telehealth services coded with the "GQ" modifier (representing "via asynchronous telecommunications system"), it shall approve/pay for these services only if the physician or practitioner is affiliated with a Federal telemedicine demonstration conducted in Alaska or Hawaii. The contractor may require the physician or practitioner at the distant site to document his or her participation in a Federal telemedicine demonstration program conducted in Alaska or Hawaii prior to paying for telehealth services provided via asynchronous, store and forward technologies.

If a contractor denies telehealth services because the physician or practitioner may not bill for them, the contractor uses MSN message 21.18: "This item or service is not covered when performed or ordered by this practitioner." The contractor uses remittance advice message 52 when denying the claim based upon MSN message 21.18.

If a service is billed with one of the telehealth modifiers and the procedure code is not designated as a covered telehealth service, the contractor denies the service using MSN message 9.4: "This item or service was denied because information required to make payment was incorrect." The remittance advice message depends on what is incorrect, e.g., B18 if procedure code or modifier is incorrect, 125 for submission billing errors, 4-12 for difference inconsistencies. The contractor uses B18 as the explanation for the denial of the claim.

The only claims from institutional facilities that FIs shall pay for telehealth services at the distant site, except for MNT services, are for physician or practitioner services when the distant site is located in a CAH that has elected Method II, and the physician or practitioner has reassigned his/her benefits to the CAH. The CAH bills its regular FI for the professional services provided at the distant site via a telecommunications system, in any of the revenue codes 096x, 097x or 098x. All requirements for billing distant site telehealth services apply.

Claims from hospitals or CAHs for MNT services are submitted to the hospital's or CAH's regular FI. Payment is based on the non-facility amount on the Medicare Physician Fee Schedule for the particular HCPCS codes.

100-4, 12, 200

Allergy Testing and Immunotherapy

B3-15050

A. Allergy Testing

The MPFSDB fee amounts for allergy testing services billed under codes 95004-95078 are established for single tests. Therefore, the number of tests must be shown on the claim.

EXAMPLE: If a physician performs 25 percutaneous tests (scratch, puncture, or prick) with allergenic extract, the physician must bill code 95004 and specify 25 in the units field of Form CMS-1500 (paper claims or electronic format). To compute payment, the Medicare carrier multiplies the payment for one test (i.e., the payment listed in the fee schedule) by the quantity listed in the units field.

B. Allergy Immunotherapy

For services rendered on or after January 1, 1995, all antigen/allergy immunotherapy services are paid for under the Medicare physician fee schedule. Prior to that date, only the antigen injection services, i.e., only codes 95115 and 95117, were paid for under the fee schedule. Codes representing antigens and their preparation and single codes representing both the antigens and their injection were paid for under the Medicare reasonable charge system. A legislative change brought all of these services under the fee schedule at the beginning of 1995 and the following policies are effective as of January 1, 1995:

1. CPT codes 95120 through 95134 are not valid for Medicare. Codes 95120 through 95134 represent complete services, i.e., services that include both the injection service as well as the antigen and its preparation.
2. Separate coding for injection only codes (i.e., codes 95115 and 95117) and/or the codes representing antigens and their preparation (i.e., codes 95144 through 95170) must be used.

   If both services are provided both codes are billed.

   This includes allergists who provide both services through the use of treatment boards.
3. If a physician bills both an injection code plus either codes 95165 or 95144, carriers pay the appropriate injection code (i.e., code 95115 or code 95117) plus the code 95165 rate. When a provider bills for codes 95115 or 95117 plus code 95144, carriers change 95144 to 95165 and pay accordingly. Code 95144 (single dose vials of antigen) should be billed only if the physician providing the antigen is providing it to be injected by some other entity. Single dose vials, which should be used only as a means of insuring proper dosage amounts for injections, are more costly than multiple dose vials (i.e., code 95165) and therefore their payment rate is higher. Allergists who prepare antigens are assumed to be able to administer proper doses from the less costly multiple dose vials. Thus, regardless of whether they use or bill for single or multiple dose vials at the same time that they are billing for an injection service, they are paid at the multiple dose vial rate.
4. The fee schedule amounts for the antigen codes (95144 through 95170) are for a single dose. When billing those codes, physicians are to specify the number of doses provided. When making payment, carriers multiply the fee schedule amount by the number of doses specified in the units field.
5. If a patient's doses are adjusted, e.g., because of patient reaction, and the antigen provided is actually more or fewer doses than originally anticipated, the physician is to make no change in the number of doses for which he or she bills. The number of doses anticipated at the time of the antigen preparation is the number of doses to be billed. This is consistent with the notes on page 30 of the Spring 1994 issue of the American Medical Association's CPT Assistant. Those notes indicate that the antigen codes mean that the physician is to identify the number of doses "prospectively planned to be provided." The physician is to "identify the number of doses scheduled when the vial is provided." This means that in cases where the patient actually gets more doses than originally anticipated (because dose amounts were decreased during treatment) and in cases where the patient gets fewer doses (because dose amounts were increased), no change is to be made in the billing. In the first case, carriers are not to pay more because the number of doses provided in the original vial(s) increased. In the second case, carriers are not to seek recoupment (if carriers have already made payment) because the number of doses is less than originally planned. This is the case for both venom and nonvenom antigen codes.
6. Venom Doses and Catch-Up Billing - Venom doses are prepared in separate vials and not mixed together - except in the case of the three vespid mix (white and yellow hornets and yellow jackets). A dose of code 95146 (the two-venom code) means getting some of two venoms. Similarly, a dose of code 95147 means getting some of three venoms; a dose of code 95148 means getting some of four venoms; and a dose of 95149 means getting some of five venoms. Some amount of each of the venoms must be provided. Questions arise when the administration of these venoms does not remain synchronized because of dosage adjustments due to patient reaction. For example, a physician prepares ten doses of code 95148 (the four venom code) in two vials - one containing 10 doses of three vespid mix and

another containing 10 doses of wasp venom. Because of dose adjustment, the three vespid mix doses last longer, i.e., they last for 15 doses. Consequently, questions arise regarding the amount of "replacement" wasp venom antigen that should be prepared and how it should be billed. Medicare pricing amounts have savings built into the use of the higher venom codes. Therefore, if a patient is in two venom, three venom, four venom or five venom therapy, the carrier objective is to pay at the highest venom level possible. This means that, to the greatest extent possible, code 95146 is to be billed for a patient in two venom therapy, code 95147 is to be billed for a patient in three venom therapy, code 95148 is to be billed for a patient in four venom therapy, and code 95149 is to be billed for a patient in five venom therapy. Thus, physicians are to be instructed that the venom antigen preparation, after dose adjustment, must be done in a manner that, as soon as possible, synchronizes the preparation back to the highest venom code possible. In the above example, the physician should prepare and bill for only 5 doses of "replacement" wasp venom - billing five doses of code 95145 (the one venom code). This will permit the physician to get back to preparing the four venoms at one time and therefore billing the doses of the "cheaper" four venom code. Use of a code below the venom treatment number for the particular patient should occur only for the purpose of "catching up."

7. Code 95165 Doses. - Code 95165 represents preparation of vials of non-venom antigens. As in the case of venoms, some non-venom antigens cannot be mixed together, i.e., they must be prepared in separate vials. An example of this is mold and pollen. Therefore, some patients will be injected at one time from one vial - containing in one mixture all of the appropriate antigens - while other patients will be injected at one time from more than one vial. In establishing the practice expense component for mixing a multidose vial of antigens, we observed that the most common practice was to prepare a 10 cc vial; we also observed that the most common use was to remove aliquots with a volume of 1 cc. Our PE computations were based on those facts. Therefore, a physician's removing 10 1cc aliquot doses captures the entire PE component for the service.

   This does not mean that the physician must remove 1 cc aliquot doses from a multidose vial. It means that the practice expenses payable for the preparation of a 10cc vial remain the same irrespective of the size or number of aliquots removed from the vial. Therefore, a physician may not bill this vial preparation code for more than 10 doses per vial; paying more than 10 doses per multidose vial would significantly overpay the practice expense component attributable to this service. (Note that this code does not include the injection of antigen(s); injection of antigen(s) is separately billable.) When a multidose vial contains less than 10cc, physicians should bill Medicare for the number of 1 cc aliquots that may be removed from the vial. That is, a physician may bill Medicare up to a maximum of 10 doses per multidose vial, but should bill Medicare for fewer than 10 doses per vial when there is less than 10cc in the vial.

   If it is medically necessary, physicians may bill Medicare for preparation of more than one multidose vial.

   EXAMPLES:

   (1) If a 10cc multidose vial is filled to 6cc with antigen, the physician may bill Medicare for 6 doses since six 1cc aliquots may be removed from the vial.

   (2) If a 5cc multidose vial is filled completely, the physician may bill Medicare for 5 doses for this vial.

   (3) If a physician removes ¬¾ cc aliquots from a 10cc multidose vial for a total of 20 doses from one vial, he/she may only bill Medicare for 10 doses. Billing for more than 10 doses would mean that Medicare is overpaying for the practice expense of making the vial.

   (4) If a physician prepares two 10cc multidose vials, he/she may bill Medicare for 20 doses. However, he/she may remove aliquots of any amount from those vials. For example, the physician may remove ¬¾ aliquots from one vial, and 1cc aliquots from the other vial, but may bill no more than a total of 20 doses.

   (5) If a physician prepares a 20cc multidose vial, he/she may bill Medicare for 20 doses, since the practice expense is calculated based on the physician's removing 1cc aliquots from a vial. If a physician removes 2cc aliquots from this vial, thus getting only 10 doses, he/she may nonetheless bill Medicare for 20 doses because the PE for 20 doses reflects the actual practice expense of preparing the vial.

   (6) If a physician prepares a 5cc multidose vial, he may bill Medicare for 5 doses, based on the way that the practice expense component is calculated. However, if the physician removes ten ¬¾ cc aliquots from the vial, he/she may still bill only 5 doses because the practice expense of preparing the vial is the same, without regard to the number of additional doses that are removed from the vial.

C. Allergy Shots and Visit Services on the Same Day

At the outset of the physician fee schedule, the question was posed as to whether visits should be billed on the same day as an allergy injection (CPT codes 95115-95117), since these codes have status indicators of A rather than T. Visits should not be billed with allergy injection services 95115 or 95117 unless the visit represents another separately identifiable service. This language parallels CPT editorial language that accompanies the allergen immunotherapy codes, which include codes 9515 and 95117. Prior to January 1, 1995, you appeared to be enforcing this policy through three (3) different means:

- Advising physician to use modifier 25 with the visit service;
- Denying payment for the visit unless documentation has been provided; and
- Paying for both the visit and the allergy shot if both are billed for.

For services rendered on or after January 1, 1995, you are to enforce the requirement that visits not be billed and paid for on the same day as an allergy injection through the following means. Effective for services rendered on or after that date, the global surgery policies will apply to all codes in the allergen immunotherapy series, including the allergy shot codes 95115 and 95117. To accomplish this, CMS changed the global surgery indicator for allergen immunotherapy codes from XXX, which meant that the global surgery concept did not apply to those codes, to 000, which means that the global surgery concept applies, but that there are no days in the postoperative global period.

Now that the global surgery policies apply to these services, you are to rely on the use of modifier 25 as the only means through which you can make payment for visit services provided on the same day as allergen immunotherapy services. In order for a physician to receive payment for a visit service provided on the same day that the physician also provides a service in the allergen immunotherapy series (i.e., any service in the series from 95115 through 95199), the physician is to bill a modifier 25 with the visit code, indicating that the patient's condition required a significant, separately identifiable visit service above and beyond the allergen immunotherapy service provided.

D. Reasonable Supply of Antigens

See CMS Manual System, Internet Only Manual, Medicare Benefits Policy Manual, CMS Pub. 100-02 Chapter 15, section 50.4.4, regarding the coverage of antigens, including what constitutes a reasonable supply of antige

100-4, 12, 210

Outpatient Mental Health Limitation

B3-2470

Regardless of the actual expenses a beneficiary incurs for treatment of mental, psychoneurotic, and personality disorders while the beneficiary is not an inpatient of a hospital at the time such expenses are incurred, the amount of those expenses that may be recognized for Part B deductible and payment purposes is limited to 62.5 percent of the Medicare allowed amount for those services. This limitation is called the outpatient mental health treatment limitation. Expenses for diagnostic services (e.g., psychiatric testing and evaluation to diagnose the patient's illness) are not subject to this limitation.

This limitation applies only to therapeutic services and to services performed to evaluate the progress of a course of treatment for a diagnosed condition.

100-4, 12, 230

Primary Care Incentive Payment Program (PCIP)

Section 5501(a) of the Affordable Care Act revises Section 1833 of the Social Security Act (the Act) by adding a new paragraph, (x), "Incentive Payments for Primary Care Services." Section 1833(x) of the Act states that in the case of primary care services furnished on or after January 1, 2011, and before January 1, 2016, there shall be a 10 percent incentive payment for such services under Part B when furnished by a primary care practitioner.

Information regarding Primary Care Incentive Payment Program (PCIP) payments made to critical access hospitals (CAHs) paid under the optional method can be found in Pub. 100-04, Chapter 4, §250.12 of this manual.

100-4, 12, 230.1

Definition of Primary Care Practitioners and Primary Care Services

Primary care practitioners are defined as:

1. A physician who has a primary specialty designation of family medicine, internal medicine, geriatric medicine, or pediatric medicine for whom primary care services accounted for at least 60 percent of the allowed charges under Part B for the practitioner in a prior period as determined appropriate by the Secretary; or
2. A nurse practitioner, clinical nurse specialist, or physician assistant for whom primary care services accounted for at least 60 percent of the allowed charges under Part B for the practitioner in a prior period as determined appropriate by the Secretary.

Primary care services are defined as HCPCS Codes:

1. 99201 through 99215 for new and established patient office or outpatient evaluation and management (E/M) visits;
2. 99304 through 99340 for initial, subsequent, discharge, and other nursing facility E/M services; new and established patient domiciliary, rest home or custodial care E/M services; and domiciliary, rest home or home care plan oversight services; and
3. 99341 through 99350 for new and established patient home E/M visits.

Practitioner Identification

Eligible practitioners will be identified on claims by the National Provider Identifier (NPI) number of the rendering practitioner. If the claim is submitted by a practitioner's group practice, the rendering practitioner's NPI must be included on the line-item for the primary care service and reflect an eligible HCPCS as identified. In order to be eligible for the PCIP, physician assistants, clinical nurse specialists, and nurse practitioners must be billing for their services under their own NPI and not furnishing services incident to physicians' services. Regardless of the specialty area in which they may be practicing, the specific nonphysician practitioners are eligible for the PCIP based on their profession and historical percentage of allowed charges as primary care services that equals or exceeds the 60 percent threshold.

Beginning in calendar year (CY) 2011, primary care practitioners will be identified based on their primary specialty of enrollment in Medicare and percentage of allowed charges for primary care services that equals or exceeds the 60 percent threshold from Medicare claims data 2 years prior to the bonus payment year.

Eligible practitioners for PCIP payments in a given calendar year (CY) will be listed by eligible NPI in the Primary Care Incentive Payment Program Eligibility File, available after January 31, of the payment year on their Medicare contractor's website. Practitioners should contact their contractor with any questions regarding their eligibility for the PCIP.

100-4, 12, 230.2

Coordination with Other Payments

Section 5501(a)(3) of the Affordable Care Act provides payment under the PCIP as an additional payment amount for specified primary care services without regard to any additional payment for the service under Section 1833(m) of the Act. Therefore, an eligible primary care physician furnishing a primary care service in a health professional shortage area (HPSA) may receive both a HPSA physician bonus payment (as described in the Medicare Claims Processing Manual, Pub. 100-04, Chapter 12, §90.4) under the HPSA physician bonus program and a PCIP incentive payment under the new program beginning in CY 2011.

100-4, 12, 230.3

Claims Processing and Payment

A. General Overview

Incentive payments will be made on a quarterly basis and shall be equal to 10 percent of the amount paid for such services under the Medicare Physician Fee Schedule (PFS) for those services furnished during the bonus payment year. For information on PCIP payments to CAHs paid under the optional method, see the Medicare Claims Processing Manual, Pub. 100-04, Chapter 4, §250.12.

On an annual basis Medicare contractors shall receive a Primary Care Incentive Payment Program Eligibility File that they shall post to their website. The file will list the NPIs of all practitioners who are eligible to receive PCIP payments for the upcoming CY.

B. Method of Payment

- Calculate and pay qualifying primary care practitioners an additional 10 percent incentive payment;
- Calculate the payment based on the amount actually paid for the services, not the Medicare approved amounts;
- Combine the PCIP incentive payments, when appropriate, with other incentive payments, including the HPSA physician bonus payment, and the HPSA Surgical Incentive Payment Program (HSIP) payment;
- Provide a special remittance form that is forwarded with the incentive payment so that physicians and practitioners can identify which type of incentive payment (HPSA physician and/or PCIP) was paid for which services.
- Practitioners should contact their contractor with any questions regarding PCIP payments.

C. Changes for Contractor Systems

The Medicare Carrier System, (MCS), Common Working File (CWF) and the National Claims History (NCH) shall be modified to accept a new PCIP indicator on the claim line. Once the type of incentive payment has been identified by the shared systems, the shared system shall modify their systems to set the indicator on the claim line as follows:

1 = HPSA;

2 = PSA;

3 = HPSA and PSA;

4 = HSIP;

5 = HPSA and HSIP;

6 = PCIP;

7 = HPSA and PCIP; and

Space = Not Applicable.

The contractor shared system shall send the HIGLAS 810 invoice for incentive payment invoices, including the new PCIP payment. The contractor shall also combine the provider's HPSA physician bonus, physician scarcity (PSA) bonus (if it should become available at a later date), HSIP payment and/or PCIP payment invoice per provider. The contractor shall receive the HIGLAS 835 payment file from HIGLAS showing a single incentive payment per provider

100-4, 13, 10

ICD-9-CM Coding for Diagnostic Tests

The ICD-9-CM Coding Guidelines for Outpatient Services (hospital-based and physician office) have instructed physicians to report diagnoses based on test results. Instructions and examples for coding specialists, contractors, physicians, hospitals, and other health care providers to use in determining the use of ICD-9-CM codes for coding diagnostic test results is found in Chapter 23.

100-4, 13, 30

Computerized Axial Tomography (CT) Procedures

Carriers do not reduce or deny payment for medically necessary multiple CT scans of different areas of the body that are performed on the same day.

The TC RVUs for CT procedures that specify "with contrast" include payment for high osmolar contrast media. When separate payment is made for low osmolar contrast media under the conditions set forth in 30.1.1, reduce payment for the contrast media as set forth in 30.1.2.

100-4, 13, 40

Magnetic Resonance Imaging (MRI) Procedures

Effective September 28, 2009

The Centers for Medicare & Medicaid Services (CMS) finds that the non-coverage of magnetic resonance imaging (MRI) for blood flow determination is no longer supported by the available evidence. CMS is removing the phrase "blood flow measurement" and local Medicare contractors will have the discretion to cover (or not cover).

Consult Publication (Pub.) 100-03, National Coverage Determinations (NCD) Manual, chapter 1, section 220.2, for specific coverage and non-coverage indications associated with MRI and MRA (Magnetic Resonance Angiography).

Prior to January 1, 2007

Carriers do not make additional payments for three or more MRI sequences. The relative value units (RVUs) reflect payment levels for two sequences.

The technical component (TC) RVUs for MRI procedures that specify "with contrast" include payment for paramagnetic contrast media. Carriers do not make separate payment under code A4647.

A diagnostic technique has been developed under which an MRI of the brain or spine is first performed without contrast material, then another MRI is performed with a standard (0.1mmol/kg) dose of contrast material and, based on the need to achieve a better image, a third MRI is performed with an additional double dosage (0.2mmol/kg) of contrast material. When the high-dose contrast technique is utilized, carriers:

- Do not pay separately for the contrast material used in the second MRI procedure;
- Pay for the contrast material given for the third MRI procedure through supply code Q9952, the replacement code for A4643, when billed with Current Procedural Terminology (CPT) codes 70553, 72156, 72157, and 72158;
- Do not pay for the third MRI procedure. For example, in the case of an MRI of the brain, if CPT code 70553 (without contrast material, followed by with contrast material(s) and further sequences) is billed, make no payment for CPT code 70551 (without contrast material(s)), the additional procedure given for the purpose of administering the double dosage, furnished during the same session. Medicare does not pay for the third procedure (as distinguished from the contrast material) because the CPT definition of code 70553 includes all further sequences; and
- Do not apply the payment criteria for low osmolar contrast media in §30.1.2 to billings for code Q9952, the replacement code for A4643.

Effective January 1, 2007

With the implementation for calendar year 2007 of a bottom-up methodology, which utilizes the direct inputs to determine the practice expense (PE) relative value units (RVUs), the cost of the contrast media is not included in the PE RVUs. Therefore, a separate payment for the contrast media used in various imaging procedures is paid. In addition to the CPT code representing the imaging procedure, separately bill the appropriate HCPCS "Q" code (Q9945–Q9954; Q9958-Q9964) for the contrast medium utilized in performing the service.

Effective February 24, 2011

Medicare will allow for coverage of MRI for beneficiaries with implanted PMs or cardioverter defibrillators (ICDs) for use in an MRI environment in a Medicare-approved clinical study as described in section 220.C.1 of the NCD manual.

Effective July 7, 2011

Medicare will allow for coverage of MRI for beneficiaries with implanted pacemakers (PMs) when the PMs are used according to the Food and Drug Administration (FDA)-approved labeling for use in an MRI environment as described in section 220.2.C.1 of the NCD Manual.

100-4, 13, 40.1.1

Magnetic Resonance Angiography (MRA) Coverage Summary

Section 1861(s)(2)(C) of the Social Security Act provides for coverage of diagnostic testing. Coverage of magnetic resonance angiography (MRA) of the head and neck, and MRA of the peripheral vessels of the lower extremities is limited as described in Publication (Pub.) 100-03, the Medicare National Coverage Determinations (NCD) Manual. This instruction has been revised as of July 1, 2003, based on a determination that coverage is reasonable and necessary in additional circumstances. Under that instruction, MRA is generally covered only to the extent that it is used as a substitute for contrast angiography, except to the extent that there are documented circumstances consistent with that instruction that demonstrates the medical necessity of both tests. Prior to June 3, 2010, there was no coverage of MRA outside of the indications and circumstances described in that instruction.

Effective for claims with dates of service on or after June 3, 2010, contractors have the discretion to cover or not cover all indications of MRA (and magnetic resonance imaging (MRI)) that are not specifically nationally covered or nationally non-covered as stated in section 220.2 of the NCD Manual.

Because the status codes for HCPCS codes 71555, 71555-TC, 71555-26, 74185, 74185-TC, and 74185-26 were changed in the Medicare Physician Fee Schedule Database from 'N' to 'R' on April 1, 1998, any MRA claims with those HCPCS codes with dates of service between April 1, 1998, and June 30, 1999, are to be processed according to the contractor's discretionary authority to determine payment in the absence of national policy.

Effective for claims with dates of service on or after February 24, 2011, Medicare will provide coverage for MRIs for beneficiaries with implanted cardiac pacemakers or implantable cardioverter defibrillators if the beneficiary is enrolled in an approved clinical study under the Coverage with Study Participation form of Coverage with Evidence Development that meets specific criteria per Pub. 100-03, the NCD Manual, chapter 1, section 220.2.C.1

100-4, 13, 60.1

Billing Instructions

A. Billing and Payment Instructions or Responsibilities for Carriers

Claims for PET scan services must be billed on Form-CMS 1500 or the electronic equivalent with the appropriate HCPCS or CPT code and diagnosis codes to the local carrier. Effective for claims received on or after July 1, 2001, PET modifiers were discontinued and are no longer a claims processing requirement for PET scan claims.

Therefore, July 1, 2001, and after the MSN messages regarding the use of PET modifiers can be discontinued. The type of service (TOS) for the new PET scan procedure codes is TOS 4, Diagnostic Radiology. Payment is based on the Medicare Physician Fee Schedule.

B. Billing and Payment Instructions or Responsibilities for FIs
Claims for PET scan procedures must be billed to the FI on Form CMS-1450 (UB-92) or the electronic equivalent with the appropriate diagnosis and HCPCS "G" code or CPT code to indicate the conditions under which a PET scan was done. These codes represent the technical component costs associated with these procedures when furnished to hospital and SNF outpatients. They are paid as follows:

- under OPPS for hospitals subject to OPPS
- under current payment methodologies for hospitals not subject to OPPS
- on a reasonable cost basis for critical access hospitals.
- on a reasonable cost basis for skilled nursing facilities.

Institutional providers bill these codes under Revenue Code 0404 (PET Scan).

Medicare contractors shall pay claims submitted for services provided by a critical access hospital (CAH) as follows: Method I technical services are paid at 101% of reasonable cost; Method II technical services are paid at 101% of reasonable cost, and professional services are paid at 115% of the Medicare Physician Fee Schedule Data Base.

C. Frequency
In the absence of national frequency limitations, for all indications covered on and after July 1, 2001, contractors can, if necessary, develop frequency limitations on any or all covered PET scan services.

D. Post-Payment Review for PET Scans
As with any claim, but particularly in view of the limitations on this coverage, Medicare may decide to conduct post-payment reviews to determine that the use of PET scans is consistent with coverage instructions. Pet scanning facilities must keep patient record information on file for each Medicare patient for whom a PET scan claim is made. These medical records can be used in any post-payment reviews and must include the information necessary to substantiate the need for the PET scan. These records must include standard information (e.g., age, sex, and height) along with sufficient patient histories to allow determination that the steps required in the coverage instructions were followed. Such information must include, but is not limited to, the date, place and results of previous diagnostic tests (e.g., cytopathology and surgical pathology reports, CT), as well as the results and reports of the PET scan(s) performed at the center. If available, such records should include the prognosis derived from the PET scan, together with information regarding the physician or institution to which the patient proceeded following the scan for treatment or evaluation. The ordering physician is responsible for forwarding appropriate clinical data to the PET scan facility.

Effective for claims received on or after July 1, 2001, CMS no longer requires paper documentation to be submitted up front with PET scan claims. Contractors shall be aware and advise providers of the specific documentation requirements for PET scans for dementia and neurodegenerative diseases. This information is outlined in section 60.12.

Documentation requirements such as physician referral and medical necessity determination are to be maintained by the provider as part of the beneficiary's medical record. This information must be made available to the carrier or FI upon request of additional documentation to determine appropriate payment of an individual claim.

100-4, 13, 60.2

Use of Gamma Cameras and Full Ring and Partial Ring PET Scanners for PET Scans

See the Medicare NCD Manual, Section 220.6, concerning 2-[F-18] Fluoro-D-Glucose (FDG) PET scanners and details about coverage.

On July 1, 2001, HCPCS codes G0210 - G0230 were added to allow billing for all currently covered indications for FDG PET. Although the codes do not indicate the type of PET scanner, these codes were used until January 1, 2002, by providers to bill for services in a manner consistent with the coverage policy.

Effective January 1, 2002, HCPCS codes G0210 - G0230 were updated with new descriptors to properly reflect the type of PET scanner used. In addition, four new HCPCS codes became effective for dates of service on and after January 1, 2002, (G0231, G0232, G0233, G0234) for covered conditions that may be billed if a gamma camera is used for the PET scan. For services performed from January 1, 2002, through January 27, 2005, providers should bill using the revised HCPCS codes G0210 - G0234.

Beginning January 28, 2005 providers should bill using the appropriate CPT code.

100-4, 13, 60.3

PET Scan Qualifying Conditions and HCPCS Code Chart

Below is a summary of all covered PET scan conditions, with effective dates.

NOTE: The G codes below except those a # can be used to bill for PET Scan services through January 27, 2005. Effective for dates of service on or after January 28, 2005, providers must bill for PET Scan services using the appropriate CPT codes. See section 60.3.1. The G codes with a # can continue to be used for billing after January 28, 2005 and these remain non-covered by Medicare. (NOTE: PET Scanners must be FDA-approved.)

Conditions	Coverage Effective Date	****HCPCS/ CPT
*Myocardial perfusion imaging (following previous PET G0030-G0047) single study, rest or stress (exercise and/or pharmacologic)	3/14/95	G0030
*Myocardial perfusion imaging (following previous PET G0030-G0047) multiple studies, rest or stress (exercise and/or pharmacologic)	3/14/95	G0031
*Myocardial perfusion imaging (following rest SPECT, 78464); single study, rest or stress (exercise and/or pharmacologic)	'3/14/95	G0032
*Myocardial perfusion imaging (following rest SPECT 78464); multiple studies, rest or stress (exercise and/or pharmacologic)	3/14/95	G0033
*Myocardial perfusion (following stress SPECT 78465); single study, rest or stress (exercise and/or pharmacologic)	3/14/95	G0034
*Myocardial Perfusion Imaging (following stress SPECT 78465); multiple studies, rest or stress (exercise and/or pharmacologic)	3/14/95	G0035
*Myocardial Perfusion Imaging (following coronary angiography 93510-93529); single study, rest or stress (exercise and/or pharmacologic)	3/14/95	G0036
*Myocardial Perfusion Imaging, (following coronary angiography), 93510-93529); multiple studies, rest or stress (exercise and/or pharmacologic)	3/14/95	G0037
*Myocardial Perfusion Imaging (following stress planar myocardial perfusion, 78460); single study, rest or stress (exercise and/or pharmacologic)	3/14/95	G0038
*Myocardial Perfusion Imaging (following stress planar myocardial perfusion, 78460); multiple studies, rest or stress (exercise and/or pharmacologic)	3/14/95	G0039
*Myocardial Perfusion Imaging (following stress echocardiogram 93350); single study, rest or stress (exercise and/or pharmacologic)	3/14/95	G0040
*Myocardial Perfusion Imaging (following stress echocardiogram, 93350); multiple studies, rest or stress (exercise and/or pharmacologic)	3/14/95	G0041
*Myocardial Perfusion Imaging (following stress nuclear ventriculogram 78481 or 78483); single study, rest or stress (exercise and/or pharmacologic)	3/14/95	G0042
*Myocardial Perfusion Imaging (following stress nuclear ventriculogram 78481 or 78483); multiple studies, rest or stress (exercise and/or pharmacologic)	3/14/95	G0043
*Myocardial Perfusion Imaging (following stress ECG, 93000); single study, rest or stress (exercise and/or pharmacologic)	3/14/95	G0044
*Myocardial perfusion (following stress ECG, 93000), multiple studies; rest or stress (exercise and/or pharmacologic)	3/14/95	G0045
*Myocardial perfusion (following stress ECG, 93015), single study; rest or stress (exercise and/or pharmacologic)	3/14/95	G0046
*Myocardial perfusion (following stress ECG, 93015); multiple studies, rest or stress (exercise and/or pharmacologic)	3/14/95	G0047
PET imaging regional or whole body; single pulmonary nodule	1/1/98	G0125
Lung cancer, non-small cell (PET imaging whole body) Diagnosis, Initial Staging, Restaging	7/1/01	G0210 G0211 G0212
Colorectal cancer (PET imaging whole body) Diagnosis, Initial Staging, Restaging	7/1/01	G0213 G0214 G0215
Melanoma (PET imaging whole body) Diagnosis, Initial Staging, Restaging	7/1/01	G0216 G0217 G0218
Melanoma for non-covered indications	7/1/01	G0219
Lymphoma (PET imaging whole body) Diagnosis, Initial Staging, Restaging	7/1/01	G0220 G0221 G0222
Head and neck cancer; excluding thyroid and CNS cancers (PET imaging whole body or regional) Diagnosis, Initial Staging, Restaging	7/1/01	G0223 G0224 G0225

* Carriers must report A4641 for the tracer Rubidium 82 when used with PET scan codes G0030 through G0047 for services performed on or before January 27, 2005

** Not FDG PET

*** For dates of service October 1, 2003, through December 31, 2003, use temporary code Q4078 for billing this radiopharmaceutical.

Conditions	Coverage Effective Date	****HCPCS/ CPT
Esophageal cancer (PET imaging whole body) Diagnosis, Initial Staging, Restaging	7/1/01	G0226 G0227 G0228
Metabolic brain imaging for pre-surgical evaluation of refractory seizures	7/1/01	G0229
Metabolic assessment for myocardial viability following inconclusive SPECT study	7/1/01	G0230
Recurrence of colorectal or colorectal metastatic cancer (PET whole body, gamma cameras only)	1/1/02	G0231
Staging and characterization of lymphoma (PET whole body, gamma cameras only)	1/1/02	G0232
Recurrence of melanoma or melanoma metastatic cancer (PET whole body, gamma cameras only)	1/1/02	G0233
Regional or whole body, for solitary pulmonary nodule following CT, or for initial staging of nonsmall cell lung cancer (gamma cameras only)	1/1/02	G0234
Non-Covered Service PET imaging, any site not otherwise specified	1/28/05	G0235
Non-Covered Service Initial diagnosis of breast cancer and/or surgical planning for breast cancer (e.g., initial staging of axillary lymph nodes), not covered (full- and partialring PET scanners only)	10/1/02	G0252
Breast cancer, staging/restaging of local regional recurrence or distant metastases, i.e., staging/restaging after or prior to course of treatment (full- and partial-ring PET scanners only)	10/1/02	G0253
Breast cancer, evaluation of responses to treatment, performed during course of treatment (full- and partial-ring PET scanners only)	10/1/02	G0254
Myocardial imaging, positron emission tomography (PET), metabolic evaluation)	10/1/02	78459
Restaging or previously treated thyroid cancer of follicular cell origin following negative I-131 whole body scan (full- and partial-ring PET scanner only)	10/1/03	G0296
Tracer Rubidium**82 (Supply of Radiopharmaceutical Diagnostic Imaging Agent) (This is only billed through Outpatient Perspective Payment System, OPPS.) (Carriers must use HCPCS Code A4641).	10/1/03	Q3000
Supply of Radiopharmaceutical Diagnostic Imaging Agent, Ammonia N-13	01/1/04	A9526
PET imaging, brain imaging for the differential diagnosis of Alzheimer's disease with aberrant features vs. fronto-temporal dementia	09/15/04	Appropriate CPT Code from section 60.3.1
PET Cervical Cancer Staging as adjunct to conventional imaging, other staging, diagnosis, restaging, monitoring	1/28/05	Appropriate CPT Code from section 60.3.1

* Carriers must report A4641 for the tracer Rubidium 82 when used with PET scan codes G0030 through G0047 for services performed on or before January 27, 2005

** Not FDG PET

*** For dates of service October 1, 2003, through December 31, 2003, use temporary code Q4078 for billing this radiopharmaceutical.

100-4, 13, 60.3.1

Appropriate CPT Codes Effective for PET Scans for Services Performed on or After January 28, 2005

NOTE: All PET scan services require the use of a radiopharmaceutical diagnostic imaging agent (tracer). The applicable tracer code should be billed when billing for a PET scan service. See section 60.3.2 below for applicable tracer codes.

CPT Code	Description
78459	Myocardial imaging, positron emission tomography (PET), metabolic evaluation
78491	Myocardial imaging, positron emission tomography (PET), perfusion, single study at rest or stress
78492	Myocardial imaging, positron emission tomography (PET), perfusion, multiple studies at rest and/or stress
78608	Brain imaging, positron emission tomography (PET); metabolic evaluation
78811	Tumor imaging, positron emission tomography (PET); limited area (eg, chest, head/neck)
78812	Tumor imaging, positron emission tomography (PET); skull base to mid-thigh
78813	Tumor imaging, positron emission tomography (PET); whole body
78814	Tumor imaging, positron emission tomography (PET) with concurrently acquired computed tomography (CT) for attenuation correction and anatomical localization; limited area (eg, chest, head/neck)
78815	Tumor imaging, positron emission tomography (PET) with concurrently acquired computed tomography (CT) for attenuation correction and anatomical localization; skull base to mid-thigh
78816	Tumor imaging, positron emission tomography (PET) with concurrently acquired computed tomography (CT) for attenuation correction and anatomical localization; whole body

100-4, 13, 60.3.2

Tracer Codes Required for PET Scans

The following tracer codes are applicable only to CPT 78491 and 78492. They can not be reported with any other code.

Institutional providers billing the fiscal intermediary

HCPCS	Description
*A9555	Rubidium Rb-82, Diagnostic, Per study dose, Up To 60 Millicuries
*Q3000 (Deleted effective 12/31/05)	Supply of Radiopharmaceutical Diagnostic Imaging Agent, Rubidium Rb-82, per dose
A9526	Nitrogen N-13 Ammonia, Diagnostic, Per study dose, Up To 40 Millicuries

NOTE: For claims with dates of service prior to 1/01/06, providers report Q3000 for supply of radiopharmaceutical diagnostic imaging agent, Rubidium Rb-82. For claims with dates of service 1/01/06 and later, providers report A9555 for radiopharmaceutical diagnostic imaging agent, Rubidium Rb-82 in place of Q3000.

Physicians / practitioners billing the carrier:

*A4641	Supply of Radiopharmaceutical Diagnostic Imaging Agent, Not Otherwise Classified
A9526	Nitrogen N-13 Ammonia, Diagnostic, Per study dose, Up To 40 Millicuries
A9555	Rubidium Rb-82, Diagnostic, Per study dose, Up To 60 Millicuries

***NOTE:** Effective January 1, 2008, tracer code A4641 is not applicable for PET Scans.

The following tracer codes are applicable only to CPT 78459, 78608, 78811-78816. They can not be reported with any other code:

Institutional providers billing the fiscal intermediary:

* A9552	Fluorodeoxyglucose F18, FDG, Diagnostic, Per study dose, Up to 45 Millicuries
* C1775 (Deleted effective 12/31/05)	Supply of Radiopharmaceutical Diagnostic Imaging Agent, Fluorodeoxyglucose F18, (2-Deoxy-2-18F Fluoro-D-Glucose), Per dose (4-40 Mci/Ml)
**A4641	Supply of Radiopharmaceutical Diagnostic Imaging Agent, Not Otherwise Classified
A9580	Sodium Fluoride F-18, Diagnostic, per study dose, up to 30 Millicuries

NOTE: For claims with dates of service prior to 1/01/06, OPPS hospitals report C1775 for supply of radiopharmaceutical diagnostic imaging agent, Fluorodeoxyglucose F18. For claims with dates of service January 1, 2006 and later, providers report A9552 for radiopharmaceutical diagnostic imaging agent, Fluorodeoxyglucose F18 in place of C1775.

** **NOTE:** Effective January 1, 2008, tracer code A4641 is not applicable for PET Scans.

*****NOTE:** Effective for claims with dates of service February 26, 2010 and later, tracer code

A9580 is applicable for PET Scans.	Physicians / practitioners billing the carrier:
A9552	Fluorodeoxyglucose F18, FDG, Diagnostic, Per study dose, Up to 45 Millicuries
*A4641	Supply of Radiopharmaceutical Diagnostic Imaging Agent, Not Otherwise Classified
A9580	Sodium Fluoride F-18, Diagnostic, per study dose, up to 30 Millicuries

***NOTE:** Effective January 1, 2008, tracer code A4641 is not applicable for PET Scans.

*****NOTE:** Effective for claims with dates of service February 26, 2010 and later, tracer code

A9580 is applicable for PET Scans.	Positron Emission Tomography Reference Table CPT

CPT	Short Descriptor	Tracer/ Code	or	Tracer/Code	Comment
78459	Myocardial imaging, positron emission tomography (PET), metabolic imaging	FDG A9552	--	--	N/A
78491	Myocardial imaging, positron emission tomography (PET), perfusion; single study at rest or stress	N-13 A9526	or	Rb-82 A9555	N/A
78492	Myocardial imaging, positron emission tomography (PET), perfusion; multiple studies at rest and/or stress	N-13 A9526	or	Rb-82 A9555	N/A
78608	Brain imaging, positron emission tomography (PET); metabolic evaluation	FDG A9552	--	--	Covered indications: Alzheimer's disease/dementias, intractable seizures Note: This code is also covered for dedicated PET brain tumor imaging.
78609	Brain imaging, positron emission tomography (PET); perfusion evaluation	--	--	--	Nationally noncovered
78811	Positron emission tomography (PET) imaging; limited area (e.g, chest, head/neck)	FDG A9552	or	NaF-18 A9580	NaF-18 PET is covered only to identify bone metastasis of cancer.

100-4, 13, 60.4

PET Scans for Imaging of the Perfusion of the Heart Using Rubidium 82 (Rb 82)(Rev. 223, Issued: 07-02-04) (Effective/Implementation: Not Applicable)

For dates of service on or after March 14, 1995, Medicare covers one PET scan for imaging of the perfusion of the heart using Rubidium 82 (Rb 82), provided that the following conditions are met:

- The PET is done at a PET imaging center with a PET scanner that has been approved by the FDA;
- The PET scan is a rest alone or rest with pharmacologic stress PET scan, used for noninvasive imaging of the perfusion of the heart for the diagnosis and management of patients with known or suspected coronary artery disease, using Rb 82; and
- Either the PET scan is used in place of, but not in addition to, a single photon emission computed tomography (SPECT) or the PET scan is used following a SPECT that was found inconclusive.

100-4, 13, 60.9

Coverage of PET Scans for Myocardial Viability

FDG PET is covered for the determination of myocardial viability following an inconclusive single photon computed tomography test (SPECT) from July 1, 2001, through September 30, 2002. Only full ring scanners are covered as the scanning medium for this service from July 1, 2001, through December 31, 2001. However, as of January 1, 2002, full and partial ring scanners are covered for myocardial viability following an inconclusive SPECT.

Beginning October 1, 2002, Medicare will cover FDG PET for the determination of myocardial viability as a primary or initial diagnostic study prior to revascularization, and will continue to cover FDG PET when used as a follow-up to an inconclusive SPECT.

However, if a patient received a FDG PET study with inconclusive results, a follow-up SPECT is not covered. FDA full and partial ring PET scanners are covered. In the event that a patient receives a SPECT with inconclusive results, a PET scan may be performed and covered by Medicare. However, a SPECT is not covered following a FDG PET with inconclusive results. See the Medicare National Coverage Determinations Manual, Section 220.6 for specific frequency limitations for Myocardial Viability following an inconclusive SPECT.

Documentation that these conditions are met should be maintained by the referring provider as part of the beneficiary's medical record.

HCPCS Code for PET Scan for Myocardial Viability

78459 Myocardial imaging, positron emission tomography (PET), metabolic evaluation

100-4, 13, 60.11

Coverage of PET Scans for Perfusion of the Heart Using Ammonia N-13

Effective for service performed on or after October 1, 2003, PET scans performed at rest or with pharmacological stress used for noninvasive imaging of the perfusion of the heart for the diagnosis and management of patients with known or suspected coronary artery disease using the FDA-approved radiopharmaceutical ammonia N-13 are covered, provided the following requirements are met.

100-4, 13, 60.12

Coverage for PET Scans for Dementia and Neurodegenerative Diseases

Effective for dates of service on or after September 15, 2004, Medicare will cover FDG PET scans for a differential diagnosis of fronto-temporal dementia (FTD) and Alzheimer's disease OR; its use in a CMS-approved practical clinical trial focused on the utility of FDG-PET in the diagnosis or treatment of dementing neurodegenerative diseases. Refer to Pub. 100-03, NCD Manual, section 220.6.13, for complete coverage conditions and clinical trial requirements and section 60.15 of this manual for claims processing information.

A. Carrier and FI Billing Requirements for PET Scan Claims for FDG-PET for the Differential Diagnosis of Fronto-temporal Dementia and Alzheimer's Disease:

- CPT Code for PET Scans for Dementia and Neurodegenerative Diseases

  Contractors shall advise providers to use the appropriate CPT code from section 60.3.1 for dementia and neurodegenerative diseases for services performed on or after January 28, 2005.

- Diagnosis Codes for PET Scans for Dementia and Neurodegenerative Diseases

  The contractor shall ensure one of the following appropriate diagnosis codes is present on claims for PET Scans for AD:

  - 290.0, 290.10 - 290.13, 290.20 - 290, 21, 290.3, 331.0, 331.11, 331.19, 331.2, 331.9, 780.93

  Medicare contractors shall use an appropriate Medicare Summary Notice (MSN) message such as 16.48, "Medicare does not pay for this item or service for this condition" to deny claims when submitted with an appropriate CPT code from section 60.3.1 and with a diagnosis code other than the range of codes listed above. Also, contractors shall use an appropriate Remittance Advice (RA) such as 11, "The diagnosis is inconsistent with the procedure."

  Medicare contractors shall instruct providers to issue an Advanced Beneficiary Notice to beneficiaries advising them of potential financial liability prior to delivering the service if one of the appropriate diagnosis codes will not be present on the claim.

- Provider Documentation Required with the PET Scan Claim

  Medicare contractors shall inform providers to ensure the conditions mentioned in the NCD Manual, section 220.6.13, have been met. The information must also be maintained in the beneficiary's medical record:

  - Date of onset of symptoms;
  - Diagnosis of clinical syndrome (normal aging, mild cognitive impairment or MCI: mild, moderate, or severe dementia);
  - Mini mental status exam (MMSE) or similar test score;
  - Presumptive cause (possible, probably, uncertain AD);
  - Any neuropsychological testing performed;
  - Results of any structural imaging (MRI, CT) performed;
  - Relevant laboratory tests (B12, thyroid hormone); and,
  - Number and name of prescribed medications.

100-4,13,60.13

Billing Requirements for PET Scans for Specific Indications of Cervical Cancer for Services Performed on or After January 28, 2005

Contractors shall accept claims for these services with the appropriate CPT code listed in section 60.3.1. Refer to Pub. 100-03, section 220.6.17, for complete coverage guidelines for this new PET oncology indication. The implementation date for these CPT codes will be April 18, 2005. Also see section 60.17, of this chapter for further claims processing instructions for cervical cancer indications.

100-4, 13, 60.15

Billing Requirements for CMS - Approved Clinical Trials and Coverage With Evidence Development Claims for PET Scans for Neurodegenerative Diseases, Previously Specified Cancer Indications, and All Other Cancer Indications Not Previously Specified

- Carriers and FIs

Effective for services on or after January 28, 2005, contractors shall accept and pay for claims for PET scans for lung cancer, esophageal cancer, colorectal cancer, lymphoma, melanoma, head & neck cancer, breast cancer, thyroid cancer, soft tissue sarcoma, brain cancer, ovarian cancer, pancreatic cancer, small cell lung cancer, and testicular cancer, as well as for neurodegenerative diseases and all other cancer indications not previously mentioned in this chapter, if these scans were performed as part of a CMS-approved clinical trial. (See Pub. 100-03, NCD Manual, sections 220.6.13 and 220.6.17.)

Contractors shall also be aware that PET scans for all cancers not previously specified at Pub. 100-03, NCD Manual, section 220.6.17, remain nationally non-covered unless performed in conjunction with a CMS-approved clinical trial.

- Carriers Only

Carriers shall pay claims for PET scans for beneficiaries participating in a CMS-approved clinical trial submitted with an appropriate CPT code from section 60.3.1, of this chapter and the -QR (Item or Service Provided in a Medicare Specified Study) modifier.

- FIs Only
In order to pay claims for PET scans on behalf of beneficiaries participating in a CMS-approved clinical trial, FIs require providers to submit claims with ICD-9 code V70.7 in the second diagnosis position on the CMS-1450 (UB-04), or the electronic equivalent, with the appropriate principal diagnosis code and an appropriate CPT code from section 60.3.1. Effective for PET scan claims for dates of service on or after January 28, 2005, FIs shall accept claims with the -QR modifier on other than inpatient claims.

NOTE: Effective for services on or after January 1, 2008, -Q0 (investigational clinical service provided in a clinical research study that is in an approved clinical research study) replaces the -QR modifier.

100-4,13,60.16

Billing and Coverage Changes for PET Scans Effective for Services on or After April 3, 2009

A. Summary of Changes
Effective for services on or after April 3, 2009, Medicare will not cover the use of FDG PET imaging to determine initial treatment strategy in patients with adenocarcinoma of the prostate.

Medicare will also not cover FDG PET imaging for subsequent treatment strategy for tumor types other than breast, cervical, colorectal, esophagus, head and neck (non-CNS/thyroid), lymphoma, melanoma, myeloma, non-small cell lung, and ovarian, unless the FDG PET is provided under the coverage with evidence development (CED) paradigm (billed with modifier -Q0, see section 60.15 of this chapter).

Last, Medicare will cover FDG PET imaging for initial treatment strategy for myeloma.

For further information regarding the changes in coverage, refer to Pub.100-03, NCD Manual, section 220.6.17.

B. New Modifiers for PET Scans
Effective for claims with dates of service on or after April 3, 2009, the following modifiers have been created for use to inform for the initial treatment strategy of biopsy-proven or strongly suspected tumors or subsequent treatment strategy of cancerous tumors:

> PI -Positron Emission Tomography (PET) or PET/Computed Tomography (CT) to inform the initial treatment strategy of tumors that are biopsy proven or strongly suspected of being cancerous based on other diagnostic testing.

Short descriptor: PET tumor init tx strat

> PS - Positron Emission Tomography (PET) or PET/Computed Tomography (CT) to inform the subsequent treatment strategy of cancerous tumors when the beneficiary's treatment physician determines that the PET study is needed to inform subsequent anti-tumor strategy.

Short descriptor: PS - PET tumor subsq tx strategy

C. Billing Changes for A/B MACs, FIs and Carriers

Effective for claims with dates of service on or after April 3, 2009, contractors shall accept FDG PET claims billed to inform initial treatment strategy with the following CPT codes AND modifier -PI: 78608, 78811, 78812, 78813, 78814, 78815, 78816.

Effective for claims with dates of service on or after April 3, 2009, contractors shall accept FDG PET claims with modifier -PS for the subsequent treatment strategy for solid tumors using a CPT code above AND an ICD-9 cancer diagnosis code.

Contractors shall also accept FDG PET claims billed to inform initial treatment strategy or subsequent treatment strategy when performed under CED with one of the PET or PET/CT CPT codes above AND modifier -PI OR modifier -PS AND an ICD-9 cancer diagnosis code AND modifier -Q0 (Investigational clinical service provided in a clinical research study that is in an approved clinical research study).

NOTE: For institutional claims continue to use diagnosis code V70.7 and condition code 30 on the claim.

D. Medicare Summary Notices, Remittance Advice Remark Codes, and Claim Adjustment Reason Codes

Effective for dates of service on or after April 3, 2009, contractors shall return as unprocessable/return to provider claims that do not include the -PI modifier with one of the PET/PET/CT CPT codes listed in subsection C. above when billing for the initial treatment strategy for solid tumors in accordance with Pub.100-03, NCD Manual, section 220.6.17.

In addition, contractors shall return as unprocessable/return to provider claims that do not include the -PS modifier with one of the CPT codes listed in subsection C. above when billing for the subsequent treatment strategy for solid tumors in accordance with Pub.100-03, NCD Manual, section 220.6.17.

The following messages apply:

> -Claim Adjustment Reason Code 4 - the procedure code is inconsistent with the modifier used or a required modifier is missing.
>
> -Remittance Advice Remark Code MA-130 - Your claim contains incomplete and/or invalid information, and no appeal rights are afforded because the claim is unprocessable. Submit a new claim with the complete/correct information.
>
> -Remittance Advice Remark Code M16 - Alert: See our Web site, mailings, or bulletins for more details concerning this policy/procedure/decision.

Also, effective for claims with dates of service on or after April 3, 2009, contractors shall return as unprocessable/return to provider FDG PET claims billed to inform initial treatment strategy or subsequent treatment strategy when performed under CED without one of the PET/PET/CT CPT codes listed in subsection C. above AND modifier -PI OR modifier -PS AND an ICD-9 cancer diagnosis code AND modifier -Q0.

The following messages apply to return as unprocessable claims:

> -Claim Adjustment Reason Code 4 - the procedure code is inconsistent with the modifier used or a required modifier is missing.
>
> -Remittance Advice Remark Code MA-130 - Your claim contains incomplete and/or invalid information, and no appeal rights are afforded because the claim is unprocessable. Submit a new claim with the complete/correct information.
>
> -Remittance Advice Remark Code M16 - Alert: See our Web site, mailings, or bulletins for more details concerning this policy/procedure/decision.

Effective April 3, 2009, contractors shall deny claims with ICD-9 diagnosis code 185 for FDG PET imaging for the initial treatment strategy of patients with adenocarcinoma of the prostate.

Contractors shall also deny claims for FDG PET imaging for subsequent treatment strategy for tumor types other than breast, cervical, colorectal, esophagus, head and neck (non-CNS/thyroid), lymphoma, melanoma, myeloma, non-small cell lung, and ovarian, unless the FDG PET is provided under CED (submitted with the -Q0 modifier) and use the following messages:

> -Medicare Summary Notice 15.4 - Medicare does not support the need for this service or item
>
> -Claim Adjustment Reason Code 50 - These are non-covered services because this is not deemed a 'medical necessity' by the payer.
>
> - Contractors shall use Group Code CO (Contractual Obligation)

If an ABN is provided with a GA modifier indicating there is a signed ABN on file, contractors shall use Group Code PR (Patient Responsibility) and the liability falls to the beneficiary.

If an ABN is provided with a GZ modifier indicating no ABN was provided, contractors shall use Group Code CO (Contractual Obligation) and the liability falls to the provider.

100-4, 13, 60.17

Billing and Coverage Changes for PET Scans for Cervical Cancer Effective for Services on or After November 10, 2009

A. Billing Changes for A/B MACs, FIs, and Carriers
Effective for claims with dates of service on or after November 10, 2009, contractors shall accept FDG PET oncologic claims billed to inform initial treatment strategy; specifically for staging in beneficiaries who have biopsy-proven cervical cancer when the beneficiary's treating physician determines the FDG PET study is needed to determine the location and/or extent of the tumor as specified in Pub 100-03, section 220.6.17.

EXCEPTION: CMS continues to non-cover FDG PET for initial diagnosis of cervical cancer related to initial treatment strategy.

NOTE: Effective for claims with dates of service on and after November 10, 2009, the -Q0 modifier is no longer necessary for FDG PET for cervical cancer.

B. Medicare Summary Notices, Remittance Advice Remark Codes, and Claim Adjustment Reason Codes
Additionally, contractors shall return as unprocessable /return to provider for FDG PET for cervical cancer for initial treatment strategy billed without the following: one of the PET/PET/ CT CPT codes listed in 60.16 C above AND modifier -PI AND an ICD-9 cervical cancer diagnosis code.

Use the following messages:

> - Claim Adjustment Reason Code 4 - the procedure code is inconsistent with the modifier used or a required modifier is missing.
>
> - Remittance Advice Remark Code MA-130 - Your claim contains incomplete and/or invalid information, and no appeal rights are afforded because the claim is unprocessable. Submit a new claim with the complete/correct information.
>
> - Remittance Advice Remark Code M16 - Alert: See our Web site, mailings, or bulletins for more details concerning this policy/procedure/decision.

100-4, 13, 60.18

100-4, 13, 60.18

Billing and Coverage Changes for PET (NaF-18) Scans to Identify Bone Metastasis of Cancer Effective for Claims With Dates of Services on or After February 26, 2010

A. Billing Changes for A/B MACs, FIs, and Carriers
Effective for claims with dates of service on and after February 26, 2010, contractors shall pay for NaF-18 PET oncologic claims to inform of initial treatment strategy (PI) or subsequent treatment strategy (PS) for suspected or biopsy proven bone metastasis ONLY in the context of a clinical study and as specified in Pub. 100-03, section 220.6. All other claims for NaF-18 PET oncology claims remain non-covered.

B. Medicare Summary Notices, Remittance Advice Remark Codes, and Claim Adjustment Reason Codes
Effective for claims with dates of service on or after February 26, 2010, contractors shall return as unprocessable NaF-18 PET oncologic claims billed with modifier TC or globally (for FIs modifier TC or globally does not apply) and HCPCS A9580 to inform the initial treatment strategy or subsequent treatment strategy for bone metastasis that do not include ALL of the following:

- PI or –PS modifier AND
- PET or PET/CT CPT code (78811, 78812, 78813, 78814, 78815, 78816) AND
- ICD-9 cancer diagnosis code AND
- Q0 modifier–Investigational clinical service provided in a clinical research study, are present on the claim.

NOTE: For institutional claims, continue to include diagnosis code V70.7 and condition code 30 to denote a clinical study.

Use the following messages:

- Claim Adjustment Reason Code 4–The procedure code is inconsistent with the modifier used or a required modifier is missing. Note: Refer to the 835 Healthcare Policy Identification Segment (loop 2110 Service Payment Information REF), if present.
- Remittance Advice Remark Code MA-130 - Your claim contains incomplete and/or invalid information, and no appeal rights are afforded because the claim is unprocessable. Submit a new claim with the complete/correct information.
- Remittance Advice Remark Code M16 - Alert: See our Web site, mailings, or bulletins for more details concerning this policy/procedure/decision.
- Claim Adjustment Reason Code 167–This (these) diagnosis(es) is (are) not covered.

Effective for claims with dates of service on or after February 26, 2010, contractors shall accept PET oncologic claims billed with modifier 26 and modifier KX to inform the initial treatment strategy or strategy or subsequent treatment strategy for bone metastasis that include the following:

- PI or –PS modifier AND
- PET or PET/CT CPT code (78811, 78812, 78813, 78814, 78815, 78816) AND
- ICD-9 cancer diagnosis code AND
- Q0 modifier–Investigational clinical service provided in a clinical research study, are present on the claim.

NOTE: If modifier KX is present on the professional component service, Contractors shall process the service as PET NaF-18 rather than PET with FDG.

Contractors shall also return as unprocessable NaF-18 PET oncologic professional component claims (i.e., claims billed with modifiers 26 and KX) to inform the initial treatment strategy or strategy or subsequent treatment strategy for bone metastasis billed with HCPCS A9580 and use the following message:

Claim Adjustment Reason Code 97–The benefit for this service is included in the payment/allowance for another service/procedure that has already been adjudicated.

NOTE: Refer to the 835 Healthcare Policy identification Segment (loop 2110 Service Payment Information REF), if present.

100-4,13,60.3.2

Tracer Codes Required for PET Scans

The following tracer codes are applicable only to CPT 78491 and 78492. They can not be reported with any other code.

Institutional providers billing the fiscal intermediary

HCPCS	*Description*
*A9555	Rubidium Rb-82, Diagnostic, Per study dose, Up To 60 Millicuries
* Q3000 (Deleted effective 12/31/05)	Supply of Radiopharmaceutical Diagnostic Imaging Agent, Rubidium Rb-82, per dose
A9526	Nitrogen N-13 Ammonia, D Diagnostic, Per study dose, Up To 40 Millicuries

NOTE: For claims with dates of service prior to 1/01/06, providers report Q3000 for supply of radiopharmaceutical diagnostic imaging agent, Rubidium Rb-82. For claims with dates of service 1/01/06 and later, providers report A9555 for radiopharmaceutical diagnostic imaging agent, Rubidium Rb-82 in place of Q3000.

Physicians / practitioners billing the carrier:

*A4641 Supply of Radiopharmaceutical Diagnostic Imaging Agent, Not Otherwise Classified

A9526 Nitrogen N-13 Ammonia, Diagnostic, Per study dose, Up To 40 Millicuries

A9555 Rubidium Rb-82, Diagnostic, Per study dose, Up To 60 Millicuries

***NOTE:** Effective January 1, 2008, tracer code A4641 is not applicable for PET Scans.

The following tracer codes are applicable only to CPT 78459, 78608, 78811-78816. They can not be reported with any other code:

Institutional providers billing the fiscal intermediary:

* A9552 Fluorodeoxyglucose F18, FDG, Diagnostic, Per study dose, Up to 45 Millicuries

* C1775 (Deleted effective 12/31/05) Supply of Radiopharmaceutical Diagnostic Imaging Agent, Fluorodeoxyglucose F18, (2-Deoxy-2-18F Fluoro-D-Glucose), Per dose (4-40 Mci/Ml)

**A4641 Supply of Radiopharmaceutical Diagnostic Imaging Agent, Not Otherwise Classified

A9580 Sodium Fluoride F-18, Diagnostic, per study dose, up to 30 Millicuries

NOTE: For claims with dates of service prior to 1/01/06, OPPS hospitals report C1775 for supply of radiopharmaceutical diagnostic imaging agent, Fluorodeoxyglucose F18. For claims with dates of service January 1, 2006 and later, providers report A9552 for radiopharmaceutical diagnostic imaging agent, Fluorodeoxyglucose F18 in place of C1775.

** **NOTE:** Effective January 1, 2008, tracer code A4641 is not applicable for PET Scans.

*****NOTE:** Effective for claims with dates of service February 26, 2010 and later, tracer code A9580 is applicable for PET Scans.

Physicians / practitioners billing the carrier:

A9552 Fluorodeoxyglucose F18, FDG, Diagnostic, Per study dose, Up to 45 Millicuries

*A4641 Supply of Radiopharmaceutical Diagnostic Imaging Agent, Not Otherwise Classified

A9580 Sodium Fluoride F-18, Diagnostic, per study dose, up to 30 Millicuries

***NOTE:** Effective January 1, 2008, tracer code A4641 is not applicable for PET Scans.

*****NOTE:** Effective for claims with dates of service February 26, 2010 and later, tracer code A9580 is applicable for PET Scans.

100-4, 13, 70.1

Weekly Radiation Therapy Management (CPT 77419 - 77430)

Carriers must pay for a physician's weekly treatment management services under code 77427. Billing entities must indicate on each claim the number of fractions for which payment is sought.

A weekly unit of treatment management is equal to five fractions or treatment sessions.

A week for the purpose of making payments under these codes is comprised of five fractions regardless of the actual time period in which the services are furnished. It is not necessary that the radiation therapist personally examine the patient during each fraction for the weekly treatment management code to be payable. Multiple fractions representing two or more treatment sessions furnished on the same day may be counted as long as there has been a distinct break in therapy sessions, and the fractions are of the character usually furnished on different days. If, at the final billing of the treatment course, there are three or four fractions beyond a multiple of five, those three or four fractions are paid for as a week. If there are one or two fractions beyond a multiple of five, payment for these services is considered as having been made through prior payments.

EXAMPLE:

18 fractions = 4 weekly services

62 fractions = 12 weekly services

8 fractions = 2 weekly services

6 fractions = 1 weekly service

If billings have occurred which indicate that the treatment course has ended (and, therefore, the number of residual fractions has been determined), but treatments resume, adjust carrier payments for the additional services consistent with the above policy.

EXAMPLE:

8 fractions = payment for 2 weeks

2 additional fractions are furnished by the same physician. No additional Medicare payment is made for the 2 additional fractions.

A. SNF Treatment Management Delivery Services

A SNF may not bill weekly treatment management services for its outpatients (codes 77419, 77420, 77425, 77430, and 77431). Instead, the SNF should bill for radiation treatment delivery (codes 77401 - 77404, 77406 - 77409, 77411 - 77414, and 77416).

Also, SNFs bill for therapeutic radiology port film (code 77417), which was previously a part of the weekly services. They enter the number of services in the units field.

100-4, 13, 70.3

Radiation Treatment Delivery (CPT 77401 - 77417)

Carriers pay for these TC services on a daily basis under CPT codes 77401-77416 for radiation treatment delivery. They do not use local codes and RVUs in paying for the TC of radiation oncology services. Multiple treatment sessions on the same day are payable as long as there has been a distinct break in therapy services, and the individual sessions are of the character usually furnished on different days. Carriers pay for CPT code 77417 (Therapeutic radiology port film(s)) on a weekly (five fractions) basis.

100-4, 13, 70.4

Clinical Brachytherapy (CPT Codes 77750 - 77799)

Carriers must apply the bundled services policy to procedures in this family of codes other than CPT code 77776. For procedures furnished in settings in which TC payments are made, carriers must pay separately for the expendable source associated with these procedures under CPT code 79900 except in the case of remote after-loading high intensity brachytherapy procedures (CPT codes 77781-77784). In the four codes cited, the expendable source is included in the RVUs for the TC of the procedures.

100-4, 13, 70.5

Radiation Physics Services (CPT Codes 77300 - 77399)

Carriers pay for the PC and TC of CPT codes 77300-77334 and 77399 on the same basis as they pay for radiologic services generally. For professional component billings in all settings, carriers presume that the radiologist participated in the provision of the service, e.g., reviewed/validated the physicist's calculation. CPT codes 77336 and 77370 are technical services only codes that are payable by carriers in settings in which only technical component is are payable.

100-4, 13, 80.1

Physician Presence

Radiologic supervision and interpretation (S&I) codes are used to describe the personal supervision of the performance of the radiologic portion of a procedure by one or more physicians and the interpretation of the findings. In order to bill for the supervision aspect of the procedure, the physician must be present during its performance. This kind of personal supervision of the performance of the procedure is a service to an individual beneficiary and differs from the type of general supervision of the radiologic procedures performed in a hospital for which FIs pay the costs as physician services to the hospital. The interpretation of the procedure may be performed later by another physician. In situations in which a cardiologist, for example, bills for the supervision (the "S") of the S&I code, and a radiologist bills for the interpretation (the "I") of the code, both physicians should use a "-52" modifier indicating a reduced service, e.g., only one of supervision and/or interpretation. Payment for the fragmented S&I code is no more than if a single physician furnished both aspects of the procedure.

100-4, 13, 80.2

Multiple Procedure Reduction

Carriers make no multiple procedure reductions in the S&I or primary non-radiologic codes in these types of procedures, or in any procedure codes for which the descriptor and RVUs reflect a multiple service reduction. For additional procedure codes that do not reflect such a reduction, carriers apply the multiple procedure reductions.

100-4, 13, 100

Interpretation of Diagnostic Tests

B3-15023

100-4, 13, 140

Bone Mass Measurements (BMMs)

Sections H1861(s)(15)H and H(rr)(1)H of the Social Security Act (the Act) (as added by 4106 of the Balanced Budget Act (BBA) of 1997) standardize Medicare coverage of medically necessary bone mass measurements by providing for uniform coverage under Medicare Part B. This coverage is effective for claims with dates of service furnished on or after July 1, 1998.

Effective for dates of service on and after January 1, 2007, the CY 2007 Physician Fee Schedule final rule expanded the number of beneficiaries qualifying for BMM by reducing the dosage requirement for glucocorticoid (steroid) therapy from 7.5 mg of prednisone per day to 5.0 mg. It also changed the definition of BMM by removing coverage for a single-photon absorptiometry as it is not considered reasonable and necessary under section 1862 (a)(1)(A) of the Act. Finally, it required that in the case of monitoring and confirmatory baseline BMMs, they be performed with a dual-energy xray absorptiometry (axial) test.

Conditions of Coverage for BMMs are located in Pub.100-02, Medicare Benefit Policy Manual, chapter 15.

100-4, 13, 140.1

Payment Methodology and HCPCS Coding

Carriers pay for BMM procedures based on the Medicare physician fee schedule. Claims from physicians, other practitioners, or suppliers where assignment was not taken are subject to the Medicare limiting charge.

The FIs pay for BMM procedures under the current payment methodologies for radiology services according to the type of provider.

Do not pay BMM procedure claims for dual photon absorptiometry, CPT procedure code 78351.

Deductible and coinsurance apply.

Any of the following CPT procedure codes may be used when billing for BMMs through December 31, 2006. All of these codes are bone densitometry measurements except code 76977, which is bone sonometry measurements. CPT procedure codes are applicable to billing FIs and carriers.

76070 76071 76075 76076 76078 76977 78350 G0130

Effective for dates of services on and after January 1, 2007, the following changes apply to BMM:

- New 2007 CPT bone mass procedure codes have been assigned for BMM. The following codes will replace current codes, however the CPT descriptors for the services remain the same:

  77078 replaces 76070

  77079 replaces 76071

  77080 replaces 76075

  77081 replaces 76076

  77083 replaces 76078
- Certain BMM tests are covered when used to screen patients for osteoporosis subject to the frequency standards described in chapter 15, section 80.5.5 of the Medicare Benefit Policy Manual.
  - Contractors will pay claims for screening tests when coded as follows:
    - Contains CPT procedure code 77078, 77079, 77080, 77081, 77083, 76977 or G0130, and
    - Contains a valid ICD-9-CM diagnosis code indicating the reason for the test is postmenopausal female, vertebral fracture, hyperparathyroidism, or steroid therapy. Contractors are to maintain local lists of valid codes for the benefit's screening categories.
  - Contractors will deny claims for screening tests when coded as follows:
    - Contains CPT procedure code 77078, 77079, 77081, 77083, 76977 or G0130, but
    - Does not contain a valid ICD-9-CM diagnosis code from the local lists of valid ICD-9-CM diagnosis codes maintained by the contractor for the benefit's screening categories indicating the reason for the test is postmenopausal female, vertebral fracture, hyperparathyroidism, or steroid therapy.
- Dual-energy x-ray absorptiometry (axial) tests are covered when used to monitor FDA-approved osteoporosis drug therapy subject to the 2-year frequency standards described in chapter 15, section 80.5.5 of the Medicare Benefit Policy Manual.
  - Contractors will pay claims for monitoring tests when coded as follows:
    - Contains CPT procedure code 77080, and
    - Contains 733.00, 733.01, 733.02, 733.03, 733.09, 733.90, or 255.0 as the ICD-9-CM diagnosis code.
  - Contractors will deny claims for monitoring tests when coded as follows:
    - Contains CPT procedure code 77078, 77079, 77081, 77083, 76977 or G0130, and
    - Contains 733.00, 733.01, 733.02, 733.03, 733.09, 733.90, or 255.0 as the ICD-9-CM diagnosis code, but
    - Does not contain a valid ICD-9-CM diagnosis code from the local lists of valid ICD-9-CM diagnosis codes maintained by the contractor for the benefit's screening categories indicating the reason for the test is postmenopausal female, vertebral fracture, hyperparathyroidism, or steroid therapy.
- Single photon absorptiometry tests are not covered. Contractors will deny CPT procedure code 78350.

The FIs are billed using the ANSI X12N 837 I or hardcopy Form CMS-1450. The appropriate bill types are: 12X, 13X, 22X, 23X, 34X, 71X (Provider-based and independent), 72X, 73X (Provider-based and freestanding), 83X, and 85X. Effective April 1, 2006, type of bill 14X is for non-patient laboratory specimens and is no longer applicable for bone mass measurements. Information regarding the claim form locators that correspond to the HCPCS/CPT code or Type of Bill and a table to crosswalk its CMS-1450 form locators to the 837 transaction are found in Chapter 25.

Providers must report HCPCS codes for bone mass measurements under revenue code 320 with number of units and line item dates of service per revenue code line for each bone mass measurement reported.

Carriers are billed for bone mass measurement procedures using the ANSI X12N 837 P or hardcopy Form CMS-1500.

100-4, 14, 10

General

Payment is made under Part B for certain surgical procedures that are furnished in ASCs and are approved for being furnished in an ASC. These procedures are those that generally do not exceed 90 minutes in length and do not require more than four hours recovery or convalescent time.

To be paid under this provision, a facility must be certified as meeting the requirements for an ASC and must enter into a written agreement with the Centers for Medicare & Medicaid Services (CMS). The certification process is described in the State Operations Manual.

Medicare will not pay an ASC for those procedures that require more than an ASC level of care, or for minor procedures that are normally performed in a physician's office.

The CMS publishes updates to the list of procedures for which an ASC may be paid each year. The complete list of procedures is available through the Public Use files (PUF) at http://www.cms.hhs.gov/researchers/. This includes applicable codes, payment groups, and payment amounts for each ASC group before adjustments for regional wage variations. Applicable wage indices are also published via program memorandum.

ASCs must accept Medicare's payment for such procedures as payment in full for the facility service with respect to those services defined as ASC facility services. The physician and anesthesiologist may bill and be paid for the professional component of the service also.

Certain other services may be performed in an ASC facility, billed by the appropriate certified provider/supplier, or in certain cases by the ASC facility itself, and paid outside of the facility rate.

100-4, 14, 40.3

Payment for Intraocular Lens (IOL)

Prior to January 1, 2008, payment for facility services furnished by an ASC for IOL insertion during or subsequent to cataract surgery includes an allowance for the lens. The procedures that include insertion of an IOL are: Payment Group 6: CPT-4 Codes 66985 and 66986 Payment Group 8: CPT-4 Codes 66982, 66983 and 66984 Physicians or suppliers are not paid for an IOL furnished to a beneficiary in an ASC after July 1, 1988. Separate claims for IOLs furnished to ASC patients beginning March 12, 1990 are denied. Also, effective March 12, 1990, procedures 66983 and 66984 are treated as single procedures for payment purposes.

Beginning January 1, 2008, the Medicare payment for the IOL is included in the Medicare ASC payment for the associated surgical procedure. Consequently, no separate payment for the IOL is made, except for a payment adjustment for NTIOLs established according to the process outlined in 42 CFR 416.185. ASCs should not report separate charges for conventional IOLs because their payment is included in the Medicare payment for the associated surgical procedure. The ASC payment system logic that excluded $150 for IOLs for purposes of the multiple surgery reduction in cases of cataract surgery prior to January 1, 2008 no longer applies, effective for dates of service on or after January 1, 2008.

Effective for dates of service on and after February 27, 2006, through February 26, 2011, Medicare pays an additional $50 for specified Category 3 NTIOLs that are provided in association with a covered ASC surgical procedure. The list of Category 3 NTIOLS is available at: http://www.cms.hhs.gov/ASCPayment/08_NTIOLs.asp#TopOfPage.

ASCs should use HCPCS code Q1003 to bill for a Category 3 NTIOL. HCPCS code Q1003, along with one of the approved surgical procedure codes (CPT codes 66982, 66983, 66984, 66985, 66986) are to be used on all NTIOL Category 3 claims associated with reduced spherical aberration from February 27, 2006, through February 26, 2011. The payment adjustment for the NTIOL is subject to beneficiary coinsurance but is not wage-adjusted.

Any subsequent IOL recognized by CMS as having the same characteristics as the first NTIOL recognized by CMS for a payment adjustment as a Category III NTIOL (those of reduced spherical aberration) will receive the same adjustment for the remainder of the 5-year period established by the first recognized IOL.

100-4, 14, 40.6

Payment for Extracorporeal Shock Wave Lithotripsy (ESWL)

A ninth ASC payment group was established in a "Federal Register" notice (56 FR 67666) published December 31, 1991. The ninth payment group amount ($1,150) was assigned to only one procedure, CPT code 50590, extracorporeal shock wave lithotripsy (ESWL). However, a court order issued March 12, 1992, has stayed the Group 9 payment rate until the Secretary publishes all information relevant to the setting of the ESWL rate, receives comments, and publishes a subsequent final notice. This has not yet been completed.

In a previous instruction (Medicare Carrier's Manual Transmittal 1435), CMS advised carriers to make payment to ASCs for ESWL services furnished after January 29, 1992, and through the date when the ASC received notice from the carrier of the court order staying the Group 9 payment rate. This was a temporary measure to avoid penalizing ASCs that furnished ESWL services in accordance with the December 31, 1991, "Federal Register" notice and that could not have been expected to know that the March 12, 1992, court order set aside the ESWL provisions of that notice. Carriers did not make Medicare payment for ESWL as an ASC procedure when such services were furnished after the date that the carrier advised an ASC of the court order.

However carriers were instructed to retain all ASC claims for ESWL with a service date after January 29, 1992, and before the date when they were notified about the court order. It may be necessary to retrieve these clams for further action at some later date.

Beginning January 1, 2008 with the revised ASC payment system, contractors may pay for any of the ESWL services that are included on the ASC list of covered surgical procedures.

100-4, 14, 40.8

40.8 - Payment When a Device is Furnished With No Cost or With Full or Partial Credit Beginning January 1, 2008

Contractors pay ASCs a reduced amount for certain specified procedures when a specified device is furnished without cost or for which either a partial or full credit is received (e.g., device recall). For specified procedure codes that include payment for a device, ASCs are required to include modifier -FB on the procedure code when a specified device is furnished without cost or for which full credit is received. If the ASC receives a partial credit of 50 percent or more of the cost of a specified device, the ASC is required to include modifier -FC on the procedure code if the procedure is on the list of specified procedures to which the -FC reduction applies. A single procedure code should not be submitted with both modifiers -FB and -FC. The pricing determination related to modifiers -FB and -FC is made prior to the application of multiple procedure payment reductions. Contractors adjust beneficiary coinsurance to reflect the reduced payment amount. Tables listing the procedures and devices to which the payment adjustments apply, and the full and partial adjustment amounts, are available on the CMS Web site.

In order to report that the receipt of a partial credit of 50 percent or more of the cost of a device, ASCs have the option of either: 1) Submitting the claim for the procedure to their Medicare contractor after the procedure's performance but prior to manufacturer acknowledgement of credit for a specified device, and subsequently contacting the contractor regarding a claims adjustment once the credit determination is made; or 2) holding the claim for the procedure until a determination is made by the manufacturer on the partial credit and submitting the claim with modifier -FC appended to the implantation procedure HCPCS code if the partial credit is 50 percent or more of the cost of the device. If choosing the first billing option, to request a claims adjustment once the credit determination is made, ASCs should keep in mind that the initial Medicare payment for the procedure involving the device is conditional and subject to adjustment.

100-4,14,40.9

Payment and Coding for Presbyopia Correcting IOLs (P-C IOLs) and Astigmatism Correcting IOLs (A-C IOLs)

(CMS payment policies and recognition of P-C IOLs and A-C IOLs are contained in Transmittal 636 (CR3927) and Transmittal 1228 (CR5527) respectively.

Effective for dates of service on and after January 1, 2008, when inserting an approved A-C IOL in an ASC concurrent with cataract extraction, HCPCS code V2787 (Astigmatism-correcting function of intraocular lens) should be billed to report the non-covered charges for the A-C IOL functionality of the inserted intraocular lens. Additionally, note that HCPCS code V2788 (Presbyopia-correcting function of intraocular lens) is no longer valid to report non-covered charges associated with the A-C IOL. However, this code continues to be valid to report non-covered charges for a P-C IOL. The payment for the conventional lens portion of the A-C IOL and P-C IOL continues to be bundled with the ASC procedure payment.

Effective for services on and after January 1, 2010, ASCs are to bill for insertion of a Category 3 new technology intraocular lens (NTIOL) that is also an approved A-C IOL or P-C IOL, concurrent with cataract extraction, using three separate codes. ASCs shall use HCPCS code V2787 or V2788, as appropriate, to report charges associated with the non-covered functionality of the A-C IOL or P-C IOL, the appropriate HCPCS code 66982 (Extracapsular cataract removal with insertion of intraocular lens prosthesis (one stage procedure), manual or mechanical technique (e.g., irrigation and aspiration or phacoemulsification), complex, requiring devices or techniques not generally used in routine cataract surgery (e.g., iris expansion device, suture support for intraocular lens, or primary posterior capsulorrhexis) or performed on patients in the amblyogenic developmental stage); 66983 (Intracapsular cataract extraction with insertion of intraocular lens prosthesis (1 stage procedure)); or 66984 (Extracapsular cataract removal with insertion of intraocular lens prosthesis (1 stage procedure), manual or mechanical technique (e.g., irrigation and aspiration or phacoemulsification)), to report the covered cataract extraction and insertion procedure; and Q1003 (New technology, intraocular lens, category 3 (reduced spherical aberration) as defined in Federal Register notice, Vol. 65, dated May 3, 2000) to report the covered NTIOL aspect of the lens on claims for insertion of an A-C IOL or P-C IOL that is also designated as an NTIOL. Listings of the CMS-approved Category 3 NTIOLs, A-C IOLs, and P-C IOLs are available on the CMS web site.

100-4, 16, 10

Background

B3-2070, B3-2070.1, B3-4110.3, B3-5114

Diagnostic X-ray, laboratory, and other diagnostic tests, including materials and the services of technicians, are covered under the Medicare program. Some clinical laboratory procedures or tests require Food and Drug Administration (FDA) approval before coverage is provided.

A diagnostic laboratory test is considered a laboratory service for billing purposes, regardless of whether it is performed in:

A physician's office, by an independent laboratory;

By a hospital laboratory for its outpatients or nonpatients;

In a rural health clinic; or

In an HMO or Health Care Prepayment Plan (HCPP) for a patient who is not a member.

When a hospital laboratory performs laboratory tests for nonhospital patients, the laboratory is functioning as an independent laboratory, and still bills the fiscal intermediary (FI). Also, when physicians and laboratories perform the same test, whether manually or with automated equipment, the services are deemed similar. Laboratory services furnished by an independent laboratory are covered under SMI if the laboratory is an approved Independent Clinical Laboratory. However, as is the case of all diagnostic services, in order to be covered these services must be related to a patient's illness or injury (or symptom or complaint) and ordered by a physician. A small number of laboratory tests can be covered as a preventive screening service.

See the Medicare Benefit Policy Manual, Chapter 15, for detailed coverage requirements.

See the Medicare Program Integrity Manual, Chapter 10, for laboratory/supplier enrollment guidelines.

See the Medicare State Operations Manual for laboratory/supplier certification requirements.

100-4, 16, 70.8

Certificate of Waiver

Effective September 1, 1992, all laboratory testing sites (except as provided in 42 CFR 493.3(b)) must have either a CLIA certificate of waiver, certificate for provider-performed microscopy procedures, certificate of registration, certificate of compliance, or certificate of accreditation to legally perform clinical laboratory testing on specimens from individuals in the United States.

The Food and Drug Administration approves CLIA waived tests on a flow basis. The CMS identifies CLIA waived tests by providing an updated list of waived tests to the Medicare contractors on a quarterly basis via a Recurring Update Notification. To be recognized as a waived test, some CLIA waived tests have unique HCPCS procedure codes and some must have a QW modifier included with the HCPCS code.

For a list of specific HCPCS codes subject to CLIA see http://www.cms.hhs.gov/CLIA/downloads/waivetbl.pdf

100-4, 17, 20.5.7

Injection Services

Where the sole purpose of an office visit was for the patient to receive an injection, payment may be made only for the injection service (if it is covered). Conversely, injection services (codes 90782, 90783, 90784, 90788, and 90799) included in the Medicare Physician Fee Schedule (MPFS) are not paid for separately, if the physician is paid for any other physician fee schedule service furnished at the same time. Pay separately for those injection services only if no other physician fee schedule service is being paid. However, pay separately for cancer chemotherapy injections (CPT codes 96400-96549) in addition to the visit furnished on the same day. In either case, the drug is separately payable. All injection claims must include the specific name of the drug and dosage. Identification of the drug enables you to pay for the services.

100-4, 18,.1.2

Table of Preventive Services

Service	CPT/HCPCS Code	Long Descriptor	USPSTF Rating	Coins /Deductible
Initial Preventive Physical Examination, IPPE	G0402	Initial preventive physical examination; face to face visits, services limited to new beneficiary during the first 12 months of Medicare enrollment	*Not Rated	WAIVED
	G0403	Electrocardiogram, routine ECG with 12 leads; performed as a screening for the initial preventive physical examination with interpretation and report		Not Waived
	G0404	Electrocardiogram, routine ECG with 12 leads; tracing only, without interpretation and report, performed as a screening for the initial preventive physical examination		Not Waived
	G0405	Electrocardiogram, routine ECG with 12 leads; interpretation and report only, performed as a screening for the initial preventive physical examination		Not Waived
Ultrasound Screening for Abdominal Aortic Aneurysm (AAA)	G0389	Ultrasound, B-scan and /or real time with image documentation; for abdominal aortic aneurysm (AAA) ultrasound screening	B	WAIVED
Cardiovascular Disease Screening	80061	Lipid panel	A	WAIVED
	82465	Cholesterol, serum or whole blood, total		WAIVED
	83718	Lipoprotein, direct measurement; high density cholesterol (hdl cholesterol)		WAIVED
	84478	Triglycerides		WAIVED
Diabetes Screening Tests	82947	Glucose; quantitative, blood (except reagent strip)	B	WAIVED
	82950	Glucose; post glucose dose (includes glucose)		WAIVED
	82951	Glucose; tolerance test (gtt), three specimens (includes glucose)	*Not Rated	WAIVED
Diabetes Self-Management Training Services (DSMT)	G0108	Diabetes outpatient self-management training services, individual, per 30 minutes	*Not Rated	Not Waived
	G0109	Diabetes outpatient self-management training services, group session (2 or more), per 30 minutes		Not Waived

Service	CPT/HCPCS Code	Long Descriptor	USPSTF Rating	Coins /Deductible
Medical Nutrition Therapy (MNT) Services	97802	Medical nutrition therapy; initial assessment and intervention, individual, face-to-face with the patient, each 15 minutes	B	WAIVED
	97803	Medical nutrition therapy; re-assessment and intervention, individual, face-to-face with the patient, each 15 minutes		WAIVED
	97804	Medical nutrition therapy; group (2 or more individual(s)), each 30 minutes		WAIVED
	G0270	Medical nutrition therapy; reassessment and subsequent intervention(s) following second referral in same year for change in diagnosis, medical condition or treatment regimen (including additional hours needed for renal disease), individual, face to face with the patient, each 15 minutes		WAIVED
	G0271	Medical nutrition therapy, reassessment and subsequent intervention(s) following second referral in same year for change in diagnosis, medical condition, or treatment regimen (including additional hours needed for renal disease), group (2 or more individuals), each 30 minutes		WAIVED
Screening Pap Test	G0123	Screening cytopathology, cervical or vaginal (any reporting system), collected in preservative fluid, automated thin layer preparation, screening by cytotechnologist under physician supervision	A	WAIVED
	G0124	Screening cytopathology, cervical or vaginal (any reporting system), collected in preservative fluid, automated thin layer preparation, requiring interpretation by physician		WAIVED
	G0141	Screening cytopathology smears, cervical or vaginal, performed by automated system, with manual rescreening, requiring interpretation by physician		WAIVED
	G0143	Screening cytopathology, cervical or vaginal (any reporting system), collected in preservative fluid, automated thin layer preparation, with manual screening and rescreening by cytotechnologist under physician supervision		WAIVED
	G0144	Screening cytopathology, cervical or vaginal (any reporting system), collected in preservative fluid, automated thin layer preparation, with screening by automated system, under physician supervision		WAIVED

Service	CPT/HCPCS Code	Long Descriptor	USPSTF Rating	Coins /Deductible
Screening Pap Test (continued)	G0145	Screening cytopathology, cervical or vaginal (any reporting system), collected in preservative fluid, automated thin layer preparation, with screening by automated system and manual rescreening under physician supervision	A	WAIVED
Screening Pap Test (continued)	G0147	Screening cytopathology smears, cervical or vaginal, performed by automated system under physician supervision	A	WAIVED
Screening Pap Test (continued)	G0148	Screening cytopathology smears, cervical or vaginal, performed by automated system with manual rescreening	A	WAIVED
Screening Pap Test (continued)	P3000	Screening papanicolaou smear, cervical or vaginal, up to three smears, by technician under physician supervision	A	WAIVED
Screening Pap Test (continued)	P3001	Screening papanicolaou smear, cervical or vaginal, up to three smears, requiring interpretation by physician	A	WAIVED
Screening Pap Test (continued)	Q0091	Screening papanicolaou smear; obtaining, preparing and conveyance of cervical or vaginal smear to laboratory	A	WAIVED
Screening Pelvic Exam	G0101	Cervical or vaginal cancer screening; pelvic and clinical breast examination	A	WAIVED
Screening Mammography	77052	Computer-aided detection (computer algorithm analysis of digital image data for lesion detection) with further physician review for interpretation, with or without digitization of film radiographic images; screening mammography (list separately in addition to code for primary procedure)	B	WAIVED
Screening Mammography	77057	Screening mammography, bilateral (2-view film study of each breast)	B	WAIVED
Screening Mammography	G0202	Screening mammography, producing direct digital image, bilateral, all views	B	WAIVED
Bone Mass Measurement	G0130	Single energy x-ray absorptiometry (sexa) bone density study, one or more sites; appendicular skeleton (peripheral) (e.g., radius, wrist, heel)	B	WAIVED
Bone Mass Measurement	77078	Computed tomography, bone mineral density study, 1 or more sites; axial skeleton (e.g., hips, pelvis, spine)	B	WAIVED
Bone Mass Measurement	77079	Computed tomography, bone mineral density study, 1 or more sites; appendicular skeleton (peripheral) (e.g., radius, wrist, heel)	B	WAIVED
Bone Mass Measurement	77080	Dual-energy x-ray absorptiometry (dxa), bone density study, 1 or more sites; axial skeleton (e.g., hips, pelvis, spine)	B	WAIVED
Bone Mass Measurement	77081	Dual-energy x-ray absorptiometry (dxa), bone density study, 1 or more sites; appendicular skeleton (peripheral) (e.g., radius, wrist, heel)	B	WAIVED

Service	CPT/HCPCS Code	Long Descriptor	USPSTF Rating	Coins /Deductible
Bone Mass Measurement (continued)	77083	Radiographic absorptiometry (e.g., photo densitometry, radiogrammetry), 1 or more sites	A	WAIVED
Bone Mass Measurement (continued)	76977	Ultrasound bone density measurement and interpretation, peripheral site(s), any method	A	WAIVED
Colorectal Cancer Screening	G0104	Colorectal cancer screening; flexible sigmoidoscopy	A	WAIVED
Colorectal Cancer Screening	G0105	Colorectal cancer screening; colonoscopy on individual at high risk	A	WAIVED
Colorectal Cancer Screening	G0106	Colorectal cancer screening; alternative to G0104, screening sigmoidoscopy, barium enema	*Not Rated	Coins. Applies & Ded. is waived
Colorectal Cancer Screening	G0120	Colorectal cancer screening; alternative to G0105, screening colonoscopy, barium enema.	A	Coins. Applies & Ded. is waived
Colorectal Cancer Screening	G0121	Colorectal cancer screening; colonoscopy on individual not meeting criteria for high risk	A	WAIVED
Colorectal Cancer Screening	82270	Blood, occult, by peroxidase activity (e.g., guaiac), qualitative; feces, consecutive	A	WAIVED
Colorectal Cancer Screening	G0328	Colorectal cancer screening; fecal occult blood test, immunoassay, 1-3 simultaneous	A	WAIVED
Prostate Cancer Screening	G0102	Prostate cancer screening; digital rectal examination	D	Not Waived
Prostate Cancer Screening	G0103	Prostate cancer screening; prostate specific antigen test (PSA)	D	WAIVED
Glaucoma Screening	G0117	Glaucoma screening for high risk patients furnished by an optometrist or ophthalmologist	I	Not Waived
Glaucoma Screening	G0118	Glaucoma screening for high risk patient furnished under the direct supervision of an optometrist or ophthalmologist	I	Not Waived
Influenza Virus Vaccine	90655	Influenza virus vaccine, split virus, preservative free, when administered to children 6-35 months of age, for intramuscular use	B	WAIVED
Influenza Virus Vaccine	90656	Influenza virus vaccine, split virus, preservative free, when administered to individuals 3 years and older, for intramuscular use	B	WAIVED
Influenza Virus Vaccine	90657	Influenza virus vaccine, split virus, when administered to children 6-35 months of age, for intramuscular use	B	WAIVED
Influenza Virus Vaccine	90660	Influenza virus vaccine, live, for intranasal use	B	WAIVED
Influenza Virus Vaccine	90662	Influenza virus vaccine, split virus, preservative free, enhanced immunogenicity via increased antigen content, for intramuscular use	B	WAIVED
Influenza Virus Vaccine	Q2035	Influenza virus vaccine, split virus, when administered to individuals 3 years of age and older, for intramuscular use (afluria)	B	WAIVED
Influenza Virus Vaccine	Q2036	Influenza virus vaccine, split virus, when administered to individuals 3 years of age and older, for intramuscular use (flulaval)	B	WAIVED

Service	CPT/HCPCS Code	Long Descriptor	USPSTF Rating	Coins /Deductible
Influenza Virus Vaccine (continued)	Q2037	Influenza virus vaccine, split virus when administered to individuals 3 years of age and older, for intramuscular use (fluvirin)	B	WAIVED
	Q2038	Influenza virus vaccine, split virus, when administered to individuals 3 years of age and older, for intramuscular use (fluzone)		WAIVED
	Q2039	Influenza virus vaccine, split virus, when administered to individuals 3 years of age and older, for intramuscular use (not otherwise specified)		WAIVED
	G0008	Administration of influenza virus vaccine		WAIVED
	G9141	Influenza A (H1N1) immunization administration (includes the physician counseling the patient/family)		WAIVED
	G9142	Influenza A (H1N1) Vaccine, any route of administration		WAIVED
Pneumococcal Vaccine	90669	Pneumococcal conjugate vaccine, polyvalent, when administered to children younger than 5 years, for intramuscular use	B	WAIVED
	90670	Pneumococcal conjugate vaccine, 13 valent, for intramuscular use.		WAIVED
	90732	Pneumococcal polysaccharide vaccine, 23-valent, adult or immunosuppressed patient dosage, when administered to individuals 2 years or older, for subcutaneous or intramuscular use		WAIVED
	G0009	Administration of pneumococcal vaccine		WAIVED
Hepatitis B Vaccine	90740	Hepatitis B vaccine, dialysis or immunosuppressed patient dosage (3 dose schedule), for intramuscular use	A	WAIVED
	90743	Hepatitis B vaccine, adolescent (2 dose schedule), for intramuscular use		WAIVED
	90744	Hepatitis B vaccine, pediatric/adolescent dosage (3 dose schedule), for intramuscular use		WAIVED
	90746	Hepatitis B vaccine, adult dosage, for intramuscular use		WAIVED
	90747	Hepatitis B vaccine, dialysis or immunosuppressed patient dosage (4 dose schedule), for intramuscular use		WAIVED
	G0010	Administration of hepatitis B vaccine		WAIVED
HIV Screening	G0432	Infectious agent antigen detection by enzyme immunoassay (EIA) technique, qualitative or semi-qualitative, multiple-step method, HIV-1 or HIV-2, screening	A	WAIVED
	G0433	Infectious agent antigen detection by enzyme-linked immunosorbent assay (ELISA) technique, antibody, HIV-1 or HIV-2, screening		WAIVED
	G0435	Infectious agent antigen detection by rapid antibody test of oral mucosa transudate, HIV-1 or HIV-2 , screening		WAIVED

Service	CPT/HCPCS Code	Long Descriptor	USPSTF Rating	Coins /Deductible
Smoking Cessation	G0436	Smoking and tobacco cessation counseling visit for the asymptomatic patient; intermediate, greater than 3 minutes, up to 10 minutes	A	WAIVED
	G0437	Smoking and tobacco cessation counseling visit for the asymptomatic patient intensive, greater than 10 minutes		WAIVED
Annual Wellness Visit	G0438	Annual wellness visit, including PPPS, first visit	*Not Rated	WAIVED
	G0439	Annual wellness visit, including PPPS, subsequent visit		WAIVED

100-4, 18, 10.2.1

Healthcare Common Procedure Coding System (HCPCS) and Diagnosis Codes

Vaccines and their administration are reported using separate codes. The following codes are for reporting the vaccines only.

HCPCS	Definition
90655	Influenza virus vaccine, split virus, preservative free, for children 6-35 months of age, for intramuscular use;
90656	Influenza virus vaccine, split virus, preservative free, for use in individuals 3 years and above, for intramuscular use;
90657	Influenza virus vaccine, split virus, for children 6-35 months of age, for intramuscular use;
90658	Influenza virus vaccine, split virus, for use in individuals 3 years of age and above, for intramuscular use;
90660	Influenza virus vaccine, live, for intranasal use;
90662	Influenza virus vaccine, split virus, preservative free, enhanced immunogenicity via increased antigen content, for intramuscular use
90669	Pneumococcal conjugate vaccine, polyvalent, for children under 5 years, for intramuscular use
90670	Pneumococcal conjugate vaccine, 13 valent, for intramuscular use
90732	Pneumococcal polysaccharide vaccine, 23-valent, adult or immunosuppressed patient dosage, for use in individuals 2 years or older, for subcutaneous or intramuscular use;
90740	Hepatitis B vaccine, dialysis or immunosuppressed patient dosage (3 dose schedule), for intramuscular use;
90743	Hepatitis B vaccine, adolescent (2 dose schedule), for intramuscular use;
90744	Hepatitis B vaccine, pediatric/adolescent dosage (3 dose schedule), for intramuscular use;
90746	Hepatitis B vaccine, adult dosage, for intramuscular use; and
90747	Hepatitis B vaccine, dialysis or immunosuppressed patient dosage (4 dose schedule), for intramuscular use.

The following codes are for reporting administration of the vaccines only. The administration of the vaccines is billed using:

HCPCS	Definition
G0008	Administration of influenza virus vaccine;
G0009	Administration of pneumococcal vaccine; and
*G0010	Administration of hepatitis B vaccine.
*90471	Immunization administration. (For OPPS hospitals billing for the hepatitis B vaccine administration)
*90472	Each additional vaccine. (For OPPS hospitals billing for the hepatitis B vaccine administration)

* **NOTE:** For claims with dates of service prior to January 1, 2006, OPPS and non-OPPS hospitals report G0010 for hepatitis B vaccine administration. For claims with dates of service January 1, 2006 and later, OPPS hospitals report 90471 or 90472 for hepatitis B vaccine administration as appropriate in place of G0010.

One of the following diagnosis codes must be reported as appropriate. If the sole purpose for the visit is to receive a vaccine or if a vaccine is the only service billed on a claim the applicable following diagnosis code may be used.

Diagnosis Code	Description
V03.82	Pneumococcus
V04.81**	Influenza
V06.6***	Pneumococcus and Influenza
V05.3	Hepatitis B

**Effective for influenza virus claims with dates of service October 1, 2003 and later.

***Effective October 1, 2006, providers may report diagnosis code V06.6 on claims for pneumococcus and/or influenza virus vaccines when the purpose of the visit was to receive both vaccines.

If a diagnosis code for pneumococcus, hepatitis B, or influenza virus vaccination is not reported on a claim, contractors may not enter the diagnosis on the claim. Contractors must follow current resolution processes for claims with missing diagnosis codes.

If the diagnosis code and the narrative description are correct, but the HCPCS code is incorrect, the carrier or intermediary may correct the HCPCS code and pay the claim. For example, if the reported diagnosis code is V04.81 and the narrative description (if annotated on the claim) says "flu shot" but the HCPCS code is incorrect, contractors may change the HCPCS code and pay for the flu vaccine. Effective October 1, 2006, carriers/AB MACs should follow the instructions in Pub. 100-04, Chapter 1, Section 80.3.2.1.1 (Carrier Data Element Requirements) for claims submitted without a HCPCS code.

Claims for hepatitis B vaccinations must report the I.D. Number of the referring physician. In addition, if a doctor of medicine or osteopathy does not order the influenza virus vaccine, the intermediary claims require:

- UPIN code SLF000 to be reported on claims submitted prior to May 23, 2008, when Medicare began accepting NPIs, only
- The provider's own NPI to be reported in the NPI field for the attending physician on claims submitted on or after May 23, 2008, when NPI requirements were implemented.

100-4, 18, 10.2.2.1

FI/AB MAC Payment for Pneumococcal Pneumonia Virus, and Hepatitis B Virus Vaccines and Their Administration

Payment for Vaccines

Payment for all of these vaccines is on a reasonable cost basis for hospitals, home health agencies (HHAs), skilled nursing facilities (SNFs), critical access hospitals (CAHs), and hospital-based renal dialysis facilities (RDFs). Payment for comprehensive outpatient rehabilitation facilities (CORFs), Indian Health Service hospitals (IHS), IHS CAHs and independent RDFs is based on 95 percent of the average wholesale price (AWP). Section 10.2.4 of this chapter contains information on payment of these vaccines when provided by RDFs or hospices. See Sec.10.2.2.2 for payment to independent and provider- based Rural Health Centers and Federally Qualified Health Clinics.

Payment for these vaccines is as follows:

Facility	Type of Bill	Payment
Hospitals, other than Indian Health Service (IHS) Hospitals and Critical Access Hospitals (CAHs)	12x, 13x	Reasonable cost
IHS Hospitals	12x, 13x, 83x	95% of AWP
IHS CAHs	85x	95% of AWP
CAHs Method I and Method II	85x	Reasonable cost
Skilled Nursing Facilities	22x, 23x	Reasonable cost
Home Health Agencies	34x	Reasonable cost
Comprehensive Outpatient Rehabilitation Facilities	75x	95% of the AWP
Independent Renal Dialysis Facilities	72x	95% of the AWP
Hospital-based Renal Dialysis Facilities	72x	Reasonable cost

Payment for Vaccine Administration

Payment for the administration of Influenza Virus and PPV vaccines is as follows:

Facility	Type of Bill	Payment
Hospitals, other than IHS Hospitals and CAHs	12x, 13x	Outpatient Prospective Payment System (OPPS) for hospitals subject to OPPS Reasonable cost for hospitals not subject to OPPS
IHS Hospitals	12x, 13x, 83x	MPFS as indicated in guidelines below.
IHS CAHs	85x	MPFS as indicated in guidelines below.
CAHs Method I and II	85x	Reasonable cost
Skilled Nursing Facilities	22x, 23x	MPFS as indicated in the guidelines below
Home Health Agencies	34x	OPPS
Comprehensive Outpatient Rehabilitation Facilities	75x	MPFS as indicated in the guidelines below
Independent RDFs	72x	MPFS as indicated in the guidelines below
Hospital-based RDFs	72x	Reasonable cost

Guidelines for pricing PPV and Influenza vaccine administration under the MPFS.

Make reimbursement based on the rate in the MPFS associated with the CPT code 90782 or 90471 as follows:

HCPCS code	Effective prior to March 1, 2003	Effective on and after March 1, 2003
G0008	90782	90471
G0009	90782	90471

See Sec.10.2.2.2 for payment to independent and provider based Rural Health Centers and Federally Qualified Health Clinics.

Payment for the administration of Hepatitis B vaccine is as follows:

Facility	Type of Bill	Payment
Hospitals other than IHS hospitals and CAHs	12x, 13x	Outpatient Prospective Payment System (OPPS) for hospitals subject to OPPS Reasonable cost for hospitals not subject to OPPS
IHS Hospitals	12x, 13x, 83x	MPFS as indicated in the guidelines below
CAHs Method I and II	85x	Reasonable cost
IHS CAHs	85x	MPFS as indicated in guidelines below.
Skilled Nursing Facilities	22x, 23x	MPFS as indicated in the chart below
Home Health Agencies	34x	OPPS
Comprehensive Outpatient Rehabilitation Facilities	75x	MPFS as indicated in the guidelines below
Independent RDFs	72x	MPFS as indicated in the chart below
Hospital-based RDFs	72x	Reasonable cost

Guidelines for pricing Hepatitis B vaccine administration under the MPFS.

Make reimbursement based on the rate in the MPFS associated with the CPT code 90782 or 90471 as follows:

HCPCS code	Effective prior to March 1, 2003	Effective on and after March 1, 2003
G0010	90782	90471

See Sec.10.2.2.2 for payment to independent and provider based Rural Health Centers and Federally Qualified Health Clinics.

100-4, 18, 10.4

CWF Edits

In order to prevent duplicate payments for influenza virus and pneumococcal vaccination claims by the local contractor/AB MAC and the centralized billing contractor, effective for claims received on or after July 1, 2002, CWF has implemented a number of edits.

NOTE: 90659 was discontinued December 31, 2003.

CWF returns information in Trailer 13 information from the history claim. The following fields are returned to the contractor:

- Trailer Code;
- Contractor Number;
- Document Control Number;
- First Service Date;
- Last Service Date;
- Provider, Physician, Supplier Number;
- Claim Type; Procedure code;
- Alert Code (where applicable); and,
- More history (where applicable.)

100-4, 18, 10.4.1

CWF Edits on FI/AB MAC Claims

In order to prevent duplicate payment by the same FI/AB MAC, CWF edits by line item on the FI/AB MAC number, the beneficiary Health Insurance Claim (HIC) number, and the date of service, the influenza virus procedure codes 90655, 90656, 90657, 90658, 90660, or 90662 and the pneumococcal procedure codes 90669, 90670, or 90732, and the administration codes G0008 or G0009.

If CWF receives a claim with either HCPCS codes 90655, 90656, 90657, 90658, 90660, or 90662 and it already has on record a claim with the same HIC number, same FI/AB MAC number, same date of service, and any one of those HCPCS codes, the second claim submitted to CWF rejects.

If CWF receives a claim with HCPCS codes 90669, 90670, or 90732 and it already has on record a claim with the same HIC number, same FI/AB MAC number, same date of service, and the same HCPCS code, the second claim submitted to CWF rejects when all four items match.

If CWF receives a claim with HCPCS administration codes G0008 or G0009 and it already has on record a claim with the same HIC number, same FI/AB MAC number, same date of service, and same procedure code, CWF rejects the second claim submitted when all four items match.

CWF returns to the FI/AB MAC a reject code "7262" for this edit. FIs/AB MACs must deny the second claim and use the same messages they currently use for the denial of duplicate claims.

100-4, 18, 10.4.2

CWF Edits on Carrier/AB MAC Claims

In order to prevent duplicate payment by the same carrier/AB MAC, CWF will edit by line item on the carrier/AB MAC number, the HIC number, the date of service, the influenza virus procedure codes 90655, 90656, 90657, 90658, 90660, or 90662; the pneumococcal procedure codes 90669, 90670, or 90732; and the administration code G0008 or G0009.

If CWF receives a claim with either HCPCS codes 90655, 90656, 90657, 90658, 90660, or 90662 and it already has on record a claim with the same HIC number, same carrier/AB MAC number, same date of service, and any one of those HCPCS codes, the second claim submitted to CWF will reject.

If CWF receives a claim with HCPCS codes 90669, 90670, or 90732 and it already has on record a claim with the same HIC number, same carrier/AB MAC number, same date of service, and the same HCPCS code, the second claim submitted to CWF will reject when all four items match.

If CWF receives a claim with HCPCS administration codes G0008 or G0009 and it already has on record a claim with the same HIC number, same carrier/AB MAC number, same date of service, and same procedure code, CWF will reject the second claim submitted.

CWF will return to the carrier/AB MAC a specific reject code for this edit. Carriers/AB MACs must deny the second claim and use the same messages they currently use for the denial of duplicate claims.

In order to prevent duplicate payment by the centralized billing contractor and local carrier/AB MAC, CWF will edit by line item for carrier number, same HIC number, same date of service, the influenza virus procedure codes 90655, 90656, 90657, 90658, 90660, or 90662; the pneumococcal procedure codes 90669, 90670, or 90732; and the administration code G0008 or G0009.

If CWF receives a claim with either HCPCS codes 90655, 90656, 90657, 90658, 90660, or 90662 and it already has on record a claim with a different carrier/AB MAC number, but same HIC number, same date of service, and any one of those same HCPCS codes, the second claim submitted to CWF will reject.

If CWF receives a claim with HCPCS codes 90669, 90670, or 90732 and it already has on record a claim with the same HIC number, different carrier/AB MAC number, same date of service, and the same HCPCS code, the second claim submitted to CWF will reject.

If CWF receives a claim with HCPCS administration codes G0008 or G0009 and it already has on record a claim with a different carrier/AB MAC number, but the same HIC number, same date of service, and same procedure code, CWF will reject the second claim submitted.

CWF will return a specific reject code for this edit. Carriers/AB MACs must deny the second claim. For the second edit, the reject code should automatically trigger the following Medicare Summary Notice (MSN) and Remittance Advice (RA) messages.

MSN: 7.2–"This is a duplicate of a claim processed by another contractor. You should receive a Medicare Summary Notice from them."

Claim adjustment reason code 18–duplicate claim or service

100-4, 18, 10.4.3

CWF A/B Crossover Edits for FI/AB MAC and Carrier/AB MAC Claims

When CWF receives a claim from the carrier/AB MAC, it will review Part B outpatient claims history to verify that a duplicate claim has not already been posted.

CWF will edit on the beneficiary HIC number; the date of service; the influenza virus procedure codes 90655, 90656, 90657, 90658, 90660, or 90662; the pneumococcal procedure codes 90669, 90670, or 90732; and the administration code G0008 or G0009.

CWF will return a specific reject code for this edit. Contractors must deny the second claim and use the same messages they currently use for the denial of duplicate claims.

100-4, 18, 20

Mammography Services (Screening and Diagnostic)

A. Screening Mammography

Beginning January 1, 1991, Medicare provides Part B coverage of screening mammographies for women. Screening mammographies are radiologic procedures for early detection of breast cancer and include a physician's interpretation of the results. A doctor's prescription or referral is not necessary for the procedure to be covered.

Whether payment can be made is determined by a woman's age and statutory frequency parameter. See Pub. 100-02, Medicare Benefit Policy Manual, chapter 15, section 280.3 for additional coverage information for a screening mammography.

Section 4101 of the Balanced Budget Act (BBA) of 1997 provides for annual screening mammographies for women over age 39 and waives the Part B deductible. Coverage applies as follows:

Age Groups	Screening Period
Under age 35	No payment allowed for screening mammography.
35-39	Baseline (pay for only one screening mammography performed on a woman between her 35thand 40thbirthday)
Over age 39	Annual (11 full months have elapsed following the month of last screening

NOTE:Count months between screening mammographies beginning the month after the date of the examination. For example, if Mrs. Smith received a screening mammography examination in January 2005, begin counting the next month (February 2005) until 11 months have elapsed. Payment can be made for another screening mammography in January 2006.

B. Diagnostic Mammography

A diagnostic mammography is a radiological mammogram and is a covered diagnostic test under the following conditions:

- A patient has distinct signs and symptoms for which a mammogram is indicated;
- A patient has a history of breast cancer; or
- A patient is asymptomatic, but based on the patient's history and other factors the physician considers significant, the physician's judgment is that a mammogram is appropriate.

Beginning January 1, 2005, Medicare Prescription Drug, Improvement, and Modernization Act (MMA) of 2003, Sec. 644, Public Law 108-173 has changed the way Medicare pays for diagnostic mammography. Medicare will pay based on the MPFS in lieu of OPPS or the lower of the actual change.

100-4, 18, 20.4

Billing Requirements - FI/A/B MAC Claims

Contractors use the weekly-updated MQSA file to verify that the billing facility is certified by the FDA to perform mammography services, and has the appropriate certification to perform the type of mammogram billed (film and/or digital). (See Sec.20.1.) FIs/A/B MACs use the provider number submitted on the claim to identify the facility and use the MQSA data file to verify the facility's certification(s). FIs/A/B MACs complete the following activities in processing mammography claims:

- If the provider number on the claim does not correspond with a certified mammography facility on the MQSA file, then intermediaries/A/B MACs deny the claim.
- When a film mammography HCPCS code is on a claim, the claim is checked for a "1" film indicator.
- If a film mammography HCPCS code comes in on a claim and the facility is certified for film mammography, the claim is paid if all other relevant Medicare criteria are met.
- If a film mammography HCPCS code is on a claim and the facility is certified for digital mammography only, the claim is denied.
- When a digital mammography HCPCS code is on a claim, the claim is checked for "2" digital indicator.
- If a digital mammography HCPCS code is on a claim and the facility is certified for digital mammography, the claim is paid if all other relevant Medicare criteria are met.
- If a digital mammography HCPCS code is on a claim and the facility is certified for film mammography only, the claim is denied.

NOTE: The Common Working File (CWF) no longer receives the mammography file for editing purposes.

Except as provided in the following sections for RHCs and FQHCs, the following procedures apply to billing for screening mammographies: The technical component portion of the screening mammography is billed on Form CMS-1450 under bill type 12X, 13X, 14X**, 22X, 23X or 85X using revenue code 0403 and HCPCS code 77057* (76092*).

The technical component portion of the diagnostic mammography is billed on Form CMS-1450 under bill type 12X, 13X, 14X**, 22X, 23X or 85X using revenue code 0401 and HCPCS code 77055* (76090*), 77056* (76091*), G0204 and G0206.

Separate bills are required for claims for screening mammographies with dates of service prior to January 1, 2002. Providers include on the bill only charges for the screening mammography. Separate bills are not required for claims for screening mammographies with dates of service on or after January 1, 2002.

See separate instructions below for rural health clinics (RHCs) and federally qualified health centers (FQHCs).

* For claims with dates of service prior to January 1, 2007, providers report CPT codes 76090, 76091, and 76092. For claims with dates of service January 1, 2007 and later, providers report CPT codes 77055, 77056, and 77057 respectively.

** For claims with dates of service April 1, 2005 and later, hospitals bill for all mammography services under the 13X type of bill or for dates of service April 1, 2007 and later, 12X or 13X as appropriate. The 14X type of bill is no longer applicable. Appropriate bill types for providers other than hospitals are 22X, 23X, and 85X.

In cases where screening mammography services are self-referred and as a result an attending physician NPI is not available, the provider shall duplicate their facility NPI in the attending physician identifier field on the claim.

100-4, 18, 20.5

Carrier Processing Requirements

Contractors use the weekly-updated file to verify that the billing facility is certified by the FDA to perform mammography services, and has the appropriate certification to perform the type of mammogram billed (film and/or digital). Carriers/B MACs match the FDA assigned, 6-digit mammography certification number on the claim to the FDA mammography certification number appearing on the file for the billing facility. Carriers/B MACs complete the following activities in processing mammography claims: If the claim does not contain the facility's 6-digit certification number, or if a 6-digit certification number is not reported in item 32 of the Form CMS-1500 for paper claims, or in the 2400 loop (REF 02 segment, where 01=EW segment) of the ASC X12N 837 professional claim format, version 4010A1, for electronic claims, then carriers/B MACs return the claim as unprocessable.

- If the claim contains a 6-digit certification number that is reported in the proper field or segment (as specified in the previous bullet) but such number does not correspond to the number specified in the MQSA file for the facility, then Carriers/B MACs deny the claim.
- When a film mammography HCPCS code is on a claim, the claim is checked for a "1" film indicator.
- If a film mammography HCPCS code comes in on a claim and the facility is certified for film mammography, the claim is paid if all other relevant Medicare criteria are met.
- If a film mammography HCPCS code is on a claim and the facility is certified for digital mammography only, the claim is denied.

- When a digital mammography HCPCS code is on a claim, the claim is checked for "2" digital indicator.
- If a digital mammography HCPCS code is on a claim and the facility is certified for digital mammography, the claim is paid if all other relevant Medicare criteria are met.
- If a digital mammography HCPCS code is on a claim and the facility is certified for film mammography only, the claim is denied.
- Process the claim to the point of payment based on the information provided on the claim and in carrier claims history.
- Identify the claim as a screening mammography claim by the CPT-4 code listed in field 24D and the diagnosis code(s) listed in field 21 of Form CMS-1500.
- Assign physician specialty code 45 to facilities that are certified to perform only screening mammography.
- Ensure that entities that bill globally for screening mammography contain a blank in modifier position #1.
- Ensure that entities that bill for the technical component use only HCPCS modifier "-TC." Ensure that physicians who bill the professional component separately use HCPCS modifier "-26." Send the mammography modifier to CWF in the first modifier position on the claim. If more than one modifier is necessary, e.g., if the service was performed in a rural Health Manpower Shortage Area (HMSA) facility, instruct providers to bill the mammography modifier in modifier position 1 and the rural (or other) modifier in modifier position 2.
- Ensure all those who are qualified include the 6-digit FDA-assigned certification number of the screening center in field 32 of Form CMS-1500 and in the REF02
- segment (where 01 = EW segment) of the 2400 loop for the ASC X12N 837 professional claim format, version 4010A1. Carriers/B MACs retain this number in their provider files.
- Waive Part B deductible and apply coinsurance for a screening mammography.
- Add diagnosis code V76.12 if a claim comes in for screening mammography without a diagnosis and the carrier file data shows this is appropriate. If there are other diagnoses on the claim, but not code V76.12, add it. (Do not change or overlay code V76.12 but ADD it). At a minimum, edit for age, frequency, and place of service (POS).
- After May 23, 2008, accept the screening mammography facility's NPI number in place of the attending/referring physician NPI number for self-referred mammography claims.

NOTE: Beginning October 1, 2003, carriers/B MACs are no longer permitted to add the ICD-9 code for a screening mammography when the screening mammography claim has no diagnosis code. Screening mammography claims with no diagnosis code must be returned as unprocessable for assigned claims. For unassigned claims, deny the claim.

Carrier Provider Education

- Educate providers that when a screening mammography turns to a diagnostic mammography on the same day for the same beneficiary, add the "-GG" modifier to the diagnostic code and bill both codes on the same claim. Both services are reimbursable by Medicare.
- Educate providers that they cannot bill an add-on code without also billing for the appropriate mammography code. If just the add-on code is billed, the service will be denied. Both the add-on code and the appropriate mammography code should be on the same claim.
- Educate providers to submit their own NPI in place of an attending/referring physician NPI in cases where screening mammography services are self-referred.

100-4, 18, 60.1

Payment

Payment (contractor) is under the MPFS except as follows:

- Fecal occult blood tests (82270* (G0107*) and G0328) are paid under the clinical diagnostic lab fee schedule except reasonable cost is paid to all non-OPPS hospitals, including CAHs, but not IHS hospitals billing on TOB 83x. IHS hospitals billing on TOB 83x are paid the ASC payment amount. Other IHS hospitals (billing on TOB 13x) are paid the OMB approved AIR, or the facility specific per visit amount as applicable. Deductible and coinsurance do not apply for these tests. See section A below for payment to Maryland waiver on TOB 13X. Payment from all hospitals for non-patient laboratory specimens on TOB 14X will be based on the clinical diagnostic fee schedule, including CAHs and Maryland waiver hospitals
- Flexible sigmoidoscopy (code G0104) is paid under OPPS for hospital outpatient departments and on a reasonable cost basis for CAHs; or current payment methodologies for hospitals not subject to OPPS.
- Colonoscopies (G0105 and G0121) and barium enemas (G0106 and G0120) are paid under OPPS for hospital outpatient departments and on a reasonable costs basis for CAHs or current payment methodologies for hospitals not subject to OPPS. Also colonoscopies may be done in an Ambulatory Surgical Center (ASC) and when done in an ASC the ASC rate applies. The ASC rate is the same for diagnostic and screening colonoscopies. The ASC rate is paid to IHS hospitals when the service is billed on TOB 83x.

Prior to January 1, 2007, deductible and coinsurance apply to HCPCS codes G0104, G0105, G0106, G0120, and G0121. Beginning with services provided on or after January 1, 2007, Section 5113 of the Deficit Reduction Act of 2005 waives the requirement of the annual Part B deductible for these screening services. Coinsurance still applies. Coinsurance and deductible applies to the diagnostic colorectal service codes listed below.

The following screening codes must be paid at rates consistent with the diagnostic codes indicated.

Screening Code	Diagnostic Code
G0104	45330
G0105 and G0121	45378
G0106 and G0120	74280

A. Special Payment Instructions for TOB 13X Maryland Waiver Hospitals
For hospitals in Maryland under the jurisdiction of the Health Services Cost Review Commission, screening colorectal services HCPCS codes G0104, G0105, G0106, 82270* (G0107*), G0120, G0121 and G0328 are paid according to the terms of the waiver, that is 94% of submitted charges minus any unmet existing deductible, co-insurance and non-covered charges. Maryland Hospitals bill TOB 13X for outpatient colorectal cancer screenings.

B. Special Payment Instructions for Non-Patient Laboratory Specimen (TOB 14X) for all hospitals
Payment for colorectal cancer screenings (82270* (G0107*) and G0328) to a hospital for a non-patient laboratory specimen (TOB 14X), is the lesser of the actual charge, the fee schedule amount, or the National Limitation Amount (NLA), (including CAHs and Maryland Waiver hospitals). Part B deductible and coinsurance do not apply.

*NOTE: For claims with dates of service prior to January 1, 2007, physicians, suppliers, and providers report HCPCS code G0107. Effective January 1, 2007, code G0107 is discontinued and replaced with CPT code 82270.

100-4, 18, 60.2

HCPCS Codes, Frequency Requirements, and Age Requirements (If Applicable)

Effective for services furnished on or after January 1, 1998, the following codes are used for colorectal cancer screening services:

- 82270* (G0107*) - Colorectal cancer screening; fecal-occult blood tests, 1-3 simultaneous determinations;
- G0104 - Colorectal cancer screening; flexible sigmoidoscopy;
- G0105 - Colorectal cancer screening; colonoscopy on individual at high risk;
- G0106 - Colorectal cancer screening; barium enema; as an alternative to G0104, screening sigmoidoscopy;
- G0120 - Colorectal cancer screening; barium enema; as an alternative to G0105, screening colonoscopy.

Effective for services furnished on or after July 1, 2001, the following codes are used for colorectal cancer screening services:

- G0121 - Colorectal cancer screening; colonoscopy on individual not meeting criteria for high risk. Note that the description for this code has been revised to remove the term "noncovered."
- G0122 - Colorectal cancer screening; barium enema (noncovered).

Effective for services furnished on or after January 1, 2004, the following code is used for colorectal cancer screening services as an alternative to 82270* (G0107*):

- G0328 - Colorectal cancer screening; immunoassay, fecal-occult blood test, 1-3 simultaneous determinations

*NOTE: For claims with dates of service prior to January 1, 2007, physicians, suppliers, and providers report HCPCS code G0107. Effective January 1, 2007, code G0107 is discontinued and replaced with CPT code 82270.

G0104 - Colorectal Cancer Screening; Flexible Sigmoidoscopy
Screening flexible sigmoidoscopies (code G0104) may be paid for beneficiaries who have attained age 50, when performed by a doctor of medicine or osteopathy at the frequencies noted below.

For claims with dates of service on or after January 1, 2002, contractors pay for screening flexible sigmoidoscopies (code G0104) for beneficiaries who have attained age 50 when these services were performed by a doctor of medicine or osteopathy, or by a physician assistant, nurse practitioner, or clinical nurse specialist (as defined in Sec.1861(aa)(5) of the Act and in the Code of Federal Regulations at42 CFR 410.74, 410.75, and410.76) at the frequencies noted above. For claims with dates of service prior to January 1, 2002, contractors pay for these services under the conditions noted only when a doctor of medicine or osteopathy performs them.

For services furnished from January 1, 1998, through June 30, 2001, inclusive:

- Once every 48 months (i.e., at least 47 months have passed following the month in which the last covered screening flexible sigmoidoscopy was done).

For services furnished on or after July 1, 2001:

- Once every 48 months as calculated above unless the beneficiary does not meet the criteria for high risk of developing colorectal cancer (refer to Sec.60.3 of this chapter) and he/she has had a screening colonoscopy (code G0121) within the preceding 10 years. If such a beneficiary has had a screening colonoscopy within the preceding 10 years, then he or she can have covered a screening flexible sigmoidoscopy only after at least 119 months have passed following the month that he/she received the screening colonoscopy (code G0121).

NOTE:If during the course of a screening flexible sigmoidoscopy a lesion or growth is detected which results in a biopsy or removal of the growth; the appropriate diagnostic procedure classified as a flexible sigmoidoscopy with biopsy or removal should be billed and paid rather than code G0104.

G0105 - Colorectal Cancer Screening; Colonoscopy on Individual at High Risk
Screening colonoscopies (code G0105) may be paid when performed by a doctor of medicine or osteopathy at a frequency of once every 24 months for beneficiaries at high risk for developing colorectal cancer (i.e., at least 23 months have passed following the month in which the last covered G0105 screening colonoscopy was performed). Refer to Sec.60.3of this chapter for the criteria to use in determining whether or not an individual is at high risk for developing colorectal cancer.

NOTE: If during the course of the screening colonoscopy, a lesion or growth is detected which results in a biopsy or removal of the growth, the appropriate diagnostic procedure classified as a colonoscopy with biopsy or removal should be billed and paid rather than code G0105.

A. Colonoscopy Cannot be Completed Because of Extenuating Circumstances

1. FIs
   When a covered colonoscopy is attempted but cannot be completed because of extenuating circumstances, Medicare will pay for the interrupted colonoscopy as long as the coverage conditions are met for the incomplete procedure. However, the frequency standards associated with screening colonoscopies will not be applied by CWF. When a covered colonoscopy is next attempted and completed, Medicare will pay for that colonoscopy according to its payment methodology for this procedure as long as coverage conditions are met, and the frequency standards will be applied by CWF. This policy is applied to both screening and diagnostic colonoscopies.

   When submitting a facility claim for the interrupted colonoscopy, providers are to suffix the colonoscopy HCPCS codes with a modifier of "-73" or" -74" as appropriate to indicate that the procedure was interrupted. Payment for covered incomplete screening colonoscopies shall be consistent with payment methodologies currently in place for complete screening colonoscopies, including those contained in42 CFR 419.44(b). In situations where a critical access hospital (CAH) has elected payment Method II for CAH patients, payment shall be consistent with payment methodologies currently in place as outlined in Chapter 3. As such, instruct CAHs that elect Method II payment to use modifier "-53" to identify an incomplete screening colonoscopy (physician professional service(s) billed in revenue code 096X, 097X, and/or 098X). Such CAHs will also bill the technical or facility component of the interrupted colonoscopy in revenue code 075X (or other appropriate revenue code) using the "-73" or "-74" modifier as appropriate.

   Note that Medicare would expect the provider to maintain adequate information in the patient's medical record in case it is needed by the contractor to document the incomplete procedure.

2. Carriers
   When a covered colonoscopy is attempted but cannot be completed because of extenuating circumstances (see Chapter 12), Medicare will pay for the interrupted colonoscopy at a rate consistent with that of a flexible sigmoidoscopy as long as coverage conditions are met for the incomplete procedure. When a covered colonoscopy is next attempted and completed, Medicare will pay for that colonoscopy according to its payment methodology for this procedure as long as coverage conditions are met. This policy is applied to both screening and diagnostic colonoscopies.

   When submitting a claim for the interrupted colonoscopy, professional providers are to suffix the colonoscopy code with a modifier of "-53" to indicate that the procedure was interrupted. When submitting a claim for the facility fee associated with this procedure, Ambulatory Surgical Centers (ASCs) are to suffix the colonoscopy code with "-73" or "-74" as appropriate. Payment for covered screening colonoscopies, including that for the associated ASC facility fee when applicable, shall be consistent with payment for diagnostic colonoscopies, whether the procedure is complete or incomplete.

   Note that Medicare would expect the provider to maintain adequate information in the patient's medical record in case it is needed by the contractor to document the incomplete procedure.

G0106 - Colorectal Cancer Screening; Barium Enema; as an Alternative to G0104, Screening Sigmoidoscopy
Screening barium enema examinations may be paid as an alternative to a screening sigmoidoscopy (code G0104). The same frequency parameters for screening sigmoidoscopies (see those codes above) apply. In the case of an individual aged 50 or over, payment may be made for a screening barium enema examination (code G0106) performed after at least 47 months have passed following the month in which the last screening barium enema or screening flexible sigmoidoscopy was performed. For example, the beneficiary received a screening barium enema examination as an alternative to a screening flexible sigmoidoscopy in January 1999. Start counts beginning February 1999. The beneficiary is eligible for another screening barium enema in January 2003. The screening barium enema must be ordered in writing after a determination that the test is the appropriate screening test. Generally, it is expected that this will be a screening double contrast enema unless the individual is unable to withstand such an exam. This means that in the case of a particular individual, the attending physician must determine that the estimated screening potential for the barium enema is equal to or greater than the screening potential that has been estimated for a screening flexible sigmoidoscopy for the same individual. The screening single contrast barium enema also requires a written order from the beneficiary's attending physician in the same manner as described above for the screening double contrast barium enema examination.

82270* (G0107*) - Colorectal Cancer Screening; Fecal-Occult Blood Test, 1-3 Simultaneous Determinations
Effective for services furnished on or after January 1, 1998, screening FOBT (code 82270* (G0107*) may be paid for beneficiaries who have attained age 50, and at a frequency of once every 12 months (i.e., at least 11 months have passed following the month in which the last covered screening FOBT was performed). This screening FOBT means a guaiac-based test for peroxidase activity, in which the beneficiary completes it by taking samples from two different sites of three consecutive stools. This screening requires a written order from the beneficiary's attending physician. (The term "attending physician" is defined to mean a doctor of medicine or osteopathy (as defined in Sec.1861(r)(1)of the Act) who is fully knowledgeable about the beneficiary's medical condition, and who would be responsible for using the results of any examination performed in the overall management of the beneficiary's specific medical problem.)

Effective for services furnished on or after January 1, 2004, payment may be made for a immunoassay-based FOBT (G0328, described below) as an alternative to the guaiacbased FOBT, 82270* (G0107*). Medicare will pay for only one covered FOBT per year, either 82270* (G0107*) or G0328, but not both.

*NOTE: For claims with dates of service prior to January 1, 2007, physicians, suppliers, and providers report HCPCS code G0107. Effective January 1, 2007, code G0107 is discontinued and replaced with CPT code 82270.

G0328 - Colorectal Cancer Screening; Immunoassay, Fecal-Occult Blood Test, 1-3 Simultaneous Determinations
Effective for services furnished on or after January 1, 2004, screening FOBT, (code G0328) may be paid as an alternative to 82270* (G0107*) for beneficiaries who have attained age 50. Medicare will pay for a covered FOBT (either 82270* (G0107*) or G0328, but not both) at a frequency of once every 12 months (i.e., at least 11 months have passed following the month in which the last covered screening FOBT was performed). Screening FOBT, immunoassay, includes the use of a spatula to collect the appropriate number of samples or the use of a special brush for the collection of samples, as determined by the individual manufacturer's instructions. This screening requires a written order from the beneficiary's attending physician. (The term "attending physician" is defined to mean a doctor of medicine or osteopathy (as defined in Sec.1861(r)(1) of the Act) who is fully knowledgeable about the beneficiary's medical condition, and who would be responsible for using the results of any examination performed in the overall management of the beneficiary's specific medical problem.)

G0120 - Colorectal Cancer Screening; Barium Enema; as an Alternative to or G0105, Screening Colonoscopy
Screening barium enema examinations may be paid as an alternative to a screening colonoscopy (code G0105) examination. The same frequency parameters for screening colonoscopies (see those codes above) apply. In the case of an individual who is at high risk for colorectal cancer, payment may be made for a screening barium enema examination (code G0120) performed after at least 23 months have passed following the month in which the last screening barium enema or the last screening colonoscopy was performed. For example, a beneficiary at high risk for developing colorectal cancer received a screening barium enema examination (code G0120) as an alternative to a screening colonoscopy (code G0105) in January 2000. Start counts beginning February 2000. The beneficiary is eligible for another screening barium enema examination (code G0120) in January 2002. The screening barium enema must be ordered in writing after a determination that the test is the appropriate screening test. Generally, it is expected that this will be a screening double contrast enema unless the individual is unable to withstand such an exam. This means that in the case of a particular individual, the attending physician must determine that the estimated screening potential for the barium enema is equal to or greater than the screening potential that has been estimated for a screening colonoscopy, for the same individual. The screening single contrast barium enema also requires a written order from the beneficiary's attending physician in the same manner as described above for the screening double contrast barium enema examination.

G0121 - Colorectal Screening; Colonoscopy on Individual Not Meeting Criteria for High Risk - Applicable On and After July 1, 2001
Effective for services furnished on or after July 1, 2001, screening colonoscopies (code G0121) performed on individuals not meeting the criteria for being at high risk for developing colorectal cancer (refer to Sec.60.3 of this chapter) may be paid under the following conditions:

- At a frequency of once every 10 years (i.e., at least 119 months have passed following the month in which the last covered G0121 screening colonoscopy was performed.)
- If the individual would otherwise qualify to have covered a G0121 screening colonoscopy based on the above but has had a covered screening flexible sigmoidoscopy (code G0104), then he or she may have covered a G0121 screening colonoscopy only after at least 47 months have passed following the month in which the last covered G0104 flexible sigmoidoscopy was performed.

NOTE: If during the course of the screening colonoscopy, a lesion or growth is detected which results in a biopsy or removal of the growth, the appropriate diagnostic procedure classified as a colonoscopy with biopsy or removal should be billed and paid rather than code G0121.

G0122 - Colorectal Cancer Screening; Barium Enema
The code is not covered by Medicare.

100-4, 18, 60.6

Billing Requirements for Claims Submitted to FIs

(Follow the general bill review instructions in Chapter 25. Hospitals use the ANSI X12N 837I to bill the FI or on the hardcopy Form CMS-1450. Hospitals bill revenue codes and HCPCS codes as follows:

Screening Test/Procedure	***Revenue Code***	***HCPCS Code***	***TOB***
Fecal Occult blood test	030X	82270*** (G0107***), G0328	12X, 13X, 14X**, 22X, 23X, 83X, 85X
Barium enema	032X	G0106, G0120, G0122	12X, 13X, 22X, 23X, 85X****
Flexible Sigmoidoscopy	*	G0104	12X, 13X, 22X, 23X, 83X, 85X****

Screening Test/Procedure	*Revenue Code*	*HCPCS Code*	*TOB*
Colonoscopy-high risk	*	G0105, G0121	12X, 13X, 22X, 23X, 83X, 85X****

* The appropriate revenue code when reporting any other surgical procedure.

** 14X is only applicable for non-patient laboratory specimens.

*** For claims with dates of service prior to January 1, 2007, physicians, suppliers, and providers report HCPCS code G0107. Effective January 1, 2007, code G0107, is discontinued and replaced with CPT code 82270.

**** CAHs that elect Method II bill revenue code 096X, 097X, and/or 098X for professional services and 075X (or other appropriate revenue code) for the technical or facility component.

Special Billing Instructions for Hospital Inpatients

When these tests/procedures are provided to inpatients of a hospital or when Part A benefits have been exhausted, they are covered under this benefit. However, the provider bills on bill type 12X using the discharge date of the hospital stay to avoid editing in the Common Working File (CWF) as a result of the hospital bundling rules.

100-4, 18, 80.2

A/B Medicare Administrative Contractor (MAC) and Contractor Billing Requirements

Effective for dates of service on and after January 1, 2005, through December 31, 2008, contractors shall recognize the HCPCS codes G0344, G0366, G0367, and G0368 shown above in §80.1 for an IPPE. The type of service (TOS) for each of these codes is as follows:

G0344: TOS = 1

G0366: TOS = 5

G0367: TOS = 5

G0368: TOS = 5

Contractors shall pay physicians or qualified nonphysician practitioners for only one IPPE performed not later than 6 months after the date the individual's first coverage begins under Medicare Part B, but only if that coverage period begins on or after January 1, 2005.

Effective for dates of service on and after January 1, 2009, contractors shall recognize the HCPCS codes G0402, G0403, G0404, and G0405 shown above in §80.1 for an IPPE. The TOS for each of these codes is as follows:

G0402: TOS = 1

G0403: TOS = 5

G0404: TOS = 5

G0405: TOS = 5

Under the MIPPA of 2008, contractors shall pay physicians or qualified nonphysician practitioners for only one IPPE performed not later than 12 months after the date the individual's first coverage begins under Medicare Part B only if that coverage period begins on or after January 1, 2009.

Contractors shall allow payment for a medically necessary Evaluation and Management (E/M) service at the same visit as the IPPE when it is clinically appropriate. Physicians and qualified nonphysician practitioners shall use CPT codes 99201-99215 to report an E/M with CPT modifier 25 to indicate that the E/M is a significant, separately identifiable service from the IPPE code reported (G0344 or G0402, whichever applies based on the date the IPPE is performed). Refer to chapter 12, § 30.6.1.1, of this manual for the physician/practitioner billing correct coding and payment policy regarding E/M services.

If the EKG performed as a component of the IPPE is not performed by the primary physician or qualified NPP during the IPPE visit, another physician or entity may perform and/or interpret the EKG. The referring physician or qualified NPP needs to make sure that the performing physician or entity bills the appropriate G code for the screening EKG, and not a CPT code in the 93000 series. Both the IPPE and the EKG should be billed in order for the beneficiary to receive the complete IPPE service. Effective for dates of service on and after January 1, 2009, the screening EKG is optional and is no longer a mandated service of an IPPE if performed as a result of a referral from an IPPE.

Should the same physician or NPP need to perform an additional medically necessary EKG in the 93000 series on the same day as the IPPE, report the appropriate EKG CPT code(s) with modifier 59, indicating that the EKG is a distinct procedural service.

Physicians or qualified nonphysician practitioners shall bill the contractor the appropriate HCPCS codes for IPPE on the Form CMS-1500 claim or an approved electronic format. The HCPCS codes for an IPPE and screening EKG are paid under the Medicare Physician Fee Schedule (MPFS). The appropriate deductible and coinsurance applies to codes G0344, G0366, G0367, G0368, G0403, G0404, and G0405. The deductible is waived for code G0402 but the coinsurance still applies.

100-4, 18, 150

Counseling to Prevent Tobacco Use

Effective for claims with dates of service on and after August 25, 2010, the Centers for Medicare & Medicaid Services (CMS) will cover counseling to prevent tobacco use services for outpatient and hospitalized Medicare beneficiaries:

1. Who use tobacco, regardless of whether they have signs or symptoms of tobacco-related disease;
2. Who are competent and alert at the time that counseling is provided; and,
3. Whose counseling is furnished by a qualified physician or other Medicare-recognized practitioner. These individuals who do not have signs or symptoms of tobacco-related disease will be covered under Medicare Part B when the above conditions of coverage are met, subject to certain frequency and other limitations.

Conditions of Medicare Part A and Medicare Part B coverage for counseling to prevent tobacco use are located in the Medicare National Coverage Determinations (NCD) Manual, Publication 100-3, chapter 1, section 210.4.1.

100-4, 18, 150.1

Healthcare Common Procedure Coding System (HCPCS) and Diagnosis Coding

The CMS has created two new G codes for billing for tobacco cessation counseling services to prevent tobacco use for those individuals who use tobacco but do not have signs or symptoms of tobacco-related disease. These are in addition to the two CPT codes 99406 and 99407 that currently are used for smoking and tobacco-use cessation counseling for symptomatic individuals.

The following HCPCS codes should be reported when billing for counseling to prevent tobacco use effective January 1, 2011:

G0436 Smoking and tobacco cessation counseling visit for the asymptomatic patient; intermediate, greater than 3 minutes, up to 10 minutes

Short descriptor: Tobacco-use counsel 3-10 min

G0437 Smoking and tobacco cessation counseling visit for the asymptomatic patient; intensive, greater than 10 minutes

Short descriptor: Tobacco-use counsel >10min

NOTE: The above G codes will not be active in contractors' systems until January 1, 2011. Therefore, contractors shall advise non-outpatient perspective payment system (OPPS) providers to use unlisted code 99199 to bill for counseling to prevent tobacco use and tobacco-related disease services during the interim period of August 25, 2010, through December 31, 2010.

On January 3, 2011, contractor's systems will accept the new G codes for services performed on or after August 25, 2010.

Two new C codes have been created for facilities paid under OPPS when billing for counseling to prevent tobacco use and tobacco-related disease services during the interim period of August 25, 2010, through December 31, 2010:

C9801 Smoking and tobacco cessation counseling visit for the asymptomatic patient, intermediate, greater than 3 minutes, up to 10 minutes

Short descriptor: Tobacco-use counsel 3-10 min

C9802 Smoking and tobacco cessation counseling visit for the asymptomatic patient, intensive, greater than 10 minutes

Short descriptor: Tobacco-use counsel >10min

Claims for smoking and tobacco use cessation counseling services G0436 and G0437 shall be submitted with diagnosis code V15.82, history of tobacco use, or 305.1, non-dependent tobacco use disorder.

Contractors shall allow payment for a medically necessary E/M service on the same day as the smoking and tobacco-use cessation counseling service when it is clinically appropriate. Physicians and qualified non-physician practitioners shall use an appropriate HCPCS code to report an E/M service with modifier -25 to indicate that the E/M service is a separately identifiable service from G0436 or G0437.

100-4, 18, 150.2

Carrier Billing Requirements

Carriers shall pay for counseling to prevent tobacco use services billed with code G0436 or G0437 for dates of service on or after January 1, 2011. Carriers shall pay for counseling services billed with code 99199 for dates of service performed on or after August 25, 2010 through December 31, 2010. The type of service (TOS) for each of the new codes is 1.

Carriers pay for counseling services billed based on the Medicare Physician Fee Schedule (MPFS). Deductible and coinsurance apply for services performed on August 25, 2010, through December 31, 2010. For claims with dates of service on and after January 1, 2011, coinsurance and deductible do not apply on G0436 and G0437.

Physicians or qualified non-physician practitioners shall bill the carrier for counseling to prevent tobacco use services on Form CMS-1500 or an approved electronic format.

NOTE: The above G codes will not be active in contractors' systems until January 1, 2011. Therefore, contractors shall advise providers to use unlisted code 99199 to bill for counseling to prevent tobacco use services during the interim period of August 25, 2010, through December 31, 2010.

100-4, 18, 150.2.1

Fiscal Intermediary (FI) Billing Requirements

The FIs shall pay for counseling to prevent tobacco use services with codes G0436 and G0437 for dates of service on or after January 1, 2011. FIs shall pay for counseling services billed with code 99199 for dates of service performed on or after August 25, 2010, through December 31, 2010. For facilities paid under OPPS, FIs shall pay for counseling services billed with codes C9801 and C9802 for dates of service performed on or after August 25, 2010, through December 31, 2010.

Claims for counseling to prevent tobacco use services should be submitted on Form CMS-1450 or its electronic equivalent.

The applicable bill types are 12X, 13X, 22X, 23X, 34X, 71X, 77X, and 85X.

Payment for outpatient services is as follows:

Type of Facility	*Method of Payment*
Rural Health Centers (RHCs) TOB 71X/Federally Qualified Health Centers (FQHCs)TOB 77X	All-inclusive rate (AIR) for the encounter
Hospitals TOBs 12X and 13X	OPPS for hospitals subject to OPPS MPFS for hospitals not subject to OPPS
Indian Health Services (IHS) Hospitals TOB 13X	AIR for the encounter
Skilled Nursing Facilities (SNFs) TOBs 22X and 23X	Medicare Physician Fee Schedule (MPFS)
Home Health Agencies (HHAs) TOB 34X	MPFS
Critical Access Hospitals (CAHs) TOB 85X	Method I: Technical services are paid at 101% of reasonable cost. Method II: technical services are paid at 101% of reasonable cost, and Professional services are paid at 115% of the MPFS Data Base
IHS CAHs TOB 85X	Based on specific rate
Maryland Hospitals	Payment is based according to the Health Services Cost Review Commission (HSCRC). That is 94% of submitted charges subject to any unmet deductible, coinsurance, and non-covered charges policies.

100-4, 18, 150.4

Common Working File (CWF)

The Common Working File (CWF) shall edit for the frequency of service limitations of counseling to prevent tobacco use sessions and smoking and tobacco-use cessation counseling services (G0436, G0437, 99406, 99407) rendered to a beneficiary for a combined total of 8 sessions within a 12-month period. The beneficiary may receive another 8 sessions during a second or subsequent year after 11 full months have passed since the first Medicare covered counseling session was performed. To start the count for the second or subsequent 12-month period, begin with the month after the month in which the first Medicare covered counseling session was performed and count until 11 full months have elapsed.

By entering the beneficiary's health insurance claim number (HICN), providers have the capability to view the number of sessions a beneficiary has received for this service via inquiry through CWF.

100-4, 20, 100.2.2

Evidence of Medical Necessity for Parenteral and Enteral Nutrition (PEN) Therapy

The PEN coverage is determined by information provided by the treating physician and the PEN supplier. A completed certification of medical necessity (CMN) must accompany and support initial claims for PEN to establish whether coverage criteria are met and to ensure that the PEN therapy provided is consistent with the attending or ordering physician's prescription.

Contractors ensure that the CMN contains pertinent information from the treating physician. Uniform specific medical data facilitate the review and promote consistency in coverage determinations and timelier claims processing.The medical and prescription information on a PEN CMN can be most appropriatelycompleted by the treating physician or from information in the patient's records by an employee of the physician for the physician's review and signature.

Although PEN suppliers sometimes may assist in providing the PEN services, they cannot complete the CMN since they do not have the same access to patient information needed to properly enter medical or prescription information. Contractors use appropriate professional relations issuances, training sessions, and meetings to ensure that all persons and PEN suppliers are aware of this limitation of their role. When properly completed, the PEN CMN includes the elements of a prescription as well as other data needed to determine whether Medicare coverage is possible. This practice will facilitate prompt delivery of PEN services and timely submittal of the related claim.

100-4, 32, 10.1

Ambulatory Blood Pressure Monitoring (ABPM) Billing Requirements

A. Coding Applicable to Local Carriers & Fiscal Intermediaries (FIs)

Effective April 1, 2002, a National Coverage Decision was made to allow for Medicare coverage of ABPM for those beneficiaries with suspected "white coat hypertension" (WCH). ABPM involves the use of a non-invasive device, which is used to measure blood pressure in 24-hour cycles. These 24-hour measurements are stored in the device and are later interpreted by a physician. Suspected "WCH" is defined as: (1) Clinic/office blood pressure >140/90 mm Hg on at least three separate clinic/office visits with two separate measurements made at each visit; (2) At least two documented separate blood pressure measurements taken outside the clinic/office which are < 140/90 mm Hg; and (3) No evidence of end-organ damage. ABPM is not covered for any other uses. Coverage policy can be found in Medicare National Coverage Determinations Manual, Chapter 1, Section 20.19. (www.cms.hhs.gov/masnuals/103 cov determ/ncd103index.asp).

The ABPM must be performed for at least 24 hours to meet coverage criteria. Payment is not allowed for institutionalized beneficiaries, such as those receiving Medicare covered skilled nursing in a facility. In the rare circumstance that ABPM needs to be performed more than once for a beneficiary, the qualifying criteria described above must be met for each subsequent ABPM test.

Effective dates for applicable Common Procedure Coding System (HCPCS) codes for ABPM for suspected WCH and their covered effective dates are as follows:

HCPCS	Definition	Effective Date
93784	ABPM, utilizing a system such as magnetic tape and/or computer disk, for 24 hours or longer; including recording, scanning analysis, interpretation and report.	04/01/2002
93786	ABPM, utilizing a system such as magnetic tape and/or computer disk, for 24 hours or longer; recording only.	04/01/2002
93788	ABPM, utilizing a system such as magnetic tape and/or computer disk, for 24 hours or longer; scanning analysis with report.	01/01/2004

HCPCS Definition Effective Date

93790	ABPM, utilizing a system such as magnetic tape and/or computer disk, for 24 hours or longer; physician review with interpretation and report.	04/01/2002

In addition, the following diagnosis code must be present:

Diagnosis Code	Description
796.2	Elevated blood pressure reading without diagnosis of hypertension.

B. FI Billing Instructions

The applicable types of bills acceptable when billing for ABPM services are 13X, 23X, 71X, 73X, 75X, and 85X. Chapter 25 of this manual provides general billing instructions that must be followed for bills submitted to FIs. The FIs pay for hospital outpatient ABPM services billed on a 13X type of bill with HCPCS 93786 and/or 93788 as follows: (1) Outpatient Prospective Payment System (OPPS) hospitals pay based on the Ambulatory Payment Classification (APC); (2) non-OPPS hospitals (Indian Health Services Hospitals, Hospitals that provide Part B services only, and hospitals located in American Samoa, Guam, Saipan and the Virgin Islands) pay based on reasonable cost, except for Maryland Hospitals which are paid based on a percentage of cost. Effective 4/1/06, type of bill 14X is for non-patient laboratory specimens and is no longer applicable for ABPM.

The FIs pay for comprehensive outpatient rehabilitation facility (CORF) ABPM services billed on a 75x type of bill with HCPCS code 93786 and/or 93788 based on the Medicare Physician Fee Schedule (MPFS) amount for that HCPCS code.

The FIs pay for ABPM services for critical access hospitals (CAHs) billed on a 85x type of bill as follows: (1) for CAHs that elected the Standard Method and billed HCPCS code 93786 and/or 93788, pay based on reasonable cost for that HCPCS code; and (2) for CAHs that elected the Optional Method and billed any combination of HCPCS codes 93786, 93788 and 93790 pay based on reasonable cost for HCPCS 93786 and 93788 and pay 115% of the MPFS amount for HCPCS 93790.

The FIs pay for ABPM services for skilled nursing facility (SNF) outpatients billed on a 23x type of bill with HCPCS code 93786 and/or 93788, based on the MPFS.

The FIs accept independent and provider-based rural health clinic (RHC) bills for visits under the all-inclusive rate when the RHC bills on a 71x type of bill with revenue code 052x for providing the professional component of ABPM services. The FIs should not make a separate payment to a RHC for the professional component of ABPM services in

addition to the all-inclusive rate. RHCs are not required to use ABPM HCPCS codes for professional services covered under the all-inclusive rate.

The FIs accept free-standing and provider-based federally qualified health center (FQHC) bills for visits under the all-inclusive rate when the FQHC bills on a 73x type of bill with revenue code 052x for providing the professional component of ABPM services.

The FIs should not make a separate payment to a FQHC for the professional component of ABPM services in addition to the all-inclusive rate. FQHCs are not required to use ABPM HCPCS codes for professional services covered under the all-inclusive rate.

The FIs pay provider-based RHCs/FQHCs for the technical component of ABPM services when billed under the base provider's number using the above requirements for that particular base provider type, i.e., a OPPS hospital based RHC would be paid for the ABPM technical component services under the OPPS using the APC for code 93786 and/or 93788 when billed on a 13x type of bill.

Independent and free-standing RHC/FQHC practitioners are only paid for providing the technical component of ABPM services when billed to the carrier following the carrier instructions.

C. Carrier Claims

Local carriers pay for ABPM services billed with diagnosis code 796.2 and HCPCS codes 93784 or for any combination of 93786, 93788 and 93790, based on the MPFS for the specific HCPCS code billed.

D. Coinsurance and Deductible
The FIs and local carriers shall apply coinsurance and deductible to payments for ABPM services except for services billed to the FI by FQHCs. For FQHCs only co-insurance applies.

100-4, 32, 12

Smoking and Tobacco-Use Cessation Counseling Services

Background: Effective for services furnished on or after March 22, 2005, a National Coverage Determination (NCD) provides for coverage of smoking and tobacco-use cessation counseling services. Conditions of Medicare Part A and Medicare Part B coverage for smoking and tobacco-use cessation counseling services are located in the Medicare National Coverage Determinations Manual, Publication 100-3, section 210.4.

100-4, 32, 12.1

HCPCS and Diagnosis Coding

The following HCPCS codes should be reported when billing for smoking and tobacco- use cessation counseling services:

99406 Smoking and tobacco-use cessation counseling visit; intermediate, greater than 3 minutes up to 10 minutes

99407 Smoking and tobacco-use cessation counseling visit; intensive, greater than 10 minutes

Note the above codes are payable for dates of service on or after January 1, 2008. Codes G0375 and G0376, below, are not valid or payable for dates of service on or after January 1, 2008.

G0375 Smoking and tobacco-use cessation counseling visit; intermediate, greater than 3 minutes up to 10 minutes

Short Descriptor: Smoke/Tobacco counseling 3-10

G0376 Smoking and tobacco-use cessation counseling visit; intensive, greater than 10 minutes

Short Descriptor: Smoke/Tobacco counseling greater than 10

NOTE: The above G codes will NOT be active in contractors' systems until July 5, 2005. Therefore, contractors shall advise providers to use unlisted code 99199 to bill for smoking and tobacco- use cessation counseling services during the interim period of March 22, 2005, through July 4, 2005, and received prior to July 5, 2005.

On July 5, 2005, contractors' systems will accept the new G codes for services performed on and after March 22, 2005.

Contractors shall allow payment for a medically necessary E/M service on the same day as the smoking and tobacco-use cessation counseling service when it is clinically appropriate. Physicians and qualified non-physician practitioners shall use an appropriate HCPCS code, such as HCPCS 99201- 99215, to report an E/M service with modifier 25 to indicate that the E/M service is a separately identifiable service from G0375 or G0376.

Contractors shall only pay for 8 Smoking and Tobacco-Use Cessation Counseling sessions in a 12-month period. The beneficiary may receive another 8 sessions during a second or subsequent year after 11 full months have passed since the first Medicare covered cessation session was performed. To start the count for the second or subsequent 12-month period, begin with the month after the month in which the first Medicare covered cessation session was performed and count until 11 full months have elapsed.

Claims for smoking and tobacco use cessation counseling services shall be submitted with an appropriate diagnosis code. Diagnosis codes should reflect: the condition the patient has that is adversely affected by tobacco use or the condition the patient is being treated for with a therapeutic agent whose metabolism or dosing is affected by tobacco use.

NOTE: This decision does not modify existing coverage for minimal cessation counseling (defined as 3 minutes or less in duration) which is already considered to be covered as part of each Evaluation and Management (E/M) visit and is not separately billable.

100-4, 32, 12.2

Carrier Billing:

Carriers shall pay for counseling services billed with codes 99406 and 99407 for dates of service on or after January 1, 2008. Carriers shall pay for counseling services billed with codes G0375 and G0376 for dates of service performed on and after March 22, 2005 through Dec. 31, 2007. The type of service (TOS) for each of the new codes is 1.

Carriers pay for counseling services billed based on the Medicare Physician Fee Schedule (MPFS). Deductible and coinsurance apply. Claims from physicians or other providers where assignment was not taken are subject to the Medicare limiting charge, which means that charges to the beneficiary may be no more than 115 percent of the allowed amount.

Physicians or qualified non-physician practitioners shall bill the carrier for smoking and tobacco-use cessation counseling services on the Form CMS-1500 or an approved electronic format.

100-4, 32, 12.3

FI Billing Requirements

The FIs shall pay for Smoking and Tobacco-Use Cessation Counseling services with codes 99406 and 99407 for dates of service on or after January 1, 2008. FIs shall pay for counseling services billed with codes G0375 and G0376 for dates of service performed on or after March 22, 2005 through December 31, 2007.

A. Claims for Smoking and Tobacco-Use Cessation Counseling Services should be submitted on Form CMS-1450 or its electronic equivalent.

The applicable bill types are 12X, 13X, 22X, 23X, 34X, 71X, 73X, 83X, and 85X. Effective 4/1/06, type of bill 14X is for non-patient laboratory specimens and is no longer applicable for Smoking and Tobacco-Use Cessation Counseling services.

Applicable revenue codes are as follows:

Provider Type	Revenue Code
Rural Health Centers (RHCs)/Federally Qualified Health Centers (FQHCs)	052X
Indian Health Services (IHS)	0510
Critical Access Hospitals (CAHs) Method II	096X, 097X, 098X
All Other Providers	0942

NOTE: When these services are provided by a clinical nurse specialist in the RHC/FQHC setting, they are considered "incident to" and do not constitute a billable visit.

Payment for outpatient services is as follows:

Type of Facility	Method of Payment
Rural Health Centers (RHCs)/Federally Qualified Health Centers (FQHCs)	All-inclusive rate (AIR) for the encounter
Indian Health Service (IHS)/Tribally owned or operated hospitals and hospital- based facilities	All-inclusive rate (AIR)
IHS/Tribally owned or operated non-hospital-based facilities	Medicare Physician Fee Schedule (MPFS)
IHS/Tribally owned or operated Critical Access Hospitals (CAHs)	Facility Specific Visit Rate
Hospitals subject to the Outpatient Prospective Payment System (OPPS)	Ambulatory Payment Classification (APC)
Hospitals not subject to OPPS	Payment is made under current methodologies
Skilled Nursing Facilities (SNFs) NOTE: Included in Part A PPS for skilled patients.	Medicare Physician Fee Schedule (MPFS)
Home Health Agencies (HHAs)	Medicare Physician Fee Schedule (MPFS)
Critical Access Hospitals (CAHs)	Method I: Technical services are paid at 101% of reasonable cost. Method II: technical services are paid at 101% of reasonable cost, and Professional services are paid at 115% of the MMPFS Data Base
Maryland Hospitals	Payment is based according to the Health Services Cost Review Commission (HSCRC). That is 94% of submitted charges subject to any unmet deductible, coinsurance, and non-covered charges policies.

NOTE: Inpatient claims submitted with Smoking and Tobacco-Use Cessation Counseling Services are processed under the current payment methodologies.

100-4, 32 ,30.1

Billing Requirements for HBO Therapy for the Treatment of Diabetic Wounds of the Lower Extremities

Hyperbaric Oxygen Therapy is a modality in which the entire body is exposed to oxygen under increased atmospheric pressure. Effective April 1, 2003, a National Coverage Decision expanded the use of HBO therapy to include coverage for the treatment of diabetic wounds of the lower extremities. For specific coverage criteria for HBO Therapy, refer to the National Coverage Determinations Manual, chapter 1, section 20.29.

NOTE: Topical application of oxygen does not meet the definition of HBO therapy as stated above. Also, its clinical efficacy has not been established. Therefore, no Medicare reimbursement may be made for the topical application of oxygen.

I. Billing Requirements for Intermediaries
Claims for HBO therapy should be submitted on Form CMS-1450 or its electronic equivalent.

a. Applicable Bill Types
The applicable hospital bill types are 11X, 13X and 85X.

b. Procedural Coding

99183 Physician attendance and supervision of hyperbaric oxygen therapy, per session.

C1300 Hyperbaric oxygen under pressure, full body chamber, per 30-minute interval.

NOTE: Code C1300 is not available for use other than in a hospital outpatient department. In skilled nursing facilities (SNFs), HBO therapy is part of the SNF PPS payment for beneficiaries in covered Part A stays.

For hospital inpatients and critical access hospitals (CAHs) not electing Method I, HBO therapy is reported under revenue code 940 without any HCPCS code. For inpatient services, show ICD-9-CM procedure code 93.59.

For CAHs electing Method I, HBO therapy is reported under revenue code 940 along with HCPCS code 99183.

c. Payment Requirements for Intermediaries
Payment is as follows:

Intermediary payment is allowed for HBO therapy for diabetic wounds of the lower extremities when performed as a physician service in a hospital outpatient setting and for inpatients. Payment is allowed for claims with valid diagnostic ICD-9 codes as shown above with dates of service on or after April 1, 2003. Those claims with invalid codes should be denied as not medically necessary.

For hospitals, payment will be based upon the Ambulatory Payment Classification (APC) or the inpatient Diagnosis Related Group (DRG). Deductible and coinsurance apply.

Payment to Critical Access Hospitals (electing Method I) is made under cost reimbursement. For Critical Access Hospitals electing Method II, the technical component is paid under cost reimbursement and the professional component is paid under the Physician Fee Schedule.

NOTE: Information regarding the form locator numbers that correspond to these data element names and a table to crosswalk UB-04 form locators to the 837 transaction is found in Chapter 25.

II. Carrier Billing Requirements
Claims for this service should be submitted on Form CMS-1500 or its electronic equivalent.

The following HCPCS code applies:

- 99183 - Physician attendance and supervision of hyperbaric oxygen therapy, per session.

a. Payment Requirements for Carriers
Payment and pricing information will occur through updates to the Medicare Physician Fee Schedule Database (MPFSDB). Pay for this service on the basis of the MPFSDB. Deductible and coinsurance apply. Claims from physicians or other practitioners where assignment was not taken, are subject to the Medicare limiting charge.

III. Medicare Summary Notices (MSNs)
Use the following MSN Messages where appropriate:

In situations where the claim is being denied on the basis that the condition does not meet our coverage requirements, use one of the following MSN Messages:

"Medicare does not pay for this item or service for this condition." (MSN Message 16.48)

The Spanish version of the MSN message should read:

"Medicare no paga por este articulo o servicio para esta afeccion."

In situations where, based on the above utilization policy, medical review of the claim results in a determination that the service is not medically necessary, use the following MSN message:

"The information provided does not support the need for this service or item." (MSN Message 15.4)

The Spanish version of the MSN message should read:

"La informacion proporcionada no confirma la necesidad para este servicio o articulo."

IV. Remittance Advice Notices
Use appropriate existing remittance advice and reason codes at the line level to express the specific reason if you deny payment for HBO therapy for the treatment of diabetic wounds of lower extremities.

100-4, 32, 40

Sacral Nerve Stimulation

A sacral nerve stimulator is a pulse generator that transmits electrical impulses to the sacral nerves through an implanted wire. These impulses cause the bladder muscles to contract, which gives the patient ability to void more properly.

100-4, 32, 40.1

Coverage Requirements

Effective January 1, 2002, sacral nerve stimulation is covered for the treatment of urinary urge incontinence, urgency-frequency syndrome and urinary retention. Sacral nerve stimulation involves both a temporary test stimulation to determine if an implantable stimulator would be effective and a permanent implantation in appropriate candidates. Both the test and the permanent implantation are covered.

The following limitations for coverage apply to all indications:

- Patient must be refractory to conventional therapy (documented behavioral, pharmacologic and/or surgical corrective therapy) and be an appropriate surgical candidate such that implantation with anesthesia can occur.
- Patients with stress incontinence, urinary obstruction, and specific neurologic diseases (e.g., diabetes with peripheral nerve involvement) that are associated with secondary manifestations of the above three indications are excluded.
- Patient must have had a successful test stimulation in order to support subsequent implantation. Before a patient is eligible for permanent implantation, he/she must demonstrate a 50% or greater improvement through test stimulation. Improvement is measured through voiding diaries.
- Patient must be able to demonstrate adequate ability to record voiding diary data such that clinical results of the implant procedure can be properly evaluated.

100-4, 32, 50

Deep Brain Stimulation for Essential Tremor and Parkinson's Disease

Deep brain stimulation (DBS) refers to high-frequency electrical stimulation of anatomic regions deep within the brain utilizing neurosurgically implanted electrodes. These DBS electrodes are stereotactically placed within targeted nuclei on one (unilateral) or both (bilateral) sides of the brain. There are currently three targets for DBS -- the thalamic ventralis intermedius nucleus (VIM), subthalamic nucleus (STN) and globus pallidus interna (GPi).

Essential tremor (ET) is a progressive, disabling tremor most often affecting the hands. ET may also affect the head, voice and legs. The precise pathogenesis of ET is unknown. While it may start at any age, ET usually peaks within the second and sixth decades. Beta-adrenergic blockers and anticonvulsant medications are usually the first line treatments for reducing the severity of tremor. Many patients, however, do not adequately respond or cannot tolerate these medications. In these medically refractory ET patients, thalamic VIM DBS may be helpful for symptomatic relief of tremor.

Parkinson's disease (PD) is an age-related progressive neurodegenerative disorder involving the loss of dopaminergic cells in the substantia nigra of the midbrain. The disease is characterized by tremor, rigidity, bradykinesia and progressive postural instability. Dopaminergic medication is typically used as a first line treatment for reducing the primary symptoms of PD. However, after prolonged use, medication can become less effective and can produce significant adverse events such as dyskinesias and other motor function complications. For patients who become unresponsive to medical treatments and/or have intolerable side effects from medications, DBS for symptom relief may be considere

100-4, 32, 60.4.1

Allowable Covered Diagnosis Codes

For services furnished on or after July 1, 2002, the applicable ICD-9-CM diagnosis code for this benefit is V43.3, organ or tissue replaced by other means; heart valve.

For services furnished on or after March 19, 2008, the applicable ICD-9-CM diagnosis codes for this benefit are:

- V43.3 (organ or tissue replaced by other means; heart valve),
- 289.81 (primary hypercoagulable state),
- 451.0-451.9 (includes 451.11, 451.19, 451.2, 451.80-451.84, 451.89) (phlebitis & thrombophlebitis),
- 453.0-453.3 (other venous embolism & thrombosis),
- 453.40-453.49 (includes 453.40-453.42, 453.8-453.9) (venous embolism and thrombosis of the deep vessels of the lower extremity, and other specified veins/unspecified sites)
- 415.11-415.12, 415.19 (pulmonary embolism & infarction) or,
- 427.31 (atrial fibrillation (established) (paroxysmal)).

100-4, 32, 60.5.2

Applicable Diagnosis Codes for Carriers

For services furnished on or after July 1, 2002, the applicable ICD-9-CM diagnosis code for this benefit is V43.3, organ or tissue replaced by other means; heart valve.

For services furnished on or after March 19, 2008, the applicable ICD-9-CM diagnosis codes for this benefit are:

- V43.3 (organ or tissue replaced by other means; heart valve),
- 289.81 (primary hypercoagulable state),
- 451.0-451.9 (includes 451.11, 451.19, 451.2, 451.80-451.84, 451.89) (phlebitis & thrombophlebitis),
- 453.0-453.3 (other venous embolism & thrombosis),
- 453.40-453.49 (includes 453.40-453.42, 453.8-453.9) (venous embolism and thrombosis of the deep vessels of the lower extremity, and other specified veins/unspecified sites)
- 415.11-415.12, 415.19 (pulmonary embolism & infarction) or,
- 427.31 (atrial fibrillation (established) (paroxysmal)).

100-4, 32, 80.8

CWF Utilization Edits

Edit 1 - Should CWF receive a claim from an FI for G0245 or G0246 and a second claim from a contractor for either G0245 or G0246 (or vice versa) and they are different dates of service and less than 6 months apart, the second claim will reject. CWF will edit to allow G0245 or G0246 to be paid no more than every 6 months for a particular beneficiary, regardless of who furnished the service. If G0245 has been paid, regardless of whether it was posted as a facility or professional claim, it must be 6 months before G0245 can be paid again or G0246 can be paid. If G0246 has been paid, regardless of whether it was posted as a facility or professional claim, it must be 6 months before G0246 can be paid again or G0245 can be paid. CWF will not impose limits on how many times each code can be paid for a beneficiary as long as there has been 6 months between each service.

The CWF will return a specific reject code for this edit to the contractors and FIs that will be identified in the CWF documentation. Based on the CWF reject code, the contractors and FIs must deny the claims and return the following messages:

MSN 18.4 -- This service is being denied because it has not been __ months since your last examination of this kind (NOTE: Insert 6 as the appropriate number of months.)

RA claim adjustment reason code 96 - Non-covered charges, along with remark code M86 - Service denied because payment already made for same/similar procedure within set time frame.

Edit 2 - The CWF will edit to allow G0247 to pay only if either G0245 or G0246 has been submitted and accepted as payable on the same date of service. CWF will return a specific reject code for this edit to the contractors and FIs that will be identified in the CWF documentation. Based on this reject code, contractors and FIs will deny the claims and return the following messages:

MSN 21.21 - This service was denied because Medicare only covers this service under certain circumstances.

RA claim adjustment reason code 107 - The related or qualifying claim/service was not identified on this claim.

Edit 3 - Once a beneficiary's condition has progressed to the point where routine foot care becomes a covered service, payment will no longer be made for LOPS evaluation and management services. Those services would be considered to be included in the regular exams and treatments afforded to the beneficiary on a routine basis. The physician or provider must then just bill the routine foot care codes, per Pub 100-02, Chapter 15, Sec.290.

The CWF will edit to reject LOPS codes G0245, G0246, and/or G0247 when on the beneficiary's record it shows that one of the following routine foot care codes were billed and paid within the prior 6 months: 11055, 11056, 11057, 11719, 11720, and/or 11721.

The CWF will return a specific reject code for this edit to the contractors and FIs that will be identified in the CWF documentation. Based on the CWF reject code, the contractors and FIs must deny the claims and return the following messages:

MSN 21.21 - This service was denied because Medicare only covers this service under certain circumstances.

The RA claim adjustment reason code 96 - Non-covered charges, along with remark code M86 - Service denied because payment already made for same/similar procedure within set time frame.

100-4, 32, 90

Stem Cell Transplantation

Stem cell transplantation is a process in which stem cells are harvested from either a patient's or donor's bone marrow or peripheral blood for intravenous infusion. Autologous stem cell transplantation (AuSCT) must be used to effect hematopoietic reconstitution following severely myelotoxic doses of chemotherapy (HDCT) and/or radiotherapy used to treat various malignancies. Allogeneic stem cell transplant may also be used to restore function in recipients having an inherited or acquired deficiency or defect.

Bone marrow and peripheral blood stem cell transplantation is a process which includes mobilization, harvesting, and transplant of bone marrow or peripheral blood stem cells and the administration of high dose chemotherapy or radiotherapy prior to the actual transplant. When bone marrow or peripheral blood stem cell transplantation is covered, all necessary steps are included in coverage. When bone marrow or peripheral blood stem cell transplantation is non-covered, none of the steps are covered.

Allogeneic and autologous stem cell transplants are covered under Medicare for specific diagnoses. See Pub. 100-03, National Coverage Determinations Manual, section 110.8.1, for a complete description of covered and noncovered conditions. The following sections contain claims processing instructions for carrier claims. For institutional claims processing instructions, please refer to Pub. 100-04, chapter 3, section 90.3.

100-4, 32, 100

Billing Requirements for Expanded Coverage of Cochlear Implantation

Effective for dates of services on and after April 4, 2005, the Centers for Medicare & Medicaid Services (CMS) has expanded the coverage for cochlear implantation to cover moderate-to-profound hearing loss in individuals with hearing test scores equal to or less than 40% correct in the best aided listening condition on tape-recorded tests of open-set sentence recognition and who demonstrate limited benefit from amplification. (See Publication 100-03, chapter 1, section 50.3, for specific coverage criteria).

In addition CMS is covering cochlear implantation for individuals with open-set sentence recognition test scores of greater than 40% to less than or equal to 60% correct but only when the provider is participating in, and patients are enrolled in, either:

A Food and Drug Administration (FDA)-approved category B investigational device exemption (IDE) clinical trial; or

A trial under the CMS clinical trial policy (see Pub. 100-03, section 310.1); or

A prospective, controlled comparative trial approved by CMS as consistent with the evidentiary requirements for national coverage analyses and meeting specific quality standards.

100-4, 32, 120.2

Coding and General Billing Requirements

Physicians and hospitals must report one of the following Current Procedural Terminology (CPT) codes on the claim:

66982 Extracapsular cataract removal with insertion of intraocular lens prosthesis (one stage procedure), manual or mechanical technique (e.g., irrigation and aspiration or phacoemulsification), complex requiring devices or techniques not generally used in routine cataract surgery (e.g., iris expansion device, suture support for intraocular lens, or primary posterior capsulorrhexis) or performed on patients in the amblyogenic development stage.

66983 Intracapsular cataract with insertion of intraocular lens prosthesis (one stage procedure)

66984 Extracapsular cataract removal with insertion of intraocular lens prosthesis (one stage procedure), manual or mechanical technique (e.g., irrigation and aspiration or phacoemulsification)

66985 Insertion of intraocular lens prosthesis (secondary implant), not associated with concurrent cataract extraction

66986 Exchange of intraocular lens

In addition, physicians inserting a P-C IOL or A-C IOL in an office setting may bill code V2632 (posterior chamber intraocular lens) for the IOL. Medicare will make payment for the lens based on reasonable cost for a conventional IOL. Place of Service (POS) = 11.

Effective for dates of service on and after January 1, 2006, physician, hospitals and ASCs may also bill the non-covered charges related to the P-C function of the IOL using HCPCS code V2788. Effective for dates of service on and after January 22, 2007 through January 1, 2008, non-covered charges related to A-C function of the IOL can be billed using HCPCS code V2788. The type of service indicator for the non-covered billed charges is Q. (The type of service is applied by the Medicare carrier and not the provider). Effective for A-C IOL insertion services on or after January 1, 2008, physicians, hospitals and ASCs should use V2787 rather than V2788 to report any additional charges that accrue.

When denying the non-payable charges submitted with V2787 or V2788, contractors shall use an appropriate Medical Summary Notice (MSN) such as 16.10 (Medicare does not pay for this item or service) and an appropriate claim adjustment reason code such as 96 (non-covered charges) for claims submitted with the non-payable charges.

Hospitals and physicians may use the proper CPT code(s) to bill Medicare for evaluation and management services usually associated with services following cataract extraction surgery, if appropriate.

A - Applicable Bill Types
The hospital applicable bill types are 12X, 13X, 83X and 85X.

B - Other Special Requirements for Hospitals
Hospitals shall continue to pay CAHs method 2 claims under current payment methodologies for conditional IOLs.

100-4, 32, 130

External Counterpulsation (ECP) Therapy

Commonly referred to as enhanced external counterpulsation, is a non-invasive outpatient treatment for coronary artery disease refractory medical and/or surgical therapy. Effective for dates of service July 1, 1999, and after, Medicare will cover ECP when its use is in patients with stable angina (Class III or Class IV, Canadian Cardiovascular Society Classification or equivalent classification) who, in the opinion of a cardiologist or cardiothoracic surgeon, are not readily amenable to surgical intervention, such as PTCA or cardiac bypass, because:

- Their condition is inoperable, or at high risk of operative complications or post-operative failure;
- Their coronary anatomy is not readily amenable to such procedures; or
- They have co-morbid states that create excessive risk.

(Refer to Publication 100-03, section 20.20 for further coverage criteria.)

100-4, 32, 130.1

Billing and Payment Requirements

Effective for dates of service on or after January 1, 2000, use HCPCS code G0166 (External counterpulsation, per session) to report ECP services. The codes for external cardiac assist (92971), ECG rhythm strip and report (93040 or 93041), pulse oximetry (94760 or 94761) and plethysmography (93922 or 93923) or other monitoring tests for examining the effects of this treatment are not clinically necessary with this service and should not be paid on the same day, unless they occur in a clinical setting not connected with the delivery of the ECP. Daily evaluation and management service, e.g., 99201-99205, 99211-99215, 99217-99220, 99241-99245, cannot be billed with the ECP treatments. Any evaluation and management service must be justified with adequate documentation of the medical necessity of the visit. Deductible and coinsurance apply.

100-4, 32, 140

Cardiac Rehabilitation Programs

Medicare covers cardiac rehabilitation exercise programs for patients who meet the following criteria:

- Have a documented diagnosis of acute myocardial infarction within the preceding 12 months; or
- Have had coronory bypass surgery; or
- Have stable angina pectoris; or
- Have had heart valve repair/replacement; or
- Have had percutaneous transluminal coronary angioplasty (PTCA) or coronary stenting; or
- Have had a heart or heart-lung transplant.

Effective for dates of services on or after March 22, 2006, services provided in connection with a cardiac rehabilitation exercise program may be considered reasonable and necessary for up to 36 sessions. Patients generally receive 2 to 3 sessions per week for 12 to 18 weeks. The contractor has discretion to cover cardiac rehabilitation services beyond 18 weeks. Coverage must not exceed a total of 72 sessions for 36 weeks.

Cardiac rehabilitation programs shall be performed incident to physician's services in outpatient hospitals, or outpatient settings such as clinics or offices. Follow the policies for services incident to the services of a physician as they apply in each setting. For example, see Pub. 100-02, chapter 6, section 2.4.1, and Pub. 100-02, chapter 15, section 60.1.

(Refer to Publication 100-03, section 20.10 for further coverage guidelines.)

100-4, 32, 140.1

Cardiac Rehabilitation Program Services Furnished On or Before Dec. 31, 2009

Medicare covers cardiac rehabilitation exercise programs for patients who meet the following criteria: Have a documented diagnosis of acute myocardial infarction within the preceding 12 months; or Have had coronary bypass surgery; or Have stable angina pectoris; or Have had heart valve repair/replacement; or Have had percutaneous transluminal coronary angioplasty (PTCA) or coronary stenting; or Have had a heart or heart-lung transplant. Effective for dates of services on or after March 22, 2006, services provided in connection with a cardiac rehabilitation exercise program may be considered reasonable and necessary for up to 36 sessions. Patients generally receive 2 to 3 sessions per week for 12 to 18 weeks. The contractor has discretion to cover cardiac rehabilitation services beyond 18 weeks. Coverage must not exceed a total of 72 sessions for 36 weeks. Cardiac rehabilitation programs shall be performed incident to physician's services in outpatient hospitals, or outpatient settings such as clinics or offices. Follow the policies for services incident to the services of a physician as they apply in each setting. For example, see Pub. 100-02, Chapter 6, Sec.2.4.1, and Pub. 100-02, Chapter 15, Sec.60.1. (Refer to Publication 100-03, Sec.20.10 for further coverage guidelines.)

100-4, 32, 140.1.1

Coding Requirements for Cardiac Rehabilitation Services Furnished On or Before Dec. 31, 2009

The following are the applicable HCPCS codes:

93797 Physician services for outpatient cardiac rehabilitation; without continuous ECG monitoring (per session); and

93798 Physician services for outpatient cardiac rehabilitation; with continuous ECG monitoring (per session).

Effective for dates of service on or after January 1, 2008 and before January 1, 2010, providers and practitioners may report more than one unit of CPT code 93797 or 93798 for a date of service if more than one cardiac rehabilitation session lasting at least 1 hour each is provided on the same day. In order to report more than one session for a given date of service, each session must last a minimum of 60 minutes. For example, if the cardiac rehabilitation services provided on a given day total 1 hour and 50 minutes, then only one session should be billed to report the cardiac rehabilitation services provided on that day.

100-4,32,140.2

Cardiac Rehabilitation Program Services Furnished On or After January 1, 2010

As specified at 42 CFR 410.49, Medicare covers cardiac rehabilitation items and services for patients who have experienced one or more of the following: An acute myocardial infarction within the preceding 12 months; or A coronary artery bypass surgery; or Current stable angina pectoris; or Heart valve repair or replacement; or Percutaneous transluminal coronary angioplasty (PTCA) or coronary stenting; or A heart or heart-lung transplant. Cardiac rehabilitation programs must include the following components:

Physician-prescribed exercise each day cardiac rehabilitation items and services are furnished; Cardiac risk factor modification, including education, counseling, and behavioral intervention at least once during the program, tailored to patients' individual needs; Psychosocial assessment; Outcomes assessment; and An individualized treatment plan detailing how components are utilized for each patient. Cardiac rehabilitation items and services must be furnished in a physician's office or a hospital outpatient setting. All settings must have a physician immediately available and accessible for medical consultations and emergencies at all time items and services are being furnished under the program. This provision is satisfied if the physician meets the requirements for the direct supervision of physician's office services as specified at 42 CFR 410.26 and for hospital outpatient therapeutic services as specified at 42 CFR 410.27.

As specified at 42 CFR 410.49(f)(1), cardiac rehabilitation program sessions are limited to a maximum of 2 1-hour sessions per day for up to 36 sessions over up to 36 weeks, with the option for an additional 36 sessions over an extended period of time if approved by the Medicare contractor.

100-4, 32, 140.2.1

Coding Requirements for Cardiac Rehabilitation Services Furnished On or After January 1, 2010

The following are the applicable CPT codes for cardiac rehabilitation services: 93797 - Physician services for outpatient cardiac rehabilitation; without continuous ECG monitoring (per session) and 93798 - Physician services for outpatient cardiac rehabilitation; with continuous ECG monitoring (per session) Effective for dates of service on or after January 1, 2010, hospitals and practitioners may report a maximum of 2 1-hour sessions per day. In order to report one session of cardiac rehabilitation services in a day, the duration of treatment must be at least 31 minutes. Two sessions of cardiac rehabilitation services may only be reported in the same day if the duration of treatment is at least 91 minutes. In other words, the first session would account for 60 minutes and the second session would account for at least 31 minutes if two sessions are reported. If several shorter periods of cardiac rehabilitation services are furnished on a given day, the minutes of service during those periods must be added together for reporting in 1-hour session increments.

Example: If the patient receives 20 minutes of cardiac rehabilitation services in the day, no cardiac rehabilitation session may be reported because less than 31 minutes of services were furnished.

Example: If a patient receives 20 minutes of cardiac rehabilitation services in the morning and 35 minutes of cardiac rehabilitation services in the afternoon of a single day, the hospital or practitioner would report 1 session of cardiac rehabilitation services under 1 unit of the appropriate CPT code for the total duration of 55 minutes of cardiac rehabilitation services on that day.

Example: If the patient receives 70 minutes of cardiac rehabilitation services in the morning and 25 minutes of cardiac rehabilitation services in the afternoon of a single day, the hospital or practitioner would report two sessions of cardiac rehabilitation services under the appropriate CPT code(s) because the total duration of cardiac rehabilitation services on that day of 95 minutes exceeds 90 minutes.

Example: If the patient receives 70 minutes of cardiac rehabilitation services in the morning and 85 minutes of cardiac rehabilitation services in the afternoon of a single day, the hospital or practitioner would report two sessions of cardiac rehabilitation services under the appropriate CPT code(s) for the total duration of cardiac rehabilitation services of 155 minutes. A maximum of two sessions per day may be reported, regardless of the total duration of cardiac rehabilitation services.

100-4, 32, 140.2.2.1

Correct Place of Service (POS) Code for CR and ICR Services on Professional Claims

Effective for claims with dates of service on and after January 1, 2010, place of service (POS) code 11 shall be used for CR and ICR services provided in a physician's office and POS 22 shall be used for services provided in a hospital outpatient setting. All other POS codes shall be denied. Contractors shall adjust their prepayment procedure edits as appropriate.

The following messages shall be used when contractors deny CR and ICR claims for POS:

Claim Adjustment Reason Code (CARC) 58 - Treatment was deemed by the payer to have been rendered in an inappropriate or invalid place of service.

NOTE: Refer to the 832 Healthcare Policy Identification Segment (loop 2110 Service payment Information REF), if present.

Remittance Advice Remark Code (RARC) N428 - Service/procedure not covered when performed in this place of service.

Medicare Summary Notice (MSN) 21.25 - This service was denied because Medicare only covers this service in certain settings.

Group Code PR (Patient Responsibility) - Where a claim is received with the GA modifier indicating that a signed ABN is on file.

Group Code CO (Contractor Responsibility) - Where a claim is received with the GZ modifier indicating that no signed ABN is on file.

100-4, 32, 140.3

Intensive Cardiac Rehabilitation Program Services Furnished On or After January 1, 2010

As specified at 42 CFR 410.49, Medicare covers intensive cardiac rehabilitation items and services for patients who have experienced one or more of the following:

An acute myocardial infarction within the preceding 12 months; or

A coronary artery bypass surgery; or

Current stable angina pectoris; or

Heart valve repair or replacement; or

Percutaneous transluminal coronary angioplasty (PTCA) or coronary stenting; or

A heart or heart-lung transplant.

Intensive cardiac rehabilitation programs must include the following components:

Physician-prescribed exercise each day cardiac rehabilitation items and services are furnished;

Cardiac risk factor modification, including education, counseling, and behavioral intervention at least once during the program, tailored to patients' individual needs;

Psychosocial assessment;

Outcomes assessment; and

An individualized treatment plan detailing how components are utilized for each patient.

Intensive cardiac rehabilitation programs must be approved by Medicare. In order to be approved, a program must demonstrate through peer-reviewed published research that it has accomplished one or more of the following for its patients:

Positively affected the progression of coronary heart disease;

Reduced the need for coronary bypass surgery; and

Reduced the need for percutaneous coronary interventions.

An intensive cardiac rehabilitation program must also demonstrate through peer-reviewed published research that it accomplished a statistically significant reduction in 5 or more of the following measures for patients from their levels before cardiac rehabilitation services to after cardiac rehabilitation services:

Low density lipoprotein;

Triglycerides;

Body mass index;

Systolic blood pressure;

Diastolic blood pressure; and

The need for cholesterol, blood pressure, and diabetes medications.

Intensive cardiac rehabilitation items and services must be furnished in a physician's office or a hospital outpatient setting. All settings must have a physician immediately available and accessible for medical consultations and emergencies at all time items and services are being furnished under the program. This provision is satisfied if the physician meets the requirements for direct supervision of physician office services as specified at 42 CFR 410.26 and for hospital outpatient therapeutic services as specified at 42 CFR 410.27.

As specified at 42 CFR 410.49(f)(2), intensive cardiac rehabilitation program sessions are limited to 72 1-hour sessions, up to 6 sessions per day, over a period of up to 18 weeks.

100-4, 32, 150.1

General

A. Covered Bariatric Surgery Procedures
Effective for services on or after February 21, 2006, Medicare has determined that the following bariatric surgery procedures are reasonable and necessary under certain conditions for the treatment of morbid obesity. The patient must have a body-mass index (BMI) >=35, have at least one co-morbidity related to obesity, and have been previously unsuccessful with medical treatment for obesity. This medical information must be documented in the patient's medical record. In addition, the procedure must be performed at an approved facility. A list of approved facilities may be found at
http://www.cms.hhs.gov/MedicareApprovedFacilitie/BSF/list.asp#TopOfPage.

Open Roux-en-Y gastric bypass (RYGBP).

Laparoscopic Roux-en-Y gastric bypass (RYGBP).

Laparoscopic adjustable gastric banding (LAGB).

Open biliopancreatic diversion with duodenal switch (BPD/DS).

Laparoscopic biliopancreatic diversion with duodenal switch (BPD/DS).

B. Non-Covered Bariatric Surgery Procedures
Effective for services on or after February 21, 2006, Medicare has determined that the following bariatric surgery procedures are not reasonable and necessary for the treatment of morbid obesity.

Open vertical banded gastroplasty.

Laparoscopic vertical banded gastroplasty.

Open sleeve gastrectomy.

Laparoscopic sleeve gastrectomy.

Open adjustable gastric banding.

Effective for services performed on and after February 12, 2009, CMS determines that open and laparoscopic Roux-en-Y gastric bypass (RYGBP), laparoscopic adjustable gastric banding (LAGB), and open and laparoscopic biliopancreatic diversion with duodenal switch (BPD/DS) in Medicare beneficiaries who have type 2 diabetes mellitus (T2DM) and a BMI <35 are not reasonable and necessary under section 1862(a)(1)(A) of the Social Security Act, and therefore are not covered.

Complete coverage guidelines can be found in the National Coverage Determination Manual (Pub. 100-03), sections 40.5 and 100.1.

100-4, 32, 150.2

HCPCS Procedure Codes for Bariatric Surgery

A. Covered HCPCS Procedure Codes
For services on or after February 21, 2006, the following HCPCS procedure codes are covered for bariatric surgery:

43770 Laparoscopy, surgical, gastric restrictive procedure; placement of adjustable gastric band (gastric band and subcutaneous port components).

43644 Laparoscopy, surgical, gastric restrictive procedure; with gastric bypass and Roux-en-Y gastroenterostomy (roux limb 150 cm or less).

43645 Laparoscopy with gastric bypass and small intestine reconstruction to limit absorption. (Do not report 43645 in conjunction with 49320, 43847.)

43845 Gastric restrictive procedure with partial gastrectomy, pylorus-preserving duodenoileostomy and ileoieostomy (50 to 100 cm common channel) to limit absorption (biliopancreatic diversion with duodenal switch).

43846 Gastric restrictive procedure, with gastric bypass for morbid obesity; with short limb (150 cm or less Roux-en-Y gastroenterostomy. (For greater than 150 cm, use 43847.) (For laparoscopic procedure, use 43644.)

43847 With small intestine reconstruction to limit absorption.

B. Noncovered HCPCS Procedure Codes
For services on or after February 21, 2006, the following HCPCS procedure codes are non-covered for bariatric surgery:

43842 Gastric restrictive procedure, without gastric bypass, for morbid obesity; vertical banded gastroplasty.

NOC code 43999 used to bill for:

- Laparoscopic vertical banded gastroplasty.
- Open sleeve gastrectomy.
- Laparoscopic sleeve gastrectomy.
- Open adjustable gastric banding.

100-4, 32, 150.6

ICD-9 Procedure Codes for Bariatric Procedures

150.6 - Claims Guidance for Payment

A. Covered Bariatric Surgery Procedures
Contractors shall process covered bariatric surgery claims as follows:

1. Identify bariatric surgery claims.
   - Contractors identify inpatient bariatric surgery claims by the presence of ICD-9-CM diagnosis code 278.01 as the primary diagnosis (for morbid obesity) and one of the covered ICD-9-CM procedure codes listed in Sec.150.3.
   - Contractors identify practitioner bariatric surgery claims by the presence of ICD-9-CM diagnosis code 278.01 as the primary diagnosis (for morbid obesity) and one of the covered HCPCS procedure codes listed in Sec.150.2.
2. Perform facility certification validation for all bariatric surgery claims on a pre-pay basis.
   - A list of approved facilities may be found at: http://www.cms.hhs.gov/MedicareApprovedFacilitie/BSF/list.asp#TopOfPage.
3. Review bariatric surgery claims data and determine whether a pre- or post-pay sample of bariatric surgery claims need further review to assure that the beneficiary has a BMI >=35 (V85.35 - V85.4), and at least one co-morbidity related to obesity.
   - The carrier/FI/A/B MAC medical director may define the appropriate method for addressing the obesity-related co-morbid requirement.

NOTE: If ICD-9-CM diagnosis code 278.01 is present, but a covered procedure code (listed in Sec.150.2 or Sec.150.3) is/are not present, the claim is not for bariatric surgery and should be processed under normal procedures.

B. Non-Covered Bariatric Surgery Procedures
Carriers, FIs and A/B MACs are to process non-covered practitioner bariatric surgery claims according to the conditions outlined below:

1. Deny claims billed with HCPCS procedure code 43842 when used for:
   - Open vertical banded gastroplasty.
2. Deny claims billed with HCPCS NOC code 43999 when used for:
   - Laparoscopic vertical banded gastroplasty.
   - Open sleeve gastrectomy.
   - Laparoscopic sleeve gastrectomy.
   - Open adjustable gastric banding.

The FIs and A/B MACs are to process non-covered inpatient bariatric surgery claims according to the conditions outlined below:

1. Reject claims billed with principal ICD-9 CM diagnosis code 278.01 and ICD-9 procedure code 44.68 when used for:
   - Open adjustable gastric banding.
   - Laparoscopic vertical banded gastroplasty.
2. Reject claims billed with principal ICD-9 CM diagnosis code 278.01 and ICD-9 procedure code 44.69 when used for:
   - Open vertical banded gastroplasty.
3. Reject claims billed with principal ICD-9 CM diagnosis code 278.01 and ICD-9 procedure code 43.89 when used for:
   - Open sleeve gastrectomy.
   - Laparoscopic sleeve gastrectomy.

NOTE: If ICD-9 procedure code 43.89 appears on the claim along with 45.51 and 45.91 to describe open or laparoscopic BPD/DS, process as a covered procedure according to Sec.150.6.A.

100-4, 32, 160.1

Category B Investigational Device Exemption (IDE) Study Coverage

Effective July 1, 2001, Medicare covers percutaneous transluminal angioplasty (PTA) of the carotid artery concurrent with stent placement when furnished in accordance with the Food and Drug Administration (FDA) protocols governing Category B Investigational Device Exemption (IDE) studies.

The billing for this procedure is based upon how the service is delivered. There are several CPT codes that may be billed depending upon how the procedure is performed. Contractor medical directors should consider what provider education information is needed to assist providers on the billing for this service.

Contractors must review their local coverage determinations to ensure that payment is provided for claims for PTA in an FDA-approved clinical study and deny any claims for services for PTA of the carotid artery when provided outside of an FDA-approved clinical study.

As a requirement for Category B IDE coverage, providers must bill a six-digit IDE Number that begins with a "G" (i.e., G123456). To identify the line as an IDE line, institutional providers must bill this IDE Number on a 0624 Revenue Code line while practitioners must bill this IDE Number along with a Q0 modifier.

100-4, 32, 160.2

Post-Approval Study Coverage

Effective October 12, 2004, Medicare covers PTA of the carotid artery concurrent with the placement of an FDA-approved carotid stent and an FDA-approved or -cleared embolic protection device (effective December 9, 2009) for an FDA-approved indication when furnished in accordance with FDA-approved protocols governing post-approval studies. Billing post-approval studies is similar to normal Category B IDE billing procedures, except that under post-approval coverage, providers must bill the Pre-Market Approval (PMA) number assigned to the stent system by the FDA. PMA numbers are like typical IDE Numbers in that they have six-digits, but they begin with a "P" (i.e., P123456) instead of a "G."

100-4, 32, 170.1

General

Effective for services performed from May 16, 2006 through August 13, 2007, the Centers for Medicare & Medicaid Services (CMS) made the decision that lumbar artificial disc replacement (LADR) with the CharitéTM lumbar artificial disc is non-covered for Medicare beneficiaries over 60 years of age. See Pub. 100-03, Medicare National Coverage Determinations Manual, section 150.10, for more information about the non-covered determination.

Effective for services performed on or after August 14, 2007, CMS made the decision that LADR with any lumbar artificial disc is non-covered for Medicare beneficiaries over 60 years of age, (i.e. on or after a beneficiary's 61st birthday).

For Medicare beneficiaries 60 years of age and younger, there is no national coverage determination for LADR, leaving such determinations to continue to be made by the local contractors.

100-4, 32, 170.2

Carrier Billing Requirements

Effective for services performed on or after May 16, 2006 through December 31, 2006, carriers shall deny claims, for Medicare beneficiaries over 60 years of age, submitted with the following Category III Codes:

0091T Single interspace, lumbar; and

0092T Each additional interspace (List separately in addition to code for primary procedure.)

Effective for services performed on or after January 1, 2007 through August 13, 2007, for Medicare beneficiaries over 60 years of age, LADR with the CharitéTM lumbar artificial disc, carriers shall deny claims submitted with the following codes:

22857 Total disc arthroplasty (artificial disc), anterior approach, including discectomy to prepare interspace (other than for decompression), lumbar, single interspace; and

0163T Total disc arthroplasty (artificial disc), anterior approach, including discectomy to prepare interspace (other than for decompression), lumbar, each additional interspace.

Carriers shall continue to follow their normal claims processing criteria for IDEs for LADR performed with an implant eligible under the IDE criteria.

For dates of service May 16, 2006 through August 13, 2007, Medicare coverage under the investigational device exemption (IDE) for LADR with a disc other than the CharitéTM lumbar disc in eligible clinical trials is not impacted.

Effective for services performed on or after August 14, 2007, carriers shall deny claims for LADR surgery, for Medicare beneficiaries over 60 years of age, (i.e. on or after a beneficiary's 61st birthday) submitted with the following codes:

22857 Total disc arthroplasty (artificial disc), anterior approach, including discectomy to prepare interspace (other than for decompression), lumbar, single interspace; and

0163T Total disc arthroplasty (artificial disc), anterior approach, including discectomy to prepare interspace (other than for decompression), lumbar, each additional interspace.

100-4, 32, 180.1

Coverage Requirements

Medicare covers cryosurgery of the prostate gland effective for claims with dates of service on or after July 1, 1999. The coverage is for:

1. Primary treatment of patients with clinically localized prostate cancer, Stages T1 - T3 (diagnosis code is 185 - malignant neoplasm of prostate).
2. Salvage therapy (effective for claims with dates of service on or after July 1, 2001 for patients:
   a. Having recurrent, localized prostate cancer;
   b. Failing a trial of radiation therapy as their primary treatment; and
   c. Meeting one of these conditions: State T2B or below; Gleason score less than 9 or; PSA less than 8 ng/ml.

100-4, 32, 180.2

Billing Requirements

Claims for cryosurgery for the prostate gland are to be submitted on the ANSI X12 ASC 837, or, in exceptional circumstances, on a hard copy Form CMS - 1450. This procedure can be rendered in an inpatient or outpatient hospital setting (types of bill (TOBs) 11x 13x, 83x, and 85x).

The FI will look for the following when processing claims with cryosurgery services:

- Diagnosis Code 185 (must be on all cryosurgical claims);
- For outpatient claims HCPCS 55873 and revenue codes 0360, 0361, or 0369 Cryosurgery ablation of localized prostate cancer, stages T1- T3 (includes ultrasonic guidance for interstitial cryosurgery probe placement, postoperative irrigations and aspiration of sloughing tissue included) must be on all outpatient claims; and
- For inpatient claims procedure code 60.62 (perineal prostatectomy- the definition includes cryoablation of prostate, cryostatectomy of prostate, and radical cryosurgical ablation of prostate) must be on the claim.

100-4, 32, 190

Billing Requirements for Extracorporeal Photopheresis

Effective for dates of services on and after December 19, 2006, Medicare has expanded coverage for extracorporeal photopheresis for patients with acute cardiac allograft rejection whose disease is refractory to standard immunosuppresive drug treatment and patients with chronic graft versus host disease whose disease is refractory to standard immunosuppresive drug treatment. (See Pub. 100-03, chapter 1, section 110.4, for complete coverage guidelines).

100-4,32,190.2

Healthcare Common Procedural Coding System (HCPCS), Applicable Diagnosis Codes and Procedure Code

The following HCPCS procedure code is used for billing extracorporeal photopheresis

36522 Photopheresis, extracorporeal

The following are the applicable ICD-9-CM diagnosis codes for the new expanded coverage:

996.83 Complications of transplanted heart, or

996.85 Complications of transplanted bone marrow.

The following is the applicable ICD-9-CM procedure code for the new expanded coverage:

99.88 Therapeutic photopheresis.

NOTE:Contractors shall edit for an appropriate oncological and autoimmune disorder diagnosis for payment of extracorporeal photopheresis according to the National Coverage Determination

100-4, 32, 220.1

220.1 - General

Effective for services on or after September 29, 2008, the Center for Medicare & Medicaid Services (CMS) made the decision that Thermal Intradiscal Procedures (TIPS) are not reasonable and necessary for the treatment of low back pain. Therefore, TIPs are non-covered. Refer to Pub.100-03, Medicare National Coverage Determination (NCD) Manual Chapter 1, Part 2, Section 150.11, for further information on the NCD.

100-4, 32, 220.2

220.2 - Contractors, A/B Medicare Administrative Contractors (MACs)

The following Healthcare Common Procedure Coding System (HCPCS) codes will be nationally non-covered by Medicare effective for dates of service on and after September 29, 2008: 22526: Percutaneous intradiscal electrothermal annuloplasty, unilateral or bilateral including fluoroscopic guidance; single level 22527: Percutaneous intradiscal electrothermal annuloplasty, unilateral or bilateral including fluoroscopic guidance; one or more additional levels 0062T: Percutaneous intradiscal annuloplasty, any method except electrothermal, unilateral or bilateral including fluoroscopic guidance; single level 0063T: Percutaneous intradiscal annuloplasty, any method except electrothermal, unilateral or bilateral including fluoroscopic guidance; one or more additional levels NOTE: The change to add the non-covered indicator for the above HCPCS codes will be part of the January 2009 Medicare Physician Fee Schedule Update. The change to the status indicator to non-cover the above HCPCS will be part of the January Integrated Outpatient Code Editor (IOCE) update.

Claims submitted with the non-covered HCPCS codes on or after September 29, 2008, will be denied by Medicare contractors

100-4, 32, 270

Claims Processing for Implantable Automatic Defibrillators

Claims Processing for Implantable Automatic Defibrillators

Claims Processing for Implantable Automatic Defibrillators

Coverage Requirements- The implantable automatic defibrillator is an electronic device designed to detect and treat life threatening tachyarrhythmias. The device consists of a pulse generator and electrodes for sensing and defibrillating.

See Sec.20.4 -Medicare National Coverage Determinations (NCD) Manual for the complete list of covered indications.

100-4, 32, 270.1

Coding Requirements for Implantable Automatic Defibrillators

The following are the applicable procedure codes for implantable automatic defibrillators:

33240- (Insertion of single or dual chamber pacing cardioverter-defibrillator pulse generator)

33241(Subcutaneous removal of single or dual chamber pacing cardioverter-defibrillator pulse generator)

33243 (Removal of single or dual chamber pacing cardioverter-defibrillator electrode(s); by thoracotomy)

33244 (Removal of single or dual chamber pacing cardioverter-defibrillator electrodes by thoracotomy)

33249- (Insertion or repositioning of electrode leads(s) for single or dual chamber pacing cardioverter-defibrillator and insertion of pulse generator)

For inpatient hospitals claims, ICD-9 CM procedure code 37.94 shall be used for to report the implantation/replacement of automatic defibrillators.

100-4, 32, 270.2

Billing Requirements for Patients Enrolled in a Data Collection System

Effective for dates of service on or after April 1, 2005, Medicare required that patients receiving a defibrillator for the primary prevention of sudden cardiac arrest be enrolled in a qualifying data collection system. Providers shall use modifier Q0 to identify patients whose data is being submitted to a data collection system.

The following ICD-9 diagnosis codes identify non-primary prevention (secondary prevention) patient or replacement implantations (e.g. due to recalled devices):

427.1	Ventricular tachycardia
427.41	Ventricular fibrillation
427.42	Ventricular flutter
427.5	Cardiac arrest
427.9	Cardiac dysrhythmia, unspecified
V12.53	Personal history of sudden cardiac arrest
996.04	Mechanical complication of cardiac device, implant, and graft, due to automatic implantable cardiac defibrillator
V53.32	Fitting and adjustment of other device, automatic implantable cardiac defibrillator

When any of the above codes appear on a claim, the Q0 modifier is not required. The Q0 modifier may be appended to claims for secondary prevention indications when data is being entered into a qualifying data collection system.

100-8, 10, 2.2.8

Cardiac Rehabilitation (CR) and Intensive Cardiac Rehabilitation (ICR)

A. General Background Information
Effective January 1, 2010, Medicare Part B covers Cardiac Rehabilitation (CR) and Intensive Cardiac Rehabilitation (ICR) program services for beneficiaries who have experienced one or more of the following:

An acute myocardial infarction within the preceding 12 months;

A coronary artery bypass surgery;

Current stable angina pectoris;

Heart valve repair or replacement;

Percutaneous transluminal coronary angioplasty or coronary stenting;

A heart or heart-lung transplant; or,

Other cardiac conditions as specified through a national coverage determination (NCD) (CR only).

ICR programs must be approved by CMS through the national coverage determination (NCD) process and must meet certain criteria for approval. Individual sites wishing to provide ICR services via an approved ICR program must enroll with their local contractor or MAC as an ICR program supplier.

B. ICR Enrollment
In order to enroll as an ICR site, a supplier must complete a Form CMS-855B, with the supplier type of "Other" selected. Contractors shall verify that the ICR program is approved by CMS through the NCD process. A list of approved ICR programs will be identified through the NCD listings, the CMS Web site and the Federal Register. Contractors shall use one of these options to verify that the ICR program has met CMS approval.

ICR suppliers shall be enrolled using specialty code 31. ICR suppliers must separately enroll each of their practice locations. Therefore, each enrolling ICR supplier can only have one practice location on its CMS-855B enrollment application and shall receive its own PTAN.

Contractors shall only accept and process reassignments (855R's) to ICR suppliers for physicians defined in 1861(r)(1) of the Act.

C. Additional Information
For more information on ICR suppliers, refer to:

42 CFR Sec.410.49;

Pub. 100-04, Medicare Claims Processing Manual, chapter 32, sections 140.2.2 - 140.2.2.6; and

Pub. 100-02, Medicare Benefit Policy Manual. chapter 15, section 232.

APPENDIX H — GLOSSARY

-centesis. Puncture, as with a needle, trocar, or aspirator; often done for withdrawing fluid from a cavity.

-ectomy. Excision, removal.

-orrhaphy. Suturing.

-ostomy. Indicates a surgically created artificial opening.

-otomy. Making an incision or opening.

-plasty. Indicates surgically formed or molded.

abdominal lymphadenectomy. Surgical removal of the abdominal lymph nodes grouping, with or without para-aortic and vena cava nodes.

ablation. Removal or destruction of a body part or tissue or its function. Ablation may be performed by surgical means, hormones, drugs, radiofrequency, heat, chemical application, or other methods.

abnormal alleles. Form of gene that includes disease-related variations.

absorbable sutures. Strands prepared from collagen or a synthetic polymer and capable of being absorbed by tissue over time. Examples include surgical gut and collagen sutures; or synthetics like polydioxanone (PDS), polyglactin 910 (Vicryl), poliglecaprone 25 (Monocryl), polyglyconate (Maxon), and polyglycolic acid (Dexon). For wound repair, see CPT codes 12001-13160. Correct code assignment is dependent upon the type of closure performed (i.e., simple, intermediate, or complex), the anatomical site, and the wound size.

acetabuloplasty. Surgical repair or reconstruction of the large cup-shaped socket in the hipbone (acetabulum) with which the head of the femur articulates.

Achilles tendon. Tendon attached to the back of the heel bone (calcaneus) that flexes the foot downward.

acromioclavicular joint. Junction between the clavicle and the scapula. The acromion is the projection from the back of the scapula that forms the highest point of the shoulder and connects with the clavicle. Trauma or injury to the acromioclavicular joint is often referred to as a dislocation of the shoulder. This is not correct, however, as a dislocation of the shoulder is a disruption of the glenohumeral joint. Synonym: AC joint.

acromionectomy. Surgical treatment for acromioclavicular arthritis in which the distal portion of the acromion process is removed.

acromioplasty. Repair of the part of the shoulder blade that connects to the deltoid muscles and clavicle.

actigraphy. Science of monitoring activity levels, particularly during sleep. In most cases, the patient wears a wristband that records motion while sleeping. The data are recorded, analyzed, and interpreted to study sleep/wake patterns and circadian rhythms.

air conduction. Transportation of sound from the air, through the external auditory canal, to the tympanic membrane and ossicular chain. Air conduction hearing is tested by presenting an acoustic stimulus through earphones or a loudspeaker to the ear.

air puff device. Instrument that measures intraocular pressure by evaluating the force of a reflected amount of air blown against the cornea.

alleles. Form of gene usually arising from a mutation responsible for a hereditary variation.

allogeneic collection. Collection of blood or blood components from one person for the use of another. Allogeneic collection was formerly termed homologous collection.

allograft. Graft from one individual to another of the same species.

amniocentesis. Surgical puncture through the abdominal wall, with a specialized needle and under ultrasonic guidance, into the interior of the pregnant uterus and directly into the amniotic sac to collect fluid for diagnostic analysis or therapeutic reduction of fluid levels.

anastomosis. Surgically created connection between ducts, blood vessels, or bowel segments to allow flow from one to the other.

anesthesia time. Time period factored into anesthesia procedures beginning with the anesthesiologist preparing the patient for surgery and ending when the patient is turned over to the recovery department.

Angelman syndrome. Early childhood emergence of a pattern of interrupted development, stiff, jerky gait, absence or impairment of speech, excessive laughter, and seizures.

angioplasty. Reconstruction or repair of a diseased or damaged blood vessel.

annuloplasty. Surgical plicaton of weakened tissue of the heart, to improve its muscular function. Annuli are thick, fibrous rings and one is found surrounding each of the cardiac chambers. The atrial and ventricular muscle fibers attach to the annuli. In annuloplasty, weakened annuli may be surgically plicated, or tucked, to improve muscular functions.

anorectal anometry. Measurement of pressure generated by anal sphincter to diagnose incontinence.

anterior chamber lenses. Lenses inserted into the anterior chamber following intracapsular cataract extraction.

applanation tonometer. Instrument that measures intraocular pressure by recording the force required to flatten an area of the cornea.

appropriateness of care. Proper setting of medical care that best meets the patient's care or diagnosis, as defined by a health care plan or other legal entity.

aqueous humor. Fluid within the anterior and posterior chambers of the eye that is continually replenished as it diffuses out into the blood. When the flow of aqueous is blocked, a build-up of fluid in the eye causes increased intraocular pressure and leads to glaucoma and blindness.

arthrotomy. Surgical incision into a joint that may include exploration, drainage, or removal of a foreign body.

ASA. American Society of Anesthesiologists. National organization for anesthesiology that maintains and publishes the guidelines and relative values for anesthesia coding.

aspirate. To withdraw fluid or air from a body cavity by suction.

atrial septal defect. Cardiac anomaly consisting of a patent opening in the atrial septum due to a fusion failure, classified as ostium secundum type, ostium primum defect, or endocardial cushion defect.

attended surveillance. Ability of a technician at a remote surveillance center or location to respond immediately to patient transmissions regarding rhythm or device alerts as they are produced and received at the remote location. These transmissions may originate from wearable or implanted therapy or monitoring devices.

auricle. External ear, which is a single elastic cartilage covered in skin and normal adnexal features (hair follicles, sweat glands, and sebaceous glands), shaped to channel sound waves into the acoustic meatus.

autogenous transplant. Tissue, such as bone, that is harvested from the patient and used for transplantation back into the same patient.

autograft. Any tissue harvested from one anatomical site of a person and grafted to another anatomical site of the same person. Most commonly, blood vessels, skin, tendons, fascia, and bone are used as autografts.

backbench preparation. Procedures performed on a donor organ following procurement to prepare the organ for transplant into the recipient. Excess fat and other tissue may be removed, the organ may be perfused, and vital arteries may be sized, repaired, or modified to fit the patient. These procedures are done on a back table in the operating room before transplantation can begin.

Bartholin's gland. Mucous-producing gland found in the vestibular bulbs on either side of the vaginal orifice and connected to the mucosal membrane at the opening by a duct.

Bartholin's gland abscess. Pocket of pus and surrounding cellulitis caused by infection of the Bartholin's gland and causing localized swelling and pain in the posterior labia majora that may extend into the lower vagina.

basic value. Relative weighted value based upon the usual anesthesia services and the relative work or cost of the specific anesthesia service assigned to each anesthesia-specific procedure code.

Berman locator. Small, sensitive tool used to detect the location of a metallic foreign body in the eye.

bifurcated. Having two branches or divisions, such as the left pulmonary veins that split off from the left atrium to carry oxygenated blood away from the heart.

biopsy. Tissue or fluid removed for diagnostic purposes through analysis of the cells in the biopsy material.

Blalock-Hanlon procedure. Excision of a segment of the right atrium, creating an atrial septal defect.

Blalock-Taussig procedure. Anastomosis of the left subclavian artery to the left pulmonary artery or the right subclavian artery to the right pulmonary artery in order to shunt some of the blood flow from the systemic to the pulmonary circulation.

blepharochalasis. Loss of elasticity and relaxation of skin of the eyelid, thickened or indurated skin on the eyelid associated with recurrent episodes of edema, and intracellular atrophy.

blepharoplasty. Plastic surgery of the eyelids to remove excess fat and redundant skin weighting down the lid. The eyelid is pulled tight and sutured to support sagging muscles.

blepharoptosis. Droop or displacement of the upper eyelid, caused by paralysis, muscle problems, or outside mechanical forces.

blepharorrhaphy. Suture of a portion or all of the opposing eyelids to shorten the palpebral fissure or close it entirely.

bone conduction. Transportation of sound through the bones of the skull to the inner ear.

bone mass measurement. Radiologic or radioisotopic procedure or other procedure approved by the FDA for identifying bone mass, detecting bone loss, or determining bone quality. The procedure includes a physician's interpretation of the results. Qualifying individuals must be an estrogen-deficient woman at clinical risk for osteoporosis with vertebral abnormalities. NCD Reference: 150.3.

brachytherapy. Form of radiation therapy in which radioactive pellets or seeds are implanted directly into the tissue being treated to deliver their dose of radiation in a more directed fashion. Brachytherapy provides radiation to the prescribed body area while minimizing exposure to normal tissue.

breakpoint. Point at which a chromosome breaks.

Bristow procedure. Anterior capsulorrhaphy prevents chronic separation of the shoulder. In this procedure, the bone block is affixed to the anterior glenoid rim with a screw.

buccal mucosa. Tissue from the mucous membrane on the inside of the cheek.

Caldwell-Luc operation. Intraoral antrostomy approach into the maxillary sinus for the removal of tooth roots or tissue, or for packing the sinus to reduce zygomatic fractures by creating a window above the teeth in the canine fossa area.

canthorrhaphy. Suturing of the palpebral fissure, the juncture between the eyelids, at either end of the eye.

canthotomy. Horizontal incision at the canthus (junction of upper and lower eyelids) to divide the outer canthus and enlarge lid margin separation.

cardio-. Relating to the heart.

cardiopulmonary bypass. Venous blood is diverted to a heart-lung machine, which mechanically pumps and oxygenates the blood temporarily so the heart can be bypassed while an open procedure on the heart or coronary arteries is performed. During bypass, the lungs are deflated and immobile.

cardioverter-defibrillator. Device that uses both low energy cardioversion or defibrillating shocks and antitachycardia pacing to treat ventricular tachycardia or ventricular fibrillation.

care plan oversight services. Physician's ongoing review and revision of a patient's care plan involving complex or multidisciplinary care modalities.

case management services. Physician case management is a process of involving direct patient care as well as coordinating and controlling access to the patient or initiating and/or supervising other necessary health care services.

cataract extraction. Surgical removal of the cataract or cloudy lens. Anterior chamber lenses are inserted in conjunction with intracapsular cataract extraction and posterior chamber lenses are inserted in conjunction with extracapsular cataract extraction.

catheter. Flexible tube inserted into an area of the body for introducing or withdrawing fluid.

Centers for Medicare and Medicaid Services. Federal agency that oversees the administration of the public health programs such as Medicare, Medicaid, and State Children's Insurance Program.

certified nurse midwife. Registered nurse who has successfully completed a program of study and clinical experience or has been certified by a recognized organization for the care of pregnant or delivering patients.

CFR. Code of Federal Regulations.

CHAMPUS. Civilian Health and Medical Program of the Uniformed Services. See Tricare.

CHAMPVA. Civilian Health and Medical Program of the Veteran's Administration.

Chiari osteotomy. Top of the femur is altered to correct a dislocated hip caused by congenital conditions or cerebral palsy. Plate and screws are often used.

chimera. Organ or anatomic structure consisting of tissues of diverse genetic constitution.

choanal atresia. Congenital, membranous, or bony closure of one or both posterior nostrils due to failure of the embryonic bucconasal membrane to rupture and open up the nasal passageway.

chondromalacia. Condition in which the articular cartilage softens, seen in various body sites but most often in the patella, and may be congenital or acquired.

chondroplasty. Surgical repair of cartilage.

chorionic villus sampling. Aspiration of a placental sample through a catheter, under ultrasonic guidance. The specialized needle is placed transvaginally through the cervix or transabdominally into the uterine cavity.

chronic pain management services. Distinct services frequently performed by anesthesiologists who have additional training in pain management procedures. Pain management services include initial and subsequent evaluation and management (E/M) services, trigger point injections, spine and spinal cord injections, and nerve blocks.

cineplastic amputation. Amputation in which muscles and tendons of the remaining portion of the extremity are arranged so that they may be utilized for motor functions. Following this type of amputation, a specially constructed prosthetic device allows the individual to execute more complex movements because the muscles and tendons are able to communicate independent movements to the device.

circadian. Relating to a cyclic, 24-hour period.

clinical social worker. Individual who possesses a master's or doctor's degree in social work and, after obtaining the degree, has performed at least two years of supervised clinical social work. A clinical social worker must be licensed by the state or, in the case of states without licensure, must completed at least two years or 3,000 hours of post-master's degree supervised clinical social work practice under the supervision of a master's level social worker.

clonal. Originating from one cell.

CMS. Centers for Medicare and Medicaid Services. Federal agency that administers the public health programs.

CO2 laser. Carbon dioxide laser that emits an invisible beam and vaporizes water-rich tissue. The vapor is suctioned from the site.

codons. Series of three adjoining bases in one polynucleotide chain of a DNA or RNA molecule that provides the codes for a specific amino acid.

colostomy. Artificial surgical opening anywhere along the length of the colon to the skin surface for the diversion of feces.

commissurotomy. Surgical division or disruption of any two parts that are joined to form a commissure in order to increase the opening. The procedure most often refers to opening the adherent leaflet bands of fibrous tissue in a stenosed mitral valve.

common variants. Nucleotide sequence differences associated with abnormal gene function. Tests are usually performed in a single series of laboratory testing (in a single, typically multiplex, assay arrangement or using more than one assay to include all variants to be examined). Variants are representative of a mutation that mainly causes a single disease, such as cystic fibrosis. Other uncommon variants could provide additional information. Tests may be performed based on society recommendations and guidelines.

community mental health center. Facility providing outpatient mental health day treatment, assessments, and education as appropriate to community members.

computerized corneal topography. Digital imaging and analysis by computer of the shape of the corneal.

conjunctiva. Mucous membrane lining of the eyelids and covering of the exposed, anterior sclera.

conjunctivodacryocystostomy. Surgical connection of the lacrimal sac directly to the conjunctival sac.

conjunctivorhinostomy. Correction of an obstruction of the lacrimal canal achieved by suturing the posterior flaps and removing any lacrimal obstruction, preserving the conjunctiva.

constitutional. Cells containing genetic code that may be passed down to future generations. May also be referred to as germline.

consultation. Advice or opinion regarding diagnosis and treatment or determination to accept transfer of care of a patient rendered by a medical professional at the request of the primary care provider.

continuous positive airway pressure device. Pressurized device used to maintain the patient's airway for spontaneous or mechanically aided breathing. Often used for patients with mild to moderate sleep apnea. Synonym: CPAP device.

core needle biopsy. Large-bore biopsy needle inserted into a mass and a core of tissue is removed for diagnostic study.

corpectomy. Removal of the body of a bone, such as a vertebra.

costochondral. Pertaining to the ribs and the scapula.

CPT. Current Procedural Terminology. Definitive procedural coding system developed by the American Medical Association that lists descriptive terms and identifying codes to provide a uniform language that describes medical, surgical, and diagnostic services for nationwide communication among physicians, patients, and third parties, used in outpatient reporting of services.

craniosynostosis. Congenital condition in which one or more of the cranial sutures fuse prematurely, creating a deformed or aberrant head shape.

craterization. Excision of a portion of bone creating a crater-like depression to facilitate drainage from infected areas of bone.

cricoid. Circular cartilage around the trachea.

CRNA. Certified registered nurse anesthetist. Nurse trained and specializing in the administration of anesthesia.

cryolathe. Tool used for reshaping a button of corneal tissue.

cryosurgery. Application of intense cold, usually produced using liquid nitrogen, to locally freeze diseased or unwanted tissue and induce tissue necrosis without causing harm to adjacent tissue.

CT. Computed tomography.

cutdown. Small, incised opening in the skin to expose a blood vessel, especially over a vein (venous cutdown) to allow venipuncture and permit a needle or cannula to be inserted for the withdrawal of blood or administration of fluids.

cytogenetic studies. Procedures in CPT that are related to the branch of genetics that studies cellular (cyto) structure and function as it relates to heredity (genetics). White blood cells, specifically T-lymphocytes, are the most commonly used specimen for chromosome analysis. NCD Reference: 190.3.

cytogenomic. Chromosomic evaluation using molecular methods.

dacryocystotome. Instrument used for incising the lacrimal duct strictures.

debride. To remove all foreign objects and devitalized or infected tissue from a burn or wound to prevent infection and promote healing.

definitive identification. Identification of microorganisms using additional tests to specify the genus or species (e.g., slide cultures or biochemical panels).

Department of Health and Human Services. Cabinet department that oversees the operating divisions of the federal government responsible for health and welfare. HHS oversees the Centers for Medicare and Medicaid Services, Food and Drug Administration, Public Health Service, and other such entities. Synonym(s): DHHS, HHS.

Department of Justice. Attorneys from DOJ and the United States Attorney's Office have, under the memorandum of understanding, the same direct access to contractor data and records as OIG and the FBI. DOJ is responsible for prosecuting the fraud and civil or criminal cases that are presented. Synonym: DOJ.

dermis. Skin layer found under the epidermis that contains a papillary upper layer and the deep reticular layer of collagen, vascular bed, and nerves.

dermis graft. Skin graft that has been separated from the epidermal tissue and the underlying subcutaneous fat, used primarily as a substitute for fascia grafts in plastic surgery.

desensitization. 1) Administration of extracts of allergens periodically to build immunity in the patient. 2) Application of medication to decrease the symptoms, usually pain, associated with a dental condition or disease.

destruction. Ablation or eradication of a structure or tissue.

diabetes outpatient self-management training services. Educational and training services furnished by a certified provider in an outpatient setting. The physician managing the individual's diabetic condition must certify that the services are needed under a comprehensive plan of care and provide the patient with the skills and knowledge necessary for therapeutic program compliance (including skills related to the self-administration of injectable drugs). The provider must meet applicable standards established by the National Diabetes Advisory or be recognized by an organization that represents individuals with diabetes as meeting standards for furnishing the services.

diagnostic procedures. Procedure performed on a patient to obtain information to assess the medical condition of the patient or to identify a disease and to determine the nature and severity of an illness or injury.

diaphragm. 1) Muscular wall separating the thorax and its structures from the abdomen. 2) Flexible disk inserted into the vagina and against the cervix as a method of birth control.

diaphysectomy. Surgical removal of a portion of the shaft of a long bone, often done to facilitate drainage from infected bone.

diathermy. Applying heat to body tissues by various methods for therapeutic treatment or surgical purposes to coagulate and seal tissue.

dilation. Artificial increase in the diameter of an opening or lumen made by medication or by instrumentation.

dissect. Cut apart or separate tissue for surgical purposes or for visual or microscopic study.

DNA marker. Specific gene sequence within a chromosome indicating the inheritance of a certain trait.

dorsal. Pertaining to the back or posterior aspect.

drugs and biologicals. Drugs and biologicals included - or approved for inclusion - in the United States Pharmacopoeia, the National Formulary, the United States Homeopathic Pharmacopoeia, in New Drugs or Accepted Dental Remedies, or approved by the pharmacy and drug therapeutics committee of the medical staff of the hospital. Also included are medically accepted and FDA approved drugs used in an anticancer chemotherapeutic regimen. The carrier determines medical acceptance based on supportive clinical evidence.

dual-lead device. Implantable cardiac device (pacemaker or implantable cardioverter-defibrillator [ICD]) in which pacing and sensing components are placed in only two chambers of the heart.

duplex scan. Noninvasive vascular diagnostic technique that uses ultrasonic scanning to identify the pattern and direction of blood flow within arteries or veins displayed in real time images. Duplex scanning combines B-mode two-dimensional pictures of the vessel structure with spectra and/or color flow Doppler mapping or imaging of the blood as it moves through the vessels.

duplication/deletion (DUP/DEL). Term used in molecular testing which examines genomic regions to determine if there are extra chromosomes (duplication) or missing chromosomes (deletions). Normal gene dosage is two copies per cell except for the sex chromosomes which have one per cell.

DuToit staple capsulorrhaphy. Reattachment of the capsule of the shoulder and glenoid labrum to the glenoid lip using staples to anchor the avulsed capsule and glenoid labrum.

Dx. Diagnosis.

DXA. Dual energy x-ray absorptiometry. Radiological technique for bone density measurement using a two-dimensional projection system in which two x-ray beams with different levels of energy are pulsed alternately and the results are given in two scores, reported as standard deviations from peak bone mass density.

dynamic mutation. Unstable or changing polynucleotides resulting in repeats related to genes that can undergo disease-producing increases or decreases in the repeats that differ within tissues or over generations.

dynamic splint. Brace that permits movement of an anatomical structure such as a hand, wrist, foot, or other part of the body after surgery or injury.

ECMO. Extracorporeal membrane oxygenation.

ectropion. Drooping of the lower eyelid away from the eye or outward turning or eversion of the edge of the eyelid, exposing the palpebral conjunctiva and causing irritation.

Eden-Hybinette procedure. Anterior shoulder repair using an anterior bone block to augment the bony anterior glenoid lip.

EDTA. Drug used to inhibit damage to the cornea by collagenase. EDTA is especially effective in alkali burns as it neutralizes soluble alkali, including lye.

effusion. Escape of fluid from within a body cavity.

electrocardiographic rhythm derived. Analysis of data obtained from readings of the heart's electrical activation, including heart rate and rhythm, variability of heart rate, ST analysis, and T-wave alternans. Other data may also be assessed when warranted.

electrocautery. Division or cutting of tissue using high-frequency electrical current to produce heat, which destroys cells.

electrode array. Electronic device containing more than one contact whose function can be adjusted during programming services. Electrodes are specialized for a particular electrochemical reaction that acts as a medium between a body surface and another instrument.

electrooculogram (EOG). Record of electrical activity associated with eye movements.

electrophysiologic studies. Electrical stimulation and monitoring to diagnose heart conduction abnormalities that predispose patients to bradyarrhythmias and to determine a patient's chance for developing ventricular and supraventricular tachyarrhythmias.

emergency. Serious medical condition or symptom (including severe pain) resulting from injury, sickness, or mental illness that arises suddenly and requires immediate care and treatment, generally received within 24 hours of onset, to avoid jeopardy to the life, limb, or health of a covered person.

empyema. Accumulation of pus within the respiratory, or pleural, cavity.

EMTALA. Emergency Medical Treatment and Active Labor Act.

endarterectomy. Removal of the thickened, endothelial lining of a diseased or damaged artery.

entropion. Inversion of the eyelid, turning the edge in toward the eyeball and causing irritation from contact of the lashes with the surface of the eye.

enucleation. Removal of a growth or organ cleanly so as to extract it in one piece.

epidermis. Outermost, nonvascular layer of skin that contains four to five differentiated layers depending on its body location: stratum corneum, lucidum, granulosum, spinosum, and basale.

epiphysiodesis. Surgical fusion of an epiphysis performed to prematurely stop further bone growth.

escharotomy. Surgical incision into the scab or crust resulting from a severe burn in order to relieve constriction and allow blood flow to the distal unburned tissue.

established patient. 1) Patient who has received professional services in a face-to-face setting within the last three years from the same physician or another physician of the same specialty who belongs to the same group practice. 2) For OPPS hospitals, patient who has been registered as an inpatient or outpatient in a hospital's provider-based clinic or emergency department within the past three years.

evacuation. Removal or purging of waste material.

evaluation and management codes. Assessment and management of a patient's health care using CPT codes 99201-99499.

evaluation and management service components. Key components of history, examination, and medical decision making that are key to selecting the correct E/M codes. Other non-key components include counseling, coordination of care, nature of presenting problem, and time.

event recorder. Portable, ambulatory heart monitor worn by the patient that makes electrocardiographic recordings of the length and frequency of aberrant cardiac rhythm to help diagnose heart conditions and to assess pacemaker functioning or programming.

exenteration. Surgical removal of the entire contents of a body cavity, such as the pelvis or orbit.

exon. One of multiple nucleic acid sequences used to encode information for a gene polypeptide or protein. Exons are separated from other exons by non-protein-coding sequences known as introns.

extended care services. Items and services provided to an inpatient of a skilled nursing facility, including nursing care, physical or occupational therapy, speech pathology, drugs and supplies, and medical social services.

external electrical capacitor device. External electrical stimulation device designed to promote bone healing. This device may also promote neural regeneration, revascularization, epiphyseal growth, and ligament maturation.

external pulsating electromagnetic field. External stimulation device designed to promote bone healing. This device may also promote neural regeneration, revascularization, epiphyseal growth, and ligament maturation.

extracorporeal. Located or taking place outside the body.

Eyre-Brook capsulorrhaphy. Reattachment of the capsule of the shoulder and glenoid labrum to the glenoid lip.

False Claims Act. Governs civil actions for filing false claims. Liability under this act pertains to any person who knowingly presents or causes to be presented a false or fraudulent claim to the government for payment or approval.

fascia. Fibrous sheet or band of tissue that envelops organs, muscles, and groupings of muscles.

fasciectomy. Excision of fascia or strips of fascial tissue.

fasciotomy. Incision or transection of fascial tissue.

fat graft. Graft composed of fatty tissue completely freed from surrounding tissue that is used primarily to fill in depressions.

FDA. Food and Drug Administration. Federal agency responsible for protecting public health by substantiating the safety, efficacy, and security of human and veterinary drugs, biological products, medical devices, national food supply, cosmetics, and items that give off radiation.

filtered speech test. Test most commonly used to identify central auditory dysfunction in which the patient is presented monosyllabic words that are low pass filtered, allowing only the parts of each word below a certain pitch to be presented. A score is given on the number of correct responses. This may be a subset of a standard battery of tests provided during a single encounter.

fissure. Deep furrow, groove, or cleft in tissue structures.

fistulization. Creation of a communication between two structures that were not previously connected.

flexor digitorum profundus tendon. Tendon originating in the proximal forearm and extending to the index finger and wrist. A thickened FDP sheath, usually caused by age, illness, or injury, can fill the carpal canal and lead to impingement of the median nerve.

fluoroscopy. Radiology technique that allows visual examination of part of the body or a function of an organ using a device that projects an x-ray image on a fluorescent screen.

focal length. Distance between the object in focus and the lens.

focused medical review. Process of targeting and directing medical review efforts on Medicare claims with the highest risk of inappropriate payment. The goal is to reduce the number of noncovered claims or unnecessary services. CMS analyzes national data such as internal billing, utilization, and payment data and provides its findings to the Medicare administrative contractor. Local medical review policies are developed identifying aberrances, abuse, and overutilized services. Providers are responsible for knowing national Medicare coverage and billing guidelines and local medical review policies and for determining whether the services provided to Medicare beneficiaries are covered by Medicare. Synonym: FMR.

fragile X syndrome. Mental retardation, enlarged testes, big jaw, high forehead, and long ears in males. In females, fragile X presents mild retardation and heterozygous sexual structures. In some families, males have shown no symptoms but carry the gene.

free flap. Tissue that is completely detached from the donor site and transplanted to the recipient site, receiving its blood supply from capillary ingrowth at the recipient site.

free microvascular flap. Tissue that is completely detached from the donor site following careful dissection and preservation of the blood vessels, then attached to the recipient site with the transferred blood vessels anastomosed to the vessels in the recipient bed.

fulguration. Destruction of living tissue by using sparks from a high-frequency electric current.

gas tamponade. Absorbable gas may be injected to force the retina against the choroid. Common gases include room air, short-acting sulfahexafluoride, intermediate-acting perfluoroethane, or long-acting perfluorooctane.

Gaucher disease. Genetic metabolic disorder in which fat deposits may accumulate in the spleen, liver, lungs, bone marrow, and brain.

gene. Basic unit of heredity that contains nucleic acid. Genes are arranged in different and unique sequences or strings that determine the gene's function. Human genes usually include multiple protein coding regions such as exons separated by introns which are nonprotein coding sections.

HCPCS. Healthcare Common Procedure Coding System. HCPCS Level I: Healthcare Common Procedure Coding System Level I. Numeric coding system used by physicians, facility outpatient departments, and ambulatory surgery centers (ASC) to code ambulatory, laboratory, radiology, and other diagnostic services for Medicare billing. This coding system contains only the American Medical Association's Physicians' Current Procedural Terminology (CPT) codes. HCPCS Level II: Healthcare Common Procedure Coding System Level II. National coding system, developed by CMS, that contains alphanumeric codes for physician and nonphysician services not included in the CPT coding system. HCPCS Level II codes cover such things as ambulance services, durable medical equipment, and orthotic and prosthetic devices. HCPCS modifiers: Two-character code (AA-ZZ) that identifies circumstances that alter or enhance the description of a service or supply. They are recognized by carriers nationally.

Hct. Hematocrit.

hemilaminectomy. Excision of a portion of the vertebral lamina.

hemodialysis. Cleansing of wastes and contaminating elements from the blood by virtue of different diffusion rates through a semipermeable membrane, which separates blood from a filtration solution that diffuses other elements out of the blood.

hemoperitoneum. Effusion of blood into the peritoneal cavity, the space between the continuous membrane lining the abdominopelvic walls and encasing the visceral organs.

heterograft. Surgical graft of tissue from one animal species to a different animal species. A common type of heterograft is porcine (pig) tissue, used for temporary wound closure.

heterotopic transplant. Tissue transplanted from a different anatomical site for usage as is natural for that tissue, for example, buccal mucosa to a conjunctival site.

HGNC. HUGO gene nomenclature committee.

HGVS. Human genome variation society.

Hickman catheter. Central venous catheter used for long-term delivery of medications, such as antibiotics, nutritional substances, or chemotherapeutic agents.

HLA. Human leukocyte antigen.

home health services. Services furnished to patients in their homes under the care of physicians. These services include part-time or intermittent skilled nursing care, physical therapy, medical social services, medical supplies, and some rehabilitation equipment. Home health supplies and services must be prescribed by a physician, and the beneficiary must be confined at home in order for Medicare to pay the benefits in full. Synonym: HHS.

homograft. Graft from one individual to another of the same species. Synonym: allogeneic graft, allograft.

hospice care. Items and services provided to a terminally ill individual by a hospice program under a written plan established and periodically reviewed by the individual's attending physician and by the medical director: Nursing care provided by or under the supervision of a registered professional nurse; Physical or occupational therapy or speech-language pathology services; Medical social services under the direction of a physician; Services of a home health aide who has successfully completed a training program; Medical supplies (including drugs and biologicals) and the use of medical appliances; Physicians' services; Short-term inpatient care (including both respite care and procedures necessary for pain control and acute and chronic symptom management) in an inpatient facility on an intermittent basis and not consecutively over longer than five days; Counseling (including dietary counseling) with respect to care of the terminally ill individual and adjustment to his death; Any item or service which is specified in the plan and for which payment may be made.

hospital. Institution that provides, under the supervision of physicians, diagnostic, therapeutic, and rehabilitation services for medical diagnosis, treatment, and care of patients. Hospitals receiving federal funds must maintain clinical records on all patients, provide 24-hour nursing services, and have a discharge planning process in place. The term "hospital" also includes religious nonmedical health care institutions and facilities of 50 beds or less located in rural areas.

HUGO. Human genome organization

IA. Intra-arterial.

ICD. Implantable cardioverter defibrillator.

ICD-10-CM. International Classification of Diseases, 10th Revision, Clinical Modification. Diagnostic coding system developed to replace ICD-9-CM in the United States. It is a clinical modification of the World Health Organization's ICD-10, already in use in much of the world, and used for mortality reporting in the United States. The implementation date for ICD-10-CM is October 1, 2013.

ICD-10-PCS. International Classification of Diseases, 10th Revision, Procedure Coding System. Effective October 1, 2013, inpatient hospital services and surgical procedures must be coded using ICD-10-PCS. This code set will replace the current ICD-9-CM, Volume 3 for procedures.

ICM. Implantable cardiovascular monitor.

ileostomy. Artificial surgical opening that brings the end of the ileum out through the abdominal wall to the skin surface for the diversion of feces through a stoma.

iliopsoas tendon. Fibrous tissue that connects muscle to bone in the pelvic region, common to the iliacus and psoas major.

ILR. Implantable loop recorder.

IM. 1) Infectious mononucleosis. 2) Internal medicine. 3) Intramuscular.

implant. Material or device inserted or placed within the body for therapeutic, reconstructive, or diagnostic purposes.

implantable cardiovascular monitor. Implantable electronic device that stores cardiovascular physiologic data such as intracardiac pressure waveforms collected from internal sensors or data such as weight and blood pressure collected from external sensors. The information stored in these devices is used as an aid in managing patients with heart failure and other cardiac conditions that are non-rhythm related. The data may be transmitted via local telemetry or remotely to a surveillance technician or an internet-based file server. Synonym: ICM.

implantable cardioverter-defibrillator. Implantable electronic cardiac device used to control rhythm abnormalities such as tachycardia, fibrillation, or bradycardia by producing high- or low-energy stimulation and pacemaker functions. It may also have the capability to provide the functions of an implantable loop recorder or implantable cardiovascular monitor. Synonym: ICD.

implantable loop recorder. Implantable electronic cardiac device that constantly monitors and records electrocardiographic rhythm. It may be triggered by the patient when a symptomatic episode occurs or activated automatically by rapid or slow heart rates. This may be the sole purpose of the device or it may be a component of another cardiac device such as a pacemaker or implantable cardioverter-defibrillator. The data can be transmitted via local telemetry or remotely to a surveillance technician or an internet-based file server. Synonym: ILR.

implantable venous access device. Catheter implanted for continuous access to the venous system for long-term parenteral feeding or for the administration of fluids or medications.

in situ. Located in the natural position or contained within the origin site, not spread into neighboring tissue.

incontinence. Inability to control urination or defecation.

infundibulectomy. Excision of the anterosuperior portion of the right ventricle of the heart.

internal direct current stimulator. Electrostimulation device placed directly into the surgical site designed to promote bone regeneration by encouraging cellular healing response in bone and ligaments.

interrogation device evaluation. Assessment of an implantable cardiac device (pacemaker, cardioverter-defibrillator, cardiovascular monitor, or loop recorder) in which collected data about the patient's heart rate and rhythm, battery and pulse generator function, and any leads or sensors present, are retrieved and evaluated. Determinations regarding device programming and appropriate treatment settings are made based on the findings. CPT provides required components for evaluation of the various types of devices.

intramedullary implants. Nail, rod, or pin placed into the intramedullary canal at the fracture site. Intramedullary implants not only provide a method of aligning the fracture, they also act as a splint and may reduce fracture pain. Implants may be rigid or flexible. Rigid implants are preferred for prophylactic treatment of diseased bone, while flexible implants are preferred for traumatic injuries.

intraocular lens. Artificial lens implanted into the eye to replace a damaged natural lens or cataract.

intravenous. Within a vein or veins.

introducer. Instrument, such as a catheter, needle, or tube, through which another instrument or device is introduced into the body.

intron. Nonprotein section of a gene that separates exons in human genes. Contains vital sequences that allow splicing of exons to produce a functional protein from a gene. Sometimes referred to as intervening sequences (IVS).

IP. 1) Interphalangeal. 2) Intraperitoneal.

irrigation. To wash out or cleanse a body cavity, wound, or tissue with water or other fluid.

Kayser-Fleischer ring. Condition found in Wilson's disease in which deposits of copper cause a pigmented ring around the cornea's outer border in the deep epithelial layers.

keratoprosthesis. Surgical procedure in which the physician creates a new anterior chamber with a plastic optical implant to replace a severely damaged cornea that cannot be repaired.

keratotomy. Surgical incision of the cornea.

krypton laser. Laser light energy that uses ionized krypton by electric current as the active source, has a radiation beam between the visible yellow-red spectrum, and is effective in photocoagulation of retinal bleeding, macular lesions, and vessel aberrations of the choroid.

lacrimal. Tear-producing gland or ducts that provides lubrication and flushing of the eyes and nasal cavities.

lacrimal punctum. Opening of the lacrimal papilla of the eyelid through which tears flow to the canaliculi to the lacrimal sac.

lacrimotome. Knife for cutting the lacrimal sac or duct.

lacrimotomy. Incision of the lacrimal sac or duct.

laparotomy. Incision through the flank or abdomen for therapeutic or diagnostic purposes.

larynx. Musculocartilaginous structure between the trachea and the pharynx that functions as the valve preventing food and other particles from entering the respiratory tract, as well as the voice mechanism. Also called the voicebox, the larynx is composed of three single cartilages: cricoid, epiglottis, and thyroid; and three paired cartilages: arytenoid, corniculate, and cuneiform.

laser surgery. Use of concentrated, sharply defined light beams to cut, cauterize, coagulate, seal, or vaporize tissue.

LEEP. Loop electrode excision procedure. Biopsy specimen or cone shaped wedge of cervical tissue is removed using a hot cautery wire loop with an electrical current running through it.

levonorgestrel. Drug inhibiting ovulation and preventing sperm from penetrating cervical mucus. It is delivered subcutaneously in polysiloxone capsules. The capsules can be effective for up to five years, and provide a cumulative pregnancy rate of less than 2 percent. The capsules are not biodegradable, and therefore must be removed. Removal is more difficult than insertion of levonorgestrel capsules because fibrosis develops around the capsules. Normal hormonal activity and a return to fertility begins immediately upon removal.

ligament. Band or sheet of fibrous tissue that connects the articular surfaces of bones or supports visceral organs.

ligation. Tying off a blood vessel or duct with a suture or a soft, thin wire.

lymphadenectomy. Dissection of lymph nodes free from the vessels and removal for examination by frozen section in a separate procedure to detect early-stage metastases.

lysis. Destruction, breakdown, dissolution, or decomposition of cells or substances by a specific catalyzing agent.

Magnuson-Stack procedure. Treatment for recurrent anterior dislocation of the shoulder that involves tightening and realigning the subscapularis tendon.

maintenance of wakefulness test. Attended study determining the patient's ability to stay awake.

Manchester colporrhaphy. Preservation of the uterus following prolapse by amputating the vaginal portion of the cervix, shortening the cardinal ligaments, and performing a colpoperineorrhaphy posteriorly.

marsupialization. Creation of a pouch in surgical treatment of a cyst in which one wall is resected and the remaining cut edges are sutured to adjacent tissue creating an open pouch of the previously enclosed cyst.

mastectomy. Surgical removal of one or both breasts.

McDonald procedure. Polyester tape is placed around the cervix with a running stitch to assist in the prevention of pre-term delivery. Tape is removed at term for vaginal delivery.

MCP. Metacarpophalangeal.

medial. Middle or midline.

medical review. Review by a Medicare administrative contractor, carrier, and/or quality improvement organization (QIO) of services and items provided by physicians, other health care practitioners, and providers of health care services under Medicare. The review determines if the items and services are reasonable and necessary and meet Medicare coverage requirements, whether the quality meets professionally recognized standards of health care, and whether the services are medically appropriate in an inpatient, outpatient, or other setting as supported by documentation.

Medicare contractor. Medicare Part A fiscal intermediary, Medicare Part B carrier, Medicare administrative contractor (MAC), or a durable medical equipment Medicare administrative contractor (DME MAC).

Medicare physician fee schedule. List of payments Medicare allows by procedure or service. Payments may vary through geographic adjustments. The MPFS is based on the resource-based relative value scale (RBRVS). A national total relative value unit (RVU) is given to each procedure (HCPCS Level I CPT, Level II national codes). Each total RVU has three components: physician work, practice expense, and malpractice insurance. Synonym: MPFS.

methylation. Mechanism used to regulate genes and protect DNA from some types of cleavage.

microarray. Small surface onto which multiple specific nucleic acid sequences can be attached to be used for analysis. Microarray may also be known as a gene chip or DNA chip. Tests can be run on the sequences for any variants that may be present.

mitral valve. Valve with two cusps that is between the left atrium and left ventricle of the heart.

moderate sedation. Medically controlled state of depressed consciousness, with or without analgesia, while maintaining the patient's airway, protective reflexes, and ability to respond to stimulation or verbal commands.

Mohs micrographic surgery. Special technique used to treat complex or ill-defined skin cancer and requires a single physician to provide two distinct services. The first service is surgical and involves the destruction of the lesion by a combination of chemosurgery and excision. The second service is that of a pathologist and includes mapping, color coding of specimens, microscopic examination of specimens, and complete histopathologic preparation.

monitored anesthesia care. Sedation, with or without analgesia, used to achieve a medically controlled state of depressed consciousness while maintaining the patient's airway, protective reflexes, and ability to respond to stimulation or verbal commands. In dental conscious sedation, the patient is rendered free of fear, apprehension, and anxiety through the use of pharmacological agents. Synonym: MAC.

monoclonal. Relating to a single clone of cells.

multiple sleep latency test (MSLT). Attended study to determine the tendency of the patient to fall asleep.

multiple-lead device. Implantable cardiac device (pacemaker or implantable cardioverter-defibrillator [ICD]) in which pacing and sensing components are placed in at least three chambers of the heart.

Mustard procedure. Corrective measure for transposition of great vessels involves an intra-atrial baffle made of pericardial tissue or synthetic material. The baffle is secured between pulmonary veins and mitral valve and between mitral and tricuspid valves. The baffle directs systemic venous flow into the left ventricle and lungs and pulmonary venous flow into the right ventricle and aorta.

mutation. Alteration in gene function that results in changes to a gene or chromosome. Can cause deficits or disease that can be inherited, can have beneficial affects, or result in no noticeable change.

mutation scanning. Process normally used on multiple polymerase chain reaction (PCR) amplicons to determine DNA sequence variants by differences in characteristics compared to normal. Specific DNA variants can then be studied further.

myasthenia gravis. Autoimmune neuromuscular disorder caused by antibodies to the acetylcholine receptors at the neuromuscular junction, interfering with proper binding of the neurotransmitter from the neuron to the target muscle, causing muscle weakness, fatigue, and exhaustion, without pain or atrophy.

myotomy. Surgical cutting of a muscle to gain access to underlying tissues or for therapeutic reasons.

myringotomy. Incision in the eardrum done to prevent spontaneous rupture precipitated by fluid pressure build-up behind the tympanic membrane and to prevent stagnant infection and erosion of the ossicles.

nasal polyp. Fleshy outgrowth projecting from the mucous membrane of the nose or nasal sinus cavity that may obstruct ventilation or affect the sense of smell.

nasal sinus. Air-filled cavities in the cranial bones lined with mucous membrane and continuous with the nasal cavity, draining fluids through the nose.

nasogastric tube. Long, hollow, cylindrical catheter made of soft rubber or plastic that is inserted through the nose down into the stomach, and is used for feeding, instilling medication, or withdrawing gastric contents.

nasolacrimal punctum. Opening of the lacrimal duct near the nose.

nasopharynx. Membranous passage above the level of the soft palate.

Nd:YAG laser. Laser light energy that uses an yttrium, aluminum, and garnet crystal doped with neodymium ions as the active source, has a radiation beam nearing the infrared spectrum, and is effective in photocoagulation, photoablation, cataract extraction, and lysis of vitreous strands.

nebulizer. Latin for mist, a device that converts liquid into a fine spray and is commonly used to deliver medicine to the upper respiratory, bronchial, and lung areas.

neurectomy. Excision of all or a portion of a nerve.

new patient. Patient who is receiving face-to-face care from a provider or another physician of the exact same specialty and subspecialty who belongs to the same group practice for the first time in three years. For OPPS hospitals, a patient who has not been registered as an inpatient or outpatient, including off-campus provider based clinic or emergency department, within the past three years.

Niemann-Pick syndrome. Accumulation of phospholipid in histiocytes in the bone marrow, liver, lymph nodes, and spleen, cerebral involvement, and red macular spots similar to Tay-Sachs disease. Most commonly found in Jewish infants.

Nissen fundoplasty. Surgical repair technique that involves the fundus of the stomach being wrapped around the lower end of the esophagus to treat reflux esophagitis.

nonabsorbable sutures. Strands of natural or synthetic material that resist absorption into living tissue and are removed once healing is under way. Nonabsorbable sutures are commonly used to close skin wounds and repair tendons or collagenous tissue.

obturator. Prosthesis used to close an acquired or congenital opening in the palate that aids in speech and chewing.

obturator nerve. Lumbar plexus nerve with anterior and posterior divisions that innervate the adductor muscles (e.g., adductor longus, adductor brevis) of the leg and the skin over the medial area of the thigh or a sacral plexus nerve with anterior and posterior divisions that innervate the superior gemellus muscles.

occult blood test. Chemical or microscopic test to determine the presence of blood in a specimen.

ocular implant. Implant inside muscular cone.

oophorectomy. Surgical removal of all or part of one or both ovaries, either as open procedure or laparoscopically. Menstruation and childbearing ability continues when one ovary is removed.

orthosis. Derived from a Greek word meaning "to make straight," it is an artificial appliance that supports, aligns, or corrects an anatomical deformity or improves the use of a moveable body part. Unlike a prosthesis, an orthotic device is always functional in nature.

osteo-. Having to do with bone.

osteogenesis stimulator. Device used to stimulate the growth of bone by electrical impulses or ultrasound.

osteotomy. Surgical cutting of a bone.

ostomy. Artificial (surgical) opening in the body used for drainage or for delivery of medications or nutrients.

pacemaker. Implantable cardiac device that controls the heart's rhythm and maintains regular beats by artificial electric discharges. This device consists of the pulse generator with a battery and the electrodes, or leads, which are placed in single or dual chambers of the heart, usually transvenously. Leads that are placed epicardially require a thoracotomy. A single chamber pacemaker has one lead in the atrium or ventricle. A dual chamber pacemaker has one lead in the right atrium and one in the right ventricle. An extra lead may be used for biventricular pacing of the left ventricle. The generator is placed in a subcutaneous pocket below the clavicle or in an abdominal location. Biventricular pacing is one key to differentiating between code choices, as is whether the leads are placed transvenously or epicardially. Some procedures may also be done on the leads alone or the generator alone. CPT provides codes for reporting implantation or replacement, removal, repair, and repositioning. NCD References: 20.8, 20.8.1, 20.8.2, 20.8.3.

palmaris longus tendon. Tendon located in the hand that flexes the wrist joint.

paratenon graft. Graft composed of the fatty tissue found between a tendon and its sheath.

passive mobilization. Pressure, movement, or pulling of a limb or body part utilizing an apparatus or device.

pedicle flap. Full-thickness skin and subcutaneous tissue for grafting that remains partially attached to the donor site by a pedicle or stem in which the blood vessels supplying the flap remain intact.

Pemberton osteotomy. Osteotomy is performed to position triradiate cartilage as a hinge for rotating the acetabular roof in cases of dysplasia of the hip in children.

penetrance. Being formed by, or pertaining to, a single clone.

percutaneous intradiscal electrothermal annuloplasty. Procedure corrects tears in the vertebral annulus by applying heat to the collagen disc walls percutaneously through a catheter. The heat contracts and thickens the wall, which may contract and close any annular tears.

percutaneous skeletal fixation. Treatment that is neither open nor closed and the injury site is not directly visualized. Fixation devices (pins, screws) are placed through the skin to stabilize the dislocation using x-ray guidance.

pericardium. Thin and slippery case in which the heart lies that is lined with fluid so that the heart is free to pulse and move as it beats.

peripheral arterial tonometry (PAT). Pulsatile volume changes in a digit are measured to determine activity in the sympathetic nervous system for respiratory analysis.

peritoneal. Space between the lining of the abdominal wall, or parietal peritoneum, and the surface layer of the abdominal organs, or visceral peritoneum. It contains a thin, watery fluid that keeps the peritoneal surfaces moist.

peritoneal dialysis. Dialysis that filters waste from blood inside the body using the peritoneum, the natural lining of the abdomen, as the semipermeable membrane across which ultrafiltration is accomplished. A special catheter is inserted into the abdomen and a dialysis solution is drained into the abdomen. This solution extracts fluids and wastes, which are then discarded when the fluid is drained. Various forms of peritoneal dialysis include CAPD, CCPD, and NIDP.

peritoneal effusion. Persistent escape of fluid within the peritoneal cavity.

pessary. Device placed in the vagina to support and reposition a prolapsing or retropositioned uterus, rectum, or vagina.

phenotype. Physical expression of a trait or characteristic as determined by an individual's genetic makeup or genotype.

photocoagulation. Application of an intense laser beam of light to disrupt tissue and condense protein material to a residual mass, used especially for treating ocular conditions.

physical status modifiers. Alphanumeric modifier used to identify the patient's health status as it affects the work related to providing the anesthesia service.

physical therapy modality. Therapeutic agent or regimen applied or used to provide appropriate treatment of the musculoskeletal system.

PICC. Peripherally inserted central catheter. PICC is inserted into one of the large veins of the arm and threaded through the vein until the tip sits in a large vein just above the heart.

PKR. Photorefractive therapy. Procedure involving the removal of the surface layer of the cornea (epithelium) by gentle scraping and use of a computer-controlled excimer laser to reshape the stroma.

pleurodesis. Injection of a sclerosing agent into the pleural space for creating adhesions between the parietal and the visceral pleura to treat a collapsed lung caused by air trapped in the pleural cavity, or severe cases of pleural effusion.

plication. Surgical technique involving folding, tucking, or pleating to reduce the size of a hollow structure or organ.

polyclonal. Containing one or more cells.

polymorphism. Genetic variation in the same species that does not harm the gene function or create disease.

polypeptide. Chain of amino acids held together by covalent bonds. Proteins are made up of amino acids.

polysomnography. Test involving monitoring of respiratory, cardiac, muscle, brain, and ocular function during sleep.

Potts-Smith-Gibson procedure. Side-to-side anastomosis of the aorta and left pulmonary artery creating a shunt that enlarges as the child grows.

Prader-Willi syndrome. Rounded face, almond-shaped eyes, strabismus, low forehead, hypogonadism, hypotonia, mental retardation, and an insatiable appetite.

presumptive identification. Identification of microorganisms using media growth, colony morphology, gram stains, or up to three specific tests (e.g., catalase, indole, oxidase, urease).

professional component. Portion of a charge for health care services that represents the physician's (or other practitioner's) work in providing the service, including interpretation and report of the procedure. This component of the service usually is charged for and billed separately from the inpatient hospital charges.

profunda. Denotes a part of a structure that is deeper from the surface of the body than the rest of the structure.

prolonged physician services. Extended pre- or post-service care provided to a patient whose condition requires services beyond the usual.

prostate. Male gland surrounding the bladder neck and urethra that secretes a substance into the seminal fluid.

prosthetic. Device that replaces all or part of an internal body organ or body part, or that replaces part of the function of a permanently inoperable or malfunctioning internal body organ or body part.

provider of services. Institution, individual, or organization that provides health care.

proximal. Located closest to a specified reference point, usually the midline.

psychiatric hospital. Specialized institution that provides, under the supervision of physicians, services for the diagnosis and treatment of mentally ill persons.

pterygium. Benign, wedge-shaped, conjunctival thickening that advances from the inner corner of the eye toward the cornea.

pterygomaxillary fossa. Wide depression on the external surface of the maxilla above and to the side of the canine tooth socket.

pulmonary artery banding. Surgical constriction of the pulmonary artery to prevent irreversible pulmonary vascular obstructive changes and overflow into the left ventricle.

Putti-Platt procedure. Realignment of the subscapularis tendon to treat recurrent anterior dislocation, thereby partially eliminating external rotation. The anterior capsule is also tightened and reinforced.

pyloroplasty. Enlargement and reconstruction of the lower portion of the stomach opening into the duodenum performed after vagotomy to speed gastric emptying and treat duodenal ulcers.

radioactive substances. Materials used in the diagnosis and treatment of disease that emit high-speed particles and energy-containing rays.

radiology services. Services that include diagnostic and therapeutic radiology, nuclear medicine, CT scan procedures, magnetic resonance imaging services, ultrasound, and other imaging procedures.

radiotherapy afterloading. Part of the radiation therapy process in which the chemotherapy agent is actually instilled into the tumor area subsequent to surgery and placement of an expandable catheter into the void remaining after tumor excision. The specialized catheter remains in place and the patient may come in for multiple treatments with radioisotope placed to treat the margin of tissue surrounding the excision. After the radiotherapy is completed, the patient returns to have the catheter emptied and removed. This is a new therapy in breast cancer treatment.

Rashkind procedure. Transvenous balloon atrial septectomy or septostomy performed by cardiac catheterization. A balloon catheter is inserted into the heart either to create or enlarge an opening in the interatrial septal wall.

repair. Surgical closure of a wound. The wound may be a result of injury/trauma or it may be a surgically created defect. Repairs are divided into three categories: simple, intermediate, and complex. Simple repair is performed when the wound is superficial and only requires simple, one layer, primary suturing. Intermediate repair is performed for wounds and lacerations in which one or more of the deeper layers of subcutaneous tissue and non-muscle fascia are repaired in addition to the skin and subcutaneous tissue. Complex repair includes repair of wounds requiring more than layered closure.

respiratory movement. Measurement of chest and abdomen movement during respiration.

respiratory airflow (ventilation). Assessment of air movement during inhalation and exhalation as measured by nasal pressure sensors and thermistor.

respiratory analysis. Assessment of components of respiration obtained by other methods such as airflow or peripheral arterial tone.

respiratory effort. Measurement of diaphragm and/or intercostal muscle for airflow using transducers to estimate thoracic and abdominal motion.

ribbons. In oncology, small plastic tubes containing radioactive sources for interstitial placement that may be cut into specific lengths tailored to the size of the area receiving ionizing radiation treatment.

Ridell sinusotomy. Frontal sinus tissue is destroyed to eliminate tumors.

RNA. Ribonucleic acid.

rural health clinic. Clinic in an area where there is a shortage of health services staffed by a nurse practitioner, physician assistant, or certified nurse midwife under physician direction that provides routine diagnostic services, including clinical laboratory services, drugs, and biologicals and that has prompt access to additional diagnostic services from facilities meeting federal requirements.

Salter osteotomy. Innominate bone of the hip is cut, removed, and repositioned to repair a congenital dislocation, subluxation, or deformity.

saucerization. Creation of a shallow, saucer-like depression in the bone to facilitate drainage of infected areas.

Schiotz tonometer. Instrument that measures intraocular pressure by recording the depth of an indentation on the cornea by a plunger of known weight.

screening mammography. Radiologic images taken of the female breast for the early detection of breast cancer.

screening pap smear. Diagnostic laboratory test consisting of a routine exfoliative cytology test (Papanicolaou test) provided to a woman for the early detection of cervical or vaginal cancer. The exam includes a clinical breast examination and a physician's interpretation of the results.

seeds. Small (1 mm or less) sources of radioactive material that are permanently placed directly into tumors.

senning procedure. Flaps of intra-atrial septum and right atrial wall are used to create two interatrial channels to divert the systemic and pulmonary venous circulation.

sensitivity tests. Number of methods of applying selective suspected allergens to the skin or mucous.

sensorineural conduction. Transportation of sound from the cochlea to the acoustic nerve and central auditory pathway to the brain.

sentinel lymph node. First node to which lymph drainage and metastasis from a cancer can occur.

separate procedures. Services commonly carried out as a fundamental part of a total service and, as such, do not usually warrant separate identification. These services are identified in CPT with the parenthetical phrase (separate procedure) at the end of the description and are payable only when performed alone.

septectomy. 1) Surgical removal of all or part of the nasal septum. 2) Submucosal resection of the nasal septum.

Shirodkar procedure. Treatment of an incompetent cervical os by placing nonabsorbent suture material in purse-string sutures as a cerclage to support the cervix.

short tandem repeat (STR)**.** Short sequences of a DNA pattern that are repeated. Can be used as genetic markers for human identity testing.

sialodochoplasty. Surgical repair of a salivary gland duct.

single-lead device. Implantable cardiac device (pacemaker or implantable cardioverter-defibrillator [ICD]) in which pacing and sensing components are placed in only one chamber of the heart.

single-nucleotide polymorphism (SNP). Single nucleotide (A, T, C, or G that is different in a DNA sequence. This difference occurs at a significant frequency in the population.

sinus of Valsalva. Any of three sinuses corresponding to the individual cusps of the aortic valve, located in the most proximal part of the aorta just above the cusps. These structures are contained within the pericardium and appear as distinct but subtle outpouchings or dilations of the aortic wall between each of the semilunar cusps of the valve.

sleep apnea. Intermittent cessation of breathing during sleep that may cause hypoxemia and pulmonary arterial hypertension.

sleep latency. Time period between lying down in bed and the onset of sleep.

sleep staging. Determination of the separate levels of sleep according to physiological measurements.

somatic. 1) Pertaining to the body or trunk. 2) In genetics acquired or occurring after birth.

speculoscopy. Viewing the cervix utilizing a magnifier and a special wavelength of light, allowing detection of abnormalities that may not be discovered on a routine Pap smear.

speech-language pathology services. Speech, language, and related function assessment and rehabilitation service furnished by a qualified speech-language pathologist. Audiology services include hearing and balance assessment services furnished by a qualified audiologist. A qualified speech pathologist and audiologist must have a master's or doctoral degree in their respective fields and be licensed to serve in the state. Speech pathologists and audiologists practicing in states without licensure must complete 350 hours of supervised clinical work and perform at least nine months of supervised full-time service after earning their degrees.

sphincteroplasty. Surgical repair done to correct, augment, or improve the muscular function of a sphincter, such as the anus or intestines.

spirometry. Measurement of the lungs' breathing capacity.

splint. Brace or support.

static splint. Brace that prevents movement and maintains support and position for an anatomical structure after surgery or injury.

stent. Tube to provide support in a body cavity or lumen.

stereotactic radiosurgery. Delivery of externally-generated ionizing radiation to specific targets for destruction or inactivation. Most often utilized in the treatment of brain or spinal tumors, high-resolution stereotactic imaging is used to identify the target and then deliver the treatment. Computer-assisted planning may also be employed. Simple and complex cranial lesions and spinal lesions are typically treated in a single planning and treatment session, although a maximum of five sessions may be required. No incision is made for stereotactic radiosurgery procedures.

stereotaxis. Three-dimensional method for precisely locating structures.

Stoffel rhizotomy. Nerve roots are sectioned to relieve pain or spastic paralysis.

strabismus. Misalignment of the eyes due to an imbalance in extraocular muscles.

surgical package. Normal, uncomplicated performance of specific surgical services, with the assumption that, on average, all surgical procedures of a given type are similar with respect to skill level, duration, and length of normal follow-up care.

symblepharopterygium. Adhesion in which the eyelid is adhered to the eyeball by a band that resembles a pterygium.

sympathectomy. Surgical interruption or transection of a sympathetic nervous system pathway.

tarso-. 1) Relating to the foot. 2) Relating to the margin of the eyelid.

tarsocheiloplasty. Plastic operation upon the edge of the eyelid for the treatment of trichiasis.

tarsorrhaphy. Suture of a portion or all of the opposing eyelids together for the purpose of shortening the palpebral fissure or closing it entirely.

technical component. Portion of a health care service that identifies the provision of the equipment, supplies, technical personnel, and costs attendant to the performance of the procedure other than the professional services.

tendon. Fibrous tissue that connects muscle to bone, consisting primarily of collagen and containing little vasculature.

tendon allograft. Allografts are tissues obtained from another individual of the same species. Tendon allografts are usually obtained from cadavers and frozen or freeze dried for later use in soft tissue repairs where the physician elects not to obtain an autogenous graft (a graft obtained from the individual on whom the surgery is being performed).

tendon suture material. Tendons are composed of fibrous tissue consisting primarily of collagen and containing few cells or blood vessels. This tissue heals more slowly than tissues with more vascularization. Because of this, tendons are usually repaired with nonabsorbable suture material. Examples include surgical silk, surgical cotton, linen, stainless steel, surgical nylon, polyester fiber, polybutester (Novafil), polyethylene (Dermalene), and polypropylene (Prolene, Surilene).

tendon transplant. Replacement of a tendon with another tendon.

tenon's capsule. Connective tissue that forms the capsule enclosing the posterior eyeball, extending from the conjunctival fornix and continuous with the muscular fascia of the eye.

tenonectomy. Excision of a portion of a tendon to make it shorter.

tenotomy. Cutting into a tendon.

TENS. Transcutaneous electrical nerve stimulator. TENS is applied by placing electrode pads over the area to be stimulated and connecting the electrodes to a transmitter box, which sends a current through the skin to sensory nerve fibers to help decrease pain in that nerve distribution.

tensilon. Edrophonium chloride. Agent used for evaluation and treatment of myasthenia gravis.

terminally ill. Individual whose medical prognosis for life expectancy is six months or less.

tetralogy of Fallot. Specific combination of congenital cardiac defects: obstruction of the right ventricular outflow tract with pulmonary stenosis, interventricular septal defect, malposition of the aorta, overriding the interventricular septum and receiving blood from both the venous and arterial systems, and enlargement of the right ventricle.

therapeutic services. Services performed for treatment of a specific diagnosis. These services include performance of the procedure, various incidental elements, and normal, related follow-up care.

thoracentesis. Surgical puncture of the chest cavity with a specialized needle or hollow tubing to aspirate fluid from within the pleural space for diagnostic or therapeutic reasons.

thoracic lymphadenectomy. Procedure to cut out the lymph nodes near the lungs, around the heart, and behind the trachea.

thoracostomy. Creation of an opening in the chest wall for drainage.

thyroglossal duct. Embryonic duct at the front of the neck, which becomes the pyramidal lobe of the thyroid gland with obliteration of the remaining duct, but may form a cyst or sinus in adulthood if it persists.

total disc arthroplasty with artificial disc. Removal of an intravertebral disc and its replacement with an implant. The implant is an artificial disc consisting of two metal plates with a weight-bearing surface of polyethylene between the plates. The plates are anchored to the vertebral immediately above and below the affected disc.

total shoulder replacement. Prosthetic replacement of the entire shoulder joint, including the humeral head and the glenoid fossa.

trabeculae carneae cordis. Bands of muscular tissue that line the walls of the ventricles in the heart.

trabeculectomy. Surgical incision between the anterior portion of the eye and the canal of Schlemm to drain the aqueous humor.

tracheostomy. Formation of a tracheal opening on the neck surface with tube insertion to allow for respiration in cases of obstruction or decreased patency. A tracheostomy may be planned or performed on an emergency basis for temporary or long-term use.

tracheotomy. Formation of a tracheal opening on the neck surface with tube insertion to allow for respiration in cases of obstruction or decreased patency. A tracheotomy may be planned or performed on an emergency basis for temporary or long-term use.

traction. Drawing out or holding tension on an area by applying a direct therapeutic pulling force.

transcranial magnetic stimulation. Application of electromagnetic energy to the brain through a coil placed on the scalp. The procedure stimulates cortical neurons and is intended to activate and normalize their processes.

transcription. Process by which messenger RNA is synthesized from a DNA template resulting in the transfer of genetic information from the DNA molecule to the messenger RNA.

translocation. Disconnection of all or part of a chromosome that reattaches to another position in the DNA sequence of the same or another chromosome. Often results in a reciprocal exchange of DNA sequences between two differently numbered chromosomes. May or may not result in a clinically significant loss of DNA.

trephine. 1) Specialized round saw for cutting circular holes in bone, especially the skull. 2) Instrument that removes small disc-shaped buttons of corneal tissue for transplanting.

tricuspid atresia. Congenital absence of the valve that may occur with other defects, such as atrial septal defect, pulmonary atresia, and transposition of great vessels.

turbinates. Scroll or shell-shaped elevations from the wall of the nasal cavity, the inferior turbinate being a separate bone, while the superior and middle turbinates are of the ethmoid bone.

tympanic membrane. Thin, sensitive membrane across the entrance to the middle ear that vibrates in response to sound waves, allowing the waves to be transmitted via the ossicular chain to the internal ear.

tympanoplasty. Surgical repair of the structures of the middle ear, including the eardrum and the three small bones, or ossicles.

unlisted procedure. Procedural descriptions used when the overall procedure and outcome of the procedure are not adequately described by an existing procedure code. Such codes are used as a last resort and only when there is not a more appropriate procedure code.

ureterorrhaphy. Surgical repair using sutures to close an open wound or injury of the ureter.

vagotomy. Division of the vagus nerves, interrupting impulses resulting in lower gastric acid production and hastening gastric emptying. Used in the treatment of chronic gastric, pyloric, and duodenal ulcers that can cause severe pain and difficulties in eating and sleeping.

variant. Nucleotide deviation from the normal sequence of a region. Variations are usually either substitutions or deletions. Substitution variations are the result of one nucleotide taking the place of another. A deletion occurs when one or more nucleotides are left out. In some cases, several in a reasonably close proximity on the same chromosome in a DNA strand. These variations result in amino acid changes in the protein made by the gene. However, the term variant does not itself imply a functional change. Intron variations are usually described in one of two ways: 1) the changed nucleotide is defined by a plus or a minus sign indicating the position relative to the first or last nucleotide to the intron, or 2) the second variant description is indicated relative to the last nucleotide of the preceding exon or first nucleotide of the following exon.

vasectomy. Surgical procedure involving the removal of all or part of the vas deferens, usually performed for sterilization or in conjunction with a prostatectomy.

ventricular septal defect. Congenital cardiac anomaly resulting in a continual opening in the septum between the ventricles that, in severe cases, causes oxygenated blood to flow back into the lungs, resulting in pulmonary hypertension.

vertebral interspace. Non-bony space between two adjacent vertebral bodies that contains the cushioning intervertebral disk.

volar. Palm of the hand (palmar) or sole of the foot (plantar).

Waterston procedure. Type of aortopulmonary shunting done to increase pulmonary blood flow where the ascending aorta is anastomosed to the right pulmonary artery.

Wharton's ducts. Salivary ducts below the mandible.

wick catheter. Device used to monitor interstitial fluid pressure, and sometimes used intraoperatively during fasciotomy procedures to evaluate the effectiveness of the decompression.

xenograft. Tissue that is nonhuman and harvested from one species and grafted to another. Pigskin is the most common xenograft for human skin and is applied to a wound as a temporary closure until a permanent option is performed.

z-plasty. Plastic surgery technique used primarily to release tension or elongate contractured scar tissue in which a Z-shaped incision is made with the middle line of the Z crossing the area of greatest tension. The triangular flaps are then rotated so that they cross the incision line in the opposite direction, creating a reversed Z.

ZPIC. Zone Program Integrity Contractor. CMS newly created entity currently being transitioned to replace the existing Program Safeguard Contractors (PSC). These contractors will be responsible for ensuring the integrity of all Medicare-related claims under Parts A and B (hospital, skilled nursing, home health, provider, and durable medical equipment claims), Part C (Medicare Advantage health plans), Part D (prescription drug plans), and coordination of Medicare-Medicaid data matches (Medi-Medi).

APPENDIX I — LISTING OF SENSORY, MOTOR, AND MIXED NERVES

This summary assigns each sensory, motor, and mixed nerve with its appropriate nerve conduction study code in order to enhance accurate reporting of codes 95900, 95903, and 95904. Each nerve constitutes one unit of service.

Motor Nerves Assigned to Codes 95900 and 95903.

I. Upper extremity, cervical plexus, and brachial plexus motor nerves
   A. Axillary motor nerve to the deltoid
   B. Long thoracic motor nerve to the serratus anterior
   C. Median nerve
      1. Median motor nerve to the abductor pollicis brevis
      2. Median motor nerve, anterior interosseous branch, to the flexor pollicis longus
      3. Median motor nerve, anterior interosseous branch, to the pronator quadratus
      4. Median motor nerve to the first lumbrical
      5. Median motor nerve to the second lumbrical
   D. Musculocutaneous motor nerve to the biceps brachii
   E. Radial nerve
      1. Radial motor nerve to the extensor carpi ulnaris
      2. Radial motor nerve to the extensor digitorum communis
      3. Radial motor nerve to the extensor indicis proprius
      4. Radial motor nerve to the brachioradialis
   F. Suprascapular nerve
      1. Suprascapular motor nerve to the supraspinatus
      2. Suprascapular motor nerve to the infraspinatus
   G. Thoracodorsal motor nerve to the latissimus dorsi
   H. Ulnar nerve
      1. Ulnar motor nerve to the abductor digiti minimi
      2. Ulnar motor nerve to the palmar interosseous
      3. Ulnar motor nerve to the first dorsal interosseous
      4. Ulnar motor nerve to the flexor carpi ulnaris
   I. Other

II. Lower extremity motor nerves
   A. Femoral motor nerve to the quadriceps
      1. Femoral motor nerve to the vastus medialis
      2. Femoral motor nerve to vastus lateralis
      3. Femoral motor nerve to vastus intermedialis
      4. Femoral motor nerve to rectus femoris
   B. Ilioinguinal motor nerve
   C. Peroneal (fibular) nerve
      1. Peroneal motor nerve to the extensor digitorum brevis
      2. Peroneal motor nerve to the peroneus brevis
      3. Peroneal motor nerve to the peroneus longus
      4. Peroneal motor nerve to the tibialis anterior
   D. Plantar motor nerve
   E. Sciatic nerve
   F. Tibial nerve
      1. Tibial motor nerve, inferior calcaneal branch, to the abductor digiti minimi
      2. Tibial motor nerve, medial plantar branch, to the abductor hallucis
      3. Tibial motor nerve, lateral plantar branch, to the flexor digiti minimi brevis
   G. Other

III. Cranial nerves and trunk
   A. Cranial nerve VII (facial motor nerve)
      1. Facial nerve to the frontalis
      2. Facial nerve to the nasalis
      3. Facial nerve to the orbicularis oculi
      4. Facial nerve to the orbicularis oris
   B. Cranial nerve XI (spinal accessory motor nerve)
   C. Cranial nerve XII (hypoglossal motor nerve)
   D. Intercostal motor nerve
   E. Phrenic motor nerve to the diaphragm
   F. Recurrent laryngeal nerve
   G. Other

IV. Nerve Roots
   A. Cervical nerve root stimulation
      1. Cervical level 5 (CT)
      2. Cervical level 6 (C6)
      3. Cervical level 7 (C7)
      4. Cervical level 8 (C8)
   B. Thoracic nerve root stimulation
      1. Thoracic level 1 (T1)
      2. Thoracic level 2 (T2)
      3. Thoracic level 3 (T3)
      4. Thoracic level 4 (T4)
      5. Thoracic level 5 (T5)
      6. Thoracic level 6 (T6)
      7. Thoracic level 7 (T7)
      8. Thoracic level 8 (T8)
      9. Thoracic level 9 (T9)
      10. Thoracic level 10 (T10)
      11. Thoracic level 11 (T11)
      12. Thoracic level 12 (T12)
   C. Lumbar nerve root stimulation
      1. Lumbar level 1 (L1)
      2. Lumbar level 2 (L2)
      3. Lumbar level 3 (L3)
      4. Lumbar level 4 (L4)
      5. Lumbar level 5 (L5)
   D. Sacral nerve root stimulation
      1. Sacral level 1 (S1)
      2. Sacral level 2 (S2)
      3. Sacral level 3 (S3)
      4. Sacral level 4 (S4)

Sensory and Mixed Nerves Assigned to Code 95904

I. Upper extremity sensory and mixed nerves
   A. Lateral antebrachial cutaneous sensory nerve
   B. Medial antebrachial cutaneous sensory nerve
   C. Medial brachial cutaneous sensory nerve
   D. Median nerve
      1. Median sensory nerve to the first digit
      2. Median sensory nerve to the second digit
      3. Median sensory nerve to the third digit
      4. Median sensory nerve to the fourth digit

5. Median palmar cutaneous sensory nerve
6. Median palmar mixed nerve

E. Posterior antebrachial cutaneous sensory nerve

F. Radial sensory nerve
1. Radial sensory nerve to the base of the thumb
2. Radial sensory nerve to digit 1

G. Ulnar nerve
1. Ulnar dorsal cutaneous sensory nerve
2. Ulnar sensory nerve to the fourth digit
3. Ulnar sensory nerve to the fifth digit
4. Ulnar palmar mixed nerve

H. Intercostal sensory nerve

I. Other

II. Lower extremity sensory and mixed nerves

A. Lateral femoral cutaneous sensory nerve

B. Medical calcaneal sensory nerve

C. Medial femoral cutaneous sensory nerve

D. Peroneal nerve
1. Deep peroneal sensory nerve
2. Superficial peroneal sensory nerve, medial dorsal cutaneous branch
3. Superficial peroneal sensory nerve, intermediate dorsal cutaneous branch

E. Posterior femoral cutaneous sensory nerve

F. Saphenous nerve
1. Saphenous sensory nerve (distal technique)
2. Saphenous sensory nerve (proximal technique)

G. Sural nerve
1. Sural sensory nerve, lateral dorsal cutaneous branch
2. Sural sensory nerve

H. Tibial sensory nerve (digital nerve to toe 1)

I. Tibial sensory nerve (medial plantar nerve)

J. Tibial sensory nerve (lateral plantar nerve)

K. Other

III. Head and trunk sensory nerves

A. Dorsal nerve of the penis

B. Greater auricular nerve

C. Ophthalmic branch of the trigeminal nerve

D. Pudendal sensory nerve

E. Suprascapular sensory nerves

F. Other

The following table provides a reasonable maximum number of studies performed per diagnostic category necessary for a physician to arrive at a diagnosis in 90% of patients with that final diagnosis. The numbers in each column represent the number of studies recommended. The appropriate number of studies to be performed is based upon the physician's discretion.

	Type of Study/Maximum Number of Studies				
		Nerve Conduction Studies (95900, 95903, 95904)		***Other EMG Studies (95934, 95936, 95937)***	
Indication	***Needle EMG (95860-95864, 95867-95870)***	***Motor NCS With and/or Without F wave***	***Sensory NCS***	***H-Reflex***	***Neuromuscular Junction Testing (Repetitive Stimulation)***
Carpal Tunnel (Unilateral)	1	3	4	—	—
Carpal Tunnel (Bilateral)	2	4	6	—	—
Radiculopathy	2	3	2	2	—
Mononeuropathy	1	3	3	2	—
Polyneuropathy/Mononeuropathy Multiplex	3	4	4	2	—
Myopathy	2	2	2	—	2
Motor Neuronopathy (e.g., ALS)	4	4	2	—	2
Plexopathy	2	4	6	2	-
Neuromuscular Junction	2	2	2	—	3
Tarsal Tunnel Syndrome (Unilateral)	1	4	4	—	—
Tarsal Tunnel Syndrome (Bilateral)	2	5	6	—	—
Weakness, Fatigue, Cramps, or Twitching (Focal)	2	3	4	—	2
Weakness, Fatigue, Cramps, or Twitching (General)	4	4	4	—	2
Pain, Numbness, or Tingling (Unilateral)	1	3	4	2	—
Pain, Numbness, or Tingling (Bilateral)	2	4	6	2	—

APPENDIX J — VASCULAR FAMILIES

This table assumes that the starting point is catheterization of the aorta. This categorization would not be accurate, for instance, if a femoral or carotid artery were catheterized with the blood's flow. The names of the arteries that appear in bold face type in the following table indicate those arteries that are most often the subject of arteriographic procedures.

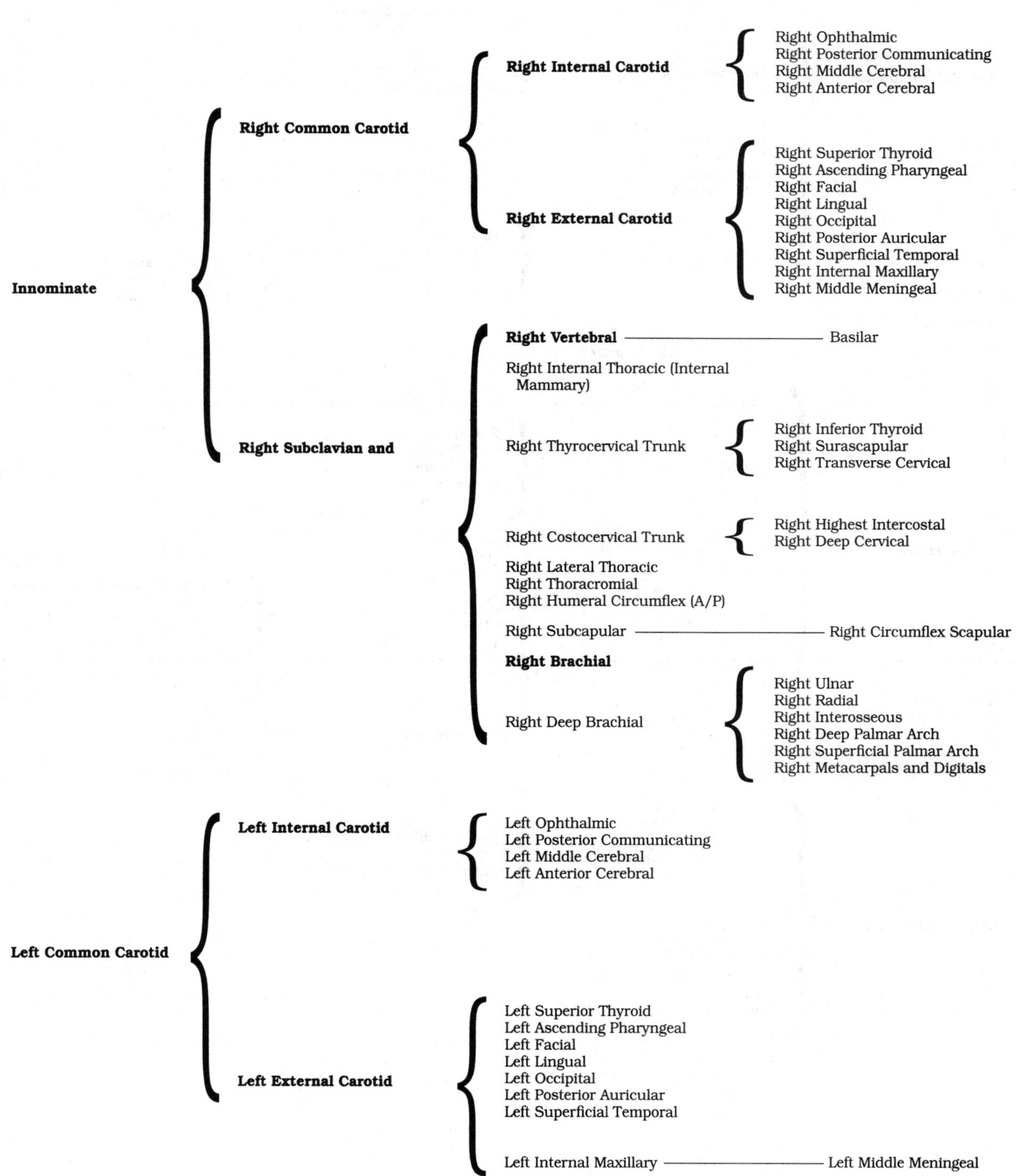

First Order	Second Order Branch	Third Order Branch	Beyond Third Order Branches
Innominate	**Right Common Carotid**	**Right Internal Carotid**	Right Ophthalmic Right Posterior Communicating Right Middle Cerebral Right Anterior Cerebral
		Right External Carotid	Right Superior Thyroid Right Ascending Pharyngeal Right Facial Right Lingual Right Occipital Right Posterior Auricular Right Superficial Temporal Right Internal Maxillary Right Middle Meningeal
	Right Subclavian and	**Right Vertebral**	Basilar
		Right Internal Thoracic (Internal Mammary)	
		Right Thyrocervical Trunk	Right Inferior Thyroid Right Surascapular Right Transverse Cervical
		Right Costocervical Trunk	Right Highest Intercostal Right Deep Cervical
		Right Lateral Thoracic Right Thoracromial Right Humeral Circumflex (A/P)	
		Right Subcapular	Right Circumflex Scapular
		Right Brachial	
		Right Deep Brachial	Right Ulnar Right Radial Right Interosseous Right Deep Palmar Arch Right Superficial Palmar Arch Right Metacarpals and Digitals
Left Common Carotid	**Left Internal Carotid**	Left Ophthalmic Left Posterior Communicating Left Middle Cerebral Left Anterior Cerebral	
	Left External Carotid	Left Superior Thyroid Left Ascending Pharyngeal Left Facial Left Lingual Left Occipital Left Posterior Auricular Left Superficial Temporal	
		Left Internal Maxillary	Left Middle Meningeal

First Order	Second Order Branch	Third Order Branch	Beyond Third Order Branches
Left Sublavian and	**Left Vertebral**		
	Left Internal Thoracic (Internal Mammary)		
	Left Thyrocervial Trunk	Left Inferior Thyroid	
		Left Suprascapular	
		Left Transverse Cervical	
	Left Costocervical Trunk	Left Hightest Intercostal	
		Left Deep Cervical	
	Left Lateral Thoracic		
	Left Thoracoacromial		
	Left Humeral Circumflex (A/P)		
	Left Subscapular	Left Circumflex Scapular	
	Left Brachial		
	Left Deep Brachial	Left Ulnar	
		Left Radial	
		Left Interosseous	Left Deep Palmar Arch
			Left Superficial Palmar Arch
			Left Metacarpals and Digitals
Intercostals			
Bronchials			
Recurrent Esophageal			
Inferior Phrenic	Superior Suprarenal		
Celiac Trunk	Left Gastric	Esphageal Branch	
	Splenic	Dorsal Pancreatic	Inferior Transverse
		Great Pancreatic	
		Caudal Pancreatic	
		Gastroepiploic	
		Short Gastrics	
	Common Hepatic	Gastroduodenal	Posterior Superior Pancreatico-duodenal
			Anterior Superior Pancreatico-duodenal
		Proper Hepatic	Left Hepatic
			Right Hepatic
			Cystic
			Gastroepiploic
			Supraduodenal
			Intermediate Hepatic
Middle Suprarenal			
Superior Mesenteric	Middle Colic		
	Inferior Pancreaticoduodenal	Posterior Infereior Pancreatico-duodenal	
		Anterior Infereior Pancreatico-duodenal	
	Jejunal		
	Ileocolic		
	Appendicular		
	Posterior Cecal		
	Anterior Cecal		
	Marginal		
	Right Colic		

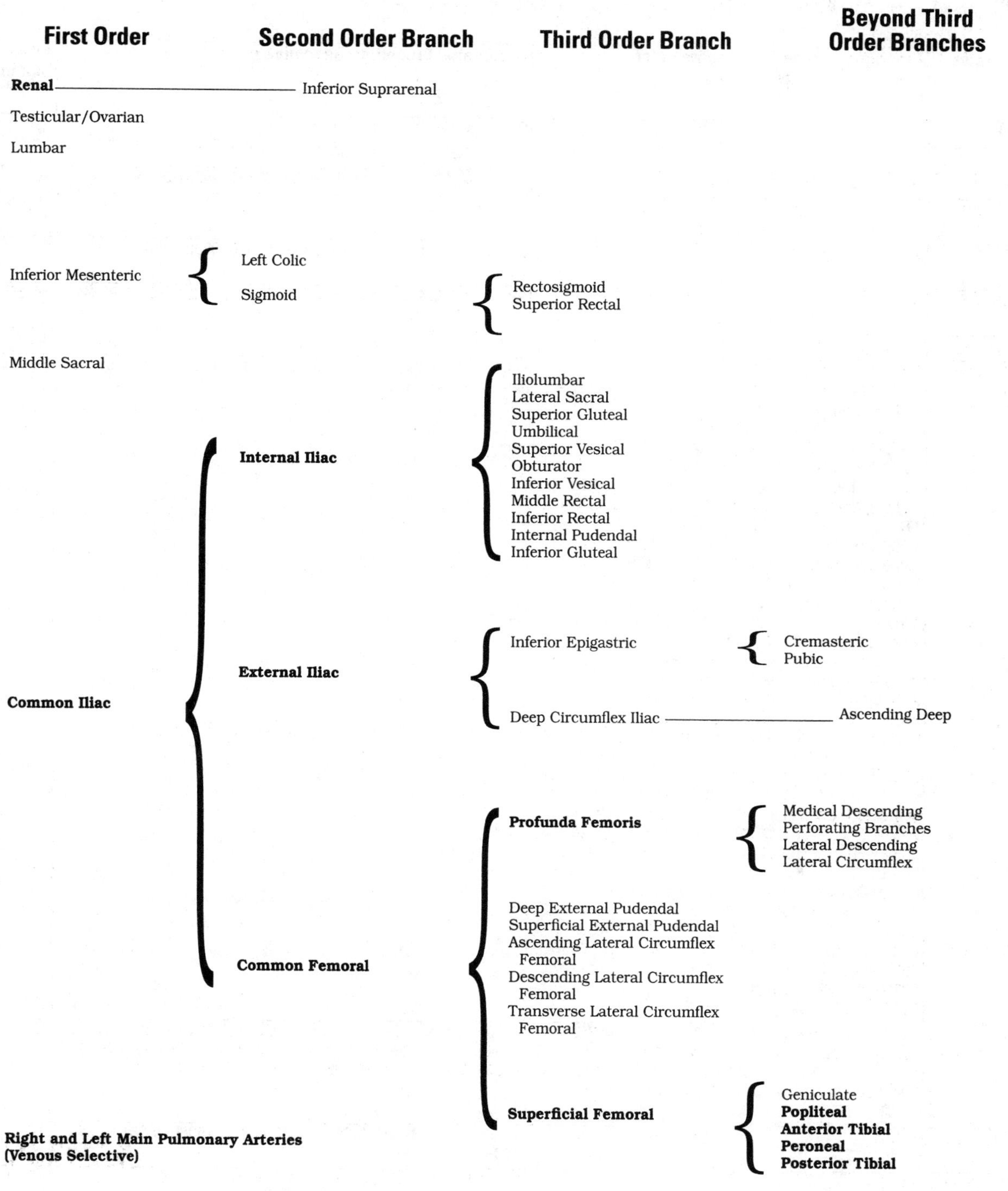

Reference: Kadir S. *Atlas of Normal and Variant Angiographic Anatomy*. Philadelphia, Pa: WB Saunders Co; 1991

APPENDIX K — PHYSICIAN QUALITY REPORTING SYSTEM (PQRS)

Numerator	Associated Diagnostic Denominator	Associated Procedure Denominator	Associated Modifiers
0014F	N/A	66982-66984	8P
0505F	585.6	90935-90937, 90957-90962	8P
0507F	585.6	90945-90947, 90965-90966, 90969-90970	8P
0509F, 1091F	307.6, 625.6, 788.30-788.31, 788.39	99201-99205, 99212-99215, 99324-99337, 99341-99350	8P
0513F, 0514F, 3281F	585.5	99201-99205, 99212-99215	8P
0517F, 3284F	365.10-365.12, 365.15	99201-99205, 99212-99215, 99307-99310, 99324-99337, 92002-92014	8P
0518F, 3288F	N/A	99201-99205, 99212-99215, 99304-99310, 99324-99337, 99341-99350, 97001-97004	1P, 8P
0520F	157.0-157.9, 162.9	77295	8P
0521F, 1125F	140.0-140.9, 141.0-141.9, 142.0-142.9, 143.0-143.9, 144.0-144.9, 145.0-145.9, 146.0-146.9, 147.0-147.9, 148.0-148.9, 149.0-149.9, 150.0-150.9, 151.0-151.9, 152.0-152.9, 153.0-153.9, 154.0-154.8, 155.0-155.2, 156.0-156.9, 157.0-157.9, 158.0-158.9, 159.0-159.9, 160.0-160.9, 161.0-161.9, 162.0-162.9, 163.0-163.9, 164.0-164.9, 165.0-165.9, 170.0-170.9, 171.0-171.9, 172.0-172.9, 173.0, 173.1, 173.2, 173.3, 173.4, 173.5, 173.6, 173.7, 173.8, 173.9, 174.0-174.9, 175.0-175.9, 176.0-179, 180.0-181, 182.0-182.8, 183.0-183.9, 184.0-185, 186.0-186.9, 187.1-187.9, 188.0-188.9, 189.0-189.9, 190.0-190.9, 191.0-191.9, 192.0-193, 194.0-194.9, 195.0-195.8, 196.0-196.9, 197.0-197.8, 198.0-198.7, 198.81-198.89, 199.0-199.2, 200.00-200.08, 200.10-200.18, 200.20-200.28, 200.30-200.38, 200.40-200.48, 200.50-200.58, 200.60-200.68, 200.70-200.78, 200.80-200.88, 201.00-201.08, 201.10-201.18, 201.20-201.28, 201.40-201.48, 201.50-201.58, 201.60-201.68, 201.70-201.78, 201.90-201.98, 202.00-202.08, 202.10-202.18, 202.20-202.28, 202.30-202.38, 202.40-202.48, 202.50-202.58, 202.60-202.68, 202.70-202.78, 202.80-202.88, 202.90-202.98, 203.00-203.02, 203.10-203.12, 203.80-203.82, 204.00-204.02, 204.10-204.12, 204.20-204.22, 204.80-204.82, 204.90-204.92, 205.00-205.02, 205.10-205.12, 205.20-205.22, 205.30-205.32, 205.80-205.82, 205.90-205.92, 206.00-206.02, 206.10-206.12, 206.20-206.22, 206.80-206.82, 206.90-206.92, 207.00-207.02, 207.10-207.12, 207.20-207.22, 207.80-207.82, 208.00-208.02, 208.10-208.12, 208.20-208.22, 208.80-208.82, 208.90-208.92, 209.00-209.03, 209.10-209.17, 209.20-209.29, 209.30-209.36, 209.70-209.79, 235.0-235.9, 236.0-236.7, 236.90-236.99, 237.0-237.6, 237.70-237.72, 237.9, 238.0-238.6, 238.71-238.77, 238.8-238.9, 239.0-239.7, 239.9	99201-99205, 99212-99215, 51720, 77427-77435, 77470, 96401-96440, 96446-96549	8P
0526F	721.3, 721.41-721.42, 721.90, 722.0, 722.10-722.2, 722.30-722.4, 722.51-722.6, 722.70-722.73, 722.80-722.83, 722.90-722.93, 723.0, 724.00-724.02, 724.09, 724.2-724.6, 724.70-724.79, 738.4-738.5, 739.3-739.4, 756.12, 846.0-846.9, 847.2	99201-99205, 99212-99215, 22210, 22214, 22220-22226, 22532-22548, 22554-22600, 22612-22632, 22818-22849, 63001-63048, 63055-63200, 97001-97002	N/A
0529F	V12.72	44388-44389, 44392-44394, 45355-45378, 45380-45381, 45383-45385	1P, 3P, 8P
0540F, 3455F, 4187F	714.0-714.2, 714.81	99201-99205, 99212-99215, 99341-99350	1P, 8P
0575F, 3494F, 3500F, 3502F, 4290F, 4293F	042, 079.53, V08	99201-99205, 99212-99215	8P
1002F	410.00-410.02, 410.10-410.12, 410.20-410.22, 410.30-410.32, 410.40-410.42, 410.50-410.52, 410.60-410.62, 410.70-410.72, 410.80-410.82, 410.90-410.92, 411.0-411.1, 411.81-412, 413.0-413.9, 414.00-414.07, 414.8-414.9, V45.82	99201-99205, 99212-99215, 99304-99310, 99324-99337, 99341-99350	8P
1005F	493.00, 493.02, 493.10, 493.12, 493.20, 493.22, 493.82, 493.90, 493.92	99201-99205, 99212-99215	8P
1006F, 1007F	715.00-715.09, 715.10-715.18, 715.20-715.28, 715.30-715.38, 715.80-715.89, 715.98	99201-99205, 99212-99215	8P

Numerator	Associated Diagnostic Denominator	Associated Procedure Denominator	Associated Modifiers
1036F	N/A	99201-99205, 99212-99215, 90801-90813, 90815, 90845, 90862, 92002-92014, 96150-96152, 97003-97004	N/A
1038F, 1039F	493.00, 493.02, 493.10, 493.12, 493.20, 493.22, 493.82, 493.90, 493.92	99201-99205, 99212-99215	N/A
1040F, 3085F	296.20-296.24, 296.34	99201-99205, 99212-99215, 90801-90815, 90845, 90862	8P
1090F	N/A	99201-99205, 99212-99215, 99324-99337, 99341-99350	1P, 8P
1100F	N/A	99201-99205, 99212-99215, 99304-99310, 99324-99337, 99341-99350, 97001-97004	N/A
1101F	N/A	99201-99205, 99212-99215, 99304-99310, 99324-99337, 99341-99350, 97001-97004	8P
1110F	N/A	99201-99205, 99212-99215, 99324-99337, 99341-99350, 90801-90815, 90845, 90862	N/A
1111F	N/A	99201-99205, 99212-99215, 99324-99337, 99341-99350, 90801-90815, 90845, 90862	8P
1116F	380.10-380.13, 380.22	99201-99205, 99212-99215, 99281-99285	1P, 8P
1119F, 1121F, 3215F, 3216F	070.51, 070.54, 070.70	99201-99205, 99212-99215	N/A
1123F	N/A	99201-99205, 99212-99215, 99218-99220, 99221-99236, 99291, 99304-99310, 99324-99337, 99341-99350	8P
1124F	N/A	99201-99205, 99212-99215, 99218-99220, 99221-99236, 99291, 99304-99310, 99324-99337, 99341-99350	N/A
1126F	140.0-140.9, 141.0-141.9, 142.0-142.9, 143.0-143.9, 144.0-144.9, 145.0-145.9, 146.0-146.9, 147.0-147.9, 148.0-148.9, 149.0-149.9, 150.0-150.9, 151.0-151.9, 152.0-152.9, 153.0-153.9, 154.0-154.8, 155.0-155.2, 156.0-156.9, 157.0-157.9, 158.0-158.9, 159.0-159.9, 160.0-160.9, 161.0-161.9, 162.0-162.9, 163.0-163.9, 164.0-164.9, 165.0-165.9, 170.0-170.9, 171.0-171.9, 172.0-172.9, 173.0, 173.1, 173.2, 173.3, 173.4, 173.5, 173.6, 173.7, 173.8, 173.9, 174.0-174.9, 175.0-175.9, 176.0-179, 180.0-181, 182.0-182.8, 183.0-183.9, 184.0-185, 186.0-186.9, 187.1-187.9, 188.0-188.9, 189.0-189.9, 190.0-190.9, 191.0-191.9, 192.0-193, 194.0-194.9, 195.0-195.8, 196.0-196.9, 197.0-197.8, 198.0-198.7, 198.81-198.89, 199.0-199.2, 200.00-200.08, 200.10-200.18, 200.20-200.28, 200.30-200.38, 200.40-200.48, 200.50-200.58, 200.60-200.68, 200.70-200.78, 200.80-200.88, 201.00-201.08, 201.10-201.18, 201.20-201.28, 201.40-201.48, 201.50-201.58, 201.60-201.68, 201.70-201.78, 201.90-201.98, 202.00-202.08, 202.10-202.18, 202.20-202.28, 202.30-202.38, 202.40-202.48, 202.50-202.58, 202.60-202.68, 202.70-202.78, 202.80-202.88, 202.90-202.98, 203.00-203.02, 203.10-203.12, 203.80-203.82, 204.00-204.02, 204.10-204.12, 204.20-204.22, 204.80-204.82, 204.90-204.92, 205.00-205.02, 205.10-205.12, 205.20-205.22, 205.30-205.32, 205.80-205.82, 205.90-205.92, 206.00-206.02, 206.10-206.12, 206.20-206.22, 206.80-206.82, 206.90-206.92, 207.00-207.02, 207.10-207.12, 207.20-207.22, 207.80-207.82, 208.00-208.02, 208.10-208.12, 208.20-208.22, 208.80-208.82, 208.90-208.92, 209.00-209.03, 209.10-209.17, 209.20-209.29, 209.30-209.36, 209.70-209.79, 235.0-235.9, 236.0-236.7, 236.90-236.99, 237.0-237.6, 237.70-237.72, 237.9, 238.0-238.6, 238.71-238.77, 238.8-238.9, 239.0-239.7, 239.9	99201-99205, 99212-99215, 51720, 77427-77435, 77470, 96401-96440, 96446-96549	N/A
1130F, 2040F, 4245F, 4248F	721.3, 721.41-721.42, 721.90, 722.0, 722.10-722.2, 722.30-722.4, 722.51-722.6, 722.70-722.73, 722.80-722.83, 722.90-722.93, 723.0, 724.00-724.02, 724.09, 724.2-724.6, 724.70-724.79, 738.4-738.5, 739.3-739.4, 756.12, 846.0-846.9, 847.2	99201-99205, 99212-99215, 22210, 22214, 22220-22226, 22532-22548, 22554-22600, 22612-22632, 22818-22849, 63001-63048, 63055-63200, 97001-97002	8P
1170F, 3470F, 3475F, 4194F	714.0-714.2, 714.81	99201-99205, 99212-99215, 99341-99350	8P
2000F, 3046F, 3048F, 3060F, 3061F, 3062F	250.00-250.03, 250.10-250.13, 250.20-250.23, 250.30-250.33, 250.40-250.43, 250.50-250.53, 250.60-250.63, 250.70-250.73, 250.80-250.83, 250.90-250.93, 357.2, 362.01-362.07, 366.41, 648.04	99201-99205, 99212-99215, 99304-99310, 99324-99337, 99341-99350, 97802-97804	8P
2010F, 2014F	481, 482.0-482.2, 482.30-482.39, 482.40-482.49, 482.81-482.9, 483.0-483.8, 485-486, 487.0	99201-99205, 99212-99215, 99281-99285, 99291, 99324-99337, 99341-99350	8P

Appendix K — Physician Quality Reporting System (PQRS)

Numerator	Associated Diagnostic Denominator	Associated Procedure Denominator	Associated Modifiers
2019F	362.52	99201-99205, 99212-99215, 99304-99310, 99324-99337, 92002-92014	1P, 2P, 8P
2021F, 5010F	362.06	99201-99205, 99212-99215, 99304-99310, 99324-99337, 92002-92014	1P, 2P, 8P
2022F, 2024F, 2026F	250.00-250.03, 250.10-250.13, 250.20-250.23, 250.30-250.33, 250.40-250.43, 250.50-250.53, 250.60-250.63, 250.70-250.73, 250.80-250.83, 250.90-250.93, 357.2, 362.01-362.07, 366.41, 648.04	99201-99205, 99212-99215, 99304-99310, 99324-99337, 99341-99350, 92002-92014, 97802-97804	8P
2027F	365.10-365.12, 365.15	99201-99205, 99212-99215, 99304-99310, 99324-99337, 92002-92014	1P, 8P
2028F	250.00-250.03, 250.10-250.13, 250.20-250.23, 250.30-250.33, 250.40-250.43, 250.50-250.53, 250.60-250.63, 250.70-250.73, 250.80-250.83, 250.90-250.93, 357.2, 362.01-362.07, 366.41, 648.04	99201-99205, 99212-99215, 99304-99310, 99324-99337, 99341-99350, 97802-97804	1P, 8P
2035F	381.10-381.19, 381.4	99201-99205, 99212-99215, 92567	1P, 2P, 8P
3014F	N/A	99201-99205, 99212-99215	1P, 8P
3016F	N/A	99201-99205, 99212-99215, 90801-90815, 90845, 90862, 96150, 96152, 97003-97004, 97802-97804, 98960-98962	1P, 8P
3017F	N/A	99201-99205, 99212-99215, 99304-99310, 99324-99337	1P, 8P
3020F, 4003F	402.01, 402.11, 402.91, 404.01, 404.03, 404.11, 404.13, 404.91, 404.93, 428.0-428.1, 428.20-428.23, 428.30-428.33, 428.9	99201-99205, 99212-99215, 99304-99310, 99324-99337, 99341-99350	8P
3021F	402.01, 402.11, 402.91, 404.01, 404.03, 404.11, 404.13, 404.91, 404.93, 428.0-428.1, 428.20-428.23, 428.30-428.33, 428.9	99201-99205, 99212-99215, 99238-99239, 99304-99310, 99324-99337, 99341-99350	8P
3022F	402.01, 402.11, 402.91, 404.01, 404.03, 404.11, 404.13, 404.91, 404.93, 428.0-428.1, 428.20-428.23, 428.30-428.33, 428.9	99201-99205, 99212-99215, 99238-99239, 99304-99310, 99324-99337, 99341-99350	N/A
3023F, 4025F	491.0-491.1, 491.20-491.9, 492.0-492.8, 496	99201-99205, 99212-99215	1P, 2P, 3P, 8P
3025F	491.0-491.1, 491.20-491.9, 492.0-492.8, 496	99201-99205, 99212-99215	8P
3027F	491.0-491.1, 491.20-491.9, 492.0-492.8, 496	99201-99205, 99212-99215	N/A
3028F, 4045F	481, 482.0-482.2, 482.30-482.39, 482.40-482.49, 482.81-482.9, 483.0-483.8, 485-486, 487.0	99201-99205, 99212-99215, 99281-99285, 99291, 99324-99337, 99341-99350	1P, 2P, 3P, 8P
3038F	N/A	32440-32488, 32503-32504, 32663	1P, 8P
3044F, 3045F, 3049F, 3050F, 3066F, 3074F, 3075F, 3077F, 3078F, 3079F, 3080F, G8506	250.00-250.03, 250.10-250.13, 250.20-250.23, 250.30-250.33, 250.40-250.43, 250.50-250.53, 250.60-250.63, 250.70-250.73, 250.80-250.83, 250.90-250.93, 357.2, 362.01-362.07, 366.41, 648.04	99201-99205, 99212-99215, 99304-99310, 99324-99337, 99341-99350, 97802-97804	N/A
3072F	250.00-250.03, 250.10-250.13, 250.20-250.23, 250.30-250.33, 250.40-250.43, 250.50-250.53, 250.60-250.63, 250.70-250.73, 250.80-250.83, 250.90-250.93, 357.2, 362.01-362.07, 366.41, 648.04	99201-99205, 99212-99215, 99304-99310, 99324-99337, 99341-99350, 92002-92014, 97802-97804	N/A
3082F, G8636, G8637, G8638	585.6	90935-90937, 90945-90947, 90957-90962, 90965-90966, 90969-90970	N/A
3083F, 3084F	585.6	90935-90937, 90945-90947, 90957-90962, 90965-90966, 90969-90970	8P
3092F	296.20-296.24, 296.34	99201-99205, 99212-99215, 90801-90815, 90845, 90862	N/A
3095F, 3096F	733.00-733.09, 805.00-805.08, 805.2, 805.4, 805.6, 805.8, 813.40-813.42, 813.44-813.45, 813.47, 813.50-813.52, 813.54, 820.00-820.09, 820.20-820.22, 820.8	99201-99205, 99212-99215, 22305-22327, 22520-22521, 22523-22524, 25600-25609, 27230-27248	1P, 2P, 3P, 8P
3100F	N/A	70498, 70547-70549, 75660-75680, 93880-93882	8P
3110F	368.12, 368.2, 386.2, 431, 433.01, 433.11, 433.21, 433.31, 433.81, 433.91, 434.01, 434.11, 434.91, 435.0-435.9, 437.7, 780.02, 781.3-781.4, 781.94, 782.0, 784.3, 784.51, 784.59	70450-70470, 70551-70553, 0042T	8P
3111F, 3112F	368.12, 368.2, 386.2, 431, 433.01, 433.11, 433.21, 433.31, 433.81, 433.91, 434.01, 434.11, 434.91, 435.0-435.9, 437.7, 780.02, 781.3-781.4, 781.94, 782.0, 784.3, 784.51, 784.59	70450-70470, 70551-70553, 0042T	N/A
3120F	413.0-413.9, 780.2, 786.59	99281-99285, 99291	1P, 2P, 8P
3155F	204.00, 204.02, 205.00, 205.02, 206.00, 206.02, 207.00, 207.02, 207.20, 207.22, 208.00, 208.02, 238.75	99201-99205, 99212-99215	1P, 2P, 3P, 8P

Numerator	Associated Diagnostic Denominator	Associated Procedure Denominator	Associated Modifiers
3160F	238.75	99201-99205, 99212-99215	3P, 8P
3170F	204.10, 204.12	99201-99205, 99212-99215	1P, 2P, 3P, 8P
3210F	034.0, 463	99201-99205, 99212-99220	1P, 8P
3218F, 4159F	070.54	99201-99205, 99212-99215	1P, 8P
3220F	070.54	99201-99205, 99212-99215	1P, 2P, 8P
3250F	153.0-153.9, 154.0-154.1, 154.8, 174.0-174.9, 175.9	88307-88309	N/A
3260F	153.0-153.9, 154.0-154.1, 154.8, 174.0-174.9, 175.9	88307-88309	1P, 8P
3265F, 4148F, 4149F	070.51, 070.54, 070.70	99201-99205, 99212-99215	1P, 2P, 8P
3266F	070.54	99201-99205, 99212-99215	8P
3269F	185	55810-55815, 55840-55845, 55866, 55873, 77427, 77776-77778, 77787	1P, 3P
3270F, 3271F, 3272F, 3273F, 3274F	185	55810-55815, 55840-55845, 55866, 55873, 77427, 77776-77778, 77787	N/A
3278F, 4051F	585.5	99201-99205, 99212-99215	1P, 2P, 8P
3279F, 3280F, 4171F, 4172F, G8476, G8477, G8478, G8639, G8640, G8641	585.5	99201-99205, 99212-99215	N/A
3285F	365.10-365.12, 365.15	99201-99205, 99212-99215, 99307-99310, 99324-99337, 92002-92014	N/A
3300F	153.0-153.9, 154.0-154.8, 174.0-174.9, V10.05-V10.06, V10.3	99201-99205, 99212-99215, 77261-77263	N/A
3301F	153.0-153.9, 154.0-154.8, 174.0-174.9, V10.05-V10.06, V10.3	99201-99205, 99212-99215, 77261-77263	8P
3315F, 3372F, 3374F, 3376F, 3378F, 3380F	174.0-174.9, V10.3	99201-99205, 99212-99215	N/A
3316F, 3370F	174.0-174.9, V10.3	99201-99205, 99212-99215	8P
3323F	150.3-150.5, 162.5	32440-32488, 32500, 32503-32504, 32657, 32663, 43107-43113, 43117-43123	1P, 8P
3328F	150.1-150.9, 151.0, 162.9	32440-32488, 32500, 32503-32504, 32657, 32663, 43107-43113, 43117-43123	8P
3340F, 3341F, 3342F, 3343F, 3344F, 3345F, 3350F, G0202	V76.12	77057	N/A
3382F	153.0-153.9, V10.05	99201-99205, 99212-99215	8P
3384F, 3386F, 3388F, 3390F	153.0-153.9, V10.05	99201-99205, 99212-99215	N/A
3471F, 3472F, 3476F, 4192F, 4193F, 4195F, 4196F	714.0-714.2, 714.81	99201-99205, 99212-99215, 99341-99350	N/A
3490F, 3492F, 3493F	042, 079.53, V08, V22.0-V22.2, V23.0-V23.3, V23.41, V23.49-V23.7, V23.81-V23.84, V23.9	99201-99205, 99212-99215	N/A
3495F, 3496F, 3503F, 4270F, 4271F	042, 079.53, V08	99201-99205, 99212-99215	N/A
3511F, 3512F	042, 079.53, V08	99201-99205, 99212-99215	2P, 8P
3570F	N/A	78300-78320	3P, 8P
4000F, 4001F	493.00, 493.02, 493.10, 493.12, 493.20, 493.22, 493.81-493.82, 493.90, 493.92	99201-99205, 99212-99220, 99341-99350	8P
4002F	410.00-410.02, 410.10-410.12, 410.20-410.22, 410.30-410.32, 410.40-410.42, 410.50-410.52, 410.60-410.62, 410.70-410.72, 410.80-410.82, 410.90-410.92, 411.0-411.1, 411.81-412, 413.0-413.9, 414.00-414.07, 414.8-414.9, V45.82	99201-99205, 99212-99215, 99304-99310, 99324-99337, 99341-99350	1P, 2P, 3P, 8P
4004F	N/A	99201-99205, 99212-99215, 90801-90813, 90815, 90845, 90862, 92002-92014, 96150-96152, 97003-97004	1P, 8P
4005F	733.09	99201-99205, 99212-99215	1P, 2P, 3P, 8P

Numerator	Associated Diagnostic Denominator	Associated Procedure Denominator	Associated Modifiers
4006F, 4011F	410.00-410.02, 410.10-410.12, 410.20-410.22, 410.30-410.32, 410.40-410.42, 410.50-410.52, 410.60-410.62, 410.70-410.72, 410.80-410.82, 410.90-410.92, 411.0-411.1, 411.81-412, 413.0-413.9, 414.00-414.07, 414.8-414.9, V45.82	99201-99205, 99212-99215, 99238-99239, 99304-99310, 99324-99337, 99341-99350	1P, 2P, 3P, 8P
4009F	402.01, 402.11, 402.91, 404.01, 404.03, 404.11, 404.13, 404.91, 404.93, 428.0-428.1, 428.20-428.23, 428.30-428.33, 428.9	99201-99205, 99212-99215, 99238-99239, 99304-99310, 99324-99337, 99341-99350	1P, 2P, 3P, 8P
4012F	402.01, 402.11, 402.91, 404.01, 404.03, 404.11, 404.13, 404.91, 404.93, 427.31, 428.0-428.1, 428.20-428.23, 428.30-428.33, 428.9	99201-99205, 99212-99215, 99304-99310, 99324-99337, 99341-99350	1P, 2P, 3P, 8P
4015F	493.00, 493.02, 493.10, 493.12, 493.20, 493.22, 493.82, 493.90, 493.92	99201-99205, 99212-99215	2P, 8P
4040F	N/A	99201-99205, 99212-99215, 99218-99220, 99324-99337, 99341-99350, 99356-99357	1P, 8P
4041F	N/A	15734, 15738, 19260-19272, 19301-19307, 19361-19369, 21627, 21632, 21740, 21750, 21805, 21825, 22325, 22524, 22554, 22558, 22600, 22612, 22630, 22800-22804, 27125-27138, 27235-27236, 27244-27245, 27269, 27440-27447, 27702-27704, 27758-27759, 27766, 27769, 27792, 27814, 28192-28193, 28293, 28415-28420, 28445, 28465, 28485, 28505, 28525, 28531, 28555, 28585, 28615, 28645, 28675-28737, 31760-31775, 31786, 31805, 32095, 32100-32150, 32215-32320, 32402, 32440-32501, 32800-32815, 32900-32940, 33020-33202, 33250-33251, 33256, 33261, 33300-33322, 33332-33411, 33413, 33416, 33422-33465, 33475, 33496, 33510-33572, 33877-33883, 33886, 33891, 34051, 34800-34805, 34825, 34830-34832, 34900, 35021, 35081, 35091, 35102, 35131, 35141, 35151, 35211-35216, 35241-35246, 35271-35276, 35301, 35311, 35526, 35601-35671, 36830, 37616, 38115, 38381, 38746, 39000-39220, 39545, 39561, 43045-43135, 43300-43313, 43320, 43325, 43327-43337, 43340-43425, 43496, 43500-43520, 43605-43634, 43640-43641, 43653, 43800-43840, 43843-43870, 44005-44010, 44020-44021, 44050-44100, 44120, 44125-44127, 44130-44136, 47420-47480, 47560-47561, 47570, 47600-47620, 47700-47800, 47802-47900, 48020-48100, 48120-48155, 48500-48548, 48554-48556, 49215, 49568, 50320, 50340-50380, 60521-60522, 61154, 61312-61313, 61315, 61510-61512, 61518, 61548, 61697, 61700, 61750-61751, 61867, 62223, 62230, 63015, 63020-63030, 63042, 63045, 63047, 63056, 63075, 63081, 63267, 63276, 64746, 0236T	1P, 8P
4042F, 4046F	N/A	15734, 15738, 19260-19272, 19301-19307, 19361-19369, 21346-21348, 21422-21423, 21432-21436, 21454-21470, 21627, 21632, 21740, 21750, 21805, 21825, 22325, 22524, 22554, 22558, 22600, 22612, 22630, 22800-22804, 27125-27138, 27235-27236, 27244-27245, 27269, 27440-27447, 27702-27704, 27758-27759, 27766, 27769, 27792, 27814, 28192-28193, 28293, 28415-28420, 28445, 28465, 28485, 28505, 28525, 28531, 28555, 28585, 28615, 28645, 28675-28737, 31360-31395, 31760-31775, 31786, 31805, 32095, 32100-32150, 32215-32320, 32402, 32440-32501, 32800-32815, 32900-32940, 33020-33208, 33212-33220, 33222-33226, 33233-33256, 33261, 33300-33322, 33332-33411, 33413, 33416, 33422-33465, 33475, 33496, 33510-33572, 33877-33883, 33886, 33891, 34051, 34800-34805, 34825, 34830-34832, 34900, 35021, 35081, 35091, 35102, 35131, 35141, 35151, 35211-35216, 35241-35246, 35271-35276, 35301, 35311, 35526, 35601-35671, 36830, 37616, 38381, 38746, 39000-39220, 39545, 39561, 41130-41155, 43045-43135, 43300-43313, 43320, 43325, 43327-43337, 43340-43425, 43496, 43500-43520, 43605-43634, 43640-43641, 43653, 43800-43840, 43843-43880, 44005-44010, 44020-44120, 44125-44127, 44130-44136, 44140-44160, 44202, 44204-44212, 44300-44346, 44615-44661, 44700, 44950, 45108-45190, 45500-45825, 47420-47480, 47560-47561, 47570, 47600-47620, 47700-47800, 47802-47900, 48020-48100, 48120-48155, 48500-48548, 48554-48556, 49215, 49568, 50320, 50340-50380, 51597, 58150-58210, 58260-58294, 60521-60522, 61154, 61312-61313, 61315, 61510-61512, 61518, 61520, 61526-61530, 61548, 61591, 61595-61596, 61598, 61606, 61616-61619, 61697, 61700, 61750-61751, 61867, 62223, 62230, 63015, 63020-63030, 63042, 63045, 63047, 63056, 63075, 63081, 63267, 63276, 64746, 69720, 69930, 69955-69970, 0236T	N/A
4043F	N/A	33120-33141, 33250-33251, 33256, 33261, 33305, 33315, 33332-33411, 33413, 33416, 33422-33465, 33475, 33496, 33510-33572	1P, 8P

Numerator	Associated Diagnostic Denominator	Associated Procedure Denominator	Associated Modifiers
4044F	N/A	19260-19272, 19301-19330, 19342-19380, 22558, 22600, 22612, 22630, 27125-27138, 27235-27236, 27244-27245, 27269, 27440-27447, 38100-38101, 38115-38120, 38571-38572, 38700-38745, 38747-38780, 39501, 39503, 39540-39561, 43020-43135, 43279-43282, 43300-43320, 43325, 43327-43337, 43340-43425, 43496, 43500-43520, 43605-43634, 43640-43645, 43651-43653, 43770-43830, 43832-43840, 43843-43880, 43886-43888, 44005-44010, 44020-44055, 44110-44120, 44125-44127, 44130, 44140-44202, 44204-44212, 44227, 44300-44346, 44602-44700, 44800-44850, 44900, 44950, 44960-44970, 45000, 45020-45190, 45395-45402, 45500-45505, 45550-45825, 46715-46762, 47010, 47100-47130, 47135-47142, 47300-47371, 47380-47382, 47400-47480, 47500-47505, 47560-47570, 47600-47900, 48000-48100, 48105-48155, 48500-48510, 48520-48548, 48554-48556, 49000-49020, 49040, 49060, 49203-49323, 49560-49566, 49570, 50020, 50220-50240, 50320, 50340-50380, 50543, 50545-50548, 50715-50728, 50760-50820, 50947-50948, 51550-51597, 51800-51820, 51900-51925, 51960, 55810-55845, 55866, 56630-56640, 58200-58240, 58285, 58951, 58953-58956, 60200-60281, 60500-60505, 60520-60650, 61313, 61510-61512, 61518, 61548, 61697, 61700, 62230, 63015, 63020, 63047, 63056, 63081, 63267, 63276	1P, 8P
4047F	N/A	00100-00103, 00120, 00140, 00145-00147, 00160-00322, 00350-00406, 00450-00500, 00528-00634, 00670-00700, 00730, 00750-00802, 00820-00832, 00840, 00844-00870, 00880-00944, 01120, 01140-01150, 01170-01190, 01202-01215, 01230-01320, 01360, 01382, 01392-01404, 01430-01444, 01464-01486, 01500-01610, 01622-01670, 01710-01716, 01732-01810, 01829-01852, 01924-01926, 01951-01953, 01961-01966, 01968-01969	8P
4048F	N/A	00100-00103, 00120, 00140, 00145-00147, 00160-00322, 00350-00406, 00450-00500, 00528-00634, 00670-00700, 00730, 00750-00802, 00820-00832, 00840, 00844-00870, 00880-00944, 01120, 01140-01150, 01170-01190, 01202-01215, 01230-01320, 01360, 01382, 01392-01404, 01430-01444, 01464-01486, 01500-01610, 01622-01670, 01710-01716, 01732-01810, 01829-01852, 01924-01926, 01951-01953, 01961-01966, 01968-01969	1P, 8P
4049F	N/A	15734, 15738, 19260-19272, 19301-19307, 19361-19369, 21346-21348, 21422-21423, 21432-21436, 21454-21470, 21627, 21632, 21740, 21750, 21805, 21825, 22325, 22524, 22554, 22558, 22600, 22612, 22630, 22800-22804, 27125-27138, 27235-27236, 27244-27245, 27269, 27440-27447, 27702-27704, 27758-27759, 27766, 27769, 27792, 27814, 28192-28193, 28293, 28415-28420, 28445, 28465, 28485, 28505, 28525, 28531, 28555, 28585, 28615, 28645, 28675-28737, 31360-31395, 31760-31775, 31786, 31805, 32095, 32100-32150, 32215-32320, 32402, 32440-32501, 32800-32815, 32900-32940, 33020-33050, 33202-33208, 33212-33220, 33222-33226, 33233-33249, 33254-33255, 33300, 33310, 33320-33322, 33877-33883, 33886, 33891, 34051, 34800-34805, 34825, 34830-34832, 34900, 35021, 35081, 35091, 35102, 35131, 35141, 35151, 35211-35216, 35241-35246, 35271-35276, 35301, 35311, 35526, 35601-35671, 36830, 37616, 38381, 38746, 39000-39220, 39545, 39561, 41130-41155, 43045-43135, 43300-43313, 43320, 43325, 43327-43337, 43340-43425, 43496, 43500-43520, 43605-43634, 43640-43641, 43653, 43800-43840, 43843-43880, 44005-44010, 44020-44120, 44125-44127, 44130-44136, 44140-44160, 44202, 44204-44212, 44300-44346, 44615-44661, 44700, 44950, 45108-45190, 45500-45825, 47420-47480, 47560-47561, 47570, 47600-47620, 47700-47800, 47802-47900, 48020-48100, 48120-48155, 48500-48548, 48554-48556, 49215, 49568, 50320, 50340-50380, 51597, 58150-58210, 58260-58294, 60521-60522, 61154, 61312-61313, 61315, 61510-61512, 61518, 61520, 61526-61530, 61548, 61591, 61595-61596, 61598, 61606, 61616-61619, 61697, 61700, 61750-61751, 61867, 62223, 62230, 63015, 63020-63030, 63042, 63045, 63047, 63056, 63075, 63081, 63267, 63276, 64746, 69720, 69930, 69955-69970, 0236T	1P, 8P
4050F	401.0-401.9, 402.00-402.01, 402.10-402.11, 402.90-402.91, 403.00-403.01, 403.10-403.11, 403.90-403.91, 404.00-404.03, 404.10-404.13, 404.93	99201-99205, 99212-99215, 99304-99310, 99324-99337, 99341-99350	8P
4070F	431, 433.01, 433.11, 433.21, 433.31, 433.81, 433.91, 434.01, 434.11, 434.91	99221-99223, 99291	1P, 2P, 8P
4073F	433.01, 433.11, 433.21, 433.31, 433.81, 433.91, 434.01, 434.11, 434.91, 435.9	99221-99223, 99238-99239	1P, 2P, 8P

Numerator	Associated Diagnostic Denominator	Associated Procedure Denominator	Associated Modifiers
4075F	427.31, 433.01, 433.11, 433.21, 433.31, 433.81, 433.91, 434.01, 434.11, 434.91, 435.9	99221-99223, 99238-99239	1P, 2P, 8P
4079F	431, 433.01, 433.11, 433.21, 433.31, 433.81, 433.91, 434.01, 434.11, 434.91	99221-99223, 99238-99239	8P
4084F	410.00-410.01, 410.10-410.11, 410.20-410.21, 410.30-410.31, 410.40-410.41, 410.50-410.51, 410.60-410.61, 410.70-410.71, 410.80-410.81, 410.91	99281-99285, 99291	1P, 2P, 8P
4090F, 4095F	238.75	99201-99205, 99212-99215	N/A
4100F	203.00, 203.02	99201-99205, 99212-99215	1P, 2P, 8P
4110F, 4115F	N/A	33510-33523, 33533-33536	1P, 8P
4120F	034.0, 460, 462-463, 465.0-465.9, 466.0	99201-99205, 99212-99220	1P
4124F	034.0, 460, 462-463, 465.0-465.9, 466.0	99201-99205, 99212-99220	N/A
4130F	380.10-380.13, 380.22	99201-99205, 99212-99215, 99281-99285	1P, 2P, 8P
4131F	380.10-380.13, 380.22	99201-99205, 99212-99215, 99281-99285	1P
4132F	380.10-380.13, 380.22	99201-99205, 99212-99215, 99281-99285	N/A
4150F, 4151F, G8458, G8459, G8460, G8461, G8462, G8463	070.54	99201-99205, 99212-99215	N/A
4153F	070.54	99201-99205, 99212-99215	1P, 2P, 3P, 8P
4158F	070.51, 070.54, 070.70	99201-99205, 99212-99215	8P
4164F	185	77427	1P, 2P, 8P
4165F	185, 197.0-197.8, 198.0-198.7, 198.89	77427	8P
4175F	360.00-360.04, 360.11-360.19, 360.20-360.29, 361.00-361.07, 362.01, 362.03-362.07, 362.12, 362.16, 362.18, 362.20-362.27, 362.31-362.32, 362.35-362.36, 362.41-362.43, 362.50-362.57, 362.70-362.76, 362.81-362.89, 363.00-363.08, 363.10-363.15, 363.20-363.22, 363.30-363.33, 363.35, 363.43, 363.50-363.57, 363.61-363.63, 363.72, 364.00-364.05, 364.10-364.11, 364.21-364.3, 365.10-365.15, 365.20-365.24, 365.31-365.32, 365.41-365.44, 365.51-365.59, 365.60-365.65, 365.81-365.9, 366.32-366.33, 368.01-368.03, 368.41, 369.00-369.08, 369.10-369.18, 370.03, 371.00-371.04, 371.20-371.23, 371.43-371.44, 371.50-371.58, 371.60-371.62, 371.70-371.73, 377.10-377.16, 377.30-377.39, 377.41, 377.51-377.54, 377.75, 379.04-379.09, 379.11-379.12, 379.51, 871.0-871.9, 921.3, 940.0-940.9, 950.9	66840-66984	8P
4177F	362.52	99201-99205, 99212-99215, 99307-99310, 99324-99337, 92002-92014	8P
4179F	174.0-174.9, V10.3	99201-99205, 99212-99215	1P, 2P, 3P, 8P
4180F	153.0-153.9, V10.05	99201-99205, 99212-99215	1P, 2P, 3P, 8P
4200F, 4201F	185, 197.0-197.8, 198.0-198.7, 198.89	77427	N/A
4250F	N/A	00100-00560, 00566, 00580-01860, 01924-01952, 01961-01966, 01968-01969	1P, 8P
4255F, 4256F	N/A	00100-00560, 00566, 00580-01860, 01924-01952, 01961-01966, 01968-01969	N/A
4267F	454.0, 454.2, 459.31, 459.33, 459.81, 707.19	99201-99205, 99212-99215	1P, 2P, 3P, 8P
4274F	585.6	90951-90959, 90963-90965	1P, 2P, 3P, 8P
4276F	042, 079.53, V08, V22.0-V22.2, V23.0-V23.3, V23.41, V23.49-V23.7, V23.81-V23.84, V23.9	99201-99205, 99212-99215	8P
4280F	042, 079.53, V08	99201-99205, 99212-99215	1P, 8P
5015F	733.00-733.09, 805.00-805.08, 805.2, 805.4, 805.6, 805.8, 813.40-813.42, 813.44-813.45, 813.47, 813.50-813.52, 813.54, 820.00-820.09, 820.20-820.22, 820.8	99201-99205, 99212-99215, 22305-22327, 22520-22521, 22523-22524, 25600-25609, 27230-27248	1P, 2P, 8P
5050F	172.9	99201-99205, 99212-99215, 11600-11646, 14000-14302, 17311, 17313	2P, 3P, 8P
6010F	431, 433.01, 433.11, 433.21, 433.31, 433.81, 433.91, 434.01, 434.11, 434.91	99221-99223	1P, 8P
6015F, 6020F	431, 433.01, 433.11, 433.21, 433.31, 433.81, 433.91, 434.01, 434.11, 434.91	99221-99223	N/A
6030F	N/A	36555-36571, 36578-36585, 93503	1P, 8P

Numerator	Associated Diagnostic Denominator	Associated Procedure Denominator	Associated Modifiers
6045F	140.0-140.9, 141.0-141.9, 142.0-142.9, 143.0-143.9, 144.0-144.9, 145.0-145.9, 146.0-146.9, 147.0-147.9, 148.0-148.9, 149.0-149.9, 150.0-150.9, 151.0-151.9, 152.0-152.9, 153.0-153.9, 154.0-154.8, 155.0-155.2, 156.0-156.9, 157.0-157.9, 158.0-158.9, 159.0-159.9, 160.0-160.9, 161.0-161.9, 162.0-162.9, 163.0-163.9, 164.0-164.9, 165.0-165.9, 170.0-170.9, 171.0-171.9, 172.0-172.9, 173.0, 173.1, 173.2, 173.3, 173.4, 173.5, 173.6, 173.7, 173.8, 173.9, 174.0-174.9, 175.0-175.9, 176.0-179, 180.0-181, 182.0-182.8, 183.0-183.9, 184.0-185, 186.0-186.9, 187.1-187.9, 188.0-188.9, 189.0-189.9, 190.0-190.9, 191.0-191.9, 192.0-193, 194.0-194.9, 195.0-195.8, 196.0-196.9, 197.0-197.8, 198.0-198.7, 198.81-198.89, 199.0-199.2, 200.00-200.08, 200.10-200.18, 200.20-200.28, 200.30-200.38, 200.40-200.48, 200.50-200.58, 200.60-200.68, 200.70-200.78, 200.80-200.88, 201.00-201.08, 201.10-201.18, 201.20-201.28, 201.40-201.48, 201.50-201.58, 201.60-201.68, 201.70-201.78, 201.90-201.98, 202.00-202.08, 202.10-202.18, 202.20-202.28, 202.30-202.38, 202.40-202.48, 202.50-202.58, 202.60-202.68, 202.70-202.78, 202.80-202.88, 202.90-202.98, 203.00-203.02, 203.10-203.12, 203.80-203.82, 204.00-204.02, 204.10-204.12, 204.20-204.22, 204.80-204.82, 204.90-204.92, 205.00-205.02, 205.10-205.12, 205.20-205.22, 205.30-205.32, 205.80-205.82, 205.90-205.92, 206.00-206.02, 206.10-206.12, 206.20-206.22, 206.80-206.82, 206.90-206.92, 207.00-207.02, 207.10-207.12, 207.20-207.22, 207.80-207.82, 208.00-208.02, 208.10-208.12, 208.20-208.22, 208.80-208.82, 208.90-208.92, 209.00-209.03, 209.10-209.17, 209.20-209.29, 209.30-209.36, 209.70-209.79, 235.0-235.9, 236.0-236.7, 236.90-236.99, 237.0-237.6, 237.70-237.72, 237.9, 238.0-238.6, 238.71-238.77, 238.8-238.9, 239.0-239.7, 239.9	99201-99205, 99212-99215, 25606, 25651, 26608, 26650, 26676, 26706, 26727, 27235, 27244-27245, 27509, 27756, 27759, 28406, 28436, 28456, 28476, 36147, 36598, 37182-37184, 37187-37188, 37210, 37225, 37227, 37229, 37231, 43260-43272, 43752, 44500, 49440-49465, 50382-50389, 50590, 51720, 61623, 62263-62264, 62280-62282, 63610, 64610, 64620, 70010-70015, 70170, 70332, 70370-70373, 70390, 71023, 71034, 71040-71090, 72240-72291, 72295, 73040, 73085, 73115, 73525, 73542, 73580, 73615, 74190-74260, 74270-74300, 74305-74363, 74425-74485, 74740-74742, 75600-75630, 75650-75756, 75791-75810, 75825-75940, 75952-75962, 75966, 75970-75984, 76000-76001, 76080, 76120, 76496, 77001-77003, 77427-77435, 77470, 92611, 93565-93568, 96401-96440, 96446-96549, 0075T, 0080T, 0234T-0235T, 0238T	8P
7010F	172.0-172.9, V10.82	99201-99205, 99212-99215	3P, 8P
7025F	V76.12	77057	8P

APPENDIX L — MEDICALLY UNLIKELY EDITS (MUES)

The Centers for Medicare & Medicaid Services (CMS) began to publish many of the edits used in the medically unlikely edits (MUE) program for the first time effective October 2008. What follows below is a list of the published CPT codes that have MUEs assigned to them and the number of units allowed with each code. CMS publishes the updates on a quarterly basis. Not all MUEs will be published, however. MUEs intended to detect and discourage any questionable payments will not be published as the agency feels the efficacy of these edits would be compromised.

The quarterly updates will be published on the CMS website at http://www.cms.gov/NationalCorrectCodInitEd/08_MUE.asp.

Professional

CPT	MUE
0019T	1
0030T	2
0042T	1
0048T	1
0050T	1
0051T	1
0052T	1
0053T	1
0054T	2
0055T	2
0071T	1
0072T	1
0073T	2
0075T	1
0076T	2
0078T	1
0079T	4
0080T	1
0081T	4
0092T	1
0095T	1
0098T	1
0099T	2
0100T	2
0101T	1
0102T	2
0103T	1
0106T	4
0107T	4
0108T	4
0109T	4
0110T	4
0111T	1
0123T	2
0124T	2
0126T	1
0159T	2
0163T	2
0164T	4
0165T	4
0169T	1
0171T	1
0172T	3
0173T	1
0174T	1
0175T	1
0179T	1
0180T	1
0181T	1
0182T	3
0183T	1
0184T	1
0190T	2
0191T	2
0192T	2
0197T	2
0198T	2
01996	1
0208T	1

CPT	MUE
0209T	1
0210T	1
0211T	1
0212T	1
0213T	1
0214T	1
0215T	1
0216T	1
0217T	1
0218T	1
0219T	1
0220T	1
0221T	1
0223T	1
0224T	1
0225T	1
0226T	1
0227T	1
0228T	2
0230T	2
0232T	1
0233T	1
0234T	2
0235T	2
0236T	1
0237T	2
0239T	1
0240T	1
0241T	1
0242T	1
0243T	1
0244T	1
0245T	1
0246T	1
0247T	1
0248T	1
0249T	1
0250T	2
0251T	1
0252T	2
0253T	1
0254T	2
0255T	2
0256T	1
0257T	1
0258T	1
0259T	1
0260T	1
0261T	1
10040	1
10060	1
10061	1
10080	1
10081	1
10180	3
11000	1
11004	1
11005	1
11006	1
11008	1

CPT	MUE
11042	1
11043	1
11044	1
11055	1
11056	1
11057	1
11100	1
11200	1
11201	1
11446	3
11450	2
11451	2
11462	2
11463	2
11471	2
11646	3
11719	1
11720	1
11721	1
11730	1
11770	1
11771	1
11772	1
11900	1
11901	1
11920	1
11921	1
11922	1
11950	1
11951	1
11952	1
11954	1
11960	3
11970	2
11971	2
11976	1
11980	1
11981	1
11982	1
11983	1
12001	1
12002	1
12004	1
12005	1
12006	1
12007	1
12011	1
12013	1
12014	1
12015	1
12016	1
12017	1
12018	1
12020	3
12021	3
12031	1
12032	1
12034	1
12035	1
12036	1

CPT	MUE
12037	1
12041	1
12042	1
12044	1
12045	1
12046	1
12047	1
12051	1
12052	1
12053	1
12054	1
12055	1
12056	1
12057	1
13100	1
13101	1
13120	1
13121	1
13131	1
13132	1
13150	1
13151	1
13152	1
13160	3
15002	1
15004	1
15040	1
15050	1
15100	1
15110	1
15115	1
15120	1
15130	1
15135	1
15150	1
15151	1
15155	1
15156	1
15170	1
15175	1
15200	1
15220	1
15240	1
15260	1
15300	1
15320	1
15330	1
15335	1
15340	1
15360	1
15365	1
15400	1
15420	1
15430	1
15570	3
15572	2
15574	2
15576	2
15600	2
15610	2

CPT	MUE
15620	2
15630	2
15650	1
15731	1
15740	3
15750	2
15756	2
15757	3
15758	3
15760	2
15770	2
15775	1
15776	1
15780	1
15781	2
15782	2
15783	2
15786	1
15787	3
15788	1
15789	1
15792	1
15793	1
15819	1
15820	1
15821	1
15822	1
15823	1
15824	1
15825	1
15826	1
15828	1
15829	1
15830	1
15832	2
15833	2
15834	2
15835	1
15836	2
15838	1
15839	2
15840	1
15841	2
15842	2
15845	2
15847	1
15851	1
15852	2
15860	1
15876	1
15877	1
15878	2
15879	2
15920	1
15922	1
15931	1
15933	1
15934	1
15935	1
15936	1

CPT	MUE
15937	1
15940	2
15941	2
15944	2
15945	2
15946	2
15950	2
15951	2
15952	2
15953	2
15956	2
15958	2
16000	1
16020	1
16025	1
16030	1
16035	1
17000	1
17003	13
17004	1
17106	1
17107	1
17108	1
17110	1
17111	1
17264	3
17266	2
17276	3
17286	3
17340	1
17360	1
17380	1
19000	2
19001	5
19020	2
19030	2
19101	3
19110	2
19112	2
19120	2
19125	2
19126	3
19260	2
19271	2
19272	2
19290	3
19296	2
19297	2
19298	2
19300	2
19301	2
19302	2
19303	2
19304	2
19305	2
19306	2
19307	2
19316	1
19318	1
19324	1

CPT	MUE
19325	1
19328	1
19330	1
19340	1
19342	1
19350	1
19355	1
19357	1
19361	1
19364	1
19366	1
19367	1
19368	1
19369	1
19370	1
19371	1
19380	1
19396	1
20100	2
20102	4
20103	4
20150	2
20200	3
20205	4
20206	3
20250	3
20251	3
20526	2
20552	1
20553	1
20555	1
20660	1
20661	1
20662	1
20663	2
20664	1
20665	1
20670	2
20680	2
20692	3
20693	2
20696	2
20697	4
20802	2
20805	2
20808	2
20824	2
20827	2
20838	2
20900	2
20910	2
20912	1
20920	2
20922	2
20924	4
20926	2
20931	1
20937	1
20938	1
20955	1

CPT	MUE
20956	1
20957	1
20962	1
20969	2
20970	2
20972	2
20973	2
20974	1
20975	1
20979	1
20982	1
20985	2
21010	1
21015	1
21025	2
21026	2
21029	1
21030	2
21031	2
21032	1
21034	1
21040	2
21044	1
21045	1
21046	2
21047	2
21048	2
21049	2
21050	1
21060	1
21070	1
21073	1
21076	1
21077	2
21079	1
21080	1
21081	1
21082	1
21083	1
21084	1
21085	1
21086	2
21087	1
21088	1
21100	1
21110	2
21116	2
21120	1
21121	1
21122	1
21123	1
21125	2
21127	2
21137	1
21138	1
21139	1
21141	1
21142	1
21143	1
21145	1

CPT	MUE
21146	1
21147	1
21150	1
21151	1
21154	1
21155	1
21159	1
21160	1
21172	1
21175	1
21179	1
21180	1
21181	1
21182	2
21183	2
21184	2
21188	1
21193	1
21194	1
21195	1
21196	1
21198	1
21199	1
21206	1
21208	2
21209	2
21210	2
21215	2
21230	2
21235	2
21240	2
21242	2
21243	2
21244	1
21245	2
21246	2
21247	2
21255	2
21256	2
21260	1
21261	1
21263	1
21267	2
21268	2
21270	2
21275	1
21280	2
21282	2
21295	2
21296	2
21310	1
21315	1
21320	1
21325	1
21330	1
21335	1
21336	1
21337	1
21338	1
21339	1
21340	1
21343	1
21344	1
21345	1
21346	1
21347	1
21348	1
21355	2
21356	2

CPT	MUE
21360	2
21365	2
21366	2
21385	2
21386	2
21387	2
21390	2
21395	2
21400	2
21401	2
21406	2
21407	2
21408	2
21421	1
21422	1
21423	1
21431	1
21432	1
21433	1
21435	1
21436	1
21440	2
21445	2
21450	1
21451	1
21452	1
21453	1
21454	1
21461	1
21462	1
21465	2
21470	1
21480	2
21485	2
21490	2
21495	1
21497	1
21501	3
21502	1
21510	1
21550	3
21556	3
21557	1
21610	2
21615	2
21616	2
21620	1
21627	1
21630	1
21632	1
21685	1
21700	2
21705	2
21720	1
21725	1
21740	1
21742	1
21743	1
21750	1
21805	3
21810	1
21820	1
21825	1
21920	3
21925	3
21935	1
22010	2
22015	2
22100	1

CPT	MUE
22101	1
22102	1
22103	3
22110	1
22112	1
22114	1
22116	3
22206	1
22207	1
22210	1
22212	1
22214	1
22216	6
22220	1
22222	1
22224	1
22305	1
22310	1
22315	1
22318	1
22319	1
22325	1
22326	1
22327	1
22328	8
22505	1
22520	1
22521	1
22522	5
22523	1
22524	1
22525	5
22532	1
22533	1
22534	3
22548	1
22551	1
22554	1
22556	1
22558	1
22585	7
22590	1
22595	1
22600	1
22610	1
22612	1
22614	15
22630	1
22632	4
22800	1
22802	1
22804	1
22808	1
22810	1
22812	1
22818	1
22819	1
22830	1
22840	1
22842	1
22843	1
22844	1
22845	1
22846	1
22847	1
22848	1
22849	1
22850	1
22851	9

CPT	MUE
22852	1
22855	1
22857	1
22862	1
22865	1
22900	3
23000	2
23020	2
23030	2
23031	2
23035	2
23040	2
23044	2
23065	2
23066	2
23075	4
23076	2
23077	1
23100	2
23101	2
23105	2
23106	2
23107	2
23120	2
23125	2
23130	2
23145	1
23146	1
23150	1
23155	1
23156	1
23170	1
23172	1
23174	1
23180	1
23182	1
23184	1
23190	1
23195	1
23200	1
23210	1
23220	1
23330	2
23331	2
23332	2
23350	2
23395	1
23397	1
23400	1
23405	2
23406	2
23410	2
23412	2
23415	2
23420	2
23430	2
23440	2
23450	2
23455	2
23460	2
23462	2
23465	2
23466	2
23470	2
23472	2
23480	2
23485	2
23490	2
23491	2

CPT	MUE
23500	2
23505	2
23515	2
23520	2
23525	2
23530	2
23532	2
23540	2
23545	2
23550	2
23552	2
23570	2
23575	2
23585	2
23600	2
23605	2
23615	2
23616	2
23620	2
23625	2
23630	2
23650	2
23655	2
23660	2
23665	2
23670	2
23675	2
23680	2
23700	2
23800	2
23802	2
23900	1
23920	2
23921	2
23930	2
23931	2
23935	2
24000	2
24006	2
24065	2
24066	2
24077	2
24100	2
24101	2
24102	2
24105	2
24110	1
24115	2
24116	1
24120	2
24125	1
24126	1
24130	2
24134	1
24136	1
24138	2
24140	2
24145	2
24147	2
24149	2
24150	1
24152	1
24155	2
24160	2
24164	2
24200	3
24201	3
24220	2
24300	2

CPT	MUE
24301	2
24305	4
24320	2
24330	2
24331	2
24332	2
24340	2
24342	2
24343	2
24344	2
24345	2
24346	2
24357	2
24358	2
24359	2
24360	2
24361	2
24362	2
24363	2
24365	2
24366	2
24400	2
24410	2
24420	2
24430	2
24435	2
24470	2
24495	2
24498	2
24500	2
24505	2
24515	2
24516	2
24530	2
24535	2
24538	2
24545	2
24546	2
24560	2
24565	2
24566	2
24575	2
24576	2
24577	2
24579	2
24582	2
24586	2
24587	2
24600	2
24605	2
24615	2
24620	2
24635	2
24640	2
24650	2
24655	2
24665	2
24666	2
24670	2
24675	2
24685	2
24800	2
24802	2
24900	2
24920	2
24925	2
24930	2
24931	2
24935	2

CPT	MUE
24940	2
25000	2
25001	2
25020	2
25023	2
25024	2
25025	2
25031	2
25035	2
25040	2
25065	5
25066	3
25076	5
25077	2
25085	2
25100	2
25101	2
25105	2
25107	2
25110	3
25111	2
25112	2
25115	2
25116	2
25119	2
25120	2
25125	1
25126	1
25130	2
25135	2
25136	2
25145	1
25150	1
25151	1
25170	1
25210	2
25215	2
25230	2
25240	2
25246	2
25248	3
25250	2
25251	2
25259	2
25275	2
25295	9
25300	2
25301	2
25315	2
25316	2
25320	2
25332	2
25335	2
25337	2
25350	2
25355	2
25360	2
25365	2
25370	2
25375	2
25390	2
25391	2
25392	2
25393	2
25394	2
25400	2
25405	2
25415	2
25420	2

CPT	MUE
25425	2
25426	2
25430	2
25431	2
25440	2
25441	2
25442	2
25443	2
25444	2
25445	2
25446	2
25449	2
25450	2
25455	2
25490	2
25491	2
25492	2
25500	2
25505	2
25515	2
25520	2
25525	2
25526	2
25530	2
25535	2
25545	2
25560	2
25565	2
25574	2
25575	2
25600	2
25605	2
25606	2
25607	2
25608	2
25609	2
25622	2
25624	2
25628	2
25630	2
25635	2
25650	2
25651	2
25652	2
25660	2
25670	2
25671	2
25675	2
25676	2
25680	2
25685	2
25690	2
25695	2
25800	2
25805	2
25810	2
25820	2
25825	2
25830	2
25900	2
25905	2
25907	2
25909	2
25915	2
25920	2
25922	2
25924	2
25927	2
25929	2

CPT	MUE
25931	2
26010	3
26011	3
26025	2
26030	2
26034	2
26035	3
26037	2
26040	2
26045	2
26070	3
26100	2
26105	2
26110	3
26117	2
26121	2
26123	2
26185	1
26205	2
26215	2
26230	3
26236	3
26250	2
26260	2
26262	2
26357	3
26358	3
26390	3
26392	3
26416	2
26428	2
26432	2
26433	2
26434	3
26494	2
26496	2
26497	2
26498	2
26508	2
26516	2
26517	2
26518	2
26548	3
26550	2
26551	2
26553	2
26554	2
26555	2
26556	2
26560	2
26561	2
26562	2
26580	2
26641	2
26645	2
26650	2
26665	2
26740	3
26742	3
26746	3
26820	2
26841	2
26842	2
26860	1
26862	1
26990	2
26991	2
26992	2
27000	2

CPT	MUE
27001	1
27003	1
27005	2
27006	2
27025	1
27027	1
27030	2
27033	2
27035	2
27036	2
27040	2
27041	3
27048	2
27049	2
27050	2
27052	2
27054	2
27057	1
27060	2
27062	2
27065	2
27066	2
27067	2
27070	2
27071	2
27075	1
27076	2
27077	2
27078	2
27080	1
27086	2
27087	2
27090	2
27091	2
27093	2
27095	2
27096	1
27097	2
27098	2
27100	2
27105	2
27110	2
27111	2
27120	2
27122	2
27125	2
27130	2
27132	2
27134	2
27137	2
27138	2
27140	2
27146	2
27147	2
27151	2
27156	2
27158	1
27161	2
27165	2
27170	2
27175	2
27176	2
27177	2
27178	2
27179	2
27181	2
27185	2
27187	2
27193	1

CPT	MUE
27194	1
27200	1
27202	1
27220	2
27222	2
27226	2
27227	2
27228	2
27230	2
27232	2
27235	2
27236	2
27238	2
27240	2
27244	2
27245	2
27246	2
27248	2
27250	2
27252	2
27253	2
27254	2
27256	2
27257	2
27258	2
27259	2
27265	2
27266	2
27267	2
27268	2
27269	2
27275	2
27280	1
27282	1
27284	2
27286	2
27290	1
27295	2
27303	2
27305	2
27306	2
27307	2
27310	2
27325	1
27326	1
27329	2
27330	2
27331	2
27332	2
27333	2
27334	2
27335	2
27340	2
27345	2
27347	2
27350	2
27355	2
27356	2
27357	2
27358	2
27365	2
27370	2
27380	2
27381	2
27385	2
27386	2
27390	2
27391	1
27392	1

CPT	MUE
27393	2
27394	1
27395	1
27396	2
27397	2
27400	2
27403	2
27405	2
27407	2
27409	2
27412	2
27415	2
27416	2
27418	2
27420	2
27422	2
27424	2
27425	2
27427	2
27428	2
27429	2
27430	2
27435	2
27437	2
27438	2
27440	2
27441	2
27442	2
27443	2
27445	2
27446	2
27447	2
27448	1
27450	1
27454	2
27455	1
27457	1
27465	2
27466	2
27468	2
27470	2
27472	2
27475	2
27477	2
27479	2
27485	2
27486	2
27487	2
27488	2
27495	2
27496	2
27497	2
27498	2
27499	2
27500	2
27501	2
27502	2
27503	2
27506	2
27507	2
27508	2
27509	2
27510	2
27511	2
27513	2
27514	2
27516	2
27517	2
27519	2

CPT	MUE
27520	2
27524	2
27530	2
27532	2
27535	2
27536	2
27538	2
27540	2
27550	2
27552	2
27556	2
27557	2
27558	2
27560	2
27562	2
27566	2
27570	2
27580	2
27590	2
27591	2
27592	2
27594	2
27596	2
27598	2
27600	2
27601	2
27602	2
27604	2
27605	2
27606	2
27607	2
27610	2
27612	2
27615	2
27620	2
27625	2
27626	2
27630	2
27635	2
27637	2
27638	2
27640	2
27641	2
27645	1
27646	1
27647	2
27648	2
27650	2
27652	2
27654	2
27656	2
27658	2
27659	2
27664	2
27665	2
27675	2
27676	2
27680	3
27681	2
27685	2
27686	2
27687	2
27690	2
27691	2
27695	2
27696	2
27698	2
27700	2
27702	2

CPT	MUE
27703	2
27704	2
27705	2
27707	2
27709	2
27712	2
27715	2
27720	2
27722	2
27724	2
27725	2
27726	2
27727	2
27730	2
27732	2
27734	2
27740	2
27742	2
27745	2
27750	2
27752	2
27756	2
27758	2
27759	2
27760	2
27762	2
27766	2
27767	2
27768	2
27769	2
27780	2
27781	2
27784	2
27786	2
27788	2
27792	2
27808	2
27810	2
27814	2
27816	2
27818	2
27822	2
27823	2
27824	2
27825	2
27826	2
27827	2
27828	2
27829	2
27830	2
27831	2
27832	2
27840	2
27842	2
27846	2
27848	2
27860	2
27870	2
27871	2
27880	2
27881	2
27882	2
27884	2
27886	2
27888	2
27889	2
27892	2
27893	2
27894	2

CPT	MUE
28001	2
28002	3
28003	2
28005	3
28035	2
28052	2
28054	2
28060	2
28062	2
28086	2
28088	2
28090	2
28092	2
28100	2
28102	2
28103	2
28106	2
28107	2
28108	2
28110	2
28111	2
28113	2
28114	2
28116	2
28118	2
28119	2
28120	2
28130	2
28171	2
28173	2
28175	2
28192	2
28193	2
28202	2
28210	2
28220	2
28222	2
28225	2
28226	2
28230	2
28238	2
28240	2
28250	2
28260	2
28261	2
28262	2
28264	2
28280	2
28286	2
28289	2
28290	2
28292	2
28293	2
28294	2
28296	2
28297	2
28298	2
28299	2
28300	2
28302	2
28304	2
28305	2
28306	2
28307	2
28309	2
28310	2
28315	2
28320	2
28322	2

CPT	MUE
28340	2
28341	2
28344	2
28360	2
28400	2
28405	2
28406	2
28415	2
28420	2
28430	2
28435	2
28436	2
28445	2
28446	2
28490	2
28495	2
28496	2
28505	2
28530	2
28531	2
28540	2
28545	2
28546	2
28555	2
28570	2
28575	2
28576	2
28585	2
28600	3
28605	3
28630	3
28705	2
28715	2
28725	2
28730	2
28735	2
28737	2
28750	2
28755	2
28760	2
28800	2
28805	2
28890	2
29000	1
29010	1
29015	1
29020	1
29025	1
29035	1
29040	1
29044	1
29046	1
29049	1
29055	1
29058	1
29065	2
29075	2
29085	2
29086	2
29105	2
29125	2
29126	2
29200	1
29240	2
29260	2
29280	2
29305	1
29325	1
29345	2

CPT	MUE	CPT	MUE	CPT	MUE	CPT	MUE	CPT	MUE	CPT	MUE	CPT	MUE	CPT	MUE
29355	2	29876	2	30802	1	31510	1	31720	1	32660	1	33254	1	33517	1
29358	2	29877	2	30901	1	31511	1	31725	1	32661	1	33255	1	33518	1
29365	2	29879	2	30903	1	31512	1	31730	1	32662	1	33256	1	33519	1
29405	2	29880	2	30905	1	31513	1	31750	1	32663	2	33257	1	33521	1
29425	2	29881	2	30906	1	31515	1	31755	1	32664	2	33258	1	33522	1
29435	2	29882	2	30915	1	31520	1	31760	1	32665	1	33259	1	33523	1
29440	2	29883	2	30920	1	31525	1	31766	1	32800	1	33261	1	33530	1
29445	2	29884	2	30930	1	31526	1	31770	2	32810	1	33265	1	33533	1
29450	1	29885	2	31000	1	31527	1	31775	1	32815	1	33266	1	33534	1
29505	2	29886	2	31002	2	31528	1	31780	1	32820	1	33282	1	33535	1
29515	2	29887	2	31020	1	31529	1	31781	1	32850	1	33284	1	33536	1
29520	2	29888	2	31030	1	31530	1	31785	1	32851	1	33300	1	33542	1
29530	2	29889	2	31032	1	31531	1	31786	1	32852	1	33305	1	33545	1
29540	2	29891	2	31040	2	31535	1	31800	1	32853	1	33310	1	33548	1
29550	2	29892	2	31050	2	31536	1	31805	1	32854	1	33315	1	33572	3
29580	2	29893	2	31051	2	31540	1	31820	1	32855	1	33320	1	33606	1
29590	2	29894	2	31070	2	31541	1	31825	1	32856	1	33321	1	33608	1
29700	2	29895	2	31075	2	31545	2	31830	1	32900	1	33322	1	33610	1
29705	2	29897	2	31080	2	31546	2	32035	2	32905	1	33330	1	33611	1
29710	2	29898	2	31081	2	31560	1	32036	2	32906	1	33332	1	33612	1
29715	1	29899	2	31084	2	31561	1	32095	2	32940	1	33335	1	33615	1
29720	1	29900	2	31085	2	31570	1	32100	1	32960	1	33400	1	33617	1
29730	2	29901	2	31086	2	31571	1	32110	2	32997	2	33401	1	33619	1
29740	1	29902	2	31087	2	31575	1	32120	1	32998	2	33403	1	33620	1
29750	1	29904	2	31090	2	31576	1	32124	2	33010	1	33404	1	33621	1
29800	2	29905	2	31200	2	31577	1	32140	1	33011	1	33405	1	33622	1
29804	2	29906	2	31201	2	31578	1	32141	1	33015	1	33406	1	33641	1
29805	2	29907	2	31205	2	31579	1	32150	1	33020	1	33410	1	33645	1
29806	2	29914	2	31225	2	31580	1	32151	1	33025	1	33411	1	33647	1
29807	2	29915	2	31230	1	31582	1	32160	1	33030	1	33412	1	33660	1
29819	2	29916	2	31231	1	31584	1	32200	2	33031	1	33413	1	33675	1
29820	2	30000	1	31233	2	31587	1	32201	2	33050	1	33414	1	33681	1
29821	2	30020	1	31235	2	31588	1	32215	2	33120	1	33415	1	33684	1
29822	2	30100	3	31237	2	31590	1	32220	2	33130	1	33416	1	33688	1
29823	2	30110	1	31238	2	31595	2	32225	2	33140	1	33417	1	33690	1
29824	2	30115	1	31239	2	31600	1	32400	2	33141	1	33420	1	33692	1
29825	2	30117	2	31240	2	31601	1	32402	2	33202	1	33422	1	33694	1
29826	2	30118	2	31254	2	31603	1	32405	2	33203	1	33425	1	33697	1
29827	2	30120	1	31255	2	31605	1	32420	2	33206	1	33426	1	33702	1
29828	2	30124	2	31256	2	31610	1	32421	3	33207	1	33427	1	33710	1
29830	2	30125	1	31267	2	31611	1	32422	3	33208	1	33430	1	33720	1
29834	2	30130	2	31276	2	31612	1	32440	1	33210	1	33460	1	33722	1
29835	2	30140	2	31287	2	31613	1	32442	1	33211	1	33463	1	33724	1
29836	2	30150	1	31288	2	31614	1	32445	1	33212	1	33464	1	33730	1
29837	2	30160	1	31290	2	31615	1	32480	2	33213	1	33465	1	33732	1
29838	2	30200	1	31291	2	31620	1	32482	1	33214	1	33468	1	33735	1
29840	2	30210	1	31292	2	31622	1	32484	2	33215	2	33470	1	33736	1
29843	2	30220	1	31293	2	31623	1	32486	1	33216	1	33471	1	33737	1
29844	2	30300	1	31294	2	31624	1	32488	1	33217	1	33472	1	33750	1
29845	2	30310	1	31295	2	31625	1	32500	2	33218	1	33474	1	33755	1
29846	2	30320	1	31296	2	31628	1	32501	1	33220	1	33475	1	33762	1
29847	2	30400	1	31297	2	31629	1	32540	1	33222	1	33476	1	33764	1
29848	2	30410	1	31300	1	31630	2	32550	2	33223	1	33478	1	33766	1
29850	2	30420	1	31320	1	31631	1	32601	1	33224	1	33496	1	33767	1
29851	2	30430	1	31360	1	31632	4	32602	1	33225	1	33500	1	33768	1
29855	2	30435	1	31365	1	31633	4	32603	1	33226	1	33501	1	33770	1
29856	2	30450	1	31367	1	31634	1	32604	1	33233	1	33502	1	33771	1
29860	2	30460	1	31368	1	31635	1	32605	1	33234	1	33503	1	33774	1
29861	2	30462	1	31370	1	31636	1	32606	1	33235	1	33504	1	33775	1
29862	2	30465	1	31375	1	31637	2	32650	2	33236	1	33505	1	33776	1
29863	2	30520	1	31380	1	31638	2	32651	2	33237	1	33506	1	33777	1
29866	2	30540	1	31382	1	31640	1	32652	2	33238	1	33507	1	33778	1
29867	2	30545	1	31390	1	31641	1	32653	1	33240	1	33508	1	33779	1
29868	2	30560	1	31395	1	31643	1	32654	2	33241	1	33510	1	33780	1
29870	2	30580	2	31400	1	31645	1	32655	2	33243	1	33511	1	33781	1
29871	2	30600	1	31420	1	31646	2	32656	2	33244	1	33512	1	33786	1
29873	2	30620	1	31500	2	31656	1	32657	2	33249	1	33513	1	33788	1
29874	2	30630	1	31502	1	31715	1	32658	1	33250	1	33514	1	33800	1
29875	2	30801	1	31505	1	31717	1	32659	1	33251	1	33516	1	33802	1

CPT	MUE
33803	1
33813	1
33814	1
33820	1
33822	1
33824	1
33840	1
33845	1
33851	1
33852	1
33853	1
33860	1
33863	1
33864	1
33870	1
33875	1
33877	1
33880	1
33881	1
33883	1
33884	3
33886	1
33889	1
33891	1
33910	1
33915	1
33916	1
33917	1
33920	1
33922	1
33924	1
33925	1
33926	1
33930	1
33933	1
33935	1
33940	1
33944	1
33945	1
33960	1
33961	1
33967	1
33968	1
33970	1
33971	1
33973	1
33974	1
33975	1
33976	1
33977	1
33978	1
33979	2
33980	2
34001	1
34051	1
34101	2
34111	2
34151	2
34201	2
34203	2
34401	1
34421	2
34451	1
34471	1
34490	2
34501	2
34510	2
34520	1
34530	2

CPT	MUE
34800	1
34802	1
34803	1
34804	1
34805	1
34806	1
34808	1
34812	1
34813	1
34820	1
34825	2
34826	4
34830	1
34831	1
34832	1
34833	1
34834	1
34900	2
35001	2
35002	2
35005	2
35011	2
35013	2
35021	2
35022	2
35045	2
35081	1
35082	1
35091	1
35092	1
35102	1
35103	1
35111	1
35112	1
35121	2
35122	1
35131	2
35132	2
35141	2
35142	2
35151	2
35152	2
35180	2
35182	2
35184	2
35188	2
35189	1
35190	2
35201	2
35206	2
35207	3
35211	3
35216	3
35221	3
35226	3
35231	2
35236	2
35241	2
35246	2
35251	2
35256	2
35261	1
35266	2
35271	2
35276	2
35281	2
35286	2
35302	2
35303	2

CPT	MUE
35304	2
35305	2
35306	2
35311	2
35321	2
35331	1
35351	2
35355	2
35361	1
35363	1
35371	2
35372	2
35390	2
35400	1
35450	2
35452	1
35458	3
35471	3
35472	1
35500	2
35501	2
35506	1
35508	1
35509	1
35510	1
35511	1
35512	1
35515	1
35516	1
35518	1
35521	2
35522	1
35523	2
35525	1
35526	3
35531	2
35533	1
35536	1
35537	1
35538	1
35539	1
35540	1
35548	1
35549	1
35551	1
35556	2
35558	2
35560	2
35563	2
35565	2
35566	2
35571	2
35572	2
35583	2
35585	2
35587	2
35600	2
35601	2
35606	1
35612	1
35616	1
35621	2
35623	2
35626	3
35636	1
35637	1
35638	1
35642	1
35645	1

CPT	MUE
35646	1
35647	1
35650	1
35651	2
35654	1
35656	2
35661	1
35663	2
35665	2
35666	2
35671	2
35681	2
35682	1
35683	1
35685	2
35686	1
35691	2
35693	2
35694	2
35695	2
35697	2
35700	2
35701	2
35721	2
35741	2
35761	2
35800	2
35820	2
35840	2
35860	2
35870	1
35875	2
35876	2
35879	2
35881	2
35883	1
35884	1
35901	1
35903	2
35905	1
35907	1
36002	2
36005	2
36010	2
36013	2
36014	2
36100	2
36120	2
36160	2
36200	2
36260	1
36261	1
36262	1
36400	1
36405	1
36406	1
36410	3
36420	2
36425	1
36430	1
36440	1
36450	1
36455	1
36468	1
36469	1
36470	2
36471	2
36475	2
36478	2

CPT	MUE
36479	2
36481	1
36510	1
36511	1
36512	1
36513	1
36514	1
36515	1
36516	1
36522	1
36555	2
36556	2
36557	2
36558	2
36560	2
36561	2
36563	2
36565	2
36566	2
36568	2
36569	2
36570	2
36571	2
36575	2
36576	2
36578	2
36580	2
36581	2
36582	2
36583	2
36584	2
36585	2
36589	2
36590	2
36592	1
36593	2
36595	2
36596	2
36597	2
36598	2
36620	3
36625	2
36640	1
36660	1
36680	1
36800	1
36810	1
36815	1
36818	1
36819	1
36820	2
36821	2
36822	1
36823	1
36825	1
36830	2
36831	1
36832	2
36833	1
36835	1
36838	2
36860	2
36861	2
36870	2
37140	1
37145	1
37160	1
37180	1
37181	1

CPT	MUE
37182	1
37183	1
37184	2
37185	2
37186	2
37187	2
37188	2
37195	1
37200	2
37201	1
37203	2
37205	1
37207	1
37209	2
37210	1
37215	2
37220	1
37221	1
37222	2
37223	2
37224	1
37225	1
37226	1
37227	1
37228	1
37229	1
37230	1
37231	1
37232	2
37233	2
37234	2
37235	2
37250	1
37500	2
37565	2
37600	1
37605	2
37606	2
37607	1
37609	2
37615	2
37616	1
37617	3
37618	2
37620	1
37650	1
37660	2
37700	1
37718	1
37722	1
37735	1
37760	1
37765	2
37766	2
37780	1
37785	1
37788	1
37790	1
38100	1
38101	1
38102	1
38115	1
38120	1
38200	1
38205	1
38206	1
38220	2
38221	2
38230	1

CPT	MUE
38240	1
38241	1
38242	1
38300	2
38305	2
38308	1
38380	1
38381	1
38382	1
38500	2
38505	3
38510	2
38520	2
38525	2
38530	2
38542	2
38550	1
38555	1
38562	1
38564	1
38570	1
38571	1
38572	1
38700	1
38720	1
38724	2
38740	2
38745	2
38746	1
38747	1
38760	1
38765	1
38770	1
38780	1
38790	1
38792	2
38794	1
38900	2
39000	1
39010	1
39200	1
39220	1
39400	1
39501	1
39503	1
39540	1
39541	1
39545	1
39560	1
39561	1
40500	2
40510	2
40520	2
40525	2
40527	2
40530	2
40650	2
40652	2
40654	2
40700	1
40701	1
40702	1
40720	1
40761	1
40800	1
40801	1
40806	2
40816	2
40818	2

CPT	MUE
40819	2
40820	2
40830	2
40831	2
40840	1
40842	1
40843	1
40844	2
40845	1
41000	1
41005	1
41006	2
41007	2
41008	2
41009	2
41010	1
41015	2
41016	1
41017	2
41018	2
41019	1
41100	3
41105	3
41108	2
41110	2
41112	2
41113	2
41114	2
41115	1
41116	3
41120	1
41130	1
41135	1
41140	1
41145	1
41150	1
41153	1
41155	1
41250	2
41251	2
41252	2
41500	1
41510	1
41512	1
41520	1
41800	2
41820	4
41822	1
41823	1
41825	2
41826	2
41827	2
41828	4
41850	2
41872	4
41874	4
42000	1
42100	3
42104	3
42106	2
42107	2
42120	1
42140	1
42145	1
42160	1
42180	1
42182	1
42200	1
42205	1

CPT	MUE
42210	1
42215	1
42220	1
42225	1
42226	1
42227	1
42235	1
42260	1
42280	1
42281	1
42300	2
42305	2
42310	2
42320	2
42330	3
42335	2
42340	2
42400	2
42405	2
42408	1
42409	1
42410	2
42415	2
42420	2
42425	2
42426	2
42440	2
42450	1
42500	2
42505	1
42507	1
42508	1
42509	1
42510	1
42550	2
42600	1
42650	2
42660	2
42665	2
42700	2
42720	1
42725	2
42800	3
42802	2
42806	1
42808	2
42809	1
42810	2
42815	2
42820	1
42821	1
42825	1
42826	1
42830	1
42831	1
42835	1
42836	1
42842	1
42844	1
42845	1
42860	1
42870	1
42890	1
42892	1
42894	1
42900	1
42950	1
42953	1
42955	1

CPT	MUE
42960	1
42961	1
42962	1
42970	1
42971	1
42972	1
43020	1
43030	1
43045	1
43100	1
43101	1
43107	1
43108	1
43112	1
43113	1
43116	1
43117	1
43118	1
43121	1
43122	1
43123	1
43124	1
43130	1
43135	1
43200	1
43201	1
43202	1
43204	1
43205	1
43215	1
43216	1
43217	1
43219	1
43220	1
43226	1
43227	2
43228	1
43231	1
43232	1
43234	1
43235	1
43236	1
43237	1
43238	1
43239	1
43240	1
43241	1
43242	1
43243	1
43244	1
43245	1
43246	1
43247	1
43248	1
43249	1
43250	1
43251	1
43255	2
43256	1
43257	1
43258	1
43259	1
43260	1
43261	1
43262	2
43263	2
43264	1
43265	1
43267	1

CPT	MUE
43268	2
43269	2
43271	1
43272	1
43273	1
43280	1
43283	1
43300	1
43305	1
43310	1
43312	1
43313	1
43314	1
43320	1
43325	1
43327	1
43328	1
43330	1
43331	1
43332	1
43333	1
43334	1
43335	1
43336	1
43337	1
43338	1
43340	1
43341	1
43350	1
43351	1
43352	1
43360	1
43361	1
43400	1
43401	1
43405	1
43410	1
43415	1
43420	1
43425	1
43450	1
43453	1
43456	1
43458	1
43460	1
43496	1
43500	1
43501	1
43502	1
43510	1
43520	1
43605	1
43610	1
43611	1
43620	1
43621	1
43622	1
43631	1
43632	1
43633	1
43634	1
43635	1
43640	1
43641	1
43644	1
43645	1
43647	1
43648	1
43651	1

CPT	MUE
43652	1
43653	1
43752	2
43753	1
43754	1
43755	1
43756	1
43757	1
43760	2
43761	2
43770	1
43771	1
43772	1
43773	1
43774	1
43800	1
43810	1
43820	1
43825	1
43830	1
43831	1
43832	1
43840	2
43843	1
43845	1
43846	1
43847	1
43848	1
43850	1
43855	1
43860	1
43865	1
43870	1
43880	1
43881	1
43882	1
43886	1
43887	1
43888	1
44005	1
44010	1
44015	1
44020	2
44021	1
44025	1
44050	1
44055	1
44100	1
44110	1
44111	1
44120	1
44125	1
44126	1
44127	1
44128	2
44132	1
44133	1
44135	1
44136	1
44137	1
44139	1
44140	2
44141	1
44143	1
44144	1
44145	1
44146	1
44147	1
44150	1

CPT	MUE
44151	1
44155	1
44156	1
44157	1
44158	1
44160	1
44180	1
44186	1
44187	1
44188	1
44202	1
44203	2
44204	2
44205	1
44206	1
44207	1
44208	1
44210	1
44211	1
44212	1
44213	1
44227	1
44300	1
44310	2
44312	1
44314	1
44316	1
44320	1
44322	1
44340	1
44345	1
44346	1
44360	1
44361	1
44363	1
44364	1
44365	1
44366	1
44369	1
44370	1
44372	1
44373	1
44376	1
44377	1
44378	1
44379	1
44380	1
44382	1
44383	1
44385	1
44386	1
44388	1
44389	1
44390	1
44391	1
44392	1
44393	1
44394	1
44397	1
44500	1
44602	1
44603	1
44604	1
44605	1
44620	2
44625	1
44626	1
44640	2
44650	2

CPT	MUE
44660	1
44661	1
44680	1
44700	1
44701	1
44715	1
44720	2
44721	2
44800	1
44820	2
44850	1
44900	1
44901	1
44950	1
44955	1
44960	1
44970	1
45000	1
45005	1
45020	1
45100	1
45108	1
45110	1
45111	1
45112	1
45113	1
45114	1
45116	1
45119	1
45120	1
45121	1
45123	1
45126	1
45130	1
45135	1
45136	1
45150	1
45160	1
45190	1
45300	1
45303	1
45305	1
45307	1
45308	1
45309	1
45315	1
45317	1
45320	1
45321	1
45327	1
45330	1
45331	1
45332	1
45333	1
45334	1
45335	1
45337	1
45338	1
45339	1
45340	1
45341	1
45342	1
45345	1
45355	1
45378	1
45379	1
45380	1
45381	1
45382	2

CPT	MUE
45383	1
45384	1
45385	1
45386	1
45387	1
45391	1
45392	1
45395	1
45397	1
45400	1
45402	1
45500	1
45505	1
45520	1
45540	1
45541	1
45550	1
45560	1
45562	1
45563	1
45800	1
45805	1
45820	1
45825	1
45900	1
45905	1
45910	1
45915	1
45990	1
46020	1
46030	1
46040	2
46045	2
46050	2
46060	2
46070	1
46080	1
46083	2
46200	1
46220	2
46221	1
46230	1
46250	1
46255	1
46257	1
46258	1
46260	1
46261	1
46262	1
46270	1
46275	1
46280	1
46285	1
46288	1
46320	2
46500	1
46505	1
46600	1
46604	1
46606	1
46608	1
46610	1
46611	1
46612	1
46614	1
46615	1
46700	1
46705	1
46706	2

CPT	MUE
46710	1
46712	1
46715	1
46716	1
46730	1
46735	1
46740	1
46742	1
46744	1
46746	1
46748	1
46750	1
46751	1
46753	1
46754	1
46760	1
46761	1
46762	1
46900	1
46910	1
46916	1
46917	1
46922	1
46924	1
46930	1
46940	1
46942	1
46945	1
46946	1
46947	1
47000	3
47001	3
47010	3
47011	3
47015	1
47100	3
47120	1
47122	1
47125	1
47130	1
47133	1
47135	1
47136	1
47140	1
47141	1
47142	1
47143	1
47144	1
47145	1
47147	3
47300	2
47350	1
47360	1
47361	1
47362	1
47370	1
47371	1
47380	1
47381	1
47382	1
47400	1
47420	1
47425	1
47460	1
47480	1
47490	1
47500	2
47505	2
47510	2

CPT	MUE
47511	2
47525	3
47530	3
47550	1
47552	1
47553	1
47554	1
47555	1
47556	1
47560	1
47561	1
47562	1
47563	1
47564	1
47570	1
47600	1
47605	1
47610	1
47612	1
47620	1
47630	1
47700	1
47701	1
47711	1
47712	1
47715	1
47720	1
47721	1
47740	1
47741	1
47760	1
47765	1
47780	1
47785	1
47800	1
47801	1
47802	1
47900	1
48000	1
48001	1
48020	1
48100	1
48102	2
48120	1
48140	1
48145	1
48146	1
48148	1
48150	1
48152	1
48153	1
48154	1
48155	1
48400	1
48500	1
48510	1
48511	1
48520	1
48540	1
48545	1
48547	1
48550	1
48551	1
48552	2
48554	1
48556	1
49000	1
49002	1
49010	1

CPT	MUE
49020	2
49021	3
49040	2
49041	3
49060	2
49061	3
49062	1
49080	1
49081	2
49180	3
49203	1
49204	1
49205	1
49215	1
49220	1
49250	1
49255	1
49320	1
49321	1
49322	1
49323	1
49324	1
49325	1
49326	1
49327	1
49400	1
49402	1
49412	1
49418	1
49419	1
49421	1
49422	1
49423	3
49424	3
49425	1
49426	1
49427	1
49428	1
49429	1
49435	1
49436	1
49440	1
49441	1
49442	1
49446	1
49450	1
49451	1
49452	1
49460	1
49465	1
49491	1
49492	1
49495	1
49496	1
49500	1
49501	1
49505	1
49507	1
49520	1
49521	1
49525	1
49540	1
49550	1
49553	1
49555	1
49557	1
49565	2
49566	2
49570	1

CPT	MUE
49572	1
49580	1
49582	1
49585	1
49587	1
49590	1
49600	1
49605	1
49606	1
49610	1
49611	1
49650	1
49651	1
49652	2
49653	2
49654	2
49655	2
49656	2
49657	2
49900	1
49904	1
49905	1
49906	1
50010	2
50020	1
50021	2
50040	2
50045	2
50060	2
50065	2
50070	2
50075	2
50080	2
50081	2
50100	2
50120	2
50125	2
50130	2
50135	2
50200	2
50205	2
50220	2
50225	2
50230	2
50234	2
50236	2
50240	2
50250	1
50280	2
50290	1
50300	1
50320	1
50323	1
50325	1
50327	3
50328	3
50329	2
50340	1
50360	1
50365	1
50370	1
50380	1
50382	1
50384	1
50385	2
50386	2
50387	1
50389	2
50390	2

CPT	MUE
50391	2
50392	2
50393	2
50394	2
50395	2
50396	2
50398	2
50400	2
50405	2
50500	1
50520	1
50525	1
50526	1
50540	1
50541	2
50542	2
50543	2
50544	2
50545	2
50546	2
50547	1
50548	2
50551	2
50553	2
50555	1
50557	2
50561	2
50562	1
50570	2
50572	2
50574	1
50575	2
50576	2
50580	1
50590	1
50592	1
50593	2
50600	2
50605	2
50610	2
50620	2
50630	2
50650	2
50660	2
50684	2
50686	2
50688	2
50690	2
50700	2
50715	1
50722	2
50725	1
50727	1
50728	1
50740	2
50750	2
50760	2
50770	1
50780	1
50782	2
50783	2
50785	1
50800	1
50810	1
50815	1
50820	1
50825	1
50830	1
50840	1

CPT	MUE
50845	1
50860	1
50900	2
50920	2
50930	2
50940	2
50945	2
50947	2
50948	2
50951	2
50953	2
50955	2
50957	2
50961	2
50970	2
50972	2
50974	2
50976	2
50980	2
51020	1
51030	1
51040	1
51045	2
51050	1
51060	2
51065	1
51080	2
51100	1
51101	1
51102	1
51500	1
51520	1
51525	1
51530	1
51535	1
51550	1
51555	1
51565	1
51570	1
51575	1
51580	1
51585	1
51590	1
51595	1
51596	1
51597	1
51600	1
51605	1
51610	1
51700	1
51701	2
51702	2
51703	2
51705	1
51710	1
51715	1
51720	1
51725	1
51726	1
51736	1
51741	1
51784	1
51785	1
51792	1
51797	1
51798	1
51800	1
51820	1
51840	1

CPT	MUE
51841	1
51845	1
51860	1
51865	1
51880	1
51900	1
51920	1
51925	1
51940	1
51960	1
51980	1
51990	1
51992	1
52000	1
52001	1
52005	2
52007	2
52010	1
52204	1
52214	1
52224	1
52234	1
52235	1
52240	1
52250	1
52260	1
52265	1
52270	1
52275	1
52276	1
52277	1
52281	1
52282	1
52283	1
52285	1
52290	1
52300	1
52301	1
52305	1
52310	1
52315	2
52317	1
52318	1
52320	2
52325	1
52327	2
52330	2
52332	1
52334	2
52341	2
52342	2
52343	2
52344	2
52345	2
52346	2
52351	1
52352	2
52353	2
52354	2
52355	2
52400	1
52402	1
52450	1
52500	1
52601	1
52630	1
52640	1
52647	1
52648	1

CPT	MUE
52649	1
52700	1
53000	1
53010	1
53020	1
53025	1
53040	1
53060	1
53080	1
53085	1
53200	1
53210	1
53215	1
53220	1
53230	1
53235	1
53240	1
53250	1
53260	1
53265	1
53270	1
53275	1
53400	1
53405	1
53410	1
53415	1
53420	1
53425	1
53430	1
53431	1
53440	1
53442	1
53444	1
53445	1
53446	1
53447	1
53448	1
53449	1
53450	1
53460	1
53500	1
53502	1
53505	1
53510	1
53515	1
53520	1
53600	1
53601	1
53605	1
53620	1
53621	1
53660	1
53661	1
53665	1
53850	1
53852	1
53860	1
54000	1
54001	1
54015	1
54050	1
54055	1
54056	1
54057	1
54060	1
54065	1
54100	3
54105	2
54110	1

CPT	MUE
54111	1
54112	1
54115	1
54120	1
54125	1
54130	1
54135	1
54150	1
54160	1
54161	1
54162	1
54163	1
54164	1
54200	1
54205	1
54220	1
54230	1
54231	1
54235	1
54240	1
54250	1
54300	1
54304	1
54308	1
54312	1
54316	1
54318	1
54322	1
54324	1
54326	1
54328	1
54332	1
54336	1
54340	1
54344	1
54348	1
54352	1
54360	1
54380	1
54385	1
54390	1
54400	1
54401	1
54405	1
54406	1
54408	1
54410	1
54411	1
54415	1
54416	1
54417	1
54420	1
54430	1
54435	1
54440	1
54450	1
54500	2
54505	1
54512	2
54520	1
54522	2
54530	2
54535	1
54550	1
54560	1
54600	2
54620	1
54640	1
54650	2

CPT	MUE
54660	1
54670	2
54680	1
54690	2
54692	2
54700	2
54800	2
54830	2
54840	2
54860	1
54861	1
54865	1
54900	1
54901	1
55000	2
55040	1
55041	1
55060	2
55100	2
55110	1
55120	1
55150	1
55175	1
55180	1
55200	1
55250	1
55300	1
55400	1
55450	1
55500	2
55520	2
55530	2
55535	2
55540	2
55550	2
55600	1
55605	2
55650	1
55680	2
55700	1
55705	1
55706	1
55720	1
55725	1
55801	1
55810	1
55812	1
55815	1
55821	1
55831	1
55840	1
55842	1
55845	1
55860	1
55862	1
55865	1
55866	1
55870	1
55873	1
55875	1
55876	1
55920	1
56405	2
56420	1
56440	1
56441	1
56442	1
56501	1
56515	1

CPT	MUE
56605	1
56620	1
56625	1
56630	1
56631	1
56632	1
56633	1
56634	1
56637	1
56640	1
56700	1
56740	2
56800	1
56805	1
56810	1
56820	1
56821	1
57000	1
57010	1
57020	1
57022	2
57023	2
57061	1
57065	1
57100	3
57105	2
57106	1
57107	1
57109	1
57110	1
57111	1
57112	1
57120	1
57130	1
57135	2
57150	1
57155	1
57156	1
57160	1
57170	1
57180	1
57200	1
57210	1
57220	1
57230	1
57240	1
57250	1
57260	1
57265	1
57267	3
57268	1
57270	1
57280	1
57282	1
57283	1
57284	1
57285	1
57287	1
57288	1
57289	1
57291	1
57292	1
57295	1
57296	1
57300	1
57305	1
57307	1
57308	1
57310	1

CPT	MUE
57311	1
57320	1
57330	1
57335	1
57400	1
57410	1
57415	1
57420	1
57421	1
57423	1
57425	1
57452	1
57454	1
57455	1
57456	1
57460	1
57461	1
57500	1
57505	1
57510	1
57511	1
57513	1
57520	1
57522	1
57530	1
57531	1
57540	1
57545	1
57550	1
57555	1
57556	1
57558	1
57700	1
57720	1
57800	1
58100	1
58110	1
58120	1
58140	1
58145	1
58146	1
58150	1
58152	1
58180	1
58200	1
58210	1
58240	1
58260	1
58262	1
58263	1
58267	1
58270	1
58275	1
58280	1
58285	1
58290	1
58291	1
58292	1
58293	1
58294	1
58301	1
58321	1
58322	1
58323	1
58340	1
58345	2
58346	1
58350	2
58353	1

CPT	MUE
58356	1
58400	1
58410	1
58520	1
58540	1
58541	1
58542	1
58543	1
58544	1
58545	1
58546	1
58548	1
58550	1
58552	1
58553	1
58554	1
58555	1
58558	1
58559	1
58560	1
58561	1
58562	1
58563	1
58565	1
58570	1
58571	1
58572	1
58573	1
58600	1
58605	1
58611	1
58615	1
58660	1
58661	1
58662	1
58670	1
58671	1
58672	1
58673	1
58700	1
58720	1
58740	1
58750	2
58752	2
58760	2
58770	2
58800	1
58805	1
58820	2
58822	2
58823	2
58825	1
58900	1
58920	1
58925	1
58940	1
58943	1
58950	1
58951	1
58952	1
58953	1
58954	1
58956	1
58957	1
58958	1
58960	1
58970	1
58974	1
58976	2

CPT	MUE
59020	1
59025	1
59050	1
59051	1
59100	1
59120	1
59121	1
59130	1
59135	1
59136	1
59140	1
59150	1
59151	1
59160	1
59200	1
59300	1
59320	1
59325	1
59350	1
59400	1
59410	1
59412	2
59414	1
59425	1
59426	1
59430	1
59510	1
59514	1
59515	1
59525	1
59610	1
59614	1
59618	1
59620	1
59622	1
59812	1
59820	1
59821	1
59830	1
59840	1
59841	1
59850	1
59851	1
59852	1
59855	1
59856	1
59857	1
59866	1
59870	1
59871	1
60000	1
60200	2
60210	1
60212	1
60220	1
60225	1
60240	1
60252	1
60254	1
60260	1
60270	1
60271	1
60280	1
60281	1
60500	1
60502	1
60505	1
60512	1
60520	1

CPT	MUE
60521	1
60522	1
60540	1
60545	2
60600	1
60605	1
60650	2
61000	1
61001	1
61020	2
61026	2
61050	1
61055	1
61070	2
61105	2
61107	2
61108	2
61120	1
61140	2
61150	2
61151	2
61154	2
61156	2
61210	1
61215	1
61250	1
61253	1
61304	1
61305	1
61312	2
61313	2
61314	2
61315	1
61316	1
61320	2
61321	2
61322	1
61323	1
61330	1
61332	2
61333	2
61334	2
61340	1
61343	1
61345	1
61440	1
61450	1
61458	1
61460	1
61470	1
61480	1
61490	1
61500	3
61501	1
61512	3
61514	2
61516	2
61517	1
61518	2
61519	2
61520	1
61521	1
61522	2
61524	2
61526	1
61530	1
61533	2
61534	1
61535	2

CPT	MUE
61536	1
61537	1
61538	1
61539	1
61540	1
61541	1
61542	1
61543	1
61544	2
61545	1
61546	1
61548	1
61550	1
61552	1
61556	1
61557	1
61558	1
61559	1
61563	2
61564	2
61566	1
61567	1
61570	2
61571	2
61575	1
61576	1
61580	1
61581	1
61582	1
61583	1
61584	1
61585	1
61586	1
61590	1
61591	1
61592	1
61595	1
61596	1
61597	1
61598	1
61600	1
61601	1
61605	1
61606	1
61607	1
61608	1
61609	1
61610	1
61611	1
61612	1
61613	1
61615	1
61616	1
61618	2
61619	2
61623	2
61624	2
61626	2
61630	2
61635	2
61680	1
61682	1
61684	1
61686	1
61690	1
61692	1
61697	3
61698	2
61700	3

CPT	MUE
61702	2
61703	1
61705	1
61708	2
61710	2
61711	1
61720	2
61735	2
61750	2
61751	3
61760	1
61770	1
61781	1
61782	1
61783	1
61790	2
61791	2
61796	1
61798	1
61800	1
61850	1
61860	1
61863	2
61864	1
61867	2
61868	2
61870	1
61875	1
61880	1
61885	2
61886	1
61888	2
62000	1
62005	1
62010	1
62100	1
62115	1
62116	1
62117	1
62120	1
62121	1
62140	1
62141	1
62142	2
62143	2
62145	2
62146	2
62147	2
62148	2
62160	1
62161	1
62162	1
62163	1
62164	1
62165	1
62180	1
62190	1
62192	1
62194	2
62200	1
62201	1
62220	1
62223	1
62225	2
62230	2
62252	2
62256	1
62258	1
62263	1

CPT	MUE
62264	1
62267	2
62268	1
62269	2
62270	2
62272	1
62273	2
62280	1
62281	1
62282	1
62284	1
62287	1
62292	1
62294	2
62310	1
62311	1
62318	1
62319	1
62350	1
62351	1
62355	1
62360	1
62361	1
62362	1
62365	1
62367	1
62368	1
63001	1
63003	1
63005	1
63011	1
63012	1
63015	1
63016	1
63017	1
63020	1
63030	1
63035	6
63040	1
63042	1
63043	6
63044	4
63045	1
63046	1
63047	1
63048	9
63050	1
63051	1
63055	1
63056	1
63057	8
63064	1
63066	3
63075	1
63076	6
63077	1
63078	5
63081	1
63082	6
63085	1
63086	6
63087	1
63088	5
63090	1
63101	1
63102	1
63170	1
63172	1
63173	1

CPT	MUE
63180	1
63182	1
63185	1
63190	1
63191	1
63194	1
63195	1
63196	1
63197	1
63198	1
63199	1
63200	1
63250	1
63251	1
63252	1
63265	1
63266	1
63267	1
63268	1
63270	1
63271	1
63272	1
63273	1
63275	1
63276	1
63277	1
63278	1
63280	1
63281	1
63282	1
63283	1
63285	1
63286	1
63287	1
63290	1
63295	1
63300	1
63301	1
63302	1
63303	1
63304	1
63305	1
63306	1
63307	1
63308	4
63600	2
63610	1
63615	1
63620	1
63621	2
63650	2
63655	1
63661	1
63662	1
63685	2
63688	2
63700	1
63702	1
63704	1
63706	1
63707	1
63709	1
63710	1
63740	1
63741	1
63744	1
63746	1
64402	2
64405	1

CPT	MUE
64408	2
64410	2
64412	2
64413	2
64415	2
64416	2
64417	2
64418	2
64420	3
64421	3
64425	2
64430	2
64435	2
64445	1
64446	2
64447	2
64448	2
64449	2
64455	1
64479	1
64483	1
64505	2
64508	2
64510	2
64517	1
64520	2
64530	2
64553	1
64555	2
64560	1
64561	2
64565	2
64566	1
64568	2
64569	2
64570	2
64575	2
64577	1
64580	2
64581	2
64585	2
64590	1
64595	1
64600	2
64605	2
64610	2
64611	1
64612	2
64613	1
64614	1
64622	1
64626	1
64630	1
64632	2
64650	1
64653	1
64680	1
64681	1
64702	2
64712	2
64713	2
64714	2
64718	2
64719	2
64721	2
64726	2
64727	3
64732	2
64734	2

CPT	MUE
64736	2
64738	2
64740	2
64742	2
64744	2
64746	2
64752	1
64755	1
64760	1
64761	1
64763	1
64766	1
64771	2
64772	2
64774	3
64776	1
64778	3
64782	2
64783	2
64786	2
64790	1
64792	2
64795	2
64802	1
64804	1
64809	1
64818	1
64821	2
64822	2
64823	2
64831	2
64834	2
64835	2
64836	2
64837	3
64840	2
64856	2
64857	3
64858	2
64859	2
64861	2
64862	2
64864	2
64865	1
64866	1
64868	1
64870	1
64872	3
64874	1
64876	1
64885	1
64886	1
64890	3
64891	2
64892	2
64893	2
64895	2
64896	2
64897	2
64898	2
64901	2
64905	1
64907	1
64910	3
64911	2
65091	2
65093	2
65101	2
65103	2

CPT	MUE
65105	2
65110	2
65112	2
65114	2
65125	2
65130	2
65135	2
65140	2
65150	2
65155	2
65175	2
65205	2
65210	2
65220	2
65222	2
65235	2
65260	2
65265	2
65270	2
65272	2
65273	2
65275	2
65280	2
65285	2
65286	2
65290	2
65400	2
65410	2
65420	2
65426	2
65430	2
65435	2
65436	2
65450	2
65600	2
65710	2
65730	2
65750	2
65755	2
65756	2
65757	2
65770	2
65772	2
65775	2
65778	2
65779	2
65780	2
65781	2
65782	2
65800	2
65805	2
65810	2
65815	2
65820	2
65850	2
65855	2
65860	2
65865	2
65870	2
65875	2
65880	2
65900	2
65920	2
65930	2
66020	2
66030	2
66130	2
66150	2
66155	2

CPT	MUE
66160	2
66165	2
66170	2
66172	2
66174	2
66175	2
66180	2
66185	2
66220	2
66225	2
66250	2
66500	2
66505	2
66600	2
66605	2
66625	2
66630	2
66635	2
66680	2
66682	2
66700	2
66710	2
66711	2
66720	2
66740	2
66761	2
66762	2
66770	2
66820	2
66821	2
66825	2
66830	2
66840	2
66850	2
66852	2
66920	2
66930	2
66940	2
66982	2
66983	2
66984	2
66985	2
66986	2
66990	2
67005	2
67010	2
67015	2
67025	2
67027	2
67028	2
67030	2
67031	2
67036	2
67039	2
67040	2
67041	2
67042	2
67043	2
67101	2
67105	2
67107	2
67108	2
67110	2
67112	2
67113	2
67115	2
67120	2
67121	2
67141	2

CPT	MUE
67145	2
67208	2
67210	2
67218	2
67220	2
67221	1
67225	1
67227	2
67228	2
67229	1
67250	2
67255	2
67311	2
67312	2
67314	2
67316	2
67318	2
67320	2
67331	2
67332	2
67334	2
67335	2
67340	2
67343	2
67345	2
67346	1
67400	2
67405	2
67412	2
67413	2
67414	2
67415	2
67420	2
67430	2
67440	2
67445	2
67450	2
67500	2
67505	2
67515	2
67550	2
67560	2
67570	2
67700	4
67710	2
67715	2
67800	1
67801	1
67805	1
67808	1
67820	2
67825	2
67830	3
67835	2
67850	4
67875	2
67880	2
67882	2
67900	2
67901	2
67902	2
67903	2
67904	2
67906	2
67908	2
67909	2
67911	4
67912	2
67914	4

CPT	MUE
67915	4
67916	4
67917	4
67921	4
67922	4
67923	4
67924	4
67930	2
67935	2
67938	2
67950	2
67961	4
67966	4
67971	2
67973	2
67974	2
67975	2
68020	2
68040	2
68100	2
68110	2
68115	2
68130	2
68135	2
68200	2
68320	2
68325	2
68326	2
68328	2
68330	2
68335	2
68340	2
68360	2
68362	2
68371	1
68400	2
68420	2
68440	2
68500	2
68505	2
68510	2
68520	2
68525	2
68530	2
68540	1
68550	1
68700	2
68705	2
68720	2
68745	2
68750	2
68760	4
68761	4
68770	2
68801	4
68810	1
68811	1
68815	1
68816	1
68840	2
68850	2
69000	2
69005	2
69020	2
69100	3
69105	2
69110	2
69120	1
69140	2

CPT	MUE
69145	2
69150	1
69155	1
69200	2
69205	2
69210	1
69220	1
69222	1
69300	1
69310	2
69320	2
69400	2
69401	2
69405	2
69420	2
69421	2
69424	1
69433	1
69436	1
69440	2
69450	2
69501	1
69502	1
69505	1
69511	1
69530	1
69535	1
69540	2
69550	1
69552	1
69554	1
69601	1
69602	1
69603	1
69604	1
69605	1
69610	2
69620	2
69631	2
69632	1
69633	1
69635	1
69636	1
69637	1
69641	1
69642	1
69643	1
69644	1
69645	1
69646	1
69650	1
69660	1
69661	1
69662	2
69666	2
69667	2
69670	1
69676	1
69700	2
69711	2
69714	2
69715	1
69717	1
69718	1
69720	2
69725	2
69740	2
69745	2
69801	1

CPT	MUE
69802	1
69805	1
69806	1
69820	1
69840	1
69905	1
69910	1
69915	1
69930	2
69950	2
69955	2
69960	2
69970	1
69990	1
70010	1
70015	1
70030	2
70100	1
70110	1
70120	2
70130	2
70134	1
70140	1
70150	1
70160	1
70170	2
70190	1
70200	1
70210	1
70220	1
70240	1
70250	1
70260	1
70300	1
70310	1
70320	1
70328	1
70330	1
70332	2
70336	1
70350	1
70355	1
70360	1
70370	1
70371	1
70373	1
70380	2
70390	2
70450	3
70460	1
70470	2
70480	1
70481	1
70482	1
70486	1
70487	1
70488	1
70490	1
70491	1
70492	1
70496	1
70498	1
70540	1
70542	1
70543	1
70544	1
70545	1
70546	1
70547	1

CPT	MUE
70548	1
70549	1
70551	1
70552	1
70553	1
70554	1
70555	1
70557	1
70558	1
70559	1
71015	2
71021	1
71022	1
71023	2
71030	2
71034	1
71035	2
71040	1
71060	1
71090	1
71100	1
71101	1
71110	1
71111	1
71120	1
71130	1
71250	1
71260	1
71270	1
71275	1
71550	1
71551	1
71552	1
71555	1
72010	1
72020	4
72040	3
72050	1
72052	1
72069	1
72070	1
72072	1
72074	1
72080	1
72090	1
72100	1
72110	1
72114	1
72120	1
72125	1
72126	1
72127	1
72128	1
72129	1
72130	1
72131	1
72132	1
72133	1
72141	1
72142	1
72146	1
72147	1
72148	1
72149	1
72156	1
72157	1
72158	1
72170	1
72190	1

CPT	MUE
72191	1
72192	1
72193	1
72194	1
72195	1
72196	1
72197	1
72198	1
72200	1
72202	1
72220	1
72240	1
72255	1
72265	1
72270	1
72275	3
72292	3
73000	2
73010	2
73020	2
73030	2
73040	2
73050	1
73060	2
73070	2
73080	2
73085	2
73090	2
73092	2
73100	2
73110	2
73115	2
73120	2
73130	2
73140	2
73200	2
73201	2
73202	2
73206	2
73218	2
73219	2
73220	2
73221	2
73222	2
73223	2
73500	2
73510	2
73520	2
73525	2
73530	2
73540	1
73542	2
73550	2
73560	2
73562	2
73564	2
73565	1
73580	2
73590	2
73592	2
73600	2
73610	2
73615	2
73620	2
73630	2
73650	2
73660	2
73700	2
73701	2

CPT	MUE
73702	2
73706	2
73718	2
73719	2
73720	2
73721	4
73722	2
73723	4
73725	2
74000	3
74010	2
74020	2
74022	2
74150	1
74160	1
74170	1
74175	1
74176	1
74177	1
74178	1
74181	1
74182	1
74183	1
74185	1
74190	1
74210	1
74220	1
74230	1
74235	1
74240	1
74241	1
74245	1
74246	1
74247	1
74249	1
74250	1
74251	1
74260	1
74270	1
74280	1
74283	1
74290	1
74291	1
74300	1
74301	2
74305	1
74320	1
74327	1
74328	1
74329	1
74330	1
74340	1
74355	1
74360	1
74363	2
74400	1
74410	1
74415	1
74420	2
74425	2
74430	1
74440	2
74445	1
74450	1
74455	1
74470	2
74475	2
74480	2
74485	2

CPT	MUE
74710	1
74740	1
74742	2
74775	1
75557	1
75559	1
75561	1
75563	1
75600	1
75605	1
75625	1
75630	1
75635	1
75650	2
75658	2
75660	1
75662	1
75665	1
75671	1
75676	1
75680	1
75685	2
75710	1
75716	1
75722	1
75724	1
75726	3
75731	1
75733	1
75736	2
75741	1
75743	1
75746	1
75756	2
75801	1
75803	1
75805	1
75807	1
75809	1
75810	1
75820	1
75822	1
75825	1
75827	1
75831	1
75833	1
75840	1
75842	1
75860	2
75870	1
75872	1
75880	2
75885	1
75887	1
75889	1
75891	1
75900	3
75901	1
75902	2
75940	1
75945	1
75952	1
75953	4
75954	2
75956	1
75957	1
75958	2
75959	1
75961	2

CPT	MUE
75962	1
75964	4
75966	1
75968	2
75970	2
75980	1
75982	2
75984	2
75989	2
76000	3
76001	2
76010	2
76080	2
76100	2
76101	1
76102	1
76120	1
76125	1
76376	2
76377	2
76380	1
76506	1
76510	2
76511	2
76512	2
76513	2
76514	1
76516	1
76519	2
76529	2
76536	1
76604	1
76645	1
76700	1
76705	2
76770	1
76775	2
76776	1
76800	1
76801	1
76802	3
76805	1
76810	3
76811	1
76812	3
76813	1
76814	3
76815	1
76817	1
76830	1
76831	1
76856	1
76857	1
76870	1
76872	1
76873	1
76881	2
76882	2
76885	1
76886	1
76930	1
76932	1
76936	2
76937	2
76940	1
76942	1
76945	1
76946	1
76948	1

CPT	MUE
76950	2
76965	2
76970	1
76975	1
76977	1
76998	1
77001	1
77002	1
77003	1
77011	1
77012	1
77013	1
77014	2
77021	1
77022	1
77053	2
77054	2
77058	1
77059	1
77071	1
77261	1
77262	1
77263	1
77280	2
77285	1
77290	1
77295	1
77301	1
77305	2
77310	2
77315	2
77321	1
77326	1
77327	1
77328	1
77332	4
77333	4
77336	1
77370	1
77371	1
77372	1
77373	1
77401	2
77402	2
77403	2
77404	2
77406	2
77407	2
77408	2
77409	2
77411	2
77412	2
77413	2
77414	2
77416	2
77417	1
77418	2
77421	2
77422	1
77423	1
77427	1
77431	1
77432	1
77435	1
77470	1
77520	1
77522	1
77523	1
77525	1

Appendix L — Medically Unlikely Edits (MUEs) — Professional

CPT	MUE
77600	1
77605	1
77610	1
77615	1
77620	1
77750	1
77761	1
77762	1
77763	1
77776	1
77777	1
77778	1
77785	3
77786	3
77787	3
77789	2
77790	2
78000	1
78001	1
78003	1
78006	1
78007	1
78010	1
78011	1
78015	1
78016	1
78018	1
78020	1
78070	1
78075	1
78102	1
78103	1
78104	1
78110	1
78111	1
78120	1
78121	1
78122	1
78130	1
78135	1
78140	1
78185	1
78190	1
78191	1
78195	1
78201	1
78202	1
78205	1
78206	1
78215	1
78216	1
78220	1
78223	1
78230	1
78231	1
78232	1
78258	1
78261	1
78262	1
78264	1
78267	1
78268	1
78270	1
78271	1
78272	1
78278	2
78282	1
78290	1
78291	1
78300	1
78305	1
78306	1
78315	1
78320	1
78414	1
78428	1
78445	1
78456	1
78457	1
78458	1
78459	1
78466	1
78468	1
78469	1
78472	1
78473	1
78481	1
78483	1
78491	1
78492	1
78494	1
78496	1
78580	1
78584	2
78585	2
78586	1
78587	1
78588	1
78591	1
78593	1
78594	1
78596	1
78600	1
78601	1
78605	1
78606	2
78607	1
78608	1
78610	1
78630	2
78635	1
78645	1
78647	1
78650	1
78660	1
78700	1
78701	2
78707	1
78708	1
78709	1
78710	1
78725	1
78730	1
78740	1
78761	1
78800	1
78801	1
78802	1
78803	1
78804	1
78805	1
78806	1
78807	1
78808	1
78811	1
78812	1
78813	1
78814	1
78815	1
78816	1
79005	1
79101	1
79200	1
79300	1
79403	1
79440	1
79445	1
80047	2
80048	2
80051	2
80053	1
80061	1
80069	1
80074	1
80076	1
80103	2
80104	1
80150	2
80152	2
80154	2
80156	2
80157	2
80158	2
80160	2
80162	2
80164	2
80166	2
80168	2
80170	2
80172	2
80173	2
80174	2
80176	1
80178	2
80182	2
80184	2
80185	2
80186	2
80188	2
80190	2
80192	2
80194	2
80195	2
80197	2
80198	2
80200	2
80201	2
80202	2
80299	3
80400	1
80402	1
80406	1
80408	1
80410	1
80412	1
80414	1
80415	1
80416	1
80417	1
80418	1
80420	1
80422	1
80424	1
80426	1
80428	1
80430	1
80432	1
80434	1
80435	1
80436	1
80438	1
80439	1
80440	1
80500	1
80502	1
81000	2
81001	2
81002	2
81003	2
81005	2
81007	1
81015	1
81020	1
81025	1
81050	2
82000	1
82003	2
82009	1
82010	4
82013	1
82016	1
82017	1
82030	1
82040	1
82042	2
82043	1
82044	1
82045	1
82055	2
82075	2
82085	1
82101	1
82103	1
82104	1
82105	1
82106	4
82107	1
82108	1
82120	1
82127	2
82128	2
82131	3
82135	1
82136	3
82139	3
82140	2
82143	2
82145	1
82150	4
82154	1
82157	1
82160	1
82163	1
82164	1
82172	3
82175	2
82180	1
82190	4
82205	1
82232	2
82239	1
82240	1
82247	2
82248	2
82252	1
82261	1
82270	1
82271	1
82272	1
82274	1
82286	1
82300	1
82306	1
82308	3
82310	2
82330	2
82331	1
82340	1
82355	3
82360	3
82365	3
82370	3
82373	1
82374	2
82375	1
82378	2
82379	1
82380	1
82382	1
82383	1
82384	2
82387	1
82390	1
82415	1
82435	2
82436	1
82438	1
82441	1
82465	1
82480	2
82482	1
82485	1
82486	2
82487	2
82488	1
82489	2
82492	2
82495	1
82507	1
82520	2
82523	1
82525	2
82528	1
82530	2
82540	1
82543	2
82544	2
82550	3
82552	3
82553	3
82554	1
82565	2
82570	3
82575	1
82585	1
82595	1
82600	1
82607	1
82608	1
82610	1
82615	1
82626	1
82627	1
82633	1
82634	2
82638	1
82646	1
82649	1
82651	1
82652	1
82654	1
82656	1
82657	3
82658	2
82666	1
82668	1
82670	2
82671	1
82672	1
82677	1
82679	1
82690	1
82693	2
82696	1
82705	1
82710	1
82715	1
82725	1
82726	1
82728	1
82731	1
82735	1
82742	1
82746	1
82747	1
82757	1
82759	1
82760	1
82775	1
82776	1
82784	6
82785	1
82787	4
82820	1
82941	1
82943	1
82946	1
82950	3
82951	1
82952	3
82953	1
82955	1
82960	1
82963	1
82965	1
82975	1
82977	1
82978	1
82979	1
82980	1
82985	1
83008	1
83009	1
83010	1
83012	1
83013	1
83014	1
83015	1
83018	7
83020	2
83021	2
83026	1
83030	1
83033	1
83036	1
83037	1
83045	1
83050	1
83051	1
83055	1
83060	1
83065	1
83068	1
83069	1
83070	1
83071	1
83080	2
83088	1
83090	2
83150	1
83491	1
83497	1
83498	2
83499	1
83500	1
83505	1
83518	2
83527	1
83528	1
83540	2
83550	1
83570	1
83582	1
83586	1
83593	1
83605	3
83615	2
83625	1
83630	1
83631	1
83632	1
83633	1
83634	1
83655	2
83661	4
83662	4
83663	4
83664	4
83670	1
83690	2
83695	1
83698	1
83700	1
83701	1
83704	1
83718	1
83719	1
83721	1
83727	1
83735	4
83775	1
83785	1
83788	3
83789	2
83805	1
83825	2
83835	2
83840	2
83857	1
83858	1
83861	2
83864	1
83866	1
83872	2
83873	1
83874	2
83880	1
83885	2
83887	2
83912	1
83915	1
83916	2
83918	2
83919	1
83921	2
83925	4
83930	2
83935	2
83937	1
83945	2
83950	1
83951	1
83970	2
83986	2
83992	2
83993	1
84022	2
84030	1
84035	1
84060	1
84061	1
84066	1
84075	2
84078	1
84080	1
84081	1
84085	1
84087	1
84100	3
84105	1
84106	1
84110	1
84112	1
84119	1
84120	1
84126	1
84127	1
84132	3
84133	2
84134	1
84135	1
84138	1
84140	1
84143	2
84144	1
84146	3
84150	2
84152	1
84153	1
84154	1
84155	1
84156	1
84157	3
84160	2
84163	1
84165	1
84166	2
84202	1
84203	1
84206	1
84207	1
84210	2

CPT	MUE
84220	1
84228	1
84233	2
84234	2
84235	1
84238	3
84252	1
84255	2
84260	1
84270	1
84275	1
84285	1
84295	3
84300	2
84302	1
84305	1
84307	1
84311	2
84315	2
84375	1
84376	1
84377	1
84378	2
84379	1
84392	1
84402	1
84403	2
84425	1
84430	1
84432	1
84436	1
84437	1
84439	1
84442	1
84445	1
84446	1
84449	1
84450	1
84460	1
84466	1
84478	1
84479	1
84480	1
84481	1
84482	1
84484	2
84485	1
84488	1
84490	1
84510	1
84512	1
84520	4
84525	1
84540	2
84545	1
84550	1
84560	2
84577	1
84578	1
84580	1
84583	1
84585	1
84586	1
84588	2
84590	1
84591	1
84597	1
84600	2
84620	1

CPT	MUE
84630	2
84702	2
84703	1
84704	1
84830	1
85002	1
85004	2
85007	1
85008	1
85009	1
85013	2
85014	2
85018	2
85025	2
85032	3
85041	2
85044	1
85045	1
85046	1
85048	2
85049	2
85055	1
85060	1
85097	2
85130	2
85170	1
85175	1
85210	2
85220	2
85230	2
85240	2
85244	2
85245	2
85246	2
85247	2
85250	2
85260	2
85270	2
85280	2
85290	2
85291	2
85292	2
85293	2
85300	2
85301	2
85302	2
85303	2
85305	2
85306	2
85307	2
85335	2
85337	1
85345	2
85348	1
85360	1
85362	2
85366	2
85370	2
85378	2
85379	2
85380	2
85384	2
85385	1
85390	3
85396	1
85400	2
85410	2
85415	2
85420	2

CPT	MUE
85421	2
85441	1
85445	1
85460	1
85461	1
85475	1
85525	2
85530	1
85536	1
85540	1
85547	1
85549	1
85555	1
85557	1
85597	1
85598	1
85611	2
85612	1
85613	1
85635	1
85651	1
85652	1
85660	1
85670	2
85675	1
85705	1
85732	4
85810	2
86021	1
86022	1
86023	2
86038	1
86039	1
86060	1
86063	1
86077	1
86078	1
86079	1
86140	1
86141	1
86146	3
86147	4
86148	1
86155	1
86156	1
86157	1
86160	4
86161	3
86162	1
86171	2
86200	1
86215	1
86225	1
86226	1
86243	1
86277	1
86280	1
86294	1
86300	2
86301	1
86304	1
86308	1
86309	1
86310	1
86316	3
86320	1
86325	2
86327	1
86332	1

CPT	MUE
86334	1
86335	2
86336	1
86337	1
86340	1
86341	1
86343	1
86344	1
86355	1
86357	1
86359	1
86360	1
86361	1
86367	1
86376	2
86378	1
86382	3
86384	1
86406	2
86430	2
86431	2
86480	1
86481	1
86485	1
86490	1
86510	1
86580	1
86590	1
86592	2
86593	2
86602	3
86603	2
86612	2
86617	2
86618	2
86619	2
86625	2
86628	3
86632	3
86641	2
86645	1
86648	2
86651	2
86652	2
86653	2
86654	2
86663	2
86664	2
86665	2
86668	2
86674	3
86677	3
86684	2
86687	2
86688	2
86689	2
86692	2
86694	2
86695	2
86696	2
86698	3
86701	2
86702	2
86703	2
86704	1
86705	1
86706	2
86707	2
86708	1

CPT	MUE
86709	1
86713	3
86720	2
86723	2
86727	2
86732	2
86738	2
86741	2
86744	2
86747	2
86750	4
86756	2
86759	2
86762	2
86768	5
86771	2
86774	2
86777	2
86778	2
86784	2
86787	2
86788	2
86789	2
86793	2
86800	1
86803	2
86804	1
86807	2
86808	1
86812	1
86813	1
86816	1
86817	1
86821	3
86822	3
86850	3
86860	2
86885	3
86906	1
86930	2
86940	1
86941	1
86945	3
86950	1
86960	3
86975	2
86976	2
86977	2
87001	1
87003	1
87045	3
87073	3
87084	2
87086	3
87103	3
87109	3
87110	2
87118	3
87143	2
87164	2
87166	2
87168	2
87169	2
87172	2
87177	3
87197	1
87207	3
87220	3
87230	3

CPT	MUE
87250	3
87255	2
87260	2
87265	2
87267	2
87269	3
87270	2
87271	2
87272	3
87273	2
87274	2
87275	2
87276	2
87277	2
87278	3
87280	2
87283	2
87285	2
87290	2
87299	2
87301	2
87305	2
87320	2
87324	3
87327	2
87328	3
87329	3
87332	2
87335	2
87336	3
87337	3
87338	1
87339	1
87340	1
87341	1
87350	1
87380	1
87385	2
87390	2
87391	2
87400	2
87420	2
87425	2
87427	3
87430	2
87449	3
87450	2
87451	2
87470	2
87471	2
87472	2
87475	2
87476	2
87477	2
87480	2
87482	2
87485	2
87486	2
87487	2
87490	2
87491	2
87492	2
87495	2
87496	2
87497	2
87498	2
87500	1
87502	1
87510	2

CPT	MUE
87511	2
87512	2
87515	2
87516	2
87517	2
87520	2
87521	2
87522	2
87525	2
87526	2
87527	2
87528	2
87529	2
87530	2
87531	2
87532	2
87533	2
87534	2
87535	2
87536	2
87537	2
87538	2
87539	2
87540	2
87541	2
87542	2
87550	2
87551	2
87552	2
87557	2
87560	2
87561	2
87562	2
87580	2
87581	2
87582	2
87590	3
87591	3
87592	2
87620	2
87621	3
87622	2
87640	2
87650	1
87651	1
87652	1
87653	1
87660	1
87797	3
87799	3
87800	2
87802	2
87803	3
87804	2
87807	2
87808	1
87810	2
87850	1
87880	2
87900	1
87901	1
87902	1
87903	1
87906	2
88104	4
88106	3
88120	2
88121	2
88125	1

CPT	MUE
88130	1
88140	1
88141	1
88142	1
88143	1
88147	1
88148	1
88150	1
88152	1
88153	1
88154	1
88155	1
88160	4
88161	4
88162	3
88164	1
88165	1
88166	1
88167	1
88172	3
88173	3
88174	1
88175	1
88177	2
88182	2
88184	1
88187	1
88188	1
88189	1
88230	2
88233	3
88239	3
88240	3
88241	3
88245	1
88248	1
88249	1
88261	2
88262	2
88263	1
88264	2
88267	2
88269	2
88273	3
88283	2
88289	1
88291	1
88300	2
88302	2
88309	3
88311	4
88318	3
88321	1
88323	1
88325	1
88329	4
88331	11
88333	4
88347	4
88348	1
88349	1
88355	1
88356	1
88358	2
88362	1
88363	1
88371	1
88372	1
88380	1

CPT	MUE
88381	1
88384	1
88385	1
88386	1
88720	1
88740	1
88741	1
89049	1
89050	2
89051	2
89055	2
89060	2
89125	2
89160	1
89190	1
89220	1
89230	1
89250	1
89251	1
89253	1
89254	1
89255	1
89257	1
89258	1
89259	1
89260	1
89261	1
89264	1
89268	1
89272	1
89280	1
89281	1
89290	1
89291	1
89300	1
89310	1
89320	1
89321	1
89322	1
89325	1
89329	1
89330	1
89331	1
89335	1
89342	1
89343	1
89344	1
89346	1
89352	1
89353	1
89354	1
89356	2
90284	1
90296	1
90375	20
90376	20
90378	3
90385	1
90396	1
90471	1
90472	4
90473	1
90474	1
90476	1
90477	1
90581	1
90585	1
90586	1
90632	1

CPT	MUE
90633	1
90634	1
90636	1
90644	1
90645	1
90646	1
90647	1
90648	1
90649	1
90650	1
90654	1
90655	1
90656	1
90657	1
90658	1
90660	1
90661	1
90662	1
90663	1
90664	1
90665	1
90666	1
90667	1
90668	1
90669	1
90675	1
90676	1
90680	1
90681	1
90690	1
90691	1
90692	1
90693	1
90696	1
90698	1
90700	1
90701	1
90702	1
90703	1
90704	1
90705	1
90706	1
90707	1
90708	1
90710	1
90712	1
90713	1
90714	1
90715	1
90716	1
90717	1
90718	1
90719	1
90720	1
90721	1
90725	1
90727	1
90732	1
90733	1
90734	1
90735	1
90736	1
90738	1
90740	2
90743	1
90744	1
90746	1
90747	2
90801	1

CPT	MUE
90802	1
90804	1
90805	1
90806	1
90807	1
90808	1
90809	1
90810	1
90811	1
90812	1
90813	1
90814	1
90815	1
90816	1
90817	1
90818	1
90819	1
90821	1
90822	1
90823	1
90824	1
90826	1
90827	1
90828	1
90829	1
90845	1
90846	1
90847	1
90849	1
90853	1
90857	1
90862	1
90865	1
90867	1
90868	1
90870	1
90880	1
90901	1
90911	1
90935	1
90937	1
90940	2
90945	1
90947	1
90951	1
90952	1
90953	1
90954	1
90955	1
90956	1
90957	1
90958	1
90959	1
90960	1
90961	1
90962	1
90963	1
90964	1
90965	1
90966	1
90967	1
90968	1
90969	1
90970	1
90989	1
90993	1
90997	1
91010	1
91013	1

CPT	MUE
91020	1
91022	1
91030	1
91034	1
91035	1
91037	1
91038	1
91040	1
91065	1
91110	1
91111	1
91117	1
91120	1
91122	1
91132	1
91133	1
92002	1
92004	1
92012	1
92014	1
92018	1
92019	1
92020	1
92025	1
92060	1
92065	1
92070	2
92081	1
92082	1
92083	1
92100	1
92120	1
92130	1
92132	1
92133	1
92134	1
92140	1
92225	2
92226	2
92227	1
92228	1
92230	2
92235	2
92240	2
92250	1
92260	1
92265	1
92270	1
92275	1
92283	1
92284	1
92285	1
92286	1
92287	1
92311	1
92312	1
92313	1
92315	1
92316	1
92317	1
92325	1
92326	2
92502	1
92504	1
92507	1
92508	1
92511	1
92512	1
92516	1

CPT	MUE
92520	1
92526	1
92541	1
92542	1
92543	4
92544	1
92545	1
92546	1
92548	1
92552	1
92553	1
92555	1
92556	1
92557	1
92561	1
92562	1
92563	1
92564	1
92565	1
92567	1
92568	1
92571	1
92572	1
92575	1
92576	1
92577	1
92579	1
92582	1
92583	1
92584	1
92585	1
92586	1
92587	1
92588	1
92596	1
92601	1
92602	1
92603	1
92604	1
92609	1
92610	1
92613	1
92615	1
92617	1
92620	1
92625	1
92626	1
92950	3
92953	2
92960	2
92961	1
92970	1
92971	1
92973	2
92974	1
92975	1
92977	1
92978	1
92979	2
92980	1
92981	2
92982	1
92984	2
92986	1
92987	1
92990	1
92992	1
92993	1
92995	1

CPT	MUE
92996	2
92997	1
92998	2
93000	3
93005	3
93015	2
93016	2
93017	2
93018	2
93024	1
93025	1
93040	3
93041	2
93042	3
93224	1
93225	1
93226	1
93227	1
93228	1
93229	1
93268	1
93270	1
93271	1
93272	1
93278	1
93279	1
93280	1
93281	1
93282	1
93283	1
93284	1
93285	1
93286	2
93287	2
93288	1
93289	1
93290	1
93291	1
93292	1
93293	1
93294	1
93295	1
93296	1
93297	1
93298	1
93299	1
93303	1
93304	1
93306	1
93307	1
93308	2
93312	2
93313	2
93314	2
93315	2
93316	2
93317	2
93318	2
93320	1
93321	1
93325	1
93350	1
93351	1
93352	1
93451	1
93452	1
93453	1
93454	1
93455	1

CPT	MUE
93456	1
93457	1
93458	1
93459	1
93460	1
93461	1
93462	1
93463	1
93464	1
93503	2
93505	1
93530	1
93531	1
93532	1
93533	1
93561	1
93562	3
93563	1
93564	1
93565	1
93566	1
93567	1
93568	1
93571	1
93572	2
93580	1
93581	1
93600	1
93602	1
93603	1
93609	1
93610	1
93612	1
93613	1
93615	1
93616	1
93618	1
93619	1
93620	1
93621	1
93622	1
93623	1
93624	1
93631	1
93640	1
93641	1
93642	1
93650	1
93651	1
93652	1
93660	1
93662	1
93701	1
93720	1
93721	1
93722	1
93724	2
93745	1
93784	1
93786	1
93788	1
93790	1
93797	2
93798	2
93875	1
93880	1
93882	1
93886	1
93888	1

CPT	MUE
93890	1
93892	1
93893	1
93922	1
93923	1
93924	1
93925	1
93926	1
93930	1
93931	1
93965	1
93970	1
93971	1
93975	1
93976	1
93978	1
93979	1
93980	1
93981	1
93982	1
93990	2
94002	1
94003	1
94004	1
94010	1
94014	1
94015	1
94016	1
94060	1
94070	1
94200	1
94240	1
94250	1
94260	1
94350	1
94360	1
94370	1
94375	1
94400	1
94450	1
94452	1
94453	1
94610	2
94620	1
94621	1
94642	1
94644	1
94645	2
94660	1
94662	1
94664	1
94667	1
94680	1
94681	1
94690	1
94720	1
94725	1
94750	1
94760	1
94761	1
94762	1
94770	1
94772	1
94775	1
94776	1
94777	1
95012	2
95056	1
95060	1

CPT	MUE
95065	1
95070	1
95071	1
95075	1
95115	1
95117	1
95250	1
95251	1
95805	1
95806	1
95807	1
95808	1
95810	1
95811	1
95812	1
95813	1
95816	1
95819	1
95822	1
95824	1
95827	1
95829	1
95830	1
95832	1
95852	1
95857	1
95860	1
95861	1
95863	1
95864	1

CPT	MUE
95865	1
95866	2
95867	1
95868	1
95869	1
95873	1
95874	1
95875	2
95921	1
95922	1
95923	1
95925	1
95926	1
95927	1
95928	1
95929	1
95930	1
95933	1
95934	1
95936	2
95950	1
95951	1
95953	1
95954	1
95955	1
95956	1
95957	1
95958	1
95961	1
95965	1

CPT	MUE
95966	1
95967	3
95970	1
95971	1
95972	1
95974	1
95975	2
95978	1
95980	1
95981	1
95982	1
95990	2
95991	2
95992	1
96000	1
96001	1
96002	1
96003	1
96004	1
96020	1
96103	1
96120	1
96125	2
96360	2
96368	2
96369	1
96371	1
96373	2
96374	2
96402	2

CPT	MUE
96405	1
96406	1
96409	2
96413	2
96416	1
96420	2
96422	2
96425	1
96440	1
96446	1
96450	1
96521	2
96522	1
96523	1
96542	1
96567	1
96570	1
96571	3
96900	1
96904	1
96910	1
96912	1
96913	1
96920	1
96921	1
96922	1
97012	1
97016	1
97018	1
97022	1

CPT	MUE
97024	1
97026	1
97028	1
97150	1
97545	1
97546	2
97597	1
97605	1
97606	1
98925	1
98926	1
98927	1
98928	1
98929	1
98940	1
98941	1
98942	1
99082	1
99143	2
99144	2
99148	2
99149	2
99170	1
99175	1
99183	1
99191	1
99192	1
99195	2
99201	1
99202	1

CPT	MUE
99203	1
99204	1
99205	1
99211	1
99212	1
99213	1
99214	1
99215	1
99217	1
99218	1
99219	1
99220	1
99221	1
99222	1
99223	1
99224	1
99225	1
99226	1
99231	1
99232	1
99233	1
99234	1
99235	1
99236	1
99238	1
99239	1
99281	1
99282	1
99283	1
99284	1

CPT	MUE
99285	1
99291	1
99304	1
99305	1
99306	1
99307	1
99308	1
99309	1
99310	1
99315	1
99316	1
99318	1
99324	1
99325	1
99326	1
99327	1
99328	1
99334	1
99335	1
99336	1
99337	1
99341	1
99342	1
99343	1
99344	1
99345	1
99347	1
99348	1
99349	1
99350	1

CPT	MUE
99354	1
99356	1
99406	1
99407	1
99455	1
99456	1
99460	1
99461	1
99462	1
99463	1
99464	1
99465	1
99466	1
99468	1
99469	1
99471	1
99472	1
99477	1
99478	1
99479	1
99480	1
99605	1
99606	1
99607	1

Appendix L — Medically Unlikely Edits (MUEs) — Professional

OPPS

CPT	MUE
0019T	1
0030T	2
0042T	1
0054T	2
0055T	2
0071T	1
0072T	1
0073T	2
0099T	2
0100T	2
0101T	1
0102T	2
0103T	1
0106T	4
0107T	4
0108T	4
0109T	4
0110T	4
0111T	1
0123T	2
0124T	2
0159T	2
0171T	1
0172T	3
0173T	1
0174T	1
0175T	1
0179T	1
0181T	1
0182T	3
0183T	1
0190T	2
0191T	2
0192T	2
0197T	2
0198T	2
0208T	1
0209T	1
0210T	1
0211T	1
0212T	1
0213T	1
0214T	1
0215T	1
0216T	1
0217T	1
0218T	1
0221T	1
0223T	1
0224T	1
0225T	1
0226T	1
0227T	1
0228T	2
0230T	2
0232T	1
0233T	1
0234T	2
0236T	1
0237T	2
0239T	1
0240T	1
0241T	1
0242T	1
0243T	1
0244T	1

CPT	MUE
0245T	1
0246T	1
0247T	1
0248T	1
0249T	1
0250T	2
0251T	1
0252T	2
0253T	1
0260T	1
0261T	1
10040	1
10060	1
10061	1
10080	1
10081	1
10180	3
11000	1
11042	1
11043	1
11044	1
11055	1
11056	1
11057	1
11100	1
11200	1
11201	1
11446	3
11450	2
11451	2
11462	2
11463	2
11471	2
11646	3
11719	1
11720	1
11721	1
11730	1
11770	1
11771	1
11772	1
11900	1
11901	1
11920	1
11921	1
11922	1
11950	1
11951	1
11952	1
11954	1
11960	3
11970	2
11971	2
11976	1
11980	1
11981	1
11982	1
11983	1
12001	1
12002	1
12004	1
12005	1
12006	1
12007	1
12011	1
12013	1
12014	1

CPT	MUE
12015	1
12016	1
12017	1
12018	1
12020	3
12021	3
12031	1
12032	1
12034	1
12035	1
12036	1
12037	1
12041	1
12042	1
12044	1
12045	1
12046	1
12047	1
12051	1
12052	1
12053	1
12054	1
12055	1
12056	1
12057	1
13100	1
13101	1
13120	1
13121	1
13131	1
13132	1
13150	1
13151	1
13152	1
13160	3
15002	1
15004	1
15040	1
15050	1
15100	1
15110	1
15115	1
15120	1
15130	1
15135	1
15150	1
15151	1
15155	1
15156	1
15170	1
15175	1
15200	1
15220	1
15240	1
15260	1
15300	1
15320	1
15330	1
15335	1
15340	1
15360	1
15365	1
15400	1
15420	1
15430	1
15570	3
15572	2

CPT	MUE
15574	2
15576	2
15600	2
15610	2
15620	2
15630	2
15650	1
15731	1
15740	3
15750	2
15760	2
15770	2
15775	1
15776	1
15780	1
15781	2
15782	2
15783	2
15786	1
15787	3
15788	1
15789	1
15792	1
15793	1
15819	1
15820	1
15821	1
15822	1
15823	1
15824	1
15825	1
15826	1
15828	1
15829	1
15830	1
15832	2
15833	2
15834	2
15835	1
15836	2
15838	1
15839	2
15840	1
15841	2
15842	2
15845	2
15847	1
15850	1
15851	1
15852	2
15860	1
15876	1
15877	1
15878	2
15879	2
15920	1
15922	1
15931	1
15933	1
15934	1
15935	1
15936	1
15937	1
15940	2
15941	2
15944	2
15945	2

CPT	MUE
15946	2
15950	2
15951	2
15952	2
15953	2
15956	2
15958	2
16000	1
16020	1
16025	1
16030	1
17000	1
17003	13
17004	1
17106	1
17107	1
17108	1
17110	1
17111	1
17264	3
17266	2
17276	3
17286	3
17340	1
17360	1
17380	1
19000	2
19001	5
19020	2
19030	2
19101	3
19110	2
19112	2
19120	2
19125	2
19126	3
19260	2
19290	3
19296	2
19297	2
19298	2
19300	2
19301	2
19302	2
19303	2
19304	2
19307	2
19316	1
19318	1
19324	1
19325	1
19328	1
19330	1
19340	1
19342	1
19350	1
19355	1
19357	1
19366	1
19370	1
19371	1
19380	1
19396	1
20100	2
20102	4
20103	4
20150	2

CPT	MUE
20200	3
20205	4
20206	3
20250	3
20251	3
20526	2
20552	1
20553	1
20555	1
20662	1
20663	2
20665	1
20670	2
20680	2
20692	3
20693	2
20696	2
20697	4
20900	2
20910	2
20912	1
20920	2
20922	2
20924	4
20926	2
20972	2
20973	2
20974	1
20975	1
20979	1
20982	1
20985	2
21010	1
21015	1
21025	2
21026	2
21029	1
21030	2
21031	2
21032	1
21034	1
21040	2
21044	1
21046	2
21047	2
21048	2
21049	2
21050	1
21060	1
21070	1
21073	1
21076	1
21077	2
21079	1
21080	1
21081	1
21082	1
21083	1
21084	1
21085	1
21086	2
21087	1
21088	1
21100	1
21110	2
21116	2
21120	1

CPT	MUE
21121	1
21122	1
21123	1
21125	2
21127	2
21137	1
21138	1
21139	1
21150	1
21175	1
21181	1
21195	1
21198	1
21199	1
21206	1
21208	2
21209	2
21210	2
21215	2
21230	2
21235	2
21240	2
21242	2
21243	2
21244	1
21245	2
21246	2
21260	1
21261	1
21263	1
21267	2
21270	2
21275	1
21280	2
21282	2
21295	2
21296	2
21310	1
21315	1
21320	1
21325	1
21330	1
21335	1
21336	1
21337	1
21338	1
21339	1
21340	1
21345	1
21355	2
21356	2
21390	2
21400	2
21401	2
21406	2
21407	2
21408	2
21421	1
21440	2
21445	2
21450	1
21451	1
21452	1
21453	1
21454	1
21461	1
21462	1

CPT	MUE
21465	2
21470	1
21480	2
21485	2
21490	2
21495	1
21497	1
21501	3
21502	1
21550	3
21556	3
21557	1
21610	2
21685	1
21700	2
21720	1
21725	1
21742	1
21743	1
21805	3
21820	1
21920	3
21925	3
21935	1
22100	1
22101	1
22102	1
22103	3
22222	1
22305	1
22310	1
22315	1
22505	1
22520	1
22521	1
22522	5
22523	1
22524	1
22525	5
22612	1
22614	15
22851	9
22900	3
23000	2
23020	2
23030	2
23031	2
23035	2
23040	2
23044	2
23065	2
23066	2
23075	4
23076	2
23077	1
23100	2
23101	2
23105	2
23106	2
23107	2
23120	2
23125	2
23130	2
23145	1
23146	1
23150	1
23155	1

CPT	MUE
23156	1
23170	1
23172	1
23174	1
23180	1
23182	1
23184	1
23190	1
23195	1
23330	2
23331	2
23350	2
23395	1
23397	1
23400	1
23405	2
23406	2
23410	2
23412	2
23415	2
23420	2
23430	2
23440	2
23450	2
23455	2
23460	2
23462	2
23465	2
23466	2
23470	2
23480	2
23485	2
23490	2
23491	2
23500	2
23505	2
23515	2
23520	2
23525	2
23530	2
23532	2
23540	2
23545	2
23550	2
23552	2
23570	2
23575	2
23585	2
23600	2
23605	2
23615	2
23616	2
23620	2
23625	2
23630	2
23650	2
23655	2
23660	2
23665	2
23670	2
23675	2
23680	2
23700	2
23800	2
23802	2
23921	2
23930	2
23931	2
23935	2

CPT	MUE
24000	2
24006	2
24065	2
24066	2
24077	2
24100	2
24101	2
24102	2
24105	2
24110	1
24115	2
24116	1
24120	2
24125	1
24126	1
24130	2
24134	1
24136	1
24138	2
24140	2
24145	2
24147	2
24149	2
24150	1
24152	1
24155	2
24160	2
24164	2
24200	3
24201	3
24220	2
24300	2
24301	2
24305	4
24320	2
24330	2
24331	2
24332	2
24340	2
24342	2
24343	2
24344	2
24345	2
24346	2
24357	2
24358	2
24359	2
24360	2
24361	2
24362	2
24363	2
24365	2
24366	2
24400	2
24410	2
24420	2
24430	2
24435	2
24470	2
24495	2
24498	2
24500	2
24505	2
24515	2
24516	2
24530	2
24535	2
24538	2
24545	2

CPT	MUE
24546	2
24560	2
24565	2
24566	2
24575	2
24576	2
24577	2
24579	2
24582	2
24586	2
24587	2
24600	2
24605	2
24615	2
24620	2
24635	2
24640	2
24650	2
24655	2
24665	2
24666	2
24670	2
24675	2
24685	2
24800	2
24802	2
24925	2
24935	2
25000	2
25001	2
25020	2
25023	2
25024	2
25025	2
25031	2
25035	2
25040	2
25065	5
25066	3
25076	5
25077	2
25085	2
25100	2
25101	2
25105	2
25107	2
25110	3
25111	2
25112	2
25115	2
25116	2
25119	2
25120	2
25125	1
25126	1
25130	2
25135	2
25136	2
25145	1
25150	1
25151	1
25170	1
25210	2
25215	2
25230	2
25240	2
25246	2
25248	3
25250	2

CPT	MUE
25251	2
25259	2
25275	2
25295	9
25300	2
25301	2
25315	2
25316	2
25320	2
25332	2
25335	2
25337	2
25350	2
25355	2
25360	2
25365	2
25370	2
25375	2
25390	2
25391	2
25392	2
25393	2
25394	2
25400	2
25405	2
25415	2
25420	2
25425	2
25426	2
25430	2
25431	2
25440	2
25441	2
25442	2
25443	2
25444	2
25445	2
25446	2
25449	2
25450	2
25455	2
25490	2
25491	2
25492	2
25500	2
25505	2
25515	2
25520	2
25525	2
25526	2
25530	2
25535	2
25545	2
25560	2
25565	2
25574	2
25575	2
25600	2
25605	2
25606	2
25607	2
25608	2
25609	2
25622	2
25624	2
25628	2
25630	2
25635	2
25650	2

CPT	MUE
25651	2
25652	2
25660	2
25670	2
25671	2
25675	2
25676	2
25680	2
25685	2
25690	2
25695	2
25800	2
25805	2
25810	2
25820	2
25825	2
25830	2
25907	2
25922	2
25929	2
25931	2
26010	3
26011	3
26025	2
26030	2
26034	2
26035	3
26037	2
26040	2
26045	2
26070	3
26100	2
26105	2
26110	3
26117	2
26121	2
26123	2
26185	1
26205	2
26215	2
26230	3
26236	3
26250	2
26260	2
26262	2
26357	3
26358	3
26390	3
26392	3
26416	2
26428	2
26432	2
26433	2
26434	3
26494	2
26496	2
26497	2
26498	2
26508	2
26516	2
26517	2
26518	2
26548	3
26550	2
26555	2
26560	2
26561	2
26562	2
26580	2

CPT	MUE
26641	2
26645	2
26650	2
26665	2
26740	3
26742	3
26746	3
26820	2
26841	2
26842	2
26860	1
26862	1
26990	2
26991	2
27000	2
27001	1
27003	1
27006	2
27027	1
27033	2
27035	2
27040	2
27041	3
27048	2
27049	2
27050	2
27052	2
27057	1
27060	2
27062	2
27065	2
27066	2
27067	2
27080	1
27086	2
27087	2
27093	2
27095	2
27096	1
27097	2
27098	2
27100	2
27105	2
27110	2
27111	2
27193	1
27194	1
27200	1
27202	1
27220	2
27230	2
27235	2
27238	2
27246	2
27250	2
27252	2
27256	2
27257	2
27265	2
27266	2
27267	2
27275	2
27305	2
27306	2
27307	2
27310	2
27325	1
27326	1
27329	2

CPT	MUE
27330	2
27331	2
27332	2
27333	2
27334	2
27335	2
27340	2
27345	2
27347	2
27350	2
27355	2
27356	2
27357	2
27358	2
27370	2
27380	2
27381	2
27385	2
27386	2
27390	2
27391	1
27392	1
27393	2
27394	1
27395	1
27396	2
27397	2
27400	2
27403	2
27405	2
27407	2
27409	2
27412	2
27415	2
27416	2
27418	2
27420	2
27422	2
27424	2
27425	2
27427	2
27428	2
27429	2
27430	2
27435	2
27437	2
27438	2
27440	2
27441	2
27442	2
27443	2
27446	2
27475	2
27496	2
27497	2
27498	2
27499	2
27500	2
27501	2
27502	2
27503	2
27508	2
27509	2
27510	2
27516	2
27517	2
27520	2
27524	2
27530	2

CPT	MUE
27532	2
27538	2
27550	2
27552	2
27560	2
27562	2
27566	2
27570	2
27594	2
27600	2
27601	2
27602	2
27604	2
27605	2
27606	2
27607	2
27610	2
27612	2
27615	2
27620	2
27625	2
27626	2
27630	2
27635	2
27637	2
27638	2
27640	2
27641	2
27647	2
27648	2
27650	2
27652	2
27654	2
27656	2
27658	2
27659	2
27664	2
27665	2
27675	2
27676	2
27680	3
27681	2
27685	2
27686	2
27687	2
27690	2
27691	2
27695	2
27696	2
27698	2
27700	2
27704	2
27705	2
27707	2
27709	2
27720	2
27722	2
27726	2
27730	2
27732	2
27734	2
27740	2
27742	2
27745	2
27750	2
27752	2
27756	2
27758	2
27759	2

Appendix L — Medically Unlikely Edits (MUEs) — OPPS

CPT	MUE
27760	2
27762	2
27766	2
27767	2
27768	2
27769	2
27780	2
27781	2
27784	2
27786	2
27788	2
27792	2
27808	2
27810	2
27814	2
27816	2
27818	2
27822	2
27823	2
27824	2
27825	2
27826	2
27827	2
27828	2
27829	2
27830	2
27831	2
27832	2
27840	2
27842	2
27846	2
27848	2
27860	2
27870	2
27871	2
27884	2
27889	2
27892	2
27893	2
27894	2
28001	2
28002	3
28003	2
28005	3
28035	2
28052	2
28054	2
28060	2
28062	2
28086	2
28088	2
28090	2
28092	2
28100	2
28102	2
28103	2
28106	2
28107	2
28108	2
28110	2
28111	2
28113	2
28114	2
28116	2
28118	2
28119	2
28120	2
28130	2
28171	2

CPT	MUE
28173	2
28175	2
28192	2
28193	2
28202	2
28210	2
28220	2
28222	2
28225	2
28226	2
28230	2
28238	2
28240	2
28250	2
28260	2
28261	2
28262	2
28264	2
28280	2
28286	2
28289	2
28290	2
28292	2
28293	2
28294	2
28296	2
28297	2
28298	2
28299	2
28300	2
28302	2
28304	2
28305	2
28306	2
28307	2
28309	2
28310	2
28315	2
28320	2
28322	2
28340	2
28341	2
28344	2
28360	2
28400	2
28405	2
28406	2
28415	2
28420	2
28430	2
28435	2
28436	2
28445	2
28446	2
28490	2
28495	2
28496	2
28505	2
28530	2
28531	2
28540	2
28545	2
28546	2
28555	2
28570	2
28575	2
28576	2
28585	2
28600	3

CPT	MUE
28605	3
28630	3
28705	2
28715	2
28725	2
28730	2
28735	2
28737	2
28750	2
28755	2
28760	2
28890	2
29000	1
29010	1
29015	1
29020	1
29025	1
29035	1
29040	1
29044	1
29046	1
29049	1
29055	1
29058	1
29065	2
29075	2
29085	2
29086	2
29105	2
29125	2
29126	2
29200	1
29240	2
29260	2
29280	2
29305	1
29325	1
29345	2
29355	2
29358	2
29365	2
29405	2
29425	2
29435	2
29440	2
29445	2
29450	1
29505	2
29515	2
29520	2
29530	2
29540	2
29550	2
29580	2
29590	2
29700	2
29705	2
29710	2
29715	1
29720	1
29730	2
29740	1
29750	1
29800	2
29804	2
29805	2
29806	2
29807	2
29819	2

CPT	MUE
29820	2
29821	2
29822	2
29823	2
29824	2
29825	2
29826	2
29827	2
29828	2
29830	2
29834	2
29835	2
29836	2
29837	2
29838	2
29840	2
29843	2
29844	2
29845	2
29846	2
29847	2
29848	2
29850	2
29851	2
29855	2
29856	2
29860	2
29861	2
29862	2
29863	2
29866	2
29867	2
29868	2
29870	2
29871	2
29873	2
29874	2
29875	2
29876	2
29877	2
29879	2
29880	2
29881	2
29882	2
29883	2
29884	2
29885	2
29886	2
29887	2
29888	2
29889	2
29891	2
29892	2
29893	2
29894	2
29895	2
29897	2
29898	2
29899	2
29900	2
29901	2
29902	2
29904	2
29905	2
29906	2
29907	2
29914	2
29915	2
29916	2

CPT	MUE
30000	1
30020	1
30100	3
30110	1
30115	1
30117	2
30118	2
30120	1
30124	2
30125	1
30130	2
30140	2
30150	1
30160	1
30200	1
30210	1
30220	1
30300	1
30310	1
30320	1
30400	1
30410	1
30420	1
30430	1
30435	1
30450	1
30460	1
30462	1
30465	1
30520	1
30540	1
30545	1
30560	1
30580	2
30600	1
30620	1
30630	1
30801	1
30802	1
30901	1
30903	1
30905	1
30906	1
30915	1
30920	1
30930	1
31000	1
31002	2
31020	1
31030	1
31032	1
31040	2
31050	2
31051	2
31070	2
31075	2
31080	2
31081	2
31084	2
31085	2
31086	2
31087	2
31090	2
31200	2
31201	2
31205	2
31231	1
31233	2
31235	2

CPT	MUE
31237	2
31238	2
31239	2
31240	2
31254	2
31255	2
31256	2
31267	2
31276	2
31287	2
31288	2
31292	2
31293	2
31294	2
31295	2
31296	2
31297	2
31300	1
31320	1
31400	1
31420	1
31500	2
31502	1
31505	1
31510	1
31511	1
31512	1
31513	1
31515	1
31520	1
31525	1
31526	1
31527	1
31528	1
31529	1
31530	1
31531	1
31535	1
31536	1
31540	1
31541	1
31545	2
31546	2
31560	1
31561	1
31570	1
31571	1
31575	1
31576	1
31577	1
31578	1
31579	1
31580	1
31582	1
31588	1
31590	1
31595	2
31600	1
31601	1
31603	1
31605	1
31610	1
31611	1
31612	1
31613	1
31614	1
31615	1
31620	1
31622	1

CPT	MUE
31623	1
31624	1
31625	1
31628	1
31629	1
31630	2
31631	1
31632	4
31633	4
31634	1
31635	1
31636	1
31637	2
31638	2
31640	1
31641	1
31643	1
31645	1
31646	2
31656	1
31715	1
31717	1
31720	2
31730	1
31750	1
31755	1
31785	1
31820	1
31825	1
31830	1
32201	2
32400	2
32405	2
32420	2
32421	3
32422	3
32550	2
32601	1
32602	1
32603	1
32604	1
32605	1
32606	1
32960	1
32998	2
33010	1
33011	1
33206	1
33207	1
33208	1
33210	1
33211	1
33212	1
33213	1
33214	1
33215	2
33216	1
33217	1
33218	1
33220	1
33222	1
33223	1
33224	1
33225	1
33226	1
33233	1
33234	1
33235	1
33240	1

CPT	MUE
33241	1
33244	1
33249	1
33282	1
33284	1
34101	2
34111	2
34201	2
34203	2
34421	2
34471	1
34490	2
34501	2
34510	2
34520	1
34530	2
35011	2
35180	2
35184	2
35188	2
35190	2
35201	2
35206	2
35207	3
35226	3
35231	2
35236	2
35256	2
35261	1
35266	2
35286	2
35321	2
35458	3
35471	3
35472	1
35500	2
35572	2
35685	2
35686	1
35761	2
35860	2
35875	2
35876	2
35879	2
35881	2
35883	1
35884	1
35903	2
36002	2
36005	2
36010	2
36013	2
36014	2
36100	2
36120	2
36160	2
36200	2
36260	1
36261	1
36262	1
36400	1
36405	1
36406	1
36410	3
36420	2
36425	3
36430	1
36440	1
36450	1

CPT	MUE
36455	1
36468	1
36469	1
36470	2
36471	2
36475	2
36478	2
36479	2
36481	1
36511	1
36512	1
36513	1
36514	1
36515	1
36516	1
36522	1
36555	2
36556	2
36557	2
36558	2
36560	2
36561	2
36563	2
36565	2
36566	2
36568	2
36569	3
36570	2
36571	2
36575	2
36576	2
36578	2
36580	2
36581	2
36582	2
36583	2
36584	2
36585	2
36589	2
36590	2
36592	1
36593	2
36595	2
36596	2
36597	2
36598	2
36620	3
36625	2
36640	1
36680	1
36800	1
36810	1
36815	1
36818	1
36819	1
36820	2
36821	2
36825	1
36830	2
36831	1
36832	2
36833	1
36835	1
36838	2
36860	2
36861	2
36870	2
37183	1
37184	2

CPT	MUE
37185	2
37186	2
37187	2
37188	2
37195	1
37200	2
37201	1
37203	2
37205	1
37207	1
37209	2
37210	1
37220	1
37221	1
37222	2
37223	2
37224	1
37225	1
37226	1
37227	1
37228	1
37229	1
37230	1
37231	1
37232	2
37233	2
37234	2
37235	2
37250	1
37500	2
37565	2
37600	1
37605	2
37606	2
37607	1
37609	2
37615	2
37620	1
37650	1
37700	1
37718	1
37722	1
37735	1
37760	1
37765	2
37766	2
37780	1
37785	1
37790	1
38120	1
38200	1
38205	1
38206	1
38220	2
38221	2
38230	1
38240	1
38241	1
38242	1
38300	2
38305	2
38308	1
38500	2
38505	3
38510	2
38520	2
38525	2
38530	2
38542	2

CPT	MUE
38550	1
38555	1
38570	1
38571	1
38572	1
38700	1
38720	1
38740	2
38745	2
38760	1
38790	1
38792	2
38794	1
38900	2
39400	1
40500	2
40510	2
40520	2
40525	2
40527	2
40530	2
40650	2
40652	2
40654	2
40700	1
40701	1
40702	1
40720	1
40761	1
40800	1
40801	1
40806	2
40816	2
40818	2
40819	2
40820	2
40830	2
40831	2
40840	1
40842	1
40843	1
40844	2
40845	1
41000	1
41005	1
41006	2
41007	2
41008	2
41009	2
41010	1
41015	2
41016	1
41017	2
41018	2
41019	1
41100	3
41105	3
41108	2
41110	2
41112	2
41113	2
41114	2
41115	1
41116	3
41120	1
41250	2
41251	2
41252	2
41500	1

CPT	MUE
41510	1
41512	1
41520	1
41800	2
41820	4
41822	1
41823	1
41825	2
41826	2
41827	2
41828	4
41850	2
41872	4
41874	4
42000	1
42100	3
42104	3
42106	2
42107	2
42120	1
42140	1
42145	1
42160	1
42180	1
42182	1
42200	1
42205	1
42210	1
42215	1
42220	1
42225	1
42226	1
42227	1
42235	1
42260	1
42280	1
42281	1
42300	2
42305	2
42310	2
42320	2
42330	3
42335	2
42340	2
42400	2
42405	2
42408	1
42409	1
42410	2
42415	2
42420	2
42425	2
42440	2
42450	1
42500	2
42505	1
42507	1
42508	1
42509	1
42510	1
42550	2
42600	1
42650	2
42660	2
42665	2
42700	2
42720	1
42725	2
42800	3

CPT	MUE
42802	2
42806	1
42808	2
42809	1
42810	2
42815	2
42820	1
42821	1
42825	1
42826	1
42830	1
42831	1
42835	1
42836	1
42842	1
42844	1
42860	1
42870	1
42890	1
42892	1
42900	1
42950	1
42955	1
42960	1
42962	1
42970	1
42972	1
43020	1
43030	1
43130	1
43200	1
43201	1
43202	1
43204	1
43205	1
43215	1
43216	1
43217	1
43219	1
43220	1
43226	1
43227	2
43228	1
43231	1
43232	1
43234	1
43235	1
43236	1
43237	1
43238	1
43239	1
43240	1
43241	1
43242	1
43243	1
43244	1
43245	1
43246	1
43247	1
43248	1
43249	1
43250	1
43251	1
43255	2
43256	1
43257	1
43258	1
43259	1
43260	1

CPT	MUE
43261	1
43262	2
43263	2
43264	1
43265	1
43267	1
43268	2
43269	2
43271	1
43272	1
43273	1
43280	1
43450	1
43453	1
43456	1
43458	1
43510	1
43647	1
43648	1
43651	1
43652	1
43653	1
43752	2
43753	1
43754	1
43755	1
43756	1
43757	1
43760	2
43761	2
43830	1
43831	1
43870	1
43886	1
43887	1
43888	1
44100	1
44180	1
44186	1
44206	1
44207	1
44208	1
44213	1
44312	1
44340	1
44360	1
44361	1
44363	1
44364	1
44365	1
44366	1
44369	1
44370	1
44372	1
44373	1
44376	1
44377	1
44378	1
44379	1
44380	1
44382	1
44383	1
44385	1
44386	1
44388	1
44389	1
44390	1
44391	1
44392	1

CPT	MUE
44393	1
44394	1
44397	1
44500	1
44701	1
44901	1
44970	1
45000	1
45005	1
45020	1
45100	1
45108	1
45150	1
45160	1
45190	1
45300	1
45303	1
45305	1
45307	1
45308	1
45309	1
45315	1
45317	1
45320	1
45321	1
45327	1
45330	1
45331	1
45332	1
45333	1
45334	1
45335	1
45337	1
45338	1
45339	1
45340	1
45341	1
45342	1
45345	1
45355	1
45378	1
45379	1
45380	1
45381	1
45382	2
45383	1
45384	1
45385	1
45386	1
45387	1
45391	1
45392	1
45500	1
45505	1
45520	1
45541	1
45560	1
45900	1
45905	1
45910	1
45915	1
45990	1
46020	1
46030	1
46040	2
46045	2
46050	2
46060	2
46070	1

CPT	MUE
46080	1
46083	2
46200	1
46220	2
46221	1
46230	1
46250	1
46255	1
46257	1
46258	1
46260	1
46261	1
46262	1
46270	1
46275	1
46280	1
46285	1
46288	1
46320	2
46500	1
46505	1
46600	1
46604	1
46606	1
46608	1
46610	1
46611	1
46612	1
46614	1
46615	1
46700	1
46706	2
46750	1
46753	1
46754	1
46760	1
46761	1
46762	1
46900	1
46910	1
46916	1
46917	1
46922	1
46924	1
46930	1
46940	1
46942	1
46945	1
46946	1
46947	1
47000	3
47001	3
47011	3
47370	1
47371	1
47382	1
47490	1
47500	2
47505	2
47510	2
47511	2
47525	3
47530	3
47552	1
47553	1
47554	1
47555	1
47556	1
47560	1

CPT	MUE
47561	1
47562	1
47563	1
47564	1
47630	1
48102	2
48511	1
49021	3
49041	3
49061	3
49080	1
49081	2
49180	3
49250	1
49320	1
49321	1
49322	1
49323	1
49324	1
49325	1
49326	1
49327	1
49400	1
49402	1
49418	1
49419	1
49421	1
49422	1
49423	3
49424	3
49426	1
49427	1
49429	1
49435	1
49436	1
49440	1
49441	1
49442	1
49446	1
49450	1
49451	1
49452	1
49460	1
49465	1
49491	1
49492	1
49495	1
49496	1
49500	1
49501	1
49505	1
49507	1
49520	1
49521	1
49525	1
49540	1
49550	1
49553	1
49555	1
49557	1
49565	2
49566	2
49570	1
49572	1
49580	1
49582	1
49585	1
49587	1
49590	1

CPT	MUE
49600	1
49650	1
49651	1
49652	2
49653	2
49654	2
49655	2
49656	2
49657	2
50020	1
50021	2
50080	2
50081	2
50200	2
50382	1
50384	1
50385	2
50386	2
50387	1
50389	2
50390	2
50391	2
50392	2
50393	2
50394	2
50395	2
50396	2
50398	2
50541	2
50542	2
50543	2
50544	2
50551	2
50553	2
50555	1
50557	2
50561	2
50562	1
50570	2
50572	2
50574	1
50575	2
50576	2
50580	1
50590	1
50592	1
50593	2
50684	2
50686	2
50688	2
50690	2
50945	2
50947	2
50948	2
50951	2
50953	2
50955	2
50957	2
50961	2
50970	2
50972	2
50974	2
50976	2
50980	2
51020	1
51030	1
51040	1
51045	2
51050	1

CPT	MUE
51065	1
51080	2
51100	1
51101	1
51102	1
51500	1
51520	1
51535	1
51600	1
51605	1
51610	1
51700	1
51701	2
51702	2
51703	2
51705	2
51710	1
51715	1
51720	1
51725	1
51726	1
51736	1
51741	1
51784	1
51785	1
51792	1
51797	1
51798	1
51880	1
51990	1
51992	1
52000	1
52001	1
52005	2
52007	2
52010	1
52204	1
52214	1
52224	1
52234	1
52235	1
52240	1
52250	1
52260	1
52265	1
52270	1
52275	1
52276	1
52277	1
52281	1
52282	1
52283	1
52285	1
52290	1
52300	1
52301	1
52305	1
52310	1
52315	2
52317	1
52318	1
52320	2
52325	1
52327	2
52330	2
52332	1
52334	2
52341	2
52342	2

CPT	MUE
52343	2
52344	2
52345	2
52346	2
52351	1
52352	2
52353	2
52354	2
52355	2
52400	1
52402	1
52450	1
52500	1
52601	1
52630	1
52640	1
52647	1
52648	1
52649	1
52700	1
53000	1
53010	1
53020	1
53025	1
53040	1
53060	1
53080	1
53085	1
53200	1
53210	1
53215	1
53220	1
53230	1
53235	1
53240	1
53250	1
53260	1
53265	1
53270	1
53275	1
53400	1
53405	1
53410	1
53420	1
53425	1
53430	1
53431	1
53440	1
53442	1
53444	1
53445	1
53446	1
53447	1
53449	1
53450	1
53460	1
53500	1
53502	1
53505	1
53510	1
53515	1
53520	1
53600	1
53601	1
53605	1
53620	1
53621	1
53660	1
53661	1

CPT	MUE
53665	1
53850	1
53852	1
53860	1
54000	1
54001	1
54015	1
54050	1
54055	1
54056	1
54057	1
54060	1
54065	1
54100	3
54105	2
54110	1
54111	1
54112	1
54115	1
54120	1
54150	1
54160	1
54161	1
54162	1
54163	1
54164	1
54200	1
54205	1
54220	1
54230	1
54231	1
54235	1
54240	1
54250	1
54300	1
54304	1
54308	1
54312	1
54316	1
54318	1
54322	1
54324	1
54326	1
54328	1
54340	1
54344	1
54348	1
54352	1
54360	1
54380	1
54385	1
54400	1
54401	1
54405	1
54406	1
54408	1
54410	1
54415	1
54416	1
54420	1
54435	1
54440	1
54450	1
54500	2
54505	1
54512	2
54520	1
54522	2
54530	2

CPT	MUE
54550	1
54560	1
54600	2
54620	1
54640	1
54660	1
54670	2
54680	1
54690	2
54692	2
54700	2
54800	2
54830	2
54840	2
54860	1
54861	1
54865	1
54900	1
54901	1
55000	2
55040	1
55041	1
55060	2
55100	2
55110	1
55120	1
55150	1
55175	1
55180	1
55200	1
55250	1
55300	1
55400	1
55450	1
55500	2
55520	2
55530	2
55535	2
55540	2
55550	2
55600	1
55680	2
55700	1
55705	1
55706	1
55720	1
55725	1
55860	1
55870	1
55873	1
55875	1
55876	1
55920	1
56405	2
56420	1
56440	1
56441	1
56442	1
56501	1
56515	1
56605	1
56620	1
56625	1
56700	1
56740	2
56800	1
56805	1
56810	1
56820	1

CPT	MUE
56821	1
57000	1
57010	1
57020	1
57022	2
57023	2
57061	1
57065	1
57100	3
57105	2
57106	1
57107	1
57109	1
57120	1
57130	1
57135	2
57150	1
57155	1
57156	1
57160	1
57170	1
57180	1
57200	1
57210	1
57220	1
57230	1
57240	1
57250	1
57260	1
57265	1
57267	3
57268	1
57282	1
57283	1
57284	1
57285	1
57287	1
57288	1
57289	1
57291	1
57292	1
57295	1
57300	1
57310	1
57320	1
57330	1
57335	1
57400	1
57410	1
57415	1
57420	1
57421	1
57423	1
57425	1
57452	1
57454	1
57455	1
57456	1
57460	1
57461	1
57500	1
57505	1
57510	1
57511	1
57513	1
57520	1
57522	1
57530	1
57550	1

CPT	MUE
57555	1
57556	1
57558	1
57700	1
57720	1
57800	1
58100	1
58110	1
58120	1
58145	1
58260	1
58262	1
58263	1
58270	1
58290	1
58291	1
58292	1
58294	1
58301	1
58321	1
58322	1
58323	1
58340	1
58345	2
58346	1
58350	2
58353	1
58356	1
58541	1
58542	1
58543	1
58544	1
58545	1
58546	1
58550	1
58552	1
58553	1
58554	1
58555	1
58558	1
58559	1
58560	1
58561	1
58562	1
58563	1
58565	1
58570	1
58571	1
58572	1
58573	1
58600	1
58615	1
58660	1
58661	1
58662	1
58670	1
58671	1
58672	1
58673	1
58770	2
58800	1
58805	1
58820	2
58823	2
58900	1
58920	1
58925	1
58970	1
58974	1

CPT	MUE
58976	2
59020	4
59025	1
59051	1
59100	1
59150	1
59151	1
59160	1
59200	1
59300	1
59320	1
59400	1
59412	2
59414	1
59425	1
59426	1
59430	1
59515	1
59812	1
59820	1
59821	1
59840	1
59841	1
59866	1
59870	1
59871	1
60000	1
60200	2
60210	1
60212	1
60220	1
60225	1
60240	1
60252	1
60260	1
60271	1
60280	1
60281	1
60500	1
60502	1
60512	1
60520	1
61000	1
61001	1
61020	2
61026	2
61050	1
61055	1
61070	2
61215	1
61330	1
61334	2
61623	2
61626	2
61720	2
61770	1
61781	1
61782	1
61783	1
61790	2
61791	2
61796	1
61798	1
61800	1
61880	1
61885	2
61886	1
61888	2
62000	1
62160	1
62194	2
62225	2
62230	2
62252	2
62263	1
62264	1
62267	2
62268	1
62269	2
62270	2
62272	2
62273	2
62280	1
62281	1
62282	1
62284	1
62287	1
62292	1
62294	2
62310	1
62311	1
62318	1
62319	1
62350	1
62351	1
62355	1
62360	1
62361	1
62362	1
62365	1
62367	1
62368	1
63001	1
63003	1
63005	1
63011	1
63012	1
63015	1
63016	1
63017	1
63020	1
63030	1
63035	6
63040	1
63042	1
63045	1
63046	1
63047	1
63048	9
63055	1
63056	1
63057	8
63064	1
63066	3
63075	1
63600	2
63610	1
63615	1
63620	1
63621	2
63650	2
63655	1
63661	1
63662	1
63685	2
63688	2
63741	1
63744	1
63746	1
64402	2
64405	1
64408	2
64410	2
64412	2
64413	2
64415	2
64416	2
64417	2
64418	2
64420	3
64421	3
64425	2
64430	2
64435	2
64445	1
64446	2
64447	2
64448	2
64449	2
64455	1
64479	1
64483	1
64505	2
64508	2
64510	2
64517	1
64520	2
64530	2
64553	1
64555	2
64560	1
64561	2
64565	2
64566	1
64568	2
64569	2
64570	2
64575	2
64577	1
64580	2
64581	2
64585	2
64590	1
64595	1
64600	2
64605	2
64610	2
64611	1
64612	2
64613	1
64614	1
64622	1
64626	1
64630	1
64632	2
64650	1
64653	1
64680	1
64681	1
64702	2
64712	2
64713	2
64714	2
64718	2
64719	2
64721	2
64726	2
64727	3
64732	2
64734	2
64736	2
64738	2
64740	2
64742	2
64744	2
64746	2
64761	1
64763	1
64766	1
64771	2
64772	2
64774	3
64776	1
64778	3
64782	2
64783	2
64786	2
64790	1
64792	2
64795	2
64802	1
64804	1
64821	2
64822	2
64823	2
64831	2
64834	2
64835	2
64836	2
64837	3
64840	2
64856	2
64857	3
64858	2
64859	2
64861	2
64862	2
64864	2
64865	1
64870	1
64872	3
64874	1
64876	1
64885	1
64886	1
64890	3
64891	2
64892	2
64893	2
64895	2
64896	2
64897	2
64898	2
64901	2
64905	1
64907	1
64910	3
64911	2
65091	2
65093	2
65101	2
65103	2
65105	2
65110	2
65112	2
65114	2
65125	2
65130	2
65135	2
65140	2
65150	2
65155	2
65175	2
65205	2
65210	2
65220	2
65222	2
65235	2
65260	2
65265	2
65270	2
65272	2
65275	2
65280	2
65285	2
65286	2
65290	2
65400	2
65410	2
65420	2
65426	2
65430	2
65435	2
65436	2
65450	2
65600	2
65710	2
65730	2
65750	2
65755	2
65756	2
65757	2
65770	2
65772	2
65775	2
65778	2
65779	2
65780	2
65781	2
65782	2
65800	2
65805	2
65810	2
65815	2
65820	2
65850	2
65855	2
65860	2
65865	2
65870	2
65875	2
65880	2
65900	2
65920	2
65930	2
66020	2
66030	2
66130	2
66150	2
66155	2
66160	2
66165	2
66170	2
66172	2
66174	2
66175	2
66180	2
66185	2
66220	2
66225	2
66250	2
66500	2
66505	2
66600	2
66605	2
66625	2
66630	2
66635	2
66680	2
66682	2
66700	2
66710	2
66711	2
66720	2
66740	2
66761	2
66762	2
66770	2
66820	2
66821	2
66825	2
66830	2
66840	2
66850	2
66852	2
66920	2
66930	2
66940	2
66982	2
66983	2
66984	2
66985	2
66986	2
66990	2
67005	2
67010	2
67015	2
67025	2
67027	2
67028	2
67030	2
67031	2
67036	2
67039	2
67040	2
67041	2
67042	2
67043	2
67101	2
67105	2
67107	2
67108	2
67110	2
67112	2
67113	2
67115	2
67120	2
67121	2
67141	2
67145	2
67208	2
67210	2
67218	2
67220	2
67221	1
67225	1
67227	2
67228	2
67229	1
67250	2
67255	2
67311	2
67312	2
67314	2
67316	2
67318	2
67320	2
67331	2
67332	2
67334	2
67335	2
67340	2
67343	2
67345	2
67346	1
67400	2
67405	2
67412	2
67413	2
67414	2
67415	2
67420	2
67430	2
67440	2
67445	2
67450	2
67500	2
67505	2
67515	2
67550	2
67560	2
67570	2
67700	4
67710	2
67715	2
67800	1
67801	1
67805	1
67808	1
67820	2
67825	2
67830	3
67835	2
67850	4
67875	2
67880	2
67882	2
67900	2
67901	2
67902	2
67903	2
67904	2
67906	2
67908	2
67909	2
67911	4
67912	2
67914	4
67915	4
67916	4
67917	4
67921	4
67922	4
67923	4
67924	4
67930	2
67935	2
67938	2
67950	2
67961	4
67966	4
67971	2
67973	2
67974	2
67975	2
68020	2
68040	2
68100	2
68110	2
68115	2
68130	2
68135	2
68200	2
68320	2
68325	2
68326	2
68328	2
68330	2
68335	2
68340	2
68360	2
68362	2
68371	1
68400	2
68420	2
68440	2
68500	2
68505	2
68510	2
68520	2
68525	2
68530	2
68540	1
68550	1
68700	2
68705	2
68720	2
68745	2
68750	2
68760	4
68761	4
68770	2
68801	4
68810	1
68811	1
68815	1
68816	1
68840	2
68850	2
69000	2
69005	2
69020	2
69100	3
69105	2
69110	2
69120	1
69140	2
69145	2
69150	1
69200	2
69205	2
69210	1

CPT	MUE
69220	1
69222	1
69300	1
69310	2
69320	2
69400	2
69401	2
69405	2
69420	2
69421	2
69424	1
69433	1
69436	1
69440	2
69450	2
69501	1
69502	1
69505	1
69511	1
69530	1
69540	2
69550	1
69552	1
69601	1
69602	1
69603	1
69604	1
69605	1
69610	2
69620	2
69631	2
69632	1
69633	1
69635	1
69636	1
69637	1
69641	1
69642	1
69643	1
69644	1
69645	1
69646	1
69650	1
69660	1
69661	1
69662	2
69666	2
69667	2
69670	1
69676	1
69700	2
69711	2
69714	2
69715	1
69717	1
69718	1
69720	2
69725	2
69740	2
69745	2
69801	1
69802	1
69805	1
69806	1
69820	1
69840	1
69905	1
69910	1
69915	1
69930	2
69955	2
69960	2
69990	1
70010	1
70015	1
70030	2
70100	1
70110	1
70120	2
70130	2
70134	1
70140	1
70150	1
70160	1
70170	2
70190	1
70200	1
70210	1
70220	1
70240	1
70250	1
70260	1
70300	1
70310	1
70320	1
70328	1
70330	1
70332	2
70336	1
70350	1
70355	1
70360	1
70370	1
70371	1
70373	1
70380	2
70390	2
70450	3
70460	1
70470	2
70480	1
70481	1
70482	1
70486	1
70487	1
70488	1
70490	1
70491	1
70492	1
70496	1
70498	1
70540	1
70542	1
70543	1
70544	1
70545	1
70546	1
70547	1
70548	1
70549	1
70551	1
70552	1
70553	1
70554	1
70555	1
70557	1
70558	1
70559	1
71015	2
71021	1
71022	1
71023	2
71030	2
71034	1
71035	2
71040	1
71060	1
71090	1
71100	1
71101	1
71110	1
71111	1
71120	1
71130	1
71250	1
71260	1
71270	1
71275	1
71550	1
71551	1
71552	1
71555	1
72010	1
72020	4
72040	3
72050	1
72052	1
72069	1
72070	1
72072	1
72074	1
72080	1
72090	1
72100	1
72110	1
72114	1
72120	1
72125	1
72126	1
72127	1
72128	1
72129	1
72130	1
72131	1
72132	1
72133	1
72141	1
72142	1
72146	1
72147	1
72148	1
72149	1
72156	1
72157	1
72158	1
72170	1
72190	1
72191	1
72192	1
72193	1
72194	1
72195	1
72196	1
72197	1
72198	1
72200	1
72202	1
72220	1
72240	1
72255	1
72265	1
72270	1
72275	3
72292	3
73000	2
73010	2
73020	2
73030	2
73040	2
73050	1
73060	2
73070	2
73080	2
73085	2
73090	2
73092	2
73100	2
73110	2
73115	2
73120	2
73130	2
73140	2
73200	2
73201	2
73202	2
73206	2
73218	2
73219	2
73220	2
73221	2
73222	2
73223	2
73500	2
73510	2
73520	2
73525	2
73530	2
73540	1
73542	2
73550	2
73560	2
73562	2
73564	2
73565	1
73580	2
73590	2
73592	2
73600	2
73610	2
73615	2
73620	2
73630	2
73650	2
73660	2
73700	2
73701	2
73702	2
73706	2
73718	2
73719	2
73720	2
73721	4
73722	2
73723	4
73725	2
74000	3
74010	2
74020	2
74022	2
74150	1
74160	1
74170	1
74175	1
74176	1
74177	1
74178	1
74181	1
74182	1
74183	1
74185	1
74190	1
74210	1
74220	1
74230	1
74235	1
74240	1
74241	1
74245	1
74246	1
74247	1
74249	1
74250	1
74251	1
74260	1
74270	1
74280	1
74283	1
74290	1
74291	1
74300	1
74301	2
74305	1
74320	1
74327	1
74328	1
74329	1
74330	1
74340	1
74355	1
74360	1
74363	2
74400	1
74410	1
74415	1
74420	2
74425	2
74430	1
74440	2
74445	1
74450	1
74455	1
74470	2
74475	2
74480	2
74485	2
74710	1
74740	1
74742	2
74775	1
75557	1
75559	1
75561	1
75563	1
75600	1
75605	1
75625	1
75630	1
75635	1
75650	2
75658	2
75660	1
75662	1
75665	1
75671	1
75676	1
75680	1
75685	2
75710	1
75716	1
75722	1
75724	1
75726	3
75731	1
75733	1
75736	2
75741	1
75743	1
75746	1
75756	2
75801	1
75803	1
75805	1
75807	1
75809	1
75810	1
75820	1
75822	1
75825	1
75827	1
75831	1
75833	1
75840	1
75842	1
75860	2
75870	1
75872	1
75880	2
75885	1
75887	1
75889	1
75891	1
75901	1
75902	2
75940	1
75945	1
75961	2
75962	1
75964	4
75966	1
75968	2
75970	2
75980	1
75982	2
75984	2
75989	2
76000	3
76001	2
76010	2
76080	2
76100	2
76101	1
76102	1
76120	1
76125	1
76376	2
76377	2
76380	2
76506	1
76510	2
76511	2
76512	2
76513	2
76514	1
76516	1
76519	2
76529	2
76536	1
76604	1
76645	1
76700	1
76705	2
76770	1
76775	2
76776	1
76800	1
76801	1
76802	3
76805	1
76810	3
76811	1
76812	3
76813	1
76814	3
76815	1
76817	1
76830	1
76831	1
76856	1
76857	1
76870	1
76872	1
76873	1
76881	2
76882	2
76885	1
76886	1
76930	1
76932	1
76936	2
76937	2
76940	1
76942	1
76945	1
76946	1
76948	1
76950	2
76965	2
76970	1
76975	1
76977	1
76998	1
77001	2
77002	1
77003	1
77011	1
77012	1
77013	1
77014	2
77021	1
77022	1
77053	2
77054	2
77058	1
77059	1
77071	1
77261	1
77262	1
77263	1
77280	2
77285	1
77290	1
77295	1
77301	1
77305	2
77310	2
77315	2
77321	1
77326	1
77327	1
77328	1
77332	4
77333	4
77336	1
77370	1
77371	1
77372	1
77373	1
77401	2
77402	2
77403	2
77404	2
77406	2
77407	2
77408	2
77409	2
77411	2
77412	2
77413	2
77414	2
77416	2
77417	1
77418	2
77421	2
77422	1
77423	1
77427	1
77435	1
77470	1
77520	1
77522	1
77523	1
77525	1
77600	1
77605	1
77610	1
77615	1
77620	1
77750	1
77761	1
77762	1
77763	1
77776	1
77777	1
77778	1
77785	3
77786	3
77787	3
77789	2
77790	2
78000	1
78001	1
78003	1

CPT	MUE
78006	1
78007	1
78010	1
78011	1
78015	1
78016	1
78018	1
78020	1
78070	1
78075	1
78102	1
78103	1
78104	1
78110	1
78111	1
78120	1
78121	1
78122	1
78130	1
78135	1
78140	1
78185	1
78190	1
78191	1
78195	1
78201	1
78202	1
78205	1
78206	1
78215	1
78216	1
78220	1
78223	1
78230	1
78231	1
78232	1
78258	1
78261	1
78262	1
78264	1
78267	1
78268	1
78270	1
78271	1
78272	1
78278	2
78282	1
78290	1
78291	1
78300	1
78305	1
78306	1
78315	1
78320	1
78414	1
78428	1
78445	1
78456	1
78457	1
78458	1
78459	1
78466	1
78468	1
78469	1
78472	1
78473	1
78481	1
78483	1
78491	1
78492	1
78494	1
78496	1
78580	1
78584	2
78585	2
78586	1
78587	1
78588	1
78591	1
78593	1
78594	1
78596	1
78600	1
78601	1
78605	1
78606	2
78607	1
78608	1
78610	1
78630	2
78635	1
78645	1
78647	1
78650	1
78660	1
78700	1
78701	2
78707	1
78708	1
78709	1
78710	1
78725	1
78730	1
78740	1
78761	1
78800	1
78801	1
78802	1
78803	1
78804	1
78805	1
78806	1
78807	1
78808	1
78811	1
78812	1
78813	1
78814	1
78815	1
78816	1
79005	1
79101	1
79200	1
79300	1
79403	1
79440	1
79445	1
80047	2
80048	2
80051	4
80053	1
80061	1
80069	1
80074	1
80076	1
80103	2
80150	2
80152	2
80154	2
80156	2
80157	2
80158	3
80160	2
80162	2
80164	2
80166	2
80168	2
80170	2
80172	2
80173	2
80174	2
80176	1
80178	2
80182	2
80184	2
80185	2
80186	2
80188	2
80190	2
80192	2
80194	2
80195	2
80197	2
80198	2
80200	2
80201	2
80202	2
80299	3
80400	1
80402	1
80406	1
80408	1
80410	1
80412	1
80414	1
80415	1
80416	1
80417	1
80418	1
80420	1
80422	1
80424	1
80426	1
80428	1
80430	1
80432	1
80434	1
80435	1
80436	1
80438	1
80439	1
80440	1
80500	1
80502	1
81000	2
81001	2
81002	2
81003	2
81005	2
81007	1
81015	1
81020	1
81025	1
81050	2
82000	1
82003	3
82009	3
82010	4
82013	1
82016	1
82017	1
82030	1
82040	1
82042	2
82043	1
82044	1
82045	2
82055	3
82075	2
82085	1
82101	1
82103	1
82104	1
82105	1
82106	4
82107	1
82108	1
82120	1
82127	2
82128	2
82131	3
82135	1
82136	3
82139	3
82140	2
82143	2
82145	1
82150	4
82154	1
82157	1
82160	1
82163	1
82164	1
82172	3
82175	2
82180	1
82190	4
82205	1
82232	2
82239	1
82240	1
82247	2
82248	2
82252	1
82261	1
82270	1
82271	3
82272	1
82274	1
82286	1
82300	1
82306	1
82308	3
82310	4
82330	4
82331	1
82340	1
82355	3
82360	3
82365	3
82370	3
82373	1
82374	3
82375	4
82378	2
82379	1
82380	1
82382	1
82383	1
82384	2
82387	1
82390	1
82415	1
82435	3
82436	1
82438	1
82441	1
82465	1
82480	2
82482	1
82485	1
82486	2
82487	2
82488	1
82489	2
82492	2
82495	1
82507	1
82520	2
82523	1
82525	2
82528	1
82530	2
82540	1
82543	2
82544	2
82550	3
82552	3
82553	3
82554	2
82565	3
82570	3
82575	1
82585	1
82595	1
82600	1
82607	1
82608	1
82610	1
82615	1
82626	1
82627	1
82633	1
82634	2
82638	1
82646	1
82649	1
82651	1
82652	1
82654	1
82656	1
82657	3
82658	2
82666	1
82668	1
82670	2
82671	1
82672	1
82677	1
82679	1
82690	1
82693	2
82696	1
82705	1
82710	1
82715	1
82725	1
82726	1
82728	1
82731	1
82735	1
82742	1
82746	1
82747	1
82757	1
82759	1
82760	1
82775	1
82776	1
82784	6
82785	1
82787	4
82820	1
82941	1
82943	1
82946	1
82950	3
82951	1
82952	3
82953	1
82955	1
82960	1
82963	1
82965	1
82975	1
82977	1
82978	1
82979	1
82980	1
82985	1
83008	1
83009	1
83010	1
83012	1
83013	1
83014	1
83015	1
83018	7
83020	2
83021	2
83026	1
83030	1
83033	1
83036	1
83037	1
83045	1
83050	4
83051	1
83055	1
83060	1
83065	1
83068	1
83069	1
83070	1
83071	1
83080	2
83088	1
83090	2
83150	1
83491	1
83497	1
83498	2
83499	1
83500	1
83505	1
83518	2
83527	1
83528	1
83540	2
83550	1
83570	1
83582	1
83586	1
83593	1
83605	3
83615	3
83625	1
83630	1
83631	1
83632	1
83633	1
83634	1
83655	2
83661	4
83662	4
83663	4
83664	4
83670	1
83690	2
83695	1
83698	1
83700	1
83701	1
83704	1
83718	1
83719	1
83721	1
83727	1
83735	4
83775	1
83785	1
83788	3
83789	2
83805	1
83825	2
83835	2
83840	2
83857	1
83858	1
83861	2
83864	1
83866	1
83872	2
83873	1
83874	4
83880	1
83885	2
83887	2
83912	1
83915	1
83916	2
83918	2
83919	1
83921	2
83925	4
83930	2
83935	2
83937	1
83945	2
83950	1
83951	1
83970	4
83986	2
83992	2
83993	1
84022	2
84030	1
84035	1
84060	1
84061	1
84066	1
84075	2
84078	1
84080	1
84081	1
84085	1
84087	1
84100	3
84105	1
84106	1
84110	1
84112	1
84119	1
84120	1
84126	1
84127	1
84132	4
84133	2
84134	1
84135	1
84138	1
84140	1
84143	2
84144	1
84146	3
84150	2
84152	1
84153	1
84154	1
84155	1
84156	1
84157	3
84160	2
84163	1
84165	1
84166	2
84202	1
84203	1
84206	1
84207	1
84210	2
84220	1
84228	1
84233	2
84234	2
84235	1
84238	3
84252	1
84255	2
84260	1
84270	1
84275	1
84285	1
84295	4
84300	2
84302	3
84305	1
84307	1
84311	2
84315	2
84375	1
84376	1

CPT	MUE
84377	1
84378	2
84379	1
84392	1
84402	1
84403	2
84425	1
84430	1
84432	1
84436	1
84437	1
84439	1
84442	1
84445	1
84446	1
84449	1
84450	1
84460	1
84466	1
84478	1
84479	1
84480	1
84481	1
84482	1
84484	3
84485	1
84488	1
84490	1
84510	1
84512	3
84520	4
84525	1
84540	2
84545	1
84550	1
84560	2
84577	1
84578	1
84580	1
84583	1
84585	1
84586	1
84588	2
84590	1
84591	1
84597	1
84600	2
84620	1
84630	2
84702	2
84703	1
84704	1
84830	1
85002	2
85004	2
85007	1
85008	2
85009	1
85013	2
85014	4
85018	4
85025	2
85032	3
85041	2
85044	1
85045	1
85046	1
85048	2
85049	2
85055	1
85060	1
85097	2
85130	2
85170	1
85175	1
85210	2
85220	2
85230	2
85240	3
85244	2
85245	2
85246	2
85247	2
85250	2
85260	2
85270	2
85280	2
85290	2
85291	2
85292	2
85293	2
85300	2
85301	2
85302	2
85303	2
85305	2
85306	2
85307	2
85335	2
85337	1
85345	2
85348	2
85360	1
85362	2
85366	2
85370	2
85378	2
85379	2
85380	2
85384	2
85385	1
85390	3
85396	1
85400	2
85410	2
85415	2
85420	2
85421	2
85441	1
85445	1
85460	1
85461	1
85475	1
85525	2
85530	1
85536	1
85540	1
85547	1
85549	1
85555	1
85557	1
85597	1
85598	1
85611	2
85612	1
85613	1
85635	1
85651	1
85652	1
85660	1
85670	2
85675	1
85705	1
85732	4
85810	2
86021	1
86022	1
86023	2
86038	1
86039	1
86060	1
86063	1
86077	1
86078	1
86079	1
86140	1
86141	1
86146	3
86147	4
86148	1
86155	1
86156	1
86157	1
86160	4
86161	3
86162	1
86171	3
86200	1
86215	1
86225	1
86226	1
86243	1
86277	1
86280	1
86294	1
86300	2
86301	1
86304	1
86308	1
86309	1
86310	1
86316	3
86320	1
86325	2
86327	1
86332	1
86334	1
86335	2
86336	1
86337	1
86340	1
86341	1
86343	1
86344	1
86355	1
86357	1
86359	1
86360	1
86361	1
86367	2
86376	2
86378	1
86382	3
86384	1
86406	2
86430	2
86431	2
86480	1
86481	1
86485	1
86490	1
86510	1
86580	1
86590	1
86592	2
86593	2
86602	3
86603	2
86612	2
86617	2
86618	2
86619	2
86625	2
86628	3
86632	3
86641	2
86645	1
86648	2
86651	2
86652	2
86653	2
86654	2
86663	2
86664	2
86665	2
86668	2
86674	3
86677	3
86684	2
86687	2
86688	2
86689	2
86692	2
86694	2
86695	2
86696	2
86698	3
86701	2
86702	2
86703	2
86704	1
86705	1
86706	2
86707	2
86708	1
86709	1
86713	3
86720	2
86723	2
86727	2
86732	2
86738	2
86741	2
86744	2
86747	2
86750	4
86756	2
86759	2
86762	2
86768	5
86771	2
86774	2
86777	2
86778	2
86784	2
86787	2
86788	2
86789	2
86793	2
86800	1
86803	2
86804	1
86807	2
86808	1
86812	1
86813	1
86816	1
86817	1
86821	3
86822	3
86850	3
86860	2
86885	3
86906	1
86930	3
86940	3
86941	3
86945	3
86950	1
86960	3
86975	2
86976	2
86977	2
87001	1
87003	1
87045	3
87073	3
87084	2
87086	3
87103	3
87109	3
87110	2
87118	3
87143	2
87164	2
87166	2
87168	2
87169	2
87172	2
87177	3
87197	1
87207	3
87220	3
87230	3
87250	3
87255	2
87260	2
87265	2
87267	2
87269	3
87270	2
87271	2
87272	3
87273	2
87274	2
87275	2
87276	2
87277	2
87278	3
87280	2
87283	2
87285	2
87290	2
87299	2
87301	2
87305	2
87320	2
87324	3
87327	2
87328	3
87329	3
87332	2
87335	2
87336	3
87337	3
87338	2
87339	1
87340	1
87341	1
87350	1
87380	1
87385	2
87390	2
87391	2
87400	2
87420	2
87425	2
87427	3
87430	2
87449	3
87450	2
87451	2
87470	2
87471	2
87472	2
87475	2
87476	2
87477	2
87480	2
87482	2
87485	2
87486	2
87487	2
87490	2
87491	2
87492	2
87495	2
87496	2
87497	2
87498	2
87500	1
87502	1
87510	2
87511	2
87512	2
87515	2
87516	2
87517	2
87520	2
87521	2
87522	2
87525	2
87526	2
87527	2
87528	2
87529	2
87530	2
87531	2
87532	2
87533	2
87534	2
87535	2
87536	2
87537	2
87538	2
87539	2
87540	2
87541	2
87542	2
87550	2
87551	2
87552	2
87557	2
87560	2
87561	2
87562	2
87580	2
87581	2
87582	2
87590	3
87591	3
87592	2
87620	2
87621	3
87622	2
87640	2
87650	1
87651	1
87652	1
87653	1
87660	1
87797	3
87799	3
87800	2
87802	2
87803	3
87804	2
87807	2
87808	1
87810	2
87850	1
87880	2
87900	1
87901	1
87902	1
87903	1
87906	2
88104	4
88106	3
88120	2
88121	2
88125	1
88130	1
88140	1
88141	1
88142	1
88143	1
88147	1
88148	1
88150	1
88152	1
88153	1
88154	1
88155	1
88160	4
88161	4
88162	3
88164	1
88165	1
88166	1
88167	1
88172	3
88173	3
88174	1
88175	1
88177	2
88182	2
88184	1
88187	1
88188	1
88189	1
88230	2
88233	2
88239	3
88240	3
88241	3
88245	1
88248	1
88249	1
88261	2
88262	2
88263	1
88264	2
88267	2
88269	2
88273	3
88283	2
88289	1
88300	2
88302	2
88309	3
88311	4
88318	3
88321	1
88323	1
88325	1
88329	4
88331	11
88333	4
88347	4
88348	1
88349	1
88355	1
88356	1
88358	2
88362	1
88363	1
88371	1
88372	1
88380	1
88381	1
88384	1
88385	1
88386	1
88720	1
88740	1
88741	1
89049	1
89050	2
89051	2
89055	2
89060	2
89125	2
89160	1
89190	1
89220	2
89230	1
89250	1
89251	1
89253	1
89254	1
89255	1

CPT	MUE
89257	1
89258	1
89259	1
89260	1
89261	1
89264	1
89268	1
89272	1
89280	1
89281	1
89290	1
89291	1
89300	1
89310	1
89320	1
89321	1
89322	1
89325	1
89329	1
89330	1
89331	1
89335	1
89342	1
89343	1
89344	1
89346	1
89352	1
89353	1
89354	1
89356	2
90375	20
90376	20
90385	1
90396	1
90471	1
90472	4
90473	1
90474	1
90476	1
90585	1
90586	1
90632	1
90633	1
90634	1
90636	1
90645	1
90646	1
90647	1
90648	1
90655	1
90656	1
90657	1
90658	1
90660	1
90665	1
90669	1
90675	1
90676	1
90680	1
90681	1
90690	1
90691	1
90692	1
90696	1
90698	1
90700	1
90701	1
90702	1
90703	1

CPT	MUE
90704	1
90705	1
90706	1
90707	1
90708	1
90710	1
90712	1
90713	1
90714	1
90715	1
90717	1
90718	1
90719	1
90720	1
90721	1
90732	1
90733	1
90734	1
90735	1
90740	2
90743	1
90744	1
90746	1
90747	2
90801	2
90802	2
90804	2
90805	2
90806	2
90807	2
90808	2
90809	2
90810	2
90811	2
90812	2
90813	2
90814	2
90815	2
90816	2
90817	2
90818	2
90819	2
90821	2
90822	2
90823	2
90824	2
90826	2
90827	2
90828	2
90829	2
90845	1
90846	1
90847	1
90849	1
90853	5
90857	5
90862	1
90865	1
90867	1
90868	1
90870	1
90880	1
90901	1
90911	1
90935	1
90937	1
90940	2
90945	1
90947	1

CPT	MUE
91010	1
91013	1
91020	1
91022	1
91030	1
91034	1
91035	1
91037	1
91038	1
91040	1
91065	1
91110	1
91111	1
91117	1
91120	1
91122	1
91132	1
91133	1
92002	1
92004	1
92012	1
92014	1
92018	1
92019	1
92020	1
92025	1
92060	1
92065	1
92070	2
92081	1
92082	1
92083	1
92100	1
92120	1
92130	1
92132	1
92133	1
92134	1
92140	1
92225	2
92226	2
92227	1
92228	1
92230	2
92235	2
92240	2
92250	1
92260	1
92265	1
92270	1
92275	1
92283	1
92284	1
92285	1
92286	1
92287	1
92311	1
92312	1
92313	1
92315	1
92316	1
92317	1
92325	1
92326	2
92502	1
92504	1
92507	1
92508	1
92511	1

CPT	MUE
92512	1
92516	1
92520	1
92526	1
92541	1
92542	1
92543	4
92544	1
92545	1
92546	1
92548	1
92552	1
92553	1
92555	1
92556	1
92557	1
92561	1
92562	1
92563	1
92564	1
92565	1
92567	1
92568	1
92571	1
92572	1
92575	1
92576	1
92577	1
92579	1
92582	1
92583	1
92584	1
92585	1
92586	1
92587	1
92588	1
92596	1
92601	1
92602	1
92603	1
92604	1
92609	1
92610	1
92613	1
92620	1
92625	1
92626	1
92950	4
92953	2
92960	2
92961	1
92973	2
92974	1
92977	1
92978	1
92979	2
92980	1
92981	2
92982	1
92984	2
92986	1
92987	1
92990	1
92995	1
92996	2
92997	1
92998	2
93005	3
93015	2

CPT	MUE
93016	1
93017	2
93018	2
93024	1
93025	1
93040	3
93041	3
93042	3
93225	1
93226	1
93229	1
93270	1
93271	1
93278	1
93279	1
93280	1
93281	1
93282	1
93283	1
93284	1
93285	1
93286	2
93287	2
93288	1
93289	1
93290	1
93291	1
93292	1
93293	1
93296	1
93299	1
93303	1
93304	1
93306	1
93307	1
93308	2
93312	2
93313	2
93314	2
93315	2
93316	2
93317	2
93318	2
93320	1
93321	1
93325	1
93350	1
93351	1
93451	1
93452	1
93453	1
93454	1
93455	1
93456	1
93457	1
93458	1
93459	1
93460	1
93461	1
93462	1
93463	1
93464	1
93503	2
93505	1
93530	1
93531	1
93532	1
93533	1
93561	1

CPT	MUE
93562	3
93563	1
93564	1
93565	1
93566	1
93567	1
93568	1
93571	1
93572	2
93580	1
93581	1
93600	1
93602	1
93603	1
93609	1
93610	1
93612	1
93613	1
93615	1
93616	1
93618	1
93619	1
93620	1
93621	1
93622	1
93623	1
93624	1
93631	1
93640	1
93641	1
93642	1
93650	1
93651	1
93652	1
93660	1
93662	1
93701	1
93720	1
93721	1
93722	1
93724	2
93740	1
93745	1
93786	1
93788	1
93797	2
93798	2
93875	1
93880	1
93882	1
93886	1
93888	1
93890	1
93892	1
93893	1
93922	1
93923	1
93924	1
93925	1
93926	1
93930	1
93931	1
93965	1
93970	1
93971	1
93975	1
93976	1
93978	1
93979	1

CPT	MUE
93980	1
93981	1
93982	1
93990	2
94002	1
94003	1
94004	1
94010	1
94014	1
94015	1
94016	1
94060	1
94070	1
94150	2
94200	1
94240	1
94250	1
94260	1
94350	1
94360	1
94370	1
94375	1
94400	1
94450	1
94452	1
94453	1
94610	2
94620	1
94621	1
94642	1
94644	1
94645	2
94660	1
94662	1
94664	1
94667	1
94680	1
94681	1
94690	1
94720	1
94725	1
94750	1
94760	1
94761	1
94762	1
94770	1
94772	1
94775	1
94776	1
95012	2
95056	1
95060	1
95065	1
95070	1
95071	1
95075	1
95115	1
95117	1
95250	1
95251	1
95805	1
95806	1
95807	1
95808	1
95810	1
95811	1
95812	1
95813	1
95816	1

CPT	MUE
95819	1
95822	1
95824	1
95827	1
95829	1
95830	1
95832	1
95852	1
95857	1
95860	1
95861	1
95863	1
95864	1
95865	1
95866	2
95867	1
95868	1
95869	1
95873	1
95874	1
95875	2
95921	1
95922	1
95923	1
95925	1
95926	1
95927	1
95928	1
95929	1
95930	1
95933	1
95934	1
95936	2
95950	1
95951	1
95953	1
95954	1
95955	1
95956	1
95957	1
95958	1
95961	1
95965	1
95966	1
95967	3
95970	1
95971	1
95972	1
95974	1
95975	2
95978	1
95980	1
95981	1
95982	1
95990	2
95991	2
95992	1
96000	1
96001	1
96002	1
96003	1
96020	1
96103	1
96120	1
96125	2
96360	2
96369	1
96371	1
96373	3

CPT	MUE
96374	2
96402	2
96405	1
96406	1
96409	2
96413	2
96416	1
96420	2
96422	2
96425	1
96440	1
96446	1
96450	1
96521	2
96522	1
96523	1
96542	1
96567	1
96570	1
96571	3
96900	1
96904	1
96910	1
96912	1
96913	1
96920	1
96921	1
96922	1
97010	1
97012	1
97016	1
97018	1
97022	1
97024	1
97026	1
97028	1
97150	1
97545	1
97546	2
97597	1
97602	1
97605	1
97606	1
98925	1
98926	1
98927	1
98928	1
98929	1
98940	1
98941	1
98942	1
99082	1
99100	3
99116	1
99135	1
99140	2
99143	2
99144	2
99148	2
99149	2
99170	1
99175	1
99183	1
99195	2
99217	1
99218	1
99219	1
99220	1
99221	1
99222	1
99223	1
99224	1
99225	1
99226	1
99231	1
99232	1
99233	1
99234	1
99235	1
99236	1
99238	1
99239	1
99281	2
99282	2
99283	2
99284	2
99285	2
99291	1
99304	1
99305	1
99306	1
99307	1
99308	1
99309	1
99310	1
99315	1
99316	1
99318	1
99324	1
99325	1
99326	1
99334	1
99335	1
99336	1
99337	1
99340	1
99341	1
99342	1
99343	1
99344	1
99345	1
99347	1
99348	1
99349	1
99350	1
99354	1
99363	1
99364	1
99366	3
99367	1
99368	3
99406	1
99407	1
99455	1
99456	1
99460	1
99463	1
99465	1

APPENDIX M — INPATIENT ONLY PROCEDURES

Inpatient Only Procedures—This appendix identifies services with the status indicator C. Medicare will not pay an OPPS hospital or ASC when they are performed on a Medicare patient as an outpatient. Physicians should refer to this list when scheduling Medicare patients for surgical procedures. CMS updates this list quarterly.

00176 Anesth pharyngeal surgery
00192 Anesth facial bone surgery
00211 Anesth cran surg hemotoma
00214 Anesth skull drainage
00215 Anesth skull repair/fract
00452 Anesth surgery of shoulder
00474 Anesth surgery of rib
00524 Anesth chest drainage
00540 Anesth chest surgery
00542 Anesth remvl pleura
00546 Anesth lung chest wall surg
00560 Anesth heart surg w/o pump
00561 Anesth heart surg < 1 yr
00562 Anesth hrt surg w/pmp age 1+
00567 Anesth cabg w/pump
00580 Anesth heart/lung transplnt
00604 Anesth sitting procedure
00622 Anesth removal of nerves
00632 Anesth removal of nerves
00670 Anesth spine cord surgery
00792 Anesth hemorr/excise liver
00794 Anesth pancreas removal
00796 Anesth for liver transplant
00802 Anesth fat layer removal
00844 Anesth pelvis surgery
00846 Anesth hysterectomy
00848 Anesth pelvic organ surg
00864 Anesth removal of bladder
00865 Anesth removal of prostate
00866 Anesth removal of adrenal
00868 Anesth kidney transplant
00882 Anesth major vein ligation
00904 Anesth perineal surgery
00908 Anesth removal of prostate
00932 Anesth amputation of penis
00934 Anesth penis nodes removal
00936 Anesth penis nodes removal
00944 Anesth vaginal hysterectomy
01140 Anesth amputation at pelvis
01150 Anesth pelvic tumor surgery
01212 Anesth hip disarticulation
01214 Anesth hip arthroplasty
01232 Anesth amputation of femur
01234 Anesth radical femur surg
01272 Anesth femoral artery surg
01274 Anesth femoral embolectomy
01402 Anesth knee arthroplasty
01404 Anesth amputation at knee
01442 Anesth knee artery surg
01444 Anesth knee artery repair
01486 Anesth ankle replacement
01502 Anesth lwr leg embolectomy
01634 Anesth shoulder joint amput
01636 Anesth forequarter amput
01638 Anesth shoulder replacement
01652 Anesth shoulder vessel surg
01654 Anesth shoulder vessel surg
01656 Anesth arm-leg vessel surg
01756 Anesth radical humerus surg
01990 Support for organ donor
11004 Debride genitalia & perineum
11005 Debride abdom wall
11006 Debride genit/per/abdom wall
11008 Remove mesh from abd wall
15756 Free myo/skin flap microvasc
15757 Free skin flap microvasc
15758 Free fascial flap microvasc
16036 Escharotomy addl incision
19271 Revision of chest wall
19272 Extensive chest wall surgery
19305 Mast radical
19306 Mast rad urban type
19361 Breast reconstr w/lat flap
19364 Breast reconstruction
19367 Breast reconstruction
19368 Breast reconstruction
19369 Breast reconstruction
20661 Application of head brace
20664 Application of halo
20802 Replantation arm complete
20805 Replant forearm complete
20808 Replantation hand complete
20816 Replantation digit complete
20824 Replantation thumb complete
20827 Replantation thumb complete
20838 Replantation foot complete
20936 Sp bone agrft local add-on
20937 Sp bone agrft morsel add-on
20938 Sp bone agrft struct add-on
20955 Fibula bone graft microvasc
20956 Iliac bone graft microvasc
20957 Mt bone graft microvasc
20962 Other bone graft microvasc
20969 Bone/skin graft microvasc
20970 Bone/skin graft iliac crest
21045 Extensive jaw surgery
21141 Reconstruct midface lefort
21142 Reconstruct midface lefort
21143 Reconstruct midface lefort
21145 Reconstruct midface lefort
21146 Reconstruct midface lefort
21147 Reconstruct midface lefort
21151 Reconstruct midface lefort
21154 Reconstruct midface lefort
21155 Reconstruct midface lefort
21159 Reconstruct midface lefort
21160 Reconstruct midface lefort
21179 Reconstruct entire forehead
21180 Reconstruct entire forehead
21182 Reconstruct cranial bone
21183 Reconstruct cranial bone
21184 Reconstruct cranial bone
21188 Reconstruction of midface
21194 Reconst lwr jaw w/graft
21196 Reconst lwr jaw w/fixation
21247 Reconstruct lower jaw bone
21255 Reconstruct lower jaw bone
21268 Revise eye sockets
21343 Treatment of sinus fracture
21344 Treatment of sinus fracture
21347 Treat nose/jaw fracture
21348 Treat nose/jaw fracture
21366 Treat cheek bone fracture
21422 Treat mouth roof fracture
21423 Treat mouth roof fracture
21431 Treat craniofacial fracture
21432 Treat craniofacial fracture
21433 Treat craniofacial fracture
21435 Treat craniofacial fracture
21436 Treat craniofacial fracture
21510 Drainage of bone lesion
21615 Removal of rib
21616 Removal of rib and nerves
21620 Partial removal of sternum
21627 Sternal debridement
21630 Extensive sternum surgery
21632 Extensive sternum surgery
21705 Revision of neck muscle/rib
21740 Reconstruction of sternum
21750 Repair of sternum separation
21810 Treatment of rib fracture(s)
21825 Treat sternum fracture
22010 I&d p-spine c/t/cerv-thor
22015 I&d p-spine l/s/ls
22110 Remove part of neck vertebra
22112 Remove part thorax vertebra
22114 Remove part lumbar vertebra
22116 Remove extra spine segment
22206 Cut spine 3 col thor
22207 Cut spine 3 col lumb
22208 Cut spine 3 col addl seg
22210 Revision of neck spine
22212 Revision of thorax spine
22214 Revision of lumbar spine
22216 Revise extra spine segment
22220 Revision of neck spine
22224 Revision of lumbar spine
22226 Revise extra spine segment
22318 Treat odontoid fx w/o graft

22319 Treat odontoid fx w/graft
22325 Treat spine fracture
22326 Treat neck spine fracture
22327 Treat thorax spine fracture
22328 Treat each add spine fx
22532 Lat thorax spine fusion
22533 Lat lumbar spine fusion
22534 Lat thor/lumb addl seg
22548 Neck spine fusion
22552 Addl neck spine fusion
22556 Thorax spine fusion
22558 Lumbar spine fusion
22585 Additional spinal fusion
22590 Spine & skull spinal fusion
22595 Neck spinal fusion
22600 Neck spine fusion
22610 Thorax spine fusion
22630 Lumbar spine fusion
22632 Spine fusion extra segment
22633 Lumbar spine fusion combined
22634 Spine fusion extra segment
22800 Fusion of spine
22802 Fusion of spine
22804 Fusion of spine
22808 Fusion of spine
22810 Fusion of spine
22812 Fusion of spine
22818 Kyphectomy 1-2 segments
22819 Kyphectomy 3 or more
22830 Exploration of spinal fusion
22840 Insert spine fixation device
22841 Insert spine fixation device
22842 Insert spine fixation device
22843 Insert spine fixation device
22844 Insert spine fixation device
22845 Insert spine fixation device
22846 Insert spine fixation device
22847 Insert spine fixation device
22848 Insert pelv fixation device
22849 Reinsert spinal fixation
22850 Remove spine fixation device
22852 Remove spine fixation device
22855 Remove spine fixation device
22856 Cerv artific diskectomy
22857 Lumbar artif diskectomy
22861 Revise cerv artific disc
22862 Revise lumbar artif disc
22864 Remove cerv artif disc
22865 Remove lumb artif disc
23200 Resect clavicle tumor
23210 Resect scapula tumor
23220 Resect prox humerus tumor
23332 Remove shoulder foreign body
23472 Reconstruct shoulder joint
23900 Amputation of arm & girdle
23920 Amputation at shoulder joint
24900 Amputation of upper arm
24920 Amputation of upper arm
24930 Amputation follow-up surgery
24931 Amputate upper arm & implant
24940 Revision of upper arm
25900 Amputation of forearm
25905 Amputation of forearm
25915 Amputation of forearm
25920 Amputate hand at wrist
25924 Amputation follow-up surgery
25927 Amputation of hand
26551 Great toe-hand transfer
26553 Single transfer toe-hand
26554 Double transfer toe-hand
26556 Toe joint transfer
26992 Drainage of bone lesion
27005 Incision of hip tendon
27025 Incision of hip/thigh fascia
27030 Drainage of hip joint
27036 Excision of hip joint/muscle
27054 Removal of hip joint lining
27070 Part remove hip bone super
27071 Part removal hip bone deep
27075 Resect hip tumor
27076 Resect hip tum incl acetabul
27077 Resect hip tum w/innom bone
27078 Rsect hip tum incl femur
27090 Removal of hip prosthesis
27091 Removal of hip prosthesis
27120 Reconstruction of hip socket
27122 Reconstruction of hip socket
27125 Partial hip replacement
27130 Total hip arthroplasty
27132 Total hip arthroplasty
27134 Revise hip joint replacement
27137 Revise hip joint replacement
27138 Revise hip joint replacement
27140 Transplant femur ridge
27146 Incision of hip bone
27147 Revision of hip bone
27151 Incision of hip bones
27156 Revision of hip bones
27158 Revision of pelvis
27161 Incision of neck of femur
27165 Incision/fixation of femur
27170 Repair/graft femur head/neck
27175 Treat slipped epiphysis
27176 Treat slipped epiphysis
27177 Treat slipped epiphysis
27178 Treat slipped epiphysis
27181 Treat slipped epiphysis
27185 Revision of femur epiphysis
27187 Reinforce hip bones
27222 Treat hip socket fracture
27226 Treat hip wall fracture
27227 Treat hip fracture(s)
27228 Treat hip fracture(s)
27232 Treat thigh fracture
27236 Treat thigh fracture
27240 Treat thigh fracture
27244 Treat thigh fracture
27245 Treat thigh fracture
27248 Treat thigh fracture
27253 Treat hip dislocation
27254 Treat hip dislocation
27258 Treat hip dislocation
27259 Treat hip dislocation
27268 Cltx thigh fx w/mnpj
27269 Optx thigh fx
27280 Fusion of sacroiliac joint
27282 Fusion of pubic bones
27284 Fusion of hip joint
27286 Fusion of hip joint
27290 Amputation of leg at hip
27295 Amputation of leg at hip
27303 Drainage of bone lesion
27365 Resect femur/knee tumor
27445 Revision of knee joint
27447 Total knee arthroplasty
27448 Incision of thigh
27450 Incision of thigh
27454 Realignment of thigh bone
27455 Realignment of knee
27457 Realignment of knee
27465 Shortening of thigh bone
27466 Lengthening of thigh bone
27468 Shorten/lengthen thighs
27470 Repair of thigh
27472 Repair/graft of thigh
27477 Surgery to stop leg growth
27485 Surgery to stop leg growth
27486 Revise/replace knee joint
27487 Revise/replace knee joint
27488 Removal of knee prosthesis
27495 Reinforce thigh
27506 Treatment of thigh fracture
27507 Treatment of thigh fracture
27511 Treatment of thigh fracture
27513 Treatment of thigh fracture
27514 Treatment of thigh fracture
27519 Treat thigh fx growth plate
27535 Treat knee fracture
27536 Treat knee fracture
27540 Treat knee fracture
27556 Treat knee dislocation
27557 Treat knee dislocation
27558 Treat knee dislocation
27580 Fusion of knee
27590 Amputate leg at thigh
27591 Amputate leg at thigh
27592 Amputate leg at thigh
27596 Amputation follow-up surgery
27598 Amputate lower leg at knee
27645 Resect tibia tumor
27646 Resect fibula tumor
27702 Reconstruct ankle joint
27703 Reconstruction ankle joint
27712 Realignment of lower leg

27715 Revision of lower leg
27724 Repair/graft of tibia
27725 Repair of lower leg
27727 Repair of lower leg
27880 Amputation of lower leg
27881 Amputation of lower leg
27882 Amputation of lower leg
27886 Amputation follow-up surgery
27888 Amputation of foot at ankle
28800 Amputation of midfoot
31225 Removal of upper jaw
31230 Removal of upper jaw
31290 Nasal/sinus endoscopy surg
31291 Nasal/sinus endoscopy surg
31360 Removal of larynx
31365 Removal of larynx
31367 Partial removal of larynx
31368 Partial removal of larynx
31370 Partial removal of larynx
31375 Partial removal of larynx
31380 Partial removal of larynx
31382 Partial removal of larynx
31390 Removal of larynx & pharynx
31395 Reconstruct larynx & pharynx
31584 Treat larynx fracture
31587 Revision of larynx
31725 Clearance of airways
31760 Repair of windpipe
31766 Reconstruction of windpipe
31770 Repair/graft of bronchus
31775 Reconstruct bronchus
31780 Reconstruct windpipe
31781 Reconstruct windpipe
31786 Remove windpipe lesion
31800 Repair of windpipe injury
31805 Repair of windpipe injury
32035 Thoracostomy w/rib resection
32036 Thoracostomy w/flap drainage
32096 Open wedge/bx lung infiltr
32097 Open wedge/bx lung nodule
32098 Open biopsy of lung pleura
32100 Exploration of chest
32110 Explore/repair chest
32120 Re-exploration of chest
32124 Explore chest free adhesions
32140 Removal of lung lesion(s)
32141 Remove/treat lung lesions
32150 Removal of lung lesion(s)
32151 Remove lung foreign body
32160 Open chest heart massage
32200 Drain open lung lesion
32215 Treat chest lining
32220 Release of lung
32225 Partial release of lung
32310 Removal of chest lining
32320 Free/remove chest lining
32440 Remove lung pneumonectomy
32442 Sleeve pneumonectomy
32445 Removal of lung extrapleural
32480 Partial removal of lung
32482 Bilobectomy
32484 Segmentectomy
32486 Sleeve lobectomy
32488 Completion pneumonectomy
32491 Lung volume reduction
32501 Repair bronchus add-on
32503 Resect apical lung tumor
32504 Resect apical lung tum/chest
32505 Wedge resect of lung initial
32506 Wedge resect of lung add-on
32507 Wedge resect of lung diag
32540 Removal of lung lesion
32650 Thoracoscopy w/pleurodesis
32651 Thoracoscopy remove cortex
32652 Thoracoscopy rem totl cortex
32653 Thoracoscopy remov fb/fibrin
32654 Thoracoscopy contrl bleeding
32655 Thoracoscopy resect bullae
32656 Thoracoscopy w/pleurectomy
32658 Thoracoscopy w/sac fb remove
32659 Thoracoscopy w/sac drainage
32661 Thoracoscopy w/pericard exc
32662 Thoracoscopy w/mediast exc
32663 Thoracoscopy w/lobectomy
32664 Thoracoscopy w/ th nrv exc
32665 Thoracoscop w/esoph musc exc
32666 Thoracoscopy w/wedge resect
32667 Thoracoscopy w/w resect addl
32668 Thoracoscopy w/w resect diag
32669 Thoracoscopy remove segment
32670 Thoracoscopy bilobectomy
32671 Thoracoscopy pneumonectomy
32672 Thoracoscopy for lvrs
32673 Thoracoscopy w/thymus resect
32674 Thoracoscopy lymph node exc
32800 Repair lung hernia
32810 Close chest after drainage
32815 Close bronchial fistula
32820 Reconstruct injured chest
32850 Donor pneumonectomy
32851 Lung transplant single
32852 Lung transplant with bypass
32853 Lung transplant double
32854 Lung transplant with bypass
32855 Prepare donor lung single
32856 Prepare donor lung double
32900 Removal of rib(s)
32905 Revise & repair chest wall
32906 Revise & repair chest wall
32940 Revision of lung
32997 Total lung lavage
33015 Incision of heart sac
33020 Incision of heart sac
33025 Incision of heart sac
33030 Partial removal of heart sac
33031 Partial removal of heart sac
33050 Resect heart sac lesion
33120 Removal of heart lesion
33130 Removal of heart lesion
33140 Heart revascularize (tmr)
33141 Heart tmr w/other procedure
33202 Insert epicard eltrd open
33203 Insert epicard eltrd endo
33236 Remove electrode/thoracotomy
33237 Remove electrode/thoracotomy
33238 Remove electrode/thoracotomy
33243 Remove eltrd/thoracotomy
33250 Ablate heart dysrhythm focus
33251 Ablate heart dysrhythm focus
33254 Ablate atria lmtd
33255 Ablate atria w/o bypass ext
33256 Ablate atria w/bypass exten
33257 Ablate atria lmtd add-on
33258 Ablate atria x10sv add-on
33259 Ablate atria w/bypass add-on
33261 Ablate heart dysrhythm focus
33265 Ablate atria lmtd endo
33266 Ablate atria x10sv endo
33300 Repair of heart wound
33305 Repair of heart wound
33310 Exploratory heart surgery
33315 Exploratory heart surgery
33320 Repair major blood vessel(s)
33321 Repair major vessel
33322 Repair major blood vessel(s)
33330 Insert major vessel graft
33332 Insert major vessel graft
33335 Insert major vessel graft
33400 Repair of aortic valve
33401 Valvuloplasty open
33403 Valvuloplasty w/cp bypass
33404 Prepare heart-aorta conduit
33405 Replacement of aortic valve
33406 Replacement of aortic valve
33410 Replacement of aortic valve
33411 Replacement of aortic valve
33412 Replacement of aortic valve
33413 Replacement of aortic valve
33414 Repair of aortic valve
33415 Revision subvalvular tissue
33416 Revise ventricle muscle
33417 Repair of aortic valve
33420 Revision of mitral valve
33422 Revision of mitral valve
33425 Repair of mitral valve
33426 Repair of mitral valve
33427 Repair of mitral valve
33430 Replacement of mitral valve
33460 Revision of tricuspid valve
33463 Valvuloplasty tricuspid
33464 Valvuloplasty tricuspid
33465 Replace tricuspid valve
33468 Revision of tricuspid valve
33470 Revision of pulmonary valve

Appendix M — Inpatient Only Procedures

33471 Valvotomy pulmonary valve
33472 Revision of pulmonary valve
33474 Revision of pulmonary valve
33475 Replacement pulmonary valve
33476 Revision of heart chamber
33478 Revision of heart chamber
33496 Repair prosth valve clot
33500 Repair heart vessel fistula
33501 Repair heart vessel fistula
33502 Coronary artery correction
33503 Coronary artery graft
33504 Coronary artery graft
33505 Repair artery w/tunnel
33506 Repair artery translocation
33507 Repair art intramural
33510 Cabg vein single
33511 Cabg vein two
33512 Cabg vein three
33513 Cabg vein four
33514 Cabg vein five
33516 Cabg vein six or more
33517 Cabg artery-vein single
33518 Cabg artery-vein two
33519 Cabg artery-vein three
33521 Cabg artery-vein four
33522 Cabg artery-vein five
33523 Cabg art-vein six or more
33530 Coronary artery bypass/reop
33533 Cabg arterial single
33534 Cabg arterial two
33535 Cabg arterial three
33536 Cabg arterial four or more
33542 Removal of heart lesion
33545 Repair of heart damage
33548 Restore/remodel ventricle
33572 Open coronary endarterectomy
33600 Closure of valve
33602 Closure of valve
33606 Anastomosis/artery-aorta
33608 Repair anomaly w/conduit
33610 Repair by enlargement
33611 Repair double ventricle
33612 Repair double ventricle
33615 Repair modified fontan
33617 Repair single ventricle
33619 Repair single ventricle
33620 Apply r&l pulm art bands
33621 Transthor cath for stent
33622 Redo compl cardiac anomaly
33641 Repair heart septum defect
33645 Revision of heart veins
33647 Repair heart septum defects
33660 Repair of heart defects
33665 Repair of heart defects
33670 Repair of heart chambers
33675 Close mult vsd
33676 Close mult vsd w/resection
33677 Cl mult vsd w/rem pul band
33681 Repair heart septum defect
33684 Repair heart septum defect
33688 Repair heart septum defect
33690 Reinforce pulmonary artery
33692 Repair of heart defects
33694 Repair of heart defects
33697 Repair of heart defects
33702 Repair of heart defects
33710 Repair of heart defects
33720 Repair of heart defect
33722 Repair of heart defect
33724 Repair venous anomaly
33726 Repair pul venous stenosis
33730 Repair heart-vein defect(s)
33732 Repair heart-vein defect
33735 Revision of heart chamber
33736 Revision of heart chamber
33737 Revision of heart chamber
33750 Major vessel shunt
33755 Major vessel shunt
33762 Major vessel shunt
33764 Major vessel shunt & graft
33766 Major vessel shunt
33767 Major vessel shunt
33768 Cavopulmonary shunting
33770 Repair great vessels defect
33771 Repair great vessels defect
33774 Repair great vessels defect
33775 Repair great vessels defect
33776 Repair great vessels defect
33777 Repair great vessels defect
33778 Repair great vessels defect
33779 Repair great vessels defect
33780 Repair great vessels defect
33781 Repair great vessels defect
33782 Nikaidoh proc
33783 Nikaidoh proc w/ostia implt
33786 Repair arterial trunk
33788 Revision of pulmonary artery
33800 Aortic suspension
33802 Repair vessel defect
33803 Repair vessel defect
33813 Repair septal defect
33814 Repair septal defect
33820 Revise major vessel
33822 Revise major vessel
33824 Revise major vessel
33840 Remove aorta constriction
33845 Remove aorta constriction
33851 Remove aorta constriction
33852 Repair septal defect
33853 Repair septal defect
33860 Ascending aortic graft
33863 Ascending aortic graft
33864 Ascending aortic graft
33870 Transverse aortic arch graft
33875 Thoracic aortic graft
33877 Thoracoabdominal graft
33880 Endovasc taa repr incl subcl
33881 Endovasc taa repr w/o subcl
33883 Insert endovasc prosth taa
33884 Endovasc prosth taa add-on
33886 Endovasc prosth delayed
33889 Artery transpose/endovas taa
33891 Car-car bp grft/endovas taa
33910 Remove lung artery emboli
33915 Remove lung artery emboli
33916 Surgery of great vessel
33917 Repair pulmonary artery
33920 Repair pulmonary atresia
33922 Transect pulmonary artery
33924 Remove pulmonary shunt
33925 Rpr pul art unifocal w/o cpb
33926 Repr pul art unifocal w/cpb
33930 Removal of donor heart/lung
33933 Prepare donor heart/lung
33935 Transplantation heart/lung
33940 Removal of donor heart
33944 Prepare donor heart
33945 Transplantation of heart
33960 External circulation assist
33961 External circulation assist
33967 Insert ia percut device
33968 Remove aortic assist device
33970 Aortic circulation assist
33971 Aortic circulation assist
33973 Insert balloon device
33974 Remove intra-aortic balloon
33975 Implant ventricular device
33976 Implant ventricular device
33977 Remove ventricular device
33978 Remove ventricular device
33979 Insert intracorporeal device
33980 Remove intracorporeal device
33981 Replace vad pump ext
33982 Replace vad intra w/o bp
33983 Replace vad intra w/bp
34001 Removal of artery clot
34051 Removal of artery clot
34151 Removal of artery clot
34401 Removal of vein clot
34451 Removal of vein clot
34502 Reconstruct vena cava
34800 Endovas aaa repr w/sm tube
34802 Endovas aaa repr w/2-p part
34803 Endovas aaa repr w/3-p part
34804 Endovas aaa repr w/1-p part
34805 Endovas aaa repr w/long tube
34806 Aneurysm press sensor add-on
34808 Endovas iliac a device addon
34812 Xpose for endoprosth femorl
34813 Femoral endovas graft add-on
34820 Xpose for endoprosth iliac
34825 Endovasc extend prosth init
34826 Endovasc exten prosth addl
34830 Open aortic tube prosth repr

34831 Open aortoiliac prosth repr
34832 Open aortofemor prosth repr
34833 Xpose for endoprosth iliac
34834 Xpose endoprosth brachial
34900 Endovasc iliac repr w/graft
35001 Repair defect of artery
35002 Repair artery rupture neck
35005 Repair defect of artery
35013 Repair artery rupture arm
35021 Repair defect of artery
35022 Repair artery rupture chest
35081 Repair defect of artery
35082 Repair artery rupture aorta
35091 Repair defect of artery
35092 Repair artery rupture aorta
35102 Repair defect of artery
35103 Repair artery rupture groin
35111 Repair defect of artery
35112 Repair artery rupture spleen
35121 Repair defect of artery
35122 Repair artery rupture belly
35131 Repair defect of artery
35132 Repair artery rupture groin
35141 Repair defect of artery
35142 Repair artery rupture thigh
35151 Repair defect of artery
35152 Repair artery rupture knee
35182 Repair blood vessel lesion
35189 Repair blood vessel lesion
35211 Repair blood vessel lesion
35216 Repair blood vessel lesion
35221 Repair blood vessel lesion
35241 Repair blood vessel lesion
35246 Repair blood vessel lesion
35251 Repair blood vessel lesion
35271 Repair blood vessel lesion
35276 Repair blood vessel lesion
35281 Repair blood vessel lesion
35301 Rechanneling of artery
35302 Rechanneling of artery
35303 Rechanneling of artery
35304 Rechanneling of artery
35305 Rechanneling of artery
35306 Rechanneling of artery
35311 Rechanneling of artery
35331 Rechanneling of artery
35341 Rechanneling of artery
35351 Rechanneling of artery
35355 Rechanneling of artery
35361 Rechanneling of artery
35363 Rechanneling of artery
35371 Rechanneling of artery
35372 Rechanneling of artery
35390 Reoperation carotid add-on
35400 Angioscopy
35450 Repair arterial blockage
35452 Repair arterial blockage
35501 Artery bypass graft
35506 Artery bypass graft
35508 Artery bypass graft
35509 Artery bypass graft
35510 Artery bypass graft
35511 Artery bypass graft
35512 Artery bypass graft
35515 Artery bypass graft
35516 Artery bypass graft
35518 Artery bypass graft
35521 Artery bypass graft
35522 Artery bypass graft
35523 Artery bypass graft
35525 Artery bypass graft
35526 Artery bypass graft
35531 Artery bypass graft
35533 Artery bypass graft
35535 Artery bypass graft
35536 Artery bypass graft
35537 Artery bypass graft
35538 Artery bypass graft
35539 Artery bypass graft
35540 Artery bypass graft
35556 Artery bypass graft
35558 Artery bypass graft
35560 Artery bypass graft
35563 Artery bypass graft
35565 Artery bypass graft
35566 Artery bypass graft
35570 Artery bypass graft
35571 Artery bypass graft
35583 Vein bypass graft
35585 Vein bypass graft
35587 Vein bypass graft
35600 Harvest art for cabg add-on
35601 Artery bypass graft
35606 Artery bypass graft
35612 Artery bypass graft
35616 Artery bypass graft
35621 Artery bypass graft
35623 Bypass graft not vein
35626 Artery bypass graft
35631 Artery bypass graft
35632 Artery bypass graft
35633 Artery bypass graft
35634 Artery bypass graft
35636 Artery bypass graft
35637 Artery bypass graft
35638 Artery bypass graft
35642 Artery bypass graft
35645 Artery bypass graft
35646 Artery bypass graft
35647 Artery bypass graft
35650 Artery bypass graft
35654 Artery bypass graft
35656 Artery bypass graft
35661 Artery bypass graft
35663 Artery bypass graft
35665 Artery bypass graft
35666 Artery bypass graft
35671 Artery bypass graft
35681 Composite bypass graft
35682 Composite bypass graft
35683 Composite bypass graft
35691 Arterial transposition
35693 Arterial transposition
35694 Arterial transposition
35695 Arterial transposition
35697 Reimplant artery each
35700 Reoperation bypass graft
35701 Exploration carotid artery
35721 Exploration femoral artery
35741 Exploration popliteal artery
35800 Explore neck vessels
35820 Explore chest vessels
35840 Explore abdominal vessels
35870 Repair vessel graft defect
35901 Excision graft neck
35905 Excision graft thorax
35907 Excision graft abdomen
36660 Insertion catheter artery
36822 Insertion of cannula(s)
36823 Insertion of cannula(s)
37140 Revision of circulation
37145 Revision of circulation
37160 Revision of circulation
37180 Revision of circulation
37181 Splice spleen/kidney veins
37182 Insert hepatic shunt (tips)
37215 Transcath stent cca w/eps
37616 Ligation of chest artery
37617 Ligation of abdomen artery
37618 Ligation of extremity artery
37660 Revision of major vein
37788 Revascularization penis
38100 Removal of spleen total
38101 Removal of spleen partial
38102 Removal of spleen total
38115 Repair of ruptured spleen
38380 Thoracic duct procedure
38381 Thoracic duct procedure
38382 Thoracic duct procedure
38562 Removal pelvic lymph nodes
38564 Removal abdomen lymph nodes
38724 Removal of lymph nodes neck
38746 Remove thoracic lymph nodes
38747 Remove abdominal lymph nodes
38765 Remove groin lymph nodes
38770 Remove pelvis lymph nodes
38780 Remove abdomen lymph nodes
39000 Exploration of chest
39010 Exploration of chest
39200 Resect mediastinal cyst
39220 Resect mediastinal tumor
39499 Chest procedure
39501 Repair diaphragm laceration
39503 Repair of diaphragm hernia

Appendix M — Inpatient Only Procedures

39540 Repair of diaphragm hernia
39541 Repair of diaphragm hernia
39545 Revision of diaphragm
39560 Resect diaphragm simple
39561 Resect diaphragm complex
39599 Diaphragm surgery procedure
41130 Partial removal of tongue
41135 Tongue and neck surgery
41140 Removal of tongue
41145 Tongue removal neck surgery
41150 Tongue mouth jaw surgery
41153 Tongue mouth neck surgery
41155 Tongue jaw & neck surgery
42426 Excise parotid gland/lesion
42845 Extensive surgery of throat
42894 Revision of pharyngeal walls
42953 Repair throat esophagus
42961 Control throat bleeding
42971 Control nose/throat bleeding
43045 Incision of esophagus
43100 Excision of esophagus lesion
43101 Excision of esophagus lesion
43107 Removal of esophagus
43108 Removal of esophagus
43112 Removal of esophagus
43113 Removal of esophagus
43116 Partial removal of esophagus
43117 Partial removal of esophagus
43118 Partial removal of esophagus
43121 Partial removal of esophagus
43122 Partial removal of esophagus
43123 Partial removal of esophagus
43124 Removal of esophagus
43135 Removal of esophagus pouch
43279 Lap myotomy heller
43282 Lap paraesoph her rpr w/mesh
43283 Lap esoph lengthening
43300 Repair of esophagus
43305 Repair esophagus and fistula
43310 Repair of esophagus
43312 Repair esophagus and fistula
43313 Esophagoplasty congenital
43314 Tracheo-esophagoplasty cong
43320 Fuse esophagus & stomach
43325 Revise esophagus & stomach
43327 Esoph fundoplasty lap
43328 Esoph fundoplasty thor
43330 Esophagomyotomy abdominal
43331 Esophagomyotomy thoracic
43332 Transab esoph hiat hern rpr
43333 Transab esoph hiat hern rpr
43334 Transthor diaphrag hern rpr
43335 Transthor diaphrag hern rpr
43336 Thorabd diaphr hern repair
43337 Thorabd diaphr hern repair
43338 Esoph lengthening
43340 Fuse esophagus & intestine
43341 Fuse esophagus & intestine
43350 Surgical opening esophagus
43351 Surgical opening esophagus
43352 Surgical opening esophagus
43360 Gastrointestinal repair
43361 Gastrointestinal repair
43400 Ligate esophagus veins
43401 Esophagus surgery for veins
43405 Ligate/staple esophagus
43410 Repair esophagus wound
43415 Repair esophagus wound
43425 Repair esophagus opening
43460 Pressure treatment esophagus
43496 Free jejunum flap microvasc
43500 Surgical opening of stomach
43501 Surgical repair of stomach
43502 Surgical repair of stomach
43520 Incision of pyloric muscle
43605 Biopsy of stomach
43610 Excision of stomach lesion
43611 Excision of stomach lesion
43620 Removal of stomach
43621 Removal of stomach
43622 Removal of stomach
43631 Removal of stomach partial
43632 Removal of stomach partial
43633 Removal of stomach partial
43634 Removal of stomach partial
43635 Removal of stomach partial
43640 Vagotomy & pylorus repair
43641 Vagotomy & pylorus repair
43644 Lap gastric bypass/roux-en-y
43645 Lap gastr bypass incl smll i
43771 Lap revise gastr adj device
43772 Lap rmvl gastr adj device
43773 Lap replace gastr adj device
43774 Lap rmvl gastr adj all parts
43800 Reconstruction of pylorus
43810 Fusion of stomach and bowel
43820 Fusion of stomach and bowel
43825 Fusion of stomach and bowel
43832 Place gastrostomy tube
43840 Repair of stomach lesion
43843 Gastroplasty w/o v-band
43845 Gastroplasty duodenal switch
43846 Gastric bypass for obesity
43847 Gastric bypass incl small i
43848 Revision gastroplasty
43850 Revise stomach-bowel fusion
43855 Revise stomach-bowel fusion
43860 Revise stomach-bowel fusion
43865 Revise stomach-bowel fusion
43880 Repair stomach-bowel fistula
43881 Impl/redo electrd antrum
43882 Revise/remove electrd antrum
44005 Freeing of bowel adhesion
44010 Incision of small bowel
44015 Insert needle cath bowel
44020 Explore small intestine
44021 Decompress small bowel
44025 Incision of large bowel
44050 Reduce bowel obstruction
44055 Correct malrotation of bowel
44110 Excise intestine lesion(s)
44111 Excision of bowel lesion(s)
44120 Removal of small intestine
44121 Removal of small intestine
44125 Removal of small intestine
44126 Enterectomy w/o taper cong
44127 Enterectomy w/taper cong
44128 Enterectomy cong add-on
44130 Bowel to bowel fusion
44132 Enterectomy cadaver donor
44133 Enterectomy live donor
44135 Intestine transplnt cadaver
44136 Intestine transplant live
44137 Remove intestinal allograft
44139 Mobilization of colon
44140 Partial removal of colon
44141 Partial removal of colon
44143 Partial removal of colon
44144 Partial removal of colon
44145 Partial removal of colon
44146 Partial removal of colon
44147 Partial removal of colon
44150 Removal of colon
44151 Removal of colon/ileostomy
44155 Removal of colon/ileostomy
44156 Removal of colon/ileostomy
44157 Colectomy w/ileoanal anast
44158 Colectomy w/neo-rectum pouch
44160 Removal of colon
44187 Lap ileo/jejuno-stomy
44188 Lap colostomy
44202 Lap enterectomy
44203 Lap resect s/intestine addl
44204 Laparo partial colectomy
44205 Lap colectomy part w/ileum
44210 Laparo total proctocolectomy
44211 Lap colectomy w/proctectomy
44212 Laparo total proctocolectomy
44227 Lap close enterostomy
44300 Open bowel to skin
44310 Ileostomy/jejunostomy
44314 Revision of ileostomy
44316 Devise bowel pouch
44320 Colostomy
44322 Colostomy with biopsies
44345 Revision of colostomy
44346 Revision of colostomy
44602 Suture small intestine
44603 Suture small intestine
44604 Suture large intestine
44605 Repair of bowel lesion
44615 Intestinal stricturoplasty
44620 Repair bowel opening
44625 Repair bowel opening

44626 Repair bowel opening
44640 Repair bowel-skin fistula
44650 Repair bowel fistula
44660 Repair bowel-bladder fistula
44661 Repair bowel-bladder fistula
44680 Surgical revision intestine
44700 Suspend bowel w/prosthesis
44715 Prepare donor intestine
44720 Prep donor intestine/venous
44721 Prep donor intestine/artery
44800 Excision of bowel pouch
44820 Excision of mesentery lesion
44850 Repair of mesentery
44899 Bowel surgery procedure
44900 Drain app abscess open
44960 Appendectomy
45110 Removal of rectum
45111 Partial removal of rectum
45112 Removal of rectum
45113 Partial proctectomy
45114 Partial removal of rectum
45116 Partial removal of rectum
45119 Remove rectum w/reservoir
45120 Removal of rectum
45121 Removal of rectum and colon
45123 Partial proctectomy
45126 Pelvic exenteration
45130 Excision of rectal prolapse
45135 Excision of rectal prolapse
45136 Excise ileoanal reservior
45395 Lap removal of rectum
45397 Lap remove rectum w/pouch
45400 Laparoscopic proc
45402 Lap proctopexy w/sig resect
45540 Correct rectal prolapse
45550 Repair rectum/remove sigmoid
45562 Exploration/repair of rectum
45563 Exploration/repair of rectum
45800 Repair rect/bladder fistula
45805 Repair fistula w/colostomy
45820 Repair rectourethral fistula
45825 Repair fistula w/colostomy
46705 Repair of anal stricture
46710 Repr per/vag pouch sngl proc
46712 Repr per/vag pouch dbl proc
46715 Rep perf anoper fistu
46716 Rep perf anoper/vestib fistu
46730 Construction of absent anus
46735 Construction of absent anus
46740 Construction of absent anus
46742 Repair of imperforated anus
46744 Repair of cloacal anomaly
46746 Repair of cloacal anomaly
46748 Repair of cloacal anomaly
46751 Repair of anal sphincter
47010 Open drainage liver lesion
47015 Inject/aspirate liver cyst
47100 Wedge biopsy of liver
47120 Partial removal of liver
47122 Extensive removal of liver
47125 Partial removal of liver
47130 Partial removal of liver
47133 Removal of donor liver
47135 Transplantation of liver
47136 Transplantation of liver
47140 Partial removal donor liver
47141 Partial removal donor liver
47142 Partial removal donor liver
47143 Prep donor liver whole
47144 Prep donor liver 3-segment
47145 Prep donor liver lobe split
47146 Prep donor liver/venous
47147 Prep donor liver/arterial
47300 Surgery for liver lesion
47350 Repair liver wound
47360 Repair liver wound
47361 Repair liver wound
47362 Repair liver wound
47380 Open ablate liver tumor rf
47381 Open ablate liver tumor cryo
47400 Incision of liver duct
47420 Incision of bile duct
47425 Incision of bile duct
47460 Incise bile duct sphincter
47480 Incision of gallbladder
47550 Bile duct endoscopy add-on
47570 Laparo cholecystoenterostomy
47600 Removal of gallbladder
47605 Removal of gallbladder
47610 Removal of gallbladder
47612 Removal of gallbladder
47620 Removal of gallbladder
47700 Exploration of bile ducts
47701 Bile duct revision
47711 Excision of bile duct tumor
47712 Excision of bile duct tumor
47715 Excision of bile duct cyst
47720 Fuse gallbladder & bowel
47721 Fuse upper gi structures
47740 Fuse gallbladder & bowel
47741 Fuse gallbladder & bowel
47760 Fuse bile ducts and bowel
47765 Fuse liver ducts & bowel
47780 Fuse bile ducts and bowel
47785 Fuse bile ducts and bowel
47800 Reconstruction of bile ducts
47801 Placement bile duct support
47802 Fuse liver duct & intestine
47900 Suture bile duct injury
48000 Drainage of abdomen
48001 Placement of drain pancreas
48020 Removal of pancreatic stone
48100 Biopsy of pancreas open
48105 Resect/debride pancreas
48120 Removal of pancreas lesion
48140 Partial removal of pancreas
48145 Partial removal of pancreas
48146 Pancreatectomy
48148 Removal of pancreatic duct
48150 Partial removal of pancreas
48152 Pancreatectomy
48153 Pancreatectomy
48154 Pancreatectomy
48155 Removal of pancreas
48400 Injection intraop add-on
48500 Surgery of pancreatic cyst
48510 Drain pancreatic pseudocyst
48520 Fuse pancreas cyst and bowel
48540 Fuse pancreas cyst and bowel
48545 Pancreatorrhaphy
48547 Duodenal exclusion
48548 Fuse pancreas and bowel
48551 Prep donor pancreas
48552 Prep donor pancreas/venous
48554 Transpl allograft pancreas
48556 Removal allograft pancreas
49000 Exploration of abdomen
49002 Reopening of abdomen
49010 Exploration behind abdomen
49020 Drain abdominal abscess
49040 Drain open abdom abscess
49060 Drain open retrop abscess
49062 Drain to peritoneal cavity
49203 Exc abd tum 5 cm or less
49204 Exc abd tum over 5 cm
49205 Exc abd tum over 10 cm
49215 Excise sacral spine tumor
49220 Multiple surgery abdomen
49255 Removal of omentum
49412 Ins device for rt guide open
49425 Insert abdomen-venous drain
49428 Ligation of shunt
49605 Repair umbilical lesion
49606 Repair umbilical lesion
49610 Repair umbilical lesion
49611 Repair umbilical lesion
49900 Repair of abdominal wall
49904 Omental flap extra-abdom
49905 Omental flap intra-abdom
49906 Free omental flap microvasc
50010 Exploration of kidney
50040 Drainage of kidney
50045 Exploration of kidney
50060 Removal of kidney stone
50065 Incision of kidney
50070 Incision of kidney
50075 Removal of kidney stone
50100 Revise kidney blood vessels
50120 Exploration of kidney
50125 Explore and drain kidney
50130 Removal of kidney stone
50135 Exploration of kidney
50205 Renal biopsy open
50220 Remove kidney open

50225 Removal kidney open complex
50230 Removal kidney open radical
50234 Removal of kidney & ureter
50236 Removal of kidney & ureter
50240 Partial removal of kidney
50250 Cryoablate renal mass open
50280 Removal of kidney lesion
50290 Removal of kidney lesion
50300 Remove cadaver donor kidney
50320 Remove kidney living donor
50323 Prep cadaver renal allograft
50325 Prep donor renal graft
50327 Prep renal graft/venous
50328 Prep renal graft/arterial
50329 Prep renal graft/ureteral
50340 Removal of kidney
50360 Transplantation of kidney
50365 Transplantation of kidney
50370 Remove transplanted kidney
50380 Reimplantation of kidney
50400 Revision of kidney/ureter
50405 Revision of kidney/ureter
50500 Repair of kidney wound
50520 Close kidney-skin fistula
50525 Repair renal-abdomen fistula
50526 Repair renal-abdomen fistula
50540 Revision of horseshoe kidney
50545 Laparo radical nephrectomy
50546 Laparoscopic nephrectomy
50547 Laparo removal donor kidney
50548 Laparo remove w/ureter
50600 Exploration of ureter
50605 Insert ureteral support
50610 Removal of ureter stone
50620 Removal of ureter stone
50630 Removal of ureter stone
50650 Removal of ureter
50660 Removal of ureter
50700 Revision of ureter
50715 Release of ureter
50722 Release of ureter
50725 Release/revise ureter
50728 Revise ureter
50740 Fusion of ureter & kidney
50750 Fusion of ureter & kidney
50760 Fusion of ureters
50770 Splicing of ureters
50780 Reimplant ureter in bladder
50782 Reimplant ureter in bladder
50783 Reimplant ureter in bladder
50785 Reimplant ureter in bladder
50800 Implant ureter in bowel
50810 Fusion of ureter & bowel
50815 Urine shunt to intestine
50820 Construct bowel bladder
50825 Construct bowel bladder
50830 Revise urine flow
50840 Replace ureter by bowel
50845 Appendico-vesicostomy
50860 Transplant ureter to skin
50900 Repair of ureter
50920 Closure ureter/skin fistula
50930 Closure ureter/bowel fistula
50940 Release of ureter
51525 Removal of bladder lesion
51530 Removal of bladder lesion
51550 Partial removal of bladder
51555 Partial removal of bladder
51565 Revise bladder & ureter(s)
51570 Removal of bladder
51575 Removal of bladder & nodes
51580 Remove bladder/revise tract
51585 Removal of bladder & nodes
51590 Remove bladder/revise tract
51595 Remove bladder/revise tract
51596 Remove bladder/create pouch
51597 Removal of pelvic structures
51800 Revision of bladder/urethra
51820 Revision of urinary tract
51840 Attach bladder/urethra
51841 Attach bladder/urethra
51865 Repair of bladder wound
51900 Repair bladder/vagina lesion
51920 Close bladder-uterus fistula
51925 Hysterectomy/bladder repair
51940 Correction of bladder defect
51960 Revision of bladder & bowel
51980 Construct bladder opening
53415 Reconstruction of urethra
53448 Remov/replc ur sphinctr comp
54125 Removal of penis
54130 Remove penis & nodes
54135 Remove penis & nodes
54390 Repair penis and bladder
54411 Remov/replc penis pros comp
54417 Remv/replc penis pros compl
54430 Revision of penis
55605 Incise sperm duct pouch
55650 Remove sperm duct pouch
55801 Removal of prostate
55810 Extensive prostate surgery
55812 Extensive prostate surgery
55815 Extensive prostate surgery
55821 Removal of prostate
55831 Removal of prostate
55840 Extensive prostate surgery
55842 Extensive prostate surgery
55845 Extensive prostate surgery
55862 Extensive prostate surgery
55865 Extensive prostate surgery
55866 Laparo radical prostatectomy
56630 Extensive vulva surgery
56631 Extensive vulva surgery
56632 Extensive vulva surgery
56633 Extensive vulva surgery
56634 Extensive vulva surgery
56637 Extensive vulva surgery
56640 Extensive vulva surgery
57110 Remove vagina wall complete
57111 Remove vagina tissue compl
57112 Vaginectomy w/nodes compl
57270 Repair of bowel pouch
57280 Suspension of vagina
57296 Revise vag graft open abd
57305 Repair rectum-vagina fistula
57307 Fistula repair & colostomy
57308 Fistula repair transperine
57311 Repair urethrovaginal lesion
57531 Removal of cervix radical
57540 Removal of residual cervix
57545 Remove cervix/repair pelvis
58140 Myomectomy abdom method
58146 Myomectomy abdom complex
58150 Total hysterectomy
58152 Total hysterectomy
58180 Partial hysterectomy
58200 Extensive hysterectomy
58210 Extensive hysterectomy
58240 Removal of pelvis contents
58267 Vag hyst w/urinary repair
58275 Hysterectomy/revise vagina
58280 Hysterectomy/revise vagina
58285 Extensive hysterectomy
58293 Vag hyst w/uro repair compl
58400 Suspension of uterus
58410 Suspension of uterus
58520 Repair of ruptured uterus
58540 Revision of uterus
58548 Lap radical hyst
58605 Division of fallopian tube
58611 Ligate oviduct(s) add-on
58700 Removal of fallopian tube
58720 Removal of ovary/tube(s)
58740 Adhesiolysis tube ovary
58750 Repair oviduct
58752 Revise ovarian tube(s)
58760 Fimbrioplasty
58822 Drain ovary abscess percut
58825 Transposition ovary(s)
58940 Removal of ovary(s)
58943 Removal of ovary(s)
58950 Resect ovarian malignancy
58951 Resect ovarian malignancy
58952 Resect ovarian malignancy
58953 Tah rad dissect for debulk
58954 Tah rad debulk/lymph remove
58956 Bso omentectomy w/tah
58957 Resect recurrent gyn mal
58958 Resect recur gyn mal w/lym
58960 Exploration of abdomen
59120 Treat ectopic pregnancy
59121 Treat ectopic pregnancy
59130 Treat ectopic pregnancy
59135 Treat ectopic pregnancy

59136 Treat ectopic pregnancy
59140 Treat ectopic pregnancy
59325 Revision of cervix
59350 Repair of uterus
59514 Cesarean delivery only
59525 Remove uterus after cesarean
59620 Attempted vbac delivery only
59830 Treat uterus infection
59850 Abortion
59851 Abortion
59852 Abortion
59855 Abortion
59856 Abortion
59857 Abortion
60254 Extensive thyroid surgery
60270 Removal of thyroid
60505 Explore parathyroid glands
60521 Removal of thymus gland
60522 Removal of thymus gland
60540 Explore adrenal gland
60545 Explore adrenal gland
60600 Remove carotid body lesion
60605 Remove carotid body lesion
60650 Laparoscopy adrenalectomy
61105 Twist drill hole
61107 Drill skull for implantation
61108 Drill skull for drainage
61120 Burr hole for puncture
61140 Pierce skull for biopsy
61150 Pierce skull for drainage
61151 Pierce skull for drainage
61154 Pierce skull & remove clot
61156 Pierce skull for drainage
61210 Pierce skull implant device
61250 Pierce skull & explore
61253 Pierce skull & explore
61304 Open skull for exploration
61305 Open skull for exploration
61312 Open skull for drainage
61313 Open skull for drainage
61314 Open skull for drainage
61315 Open skull for drainage
61316 Implt cran bone flap to abdo
61320 Open skull for drainage
61321 Open skull for drainage
61322 Decompressive craniotomy
61323 Decompressive lobectomy
61332 Explore/biopsy eye socket
61333 Explore orbit/remove lesion
61340 Subtemporal decompression
61343 Incise skull (press relief)
61345 Relieve cranial pressure
61440 Incise skull for surgery
61450 Incise skull for surgery
61458 Incise skull for brain wound
61460 Incise skull for surgery
61470 Incise skull for surgery
61480 Incise skull for surgery
61490 Incise skull for surgery
61500 Removal of skull lesion
61501 Remove infected skull bone
61510 Removal of brain lesion
61512 Remove brain lining lesion
61514 Removal of brain abscess
61516 Removal of brain lesion
61517 Implt brain chemotx add-on
61518 Removal of brain lesion
61519 Remove brain lining lesion
61520 Removal of brain lesion
61521 Removal of brain lesion
61522 Removal of brain abscess
61524 Removal of brain lesion
61526 Removal of brain lesion
61530 Removal of brain lesion
61531 Implant brain electrodes
61533 Implant brain electrodes
61534 Removal of brain lesion
61535 Remove brain electrodes
61536 Removal of brain lesion
61537 Removal of brain tissue
61538 Removal of brain tissue
61539 Removal of brain tissue
61540 Removal of brain tissue
61541 Incision of brain tissue
61542 Removal of brain tissue
61543 Removal of brain tissue
61544 Remove & treat brain lesion
61545 Excision of brain tumor
61546 Removal of pituitary gland
61548 Removal of pituitary gland
61550 Release of skull seams
61552 Release of skull seams
61556 Incise skull/sutures
61557 Incise skull/sutures
61558 Excision of skull/sutures
61559 Excision of skull/sutures
61563 Excision of skull tumor
61564 Excision of skull tumor
61566 Removal of brain tissue
61567 Incision of brain tissue
61570 Remove foreign body brain
61571 Incise skull for brain wound
61575 Skull base/brainstem surgery
61576 Skull base/brainstem surgery
61580 Craniofacial approach skull
61581 Craniofacial approach skull
61582 Craniofacial approach skull
61583 Craniofacial approach skull
61584 Orbitocranial approach/skull
61585 Orbitocranial approach/skull
61586 Resect nasopharynx skull
61590 Infratemporal approach/skull
61591 Infratemporal approach/skull
61592 Orbitocranial approach/skull
61595 Transtemporal approach/skull
61596 Transcochlear approach/skull
61597 Transcondylar approach/skull
61598 Transpetrosal approach/skull
61600 Resect/excise cranial lesion
61601 Resect/excise cranial lesion
61605 Resect/excise cranial lesion
61606 Resect/excise cranial lesion
61607 Resect/excise cranial lesion
61608 Resect/excise cranial lesion
61609 Transect artery sinus
61610 Transect artery sinus
61611 Transect artery sinus
61612 Transect artery sinus
61613 Remove aneurysm sinus
61615 Resect/excise lesion skull
61616 Resect/excise lesion skull
61618 Repair dura
61619 Repair dura
61624 Transcath occlusion cns
61630 Intracranial angioplasty
61635 Intracran angioplsty w/stent
61680 Intracranial vessel surgery
61682 Intracranial vessel surgery
61684 Intracranial vessel surgery
61686 Intracranial vessel surgery
61690 Intracranial vessel surgery
61692 Intracranial vessel surgery
61697 Brain aneurysm repr complx
61698 Brain aneurysm repr complx
61700 Brain aneurysm repr simple
61702 Inner skull vessel surgery
61703 Clamp neck artery
61705 Revise circulation to head
61708 Revise circulation to head
61710 Revise circulation to head
61711 Fusion of skull arteries
61735 Incise skull/brain surgery
61750 Incise skull/brain biopsy
61751 Brain biopsy w/ct/mr guide
61760 Implant brain electrodes
61850 Implant neuroelectrodes
61860 Implant neuroelectrodes
61863 Implant neuroelectrode
61864 Implant neuroelectrde addl
61867 Implant neuroelectrode
61868 Implant neuroelectrde addl
61870 Implant neuroelectrodes
61875 Implant neuroelectrodes
62005 Treat skull fracture
62010 Treatment of head injury
62100 Repair brain fluid leakage
62115 Reduction of skull defect
62116 Reduction of skull defect
62117 Reduction of skull defect
62120 Repair skull cavity lesion
62121 Incise skull repair
62140 Repair of skull defect
62141 Repair of skull defect
62142 Remove skull plate/flap

62143 Replace skull plate/flap
62145 Repair of skull & brain
62146 Repair of skull with graft
62147 Repair of skull with graft
62148 Retr bone flap to fix skull
62161 Dissect brain w/scope
62162 Remove colloid cyst w/scope
62163 Zneuroendoscopy w/fb removal
62164 Remove brain tumor w/scope
62165 Remove pituit tumor w/scope
62180 Establish brain cavity shunt
62190 Establish brain cavity shunt
62192 Establish brain cavity shunt
62200 Establish brain cavity shunt
62201 Brain cavity shunt w/scope
62220 Establish brain cavity shunt
62223 Establish brain cavity shunt
62256 Remove brain cavity shunt
62258 Replace brain cavity shunt
63043 Laminotomy addl cervical
63044 Laminotomy addl lumbar
63050 Cervical laminoplasty
63051 C-laminoplasty w/graft/plate
63077 Spine disk surgery thorax
63078 Spine disk surgery thorax
63081 Removal of vertebral body
63082 Remove vertebral body add-on
63085 Removal of vertebral body
63086 Remove vertebral body add-on
63087 Removal of vertebral body
63088 Remove vertebral body add-on
63090 Removal of vertebral body
63091 Remove vertebral body add-on
63101 Removal of vertebral body
63102 Removal of vertebral body
63103 Remove vertebral body add-on
63170 Incise spinal cord tract(s)
63172 Drainage of spinal cyst
63173 Drainage of spinal cyst
63180 Revise spinal cord ligaments
63182 Revise spinal cord ligaments
63185 Incise spinal column/nerves
63190 Incise spinal column/nerves
63191 Incise spinal column/nerves
63194 Incise spinal column & cord
63195 Incise spinal column & cord
63196 Incise spinal column & cord
63197 Incise spinal column & cord
63198 Incise spinal column & cord
63199 Incise spinal column & cord
63200 Release of spinal cord
63250 Revise spinal cord vessels
63251 Revise spinal cord vessels
63252 Revise spinal cord vessels
63265 Excise intraspinal lesion
63266 Excise intraspinal lesion
63267 Excise intraspinal lesion
63268 Excise intraspinal lesion
63270 Excise intraspinal lesion
63271 Excise intraspinal lesion
63272 Excise intraspinal lesion
63273 Excise intraspinal lesion
63275 Biopsy/excise spinal tumor
63276 Biopsy/excise spinal tumor
63277 Biopsy/excise spinal tumor
63278 Biopsy/excise spinal tumor
63280 Biopsy/excise spinal tumor
63281 Biopsy/excise spinal tumor
63282 Biopsy/excise spinal tumor
63283 Biopsy/excise spinal tumor
63285 Biopsy/excise spinal tumor
63286 Biopsy/excise spinal tumor
63287 Biopsy/excise spinal tumor
63290 Biopsy/excise spinal tumor
63295 Repair of laminectomy defect
63300 Removal of vertebral body
63301 Removal of vertebral body
63302 Removal of vertebral body
63303 Removal of vertebral body
63304 Removal of vertebral body
63305 Removal of vertebral body
63306 Removal of vertebral body
63307 Removal of vertebral body
63308 Remove vertebral body add-on
63700 Repair of spinal herniation
63702 Repair of spinal herniation
63704 Repair of spinal herniation
63706 Repair of spinal herniation
63707 Repair spinal fluid leakage
63709 Repair spinal fluid leakage
63710 Graft repair of spine defect
63740 Install spinal shunt
64752 Incision of vagus nerve
64755 Incision of stomach nerves
64760 Incision of vagus nerve
64809 Remove sympathetic nerves
64818 Remove sympathetic nerves
64866 Fusion of facial/other nerve
64868 Fusion of facial/other nerve
65273 Repair of eye wound
69155 Extensive ear/neck surgery
69535 Remove part of temporal bone
69554 Remove ear lesion
69950 Incise inner ear nerve
75900 Intravascular cath exchange
75952 Endovasc repair abdom aorta
75953 Abdom aneurysm endovas rpr
75954 Iliac aneurysm endovas rpr
75956 Xray endovasc thor ao repr
75957 Xray endovasc thor ao repr
75958 Xray place prox ext thor ao
75959 Xray place dist ext thor ao
92970 Cardioassist internal
92971 Cardioassist external
92975 Dissolve clot heart vessel
92992 Revision of heart chamber
92993 Revision of heart chamber
99190 Special pump services
99191 Special pump services
99192 Special pump services
99356 Prolonged service inpatient
99357 Prolonged service inpatient
99462 Sbsq nb em per day hosp
99468 Neonate crit care initial
99469 Neonate crit care subsq
99471 Ped critical care initial
99472 Ped critical care subsq
99475 Ped crit care age 2-5 init
99476 Ped crit care age 2-5 subsq
99477 Init day hosp neonate care
99478 Ic lbw inf < 1500 gm subsq
99479 Ic lbw inf 1500-2500 g subsq
99480 Ic inf pbw 2501-5000 g subsq
0048T Implant ventricular device
0050T Removal circulation assist
0051T Implant total heart system
0052T Replace component heart syst
0053T Replace component heart syst
0075T Perq stent/chest vert art
0076T S&i stent/chest vert art
0078T Endovasc aort repr w/device
0079T Endovasc visc extnsn repr
0080T Endovasc aort repr rad s&i
0081T Endovasc visc extnsn s&i
0092T Artific disc addl
0095T Artific diskectomy addl
0098T Rev artific disc addl
0163T Lumb artif diskectomy addl
0164T Remove lumb artif disc addl
0165T Revise lumb artif disc addl
0169T Place stereo cath brain
0195T Arthrod presac interbody
0196T Arthrod presac interbody eac
0202T Post vert arthrplst 1 lumbar
0219T Plmt post facet implt cerv
0220T Plmt post facet implt thor
0235T Trluml perip athrc visceral
0254T Evasc rpr iliac art bifur
0255T Evasc rpr iliac art bifr s&i
0256T Evasc aortic hrt valve
0257T Opn tthrc aortic hrt valve
0258T Aortic hrt valv w/o card byp
0259T Aortic hrt valve w/card byp
0262T Impltj pulm vlv evasc appr
0266T Implt/rpl crtd sns dev total
0281T Laa closure w/implant
0293T Ins lt atrl press monitor

NOTES

NOTES

NOTES

NOTES